KAPLAN & SADOCK

Concise
Textbook of Clinical Psychiatry

Fourth 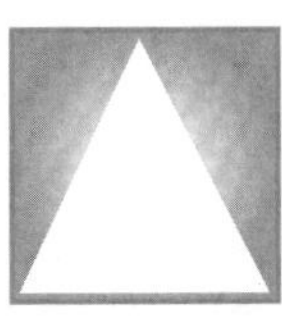 Edition

KAPLAN & SADOCK'S

Concise
Textbook of Clinical Psychiatry

Fourth 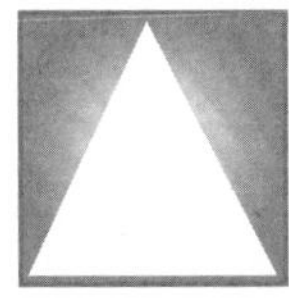 Edition

Benjamin James Sadock, M.D.

Menas S. Gregory Professor of Psychiatry
Department of Psychiatry
New York University School of Medicine
Attending Psychiatrist, Tisch Hospital
Attending Psychiatrist, Bellevue Hospital Center
New York, New York

Virginia Alcott Sadock, M.D.

Professor of Psychiatry
Department of Psychiatry
New York University School of Medicine
Attending Psychiatrist, Tisch Hospital
Attending Psychiatrist, Bellevue Hospital Center
New York, New York

Pedro Ruiz, M.D.

Clinical Professor
Menninger Department of Psychiatry and Behavioral Sciences
Baylor College of Medicine
Houston, Texas

Wolters Kluwer

Philadelphia • Baltimore • New York • London
Buenos Aires • Hong Kong • Sydney • Tokyo

Acquisitions Editor: Chris Teja
Product Development Editor: Andrea Vosburgh
Marketing Manager: Rachel Mante Leung
Production Project Manager: Bridgett Dougherty
Design Coordinator: Elaine Kasmer
Senior Manufacturing Coordinator: Beth Welsh
Prepress Vendor: Aptara, Inc.

Fourth Edition

9 8 7 6 5 4 3 2 1

Printed in China

Library of Congress Cataloging-in-Publication Data
Names: Sadock, Benjamin J., author. | Sadock, Virginia A., author. | Ruiz, Pedro, author. | Abridgement of (work): Sadock, Benjamin J., Kaplan & Sadock's synopsis of psychiatry. Eleventh edition.
Title: Kaplan & Sadock's concise textbook of clinical psychiatry / Benjamin James Sadock, Virginia Alcott Sadock, Pedro Ruiz.
Other titles: Kaplan and Sadock's concise textbook of clinical psychiatry | Concise textbook of clinical psychiatry
Description: Fourth edition. | Philadelphia : Wolters Kluwer, [2017] | Includes index. | Abridgement of Kaplan & Sadock's synopsis of psychiatry / Benjamin James Sadock, Virginia Alcott Sadock, Pedro Ruiz. 11th edition. 2015.
Identifiers: LCCN 2016039138 | ISBN 9781496345257
Subjects: | MESH: Mental Disorders
Classification: LCC RC437.5 | NLM WM 140 | DDC 616.89–dc23
LC record available at https://lccn.loc.gov/2016039138

LWW.com

CCS1216

To
Our Grandchildren

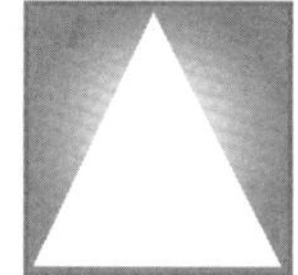

Preface

This *Concise Textbook of Clinical Psychiatry* covers the diagnosis and treatment of mental disorders in adults and children. It evolved from our experience editing a larger volume, *Kaplan & Sadock's Synopsis of Psychiatry,* eleventh edition, which covers both the behavioral sciences and the diagnosis and treatment of psychiatric disorders. The elimination of the sections on the behavioral sciences accounts for this book's smaller and more manageable size. It is designed to meet the needs of readers who require a compact but thorough coverage of all of clinical psychiatry.

Since its beginning, the goal of this book has been to foster professional competence and ensure the highest quality care to those with mental disorders. An eclectic, multidisciplinary approach has been its hallmark; thus, biological, psychological, and sociological factors are equitably presented as they affect the person in health and disease. Each edition is thoroughly updated and the textbook has the reputation of being an independent, consistent, accurate, objective, and reliable compendium of new events in the field of psychiatry.

The text is organized to serve diverse professional groups: psychiatrists and nonpsychiatric physicians, medical students, psychologists, social workers, psychiatric nurses, and other mental health professionals, such as occupational and art therapists, among others. We have been extremely gratified by its wide acceptance and use, both in the United States and around the world.

CLASSIFICATION OF DISORDERS: DSM-5

A fifth edition of the *American Psychiatric Association Diagnostic and Statistical Manual of Mental Disorders* (DSM-5) was published in 2013. That book contains the official nomenclature used by psychiatrists and other mental health professionals in the United States; the psychiatric disorders discussed in this textbook are consistent with and follow that nosology. Every section dealing with clinical disorders has been updated thoroughly and completely to include the revisions contained in the DSM-5.

CASE HISTORIES

Case histories are an integral part of this text and are used extensively to add clarity and bring life to the clinical disorders described. Cases come from various sources, including the contributors to the current and previous editions of the *Comprehensive Textbook of Psychiatry* and our hospital colleagues, all of whom we thank for their contributions. Some also come from the authors' clinical experience at Bellevue Hospital in New York. Cases appear in tinted type to help the reader find them easily.

NEW AND UPDATED SECTIONS

The introduction of the DSM-5 in 2013 reframed psychiatric nosology, and the reader will find every section of this text revised and updated to reflect those changes. The chapter on *Classification in Psychiatry* provides a concise overview and definition of every psychiatric disorder listed in the DSM-5. In the rest of the book, each of these disorders is discussed in great detail in separate chapters and sections.

There are several sections that cover end-of-life issues and reflect the important role psychiatrists have in the clinical specialty of palliative medicine. Pain control, which is a relatively new but important area in which psychiatrists play a significant role, is also covered as is the proper use of opioids in controlling pain. In the chapter entitled *Gender Dysphoria*—a new diagnostic category included in the DSM-5—special attention is given to issues that affect gay, lesbian, bisexual, and transgender persons. The chapter *Psychiatry and Reproductive Medicine* was revised extensively to keep pace with advances in women's health issues. The chapter *Ethics in Psychiatry* was updated to include an extensive discussion of physician-assisted suicide. This topic is also given special attention in the section entitled *Euthanasia.* In the last edition, the section on *Posttraumatic Stress Disorder* covered the tragic events of September 11, 2001, involving the World Trade Center in New York and the Pentagon in Washington. Regrettably, other disasters such as Hurricane Sandy and the Newtown killings have occurred since then. The psychological effects of those events are covered, as are the effects of the wars in Iraq and Afghanistan on the mental health of the veterans of those wars. Related to that is new coverage of the effects of terrorism and torture, two areas rarely covered in textbooks of psychiatry, but of extreme importance to psychiatrists who treat its victims.

Two new chapters, *Public Psychiatry* and *World Aspects of Psychiatry,* have been added to this edition, both of which reflect the national and global scope of psychiatry and the need for clinicians to understand disorders that appear around the world. A new section covers brain stimulation methods and such new advances as transmagnetic and deep brain stimulation developed to restore health to those patients who have not responded to conventional therapies and who are among the most severely mentally ill. The chapter on psychotherapy has been expanded to include newer treatments such as *Mentalization* and *Mindfulness*, both of which are covered in a newly written section. Finally, every chapter covering clinical disorders has been revised and updated to reflect the latest advances in the field.

PSYCHOPHARMACOLOGY

The authors are committed to classifying drugs used to treat mental disorders according to their pharmacological activity and mechanism of action rather than using such categories as antidepressants, antipsychotics, anxiolytics, and mood stabilizers, which are overly broad and do not reflect, scientifically, the clinical use of psychotropic medication. For example, many antidepressant drugs are used to treat anxiety disorders; some anxiolytics are used to treat depression and bipolar disorders; and drugs from all categories are used to treat other clinical problems, such as eating disorders, panic disorders, and impulse-control disorders. Many drugs are also used to treat a variety of mental disorders that do not fit into any broad classification. Information about all pharmacological agents used in psychiatry, including pharmacodynamics, pharmacokinetics, dosages, adverse effects, and drug–drug interactions, has been thoroughly updated to reflect recent research.

CHILDHOOD DISORDERS

The chapters covering childhood disorders have been extensively revised to include important new material. The DSM-5 introduced some new childhood diagnostic categories and eliminated others. For example, diagnoses such as *Pervasive Developmental Disorder, Rett's Disorder,* and *Asperger's Disorder* are now subsumed under the rubric of *Autism Spectrum Disorder,* and *Disruptive Mood Dysregulation Disorder* and *Attenuated Psychosis Syndrome* were added as new diagnostic entities. These and other changes are reflected in the expanded coverage of disorders that usually begin in childhood and adolescence. The section dealing with the impact of terrorism has been updated to reflect new information about posttraumatic stress disorders in children, including the latest data on the psychological effects on children exposed to natural and man-made disasters. The section *Anxiety Disorders* was reorganized and updated thoroughly and *Obsessive–Compulsive Disorder* is now a separate chapter. The section that deals with the use of pharmacological agents in children was updated extensively to reflect the many changes in the use of medications to treat disorders of childhood that have occurred since the last edition of this book was published.

GLOSSARY

Unique to this edition is a new and updated comprehensive glossary of psychiatric signs and symptoms. Psychiatry is a descriptive science and the knowledge and accurate usage of the many terms available to the clinician is crucial to successful diagnosis and treatment. We hope readers find this addition to the textbook of use.

REFERENCES

References have been eliminated in this text to conserve space and readers are directed to our other textbooks, the *Synopsis of Psychiatry* and the *Comprehensive Textbook of Psychiatry,* for that information. More important than space constraints, however, is the fact that modern-day readers consult internet databases such as *PubMed* and *Google Scholar* to stay abreast of the most current literature, and we encourage that trend. References in textbooks tend to lag behind the most current literature and internet resources make up for that deficiency.

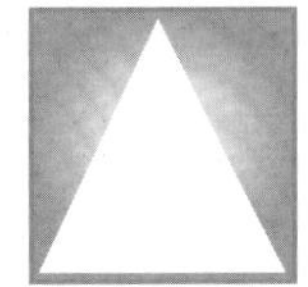

Acknowledgments

We deeply appreciate and are profoundly grateful for the work of our distinguished Contributing Editors, Caroly Pataki, M.D., Norman Sussman, M.D., and Samoon Ahmad, M.D., who gave generously of their time and expertise in the preparation of the parent textbook from which this book is derived, *Synopsis of Psychiatry.* Dr. Pataki was responsible for updating and revising the section on childhood and adolescent disorders and also served with distinction as Contributing Editor of child psychiatry in the *Comprehensive Textbook of Psychiatry* for many editions. Dr. Sussman was the Contributing Editor in the section on psychopharmacology in *Syno*psis and also served as Contributing Editor for the *Comprehensive Textbook* in that area.

We especially want to thank Dr. Ahmad, in his capacity of Contributing and Consulting Editor for this book and who updated the many advances in the field of psychopharmacology that occurred since the last edition of this book was published. He is an experienced psychiatrist and psychopharmacologist whose help we value immensely.

We also wish to thank Dorice Viera, Associate Curator of the Frederick L. Ehrman Medical Library at the New York University School of Medicine, for her valuable assistance.

We express our deep thanks to Nitza Jones-Sepulveda and Hayley Weinberg, who worked on this and many other *Kaplan & Sadock* books. Special thanks are also extended to Heidi-ann Grech, who worked on this textbook with intelligence and alacrity. We also acknowledge and thank Gladys Robles, who was of invaluable assistance to all of the authors, especially Dr. Ruiz.

Among the many others to thank are Seeba Anam, M.D., René Robinson, M.D., Nora Oberfield, M.D., Marissa Kaminsky, M.D., Caroline Press, M.D., Michael Stanger, M.D., Rajan Bahl, M.D., Jay K. Kantor, Ph.D., James Sadock, M.D., Victoria Sadock Gregg, M.D., Kristel Carrington, M.D., Rubiahna Vaughn, M.D., Samuel Lipkin, M.D., and Melissa Chang M.D. Laura Erikson-Schroth, M.D. deserves special thanks for her expert help in the section on *Gender Dysphoria*.

We thank Alan and Marilyn Zublatt for their generous support of this and other *Kaplan & Sadock* textbooks. Over the years they have been unselfish benefactors to many educational, clinical, and research projects at the NYU Medical Center.

Lippincott Williams & Wilkins has been our publisher for nearly half a century and as always, their staff was most efficient. At LWW we wish to thank Andrea Vosburgh, Product Development Editor at LWW, who helped in ways too numerous to mention. And we also wish to congratulate her on the birth of her son Samuel, who was born shortly before this book went to press. Franny Murphy deserves special thanks for stepping in at a crucial time in the production of several of our texts in both production and editing. Chris Miller at Aptara also deserves thanks for her work on this and other *Kaplan & Sadock* titles.

Finally, we want to express our deep thanks to Charles Marmar, M.D., Professor and Chairman of the Department of Psychiatry at New York University School of Medicine, who gave us his full support throughout the project. He has guided the department into the 21st century with dedication, skill, and enthusiasm. Under his leadership, NYU has become one of the leading centers of psychiatry and neuroscience both in this country and around the world.

Benjamin Sadock, M.D.
Virginia Sadock, M.D.
Pedro Ruiz, M.D.

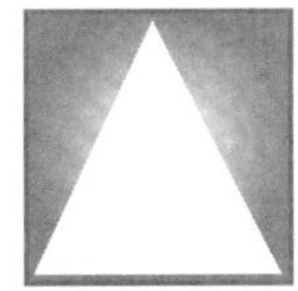

Contents

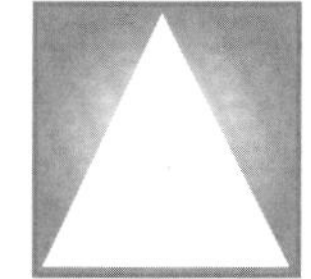

About the Authors

Benjamin J. Sadock, M.D. Benjamin James Sadock, M.D. is the Menas S. Gregory Professor of Psychiatry in the Department of Psychiatry at the New York University (NYU) School of Medicine. He is a graduate of Union College, received his M.D. degree from New York Medical College, and completed his internship at Albany Hospital. He completed his residency at Bellevue Psychiatric Hospital and then entered military service as Captain US Air force, where he served as Acting Chief of Neuropsychiatry at Sheppard Air Force Base in Texas. He has held faculty and teaching appointments at Southwestern Medical School and Parkland Hospital in Dallas and at New York Medical College, St. Luke's Hospital, the New York State Psychiatric Institute, and Metropolitan Hospital in New York City. Dr. Sadock joined the faculty of the NYU School of Medicine in 1980 and served in various positions: Director of Medical Student Education in Psychiatry, Co-Director of the Residency Training Program in Psychiatry, and Director of Graduate Medical Education. Currently, Dr. Sadock is Co-Director of Student Mental Health Services, Psychiatric Consultant to the Admissions Committee, and Co-Director of Continuing Education in Psychiatry at the NYU School of Medicine. Dr. Sadock is a Diplomate of the American Board of Psychiatry and Neurology and served as an Associate Examiner for the Board for more than a decade. He is a Distinguished Life Fellow of the American Psychiatric Association, a Fellow of the American College of Physicians, a Fellow of the New York Academy of Medicine, and a member of Alpha Omega Alpha Honor Society. He is active in numerous psychiatric organizations and was president and founder of the NYU-Bellevue Psychiatric Society. Dr. Sadock was a member of the National Committee in Continuing Education in Psychiatry of the American Psychiatric Association, served on the Ad Hoc Committee on Sex Therapy Clinics of the American Medical Association, was a Delegate to the Conference on Recertification of the American Board of Medical Specialists, and was a representative of the American Psychiatric Association Task Force on the National Board of Medical Examiners and the American Board of Psychiatry and Neurology. In 1985, he received the Academic Achievement Award from New York Medical College and was appointed Faculty Scholar at NYU School of Medicine in 2000. He is the author or editor of more than 100 publications (including 49 books), a reviewer for psychiatric journals, and lectures on a broad range of topics in general psychiatry. Dr. Sadock maintains a private practice for diagnostic consultations and psychiatric treatment. He has been married to Virginia Alcott Sadock, M.D., Professor of Psychiatry at NYU School of Medicine, since completing his residency. Dr. Sadock enjoys opera, golf, traveling, and is an enthusiastic fly fisherman.

Virginia A. Sadock, M.D. Virginia Alcott Sadock, M.D. joined the faculty of the New York University (NYU) School of Medicine in 1980, where she is currently Professor of Psychiatry and Attending Psychiatrist at the Tisch Hospital and Bellevue Hospital. She is Director of the Program in Human Sexuality at the NYU Langone Medical Center, one of the largest treatment and training programs of its kind in the United States. She is the author of more than 50 articles and chapters on sexual behavior and was the developmental editor of *The Sexual Experience*, one of the first major textbooks on human sexuality, published by Williams & Wilkins. She serves as a referee and book reviewer for several medical journals, including the *American Journal of Psychiatry* and the *Journal of the American Medical Association*. She has long been interested in the role of women in medicine and psychiatry and was a founder of the Committee on Women in Psychiatry of the New York County District Branch of the American Psychiatric Association. She is active in academic matters, served as an Assistant and Associate Examiner for the American Board of Psychiatry and Neurology for more than 20 years, and was also a member of the Test Committee in Psychiatry for both the American Board of Psychiatry and the Psychiatric Knowledge and Self-Assessment Program (PKSAP) of the American Psychiatric Association. She has chaired the Committee on Public Relations of the New York County District Branch of the American Psychiatric Association, has been a regional council member of the American Association of Sex Education Counselors and Therapists, a founding member of the Society of Sex Therapy and Research, and is President of the NYU Alumni Association of Sex Therapists. She has participated in the National Medical Television Network series *Women in Medicine* and the Emmy Award–winning PBS television documentary *Women and Depression* and currently hosts the radio program *Sexual Health and Well-being* (Sirius-XM) at NYU Langone Medical Center. She lectures extensively both in this country and abroad on sexual dysfunction, relational problems, and depression and anxiety disorders. She is a Distinguished Fellow of the American Psychiatric Association, a Fellow of the New York Academy of Medicine, and a Diplomate of the American Board of Psychiatry and Neurology. Dr. Sadock is a graduate of Bennington College, received her M.D. degree from New York Medical College, and trained in psychiatry at Metropolitan Hospital. She lives in Manhattan with her husband, Dr. Benjamin Sadock, where she maintains an active practice that includes individual psychotherapy, couples and marital therapy, sex therapy, psychiatric consultation, and pharmacotherapy. She and her husband have two children, James and Victoria, both emergency physicians, and three grandchildren, Emily, Celia, and Oliver. In her leisure time, Dr. Sadock enjoys theater, film, golf, reading fiction, and travel.

Pedro Ruiz, M.D. Pedro Ruiz, M.D. is Clinical Professor at the Menninger Department of Psychiatry and Behavioral Sciences of the Baylor College of Medicine in Houston, Texas. He graduated from medical School at the University of Paris in France. He conducted his residency training in psychiatry at the University of Miami Miller School of Medicine in Florida. He has held faculty appointments at a professorial level at Albert Einstein College of Medicine of Yeshiva University in New York City, at Baylor College of Medicine and the University of Texas Medical School both at Houston, and at the University of Miami Miller School of Medicine in Miami. He has also served in various academic positions: Director of the Lincoln Hospital Community Mental Health Center, Director of the Bronx Psychiatric Center, Assistant Dean and Vice Chair of the Department of Psychiatry, all at Albert Einstein College of Medicine in New York City; Chief of Psychiatry Service at Ben Taub General Hospital and Vice-Chair of the Department of Psychiatry and Behavioral Sciences at Baylor College of Medicine in Houston, Texas; Acting Chair, Vice Chair and Medical Director of the Mental Sciences Institute, all at the University of Texas Medical School at Houston in Houston, Texas; and Professor and Executive Vice Chair and Directors of Clinical Programs in the Department of Psychiatry and Behavioral Sciences of the University of Miami Miller Scholl of Medicine in Miami, Florida. Dr. Ruiz is a Distinguish Life Fellow of the American Psychiatric Association; a Fellow of the American College of Psychiatrists, the American Association for Social Psychiatry, the Benjamin Rush Society and the American Group Psychotherapy Association; and an Honorary Fellow of the World Psychiatric Association; Dr. Ruiz was also President of the American College of Psychiatrists (2000–2001), American Association for Social Psychiatry (2000–2002), American Board of Psychiatry and Neurology (2002–2003), American Psychiatric Association (2006–2007), the World Psychiatric Association (2011–2014) and the World Association on Dual Disorders (2015–2018); Dr. Ruiz has served in 56 Editorial Boards, among them The American Journal of Psychiatry, Psychiatric Services, Addictive Disorders and Their Treatment and The Journal of Nervous and Mental Disease. Dr. Ruiz has also received 96 awards and honors; Dr. Ruiz has also published 28 books, 263 original articles and editorials and 120 book chapters; Dr. Ruiz has also delivered 270 Grand Rounds and Invited Lectures, and has also attended and presented at 514 international congresses. Dr. Ruiz and his wife Angela have two children, Pedro Pablo and Angela Maria and four grandchildren: Francisco Antonio, Pedro Pablo Jr., Omar Joseph III, and Pablo Antonio. Dr. Ruiz enjoys reading literary novels, theater and literary movies, traveling internationally and fishing.

1 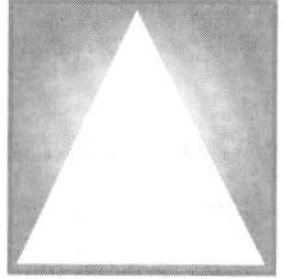

Classification in Psychiatry

Systems of classification for psychiatric diagnoses have several purposes: to distinguish one psychiatric diagnosis from another, so that clinicians can offer the most effective treatment; to provide a common language among health care professionals; and to explore the still unknown causes of many mental disorders. The two most important psychiatric classifications are the *Diagnostic and Statistical Manual of Mental Disorders* (DSM) developed by the American Psychiatric Association in collaboration with other groups of mental health professionals, and the *International Classification of Diseases* (ICD) developed by the World Health Organization.

HISTORY

The various classification systems used in psychiatry date back to Hippocrates, who introduced the terms *mania* and *hysteria* as forms of mental illness in the fifth century BC. Since then, each era has introduced its own psychiatric classification. The first US classification was introduced in 1869 at the annual meeting of the American Medico-Psychological Association, which later became the American Psychiatric Association. In 1952, the American Psychiatric Association's Committee on Nomenclature and Statistics published the first edition of DSM (DSM-I). Six editions have been published since then: DSM-II (1968); DSM-III (1980); a revised DSM-III, DSM-III-R (1987); DSM-IV (1994); DSM-IV-TR (TR stands for Text Revision) (2000); and DSM-5 published in 2013 (the roman numerals no longer used). This textbook uses the latest DSM-5 nosology throughout.

DSM-5 CLASSIFICATION

The DSM-5 lists 22 major categories of mental disorders, comprising more than 150 discrete illnesses. All of the disorders listed in DSM-5 are described in detail in the sections of the book that follow and cover epidemiology, etiology, diagnosis, differential diagnoses, clinical features, and treatment of each disorder. In this section, only a brief description of the disorders is provided to give the reader an overview of psychiatric classification including some of the changes made from DSM-IV to DSM-5.

NEURODEVELOPMENTAL DISORDERS

These disorders are usually first diagnosed in infancy, childhood, or adolescence.

Intellectual Disability or Intellectual Developmental Disorder (previously called Mental Retardation in DSM-IV). Intellectual disability (ID) is characterized by significant, below average intelligence and impairment in adaptive functioning. Adaptive functioning refers to how effective individuals are in achieving age-appropriate common demands of life in areas such as communication, self-care, and interpersonal skills. In DSM-5, ID is classified as mild, moderate, severe, or profound based on overall functioning; in DSM-IV, it was classified according to intelligence quotient (IQ) as mild (50–55 to 70), moderate (35–40 to 50–55), severe (20–25 to 35–40), or profound (below 20–25). A variation of ID called *Global Developmental Delay* is for children under 5 years with severe defects exceeding those above. *Borderline Intellectual Functioning* is used in DSM-5 but is not clearly differentiated from mild ID. In DSM-IV, it meant an IQ of about 70, whereas in DSM-5 it is categorized as a condition that may be the focus of clinical attention but no criteria are given.

COMMUNICATION DISORDERS. There are four types of communication disorders that are diagnosed when problems in communication cause significant impairment in functioning: (1) *Language Disorder* is characterized by a developmental impairment in vocabulary resulting in difficulty producing age-appropriate sentences; (2) *Speech Sound Disorder* is marked by difficulty in articulation; (3) *Childhood-Onset Fluency Disorder or Stuttering* is characterized by difficulty in fluency, rate, and rhythm of speech; and (4) *Social or Pragmatic Communication Disorder* is a profound difficulty in social interaction and communication with peers.

AUTISM SPECTRUM DISORDER. The autistic spectrum includes a range of behaviors characterized by severe difficulties in multiple developmental areas, including social relatedness, communication, and range of activity and repetitive and stereotypical patterns of behavior, including speech. They are divided into three levels: Level 1 is characterized by the ability to speak with reduced social interaction (this level resembles Asperger's disorder which is no longer part of DSM-5); Level 2 which is characterized by minimal speech and minimal social interaction (diagnosed as Rett's disorder in DSM-IV, but not part of DSM-5); and Level 3, marked by a total lack of speech and no social interaction.

ATTENTION-DEFICIT/HYPERACTIVITY DISORDER. Since the 1990s, Attention-deficit/Hyperactivity disorder (ADHD) has been one of the most frequently discussed psychiatric disorders in the lay media because of the sometimes unclear line between age-appropriate normal and disordered behavior and because of the concern that children without the disorder are being misdiagnosed and treated with medication. The central features of the disorder are persistent inattention, or hyperactivity and impulsivity, or both, that cause clinically significant impairment in functioning.

SPECIFIC LEARNING DISORDERS. These are maturational deficits in development that are associated with difficulty in acquiring specific skills in *reading* (also known as dyslexia); in *written expression;* or in *mathematics* (also known as dyscalculia).

MOTOR DISORDERS. Analogous to learning disorders, motor disorders are diagnosed when motor coordination is substantially below expectations based on age and intelligence, and when coordination problems significantly interfere with functioning. There are three major types of motor disorders: (1) *Developmental Coordination Disorder* is an impairment in the development of motor coordination, for example, delays in crawling or walking, dropping things, or poor sports performance; (2) *Stereotypic Movement Disorder* consists of repetitive motion activity, for example, head banging and body rocking; and (3) *Tic Disorder* is characterized by sudden involuntary, recurrent, and stereotyped movement or vocal sounds. There are two types of tic disorders; the first is *Tourette's Disorder,* characterized by motor and vocal tics including coprolalia, and the second is *Persistent Chronic Motor or Vocal Tic Disorders* marked by a single motor or vocal tic.

SCHIZOPHRENIA SPECTRUM AND OTHER PSYCHOTIC DISORDERS

The section on schizophrenia and other psychotic disorders includes eight specific disorders (schizophrenia, schizophreniform disorder, schizoaffective disorder, delusional disorder, brief psychotic disorder, substance/medication-induced psychotic disorder, psychotic disorder due to another medical condition, and catatonia) in which psychotic symptoms are prominent features of the clinical picture. The grouping of disorders in DSM-5 under this heading includes schizotypal personality disorder which is not a psychotic disorder; but which sometimes precedes full-blown schizophrenia. In *Synopsis* this is discussed under personality disorders (see Chapter 18).

SCHIZOPHRENIA. Schizophrenia is a chronic disorder in which prominent hallucinations or delusions are usually present. The individual must be ill for at least 6 months, although he or she need not be actively psychotic during all of that time. Three phases of the disorder are recognized by clinicians although they are not included in DSM-5 as discrete phases. The *prodrome phase* refers to deterioration in function before the onset of the active psychotic phase. The *active phase* symptoms (delusions, hallucinations, disorganized speech, grossly disorganized behavior, or negative symptoms such as flat affect, avolition, and alogia) must be present for at least 1 month. The *residual phase* follows the active phase. The features of the residual and prodromal phases include functional impairment and abnormalities of affect, cognition, and communication. In DSM-IV, schizophrenia was subtyped according to the most prominent symptoms present at the time of the evaluation (paranoid, disorganized, catatonic, undifferentiated, and residual types); however, those subtypes are no longer part of the official DSM-5 nomenclature. Nevertheless they are phenomenological accurate and are included in ICD-10. The subtypes remain useful descriptions that clinicians still find helpful when communicating with one another.

DELUSIONAL DISORDER. Delusional disorder is characterized by persistent delusions, for example, erotomanic, grandiose, jealous, persecutory, somatic, mixed, and unspecified. In general, the delusions are about situations that could occur in real life such as infidelity, being followed, or having an illness, which are categorized as nonbizarre beliefs. Within this category one finds what was termed in DSM-IV *shared delusional disorder* (also known as *folie à deux*) but has been renamed as *delusional symptoms in partner with delusional disorder* in DSM-5 and is characterized by a delusional belief that develops in a person who has a close relationship with another person with the delusion, the content of which is similar. *Paranoia* (a term not included in DSM-5) is a rare condition characterized by the gradual development of an elaborate delusional system, usually with grandiose ideas; it has a chronic course and the rest of the personality remains intact.

BRIEF PSYCHOTIC DISORDER. Brief psychotic disorder requires the presence of delusions, hallucinations, disorganized speech, grossly disorganized behavior, or catatonic behavior for at least 1 day but less than 1 month. It may be precipitated by an external life stress. After the episodes, the individual returns to his or her usual level of functioning.

SCHIZOPHRENIFORM DISORDER. Schizophreniform disorder is characterized by the same active phase symptoms of schizophrenia (delusions, hallucinations, disorganized speech, grossly disorganized behavior, or negative symptoms), but it lasts between 1 and 6 months and has no prodromal or residual phase features of social or occupational impairment.

SCHIZOAFFECTIVE DISORDER. Schizoaffective disorder is also characterized by the same active phase symptoms of schizophrenia (delusions, hallucinations, disorganized speech, grossly disorganized behavior, or negative symptoms), as well as the presence of a manic or depressive syndrome that is not brief relative to the duration of the psychosis. Individuals with schizoaffective disorder, in contrast to a mood disorder with psychotic features, have delusions or hallucinations for at least 2 weeks without coexisting prominent mood symptoms.

SUBSTANCE/MEDICATION-INDUCED PSYCHOTIC DISORDER. These are disorders with symptoms of psychosis caused by psychoactive or other substances, for example, hallucinogens and cocaine.

PSYCHOTIC DISORDER DUE TO ANOTHER MEDICAL CONDITION. This disorder is characterized by hallucinations or delusions that result from a medical illness, for example, temporal lobe epilepsy, avitaminosis, and meningitis.

CATATONIA. Catatonia is characterized by motor abnormalities such as catalepsy (waxy flexibility), mutism, posturing, and negativism. It can be associated with *another mental disorder,* for example, schizophrenia or bipolar disorder or *due to another medical condition,* for example, neoplasm, head trauma, and hepatic encephalopathy.

BIPOLAR AND RELATED DISORDERS

Bipolar disorder is characterized by severe mood swings between depression and elation and by remission and recurrence. There are four variants: bipolar I disorder, bipolar II disorder, cyclothymic disorder, and bipolar disorder due to substance/medication or another medical condition.

BIPOLAR I DISORDER. The necessary feature of bipolar I disorder is a history of a manic or mixed manic and depressive episode. Bipolar I disorder is subtyped in many ways: type of current episode (manic, hypomanic depressed, or mixed), severity and remission status (mild, moderate, severe without psychosis, severe with psychotic features, partial remission, or full remission), and whether the recent course is characterized by rapid cycling (at least four episodes in 12 months).

BIPOLAR II DISORDER. Bipolar II disorder is characterized by a history of hypomanic and major depressive episodes. The symptom criteria for a hypomanic episode are the same as those for a manic episode, although hypomania only requires a minimal duration of 4 days. The major difference between mania and hypomania is the severity of the impairment associated with the syndrome.

CYCLOTHYMIC DISORDER. This is the bipolar equivalent of dysthymic disorder (see below). Cyclothymic disorder is a mild, chronic mood disorder with numerous depressive and hypomanic episodes over the course of at least 2 years.

BIPOLAR DISORDER DUE TO ANOTHER MEDICAL CONDITION. Bipolar disorder caused by a general medical condition is diagnosed when evidence indicates that a significant mood disturbance is the direct consequence of a general medical condition, for example, frontal lobe tumor.

SUBSTANCE/MEDICATION INDUCED BIPOLAR DISORDER. Substance-induced mood disorder is diagnosed when the cause of the mood disturbance is substance intoxication, withdrawal, or medication, for example, amphetamine.

DEPRESSIVE DISORDERS

Depressive disorders are characterized by depression, sadness, irritability, psychomotor retardation, and, in severe cases, suicidal ideation. They include a number of conditions described below.

MAJOR DEPRESSIVE DISORDER. The necessary feature of major depressive disorder is depressed mood or loss of interest or pleasure in usual activities. All symptoms must be present nearly every day, except suicidal ideation or thoughts of death, which need only be recurrent. The diagnosis is excluded if the symptoms are the result of a normal bereavement and if psychotic symptoms are present in the absence of mood symptoms.

PERSISTENT DEPRESSIVE DISORDER OR DYSTHYMIA. Dysthymia is a mild, chronic form of depression that lasts for at least 2 years, during which, on most days, the individual experiences depressed mood for most of the day and at least two other symptoms of depression.

PREMENSTRUAL DYSPHORIC DISORDER. Premenstrual dysphoric disorder occurs about 1 week before the menses and is characterized by irritability, emotional lability, headache, and anxiety or depression that remits after the menstrual cycle is over.

SUBSTANCE/MEDICATION-INDUCED DEPRESSIVE DISORDER. This disorder is characterized by a depressed mood that is due to a substance, for example, alcohol or medication such as barbiturate.

DEPRESSIVE DISORDER DUE TO ANOTHER MEDICAL CONDITION. This condition is a state of depression secondary to a medical disorder, for example, hypothyroidism, Cushing's syndrome.

OTHER SPECIFIED DEPRESSIVE DISORDER. This diagnostic category includes two subtypes: (1) *Recurrent Depressive Episode* which is a depression that lasts between 2 and 13 days and that occurs at least once a month; and (2) *Short-Duration Depressive Episode* which is a depressed mood lasting between 4 and 14 days and which is nonrecurrent.

UNSPECIFIED DEPRESSIVE DISORDER. This diagnostic category includes four major subtypes: (1) *Melancholia* which is a severe form of major depression characterized by hopelessness, anhedonia, psychomotor retardation, and which also carries with it a high risk of suicide; (2) *Atypical Depression* which is marked by a depressed mood that is associated with weight gain instead of weight loss and with hypersomnia instead of insomnia; (3) *Peripartum Depression* is a depression that occurs around parturition, or within one month after giving birth (called postpartum depression in DSM-IV); and (4) *Seasonal Pattern* which is a depressed mood that occurs at a particular time of the year, usually winter (also known as seasonal affective disorder [SAD]).

DISRUPTIVE MOOD DYSREGULATION DISORDER. This is a new diagnosis listed as a depressive disorder that is diagnosed in children over the age of six and under the age of 18 and is characterized by severe temper tantrums, chronic irritability, and angry mood.

ANXIETY DISORDERS

The section on anxiety disorders includes nine specific disorders (panic disorder, agoraphobia, specific phobia, social anxiety disorder or social phobia, generalized anxiety disorder, anxiety disorder caused by a general medical condition, and substance-induced anxiety disorder) in which anxious symptoms are a prominent feature of the clinical picture. Because separation anxiety disorder and selective mutism occur in childhood, they are discussed in the childhood disorders section of this book.

PANIC DISORDER. A panic attack is characterized by feelings of intense fear or terror that come on suddenly in situations where there is nothing to fear. It is accompanied by heart racing or pounding, chest pain, shortness of breath or choking, dizziness, trembling or shaking, feeling faint or lightheaded, sweating, and nausea.

AGORAPHOBIA. Agoraphobia is a frequent consequence of panic disorder, although it can occur in the absence of panic attacks. Persons with agoraphobia avoid (or try to avoid) situations that they think might trigger a panic attack (or panic-like symptoms) or situations from which they think escape might be difficult if they have a panic attack.

SPECIFIC PHOBIA. Specific phobia is characterized by an excessive, unreasonable fear of specific objects or situations that almost always occurs on exposure to the feared stimulus. The phobic stimulus is avoided, or, when not avoided, the individual feels severely anxious or uncomfortable.

SOCIAL ANXIETY DISORDER OR SOCIAL PHOBIA. Social phobia is characterized by the fear of being embarrassed or humiliated in front of others. Similar to specific phobia, the phobic stimuli are avoided, or, when not avoided, the individual feels severely anxious and uncomfortable. When the phobic stimuli include most social situations, then it is specified as *generalized social phobia.*

GENERALIZED ANXIETY DISORDER. Generalized anxiety disorder is characterized by chronic excessive worry that occurs more days than not and is difficult to control. The worry is associated with symptoms, such as concentration problems, insomnia, muscle tension, irritability, and physical restlessness, and causes clinically significant distress or impairment.

ANXIETY DISORDER DUE TO ANOTHER MEDICAL CONDITION. Anxiety disorder caused by a general medical condition is diagnosed when evidence indicates that significant anxiety is the direct consequence of a general medical condition, for example, hyperthyroidism.

SUBSTANCE/MEDICATION-INDUCED ANXIETY DISORDER. Substance-induced anxiety disorder is diagnosed when the cause of the anxiety is a substance, for example, cocaine, or is the result of a medication such as cortisol.

SEPARATION ANXIETY DISORDER. Separation anxiety disorder occurs in children and is characterized by excessive anxiety about separating from home or loved ones beyond the expected child's developmental level.

SELECTIVE MUTISM. Selective mutism is characterized by persistent refusal to speak in specific situations despite the demonstration of speaking ability in other situations.

OBSESSIVE-COMPULSIVE AND RELATED DISORDERS

There are eight categories of disorders listed in this section, all of which have associated obsessions (repeated thoughts) or compulsions (repeated activities).

OBSESSIVE COMPULSIVE DISORDER. Obsessive Compulsive Disorder (OCD) is characterized by repetitive and intrusive thoughts or images that are unwelcome (obsessions) or repetitive behaviors that the person feels compelled to do (compulsions), or both. Most often, the compulsions are done to reduce the anxiety associated with the obsessive thought.

BODY DYSMORPHIC DISORDER. Body dysmorphic disorder is characterized by a distressing and impairing preoccupation with an imagined or slight defect in appearance. If the belief is held with delusional intensity, then delusional disorder, somatic type, might be diagnosed.

HOARDING DISORDER. Hoarding disorder is a behavioral pattern of accumulating items in a compulsive manner that may or may not have any utility to the person. The person is unable to get rid of those items even though they may create hazardous situations in the home such as risk of fire.

TRICHOTILLOMANIA OR HAIR-PULLING DISORDER. Trichotillomania is characterized by repeated hair pulling causing noticeable hair loss. It may occur anywhere on the body, for example, head, eyebrows, pubic area.

EXCORIATION OR SKIN-PICKING DISORDER. Skin-picking disorder is marked by the compulsive need to pick at ones skin to the point of doing physical harm.

SUBSTANCE/MEDICATION-INDUCED OBSESSIVE-COMPULSIVE DISORDER. This disorder is characterized by obsessive or compulsive behavior that is secondary to the use of a medication or a substance such as abuse of cocaine which can cause compulsive skin-picking (called formication).

OBSESSIVE-COMPULSIVE DISORDER DUE TO ANOTHER MEDICAL CONDITION. The cause of either obsessive or compulsive behavior is due to a medical condition, as sometimes may occur after a streptococcal infection.

OTHER SPECIFIED OBSESSIVE-COMPULSIVE AND RELATED DISORDERS. This category includes a group of disorders such as *obsessional jealousy* in which one person has repeated thoughts about infidelity in the spouse or partner. It must be distinguished from a delusional belief such as *Koro,* which is a disorder found in South and East Asia in which the person believes the genitalia are shrinking and disappearing into the body; and *Body-Focused Repetitive Behavior Disorder* in which the person engages in a compulsive behavioral pattern such as nail biting or lip chewing.

TRAUMA OR STRESSOR-RELATED DISORDER

This group of disorders is caused by exposure to a natural or man-made disaster or to a significant life stressor such as experiencing abuse. There are six conditions that fall under this category in DSM-5.

REACTIVE ATTACHMENT DISORDER. This disorder appears in infancy or early childhood and is characterized by a severe impairment in the ability to relate because of grossly pathological caregiving.

DISINHIBITED SOCIAL ENGAGEMENT DISORDER. This is a condition in which the child or adolescent has a deep seated fear of interacting with strangers, especially adults, usually as a result of traumatic upbringing.

POSTTRAUMATIC STRESS DISORDER. Posttraumatic stress disorder (PTSD) occurs after a traumatic event in which the individual believes that he or she is in physical danger or that his or her life is in jeopardy. PTSD can also occur after witnessing a violent or life-threatening event happening to someone else. The symptoms of PTSD usually occur soon after the traumatic event, although, in some cases, the symptoms develop months or even years after the trauma. PTSD is diagnosed when a person reacts to the traumatic event with fear and re-experiences symptoms over time or has symptoms of avoidance and hyperarousal. The symptoms persist for at least one month and cause clinically significant impairment in functioning or distress.

ACUTE STRESS DISORDER. Acute stress disorder occurs after the same type of stressors that precipitate PTSD however acute stress disorder is not diagnosed if the symptoms last beyond one month.

ADJUSTMENT DISORDERS. Adjustment disorders are maladaptive reactions to clearly defined life stress. They are divided into subtypes depending on symptoms—with *anxiety,* with *depressed mood,* with *mixed anxiety and depressed mood, disturbance of conduct,* and *mixed disturbance of emotions and conduct.*

PERSISTENT COMPLEX BEREAVEMENT DISORDER. Chronic and persistent grief that is characterized by bitterness, anger, or ambivalent feelings toward the dead accompanied by intense and prolonged withdrawal characterizes persistent complex bereavement disorder (also known as complicated grief or complicated bereavement). This must be distinguished from normal grief or bereavement.

DISSOCIATIVE DISORDERS

The section on dissociative disorders includes four specific disorders (dissociative amnesia, dissociative fugue, dissociative identity disorder, and depersonalization/derealization disorder) characterized by a disruption in the usually integrated functions of consciousness, memory, identity, or perception.

DISSOCIATIVE AMNESIA. Dissociative amnesia is characterized by memory loss of important personal information that is usually traumatic in nature.

DISSOCIATIVE FUGUE. Dissociative fugue is characterized by sudden travel away from home associated with partial or complete memory loss about one's identity.

DISSOCIATIVE IDENTITY DISORDER. Formerly called multiple personality disorder, the essential feature of dissociative identity disorder is the presence of two or more distinct identities that assume control of the individual's behavior.

DEPERSONALIZATION/DEREALIZATION DISORDER. The essential feature of depersonalization/derealization disorder is persistent or recurrent episodes of depersonalization (an altered sense of one's physical being, including feeling that one is outside of one's body, physically cut off or distanced from people, floating, observing oneself from a distance, as though in a dream), or derealization (experiencing the environment as unreal or distorted).

SOMATIC SYMPTOM AND RELATED DISORDERS (PREVIOUSLY CALLED SOMATOFORM DISORDERS IN DSM-IV)

This group of disorders is characterized by marked preoccupation with the body and fears of disease or consequences of disease, for example, death.

SOMATIC SYMPTOM DISORDER. Somatic symptom disorder is characterized by high levels of anxiety and persistent worry about somatic signs and symptoms that are misinterpreted as having a known medical disorder, also known as hypochondriasis.

ILLNESS ANXIETY DISORDER. Illness anxiety disorder is the fear of being sick with few or no somatic symptoms. A new diagnosis in DSM-5.

FUNCTIONAL NEUROLOGICAL SYMPTOM DISORDER. Formerly known as conversion disorder in DSM-IV, this condition is characterized by unexplained voluntary or motor sensory deficits that suggest the presence of a neurological or other general medical condition. Psychological conflict is determined to be responsible for the symptoms.

PSYCHOLOGICAL FACTORS AFFECTING OTHER MEDICAL CONDITIONS. This category is for psychological problems that negatively affect a medical condition by increasing the risk of an adverse outcome.

FACTITIOUS DISORDER. Factitious disorder, also called Munchausen syndrome, refers to the deliberate feigning of physical or psychological symptoms to assume the sick role. *Factitious Disorder Imposed on Another* (previously called Factitious Disorder by Proxy) is when one person presents the other person as ill, most often mother and child. Factitious disorder is distinguished from malingering in which symptoms are also falsely reported; however, the motivation in malingering is external incentives, such as avoidance of responsibility, obtaining financial compensation, or obtaining substances.

OTHER SPECIFIED SOMATIC SYMPTOM AND RELATED DISORDER. This category is for disorders that are not classified above. One such disorder is *Pseudocyesis* in which a person believes falsely that she (or he in rare instances) is pregnant.

FEEDING AND EATING DISORDERS

Feeding and eating disorders are characterized by a marked disturbance in eating behavior.

ANOREXIA NERVOSA. Anorexia nervosa is an eating disorder characterized by loss of body weight and refusal to eat. Appetite is usually intact.

BULIMIA NERVOSA. Bulimia Nervosa is an eating disorder characterized by recurrent and frequent binge eating with or without vomiting.

BINGE EATING DISORDER. Binge eating disorder is a variant of bulimia nervosa with occasional, once a week, binge eating.

PICA. Pica is the eating of nonnutritional substances, for example, starch.

RUMINATION DISORDER. The essential feature of rumination disorder is the repeated regurgitation of food, usually beginning in infancy or childhood.

AVOIDANT/RESTRICTIVE FOOD INTAKE DISORDER. Previously called feeding disorder of infancy or childhood in DSM-IV, the main feature of this disorder is a lack of interest in food or eating resulting in failure to thrive.

ELIMINATION DISORDERS

These are disorders of elimination caused by physiological or psychological factors. There are two types of elimination disorders: *Encopresis,* which is the inability to maintain bowel control, and *Enuresis,* which is the inability to maintain bladder control.

SLEEP–WAKE DISORDERS

Sleep–wake disorders involve disruptions in sleep quality, timing, and amount that result in daytime impairment and distress. They include the following disorders or disorder groups in DSM-5.

INSOMNIA DISORDER. Difficulty falling asleep or staying asleep is characteristic of insomnia disorder. Insomnia can be an independent condition or it can be comorbid with another mental disorder, another sleep disorder, or another medical condition.

HYPERSOMNOLENCE DISORDER. Hypersomnolence disorder, or hypersomnia, occurs when a person sleeps too much and feels excessively tired in spite of normal or because of prolonged quantity of sleep.

PARASOMNIAS. Parasomnias are marked by unusual behavior, experiences, or physiological events during sleep. This category is divided into three subtypes: *Non-Rem Movement Sleep Arousal Disorders* involve incomplete awakening from sleep accompanied by either sleepwalking or sleep terror disorder; *Nightmare Disorder* in which nightmares induce awakening repeatedly and cause distress and impairment; and *REM Sleep Behavior Disorder* which is characterized by vocal or motor behavior during sleep.

NARCOLEPSY. Narcolepsy is marked by sleep attacks, usually with loss of muscle tone (cataplexy).

BREATHING-RELATED SLEEP DISORDERS. There are three subtypes of breathing-related sleep disorders. The most common of the three is *Obstructive Sleep Apnea Hypopnea* in which apneas (absence of airflow) and hypopneas (reduction in airflow) occur repeatedly during sleep, causing snoring and daytime sleepiness. *Central Sleep Apnea* is the presence of Cheyne–Stokes breathing in addition to apneas and hypopneas. Finally, *Sleep-Related Hypoventilation* causes elevated CO_2 levels from decreased respiration.

RESTLESS LEGS SYNDROME. Restless legs syndrome is the compulsive movement of legs during sleep.

SUBSTANCE/MEDICATION INDUCED SLEEP DISORDER. This category includes sleep disorders that are caused by a drug or medication, for example, alcohol, caffeine.

CIRCADIAN RHYTHM SLEEP–WAKE DISORDERS. Underlying these disorders is a pattern of sleep disruption that alters or misaligns a person's circadian system, resulting in insomnia or excessive sleepiness. There are six types: (1) *Delayed sleep phase type* is characterized by sleep–wake times that are several hours later than desired or conventional times, (2) *Advanced sleep phase type* is characterized by earlier than usual sleep-onset and wake-up times, (3) *Irregular sleep–wake type* is characterized by fragmented sleep throughout the 24-hour day with no major sleep period and no discernible sleep–wake circadian rhythm, (4) *Non–24-hour sleep–wake type* is a circadian period that is not aligned to the external 24-hour environment, most common among blind or visually impaired individuals, (5) *Shift work type* is caused by working in a night schedule on a regular basis, and (6) *Unspecified type* that does not meet any of the above criteria.

SEXUAL DYSFUNCTIONS

Sexual dysfunctions are divided into 10 disorders that are related to change in sexual desire or performance.

DELAYED EJACULATION. Delayed ejaculation is the inability or marked delay in the ability to ejaculate during coitus or masturbation.

ERECTILE DISORDER. Erectile disorder is the inability to achieve or maintain an erection sufficient for coital penetration.

FEMALE ORGASMIC DISORDER. Female orgasmic disorder is the absence of the ability to achieve orgasm and/or a significant reduction in intensity of orgasmic sensations during masturbation or coitus.

FEMALE SEXUAL INTEREST/AROUSAL DISORDER. Female sexual interest/arousal disorder is absent or decreased interest in sexual fantasy or behavior which causes distress in the individual.

GENITOPELVIC PAIN/PENETRATION DISORDER. Genitopelvic pain/penetration disorder replaces the terms vaginismus and dyspareunia (vaginal spasm and pain interfering with coitus). It is the anticipation of or actual pain during sex activities, particularly related to intromission.

MALE HYPOACTIVE SEXUAL DESIRE DISORDER. Male hypoactive sexual desire disorder is absent or reduced sexual fantasy or desire in males.

PREMATURE OR EARLY EJACULATION. Premature ejaculation is manifested by ejaculation that occurs before or immediately after intromission during coitus.

SUBSTANCE/MEDICATION INDUCED SEXUAL DYSFUNCTION. Substance/medication induced sexual dysfunction is impaired function due to substances, for example, fluoxetine.

OTHER UNSPECIFIED SEXUAL DYSFUNCTIONS. These dysfunctions include sexual disorder due to a medical condition, for example, multiple sclerosis.

GENDER DYSPHORIA

Gender dysphoria is characterized by a persistent discomfort with one's biological sex and in some cases, the desire to have sex organs of the opposite sex. It is subdivided into *gender dysphoria in children* and *gender dysphoria in adolescents and adults.*

DISRUPTIVE, IMPULSE-CONTROL, AND CONDUCT DISORDERS

Included in this category are conditions involving problems in the self-control of emotions and behaviors.

OPPOSITIONAL DEFIANT DISORDER. Oppositional defiant disorder is diagnosed in children and adolescents. Symptoms include anger, irritability, defiance, and refusal to comply with regulations.

INTERMITTENT EXPLOSIVE DISORDER. Intermittent explosive disorder involves uncontrolled outbursts of aggression.

CONDUCT DISORDER. Conduct disorder is diagnosed in children and adolescents and is characterized by fighting and bullying.

PYROMANIA. Repeated fire-setting is the distinguishing feature of pyromania.

KLEPTOMANIA. Repeated stealing is the distinguishing feature of kleptomania.

SUBSTANCE RELATED DISORDERS

Substance-Induced Disorders. Psychoactive and other substances may cause intoxication and withdrawal syndrome and induce psychiatric disorders including bipolar and related disorders, obsessive-compulsive and related disorders, sleep disorders, sexual dysfunction, delirium, and neurocognitive disorders.

SUBSTANCE USE DISORDERS. Sometimes referred to as addiction, this is a group of disorders diagnosed by the substance abused—alcohol, cocaine, cannabis, hallucinogens, inhalants, opioids, sedative, stimulant, or tobacco.

ALCOHOL RELATED DISORDERS. Alcohol related disorders result in impairment caused by excessive use of alcohol. They include *alcohol use disorder* which is recurrent alcohol use with developing tolerance and withdrawal and *alcohol intoxication* which is simple drunkenness, and *alcohol withdrawal* which can involve delirium tremens (DTs).

OTHER ALCOHOL INDUCED DISORDERS. This group of disorders includes psychotic, bipolar, depressive, anxiety, sleep, sexual, or neurocognitive disorders including amnestic disorder (also known as Korsakoff's syndrome). Wernicke's encephalopathy, a neurological condition of ataxia, ophthalmoplegia, and confusion develops from chronic alcohol use. The two may coexist (Wernicke–Korsakoff's syndrome). *Alcohol-induced persisting dementia* is differentiated from Korsakoff's syndrome by multiple cognitive deficits.

Similar categories (intoxication, withdrawal, and induced disorders) exist for caffeine, cannabis, phencyclidine, other hallucinogens, inhalants, opioids, sedative, hypnotic, or anxiolytics, stimulants, and tobacco.

GAMBLING DISORDER. Gambling disorder is classified as a *non–substance-related disorder.* It involves compulsive gambling with an inability to stop or cut down, leading to social and financial difficulties. Some clinicians believe sexual addiction should be classified in the same way; but it is not a DSM-5 diagnosis.

NEUROCOGNITIVE DISORDERS (PREVIOUSLY CALLED DEMENTIA, DELIRIUM, AMNESTIC AND OTHER COGNITIVE DISORDERS IN DSM-IV)

These are disorders characterized by changes in brain structure and function that result in impaired learning, orientation judgment, memory, and intellectual functions. They are divided into three categories.

DELIRIUM. Delirium is marked by short-term confusion and cognition caused by substance intoxication or withdrawal (cocaine, opioids, phencyclidine), medication (cortisol), general medical condition (infection), or other causes (sleep deprivation).

MILD NEUROCOGNITIVE DISORDER. Mild neurocognitive disorder is a mild or modest decline in cognitive function. It must be distinguished from normal age related cognitive change (normal age-related senescence).

MAJOR NEUROCOGNITIVE DISORDER. Major neurocognitive disorder (a term that may be used synonymously with dementia which is still preferred by most psychiatrists) is marked by severe impairment in memory, judgment, orientation, and cognition. There are 13 subtypes (Table 1–1): *Alzheimer's disease* which usually occurs in persons over the age of 65 and is manifested by progressive intellectual deterioration and dementia; *vascular dementia* which is a stepwise progression in cognitive deterioration caused by vessel thrombosis or hemorrhage; *frontotemporal lobar degeneration* which is marked by behavioral inhibition (also known as Picks disease); *Lewy body disease* which involves hallucinations with dementia; *Traumatic Brain Injury* from physical trauma; *HIV disease; Prion disease* which is caused by slow-growing transmissible prion protein; *Parkinson's disease; Huntington's disease; caused by a medical condition; substance/medication induced,* for example, alcohol causing Korsakoff's syndrome; *multiple etiologies* and *unspecified dementia.*

PERSONALITY DISORDERS

Personality disorders are characterized by deeply engrained, generally lifelong maladaptive patterns of behavior that are usually recognizable at adolescence or earlier.

Table 1–1
Major Subtypes of Neurocognitive Disorder (Dementia)

Alzheimer's disease
Vascular dementia
Lewy body disease
Parkinson's disease
Frontotemporal dementia (Pick's disease)
Traumatic brain injury
HIV infection
Substance/medication-induced dementia
Huntington's disease
Prion disease
Other medical condition (known as Amnestic syndrome in DSM-IV-TR)
Multiple etiologies
Unspecified dementia

PARANOID PERSONALITY DISORDER. Paranoid personality disorder is characterized by unwarranted suspicion, hypersensitivity, jealousy, envy, rigidity, excessive self-importance, and a tendency to blame and ascribe evil motives to others.

SCHIZOID PERSONALITY DISORDER. Schizoid personality disorder is characterized by shyness, oversensitivity, seclusiveness, avoidance of close or competitive relationships, eccentricity, no loss of capacity to recognize reality, daydreaming, and an ability to express hostility and aggression.

SCHIZOTYPAL PERSONALITY DISORDER. Schizotypal personality disorder is similar to schizoid personality disorder, but the person also exhibits slight losses of reality testing, has odd beliefs, and is aloof and withdrawn.

OBSESSIVE-COMPULSIVE PERSONALITY DISORDER. Obsessive-compulsive personality disorder (OCPD) is characterized by excessive concern with conformity and standards of conscience; patient may be rigid, overconscientious, over dutiful, over inhibited, and unable to relax (three *Ps*—punctual, parsimonious, precise).

HISTRIONIC PERSONALITY DISORDER. Histrionic personality disorder is characterized by emotional instability, excitability, over reactivity, vanity, immaturity, dependency, and self-dramatization that is attention seeking and seductive.

AVOIDANT PERSONALITY DISORDER. Avoidant personality disorder is characterized by low levels of energy, easy fatigability, lack of enthusiasm, inability to enjoy life, and oversensitivity to stress.

ANTISOCIAL PERSONALITY DISORDER. Antisocial personality disorder covers persons in conflict with society. They are incapable of loyalty, selfish, callous, irresponsible, impulsive, and unable to feel guilt or learn from experience; they have low level of frustration tolerance and a tendency to blame others.

NARCISSISTIC PERSONALITY DISORDER. Narcissistic personality disorder is characterized by grandiose feelings, sense of entitlement, lack of empathy, envy, manipulativeness, and need for attention and admiration.

BORDERLINE PERSONALITY DISORDER. Borderline personality disorder is characterized by instability, impulsiveness, chaotic sexuality, suicidal acts, self-mutilating behavior, identity problems, ambivalence, and feeling of emptiness and boredom.

DEPENDENT PERSONALITY DISORDER. This is characterized by passive and submissive behavior; person is unsure of himself or herself and becomes entirely dependent on others.

PERSONALITY CHANGES DUE TO ANOTHER MEDICAL CONDITION. This category includes alterations to a person's personality due to a medical condition, for example, brain tumor.

UNSPECIFIED PERSONALITY DISORDER. This category involves other personality traits that do not fit any of the patterns described above.

PARAPHILIC DISORDERS AND PARAPHILIA

In *paraphilia,* a person's sexual interests are directed primarily toward objects rather than toward people, toward sexual acts not usually associated with coitus, or toward coitus performed under bizarre circumstances. A *paraphilic disorder* is acted out sexual behavior that can cause possible harm to another person. Included are: *exhibitionism* (genital exposure); *voyeurism* (watching sexual acts); *frotteurism* (rubbing against another person); *pedophilia* (sexual attraction toward children); *sexual masochism* (receiving pain); *sexual sadism* (inflicting pain); *fetishism* (arousal from an inanimate object); and *transvestism* (cross-dressing).

OTHER MENTAL DISORDERS

This is a residual category that includes four disorders that do not meet the full criteria for any of the previously described mental disorders: (1) *Other specified mental disorder due to another medical condition,* for example, dissociative symptoms secondary to temporal lobe epilepsy; (2) *Unspecified mental disorder due to another medical condition,* for example, temporal lobe epilepsy producing unspecified symptoms; (3) *Other specified mental disorder* in which symptoms are present but subthreshold for a specific mental illness; and (4) *Unspecified mental disorder* in which symptoms are present but subthreshold for any mental disorder.

Some clinicians use the term ***forme fruste*** (French, "unfinished form") to describe atypical or attenuated manifestation of a disease or syndrome, with the implication of incompleteness or partial presence of the condition or disorder. This term might apply to 3 and 4 above.

MEDICATION-INDUCED MOVEMENT DISORDERS AND OTHER ADVERSE EFFECTS OF MEDICATION

Ten disorders are included in this category: (1) *Neuroleptic or other medication-induced Parkinsonism* presents as rhythmic tremor, rigidity, akinesia, or bradykinesia that is reversible when the causative drug is withdrawn or its dosage reduced; (2) *Neuroleptic malignant syndrome* presents as muscle rigidity, dystonia, or hyperthermia; (3) *Medication-induced acute dystonia* consists of slow, sustained contracture of musculature causing postural deviations; (4) *Medication-induced acute akathisia* presents as motor restlessness with constant movement; (5) *Tardive dyskinesia* is characterized by involuntary movement of the lips, jaw, tongue, and by other involuntary dyskinetic movements; (6) *Tardive dystonia or akathisia* is a variant of tardive dyskinesia that involves extrapyramidal syndrome; (7) *Medication-induced postural tremor* is a fine tremor, usually at rest, that is caused by medication; (8) *Other medication-induced movement disorder* describes atypical extrapyramidal syndrome from a medication; (9) *Antidepressant discontinuation syndrome* is a withdrawal syndrome that arises after abrupt cessation of antidepressant drugs, for example, fluoxetine; and (10) *Other adverse effect of medication* includes changes in blood pressure, diarrhea etc. due to medication.

OTHER CONDITIONS THAT MAY BE A FOCUS OF CLINICAL ATTENTION

These are conditions that may interfere with overall functioning but are not severe enough to warrant a psychiatric diagnosis. These conditions are not mental disorders but may aggravate an existing mental disorder.

A broad range of life problems and stressors are included in this section among which are: (1) *Relational Problems* including *Problems Related to Family Upbringing,* such as problems with siblings or upbringing away from parents, and *Problems Related to Primary Support Group,* such as problems with a spouse or intimate partner, separation or divorce, family expressed emotion (EE), or uncomplicated bereavement; and (2) *Abuse and Neglect,* which includes *Child Maltreatment and Neglect Problems,* such as physical abuse, sexual abuse, neglect, or psychological abuse; and *Adult Maltreatment and Neglect Problems,* which involves spouse or partner physical, sexual, and psychological violence and neglect, or adult abuse by a nonspouse or nonpartner. Borderline intellectual functioning is included here in DSM-5.

CONDITIONS FOR FURTHER STUDY

In addition to the diagnostic categories listed above, other categories of illness are listed in DSM-5 that requires further study before they become part of the official nomenclature. Some of these disorders are controversial.

There are eight disorders in this group: (1) *Attenuated Psychosis Syndrome* refers to sub-threshold signs and symptoms of psychosis that develop in adolescence; (2) *Depressive Episodes With Short-duration Hypomania* are short episodes (2 to 3 days) of hypomania that occur with major depression; (3) *Persistent Complex Bereavement Disorder* is bereavement that persists over one year after loss; (4) *Caffeine Use Disorder* is dependence on caffeine with withdrawal syndrome; (5) *Internet Gaming Disorder* is the excessive use of internet that disrupts normal living; (6) *Neurobehavioral Disorder Associated With Prenatal Alcohol Exposure* covers all developmental disorders that occur in utero due to excessive alcohol use by mother, for example, fetal alcohol syndrome; (7) *Suicidal Behavior Disorder* is repeated suicide attempts that occur irrespective of diagnostic category of mental illness; and (8) *Non-Suicidal Self-Injury* is skin-cutting and other self-harm without suicidal intent.

2

Psychiatric Interview, History, and Mental Status Examination

The psychiatric interview is the most important element in the evaluation and care of persons with mental illness. A major purpose of the initial psychiatric interview is to obtain information that will establish a criteria-based diagnosis. This process, helpful in the prediction of the course of the illness and the prognosis, leads to treatment decisions. A well-conducted psychiatric interview results in a multidimensional understanding of the biopsychosocial elements of the disorder and provides the information necessary for the psychiatrist, in collaboration with the patient, to develop a person-centered treatment plan.

The two overarching elements of the psychiatric interview are the psychiatric history and the mental status examination. The history is based on the subjective report of the patient and in some cases the report of collaterals including other health care providers, family, and other caregivers. The mental status examination is the interviewer's objective tool similar to the physical examination in other areas of medicine. The physical examination, although not part of the interview itself, is included because of its potential relevance in the psychiatric diagnosis and also because it usually is included as part of the psychiatric evaluation especially in the inpatient setting. (In addition, much relevant information can be verbally obtained by the physician as parts of the physical examination are performed.) Similarly, the formulation, diagnosis, and treatment plan are included because they are products of the interview and also influence the course of the interview in a dynamic fashion as the interview moves back and forth pursuing, for example, whether certain diagnostic criteria are met or whether potential elements of the treatment plan are realistic.

IDENTIFYING DATA

This section is brief, one or two sentences, and typically includes the patient's name, age, gender, marital status (or significant other relationship), race or ethnicity, and occupation. Often the referral source is also included.

It is important to clarify where the information has come from, especially if others have provided information and/or records reviewed, and the interviewer's assessment of how reliable the data is.

CHIEF COMPLAINT (CC)

This should be the patient's presenting complaint, ideally in their own words. Examples include, "I'm depressed," or, "I have a lot of anxiety."

A 64-year-old man presented in a psychiatric emergency room with a chief complaint, "I'm melting away like a snowball." He had become increasingly depressed over 3 months. Four weeks before the ER visit, he had seen his primary care physician who had increased his antidepressant medication (imipramine) from 25 to 75 mg, and also added hydrochlorothiazide (50 mg) because of mild hypertension and slight pedal edema. Over the ensuing 4 weeks, the patient's condition deteriorated. In the emergency room he was noted to have depressed mood, hopelessness, weakness, significant weight loss, and psychomotor retardation and was described as appearing "depleted." He also appeared dehydrated, and blood work indicated he was hypokalemic. Examination of his medication revealed that the medication bottles had been mislabeled; he was taking 25 mg of imipramine (generally a nontherapeutic dose) and 150 mg of hydrochlorothiazide. He was indeed, "melting away like a snowball." Fluid and potassium replacement and a therapeutic dose of an antidepressant resulted in significant improvement.

HISTORY OF PRESENT ILLNESS (HPI)

The present illness is a chronological description of the evolution of the symptoms of the current episode. In addition, the account should also include any other changes that have occurred during this same time period in the patient's interests, interpersonal relationships, behaviors, personal habits, and physical health. As noted above, the patient may provide much of the essential information for this section in response to an open-ended question such as, "Can you tell me in your own words what brings you here today?" Other times the clinician may have to lead the patient through parts of the presenting problem. Details that should be gathered include the length of time that the current symptoms have been present and whether there have been fluctuations in the nature or severity of those symptoms over time. ("I have been depressed for the last 2 weeks" vs. "I've had depression all my life.") The presence or absence of stressors should be established, and these may include situations at home, work, school, legal issues, medical comorbidities, and interpersonal difficulties. Also important are factors that alleviate or exacerbate symptoms such as medications, support, coping skills, or time of day. The essential questions to be answered in the history of the present illness include what (symptoms), how much (severity), how long, and associated factors. It is also important to identify why the patient is seeking help now, what are the "triggering" factors. "I'm here now because my girlfriend told me if I don't get help with this nervousness she is going to leave me." Identifying the setting in which the illness began can be revealing and helpful in understanding the etiology of, or significant contributors to, the condition. If any treatment has been received for the current episode, it should be defined in terms of who saw the patient and how often, what was done (e.g., psychotherapy or medication), and the specifics of the modality used. Also, is that treatment continuing and, if not, why not? The psychiatrist should be alert for any hints of abuse by former therapists as this experience, unless addressed, can be a major impediment to a healthy and helpful therapeutic alliance.

PAST PSYCHIATRIC HISTORY (PH)

In the past psychiatric history (PH), the clinician should obtain information about all psychiatric illnesses and their course over the patient's lifetime, including symptoms and treatment. Because comorbidity is the rule rather than the exception, in addition to prior episodes of the same illness (e.g., past episodes of depression in an individual who has a major depressive disorder) the psychiatrist should also be alert for the signs and symptoms of other psychiatric disorders. Description of past symptoms should include when they occurred, how long they lasted, and the frequency and severity of episodes.

Past treatment episodes should be reviewed in detail. These include outpatient treatment such as psychotherapy (individual, group, couple, or family), day treatment or partial hospitalization, inpatient treatment, including voluntary or involuntary and what precipitated the need for the higher level of care, support groups, or other forms of treatment such as vocational training. Medications and other modalities such as electroconvulsive therapy, light therapy, or alternative treatments should be carefully reviewed. One should explore what was prescribed (may have to offer lists of names to patients), how long and at what doses they were used (to establish adequacy of the trials), and why they were stopped. Important questions include what was the response to the medication/modality and whether there were side effects. It is also helpful to establish whether there was reasonable compliance with the recommended treatment. The psychiatrist should also inquire whether a diagnosis was made, what it was, and who made the diagnosis. Although a diagnosis made by another clinician should not be automatically accepted as valid, it is important information that can be used by the psychiatrist in forming his or her opinion.

Special consideration should be given to establishing a lethality history that is important in the assessment of current risk. Past suicidal ideation, intent, plan, and attempts should be reviewed including the nature of attempts, perceived lethality of the attempts, save potential, suicide notes, giving away things, or other death preparations. Because many patients will withhold specific information about recent suicidal behaviors or suicidal ideation, Shawn Shea recommends a technique of several specific behavioral questions to determine how close the patient was to a lethal attempt. Violence and homicidality history will include any violent actions or intent. Specific questions about domestic violence, legal complications, and outcome of the victim may be helpful in defining this history more clearly. History of nonsuicidal self-injurious behavior should also be covered including any history of cutting, burning, banging head, and biting oneself. The feelings, including relief of distress, that accompany or follow the behavior should also be explored as well as the degree to which the patient has gone to hide the evidence of these behaviors.

SUBSTANCE USE/ABUSE AND ADDICTIONS

A careful review of substance use, abuse, and addictions is essential to the psychiatric interview. The clinician should keep in mind that this information may be difficult for the patient to discuss, and a nonjudgmental style will elicit more accurate information. If the patient seems reluctant to share such information, specific questions may be helpful (e.g., "Have you ever used marijuana?" or "Do you typically drink alcohol every day?"). History of use should include what substances have been used including alcohol, drugs, medications (prescribed or not prescribed to the patient), and routes of use (oral, snorting, or intravenous). The frequency and amount of use should be determined keeping in mind the tendency for patients to minimize or deny use that may be perceived as socially unacceptable. Also, there are many misconceptions about alcohol that can lead to erroneous data. The definition of alcohol may be misunderstood. "No, I don't use alcohol." Later in same interview, "I drink a fair amount of beer." Also the amount of alcohol can be confused with the volume of the drink. "I'm not worried about my alcohol use. I mix my own drinks and I add a lot of water." In response to a follow-up question, "How much bourbon? Probably three or four shots." Tolerance, the need for increasing amounts of use, and any withdrawal symptoms should be established to help determine abuse versus dependence. Impact of use on social interactions, work, school, legal consequences, driving while intoxicated (DWI), should be covered.

Any periods of sobriety should be noted including length of time and setting such as in jail, legally mandated, etc. A history of treatment episodes should be explored including inpatient detoxification or rehabilitation, outpatient treatment, group therapy, other settings including self-help groups, Alcoholics Anonymous (AA) or Narcotics Anonymous (NA), halfway houses, or group homes.

Current substance abuse or dependence can have a significant impact on psychiatric symptoms and treatment course. The patient's readiness for change should be determined including whether they are in the precontemplative, contemplative, or action phases. Referral to the appropriate treatment setting should be considered.

Other important substances and addictions that should be covered in this section include tobacco and caffeine use, gambling, eating behaviors, and internet use. Exploration of tobacco use is especially important because persons abusing substances are more likely to die as a result of tobacco use than because of the identified abused substance. Gambling history should include casino visits, horse racing, lottery and scratch cards, and sports betting. Addictive type eating may include binge eating disorder. Overeaters Anonymous (OA) and Gamblers Anonymous (GA) are 12-step programs, similar to AA, for patients with addictive eating behaviors and gambling addictions.

PAST MEDICAL HISTORY

The past medical history includes an account of major medical illnesses and conditions as well as treatments, both past and present. Any past surgeries should also be reviewed. The patient's reaction to these illnesses and coping skills employed are important to understand. The past medical history is an important consideration when determining potential causes of mental illness as well as comorbid or confounding factors and may dictate potential treatment options or limitations. Medical illnesses can precipitate a psychiatric disorder (e.g., anxiety disorder in an individual recently diagnosed with cancer), mimic a psychiatric disorder (hyperthyroidism resembling an anxiety disorder), be precipitated by a psychiatric disorder or its treatment (metabolic syndrome in a patient on a second-generation antipsychotic medication), or influence the choice of treatment of a psychiatric disorder (renal disorder and the use of lithium carbonate). It is important to pay special attention to neurological issues including seizures, head injury, and pain disorder. Any known history of prenatal or birthing problems or issues with developmental milestones should be noted. In women, a reproductive and menstrual history is important as well as a careful assessment of potential for current or future pregnancy. ("How do you know you are not pregnant?" may be answered with "because I have had my tubes tied," or "I just hope I'm not.")

A careful review of all current medications is very important. This should include all current psychiatric medications with attention to how long they have been used, compliance with schedules, effect of the medications, and any side effects. It is often helpful to be very specific in determining compliance and side effects including asking questions such as, "how many days out of the week are you able to actually take this medication?," or, "have you noticed any change in your sexual function since starting this medication?," as the patient may not spontaneously offer this information that may be embarrassing or perceived to be treatment interfering.

Nonpsychiatric medications, over-the-counter medications, sleep aids, herbal, and alternative medications should also be reviewed. These can all potentially have psychiatric implications including side effects or producing symptoms as well as potential medication interactions dictating treatment options. Optimally the patient should be asked to bring all medications, prescribed or not, over-the-counter preparations, vitamins, and herbs with them to the interview.

Allergies to medications must be covered including which medication and the nature of, the extent of, and the treatment of the allergic response. Psychiatric patients should be encouraged to have adequate and regular medical care. The sharing of appropriate information between the primary care physicians, other medical specialists, and the psychiatrist can be very helpful for optimal patient care. The initial interview is an opportunity to reinforce that concept with the patient. At times a patient may not want information to be shared with their primary care physician. This wish should be respected although it may be useful to explore if there is some information that can be shared. Often patients want to restrict certain social or family information (e.g., an extramarital affair) but are comfortable with other information (medication prescribed) being shared.

FAMILY HISTORY

Because many psychiatric illnesses are familial and a significant number of those have a genetic predisposition, if not cause, a careful review of family history is an essential part of the psychiatric assessment. Furthermore, an accurate family history helps not only in defining a patient's potential risk factors for specific illnesses but also the formative psychosocial background of the patient. Psychiatric diagnoses, medications, hospitalizations, substance-use disorders, and lethality history should all be covered. The importance of these issues is highlighted, for example, by the evidence that, at times, there appears to be a familial response to medications and a family history of suicide is a significant risk factor for suicidal behaviors in the patient. The interviewer must keep in mind that the diagnosis ascribed to a family member may or may not be accurate and some data about the presentation and treatment of that illness may be helpful. Medical illnesses present in family histories may also be important in both the diagnosis and the treatment of the patient. An example is a family history of diabetes or hyperlipidemia affecting the choice of antipsychotic medication that may carry a risk for development of these illnesses in the patient. Family traditions, beliefs, and expectations may also play a significant role in the development, expression, or course of the illness. Also the family history is important in identifying potential support as well as stresses for the patient and depending on the degree of disability of the patient the availability and adequacy of potential caregivers.

DEVELOPMENTAL AND SOCIAL HISTORY

The developmental and social history reviews the stages of the patient's life. It is an important tool in determining the context of psychiatric symptoms and illnesses and may, in fact, identify some of the major factors in the evolution of the disorder. Frequently, current psychosocial stressors will be revealed in the course of obtaining a social history. It can often be helpful to review the social history chronologically to ensure all information is covered.

Any available information concerning prenatal or birthing history and developmental milestones should be noted. For the large majority of adult patients such information is not readily available and when it is it may not be fully accurate. Childhood history will include childhood home environment including members of the family and social environment including the number and quality of friendships. A detailed school history including how far the patient went in school and how old they were at that level, any special education circumstances or learning disorders, behavioral problems at school, academic performance, and extracurricular activities should be obtained. Childhood physical and sexual abuse should be carefully queried.

Work history will include types of jobs, performance at jobs, reasons for changing jobs, and current work status. The nature of the patient's relationships with supervisors and coworkers should be reviewed. The patient's income, financial issues, and insurance coverage including pharmacy benefits are often important issues.

Military history, where applicable, should be noted including rank achieved, combat exposure, disciplinary actions, and discharge status. Marriage and relationship history including sexual preferences and current family structure should be explored. This should include the patient's capacity to develop and maintain stable and mutually satisfying relationships as well as issues of intimacy and sexual behaviors. Current relationships with parents, grandparents, children, and grandchildren are an important part of the social history. Legal history is also relevant, especially any pending charges or lawsuits. The social history also includes hobbies, interests, pets, and leisure time activities and how this has fluctuated over time. It is important to identify cultural and religious influences on the patient's life and current religious beliefs and practices.

A brief overview of the sexual history is given in Table 2–1.

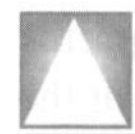

Table 2–1
Sexual History

1. Screening questions
   a. Are you sexually active?
   b. Have you noticed any changes or problems with sex recently?
2. Developmental
   a. Acquisition of sexual knowledge
   b. Onset of puberty/menarche
   c. Development of sexual identity and orientation
   d. First sexual experiences
   e. Sex in romantic relationship
   f. Changing experiences or preferences over time
   g. Sex and advancing age
3. Clarification of sexual problems
   a. Desire phase
      Presence of sexual thoughts or fantasies
      When do they occur and what is their object?
      Who initiates sex and how?
   b. Excitement phase
      Difficulty in sexual arousal (achieving or maintaining erections, lubrication), during foreplay and preceding orgasm
   c. Orgasm phase
      Does orgasm occur?
      Does it occur too soon or too late?
      How often and under what circumstances does orgasm occur?
      If orgasm does not occur, is it because of not being excited or lack of orgasm despite being aroused?
   d. Resolution phase
      What happens after sex is over (e.g., contentment, frustration, continued arousal)?

REVIEW OF SYSTEMS

The review of systems attempts to capture any current physical or psychological signs and symptoms not already identified in the present illness. Particular attention is paid to neurological and systemic symptoms (e.g., fatigue or weakness). Illnesses that might contribute to the presenting complaints or influence the choice of therapeutic agents should be carefully considered (e.g., endocrine, hepatic, or renal disorders). Generally, the review of systems is organized by the major systems of the body.

MENTAL STATUS EXAMINATION

The mental status examination (MSE) is the psychiatric equivalent of the physical examination in the rest of medicine. The MSE explores all the areas of mental functioning and denotes evidence of signs and symptoms of mental illnesses. Data are gathered for the mental status examination throughout the interview from the initial moments of the interaction including what the patient is wearing and their general presentation. Most of the information does not require direct questioning, and the information gathered from observation may give the clinician a different dataset than patient responses. Direct questioning augments and rounds out the MSE. The MSE gives the clinician a snapshot of the patient's mental status at the time of the interview and is useful for subsequent visits to compare and monitor changes over time. The psychiatric mental status examination includes cognitive screening (discussed below under *Cognition*).

APPEARANCE AND BEHAVIOR. This section consists of a general description of how the patient looks and acts during the interview. Does the patient appear to be their stated age, younger or older? Is this related to their style of dress, physical features, or style of interaction? Items to be noted include what the patient is wearing, including body jewelry, and whether it is appropriate for the context. For example, a patient in a hospital gown would be appropriate in the emergency room or inpatient unit but not in an outpatient clinic. Distinguishing features, including disfigurations, scars, and tattoos are noted. Grooming and hygiene are also included in the overall appearance and can be clues to the patient's level of functioning.

The description of a patient's behavior includes a general statement about whether they are exhibiting acute distress and then a more specific statement about the patient's approach to the interview. The patient may be described as cooperative, agitated, disinhibited, disinterested, etc. Once again, appropriateness is an important factor to consider in the interpretation of the observation. If a patient is brought involuntarily for examination, it may be appropriate, certainly understandable, that he or she is somewhat uncooperative, especially at the beginning of the interview.

MOTOR ACTIVITY. Motor activity may be described as normal, slowed (bradykinesia), or agitated (hyperkinesia). This can give clues to diagnoses (e.g., depression vs. mania) as well as confounding neurological or medical issues. Gait, freedom of movement, any unusual or sustained postures, pacing, and hand wringing are described. The presence or absence of any tics should be noted, as should be jitteriness, tremor, apparent restlessness, lip smacking, and tongue protrusions. These can be clues to adverse reactions or side effects of medications such as tardive dyskinesia, akathisia, or parkinsonian features from antipsychotic medications or suggestion of symptoms of illnesses such as attention-deficit/hyperactivity disorder.

SPEECH. Evaluation of speech is an important part of the MSE. Elements considered include fluency, amount, rate, tone, and volume. Fluency can refer to whether the patient has full command of the English language as well as potentially more subtle fluency issues such as stuttering, word finding difficulties, or paraphasic errors. (A Spanish-speaking patient with an interpreter would be considered not fluent in English but an attempt should be made to establish whether he or she is fluent in Spanish.) The evaluation of the amount of speech refers to whether it is normal, increased, or decreased. Decreased amounts of speech may suggest several different things ranging from anxiety or disinterest to thought blocking or psychosis. Increased amounts of speech often (but not always) are suggestive of mania or hypomania. A related element is the speed or rate of speech. Is it slowed or rapid (pressured)? Finally speech can be evaluated for its tone and volume. Descriptive terms for these elements include irritable, anxious, dysphoric, loud, quiet, timid, angry, or childlike.

MOOD. The terms mood and affect vary in their definition, and a number of authors have recommended combining the two elements into a new label "emotional expression." Traditionally, mood is defined as the patient's internal and sustained emotional state. Its experience is subjective, and hence it is best to use the patient's own words in describing their mood. Terms such as "sad," "angry," "guilty," or "anxious" are common descriptions of mood.

AFFECT. Affect differs from mood in that affect is the expression of mood or what the patient's mood appears to be to the clinician. Affect is often described with the following elements: Quality, quantity, range, appropriateness, and congruence. Terms used to describe the quality (or tone) of a patient's affect include dysphoric, happy, euthymic, irritable, angry, agitated, tearful, sobbing, and flat. Speech is often an important clue to the assessment of affect but not exclusive. Quantity of affect is a measure of its intensity. Two patients both described as having depressed affect can be very different if one is described as mildly depressed and the other as severely depressed. Range can be restricted, normal, or labile. "Flat" is a term that has been used for severely restricted range of affect that is described in some patients with schizophrenia. Appropriateness of affect refers to how the affect correlates to the setting. A patient who is laughing at a solemn moment of a funeral service is described as having inappropriate affect. Affect can also be congruent or incongruent with the patient's described mood or thought content. A patient may report feeling depressed or describe a depressive theme but do so with laughter, smiling, and no suggestion of sadness.

Thought Content

Thought content is essentially what thoughts are occurring to the patient. This is inferred by what the patient spontaneously expresses, as well as responses to specific questions aimed at eliciting particular pathology. Some patients may perseverate or ruminate on specific content or thoughts. They may focus on material that is considered obsessive or compulsive. Obsessional thoughts are unwelcome and repetitive thoughts that intrude into the patient's consciousness. They are generally ego-alien and resisted by the patient. Compulsions are repetitive, ritualized behaviors that patients feel compelled to perform to avoid an increase in anxiety or some dreaded outcome. Another large category of thought content pathology is delusions. Delusions are false, fixed ideas that are not shared by others and can be divided into bizarre and nonbizarre (nonbizarre delusions refer to thought content that is not true but is not out of the realm of possibility).

Common delusions include grandiose, erotomanic, jealous, somatic, and persecutory. It is often helpful to suggest delusional content to patients who may have learned to not spontaneously discuss them. Questions that can be helpful include, "do you ever feel like someone is following you or out to get you," and "do you feel like the TV or radio has a special message for you?" An affirmative answer to the latter question indicates an "idea of reference." Paranoia can be closely related to delusional material and can range from "soft" paranoia such as general suspiciousness to more severe forms that impact daily functioning. Questions that can elicit paranoia can include asking about the patient worrying about cameras, microphones, or the government.

Suicidality and homicidality fall under the category of thought content but here are discussed separately because of their particular importance in being addressed in every initial psychiatric interview. Simply asking if someone is suicidal or homicidal is not adequate. One must get a sense of ideation, intent, plan, and preparation. While completed suicide is extremely difficult to accurately predict, there are identified risk factors, and these can be used in conjunction with an evaluation of the patient's intent and plan for acting on thoughts of suicide.

Thought Process

Thought process differs from thought content in that it does not describe what the person is thinking rather how the thoughts are formulated, organized, and expressed. A patient can have normal thought process with significantly delusional thought content. Conversely, there may be generally normal thought content but significantly impaired thought process. Normal thought process is typically described as linear, organized, and goal-directed. With flight of ideas, the patient rapidly moves from one thought to another, at a pace that is difficult for the listener to keep up with, but all of the ideas are logically connected. The circumstantial patient often includes details and material that is not directly relevant to the subject or answer to the question but does eventually returns to address the subject or answer the question. Typically the examiner can follow a circumstantial train of thought, seeing connections between the sequential statements. Tangential thought process may at first appear similar, but the patient never returns to the original point or question. The tangential thoughts are seen as irrelevant and related in a minor, insignificant manner. Loose thoughts or associations differ from circumstantial and tangential thoughts in that with loose thoughts it is difficult or impossible to see the connections between the sequential content. Perseveration is the tendency to focus on a specific idea or content without the ability to move on to other topics. The perseverative patient will repeatedly come back to the same topic despite the interviewer's attempts to change the subject. Thought blocking refers to a disordered thought process in which the patient appears to be unable to complete a thought. The patient may stop midsentence or midthought and leave the interviewer waiting for the completion. When asked about this, patients will often remark that they don't know what happened and may not remember what was being discussed. Neologisms refer to a new word or condensed combination of several words that is not a true word and is not readily understandable although sometimes the intended meaning or partial meaning may be apparent. Word salad is speech characterized by confused, and often repetitious, language with no apparent meaning or relationship attached to it.

Perceptual Disturbances

Perceptual disturbances include hallucinations, illusions, depersonalization, and derealization. Hallucinations are perceptions in the absence of stimuli to account for them. Auditory hallucinations are the hallucinations most frequently encountered in the psychiatric setting. Other hallucinations can include visual, tactile, olfactory, and gustatory (taste). The interviewer should make a distinction between a true hallucination and a misperception of stimuli (illusion). Hearing the wind rustle through the trees outside one's bedroom and thinking a name is being called is an illusion. Hypnagogic hallucinations (at the interface of wakefulness and sleep) may be normal phenomena. At times patients without psychosis may hear their name called or see flashes or shadows out of the corner of their eyes. In describing hallucinations, the interviewer should include what the patient is experiencing, when it occurs, how often it occurs, and whether it is uncomfortable (ego dystonic) or not. In the case of auditory hallucinations it can be useful to learn if the patient hears words, commands, or conversations and whether the voice is recognizable to the patient.

Depersonalization is a feeling that one is not oneself or that something has changed. Derealization is a feeling that one's environment has changed in some strange way that is difficult to describe.

Cognition

The elements of cognitive functioning that should be assessed are alertness, orientation, concentration, memory (both short and long term), calculation, fund of knowledge, abstract reasoning, insight, and judgment.

Note should be made of the patient's level of alertness. The amount of detail in assessing cognitive function will depend on the purpose of the examination and also what has already been learned in the interview about the patient's level of functioning, performance at work, handling daily chores, balancing one's checkbook, etc. In addition, the psychiatrist will have already elicited data concerning the patient's memory for both remote and recent past. A general sense of intellectual level and how much schooling the patient has had can help distinguish intelligence and educational issues versus cognitive impairment that might be seen in delirium or dementia. See Table 2–2 for an overview of questions used to test cognitive function in the mental status examination.

Abstract Reasoning

Abstract reasoning is the ability to shift back and forth between general concepts and specific examples. Having the patient identify similarities between like objects or concepts (apple and pear, bus and airplane, or a poem and a painting) as well as interpreting proverbs can be useful in assessing one's ability to abstract. Cultural and educational factors and limitations should be kept in mind when assessing ability to abstract. Occasionally, the inability to abstract or the idiosyncratic manner of grouping items can be dramatic.

Table 2–2
Questions Used to Test Cognitive Functions in the Sensorium Section of the Mental Status Examination

1.	Alertness	(Observation)
2.	Orientation	What is your name? Who am I? What place is this? Where is it located? What city are we in?
3.	Concentration	Starting at 100, count backward by 7 (or 3). Say the letters of the alphabet backward starting with Z. Name the months of the year backward starting with December.
4.	Memory Immediate	Repeat these numbers after me: 1, 4, 9, 2, 5.
	Recent	What did you have for breakfast? What were you doing before we started talking this morning? I want you to remember these three things: a yellow pencil, a cocker spaniel, and Cincinnati. After a few minutes I'll ask you to repeat them.
	Long term	What was your address when you were in the third grade? Who was your teacher? What did you do during the summer between high school and college?
5.	Calculations	If you buy something that costs \$3.75 and you pay with a \$5 bill, how much change should you get? What is the cost of three oranges if a dozen oranges cost \$4.00?
6.	Fund of knowledge	What is the distance between New York and Los Angeles? What body of water lies between South America and Africa?
7.	Abstract reasoning	Which one does not belong in this group: a pair of scissors, a canary, and a spider? Why? How is an apple and an orange alike?

Insight

Insight, in the psychiatric evaluation, refers to the patient's understanding of how they are feeling, presenting, and functioning as well as what the potential causes of their psychiatric presentation may be. The patient may have no insight, partial insight, or full insight. A component of insight often is reality testing in the case of a patient with psychosis. An example of intact reality testing would be, "I know that there are not really little men talking to me when I am alone, but I feel like I can see them and hear their voices." As indicated by this example, the amount of insight is not an indicator of the severity of the illness. A person with psychosis may have good insight while a person with a mild anxiety disorder may have little or no insight.

Judgment

Judgment refers to the person's capacity to make good decisions and act on them. The level of judgment may or may not correlate to the level of insight. A patient may have no insight into their illness but have good judgment. It has been traditional to use hypothetical examples to test judgment. For example, "What would you do if you found a stamped envelope on the sidewalk?" It is better to use real situations from the patient's own experience to test judgment. The important issues in assessing judgment include whether a patient is doing things that are dangerous or going to get them into trouble and whether the patient is able to effectively participate in their own care. Significantly impaired judgment may be cause for considering a higher level of care or more restrictive setting such as inpatient hospitalization.

See Table 2–2 for common questions the examiner can ask to elicit data for the psychiatric history and mental status, and for some useful clinical hints.

PHYSICAL EXAMINATION

The inclusion and extent of physical examination will depend on the nature and setting of the psychiatric interview. In the outpatient setting, little or no physical examination may be routinely performed while in the emergency room or inpatient setting a more complete physical examination is warranted. Vital signs, weight, waist circumference, body mass index, and height may be important measurements to follow particularly given the potential effects of psychiatric medications or illnesses on these parameters. The Abnormal Involuntary Movement Scale (AIMS) is an important screening test to be followed when using antipsychotic medication to monitor for potential side effects such as tardive dyskinesia. A focused neurological evaluation is an important part of the psychiatric assessment.

In those instances where a physical examination is not performed, the psychiatrist should ask the patient when the last physical examination was performed and by whom. As part of the communication with that physician, the psychiatrist should enquire about any abnormal findings.

FORMULATION

The culmination of the data gathering aspect of the psychiatric interview is developing a formulation and diagnosis (diagnoses) as well as recommendations and treatment planning. In this part of the evaluation process, the data gathering is supplanted by data processing where the various themes contribute to a biopsychosocial understanding of the patient's illness. Although the formulation is placed near the end of the reported or written evaluation, actually it is developed as part of a dynamic process throughout the interview as new hypotheses are created and tested by further data that is elicited. The formulation should include a brief summary of the patient's history, presentation, and current status. It should include discussion of biological factors (medical, family, and medication history) as well as psychological factors such as childhood circumstances, upbringing, and past interpersonal interactions and social factors including stressors, and contextual circumstances such as finances, school, work, home, and interpersonal relationships. These elements should lead to a differential diagnosis of the patient's illness (if any) as well as a provisional diagnosis. Finally, the formulation should include a summary of the safety assessment, which contributes to the determination of level of care recommended or required.

TREATMENT PLANNING

The assessment and formulation will appear in the written note correlating to the psychiatric interview, but the discussion with the patient may only be a summary of this assessment geared towards the patient's ability to understand and interpret the information. Treatment planning and recommendations in contrast are an integral part of the psychiatric interview and should be explicitly discussed with the patient in detail.

The first part of treatment planning involves determining whether a treatment relationship is to be established between the interviewer and patient. Cases where this may not be the case include if the interview was done in consultation, for a legal matter or as a third party review, or in the emergency room or other acute setting. If a treatment relationship is not being started, then the patient should be informed as to what the recommended treatment is (if any). In certain cases this may not be voluntary (as in the case of an involuntary hospitalization). In most cases, there should be a discussion of the options available so that the patient can participate in the decisions about next steps. If a treatment relationship is being initiated, then the structure of that treatment should be discussed. Will the main focus be on medication management, psychotherapy, or both? What will the frequency of visits be? How will the clinician be paid for service and what are the expectations for the patient to be considered engaged in treatment?

Medication recommendations should include a discussion of possible therapeutic medications, the risks and benefits of no medication treatment, and alternative treatment options. The prescriber must obtain informed consent from the patient for any medications (or other treatments) initiated.

Other clinical treatment recommendations may include referral for psychotherapy, group therapy, chemical dependency evaluation or treatment, or medical assessment. There also may be recommended psychosocial interventions including case management, group home or assisted living, social clubs, support groups such as a mental health alliance, the National Alliance for the Mentally Ill, and AA.

Collaboration with primary care doctors, specialists, or other clinicians should always be a goal, and proper patient consent must be obtained for this. Similarly, family involvement in a patient's care can often be a useful and integral part of treatment and requires proper patient consent.

A thorough discussion of safety planning and contact information should occur during the psychiatric interview. The clinician's contact information as well as after-hours coverage scheme should be reviewed. The patient needs to be informed what they should do in the case of an emergency including using the emergency room or calling 911 or crisis hotlines that are available.

3 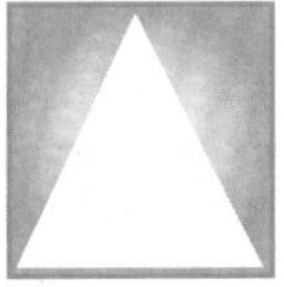

Medical Assessment and Laboratory Testing in Psychiatry

Two recent issues have pushed medical assessment and laboratory testing in psychiatric patients to the forefront of attention for most clinicians: the widespread recognition of the pervasive problem of metabolic syndrome in clinical psychiatry and the shorter life expectancy of psychiatric patients compared to that of the general population. Factors that may contribute to medical comorbidity include abuse of tobacco, alcohol and drugs, poor dietary habits, and obesity. Further, many psychotropic medications are associated with health risks that include obesity, metabolic syndrome, and hyperprolactinemia. Consequently, monitoring the physical health of psychiatric patients has become a more prominent issue.

A logical and systematic approach to the use of medical assessment and laboratory testing by the psychiatrist is vital to achieving the goals of arriving at accurate diagnoses, identifying medical comorbidities, implementing appropriate treatment, and delivering cost-effective care. With respect to the diagnosis or management of medical disease, consultation with colleagues in other specialties is important. Good clinicians recognize the limits of their expertise and the need for consultation with their nonpsychiatric colleagues.

PHYSICAL HEALTH MONITORING

Monitoring the physical health of psychiatric patients has two goals: to provide appropriate care for existing illnesses and protect the patient's current health from possible future impairment. Disease prevention should begin with a clear concept of the condition to be avoided. Ideally, in psychiatry this would be a focus on commonly found conditions that could be a significant source of morbidity or mortality. It is clear that in psychiatry a small number of clinical problems underlie a significant number of impairments and premature deaths.

ROLE OF HISTORY AND PHYSICAL EXAMINATION

A thorough history, including a review of systems, is the basis for a comprehensive patient assessment. The history guides the clinician in the selection of laboratory studies that are relevant for a specific patient. Many psychiatric patients, owing to their illnesses, are not capable of providing sufficiently detailed information. Collateral sources of information, including family members and prior clinicians and their medical records, may be particularly helpful in the assessment of such patients.

The patient's medical history is an important component of the history. It should include notation of prior injuries and, in particular, head injuries that resulted in loss of consciousness and other causes of unconsciousness. The patient's medical history should also note pain conditions, ongoing medical problems, prior hospitalizations, prior surgeries, and a list of the patient's current medications. Toxic exposures are another important component of the medical history. Such exposures are often workplace related.

The social history contains many of the details relevant to the assessment of character pathology, including risk factors for personality disorders, as well as information relevant to the assessment of major disorders. Commonly, the social history includes a legal history, information about family and other significant relationships, and an occupational history.

In evaluating patients who appear demented, the role of the physical examination is to elucidate possible causative factors such as the cogwheel rigidity and tremor associated with Parkinson's disease or neurological deficits suggestive of prior strokes. Standard laboratory studies commonly assessed in dementia patients include a complete blood count (CBC), serum electrolytes, liver function tests, blood urea nitrogen (BUN), creatinine (Cr), thyroid function tests, serum B_{12} and folate levels, Venereal Disease Research Laboratory (VDRL) test, and a urinalysis. Currently there is no clear clinical indication for testing for the apolipoprotein E epsilon 4 allele. Often, a computed tomography (CT) scan is performed if there are focal neurological findings, and an EEG may be performed if there is delirium. When patients are delirious, the neurological examination may be complicated by inattention due to altered levels of consciousness. Delirium workup often includes the same laboratory workup described above for dementia. Urine or blood cultures, chest radiograph, neuroimaging studies, or EEG also may be appropriate.

IMAGING OF THE CENTRAL NERVOUS SYSTEM

Imaging of the central nervous system (CNS) can be broadly divided into two domains: structural and functional. Structural imaging provides detailed, noninvasive visualization of the morphology of the brain. Functional imaging provides a visualization of the spatial distribution of specific biochemical processes. Structural imaging includes x-ray CT and magnetic resonance imaging (MRI). Functional imaging includes positron emission tomography (PET), single photon emission computed tomography (SPECT), functional MRI (fMRI), and magnetic resonance spectroscopy (MRS). With the limited exception of PET scanning, functional imaging techniques are still research tools that are not yet ready for routine clinical use.

Magnetic Resonance Imaging

MRI scans are used to distinguish structural brain abnormalities that may be associated with a patient's behavioral changes. These studies provide the clinician with images of anatomical structures viewed from cross-sectional, coronal, or oblique perspectives. MRI scans can detect a large variety of structural abnormalities. The MRI is particularly useful in examining the temporal lobes, the cerebellum, and deep subcortical structures. It is unique in its ability to identify periventricular white matter hyperintensities. MRI scans are useful in examining the patient for particular diseases, such as nonmeningeal neoplasms, vascular malformations, seizure foci, demyelinating disorders, neurodegenerative disorders, and infarctions. Advantages of MRI include the absence of ionizing radiation and the absence of iodine-based contrast agents. MRI scans are contraindicated when the patient has a pacemaker, aneurysm clips, or ferromagnetic foreign bodies.

Computed Tomography

CT scans are used to identify structural brain abnormalities that may contribute to a patient's behavioral abnormalities. These studies provide the clinician with cross-sectional x-ray images of the brain. CT scans can detect a large variety of structural abnormalities in the cortical and subcortical regions of the brain. CT scans are useful when a clinician is looking for evidence of a stroke, subdural hematoma, tumor, or abscess. These studies also permit visualization of skull fractures. CT scans are the preferred modality when there is suspicion of a meningeal tumor, calcified lesions, acute subarachnoid or parenchymal hemorrhage, or acute parenchymal infarction.

CT scans may be performed with or without contrast. The purpose of contrast is to enhance the visualization of diseases that alter the blood–brain barrier, such as tumors, strokes, abscesses, and other infections.

Positron Emission Tomography

PET scans are performed predominately at university medical centers. PET scans require a positron emission tomograph (the scanner) and a cyclotron to create the relevant isotopes. This type of scan involves the detection and measurement of emitted positron radiation after the injection of a compound that has been tagged with a positron-emitting isotope. Typically, PET scans use fluorodeoxyglucose (FDG) to measure regional brain glucose metabolism. Glucose is the principal energy source for the brain. These scans can provide information about the relative activation of brain regions because regional glucose metabolism is directly proportionate to neuronal activity. Brain FDG scans are useful in the differential diagnosis of dementing disease. The most consistent finding in the PET literature is the pattern of temporal–parietal glucose hypometabolism in patients with Alzheimer's type dementia.

PET scanning also has the ability to differentiate between normal aging, mild cognitive impairment, and Alzheimer's disease by determining regional cerebral patterns of plaques and tangles associated with Alzheimer's disease. A compound known as FDDNP binds to the amyloid senile plaques and tau neurofibrillary tangles. FDDNP appears to be superior to FDG PET in differentiating Alzheimer's patients from those with mild cognitive impairment and subjects with normal aging and no cognitive impairment.

Single Photon Emission Computed Tomography

SPECT is available in most hospitals but is rarely used to study the brain. SPECT is more commonly used to study other organs, such as the heart, liver, and spleen. Some recent work, however, attempts to correlate SPECT brain imaging with mental disorders.

Functional Magnetic Resonance Imaging

fMRI is a research scan used to measure regional cerebral blood flow. Often, fMRI data are superimposed on conventional MRI images, resulting in detailed brain maps of brain structure and function. The measurement of blood flow involves the use of the heme molecule as an endogenous contrast agent. The rate of flow of heme molecules can be measured, resulting in an assessment of regional cerebral metabolism.

Magnetic Resonance Spectroscopy

MRS is another research method to measure regional brain metabolism. MRS scans are performed on conventional MRI devices that have had specific upgrades to their hardware and software. The upgrades permit the signal from protons to be suppressed and other compounds to be measured. (Conventional MRI images are, in reality, a map of the spatial distribution of protons found in water and fat.)

Magnetic Resonance Angiography

Magnetic resonance angiography (MRA) is a method for creating three-dimensional maps of cerebral blood flow. Neurologists and neurosurgeons more commonly use this test. It is rarely used by psychiatrists.

TOXICOLOGY STUDIES

Urine drugs of abuse screens are immunoassays that detect barbiturates, benzodiazepines, cocaine metabolites, opiates, phencyclidine, tetrahydrocannabinol, and tricyclic antidepressants. These rapid tests provide results within an hour. However, they are screening tests. Additional testing is required to confirm the results of this screen.

Testing to determine blood concentrations of certain psychotropic medications enables the clinician to ascertain whether blood levels of medications are at therapeutic, subtherapeutic, or toxic levels. Psychiatric symptoms are not uncommon when prescribed medications are at toxic levels. In the debilitated and the elderly, pathological symptoms may occur at therapeutic concentrations. The normal reference range varies between laboratories. It is important to check with the laboratory performing the test to obtain the normal reference range for that laboratory.

Testing for drugs of abuse usually is performed on urine specimens. It also may be performed on specimens of blood, breath (alcohol), hair, saliva, and sweat. Urine screens provide information about recent use of frequently abused drugs such as alcohol, amphetamines, cocaine, marijuana, opioids, and phencyclidine along with 3,4-methylenedioxymethamphetamine (MDMA) (ecstasy). Many substances may produce false positives with urine drug screening tests. When a false positive is suspected a confirmatory test may be requested.

Comprehensive qualitative toxicology screening is usually performed by liquid and gas chromatography. This may require many hours to perform and is rarely done in routine clinical situations. It is usually performed in patients with unexplained toxicity and an atypical clinical picture.

Qualitative toxicology assessments may be useful in managing patients who have overdosed, when combined with clinical assessment and knowledge of when the ingestion occurred.

Drug Abuse

Patients are frequently unreliable when reporting their drug abuse history. Drug-induced mental disorders often resemble primary psychiatric disorders. Furthermore, substance abuse can exacerbate preexisting mental illness. Indications for ordering a drug abuse screen include unexplained behavioral symptoms, a history of illicit drug use or dependence in a new patient evaluation, or a high-risk background (e.g., criminal record, adolescents, and prostitutes). A drug abuse screen also is frequently used to monitor patient abstinence during treatment of substance abuse. Such tests can be ordered on a scheduled or random basis. Many clinicians believe random testing may be more accurate in the assessment of abstinence. The tests may also help to motivate the patient.

Other laboratory data may suggest a problem with substance abuse. An increase in the mean corpuscular volume is associated with alcohol abuse. Liver enzymes may be increased with alcohol abuse or from hepatitis B or C acquired from IV drug abuse. Serological testing for hepatitis B or C can confirm that diagnosis. IV drug abusers are at risk for bacterial endocarditis. If bacterial endocarditis is suspected, then further medical workup is indicated.

TESTED SUBSTANCES. Routine tests are available for phencyclidine (PCP), cocaine, tetrahydrocannabinol (THC) (also known as *marijuana*), benzodiazepines, methamphetamine and its metabolite amphetamine, morphine (Duramorph), codeine, methadone (Dolophine), propoxyphene (Darvon), barbiturates, lysergic acid diethylamide (LSD), and MDMA (also known as *ecstasy*).

Drug screening tests may have high false-positive rates. This is often due to the interaction of prescribed medication with the test, resulting in false-positive results, and lack of confirmatory testing. False-negative tests are common as well. False-negative results may be due to problems with specimen collection and storage.

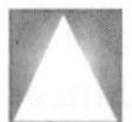

Table 3–1
Drugs of Abuse That Can Be Detected in Urine

Drug	Length of Time Detected in Urine
Alcohol	7–12 hours
Amphetamine	48–72 hours
Barbiturate	24 hours (short acting); 3 weeks (long acting)
Benzodiazepine	3 days
Cocaine	6–8 hours (metabolites 2–4 days)
Codeine	48 hours
Heroin	36–72 hours
Marijuana	2–7 days
Methadone	3 days
Methaqualone	7 days
Morphine	48–72 hours

Testing is most commonly performed on urine, although serum testing is also possible for most agents. Hair and saliva testing are also available in some laboratories. Alcohol can also be detected in the breath (breathalyzer). With the exception of alcohol, drug levels are not usually determined. Instead, only the presence or absence of the drug is determined. There is usually not a meaningful or useful correlation between the level of the drug and clinical behavior. The length of time that a substance can be detected in the urine is listed in Table 3–1.

Alcohol

There is no single test or finding on physical examination that is diagnostic for alcohol abuse. The history of the pattern of alcohol ingestion is most important in making the diagnosis. Laboratory test results and findings on physical examination may help to confirm the diagnosis. In patients with acute alcohol intoxication, a blood alcohol level (BAL) may be useful. A high BAL in a patient who clinically does not show significant intoxication is consistent with tolerance. Significant clinical evidence of intoxication with a low BAL should suggest intoxication with additional agents. Intoxication is commonly found with levels between 100 and 300 mg/dL. The degree of alcohol intoxication can also be assessed using the concentration of alcohol in expired respirations (breathalyzer). Chronic alcohol use is commonly associated with other laboratory abnormalities, including elevation in liver enzymes, such as AST, which is usually greater than serum ALT. Bilirubin also is often elevated. Total protein and albumin may be low, and prothrombin time (PT) may be increased. A macrocytic anemia may be present.

Alcohol abuse may be associated with rhinophyma, telangiectasias, hepatomegaly, and evidence of trauma on physical examination. In withdrawal, patients may have hypertension, tremulousness, and tachycardia.

Laboratory studies in patients who abuse alcohol may reveal macrocytosis. This occurs in most patients who consume four or more drinks per day. Alcoholic liver disease is characterized by elevations in AST and ALT, typically in a ratio of AST to ALT of 2:1 or greater. GGT may be elevated. Carbohydrate-deficient transferrin (CDT) may be helpful in the identification of chronic heavy alcohol use. It has a sensitivity of 60 to 70 percent and a specificity of 80 to 90 percent.

BAL is used to legally define intoxication in the determination of whether an individual is driving under the influence. The legal limit in many states is 80 mg/dL. However, clinical manifestations of intoxication vary with an individual's degree of alcohol tolerance. At the same BAL, an individual who chronically abuses alcohol may exhibit less impairment than an alcohol naive individual. Generally a BAL in the range of 50 to 100 mg/dL is associated with impaired judgment and coordination, and levels greater than 100 mg/dL produce ataxia.

Environmental Toxins

Specific toxins are associated with a variety of behavioral abnormalities. Exposure to toxins commonly occurs through occupation or hobbies.

Aluminum intoxication can cause a dementialike condition. Aluminum can be detected in the urine or blood.

Arsenic intoxication may cause fatigue, loss of consciousness, anemia, and hair loss. Arsenic can be detected in urine, blood, and hair.

Manganese intoxication may present with delirium, confusion, and a parkinsonian syndrome. Manganese may be detected in urine, blood, and hair.

Symptoms of mercury intoxication include apathy, poor memory, lability, headache, and fatigue. Mercury can be detected in urine, blood, and hair.

Manifestations of lead intoxication include encephalopathy, irritability, apathy, and anorexia. Lead can be detected in blood or urine. Lead levels typically are assessed by collecting a 24-hour urine sample. The free erythrocyte protoporphyrin test is a screening test for chronic lead intoxication. This test is commonly coupled with a blood lead level. The Centers for Disease Control specify that a lead level greater than 25 μg/dL is significant for children. The incidence of lead toxicity in children has been falling recently.

Significant exposure to organic compounds, such as insecticides, may produce behavioral abnormalities. Many insecticides have strong anticholinergic effects. There are no readily available laboratory tests to detect these compounds. Poison control centers may assist in the identification of appropriate testing facilities.

Volatile Solvent Inhalation

Volatile substances produce vapors that are inhaled for their psychoactive effect. The most commonly abused volatile solvents include gasoline, glue, paint thinner, and correction fluid. The aerosol propellants from cleaning sprays, deodorant sprays, and whipped cream containers may be abused. Nitrites, such as amyl nitrite ("poppers") and butyl nitrite vials ("rush"), and anesthetic gases, such as chloroform, ether, and nitrous oxide, are also abused.

Chronic abuse of volatile solvents is associated with damage to the brain, liver, kidneys, lung, heart, bone marrow, and blood. Abuse may produce hypoxia or anoxia. Signs of abuse include short-term memory loss, cognitive impairment, slurred and "scanning" speech, and tremor. Cardiac arrhythmias may occur. Exposure to toluene, which is present in many cleaning solutions, paints, and glues, has been associated with loss of clear gray–white matter differentiation and with brain atrophy on MRI scans. Methemoglobinemia has occurred with butyl nitrite abuse. Chronic use of volatile solvents is associated with the production of panic attacks and an organic personality disorder. Chronic use may also produce impairment in working memory and executive cognitive function.

SERUM MEDICATION CONCENTRATIONS

Serum concentrations of psychotropic medications are assessed to minimize the risk of toxicity to patients receiving these medications and to ensure the administration of amounts sufficient to produce therapeutic response. This is particularly true for medications with therapeutic blood levels. Medication levels are often influenced by hepatic metabolism. This metabolism occurs via the action of enzymes in the liver.

Acetaminophen

Acetaminophen may produce hepatic necrosis, which in some cases may be fatal. Acetaminophen is one of the most frequently used agents in intentional drug overdoses and is a common cause of overdose-related deaths. Toxicity is associated with levels greater than 5 mg/dL (>330 μmol/L) in patients without preexisting liver disease. Chronic abusers of alcohol are particularly vulnerable to the effects of overdose. Acetylcysteine (Mucomyst) treatment must occur promptly after overdose to prevent hepatotoxicity.

Salicylate Toxicity

Aspirin is frequently ingested in overdose. Consequently, serum salicylate levels often are obtained in overdose cases. Some rheumatic patients may chronically ingest large amounts of salicylate for therapeutic reasons. Ingestion of 10 to 30 g of aspirin may be fatal. Most patients will develop symptoms of toxicity when salicylate levels are greater than 40 mg/dL (2.9 mmol/L). Common symptoms of toxicity include acid–base abnormalities, tachypnea, tinnitus, nausea, and vomiting. In cases of severe toxicity, symptoms may include hyperthermia, altered mental status, pulmonary edema, and death.

Antipsychotic agents

Clozapine. Clozapine (Clozaril) levels are trough levels determined in the morning before administration of the morning dose of medication. A therapeutic range for clozapine has not been established; however, a level of 100 mg/mL is widely considered to be the minimum therapeutic threshold. At least 350 mg/mL of clozapine is considered to be necessary to achieve therapeutic response in patients with refractory schizophrenia. The likelihood of seizures and other side effects increases with clozapine levels greater than 1,200 mg/mL or dosages greater than 600 mg per day or both. Clozapine is a common cause of a leukopenia in psychiatry. When moderate to severe leucopenia develops, clozapine treatment must be interrupted, but patients may be retreated with clozapine in the future.

Mood Stabilizers

Carbamazepine. Carbamazepine (Tegretol) may produce changes in the levels of white blood cells, platelets, and, under rare circumstances, red blood cells. Anemia, aplastic anemia, leucopenia, and thrombocytopenia may all occur but are rare. Pretreatment evaluations typically include CBC.

Carbamazepine may produce hyponatremia. This hyponatremia is usually mild and does not produce clinical symptoms. However, carbamazepine may cause the syndrome of inappropriate secretion of antidiuretic hormone (SIADH). Carbamazepine may produce a variety of congenital abnormalities, including spina bifida and anomalies of the fingers.

Manifestations of toxicity may include nausea, vomiting, urinary retention, ataxia, confusion, drowsiness, agitation, or nystagmus. At very high levels, symptoms may also include cardiac dysrhythmias, seizures, and respiratory depression.

Lithium. Lithium (Eskalith) has a narrow therapeutic index. Consequently, blood levels of lithium must be monitored to achieve therapeutic dosing and avoid toxicity. Side effects are dose dependent. Symptoms of toxicity include tremors, sedation, and confusions. At higher levels delirium, seizures, and coma may occur. Symptoms of toxicity may begin to manifest with serum levels of greater than 1.2 mEq/L and are common with levels greater than 1.4 mEq/L. Elderly or debilitated patients may show signs of toxicity with levels less than 1.2 mEq/L.

Valproate. Because of the risk of hepatotoxicity, ranging from mild dysfunction to hepatic necrosis, pretreatment liver function tests are usually obtained. More commonly valproate (valproic acid [Depakene] and divalproex [Depakote]) may cause a sustained elevation in liver transaminase levels of as much as three times the upper limit of normal.

Valproate may increase the risk of birth defects. A pretreatment urine pregnancy test is usually obtained in women of childbearing years. Women should be cautioned to use adequate contraception.

Hematological abnormalities are also possible and include leucopenia and thrombocytopenia. Treatment with valproate may increase serum ammonia levels. It is prudent to obtain an ammonia level in a patient undergoing valproate treatment who present with altered mental status or lethargy. Acute pancreatitis may also occur.

Antidepressants

Monoamine Oxidase Inhibitors. Treatment with monoamine oxidase inhibitors (MAOIs) can cause orthostasis and, rarely, hypertensive crisis. Baseline blood pressure measurement should be obtained before the initiation of treatment, and blood pressure should be monitored during treatment.

There are no meaningful blood levels for MAOIs, and direct monitoring of MAOI blood levels is not clinically indicated. Treatment with MAOIs is occasionally associated with hepatotoxicity. For this reason, liver function tests usually are obtained at the initiation of treatment and periodically after.

Tricyclic and Tetracyclic Antidepressants. Routine laboratory studies obtained before initiation of tricyclic or tetracyclic antidepressants (TCAs) typically include CBC, serum electrolytes, and liver function tests. Because TCAs affect cardiac conduction, clinicians also may obtain an ECG to assess for the presence of abnormal cardiac rhythms and prolonged PR, QRS, and QTc complexes before initiation of these medications.

NEUROLEPTIC MALIGNANT SYNDROME

Neuroleptic malignant syndrome (NMS) is a rare, potentially fatal, consequence of neuroleptic administration. The syndrome consists of autonomic instability, hyperpyrexia, severe extrapyramidal symptoms (i.e., rigidity), and delirium. Sustained muscle contraction results in peripheral heat generation and muscle breakdown. Muscle breakdown contributes to elevated levels of creatine kinase (CK). Peripheral heat generation with impaired central mechanisms of thermoregulation results in hyperpyrexia. Myoglobinuria and leukocytosis are common. Hepatic and renal failure may occur. Liver enzymes become elevated with liver failure. Patients may die from hyperpyrexia, aspiration pneumonia, renal failure, hepatic failure, respiratory arrest, or cardiovascular collapse. Treatment includes discontinuation of the neuroleptic, hydration, administration of muscle relaxants, and general supportive nursing care.

A typical laboratory workup of NMS includes a CBC, serum electrolytes, BUN, Cr, and CK. A urinalysis, including an assessment of urine myoglobin, is also usually performed. As part of the differential diagnosis, blood and urine cultures are performed as part of a fever workup. Pronounced elevations in the WBC may occur in NMS. White blood cell counts are typically in the range from 10,000 to 40,000 per mm^3.

Muscle Injury

Serum CK levels may rise in response to repeated intramuscular (IM) injections, prolonged or agitated periods in restraint, or NMS. Dystonic reactions from neuroleptic administration may also result in elevated levels of CK.

ELECTROCONVULSIVE THERAPY

Electroconvulsive therapy (ECT) is usually reserved for patients with the most treatment-resistant depression. Typical laboratory tests obtained before the administration of ECT include a CBC, serum electrolytes, urinalysis, and liver function tests. However, no specific laboratory tests are required in the pre-ECT evaluation. Usually, an ECG is also obtained. A spinal x-ray series is no longer considered routinely indicated because of the low risk of spinal injury associated with modern administration techniques that use paralyzing agents. A comprehensive medical history and physical examination are useful screening tools to identify possible conditions that could complicate treatment.

ENDOCRINE EVALUATIONS

Endocrine disease is of great relevance to psychiatry. Management of psychiatric illness is complicated by comorbid endocrine disease. Endocrine illness frequently has psychiatric manifestations. For these reasons, screening for endocrine disease often is of relevance to the psychiatrist.

Adrenal Disease

Adrenal disease may have psychiatric manifestations, including depression, anxiety, mania, dementia, psychosis, and delirium. However, patients with adrenal disease rarely come to the attention of psychiatrists. Assessment and management of these patients are best done in conjunction with specialists.

Low plasma levels of cortisol are found in Addison's disease. These patients may have symptoms that are also common in psychiatric conditions including fatigue, anorexia, weight loss, and malaise. Patients may also have memory impairment, confusion, or delirium. Depression or psychosis with hallucinations and delusions may occur.

Elevated levels of cortisol are seen in Cushing's syndrome. About half of all patients with Cushing's syndrome develop psychiatric symptoms. These symptoms may include lability, irritability, anxiety, panic attacks, depressed mood, euphoria, mania, or paranoia. Cognitive dysfunctions may include cognitive slowing and poor short-term memory. Symptoms usually improve when cortisol normalizes. If not, or if symptoms are severe, then psychiatric treatment may be necessary.

Cortisol levels have not been found to be useful in the assessment or management of primary psychiatric disease. In particular, the dexamethasone-suppression test (DST) remains a research tool in psychiatry that is not used in routine clinical care.

Anabolic Steroid Use

Use of anabolic steroids has been associated with irritability, aggression, depression, and psychosis. Athletes and bodybuilders are common abusers of anabolic steroids. Urine specimens can be used to screen for these agents. Because so many compounds have been synthesized, a variety of tests may be required to confirm the diagnosis, depending upon the compound that has been used. Consultation with a specialist is advised. Generally, androgens other than testosterone can be detected by gas chromatography and mass spectroscopy.

Antidiuretic Hormone

Arginine vasopressin (AVP), also called antidiuretic hormone (ADH), is decreased in central diabetes insipidus (DI). DI may be central (due to the pituitary or hypothalamus) or nephrogenic. Nephrogenic DI may be acquired or due to an inherited X-linked condition. Lithium-induced DI is an example of an acquired form of DI. Lithium has been shown to decrease the sensitivity of renal tubules to AVP. Patients with central DI respond to the administration of vasopressin with a decrease in urine output. Secondary central DI may develop in response to head trauma that produces damage in the pituitary or hypothalamus.

About one-fifth of patients taking lithium develop polyuria, and a larger amount may have some degree of impairment in concentrating urine. Chronic treatment with lithium is a common cause of nephrogenic diabetes insipidus. However, there are other causes of polyuria in lithium-treated patients in addition to nephrogenic diabetes insipidus. Primary polydipsia is common and is often associated with the dry mouth associated with many psychiatric medications. Central diabetes has also been associated with lithium treatment.

Excessive secretion of AVP results in increased retention of fluid in the body. This condition is called SIADH. Water retention in SIADH causes hyponatremia. SIADH may develop in response to injury to the brain or from medication administration (including phenothiazines, butyrophenones, carbamazepine, and oxcarbazepine). The hyponatremia associated with this condition may produce delirium.

Human Chorionic Gonadotropin

Human chorionic gonadotropin (hCG) can be assessed in the urine and blood. The urine test for hCG is the basis for the commonly used urine pregnancy test. This immunometric test is able to detect pregnancy approximately 2 weeks after an expected menstrual period has passed. Routine tests are most accurate when performed 1 to 2 weeks after a missed period and are not reliably accurate until the 2-week period has passed. However, there are ultrasensitive urine hCG tests that can accurately detect pregnancy 7 days after fertilization. Pregnancy tests are often obtained before initiating certain psychotropic medications, such as lithium, carbamazepine, and valproic acid, which are associated with congenital anomalies.

Parathormone

Parathormone (parathyroid hormone) modulates serum concentrations of calcium and phosphorus. Dysregulation in this hormone and the resulting production of abnormalities in calcium and phosphorus may produce depression or delirium.

Prolactin

Prolactin levels may become elevated in response to the administration of antipsychotic agents. Elevations in serum prolactin result from the blockade of dopamine receptors in the pituitary. This blockade produces an increase in prolactin synthesis and release.

Cerebral MRI is not usually performed if the patient is taking an antipsychotic drug known to cause hyperprolactinemia and the magnitude of the prolactin elevation is consistent with drug-induced causes.

4 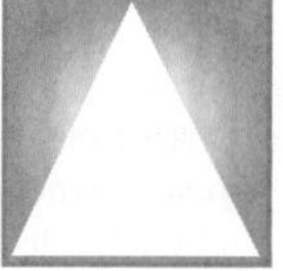

Schizophrenia Spectrum and Other Psychotic Disorders

▲ 4.1 Schizophrenia

Although schizophrenia is discussed as if it is a single disease, it probably comprises a group of disorders with heterogeneous etiologies, and it includes patients whose clinical presentations, treatment response, and courses of illness vary. Signs and symptoms are variable and include changes in perception, emotion, cognition, thinking, and behavior. The expression of these manifestations varies across patients and over time, but the effect of the illness is always severe and is usually long lasting. The disorder usually begins before age 25 years, persists throughout life, and affects persons of all social classes. Both patients and their families often suffer from poor care and social ostracism because of widespread ignorance about the disorder. Schizophrenia is one of the most common of the serious mental disorders, but its essential nature remains to be clarified; thus, it is sometimes referred to as a syndrome, as the group of schizophrenias, or, the schizophrenia spectrum. Clinicians should appreciate that the diagnosis of schizophrenia is based entirely on the psychiatric history and mental status examination. There is no laboratory test for schizophrenia, nor is there a pathognomonic sign.

HISTORY

Written descriptions of symptoms commonly observed today in patients with schizophrenia are found throughout history. Early Greek physicians described delusions of grandeur, paranoia, and deterioration in cognitive functions and personality. It was not until the 19th century, however, that schizophrenia emerged as a medical condition worthy of study and treatment. Two major figures in psychiatry and neurology who studied the disorder were Emil Kraepelin (1856–1926) and Eugene Bleuler (1857–1939). Earlier, Benedict Morel (1809–1873), a French psychiatrist, had used the term *démence précoce* to describe deteriorated patients whose illnesses began in adolescence.

EMIL KRAEPELIN. Kraepelin translated Morel's *démence précoce* into *dementia precox,* a term that emphasized the change in cognition (dementia) and early onset (precox) of the disorder. Patients with dementia precox were described as having a long-term deteriorating course and the clinical symptoms of hallucinations and delusions. Kraepelin distinguished these patients from those who underwent distinct episodes of illness alternating with periods of normal functioning, which he classified as having manic-depressive psychosis. Another separate condition called *paranoia* was characterized by persistent persecutory delusions. These patients lacked the deteriorating course of dementia precox and the intermittent symptoms of manic-depressive psychosis.

EUGENE BLEULER. Bleuler coined the term *schizophrenia,* which replaced *dementia precox* in the literature. He chose the term to express the presence of schisms among thought, emotion, and behavior in patients with the disorder. Bleuler stressed that, unlike Kraepelin's concept of dementia precox, schizophrenia need not have a deteriorating course. This term is often misconstrued, especially by lay people, to mean split personality. Split personality, called dissociative identity disorder, differs completely from schizophrenia.

THE FOUR AS. Bleuler identified specific fundamental (or primary) symptoms of schizophrenia to develop his theory about the internal mental schisms of patients. These symptoms included associational disturbances of thought, especially looseness, affective disturbances, autism, and ambivalence, summarized as the four As: associations, affect, autism, and ambivalence. Bleuler also identified accessory (secondary) symptoms, which included the symptoms that Kraepelin saw as major indicators of dementia precox: hallucinations and delusions.

OTHER THEORISTS

ERNST KRETSCHMER (1888–1926). Kretschmer compiled data to support the idea that schizophrenia occurred more often among persons with asthenic (i.e., slender, lightly muscled physiques), athletic, or dysplastic body types rather than among persons with pyknic (i.e., short, stocky physiques) body types. He thought the latter were more likely to incur bipolar disorders. His observations may seem strange, but they are not inconsistent with a superficial impression of the body types in many persons with schizophrenia.

KURT SCHNEIDER (1887–1967). Schneider contributed a description of first-rank symptoms, which, he stressed, were not specific for schizophrenia and were not to be rigidly applied but were useful for making diagnoses. He emphasized that in patients who showed no first-rank symptoms, the disorder could be diagnosed exclusively on the basis of second-rank symptoms and an otherwise typical clinical appearance. Clinicians frequently ignore his warnings and sometimes see the absence of first-rank symptoms during a single interview as evidence that a person does not have schizophrenia.

KARL JASPERS (1883–1969). Jaspers, a psychiatrist and philosopher, played a major role in developing existential psychoanalysis. He was interested in the phenomenology of mental illness and the subjective feelings of patients with mental illness. His work paved the way toward trying to understand the psychological meaning of schizophrenic signs and symptoms such as delusions and hallucinations.

ADOLF MEYER (1866–1950). Meyer, the founder of psychobiology, saw schizophrenia as a reaction to life stresses. It was a maladaptation that was understandable in terms of the patient's life experiences. Meyer's view was represented in the nomenclature of the 1950s, which referred to the schizophrenic reaction. In later editions of DSM, the term reaction was dropped.

EPIDEMIOLOGY

In the United States, the lifetime prevalence of schizophrenia is about 1 percent, which means that about 1 person in 100 will develop schizophrenia during their lifetime. The Epidemiologic Catchment Area study sponsored by the National Institute of Mental Health reported a lifetime prevalence of 0.6 to 1.9 percent. In the United States, about 0.05 percent of the total population is treated for schizophrenia in any single year, and only about half of all patients with schizophrenia obtain treatment, despite the severity of the disorder.

Gender and Age

Schizophrenia is equally prevalent in men and women. The two genders differ, however, in the onset and course of illness. Onset is earlier in men than in women. More than half of all male schizophrenia patients, but only one-third of all female schizophrenia patients, are first admitted to a psychiatric hospital before age 25 years. The peak ages of onset are 10 to 25 years for men and 25 to 35 years for women. Unlike men, women display a bimodal age distribution, with a second peak occurring in middle age. Approximately 3 to 10 percent of women with schizophrenia present with disease onset after age 40 years. About 90 percent of patients in treatment for schizophrenia are between 15 and 55 years old. Onset of schizophrenia before age 10 years or after age 60 years is extremely rare. Some studies have indicated that men are more likely to be impaired by negative symptoms (described later) than are women and that women are more likely to have better social functioning than are men before disease onset. In general, the outcome for female schizophrenia patients is better than that for male schizophrenia patients. When onset occurs after age 45 years, the disorder is characterized as late-onset schizophrenia.

Reproductive Factors

The use of psychopharmacological drugs, the open-door policies in hospitals, the deinstitutionalization in state hospitals, and the emphasis on rehabilitation and community-based care for patients have all led to an increase in the marriage and fertility rates among persons with schizophrenia. Because of these factors, the number of children born to parents with schizophrenia is continually increasing. The fertility rate for persons with schizophrenia is close to that for the general population. First-degree biological relatives of persons with schizophrenia have a 10 times greater risk for developing the disease than the general population.

Medical Illness

Persons with schizophrenia have a higher mortality rate from accidents and natural causes than the general population. Institution- or treatment-related variables do not explain the increased mortality rate, but the higher rate may be related to the fact that the diagnosis and treatment of medical and surgical conditions in schizophrenia patients can be clinical challenges. Several studies have shown that up to 80 percent of all schizophrenia patients have significant concurrent medical illnesses and that up to 50 percent of these conditions may be undiagnosed.

Infection and Birth Season

Persons who develop schizophrenia are more likely to have been born in the winter and early spring and less likely to have been born in late spring and summer. In the Northern Hemisphere, including the United States, persons with schizophrenia are more often born in the months from January to April. In the Southern Hemisphere, persons with schizophrenia are more often born in the months from July to September. Season-specific risk factors, such as a virus or a seasonal change in diet, may be operative. Another hypothesis is that persons with a genetic predisposition for schizophrenia have a decreased biological advantage to survive season-specific insults.

Studies have pointed to gestational and birth complications, exposure to influenza epidemics, maternal starvation during pregnancy, Rhesus factor incompatibility, and an excess of winter births in the etiology of schizophrenia. The nature of these factors suggests a neurodevelopmental pathological process in schizophrenia, but the exact pathophysiological mechanism associated with these risk factors is not known.

Epidemiological data show a high incidence of schizophrenia after prenatal exposure to influenza during several epidemics of the disease. Some studies show that the frequency of schizophrenia is increased after exposure to influenza—which occurs in the winter—during the second trimester of pregnancy. Other data supporting a viral hypothesis are an increased number of physical anomalies at birth, an increased rate of pregnancy and birth complications, seasonality of birth consistent with viral infection, geographical clusters of adult cases, and seasonality of hospitalizations.

Viral theories stem from the fact that several specific viral theories have the power to explain the particular localization of pathology necessary to account for a range of manifestations in schizophrenia without overt febrile encephalitis.

Substance Abuse

Substance abuse is common in schizophrenia. The lifetime prevalence of any drug abuse (other than tobacco) is often greater than 50 percent. For all drugs of abuse (other than tobacco), abuse is associated with poorer function. In one population-based study, the lifetime prevalence of alcohol within schizophrenia was 40 percent. Alcohol abuse increases risk of hospitalization and, in some patients, may increase psychotic symptoms. People with schizophrenia have an increased prevalence of abuse of common street drugs. There has been particular interest in the association between cannabis and schizophrenia. Those reporting high levels of cannabis use (more than 50 occasions) were at sixfold increased risk of schizophrenia compared with nonusers. The use of amphetamines, cocaine, and similar drugs should raise particular concern because of their marked ability to increase psychotic symptoms.

Nicotine

Up to 90 percent of schizophrenia patients may be dependent on nicotine. Apart from smoking-associated mortality, nicotine decreases the blood concentrations of some antipsychotics. There are suggestions that the increased prevalence in smoking is due, at least in part, to brain abnormalities in nicotinic receptors. A specific polymorphism in a nicotinic receptor has been linked to a genetic risk for schizophrenia. Nicotine administration appears to improve some cognitive impairments and parkinsonism in schizophrenia, possibly because of nicotine-dependent activation of dopamine neurons. Recent studies have also demonstrated that nicotine may decrease positive symptoms such as hallucinations in schizophrenia patients by its effect on nicotine receptors in the brain that reduce the perception of outside stimuli, especially noise. In that sense, smoking is a form of self-medication.

Population Density

The prevalence of schizophrenia has been correlated with local population density in cities with populations of more than 1 million people. The correlation is weaker in cities of 100,000 to 500,000 people and is absent in cities with fewer than 10,000 people. The effect of population density is consistent with the observation that the incidence of schizophrenia in children of either one or two parents with schizophrenia is twice as high in cities as in rural communities. These observations suggest that social stressors in urban settings may affect the development of schizophrenia in persons at risk.

Socioeconomic and Cultural Factors

Economics. Because schizophrenia begins early in life; causes significant and long-lasting impairments; makes heavy demands for hospital care; and requires ongoing clinical care, rehabilitation, and support services, the financial cost of the illness in the United States is estimated to exceed that of all cancers combined. Patients with a diagnosis of schizophrenia are reported to account for 15 to 45 percent of homeless Americans.

Hospitalization. The development of effective antipsychotic drugs and changes in political and popular attitudes toward the treatment and the rights of persons who are mentally ill have dramatically changed the patterns of hospitalization for schizophrenia patients since the mid-1950s. Even with antipsychotic medication, however, the probability of readmission within 2 years after discharge from the first hospitalization is about 40 to 60 percent. Patients with schizophrenia occupy about 50 percent of all mental hospital beds and account for about 16 percent of all psychiatric patients who receive any treatment.

ETIOLOGY

Genetic Factors

There is a genetic contribution to some, perhaps all, forms of schizophrenia, and a high proportion of the variance in liability to schizophrenia is due to additive genetic effects. For example, schizophrenia and schizophrenia-related disorders (e.g., schizotypal personality disorder) occur at an increased rate among the biological relatives of patients with schizophrenia. The likelihood of a person having schizophrenia is correlated with the closeness of the relationship to an affected relative (e.g., first- or second-degree relative). In the case of monozygotic twins who have identical genetic endowment, there is an approximately 50 percent concordance rate for schizophrenia. This rate is four to five times the concordance rate in dizygotic twins or the rate of occurrence found in other first-degree relatives (i.e., siblings, parents, or offspring). The role of genetic factors is further reflected in the drop-off in the occurrence of schizophrenia among second- and third-degree relatives, in whom one would hypothesize a decreased genetic loading. The finding of a higher rate of schizophrenia among the biological relatives of an adopted-away person who develops schizophrenia, compared with the adoptive, nonbiological relatives who rear the patient, provides further support to the genetic contribution in the etiology of schizophrenia. Nevertheless, the monozygotic twin data clearly demonstrate the fact that individuals who are genetically vulnerable to schizophrenia do not inevitably develop schizophrenia; other factors (e.g., environment) must be involved in determining a schizophrenia outcome. If a vulnerability–liability model of schizophrenia is correct in its postulation of an environmental influence, then other biological or psychosocial environment factors may prevent or cause schizophrenia in the genetically vulnerable individual.

Some data indicate that the age of the father has a correlation with the development of schizophrenia. In studies of schizophrenia patients with no history of illness in either the maternal or paternal line, it was found that those born from fathers older than the age of 60 years were vulnerable to developing the disorder. Presumably, spermatogenesis in older men is subject to greater epigenetic damage than in younger men.

The modes of genetic transmission in schizophrenia are unknown, but several genes appear to make a contribution to schizophrenia vulnerability. Linkage and association genetic studies have provided strong evidence for nine linkage sites: 1q, 5q, 6p, 6q, 8p, 10p, 13q, 15q, and 22q. Further analyses of these chromosomal sites have led to the identification of specific candidate genes, and the best current candidates are α-7 nicotinic receptor, *DISC 1, GRM 3, COMT, NRG 1, RGS 4,* and *G 72.* Recently, mutations of the genes dystrobrevin (DTNBP1) and neureglin 1 have been found to be associated with negative features of schizophrenia.

Biochemical Factors

Dopamine Hypothesis. The simplest formulation of the dopamine hypothesis of schizophrenia posits that schizophrenia results from too much dopaminergic activity. The theory evolved from two observations. First, the efficacy and the potency of many antipsychotic drugs (i.e., the dopamine receptor antagonists [DRAs]) are correlated with their ability to act as antagonists of the dopamine type 2 (D_2) receptor. Second, drugs that increase dopaminergic activity, notably cocaine and amphetamine, are psychotomimetic. The basic theory does not elaborate on whether the dopaminergic hyperactivity is due to too much release of dopamine, too many dopamine receptors, hypersensitivity of the dopamine receptors to dopamine, or a combination of these mechanisms. Which dopamine tracts in the brain are involved is also not specified in the theory, although the mesocortical and mesolimbic tracts are most often implicated. The dopaminergic neurons in these tracts project from their cell bodies in the midbrain to dopaminoceptive neurons in the limbic system and the cerebral cortex.

Excessive dopamine release in patients with schizophrenia has been linked to the severity of positive psychotic symptoms. Position emission tomography studies of dopamine receptors document an increase in D_2 receptors in the caudate nucleus of drug-free patients with schizophrenia. There have also been reports of increased dopamine concentration in the amygdala, decreased density of the dopamine transporter, and increased numbers of dopamine type 4 receptors in the entorhinal cortex.

SEROTONIN. Current hypotheses posit serotonin excess as a cause of both positive and negative symptoms in schizophrenia. The robust serotonin antagonist activity of clozapine and other second-generation antipsychotics coupled with the effectiveness of clozapine to decrease positive symptoms in chronic patients has contributed to the validity of this proposition.

NOREPINEPHRINE. Anhedonia—the impaired capacity for emotional gratification and the decreased ability to experience pleasure—has long been noted to be a prominent feature of schizophrenia. A selective neuronal degeneration within the norepinephrine reward neural system could account for this aspect of schizophrenic symptomatology. However, biochemical and pharmacological data bearing on this proposal are inconclusive.

GABA. The inhibitory amino acid neurotransmitter γ-aminobutyric acid (GABA) has been implicated in the pathophysiology of schizophrenia based on the finding that some patients with schizophrenia have a loss of GABAergic neurons in the hippocampus. GABA has a regulatory effect on dopamine activity, and the loss of inhibitory GABAergic neurons could lead to the hyperactivity of dopaminergic neurons.

NEUROPEPTIDES. Neuropeptides, such as substance P and neurotensin, are localized with the catecholamine and indolamine neurotransmitters and influence the action of these neurotransmitters. Alteration in neuropeptide mechanisms could facilitate, inhibit, or otherwise alter the pattern of firing these neuronal systems.

GLUTAMATE. Glutamate has been implicated because ingestion of phencyclidine, a glutamate antagonist, produces an acute syndrome similar to schizophrenia. The hypotheses proposed about glutamate include those of hyperactivity, hypoactivity, and glutamate-induced neurotoxicity.

ACETYLCHOLINE AND NICOTINE. Postmortem studies in schizophrenia have demonstrated decreased muscarinic and nicotinic receptors in the caudate-putamen, hippocampus, and selected regions of the prefrontal cortex. These receptors play a role in the regulation of neurotransmitter systems involved in cognition, which is impaired in schizophrenia.

Neuropathology

In the 19th century, neuropathologists failed to find a neuropathological basis for schizophrenia, and thus they classified schizophrenia as a functional disorder. By the end of the 20th century, however, researchers had made significant strides in revealing a potential neuropathological basis for schizophrenia, primarily in the limbic system and the basal ganglia, including neuropathological or neurochemical abnormalities in the cerebral cortex, the thalamus, and the brainstem. The loss of brain volume widely reported in schizophrenic brains appears to result from reduced density of the axons, dendrites, and synapses that mediate associative functions of the brain. Synaptic density is highest at age 1 year and then is pared down to adult values in early adolescence. One theory, based in part on the observation that patients often develop schizophrenic symptoms during adolescence, holds that schizophrenia results from excessive pruning of synapses during this phase of development.

Cerebral Ventricles.

Computed tomography (CT) scans of patients with schizophrenia have consistently shown lateral and third ventricular enlargement and some reduction in cortical volume. Reduced volumes of cortical gray matter have been demonstrated during the earliest stages of the disease. Several investigators have attempted to determine whether the abnormalities detected by CT are progressive or static. Some studies have concluded that the lesions observed on CT scan are present at the onset of the illness and do not progress. Other studies, however, have concluded that the pathological process visualized on CT scan continues to progress during the illness. Thus, whether an active pathological process is continuing to evolve in schizophrenia patients is still uncertain.

Reduced Symmetry.

There is a reduced symmetry in several brain areas in schizophrenia, including the temporal, frontal, and occipital lobes. This reduced symmetry is believed by some investigators to originate during fetal life and to be indicative of a disruption in brain lateralization during neurodevelopment.

Limbic System.

Because of its role in controlling emotions, the limbic system has been hypothesized to be involved in the pathophysiology of schizophrenia. Studies of postmortem brain samples from schizophrenia patients have shown a decrease in the size of the region, including the amygdala, the hippocampus, and the parahippocampal gyrus. This neuropathological finding agrees with the observation made by magnetic resonance imaging studies of patients with schizophrenia. The hippocampus is not only smaller in size in schizophrenia but is also functionally abnormal as indicated by disturbances in glutamate transmission. Disorganization of the neurons within the hippocampus has also been seen in brain tissue sections of schizophrenia patients compared with healthy control participants without schizophrenia.

Prefrontal Cortex.

There is considerable evidence from postmortem brain studies that supports anatomical abnormalities in the prefrontal cortex in schizophrenia. Functional deficits in the prefrontal brain imaging region have also been demonstrated. It has long been noted that several symptoms of schizophrenia mimic those found in persons with prefrontal lobotomies or *frontal lobe syndromes*.

Thalamus.

Some studies of the thalamus show evidence of volume shrinkage or neuronal loss, in particular subnuclei. The medial dorsal nucleus of the thalamus, which has reciprocal connections with the prefrontal cortex, has been reported to contain a reduced number of neurons. The total number of neurons, oligodendrocytes, and astrocytes is reduced by 30 to 45 percent in schizophrenia patients. This putative finding does not appear to be due to the effects of antipsychotic drugs because the volume of the thalamus is similar in size between patients with schizophrenia treated chronically with medication and neuroleptic-naive subjects.

Basal Ganglia and Cerebellum. The basal ganglia and cerebellum have been of theoretical interest in schizophrenia for at least two reasons. First, many patients with schizophrenia show odd movements, even in the absence of medication-induced movement disorders (e.g., tardive dyskinesia). The odd movements can include an awkward gait, facial grimacing, and stereotypies. Because the basal ganglia and cerebellum are involved in the control of movement, disease in these areas is implicated in the pathophysiology of schizophrenia. Second, the movement disorders involving the basal ganglia (e.g., Huntington's disease, Parkinson's disease) are the ones most commonly associated with psychosis. Neuropathological studies of the basal ganglia have produced variable and inconclusive reports about cell loss or the reduction of volume of the globus pallidus and the substantia nigra. Studies have also shown an increase in the number of D_2 receptors in the caudate, the putamen, and the nucleus accumbens. The question remains, however, whether the increase is secondary to the patient having received antipsychotic medications. Some investigators have begun to study the serotonergic system in the basal ganglia; a role for serotonin in psychotic disorder is suggested by the clinical usefulness of antipsychotic drugs that are serotonin antagonists (e.g., clozapine, risperidone).

Neural Circuits

There has been a gradual evolution from conceptualizing schizophrenia as a disorder that involves discrete areas of the brain to a perspective that views schizophrenia as a disorder of brain neural circuits. For example, as mentioned previously, the basal ganglia and cerebellum are reciprocally connected to the frontal lobes, and the abnormalities in frontal lobe function seen in some brain imaging studies may be due to disease in either area rather than in the frontal lobes themselves. It is also hypothesized that an early developmental lesion of the dopaminergic tracts to the prefrontal cortex results in the disturbance of prefrontal and limbic system function and leads to the positive and negative symptoms and cognitive impairments observed in patients with schizophrenia.

Of particular interest in the context of neural circuit hypotheses linking the prefrontal cortex and limbic system are studies demonstrating a relationship between hippocampal morphological abnormalities and disturbances in prefrontal cortex metabolism or function (or both). Data from functional and structural imaging studies in humans suggest that whereas dysfunction of the anterior cingulate basal ganglia thalamocortical circuit underlies the production of positive psychotic symptoms, dysfunction of the dorsolateral prefrontal circuit underlies the production of primary, enduring, negative, or deficit symptoms. There is a neural basis for cognitive functions that is impaired in patients with schizophrenia. The observation of the relationship among impaired working memory performance, disrupted prefrontal neuronal integrity, altered prefrontal, cingulate, and inferior parietal cortex, and altered hippocampal blood flow provides strong support for disruption of the normal working memory neural circuit in patients with schizophrenia. The involvement of this circuit, at least for auditory hallucinations, has been documented in a number of functional imaging studies that contrast hallucinating and nonhallucinating patients.

Brain Metabolism

Studies using magnetic resonance spectroscopy, a technique that measures the concentration of specific molecules in the brain, found that patients with schizophrenia had lower levels of phosphomonoester and inorganic phosphate and higher levels of phosphodiester than a control group. Furthermore, concentrations of N-acetyl aspartate, a marker of neurons, were lower in the hippocampus and frontal lobes of patients with schizophrenia.

Applied Electrophysiology

Electroencephalographic studies indicate that many schizophrenia patients have abnormal records, increased sensitivity to activation procedures (e.g., frequent spike activity after sleep deprivation), decreased alpha activity, increased theta and delta activity, possibly more epileptiform activity than usual, and possibly more left-sided abnormalities than usual. Schizophrenia patients also exhibit an inability to filter out irrelevant sounds and are extremely sensitive to background noise. The flooding of sound that results makes concentration difficult and may be a factor in the production of auditory hallucinations. This sound sensitivity may be associated with a genetic defect.

Complex Partial Epilepsy. Schizophrenia-like psychoses have been reported to occur more frequently than expected in patients with complex partial seizures, especially seizures involving the temporal lobes. Factors associated with the development of psychosis in these patients include a left-sided seizure focus, medial temporal location of the lesion, and an early onset of seizures. The first-rank symptoms described by Schneider may be similar to symptoms of patients with complex partial epilepsy and may reflect the presence of a temporal lobe disorder when seen in patients with schizophrenia.

Evoked Potentials. A large number of abnormalities in evoked potential among patients with schizophrenia have been described. The P300 has been most studied and is defined as a large, positive evoked-potential wave that occurs about 300 milliseconds after a sensory stimulus is detected. The major source of the P300 wave may be located in the limbic system structures of the medial temporal lobes. In patients with schizophrenia, the P300 has been reported to be statistically smaller than in comparison groups. Abnormalities in the P300 wave have also been reported to be more common in children who, because they have affected parents, are at high risk for schizophrenia. Whether the characteristics of the P300 represent a state or a trait phenomenon remains controversial. Other evoked potentials reported to be abnormal in patients with schizophrenia are the N100 and the contingent negative variation. The N100 is a negative wave that occurs about 100 milliseconds after a stimulus, and the contingent negative variation is a slowly developing, negative-voltage shift following the presentation of a sensory stimulus that is a warning for an upcoming stimulus. The evoked-potential data have been interpreted as indicating that although patients with schizophrenia are unusually sensitive to a sensory stimulus (larger early evoked potentials), they compensate for the increased sensitivity by blunting the processing of information at higher cortical levels (indicated by smaller late evoked potentials).

Eye Movement Dysfunction

The inability to follow a moving visual target accurately is the defining basis for the disorders of smooth visual pursuit and disinhibition of saccadic eye movements seen in patients with schizophrenia. Eye movement dysfunction may be a trait marker for schizophrenia; it is independent of drug treatment and clinical state and is also seen in first-degree relatives of probands with schizophrenia. Various studies have reported abnormal eye movements in 50 to 85 percent of patients with schizophrenia compared with about 25 percent in psychiatric patients without schizophrenia and fewer than 10 percent in nonpsychiatrically ill control participant.

Psychoneuroimmunology

Several immunological abnormalities have been associated with patients who have schizophrenia. The abnormalities include decreased T-cell interleukin-2 production, reduced number and responsiveness of peripheral lymphocytes, abnormal cellular and humoral reactivity to neurons, and the presence of brain-directed (antibrain) antibodies. The data can be interpreted variously as representing the effects of a neurotoxic virus or of an endogenous autoimmune disorder. Most carefully conducted investigations that have searched for evidence of neurotoxic viral infections in schizophrenia have had negative results, although epidemiological data show a high incidence of schizophrenia after prenatal exposure to influenza during several epidemics of the disease. Other data supporting a viral hypothesis are an increased number of physical anomalies at birth, an increased rate of pregnancy and birth complications, seasonality of birth consistent with viral infection, geographical clusters of adult cases, and seasonality of hospitalizations. Nonetheless, the inability to detect genetic evidence of viral infection reduces the significance of all circumstantial data. The possibility of autoimmune brain antibodies has some data to support it; the pathophysiological process, if it exists, however, probably explains only a subset of the population with schizophrenia.

Psychoneuroendocrinology

Many reports describe neuroendocrine differences between groups of patients with schizophrenia and groups of control subjects. For example, results of the dexamethasone-suppression test have been reported to be abnormal in various subgroups of patients with schizophrenia, although the practical or predictive value of the test in schizophrenia has been questioned. One carefully done report, however, has correlated persistent nonsuppression on the dexamethasone-suppression test in schizophrenia with a poor long-term outcome.

Some data suggest decreased concentrations of luteinizing hormone or follicle-stimulating hormone, perhaps correlated with age of onset and length of illness. Two additional reported abnormalities may be correlated with the presence of negative symptoms: a blunted release of prolactin and growth hormone on gonadotropin-releasing hormone or thyrotropin-releasing hormone stimulation and a blunted release of growth hormone on apomorphine stimulation.

Psychosocial and Psychoanalytic Theories

If schizophrenia is a disease of the brain, it is likely to parallel diseases of other organs (e.g., myocardial infarctions, diabetes) whose courses are affected by psychosocial stress. Thus, clinicians should consider both psychosocial and biological factors affecting schizophrenia.

The disorder affects individual patients, each of whom has a unique psychological makeup. Although many psychodynamic theories about the pathogenesis of schizophrenia seem outdated, perceptive clinical observations can help contemporary clinicians understand how the disease may affect a patient's psyche.

Psychoanalytic Theories

Sigmund Freud postulated that schizophrenia resulted from developmental fixations early in life. These fixations produce defects in ego development, and he postulated that such defects contributed to the symptoms of schizophrenia. Ego disintegration in schizophrenia represents a return to the time when the ego was not yet developed or had just begun to be established. Because the ego affects the interpretation of reality and the control of inner drives, such as sex and aggression, these ego functions are impaired. Thus, intrapsychic conflict arising from the early fixations and the ego defect, which may have resulted from poor early object relations, fuel the psychotic symptoms.

As described by Margaret Mahler, there are distortions in the reciprocal relationship between the infant and the mother. The child is unable to separate from, and progress beyond, the closeness and complete dependence that characterize the mother–child relationship in the oral phase of development. As a result, the person's identity never becomes secure.

Paul Federn hypothesized that the defect in ego functions permits intense hostility and aggression to distort the mother–infant relationship, which leads to eventual personality disorganization and vulnerability to stress. The onset of symptoms during adolescence occurs when teenagers need a strong ego to function independently, to separate from the parents, to identify tasks, to control increased internal drives, and to cope with intense external stimulation.

Harry Stack Sullivan viewed schizophrenia as a disturbance in interpersonal relatedness. The patient's massive anxiety creates a sense of unrelatedness that is transformed into parataxic distortions, which are usually, but not always, persecutory. To Sullivan, schizophrenia is an adaptive method used to avoid panic, terror, and disintegration of the sense of self. The source of pathological anxiety results from cumulative experiential traumas during development.

Psychoanalytic theory also postulates that the various symptoms of schizophrenia have symbolic meaning for individual patients. For example, fantasies of the world coming to an end may indicate a perception that a person's internal world has broken down. Feelings of inferiority are replaced by delusions of grandeur and omnipotence. Hallucinations may be substitutes for a patient's inability to deal with objective reality and may represent inner wishes or fears. Delusions, similar to hallucinations, are regressive, restitutive attempts to create a new reality or to express hidden fears or impulses.

Regardless of the theoretical model, all psychodynamic approaches are founded on the premise that psychotic symptoms have meaning in schizophrenia. Patients, for example, may become grandiose after an injury to their self-esteem. Similarly, all theories recognize that human relatedness may be terrifying for persons with schizophrenia. Although research on the efficacy of psychotherapy with schizophrenia shows mixed results, concerned persons who offer compassion and a sanctuary in the confusing world of schizophrenia must be a cornerstone of any overall treatment plan. Long-term follow-up studies show that some patients who bury psychotic episodes probably do not benefit from exploratory psychotherapy, but those who are able to integrate the psychotic experience into their lives may benefit from some insight-oriented approaches. There is renewed interest in the use of long-term individual psychotherapy in the treatment of schizophrenia, especially when combined with medication.

Learning Theories

According to learning theorists, children who later have schizophrenia learn irrational reactions and ways of thinking by imitating parents who have their own significant emotional problems. In learning theory, the poor interpersonal relationships of persons with schizophrenia develop because of poor models for learning during childhood.

Family Dynamics

In a study of British 4-year-old children, those who had a poor mother–child relationship had a sixfold increase in the risk of developing schizophrenia, and offspring from schizophrenic mothers who were adopted away at birth were more likely to develop the illness if they were reared in adverse circumstances compared with those raised in loving homes by stable adoptive parents. Nevertheless, no well-controlled evidence indicates that a specific family pattern plays a causative role in the development of schizophrenia. Some patients with schizophrenia do come from dysfunctional families, just as do many nonpsychiatrically ill persons. It is important, however, not to overlook pathological family behavior that can significantly increase the emotional stress with which a vulnerable patient with schizophrenia must cope.

Double Bind

The double-bind concept was formulated by Gregory Bateson and Donald Jackson to describe a hypothetical family in which children receive conflicting parental messages about their behavior, attitudes, and feelings. In Bateson's hypothesis, children withdraw into a psychotic state to escape the unsolvable confusion of the double bind. Unfortunately, the family studies that were conducted to validate the theory were seriously flawed methodologically. The theory has value only as a descriptive pattern, not as a causal explanation of schizophrenia. An example of a double bind is a parent who tells a child to provide cookies for his or her friends and then chastises the child for giving away too many cookies to playmates.

SCHISMS AND SKEWED FAMILIES. Theodore Lidz described two abnormal patterns of family behavior. In one family type, with a prominent schism between the parents, one parent is overly close to a child of the opposite gender. In the other family type, a skewed relationship between a child and one parent involves a power struggle between the parents and the resulting dominance of one parent. These dynamics stress the tenuous adaptive capacity of the person with schizophrenia.

PSEUDOMUTUAL AND PSEUDOHOSTILE FAMILIES. As described by Lyman Wynne, some families suppress emotional expression by consistently using pseudomutual or pseudohostile verbal communication. In such families, a unique verbal communication develops, and when a child leaves home and must relate to other persons, problems may arise. The child's verbal communication may be incomprehensible to outsiders.

EXPRESSED EMOTION. Parents or other caregivers may behave with overt criticism, hostility, and overinvolvement toward a person with schizophrenia. Many studies have indicated that in families with high levels of expressed emotion, the relapse rate for schizophrenia is high. The assessment of expressed emotion involves analyzing both what is said and the manner in which it is said.

DIAGNOSIS

According to DSM-5 there are five key signs and symptoms that characterize schizophrenia: (1) hallucinations; (2) delusions; (3) disorganized speech, for example, loose associations; (4) disorganized behavior (which may manifest as catatonia); and (5) negative symptoms such as apathy, abulia, and anhedonia (see Table 4.1–1 for a list of negative symptoms associated with schizophrenia). Not all of the signs and symptoms mentioned above need be present to make the diagnosis; but the diagnosis cannot be made unless one of the following is present: delusions, hallucinations, or disorganized speech. This is consistent with what Bleuler mentioned (see above): delusions and hallucinations are not always present in schizophrenia. Finally, signs and symptoms must be present for at least 6 months before a diagnosis of schizophrenia can be made.

Subtypes

Five subtypes of schizophrenia have been described based predominantly on clinical presentation: paranoid, disorganized, catatonic, undifferentiated, and residual. DSM-5 no longer uses these subtypes but they are listed in the 10th revision of the *International Statistical Classification of Diseases and Related Health Problems* (ICD-10). They are included in this text because the authors believe them to be of clinical significance and they are still used by most clinicians in the United States and around the world to describe the phenomenology of schizophrenia.

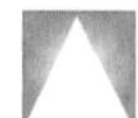

Table 4.1–1
Negative Symptoms in Schizophrenia

I. Affective flattening or blunting
   a. Unchanging facial expressions
   b. Decreased spontaneous movement
   c. Paucity of expressive gesture
   d. Poor eye contact
   e. Affective nonresponsivity
   f. Inappropriate affect
   g. Lack of vocal inflections
II. Alogia
   a. Poverty of speech
   b. Poverty of content of speech
   c. Blocking
   d. Increased latency of response
III. Avolition—apathy
   a. Grooming and hygiene
   b. Impersistence at work or school
   c. Physical anergia
IV. Anhedonia—asociality
   a. Recreational interests and activities
   b. Sexual interest and activities
   c. Intimacy and closeness
   d. Relationships with friends
V. Attention
   a. Social inattentiveness
   b. Inattentiveness during testing

Courtesy of Carol Tamminga, MD.

Paranoid Type

The paranoid type of schizophrenia is characterized by preoccupation with one or more delusions or frequent auditory hallucinations. Classically, the paranoid type of schizophrenia is characterized mainly by the presence of delusions of persecution or grandeur. Patients with paranoid schizophrenia usually have their first episode of illness at an older age than do patients with catatonic or disorganized schizophrenia. Patients in whom schizophrenia occurs in the late 20s or 30s have usually established a social life that may help them through their illness, and the ego resources of paranoid patients tend to be greater than those of patients with catatonic and disorganized schizophrenia. Patients with the paranoid type of schizophrenia show less regression of their mental faculties, emotional responses, and behavior than do patients with other types of schizophrenia.

Patients with paranoid schizophrenia are typically tense, suspicious, guarded, reserved, and sometimes hostile or aggressive, but they can occasionally conduct themselves adequately in social situations. Their intelligence in areas not invaded by their psychosis tends to remain intact.

Disorganized Type

The disorganized type of schizophrenia is characterized by a marked regression to primitive, disinhibited, and unorganized behavior and by the absence of symptoms that meet the criteria for the catatonic type. The onset of this subtype is generally early, occurring before age 25 years. Disorganized patients are usually active but in an aimless, nonconstructive manner. Their thought disorder is pronounced, and their contact with reality is poor. Their personal appearance is disheveled, and their social behavior and their emotional responses are inappropriate. They often burst into laughter without any apparent reason. Incongruous grinning and grimacing are common in these patients, whose behavior is best described as silly or fatuous.

Patient AB, a 32-year-old woman, began to lose weight and became careless about her work, which deteriorated in quality and quantity. She believed that other women at her place of employment were circulating slanderous stories concerning her and complained that a young man employed in the same plant had put his arm around her and insulted her. Her family demanded that the charge be investigated, which showed not only that the charge was without foundation but also that the man in question had not spoken to her for months. One day she returned home from work, and as she entered the house, she laughed loudly, watched her sister-in-law suspiciously, refused to answer questions, and at the sight of her brother began to cry. She refused to go to the bathroom, saying that a man was looking in the windows at her. She ate no food, and the next day she declared that her sisters were "bad women," that everyone was talking about her, and that someone had been having sexual relations with her, and although she could not see him, he was "always around."

The patient was admitted to a public psychiatric hospital. As she entered the admitting office, she laughed loudly and repeatedly screamed in a loud tone, "She cannot stay here; she's got to go home!" She grimaced and performed various stereotyped movements of her hands. When seen on the ward an hour later, she paid no attention to questions, although she talked to herself in a childish tone. She moved about constantly, walked on her toes in a dancing manner, pointed aimlessly about, and put out her tongue and sucked her lips in the manner of an infant. At times she moaned and cried like a child but shed no tears. As the months passed, she remained silly, childish, preoccupied, and inaccessible, grimacing, gesturing, pointing at objects in a stereotyped way, and usually chattering to herself in a peculiar high-pitched voice, with little of what she said being understood. Her condition continued to deteriorate, she remained unkempt, and she presented a picture of extreme introversion and regression, with no interest either in the activities of the institution or in her relatives who visited her. *(Adapted from case of Arthur P. Noyes, M.D., and Lawrence C. Kolb, M.D.)*

Catatonic Type

The catatonic type of schizophrenia, which was common several decades ago, has become rare in Europe and North America. The classic feature of the catatonic type is a marked disturbance in motor function; this disturbance may involve stupor, negativism, rigidity, excitement, or posturing. Sometimes the patient shows a rapid alteration between extremes of excitement and stupor. Associated features include stereotypies, mannerisms, and waxy flexibility. Mutism is particularly common. During catatonic excitement, patients need careful supervision to prevent them from hurting themselves or others. Medical care may be needed because of malnutrition, exhaustion, hyperpyrexia, or self-inflicted injury.

AC, age 32 years, was admitted to the hospital. On arrival, he was noted to be an asthenic, poorly nourished man with dilated pupils, hyperactive tendon reflexes, and a pulse rate of 120 beats/min. He showed many mannerisms, laid down on the floor, pulled at his foot, made undirected violent striking movements, struck attendants, grimaced, assumed rigid and strange postures, refused to speak, and appeared to be having auditory hallucinations. When seen later in the day, he was found to be in a stuporous state. His face was without expression, he was mute and rigid, and he paid no attention to those about him or to their questions. His eyes were closed, and his eyelids could be separated only with effort. There was no response to pinpricks or other painful stimuli.

He gradually became accessible, and when asked concerning himself, he referred to his stuporous period as sleep and maintained that he had no recollection of any events occurring during it. He said, "I didn't know anything. Everything seemed to be dark as far as my mind is concerned. Then I began to see a little light, like the shape of a star. Then my head got through the star gradually. I saw more and more light until I saw everything in a perfect form a few days ago." He explained his mutism by saying that he had been afraid he would "say the wrong thing" and that he "didn't know exactly what to talk about." From his obviously inadequate emotional response and his statement that he was "a scientist and an inventor of the most extraordinary genius of the 20th century," it was plain that he was still far from well. *(Adapted from case of Arthur P. Noyes, M.D., and Lawrence C. Kolb, M.D.)*

Undifferentiated Type

Frequently, patients who clearly have schizophrenia cannot be easily fit into one type or another. These patients are classified as having schizophrenia of the undifferentiated type.

Residual Type

The residual type of schizophrenia is characterized by continuing evidence of the schizophrenic disturbance in the absence of a complete set of active symptoms or of sufficient symptoms to meet the diagnosis of another type of schizophrenia. Emotional blunting, social withdrawal, eccentric behavior, illogical thinking, and mild loosening of associations commonly appear in the residual type. When delusions or hallucinations occur, they are neither prominent nor accompanied by strong affect.

Other Subtypes

The subtyping of schizophrenia has had a long history; other subtyping schemes appear in the literature, especially literature from countries outside of the United States.

Bouffée Délirante (Acute Delusional Psychosis)

This French diagnostic concept differs from a diagnosis of schizophrenia primarily on the basis of symptom duration of less than 3 months. The diagnosis is similar to the DSM-5 diagnosis of schizophreniform disorder. French clinicians report that about 40 percent of patients with a diagnosis of *bouffée délirante* progress in their illness and are eventually classified as having schizophrenia.

Latent. The concept of latent schizophrenia was developed during a time when theorists conceived of the disorder in broad diagnostic terms. Currently, patients must be very mentally ill to warrant a diagnosis of schizophrenia, but with a broad diagnostic concept of schizophrenia, the condition of patients who would not currently be thought of as severely ill could have received a diagnosis of schizophrenia. Latent schizophrenia, for example, was often the diagnosis used for what are now called borderline, schizoid, and schizotypal personality disorders. These patients may occasionally show peculiar behaviors or thought disorders but do not consistently manifest psychotic symptoms. In the past, the syndrome was also termed *borderline schizophrenia.*

Oneiroid. The oneiroid state refers to a dream-like state in which patients may be deeply perplexed and not fully oriented in time and place. The term *oneiroid schizophrenia* has been used for patients who are engaged in their hallucinatory experiences to the exclusion of involvement in the real world. When an oneiroid state is present, clinicians should be particularly careful to examine patients for medical or neurological causes of the symptoms.

After a 20-year-old female college student had recovered from her schizophrenic breakdown, she wrote the following description of her experiences during the oneiroid phase:

This is how I remember it. The road has changed. It is twisted and it used to be straight. Nothing is constant—all is in motion. The trees are moving. They do not remain at rest. How is it my mother does not bump into the trees that are moving? I follow my mother. I am afraid, but I follow. I have to share my strange thoughts with someone. We are sitting on a bench. The bench seems low. It, too, has moved. "The bench is low," I say. "Yes," says my mother. "This isn't how it used to be. How come there are no people around? There are usually lots of people and it is Sunday and there are no people. This is strange." All these strange questions irritate my mother who then says she must be going soon. While I continue thinking I'm in a kind of nowhere....

There are no days; no nights; sometimes it is darker than other times—that's all. It is never quite black, just dark gray. There is no such thing as time—there is only eternity. There is no such thing as death—nor heaven and hell—there is only a timeless—hateful—spaceless—worsening of things. You can never go forward; you must always regress into this horrific mess....

The outside was moving rather swiftly, everything seemed topsy-turvy—things were flying about. It was very strange. I wanted to get back to the quiet very badly but when I got back I couldn't remember where anything was (e.g., the bathroom).... *(Courtesy of Heinz E. Lehmann, M.D.)*

Paraphrenia. The term *paraphrenia* is sometimes used as a synonym for paranoid schizophrenia or for either a progressively deteriorating course of illness or the presence of a well-systemized delusional system. The multiple meanings of the term render it ineffectual in communicating information.

Pseudoneurotic Schizophrenia. Occasionally, patients who initially have such symptoms as anxiety, phobias, obsessions, and compulsions later reveal symptoms of thought disorder and psychosis. These patients are characterized by symptoms of pananxiety, panphobia, panambivalence, and sometimes chaotic sexuality. Unlike persons with anxiety disorders, pseudoneurotic patients have free-floating anxiety that rarely subsides. In clinical descriptions, the patients seldom become overtly and severely psychotic. This condition is currently diagnosed as borderline personality disorder.

Simple Deteriorative Disorder (Simple Schizophrenia). Simple deteriorative disorder is characterized by a gradual, insidious loss of drive and ambition. Patients with the disorder are usually not overtly psychotic and do not experience persistent hallucinations or delusions. Their primary symptom is withdrawal from social and work-related situations. The syndrome must be differentiated from depression, a phobia, a dementia, or an exacerbation of personality traits. Clinicians should be sure that patients truly meet the diagnostic criteria for schizophrenia before making the diagnosis.

An unmarried man, 27 years old, was brought to the mental hospital because he had on several occasions become violent toward his father. For a few weeks, he had hallucinations and heard voices. The voices eventually ceased, but he then adopted a strange way of life. He would sit up all night, sleep all day, and become very angry when his father tried to get him out of bed. He did not shave or wash for weeks, smoked continuously, ate very irregularly, and drank enormous quantities of tea.

In the hospital, he adjusted rapidly to the new environment and was found to be generally cooperative. He showed no marked abnormalities of mental state or behavior, except for his lack of concern for just about anything. He kept to himself as much as possible and conversed little with patients or staff. His personal hygiene had to be supervised by the nursing staff; otherwise, he would quickly become dirty and untidy.

Six years after his admission to the hospital, he is described as shiftless and careless, sullen and unreasonable. He lies on a couch all day long. Although many efforts have been made to get the patient to accept therapeutic work assignments, he refuses to consider any kind of regular occupation. In the summer, he wanders about the hospital grounds or lies under a tree. In the winter, he wanders through the tunnels connecting the various hospital buildings and is often seen stretched out for hours under the warm pipes that carry the steam through the tunnels. *(Courtesy of Heinz E. Lehmann, M.D.)*

Postpsychotic Depressive Disorder of Schizophrenia. After an acute schizophrenia episode, some patients become depressed. The symptoms of postpsychotic depressive disorder of schizophrenia can closely resemble the symptoms of the residual phase of schizophrenia and the adverse effects of commonly used antipsychotic medications. The diagnosis should not be made if they are substance induced or part of a mood disorder due to a general medical condition. These depressive states occur in up to 25 percent of patients with schizophrenia and are associated with an increased risk of suicide.

Early-Onset Schizophrenia. A small minority of patients manifest schizophrenia in childhood. Such children may at first present diagnostic problems, particularly with differentiation from mental retardation and autistic disorder. Recent studies have established that the diagnosis of childhood schizophrenia may be based on the same symptoms used for adult schizophrenia. Its onset is usually insidious, its course tends to be chronic, and the prognosis is mostly unfavorable.

Late-Onset Schizophrenia. Late-onset schizophrenia is clinically indistinguishable from schizophrenia but has an onset after age 45 years. This condition tends to appear more frequently in women and tends to be characterized by a predominance of paranoid symptoms. The prognosis is favorable, and these patients usually do well on antipsychotic medication.

Deficit Schizophrenia

In the 1980s, criteria were promulgated for a subtype of schizophrenia characterized by enduring, idiopathic negative symptoms. These patients were said to exhibit the deficit syndrome. This group of patients is now said to have deficit. Patients with schizophrenia with positive symptoms are said to have nondeficit schizophrenia. The symptoms used to define deficit schizophrenia are strongly interrelated, although various combinations of the six negative symptoms in the criteria can be found.

Deficit patients have a more severe course of illness than nondeficit patients, with a higher prevalence of abnormal involuntary movements before administration of antipsychotic drugs and poorer social function before the onset of psychotic symptoms. The onset of the first psychotic episode is more often insidious, and these patients show less long-term recovery of function than do nondeficit patients. Deficit patients are also less likely to marry than are other patients with schizophrenia. However, despite their poorer level of function and greater social isolation, both of which should increase a patient's stress and, therefore, the risk of serious depression, deficit patients appear to have a decreased risk of major depression and probably have a decreased risk of suicide as well.

The risk factors of deficit patients differ from those of nondeficit patients; whereas deficit schizophrenia is associated with an excess of summer births, nondeficit patients have an excess of winter births. Deficit schizophrenia may also be associated with a greater familial risk of schizophrenia and of mild, deficit-like features in the nonpsychotic relatives of deficit probands. Within a family with multiple affected siblings, the deficit–nondeficit categorization tends to be uniform. The deficit group also has a higher prevalence of men.

The psychopathology of deficit patients impacts treatment; their lack of motivation, lack of distress, greater cognitive impairment, and asocial nature undermine the efficacy of psychosocial interventions, as well as their adherence to medication regimens. Their cognitive impairment, which is greater than that of nondeficit subjects, also contributes to this lack of efficacy.

Psychological Testing. Patients with schizophrenia generally perform poorly on a wide range of neuropsychological tests. Vigilance, memory, and concept formation are most affected and consistent with pathological involvement in the frontotemporal cortex.

Objective measures of neuropsychological performance, such as the Halstead–Reitan battery and the Luria–Nebraska battery, often give abnormal findings, such as bilateral frontal and temporal lobe dysfunction, including impairments in attention, retention time, and problem-solving ability. Motor ability is also impaired, possibly related to brain asymmetry.

Intelligence Tests. When groups of patients with schizophrenia are compared with groups of psychiatric patients without schizophrenia or with the general population, the schizophrenia patients tend to score lower on intelligence tests. Statistically, the evidence suggests that low intelligence is often present at the onset, and intelligence may continue to deteriorate with the progression of the disorder.

Projective and Personality Tests. Projective tests, such as the Rorschach test and the Thematic Apperception test, may indicate bizarre ideation. Personality inventories, such as the Minnesota Multiphasic Personality Inventory, often give abnormal results in schizophrenia, but the contribution to diagnosis and treatment planning is minimal.

CLINICAL FEATURES

A discussion of the clinical signs and symptoms of schizophrenia raises three key issues. First, no clinical sign or symptom is pathognomonic for schizophrenia; every sign or symptom seen in schizophrenia occurs in other psychiatric and neurological disorders. This observation is contrary to the often-heard clinical opinion that certain signs and symptoms are diagnostic of schizophrenia. Therefore, a patient's history is essential for the diagnosis of schizophrenia; clinicians cannot diagnose schizophrenia simply by results of a mental status examination, which may vary. Second, a patient's symptoms change with time. For example, a patient may have intermittent hallucinations and a varying ability to perform adequately in social situations, or significant symptoms of a mood disorder may come and go during the course of schizophrenia. Third, clinicians must take into account the patient's educational level, intellectual ability, and cultural and subcultural membership. An impaired ability to understand abstract concepts, for example, may reflect either the patient's education or his or her intelligence. Religious organizations and cults may have customs that seem strange to outsiders but are normal to those within the cultural setting.

Premorbid Signs and Symptoms

In theoretical formulations of the course of schizophrenia, premorbid signs and symptoms appear before the prodromal phase of the illness. The differentiation implies that premorbid signs and symptoms exist before the disease process evidences itself and that the prodromal signs and symptoms are parts of the evolving disorder. In the typical, but not invariable, premorbid history of schizophrenia, patients had schizoid or schizotypal personalities characterized as quiet, passive, and introverted; as children, they had few friends. Preschizophrenic adolescents may have no close friends and no dates and may avoid team sports. They may enjoy watching movies and television, listening to music, or playing computer games to the exclusion of social activities. Some adolescent patients may show a sudden onset of obsessive-compulsive behavior as part of the prodromal picture.

The validity of the prodromal signs and symptoms, almost invariably recognized after the diagnosis of schizophrenia has been made, is uncertain; after schizophrenia is diagnosed, the retrospective remembrance of early signs and symptoms is affected. Nevertheless, although the first hospitalization is often believed to mark the beginning of the disorder, signs and symptoms have often been present for months or even years. The signs may have started with complaints about somatic symptoms, such as headache, back and muscle pain, weakness, and digestive problems. The initial diagnosis may be malingering, chronic fatigue syndrome, or somatization disorder. Family and friends may eventually notice that the person has changed and is no longer functioning well in occupational, social, and personal activities. During this stage, a patient may begin to develop an interest in abstract ideas, philosophy, and the occult or religious questions. Additional prodromal signs and symptoms can include markedly peculiar behavior, abnormal affect, unusual speech, bizarre ideas, and strange perceptual experiences.

Mental Status Examination

General Description. The appearance of a patient with schizophrenia can range from that of a completely disheveled, screaming, agitated person to an obsessively groomed, completely silent, and immobile person. Between these two poles, patients may be talkative and may exhibit bizarre postures. Their behavior may become agitated or violent, apparently in an unprovoked manner, but usually in response to hallucinations. In contrast, in catatonic stupor, often referred to as catatonia, patients seem completely lifeless and may exhibit such signs as muteness, negativism, and automatic obedience. Waxy flexibility, once a common sign in catatonia, has become rare, as has manneristic behavior. A person with a less extreme subtype of catatonia may show marked social withdrawal and egocentricity, a lack of spontaneous speech or movement, and an absence of goal-directed behavior. Patients with catatonia may sit immobile and speechless in their chairs, respond to questions with only short answers, and move only when directed to move. Other obvious behavior may include odd clumsiness or stiffness in body movements, signs now seen as possibly indicating a disease process in the basal ganglia. Patients with schizophrenia are often poorly groomed, fail to bathe, and dress much too warmly for the prevailing temperatures. Other odd behaviors include tics; stereotypies; mannerisms; and, occasionally, echopraxia, in which patients imitate the posture or the behavior of the examiner.

Precox feeling. Some experienced clinicians report a precox feeling, an intuitive experience of their inability to establish an emotional rapport with a patient. Although the experience is common, no data indicate that it is a valid or reliable criterion in the diagnosis of schizophrenia.

Mood, Feelings, and Affect

Two common affective symptoms in schizophrenia are reduced emotional responsiveness, sometimes severe enough to warrant the label of anhedonia, and overly active and inappropriate emotions such as extremes of rage, happiness, and anxiety. A flat or blunted affect can be a symptom of the illness itself, of the parkinsonian adverse effects of antipsychotic medications, or of depression, and differentiating these symptoms can be a clinical challenge. Overly emotional patients may describe exultant feelings of omnipotence, religious ecstasy, terror at the disintegration of their souls, or paralyzing anxiety about the destruction of the universe. Other feeling tones include perplexity, a sense of isolation, overwhelming ambivalence, and depression.

Perceptual Disturbances

HALLUCINATIONS. Any of the five senses may be affected by hallucinatory experiences in patients with schizophrenia. The most common hallucinations, however, are auditory, with voices that are often threatening, obscene, accusatory, or insulting. Two or more voices may converse among themselves, or a voice may comment on the patient's life or behavior. Visual hallucinations are common, but tactile, olfactory, and gustatory hallucinations are unusual; their presence should prompt the clinician to consider the possibility of an underlying medical or neurological disorder that is causing the entire syndrome.

> A 48-year-old man, who had been diagnosed with schizophrenia while in the army at age 21 years, led an isolated and often frightened existence, living alone and supported by disability payments. Although he would confirm that he had chronic auditory hallucinations, he was never comfortable with discussing the content of these hallucinations, and a review of records showed this was a long-term pattern for the patient. Otherwise the patient had good rapport with his psychiatrist and was enthusiastic about the possibility of participating in a study of a novel antipsychotic agent. During the informed consent procedure, the patient asked about the possibility that the new medication might decrease his chronic auditory hallucinations. When it was acknowledged that any response was possible, including decreases in his hallucinations, the patient broke off the discussion abruptly and left the office. At a later visit, he reported that his most reliable pleasure in life was nightly discussions of gossip with hallucinations of voices he believed belonged to 17th-century French courtiers, and the chance that he might lose these conversations and the companionship they offered was too frightening for him to consider. *(Adapted from Stephen Lewis, M.D., P. Rodrigo Escalona, M.D., and Samuel J. Keith, M.D.)*

Cenesthetic Hallucinations. Cenesthetic hallucinations are unfounded sensations of altered states in bodily organs. Examples of cenesthetic hallucinations include a burning sensation in the brain, a pushing sensation in the blood vessels, and a cutting sensation in the bone marrow. Bodily distortions may also occur.

Illusions. As differentiated from hallucinations, whereas illusions are distortions of real images or sensations, hallucinations are not based on real images or sensations. Illusions can occur in schizophrenia patients during active phases, but they can also occur during the prodromal phases and during periods of remission. Whenever illusions or hallucinations occur, clinicians should consider the possibility of a substance-related cause for the symptoms, even when patients have already received a diagnosis of schizophrenia.

Thought. Disorders of thought are the most difficult symptoms for many clinicians and students to understand, but they may be the core symptoms of schizophrenia. Dividing the disorders of thought into disorders of thought content, form of thought, and thought process is one way to clarify them.

Thought Content. Disorders of thought content reflect the patient's ideas, beliefs, and interpretations of stimuli. Delusions, the most obvious example of a disorder of thought content, are varied in schizophrenia and may assume persecutory, grandiose, religious, or somatic forms.

Patients may believe that an outside entity controls their thoughts or behavior or, conversely, that they control outside events in an extraordinary fashion (such as causing the sun to rise and set or by preventing earthquakes). Patients may have an intense and consuming preoccupation with esoteric, abstract, symbolic, psychological, or philosophical ideas. Patients may also worry about allegedly life-threatening but bizarre and implausible somatic conditions, such as the presence of aliens inside the patient's testicles affecting his ability to father children.

The phrase *loss of ego boundaries* describes the lack of a clear sense of where the patient's own body, mind, and influence end and where those of other animate and inanimate objects begin. For example, patients may think that other persons, the television, or the newspapers are referring to them (*ideas of reference*). Other symptoms of the loss of ego boundaries include the sense that the patient has physically fused with an outside object (e.g., a tree or another person) or that the patient has disintegrated and fused with the entire universe (*cosmic identity*). With such a state of mind, some patients with schizophrenia doubt their gender or their sexual orientation. These symptoms should not be confused with transvestism, transsexuality, or other gender identity problems.

Form of Thought. Disorders of the form of thought are objectively observable in patients' spoken and written language. The disorders include looseness of associations, derailment, incoherence, tangentiality, circumstantiality, neologisms, echolalia, verbigeration, word salad, and mutism. Although looseness of associations was once described as pathognomonic for schizophrenia, the symptom is frequently seen in mania. Distinguishing between looseness of associations and tangentiality can be difficult for even the most experienced clinicians.

The following sample is taken from a memo typed by a secretary with schizophrenia who was still able to work part time in an office. Note her preoccupation with the mind, the Trinity, and other esoteric matters. Also note that peculiar restructuring of concepts by hyphenating the words germ-any (the patient had a distinct fear of germs) and infer-no (inferring that there will be no salvation). The "chain reaction" is a reference to atomic piles.

> Mental health is the Blessed Trinity, and as man cannot be without God, it is futile to deny His Son. For the Creation understand germ-any in Voice New Order, not lie of chained reaction, spawning mark in temple Cain with Babel grave'n image to wanton V day "Israel." Lucifer fell Jew prostitute and lambeth walks by roam to sex ritual, in Bible six million of the Babylon woman, infer-no Salvation.

The one common factor in the thought process above is a preoccupation with invisible forces, radiation, witchcraft, religion, philosophy, and psychology and a leaning toward the esoteric, the abstract, and the symbolic. Consequently, the thinking of a person with schizophrenia is characterized simultaneously by both an overly concrete and an overly symbolic nature.

Thought Process. Disorders in thought process concern the way ideas and languages are formulated. The examiner infers a disorder from what and how the patient speaks, writes, or draws. The examiner may also assess the patient's thought process by observing his or her behavior, especially in carrying out discrete tasks (e.g., in occupational therapy). Disorders of thought process include flight of ideas, thought blocking, impaired attention, poverty of thought content, poor abstraction abilities, perseveration, idiosyncratic associations (e.g., identical predicates, clang associations), overinclusion, and circumstantiality. *Thought control,* in which outside forces are controlling what the patient thinks or feels, is common, as is *thought broadcasting,* in which patients think others can read their minds or that their thoughts are broadcast through television sets or radios.

Impulsiveness, Violence, Suicide, and Homicide. Patients with schizophrenia may be agitated and have little impulse control when ill. They may also have decreased social sensitivity and appear to be impulsive when, for example, they grab another patient's cigarettes, change television channels abruptly, or throw food on the floor. Some apparently impulsive behavior, including suicide and homicide attempts, may be in response to hallucinations commanding the patient to act.

VIOLENCE. Violent behavior (excluding homicide) is common among untreated schizophrenia patients. Delusions of a persecutory nature, previous episodes of violence, and neurological deficits are risk factors for violent or impulsive behavior. Management includes appropriate antipsychotic medication. Emergency treatment consists of restraints and seclusion. Acute sedation with lorazepam (Ativan), 1 to 2 mg intramuscularly, repeated every hour as needed, may be necessary to prevent the patient from harming others. If a clinician feels fearful in the presence of a schizophrenia patient, it should be taken as an internal clue that the patient may be on the verge of acting out violently. In such cases, the interview should be terminated or be conducted with an attendant at the ready.

SUICIDE. Suicide is the single leading cause of premature death among people with schizophrenia. Suicide attempts are made by 20 to 50 percent of the patients, with long-term rates of suicide estimated to be 10 to 13 percent. According to DSM-5 approximately 5 to 6 percent of schizophrenic patients die by suicide, but this is probably an underestimation. Often, suicide in schizophrenia seems to occur "out of the blue," without prior warnings or expressions of verbal intent. The most important factor is the presence of a major depressive episode. Epidemiological studies indicate that up to 80 percent of schizophrenia patients may have a major depressive episode at some time in their lives. Some data suggest that those patients with the best prognosis (few negative symptoms, preservation of capacity to experience affects, better abstract thinking) can paradoxically also be at highest risk for suicide. The profile of the patient at greatest risk is a young man who once had high expectations, declined from a higher level of functioning, realizes that his dreams are not likely to come true, and has lost faith in the effectiveness of treatment. Other possible contributors to the high rate of suicide include command hallucinations and drug abuse. Two-thirds or more of schizophrenic patients who commit suicide have seen an apparently unsuspecting clinician within 72 hours of death. A large pharmacological study suggests that clozapine (Clozaril) may have particular efficacy in reducing suicidal ideation in schizophrenia patients with prior hospitalizations for suicidality. Adjunctive antidepressant medications have been shown to be effective in alleviating co-occurring major depression in schizophrenia.

The following is an example of an unpredictable suicide in a patient with schizophrenia who had been responding to psychiatric treatment:

> The patient had been an autistic child and did not speak until he was 7 years old. He had responded well to psychiatric treatment, and at age 13 his IQ was reported as 122. At age 17 he became violent toward his parents, shaved all his hair off, and made such statements as, "I like bank robbers knocking people unconscious" and "I think tough gangs are funny because they beat down people." While saying this, he laughed loudly. He was admitted to a mental hospital, where he responded with definite improvement to pharmacotherapy and psychotherapy, and he went home regularly for weekends.
>
> He left various notes on his desk before committing suicide. Among these notes was an eight-page list giving 211 "inexcusable mistakes throughout my life." Each one was dated, for example, "1952, 2nd of November: throwing up in my friend's house on a shoe-box. 1953, 17th August: accidentally wearing a watch that wasn't water-proof in the bath-tub. 1956, 23rd of September: slamming back-door of Meteor after getting in."
>
> He then proceeded in his notes to give "the causes of the mistakes:" "Montreal having a mountain; I have a receding hair-line; my height since I was nine years old; Canada having two languages...." He also wrote: "My feelings of tension since 1962 is getting worse most of the time. I planned the date of my death without the slightest trace of emotion...."
>
> The boy hanged himself at age 18 in the family garage. An experienced psychiatrist who had repeatedly interviewed him noted no signs of depression only a week before. *(Courtesy of Heinz E. Lehmann, M.D.)*

HOMICIDE. Despite the sensational attention that the news media provides when a patient with schizophrenia murders someone, the available data indicate that these patients are no more likely to commit homicide than is a member of the general population. When a patient with schizophrenia does commit homicide, it may be for unpredictable or bizarre reasons based on hallucinations or delusions. Possible predictors of homicidal activity are a history of previous violence, dangerous behavior while hospitalized, and hallucinations or delusions involving such violence.

Sensorium and Cognition

Orientation. Patients with schizophrenia are usually oriented to person, time, and place. The lack of such orientation should prompt clinicians to investigate the possibility of a medical or neurological brain disorder. Some patients with schizophrenia may give incorrect or bizarre answers to questions about orientation, for example, "I am Christ; this is heaven; and it is AD 35."

Memory. Memory, as tested in the mental status examination, is usually intact, but there can be minor cognitive deficiencies. It may not be possible, however, to get the patient to attend closely enough to the memory tests for the ability to be assessed adequately.

Cognitive Impairment. An important development in the understanding of the psychopathology of schizophrenia is an appreciation of the importance of cognitive impairment in the disorder. In outpatients, cognitive impairment is a better predictor of level of function than is the severity of psychotic symptoms. Patients with schizophrenia typically exhibit subtle cognitive dysfunction in the domains of attention, executive function, working memory, and episodic memory. Although a substantial percentage of patients have normal intelligence quotients, it is possible that every person who has schizophrenia has cognitive dysfunction compared with what he or she would be able to do without the disorder. Although these impairments cannot function as diagnostic tools, they are strongly related to the functional outcome of the illness and, for that reason, have clinical value as prognostic variables, as well as for treatment planning.

The cognitive impairment seems already to be present when patients have their first episode and appears largely to remain stable over the course of early illness. (There may be a small subgroup of patients who have a true dementia in late life that is not due to other cognitive disorders, such as Alzheimer's disease.) Cognitive impairments are also present in attenuated forms in nonpsychotic relatives of schizophrenia patients.

The cognitive impairments of schizophrenia have become the target of pharmacological and psychosocial treatment trials. It is likely that effective treatments will become widely available within a few years, and these are likely to lead to an improvement in the quality of life and level of functioning of people with schizophrenia.

Judgment and Insight. Classically, patients with schizophrenia are described as having poor insight into the nature and the severity of their disorder. The so-called lack of insight is associated with poor compliance with treatment. When examining schizophrenia patients, clinicians should carefully define various aspects of insight, such as awareness of symptoms, trouble getting along with people, and the reasons for these problems. Such information can be clinically useful in tailoring a treatment strategy and theoretically useful in postulating what areas of the brain contribute to the observed lack of insight (e.g., the parietal lobes).

Reliability. A patient with schizophrenia is no less reliable than any other psychiatric patient. The nature of the disorder, however, requires the examiner to verify important information through additional sources.

Somatic Comorbidity

Neurological Findings. Localizing and nonlocalizing neurological signs (also known as hard and soft signs, respectively) have been reported to be more common in patients with schizophrenia than in other psychiatric patients. Nonlocalizing signs include dysdiadochokinesia, astereognosis, primitive reflexes, and diminished dexterity. The presence of neurological signs and symptoms correlates with increased severity of illness, affective blunting, and a poor prognosis. Other abnormal neurological signs include tics, stereotypies, grimacing, impaired fine motor skills, abnormal motor tone, and abnormal movements. One study has found that only about 25 percent of patients with schizophrenia are aware of their own abnormal involuntary movements and that the lack of awareness is correlated with a lack of insight about the primary psychiatric disorder and the duration of illness.

Eye Examination. In addition to the disorder of smooth ocular pursuit (saccadic movement), patients with schizophrenia have an elevated blink rate. The elevated blink rate is believed to reflect hyperdopaminergic activity. In primates, blinking can be increased by dopamine agonists and reduced by dopamine antagonists.

Speech. Although the disorders of speech in schizophrenia (e.g., looseness of associations) are classically considered to indicate a thought disorder, they may also indicate a *forme fruste* of aphasia, perhaps implicating the dominant parietal lobe. The inability of schizophrenia patients to perceive the prosody of speech or to inflect their own speech can be seen as a neurological symptom of a disorder in the nondominant parietal lobe. Other parietal lobe–like symptoms in schizophrenia include the inability to carry out tasks (i.e., apraxia), right–left disorientation, and lack of concern about the disorder.

Other Comorbidity

Obesity. Patients with schizophrenia appear to be more obese, with higher body mass indexes (BMIs) than age- and gender-matched cohorts in the general population. This is due, at least in part, to the effect of many antipsychotic medications, as well as poor nutritional balance and decreased motor activity. This weight gain, in turn, contributes to an increased risk of cardiovascular morbidity and mortality, an increased risk of diabetes, and other obesity-related conditions such as hyperlipidemia and obstructive sleep apnea.

Diabetes Mellitus. Schizophrenia is associated with an increased risk of type II diabetes mellitus. This is probably due, in part, to the association with obesity noted previously, but there is also evidence that some antipsychotic medications cause diabetes through a direct mechanism.

Cardiovascular Disease. Many antipsychotic medications have direct effects on cardiac electrophysiology. In addition, obesity; increased rates of smoking, diabetes, hyperlipidemia; and a sedentary lifestyle all independently increase the risk of cardiovascular morbidity and mortality.

HIV. Patients with schizophrenia appear to have a risk of HIV infection that is 1.5 to 2 times that of the general population. This association is thought to be due to increased risk behaviors, such as unprotected sex, multiple partners, and increased drug use.

Chronic Obstructive Pulmonary Disease. Rates of chronic obstructive pulmonary disease are reportedly increased in schizophrenia compared with the general population. The increased prevalence of smoking is an obvious contributor to this problem and may be the only cause.

Rheumatoid Arthritis. Patients with schizophrenia have approximately one-third the risk of rheumatoid arthritis that is found in the general population. This inverse association has been replicated several times, the significance of which is unknown.

DIFFERENTIAL DIAGNOSIS

Secondary Psychotic Disorders

A wide range of nonpsychiatric medical conditions and a variety of substances can induce symptoms of psychosis and catatonia (Table 4.1–2). The most appropriate diagnosis for such psychosis or catatonia is psychotic disorder due to a general medical condition, catatonic disorder due to a general medical condition, or substance-induced psychotic disorder.

When evaluating a patient with psychotic symptoms, clinicians should follow the general guidelines for assessing nonpsychiatric conditions. First, clinicians should aggressively pursue an undiagnosed nonpsychiatric medical condition when a patient exhibits any unusual or rare symptoms or any variation in the level of consciousness. Second, clinicians should attempt to obtain a complete family history, including a history of medical, neurological, and psychiatric disorders. Third, clinicians should consider the possibility of a nonpsychiatric medical condition, even in patients with previous diagnoses of schizophrenia. A patient with schizophrenia is just as likely to have a brain tumor that produces psychotic symptoms as is a patient without schizophrenia.

Other Psychotic Disorders

The psychotic symptoms of schizophrenia can be identical with those of schizophreniform disorder, brief psychotic disorder, schizoaffective disorder, and delusional disorders. *Schizophreniform disorder* differs from schizophrenia in that the symptoms have a duration of at least 1 month but less than 6 months. *Brief psychotic disorder* is the appropriate diagnosis when the symptoms have lasted at least 1 day but less than 1 month and when the patient has not returned to the premorbid state of functioning within that time. There may also be a precipitating traumatic event. When a manic or depressive syndrome develops concurrently with the major symptoms of schizophrenia, *schizoaffective disorder* is the appropriate diagnosis. Nonbizarre delusions present for at least 1 month without other symptoms of schizophrenia or a mood disorder warrant the diagnosis of *delusional disorder*.

Mood Disorders

A patient with a major depressive episode may present with delusions and hallucinations, whether the patient has unipolar or

Table 4.1–2
Differential Diagnosis of Schizophrenia-Like Symptoms

Medical and Neurological
- Substance induced—amphetamine, hallucinogens, belladonna alkaloids, alcohol hallucinosis, barbiturate withdrawal, cocaine, phencyclidine
- Epilepsy—especially temporal lobe epilepsy
- Neoplasm, cerebrovascular disease, or trauma—especially frontal or limbic
- Other conditions
- Acute intermittent porphyria
- AIDS
- Vitamin B_{12} deficiency
- Carbon monoxide poisoning
- Cerebral lipoidosis
- Creutzfeldt-Jakob disease
- Fabry's disease
- Fahr's disease
- Hallervorden–Spatz disease
- Heavy metal poisoning
- Herpes encephalitis
- Homocystinuria
- Huntington's disease
- Metachromatic leukodystrophy
- Neurosyphilis
- Normal pressure hydrocephalus
- Pellagra
- Systemic lupus erythematosus
- Wernicke–Korsakoff syndrome
- Wilson's disease

Psychiatric
- Atypical psychosis
- Autistic disorder
- Brief psychotic disorder
- Delusional disorder
- Factitious disorder with predominantly psychological signs and symptoms
- Malingering
- Mood disorders
- Normal adolescence
- Obsessive-compulsive disorder
- Personality disorders—schizotypal, schizoid, borderline, paranoid
- Schizoaffective disorder
- Schizophrenia
- Schizophreniform disorder

bipolar mood disorder. Delusions seen with psychotic depression are typically mood congruent and involve themes such as guilt, self-depreciation, deserved punishment, and incurable illnesses. In mood disorders, psychotic symptoms resolve completely with the resolution of depression. A depressive episode that is this severe may also result in loss of functioning, decline in self-care, and social isolation, but these are secondary to the depressive symptoms and should not be confused with the negative symptoms of schizophrenia.

A full-blown manic episode often presents with delusions and sometimes hallucinations. Delusions in mania are most often mood congruent and typically involve grandiose themes. The flight of ideas seen in mania may, at times, be confused with the thought disorder of schizophrenia. Special attention during mental status examination of a patient with a flight of ideas is required to note whether the associative links between topics are conserved, although the conversation is difficult for the observer to follow because of the patient's accelerated rate of thinking.

Personality Disorders

Various personality disorders may have some features of schizophrenia. Schizotypal, schizoid, and borderline personality disorders are the personality disorders with the most similar symptoms. Severe obsessive-compulsive personality disorder may mask an underlying schizophrenic process. Personality disorders, unlike schizophrenia, have mild symptoms and a history of occurring throughout a patient's life; they also lack an identifiable date of onset.

Malingering and Factitious Disorders

For a patient who imitates the symptoms of schizophrenia but does not actually have the disorder, either malingering or factitious disorder may be an appropriate diagnosis. Persons have faked schizophrenic symptoms and have been admitted into and treated at psychiatric hospitals. The condition of patients who are completely in control of their symptom production may qualify for a diagnosis of malingering; such patients usually have some obvious financial or legal reason to want to be considered mentally ill. The condition of patients who are less in control of their falsification of psychotic symptoms may qualify for a diagnosis of factitious disorder. Some patients with schizophrenia, however, may falsely complain of an exacerbation of psychotic symptoms to obtain increased assistance benefits or to gain admission to a hospital.

COURSE AND PROGNOSIS

Course

A premorbid pattern of symptoms may be the first evidence of illness, although the importance of the symptoms is usually recognized only retrospectively. Characteristically, the symptoms begin in adolescence and are followed by the development of prodromal symptoms in days to a few months. Social or environmental changes, such as going away to college, using a substance, or a relative's death, may precipitate the disturbing symptoms, and the prodromal syndrome may last a year or more before the onset of overt psychotic symptoms.

The classic course of schizophrenia is one of exacerbations and remissions. After the first psychotic episode, a patient gradually recovers and may then function relatively normally for a long time. Patients usually relapse, however, and the pattern of illness during the first 5 years after the diagnosis generally indicates the patient's course. Further deterioration in the patient's baseline functioning follows each relapse of the psychosis. This failure to return to baseline functioning after each relapse is the major distinction between schizophrenia and the mood disorders. Sometimes a clinically observable postpsychotic depression follows a psychotic episode, and the schizophrenia patient's vulnerability to stress is usually lifelong. Positive symptoms tend to become less severe with time, but the socially debilitating negative or deficit symptoms may increase in severity. Although about one-third of all schizophrenia patients have some marginal or integrated social existence, most have lives characterized by aimlessness; inactivity; frequent hospitalizations; and, in urban settings, homelessness and poverty.

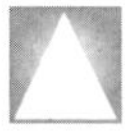

Table 4.1–3
Features Weighting Toward Good to Poor Prognosis in Schizophrenia

Good Prognosis	Poor Prognosis
Late onset	Young onset
Obvious precipitating factors	No precipitating factors
Acute onset	Insidious onset
Good premorbid social, sexual, and work histories	Poor premorbid social, sexual, and work histories
Mood disorder symptoms (especially depressive disorders)	Withdrawn, autistic behavior
Married	Single, divorced, or widowed
Family history of mood disorders	Family history of schizophrenia
Good support systems	Poor support systems
Positive symptoms	Negative symptoms
	Neurological signs and symptoms
	History of perinatal trauma
	No remissions in 3 years
	Many relapses
	History of assaultiveness

Prognosis

Several studies have shown that over the 5- to 10-year period after the first psychiatric hospitalization for schizophrenia, only about 10 to 20 percent of patients can be described as having a good outcome. More than 50 percent of patients can be described as having a poor outcome, with repeated hospitalizations, exacerbations of symptoms, episodes of major mood disorders, and suicide attempts. Despite these glum figures, schizophrenia does not always run a deteriorating course, and several factors have been associated with a good prognosis (Table 4.1–3).

Reported remission rates range from 10 to 60 percent, and a reasonable estimate is that 20 to 30 percent of all schizophrenia patients are able to lead somewhat normal lives. About 20 to 30 percent of patients continue to experience moderate symptoms, and 40 to 60 percent of patients remain significantly impaired by their disorder for their entire lives. Patients with schizophrenia do much poorer than patients with mood disorders, although 20 to 25 percent of mood disorder patients are also severely disturbed at long-term follow-up.

TREATMENT

Although antipsychotic medications are the mainstay of the treatment for schizophrenia, research has found that psychosocial interventions, including psychotherapy, can augment the clinical improvement. Just as pharmacological agents are used to treat presumed chemical imbalances, nonpharmacological strategies must treat nonbiological issues. The complexity of schizophrenia usually renders any single therapeutic approach inadequate to deal with the multifaceted disorder. Psychosocial modalities should be integrated into the drug treatment regimen and should support it. Patients with schizophrenia benefit more from the combined use of antipsychotic drugs and psychosocial treatment than from either treatment used alone.

Hospitalization

Hospitalization is indicated for diagnostic purposes; for stabilization of medications; for patients' safety because of suicidal or homicidal ideation; and for grossly disorganized or inappropriate behavior, including the inability to take care of basic needs such as food, clothing, and shelter. Establishing an effective association between patients and community support systems is also a primary goal of hospitalization.

Short stays of 4 to 6 weeks are just as effective as long-term hospitalizations, and hospital settings with active behavioral approaches produce better results than do custodial institutions. Hospital treatment plans should be oriented toward practical issues of self-care, quality of life, employment, and social relationships. During hospitalization, patients should be coordinated with aftercare facilities, including their family homes, foster families, board-and-care homes, and halfway houses. Day care centers and home visits by therapists or nurses can help patients remain out of the hospital for long periods and can improve the quality of their daily lives.

Pharmacotherapy

The introduction of chlorpromazine (Thorazine) in 1952 may be the most important single contribution to the treatment of a psychiatric illness. Henri Laborit, a surgeon in Paris, noticed that administering chlorpromazine to patients before surgery resulted in an unusual state in which they seemed less anxious regarding the procedure. Chlorpromazine was subsequently shown to be effective at reducing hallucinations and delusions, as well as excitement. It was also noted that it caused side effects that appeared similar to parkinsonism.

Antipsychotics diminish psychotic symptom expression and reduce relapse rates. Approximately 70 percent of patients treated with any antipsychotic achieve remission.

The drugs used to treat schizophrenia have a wide variety of pharmacological properties, but all share the capacity to antagonize postsynaptic dopamine receptors in the brain. Antipsychotics can be categorized into two main groups: the older conventional antipsychotics, which have also been called *first-generation antipsychotics* or DRAs, and the newer drugs, which have been called *second-generation antipsychotics or serotonin dopamine antagonists (SDAs).*

Clozapine (Clozaril), the first effective antipsychotic with negligible extrapyramidal side effects, was discovered in 1958 and first studied during the 1960s. However, in 1976, it was noted that clozapine was associated with a substantial risk of agranulocytosis. This property resulted in delays in the introduction of clozapine. In 1990, clozapine finally became available in the United States, but its use was restricted to patients who responded poorly to other agents.

PHASES OF TREATMENT IN SCHIZOPHRENIA

Treatment of Acute Psychosis

Acute psychotic symptoms require immediate attention. Treatment during the acute phase focuses on alleviating the most severe psychotic symptoms. This phase usually lasts from 4 to

8 weeks. Acute schizophrenia is typically associated with severe agitation, which can result from such symptoms as frightening delusions, hallucinations, or suspiciousness, or from other causes (including stimulant abuse). Patients with akathisia can appear agitated when they experience a subjective feeling of motor restlessness. Differentiating akathisia from psychotic agitation can be difficult, particularly when patients are incapable of describing their internal experience. If patients are receiving an agent associated with extrapyramidal side effects, usually a first-generation antipsychotic, a trial with an anticholinergic anti-Parkinson medication, benzodiazepine, or propranolol (Inderal) may be helpful in making the discrimination.

Clinicians have a number of options for managing agitation that result from psychosis. Antipsychotics and benzodiazepines can result in relatively rapid calming of patients. With highly agitated patients, intramuscular administration of antipsychotics produces a more rapid effect. An advantage of an antipsychotic is that a single intramuscular injection of haloperidol (Haldol), fluphenazine (Prolixin, Permitil), olanzapine (Zyprexa), or ziprasidone (Geodon) will often result in calming effect without excessive sedation. Low-potency antipsychotics are often associated with sedation and postural hypotension, particularly when they are administered intramuscularly. Intramuscular ziprasidone and olanzapine are similar to their oral counterparts in not causing substantial extrapyramidal side effects during acute treatment. This can be an important advantage over haloperidol or fluphenazine, which can cause frightening dystonias or akathisia in some patients. A rapidly dissolving oral formulation of olanzapine (Zydis) may also be helpful as an alternative to an intramuscular injection.

Benzodiazepines are also effective for agitation during acute psychosis. Lorazepam (Ativan) has the advantage of reliable absorption when it is administered either orally or intramuscularly. The use of benzodiazepines may also reduce the amount of antipsychotic that is needed to control psychotic patients.

Treatment during Stabilization and Maintenance Phase

In the stable or maintenance phase, the illness is in a relative stage of remission. The goals during this phase are to prevent psychotic relapse and to assist patients in improving their level of functioning. As newer medications have been introduced with a substantively reduced risk of tardive dyskinesia, one of the major concerns about long-term treatment has been diminished. During this phase, patients are usually in a relative state of remission with only minimal psychotic symptoms. Stable patients who are maintained on an antipsychotic have a much lower relapse rate than patients who have their medications discontinued. Data suggest that 16 to 23 percent of patients receiving treatment will experience a relapse within 1 year, and 53 to 72 percent will relapse without medications. Even patients who have had only one episode have a four in five chance of relapsing at least once over the following 5 years. Stopping medication increases this risk fivefold. Although published guidelines do not make definitive recommendations about the duration of maintenance treatment after the first episode, recent data suggest that 1 or 2 years might not be adequate. This is a particular concern when patients have achieved good employment status or are involved in educational programs because they have a lot to lose if they experience another psychotic decompensation.

It is generally recommended that multiepisode patients receive maintenance treatment for at least 5 years, and many experts recommend pharmacotherapy on an indefinite basis.

Noncompliance. Noncompliance with long-term antipsychotic treatment is very high. An estimated 40 to 50 percent of patients become noncompliant within 1 or 2 years. Compliance increases when long-acting medication is used instead of oral medication.

When beginning long-acting drugs, some oral supplementation is necessary while peak plasma levels are being achieved. Fluphenazine and haloperidol have been formulated as long-acting injectables. Long-acting forms of risperidone, paliperidone, aripiprazole, and olanzapine are also available.

There are a number of advantages to using long-acting injectable medication. Clinicians know immediately when noncompliance occurs and have some time to initiate appropriate interventions before the medication effect dissipates; there is less day-to-day variability in blood levels, making it easier to establish a minimum effective dose; and finally, many patients prefer it to having to remember dosage schedules of daily oral preparations.

STRATEGIES FOR POOR RESPONDERS

When patients with acute schizophrenia are administered an antipsychotic medication, approximately 60 percent will improve to the extent that they will achieve a complete remission or experience only mild symptoms; the remaining 40 percent of patients will improve but still demonstrate variable levels of positive symptoms that are resistant to the medications. Rather than categorizing patients into responders and nonresponders, it is more accurate to consider the degree to which the illness is improved by medication. Some resistant patients are so severely ill that they require chronic institutionalization. Others respond to an antipsychotic with substantial suppression of their psychotic symptoms but demonstrate persistent symptoms, such as hallucinations or delusions.

Before considering a patient a poor responder to a particular drug, it is important to assure that they received an adequate trial of the medication. A 4- to 6-week trial on an adequate dose of an antipsychotic represents a reasonable trial for most patients. Patients who demonstrate even a mild amount of improvement during this period may continue to improve at a steady rate for 3 to 6 months. It may be helpful to confirm that the patient is receiving an adequate amount of the drug by monitoring the plasma concentration. This information is available for a number of antipsychotics, including haloperidol, clozapine, fluphenazine, trifluoperazine (Stelazine), and perphenazine (Trilafon). A very low plasma concentration may indicate that the patient has been noncompliant or, more commonly, only partially compliant. It may also suggest that the patient is a rapid metabolizer of the antipsychotic or that the drug is not being adequately absorbed. Under these conditions, raising the dose may be helpful. If the level is relatively high, clinicians should consider whether side effects may be interfering with therapeutic response.

If the patient is responding poorly, one may increase the dose above the usual therapeutic level; however, higher doses are not usually associated with greater improvement than conventional doses. Changing to another drug is preferable to titrating to a high dose.

If a patient has responded poorly to a conventional DRA, it is unlikely that this individual will do well on another DRA. Changing to an SDA is more likely to be helpful.

Clozapine is effective for patients who respond poorly to DRAs. Double-blind studies comparing clozapine with other antipsychotics indicated that clozapine had the clearest advantage over conventional drugs in patients with the most severe psychotic symptoms, as well as in those who had previously responded poorly to other antipsychotics. When clozapine was compared with chlorpromazine in a severely psychotic group of individuals who had failed in trials with at least three antipsychotics, clozapine was significantly more effective in nearly every dimension of psychopathology, including both positive symptoms and negative symptoms.

MANAGING SIDE EFFECTS

Patients frequently experience side effects of an antipsychotic before they experience clinical improvement. Whereas a clinical response may be delayed for days or weeks after drugs are started, side effects may begin almost immediately. For low-potency drugs, these side effects are likely to include sedation, postural hypotension, and anticholinergic effects, whereas high-potency drugs are likely to cause extrapyramidal side effects.

Extrapyramidal Side Effects

Clinicians have a number of alternatives for treating extrapyramidal side effects. These include reducing the dose of the antipsychotic (which is most commonly a DRA), adding an anti-Parkinson medication, and changing the patient to an SDA that is less likely to cause extrapyramidal side effects. The most effective anti-Parkinson medications are the anticholinergic anti-Parkinson drugs. However, these medications have their own side effects, including dry mouth; constipation; blurred vision; and, often, memory loss. Also, these medications are often only partially effective, leaving patients with substantial amounts of lingering extrapyramidal side effects. Centrally acting β-blockers, such as propranolol, are also often effective for treating akathisia. Most patients respond to dosages between 30 and 90 mg per day.

If conventional antipsychotics are being prescribed, clinicians may consider prescribing prophylactic anti-Parkinson medications for patients who are likely to experience disturbing extrapyramidal side effects. These include patients who have a history of extrapyramidal side effect sensitivity and those who are being treated with relatively high doses of high-potency drugs. Prophylactic anti-Parkinson medications may also be indicated when high-potency drugs are prescribed for young men who tend to have an increased vulnerability for developing dystonias. Again, these patients should be candidates for newer drugs.

Some individuals are highly sensitive to extrapyramidal side effects at the dose that is necessary to control their psychosis. For many of these patients, medication side effects may seem worse than the illness itself. These patients should be treated routinely with an SDA because these agents result in substantially fewer extrapyramidal side effects than the DRAs. However, these highly sensitive individuals may even experience extrapyramidal side effects on an SDA. Risperidone may cause extrapyramidal side effects even at low doses—for example, 0.5 mg—but the severity and risk are increased at higher doses—for example, more than 6 mg. Olanzapine and ziprasidone are also associated with dose-related parkinsonism and akathisia.

Tardive Dyskinesia

About 20 to 30 percent of patients on long-term treatment with a conventional DRA will exhibit symptoms of tardive dyskinesia. About 3 to 5 percent of young patients receiving a DRA develop tardive dyskinesia each year. The risk in elderly patients is much higher. Although seriously disabling dyskinesia is uncommon, it can affect walking, breathing, eating, and talking when it occurs. Individuals who are more sensitive to acute extrapyramidal side effects appear to be more vulnerable to developing tardive dyskinesia. Patients with comorbid cognitive or mood disorders may also be more vulnerable to tardive dyskinesia than those with only schizophrenia.

The onset of the abnormal movements usually occurs either while the patient is receiving an antipsychotic or within 4 weeks of discontinuing an oral antipsychotic or 8 weeks after the withdrawal of a depot antipsychotic. There is a slightly lower risk of tardive dyskinesia with new-generation drugs. However, the risk of tardive dyskinesia is not absent with the SDAs.

Recommendations for preventing and managing tardive dyskinesia include (1) using the lowest effective dose of antipsychotic; (2) prescribing cautiously with children, elderly patients, and patients with mood disorders; (3) examining patients on a regular basis for evidence of tardive dyskinesia; (4) considering alternatives to the antipsychotic being used and considering dosage reduction when tardive dyskinesia is diagnosed; and (5) considering a number of options if the tardive dyskinesia worsens, including discontinuing the antipsychotic or switching to a different drug. Clozapine has been shown to be effective in reducing severe tardive dyskinesia or tardive dystonia.

Other Side Effects

Sedation and postural hypotension can be important side effects for patients who are being treated with low-potency DRAs, such as perphenazine. These effects are often most severe during the initial dosing with these medications. As a result, patients treated with these medications—particularly clozapine—may require weeks to reach a therapeutic dose. Although most patients develop tolerance to sedation and postural hypotension, sedation may continue to be a problem. In these patients, daytime drowsiness may interfere with a patient's attempts to return to community life.

All DRAs, as well as SDAs, elevate prolactin levels, which can result in galactorrhea and irregular menses. Long-term elevations in prolactin and the resultant suppression in gonadotropin-releasing hormone can cause suppression in gonadal hormones. These, in turn, may have effects on libido and sexual functioning. There is also concern that elevated prolactin may cause decreases in bone density and lead to osteoporosis. The concerns about hyperprolactinemia, sexual functioning, and bone density are based on experiences with prolactin elevations related to tumors and other causes. It is unclear if these risks are also associated with the lower elevations that occur with prolactin-elevating drugs.

Health Monitoring in Patients Receiving Antipsychotics

Because of the effects of the SDAs on insulin metabolism, psychiatrists should monitor a number of health indicators, including BMI, fasting blood glucose, and lipid profiles. Patients should be weighed and their BMIs calculated for every visit for 6 months after a medication change.

Side Effects of Clozapine

Clozapine has a number of side effects that make it a difficult drug to administer. The most serious is a risk of agranulocytosis. This potentially fatal condition occurs in approximately 0.3 percent of patients treated with clozapine during the first year of exposure. Subsequently, the risk is substantially lower. As a result, patients who receive clozapine in the United States are required to be in a program of weekly blood monitoring for the first 6 months and biweekly monitoring for the next 6 months. After 1 year of treatment without hematological problems, monitoring can be performed monthly.

Clozapine is also associated with a higher risk of seizures than other antipsychotics. The risk reaches nearly 5 percent at doses of more than 600 mg. Patients who develop seizures with clozapine can usually be managed by reducing the dose and adding an anticonvulsant, usually valproate (Depakene). Myocarditis has been reported to occur in approximately 5 patients per 100,000 patient-years. Other side effects with clozapine include hypersalivation, sedation, tachycardia, weight gain, diabetes, fever, and postural hypotension.

OTHER BIOLOGICAL THERAPIES

Electroconvulsive therapy (ECT) has been studied in both acute and chronic schizophrenia. Studies in recent-onset patients indicate that ECT is about as effective as antipsychotic medications and more effective than psychotherapy. Other studies suggest that supplementing antipsychotic medications with ECT is more effective than antipsychotic medications alone. Antipsychotic medications should be administered during and after ECT treatment. Although psychosurgery is no longer considered an appropriate treatment, it is practiced on a limited experimental basis for severe, intractable cases.

PSYCHOSOCIAL THERAPIES

Psychosocial therapies include a variety of methods to increase social abilities, self-sufficiency, practical skills, and interpersonal communication in schizophrenia patients. The goal is to enable persons who are severely ill to develop social and vocational skills for independent living. Such treatment is carried out at many sites, including hospitals, outpatient clinics, mental health centers, day hospitals, and home or social clubs.

Social Skills Training

Social skills training is sometimes referred to as behavioral skills therapy. Along with pharmacological therapy, this therapy can be directly supportive and useful to the patient. In addition to the psychotic symptoms seen in patients with schizophrenia, other noticeable symptoms involve the way the person relates to others, including poor eye contact, unusual delays in response, odd facial expressions, lack of spontaneity in social situations, and inaccurate perception or lack of perception of emotions in other people. Behavioral skills training addresses these behaviors through the use of videotapes of others and of the patient, role playing in therapy, and homework assignments for the specific skills being practiced. Social skills training has been shown to reduce relapse rates as measured by the need for hospitalization.

Family-Oriented Therapies

Because patients with schizophrenia are often discharged in an only partially remitted state, a family to which a patient returns can often benefit from a brief but intensive (as often as daily) course of family therapy. The therapy should focus on the immediate situation and should include identifying and avoiding potentially troublesome situations. When problems do emerge with the patient in the family, the aim of the therapy should be to resolve the problem quickly.

In wanting to help, family members often encourage a relative with schizophrenia to resume regular activities too quickly, both from ignorance about the disorder and from denial of its severity. Without being overly discouraging, therapists must help both the family and the patient understand and learn about schizophrenia and must encourage discussion of the psychotic episode and the events leading up to it. Ignoring the psychotic episode, a common occurrence, often increases the shame associated with the event and does not exploit the freshness of the episode to understand it better. Psychotic symptoms often frighten family members, and talking openly with the psychiatrist and with the relative with schizophrenia often eases all parties. Therapists can direct later family therapy toward long-range application of stress-reducing and coping strategies and toward the patient's gradual reintegration into everyday life.

Therapists must control the emotional intensity of family sessions with patients with schizophrenia. The excessive expression of emotion during a session can damage a patient's recovery process and undermine potentially successful future family therapy. Several studies have shown that family therapy is especially effective in reducing relapses.

National Alliance on Mental Illness. The National Alliance on Mental Illness (NAMI) and similar organizations offer support groups for family members and friends of patients who are mentally ill and for patients themselves. These organizations offer emotional and practical advice about obtaining care in the sometimes complex health care delivery system and are useful sources to which to refer family members. NAMI has also waged a campaign to destigmatize mental illness and to increase government awareness of the needs and rights of persons who are mentally ill and their families.

Case Management

Because a variety of professionals with specialized skills, such as psychiatrists, social workers, and occupational therapists, among others, are involved in a treatment program, it is helpful to have one person aware of all the forces acting on the patient. The case manager ensures that their efforts are coordinated and that the patient keeps appointments and complies with treatment plans; the case manager may make home visits and even accompany the patient to work. The success of the program depends on the educational background, training, and competence of the individual case manager, which vary. Case managers often have too many cases to manage effectively. The ultimate benefits of the program have yet to be demonstrated.

Assertive Community Treatment

The Assertive Community Treatment (ACT) program was originally developed by researchers in Madison, Wisconsin, in the 1970s, for the delivery of services for persons with chronic mental illness. Patients are assigned to one multidisciplinary team (e.g., case manager, psychiatrist, nurse, general physicians). The team has a fixed caseload of patients and delivers all services when and where needed by the patient, 24 hours a day, 7 days a week. This is mobile and intensive intervention that provides treatment, rehabilitation, and support activities. These include home delivery of medications, monitoring of mental and physical health, in vivo social skills, and frequent contact with family members. There is a high staff-to-patient ratio (1:12). ACT programs can effectively decrease the risk of rehospitalization for persons with schizophrenia, but they are labor-intensive and expensive programs to administer.

Group Therapy

Group therapy for persons with schizophrenia generally focuses on real-life plans, problems, and relationships. Groups may be behaviorally oriented, psychodynamically or insight oriented, or supportive. Some investigators doubt that dynamic interpretation and insight therapy are valuable for typical patients with schizophrenia. But group therapy is effective in reducing social isolation, increasing the sense of cohesiveness, and improving reality testing for patients with schizophrenia. Groups led in a supportive manner appear to be most helpful for schizophrenia patients.

Cognitive Behavioral Therapy

Cognitive behavioral therapy has been used in schizophrenia patients to improve cognitive distortions, reduce distractibility, and correct errors in judgment. There are reports of ameliorating delusions and hallucinations in some patients using this method. Patients who might benefit generally have some insight into their illness.

Individual Psychotherapy

Studies of the effects of individual psychotherapy in the treatment of schizophrenia have provided data that the therapy is helpful and that the effects are additive to those of pharmacological treatment. In psychotherapy with a schizophrenia patient, developing a therapeutic relationship that the patient experiences as safe is critical. The therapist's reliability, the emotional distance between the therapist and the patient, and the genuineness of the therapist as interpreted by the patient all affect the therapeutic experience. Psychotherapy for a schizophrenia patient should be thought of in terms of decades, rather than sessions, months, or even years.

Some clinicians and researchers have emphasized that the ability of a patient with schizophrenia to form a therapeutic alliance with a therapist is predictive of the outcome. Schizophrenia patients who are able to form a good therapeutic alliance are likely to remain in psychotherapy, to remain compliant with their medications, and to have good outcomes at 2-year follow-up evaluations.

The relationship between clinicians and patients differs from that encountered in the treatment of nonpsychotic patients. Establishing a relationship is often difficult. Persons with schizophrenia are desperately lonely, yet defend against closeness and trust; they are likely to become suspicious, anxious, or hostile or to regress when someone attempts to draw close. Therapists should scrupulously respect a patient's distance and privacy and should demonstrate simple directness, patience, sincerity, and sensitivity to social conventions in preference to premature informality and the condescending use of first names. The patient is likely to perceive exaggerated warmth or professions of friendship as attempts at bribery, manipulation, or exploitation.

In the context of a professional relationship, however, flexibility is essential in establishing a working alliance with the patient. A therapist may have meals with the patient, sit on the floor, go for a walk, eat at a restaurant, accept and give gifts, play table tennis, remember the patient's birthday, or just sit silently with the patient. The major aim is to convey the idea that the therapist is trustworthy, wants to understand the patient and tries to do so, and has faith in the patient's potential as a human, no matter how disturbed, hostile, or bizarre the patient may be at the moment.

Personal Therapy

A flexible type of psychotherapy called personal therapy is a recently developed form of individual treatment for schizophrenia patients. Its objective is to enhance personal and social adjustment and to forestall relapse. It is a selected method using social skills and relaxation exercises, psychoeducation, self-reflection, self-awareness, and exploration of individual vulnerability to stress. The therapist provides a setting that stresses acceptance and empathy. Patients receiving personal therapy show improvement in social adjustment (a composite measure that includes work performance, leisure, and interpersonal relationships) and have a lower relapse rate after 3 years than patients not receiving personal therapy.

Dialectical Behavior Therapy

This form of therapy, which combines cognitive and behavioral theories in both individual and group settings, has proved useful in borderline states and may have benefit in schizophrenia. Emphasis is placed on improving interpersonal skills in the presence of an active and empathic therapist.

Vocational Therapy

A variety of methods and settings are used to help patients regain old skills or develop new ones. These include sheltered workshops, job clubs, and part-time or transitional employment programs. Enabling patients to become gainfully employed is both a means toward, and a sign of, recovery. Many schizophrenia patients are capable of performing high-quality work despite their illness. Others may exhibit exceptional skill or even brilliance in a limited field as a result of some idiosyncratic aspect of their disorder.

Art Therapy

Many schizophrenia patients benefit from art therapy, which provides them with an outlet for their constant bombardment of imagery. It helps them communicate with others and share their inner, often frightening world with others.

Cognitive Training

Cognitive training or cognitive remediation is a technique introduced recently for the treatment of schizophrenia. Utilizing computer-generated exercises, neural networks are influenced in such a way that cognition, including working memory, is improved which translates into more effective social functioning. The field is in its infancy and further work and replication of studies is needed; however, it is a technique that is easily learned and administered and holds great promise.

▲ 4.2 Schizoaffective Disorder

Schizoaffective disorder has features of both schizophrenia and mood disorders. In current diagnostic systems, patients can receive the diagnosis of schizoaffective disorder if they fit into one of the following six categories: (1) patients with schizophrenia who have mood symptoms, (2) patients with mood disorder who have symptoms of schizophrenia, (3) patients with both mood disorder and schizophrenia, (4) patients with a third psychosis unrelated to schizophrenia and mood disorder, (5) patients whose disorder is on a continuum between schizophrenia and mood disorder, and (6) patients with some combination of the above.

George H. Kirby, in 1913, and August Hoch, in 1921, both described patients with mixed features of schizophrenia and affective (mood) disorders. Because their patients did not have the deteriorating course of dementia precox, Kirby and Hoch classified them in Emil Kraepelin's manic-depressive psychosis group.

In 1933, Jacob Kasanin introduced the term *schizoaffective disorder* to refer to a disorder with symptoms of both schizophrenia and mood disorders. In patients with the disorder, the onset of symptoms was sudden and often occurred in adolescence. Patients tended to have a good premorbid level of functioning, and often a specific stressor preceded the onset of symptoms. The family histories of the patients often included a mood disorder. Because Eugen Bleuler's broad concept of schizophrenia had eclipsed Kraepelin's narrow concept, Kasanin believed that the patients had a type of schizophrenia. From 1933 to about 1970, patients whose symptoms were similar to those of Kasanin's patients were variously classified as having schizoaffective disorder, atypical schizophrenia, good-prognosis schizophrenia, remitting schizophrenia, and cycloid psychosis—terms that emphasized a relation to schizophrenia.

Around 1970, two sets of data shifted the view of schizoaffective disorder from a schizophrenic illness to a mood disorder. First, lithium carbonate (Eskalith) was shown to be an effective and specific treatment for both bipolar disorders and some cases of schizoaffective disorder. Second, the United States–United Kingdom study published in 1968 by John Cooper and his colleagues showed that the variation in the number of patients classified as schizophrenic in the United States and in the United Kingdom resulted from an overemphasis in the United States on the presence of psychotic symptoms as a diagnostic criterion for schizophrenia.

EPIDEMIOLOGY

The lifetime prevalence of schizoaffective disorder is less than 1 percent, possibly in the range of 0.5 to 0.8 percent. These figures, however, are estimates; various studies of schizoaffective disorder have used varying diagnostic criteria. In clinical practice, a preliminary diagnosis of schizoaffective disorder is frequently used when a clinician is uncertain of the diagnosis.

Gender and Age Differences

Sex differences in the rates of schizoaffective disorder in clinical samples generally parallel sex differences seen in mood disorders, with approximately equal numbers of men and women who have the bipolar subtype and are more than twofold female to male predominance among individuals with the depressed subtype of schizoaffective disorder. The depressive type of schizoaffective disorder may be more common in older persons than in younger persons, and the bipolar type may be more common in young adults than in older adults. The age of onset for women is later than that for men, as in schizophrenia. Men with schizoaffective disorder are likely to exhibit antisocial behavior and to have a markedly flat or inappropriate affect.

ETIOLOGY

The cause of schizoaffective disorder is unknown. The disorder may be a type of schizophrenia, a type of mood disorder, or the simultaneous expression of each. Schizoaffective disorder may also be a distinct third type of psychosis, one that is unrelated to either schizophrenia or a mood disorder. The most likely possibility is that schizoaffective disorder is a heterogeneous group of disorders encompassing all of these possibilities.

Studies designed to explore the etiology have examined family histories, biological markers, short-term treatment responses, and long-term outcomes. Most studies have considered patients with schizoaffective disorder to be a homogeneous group, but recent studies have examined the bipolar and depressive types of schizoaffective disorder separately.

Although much of the family and genetic research in schizoaffective disorder is based on the premise that schizophrenia and the mood disorders are completely separate entities, some data indicate that they may be genetically related. Studies of the disrupted in schizophrenia 1 (*DISC1*) gene, located on chromosome 1q42, suggest its possible involvement in schizoaffective disorder as well as schizophrenia and bipolar disorder.

As a group, patients with schizoaffective disorder have a better prognosis than patients with schizophrenia and a worse prognosis than patients with mood disorders. Also, as a group, patients with schizoaffective disorder tend to have a nondeteriorating course and respond better to lithium than do patients with schizophrenia.

Consolidation of Data

A reasonable conclusion from the available data is that patients with schizoaffective disorder are a heterogeneous group: some have schizophrenia with prominent affective symptoms, others have a mood disorder with prominent schizophrenic symptoms, and still others have a distinct clinical syndrome. The hypothesis that patients with schizoaffective disorder have both schizophrenia and a mood disorder is untenable because the calculated co-occurrence of the two disorders is much lower than the incidence of schizoaffective disorder.

DIAGNOSIS AND CLINICAL FEATURES

According to the fifth edition of the *Diagnostic and Statistical Manual of Mental Disorders* (DSM-5) schizoaffective disorder combines features of both schizophrenia and affective or mood disorder. Thus, delusions or hallucinations will be present in addition to a disturbance of mood. If the mood is one of mania, it is called bipolar type of schizoaffective disorder; if the mood is one of depression, it is called depressive type. The clinician must accurately diagnose the affective illness, making sure it meets the criteria of either a manic or a depressive episode. In addition, the mood component should be present for the majority (>50 percent) of the total illness. As with most psychiatric diagnoses, schizoaffective disorder should not be used if the symptoms are caused by substance abuse or a secondary medical condition.

Mr. C was 24 years old with no previous psychiatric history. Pregnancy, birth, early development, and adjustment through army service as a paramedic were normal. After discharge from the army, he began to study law but then quit school and traveled in Asia, where he used cannabis. Family members who saw him during this time noticed several changes: He insisted on changing his name, he began to isolate himself, and he believed that he was the heir of the Dali Lama. When he became aggressive and argumentative, he was brought home and hospitalized. On admission, he was dressed like a Tibetan monk, with his head shaved. Although oriented to time and place, he had delusions of grandeur, stating that he was the most clever man on the planet and was the ancestor of the Messiah. He was also suspicious, arrogant, and argumentative. On laboratory assessment, he was also found to have hepatitis A. He was treated with perphenazine 28 mg per day and ultimately discharged to outpatient treatment. He tried again to attend law school but could not persist for more than a year before quitting. When his psychiatrist agreed to stop his antipsychotic medications, he relapsed a month later. His second admission occurred following a manic episode during which he spent money lavishly, had angry outbursts, was excessively talkative, was hyperactive, and believed he was the Messiah. He was treated with haloperidol 5 mg per day and lithium (Eskalith) 1,200 mg. After discharge and another attempt at law school, he traveled to India. He was brought home, rehospitalized with another manic episode, and discharged on depot antipsychotic medications. After being rehospitalized because of extrapyramidal side effects, he was prescribed olanzapine 20 mg per day and valproic acid (Depakene) 1,000 mg per day. During that hospitalization, his mood seemed more depressed, but he did not meet the criteria for an episode of major depressive disorder. During the subsequent 5 years, he remained out of the hospital and had no episodes of mood disorder. He was careful to avoid using cannabis or other substances. He does not work but functions well as a husband and father. From time to time he has thoughts that he might be hurt by other people inflicting injury on his liver, but these thoughts never last more than a few days.

The first aspect of establishing a differential diagnosis was determining whether the psychosis was due to a general medical condition or a substance-use disorder. These possibilities seemed unlikely because hepatitis would rarely be associated with the development of an acute manic syndrome. Although cannabis use can precipitate psychosis, the patient's psychotic symptoms and mood disturbance also occurred in the absence of substance use. In addition, the patient's longitudinal course was not consistent with either a substance-induced disorder or a psychosis due to a general medical condition. Mr. C's mood episodes were distinct, but he also had clear psychotic symptoms in the absence of a mood episode, making schizoaffective disorder a more appropriate diagnosis than bipolar disorder with psychotic features. His course also showed a lack of return to his premorbid level of function despite reasonable control of his symptoms with an antipsychotic and a mood stabilizing anticonvulsant. The duration of his mood symptoms relative to the total illness duration was significant and consistent with a diagnosis of schizoaffective disorder.

Mrs. P is a 47-year-old, divorced, unemployed woman who lived alone and who experienced chronic psychotic symptoms despite treatment with olanzapine 20 mg per day and citalopram (Celexa) 20 mg per day. She believed that she was getting messages from God and the police department to go on a mission to fight against drugs. She also believed that an organized crime group was trying to stop her in this pursuit. The onset of her illness began at age 20 years when she experienced the first of several depressive episodes. She also described periods when she felt more energetic and talkative; had a decreased need for sleep; and was more active, sometimes cleaning her house throughout the night. About 4 years after the onset of her symptoms, she began to hear "voices" that became stronger when she was depressed but were still present and disturbed her even when her mood was euthymic. About 10 years after her illness began, she developed the belief that policemen were everywhere and that the neighbors were spying on her. She was hospitalized voluntarily. Two years later, she had another depressive episode, and the auditory hallucinations told her she could not live in her apartment. She was tried on lithium, antidepressants, and antipsychotic medications but continued to be chronically symptomatic with mood symptoms as well as psychosis.

Mrs. P demonstrates a "classic" presentation of schizoaffective disorder in which clear depressive and hypomanic episodes are present in combination with continuous psychotic illness and first-rank symptoms. Her course is typical of many individuals with schizoaffective disorder.

DIFFERENTIAL DIAGNOSIS

The psychiatric differential diagnosis includes all the possibilities usually considered for mood disorders and for schizophrenia. In any differential diagnosis of psychotic disorders, a complete medical workup should be performed to rule out organic causes for the symptoms. A history of substance use (with or without positive results on a toxicology screening test) may indicate a substance-induced disorder. Pre-existing medical conditions, their treatment, or both can cause psychotic and mood disorders. Any suspicion of a neurological abnormality warrants consideration of a brain scan to rule out anatomical pathology and an electroencephalogram to determine any possible seizure disorders (e.g., temporal lobe epilepsy). Psychotic disorder caused by seizure disorder is more common than that seen in the general population. It tends to be characterized by paranoia, hallucinations, and ideas of reference. Patients with epilepsy with psychosis are believed to have a better level of function than patients with schizophrenic spectrum disorders. Better control of the seizures can reduce the psychosis.

COURSE AND PROGNOSIS

Considering the uncertainty and evolving diagnosis of schizoaffective disorder, it is difficult to determine the long-term course and prognosis. Given the definition of the diagnosis, patients with schizoaffective disorder might be expected to have a course similar to an episodic mood disorder, a chronic schizophrenic course, or some intermediate outcome. It has been presumed that an increasing presence of schizophrenic symptoms predicted a worse prognosis. After 1 year, patients with schizoaffective disorder had different outcomes, depending on whether their predominant symptoms were affective (better prognosis) or schizophrenic (worse prognosis). One study that followed patients diagnosed with schizoaffective disorder for 8 years found that the outcomes of these patients more closely resembled schizophrenia than a mood disorder with psychotic features.

TREATMENT

Mood stabilizers are a mainstay of treatment for bipolar disorders and would be expected to be important in the treatment of patients with schizoaffective disorder. One study that compared lithium with carbamazepine (Tegretol) found that carbamazepine was superior for schizoaffective disorder, depressive type, but found no difference in the two agents for the bipolar type. In practice, however, these medications are used extensively alone, in combination with each other, or with an antipsychotic agent. In manic episodes, patients who are schizoaffective should be treated aggressively with dosages of a mood stabilizer in the middle to high therapeutic blood concentration range. As the patient enters maintenance phase, the dosage can be reduced to a low to middle range to avoid adverse effects and potential effects on organ systems (e.g., thyroid and kidney) and to improve ease of use and compliance. Laboratory monitoring of plasma drug concentrations and periodic screening of thyroid, kidney, and hematological functioning should be performed.

By definition, many patients who are schizoaffective have major depressive episodes. Treatment with antidepressants mirrors treatment of bipolar depression. Care should be taken not to precipitate a cycle of rapid switches from depression to mania with the antidepressant. The choice of antidepressant should take into account previous antidepressant successes or failures. Selective serotonin reuptake inhibitors (e.g., fluoxetine [Prozac] and sertraline [Zoloft]) are often used as first-line agents because they have less effect on cardiac status and have a favorable overdose profile. Agitated or insomniac patients, however, may benefit from a tricyclic drug. As in all cases of intractable mania, the use of ECT should be considered. As mentioned, antipsychotic agents are important in the treatment of the psychotic symptoms of schizoaffective disorder.

Psychosocial Treatment

Patients benefit from a combination of family therapy, social skills training, and cognitive rehabilitation. Because the psychiatric field has had difficulty deciding on the exact diagnosis and prognosis of schizoaffective disorder, this uncertainty must be explained to the patient. The range of symptoms can be vast because patients contend with both ongoing psychosis and varying mood states. It can be very difficult for family members to keep up with the changing nature and needs of these patients. Medication regimens can be complicated, with multiple medications from all classes of drugs.

▲ 4.3 Schizophreniform Disorder

The concept of schizophreniform disorder was introduced in 1939 by Gabriel Langfeldt (1895–1983) to describe a condition with a sudden onset and benign course associated with mood symptoms and clouding of consciousness. The symptoms of schizophreniform are similar to those of schizophrenia; however, with schizophreniform disorder, the symptoms last for at least 1 month but less than 6 months. In contrast, for a patient to meet the diagnostic criteria for schizophrenia, the symptoms must have been present for at least 6 months. Patients with schizophreniform disorder return to their baseline level of functioning after the disorder has resolved.

EPIDEMIOLOGY

Little is known about the incidence, prevalence, and sex ratio of schizophreniform disorder. The disorder is most common in adolescents and young adults and is less than half as common as schizophrenia. A fivefold greater rate of schizophreniform disorder has been found in men than in women. A 1-year prevalence rate of 0.09 percent and a lifetime prevalence rate of 0.11 percent have been reported.

Several studies have shown that the relatives of patients with schizophreniform disorder are at high risk of having other psychiatric disorders, but the distribution of the disorders differs from the distribution seen in the relatives of patients with schizophrenia and bipolar disorders. Specifically, the relatives of patients with schizophreniform disorders are more likely to have mood disorders than are the relatives of patients with schizophrenia. In addition, the relatives of patients with schizophreniform disorder are more likely to have a diagnosis of a psychotic mood disorder than are the relatives of patients with bipolar disorders.

ETIOLOGY

The cause of schizophreniform disorder is not known. As Langfeldt noted in 1939, patients with this diagnostic label are likely to be heterogeneous. In general, whereas some patients have a disorder similar to schizophrenia, others have a disorder similar to a mood disorder. Because of the generally good outcome, the disorder probably has similarities to the episodic nature of mood disorders. Some data, however, indicate a close relation to schizophrenia.

In support of the relation to mood disorders, several studies have shown that patients with schizophreniform disorder, as a group, have more affective symptoms (especially mania) and a better outcome than patients with schizophrenia. Also, the increased occurrence of mood disorders in the relatives of patients with schizophreniform disorder indicates a relation to mood disorders. Thus, the biological and epidemiological data are most consistent with the hypothesis that the current diagnostic category defines a group of patients, some of whom have a disorder similar to schizophrenia; others have a disorder resembling a mood disorder.

Brain Imaging

A relative activation deficit in the inferior prefrontal region of the brain while the patient is performing a region-specific psychological task (the Wisconsin Card Sorting Test), as reported for patients with schizophrenia, has been reported in patients with schizophreniform disorder. One study showed the deficit to be limited to the left hemisphere and found impaired striatal activity suppression limited to the left hemisphere during the activation procedure. The data can be interpreted to indicate a physiological similarity between the psychosis of schizophrenia and the psychosis of schizophreniform disorder. Additional central nervous system factors, as yet unidentified, may lead to either the long-term course of schizophrenia or the foreshortened course of schizophreniform disorder.

Although some data indicate that patients with schizophreniform disorder may have enlarged cerebral ventricles, as determined by computed tomography and magnetic resonance imaging, other data indicate that, unlike the enlargement seen in schizophrenia, the ventricular enlargement in schizophreniform disorder is not correlated with either outcome or other biological measures.

Other Biological Measures

Although brain imaging studies point to a similarity between schizophreniform disorder and schizophrenia, at least one study of electrodermal activity indicated a difference. Patients with schizophrenia who were born during the winter and spring months (a period of high risk for the birth of these patients) had hyporesponsive skin conductances, but this association was absent in patients with schizophreniform disorder. The significance and the meaning of this single study are difficult to interpret, but the results do suggest caution in assuming similarity between patients with schizophrenia and those with schizophreniform disorder. Data from at least one study of eye tracking in the two groups also indicate that they may differ in some biological measures.

DIAGNOSTIC AND CLINICAL FEATURES

Schizophreniform disorder is an acute psychotic disorder that has a rapid onset and lacks a long prodromal phase. Although many patients with schizophreniform disorder may experience functional impairment at the time of an episode, they are unlikely to report a progressive decline in social and occupational functioning. The initial symptom profile is the same as that of schizophrenia in that two or more psychotic symptoms (hallucinations, delusions, disorganized speech and behavior, or negative symptoms) must be present. Schneiderian first-rank symptoms are frequently observed. Also an increased likelihood is found of emotional turmoil and confusion, the presence of which may indicate a good prognosis. Although negative symptoms may be present, they are relatively uncommon in schizophreniform disorder and are considered poor prognostic features. In a small series of first-admission patients with schizophreniform, one-fourth had moderate to severe negative symptoms. Almost all were initially categorized as having "schizophreniform disorder without good prognostic features," and 2 years later, 73 percent were rediagnosed with schizophrenia compared with 38 percent of those with "good prognostic features."

By definition, patients with schizophreniform disorder return to their baseline state within 6 months. In some instances, the illness is episodic, with more than one episode occurring after long periods of full remission. If the combined duration of symptomatology exceeds 6 months, however, then schizophrenia should be considered.

Mr. C, a 28-year-old accountant, was brought to the emergency department by the police in handcuffs. He was disheveled, and shouted and struggled with the police officers. It was apparent that he was hearing voices because he would respond to them with shouts such as, "Shut up! I told you I won't do it!" However, when confronted about the voices, he denied hearing anything. Mr. C had a hypervigilant stare and jumped at the slightest noise. He stated that he must run away quickly because he knew he would be killed shortly otherwise.

Mr. C was functioning well until 2 months before hospitalization. He was an accountant at a prestigious company and had close friends and a live-in girlfriend. Most people who knew him would describe him as friendly, but he was occasionally quarrelsome.

When his girlfriend suddenly broke off the relationship and moved out of their apartment, Mr. C was distressed. However, he was convinced that he could win her back, so he began to "accidentally" run into her at her job or her new apartment with flowers and various gifts. When she strongly told him that she wanted nothing more to do with him and requested that he leave her alone, Mr. C was convinced that she wanted him dead. He became so preoccupied with this notion that his work began to suffer. Out of fear for his life, Mr. C took off from work frequently, and when he did report to work, he was often tardy and did subpar work, making many errors. His supervisor confronted Mr. C about his behavior, threatening termination if it continued. Mr. C was embarrassed and resented his supervisor for the confrontation. He believed that his ex-girlfriend had hired the supervisor to kill him.

His beliefs were confirmed by a voice that would mock him. The voice told him time and again that he should quit his job, relocate to another city, and forget about his ex-girlfriend, but Mr. C refused, believing it would give them "more satisfaction than they deserved." He continued working, albeit cautiously, all the while fearing for his life.

Through it all, Mr. C believed himself to be the lone victim. He would awake abruptly at night from nightmares but would be able to fall right back to sleep. He had not lost any weight and had no other vegetative symptoms. His affect alternated between rage and terror. His mind was unusually alert and active, but he was not otherwise hyperactive, excessively energetic, or expansive. He did not display any formal thought disorder.

Mr. C was hospitalized and treated with antipsychotic medication. His symptoms remitted after several weeks of treatment, and he was well and able to return to work shortly after discharge.

DIFFERENTIAL DIAGNOSIS

It is important to first differentiate schizophreniform disorder from psychoses that can arise from medical conditions. This is accomplished by taking a detailed history and physical examination and, when indicated, performing laboratory tests or imaging studies. A detailed history of medication use, including over-the-counter medications and herbal products, is essential because many therapeutic agents can also produce an acute psychosis. Although it is not always possible to distinguish substance-induced psychosis from other psychotic disorders cross-sectionally, a rapid onset of psychotic symptoms in a patient with a significant substance history should raise the suspicion of a substance-induced psychosis. A detailed substance use history and toxicological screen are also important for treatment planning in an individual with a new onset of psychosis.

The duration of psychotic symptoms is one factor that distinguishes schizophreniform disorder from other syndromes. Schizophrenia is diagnosed if the duration of the prodromal, active, and residual phases lasts for more than 6 months; symptoms that occur for less than 1 month indicate a brief psychotic disorder. In general, a diagnosis of brief psychotic disorder does not require that a major stressor be present.

Distinguishing mood disorders with psychotic features from schizophreniform disorder is sometimes difficult. Furthermore, schizophreniform disorder and schizophrenia can be highly comorbid with mood and anxiety disorders. Additional confounds are that mood symptoms, such as loss of interest and pleasure, may be difficult to distinguish from negative symptoms, avolition, and anhedonia. Some mood symptoms may also be present during the early course of schizophrenia. A thorough longitudinal history is important in elucidating the diagnosis because the presence of psychotic symptoms exclusively during periods of mood disturbance is an indication of a primary mood disorder.

COURSE AND PROGNOSIS

The course of schizophreniform disorder, for the most part, is defined in the criteria. It is a psychotic illness lasting more than 1 month and less than 6 months. The real issue is what happens to persons with this illness over time. Most estimates of progression to schizophrenia range between 60 and 80 percent. What happens to the other 20 to 40 percent is currently not known. Some will have a second or third episode during which they will deteriorate into a more chronic condition of schizophrenia. A few, however, may have only this single episode and then continue on with their lives, which is clearly the outcome desired by all clinicians and family members, although it is probably a rare occurrence and should not be held out as likely.

TREATMENT

Hospitalization, which is often necessary in treating patients with schizophreniform disorder, allows effective assessment, treatment, and supervision of a patient's behavior. The psychotic symptoms can usually be treated by a 3- to 6-month course of antipsychotic drugs (e.g., risperidone). Several studies have shown that patients with schizophreniform disorder respond to antipsychotic treatment much more rapidly than patients with schizophrenia. In one study, about 75 percent of patients with schizophreniform disorder and only 20 percent of the patients with schizophrenia responded to antipsychotic medications within 8 days. A trial of lithium (Eskalith), carbamazepine (Tegretol), or valproate (Depakene) may be warranted for treatment and prophylaxis if a patient has a recurrent episode. Psychotherapy is usually necessary to help patients integrate the psychotic experience into their understanding of their own minds and lives. ECT may be indicated for some patients, especially those with marked catatonic or depressed features.

Finally, most patients with schizophreniform disorder progress to full-blown schizophrenia despite treatment. In those cases, a course of management consistent with a chronic illness must be formulated.

▲ 4.4 Delusional Disorder and Shared Psychotic Disorder

Delusions are false fixed beliefs not in keeping with the culture. They are among the most interesting of psychiatric symptoms because of the great variety of false beliefs that can be held by so many people and because they are so difficult to treat. The diagnosis of delusional disorder is made when a person exhibits delusions of at least 1 month's duration that cannot be attributed to other psychiatric disorders. The delusions must be about situations that can occur in real life, such as being followed, infected, loved at a distance, and so on; that is, they usually have to do with phenomena that, although not real, are nonetheless possible. These types of delusions have been called nonbizarre for that reason opposed to delusions with bizarre content, for example, being impregnated by aliens. Bizarre delusions are usually found in schizophrenia. Several types of delusions may be present (see below) and the predominant type is specified when the diagnosis is made.

EPIDEMIOLOGY

An accurate assessment of the epidemiology of delusional disorder is hampered by the relative rareness of the disorder, as well as by its changing definitions in recent history. Moreover, delusional disorder may be underreported because delusional patients rarely seek psychiatric help unless forced to do so by their families or by the courts. Even with these limitations, however, the literature does support the contention that delusional disorder, although uncommon, has a relatively steady rate.

The prevalence of delusional disorder in the United States is currently estimated to be 0.2 to 0.3 percent. Thus, delusional disorder is much rarer than schizophrenia, which has a prevalence of about 1 percent, and the mood disorders, which have a prevalence of about 5 percent. The annual incidence of delusional disorder is 1 to 3 new cases per 100,000 persons. The mean age of onset is about 40 years, but the range for age of onset runs from 18 years of age to the 90s. A slight preponderance of female patients exists. Men are more likely to develop paranoid delusions than women, who are more likely to develop delusions of erotomania. Many patients are married and employed, but some association is seen with recent immigration and low socioeconomic status.

ETIOLOGY

As with all major psychiatric disorders, the cause of delusional disorder is unknown. Moreover, patients currently classified as having delusional disorder probably have a heterogeneous group of conditions with delusions as the predominant symptom. The central concept about the cause of delusional disorder is its distinctness from schizophrenia and the mood disorders. Delusional disorder is much rarer than either schizophrenia or mood disorders, with a later onset than schizophrenia and a much less pronounced female predominance than the mood disorders. The most convincing data come from family studies that report an increased prevalence of delusional disorder and related personality traits (e.g., suspiciousness, jealousy, and secretiveness) in the relatives of delusional disorder probands. Family studies have reported neither an increased incidence of schizophrenia and mood disorders in the families of delusional disorder probands nor an increased incidence of delusional disorder in the families of probands with schizophrenia. Long-term follow-up of patients with delusional disorder indicates that the diagnosis of delusional disorder is relatively stable, with fewer than one-fourth of the patients eventually being reclassified as having schizophrenia and fewer than 10 percent of patients eventually being reclassified as having a mood disorder. These data indicate that delusional disorder is not simply an early stage in the development of one or both of these two more common disorders.

Biological Factors

A wide range of nonpsychiatric medical conditions and substances, including clear-cut biological factors, can cause delusions, but not everyone with a brain tumor, for example, has delusions. Unique, and not yet understood, factors in a patient's brain and personality are likely to be relevant to the specific pathophysiology of delusional disorder.

The neurological conditions most commonly associated with delusions affect the limbic system and the basal ganglia. Patients whose delusions are caused by neurological diseases and who show no intellectual impairment tend to have complex delusions similar to those in patients with delusional disorder. Conversely, patients with neurological disorder with intellectual impairments often have simple delusions unlike those in patients with delusional disorder. Thus, delusional disorder may involve the limbic system or basal ganglia in patients who have intact cerebral cortical functioning.

Delusional disorder can arise as a normal response to abnormal experiences in the environment, the peripheral nervous system, or the central nervous system (CNS). Thus, if patients have erroneous sensory experiences of being followed (e.g., hearing footsteps), they may come to believe that they are actually being followed. This hypothesis hinges on the presence of hallucinatory-like experiences that need to be explained. The presence of such hallucinatory experiences in delusional disorder has not been proved.

Psychodynamic Factors

Practitioners have a strong clinical impression that many patients with delusional disorder are socially isolated and have attained less than expected levels of achievement. Specific psychodynamic theories about the cause and the evolution of delusional symptoms involve suppositions regarding hypersensitive persons and specific ego mechanisms, which are reaction formation, projection, and denial.

Freud's Contributions. Sigmund Freud believed that delusions, rather than being symptoms of the disorder, are part of a healing process. In 1896, he described projection as the main defense mechanism in paranoia. Later, Freud read *Memories of My Nervous Illness,* an autobiographical account by Daniel Paul Schreber. Although he never met Schreber, Freud theorized from his review of the autobiography that unconscious homosexual tendencies are defended against by denial and projection. According to classic psychodynamic theory, the dynamics underlying the formation of delusions for a female patient are the same as for a male patient. Careful studies of patients with delusions have been unable to corroborate Freud's theories, although they may be relevant in individual cases. Overall, no higher incidence of homosexual ideation or activity is found in patients with delusions than in other groups. Freud's major contribution, however, was to demonstrate the role of projection in the formation of delusional thought.

Paranoid Pseudocommunity. Norman Cameron described seven situations that favor the development of delusional disorders: an increased expectation of receiving sadistic treatment, situations that increase distrust and suspicion, social isolation, situations that increase envy and jealousy, situations that lower self-esteem, situations that cause persons to see their own defects in others, and situations that increase the potential for rumination over probable meanings and motivations. When frustration from any combination of these conditions exceeds the tolerable limit, persons become withdrawn and anxious; they realize that something is wrong, seek an explanation for the problem, and crystallize a delusional system as a solution. Elaboration of the delusion to include imagined persons and attribution of malevolent motivations to both real and imagined persons results in the organization of the *pseudocommunity*—a perceived community of plotters. This delusional entity hypothetically binds together projected fears and wishes to justify the patient's aggression and to provide a tangible target for the patient's hostilities.

Other Psychodynamic Factors. Clinical observations indicate that many, if not all, paranoid patients experience a lack of trust in relationships. A hypothesis relates this distrust to a consistently hostile family environment, often with an overcontrolling mother and a distant or sadistic father. Erik Erikson's concept of trust versus mistrust in early development is a useful model to explain the suspiciousness of a paranoid individual who never went through the healthy experience of having his or her needs satisfied by what Erikson termed the "outer-providers." Thus, they have a general distrust of their environment.

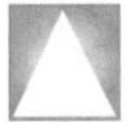

Table 4.4–1
Risk Factors Associated with Delusional Disorder

Advanced age
Sensory impairment or isolation
Family history
Social isolation
Personality features (e.g., unusual interpersonal sensitivity)
Recent immigration

Defense Mechanisms. Patients with delusional disorder use primarily the defense mechanisms of reaction formation, denial, and projection. They use reaction formation as a defense against aggression, dependence needs, and feelings of affection and transform the need for dependence into staunch independence. Patients use denial to avoid awareness of painful reality. Consumed with anger and hostility and unable to face responsibility for the rage, they project their resentment and anger onto others and use projection to protect themselves from recognizing unacceptable impulses in themselves.

Other Relevant Factors. Delusions have been linked to a variety of additional factors such as social and sensory isolation, socioeconomic deprivation, and personality disturbance. Deaf and visually impaired individuals and possibly immigrants with limited ability in a new language may be more vulnerable to delusion formation than the normal population. Vulnerability is heightened with advanced age. Delusional disturbance and other paranoid features are common in elderly adults. In short, multiple risk factors are associated with the formation of delusions, and the source and pathogenesis of delusional disorders per se have yet to be specified (Table 4.4–1).

DIAGNOSIS AND CLINICAL FEATURES

The fifth edition of the *Diagnostic and Statistical Manual of Mental Disorders* (DSM-5) criteria for delusional disorder require the presents of one or more delusions which are present for at least 1 month.

Mental Status

General Description. Patients are usually well groomed and well dressed, without evidence of gross disintegration of personality or of daily activities, yet they may seem eccentric, odd, suspicious, or hostile. They are sometimes litigious and may make this inclination clear to the examiner. The most remarkable feature of patients with delusional disorder is that the mental status examination shows them to be quite normal except for a markedly abnormal delusional system. Patients may attempt to engage clinicians as allies in their delusions, but a clinician should not pretend to accept the delusion; this collusion further confounds reality and sets the stage for eventual distrust between the patient and the therapist.

Mood, Feelings, and Affect. Patients' moods are consistent with the content of their delusions. A patient with grandiose delusions is euphoric; one with persecutory delusions is suspicious. Whatever the nature of the delusional system, the examiner may sense some mild depressive qualities.

Perceptual Disturbances. By definition, patients with delusional disorder do not have prominent or sustained hallucinations. A few delusional patients have other hallucinatory experiences—virtually always auditory rather than visual.

Thought. Disorder of thought content, in the form of delusions, is the key symptom of the disorder. The delusions are usually systematized and are characterized as being possible (e.g., delusions of being persecuted, having an unfaithful spouse, being infected with a virus, or being loved by a famous person). These examples of delusional content contrast with the bizarre and impossible delusional content in some patients with schizophrenia. The delusional system itself can be complex or simple. Patients lack other signs of thought disorder, although some may be verbose, circumstantial, or idiosyncratic in their speech when they talk about their delusions. Clinicians should not assume that all unlikely scenarios are delusional; the veracity of a patient's beliefs should be checked before deeming their content to be delusional.

Sensorium and Cognition

ORIENTATION. Patients with delusional disorder usually have no abnormality in orientation unless they have a specific delusion about a person, place, or time.

MEMORY. Memory and other cognitive processes are intact in patients with delusional disorder.

Impulse Control. Clinicians must evaluate patients with delusional disorder for ideation or plans to act on their delusional material by suicide, homicide, or other violence. Although the incidence of these behaviors is not known, therapists should not hesitate to ask patients about their suicidal, homicidal, or other violent plans. Destructive aggression is most common in patients with a history of violence; if aggressive feelings existed in the past, therapists should ask patients how they managed those feelings. If patients cannot control their impulses, hospitalization is probably necessary. Therapists can sometimes help foster a therapeutic alliance by openly discussing how hospitalization can help patients gain additional control of their impulses.

Judgment and Insight. Patients with delusional disorder have virtually no insight into their condition and are almost always brought to the hospital by the police, family members, or employers. Judgment can best be assessed by evaluating the patient's past, present, and planned behavior.

Reliability. Patients with delusional disorder are usually reliable in their information, except when it impinges on their delusional system.

TYPES

Persecutory Type

The delusion of persecution is a classic symptom of delusional disorder; persecutory-type and jealousy-type delusions are probably the forms seen most frequently by psychiatrists. Patients with this subtype are convinced that they are being persecuted or harmed. The persecutory beliefs are often associated with querulousness, irritability, and anger, and the individual who acts out his or her anger may at times be assaultive or even homicidal. At other times, such individuals may become preoccupied with formal litigation against their perceived persecutors. In contrast to persecutory delusions in schizophrenia, the clarity, logic, and systematic elaboration of the persecutory theme in delusional disorder leave a remarkable stamp on this condition. The absence of other psychopathology, of deterioration in personality, or of deterioration in most areas of functioning also contrasts with the typical manifestations of schizophrenia.

Mrs. S, 62 years old, was referred to a psychiatrist because of reports of being unable to sleep. She had previously worked full time taking care of children, and she played tennis almost every day and managed her household chores. However, she had now become preoccupied with the idea that her downstairs neighbor was doing a variety of things to harass her and wanted to get her to move away. At first, Mrs. S based her belief on certain looks that he gave her and damage done to her mailbox, but later she felt he might be leaving empty bottles of cleaning solutions in the basement so she would be overcome by fumes. As a result, the patient was fearful of falling asleep, convinced that she might be asphyxiated and unable to awaken in time to get help. She felt somewhat depressed and thought her appetite might be decreased from the stress of being harassed. However, she had not lost weight and still enjoyed playing tennis and going out with friends. At one point she considered moving to another apartment but then decided to fight back. The episode had gone on for 8 months when her daughter persuaded her to have a psychiatric assessment. In the interview, Mrs. S was pleasant and cooperative. Except for mild depressive symptoms and the specific delusion about being harassed by her neighbor, her mental status was normal.

Mrs. S had a past history of depression 30 years before, which followed the death of a close friend. She saw a counselor for several months and found this helpful, but she was not treated with medication. For the current episode, she agreed to take medications, although she believed her neighbor was more in need of treatment than she was. Her symptoms improved somewhat with risperidone (Risperdal) 2 mg at bedtime and clonazepam (Klonopin) 0.5 mg every morning and at bedtime.

This patient presented with a single delusion regarding her neighbor that was within the realm of possibility (i.e., not bizarre). Other areas of her functioning were normal. Although mild depressive symptoms were present, she did not meet criteria for major depressive disorder. Her prior symptoms of depression appeared to be related to a normal bereavement reaction and had not required pharmacotherapy or hospitalization. Thus, her current presentation is one of delusional disorder, persecutory type and not major depressive disorder with psychotic features. In terms of treatment, the ability to create a working alliance with the patient; avoiding the discussion of the veracity of her delusion; and focusing on her anxiety, depression, and difficulty falling asleep enabled her psychiatrist to introduce the medications with beneficial results. *(Courtesy of Laura J. Fochtmann, M.D., Ramin Mojtabai, M.D., Ph.D., M.P.H., and Evelyn J. Bromet, Ph.D.)*

Jealous Type

Delusional disorder with delusions of infidelity has been called *conjugal paranoia* when it is limited to the delusion that a spouse has been unfaithful. The eponym *Othello syndrome* has been used to describe morbid jealousy that can arise from multiple concerns. The delusion usually affects men, often those with no prior psychiatric illness. It may appear suddenly and serve to explain a host of present and past events involving the spouse's behavior. The condition is difficult to treat and may diminish only on separation, divorce, or death of the spouse.

Marked jealousy (usually termed *pathological* or *morbid jealousy*) is thus a symptom of many disorders—including schizophrenia (in which female patients more commonly display this feature), epilepsy, mood disorders, drug abuse, and alcoholism—for which treatment is directed at the primary disorder. Jealousy is a powerful emotion; when it occurs in delusional disorder or as part of another condition, it can be potentially dangerous and has been associated with violence, notably both suicide and homicide. The forensic aspects of the symptom have been noted repeatedly, especially its role as a motive for murder. Physical and verbal abuse occur more frequently, however, than do extreme actions among individuals with this symptom. Caution and care in deciding how to deal with such presentations are essential not only for diagnosis but also from the point of view of safety.

Mr. M was a 51-year-old married white man who lived with his wife in their own home and who worked full time driving a sanitation truck. Before his hospitalization, he became concerned that his wife was having an affair. He began to follow her, kept notes on his observations, and badgered her constantly about this, often waking her up in the middle of the night to make accusations. Shortly before admission, these arguments led to physical violence, and he was brought to the hospital by police. In addition to concerns about his wife's fidelity, Mr. M reported feelings of depression over his wife's "betrayal of [their] marriage vows," but he noted no changes in sleep, appetite, or work-related functioning. He was treated with a low dose of an antipsychotic medication and described being less concerned about his wife's behavior. After discharge, he remained on medications and was seen by a psychiatrist monthly, but 10 years later, he continued to believe that his wife was unfaithful. His wife noted that he sometimes became upset about the delusion but that he had not become aggressive or required readmission.

This patient experienced a fixed, encapsulated delusion of jealousy that did not interfere with his other activities and that showed a partial response to antipsychotic medications. Although he initially reported feeling somewhat depressed over his wife's perceived infidelity, he did not have other symptoms suggestive of a major depressive episode. *(Courtesy of Laura J. Fochtmann, M.D., Ramin Mojtabai, M.D., Ph.D., M.P.H., and Evelyn J. Bromet, Ph.D.)*

Erotomanic Type

In erotomania, which has also been referred to as *de Clérambault syndrome* or *psychose passionelle,* the patient has the delusional conviction that another person, usually of higher status, is in love with him or her. Such patients also tend to be solitary, withdrawn, dependent, and sexually inhibited as well as to have poor levels of social or occupational functioning. The following operational criteria for the diagnosis of erotomania have been suggested: (1) a delusional conviction of amorous communication, (2) object of much higher rank, (3) object being the first to fall in love, (4) object being the first to make advances, (5) sudden onset (within a 7-day period), (6) object remains unchanged, (7) patient rationalizes paradoxical behavior of the object, (8) chronic course, and (9) absence of hallucinations. Besides being the key symptom in some cases of delusional disorder, it is known to occur in schizophrenia, mood disorder, and other organic disorders.

Patients with erotomania frequently show certain characteristics: They are generally unattractive women in low-level jobs who lead withdrawn, lonely lives; they are single and have few sexual contacts. They select secret lovers who differ substantially from them. They exhibit what has been called *paradoxical conduct,* the delusional phenomenon of interpreting all denials of love, no matter how clear, as secret affirmations of love. The course may be chronic, recurrent, or brief. Separation from the love object may be the only satisfactory intervention. Although men are less commonly affected by this condition than women, they may be more aggressive and possibly violent in their pursuit of love. Hence, in forensic populations, men with this condition predominate. The object of aggression may not be the loved individual but companions or protectors of the love object who are viewed as trying to come between the lovers. The tendency toward violence among men with erotomania may lead initially to police, rather than psychiatric, contact. In certain cases, resentment and rage in response to an absence of reaction from all forms of love communication may sufficiently escalate to put the love object in danger. The so-called stalkers, who continually follow their perceived lovers, frequently have delusions. Although most stalkers are men, women also stalk, and both groups have a high potential for violence.

Mrs. D was a 32-year-old nurse who was married and had two children. She had worked in the hospital for 12 years and functioned well in her job. She had previously believed that one of the hospital's attending physicians was in love with her. Now she was referred by her supervisor for a psychiatric evaluation after she had assaulted one of the residents, claiming he was in love with her. Her current delusion began when the young physician entered a room where she was lying in bed after cosmetic surgery and pointed at her. She had not known him before, but at that moment she became convinced that he was in love with her. She tried to approach him several times by letter and phone, and although he did not respond, she was convinced that he was trying to transmit his love through looks he gave her and through the tone of his voice. She did not report any associated hallucinatory experiences. The resident met her and denied being in love with her, but she began stalking him, culminating in the assault and the request for consultation.

Mrs. D initially refused to take any medications. She was treated with psychotherapy for several months, during which she continued to work and was able to avoid contact with the resident. The therapist arranged a three-way meeting with himself, the patient, and the resident. After this meeting, there was a small reduction in the intensity of Mrs. D's belief, but she continued to maintain it nonetheless. She subsequently agreed to take antipsychotic medications and was given perphenazine 16 mg per day, but there was no improvement. The delusion subsided only after the resident moved to another hospital.

This patient's presentation demonstrates a number of the features of the erotomanic type of delusional disorder. In particular, her delusion began abruptly with what she perceived to be a specific response to her by the resident. Her delusional conviction that he was in love with her persisted even after being confronted, and she rationalized his lack of apparent interest in her. The presence of a previous episode and the poor response to antipsychotic medications are consistent with the often chronic nature of the disorder, albeit with a different person being the object of her delusions. The absence of hallucinations and the preservation of her ability to function suggest a diagnosis of delusional disorder rather than schizophrenia. *(Example provided by S. Fennig and originally published in Fennig S, Fochtmann LJ, Bromet EJ. Delusional disorder and shared psychotic disorder. In: Sadock BJ, Sadock VA, eds. Kaplan and Sadock's Comprehensive Textbook of Psychiatry. 8th edition. Philadelphia: Lippincott Williams & Wilkins; 2005:1525.)*

Somatic Type

Delusional disorder with somatic delusions has been called *monosymptomatic hypochondriacal psychosis.* The condition differs from other conditions with hypochondriacal symptoms in the degree of reality impairment. In delusional disorder, the delusion is fixed, unarguable, and presented intensely because the patient is totally convinced of the physical nature of the disorder. In contrast, persons with hypochondriasis often admit that their fear of illness is largely groundless. The content of the somatic delusion can vary widely from case to case. The three main types are (1) delusions of infestation (including parasitosis); (2) delusions of dysmorphophobia, such as of misshapenness, personal ugliness, or exaggerated size of body parts (this category seems closest to that of body dysmorphic disorder); and (3) delusions of foul body odors or halitosis. This third category, sometimes referred to as *olfactory reference syndrome,* appears somewhat different from the category of delusions of infestation in that patients with the former have an earlier age of onset (mean, 25 years), male predominance, single status, and absence of past psychiatric treatment. Otherwise, the three groups, although individually low in prevalence, appear to overlap.

The onset of symptoms with the somatic type of delusional disorder may be gradual or sudden. In most patients, the illness is unremitting, although the delusion severity may fluctuate. Hyperalertness and high anxiety also characterize patients with this subtype. Some themes recur, such as concerns about infestation in delusional parasitosis, preoccupation with body features with the dysmorphic delusions, and delusional concerns about body odor, which are sometimes referred to as *bromosis.* In delusional parasitosis, tactile sensory phenomena are often linked to the delusional beliefs.

Patients with the somatic type of delusional disorder rarely present for psychiatric evaluation, and when they do, it is usually in the context of a psychiatric consultation or liaison service. Instead, patients generally present to a specific medical specialist for evaluation. Thus, these individuals are more often encountered by dermatologists, plastic surgeons, urologists, acquired immune deficiency syndrome (AIDS) specialists, and sometimes dentists or gastroenterologists.

Mrs. G. was a 56-year-old homemaker and mother of two who was hospitalized in the burn unit for wound care and skin grafting after sustaining chemical burns to her trunk and extremities. Six months before admission, Mrs. G had become increasingly convinced that tiny bugs had burrowed underneath her skin. She tried to rid herself of them by washing multiple times each day with medicated soap and lindane shampoo. She also visited several dermatologists and had provided samples of "dead bugs" for them to examine under the microscope. All told her there was nothing wrong with her and suggested that her problems were psychiatric in nature. She became increasingly distressed by the infestation and worried that the bugs might invade her other organs if not eradicated. Consequently, she decided to asphyxiate the bugs by covering her body with gasoline and holding it against her skin with plastic wrap. She noted that her skin became red and felt as though it were burning, but she viewed this as a positive sign that the bugs were being killed and writhing around as they died. Several hours after she had applied the gasoline, her daughter came to the house, saw Mrs. G's condition, and took her to the hospital. When evaluated in the burn unit, Mrs. G spoke openly of her concerns about the bugs and was still unsure whether they were present or not. At the same time, she recognized that it had been a mistake to try to kill them with gasoline. She was oriented to person, place, and time and had no other delusional beliefs or auditory or visual hallucinations. She said her mood was "okay," although she was realistically concerned about the extensive treatment that she would require and the difficult process of recovering from her injury. She reported no suicidal ideas or intent before admission and had no history of psychiatric treatment. She also did not report any use of substances except for drinking several beers socially about twice each month. During her stay in the hospital, she was treated with haloperidol in doses of up to 5 mg per day with improvement in her delusions.

This patient demonstrates a classic presentation of delusional parasitosis, including the repeated visits to other physicians, the absolute conviction that an infestation is present, and the collection of "evidence" to support this belief. The lack of a significant history of alcohol or substance use suggests that the sensation of bugs crawling on her skin was not associated with substance intoxication or withdrawal. She also did not have disorientation or fluctuations in her level of consciousness that would suggest delirium, other psychotic symptoms that would suggest schizophrenia, or depressive symptoms that would suggest major depressive disorder with psychotic features. *(Courtesy of Laura J. Fochtmann, M.D., Ramin Mojtabai, M.D., Ph.D., M.P.H., and Evelyn J. Bromet, Ph.D.)*

Grandiose Type

Delusions of grandeur (megalomania) have been noted for years. They were first described by Kraepelin.

A 51-year-old man was arrested for disturbing the peace. Police had been called to a local park to stop him from carving his initials and those of a recently formed religious cult into various trees surrounding a pond in the park. When confronted, he had scornfully argued that having been chosen to begin a new town-wide religious revival, it was necessary for him to publicize his intent in a permanent fashion. The police were unsuccessful in preventing the man from cutting another tree and arrested him. Psychiatric examination was ordered at the state hospital, and the patient was observed there for several weeks. He denied any emotional difficulty and had never received psychiatric treatment. He had no history of euphoria or mood swings. The patient was angry about being hospitalized and only gradually permitted the doctor to interview him. In a few days, however, he was busy preaching to his fellow patients and letting them know that he had been given a special mandate from God to bring in new converts through his ability to heal. Eventually, his preoccupation with special powers diminished, and no other evidence of psychopathology was observed. The patient was discharged, having received no medication at all. Two months later he was arrested at a local theater, this time for disrupting the showing of a film that depicted subjects he believed to be satanic.

Mixed Type

The category mixed type applies to patients with two or more delusional themes. This diagnosis should be reserved for cases in which no single delusional type predominates.

Unspecified Type

The category unspecified type is reserved for cases in which the predominant delusion cannot be subtyped within the previous categories. A possible example is certain delusions of misidentification, for example, Capgras syndrome, named for the French psychiatrist who described the *illusion des sosies,* or the illusion of doubles. The delusion in Capgras syndrome is the belief that a familiar person has been replaced by an impostor. Others have described variants of the Capgras syndrome, namely, the delusion that persecutors or familiar persons can assume the guise of strangers (*Frégoli's phenomenon*) and the very rare delusion that familiar persons can change themselves into other persons at will (*intermetamorphosis*). Each disorder is not only rare but may also be associated with schizophrenia, dementia, epilepsy, and other organic disorders. Reported cases have been predominantly in women, have had associated paranoid features, and have included feelings of depersonalization or derealization. The delusion may be short lived, recurrent, or persistent. It is unclear whether delusional disorder can appear with such a delusion. Certainly, the Frégoli and intermetamorphosis delusions have bizarre content and are unlikely, but the delusion in Capgras syndrome is a possible candidate for delusional disorder. The role of hallucination or perceptual disturbance in this condition needs to be explicated. Cases have appeared after sudden brain damage.

In the 19th century, the French psychiatrist Jules Cotard described several patients with a syndrome called *délire de négation,* sometimes referred to as *nihilistic delusional disorder* or *Cotard syndrome.* Patients with the syndrome complain of having lost not only possessions, status, and strength but also their heart, blood, and intestines. The world beyond them is reduced to nothingness. This relatively rare syndrome is usually considered a precursor to a schizophrenic or depressive episode. With the common use today of antipsychotic drugs, the syndrome is seen even less frequently than in the past.

SHARED PSYCHOTIC DISORDER

Shared psychotic disorder (also referred to over the years as *shared paranoid disorder, induced psychotic disorder, folie impose,* and *double insanity*) was first described by two French psychiatrists, Lasegue and Falret, in 1877, who named it *folie á deux.* In DSM-5, this disorder is referred to as "Delusional Symptoms in Partner of Individual with Delusional Disorder," an unnecessary nomenclature change in the view of most psychiatrists. It is probably rare, but incidence and prevalence figures are lacking, and the literature consists almost entirely of case reports.

The disorder is characterized by the transfer of delusions from one person to another. Both persons are closely associated for a long time and typically live together in relative social isolation. In its most common form, the individual who first has the delusion (the primary case) is often chronically ill and typically is the influential member of a close relationship with a more suggestible person (the secondary case) who also develops the delusion. The person in the secondary case is frequently less intelligent, more gullible, more passive, or more lacking in self-esteem than the person in the primary case. If the pair separates, the secondary person may abandon the delusion, but this outcome is not seen uniformly. The occurrence of the delusion is attributed to the strong influence of the more dominant member. Old age, low intelligence, sensory impairment, cerebrovascular disease, and alcohol abuse are among the factors associated with this peculiar form of psychotic disorder. A genetic predisposition to idiopathic psychoses has also been suggested as a possible risk factor.

Other special forms have been reported, such as *folie simultanée,* in which two persons become psychotic simultaneously and share the same delusion. Occasionally, more than two individuals are involved (e.g., *folie á trois, quatre, cinq;* also *folie á famille*), but such cases are especially rare. The most common relationships in shared psychotic disorder are sister–sister, husband–wife, and mother–child, but other combinations have also been described. Almost all cases involve members of a single family.

A 52-year-old man was referred by the court for inpatient psychiatric examination, charged with disturbing the peace. He had been arrested for disrupting a trial, complaining of harassment by various judges. He had walked into a courtroom, marched to the bench, and begun to berate the probate judge. While in the hospital, he related a detailed account of conspiratorial goings-on in the local judiciary. A target of certain judges, he claimed he had been singled out for a variety of reasons for many years: he knew what was going on; he had kept records of wrongdoings; and he understood the significance of the whole matter. He refused to elaborate on the specific nature of the conspiracy. He had responded to it with frequent letters to newspapers, the local bar association, and even to a Congressional subcommittee. His mental state, apart from his story and a mildly depressed mood, was entirely normal.

A family interview revealed that his wife and several grown children shared the belief in a judicial conspiracy directed against the patient. There was no change in delusional thinking in the patient or the family after ten days of observation. The patient refused follow-up.

In this case, protection is provided by others who share the delusion and believe in the reasonableness of the response; such cases are uncommon, if not rare. *(Courtesy of TC Manschreck, M.D.)*

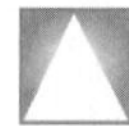

Table 4.4–2
Potential Medical Etiologies of Delusional Syndromes

Disease or Disorder Class	Examples
Neurodegenerative disorders	Alzheimer's disease, Pick's disease, Huntington's disease, basal ganglia calcification, multiple sclerosis, metachromatic leukodystrophy
Other central nervous system disorders	Brain tumors, especially temporal lobe and deep hemispheric tumors; epilepsy, especially complex partial seizure disorder; head trauma (subdural hematoma); anoxic brain injury; fat embolism
Vascular disease	Atherosclerotic vascular disease, especially when associated with diffuse, temporoparietal, or subcortical lesions; hypertensive encephalopathy; subarachnoid hemorrhage, temporal arteritis
Infectious disease	Human immunodeficiency virus or acquired immune deficiency syndrome, encephalitis lethargica, Creutzfeldt–Jakob disease, syphilis, malaria, acute viral encephalitis
Metabolic disorder	Hypercalcemia, hyponatremia, hypoglycemia, uremia, hepatic encephalopathy, porphyria
Endocrinopathies	Addison's disease, Cushing's syndrome, hyper- or hypothyroidism, panhypopituitarism
Vitamin deficiencies	Vitamin B_{12} deficiency, folate deficiency, thiamine deficiency, niacin deficiency
Medications	Adrenocorticotropic hormones, anabolic steroids, corticosteroids, cimetidine, antibiotics (cephalosporins, penicillin), disulfiram, anticholinergic agents
Substances	Amphetamines, cocaine, alcohol, cannabis, hallucinogens
Toxins	Mercury, arsenic, manganese, thallium

DIFFERENTIAL DIAGNOSIS

Medical Conditions

In making a diagnosis of delusional disorder, the first step is to eliminate medical disorders as a potential cause of delusions. Many medical conditions can be associated with the development of delusions (Table 4.4–2), at times accompanying a delirious state.

Toxic-metabolic conditions and disorders affecting the limbic system and basal ganglia are most often associated with the emergence of delusional beliefs. Complex delusions occur more frequently in patients with subcortical pathology. In Huntington's disease and in individuals with idiopathic basal ganglia calcifications, for example, more than 50 percent of patients demonstrated delusions at some point in their illness. After right cerebral infarction, types of delusions that are more prevalent include anosognosia and reduplicative paramnesia (i.e., individuals believing they are in different places at the same time). Capgras syndrome has been observed in a number of medical disorders, including CNS lesions, vitamin B_{12} deficiency, hepatic encephalopathy, diabetes, and hypothyroidism. Focal syndromes have more often involved the right rather than the left hemisphere. Delusions of infestation, lycanthropy (i.e., the false belief that the patient is an animal, often a wolf or "werewolf"), heutoscopy (i.e., the false belief that one has a double), and erotomania have been reported in small numbers of patients with epilepsy, CNS lesions, or toxic-metabolic disorders.

Delirium, Dementia, and Substance-Related Disorders

Delirium and dementia should be considered in the differential diagnosis of a patient with delusions. Delirium can be differentiated by the presence of a fluctuating level of consciousness or impaired cognitive abilities. Delusions early in the course of a dementing illness, as in dementia of the Alzheimer's type, can give the appearance of a delusional disorder; however, neuropsychological testing usually detects cognitive impairment. Although alcohol abuse is an associated feature for patients with delusional disorder, delusional disorder should be distinguished from alcohol-induced psychotic disorder with hallucinations. Intoxication with sympathomimetics (including amphetamine), marijuana, or L-dopa is likely to result in delusional symptoms.

Other Disorders

The psychiatric differential diagnosis for delusional disorder includes malingering and factitious disorder with predominantly psychological signs and symptoms. The nonfactitious disorders in the differential diagnosis are schizophrenia, mood disorders, obsessive-compulsive disorder, somatoform disorders, and paranoid personality disorder. Delusional disorder is distinguished from schizophrenia by the absence of other schizophrenic symptoms and by the nonbizarre quality of the delusions; patients with delusional disorder also lack the impaired functioning seen in schizophrenia. The somatic type of delusional disorder may resemble a depressive disorder or a somatoform disorder. The somatic type of delusional disorder is differentiated from depressive disorders by the absence of other signs of depression and the lack of a pervasive quality to the depression. Delusional disorder can be differentiated from somatoform disorders by the degree to which the somatic belief is held by the patient. Patients with somatoform disorders allow for the possibility that their disorder does not exist, but patients with delusional disorder do not doubt its reality. Separating paranoid personality disorder from delusional disorder requires the sometimes difficult clinical distinction between extreme suspiciousness and frank delusion. In general, if clinicians doubt that a symptom is a delusion, the diagnosis of delusional disorder should not be made.

COURSE AND PROGNOSIS

Some clinicians and some research data indicate that an identifiable psychosocial stressor often accompanies the onset of delusional disorder. The nature of the stressor, in fact, may warrant some suspicion or concern. Examples of such stressors are recent immigration, social conflict with family members or friends, and social isolation. A sudden onset is generally thought to be more common than an insidious onset. Some clinicians believe that a person with delusional disorder is likely to have below-average intelligence and that the premorbid personality of such a person is likely to be extroverted, dominant, and hypersensitive. The person's initial suspicions or concerns gradually become elaborate, consume much of the person's attention, and finally become delusional. Persons may begin quarreling with coworkers; may seek protection from the Federal Bureau of Investigation (FBI) or the police; or may begin visiting many medical or surgical physicians to seek consultations, lawyers about suits, or police about delusional suspicions.

As mentioned, delusional disorder is considered a fairly stable diagnosis. About 50 percent of patients have recovered at long-term follow-up, 20 percent show decreased symptoms, and 30 percent exhibit no change. The following factors correlate with a good prognosis: high levels of occupational, social, and functional adjustments; female sex; onset before age 30 years; sudden onset; short duration of illness; and the presence of precipitating factors. Although reliable data are limited, patients with persecutory, somatic, and erotic delusions are thought to have a better prognosis than patients with grandiose and jealous delusions.

TREATMENT

Delusional disorder was generally regarded as resistant to treatment, and interventions often focused on managing the morbidity of the disorder by reducing the impact of the delusion on the patient's (and family's) life. In recent years, however, the outlook has become less pessimistic or restricted in planning effective treatment. The goals of treatment are to establish the diagnosis, to decide on appropriate interventions, and to manage complications (Table 4.4–3). The success of these goals depends on an effective and therapeutic doctor–patient relationship, which is far from easy to establish. The patients do not complain about psychiatric symptoms and often enter treatment against their will; even psychiatrists may be drawn into their delusional nets.

In shared psychiatric disorder, the patients must be separated. If hospitalization is indicated, they should be placed on different units and have no contact. In general, the healthier of the two will give up the delusional belief (sometimes without any other therapeutic intervention). The sicker of the two will maintain the false fixed belief.

Psychotherapy

The essential element in effective psychotherapy is to establish a relationship in which patients begin to trust a therapist. Individual therapy seems to be more effective than group therapy; insight-oriented, supportive, cognitive, and behavioral therapies are often effective. Initially, a therapist should neither agree with nor challenge a patient's delusions. Although therapists must ask about a delusion to establish its extent, persistent questioning about it should probably be avoided. Physicians may stimulate

Table 4.4-3
Diagnosis and Management of Delusional Disorder

Rule out other causes of paranoid features
Confirm the absence of other psychopathology
Assess consequences of delusion-related behavior
Demoralization
Despondency
Anger, fear
Depression
Impact of search for "medical diagnosis," "legal solution," "proof of infidelity," and so on (e.g., financial, legal, personal, occupational)
Assess anxiety and agitation
Assess potential for violence, suicide
Assess need for hospitalization
Institute pharmacological and psychological therapies
Maintain connection through recovery

the motivation to receive help by emphasizing a willingness to help patients with their anxiety or irritability without suggesting that the delusions be treated, but therapists should not actively support the notion that the delusions are real.

The unwavering reliability of therapists is essential in psychotherapy. Therapists should be on time and make appointments as regularly as possible, with the goal of developing a solid and trusting relationship with a patient. Overgratification may actually increase patients' hostility and suspiciousness because ultimately they must realize that not all demands can be met. Therapists can avoid overgratification by not extending the designated appointment period, by not giving extra appointments unless absolutely necessary, and by not being lenient about the fee.

Therapists should avoid making disparaging remarks about a patient's delusions or ideas but can sympathetically indicate to patients that their preoccupation with their delusions is both distressing to themselves and interferes with a constructive life. When patients begin to waver in their delusional beliefs, therapists may increase reality testing by asking the patients to clarify their concerns.

A useful approach in building a therapeutic alliance is to empathize with the patient's internal experience of being overwhelmed by persecution. It may be helpful to make such comments as, "You must be exhausted, considering what you have been through." Without agreeing with every delusional misperception, a therapist can acknowledge that from the patient's perspective, such perceptions create much distress. The ultimate goal is to help patients entertain the possibility of doubt about their perceptions. As they become less rigid, feelings of weakness and inferiority, associated with some depression, may surface. When a patient allows feelings of vulnerability to enter into the therapy, a positive therapeutic alliance has been established, and constructive therapy becomes possible.

When family members are available, clinicians may decide to involve them in the treatment plan. Without being delusionally seen as siding with the enemy, a clinician should attempt to enlist the family as allies in the treatment process. Consequently, both the patient and the family need to understand that the therapist maintains physician–patient confidentiality and that communications from relatives are discussed with the patient. The family may benefit from the therapist's support and thus may support the patient.

A good therapeutic outcome depends on a psychiatrist's ability to respond to the patient's mistrust of others and the resulting interpersonal conflicts, frustrations, and failures. The mark of successful treatment may be a satisfactory social adjustment rather than abatement of the patient's delusions.

Hospitalization

Patients with delusional disorder can generally be treated as outpatients, but clinicians should consider hospitalization for several reasons. First, patients may need a complete medical and neurological evaluation to determine whether a nonpsychiatric medical condition is causing the delusional symptoms. Second, patients need an assessment of their ability to control violent impulses (e.g., to commit suicide or homicide) that may be related to the delusional material. Third, patients' behavior about the delusions may have significantly affected their ability to function within their family or occupational settings; they may require professional intervention to stabilize social or occupational relationships.

If a physician is convinced that a patient would receive the best treatment in a hospital, then the physician should attempt to persuade the patient to accept hospitalization; failing that, legal commitment may be indicated. If a physician convinces a patient that hospitalization is inevitable, the patient often voluntarily enters a hospital to avoid legal commitment.

Pharmacotherapy

In an emergency, severely agitated patients should be given an antipsychotic drug intramuscularly. Although no adequately conducted clinical trials with large numbers of patients have been conducted, most clinicians consider antipsychotic drugs the treatment of choice for delusional disorder. Patients are likely to refuse medication because they can easily incorporate the administration of drugs into their delusional systems; physicians should not insist on medication immediately after hospitalization but, rather, should spend a few days establishing rapport with the patient. Physicians should explain potential adverse effects to patients, so that they do not later suspect that the physician lied.

A patient's history of medication response is the best guide to choosing a drug. A physician should often start with low doses (e.g., 2 mg of haloperidol [Haldol] or 2 mg of risperidone [Risperdal]) and increase the dose slowly. If a patient fails to respond to the drug at a reasonable dosage in a 6-week trial, antipsychotic drugs from other classes should be tried. Some investigators have indicated that pimozide may be particularly effective in delusional disorder, especially in patients with somatic delusions. A common cause of drug failure is noncompliance, which should also be evaluated. Concurrent psychotherapy facilitates compliance with drug treatment.

If the patient receives no benefit from antipsychotic medication, discontinue use of the drug. In patients who do respond to antipsychotic drugs, some data indicate that maintenance doses can be low. Although essentially no studies evaluate the use of antidepressants, lithium (Eskalith), or anticonvulsants (e.g., carbamazepine [Tegretol] and valproate [Depakene]) in the treatment of delusional disorder, trials with these drugs may be warranted in patients who do not respond to antipsychotic drugs. Trials of these drugs should also be considered when a patient has either the features of a mood disorder or a family history of mood disorders.

▲ 4.5 Brief Psychotic Disorder, Other Psychotic Disorders, and Catatonia

BRIEF PSYCHOTIC DISORDER

Brief psychotic disorder is defined as a psychotic condition that involves the sudden onset of psychotic symptoms, which lasts 1 day or more but less than 1 month. Remission is full, and the individual returns to the premorbid level of functioning. Brief psychotic disorder is an acute and transient psychotic syndrome.

History

Brief psychotic disorder has been poorly studied in psychiatry in the United States, partly because of the frequent changes in diagnostic criteria during the past 15 years. The diagnosis has been better appreciated and more completely studied in Scandinavia and other Western European countries than in the United States. Patients with disorders similar to brief psychotic disorder were previously classified as having reactive, hysterical, stress, and psychogenic psychoses.

Reactive psychosis was often used as a synonym for good-prognosis schizophrenia, but a diagnosis of brief psychotic disorder is not meant to imply a relation with schizophrenia. In 1913, Karl Jaspers described several essential features for the diagnosis of reactive psychosis, including an identifiable and extremely traumatic stressor, a close temporal relation between the stressor and the development of the psychosis, and a generally benign course for the psychotic episode. Jaspers also stated that the content of the psychosis often reflected the nature of the traumatic experience and that the development of the psychosis seemed to serve a purpose for the patient, often as an escape from a traumatic condition.

Epidemiology

The exact incidence and prevalence of brief psychotic disorder is not known, but it is generally considered uncommon. According to DSM-5, 9 percent of first-episode psychoses can be diagnosed as a brief psychotic episode. The disorder occurs more often among younger patients (20s and 30s) than among older patients. Brief psychotic disorder is more common in women than in men. Such epidemiological patterns are sharply distinct from those of schizophrenia. Some clinicians indicate that the disorder may be seen most frequently in patients from low socioeconomic classes and in those who have experienced disasters or major cultural changes (e.g., immigrants). The age of onset in industrialized settings may be higher than in developing countries. Persons who have gone through major psychosocial stressors may be at greater risk for subsequent brief psychotic disorder.

Comorbidity

The disorder is often seen in patients with personality disorders (most commonly, histrionic, narcissistic, paranoid, schizotypal, and borderline personality disorders).

Etiology

The cause of brief psychotic disorder is unknown. Patients who have a personality disorder may have a biological or psychological vulnerability for the development of psychotic symptoms, particularly those with borderline, schizoid, schizotypal, or paranoid qualities. Some patients with brief psychotic disorder have a history of schizophrenia or mood disorders in their families, but this finding is nonconclusive. Psychodynamic formulations have emphasized the presence of inadequate coping mechanisms and the possibility of secondary gain for patients with psychotic symptoms. Additional psychodynamic theories suggest that the psychotic symptoms are a defense against a prohibited fantasy, the fulfillment of an unattained wish, or an escape from a stressful psychosocial situation.

Diagnosis

A diagnosis of brief psychotic disorder is appropriate when psychotic symptoms last at least 1 day but less than 1 month and are not associated with a mood disorder, a substance-related disorder, or a psychotic disorder caused by a general medical condition. There are three subtypes of brief psychotic disorder: (1) the presence of a stressor, (2) the absence of a stressor, and (3) a postpartum onset. As with other acutely ill psychiatric patients, the history necessary to make the diagnosis may not be obtainable solely from the patient. Although psychotic symptoms may be obvious, information about prodromal symptoms, previous episodes of a mood disorder, and a recent history of ingestion of a psychotomimetic substance may not be available from the clinical interview alone. In addition, clinicians may not be able to obtain accurate information about the presence or absence of precipitating stressors. Such information is usually best and most accurately obtained from a relative or a friend.

Clinical Features

The symptoms of brief psychotic disorder always include at least one major symptom of psychosis, such as hallucinations, delusions, and disorganized thoughts, usually with an abrupt onset, but do not always include the entire symptom pattern seen in schizophrenia. Some clinicians have observed that labile mood, confusion, and impaired attention may be more common at the onset of brief psychotic disorder than at the onset of eventually chronic psychotic disorders. Characteristic symptoms in brief psychotic disorder include emotional volatility, strange or bizarre behavior, screaming or muteness, and impaired memory of recent events. Some of the symptoms suggest a diagnosis of delirium and warrant a medical workup, especially to rule out adverse reactions to drugs.

Scandinavian and other European literature describes several characteristic symptom patterns in brief psychotic disorder, although these may differ somewhat in Europe and America. The symptom patterns include acute paranoid reactions and reactive confusion, excitation, and depression. Some data suggest that, in the United States, paranoia is often the predominant symptom in the disorder. In French psychiatry, *bouffée délirante* (discussed in Section 4.1) is similar to brief psychotic disorder.

Precipitating Stressors. The clearest examples of precipitating stressors are major life events that would cause any person significant emotional upset. Such events include the loss of a close family member or a severe automobile accident. Some clinicians argue that the severity of the event must be considered in relation to the patient's life. This view, although reasonable, may broaden the definition of precipitating stressor to include events unrelated to the psychotic episode. Others have argued that the stressor may be a series of modestly stressful events rather than a single markedly stressful event, but evaluating the amount of stress caused by a sequence of events calls for an almost impossibly high degree of clinical judgment.

A 20-year-old man was admitted to the psychiatric ward of a hospital shortly after starting military duty. During the first week after his arrival to the military base, he thought the other recruits looked at him in a strange way. He watched the people around him to see whether they were out "to get" him. He heard voices calling his name several times. He became increasingly suspicious and after another week had to be admitted for psychiatric evaluation. There he was guarded, scowling, skeptical, and depressed. He gave the impression of being very shy and inhibited. His psychotic symptoms disappeared rapidly when he was treated with an antipsychotic drug. However, he had difficulties in adjusting to hospital light. Transfer to a long-term medical hospital was considered, but after 3 months, a decision was made to discharge him to his home. He was subsequently judged unfit to return to military services.

The patient was the eldest of five siblings. His father was an intemperate drinker who became angry and brutal when drunk. The family was poor, and there were constant fights between the parents. As a child, the patient was inhibited and fearful and often ran into the woods when troubled. He had academic difficulties.

When the patient got older, he preferred to spend time alone and disliked being with people. He occasionally took part in local parties. Although he was never a heavy drinker, he often got into fights when he had a drink or two.

The patient was reinterviewed by hospital personnel at 4 years, 7 years, and 23 years after his admission. He has had no recurrences of any psychotic symptoms and has been fully employed since 6 months after he left the hospital. He married, and at the last follow-up, he had two grown children.

After leaving the hospital, the patient worked for 2 years in a factory. For the past 20 years, he has managed a small business, and it has run well. He has been very happy at work and in his family life. He has made an effort to overcome his tendency toward isolation and has several friends.

The patient believes that his natural tendency is to be socially isolated and that his disorder was connected with the fact that in the military, he was forced to deal with other people. *(Adapted from Laura J. Fochtmann, M.D., Ramin Mojtabai, M.D., Ph.D., M.P.H., and Evelyn J. Bromet, Ph.D.)*

Differential Diagnosis

Clinicians must not assume that the correct diagnosis for a patient who is briefly psychotic is brief psychotic disorder, even when a clear precipitating psychosocial factor is identified. Such a factor may be merely coincidental. If psychotic symptoms are present longer than 1 month, the diagnoses of schizophreniform disorder, schizoaffective disorder, schizophrenia, mood disorders with psychotic features, delusional disorder, and psychotic disorder not otherwise specified must be entertained. If psychotic symptoms of sudden onset are present for less than 1 month in response to an obvious stressor, however, the diagnosis of brief psychotic disorder is strongly suggested. Other diagnoses to consider in the differential diagnosis include factitious disorder with predominantly psychological signs and symptoms, malingering, psychotic disorder caused by a general medical condition, and substance-induced psychotic disorder. In factitious disorder, symptoms are intentionally produced; in malingering, a specific goal is involved in appearing psychotic (e.g., to gain admission to the hospital); and when associated with a medical condition or drugs, the cause becomes apparent with proper medical or drug workups. If the patient admits to using illicit substances, the clinician can make the assessment of substance intoxication or substance withdrawal without the use of laboratory testing. Patients with epilepsy or delirium can also show psychotic symptoms that resemble those seen in brief psychotic disorder. Additional psychiatric disorders to be considered in the differential diagnosis include dissociative identity disorder and psychotic episodes associated with borderline and schizotypal personality disorders.

Course and Prognosis

By definition, the course of brief psychotic disorder is less than 1 month. Nonetheless, the development of such a significant psychiatric disorder may signify a patient's mental vulnerability. Approximately half of patients who are first classified as having brief psychotic disorder later display chronic psychiatric syndromes such as schizophrenia and mood disorders. Patients with brief psychotic disorder, however, generally have good prognoses, and European studies have indicated that 50 to 80 percent of all patients have no further major psychiatric problems.

The length of the acute and residual symptoms is often just a few days. Occasionally, depressive symptoms follow the resolution of the psychotic symptoms. Suicide is a concern during both the psychotic phase and the postpsychotic depressive phase. Several indicators have been associated with a good prognosis (Table 4.5–1).

Treatment

Hospitalization. A patient who is acutely psychotic may need brief hospitalization for both evaluation and protection. Evaluation requires close monitoring of symptoms and assessment of the patient's level of danger to self and others. In addition, the quiet, structured setting of a hospital may help patients regain their sense of reality. While clinicians wait for the setting or the drugs to have their effects, seclusion, physical restraints, or one-to-one monitoring of the patient may be necessary.

Pharmacotherapy. The two major classes of drugs to be considered in the treatment of brief psychotic disorder are the antipsychotic drugs and the benzodiazepines. When an antipsychotic drug is chosen, a high-potency antipsychotic drug, such as haloperidol, or a serotonin dopamine agonist such as ziprasidone may be used. In patients who are at high risk for the development of extrapyramidal adverse effects (e.g., young men), a serotonin dopamine antagonist drug should be administered as prophylaxis against medication-induced movement disorder symptoms.

Table 4.5–1
Good Prognostic Features for Brief Psychotic Disorder

Good premorbid adjustment
Few premorbid schizoid traits
Severe precipitating stressor
Sudden onset of symptoms
Affective symptoms
Confusion and perplexity during psychosis
Little affective blunting
Short duration of symptoms
Absence of relatives with schizophrenia

Alternatively, benzodiazepines can be used in the short-term treatment of psychosis. Although benzodiazepines have limited or no usefulness in the long-term treatment of psychotic disorders, they can be effective for a short time and are associated with fewer adverse effects than the antipsychotic drugs. In rare cases, the benzodiazepines are associated with increased agitation and, more rarely still, with withdrawal seizures, which usually occur only with the sustained use of high dosages. The use of other drugs in the treatment of brief psychotic disorder, although reported in case studies, has not been supported in any large-scale studies. Anxiolytic medications, however, are often useful during the first 2 to 3 weeks after the resolution of the psychotic episode. Clinicians should avoid long-term use of any medication in the treatment of the disorder. If maintenance medication is necessary, a clinician may have to reconsider the diagnosis.

Psychotherapy. Although hospitalization and pharmacotherapy are likely to control short-term situations, the difficult part of treatment is the psychological integration of the experience (and possibly the precipitating trauma, if one was present) into the lives of the patients and their families. Psychotherapy is of use in providing an opportunity to discuss the stressors and the psychotic episode. Exploration and development of coping strategies are the major topics in psychotherapy. Associated issues include helping patients deal with the loss of self-esteem and to regain self-confidence. An individualized treatment strategy based on increasing problem-solving skills while strengthening the ego structure through psychotherapy appears to be the most efficacious. Family involvement in the treatment process may be crucial to a successful outcome.

PSYCHOTIC DISORDER NOT OTHERWISE SPECIFIED

Under the umbrella of psychosis not otherwise specified is a variety of clinical presentations that do not fit within current diagnostic rubrics. It includes psychotic symptomatology (i.e., delusions, hallucinations, disorganized speech, grossly disorganized or catatonic behavior) about which there is inadequate information to make a specific diagnosis or about which there is contradictory information. It also includes disorders with psychotic symptoms that do not meet the criteria for any specific psychotic disorder, such as patients who present to hospital with persistent auditory hallucinations that are not accompanied by mood disturbances and that are not pathognomonic for schizophrenia.

Autoscopic Psychosis

Although not included in DSM-5, autoscopic psychosis is of clinical interest. The characteristic symptom of autoscopic psychosis is a visual hallucination of all or part of the person's own body. The hallucinatory perception, which is called a *phantom,* is usually colorless and transparent, and because the phantom imitates the person's movements, it is perceived as though appearing in a mirror. The phantom tends to appear suddenly and without warning.

Epidemiology. Autoscopy is a rare phenomenon. Some persons have an autoscopic experience only once or a few times; others have the experience more often. Although the data are limited, sex, age, heredity, and intelligence do not seem to be related to the occurrence of the syndrome.

Etiology. The cause of the autoscopic phenomenon is unknown. A biological hypothesis is that abnormal, episodic activity in areas of the temporoparietal lobes is involved with the sense of self, perhaps combined with abnormal activity in parts of the visual cortex. Psychological theories have associated the syndrome with personalities characterized by imagination; visual sensitivity; and, possibly, narcissistic personality disorder traits. Such persons may likely experience autoscopic phenomena during periods of stress.

Course and Prognosis. The classic descriptions of the phenomenon indicate that, in most cases, the syndrome is neither progressive nor incapacitating. Affected persons usually maintain some emotional distance from the phenomenon, an observation that suggests a specific neuroanatomical lesion. Rarely do the symptoms reflect the onset of schizophrenia or other psychotic disorders.

Treatment. Patients usually respond to antianxiety medication. In severe cases, antipsychotic medications may be needed.

Motility Psychosis

Motility psychosis is not considered an "official" DSM-5 diagnosis but is of clinical significance. It is probably a variant of brief psychotic disorder. The two forms of motility psychosis are akinetic and hyperkinetic. The akinetic form of motility psychosis has a clinical presentation similar to that of catatonic stupor. In contrast to the catatonic type of schizophrenia, however, akinetic motility psychosis has a rapidly resolving and favorable course that does not lead to personality deterioration. In its hyperkinetic form, motility psychosis can resemble manic or catatonic excitement. As with the akinetic form, the hyperkinetic form usually has a rapidly resolving and favorable course. Patients may switch from the akinetic to hyperkinetic form rapidly and may represent a danger to others during the excited phase. Mood is extremely labile in these patients.

Postpartum Psychosis

Postpartum psychosis (sometimes called *puerperal psychosis*) is an example of psychotic disorder not otherwise specified that occurs in women who have recently delivered a baby; the syndrome is most often characterized by the mother's depression, delusions, and thoughts of harming either her infant or herself. For a more detailed discussion see Chapter 21.

PSYCHOTIC DISORDERS DUE TO A GENERAL MEDICAL CONDITION AND SUBSTANCE- OR MEDICATION-INDUCED PSYCHOTIC DISORDER

The evaluation of a patient with psychotic disorders requires consideration of the possibility that the psychotic symptoms result from a general medical condition such as a brain tumor or the ingestion of a substance such as phencyclidine (PCP) or medication such as cortisol.

Epidemiology

Relevant epidemiological data about psychotic disorder caused by a general medical condition and substance-induced psychotic disorder are lacking. The disorders are most often encountered in patients who abuse alcohol or other substances on a long-term basis. The delusional syndrome that may accompany complex partial seizures is more common in women than in men.

Etiology

Physical conditions such as cerebral neoplasms, particularly of the occipital or temporal areas, can cause hallucinations. Sensory deprivation, as in people who are blind or deaf, can also result in hallucinatory or delusional experiences. Lesions involving the temporal lobe and other cerebral regions, especially the right hemisphere and the parietal lobe, are associated with delusions.

Psychoactive substances are common causes of psychotic syndromes. The most commonly involved substances are alcohol, indole hallucinogens, such as lysergic acid diethylamide (LSD), amphetamine, cocaine, mescaline, PCP, and ketamine. Many other substances, including steroids and thyroxine, can produce hallucinations.

Diagnosis

Psychotic Disorder due to a General Medical Condition. The diagnosis of psychotic disorder due to a general medical condition is defined by specifying the predominant symptoms. When the diagnosis is used, the medical condition, along with the predominant symptoms pattern, should be included in the diagnosis (e.g., psychotic disorder due to a brain tumor, with delusions). The disorder does not occur exclusively while a patient is delirious or demented, and the symptoms are not better accounted for by another mental disorder.

Substance- or Medication-Induced Psychotic Disorder. The diagnostic category of substance-induced psychotic disorder is reserved for those with psychotic symptoms and impaired reality testing caused by substances or medications. People with substance-induced psychotic symptoms (e.g., hallucinations, delusions) but with intact reality testing should be classified as having a substance-related disorder (e.g., PCP intoxication with perceptual disturbances). The full diagnosis of substance-induced psychotic disorder should include the type of substance or medication involved, the stage of substance use when the disorder began (e.g., during intoxication or withdrawal), and the clinical phenomena (e.g., hallucinations or delusions). Typical substances include alcohol, sedatives, cannabis, phencyclidine, acetaminophen, and cocaine among others.

Clinical Features

Hallucinations. Hallucinations can occur in one or more sensory modalities. Tactile hallucinations (e.g., a sensation of bugs crawling on the skin) are characteristic of cocaine use. Auditory hallucinations are usually associated with psychoactive substance abuse; auditory hallucinations can also occur in persons who are deaf. Olfactory hallucinations can result from temporal lobe epilepsy; visual hallucinations can occur in persons who are blind because of cataracts. Hallucinations are either recurrent or persistent and are experienced in a state of full wakefulness and alertness; a hallucinating patient shows no significant changes in cognitive functions. Visual hallucinations often take the form of scenes involving diminutive (lilliputian) human figures or small animals. Rare musical hallucinations typically feature religious songs. Patients with psychotic disorder caused by a general medical condition and substance-induced psychotic disorder may act on their hallucinations. In alcohol-related hallucinations, threatening, critical, or insulting third-person voices speak about the patients and may tell them to harm either themselves or others. Such patients are dangerous and are at significant risk for suicide or homicide. Patients may or may not believe that the hallucinations are real.

Delusions. Secondary and substance-induced delusions are usually present in a state of full wakefulness. Patients experience no change in the level of consciousness, although mild cognitive impairment may be observed. Patients may appear confused, disheveled, or eccentric, with tangential or even incoherent speech. Hyperactivity and apathy may be present, and an associated dysphoric mood is thought to be common. The delusions can be systematized or fragmentary, with varying content, but persecutory delusions are the most common.

Differential Diagnosis. Psychotic disorder due to a general medical condition and substance- or medication-induced psychotic disorder must be distinguished from delirium (in which patients have a clouded sensorium), from dementia (in which patients have major intellectual deficits), and from schizophrenia (in which patients have other symptoms of thought disorder and impaired functioning). Psychotic disorder due to a general medical condition and substance-induced psychotic disorder must also be differentiated from psychotic mood disorders (in which other affective symptoms are pronounced).

Treatment

Treatment involves identifying the general medical condition or the particular substance involved. At that point, treatment is directed toward the underlying condition and the patient's immediate behavioral control. Hospitalization may be necessary to evaluate patients completely and to ensure their safety. Antipsychotic agents (e.g., olanzapine [Zyprexa] or haloperidol) may be necessary for immediate and short-term control of psychotic or aggressive behavior, although benzodiazepines may also be useful for controlling agitation and anxiety.

CATATONIC DISORDER

Catatonia is a new diagnostic category in DSM-5 introduced because it can occur over a broad spectrum of mental disorders, most often in severe psychotic and mood disorders. It can also be caused by an underlying medical condition or induced by a substance.

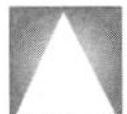

Table 4.5–2
Signs and Symptoms of Catatonic Disorder

Stupor
Catalepsy
Waxy flexibility
Mutism
Negativism
Posturing
Mannerism
Stereotypy
Agitation
Grimacing
Echolalia
Echopraxia

See glossary for the definitions of signs and symptoms.

Diagnosis

Catatonia is a clinical syndrome characterized by striking behavioral abnormalities that may include motoric immobility or excitement, profound negativism, or echolalia (mimicry of speech) or echopraxia (mimicry of movement). A diagnosis of catatonic disorder due to a general medical condition can be made if there is evidence that the condition is due to the physiological effects of a general medical condition. The diagnosis is not made if the catatonia is better explained by a primary mental disorder, such as schizophrenia or psychotic depression, or if catatonic symptoms occur exclusively within the course of delirium (Table 4.5–2).

Epidemiology

Catatonia is an uncommon condition mostly seen in advanced primary mood or psychotic illnesses. Among inpatients with catatonia, 25 to 50 percent are related to mood disorders (e.g., major depressive episode, recurrent, with catatonic features), and approximately 10 percent are associated with schizophrenia. The prevalence of catatonia due to medical conditions of substances is unknown.

Etiology

Medical conditions that can cause catatonia include neurological disorders (e.g., nonconvulsive status epilepticus, and head trauma), infections (e.g., encephalitis), and metabolic disturbances (e.g., hepatic encephalopathy, hyponatremia, and hypercalcemia).

Medications that can cause catatonia include corticosteroids, immunosuppressants, and antipsychotic (i.e., neuroleptic) agents. Catatonic symptoms may be seen in extreme forms of neuroleptic-induced parkinsonism or neuroleptic malignant syndrome, a rare, potentially life-threatening disorder associated with fever, autonomic instability, impaired consciousness, and rigidity.

Diagnosis and Clinical Features

DSM-5 criteria for the diagnosis of catatonic disorder due to a general medical condition include behavioral changes characteristic of catatonia, evidence of a physiological basis for the symptoms, and exclusion of primary mental disorders and delirium. The diagnosis of catatonia due to a mental disorder is used when the disorder occurs in a psychiatric rather than another medical condition. In either case, the signs and symptoms of catatonia are similar; it is the etiology that differs. Behavioral changes may include motoric immobility or excessive activity, extreme negativism or mutism, peculiarities of voluntary movement, and echolalia or echopraxia. Waxy flexibility, a form of artificial posturing often evident on physical examination, may be present. Lethal catatonia is a rare advanced stage of the disorder that features fever and autonomic instability and may be fatal.

For catatonia secondary to antipsychotic agents, the diagnoses of neuroleptic-induced parkinsonism and neuroleptic malignant syndrome may be appropriate. For catatonia due to nonneuroleptic substances, the diagnosis of medication-induced movement disorder not otherwise specified is available.

Laboratory Examination

There are no pathognomonic laboratory findings in catatonia. The laboratory evaluation should be used to rule out an underlying medical condition. Appropriate medical tests may include complete blood counts, electrolytes, brain imaging, and electroencephalography (if seizures are suspected). In addition, serum creatinine phosphokinase, white blood cell count, and serum transaminases should be checked because the results of laboratory tests are elevated in patients with neuroleptic malignant syndrome.

Differential Diagnosis

Differential diagnoses include hypoactive delirium, end-stage dementia, and akinetic mutism, as well as catatonia due to a primary psychiatric disorder. It is important to identify cases of catatonia occurring in the setting of neuroleptic malignant syndrome because the latter diagnosis can be fatal. Features suggesting neuroleptic malignant syndrome include autonomic instability and delirium in addition to elevated serum creatinine phosphokinase, white blood cell count, and serum transaminases.

Course and Treatment

Catatonia impairs a person's ability to care for him- or herself and therefore requires hospitalization. In an excited state, the catatonic patient may represent a danger to others; hence, close supervision is needed. Fluid and nutrient intake must be maintained, often with intravenous lines or feeding tubes. The catatonic individual must be assisted with hygiene.

The primary treatment modality is identifying and correcting the underlying medical or pharmacological cause. Offending substances must be removed or minimized.

Benzodiazepines can provide temporary improvement in symptoms, and their use may improve patients' ability to communicate and to care for themselves. ECT is appropriate for catatonia due to a general medical condition, especially if the catatonia is life threatening (e.g., inability to eat) or has developed into lethal (malignant) catatonia. The mechanism behind the efficacy of ECT is unknown.

5 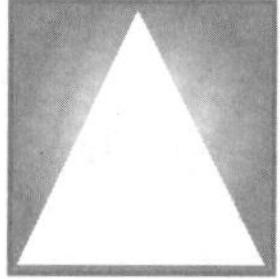

Mood Disorders

▲ 5.1 Major Depression and Bipolar Disorder

Mood can be defined as a pervasive and sustained emotion or feeling tone that influences a person's behavior and colors his or her perception of being in the world. Disorders of mood—sometimes called affective disorders—make up an important category of psychiatric illness consisting of depressive disorder, bipolar disorder, and other disorders, which are discussed in this section and in the section that follows.

A variety of adjectives are used to describe mood: depressed, sad, empty, melancholic, distressed, irritable, disconsolate, elated, euphoric, manic, gleeful, and many others, all descriptive in nature. Some can be observed by the clinician (e.g., an unhappy visage), and others can be felt only by the patient (e.g., hopelessness). Mood can be labile, fluctuating, or alternating rapidly between extremes (e.g., laughing loudly and expansively one moment, tearful and despairing the next). Other signs and symptoms of mood disorders include changes in activity level, cognitive abilities, speech, and vegetative functions (e.g., sleep, appetite, sexual activity, and other biological rhythms). These disorders virtually always result in impaired interpersonal, social, and occupational functioning.

It is tempting to consider disorders of mood on a continuum with normal variations in mood. Patients with mood disorders, however, often report an ineffable, but distinct, quality to their pathological state. The concept of a continuum, therefore, may represent the clinician's overidentification with the pathology, thus possibly distorting his or her approach to patients with mood disorder.

Patients with only major depressive episodes are said to have *major depressive disorder* or *unipolar depression*. Patients with both manic and depressive episodes or patients with manic episodes alone are said to have *bipolar disorder*. The terms "unipolar mania" and "pure mania" are sometimes used for patients who are bipolar but who do not have depressive episodes.

Three additional categories of mood disorders are hypomania, cyclothymia, and dysthymia. Hypomania is an episode of manic symptoms that does not meet the criteria for manic episode. Cyclothymia and dysthymia as disorders that represent less severe forms of bipolar disorder and major depression, respectively.

The field of psychiatry has considered major depression and bipolar disorder to be two separate disorders, particularly in the past 20 years. The possibility that bipolar disorder is actually a more severe expression of major depression has been reconsidered recently, however. Many patients given a diagnosis of a major depressive disorder reveal, on careful examination, past episodes of manic or hypomanic behavior that have gone undetected. Many authorities see considerable continuity between recurrent depressive and bipolar disorders. This has led to widespread discussion and debate about the bipolar spectrum, which incorporates classic bipolar disorder, bipolar II, and recurrent depressions.

HISTORY

The Old Testament story of King Saul describes a depressive syndrome, as does the story of Ajax's suicide in Homer's *Iliad.* About 400 BC, Hippocrates used the terms *mania* and *melancholia* to describe mental disturbances. Around 30 AD, the Roman physician Celsus described melancholia (from Greek *melan* ["black"] and *chole* ["bile"]) in his work *De re medicina* as a depression caused by black bile. The first English text entirely related to depression was Robert Burton's *Anatomy of Melancholy,* published in 1621.

In 1854, Jules Falret described a condition called *folie circulaire,* in which patients experience alternating moods of depression and mania. In 1882, the German psychiatrist Karl Kahlbaum, using the term *cyclothymia,* described mania and depression as stages of the same illness. In 1899, Emil Kraepelin, building on the knowledge of previous French and German psychiatrists, described manic-depressive psychosis using most of the criteria that psychiatrists now use to establish a diagnosis of bipolar I disorder. According to Kraepelin, the absence of a dementing and deteriorating course in manic-depressive psychosis differentiated it from dementia precox (as schizophrenia was then called). Kraepelin also described a depression that came to be known as involutional melancholia, which has since come to be viewed as a severe form of mood disorder that begins in late adulthood.

Depression

A major depressive disorder occurs without a history of a manic, mixed, or hypomanic episode. A major depressive episode must last at least 2 weeks, and typically a person with a diagnosis of a major depressive episode also experiences at least four symptoms from a list that includes changes in appetite and weight, changes in sleep and activity, lack of energy, feelings of guilt, problems thinking and making decisions, and recurring thoughts of death or suicide.

Mania

A manic episode is a distinct period of an abnormally and persistently elevated, expansive, or irritable mood lasting for at least 1 week or less if a patient must be hospitalized. A hypomanic episode lasts at least 4 days and is similar to a manic episode except that it is not sufficiently severe to cause impairment in social or occupational functioning, and no psychotic features are present. Both mania and hypomania are associated with inflated self-esteem, a decreased need for sleep, distractibility, great physical and mental activity, and overinvolvement in pleasurable behavior. Bipolar I disorder is defined as having a clinical course of one or more manic episodes and, sometimes, major depressive episodes. A mixed episode is a period of at least 1 week in which both a manic episode and a major depressive episode occur almost daily. A variant of bipolar disorder characterized by episodes of major depression and hypomania rather than mania is known as *bipolar II disorder.*

Dysthymia and Cyclothymia

Two additional mood disorders, dysthymic disorder and cyclothymic disorder (discussed fully in Section 8.2) have also been discussed clinically for some time. Dysthymic disorder and cyclothymic disorder are characterized by the presence of symptoms that are less severe than those of major depressive disorder and bipolar I disorder, respectively. Dysthymic disorder is characterized by at least 2 years of depressed mood that is not sufficiently severe to fit the diagnosis of major depressive episode. Cyclothymic disorder is characterized by at least 2 years of frequently occurring hypomanic symptoms that cannot fit the diagnosis of manic episode and of depressive symptoms that cannot fit the diagnosis of major depressive episode.

EPIDEMIOLOGY

Incidence and Prevalence

Mood disorders are common. In the most recent surveys, major depressive disorder has the highest lifetime prevalence (almost 17 percent) of any psychiatric disorder. The lifetime prevalence rate of different forms of depressive disorder, according to community surveys, are shown in Table 5.1–1. The lifetime prevalence rate for major depression is 5 to 17 percent. The lifetime prevalence rates of different clinical forms of bipolar disorder are shown in Table 5.1–2. The annual incidence of bipolar illness is considered generally to be less than 1 percent, but it is difficult to estimate because milder forms of bipolar disorder are often missed.

Table 5.1–1
Lifetime Prevalence Rates of Depressive Disorders

	Type	Lifetime
Major depressive episode	Range	5–17
	Average	12
Dysthymic disorder	Range	3–6
	Average	5
Minor depressive disorder	Range	10
	Average	—
Recurrent brief depressive disorder	Range	16

Adapted from Rihmer Z, Angst A. Mood Disorders: Epidemiology. In: Sadock BJ, Sadock VA, eds. *Comprehensive Textbook of Psychiatry.* 8th ed. Baltimore, MD: Lippincott Williams & Wilkins; 2004.

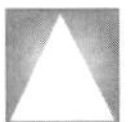

Table 5.1–2
Lifetime Prevalence Rates of Bipolar I Disorder, Bipolar II Disorder, Cyclothymic Disorder, and Hypomania

	Lifetime Prevalence (%)
Bipolar I disorder	0–2.4
Bipolar II disorder	0.3–4.8
Cyclothymia	0.5–6.3
Hypomania	2.6–7.8

Adapted from Rihmer Z, Angst A. Mood disorders: Epidemiology. In: Sadock BJ, Sadock VA, eds. *Comprehensive Textbook of Psychiatry.* 8th ed. Baltimore, MD: Lippincott Williams & Wilkins; 2004.

Sex

An almost universal observation, independent of country or culture, is the twofold greater prevalence of major depressive disorder in women than in men. The reasons for the difference are hypothesized to involve hormonal differences, the effects of childbirth, differing psychosocial stressors for women and for men, and behavioral models of learned helplessness. In contrast to major depressive disorder, bipolar I disorder has an equal prevalence among men and women. Manic episodes are more common in men, and depressive episodes are more common in women. When manic episodes occur in women, they are more likely than men to present a mixed picture (e.g., mania and depression). Women also have a higher rate of being rapid cyclers, defined as having four or more manic episodes in a one-year period.

Age

The onset of bipolar I disorder is earlier than that of major depressive disorder. The age of onset for bipolar I disorder ranges from childhood (as early as age of 5 or 6 years) to 50 years or even older in rare cases, with a mean age of 30 years. The mean age of onset for major depressive disorder is about 40 years, with 50 percent of all patients having an onset between the ages of 20 and 50 years. Major depressive disorder can also begin in childhood or in old age. Recent epidemiological data suggest that the incidence of major depressive disorder may be increasing among people younger than 20 years of age. This may be related to the increased use of alcohol and drugs of abuse in this age group.

Marital Status

Major depressive disorder occurs most often in persons without close interpersonal relationships and in those who are divorced or separated. Bipolar I disorder is more common in divorced and single persons than among married persons, but this difference may reflect the early onset and the resulting marital discord characteristic of the disorder.

Socioeconomic and Cultural Factors

No correlation has been found between socioeconomic status and major depressive disorder. A higher than average incidence of bipolar I disorder is found among the upper socioeconomic groups. Bipolar I disorder is more common in persons who did not graduate from college than in college graduates, however, which may also reflect the relatively early age of onset for the disorder. Depression is more common in rural areas than in urban areas. The prevalence of mood disorder does not differ among races. A tendency exists, however, for examiners to underdiagnose mood disorder and over diagnose schizophrenia in patients whose racial or cultural background differs from theirs.

COMORBIDITY

Individuals with major mood disorders are at an increased risk of having one or more additional comorbid disorders. The most frequent disorders are alcohol abuse or dependence, panic disorder, obsessive-compulsive disorder (OCD), and social anxiety disorder. Conversely, individuals with substance use disorders and anxiety disorders also have an elevated risk of lifetime or current comorbid mood disorder. In both unipolar and bipolar disorder, whereas men more frequently present with substance use disorders, women more frequently present with comorbid anxiety and eating disorders. In general, patients who are bipolar more frequently show comorbidity of substance use and anxiety disorders than do patients with unipolar major depression. In the Epidemiological Catchment Area (ECA) study, the lifetime history of substance use disorders, panic disorder, and OCD was approximately twice as high among patients with bipolar I disorder (61 percent, 21 percent, and 21 percent, respectively) than in patients with unipolar major depression (27 percent, 10 percent, and 12 percent, respectively). Comorbid substance use disorders and anxiety disorders worsen the prognosis of the illness and markedly increase the risk of suicide among patients who are unipolar major depressive and bipolar.

ETIOLOGY

Biological Factors

Many studies have reported biological abnormalities in patients with mood disorders. Until recently, the monoamine neurotransmitters—norepinephrine (NE), dopamine, serotonin, and histamine—were the main focus of theories and research about the etiology of these disorders. A progressive shift has occurred from focusing on disturbances of single neurotransmitter systems in favor of studying neurobehavioral systems, neural circuits, and more intricate neuroregulatory mechanisms. The monoaminergic systems, thus, are now viewed as broader, neuromodulatory systems, and disturbances are as likely to be secondary or epiphenomenal effects as they are directly or causally related to etiology and pathogenesis.

Biogenic Amines. Of the biogenic amines, NE and serotonin are the two neurotransmitters most implicated in the pathophysiology of mood disorders.

NOREPINEPHRINE. The correlation suggested by basic science studies between the downregulation or decreased sensitivity of β-adrenergic receptors and clinical antidepressant responses is probably the single most compelling piece of data indicating a direct role of the noradrenergic system in depression. Other evidence has also implicated the presynaptic β_2-receptors in depression because activation of these receptors results in a decrease of the amount of NE released. Presynaptic β_2-receptors are also located on serotonergic neurons and regulate the amount of serotonin released. The clinical effectiveness of antidepressant drugs with noradrenergic effects—for example, venlafaxine (Effexor)—further supports a role for NE in the pathophysiology of at least some of the symptoms of depression.

SEROTONIN. With the huge effect that the selective serotonin reuptake inhibitors (SSRIs)—for example, fluoxetine (Prozac)—have made on the treatment of depression, serotonin has become the biogenic amine neurotransmitter most commonly associated with depression. The identification of multiple serotonin receptor subtypes has also increased the excitement within the research community about the development of even more specific treatments for depression. Besides that SSRIs and other serotonergic antidepressants are effective in the treatment of depression, other data indicate that serotonin is involved in the pathophysiology of depression. Depletion of serotonin may precipitate depression, and some patients with suicidal impulses have low cerebrospinal fluid (CSF) concentrations of serotonin metabolites and low concentrations of serotonin uptake sites on platelets.

DOPAMINE. Although NE and serotonin are the biogenic amines most often associated with the pathophysiology of depression, dopamine has also been theorized to play a role. The data suggest that dopamine activity may be reduced in depression and increased in mania. The discovery of new subtypes of the dopamine receptors and an increased understanding of the presynaptic and postsynaptic regulation of dopamine function have further enriched research into the relation between dopamine and mood disorders. Drugs that reduce dopamine concentrations—for example, reserpine (Serpasil)—and diseases that reduce dopamine concentrations (e.g., Parkinson's disease) are associated with depressive symptoms. In contrast, drugs that increase dopamine concentrations, such as tyrosine, amphetamine, and bupropion (Wellbutrin), reduce the symptoms of depression. Two recent theories about dopamine and depression are that the mesolimbic dopamine pathway may be dysfunctional in depression and that the dopamine D_1 receptor may be hypoactive in depression.

Other Neurotransmitter Disturbances. Acetylcholine (ACh) is found in neurons that are distributed diffusely throughout the cerebral cortex. Cholinergic neurons have reciprocal or interactive relationships with all three monoamine systems. Abnormal levels of choline, which is a precursor to ACh, have been found at autopsy in the brains of some depressed patients, perhaps reflecting abnormalities in cell phospholipid composition. Cholinergic agonist and antagonist drugs have differential clinical effects on depression and mania. Agonists can produce lethargy, anergia, and psychomotor retardation in healthy subjects, can exacerbate symptoms in depression, and can reduce symptoms in mania. These effects generally are not sufficiently robust to have clinical applications, and adverse effects are problematic. In an animal model of depression, strains of mice that are super- or subsensitive to cholinergic agonists have been found susceptible or more resistant to developing learned helplessness (discussed later). Cholinergic agonists can induce changes in hypothalamic–pituitary adrenal (HPA) activity and sleep that mimic those associated with severe depression. Some patients with mood disorders in remission, as well as their never-ill first-degree relatives, have a trait-like increase in sensitivity to cholinergic agonists.

γ-Aminobutyric acid (GABA) has an inhibitory effect on ascending monoamine pathways, particularly the mesocortical and mesolimbic systems. Reductions of GABA have been observed in plasma, CSF, and brain GABA levels in depression.

Animal studies have also found that chronic stress can reduce and eventually deplete GABA levels. By contrast, GABA receptors are upregulated by antidepressants, and some GABAergic medications have weak antidepressant effects.

The amino acids glutamate and glycine are the major excitatory and inhibitory neurotransmitters in the CNS. Glutamate and glycine bind to sites associated with the N-methyl-D-aspartate (NMDA) receptor, and an excess of glutamatergic stimulation can cause neurotoxic effects. Importantly, a high concentration of NMDA receptors exists in the hippocampus. Glutamate, thus, may work in conjunction with hypercortisolemia to mediate the deleterious neurocognitive effects of severe recurrent depression. Emerging evidence suggests that drugs that antagonize NMDA receptors have antidepressant effects.

Second Messengers and Intracellular Cascades. The binding of a neurotransmitter and a postsynaptic receptor triggers a cascade of membrane-bound and intracellular processes mediated by second messenger systems. Receptors on cell membranes interact with the intracellular environment via guanine nucleotide-binding proteins (G proteins). The G proteins, in turn, connect to various intracellular enzymes (e.g., adenylate cyclase, phospholipase C, and phosphodiesterase) that regulate utilization of energy and formation of second messengers, such as cyclic nucleotide (e.g., cyclic adenosine monophosphate [cAMP] and cyclic guanosine monophosphate [cGMP]), as well as phosphatidylinositols (e.g., inositol triphosphate and diacylglycerol) and calcium-calmodulin. Second messengers regulate the function of neuronal membrane ion channels. Increasing evidence also indicates that mood-stabilizing drugs act on G proteins or other second messengers.

Alterations of Hormonal Regulation. Lasting alterations in neuroendocrine and behavioral responses can result from severe early stress. Animal studies indicate that even transient periods of maternal deprivation can alter subsequent responses to stress. Activity of the gene coding for the neurokinin brain-derived neurotrophic growth factor (BDNF) is decreased after chronic stress, as is the process of neurogenesis. Protracted stress thus can induce changes in the functional status of neurons and, eventually, cell death. Recent studies in depressed humans indicate that a history of early trauma is associated with increased HPA activity accompanied by structural changes (i.e., atrophy or decreased volume) in the cerebral cortex.

Elevated HPA activity is a hallmark of mammalian stress responses and one of the clearest links between depression and the biology of chronic stress. Hypercortisolema in depression suggests one or more of the following central disturbances: decreased inhibitory serotonin tone; increased drive from NE, ACh, or corticotropin-releasing hormone (CRH); or decreased feedback inhibition from the hippocampus.

Evidence of increased HPA activity is apparent in 20 to 40 percent of depressed outpatients and 40 to 60 percent of depressed inpatients.

Elevated HPA activity in depression has been documented via excretion of urinary-free cortisol (UFC), 24-hour (or shorter time segments) intravenous (IV) collections of plasma cortisol levels, salivary cortisol levels, and tests of the integrity of feedback inhibition. A disturbance of feedback inhibition is tested by administration of dexamethasone (Decadron) (0.5 to 2.0 mg), a potent synthetic glucocorticoid, which normally suppresses HPA axis activity for 24 hours. Nonsuppression of cortisol secretion at 8:00 AM the following morning or subsequent escape from suppression at 4:00 PM or 11:00 PM is indicative of impaired feedback inhibition. Hypersecretion of cortisol and dexamethasone nonsuppression are imperfectly correlated (approximately 60 percent concordance). A more recent development to improve the sensitivity of the test involves infusion of a test dose of CRH after dexamethasone suppression.

These tests of feedback inhibition are not used as diagnostic tests because adrenocortical hyperactivity (albeit usually less prevalent) is observed in mania, schizophrenia, dementia, and other psychiatric disorders.

THYROID AXIS ACTIVITY. Approximately 5 to 10 percent of people evaluated for depression have previously undetected thyroid dysfunction, as reflected by an elevated basal thyroid-stimulating hormone (TSH) level or an increased TSH response to a 500-mg infusion of the hypothalamic neuropeptide thyroid-releasing hormone (TRH). Such abnormalities are often associated with elevated antithyroid antibody levels and, unless corrected with hormone replacement therapy, can compromise response to treatment. An even larger subgroup of depressed patients (e.g., 20 to 30 percent) shows a blunted TSH response to TRH challenge. To date, the major therapeutic implication of a blunted TSH response is evidence of an increased risk of relapse despite preventive antidepressant therapy. Of note, unlike the dexamethasone-suppression test (DST), blunted TSH response to TRH does not usually normalize with effective treatment.

GROWTH HORMONE. Growth hormone (GH) is secreted from the anterior pituitary after stimulation by NE and dopamine. Secretion is inhibited by somatostatin, a hypothalamic neuropeptide, and CRH. Decreased CSF somatostatin levels have been reported in depression, and increased levels have been observed in mania.

PROLACTIN. Prolactin is released from the pituitary by serotonin stimulation and inhibited by dopamine. Most studies have not found significant abnormalities of basal or circadian prolactin secretion in depression, although a blunted prolactin response to various serotonin agonists has been described. This response is uncommon among premenopausal women, suggesting that estrogen has a moderating effect.

Alterations of Sleep Neurophysiology. Depression is associated with a premature loss of deep (slow-wave) sleep and an increase in nocturnal arousal. The latter is reflected by four types of disturbance: (1) an increase in nocturnal awakenings, (2) a reduction in total sleep time, (3) increased phasic rapid eye movement (REM) sleep, and (4) increased core body temperature. The combination of increased REM drive and decreased slow-wave sleep results in a significant reduction in the first period of non-REM (NREM) sleep, a phenomenon referred to as *reduced REM latency.* Reduced REM latency and deficits of slow-wave sleep typically persist after recovery of a depressive episode. Blunted secretion of GH after sleep onset is associated with decreased slow-wave sleep and shows similar state-independent or trait-like behavior. The combination of reduced REM latency, increased REM density, and decreased sleep maintenance identifies approximately 40 percent of depressed outpatients and

80 percent of depressed inpatients. False-negative findings are commonly seen in younger, hypersomnolent patients, who may actually experience an increase in slow-wave sleep during episodes of depression. Approximately 10 percent of otherwise healthy individuals have abnormal sleep profiles, and, as with dexamethasone nonsuppression, false-positive cases are not uncommonly seen in other psychiatric disorders.

Patients manifesting a characteristically abnormal sleep profile have been found to be less responsive to psychotherapy and have a greater risk of relapse or recurrence and may benefit preferentially from pharmacotherapy.

Immunological Disturbance. Depressive disorders are associated with several immunological abnormalities, including decreased lymphocyte proliferation in response to mitogens and other forms of impaired cellular immunity. These lymphocytes produce neuromodulators, such as corticotropin-releasing factor (CRF), and cytokines, peptides known as *interleukins*. There appears to be an association with clinical severity, hypercortisolism, and immune dysfunction, and the cytokine interleukin-1 may induce gene activity for glucocorticoid synthesis.

Structural and Functional Brain Imaging. Computed axial tomography (CAT) and magnetic resonance imaging (MRI) scans have permitted sensitive, noninvasive methods to assess the living brain, including cortical and subcortical tracts, as well as white matter lesions. The most consistent abnormality observed in the depressive disorders is increased frequency of abnormal hyperintensities in subcortical regions, such as periventricular regions, the basal ganglia, and the thalamus. More common in bipolar I disorder and among elderly adults, these hyperintensities appear to reflect the deleterious neurodegenerative effects of recurrent affective episodes. Ventricular enlargement, cortical atrophy, and sulcal widening have also been reported in some studies. Some depressed patients may also have reduced hippocampal or caudate nucleus volumes, or both, suggesting more focal defects in relevant neurobehavioral systems. Diffuse and focal areas of atrophy have been associated with increased illness severity, bipolarity, and increased cortisol levels.

The most widely replicated positron emission tomography (PET) finding in depression is decreased anterior brain metabolism, which is generally more pronounced on the left side. From a different vantage point, depression may be associated with a relative increase in nondominant hemispheric activity. Furthermore, a reversal of hypofrontality occurs after shifts from depression into hypomania, such that greater left hemisphere reductions are seen in depression compared with greater right hemisphere reductions in mania. Other studies have observed more specific reductions of reduced cerebral blood flow or metabolism, or both, in the dopaminergically innervated tracts of the mesocortical and mesolimbic systems in depression. Again, evidence suggests that antidepressants at least partially normalize these changes.

In addition to a global reduction of anterior cerebral metabolism, increased glucose metabolism has been observed in several limbic regions, particularly among patients with relatively severe recurrent depression and a family history of mood disorder. During episodes of depression, increased glucose metabolism is correlated with intrusive ruminations.

Neuroanatomical Considerations. Both the symptoms of mood disorders and biological research findings support the hypothesis that mood disorders involve pathology of the brain. Modern affective neuroscience focuses on the importance of four brain regions in the regulation of normal emotions: the prefrontal cortex (PFC), the anterior cingulate, the hippocampus, and the amygdala. The PFC is viewed as the structure that holds representations of goals and appropriate responses to obtain these goals. Such activities are particularly important when multiple, conflicting behavioral responses are possible or when it is necessary to override affective arousal. Evidence indicates some hemispherical specialization in PFC function. For example, whereas left-sided activation of regions of the PFC is more involved in goal-directed or appetitive behaviors, regions of the right PFC are implicated in avoidance behaviors and inhibition of appetitive pursuits. Subregions in the PFC appear to localize representations of behaviors related to reward and punishment.

The anterior cingulate cortex (ACC) is thought to serve as the point of integration of attentional and emotional inputs. Two subdivisions have been identified: an affective subdivision in the rostral and ventral regions of the ACC and a cognitive subdivision involving the dorsal ACC. The former subdivision shares extensive connections with other limbic regions, and the latter interacts more with the PFC and other cortical regions. It is proposed that activation of the ACC facilitates control of emotional arousal, particularly when goal attainment has been thwarted or when novel problems have been encountered.

The hippocampus is most clearly involved in various forms of learning and memory, including fear conditioning, as well as inhibitory regulation of the HPA axis activity. Emotional or contextual learning appears to involve a direct connection between the hippocampus and the amygdala.

The amygdala appears to be a crucial way station for processing novel stimuli of emotional significance and coordinating or organizing cortical responses. Located just above the hippocampi bilaterally, the amygdala has long been viewed as the heart of the limbic system. Although most research has focused on the role of the amygdala in responding to fearful or painful stimuli, it may be ambiguity or novelty, rather than the aversive nature of the stimulus per se, that brings the amygdala on line.

Genetic Factors

Numerous family, adoption, and twin studies have long documented the heritability of mood disorders. Recently, however, the primary focus of genetic studies has been to identify specific susceptibility genes using molecular genetic methods.

Family Studies. Family studies address the question of whether a disorder is familial. More specifically, is the rate of illness in the family members of someone with the disorder greater than that of the general population? Family data indicate that if one parent has a mood disorder, a child will have a risk of between 10 and 25 percent for mood disorder. If both parents are affected, this risk roughly doubles. The more members of the family who are affected, the greater the risk is to a child. The risk is greater if the affected family members are first-degree relatives rather than more distant relatives. A family history of bipolar disorder conveys a greater risk for mood disorders in general and, specifically, a much greater risk for bipolar disorder. Unipolar disorder is typically the most common form of mood disorder in families of bipolar probands. This familial overlap suggests some degree of common genetic underpinnings between these two forms of mood disorder. The presence of more severe illness in the family also conveys a greater risk.

Adoption Studies. Adoption studies provide an alternative approach to separating genetic and environmental factors in familial transmission. Only a limited number of such studies have been reported, and their results have been mixed. One large study found a threefold increase in the rate of bipolar disorder and a twofold increase in unipolar disorder in the biological relatives of bipolar probands. Similarly, in a Danish sample, a threefold increase in the rate of unipolar disorder and a sixfold increase in the rate of completed suicide in the biological relatives of affectively ill probands were reported. Other studies, however, have been less convincing and have found no difference in the rates of mood disorders.

Twin Studies. Twin studies provide the most powerful approach to separating genetic from environmental factors, or "nature" from "nurture." The twin data provide compelling evidence that genes explain only 50 to 70 percent of the etiology of mood disorders. Environment or other nonheritable factors must explain the remainder. Therefore, it is a predisposition or susceptibility to disease that is inherited. Considering unipolar and bipolar disorders together, these studies find a concordance rate for mood disorder in the monozygotic (MZ) twins of 70 to 90 percent compared with the same-sex dizygotic (DZ) twins of 16 to 35 percent. This is the most compelling data for the role of genetic factors in mood disorders.

Linkage Studies. DNA markers are segments of DNA of known chromosomal location, which are highly variable among individuals. They are used to track the segregation of specific chromosomal regions within families affected with a disorder. When a marker is identified with disease in families, the disease is said to be *genetically linked* (Table 5.1–3). Chromosomes 18q and 22q are the two regions with strongest evidence for linkage to bipolar disorder. Several linkage studies have found evidence for the involvement of specific genes in clinical subtypes. For example, the linkage evidence on 18q has been shown to be derived largely from bipolar II—bipolar II sibling pairs and from families in which the probands had panic symptoms.

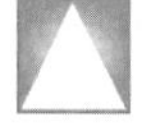

Table 5.1–3
Selected Chromosomal Regions with Evidence of Linkage to Bipolar Disorder

Chromosome 18	Data suggest the presence of as many as four different loci on this one chromosome. Studies have found linkage to 18q to preferentially occur in families in which affective illness was transmitted through the mother, suggesting a possible parent-of-origin effect.
Chromosome 21q	Regions have shown linkage or association to both schizophrenia and bipolar disorder.
Chromosome 22q	The breakpoint cluster region (BCR) gene is located on chromosome 22q11. The BCR gene encodes an activating protein, which is known to play important roles in neuron growth and axonal guidance.

Gene-mapping studies of unipolar depression have found very strong evidence of linkage to the locus for cAMP response element-binding protein (CREB1) on chromosome 2. Eighteen other genomic regions were found to be linked; some of these displayed interactions with the CREB1 locus. Another study has reported evidence for a gene–environment interaction in the development of major depression. Subjects who underwent adverse life events were shown, in general, to be at an increased risk for depression. Of such subjects, however, those with a variant in the serotonin transporter gene showed the greatest increase in risk. This is one of the first reports of a specific gene–environment interaction in a psychiatric disorder.

Psychosocial Factors

Life Events and Environmental Stress. A long-standing clinical observation is that stressful life events more often precede first, rather than subsequent, episodes of mood disorders. This association has been reported for both patients with major depressive disorder and patients with bipolar I disorder. One theory proposed to explain this observation is that the stress accompanying the first episode results in long-lasting changes in the brain's biology. These long-lasting changes may alter the functional states of various neurotransmitter and intraneuronal signaling systems, changes that may even include the loss of neurons and an excessive reduction in synaptic contacts. As a result, a person has a high risk of undergoing subsequent episodes of a mood disorder, even without an external stressor.

Some clinicians believe that life events play the primary or principal role in depression; others suggest that life events have only a limited role in the onset and timing of depression. The most compelling data indicate that the life event most often associated with development of depression is losing a parent before the age of 11 years. The environmental stressor most often associated with the onset of an episode of depression is the loss of a spouse. Another risk factor is unemployment; persons out of work are three times more likely to report symptoms of an episode of major depression than those who are employed. Guilt may also play a role.

Ms. C, a 23-year-old woman, became acutely depressed when she was accepted to a prestigious graduate school. Ms. C had been working diligently toward this acceptance for the past 4 years. She reported being "briefly happy, for about 20 minutes" when she learned the good news but rapidly slipped into a hopeless state in which she recurrently pondered the pointlessness of her aspirations, cried constantly, and had to physically stop herself from taking a lethal overdose of her roommate's insulin. In treatment, she focused on her older brother, who had regularly insulted her throughout the course of her life, and how "he's not doing well." She found herself very worried about him. She mentioned that she was not used to being the "successful" one of the two of them. In connection with her depression, it emerged that Ms. C's brother had had a severe, life-threatening, and disfiguring pediatric illness that had required much family time and attention throughout their childhood. Ms. C had become "used to" his insulting manner toward her. In fact, it seemed that she required her brother's abuse of her in order not to feel overwhelmed by survivor guilt about being the "healthy, normal" child. "He might insult me, but I look up to him. I adore him. Any attention he pays to me is like a drug," she said. Ms. C's acceptance to graduate school had challenged her defensive and essential compensatory image of herself as being less successful, or damaged, in comparison with her brother, thereby overwhelming her with guilt. Her depression remitted in psychodynamic psychotherapy as she better understood her identification with and fantasy submission to her brother. *(Courtesy of JC Markowitz, M.D. and BL Milrod, M.D.)*

Personality Factors. No single personality trait or type uniquely predisposes a person to depression; all humans, of whatever personality pattern, can and do become depressed under appropriate circumstances. Persons with certain personality disorders—OCD, histrionic, and borderline—may be at greater risk for depression than persons with antisocial or paranoid personality disorder. The latter can use projection and other externalizing defense mechanisms to protect themselves from their inner rage. No evidence indicates that any particular personality disorder is associated with later development of bipolar I disorder; however, patients with dysthymic disorder and cyclothymic disorder are at risk of later developing major depression or bipolar I disorder.

Recent stressful events are the most powerful predictors of the onset of a depressive episode. From a psychodynamic perspective, the clinician is always interested in the meaning of the stressor. Research has demonstrated that stressors that the patient experience as reflecting negatively on his or her self-esteem are more likely to produce depression. Moreover, what may seem to be a relatively mild stressor to outsiders may be devastating to the patient because of particular idiosyncratic meanings attached to the event.

Psychodynamic Factors in Depression. The psychodynamic understanding of depression defined by Sigmund Freud and expanded by Karl Abraham is known as the classic view of depression. That theory involves four key points: (1) disturbances in the infant–mother relationship during the oral phase (the first 10 to 18 months of life) predispose to subsequent vulnerability to depression; (2) depression can be linked to real or imagined object loss; (3) introjection of the departed objects is a defense mechanism invoked to deal with the distress connected with the object's loss; and (4) because the lost object is regarded with a mixture of love and hate, feelings of anger are directed inward at the self.

Ms. E, a 21-year-old college student, presented with major depression and panic disorder since early adolescence. She reported hating herself, crying constantly, and feeling profoundly hopeless in part because of the chronicity of her illness. Even at the time of presentation, she noted her sensitivity to her mother's moods. "My mother's just always depressed, and it makes me so miserable. I just don't know what to do," she said. "I always want something from her, I don't even know what, but I never get it. She always says the wrong thing, talks about how disturbed I am, stuff like that, makes me feel bad about myself." In one session, Ms. E poignantly described her childhood: "I spent a lot of time with my mother, but she was always too tired, she never wanted to do anything or play with me. I remember building a house with blankets over the coffee table and peeking out, spying on her. She was always depressed and negative, like a negative sink in the room, making it empty and sad. I could never get her to do anything." This patient experienced extreme guilt in her psychotherapy when she began to talk about her mother's depression. "I feel so bad," she sobbed. "It's like I'm saying bad things about her. And I love her so much, and I know she loves me. I feel it's so disloyal of me." Her depression remitted in psychodynamic psychotherapy as she became more aware of and better able to tolerate her feelings of rage and disappointment with her mother. *(Courtesy of JC Markowitz, M.D. and BL Milrod, M.D.)*

Melanie Klein understood depression as involving the expression of aggression toward loved ones, much as Freud did. Edward Bibring regarded depression as a phenomenon that sets in when a person becomes aware of the discrepancy between extraordinarily high ideals and the inability to meet those goals. Edith Jacobson saw the state of depression as similar to a powerless, helpless child victimized by a tormenting parent. Silvano Arieti observed that many depressed people have lived their lives for someone else rather than for themselves. He referred to the person for whom depressed patients live as the dominant other, which may be a principle, an ideal, or an institution, as well as an individual. Depression sets in when patients realize that the person or ideal for which they have been living is never going to respond in a manner that will meet their expectations. Heinz Kohut's conceptualization of depression, derived from his self-psychological theory, rests on the assumption that the developing self has specific needs that must be met by parents to give the child a positive sense of self-esteem and self-cohesion. When others do not meet these needs, there is a massive loss of self-esteem that presents as depression. John Bowlby believed that damaged early attachments and traumatic separation in childhood predispose to depression. Adult losses are said to revive the traumatic childhood loss and so precipitate adult depressive episodes.

Psychodynamic Factors in Mania. Most theories of mania view manic episodes as a defense against underlying depression. Abraham, for example, believed that the manic episodes may reflect an inability to tolerate a developmental tragedy, such as the loss of a parent. The manic state may also result from a tyrannical superego, which produces intolerable self-criticism that is then replaced by euphoric self-satisfaction. Bertram Lewin regarded the manic patient's ego as overwhelmed by pleasurable impulses, such as sex, or by feared impulses, such as aggression. Klein also viewed mania as a defensive reaction to depression, using manic defenses such as omnipotence, in which the person develops delusions of grandeur.

Ms. G, a 42-year-old housewife and mother of a 4-year-old boy, developed symptoms of hypomania and later of frank mania without psychosis, when her only son was diagnosed with acute lymphocytic leukemia. A profoundly religious woman who had experienced 10 years of difficulty with conception, Ms. G was a devoted mother. She reported that she was usually rather down. Before her son's illness, she used to joke that she had become pregnant with him by divine intervention. When her son was diagnosed and subsequently hospitalized, he required painful medical tests and emergency chemotherapy, which made him very ill. The doctors regularly barraged Ms. G with bad news about his prognosis during the first few weeks of his illness.

Ms. G was ever present with her son at the hospital, never sleeping, always caring for him, yet the pediatricians noted that as the child became more debilitated and the prognosis more grim, she seemed to bubble over with renewed cheerfulness, good humor, and high spirits. She could not seem to stop herself from cracking jokes to the hospital staff during her son's painful procedures, and as the jokes became louder and more inappropriate, the staff grew more concerned. During her subsequent psychiatric consultation (requested by the pediatric staff), Ms. G reported that her current "happiness and optimism" were justified by her sense of "oneness" with Mary, the mother of God. "We are together now, she and I, and she has become a part of me. We have a special relationship," she winked. Despite these statements, Ms. G was not psychotic and said that she was "speaking metaphorically, of course, only as a good Catholic would." Her mania resolved when her son achieved remission and was discharged from the hospital. *(Courtesy of JC Markowitz, M.D. and BL Milrod, M.D.)*

Other Formulations of Depression

Cognitive Theory. According to cognitive theory, depression results from specific cognitive distortions present in persons susceptible to depression. These distortions, referred to as *depressogenic schemata,* are cognitive templates that perceive both internal and external data in ways that are altered by early experiences. Aaron Beck postulated a cognitive triad of depression that consists of (1) views about the self—a negative self-precept, (2) about the environment—a tendency to experience the world as hostile and demanding, and (3) about the future—the expectation of suffering and failure. Therapy consists of modifying these distortions. The elements of cognitive theory are summarized in Table 5.1–4.

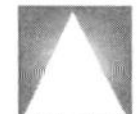

Table 5.1–4
Elements of Cognitive Theory

Element	Definition
Cognitive triad	Beliefs about oneself, the world, and the future
Schemas	Ways of organizing and interpreting experiences
Cognitive distortions	
Arbitrary inference	Drawing a specific conclusion without sufficient evidence
Specific abstraction	Focus on a single detail while ignoring other, more important aspects of an experience
Overgeneralization	Forming conclusions based on too little and too narrow experience
Magnification and minimization	Over- or undervaluing the significance of a particular event
Personalization	Tendency to self-reference external events without basis
Absolutist, dichotomous thinking	Tendency to place experience into all-or-none categories

(Courtesy of Robert M.A. Hirschfeld, MD and M. Tracie Shea, PhD.)

Learned Helplessness. The learned helplessness theory of depression connects depressive phenomena to the experience of uncontrollable events. For example, when dogs in a laboratory were exposed to electrical shocks from which they could not escape, they showed behaviors that differentiated them from dogs that had not been exposed to such uncontrollable events. The dogs exposed to the shocks would not cross a barrier to stop the flow of electric shock when put in a new learning situation. They remained passive and did not move. According to the learned helplessness theory, the shocked dogs learned that outcomes were independent of responses, so they had both cognitive motivational deficit (i.e., they would not attempt to escape the shock) and emotional deficit (indicating decreased reactivity to the shock). In the reformulated view of learned helplessness as applied to human depression, internal causal explanations are thought to produce a loss of self-esteem after adverse external events. Behaviorists who subscribe to the theory stress that improvement of depression is contingent on the patient's learning a sense of control and mastery of the environment.

Diagnosis

Major Depressive Disorder, Single Episode. Depression may occur as a single episode or may be recurrent. Differentiation between these patients and those who have two or more episodes of major depressive disorder is justified because of the uncertain course of the former patients' disorder. Several studies have reported data consistent with the notion that major depression covers a heterogeneous population of disorders. One type of study assessed the stability of a diagnosis of major depression in a patient over time. The study found that 25 to 50 percent of the patients were later reclassified as having a different psychiatric condition or a nonpsychiatric medical condition with psychiatric symptoms. A second type of study evaluated first-degree relatives of affectively ill patients to determine the presence and types of psychiatric diagnoses for these relatives over time. Both types of studies found that depressed patients with more depressive symptoms are more likely to have stable diagnoses over time and are more likely to have affectively ill relatives than are depressed patients with fewer depressive symptoms. Also, patients with bipolar I disorder and those with bipolar II disorder (recurrent major depressive episodes with hypomania) are likely to have stable diagnoses over time.

Major Depressive Disorder, Recurrent

Patients who are experiencing at least a second episode of depression are classified as having major depressive disorder, recurrent. The essential problem with diagnosing recurrent episodes of major depressive disorder is choosing the criteria to designate the resolution of each period. Two variables are the degree of resolution of the symptoms and the length of the resolution. DSM-5 requires that distinct episodes of depression be separated by at least 2 months during which a patient has no significant symptoms of depression.

Bipolar I Disorder

The DSM-5 criteria for a bipolar I disorder requires the presence of a distinct period of abnormal mood lasting at least 1 week and includes separate bipolar I disorder diagnoses for a single manic episode and a recurrent episode based on the symptoms of the most recent episode as described below.

The designation bipolar I disorder is synonymous with what was formerly known as bipolar disorder—a syndrome in which a complete set of mania symptoms occurs during the course of the disorder. The diagnostic criteria for bipolar II disorder is characterized by depressive episodes and hypomanic episodes during the course of the disorder, but the episodes of manic-like symptoms do not quite meet the diagnostic criteria for a full manic syndrome.

Manic episodes clearly precipitated by antidepressant treatment (e.g., pharmacotherapy, electroconvulsive therapy [ECT]) do not indicate bipolar I disorder.

Bipolar I Disorder, Single Manic Episode. According to DSM-5, patients must be experiencing their first manic episode to meet the diagnostic criteria for bipolar I disorder, single manic episode. This requirement rests on the fact that patients who are having their first episode of bipolar I disorder depression cannot be distinguished from patients with major depressive disorder.

Bipolar I Disorder, Recurrent. The issues about defining the end of an episode of depression also apply to defining the end of an episode of mania. Manic episodes are considered distinct when they are separated by at least 2 months without significant symptoms of mania or hypomania.

Bipolar II Disorder

The diagnostic criteria for bipolar II disorder specify the particular severity, frequency, and duration of the hypomanic symptoms. The diagnostic criteria for a hypomanic episode are listed together with the criteria for bipolar II disorder. The criteria have been established to decrease over diagnosis of hypomanic episodes and the incorrect classification of patients with major depressive disorder as patients with bipolar II disorder. Clinically, psychiatrists may find it difficult to distinguish euthymia from hypomania in a patient who has been chronically depressed for many months or years. As with bipolar I disorder, antidepressant-induced hypomanic episodes are not diagnostic of bipolar II disorder.

Specifiers (Symptom Features)

In addition to the severity, psychotic, and remission descriptions, additional symptom features (specifiers) can be used to describe patients with various mood disorders.

With Psychotic Features. The presence of psychotic features in major depressive disorder reflects severe disease and is a poor prognostic indicator. A review of the literature comparing psychotic with nonpsychotic major depressive disorders indicates that the two conditions may be distinct in their pathogenesis. One difference is that bipolar I disorder is more common in the families of probands with psychotic depression than in the families of probands with nonpsychotic depression.

The psychotic symptoms themselves are often categorized as either mood congruent, that is, in harmony with the mood disorder ("I deserve to be punished because I am so bad"), or mood incongruent, not in harmony with the mood disorder. Patients with mood disorder with mood-congruent psychoses have a psychotic type of mood disorder; however, patients with mood disorder with mood-incongruent psychotic symptoms may have schizoaffective disorder or schizophrenia.

The following factors have been associated with a poor prognosis for patients with mood disorders: long duration of episodes, temporal dissociation between the mood disorder and the psychotic symptoms, and a poor premorbid history of social adjustment. The presence of psychotic features also has significant treatment implications. These patients typically require antipsychotic drugs in addition to antidepressants or mood stabilizers and may need ECT to obtain clinical improvement.

With Melancholic Features. *Melancholia* is one of the oldest terms used in psychiatry, dating back to Hippocrates in the fourth century to describe the dark mood of depression. It is still used to refer to a depression characterized by severe anhedonia, early morning awakening, weight loss, and profound feelings of guilt (often over trivial events). It is not uncommon for patients who are melancholic to have suicidal ideation. Melancholia is associated with changes in the autonomic nervous system and in endocrine functions. For that reason, melancholia is sometimes referred to as "endogenous depression" or depression that arises in the absence of external life stressors or precipitants. The DSM-5 melancholic features can be applied to major depressive episodes in major depressive disorder, bipolar I disorder, or bipolar II disorder.

With Atypical Features. The introduction of a formally defined depression with atypical features is a response to research and clinical data indicating that patients with atypical features have specific, predictable characteristics: overeating and oversleeping. These symptoms have sometimes been referred to as *reversed vegetative symptoms,* and the symptom pattern has sometimes been called *hysteroid dysphoria.* When patients with major depressive disorder with atypical features are compared with patients with typical depression features, the patients with atypical features are found to have a younger age of onset; more severe psychomotor slowing; and more frequent coexisting diagnoses of panic disorder, substance abuse or dependence, and somatization disorder. The high incidence and severity of anxiety symptoms in patients with atypical features have sometimes been correlated with the likelihood of their being misclassified as having an anxiety disorder rather than a mood disorder. Patients with atypical features may also have a long-term course, a diagnosis of bipolar I disorder, or a seasonal pattern to their disorder.

The DSM-5 atypical features can be applied to the most recent major depressive episode in major depressive disorder, bipolar I disorder, bipolar II disorder, or dysthymic disorder. Atypical depression may mask manic symptoms as in the following case.

> Kevin, a 15-year-old adolescent, was referred to a sleep center to rule out narcolepsy. His main complaints were fatigue, boredom, and a need to sleep all the time. Although he had always started the day somewhat slowly, he now could not get out of bed to go to school. That alarmed his mother, prompting sleep consultation.

Formerly a B student, he had been failing most of his courses in the 6 months before referral. Psychological counseling, predicated on the premise that his family's recent move from another city had led to Kevin's isolation, had not been beneficial. Extensive neurological and general medical workup findings had also proven negative. He slept 12 to 15 hours per day but denied cataplexy, sleep paralysis, and hypnagogic hallucinations. During psychiatric interview, he denied being depressed but admitted that he had lost interest in everything except his dog. He had no drive, participated in no activities, and had gained 30 pounds in 6 months. He believed that he was "brain damaged" and wondered whether it was worth living like that. The question of suicide disturbed him because it was contrary to his religious beliefs. These findings led to the prescription of desipramine (Norpramin) in a dosage that was gradually increased to 200 mg per day over 3 weeks. Not only did desipramine reverse the presenting complaints, but it also pushed him to the brink of a manic episode. *(Courtesy of HS Akiskal, M.D.)*

With Catatonic Features. As a symptom, catatonia can be present in several mental disorders, most commonly, schizophrenia and the mood disorders. The presence of catatonic features in patients with mood disorders may have prognostic and treatment significance.

The hallmark symptoms of catatonia—stuporousness, blunted affect, extreme withdrawal, negativism, and marked psychomotor retardation—can be seen in both catatonic and noncatatonic schizophrenia, major depressive disorder (often with psychotic features), and medical and neurological disorders. Clinicians often do not associate catatonic symptoms with bipolar I disorder because of the marked contrast between the symptoms of stuporous catatonia and the classic symptoms of mania. Because catatonic symptoms are a behavioral syndrome appearing in several medical and psychiatric conditions, catatonic symptoms do not imply a single diagnosis. Catatonia is discussed in detail in Section 4.5.

Postpartum Onset. DSM-5 allows the specification of a postpartum mood disturbance if the onset of symptoms is within 4 weeks postpartum. Postpartum mental disorders commonly include psychotic symptoms. Postpartum disorders are discussed in Chapter 23.

Rapid Cycling. Patients with rapid cycling bipolar I disorder are likely to be female and to have had depressive and hypomanic episodes. No data indicate that rapid cycling has a familial pattern of inheritance; thus, an external factor such as stress or drug treatment may be involved in the pathogenesis of rapid cycling. The DSM-5 criteria specify that the patient must have at least four episodes within a 12-month period.

Seasonal Pattern. Patients with a seasonal pattern to their mood disorders tend to experience depressive episodes during a particular season, most commonly winter. The pattern has become known as seasonal affective disorder (SAD), although this term is not used in DSM-5. Two types of evidence indicate that the seasonal pattern may represent a separate diagnostic entity. First, the patients are likely to respond to treatment with light therapy, although no studies with controls to evaluate light therapy in nonseasonally depressed patients have been conducted. Second, research has shown that patients evince decreased metabolic activity in the orbital frontal cortex and in the left inferior parietal lobe. Further studies are necessary to differentiate depressed persons with seasonal pattern from other depressed persons. This disorder is discussed further in Section 12.2 on Sleep–Wake Disorders.

Non–DSM-5 Types. Other systems that identify types of patients with mood disorders usually separate patients with good and poor prognoses or patients who may respond to one treatment or another. They also differentiate endogenous-reactive and primary-secondary schemes.

The endogenous-reactive continuum is a controversial division. It implies that endogenous depressions are biological and that reactive depressions are psychological, primarily on the basis of the presence or absence of an identifiable precipitating stress. Other symptoms of endogenous depression have been described as diurnal variation, delusions, psychomotor retardation, early morning awakening, and feelings of guilt; thus, endogenous depression is similar to the DSM-5 diagnosis of major depressive disorder with psychotic features, melancholic features, or both. Symptoms of reactive depression included initial insomnia, anxiety, emotional lability, and multiple somatic complaints.

Primary depressions are what DSM-5 refers to as mood disorders, except for the diagnoses of mood disorder caused by a general medical condition and substance-induced mood disorder, which are considered secondary depressions. Double depression is the condition in which major depressive disorder is superimposed on dysthymic disorder. A depressive equivalent is a symptom or syndrome that may be a *forme fruste* of a depressive episode. For example, a triad of truancy, alcohol abuse, and sexual promiscuity in a formerly well-behaved adolescent may constitute a depressive equivalent.

CLINICAL FEATURES

The two basic symptom patterns in mood disorders are depression and mania. Depressive episodes can occur in both major depressive disorder and bipolar I disorder. Researchers have attempted to find reliable differences between bipolar I disorder depressive episodes and episodes of major depressive disorder, but the differences are elusive. In a clinical situation, only the patient's history, family history, and future course can help differentiate the two conditions. Some patients with bipolar I disorder have mixed states with both manic and depressive features, and some seem to experience brief—minutes to a few hours—episodes of depression during manic episodes.

Depressive Episodes

A depressed mood and a loss of interest or pleasure are the key symptoms of depression. Patients may say that they feel blue, hopeless, in the dumps, or worthless. For a patient, the depressed mood often has a distinct quality that differentiates it from the normal emotion of sadness or grief. Patients often describe the symptom of depression as one of agonizing emotional pain and sometimes complain about being unable to cry, a symptom that resolves as they improve.

About two-thirds of all depressed patients contemplate suicide, and 10 to 15 percent commit suicide. Those recently hospitalized with a suicide attempt or suicidal ideation have a higher lifetime risk of successful suicide than those never hospitalized for suicidal ideation. Some depressed patients sometimes seem unaware of their depression and do not complain of a mood disturbance even though they exhibit withdrawal from family, friends, and activities that previously interested them. Almost all depressed patients (97 percent) complain about reduced energy; they have difficulty finishing tasks, are impaired at school and work, and have less motivation to undertake new projects. About 80 percent of patients complain of trouble sleeping, especially early morning awakening (i.e., terminal insomnia) and multiple awakenings at night, during which they ruminate about their problems. Many patients have decreased appetite and weight loss, but others experience increased appetite and weight gain and sleep longer than usual. These patients are classified as having atypical features.

Anxiety, a common symptom of depression, affects as many as 90 percent of all depressed patients. The various changes in food intake and rest can aggravate coexisting medical illnesses such as diabetes, hypertension, chronic obstructive lung disease, and heart disease. Other vegetative symptoms include abnormal menses and decreased interest and performance in sexual activities. Sexual problems can sometimes lead to inappropriate referrals, such as to marital counseling and sex therapy, when clinicians fail to recognize the underlying depressive disorder. Anxiety (including panic attacks), alcohol abuse, and somatic complaints (e.g., constipation and headaches) often complicate the treatment of depression. About 50 percent of all patients describe a diurnal variation in their symptoms, with increased severity in the morning and lessening of symptoms by evening. Cognitive symptoms include subjective reports of an inability to concentrate (84 percent of patients in one study) and impairments in thinking (67 percent of patients in another study).

Depression in Children and Adolescents. School phobia and excessive clinging to parents may be symptoms of depression in children. Poor academic performance, substance abuse, antisocial behavior, sexual promiscuity, truancy, and running away may be symptoms of depression in adolescents.

Depression in Older People. Depression is more common in older persons than it is in the general population. Various studies have reported prevalence rates ranging from 25 percent to almost 50 percent, although the percentage of these cases that are caused by major depressive disorder is uncertain. Several studies indicate that depression in older persons may be correlated with low socioeconomic status, the loss of a spouse, a concurrent physical illness, and social isolation. Other studies have indicated that depression in older persons is underdiagnosed and undertreated, perhaps particularly by general practitioners. The underrecognition of depression in older persons may occur because the disorder appears more often with somatic complaints in older, than in younger, age groups. Further, ageism may influence and cause clinicians to accept depressive symptoms as normal in older patients.

Manic Episodes

An elevated, expansive, or irritable mood is the hallmark of a manic episode. The elevated mood is euphoric and often infectious and can even cause a countertransferential denial of illness by an inexperienced clinician. Although uninvolved persons may not recognize the unusual nature of a patient's mood, those who know the patient recognize it as abnormal. Alternatively, the mood may be irritable, especially when a patient's overtly ambitious plans are thwarted. Patients often exhibit a change of predominant mood from euphoria early in the course of the illness to later irritability.

The treatment of manic patients in an inpatient ward can be complicated by their testing of the limits of ward rules, tendency to shift responsibility for their acts onto others, exploitation of the weaknesses of others, and propensity to create conflicts among staff members. Outside the hospital, manic patients often drink alcohol excessively, perhaps in an attempt to self-medicate. Their disinhibited nature is reflected in excessive use of the telephone, especially in making long-distance calls during the early morning hours.

Pathological gambling, a tendency to disrobe in public places, wearing clothing and jewelry of bright colors in unusual or outlandish combinations, and inattention to small details (e.g., forgetting to hang up the telephone) are also symptomatic of the disorder. Patients act impulsively and at the same time with a sense of conviction and purpose. They are often preoccupied by religious, political, financial, sexual, or persecutory ideas that can evolve into complex delusional systems. Occasionally, manic patients become regressed and play with their urine and feces.

Mania in Adolescents. Mania in adolescents is often misdiagnosed as antisocial personality disorder or schizophrenia. Symptoms of mania in adolescents may include psychosis, alcohol or other substance abuse, suicide attempts, academic problems, philosophical brooding, OCD symptoms, multiple somatic complaints, marked irritability resulting in fights, and other antisocial behaviors. Although many of these symptoms are seen in normal adolescents, severe or persistent symptoms should cause clinicians to consider bipolar I disorder in the differential diagnosis.

Bipolar II Disorder

The clinical features of bipolar II disorder are those of major depressive disorder combined with those of a hypomanic episode. Although the data are limited, a few studies indicate that bipolar II disorder is associated with more marital disruption and with onset at an earlier age than bipolar I disorder. Evidence also indicates that patients with bipolar II disorder are at greater risk of both attempting and completing suicide than patients with bipolar I disorder and major depressive disorder.

Coexisting Disorders

Anxiety. In the anxiety disorders, DSM-5 notes the existence of mixed anxiety–depressive disorder. Significant symptoms of anxiety can and often do coexist with significant symptoms of depression. Whether patients who exhibit significant symptoms of both anxiety and depression are affected by two distinct disease processes or by a single disease process that produces both sets of symptoms is not yet resolved. Patients of both types may constitute the group of patients with mixed anxiety–depressive disorder.

Alcohol Dependence. Alcohol dependence frequently coexists with mood disorders. Both patients with major depressive disorder and those with bipolar I disorder are likely to meet the diagnostic criteria for an alcohol use disorder. The available data indicate that alcohol dependence is more strongly associated with a coexisting diagnosis of depression in women than in men. In contrast, the genetic and family data about men who have both mood disorder and alcohol dependence indicate that they are likely to have two genetically distinct disease processes.

Other Substance-Related Disorders. Substance-related disorders other than alcohol dependence are also commonly associated with mood disorders. The abuse of substances may be involved in precipitating an episode of illness or, conversely, may represent patients' attempts to treat their own illnesses. Although manic patients seldom use sedatives to dampen their euphoria, depressed patients often use stimulants, such as cocaine and amphetamines, to relieve their depression.

Medical Conditions. Depression commonly coexists with medical conditions, especially in older persons. When depression and medical conditions coexist, clinicians must try to determine whether the underlying medical condition is pathophysiologically related to the depression or whether any drugs that the patient is taking for the medical condition are causing the depression. Many studies indicate that treatment of a coexisting major depressive disorder can improve the course of the underlying medical disorder, including cancer.

MENTAL STATUS EXAMINATION

General Description

Generalized psychomotor retardation is the most common symptom of depression, although psychomotor agitation is also seen, especially in older patients. Hand wringing and hair pulling are the most common symptoms of agitation. Classically, a depressed patient has a stooped posture, no spontaneous movements, and a downcast, averted gaze. On clinical examination, depressed patients exhibiting gross symptoms of psychomotor retardation may appear identical to patients with catatonic schizophrenia.

> Ms. A, a 34-year-old literature professor, presented to a mood clinic with the following complaint: "I am in a daze, confused, disoriented, staring. My thoughts do not flow, my mind is arrested.... I seem to lack any sense of direction, purpose.... I have such an inertia, I cannot assert myself. I cannot fight; I have no will."

Mood, Affect, and Feelings

Depression is the key symptom, although about 50 percent of patients deny depressive feelings and do not appear to be particularly depressed. Family members or employers often bring or send these patients for treatment because of social withdrawal and generally decreased activity.

Speech

Many depressed patients have decreased rate and volume of speech; they respond to questions with single words and exhibit delayed responses to questions. The examiner may literally have to wait 2 or 3 minutes for a response to a question.

Perceptual Disturbances

Depressed patients with delusions or hallucinations are said to have a major depressive episode with psychotic features. Even in the absence of delusions or hallucinations, some clinicians use the term *psychotic depression* for grossly regressed depressed patients—mute, not bathing, soiling. Such patients are probably better described as having catatonic features.

Delusions and hallucinations that are consistent with a depressed mood are said to be mood congruent. Mood-congruent delusions in a depressed person include those of guilt, sinfulness, worthlessness, poverty, failure, persecution, and terminal somatic illnesses (such as cancer and a "rotting" brain). The content of mood-incongruent delusions or hallucinations is not consistent with a depressed mood. For example, a mood-incongruent delusion in a depressed person might involve grandiose themes of exaggerated power, knowledge, and worth. When that occurs, a schizophrenic disorder should be considered.

> A 42-year-old civil servant said that she was so paralyzed by depression that she felt that she had no personal initiative and volition left; she believed that some malignant force had taken over her actions and that it was commenting on every action that she was undertaking. The patient recovered fully with thymoleptic medication. There is no reason to believe that, in this patient, the feelings of somatic passability and running commentary indicated a schizophrenic process.

Thought

Depressed patients customarily have negative views of the world and of themselves. Their thought content often includes nondelusional ruminations about loss, guilt, suicide, and death. About 10 percent of all depressed patients have marked symptoms of a thought disorder, usually thought blocking and profound poverty of content.

Sensorium and Cognition

Orientation. Most depressed patients are oriented to person, place, and time, although some may not have sufficient energy or interest to answer questions about these subjects during an interview.

Memory. About 50 to 75 percent of all depressed patients have a cognitive impairment, sometimes referred to as *depressive pseudodementia.* Such patients commonly complain of impaired concentration and forgetfulness.

Impulse Control

About 10 to 15 percent of all depressed patients commit suicide, and about two-thirds have suicidal ideation. Depressed patients with psychotic features occasionally consider killing a person as a result of their delusional systems, but the most severely depressed patients often lack the motivation or the energy to act in an impulsive or violent way. Patients with depressive disorders are at increased risk of suicide as they begin to improve and regain the energy needed to plan and carry out a suicide (paradoxical suicide). It is usually clinically unwise to give a depressed patient a large prescription for a large number of antidepressants, especially tricyclic drugs, at the time of their discharge from the hospital. Similarly, drugs that may be activating, such as fluoxetine, may be prescribed in such a way that the energizing qualities are minimized (e.g., be given a benzodiazepine at the same time).

Judgment and Insight

Judgment is best assessed by reviewing patients' actions in the recent past and their behavior during the interview. Depressed patients' descriptions of their disorder are often hyperbolic; they overemphasize their symptoms, their disorder, and their life problems. It is difficult to convince such patients that improvement is possible.

Reliability

In interviews and conversations, depressed patients overemphasize the bad and minimize the good. A common clinical mistake is to unquestioningly believe a depressed patient who states that a previous trial of antidepressant medications did not work. Such statements may be false, and they require confirmation from another source. Psychiatrists should not view patients' misinformation as an intentional fabrication; the admission of any hopeful information may be impossible for a person in a depressed state of mind.

Objective Rating Scales for Depression

Objective rating scales for depression can be useful in clinical practice for documenting the depressed patient's clinical state.

ZUNG. The Zung Self-Rating Depression Scale is a 20-item report scale. A normal score is 34 or less; a depressed score is 50 or more. The scale provides a global index of the intensity of a patient's depressive symptoms, including the affective expression of depression.

RASKIN. The Raskin Depression Scale is a clinician-rated scale that measures the severity of a patient's depression, as reported by the patient and as observed by the physician, on a 5-point scale of three dimensions: verbal report, displayed behavior, and secondary symptoms. The scale has a range of 3 to 13; a normal score is 3, and a depressed score is 7 or more.

HAMILTON. The Hamilton Rating Scale for Depression (HAM-D) is a widely used depression scale with up to 24 items, each of which is rated 0 to 4 or 0 to 2, with a total score of 0 to 76. The clinician evaluates the patient's answers to questions about feelings of guilt, thoughts of suicide, sleep habits, and other symptoms of depression, and the ratings are derived from the clinical interview.

Manic Episodes

Manic patients are excited, talkative, sometimes amusing, and frequently hyperactive. At times, they are grossly psychotic and disorganized and require physical restraints and the intramuscular injection of sedating drugs.

Mood, Affect, and Feelings

Manic patients classically are euphoric, but they can also be irritable, especially when mania has been present for some time. They also have a low frustration tolerance, which can lead to feelings of anger and hostility. Manic patients may be emotionally labile, switching from laughter to irritability to depression in minutes or hours.

Speech

Manic patients cannot be interrupted while they are speaking, and they are often intrusive nuisances to those around them. Their speech is often disturbed. As the mania gets more intense, speech becomes louder, more rapid, and difficult to interpret. As the activated state increases, their speech is filled with puns, jokes, rhymes, plays on words, and irrelevancies. At a still greater activity level, associations become loosened, the ability to concentrate fades, and flight of ideas, clanging, and neologisms appear. In acute manic excitement, speech can be totally incoherent and indistinguishable from that of a person with schizophrenia.

Perceptual Disturbances

Delusions occur in 75 percent of all manic patients. Mood-congruent manic delusions are often concerned with great wealth, extraordinary abilities, or power. Bizarre and mood-incongruent delusions and hallucinations also appear in mania.

A 29-year-old female college graduate, mother of two children, and wife of a bank president, had experienced several manic and retarded depressive episodes that had responded to lithium carbonate. She was referred to the author because she had developed the delusion that she had been involved in an international plot. Careful probing revealed that the delusion represented further elaboration, in a rather fantastic fashion, of a grandiose delusion that she had experienced during her last postpartum manic episode. She believed that she had played an important role in uncovering the plot, thereby becoming a national hero. Nobody knew about it, she contended, because the circumstances of the plot were top secret. She further believed that she had saved her country from the international scheme and suspected that she was singled out for persecution by the perpetrators of the plot. At one point, she had even entertained the idea that the plotters sent special radio communications to intercept and interrupt her thoughts. As is typical in such cases, she was on a heavy dosage of a lithium–antipsychotic combination. The consultation was requested because the primary mood symptoms were under control, yet, she had not given up her grandiose delusion. She flippantly remarked, "I must be crazy to believe in my involvement in an international plot," but she could not help but believe in it. Over several months, seen typically in 60-minute sessions weekly, the patient had developed sufficient trust that the author could gently challenge her beliefs.

She was, in effect, told that her self-professed role in the international scheme was highly implausible and that someone with her superior education and high social standing could not entertain a belief, to use her own words, "as crazy as that." She eventually broke into tears, saying that everyone in her family was so accomplished and famous that to keep up with them she had to be involved in something grand; in effect, the international scheme, she said, was her only claim to fame: "Nobody ever gives me credit for raising two kids, and throwing parties for my husband's business colleagues: My mother is a dean, my older brother holds high political office; my sister is a medical researcher with five discoveries to her credit [all true], and who am I? Nothing. Now, do you understand why I need to be a national hero?" As she alternated, over subsequent months, between such momentary flashes of insight and delusional denial, antipsychotic medication was gradually discontinued. Maintained on lithium, she now only makes passing reference to the grand scheme. She was encouraged to pursue her career goal toward a master's degree in library science. *(Courtesy of HS Akiskal, M.D.)*

Thought. The manic patient's thought content includes themes of self-confidence and self-aggrandizement. Manic patients are often easily distracted, and their cognitive functioning in the manic state is characterized by an unrestrained and accelerated flow of ideas.

Sensorium and Cognition. Although the cognitive deficits of patients with schizophrenia have been much discussed, less has been written about similar deficits in patients with bipolar I disorder. These deficits can be interpreted as reflecting diffuse cortical dysfunction; subsequent work may localize the abnormal areas. Grossly, orientation and memory are intact, although some manic patients may be so euphoric that they answer questions testing orientation incorrectly. Emil Kraepelin called the symptom "delirious mania."

Impulse Control. About 75 percent of all manic patients are assaultive or threatening. Manic patients do attempt suicide and homicide, but the incidence of these behaviors is unknown.

Judgment and Insight. Impaired judgment is a hallmark of manic patients. They may break laws about credit cards, sexual activities, and finances and sometimes involve their families in financial ruin. Manic patients also have little insight into their disorder.

Reliability. Manic patients are notoriously unreliable in their information. Because lying and deceit are common in mania, inexperienced clinicians may treat manic patients with inappropriate disdain.

DIFFERENTIAL DIAGNOSIS

Major Depressive Disorder

Medical Disorders. The diagnosis of mood disorder due to a general medical condition must be considered. Failure to obtain a good clinical history or to consider the context of a patient's current life situation can lead to diagnostic errors. Clinicians should have depressed adolescents tested for mononucleosis, and patients who are markedly overweight or underweight should be tested for adrenal and thyroid dysfunctions. Homosexuals, bisexual men, prostitutes, and persons who abuse a substance intravenously should be tested for acquired immune deficiency syndrome (AIDS). Older patients should be evaluated for viral pneumonia and other medical conditions.

Many neurological and medical disorders and pharmacological agents can produce symptoms of depression. Patients with depressive disorders often first visit their general practitioners with somatic complaints. Most medical causes of depressive disorders can be detected with a comprehensive medical history, a complete physical and neurological examination, and routine blood and urine tests. The workup should include tests for thyroid and adrenal functions because disorders of both of these endocrine systems can appear as depressive disorders. In substance-induced mood disorder, a reasonable rule of thumb is that any drug a depressed patient is taking should be considered a potential factor in the mood disorder. Cardiac drugs, antihypertensives, sedatives, hypnotics, antipsychotics, antiepileptics, antiparkinsonian drugs, analgesics, antibacterials, and antineoplastics are all commonly associated with depressive symptoms.

NEUROLOGICAL CONDITIONS. The most common neurological problems that manifest depressive symptoms are Parkinson's disease, dementing illnesses (including dementia of the Alzheimer's type), epilepsy, cerebrovascular diseases, and tumors. About 50 to 75 percent of all patients with Parkinson's disease have marked symptoms of depressive disorder that do not correlate with the patient's physical disability, age, or duration of illness but do correlate with the presence of abnormalities found on neuropsychological tests. The symptoms of depressive disorder can be masked by the almost identical motor symptoms of Parkinson's disease. Depressive symptoms often respond to antidepressant drugs or ECT. The interictal changes associated with temporal lobe epilepsy can mimic a depressive disorder, especially if the epileptic focus is on the right side. Depression is a common complicating feature of cerebrovascular diseases, particularly in the 2 years after the episode. Depression is more common in anterior brain lesions than in posterior brain lesions and, in both cases, often responds to antidepressant medications. Tumors of the diencephalic and temporal regions are particularly likely to be associated with depressive disorder symptoms.

PSEUDODEMENTIA. Clinicians can usually differentiate the pseudodementia of major depressive disorder from the dementia of a disease, such as dementia of the Alzheimer's type, on clinical grounds. The cognitive symptoms in major depressive disorder have a sudden onset, and other symptoms of the disorder, such as self-reproach, are also present. A diurnal variation in the cognitive problems, which is not seen in primary dementias, may occur. Whereas depressed patients with cognitive difficulties often do not try to answer questions ("I don't know"), patients with dementia may confabulate. During an interview, depressed patients can sometimes be coached and encouraged into remembering, an ability that demented patients lack.

Mental Disorders

Depression can be a feature of virtually any mental disorder, but the mental disorders listed in Table 5.1–5 deserve particular consideration in the differential diagnosis.

OTHER MOOD DISORDERS. Clinicians must consider a range of diagnostic categories before arriving at a final diagnosis.

Table 5.1–5
Mental Disorders That Commonly Have Depressive Features

Adjustment disorder with depressed mood
Alcohol use disorders
Anxiety disorders
Generalized anxiety disorder
Mixed anxiety–depressive disorder
Panic disorder
Posttraumatic stress disorder
Obsessive-compulsive disorder
Eating disorders
Anorexia nervosa
Bulimia nervosa
Mood disorders
Bipolar I disorder
Bipolar II disorder
Cyclothymic disorder
Dysthymic disorder
Major depressive disorder
Minor depressive disorder
Mood disorder due to a general medical condition
Recurrent brief depressive disorder
Substance-induced mood disorder
Schizophrenia
Schizophreniform disorder
Somatoform disorders (especially somatization disorder)

Mood disorder caused by a general medical condition and substance-induced mood disorder must be ruled out. Clinicians must also determine whether a patient has had episodes of mania-like symptoms, indicating bipolar I disorder (complete manic and depressive syndromes), bipolar II disorder (recurrent major depressive episodes with hypomania), or cyclothymic disorder (incomplete depressive and manic syndromes). If a patient's symptoms are limited to those of depression, clinicians must assess the severity and duration of the symptoms to differentiate among major depressive disorder (complete depressive syndrome for 2 weeks), minor depressive disorder (incomplete but episodic depressive syndrome), recurrent brief depressive disorder (complete depressive syndrome but for less than 2 weeks per episode), and dysthymic disorder (incomplete depressive syndrome without clear episodes).

OTHER MENTAL DISORDERS. Substance-related disorders, psychotic disorders, eating disorders, adjustment disorders, somatoform disorders, and anxiety disorders are all commonly associated with depressive symptoms and should be considered in the differential diagnosis of a patient with depressive symptoms. Perhaps the most difficult differential is that between anxiety disorders with depression and depressive disorders with marked anxiety. An abnormal result on the dexamethasone-suppression test, the presence of shortened REM latency on a sleep electroencephalogram (EEG), and a negative lactate infusion test result support a diagnosis of major depressive disorder in particularly ambiguous cases.

UNCOMPLICATED BEREAVEMENT. Uncomplicated bereavement is not considered a mental disorder even though about one-third of all bereaved spouses for a time meet the diagnostic criteria for major depressive disorder. Some patients with uncomplicated bereavement do develop major depressive disorder, but the diagnosis is not made unless no resolution of the grief occurs. The differentiation is based on the symptoms' severity and length. In major depressive disorder, common symptoms that evolve from unresolved bereavement are a morbid preoccupation with worthlessness; suicidal ideation; feelings that the person has committed an act (not just an omission) that caused the spouse's death; mummification (keeping the deceased's belongings exactly as they were); and a particularly severe anniversary reaction, which sometimes includes a suicide attempt.

In severe forms of bereavement depression, the patient simply pines away, unable to live without the departed person, usually a spouse. Such persons do have a serious medical condition. Their immune function is often depressed, and their cardiovascular status is precarious. Death can ensue within a few months of that of a spouse, especially among elderly men. Such considerations suggest that it would be clinically unwise to withhold antidepressants from many persons experiencing such an intense mourning.

A 75-year-old widow was brought to treatment by her daughter because of severe insomnia and total loss of interest in daily routines after her husband's death 1 year before. She had been agitated for the first 2 to 3 months and thereafter "sank into total inactivity—not wanting to get out of bed, not wanting to do anything, not wanting to go out." According to her daughter, she was married at 21 years of age, had four children, and had been a housewife until her husband's death from a heart attack. Her past psychiatric history was negative; premorbid adjustment had been characterized by compulsive traits. During the interview, she was dressed in black; appeared moderately slowed; and sobbed intermittently, saying "I search everywhere for him.... I don't find him." When asked about life, she said, "Everything I see is black." Although she expressed no interest in food, she did not seem to have lost an appreciable amount of weight. Her DST [dexamethasone suppression test] result was 18 mg/dL. The patient declined psychiatric care, stating that she "preferred to join her husband rather than get well." She was too religious to commit suicide, but by refusing treatment, she felt that she would "pine away... find relief in death and reunion." *(Courtesy of HS Akiskal, M.D.)*

Schizophrenia. Much has been published about the clinical difficulty of distinguishing a manic episode from schizophrenia. Although difficult, a differential diagnosis is possible. Merriment, elation, and infectiousness of mood are much more common in manic episodes than in schizophrenia. The combination of a manic mood, rapid or pressured speech, and hyperactivity weighs heavily toward a diagnosis of a manic episode. The onset in a manic episode is often rapid and is perceived as a marked change from a patient's previous behavior. Half of all patients with bipolar I disorder have a family history of mood disorder. Catatonic features may be part of a depressive phase of bipolar I disorder. When evaluating patients with catatonia, clinicians should look carefully for a past history of manic or depressive episodes and for a family history of mood disorders. Manic symptoms in persons from minority groups (particularly blacks and Hispanics) are often misdiagnosed as schizophrenic symptoms.

Medical Conditions. In contrast to depressive symptoms, which are present in many psychiatric disorders, manic symptoms are more distinctive, although they can be caused by a wide range of medical and neurological conditions and substances.

Antidepressant treatment can also be associated with the precipitation of mania in some patients.

Bipolar I Disorder

When a patient with bipolar I disorder has a depressive episode, the differential diagnosis is the same as that for a patient being considered for a diagnosis of major depressive disorder. When a patient is manic, however, the differential diagnosis includes bipolar I disorder, bipolar II disorder, cyclothymic disorder, mood disorder caused by a general medical condition, and substance-induced mood disorder. For manic symptoms, borderline, narcissistic, histrionic, and antisocial personality disorders need special consideration.

Bipolar II Disorder

The differential diagnosis of patients being evaluated for a mood disorder should include the other mood disorders, psychotic disorders, and borderline disorder. The differentiation between major depressive disorder and bipolar I disorder, on one hand, and bipolar II disorder, on the other hand, rests on the clinical evaluation of the mania-like episodes. Clinicians should not mistake euthymia in a chronically depressed patient for a hypomanic or manic episode. Patients with borderline personality disorder often have a severely disrupted life, similar to that of patients with bipolar II disorder, because of the multiple episodes of significant mood disorder symptoms.

Major Depressive Disorder versus Bipolar Disorder

The question of whether a patient has major depressive disorder or bipolar disorder has emerged as a major challenge in clinical practice. Numerous studies have shown that bipolar disorder is not only confused with personality, substance use, and schizophrenic disorders but also with depressive and anxiety disorders. Certain features—especially in combination—are predictive of bipolar disorder (Table 5.1–6).

Table 5.1–6
Clinical Features Predictive of Bipolar Disorder

- Early age at onset
- Psychotic depression before 25 years of age
- Postpartum depression, especially one with psychotic features
- Rapid onset and offset of depressive episodes of short duration (<3 months)
- Recurrent depression (more than five episodes)
- Depression with marked psychomotor retardation
- Atypical features (reverse vegetative signs)
- Seasonality
- Bipolar family history
- High-density, three-generation pedigrees
- Trait mood lability (cyclothymia)
- Hyperthymic temperament
- Hypomania associated with antidepressants
- Repeated (at least three times) loss of efficacy of antidepressants after initial response
- Depressive mixed state (with psychomotor excitement, irritable hostility, racing thoughts, and sexual arousal *during* major depression)

More broad indicators of bipolarity include the following conditions, none of which, by itself, confirms a bipolar diagnosis, but should raise clinical suspicion in that direction: agitated depression, cyclical depression, episodic sleep dysregulation, or a combination of these; refractory depression (failed antidepressants from three different classes); depression in someone with an extroverted profession, periodic impulsivity, such as gambling, sexual misconduct, and wanderlust, or periodic irritability, suicidal crises, or both; and depression with erratic personality disorders.

COURSE AND PROGNOSIS

Studies of the course and prognosis of mood disorders have generally concluded that mood disorders tend to have long courses and that patients tend to have relapses. Although mood disorders are often considered benign in contrast to schizophrenia, they exact a profound toll on affected patients.

Major Depressive Disorder

Course

ONSET. About 50 percent of patients having their first episode of major depressive disorder exhibited significant depressive symptoms before the first identified episode. Therefore, early identification and treatment of early symptoms may prevent the development of a full depressive episode. Although symptoms may have been present, patients with major depressive disorder usually have not had a premorbid personality disorder. The first depressive episode occurs before the age of 40 years in about 50 percent of patients. A later onset is associated with the absence of a family history of mood disorders, antisocial personality disorder, and alcohol abuse.

DURATION. An untreated depressive episode lasts 6 to 13 months; most treated episodes last about 3 months. The withdrawal of antidepressants before 3 months has elapsed almost always results in the return of the symptoms. As the course of the disorder progresses, patients tend to have more frequent episodes that last longer. Over a 20-year period, the mean number of episodes is five or six.

DEVELOPMENT OF MANIC EPISODES. About 5 to 10 percent of patients with an initial diagnosis of major depressive disorder have a manic episode 6 to 10 years after the first depressive episode. The mean age for this switch is 32 years, and it often occurs after two to four depressive episodes. Although the data are inconsistent and controversial, some clinicians report that the depression of patients who are later classified as having bipolar I disorder is often characterized by hypersomnia, psychomotor retardation, psychotic symptoms, a history of postpartum episodes, a family history of bipolar I disorder, and a history of antidepressant-induced hypomania.

Prognosis. Major depressive disorder is not a benign disorder. It tends to be chronic, and patients tend to relapse. Patients who have been hospitalized for a first episode of major depressive disorder have about a 50 percent chance of recovering in the first year. The percentage of patients recovering after repeated hospitalization decreases with passing time. Many unrecovered patients remain affected with dysthymic disorder. About 25 percent of patients experience a recurrence of major depressive disorder in the first 6 months after release from a hospital, about 30 to 50 percent in the following 2 years, and about 50 to 75 percent in 5 years. The incidence of relapse is lower than these figures in patients who continue prophylactic psychopharmacological treatment and in patients who have had only one or two depressive episodes. Generally, as a patient experiences more and more depressive episodes, the time between the episodes decreases, and the severity of each episode increases.

PROGNOSTIC INDICATORS. Many studies have focused on identifying both good and bad prognostic indicators in the course of major depressive disorder. Mild episodes, the absence of psychotic symptoms, and a short hospital stay are good prognostic indicators. Psychosocial indicators of a good course include a history of solid friendships during adolescence, stable family functioning, and generally sound social functioning for the 5 years preceding the illness. Additional good prognostic signs are the absence of a comorbid psychiatric disorder and of a personality disorder, no more than one previous hospitalization for major depressive disorder, and an advanced age of onset. The possibility of a poor prognosis is increased by coexisting dysthymic disorder, abuse of alcohol and other substances, anxiety disorder symptoms, and a history of more than one previous depressive episode. Men are more likely than women to experience a chronically impaired course.

Bipolar I Disorder

Course. The natural history of bipolar I disorder is such that it is often useful to make a graph of a patient's disorder and to keep it up to date as treatment progresses. Although cyclothymic disorder is sometimes diagnosed retrospectively in patients with bipolar I disorder, no identified personality traits are specifically associated with bipolar I disorder.

Bipolar I disorder most often starts with depression (75 percent of the time in women, 67 percent in men) and is a recurring disorder. Most patients experience both depressive and manic episodes, although 10 to 20 percent experience only manic episodes. The manic episodes typically have a rapid onset (hours or days) but may evolve over a few weeks. An untreated manic episode lasts about 3 months; therefore, clinicians should not discontinue giving drugs before that time. Of persons who have a single manic episode, 90 percent are likely to have another. As the disorder progresses, the time between episodes often decreases. After about five episodes, however, the interepisode interval often stabilizes at 6 to 9 months. Of persons with bipolar disorder, 5 to 15 percent have four or more episodes per year and can be classified as rapid cyclers.

Bipolar I Disorder in Children and Older Persons.

Bipolar I disorder can affect both the very young and older persons. The incidence of bipolar I disorder in children and adolescents is about 1 percent, and the onset can be as early as age 8 years. Common misdiagnoses are schizophrenia and oppositional defiant disorder.

Bipolar I disorder with such an early onset is associated with a poor prognosis. Manic symptoms are common in older persons, although the range of causes is broad and includes nonpsychiatric medical conditions, dementia, and delirium, as well as bipolar I disorder. The onset of true bipolar I disorder in older persons is relatively uncommon.

Prognosis. Patients with bipolar I disorder have a poorer prognosis than do patients with major depressive disorder. About 40 to 50 percent of patients with bipolar I disorder may have a second manic episode within 2 years of the first episode. Although lithium prophylaxis improves the course and prognosis of bipolar I disorder, probably only 50 to 60 percent of patients achieve significant control of their symptoms with lithium. One 4-year follow-up study of patients with bipolar I disorder found that a premorbid poor occupational status, alcohol dependence, psychotic features, depressive features, interepisode depressive features, and male gender were all factors that contributed to a poor prognosis. Short duration of manic episodes, advanced age of onset, few suicidal thoughts, and few coexisting psychiatric or medical problems predict a better outcome.

About 7 percent of patients with bipolar I disorder do not have a recurrence of symptoms; 45 percent have more than one episode, and 40 percent have a chronic disorder. Patients may have from 2 to 30 manic episodes, although the mean number is about nine. About 40 percent of all patients have more than ten episodes. On long-term follow-up, 15 percent of all patients with bipolar I disorder are well, 45 percent are well but have multiple relapses, 30 percent are in partial remission, and 10 percent are chronically ill. One-third of all patients with bipolar I disorder have chronic symptoms and evidence of significant social decline.

Bipolar II Disorder

The course and prognosis of bipolar II disorder indicate that the diagnosis is stable because there is a high likelihood that patients with bipolar II disorder will have the same diagnosis up to 5 years later. Bipolar II disorder is a chronic disease that warrants long-term treatment strategies.

TREATMENT

Treatment of patients with mood disorders should be directed toward several goals. First, the patient's safety must be guaranteed. Second, a complete diagnostic evaluation of the patient is necessary. Third, a treatment plan that addresses not only the immediate symptoms but also the patient's prospective well-being should be initiated. Although current treatment emphasizes pharmacotherapy and psychotherapy addressed to the individual patient, stressful life events are also associated with increases in relapse rates. Thus, treatment should address the number and severity of stressors in patients' lives.

Overall, the treatment of mood disorders is rewarding for psychiatrists. Specific treatments are now available for both manic and depressive episodes, and data indicate that prophylactic treatment is also effective. Because the prognosis for each episode is good, optimism is always warranted and is welcomed by both the patient and the patient's family. Mood disorders are chronic, however, and the psychiatrist must educate the patient and the family about future treatment strategies.

Hospitalization

The first and most critical decision a physician must make is whether to hospitalize a patient or attempt outpatient treatment. Clear indications for hospitalization are the risk of suicide or homicide, a patient's grossly reduced ability to get food and shelter, and the need for diagnostic procedures. A history of rapidly progressing symptoms and the rupture of a patient's usual support systems are also indications for hospitalization.

A physician may safely treat mild depression or hypomania in the office if he or she evaluates the patient frequently. Clinical signs of impaired judgment, weight loss, or insomnia should be minimal. The patient's support system should be strong, neither overinvolved nor withdrawing from the patient. Any adverse changes in the patient's symptoms or behavior or the attitude of the patient's support system may suffice to warrant hospitalization.

Patients with mood disorders are often unwilling to enter a hospital voluntarily and may have to be involuntarily committed. These patients often cannot make decisions because of their slowed thinking, negative *Weltanschauung* (world view), and hopelessness. Patients who are manic often have such a complete lack of insight into their disorder that hospitalization seems absolutely absurd to them.

Psychosocial Therapy

Although most studies indicate—and most clinicians and researchers believe—that a combination of psychotherapy and pharmacotherapy is the most effective treatment for major depressive disorder, some data suggest another view: Either pharmacotherapy or psychotherapy alone is effective, at least in patients with mild major depressive episodes, and the regular use of combined therapy adds to the cost of treatment and exposes patients to unnecessary adverse effects.

Three types of short-term psychotherapies—cognitive therapy, interpersonal therapy, and behavior therapy—have been studied to determine their efficacy in the treatment of major depressive disorder. Although its efficacy in treating major depressive disorder is not as well researched as these three therapies, psychoanalytically oriented psychotherapy has long been used for depressive disorders, and many clinicians use the technique as their primary method. What differentiates the three short-term psychotherapy methods from the psychoanalytically oriented approach are the active and directive roles of the therapist, the directly recognizable goals, and the end points for short-term therapy.

Accumulating evidence is encouraging about the efficacy of dynamic therapy. In a randomized, controlled trial comparing psychodynamic therapy with cognitive behavior therapy, the outcome of the depressed patients was the same in the two treatments.

The National Institute of Mental Health (NIMH) Treatment of Depression Collaborative Research Program found the following predictors of response to various treatments: low social dysfunction suggested a good response to interpersonal therapy, low cognitive dysfunction suggested a good response to cognitive-behavioral therapy and pharmacotherapy, high work dysfunction suggested a good response to pharmacotherapy, and high depression severity suggested a good response to interpersonal therapy and pharmacotherapy.

Cognitive Therapy. Cognitive therapy, originally developed by Aaron Beck, focuses on the cognitive distortions postulated to be present in major depressive disorder. Such distortions include selective attention to the negative aspects of circumstances and unrealistically morbid inferences about consequences. For example, apathy and low energy result from a patient's expectation of failure in all areas. The goal of cognitive therapy is to alleviate depressive episodes and prevent their recurrence by helping patients identify and test negative cognitions; develop alternative, flexible, and positive ways of thinking; and rehearse new cognitive and behavioral responses.

Studies have shown that cognitive therapy is effective in the treatment of major depressive disorder. Most studies found that cognitive therapy is equal in efficacy to pharmacotherapy and is associated with fewer adverse effects and better follow-up than pharmacotherapy. Some of the best controlled studies have indicated that the combination of cognitive therapy and pharmacotherapy is more efficacious than either therapy alone, although other studies have not found that additive effect. At least one study, the NIMH Treatment of Depression Collaborative Research Program, found that pharmacotherapy, either alone or with psychotherapy, may be the treatment of choice for patients with severe major depressive episodes.

Interpersonal Therapy. Interpersonal therapy, developed by Gerald Klerman, focuses on one or two of a patient's current interpersonal problems. This therapy is based on two assumptions. First, current interpersonal problems are likely to have their roots in early dysfunctional relationships. Second, current interpersonal problems are likely to be involved in precipitating or perpetuating the current depressive symptoms. Controlled trials have indicated that interpersonal therapy is effective in the treatment of major depressive disorder and, not surprisingly, may be specifically helpful in addressing interpersonal problems. Some studies indicate that interpersonal therapy may be the most effective method for severe major depressive episodes when the treatment choice is psychotherapy alone.

The interpersonal therapy program usually consists of 12 to 16 weekly sessions and is characterized by an active therapeutic approach. Intrapsychic phenomena, such as defense mechanisms and internal conflicts, are not addressed. Discrete behaviors—such as lack of assertiveness, impaired social skills, and distorted thinking—may be addressed but only in the context of their meaning in, or their effect on, interpersonal relationships.

Behavior Therapy. Behavior therapy is based on the hypothesis that maladaptive behavioral patterns result in a person's receiving little positive feedback and perhaps outright rejection from society. By addressing maladaptive behaviors in therapy, patients learn to function in the world in such a way that they receive positive reinforcement. Behavior therapy for major depressive disorder has not yet been the subject of many controlled studies. The limited data indicate that it is an effective treatment for major depressive disorder.

Psychoanalytically Oriented Therapy. The psychoanalytic approach to mood disorders is based on psychoanalytic theories about depression and mania. The goal of psychoanalytic psychotherapy is to effect a change in a patient's personality structure or character, not simply to alleviate symptoms.

Improvements in interpersonal trust, capacity for intimacy, coping mechanisms, the capacity to grieve, and the ability to experience a wide range of emotions are some of the aims of psychoanalytic therapy. Treatment often requires the patient to experience periods of heightened anxiety and distress during the course of therapy, which may continue for several years.

Family Therapy. Family therapy is not generally viewed as a primary therapy for the treatment of major depressive disorder, but increasing evidence indicates that helping a patient with a mood disorder to reduce and cope with stress can lessen the chance of a relapse. Family therapy is indicated if the disorder jeopardizes a patient's marriage or family functioning or if the mood disorder is promoted or maintained by the family situation. Family therapy examines the role of the mood-disordered member in the overall psychological well-being of the whole family; it also examines the role of the entire family in the maintenance of the patient's symptoms. Patients with mood disorders have a high rate of divorce, and about 50 percent of all spouses report that they would not have married or had children if they had known that the patient was going to develop a mood disorder.

Vagal Nerve Stimulation

Experimental stimulation of the vagus nerve in several studies designed for the treatment of epilepsy found that patients showed improved mood. This observation led to the use of left vagal nerve stimulation (VNS) using an electronic device implanted in the skin, similar to a cardiac pacemaker. Preliminary studies have shown that a number of patients with chronic, recurrent major depressive disorder went into remission when treated with VNS. The mechanism of action of VNS to account for improvement is unknown. The vagus nerve connects to the enteric nervous system and, when stimulated, may cause release of peptides that act as neurotransmitters. Extensive clinical trials are being conducted to determine the efficacy of VNS.

Transcranial Magnetic Stimulation

Transcranial magnetic stimulation (TMS) shows promise as a treatment for depression. It involves the use of very short pulses of magnetic energy to stimulate nerve cells in the brain. It is specifically indicated for the treatment of depression in adult patients who have failed to achieve satisfactory improvement from one prior antidepressant medication at or above the minimal effective dose and duration in the current episode.

Repetitive transcranial magnetic stimulation (rTMS) produces focal secondary electrical stimulation of targeted cortical regions. It is nonconvulsive, requires no anesthesia, has a safe side effect profile, and is not associated with cognitive side effects.

The patients do not require anesthesia or sedation and remain awake and alert. It is a 40-minute outpatient procedure that is prescribed by a psychiatrist and performed in a psychiatrist's office. The treatment is typically administered daily for 4 to 6 weeks. The most common adverse event related to treatment was scalp pain or discomfort.

TMS therapy is contraindicated in patients with implanted metallic devices or nonremovable metallic objects in or around the head.

Sleep Deprivation

Mood disorders are characterized by sleep disturbance. Mania tends to be characterized by a decreased need for sleep, but depression can be associated with either hypersomnia or insomnia. Sleep deprivation may precipitate mania in patients with bipolar I disorder and temporarily relieve depression in those who have unipolar depression. Approximately 60 percent of patients with depressive disorders exhibit significant but transient benefits from total sleep deprivation. The positive results are typically reversed by the next night of sleep. Several strategies have been used in an attempt to achieve a more sustained response to sleep deprivation. One method used serial total sleep deprivation with a day or two of normal sleep in between. This method does not achieve a sustained antidepressant response because the depression tends to return with normal sleep cycles. Another approach used phase delay in the time patients go to sleep each night, or partial sleep deprivation. In this method, patients may stay awake from 2 AM to 10 PM daily. Up to 50 percent of patients get same-day antidepressant effects from partial sleep deprivation, but this benefit also tends to wear off in time. In some reports, however, serial partial sleep deprivation has been used successfully to treat insomnia associated with depression. The third, and probably most effective, strategy combines sleep deprivation with pharmacological treatment of depression. A number of studies have suggested that total and partial sleep deprivation followed by immediate treatment with an antidepressant or lithium (Eskalith) sustains the antidepressant effects of sleep deprivation. Likewise, several reports have suggested that sleep deprivation accelerates the response to antidepressants, including fluoxetine (Prozac) and nortriptyline (Aventyl, Pamelor). Sleep deprivation has also been noted to improve premenstrual dysphoria. (Premenstrual dysphoric disorder, which is classified as a depressive disorder in DSM-5, is discussed in detail in Section 26.1, Psychiatry and Reproductive Medicine.)

Phototherapy

Phototherapy (light therapy) was introduced in 1984 as a treatment for SAD (mood disorder with seasonal pattern). In this disorder, patients typically experience depression as the photoperiod of the day decreases with advancing winter. Women represent at least 75 percent of all patients with seasonal depression, and the mean age of presentation is 40 years. Patients rarely present older than the age of 55 years with seasonal affective disorder.

Phototherapy typically involves exposing the affected patient to bright light in the range of 1,500 to 10,000 lux or more, typically with a light box that sits on a table or desk. Patients sit in front of the box for approximately 1 to 2 hours before dawn each day, although some patients may also benefit from exposure after dusk. Alternatively, some manufacturers have developed light visors, with a light source built into the brim of the hat. These light visors allow mobility, but recent controlled studies have questioned the use of this type of light exposure. Trials have typically lasted 1 week, but longer treatment durations may be associated with greater response.

Phototherapy tends to be well tolerated. Newer light sources tend to use lower light intensities and come equipped with filters; patients are instructed not to look directly at the light source. As with any effective antidepressant, phototherapy, on rare occasions, has been implicated in switching some depressed patients into mania or hypomania.

In addition to seasonal depression, the other major indication for phototherapy may be in sleep disorders. Phototherapy has been used to decrease the irritability and diminished functioning associated with shift work. Sleep disorders in geriatric patients have reportedly improved with exposure to bright light during the day. Likewise, some evidence suggests that jet lag might respond to light therapy. Preliminary data indicate that phototherapy may benefit some patients with OCD that has a seasonal variation.

Pharmacotherapy

After a diagnosis has been established, a pharmacological treatment strategy can be formulated. Accurate diagnosis is crucial because unipolar and bipolar spectrum disorders require different treatment regimens.

The objective of pharmacologic treatment is symptom remission, not just symptom reduction. Patients with residual symptoms, as opposed to full remission, are more likely to experience a relapse or recurrence of mood episodes and to experience ongoing impairment of daily functioning.

Major Depressive Disorder.

The use of specific pharmacotherapy approximately doubles the chances that a depressed patient will recover in 1 month. All currently available antidepressants may take up to 3 to 4 weeks to exert significant therapeutic effects, although they may begin to show their effects earlier. Choice of antidepressants is determined by the side effect profile least objectionable to a given patient's physical status, temperament, and lifestyle. That numerous classes of antidepressants (Table 5.1–7) are available, many with different mechanisms of action, represents indirect evidence for heterogeneity of putative biochemical lesions. Although the first antidepressant drugs, the monoamine oxidase inhibitors (MAOIs) and tricyclic antidepressants (TCAs), are still in use, newer compounds have made the treatment of depression more "clinician and patient friendly."

GENERAL CLINICAL GUIDELINES. The most common clinical mistake leading to an unsuccessful trial of an antidepressant drug is the use of too low a dosage for too short a time. Unless adverse events prevent it, the dosage of an antidepressant should be raised to the maximum recommended level and maintained at that level for at least 4 or 5 weeks before a drug trial is considered unsuccessful. Alternatively, if a patient is improving clinically on a low dosage of the drug, this dosage should not be raised unless clinical improvement stops before maximal benefit is obtained. When a patient does not begin to respond to appropriate dosages of a drug after 2 or 3 weeks, clinicians may decide to obtain a plasma concentration of the drug if the test is available for the particular drug being used. The test may indicate either noncompliance or particularly unusual pharmacokinetic disposition of the drug and may thereby suggest an alternative dosage.

DURATION AND PROPHYLAXIS. Antidepressant treatment should be maintained for at least 6 months or the length of a previous episode, whichever is greater. Prophylactic treatment with antidepressants is effective in reducing the number and severity of recurrences. One study concluded that when episodes are less than $2^1/_2$ years apart, prophylactic treatment for 5 years is probably indicated. Another factor suggesting prophylactic treatment is the seriousness of previous depressive episodes. Episodes that have involved significant suicidal ideation or impairment of psychosocial functioning may indicate that clinicians should consider prophylactic treatment. When antidepressant treatment is stopped, the drug dose should be tapered gradually over 1 to 2 weeks, depending on the half-life of the particular compound. Several studies indicate that maintenance antidepressant medication appears to be safe and effective for the treatment of chronic depression.

Prevention of new mood episodes (i.e., recurrences) is the aim of the maintenance phase of treatment. Only patients with recurrent or chronic depressions are candidates for maintenance treatment.

INITIAL MEDICATION SELECTION. The available antidepressants do not differ in overall efficacy, speed of response, or long-term effectiveness. Antidepressants, however, do differ in their pharmacology, drug–drug interactions, short- and long-term side effects, likelihood of discontinuation symptoms, and ease of dose adjustment. Failure to tolerate or to respond to one medication does not imply that other medications will also fail. Selection of the initial treatment depends on the chronicity of the condition, course of illness (a recurrent or chronic course is associated with increased likelihood of subsequent depressive symptoms without treatment), family history of illness and treatment response, symptom severity, concurrent general medical or other psychiatric conditions, prior treatment responses to other acute phase treatments, potential drug–drug interactions, and patient preference. In general, approximately 45 to 60 percent of all outpatients with uncomplicated (i.e., minimal psychiatric and general medical comorbidity), nonchronic, nonpsychotic major depressive disorder who begin treatment with medication respond (i.e., achieve at least a 50 percent reduction in baseline symptoms); however, only 35 to 50 percent achieve remission (i.e., the virtual absence of depressive symptoms).

TREATMENT OF DEPRESSIVE SUBTYPES. Clinical types of major depressive episodes may have varying responses to particular antidepressants or to drugs other than antidepressants. Patients with major depressive disorder with atypical features may preferentially respond to treatment with MAOIs or SSRIs. Antidepressants with dual action on both serotonergic and noradrenergic receptors demonstrate greater efficacy in melancholic depressions. Patients with seasonal winter depression can be treated with light therapy. Treatment of major depressive episodes with psychotic features may require a combination of an antidepressant and an atypical antipsychotic. Several studies have also shown that ECT is effective for this indication—perhaps more effective than pharmacotherapy. For those with atypical symptom features, strong evidence exists for the effectiveness of MAOIs. SSRIs and bupropion (Wellbutrin) are also of use in atypical depression.

COMORBID DISORDERS. The concurrent presence of another disorder can affect initial treatment selection. For example, the successful treatment of OCD associated with depressive symptoms usually results in remission of the depression. Similarly, when panic disorder occurs with major depression, medications

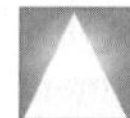

Table 5.1–7
Antidepressant Medications

Generic (Brand) Name	Usual Daily Dose (mg)	Common Side Effects	Clinical Caveats
NE Reuptake Inhibitors			
Desipramine (Norpramin, Pertofrane)	75–300	Drowsiness, insomnia, OSH, agitation, CA, weight ↑, anticholinergic[a]	Overdose may be fatal. Dose titration is needed.
Protriptyline (Vivactil)	20–60	Drowsiness, insomnia, OSH, agitation, CA, anticholinergic[a]	Overdose may be fatal. Dose titration is needed.
Nortriptyline (Aventyl, Pamelor)	40–200	Drowsiness, OSH, CA, weight ↑, anticholinergic[a]	Overdose may be fatal. Dose titration is needed.
Maprotiline (Ludiomil)	100–225	Drowsiness, CA, weight ↑, anticholinergic[a]	Overdose may be fatal. Dose titration is needed.
5-HT Reuptake Inhibitors			
Citalopram (Celexa)	20—60	All SSRIs may cause insomnia, agitation, sedation, GI distress, and sexual dysfunction	Many SSRIs inhibit various cytochrome P450 isoenzymes. They are better tolerated than tricyclics and have high safety in overdose. Shorter half-life SSRIs may be associated with discontinuation symptoms when abruptly stopped.
Escitalopram (Lexapro)	10—20		
Fluoxetine (Prozac)	10—40		
Fluvoxamine (Luvox)[b]	100—300		
Paroxetine (Paxil)	20—50		
Sertraline (Zoloft)	50—150		
Vortioxetine (Brintellix)	10–20		
NE and 5-HT Reuptake Inhibitors			
Amitriptyline (Elavil, Endep)	75–300	Drowsiness, OSH, CA, weight ↑, anticholinergic[a]	Overdose may be fatal. Dose titration is needed.
Doxepin (Triadapin, Sinequan)	75–300	Drowsiness, OSH, CA, weight ↑, anticholinergic[a]	Overdose may be fatal.
Imipramine (Tofranil)	75–300	Drowsiness, insomnia and agitation, OSH, CA, GI distress, weight ↑, anticholinergic[a]	Overdose may be fatal. Dose titration needed.
Trimipramine (Surmontil)	75–300	Drowsiness, OSH, CA, weight ↑, anticholinergic[a]	—
Venlafaxine (Effexor)	150–375	Sleep changes, GI distress, discontinuation syndrome	Higher doses may cause hypertension. Dose titration is needed. Abrupt discontinuation may result in discontinuation symptoms.
Duloxetine (Cymbalta)	30–60	GI distress, discontinuation syndrome	
Pre- and Postsynaptic Active Agents			
Nefazodone	300–600	Sedation	Dose titration is needed. No sexual dysfunction.
Mirtazapine (Remeron)	15–30	Sedation, weight ↑	No sexual dysfunction.
Dopamine Reuptake Inhibitor			
Bupropion (Wellbutrin)	200–400	Insomnia or agitation, GI distress	Twice-a-day dosing with sustained release. No sexual dysfunction or weight gain.
Mixed Action Agents			
Amoxapine (Asendin)	100–600	Drowsiness, insomnia or agitation, CA, weight ↑, OSH, anticholinergic[a]	Movement disorders may occur. Dose titration is needed.
Clomipramine (Anafranil)	75–300	Drowsiness, weight ↑	Dose titration is needed.
Trazodone (Desyrel)	150–600	Drowsiness, OSH, CA, GI distress, weight ↑	Priapism is possible.

Note: Dose ranges are for adults in good general medical health, taking no other medications, and age 18 to 60 years. Doses vary depending on the agent, concomitant medications, the presence of general medical or surgical conditions, age, genetic constitution, and other factors. Brand names are those used in the United States.

CA, cardiac arrhythmia; 5-HT, serotonin; GI, gastrointestinal; NE, norepinephrine; OSH, orthostatic hypotension; SSRI, selective serotonin reuptake inhibitor.

[a]Dry mouth, blurred vision, urinary hesitancy, and constipation.

[b]Not approved as an antidepressant in the United States by the U.S. Food and Drug Administration.

with demonstrated efficacy in both conditions are preferred (e.g., tricyclics and SSRIs). In general, the nonmood disorder dictates the choice of treatment in comorbid states.

Concurrent substance abuse raises the possibility of a substance-induced mood disorder, which must be evaluated by history or by requiring abstinence for several weeks. Abstinence often results in remission of depressive symptoms in substance-induced mood disorders. For those with continuing significant depressive symptoms, even with abstinence, an independent mood disorder is diagnosed and treated.

General medical conditions are established risk factors in the development of depression. The presence of a major depressive episode is associated with increased morbidity or mortality of many general medical conditions (e.g., cardiovascular disease, diabetes, cerebrovascular disease, and cancer).

THERAPEUTIC USE OF SIDE EFFECTS. Choosing more sedating antidepressants (e.g., amitriptyline [Elavil, Endep]) for more anxious, depressed patients or more activating agents (e.g., desipramine) for more psychomotor-retarded patients is not generally helpful. For example, any short-term benefits with paroxetine, mirtazapine, or amitriptyline (more sedating drugs) on symptoms of anxiety or insomnia may become liabilities over time. These drugs often continue to be sedating in the longer run, which can lead to patients prematurely discontinuing medication and increase the risk of relapse or recurrence. Some practitioners use adjunctive medications (e.g., sleeping pills or anxiolytics) combined with antidepressants to provide more immediate symptom relief or to cover those side effects to which most patients ultimately adapt.

A patient's prior treatment history is important because an earlier response typically predicts current response. A documented failure on a properly conducted trial of a particular antidepressant class (e.g., SSRIs, tricyclics, or MAOIs) suggests choosing an agent from an alternative class. The history of a first-degree relative responding to a particular drug is associated with a good response to the same class of agents in the patient.

ACUTE TREATMENT FAILURES. Patients may not respond to a medication, because (1) they cannot tolerate the side effects, even in the face of a good clinical response; (2) an idiosyncratic adverse event may occur; (3) the clinical response is not adequate; or (4) the wrong diagnosis has been made. Acute phase medication trials should last 4 to 6 weeks to determine if meaningful symptom reduction is attained. Most (but not all) patients who ultimately respond fully show at least a partial response (i.e., at least a 20 to 25 percent reduction in pretreatment depressive symptom severity) by week 4 if the dose is adequate during the initial weeks of treatment. Lack of a partial response by 4 to 6 weeks indicates that a treatment change is needed. Longer time periods—8 to 12 weeks or longer—are needed to define the ultimate degree of symptom reduction achievable with a medication. Approximately half of patients require a second medication treatment trial because the initial treatment is poorly tolerated or ineffective.

SELECTING SECOND TREATMENT OPTIONS. When the initial treatment is unsuccessful, switching to an alternative treatment or augmenting the current treatment is a common option. The choice between switching from the initial single treatment to a new single treatment (as opposed to adding a second treatment to the first one) rests on the patient's prior treatment history, the degree of benefit achieved with the initial treatment, and patient preference. As a rule, switching rather than augmenting is preferred after an initial medication failure. On the other hand, augmentation strategies are helpful with patients who have gained some benefit from the initial treatment but who have not achieved remission. The best-documented augmentation strategies involve lithium (Eskalith) or thyroid hormone. A combination of an SSRI and bupropion (Wellbutrin) is also widely used. In fact, no combination strategy has been conclusively shown to be more effective than another. ECT is effective in psychotic and nonpsychotic forms of depression but is recommended generally only for repeatedly nonresponsive cases or in patients with very severe disorders.

A new therapy involves the use of the anesthetic agent ketamine, which has been shown to be effective in treatment resistant depression. It has a mechanism of action that inhibits the postsynaptic glutamate binding protein NDMA receptor. Because abnormalities in glutamatergic signaling have been implicated in major depressive disorder, this may account for its efficacy. Patients usually receive a single infusion of ketamine over a 30-minute period at a concentration of 0.5 mg/kg. A positive response is usually seen within 24 hours, and improved mood lasts for about 2 to 7 days. The most common side effects are dizziness, headache, and poor coordination, which are transitory. Dissociative symptoms, including hallucinations, may also occur.

COMBINED TREATMENT. Medication and formal psychotherapy are often combined in practice. If physicians view mood disorders as fundamentally evolving from psychodynamic issues, their ambivalence about the use of drugs may result in a poor response, noncompliance and probably inadequate dosages for a too short treatment period. Alternatively, if physicians ignore the psychosocial needs of a patient, the outcome of pharmacotherapy may be compromised. Several trials of a combination of pharmacotherapy and psychotherapy for chronically depressed outpatients have shown a higher response and higher remission rates for the combination than for either treatment used alone.

Bipolar Disorders. The pharmacological treatment of bipolar disorders is divided into both acute and maintenance phases. Bipolar treatment, however, also involves the formulation of different strategies for the patient who is experiencing mania or hypomania or depression. Lithium and its augmentation by antidepressants, antipsychotics, and benzodiazepines has been the major approach to the illness, but three anticonvulsant mood stabilizers—carbamazepine (Tegretol), valproate (Depakene), and lamotrigine (Lamictal)—have been added more recently, as well as a series of atypical antipsychotics, most of which are approved for the treatment of acute mania, for monotherapy of acute depression, and for prophylactic treatment. Each of these medications is associated with a unique side effect and safety profile, and no one drug is predictably effective for all patients. Often, it is necessary to try different medications before an optimal treatment is found.

TREATMENT OF ACUTE MANIA. The treatment of acute mania, or hypomania, usually is the easiest phases of bipolar disorders to treat. Agents can be used alone or in combination to bring the patient down from a high. Patients with severe mania are best treated in the hospital where aggressive dosing is possible and an adequate response can be achieved within days or weeks. Adherence to treatment, however, is often a problem because patients with mania frequently lack insight into their illness and refuse to take medication. Because impaired judgment, impulsivity, and aggressiveness combine to put the patient or others at risk, many patients in the manic phase are medicated to protect themselves and others from harm.

Lithium Carbonate. Lithium carbonate is considered the prototypical "mood stabilizer." Yet because the onset of antimanic action with lithium can be slow, it usually is supplemented in the early phases of treatment by atypical antipsychotics, mood-stabilizing anticonvulsants, or high-potency benzodiazepines. Therapeutic lithium levels are between 0.6 and 1.2 mEq/L. The introduction of newer drugs with more favorable side effects, lower toxicity, and less need for frequent laboratory testing has resulted in a decline in lithium use. For many patients, however, its clinical benefits can be remarkable.

Valproate. Valproate (valproic acid [Depakene] or divalproex sodium [Depakote]) has surpassed lithium in use for acute mania. Unlike lithium, valproate is only indicated for acute mania, although most experts agree it also has prophylactic effects. Typical dose levels of valproic acid are 750 to 2,500 mg per day, achieving blood levels between 50 and 120 μg/mL. Rapid oral loading with 15 to 20 mg/kg of divalproex sodium from day 1 of treatment has been well tolerated and associated with a rapid onset of response. A number of laboratory tests are required during valproate treatment.

Carbamazepine and Oxcarbazepine. Carbamazepine has been used worldwide for decades as a first-line treatment for acute mania but has only gained approval in the United States in 2004. Typical doses of carbamazepine to treat acute mania range between 600 and 1,800 mg per day associated with blood levels of between 4 and 12 μg/mL. The keto congener of carbamazepine, oxcarbazepine, may possess similar antimanic properties. Higher doses than those of carbamazepine are required because 1,500 mg of oxcarbazepine approximates 1,000 mg of carbamazepine.

Clonazepam and Lorazepam. The high-potency benzodiazepine anticonvulsants used in acute mania include clonazepam (Klonopin) and lorazepam (Ativan). Both may be effective and are widely used for adjunctive treatment of acute manic agitation, insomnia, aggression, and dysphoria, as well as panic. The safety and the benign side effect profile of these agents render them ideal adjuncts to lithium, carbamazepine, or valproate.

Atypical and Typical Antipsychotics. All of the atypical antipsychotics have demonstrated antimanic efficacy and are approved by the Food and Drug Administration for this indication. Compared with older agents, such as haloperidol (Haldol) and chlorpromazine (Thorazine), atypical antipsychotics have a lesser liability for excitatory postsynaptic potential and tardive dyskinesia; many do not increase prolactin. However, they have a wide range of substantial to no risk for weight gain with its associated problems of insulin resistance, diabetes, hyperlipidemia, hypercholesterolemia, and cardiovascular impairment. Some patients, however, require maintenance treatment with an antipsychotic medication.

TREATMENT OF ACUTE BIPOLAR DEPRESSION. The relative usefulness of standard antidepressants in bipolar illness, in general, and in rapid cycling and mixed states, in particular, remains controversial because of their propensity to induce cycling, mania, or hypomania. Accordingly, antidepressant drugs are often enhanced by a mood stabilizer in the first-line treatment for a first or isolated episode of bipolar depression. A fixed combination of olanzapine and fluoxetine (Symbyax) has been shown to be effective in treating acute bipolar depression for an 8-week period without inducing a switch to mania or hypomania.

Paradoxically, many patients who are bipolar in the depressed phase do not respond to treatment with standard antidepressants. In these instances, lamotrigine or low-dose ziprasidone (20 to 80 mg per day) may prove effective. Quetiapine or lurasidone may also be used.

Electroconvulsive therapy may also be useful for patients with bipolar depression who do not respond to lithium or other mood stabilizers and their adjuncts, particularly in cases in which intense suicidal tendency presents as a medical emergency.

Other Agents. When standard treatments fail, other types of compounds may prove effective. The calcium channel antagonist verapamil (Calan, Isoptin) has acute antimanic efficacy. Gabapentin, topiramate, zonisamide, levetiracetam, and tiagabine have not been shown to have acute antimania effects, although some patients may benefit from a trial of these agents when standard therapies have failed. Lamotrigine does not possess acute antimanic properties but does help prevent recurrence of manic episodes. Small studies suggest the potential acute antimanic and prophylactic efficacy of phenytoin. ECT is effective in acute mania. Bilateral treatments are required because unilateral, nondominant treatments have been reported to be ineffective or even to exacerbate manic symptoms. ECT is reserved for patients with rare refractory mania and for patients with medical complications, as well as extreme exhaustion (malignant hyperthermia or lethal catatonia).

MAINTENANCE TREATMENT OF BIPOLAR DISORDER. Preventing recurrences of mood episodes is the greatest challenge facing clinicians. Not only must the chosen regimen achieve its primary goal—sustained euthymia—but the medications should not produce unwanted side effects that affect functioning. Sedation, cognitive impairment, tremor, weight gain, and rash are some side effects that lead to treatment discontinuation.

Lithium, carbamazepine, and valproic acid, alone or in combination, are the most widely used agents in the long-term treatment of patients with bipolar disorder. Lamotrigine has prophylactic antidepressant and, potentially, mood-stabilizing properties. Patients with bipolar I disorder depression taking lamotrigine exhibit a rate of switch into mania that is the same as the rate with placebo. Lamotrigine appears to have superior acute and prophylactic antidepressant properties compared with antimanic properties. Given that breakthrough depressions are a difficult problem during prophylaxis, lamotrigine has a unique therapeutic role. Very slow increases of lamotrigine help avoid the rare side effect of lethal rash. A dose of 200 mg per day appears to be the average in many studies. The incidence of severe rash (i.e., Stevens–Johnson syndrome, a toxic epidermal necrolysis) is now thought to be approximately two in 10,000 adults and four in 10,000 children.

Thyroid supplementation is frequently necessary during long-term treatment. Many patients treated with lithium develop hypothyroidism, and many patients with bipolar disorder have idiopathic thyroid dysfunction. T_3 (25 to 50 μg per day), because of its short half-life, is often recommended for acute augmentation strategies, but T_4 is frequently used for long-term maintenance. In some centers, hypermetabolic doses of thyroid hormone are used. Data indicate improvement in both manic and depressive phases with hypermetabolic T_4-augmenting strategies. Table 5.1–8 summarizes the principles of treatment of bipolar disorders.

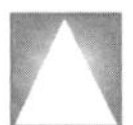

Table 5.1–8
Principles in the Treatment of Bipolar Disorders

Maintain dual treatment focus: (1) acute short term and (2) prophylaxis.
Chart illness retrospectively and prospectively.
Mania as medical emergency: Treat first; chemistries later.
Load valproate and lithium (Eskalith); titrate lamotrigine (Lamictal) slowly.
Careful combination treatment can decrease adverse effects.
Augment rather than substitute in treatment-resistant patient.
Retain lithium in regimen for its antisuicide and neuroprotective effects.
Taper lithium slowly, if at all.
Educate patient and family about illness and risk-to-benefit ratios of acute and prophylactic treatments.
Give statistics (i.e., 50% relapse in first 5 months off lithium).
Assess compliance and suicidality regularly.
Develop an early warning system for identification and treatment of emergent symptoms.
Contract with patient as needed for suicide and substance use avoidance.
Use regular visits; monitor course and adverse effects.
Arrange for interval phone contact when needed.
Develop fire drill for mania reemergence.
Inquire about and address comorbid alcohol and substance abuse.
Targeted psychotherapy; use medicalization of illness.
Treat patient as a coinvestigator in the development of effective clinical approaches to the illness.
If treatment is successful, be conservative in making changes, maintain the course, and continue full-dose pharmacoprophylaxis in absence of side effects.
If treatment response is inadequate, be aggressive in searching for more effective alternatives.

▲ 5.2 Dysthymia and Cyclothymia

DYSTHYMIA (Persistant Depressive Disorder)

The most typical features of dysthymia, also known as persistent depressive disorder in DSM-5, is the presence of a depressed mood that lasts most of the day and is present almost continuously. There are associated feelings of inadequacy, guilt, irritability, and anger; withdrawal from society; loss of interest; and inactivity and lack of productivity. The term *dysthymia,* which means "ill humored," was introduced in 1980. Before that time, most patients now classified as having dysthymia were classified as having depressive neurosis (also called neurotic depression).

Dysthymia is distinguished from major depressive disorder by the fact that patients complain that they have always been depressed. Thus, most cases are of early onset, beginning in childhood or adolescence and certainly occurring by the time patients reach their 20s. A late-onset subtype, much less prevalent and not well characterized clinically, has been identified among middle-aged and geriatric populations, largely through epidemiological studies in the community.

Although dysthymia can occur as a secondary complication of other psychiatric disorders, the core concept of dysthymia refers to a subaffective or subclinical depressive disorder with (1) low-grade chronicity for at least 2 years; (2) insidious onset, with origin often in childhood or adolescence; and (3) a persistent or intermittent course. The family history of patients with dysthymia is typically replete with both depressive and bipolar disorders, which is one of the more robust findings supporting its link to primary mood disorder.

Epidemiology

Dysthymia is common among the general population and affects 5 to 6 percent of all persons. It is seen among patients in general psychiatric clinics, where it affects between half and one-third of all patients. No gender differences are seen for incidence rates. The disorder is more common in women younger than 64 years of age than in men of any age and is more common among unmarried and young persons and in those with low incomes. Dysthymia frequently coexists with other mental disorders, particularly major depressive disorder, and in persons with major depressive disorder, there is less likelihood of full remission between episodes. The patients may also have coexisting anxiety disorders (especially panic disorder), substance abuse, and borderline personality disorder. The disorder is more common among those with first-degree relatives with major depressive disorder. Patients with dysthymia are likely to be taking a wide range of psychiatric medications, including antidepressants, antimanic agents such as lithium (Eskalith) and carbamazepine (Tegretol), and sedative-hypnotics.

Etiology

Biological Factors.

The biological basis for the symptoms of dysthymia and major depressive disorder are similar, but the biological bases for the underlying pathophysiology in the two disorders differ.

SLEEP STUDIES. Decreased rapid eye movement (REM) latency and increased REM density are two state markers of depression in major depressive disorder that also occur in a significant proportion of patients with dysthymia.

NEUROENDOCRINE STUDIES. The two most studied neuroendocrine axes in major depressive disorder and dysthymia are the adrenal axis and the thyroid axis, which have been tested by using the dexamethasone-suppression test (DST) and the thyrotropin-releasing hormone (TRH)-stimulation test, respectively. Although the results of studies are not absolutely consistent, most indicate that patients with dysthymia are less likely to have abnormal results on a DST than are patients with major depressive disorder.

Psychosocial Factors.

Psychodynamic theories about the development of dysthymia posit that the disorder results from personality and ego development and culminates in difficulty adapting to adolescence and young adulthood. Karl Abraham, for example, thought that the conflicts of depression center on oral- and anal-sadistic traits. Anal traits include excessive orderliness, guilt, and concern for others; they are postulated to be a defense against preoccupation with anal matter and with disorganization, hostility, and self-preoccupation. A major defense mechanism used is reaction formation. Low self-esteem, anhedonia, and introversion are often associated with the depressive character.

FREUD. In *Mourning and Melancholia,* Sigmund Freud asserted that an interpersonal disappointment early in life can cause a vulnerability to depression that leads to ambivalent love relationships as an adult; real or threatened losses in adult life then trigger depression. Persons susceptible to depression are orally dependent and require constant narcissistic gratification. When deprived of love, affection, and care, they become clinically depressed; when they experience a real loss, they internalize or introject the lost object and turn their anger on it and thus on themselves.

COGNITIVE THEORY. The cognitive theory of depression also applies to dysthymia. It holds that a disparity between actual and fantasized situations leads to diminished self-esteem and a sense of helplessness. The success of cognitive therapy in the treatment of some patients with dysthymia may provide some support for the theoretical model.

Diagnosis and Clinical Features

The DSM-5 diagnosis criteria for dysthymia stipulate the presence of a depressed mood most of the time for at least 2 years (or 1 year for children and adolescents). To meet the diagnostic criteria, a patient should not have symptoms that are better accounted for as major depressive disorder and should never have had a manic or hypomanic episode. DSM-5 allows clinicians to specify whether the onset was early (before the age of 21 years) or late (age of 21 years or older). DSM-5 also allows specification of atypical features in dysthymia.

The profile of dysthymia overlaps with that of major depressive disorder but differs from it in that symptoms tend to outnumber signs (more subjective than objective depression). This means that disturbances in appetite and libido are uncharacteristic, and psychomotor agitation or retardation is not observed. This all translates into a depression with attenuated symptomatology. Subtle endogenous features are observed, however, including inertia, lethargy, and anhedonia that are characteristically worse in the morning. Because patients presenting clinically often fluctuate in and out of a major depression, the core DSM-5 criteria for dysthymia tend to emphasize vegetative dysfunction; however, cognitive symptoms are often present (Table 5.2–1).

Dysthymia is quite heterogeneous. Anxiety is not a necessary part of its clinical picture, yet dysthymia is often diagnosed in patients with anxiety and phobic disorders. That clinical situation is sometimes diagnosed as mixed anxiety depressive disorder. For greater operational clarity, it is best to restrict dysthymia to a primary disorder, one that cannot be explained by another psychiatric disorder. The essential features of such primary dysthymia include habitual gloom, brooding, lack of joy in life, and preoccupation with inadequacy. Dysthymia then is best characterized as long-standing, fluctuating, low-grade depression, experienced as part of the habitual self and representing an accentuation of traits observed in the depressive temperament. The clinical picture of dysthymia is varied, with some patients proceeding to major depression and others manifesting the pathology largely at the personality level.

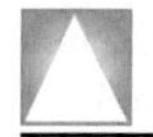

Table 5.2–1
Diagnostic Features of Dysthymia

1. Easily depressed
2. Little joy in living
3. Inclined to be gloomy and morbid
4. Pessimistic, self-deprecatory
5. Low self-esteem
6. Fearful of disapproval, indecisive
7. May be suspicious of others

A 27-year-old male grade-school teacher presented with the chief complaint that life was a painful duty that had always lacked luster for him. He said that he felt "enveloped by a sense of gloom" that was nearly always with him. Although he was respected by his peers, he felt "like a grotesque failure, a self-concept I have had since childhood." He stated that he merely performed his responsibilities as a teacher and that he had never derived any pleasure from anything he had done in life. He said that he had never had any romantic feelings; sexual activity, in which he had engaged with two different women, had involved pleasureless orgasm. He said that he felt empty, going through life without any sense of direction, ambition, or passion, a realization that itself was tormenting. He had bought a pistol to put an end to what he called his "useless existence" but did not carry out suicide, believing that it would hurt his students and the small community in which he lived. *(Courtesy of HS Akiskal, M.D.)*

Dysthymic Variants. Dysthymia is common in patients with chronically disabling physical disorders, particularly among elderly adults. Dysthymia-like, clinically significant, subthreshold depression lasting 6 or more months has also been described in neurological conditions, including stroke. According to a recent World Health Organization (WHO) conference, this condition aggravates the prognosis of the underlying neurological disease and therefore deserves pharmacotherapy.

Prospective studies on children have revealed an episodic course of dysthymia with remissions, exacerbations, and eventual complications by major depressive episodes, 15 to 20 percent of which might even progress to hypomanic, manic, or mixed episodes postpuberty. Persons with dysthymia presenting clinically as adults tend to pursue a chronic unipolar course that may or may not be complicated by major depression. They rarely develop spontaneous hypomania or mania. When treated with antidepressants, however, some of them may develop brief hypomanic switches that typically disappear when the antidepressant dose is decreased.

Differential Diagnosis

The differential diagnosis for dysthymia is essentially identical to that for major depressive disorder. Many substances and medical illnesses can cause chronic depressive symptoms. Two disorders are particularly important to consider in the differential diagnosis of dysthymia—minor depressive disorder and recurrent brief depressive disorder.

Minor Depressive Disorder. Minor depressive disorder (discussed in Section 8.1) is characterized by episodes of depressive symptoms that are less severe than those seen in major depressive disorder. The difference between dysthymia and minor depressive disorder is primarily the episodic nature of the symptoms in the latter. Between episodes, patients with minor depressive disorder have a euthymic mood, but patients with dysthymia have virtually no euthymic periods.

Recurrent Brief Depressive Disorder. Recurrent brief depressive disorder (discussed in Section 8.1) is characterized by brief periods (less than 2 weeks) during which depressive episodes are present. Patients with the disorder would meet the diagnostic criteria for major depressive disorder if their episodes lasted longer. Patients with recurrent brief depressive disorder differ from patients with dysthymia on two counts: They have an episodic disorder, and their symptoms are more severe.

Double Depression. An estimated 40 percent of patients with major depressive disorder also meet the criteria for dysthymia, a combination often referred to as *double depression.* Available data support the conclusion that patients with double depression have a poorer prognosis than patients with only major depressive disorder. The treatment of patients with double depression should be directed toward both disorders because the resolution of the symptoms of major depressive episode still leaves these patients with significant psychiatric impairment.

Alcohol and Substance Abuse. Patients with dysthymia commonly meet the diagnostic criteria for a substance-related disorder. This comorbidity can be logical; patients with dysthymia tend to develop coping methods for their chronically depressed state that involve substance abuse. Therefore, they are likely to use alcohol, stimulants such as cocaine, or marijuana, the choice perhaps depending primarily on a patient's social context. The presence of a comorbid diagnosis of substance abuse presents a diagnostic dilemma for clinicians; the long-term use of many substances can result in a symptom picture indistinguishable from that of dysthymia.

Course and Prognosis

About 50 percent of patients with dysthymia experience an insidious onset of symptoms before 25 years of age. Despite the early onset, patients often suffer with the symptoms for a decade before seeking psychiatric help and may consider early-onset dysthymia simply part of life. Patients with an early onset of symptoms are at risk for either major depressive disorder or bipolar I disorder in the course of their disorder. Studies of patients with the diagnosis of dysthymia indicate that about 20 percent progressed to major depressive disorder, 15 percent to bipolar II disorder, and fewer than 5 percent to bipolar I disorder.

The prognosis for patients with dysthymia varies. Antidepressive agents and specific types of psychotherapies (e.g., cognitive and behavior therapies) have positive effects on the course and prognosis of dysthymia. The available data about previously available treatments indicate that only 10 to 15 percent of patients are in remission 1 year after the initial diagnosis. About 25 percent of all patients with dysthymia never attain a complete recovery. Overall, however, the prognosis is good with treatment.

Treatment

Historically, patients with dysthymia either received no treatment or were seen as candidates for long-term, insight-oriented psychotherapy. Contemporary data offer the most objective support for cognitive therapy, behavior therapy, and pharmacotherapy. The combination of pharmacotherapy and some form of psychotherapy may be the most effective treatment for the disorder.

Cognitive Therapy. Cognitive therapy is a technique in which patients are taught new ways of thinking and behaving to replace faulty negative attitudes about themselves, the world, and the future. It is a short-term therapy program oriented toward current problems and their resolution.

Behavior Therapy. Behavior therapy for depressive disorders is based on the theory that depression is caused by a loss of positive reinforcement as a result of separation, death, or sudden environmental change. The various treatment methods focus on specific goals to increase activity, to provide pleasant experiences, and to teach patients how to relax. Altering personal behavior in depressed patients is believed to be the most effective way to change the associated depressed thoughts and feelings. Behavior therapy is often used to treat the learned helplessness of some patients who seem to meet every life challenge with a sense of impotence.

Insight-Oriented (Psychoanalytic) Psychotherapy. Individual insight-oriented psychotherapy is the most common treatment method for dysthymia, and many clinicians consider it the treatment of choice. The psychotherapeutic approach attempts to relate the development and maintenance of depressive symptoms and maladaptive personality features to unresolved conflicts from early childhood. Insight into depressive equivalents (e.g., substance abuse) or into childhood disappointments as antecedents to adult depression can be gained through treatment. Ambivalent current relationships with parents, friends, and others in the patient's current life are examined. Patients' understanding of how they try to gratify an excessive need for outside approval to counter low self-esteem and a harsh superego is an important goal of this therapy.

Interpersonal Therapy. In interpersonal therapy for depressive disorders, a patient's current interpersonal experiences and ways of coping with stress are examined to reduce depressive symptoms and to improve self-esteem. Interpersonal therapy lasts for about 12 to 16 weekly sessions and can be combined with antidepressant medication.

Family and Group Therapies. Family therapy may help both the patient and the patient's family deal with the symptoms of the disorder, especially when a biologically based subaffective syndrome seems to be present. Group therapy may help withdrawn patients learn new ways to overcome their interpersonal problems in social situations.

Pharmacotherapy. Because of long-standing and commonly held theoretical beliefs that dysthymia is primarily a psychologically determined disorder, many clinicians avoid prescribing antidepressants for patients; however, many studies have shown therapeutic success with antidepressants. The data generally indicate that selective serotonin reuptake inhibitors (SSRIs) venlafaxine and bupropion are an effective treatment for patients with dysthymia. Monoamine oxidase inhibitors (MAOIs) are effective in a subgroup of patients with the disorder, a group who may also respond to the judicious use of amphetamines.

Hospitalization. Hospitalization is usually not indicated for patients with dysthymia, but particularly severe symptoms, marked social or professional incapacitation, the need for extensive diagnostic procedures, and suicidal ideation are all indications for hospitalization.

CYCLOTHYMIC DISORDER

Cyclothymic disorder is symptomatically a mild form of bipolar II disorder, characterized by episodes of hypomania and mild depression. In DSM-5, cyclothymic disorder is defined as a "chronic, fluctuating mood disturbance" with many periods of hypomania and of depression. The disorder is differentiated from bipolar II disorder, which is characterized by the presence of major (not minor) depressive and hypomanic episodes. As with dysthymia, the inclusion of cyclothymic disorder with the mood disorders implies a relation, probably biological, to bipolar I disorder. Some psychiatrists, however, consider cyclothymic disorder to have no biological component and to result from chaotic object relations early in life.

Contemporary conceptualization of cyclothymic disorder is based to some extent on the observations of Emil Kraepelin and Kurt Schneider that one-third to two-thirds of patients with mood disorders exhibit personality disorders. Kraepelin described four types of personality disorders: depressive (gloomy), manic (cheerful and uninhibited), irritable (labile and explosive), and cyclothymic. He described the irritable personality as simultaneously depressive and manic and the cyclothymic personality as the alternation of the depressive and manic personalities.

Epidemiology

Patients with cyclothymic disorder may constitute from 3 to 5 percent of all psychiatric outpatients, perhaps particularly those with significant complaints about marital and interpersonal difficulties. In the general population, the lifetime prevalence of cyclothymic disorder is estimated to be about 1 percent. This figure is probably lower than the actual prevalence because, as with patients with bipolar I disorder, the patients may not be aware that they have a psychiatric problem. Cyclothymic disorder, as with dysthymia, frequently coexists with borderline personality disorder. An estimated 10 percent of outpatients and 20 percent of inpatients with borderline personality disorder have a coexisting diagnosis of cyclothymic disorder. The female-to-male ratio in cyclothymic disorder is about 3 to 2, and 50 to 75 percent of all patients have an onset between ages 15 and 25 years. Families of persons with cyclothymic disorder often contain members with substance-related disorder.

Etiology

As with dysthymia, controversy exists about whether cyclothymic disorder is related to the mood disorders, either biologically or psychologically. Some researchers have postulated that cyclothymic disorder has a closer relation to borderline personality disorder than to the mood disorders. Despite these controversies, the preponderance of biological and genetic data favors the idea of cyclothymic disorder as a bona fide mood disorder.

Biological Factors. About 30 percent of all patients with cyclothymic disorder have positive family histories for bipolar I disorder; this rate is similar to the rate for patients with bipolar I disorder. Moreover, the pedigrees of families with bipolar I disorder often contain generations of patients with bipolar I disorder linked by a generation with cyclothymic disorder. Conversely, the prevalence of cyclothymic disorder in the relatives of patients with bipolar I disorder is much higher than the prevalence of cyclothymic disorder either in the relatives of patients with other mental disorders or in persons who are mentally healthy. The observations that about one-third of patients with cyclothymic disorder subsequently have major mood disorders, that they are particularly sensitive to antidepressant-induced hypomania, and that about 60 percent respond to lithium add further support to the idea of cyclothymic disorder as a mild or attenuated form of bipolar II disorder.

Psychosocial Factors. Most psychodynamic theories postulate that the development of cyclothymic disorder lies in traumas and fixations during the oral stage of infant development. Freud hypothesized that the cyclothymic state is the ego's attempt to overcome a harsh and punitive superego. Hypomania is explained psychodynamically as the lack of self-criticism and an absence of inhibitions occurring when a depressed person throws off the burden of an overly harsh superego. The major defense mechanism in hypomania is denial, by which the patient avoids external problems and internal feelings of depression.

Patients with cyclothymic disorder are characterized by periods of depression alternating with periods of hypomania. Psychoanalytic exploration reveals that such patients defend themselves against underlying depressive themes with their euphoric or hypomanic periods. Hypomania is frequently triggered by a profound interpersonal loss. The false euphoria generated in such instances is a patient's way to deny dependence on love objects and simultaneously disavowing any aggression or destructiveness that may have contributed to the loss of the loved person.

Diagnosis and Clinical Features

Although many patients seek psychiatric help for depression, their problems are often related to the chaos that their manic episodes have caused. Clinicians must consider a diagnosis of cyclothymic disorder when a patient appears with what may seem to be sociopathic behavioral problems. Marital difficulties and instability in relationships are common complaints because patients with cyclothymic disorder are often promiscuous and irritable while in manic and mixed states. Although there are anecdotal reports of increased productivity and creativity when patients are hypomanic, most clinicians report that their patients become disorganized and ineffective in work and school during these periods.

The DSM-5 diagnostic criteria for cyclothymic disorder stipulate that a patient has never met the criteria for a major depressive episode and did not meet the criteria for a manic episode during the first 2 years of the disturbance. They are hypomanic rather than manic (see Table 5.2–2). The criteria also require the more or less constant presence of symptoms for 2 years (or 1 year for children and adolescents).

Signs and Symptoms. The symptoms of cyclothymic disorder are identical to the symptoms of bipolar II disorder except that they are generally less severe. On occasion, however, the symptoms may be equally severe but of shorter duration than those seen in bipolar II disorder. About half of all patients with

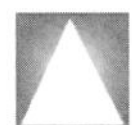

Table 5.2–2
Diagnostic Features of Hypomania

1. Cheerful tendencies, sometimes inappropriately so
2. Lack of inhibition, sometimes impulsive
3. Confident, aggressive, optimistic
4. Energetic
5. Easily influenced by others
6. Blustering, gregarious
7. Argumentative, hypercritical
8. Resentful of controls and easily frustrated

cyclothymic disorder have depression as their major symptom, and these patients are most likely to seek psychiatric help while depressed. Some patients with cyclothymic disorder have primarily hypomanic symptoms and are less likely to consult a psychiatrist than primarily depressed patients. Almost all patients with cyclothymic disorder have periods of mixed symptoms with marked irritability.

Most patients with cyclothymic disorder seen by psychiatrists have not succeeded in their professional and social lives as a result of their disorder, but a few have become high achievers who have worked especially long hours and have required little sleep. Some persons' ability to control the symptoms of the disorder successfully depends on multiple individual, social, and cultural attributes.

The lives of most patients with cyclothymic disorder are difficult. The cycles of the disorder tend to be much shorter than those in bipolar I disorder. In cyclothymic disorder, the changes in mood are irregular and abrupt and sometimes occur within hours. The unpredictable nature of the mood changes produces great stress. Patients often feel that their moods are out of control. In irritable, mixed periods, they may become involved in unprovoked disagreements with friends, family, and coworkers.

Mr. B, a 25-year-old single man, came for evaluation due to irritability, insomnia, jumpiness, and excessive energy. He reported that such episodes lasted from a few days to a few weeks and alternated with longer periods of feeling hopeless, dejected, and worn out with thoughts of suicide. Mr. B reported having been this way for as long as he could remember. He had never been treated for his symptoms. He denied using drugs and said he had "only the occasional drink to relax."

As a child, Mr. B went from one foster family to another and was an irresponsible and trouble-making child. He frequently ran away from home, was absent from school, and committed minor crimes. He ran away from his last foster family at the age of 16 years and drifted ever since, taking occasional odd jobs. When he became restless at one location or job, he quickly moved on to the next. He did not have close friends because he would form and end friendships quickly.

Substance Abuse. Alcohol abuse and other substance abuse are common in patients with cyclothymic disorder, who use substances either to self-medicate (with alcohol, benzodiazepines, and marijuana) or to achieve even further stimulation (with cocaine, amphetamines, and hallucinogens) when they are manic. About 5 to 10 percent of all patients with cyclothymic disorder have substance dependence. Persons with this disorder often have a history of multiple geographical moves, involvements in religious cults, and dilettantism.

Differential Diagnosis

When a diagnosis of cyclothymic disorder is under consideration, all the possible medical and substance-related causes of depression and mania, such as seizures and particular substances (cocaine, amphetamine, and steroids), must be considered. Borderline, antisocial, histrionic, and narcissistic personality disorders should also be considered in the differential diagnosis. Attention-deficit/hyperactivity disorder (ADHD) can be difficult to differentiate from cyclothymic disorder in children and adolescents. A trial of stimulants helps most patients with ADHD and exacerbates the symptoms of most patients with cyclothymic disorder. The diagnostic category of bipolar II disorder (discussed in Section 5.1) is characterized by the combination of major depressive and hypomanic episodes.

Course and Prognosis

Some patients with cyclothymic disorder are characterized as having been sensitive, hyperactive, or moody as young children. The onset of frank symptoms of cyclothymic disorder often occurs insidiously in the teens or early 20s. The emergence of symptoms at that time hinders a person's performance in school and the ability to establish friendships with peers. The reactions of patients to such a disorder vary; patients with adaptive coping strategies or ego defenses have better outcomes than patients with poor coping strategies. About one-third of all patients with cyclothymic disorder develop a major mood disorder, most often bipolar II disorder.

Treatment

Biological Therapy. The mood stabilizers and antimanic drugs are the first line of treatment for patients with cyclothymic disorder. Although the experimental data are limited to studies with lithium, other antimanic agents—for example, carbamazepine and valproate (Depakene)—are reported to be effective. Dosages and plasma concentrations of these agents should be the same as those in bipolar I disorder. Antidepressant treatment of depressed patients with cyclothymic disorder should be done with caution because these patients have increased susceptibility to antidepressant-induced hypomanic or manic episodes. About 40 to 50 percent of all patients with cyclothymic disorder who are treated with antidepressants experience such episodes.

Psychosocial Therapy. Psychotherapy for patients with cyclothymic disorder is best directed toward increasing patients' awareness of their condition and helping them develop coping mechanisms for their mood swings. Therapists usually need to help patients repair any damage, both work and family related, done during episodes of hypomania. Because of the long-term nature of cyclothymic disorder, patients often require lifelong treatment. Family and group therapies may be supportive, educational, and therapeutic for patients and for those involved in their lives. The psychiatrist conducting psychotherapy is able to evaluate the degree of cyclothymia and so provide an early warning system to prevent full-blown manic attacks before they occur.

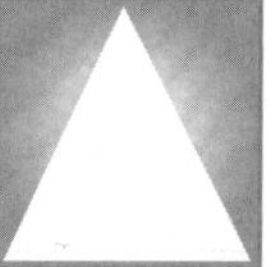

6 Anxiety Disorders

▲ 6.1 Overview

Anxiety represents a core phenomenon around which considerable psychiatric theory has been organized. Thus, the term "anxiety" has played a central role in psychodynamic theory, as well as in neuroscience-focused research and various schools of thought heavily influenced by cognitive-behavioral principles. Anxiety disorders are associated with significant morbidity and often are chronic and resistant to treatment. Anxiety disorders can be viewed as a family of related but distinct mental disorders, which include (1) panic disorder, (2) agoraphobia, (3) specific phobia, (4) social anxiety disorder or phobia, and (5) generalized anxiety disorder. Each of these disorders is discussed in detail in the sections that follow.

A fascinating aspect of anxiety disorders is the exquisite interplay of genetic and experiential factors. Little doubt exists that abnormal genes predispose to pathological anxiety states; however, evidence clearly indicates that traumatic life events and stress are also etiologically important. Thus, the study of anxiety disorders presents a unique opportunity to understand the relation between nature and nurture in the etiology of mental disorders.

NORMAL ANXIETY

Everyone experiences anxiety. It is characterized most commonly as a diffuse, unpleasant, vague sense of apprehension, often accompanied by autonomic symptoms such as headache, perspiration, palpitations, tightness in the chest, mild stomach discomfort, and restlessness, indicated by an inability to sit or stand still for long. The particular constellation of symptoms present during anxiety tends to vary among persons (Table 6.1–1).

Fear versus Anxiety

Anxiety is an alerting signal; it warns of impending danger and enables a person to take measures to deal with a threat. Fear is a similar alerting signal, but it should be differentiated from anxiety. Fear is a response to a known, external, definite, or nonconflictual threat; anxiety is a response to a threat that is unknown, internal, vague, or conflictual.

This distinction between fear and anxiety arose accidentally. When Freud's early translator mistranslated *angst,* the German word for "fear," as anxiety, Freud himself generally ignored the distinction that associates anxiety with a repressed, unconscious object and fear with a known, external object. The distinction may be difficult to make because fear can also be caused by an unconscious, repressed, internal object displaced to another object in the external world. For example, a boy may fear barking dogs because he actually fears his father and unconsciously associates his father with barking dogs.

Nevertheless, according to post-freudian psychoanalytic formulations, the separation of fear and anxiety is psychologically justifiable. The emotion caused by a rapidly approaching car as a person crosses the street differs from the vague discomfort a person may experience when meeting new persons in a strange setting. The main psychological difference between the two emotional responses is the suddenness of fear and the insidiousness of anxiety.

In 1896, Charles Darwin gave the following psychophysiological description of acute fear merging into terror:

> Fear is often preceded by astonishment, and is so far akin to it, that both lead to the senses of sight and learning being instantly aroused. In both cases the eyes and mouth are widely opened, and the eyebrows raised. The frightened man at first stands like a statue motionless and breathless, or crouches down as if instinctively to escape observation. The heart beats quickly and violently, so that it palpitates or knocks against the ribs; but it is very doubtful whether it then works more efficiently than usual, so as to send a greater supply of blood to all parts of the body; for the skin instantly becomes pale, as during incipient faintness. This paleness of the surface, however, is probably in large part, or exclusively, due to the vasomotor center being affected in such a manner as to cause the contraction of the small arteries of the skin. That the skin is much affected under the sense of great fear, we see in the marvelous and inexplicable manner in which perspiration immediately exudes from it. This exudation is all the more remarkable, as the surface is then cold, and hence the term a cold sweat; whereas, the sudorific glands are properly excited into action when the surface is heated. The hairs also on the skin stand erect; and the superficial muscles shiver. In connection with the disturbed action of the heart, the breathing is hurried. The salivary glands act imperfectly; the mouth becomes dry, and is often opened and shut. I have also noticed that under slight fear there is a strong tendency to yawn. One of the best-marked symptoms is the trembling of all the muscles of the body; and this is often first seen in the lips. From this cause, and from the dryness of the mouth, the voice becomes husky or indistinct, or may altogether fail....
>
> As fear increases into an agony of terror, we behold, as under all violent emotions, diversified results. The heart beats wildly or may fail to act and faintness ensues; there is a deathlike pallor; the breathing is labored; the wings of the nostrils are widely dilated; there is a gasping and convulsive motion on the lips, a tremor on the hollow cheek, a gulping and catching of the throat; the uncovered and protruding eyeballs are fixed on the object of terror; or they may roll restlessly from side to

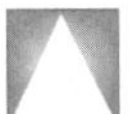

Table 6.1–1
Peripheral Manifestations of Anxiety

Diarrhea
Dizziness, lightheadedness
Hyperhidrosis
Hyperreflexia
Palpitations
Pupillary mydriasis
Restlessness (e.g., pacing)
Syncope
Tachycardia
Tingling in the extremities
Tremors
Upset stomach ("butterflies")
Urinary frequency, hesitancy, urgency

side. The pupils are said to be enormously dilated. All the muscles of the body may become rigid, or may be thrown into convulsive movements. The hands are alternately clenched and opened, often with a twitching movement. The arms may be protruded, as if to avert some dreadful danger, or may be thrown wildly over the head.... In other cases there is a sudden and uncontrollable tendency to headlong flight; and so strong is this, that the boldest soldiers may be seized with a sudden panic.

Is Anxiety Adaptive?

Anxiety and fear both are alerting signals and act as a warning of an internal and external threat. Anxiety can be conceptualized as a normal and adaptive response that has lifesaving qualities and warns of threats of bodily damage, pain, helplessness, possible punishment, or the frustration of social or bodily needs; of separation from loved ones; of a menace to one's success or status; and ultimately of threats to unity or wholeness. It prompts a person to take the necessary steps to prevent the threat or to lessen its consequences. This preparation is accompanied by increased somatic and autonomic activity controlled by the interaction of the sympathetic and parasympathetic nervous systems. Examples of a person warding off threats in daily life include getting down to the hard work of preparing for an examination, dodging a ball thrown at the head, sneaking into the dormitory after curfew to prevent punishment, and running to catch the last commuter train. Thus, anxiety prevents damage by alerting the person to carry out certain acts that forestall the danger.

Stress and Anxiety

Whether an event is perceived as stressful depends on the nature of the event and on the person's resources, psychological defenses, and coping mechanisms. All involve the ego, a collective abstraction for the process by which a person perceives, thinks, and acts on external events or internal drives. A person whose ego is functioning properly is in adaptive balance with both external and internal worlds; if the ego is not functioning properly and the resulting imbalance continues sufficiently long, the person experiences chronic anxiety.

Whether the imbalance is external, between the pressures of the outside world and the person's ego, or internal, between the person's impulses (e.g., aggressive, sexual, and dependent impulses) and conscience, the imbalance produces a conflict. Whereas externally caused conflicts are usually interpersonal, those that are internally caused are intrapsychic or intrapersonal. A combination of the two is possible, as in the case of employees whose excessively demanding and critical boss provokes impulses that they must control for fear of losing their jobs. Interpersonal and intrapsychic conflicts, in fact, are usually intertwined. Because human beings are social, their main conflicts are usually with other persons.

Symptoms of Anxiety

The experience of anxiety has two components: the awareness of the physiological sensations (e.g., palpitations and sweating) and the awareness of being nervous or frightened. A feeling of shame may increase anxiety—"Others will recognize that I am frightened." Many persons are astonished to find out that others are not aware of their anxiety or, if they are, do not appreciate its intensity.

In addition to motor and visceral effects, anxiety affects thinking, perception, and learning. It tends to produce confusion and distortions of perception, not only of time and space but also of persons and the meanings of events. These distortions can interfere with learning by lowering concentration, reducing recall, and impairing the ability to relate one item to another—that is, to make associations.

An important aspect of emotions is their effect on the selectivity of attention. Anxious persons likely select certain things in their environment and overlook others in their effort to prove that they are justified in considering the situation frightening. If they falsely justify their fear, they augment their anxieties by the selective response and set up a vicious circle of anxiety, distorted perception, and increased anxiety. If, alternatively, they falsely reassure themselves by selective thinking, appropriate anxiety may be reduced, and they may fail to take necessary precautions.

PATHOLOGICAL ANXIETY

Epidemiology

The anxiety disorders make up one of the most common groups of psychiatric disorders. The National Comorbidity Study reported that one of four persons met the diagnostic criteria for at least one anxiety disorder and that there is a 12-month prevalence rate of 17.7 percent. Women (30.5 percent lifetime prevalence) are more likely to have an anxiety disorder than are men (19.2 percent lifetime prevalence). The prevalence of anxiety disorders decreases with higher socioeconomic status.

Contributions of Psychological Sciences

Three major schools of psychological theory—psychoanalytic, behavioral, and existential—have contributed theories about the causes of anxiety. Each theory has both conceptual and practical usefulness in treating anxiety disorders.

Psychoanalytic Theories. Although Freud originally believed that anxiety stemmed from a physiological buildup of libido, he ultimately redefined anxiety as a signal of the presence of danger in the unconscious. Anxiety was viewed as the result of psychic conflict between unconscious sexual or aggressive wishes and corresponding threats from the superego or external reality. In response to this signal, the ego mobilized defense mechanisms to prevent unacceptable thoughts and feelings from emerging into conscious awareness. In his classic paper "Inhibitions, Symptoms, and Anxiety," Freud states that "it was anxiety which produced repression and not, as I formerly believed, repression which produced anxiety." Today, many neurobiologists continue to substantiate many of Freud's original ideas and theories. One example is the role of the amygdala, which subserves the fear response without any reference to conscious memory and substantiates Freud's concept of an unconscious memory system for anxiety responses. One of the unfortunate consequences of regarding the symptom of anxiety as a disorder rather than a signal is that the underlying sources of the anxiety may be ignored. From a psychodynamic perspective, the goal of therapy is not necessary to eliminate all anxiety but to increase anxiety tolerance—that is, the capacity to experience anxiety—and use it as a signal to investigate the underlying conflict that has created it. Anxiety appears in response to various situations during the life cycle, and although psychopharmacological agents may ameliorate symptoms, they may do nothing to address the life situation or its internal correlates that have induced the state of anxiety. In the following case, a disturbing fantasy precipitated an anxiety attack.

A married man 32 years of age was referred for therapy for severe and incapacitating anxiety, which was clinically manifested as repeated outbreaks of acute attacks of panic. Initially, he had absolutely no idea what had precipitated his attacks, nor were they associated with any conscious mental content. In the early weeks of treatment, he spent most of his time trying to impress the doctor with how hard he had worked and how effectively he had functioned before he was taken ill. At the same time, he described how fearful he was that he would fail at a new business venture he had embarked on. One day, with obvious acute anxiety that practically prevented him from talking, he revealed a fantasy that had suddenly popped into his mind a day or two before and had led to the outbreak of a severe anxiety attack. He had had the image of a large spike being driven through his penis. He also recalled that, as a child of 7, he was fascinated by his mother's clothing and that, on occasion, when she was out of the house, he dressed himself up in them. As an adult, he was fascinated by female lingerie and would sometimes find himself impelled by a desire to wear women's clothing. He had never yielded to the impulse, but on those occasions when the idea entered his consciousness, he became overwhelmed by acute anxiety and panic.

To understand fully a particular patient's anxiety from a psychodynamic view, it is often useful to relate the anxiety to developmental issues. At the earliest level, disintegration anxiety may be present. This anxiety derives from the fear that the self will fragment because others are not responding with needed affirmation and validation. Persecutory anxiety can be connected with the perception that the self is being invaded and annihilated by an outside malevolent force. Another source of anxiety involves a child who fears losing the love or approval of a parent or loved object. Freud's theory of castration anxiety is linked to the oedipal phase of development in boys, in which a powerful parental figure, usually the father, may damage the little boy's genitals or otherwise cause bodily harm. At the most mature level, superego anxiety is related to guilt feelings about not living up to internalized standards of moral behavior derived from the parents. Often, a psychodynamic interview can elucidate the principal level of anxiety with which a patient is dealing. Some anxiety is obviously related to multiple conflicts at various developmental levels.

Behavioral Theories. The behavioral or learning theories of anxiety postulate that anxiety is a conditioned response to a specific environmental stimulus. In a model of classic conditioning, a girl raised by an abusive father, for example, may become anxious as soon as she sees the abusive father. Through generalization, she may come to distrust all men. In the social learning model, a child may develop an anxiety response by imitating the anxiety in the environment, such as in anxious parents.

Existential Theories. Existential theories of anxiety provide models for generalized anxiety, in which no specifically identifiable stimulus exists for a chronically anxious feeling. The central concept of existential theory is that persons experience feelings of living in a purposeless universe. Anxiety is their response to the perceived void in existence and meaning. Such existential concerns may have increased since the development of nuclear weapons and bioterrorism.

Contributions of Biological Sciences

Autonomic Nervous System. Stimulation of the autonomic nervous system causes certain symptoms—cardiovascular (e.g., tachycardia), muscular (e.g., headache), gastrointestinal (e.g., diarrhea), and respiratory (e.g., tachypnea). The autonomic nervous systems of some patients with anxiety disorder, especially those with panic disorder, exhibit increased sympathetic tone, adapt slowly to repeated stimuli, and respond excessively to moderate stimuli.

Neurotransmitters. The three major neurotransmitters associated with anxiety on the bases of animal studies and responses to drug treatment are norepinephrine (NE), serotonin, and γ-aminobutyric acid (GABA). Much of the basic neuroscience information about anxiety comes from animal experiments involving behavioral paradigms and psychoactive agents. One such experiment to study anxiety was the conflict test, in which the animal is simultaneously presented with stimuli that are positive (e.g., food) and negative (e.g., electric shock). Anxiolytic drugs (e.g., benzodiazepines) tend to facilitate the adaptation of the animal to this situation, but other drugs (e.g., amphetamines) further disrupt the animal's behavioral responses.

NOREPINEPHRINE. Chronic symptoms experienced by patients with anxiety disorder, such as panic attacks, insomnia, startle, and autonomic hyperarousal, are characteristic of increased noradrenergic function. The general theory about the role of NE in anxiety disorders is that affected patients may have a poorly regulated noradrenergic system with occasional bursts of activity. The cell bodies of the noradrenergic system are primarily localized to the locus coeruleus in the rostral pons, and they project their axons to the cerebral cortex, the limbic system, the brainstem, and the spinal cord. Experiments in primates have demonstrated that stimulation of the locus coeruleus produces a fear response in the animals and that ablation of the same area inhibits or completely blocks the ability of the animals to form a fear response.

Human studies have found that in patients with panic disorder, β-adrenergic receptor agonists (e.g., isoproterenol [Isuprel]) and α_2-adrenergic receptor antagonists (e.g., yohimbine [Yocon]) can provoke frequent and severe panic attacks. Conversely, clonidine (Catapres), an α_2-receptor agonist, reduces anxiety symptoms in some experimental and therapeutic situations. A less consistent finding is that patients with anxiety disorders, particularly panic disorder, have elevated cerebrospinal fluid (CSF) or urinary levels of the noradrenergic metabolite 3-methoxy-4-hydroxyphenylglycol (MHPG).

HYPOTHALAMIC–PITUITARY–ADRENAL AXIS. Consistent evidence indicates that many forms of psychological stress increase the synthesis and release of cortisol. Cortisol serves to mobilize and to replenish energy stores and contributes to increased arousal, vigilance, focused attention, and memory formation; inhibition of the growth and reproductive system; and containment of the immune response. Excessive and sustained cortisol secretion can have serious adverse effects, including hypertension, osteoporosis, immunosuppression, insulin resistance, dyslipidemia, dyscoagulation, and, ultimately, atherosclerosis and cardiovascular disease. Alterations in hypothalamic–pituitary–adrenal (HPA) axis function have been demonstrated in PTSD. In patients with panic disorder, blunted adrenocorticoid hormone (ACTH) responses to corticotropin-releasing factor (CRF) have been reported in some studies and not in others.

CORTICOTROPIN-RELEASING HORMONE. One of the most important mediators of the stress response, corticotropin-releasing hormone (CRH) coordinates the adaptive behavioral and physiological changes that occur during stress. Hypothalamic levels of CRH are increased by stress, resulting in activation of the HPA axis and increased release of cortisol and dehydroepiandrosterone (DHEA). CRH also inhibits a variety of neurovegetative functions, such as food intake, sexual activity, and endocrine programs for growth and reproduction.

SEROTONIN. The identification of many serotonin receptor types has stimulated the search for the role of serotonin in the pathogenesis of anxiety disorders. Different types of acute stress result in increased 5-hydroxytryptamine (5-HT) turnover in the prefrontal cortex, nucleus accumbens, amygdala, and lateral hypothalamus. The interest in this relation was initially motivated by the observation that serotonergic antidepressants have therapeutic effects in some anxiety disorders—for example, clomipramine (Anafranil) in obsessive-compulsive disorder (OCD). The effectiveness of buspirone (BuSpar), a serotonin 5-HT_{1A} receptor agonist, in the treatment of anxiety disorders also suggests the possibility of an association between serotonin and anxiety. The cell bodies of most serotonergic neurons are located in the raphe nuclei in the rostral brainstem and project to the cerebral cortex, the limbic system (especially, the amygdala and the hippocampus), and the hypothalamus. Several reports indicate that meta-chlorophenylpiperazine (mCPP), a drug with multiple serotonergic and nonserotonergic effects, and fenfluramine (Pondimin), which causes the release of serotonin, do cause increased anxiety in patients with anxiety disorders; and many anecdotal reports indicate that serotonergic hallucinogens and stimulants—for example, lysergic acid diethylamide (LSD) and 3,4-methylenedioxymethamphetamine (MDMA)—are associated with the development of both acute and chronic anxiety disorders in persons who use these drugs. Clinical studies of 5-HT function in anxiety disorders have had mixed results. One study found that patients with panic disorder had lower levels of circulating 5-HT compared with control participants. Thus, no clear pattern of abnormality in 5-HT function in panic disorder has emerged from analysis of peripheral blood elements.

GABA. A role of GABA in anxiety disorders is most strongly supported by the undisputed efficacy of benzodiazepines, which enhance the activity of GABA at the GABA type A ($GABA_A$) receptor, in the treatment of some types of anxiety disorders. Although low-potency benzodiazepines are most effective for the symptoms of generalized anxiety disorder, high-potency benzodiazepines, such as alprazolam (Xanax), and clonazepam are effective in the treatment of panic disorder. Studies in primates have found that autonomic nervous system symptoms of anxiety disorders are induced when a benzodiazepine inverse agonist, β-carboline-3-carboxylic acid (BCCE), is administered. BCCE also causes anxiety in normal control volunteers. A benzodiazepine antagonist, flumazenil (Romazicon), causes frequent severe panic attacks in patients with panic disorder. These data have led researchers to hypothesize that some patients with anxiety disorders have abnormal functioning of their $GABA_A$ receptors, although this connection has not been shown directly.

APLYSIA. A neurotransmitter model for anxiety disorders is based on the study of *Aplysia californica* by Nobel Prize winner Eric Kandel, M.D. *Aplysia* is a sea snail that reacts to danger by moving away, withdrawing into its shell, and decreasing its feeding behavior. These behaviors can be classically conditioned, so that the snail responds to a neutral stimulus as if it were a dangerous stimulus. The snail can also be sensitized by random shocks, so that it exhibits a flight response in the absence of real danger. Parallels have previously been drawn between classic conditioning and human phobic anxiety. The classically conditioned *Aplysia* shows measurable changes in presynaptic facilitation, resulting in the release of increased amounts of neurotransmitter. Although the sea snail is a simple animal, this work shows an experimental approach to complex neurochemical processes potentially involved in anxiety disorders in humans.

NEUROPEPTIDE Y. Neuropeptide Y (NPY) is a highly conserved 36-amino acid peptide, which is among the most abundant peptides found in mammalian brain. Evidence suggesting the involvement of the amygdala in the anxiolytic effects of NPY is robust, and it probably occurs via the NPY-Y1 receptor. NPY has counterregulatory effects on corticotropin-releasing hormone (CRH) and locus coeruleus-NE systems at brain sites that are important in the expression of anxiety, fear, and depression. Preliminary studies in special operations soldiers under extreme training stress indicate that high NPY levels are associated with better performance.

GALANIN. Galanin is a peptide that, in humans, contains 30 amino acids. It has been demonstrated to be involved in a number of physiological and behavioral functions, including learning and memory, pain control, food intake, neuroendocrine control, cardiovascular regulation, and, most recently, anxiety. A dense galanin immunoreactive fiber system originating in the locus coeruleus innervates forebrain and midbrain structures, including the hippocampus, hypothalamus, amygdala, and prefrontal cortex. Studies in rats have shown that galanin administered centrally modulates anxiety-related behaviors. Galanin and NPY receptor agonists may be novel targets for antianxiety drug development.

Brain Imaging Studies. A range of brain imaging studies, almost always conducted with a specific anxiety disorder, has produced several possible leads in the understanding of anxiety disorders. Structural studies—for example, computed tomography (CT) and magnetic resonance imaging (MRI)—occasionally show some increase in the size of cerebral ventricles. In one study, the increase was correlated with the length of time patients had been taking benzodiazepines. In one MRI study, a specific defect in the right temporal lobe was noted in patients with panic disorder. Several other brain imaging studies have reported abnormal findings in the right hemisphere but not the left hemisphere; this finding suggests that some types of cerebral asymmetries may be important in the development of anxiety disorder symptoms in specific patients. Functional brain imaging studies—for example, positron emission tomography (PET), single-photon emission computed tomography (SPECT), and electroencephalography (EEG)—of patients with anxiety disorder have variously reported abnormalities in the frontal cortex; the occipital and temporal areas; and, in a study of panic disorder, the parahippocampal gyrus. Several functional neuroimaging studies have implicated the caudate nucleus in the pathophysiology of OCD. In posttraumatic stress disorder, Functional magnetic brain imaging (fMRI) studies have found increased activity in the amygdala, a brain region associated with fear. A conservative interpretation of these data is that some patients with anxiety disorders have a demonstrable functional cerebral pathological condition and that the condition may be causally relevant to their anxiety disorder symptoms.

Genetic Studies. Genetic studies have produced solid evidence that at least some genetic component contributes to the development of anxiety disorders. Heredity has been recognized as a predisposing factor in the development of anxiety disorders. Almost half of all patients with panic disorder have at least one affected relative. The figures for other anxiety disorders, although not as high, also indicate a higher frequency of the illness in first-degree relatives of affected patients than in the relatives of nonaffected persons. Although adoption studies with anxiety disorders have not been reported, data from twin registries also support the hypothesis that anxiety disorders are at least partially genetically determined. Clearly, a linkage exists between genetics and anxiety disorders, but no anxiety disorder is likely to result from a simple mendelian abnormality. One report has attributed about 4 percent of the intrinsic variability of anxiety within the general population to a polymorphic variant of the gene for the serotonin transporter, which is the site of action of many serotonergic drugs. Persons with the variant produce less transporter and have higher levels of anxiety.

In 2005, a scientific team, led by National Institute of Mental Health grantee and Noble Laureate Dr. Eric Kandel demonstrated that knocking out a gene in the brain's fear hub creates mice unperturbed by situations that would normally trigger instinctive or learned fear responses. The gene codes for *stathmin,* a protein that is critical for the amygdala to form fear memories. Stathmin knockout mice showed less anxiety when they heard a tone that had previously been associated with a shock, indicating less learned fear. The knockout mice also were more susceptible to explore novel open space and maze environments, a reflection of less innate fear. Kandel suggests that stathmin knockout mice can be used as a model of anxiety states of mental disorders with innate and learned fear components: these animals could be used to develop new antianxiety agents. Whether stathmin is similarly expressed and pivotal for anxiety in the human amygdala remains to be confirmed.

Neuroanatomical Considerations. The locus coeruleus and the raphe nuclei project primarily to the limbic system and the cerebral cortex. In combination with the data from brain imaging studies, these areas have become the focus of much hypothesis-forming about the neuroanatomical substrates of anxiety disorders.

LIMBIC SYSTEM. In addition to receiving noradrenergic and serotonergic innervation, the limbic system also contains a high concentration of $GABA_A$ receptors. Ablation and stimulation studies in nonhuman primates have also implicated the limbic system in the generation of anxiety and fear responses. Two areas of the limbic system have received special attention in the literature: increased activity in the septohippocampal pathway, which may lead to anxiety; and the cingulate gyrus, which has been implicated particularly in the pathophysiology of OCD.

CEREBRAL CORTEX. The frontal cerebral cortex is connected with the parahippocampal region, the cingulate gyrus, and the hypothalamus and thus may be involved in the production of anxiety disorders. The temporal cortex has also been implicated as a pathophysiological site in anxiety disorders. This association is based in part on the similarity in clinical presentation and electrophysiology between some patients with temporal lobe epilepsy and patients with OCD.

▲ 6.2 Panic Disorder

An acute intense attack of anxiety accompanied by feelings of impending doom is known as *panic disorder.* The anxiety is characterized by discrete periods of intense fear that can vary from several attacks during one day to only a few attacks during a year. Patients with panic disorder present with a number of comorbid conditions, most commonly agoraphobia, which refers to a fear of or anxiety regarding places from which escape might be difficult.

HISTORY

The idea of panic disorder may have its roots in the concept of irritable heart syndrome, which the physician Jacob Mendes DaCosta (1833–1900) noted in soldiers in the American Civil War. DaCosta's syndrome included many psychological and somatic symptoms that have since been included among the diagnostic criteria for panic disorder. In 1895, Sigmund Freud introduced the concept of anxiety neurosis, consisting of acute and chronic psychological and somatic symptoms.

EPIDEMIOLOGY

The lifetime prevalence of panic disorder is in the 1 to 4 percent range, with 6-month prevalence approximately 0.5 to 1.0 percent and 3 to 5.6 percent for panic attacks. Women are two to three times more likely to be affected than men, although underdiagnosis of panic disorder in men may contribute to the skewed distribution. The differences among Hispanics, whites, and blacks are few. The only social factor identified as contributing to the development of panic disorder is a recent history of divorce or separation. Panic disorder most commonly develops in young adulthood—the mean age of presentation is about 25 years—but both panic disorder and agoraphobia can develop at any age. Panic disorder has been reported in children and adolescents, and it is probably underdiagnosed in these age groups.

COMORBIDITY

Of patients with panic disorder, 91 percent have at least one other psychiatric disorder. About one-third of persons with panic disorders have major depressive disorder before onset; about two-thirds first experience panic disorder during or after the onset of major depression.

Other disorders also commonly occur in persons with panic disorder. Of persons with panic disorder, 15 to 30 percent also have social anxiety disorder or social phobia, 2 to 20 percent have specific phobia, 15 to 30 percent have generalized anxiety disorder, 2 to 10 percent have PTSD, and up to 30 percent have OCD. Other common comorbid conditions are hypochondriasis or illness anxiety disorder, personality disorders, and substance-related disorders.

ETIOLOGY

Biological Factors

Research on the biological basis of panic disorder has produced a range of findings; one interpretation is that the symptoms of panic disorder are related to a range of biological abnormalities in brain structure and function. Most work has used biological stimulants to induce panic attacks in patients with panic disorder. Considerable evidence indicates that abnormal regulation of brain noradrenergic systems is also involved in the pathophysiology of panic disorder. These and other studies have produced hypotheses implicating both peripheral and central nervous system (CNS) dysregulation in the pathophysiology of panic disorder. The autonomic nervous systems of some patients with panic disorder have been reported to exhibit increased sympathetic tone, to adapt slowly to repeated stimuli, and to respond excessively to moderate stimuli. Studies of the neuroendocrine status of these patients have shown several abnormalities, although the studies have been inconsistent in their findings.

The major neurotransmitter systems that have been implicated are those for norepinephrine, serotonin, and GABA. Serotonergic dysfunction is quite evident in panic disorder, and various studies with mixed serotonin agonist–antagonist drugs have demonstrated increased rates of anxiety. Such responses may be caused by postsynaptic serotonin hypersensitivity in panic disorder. Preclinical evidence suggests that attenuation of local inhibitory GABAergic transmission in the basolateral amygdala, midbrain, and hypothalamus can elicit anxiety-like physiological responses. The biological data have led to a focus on the brainstem (particularly the noradrenergic neurons of the locus coeruleus and the serotonergic neurons of the median raphe nucleus), the limbic system (possibly responsible for the generation of anticipatory anxiety), and the prefrontal cortex (possibly responsible for the generation of phobic avoidance). Among the various neurotransmitters involved, the noradrenergic system has also attracted much attention, with the presynaptic α_2-adrenergic receptors, particularly, playing a significant role. Patients with panic disorder are sensitive to the anxiogenic effects of yohimbine in addition to having exaggerated MHPG, cortisol, and cardiovascular responses. They have been identified by pharmacological challenges with the α_2-receptor agonist clonidine (Catapres) and the α_2-receptor antagonist yohimbine (Yocon), which stimulates firing of the locus coeruleus and elicits high rates of panic-like activity in those with panic disorder.

Panic-Inducing Substances. Panic-inducing substances (sometimes called *panicogens*) induce panic attacks in most patients with panic disorder and in a much smaller proportion of persons without panic disorder or a history of panic attacks. So-called respiratory panic-inducing substances cause respiratory stimulation and a shift in the acid–base balance. These substances include carbon dioxide (5 to 35 percent mixtures), sodium lactate, and bicarbonate. Neurochemical panic-inducing substances that act through specific neurotransmitter systems include yohimbine, an α_2-adrenergic receptor antagonist; mCPP, an agent with multiple serotonergic effects; m-Caroline drugs; $GABA_B$ receptor inverse agonists; flumazenil (Romazicon), a $GABA_B$ receptor antagonist; cholecystokinin; and caffeine. Isoproterenol (Isuprel) is also a panic-inducing substance, although its mechanism of action in inducing panic attacks is poorly understood. The respiratory panic-inducing substances may act initially at the peripheral cardiovascular baroreceptors and relay their signal by vagal afferents to the nucleus tractus solitarii and then on to the nucleus paragigantocellularis of the medulla. The hyperventilation in patients with panic disorder may be caused by a hypersensitive suffocation alarm system whereby increasing PCO_2 and brain lactate concentrations prematurely activate a physiological asphyxia monitor. The neurochemical panic-inducing substances are presumed to primarily affect the noradrenergic, serotonergic, and GABA receptors of the CNS directly.

Brain Imaging. Structural brain imaging studies, for example, MRI, in patients with panic disorder have implicated pathological involvement in the temporal lobes, particularly the hippocampus and the amygdala. One MRI study reported abnormalities, especially cortical atrophy, in the right temporal lobe of these patients. Functional brain imaging studies, for example, positron emission tomography (PET), have implicated dysregulation of cerebral blood flow (smaller increase or an actual decrease in cerebral blood flow). Specifically, anxiety disorders and panic attacks are associated with cerebral vasoconstriction, which may result in CNS symptoms, such as dizziness, and in peripheral nervous system symptoms that may be induced by hyperventilation and hypocapnia. Most functional brain imaging studies have used a specific panic-inducing substance (e.g., lactate, caffeine, or yohimbine) in combination with PET or SPECT to assess the effects of the panic-inducing substance and the induced panic attack on cerebral blood flow.

Mitral Valve Prolapse. Although great interest was formerly expressed in an association between mitral valve prolapse and panic disorder, research has almost completely erased any clinical significance or relevance to the association. Mitral valve prolapse is a heterogeneous syndrome consisting of the prolapse of one of the mitral valve leaflets, resulting in a midsystolic click on cardiac auscultation. Studies have found that the prevalence of panic disorder in patients with mitral valve prolapse is the same as the prevalence of panic disorder in patients without mitral valve prolapse.

Genetic Factors

Various studies have found that the first-degree relatives of patients with panic disorder have a four- to eightfold higher risk for panic disorder than first-degree relatives of other psychiatric patients. The twin studies conducted to date have generally reported that monozygotic twins are more likely to be concordant for panic disorder than are dizygotic twins. At this point, no data exist indicating an association between a specific chromosomal location or mode of transmission and this disorder.

Psychosocial Factors

Psychoanalytic theories have been developed to explain the pathogenesis of panic disorder. Psychoanalytic theories conceptualize panic attacks as arising from an unsuccessful defense against anxiety-provoking impulses. What was previously a mild signal anxiety becomes an overwhelming feeling of apprehension, complete with somatic symptoms.

Many patients describe panic attacks as coming out of the blue, as though no psychological factors were involved, but psychodynamic exploration frequently reveals a clear psychological trigger for the panic attack. Although panic attacks are correlated neurophysiologically with the locus coeruleus, the onset of panic is generally related to environmental or psychological factors. Patients with panic disorder have a higher incidence of stressful life events (particularly loss) than control subjects in the months before the onset of panic disorder. Moreover, the patients typically experience greater distress about life events than control subjects do.

The hypothesis that stressful psychological events produce neurophysiological changes in panic disorder is supported by a study of female twins. Separation from the mother early in life was clearly more likely to result in panic disorder than was paternal separation in the cohort of 1,018 pairs of female twins. Another etiological factor in adult female patients appears to be childhood physical and sexual abuse. Approximately 60 percent of women with panic disorder have a history of childhood sexual abuse compared with 31 percent of women with other anxiety disorders. Further support for psychological mechanisms in panic disorder can be inferred from a study of panic disorder in which patients received successful treatment with cognitive therapy. Before the therapy, the patients responded to panic attack induction with lactate. After successful cognitive therapy, lactate infusion no longer produced a panic attack.

The research indicates that the cause of panic attacks is likely to involve the unconscious meaning of stressful events and that the pathogenesis of the panic attacks may be related to neurophysiological factors triggered by the psychological reactions. Psychodynamic clinicians should always thoroughly investigate possible triggers whenever assessing a patient with panic disorder. The psychodynamics of panic disorder are summarized in Table 6.2–1.

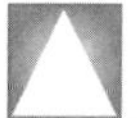

Table 6.2–1
Psychodynamic Themes in Panic Disorder

1. Difficulty tolerating anger
2. Physical or emotional separation from significant person both in childhood and in adult life
3. May be triggered by situations of increased work responsibilities
4. Perception of parents as controlling, frightening, critical, and demanding
5. Internal representations of relationships involving sexual or physical abuse
6. A chronic sense of feeling trapped
7. Vicious cycle of anger at parental rejecting behavior followed by anxiety that the fantasy will destroy the tie to parents
8. Failure of signal anxiety function in ego related to self-fragmentation and self-other boundary confusion
9. Typical defense mechanisms: reaction formation, undoing, somatization, and externalization

DIAGNOSIS

Panic Attacks

A panic attack is a sudden period of intense fear or apprehension that may last from minutes to hours. Panic attacks can occur in mental disorders other than panic disorder, particularly in specific phobia, social phobia, and PTSD. Unexpected panic attacks occur at any time and are not associated with any identifiable situational stimulus, but panic attacks need not be unexpected. Attacks in patients with social and specific phobias are usually expected or cued to a recognized or specific stimulus. Some panic attacks do not fit easily into the distinction between unexpected and expected, and these attacks are referred to as *situationally predisposed panic attacks.* They may or may not occur when a patient is exposed to a specific trigger, or they may occur either immediately after exposure or after a considerable delay.

Panic Disorder

The fifth edition of the *Diagnostic and Statistical Manual of Mental Disorders* (DSM-5) diagnostic criteria for panic disorder specifies that a panic attack is "an abrupt surge of intense fear or intense discomfort." In addition, there are a multitude of signs and symptoms as described in the overview section of this chapter among which are rapid heartbeat, palpitations, shortness of breath, dizziness, and a fear of impending death among others (see below under Clinical Features).

Some community surveys have indicated that panic attacks are common, and a major issue in developing diagnostic criteria for panic disorder was determining a threshold number or frequency of panic attacks required to meet the diagnosis. Setting the threshold too low results in the diagnosis of panic disorder in patients who do not have an impairment from an occasional panic attack; setting the threshold too high results in a situation in which patients who are impaired by their panic attacks do not meet the diagnostic criteria. DSM specifies that at least one of the attacks must be followed within one month by either a fear of another attack or a change in behavior to avoid the feared attack or both.

CLINICAL FEATURES

The first panic attack is often completely spontaneous, although panic attacks occasionally follow excitement, physical exertion, sexual activity, or moderate emotional trauma. Clinicians should attempt to ascertain any habit or situation that commonly precedes a patient's panic attacks. Such activities may include the use of caffeine, alcohol, nicotine, or other substances; unusual patterns of sleeping or eating; and specific environmental settings, such as harsh lighting at work.

The attack often begins with a 10-minute period of rapidly increasing symptoms. The major mental symptoms are extreme fear and a sense of impending death and doom. Patients usually cannot name the source of their fear; they may feel confused and have trouble concentrating. The physical signs often include tachycardia, palpitations, dyspnea, and sweating. Patients often try to leave whatever situation they are in to seek help. The attack generally lasts 20 to 30 minutes and rarely more than an hour. A formal mental status examination during a panic attack may reveal rumination, difficulty speaking (e.g., stammering), and impaired memory. Patients may experience depression or depersonalization during an attack. The symptoms can disappear quickly or gradually. Between attacks, patients may have anticipatory anxiety about having another attack. The differentiation between anticipatory anxiety and generalized anxiety disorder can be difficult, although patients with pain disorder with anticipatory anxiety can name the focus of their anxiety.

Somatic concerns of death from a cardiac or respiratory problem may be the major focus of patients' attention during panic attacks. Patients may believe that the palpitations and chest pain indicate that they are about to die. As many as 20 percent of such patients actually have syncopal episodes during a panic attack. The patients may be seen in emergency departments as young (20s), physically healthy persons who nevertheless insist that they are about to die from a heart attack. Rather than immediately diagnosing hypochondriasis, the emergency department physician should consider a diagnosis of panic disorder. Hyperventilation can produce respiratory alkalosis and other symptoms. The age-old treatment of breathing into a paper bag sometimes helps because it decreases alkalosis.

Mrs. K was a 35-year-old woman who initially presented for treatment at the medical emergency department at a large university-based medical center. She reported that while sitting at her desk at her job, she had suddenly experienced difficulty breathing, dizziness, tachycardia, shakiness, and a feeling of terror that she was going to die of a heart attack. A colleague drove her to the emergency department, where she received a full medical evaluation, including electrocardiography and routine blood work, which revealed no sign of cardiovascular, pulmonary, or other illness. She was subsequently referred for psychiatric evaluation, where she revealed that she had experienced two additional episodes over the past month, once when driving home from work and once when eating breakfast. However, she had not presented for medical treatment because the symptoms had resolved relatively quickly each time, and she worried that if she went to the hospital without ongoing symptoms, "people would think I'm crazy." Mrs. K reluctantly took the phone number of a local psychiatrist but did not call until she experienced a fourth episode of a similar nature. *(Courtesy of Erin B. McClure-Tone, Ph.D. and Daniel S. Pine, M.D.)*

Associated Symptoms

Depressive symptoms are often present in panic disorder, and in some patients, a depressive disorder coexists with the panic disorder. Some studies have found that the lifetime risk of suicide in persons with panic disorder is higher than it is in persons with no mental disorder. Clinicians should be alert to the risk of suicide. In addition to agoraphobia, other phobias and OCD can coexist with panic disorder. The psychosocial consequences of panic disorder, in addition to marital discord, can include time lost from work, financial difficulties related to the loss of work, and alcohol and other substance abuse.

DIFFERENTIAL DIAGNOSIS

Panic Disorder

The differential diagnosis for a patient with panic disorder includes many medical disorders (Table 6.2–2), as well as many mental disorders.

Medical Disorders

Panic disorder must be differentiated from a number of medical conditions that produce similar symptomatology. Panic attacks are associated with a variety of endocrinological disorders, including both hypo- and hyperthyroid states, hyperparathyroidism, and pheochromocytomas. Episodic hypoglycemia associated with insulinomas can also produce panic-like states, as can primary neuropathological processes. These include seizure disorders, vestibular dysfunction, neoplasms, or the effects of both

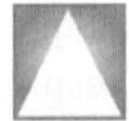

Table 6.2–2
Differential Diagnosis for Panic Disorder

Cardiovascular Diseases	
Anemia	Hypertension
Angina	Mitral valve prolapse
Congestive heart failure	Myocardial infarction
Hyperactive β-adrenergic state	Paradoxical atrial tachycardia
Pulmonary Diseases	
Asthma	Pulmonary embolus
Hyperventilation	
Neurological Diseases	
Cerebrovascular disease	Migraine
Epilepsy	Multiple sclerosis
Huntington's disease	Transient ischemic attack
Infection	Tumor
Ménière's disease	Wilson's disease
Endocrine Diseases	
Addison's disease	Hypoglycemia
Carcinoid syndrome	Hypoparathyroidism
Cushing's syndrome	Menopausal disorders
Diabetes	Pheochromocytoma
Hyperthyroidism	Premenstrual syndrome
Drug Intoxications	
Amphetamine	Hallucinogens
Amyl nitrite	Marijuana
Anticholinergics	Nicotine
Cocaine	Theophylline
Drug Withdrawal	
Alcohol	Opiates and opioids
Antihypertensives	Sedative–hypnotics
Other Conditions	
Anaphylaxis	Systemic infections
B_{12} deficiency	Systemic lupus erythematosus
Electrolyte disturbances	Temporal arteritis
Heavy metal poisoning	Uremia

prescribed and illicit substances on the CNS. Finally, disorders of the cardiac and pulmonary systems, including arrhythmias, chronic obstructive pulmonary disease, and asthma, can produce autonomic symptoms and accompanying crescendo anxiety that can be difficult to distinguish from panic disorder. Clues of an underlying medical etiology to panic-like symptoms include the presence of atypical features during panic attacks, such as ataxia, alterations in consciousness, or bladder dyscontrol; onset of panic disorder relatively late in life; or physical signs or symptoms indicative of an underlying medical disorder.

Mental Disorders

Panic disorder also must be differentiated from a number of psychiatric disorders, particularly other anxiety disorders. Panic attacks occur in many anxiety disorders, including social and specific phobia, Panic may also occur in PTSD and OCD. The key to correctly diagnosing panic disorder and differentiating the condition from other anxiety disorders involves the documentation of recurrent spontaneous panic attacks at some point in the illness. Differentiation from generalized anxiety disorder can also be difficult. Classically, panic attacks are characterized by their rapid onset (within minutes) and short duration (usually less than 10 to 15 minutes), in contrast to the anxiety associated with generalized anxiety disorder, which emerges and dissipates more slowly. Making this distinction can be difficult, however, because the anxiety surrounding panic attacks can be more diffuse and slower to dissipate than is typical. Because anxiety is a frequent concomitant of many other psychiatric disorders, including the psychoses and affective disorders, discrimination between panic disorder and a multitude of disorders can also be difficult.

Specific and Social Phobias

Sometimes it is difficult to distinguish between panic disorder, on the one hand, and specific and social phobias, on the other hand. Some patients who experience a single panic attack in a specific setting (e.g., an elevator) may go on to have long-lasting avoidance of the specific setting, regardless of whether they ever have another panic attack. These patients meet the diagnostic criteria for a specific phobia, and clinicians must use their judgment about what is the most appropriate diagnosis. In another example, a person who experiences one or more panic attacks may then fear speaking in public. Although the clinical picture is almost identical to the clinical picture in social phobia, a diagnosis of social phobia is excluded because the avoidance of the public situation is based on fear of having a panic attack rather than on fear of the public speaking itself.

COURSE AND PROGNOSIS

Panic disorder usually has its onset in late adolescence or early adulthood, although onset during childhood, early adolescence, and midlife does occur. Some data implicate increased psychosocial stressors with the onset of panic disorder, although no psychosocial stressor can be definitely identified in most cases.

Panic disorder, in general, is a chronic disorder, although its course is variable, both among patients and within a single patient. The available long-term follow-up studies of panic disorder are difficult to interpret because they have not controlled for the effects of treatment. Nevertheless, about 30 to 40 percent of patients seem to be symptom free at long-term follow-up, about 50 percent have symptoms that are sufficiently mild not to affect their lives significantly, and about 10 to 20 percent continue to have significant symptoms.

After the first one or two panic attacks, patients may be relatively unconcerned about their condition; with repeated attacks, however, the symptoms may become a major concern. Patients may attempt to keep the panic attacks secret and thereby cause their families and friends concern about unexplained changes in behavior. The frequency and severity of the attacks can fluctuate. Panic attacks can occur several times in a day or less than once a month. Excessive intake of caffeine or nicotine can exacerbate the symptoms.

Depression can complicate the symptom picture in anywhere from 40 to 80 percent of all patients, as estimated by various studies. Although the patients do not tend to talk about suicidal ideation, they are at increased risk for committing suicide. Alcohol and other substance dependence occur in about 20 to 40 percent of all patients, and OCD may also develop. Family interactions and performance in school and at work commonly suffer. Patients with good premorbid functioning and symptoms of brief duration tend to have good prognoses.

TREATMENT

With treatment, most patients exhibit dramatic improvement in the symptoms of panic disorder and agoraphobia. The two most effective treatments are pharmacotherapy and cognitive-behavioral therapy. Family and group therapy may help affected patients and their families adjust to the patient's disorder and to the psychosocial difficulties that the disorder may have precipitated.

Pharmacotherapy

Overview. Alprazolam (Xanax) and paroxetine (Paxil) are the two drugs approved by the U.S. Food and Drug Administration (FDA) for the treatment of panic disorder. In general, experience is showing superiority of the selective serotonin reuptake inhibitors (SSRIs) and clomipramine (Anafranil) over the benzodiazepines, monoamine oxidase inhibitors (MAOIs), and tricyclic and tetracyclic drugs in terms of effectiveness and tolerance of adverse effects. Some reports have suggested a role for venlafaxine (Effexor), and buspirone (BuSpar) has been suggested as an additive medication in some cases. Venlafaxine is approved by the FDA for treatment of generalized anxiety disorder and may be useful in panic disorder combined with depression. β-Adrenergic receptor antagonists have not been found to be particularly useful for panic disorder. A conservative approach is to begin treatment with paroxetine, sertraline (Zoloft), citalopram (Celexa), or fluvoxamine (Luvox) in isolated panic disorder. If rapid control of severe symptoms is desired, a brief course of alprazolam should be initiated concurrently with the SSRI followed by slowly tapering use of the benzodiazepine. In long-term use, fluoxetine (Prozac) is an effective drug for panic with comorbid depression, although its initial activating properties may mimic panic symptoms for the first several weeks, and it may be poorly tolerated on this basis. Clonazepam (Klonopin) can be prescribed for patients who anticipate a situation in which panic may occur (0.5 to 1 mg as required). Common dosages for antipanic drugs are listed in Table 6.2–3.

Table 6.2–3
Recommended Dosages for Commonly Used Antipanic Drugs (Daily Unless Indicated Otherwise)

Drug	Starting (mg)	Maintenance (mg)
SSRIs		
Paroxetine	5–10	20–60
Paroxetine CR	12.5–25	62.5
Fluoxetine	2–5	20–60
Sertraline	12.5–25	50–200
Fluvoxamine	12.5	100–150
Citalopram	10	20–40
Escitalopram	10	20
Tricyclic Antidepressants		
Clomipramine	5–12.5	50–125
Imipramine	10–25	150–500
Desipramine	10–25	150–200
Benzodiazepines		
Alprazolam	0.25–0.5 tid	0.5–2 tid
Clonazepam	0.25–0.5 bid	0.5–2 bid
Diazepam	2–5 bid	5–30 bid
Lorazepam	0.25–0.5 bid	0.5–2 bid
MAOIs		
Phenelzine	15 bid	15–45 bid
Tranylcypromine	10 bid	10–30 bid
RIMAs		
Moclobemide	50	300–600
Brofaromine	50	150–200
Atypical Antidepressants		
Venlafaxine	6.25–25	50–150
Venlafaxine XR	37.5	150–225
Other Agents		
Valproic acid	125 bid	500–750 bid
Inositol	6,000 bid	6,000 bid

bid, twice a day; MAOI, monoamine oxidase inhibitors; RIMA, reversible inhibitor of monoamine oxidase type A; SSRIs, selective serotonin reuptake inhibitor; tid, three times a day.

Selective Serotonin Reuptake Inhibitors. All SSRIs are effective for panic disorder. Paroxetine and paroxetine CR have sedative effects and tend to calm patients immediately, which lead to greater compliance and less discontinuation, but this must be weighed against its weight gain potential. Citalopram, escitalopram (Lexapro), fluvoxamine, and sertraline are the next best tolerated. Anecdotal reports suggest that patients with panic disorder are particularly sensitive to the activating effects of SSRIs, particularly fluoxetine, so they should be given initially at small dosages and titrated up slowly. At therapeutic dosages—for example, 20 mg a day of paroxetine—some patients may experience increased sedation. One approach for patients with panic disorder is to give 5 or 10 mg a day of paroxetine or 12.5 to 25 mg of paroxetine CR for 1 to 2 weeks and then increase the dosage by 10 mg of paroxetine or 12.5 mg of paroxetine CR a day every 1 to 2 weeks to a maximum of 60 mg of paroxetine or 62.5 mg of paroxetine CR. If sedation becomes intolerable, then taper the paroxetine dosage down to 10 mg a day of paroxetine or 12.5 mg of paroxetine CR and switch to fluoxetine at 10 mg a day and titrate upward slowly. Other strategies can be used based on the experience of the clinician.

Benzodiazepines. Benzodiazepines have the most rapid onset of action against panic, often within the first week, and they can be used for long periods without the development of tolerance to the antipanic effects. Alprazolam has been the most widely used benzodiazepine for panic disorder, but controlled studies have demonstrated equal efficacy for lorazepam (Ativan), and case reports have also indicated that clonazepam may be effective. Some patients use benzodiazepines as needed when faced with a phobic stimulus. Benzodiazepines can reasonably be used as the first agent for treatment of panic disorder while a serotonergic drug is being slowly titrated to a therapeutic dose. After 4 to 12 weeks, benzodiazepine use can be slowly tapered (over 4 to 10 weeks) while the serotonergic drug is continued. The major reservation among clinicians regarding the use of benzodiazepines for panic disorder is the potential for dependence, cognitive impairment, and abuse, especially after long-term use. Patients should be instructed not to drive, abstain from alcohol or other CNS depressant medications, and avoid operating dangerous equipment while taking benzodiazepines. Whereas benzodiazepines elicit a sense of well-being, discontinuation of benzodiazepines produces a well-documented and unpleasant withdrawal syndrome. Anecdotal reports and small case series have indicated that addiction to alprazolam is one of the most difficult to overcome, and it may require a comprehensive program of detoxification. Benzodiazepine dosage should be tapered slowly, and all anticipated withdrawal effects should be thoroughly explained to the patient.

Tricyclic and Tetracyclic Drugs. At the present time, SSRIs are considered the first-line agents for the treatment of panic disorder. Data, however, show that among tricyclic drugs, clomipramine and imipramine (Tofranil) are the most effective in the treatment of panic disorder. Clinical experience indicates that the dosages must be titrated slowly upward to avoid overstimulation and that the full clinical benefit requires full dosages and may not be achieved for 8 to 12 weeks. Some data support the efficacy of desipramine (Norpramin), and less evidence suggests a role for maprotiline (Ludiomil), trazodone (Desyrel), nortriptyline (Pamelor), amitriptyline (Elavil), and doxepin (Adapin). Tricyclic drugs are less widely used than SSRIs because the tricyclic drugs generally have more severe adverse effects at the higher dosages required for effective treatment of panic disorder.

Monoamine Oxidase Inhibitors. The most robust data support the effectiveness of phenelzine (Nardil), and some data also support the use of tranylcypromine (Parnate). MAOIs appear less likely to cause overstimulation than either SSRIs or tricyclic drugs, but they may require full dosages for at least 8 to 12 weeks to be effective. The need for dietary restrictions has limited the use of MAOIs, particularly since the appearance of the SSRIs.

Treatment Nonresponse. If patients fail to respond to one class of drugs, another should be tried. Recent data support the effectiveness of venlafaxine. The combination of an SSRI or a tricyclic drug and a benzodiazepine or of an SSRI and lithium or a tricyclic drug can be tried. Case reports have suggested the effectiveness of carbamazepine (Tegretol), valproate (Depakene), and calcium channel inhibitors. Buspirone may have a role in the augmentation of other medications but has little effectiveness by itself. Clinicians should reassess the patient, particularly to establish the presence of comorbid conditions such as depression, alcohol use, or other substance use.

Duration of Pharmacotherapy. When it becomes effective, pharmacological treatment should generally continue for 8 to 12 months. Data indicate that panic disorder is a chronic, perhaps lifelong, condition that recurs when treatment is discontinued. Studies have reported that 30 to 90 percent of patients with panic disorder who have had successful treatment have a relapse when their medication is discontinued. Patients may be likely to relapse if they have been given benzodiazepines and the benzodiazepine therapy is terminated in a way that causes withdrawal symptoms.

Cognitive and Behavior Therapies

Cognitive and behavior therapies are effective treatments for panic disorder. Various reports have concluded that cognitive and behavior therapies are superior to pharmacotherapy alone; other reports have concluded the opposite. Several studies and reports have found that the combination of cognitive or behavior therapy with pharmacotherapy is more effective than either approach alone. Several studies that included long-term follow-up of patients who received cognitive or behavior therapy indicate that the therapies are effective in producing long-lasting remission of symptoms.

Cognitive Therapy. The two major foci of cognitive therapy for panic disorder are instruction about a patient's false beliefs and information about panic attacks. The instruction about false beliefs centers on the patient's tendency to misinterpret mild bodily sensations as indicating impending panic attacks, doom, or death. The information about panic attacks includes explanations that when panic attacks occur, they are time limited and not life-threatening.

Dynamic Psychotherapy. Cognitive and behavioral therapy have replaced the dynamic psychotherapies as the first line of therapy. Nevertheless, in those instances where there has been no response an understanding of conscious and unconscious conflicts that contribute to both anxiety and panic may be useful in selected cases.

▲ 6.3 Agoraphobia

Agoraphobia refers to a fear of or anxiety regarding places from which escape might be difficult. It can be the most disabling of the phobias because it can significantly interfere with a person's ability to function in work and social situations outside the home. In the United States, most researchers of panic disorder believe that agoraphobia almost always develops as a complication in patients with panic disorder. That is, the fear of having a panic attack in a public place from which escape would be formidable is thought to cause the agoraphobia. Although agoraphobia often coexists with panic disorder, DSM-5 classifies agoraphobia as a separate condition that may or may not be comorbid with panic disorder.

HISTORY

The term *agoraphobia* was coined in 1871 to describe the condition of patients who were afraid to venture alone into public places. The term is derived from the Greek words *agora* and *phobos,* meaning "fear of the marketplace."

EPIDEMIOLOGY

The lifetime prevalence of agoraphobia is somewhat controversial, varying between 2 to 6 percent across studies. According to the DSM-5, persons older than age 65 years have a 0.4 percent prevalence rate of agoraphobia, but this may be a low estimate. The major factor leading to this wide range of estimates relates to disagreement about the conceptualization of agoraphobia's relationship to panic disorder. Although studies of agoraphobia in psychiatric settings have reported that at least three fourths of the affected patients have panic disorder as well, studies of agoraphobia in community samples have found that as many as half the patients have agoraphobia without panic disorder. The reasons for these divergent findings are unknown but probably involve differences in ascertainment techniques. In many cases, the onset of agoraphobia follows a traumatic event.

DIAGNOSIS AND CLINICAL FEATURES

The DSM-5 diagnostic criteria for agoraphobia stipulates marked fear or anxiety about at least one situation from two or more of five situation groups: (1) using public transportation (e.g., bus, train, cars, planes), (2) in an open space (e.g., park, shopping center, parking lot), (3) in an enclosed space (e.g., stores, elevators, theaters), (4) in a crowd or standing in line, or (5) alone outside of the home. The fear or anxiety must be persistent and last at least 6 months. Patients with agoraphobia rigidly avoid situations in which it would be difficult to obtain help. They prefer to be accompanied by a friend or a family member in busy streets, crowded stores, closed-in spaces (e.g., tunnels, bridges, and elevators), and closed-in vehicles (e.g., subways, buses, and airplanes). Patients may insist that they be accompanied every time they leave the house. The behavior can result in marital discord, which may be misdiagnosed as the primary problem. Severely affected patients may simply refuse to leave the house. Particularly before a correct diagnosis is made, patients may be terrified that they are going crazy.

Mrs. W was a 33-year-old married woman. She visited an anxiety clinic reporting that she felt like she was having a heart attack whenever she left her home. Her disorder began 8 years earlier while attending a yoga class when she suddenly noticed a dramatic increase in her heartbeat, felt stabbing pains in her chest, and had difficulty breathing. She began sweating and trembling and felt dizzy. She immediately went to the emergency department, where an electrocardiogram was performed. No abnormalities were detected. Over the next few months, Mrs. W experienced similar attacks of 15 to 30 minutes' duration about four times per month. She often sought medical advice after each episode, and each time no physical abnormalities were detected. After experiencing a few of these attacks, Mrs. W became afraid of having an attack away from home and would not leave her home unless absolutely necessary, in which case she needed to have her cell phone or be accompanied by someone. Even so, she avoided crowded places such as malls, movie theaters, and banks, where rapid escape is sometimes blocked. Her symptoms and avoidance dominated her life, although she was aware that they were irrational and excessive. She experienced mild depression and restlessness and had difficulty sleeping.

DIFFERENTIAL DIAGNOSIS

The differential diagnosis for agoraphobia includes all the medical disorders that can cause anxiety or depression. The psychiatric differential diagnosis includes major depressive disorder, schizophrenia, paranoid personality disorder, avoidance personality disorder, and dependent personality disorder.

COURSE AND PROGNOSIS

Most cases of agoraphobia are thought to be caused by panic disorder. When the panic disorder is treated, the agoraphobia often improves with time. For rapid and complete reduction of agoraphobia, behavior therapy is sometimes indicated. Agoraphobia without a history of panic disorder is often incapacitating and chronic, and depressive disorders and alcohol dependence often complicate its course.

TREATMENT

Pharmacotherapy

Benzodiazepines. Benzodiazepines have the most rapid onset of action against panic. Some patients use them as needed when faced with a phobic stimulus. Alprazolam (Xanax) and lorazepam (Ativan) are the most commonly prescribed benzodiazepines. Clonazepam (Klonopin) has also been shown to be effective. The major reservations among clinicians regarding the use of benzodiazepines are the potential for dependence, cognitive impairment, and abuse, particularly with long-term use. However, when used appropriately under medical supervision, benzodiazepines are efficacious and generally well-tolerated. The most common side effects are mild dizziness and sedation, both of which are generally attenuated by time or change of dose. Caution must be exercised when using heavy or dangerous machinery or when driving, especially when first starting the medication or when the dose is changed. Benzodiazepines should not be used in combination with alcohol because they can intensify its effects. Benzodiazepines are also best avoided in individuals with histories of alcohol or substance abuse unless there are compelling reasons, such as failure to respond to other classes of medications.

Selective Serotonin Reuptake Inhibitors. SSRIs have been shown to help reduce or prevent relapse from various forms of anxiety, including agoraphobia. Effective doses are essentially the same as for the treatment of depression, although it is customary to start with lower initial doses than in depression to minimize an initial anxiolytic effect, which is almost always short lived, and to titrate upward somewhat slower toward a therapeutic dose. The main advantages of SSRIs antidepressants include their improved safety profile in overdose and more tolerable side-effect burden. Common side effects of most SSRIs are sleep disturbance, drowsiness, lightheadedness, nausea, and diarrhea; many of these adverse effects improve with continued use. Another commonly reported side effect of SSRIs is sexual dysfunction (i.e., decreased libido, delayed ejaculation in men, delayed orgasm in women), which rarely improves with time or switching among SSRIs (or from an SSRI to a serotonin–norepinephrine reuptake inhibitor [SNRI]). Proposed strategies to combat sexual dysfunction in patients taking SSRIs include adjunctive use of yohimbine (Yocon), bupropion (Wellbutrin), or mirtazapine (Remeron); dose reduction; or adjunctive use of sildenafil (Viagra). Another issue to be considered when prescribing an SSRI is the possibility of a discontinuation syndrome if these medications are stopped abruptly. Commonly reported symptoms of this condition, which tend to occur 2 to 4 days after medication cessation, include increased anxiety, irritability, tearfulness, dizziness or lightheadedness, malaise, sleep disturbance, and concentration difficulties. This discontinuation syndrome is most common among SSRIs with shorter half-lives (e.g., paroxetine [Paxil]).

Tricyclic and Tetracyclic Drugs. Although SSRIs are considered the first-line agents for treatment of panic disorders with or without agoraphobia, the tricyclic drugs clomipramine (Anafranil) and imipramine (Tofranil) are the most effective in the treatment of these disorders. Dosages must be titrated slowly upward to avoid overstimulation (e.g., "jitteriness" syndrome), and the full clinical benefit requires full dosages and may not be achieved for 8 to 12 weeks. Therapeutic drug monitoring (TDM) may be useful to ensure that the patient is on an adequate dose of medication while avoiding issues of toxicity. The other adverse effects to these antidepressants are related to their effects on seizure threshold, as well as anticholinergic and potentially harmful cardiac effects, particularly in overdose.

Psychotherapy

Supportive Psychotherapy. Supportive psychotherapy involves the use of psychodynamic concepts and a therapeutic alliance to promote adaptive coping. Adaptive defenses are encouraged and strengthened, and maladaptive ones are discouraged. The therapist assists in reality testing and may offer advice regarding behavior.

Insight-Oriented Psychotherapy. In insight-oriented psychotherapy, the goal is to increase the patient's development of insight into psychological conflicts that, if unresolved, can manifest as symptomatic behavior.

Behavior Therapy. In behavior therapy, the basic assumption is that change can occur without the development of psychological insight into underlying causes. Techniques include positive and negative reinforcement, systematic desensitization, flooding, implosion, graded exposure, response prevention, stop thought, relaxation techniques, panic control therapy, self-monitoring, and hypnosis.

Cognitive Therapy. This is based on the premise that maladaptive behavior is secondary to distortions in how people perceive themselves and in how other perceive them. Treatment is short term and interactive, with assigned homework and tasks to be performed between sessions that focus on correcting distorted assumptions and cognitions. The emphasis is on confronting and examining situations that elicit interpersonal anxiety and associated mild depression.

Virtual Therapy. Computer programs have been developed that allow patients to see themselves as avatars who are then placed in open or crowded spaces (e.g., a supermarket). As they identify with the avatars in repeated computer sessions, they are able to master their anxiety through deconditioning.

▲ 6.4 Specific Phobia

The term *phobia* refers to an excessive fear of a specific object, circumstance, or situation. A specific phobia is a strong, persisting fear of an object or situation. The diagnosis of specific phobia requires the development of intense anxiety, even to the point of panic, when exposed to the feared object. Persons with specific phobias may anticipate harm, such as being bitten by a dog, or may panic at the thought of losing control; for instance, if they fear being in an elevator, they may also worry about fainting after the door closes.

EPIDEMIOLOGY

Phobias are one of the most common mental disorders in the United States, where approximately 5 to 10 percent of the population is estimated to have these troubling and sometimes disabling disorders. The lifetime prevalence of specific phobia is about 10 percent. Specific phobia is the most common mental disorder among women and the second most common among men, second only to substance-related disorders. The 6-month prevalence of specific phobia is about 5 to 10 per 100 persons (Table 6.4–1). The rates of specific phobias in women (14 to 16 percent) were double those of men (5 to 7 percent), although the ratio is closer to 1 to 1 for the fear of blood, injection, or injury type. (Types of phobias are discussed below in this section.) The peak age of onset for the natural environment type and the blood–injection–injury type is in the range of 5 to 9 years, although onset also occurs at older ages. In contrast, the peak age of onset for the situational type (except fear of heights) is higher, in the mid-20s, which is closer to the age of onset for agoraphobia. The feared objects and situations in specific phobias (listed in descending frequency of appearance) are animals, storms, heights, illness, injury, and death.

COMORBIDITY

Reports of comorbidity in specific phobia range from 50 to 80 percent. Common comorbid disorders with specific phobia include anxiety, mood, and substance-related disorders.

ETIOLOGY

General Principles of Phobias

Behavioral Factors. In 1920, John B. Watson wrote an article called "Conditioned Emotional Reactions," in which he recounted his experiences with Little Albert, an infant with a fear of rats and rabbits. Unlike Sigmund Freud's case of Little Hans, who had phobic symptoms (of horses) in the natural course of his maturation, Little Albert's difficulties were the direct result of the scientific experiments of two psychologists

Table 6.4–1
Lifetime Prevalence Rates of Specific Phobia

Site	Men (%)	Women (%)	Total (%)
United States (National Comorbidity Survey)	6.7	15.7	11.3
United States (Epidemiological Catchment Area Study)	7.7	14.4	11.2
Puerto Rico	7.6	9.6	8.6
Edmonton, Canada	4.6	9.8	7.2
Korea	2.6	7.9	5.4
Zurich, Switzerland	5.2	16.1	10.7
Netherlands	6.6	13.6	10.1

who used techniques that had successfully induced conditioned responses in laboratory animals.

Watson's hypothesis invoked the traditional pavlovian stimulus–response model of the conditioned reflex to account for the creation of the phobia: Anxiety is aroused by a naturally frightening stimulus that occurs in contiguity with a second inherently neutral stimulus. As a result of the contiguity, especially when the two stimuli are paired on several successive occasions, the originally neutral stimulus becomes capable of arousing anxiety by itself. The neutral stimulus, therefore, becomes a conditioned stimulus for anxiety production.

In the classic stimulus–response theory, the conditioned stimulus gradually loses its potency to arouse a response if it is not reinforced by periodic repetition of the unconditioned stimulus. In phobias, attenuation of the response to the stimulus does not occur; the symptom may last for years without any apparent external reinforcement. Operant conditioning theory provides a model to explain this phenomenon: Anxiety is a drive that motivates the organism to do whatever it can to obviate a painful affect. In the course of its random behavior, the organism learns that certain actions enable it to avoid the anxiety-provoking stimulus. These avoidance patterns remain stable for long periods as a result of the reinforcement they receive from their capacity to diminish anxiety. This model is readily applicable to phobias in that avoidance of the anxiety-provoking object or situation plays a central part. Such avoidance behavior becomes fixed as a stable symptom because of its effectiveness in protecting the person from the phobic anxiety.

Learning theory, which is particularly relevant to phobias, provides simple and intelligible explanations for many aspects of phobic symptoms. Critics contend, however, that learning theory deals mostly with surface mechanisms of symptom formation and is less useful than psychoanalytic theories in clarifying some of the complex underlying psychic processes involved.

Psychoanalytic Factors. Sigmund Freud's formulation of phobic neurosis is still the analytic explanation of specific phobia and social phobia. Freud hypothesized that the major function of anxiety is to signal the ego that a forbidden unconscious drive is pushing for conscious expression and to alert the ego to strengthen and marshal its defenses against the threatening instinctual force. Freud viewed the phobia—anxiety hysteria, as he continued to call it—as a result of conflicts centered on an unresolved childhood oedipal situation. Because sex drives continue to have a strong incestuous coloring in adults, sexual arousal can kindle an anxiety that is characteristically a fear of castration. When repression fails to be entirely successful, the ego must call on auxiliary defenses. In patients with phobias, the primary defense involved is displacement; that is, the sexual conflict is displaced from the person who evokes the conflict to a seemingly unimportant, irrelevant object or situation, which then has the power to arouse a constellation of affects, one of which is called *signal anxiety*. The phobic object or situation may have a direct associative connection with the primary source of the conflict and thus symbolizes it (the defense mechanism of symbolization).

Furthermore, the situation or the object is usually one that the person can avoid; with the additional defense mechanism of avoidance, the person can escape suffering serious anxiety. The end result is that the three combined defenses (repression, displacement, and symbolization) may eliminate the anxiety. The anxiety is controlled at the cost of creating a phobic neurosis, however. Freud first discussed the theoretical formulation of phobia formation in his famous case history of Little Hans, a 5-year-old boy who feared horses.

Although psychiatrists followed Freud's thought that phobias resulted from castration anxiety, recent psychoanalytic theorists have suggested that other types of anxiety may be involved. In agoraphobia, for example, separation anxiety clearly plays a leading role, and in erythrophobia (a fear of red that can be manifested as a fear of blushing), the element of shame implies the involvement of superego anxiety. Clinical observations have led to the view that anxiety associated with phobias has a variety of sources and colorings.

Phobias illustrate the interaction between a genetic constitutional diathesis and environmental stressors. Longitudinal studies suggest that certain children are constitutionally predisposed to phobias because they are born with a specific temperament known as behavioral inhibition to the unfamiliar, but a chronic environmental stress must act on a child's temperamental disposition to create a full-blown phobia. Stressors, such as the death of a parent, separation from a parent, criticism or humiliation by an older sibling, and violence in the household, may activate the latent diathesis within the child, who then becomes symptomatic. An overview of psychodynamic aspects of phobias is summarized in Table 6.4–2.

Counterphobic Attitude. Otto Fenichel called attention to the fact that phobic anxiety can be hidden behind attitudes and behavior patterns that represent a denial, either that the dreaded object or situation is dangerous or that the person is afraid of it. Instead of being a passive victim of external circumstances, a person reverses the situation and actively attempts to confront and master whatever is feared. Persons with counterphobic attitudes seek out situations of danger and rush enthusiastically toward them. Devotees of potentially dangerous sports, such as parachute jumping and rock climbing, may be exhibiting counterphobic behavior. Such patterns may be secondary to phobic anxiety or may be normal means of dealing with a realistically dangerous situation. Children's play may exhibit counterphobic elements, as when children play doctor and give

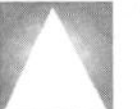

Table 6.4–2
Psychodynamic Themes in Phobias

- ▲ Principal defense mechanisms include displacement, projection, and avoidance.
- ▲ Environmental stressors, including humiliation and criticism from an older sibling, parental fights, or loss and separation from parents, interact with a genetic-constitutional diathesis.
- ▲ A characteristic pattern of internal object relations is externalized in social situations in the case of social phobia.
- ▲ Anticipation of humiliation, criticism, and ridicule is projected onto individuals in the environment.
- ▲ Shame and embarrassment are the principal affect states.
- ▲ Family members may encourage phobic behavior and serve as obstacles to any treatment plan.
- ▲ Self-exposure to the feared situation is a basic principle of all treatment.

a doll the shot they received earlier that day in the pediatrician's office. This pattern of behavior may involve the related defense mechanism of identifying with the aggressor.

Specific Phobia

The development of specific phobia may result from the pairing of a specific object or situation with the emotions of fear and panic. Various mechanisms for the pairing have been postulated. In general, a nonspecific tendency to experience fear or anxiety forms the backdrop; when a specific event (e.g., driving) is paired with an emotional experience (e.g., an accident), the person is susceptible to a permanent emotional association between driving or cars and fear or anxiety. The emotional experience itself can be in response to an external incident, as a traffic accident, or to an internal incident, most commonly a panic attack. Although a person may never again experience a panic attack and may not meet the diagnostic criteria for panic disorder, he or she may have a generalized fear of driving, not an expressed fear of having a panic attack while driving. Other mechanisms of association between the phobic object and the phobic emotions include modeling, in which a person observes the reaction in another (e.g., a parent), and information transfer, in which a person is taught or warned about the dangers of specific objects (e.g., venomous snakes).

Genetic Factors. Specific phobia tends to run in families. The blood–injection–injury type has a particularly high familial tendency. Studies have reported that two-thirds to three-fourths of affected probands have at least one first-degree relative with specific phobia of the same type, but the necessary twin and adoption studies have not been conducted to rule out a significant contribution by nongenetic transmission of specific phobia.

DIAGNOSIS

The DSM-5 includes distinctive types of specific phobia: animal type, natural environment type (e.g., storms), blood–injection–injury type (e.g., needles), situational type (e.g., cars, elevators, planes), and other type (for specific phobias that do not fit into the previous four types). The key feature of each type of phobia is that fear symptoms occur only in the presence of a specific object. The blood–injection–injury type is differentiated from the others in that bradycardia and hypotension often follow the initial tachycardia that is common to all phobias. The blood–injection–injury type of specific phobia is particularly likely to affect many members and generations of a family. One type of phobia of recently reported phobia is space phobia, in which persons fear falling when there is no nearby support, such as a wall or a chair. Some data indicate that affected persons may have abnormal right hemisphere function, possibly resulting in visual–spatial impairment. Balance disorders should be ruled out in such patients.

Phobias have traditionally been classified according to specific fear by means of Greek or Latin prefixes, as indicated in Table 6.4–3. Other phobias that are related to changes in the society are the fear of electromagnetic fields, of microwaves, and of society as a whole (amaxophobia).

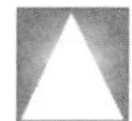

Table 6.4–3
Phobias

Acrophobia	Fear of heights
Agoraphobia	Fear of open places
Ailurophobia	Fear of cats
Hydrophobia	Fear of water
Claustrophobia	Fear of closed spaces
Cynophobia	Fear of dogs
Mysophobia	Fear of dirt and germs
Pyrophobia	Fear of fire
Xenophobia	Fear of strangers
Zoophobia	Fear of animals

Mr. S was a successful lawyer who presented for treatment after his firm, to which he had previously been able to walk from home, moved to a new location that he could only reach by driving. Mr. S reported that he was "terrified" of driving, particularly on highways. Even the thought of getting into a car led him to worry that he would die in a fiery crash. His thoughts were associated with intense fear and numerous somatic symptoms, including a racing heart, nausea, and sweating. Although the thought of driving was terrifying in and of itself, Mr. S became nearly incapacitated when he drove on busy roads, often having to pull over to vomit. *(Courtesy of Erin B. McClure-Tone, Ph.D. and Daniel S. Pine, M.D.)*

CLINICAL FEATURES

Phobias are characterized by the arousal of severe anxiety when patients are exposed to specific situations or objects or when patients even anticipate exposure to the situations or objects. Exposure to the phobic stimulus or anticipation of it almost invariably results in a panic attack in a person who is susceptible to them.

Persons with phobias, by definition, try to avoid the phobic stimulus; some go to great trouble to avoid anxiety-provoking situations. For example, a patient with a phobia may take a bus across the United States, rather than fly, to avoid contact with the object of the patient's phobia, an airplane. Perhaps as another way to avoid the stress of the phobic stimulus, many patients have substance-related disorders, particularly alcohol use disorders. Moreover, an estimated one-third of patients with social phobia have major depressive disorder.

The major finding on the mental status examination is the presence of an irrational and ego-dystonic fear of a specific situation, activity, or object; patients are able to describe how they avoid contact with the phobia. Depression is commonly found on the mental status examination and may be present in as many as one-third of all patients with phobia.

DIFFERENTIAL DIAGNOSIS

Nonpsychiatric medical conditions that can result in the development of a phobia include the use of substances (particularly hallucinogens and sympathomimetics), CNS tumors, and cerebrovascular diseases. Phobic symptoms in these instances are unlikely in the absence of additional suggestive findings on physical, neurological, and mental status examinations. Schizophrenia is also in the differential diagnosis of specific phobia because patients with schizophrenia can have phobic symptoms as part of their psychoses. Unlike patients with schizophrenia, however, patients with phobia have insight into the irrationality of their fears and lack the bizarre quality and other psychotic symptoms that accompany schizophrenia.

In the differential diagnosis of specific phobia, clinicians must consider panic disorder, agoraphobia, and avoidant personality disorder. Differentiation among panic disorder, agoraphobia, social phobia, and specific phobia can be difficult in individual cases. In general, however, patients with specific phobia tend to experience anxiety immediately when presented with the phobic stimulus. Furthermore, the anxiety or panic is limited to the identified situation; patients are not abnormally anxious when they are neither confronted with the phobic stimulus nor caused to anticipate the stimulus.

Other diagnoses to consider in the differential diagnosis of specific phobia are hypochondriasis, OCD, and paranoid personality disorder. Whereas hypochondriasis is the fear of having a disease, specific phobia of the illness type is the fear of contracting the disease. Some patients with OCD manifest behavior indistinguishable from that of a patient with specific phobia. For example, whereas patients with OCD may avoid knives because they have compulsive thoughts about killing their children, patients with specific phobia about knives may avoid them for fear of cutting themselves. Patients with paranoid personality disorder have generalized fear that distinguishes them from those with specific phobia.

COURSE AND PROGNOSIS

Specific phobia exhibits a bimodal age of onset, with a childhood peak for animal phobia, natural environment phobia, and blood–injection–injury phobia and an early adulthood peak for other phobias, such as situational phobia. Limited prospective epidemiological data are available that chart the natural course of specific phobia. Because patients with isolated specific phobia rarely present for treatment, there is also little research on the course of the disorder in the clinic. The limited information that is available suggests that most specific phobias that begin in childhood and persist into adulthood will continue to persist for many years. The severity of the condition is believed to remain relatively constant, which contrasts with the waxing and waning course seen in other anxiety disorders.

TREATMENT

Phobias

Behavior Therapy. The most studied and most effective treatment for phobias is probably behavior therapy. The key aspects of successful treatment are (1) the patient's commitment to treatment; (2) clearly identified problems and objectives; and (3) available alternative strategies for coping with the feelings. A variety of behavioral treatment techniques have been used, the most common being systematic desensitization, a method pioneered by Joseph Wolpe. In this method, the patient is exposed serially to a predetermined list of anxiety-provoking stimuli graded in a hierarchy from the least to the most frightening. Through the use of antianxiety drugs, hypnosis, and instruction in muscle relaxation, patients are taught how to induce in themselves both mental and physical repose. After they have mastered the techniques, patients are taught to use them to induce relaxation in the face of each anxiety-provoking stimulus. As they become desensitized to each stimulus in the scale, the patients move up to the next stimulus until, ultimately, what previously produced the most anxiety no longer elicits the painful affect.

Other behavioral techniques that have been used more recently involve intensive exposure to the phobic stimulus through either imagery or desensitization in vivo. In imaginal flooding, patients are exposed to the phobic stimulus for as long as they can tolerate the fear until they reach a point at which they can no longer feel it. Flooding (also known as implosion) in vivo requires patients to experience similar anxiety through exposure to the actual phobic stimulus.

Insight-Oriented Psychotherapy. Early in the development of psychoanalysis and the dynamically oriented psychotherapies, theorists believed that these methods were the treatments of choice for phobic neurosis, which was then thought to stem from oedipal–genital conflicts. Soon, however, therapists recognized that, despite progress in uncovering and analyzing unconscious conflicts, patients frequently failed to lose their phobic symptoms. Moreover, by continuing to avoid phobic situations, patients excluded a significant degree of anxiety and its related associations from the analytic process. Both Freud and his pupil Sándor Ferenczi recognized that if progress in analyzing these symptoms was to be made, therapists had to go beyond their analytic roles and actively urge patients with phobia to seek the phobic situation and experience the anxiety and resultant insight. Since then, psychiatrists have generally agreed that a measure of activity on the therapist's part is often required to treat phobic anxiety successfully. The decision to apply the techniques of psychodynamic insight-oriented therapy should be based not on the presence of phobic symptoms alone but on positive indications from the patient's ego structure and life patterns for the use of this method of treatment. Insight-oriented therapy enables patients to understand the origin of the phobia, the phenomenon of secondary gain, and the role of resistance and enables them to seek healthy ways of dealing with anxiety-provoking stimuli.

Virtual Therapy. A number of computer-generated simulations of phobic disorders have been developed. Patients are exposed to or interact with the phobic object or situation on the computer screen. Countless numbers of such programs are available, and others are in continual development. Variable success rates have been reported, but virtual therapy for phobic disorder is on the cutting edge of using computers to treat mental illness.

Other Therapeutic Modalities. Hypnosis, supportive therapy, and family therapy may be useful in the treatment of phobic disorders. Hypnosis is used to enhance the therapist's suggestion that the phobic object is not dangerous, and self-hypnosis can be taught to the patient as a method of relaxation when confronted with the phobic object. Supportive psychotherapy and family therapy are often useful in helping the patient actively confront the phobic object during treatment. Not only can family therapy enlist the aid of the family in treating the patient, but it may also help the family understand the nature of the patient's problem.

Specific Phobia

A common treatment for specific phobia is exposure therapy. In this method, therapists desensitize patients by using a series of gradual, self-paced exposures to the phobic stimuli, and they teach patients various techniques to deal with anxiety, including relaxation, breathing control, and cognitive approaches. The cognitive–behavioral approaches include reinforcing the realization that the phobic situation is, in fact, safe. The key aspects of successful behavior therapy are the patient's commitment to treatment, clearly identified problems and objectives, and alternative strategies for coping with the patient's feelings. In the special situation of blood–injection–injury phobia, some therapists recommend that patients tense their bodies and remain seated during the exposure to help avoid the possibility of fainting from a vasovagal reaction to the phobic stimulation. β-Adrenergic receptor antagonists may be useful in the treatment of specific phobia, especially when the phobia is associated with panic attacks. Pharmacotherapy (e.g., benzodiazepines), psychotherapy, or combined therapy directed to the attacks may also be of benefit.

▲ 6.5 Social Anxiety Disorder (Social Phobia)

Social anxiety disorder (also referred to as social phobia) involves the fear of social situations, including situations that involve scrutiny or contact with strangers. The term *social anxiety* reflects the distinct differentiation of social anxiety disorder from specific phobia, which is the intense and persistent fear of an object or situation. Persons with social anxiety disorder are fearful of embarrassing themselves in social situations (i.e., social gatherings, oral presentations, meeting new people). They may have specific fears about performing specific activities such as eating or speaking in front of others, or they may experience a vague, nonspecific fear of "embarrassing oneself." In either case, the fear in social anxiety disorder is of the embarrassment that may occur in the situation, not of the situation itself.

EPIDEMIOLOGY

Various studies have reported a lifetime prevalence ranging from 3 to 13 percent for social anxiety disorder. The 6-month prevalence is about 2 to 3 per 100 persons (Table 6.5–1). In epidemiological studies, females are affected more often than males, but in clinical samples, the reverse is often true. The reasons for these varying observations are unknown. The peak age of onset for social anxiety disorder is in the teens, although onset is common as young as 5 years of age and as old as 35 years.

COMORBIDITY

Persons with social anxiety disorder may have a history of other anxiety disorders, mood disorders, substance-related disorders, and bulimia nervosa.

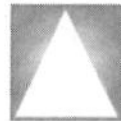

Table 6.5–1
Lifetime Prevalence Rates of Social Anxiety Disorder

Site	Men (%)	Women (%)	Total (%)
United States (National Comorbidity Survey)	11.1	15.5	13.3
United States (Epidemiological Catchment Area Study)	2.1	3.1	2.6
Edmonton, Canada	1.3	2.1	1.7
Puerto Rico	0.8	1.1	1.0
Korea	0.1	1.0	0.5
Zurich, Switzerland	3.7	7.3	5.6
Taiwan	0.2	1.0	0.6
Netherlands	5.9	9.7	7.8

ETIOLOGY

Several studies have reported that some children possibly have a trait characterized by a consistent pattern of behavioral inhibition. This trait may be particularly common in the children of parents who are affected with panic disorder, and it may develop into severe shyness as the children grow older. At least some persons with social anxiety disorder may have exhibited behavioral inhibition during childhood. Perhaps associated with this trait, which is thought to be biologically based, are the psychologically based data indicating that the parents of persons with social anxiety disorder, as a group, were less caring, more rejecting, and more overprotective of their children than were other parents. Some social anxiety disorder research has referred to the spectrum from dominance to submission observed in the animal kingdom. For example, whereas dominant humans may tend to walk with their chins in the air and to make eye contact, submissive humans may tend to walk with their chins down and to avoid eye contact.

Neurochemical Factors

The success of pharmacotherapies in treating social anxiety disorder has generated two specific neurochemical hypotheses about two types of social anxiety disorder. Specifically, the use of β-adrenergic receptor antagonists—for example, propranolol (Inderal)—for performance phobias (e.g., public speaking) has led to the development of an adrenergic theory for these phobias. Patients with performance phobias may release more norepinephrine or epinephrine, both centrally and peripherally, than do nonphobic persons, or such patients may be sensitive to a normal level of adrenergic stimulation. The observation that MAOIs may be more effective than tricyclic drugs in the treatment of generalized social anxiety disorder, in combination with preclinical data, has led some investigators to hypothesize that dopaminergic activity is related to the pathogenesis of the disorder. One study has shown significantly lower homovanillic acid concentrations. Another study using SPECT demonstrated decreased striatal dopamine reuptake site density. Thus, some evidence suggests dopaminergic dysfunction in social anxiety disorder.

Genetic Factors

First-degree relatives of persons with social anxiety disorder are about three times more likely to be affected with social anxiety disorder than are first-degree relatives of those without mental disorders. And some preliminary data indicate that monozygotic twins are more often concordant than are dizygotic twins, although in social anxiety disorder, it is particularly important to study twins reared apart to help control for environmental factors.

DIAGNOSIS AND CLINICAL FEATURES

Social anxiety disorder is diagnosed when the person has a debilitating fear of one or more social situations such as public speaking or performing, e.g., acting or playing a musical instrument, in which they are observed by others. The clinician should recognize that at least some degree of social anxiety or self-consciousness is common in the general population. Community studies suggest that roughly one-third of all persons consider themselves to be far more anxious than other people in social situations. Moreover, such concerns may appear particularly heightened during certain developmental stages, such as adolescence, or after life transitions, such as marriage or occupation changes, associated with new demands for social interaction. Such anxiety only becomes social anxiety disorder when the anxiety either prevents an individual from participating in desired activities or causes marked distress during such activities.

Ms. B was a 29-year-old computer programmer who presented for treatment after she was offered promotion to a managerial position at her firm. Although she wanted the raise and the increased responsibility that would come with the new job, which she had agreed to try on a probationary basis, Ms. B reported that she was reluctant to accept the position because it required frequent interactions with employees from other divisions of the company, as well as occasional public speaking. She stated that she had always felt nervous around new people, whom she worried would ridicule her for "saying stupid things" or committing social faux pas. She also reported feeling "terrified" to speak before groups. These fears had not previously interfered with her social life and job performance. However, since starting her probationary job, Ms. B reported that they had become problematic. She noted that when she had to interact with others, her heart started racing, her mouth became dry, and she felt sweaty. At meetings, she had sudden thoughts that she would say something very foolish or commit a terrible social gaffe that would cause people to laugh. As a consequence, she had skipped several important meetings and left others early. *(Courtesy of Erin B. McClure-Tone, Ph.D. and Daniel S. Pine, M.D.)*

DIFFERENTIAL DIAGNOSIS

Social anxiety disorder needs to be differentiated from appropriate fear and normal shyness, respectively. Differential diagnostic considerations for social anxiety disorder are agoraphobia, panic disorder, avoidant personality disorder, major depressive disorder, and schizoid personality disorder. A patient with agoraphobia is often comforted by the presence of another person in an anxiety-provoking situation, but a patient with social anxiety disorder is made more anxious by the presence of other people. Whereas breathlessness, dizziness, a sense of suffocation, and a fear of dying are common in panic disorder and agoraphobia, the symptoms associated with social anxiety disorder usually involve blushing, muscle twitching, and anxiety about scrutiny (Table 6.5–2). Differentiation between social anxiety disorder and avoidant personality disorder can be difficult and can require extensive interviews and psychiatric histories.

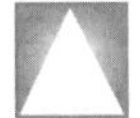

Table 6.5–2
Signs and Symptoms upon Exposure to the Phobic Situation

Anxiety
Fatigue
Palpitations
Nausea
Tremor
Sweating
Panic attack
Urinary frequency
Withdrawal from feared situation

The avoidance of social situations can often be a symptom in depression, but a psychiatric interview with the patient is likely to elicit a broad constellation of depressive symptoms. In patients with schizoid personality disorder, the lack of interest in socializing, not the fear of socializing, leads to the avoidant social behavior.

COURSE AND PROGNOSIS

Social anxiety disorder tends to have its onset in late childhood or early adolescence. Existing prospective epidemiological findings indicate that social anxiety disorder is typically chronic, although patients whose symptoms do remit tend to stay well. Both retrospective epidemiological studies and prospective clinical studies suggest that the disorder can profoundly disrupt the life of an individual over many years. This can include disruption in school or academic achievement and interference with job performance and social development.

TREATMENT

Both psychotherapy and pharmacotherapy are useful in treating social anxiety disorder. Some studies indicate that the use of both pharmacotherapy and psychotherapy produces better results than either therapy alone, although the finding may not be applicable to all situations and patients.

Effective drugs for the treatment of social anxiety disorder include (1) SSRIs, (2) the benzodiazepines, (3) venlafaxine (Effexor), and (4) buspirone (BuSpar). Most clinicians consider SSRIs the first-line treatment choice for patients with more generalized forms of social anxiety disorder. The benzodiazepines alprazolam (Xanax) and clonazepam (Klonopin) are also efficacious in social anxiety disorder. Buspirone has shown additive effects when used to augment treatment with SSRIs.

In severe cases, successful treatment of social anxiety disorder with both irreversible MAOIs such as phenelzine (Nardil) and reversible inhibitors of monoamine oxidase such as moclobemide (Aurorix) and brofaromine (Consonar), which are not available in the United States, has been reported. Therapeutic dosages of phenelzine range from 45 to 90 mg a day, with response rates ranging from 50 to 70 percent; approximately 5 to 6 weeks is needed to assess the efficacy.

The treatment of social anxiety disorder associated with performance situations frequently involves the use of β-adrenergic receptor antagonists shortly before exposure to a phobic stimulus. The two compounds most widely used are atenolol (Tenormin) 50 to 100 mg taken about 1 hour before the performance, or propranolol, 20 to 40 mg.

There have been anecdotal reports of persons having severe arrhythmias or heart attacks during or shortly after a public performance such as giving a speech. Tachycardia from anxiety in a person with compromised cardiac status may be the cause. In such situations the prophylactic use of β-adrenergic receptor antagonists which cause bradycardia may be life-saving.

Another option to help with performance anxiety is a relatively short- or intermediate-acting benzodiazepine, such as lorazepam or alprazolam. Cognitive, behavioral, and exposure techniques are also useful in performance situations.

Psychotherapy for social anxiety disorder usually involves a combination of behavioral and cognitive methods, including cognitive retraining, desensitization, rehearsal during sessions, and a range of homework assignments.

▲ 6.6 Generalized Anxiety Disorder

Anxiety can be conceptualized as a normal and adaptive response to threat that prepares the organism for flight or fight. Persons who seem to be anxious about almost everything, however, are likely to be classified as having generalized anxiety disorder. Generalized anxiety disorder is defined as excessive anxiety and worry about several events or activities for most days during at least a 6-month period. The worry is difficult to control and is associated with somatic symptoms, such as muscle tension, irritability, difficulty sleeping, and restlessness. The anxiety is not focused on features of another disorder, is not caused by substance use or a general medical condition, and does not occur only during a mood or psychiatric disorder. The anxiety is difficult to control, is subjectively distressing, and produces impairment in important areas of a person's life.

EPIDEMIOLOGY

Generalized anxiety disorder is a common condition; reasonable estimates for its 1-year prevalence range from 3 to 8 percent. The ratio of women to men with the disorder is about 2 to 1, but the ratio of women to men who are receiving inpatient treatment for the disorder is about 1 to 1. A lifetime prevalence is close to 5 percent with the Epidemiological Catchment Area (ECA) study suggesting a lifetime prevalence as high as 8 percent. In anxiety disorder clinics, about 25 percent of patients have generalized anxiety disorder. The disorder usually has its onset in late adolescence or early adulthood, although cases are commonly seen in older adults. Also, some evidence suggests that the prevalence of generalized anxiety disorder is particularly high in primary care settings.

COMORBIDITY

Generalized anxiety disorder is probably the disorder that most often coexists with another mental disorder, usually social phobia, specific phobia, panic disorder, or a depressive disorder. Perhaps 50 to 90 percent of patients with generalized anxiety disorder have another mental disorder. As many as 25 percent of patients eventually experience panic disorder. Generalized anxiety disorder is differentiated from panic disorder by the absence of spontaneous panic attacks. An additional high percentage of patients are likely to have major depressive disorder. Other common disorders associated with generalized anxiety disorder are dysthymic disorder and substance-related disorders.

ETIOLOGY

The cause of generalized anxiety disorder is not known. As currently defined, generalized anxiety disorder probably affects a heterogeneous group of persons. Perhaps because a certain degree of anxiety is normal and adaptive, differentiating normal anxiety from pathological anxiety and differentiating biological causative factors from psychosocial factors are difficult. Biological and psychological factors probably work together.

Biological Factors

The therapeutic efficacies of benzodiazepines and the azapirones (e.g., buspirone [BuSpar]) have focused biological research efforts on the γ-aminobutyric acid and serotonin neurotransmitter systems. Whereas benzodiazepines (which are benzodiazepine receptor agonists) are known to reduce anxiety, flumazenil (Romazicon) (a benzodiazepine receptor antagonist) and the β-carbolines (benzodiazepine receptor reverse agonists) are known to induce anxiety. Although no convincing data indicate that the benzodiazepine receptors are abnormal in patients with generalized anxiety disorder, some researchers have focused on the occipital lobe, which has the highest concentrations of benzodiazepine receptors in the brain. Other brain areas hypothesized to be involved in generalized anxiety disorder are the basal ganglia, the limbic system, and the frontal cortex. Because buspirone is an agonist at the serotonin 5-HT_{1A} receptor, there is the hypothesis that the regulation of the serotonergic system in generalized anxiety disorder is abnormal. Other neurotransmitter systems that have been the subject of research in generalized anxiety disorder include the norepinephrine, glutamate, and cholecystokinin systems. Some evidence indicates that patients with generalized anxiety disorder may have subsensitivity of their α_2-adrenergic receptors, as indicated by a blunted release of growth hormone after clonidine (Catapres) infusion.

Brain imaging studies of patients with generalized anxiety disorder have revealed significant findings. One PET study reported a lower metabolic rate in basal ganglia and white matter in patients with generalized anxiety disorder than in normal control subjects. A few genetic studies have also been conducted in the field. One study found that a genetic relation might exist between generalized anxiety disorder and major depressive disorder in women. Another study showed a distinct, but difficult-to-quantitate, genetic component in generalized anxiety disorder. About 25 percent of first-degree relatives of patients with generalized anxiety disorder are also affected.

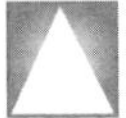

Table 6.6–1
Familial Relative Risks in Selected Anxiety Disorders

Disorder	Population Prevalence (%)	Familial Relative Risk[a]
Panic disorder	1–3	2–20
Generalized anxiety disorder	3–5	6
Obsessive-compulsive disorder	1–3	3–5

[a]Ratio of risk to relatives of cases versus risk to relatives of controls.

Male relatives are likely to have an alcohol use disorder. Some twin studies report a concordance rate of 50 percent in monozygotic twins and 15 percent in dizygotic twins. Table 6.6-1 lists relative genetic risks in selected anxiety disorders.

A variety of electroencephalogram (EEG) abnormalities has been noted in alpha rhythm and evoked potentials. Sleep EEG studies have reported increased sleep discontinuity, decreased delta sleep, decreased stage 1 sleep, and reduced rapid eye movement sleep. These changes in sleep architecture differ from the changes seen in depressive disorders.

Psychosocial Factors

The two major schools of thought about psychosocial factors leading to the development of generalized anxiety disorder are the cognitive–behavioral school and the psychoanalytic school. According to the cognitive–behavioral school, patients with generalized anxiety disorder respond to incorrectly and inaccurately perceived dangers. The inaccuracy is generated by selective attention to negative details in the environment, by distortions in information processing, and by an overly negative view of the person's own ability to cope. The psychoanalytic school hypothesizes that anxiety is a symptom of unresolved, unconscious conflicts. Sigmund Freud first presented this psychological theory in 1909 with his description of Little Hans; before then, Freud had conceptualized anxiety as having a physiological basis. An example of Freudian theory as applied to general anxiety can be seen in the following case:

Mrs. B, a 26-year-old married woman, was admitted to the hospital for the evaluation of persistent anxiety that had begun 8 months earlier and was becoming increasingly disabling. Especially disturbing to the patient was the spontaneous intrusion of intermittent images in her mind's eye of her father and herself locked in a naked sexual embrace. The images were not only frightening, but they puzzled her greatly because she had always disliked her father intensely. Not only was he "poison" to her, but she tried to avoid any contact with him and found it difficult to talk to him if she was forced to be in his company.

As the patient described the difficulty of her relationship with her father, she suddenly recalled that her anxiety had begun at a time when her father was seemingly being more intrusive than ever as he tried to help her and her husband over a period of financial difficulty.

As the patient continued to revile her father, she suddenly commented that her mother had told her that her father "had been good to me when I was little and he used to sing songs to me and take me on his lap, but I don't remember. I only remember when he was mean to me. I just am glad when he keeps on talking mean to me the way he always has. I just wouldn't know what to do if he was nice to me." When asked by the interviewer if there might have been a time when she had wanted him to be nice to her, the patient replied, "When I was little, I just wanted to know that he did love me a little. I guess I always wanted him to be nice to me. But when I stop to think about it, I guess I didn't want him to be nice to me." The doctor then commented, "It sounds as if a part of you wants to be close to your father." In response, the patient burst into agitated sobs and blurted out, "I don't know how to be close to my father! I am too old to care about my father now!"

When the patient regained her composure, she recalled the memory of an event she had not thought of since it had occurred 15 years earlier. When she was 11 years old, she reported, while in the living room with her father, she had suddenly had the mental image of being in a sexual embrace with him. Terrified, she had run into the kitchen to find her mother. There had been no recurrence of that image until the onset of the current illness, and the incident had remained forgotten until its recall during the interview. Its emergence into consciousness amplified the history of the patient's illness and disclosed an earlier transient outbreak of the same symptoms she had experienced as an adult. After the patient had recovered her composure, she recalled further hitherto forgotten memories. She had slept in her parents' bedroom until she was 6, during which period her father, on one occasion, had taken her into bed and told her stories and, on another, had yelled at her very angrily as she lay in her crib.

During a clinical interview the next day, the patient revealed a fact that she had forgotten in her earlier account of her illness: At the end of the period during which her father had been making the friendly overtures that had so deeply troubled her, and the night before the sudden onset of her symptoms, she had had a nightmare. She was, she dreamed, at a zoo. It was night, and she heard strange noises in the darkness. She asked an attendant standing next to her what the noises were. "Oh," the attendant replied casually, "that's only the animals mating." She then noticed a large, gray elephant lying on its right side in the grass in front of her. As she watched, she noticed the creature moving its left hind leg up and down as if it were trying to get to its feet. At that point she awoke from the dream with a feeling of terror and, afterward, during the morning, experienced the first episode of the frightening imagery of sexual activity with her father.

In direct association to the dream, the patient recalled a long-forgotten childhood memory of an incident that had occurred during her fourth or fifth year. She had awoken one night while in her crib in her parents' bedroom to observe her parents having sexual intercourse. They suddenly became aware of her watching them and sprang apart. The patient remembered seeing her mother hastily pulling up the bedclothes around her to cover her nakedness. Her father, meanwhile, rolled over half on his back, half on his left side. The patient noticed his erection and then saw him lift up his left leg as he sat up and yelled at her angrily to go to sleep.

It was not easy for the patient to communicate these memories. She spoke haltingly in a low voice and was visibly ashamed and anxious throughout the whole recital of the dream and its associations. She discharged a great quantity of affect, but after doing so, appeared considerably relaxed, relieved, and composed. On her return to the psychiatric ward, she was observed to be cheerful and outgoing with the ward personnel and other patients. Of particular note was that she no longer experienced any anxiety and had no recurrence of the sexual images involving her father that had previously been so deeply distressing. The patient was discharged a short while later after a further series of psychotherapeutic interviews, and when seen for a follow-up visit 2 months later, she reported continued emotional calm and comfort, without recurrence of psychiatric symptoms.

DIAGNOSIS

Generalized anxiety disorder is characterized by a pattern of frequent, persistent worry and anxiety that is out of proportion to the impact of the event or circumstance that is the focus of the worry. The distinction between generalized anxiety disorder and normal anxiety is emphasized by the use of the word "excessive" in the criteria and by the specification that the symptoms cause significant impairment or distress. Signs and symptoms for generalized anxiety disorder are listed in Table 6.6–2.

CLINICAL FEATURES

The essential characteristics of generalized anxiety disorder are sustained and excessive anxiety and worry accompanied by either motor tension or restlessness. The anxiety is excessive and interferes with other aspects of a person's life. This pattern must occur more days than not for at least 3 months. The motor tension is most commonly manifested as shakiness, restlessness, and headaches.

Patients with generalized anxiety disorder usually seek out a general practitioner or internist for help with a somatic symptom. Alternatively, the patients go to a specialist for a specific symptom (e.g., chronic diarrhea). A specific nonpsychiatric medical disorder is rarely found, and patients vary in their doctor-seeking behavior. Some patients accept a diagnosis of generalized anxiety disorder and the appropriate treatment; others seek additional medical consultations for their problems.

Mr. G was a successful, married, 28-year-old teacher who presented for a psychiatric evaluation to treat mounting symptoms of worry and anxiety. Mr. G noted that for the preceding year, he had become more and more worried about his job performance. For example, although he had always been a respected and popular lecturer, he found himself worrying more and more about his ability to engage students and convey material effectively. Similarly, although he had always been financially secure, he increasingly worried that he was going to lose his wealth due to unexpected expenses. Mr. G noted frequent somatic symptoms that accompanied his worries. For example, he often felt tense and irritable while he worked and spent time with his family, and he had difficulty distracting himself from worries about the upcoming challenges for the next day. He reported feeling increasingly restless, especially at night, when his worries kept him from falling asleep. *(Courtesy of Erin B. McClure-Tone, Ph.D. and Daniel S. Pine, M.D.)*

Table 6.6–2
Signs and Symptoms of Generalized Anxiety

Feeling of being nervous
Muscular spasm or tension
Tremors or generalized trembling
Sweating
Vertigo
Precordial discomfort or pain
Apprehension
Dry mouth
Difficulty concentrating
Sense of impending doom

DIFFERENTIAL DIAGNOSIS

As with other anxiety disorders, generalized anxiety disorder must be differentiated from both medical and psychiatric disorders. Neurological, endocrinological, metabolic, and medication-related disorders similar to those considered in the differential diagnosis of panic disorder must be considered in the differential diagnosis of generalized anxiety disorder. Common co-occurring anxiety disorders also must be considered, including panic disorder, phobias, OCD, and PTSD. To meet criteria for generalized anxiety disorder, patients must both exhibit the full syndrome, and their symptoms also cannot be explained by the presence of a comorbid anxiety disorder. To diagnose generalized anxiety disorder in the context of other anxiety disorders, it is most important to document anxiety or worry related to circumstances or topics that are either unrelated, or only minimally related, to other disorders. Proper diagnosis involves both definitively establishing the presence of generalized anxiety disorder and properly diagnosing other anxiety disorders. Patients with generalized anxiety disorder frequently develop major depressive disorder. As a result, this condition must also be recognized and distinguished. The key to making a correct diagnosis is documenting anxiety or worry that is unrelated to the depressive disorder.

COURSE AND PROGNOSIS

The age of onset is difficult to specify; most patients with the disorder report that they have been anxious for as long as they can remember. Patients usually come to a clinician's attention in their 20s, although the first contact with a clinician can occur at virtually any age. Only one-third of patients who have generalized anxiety disorder seek psychiatric treatment. Many go to general practitioners, internists, cardiologists, pulmonary specialists, or gastroenterologists, seeking treatment for the somatic component of the disorder. Because of the high incidence of comorbid mental disorders in patients with generalized anxiety disorder, the clinical course and prognosis of the disorder are difficult to predict. Nonetheless, some data indicate that life events are associated with the onset of generalized anxiety disorder: The occurrence of several negative life events greatly increases the likelihood that the disorder will develop. By definition, generalized anxiety disorder is a chronic condition that may well be lifelong.

TREATMENT

The most effective treatment of generalized anxiety disorder is probably one that combines psychotherapeutic, pharmacotherapeutic, and supportive approaches. The treatment may take a significant amount of time for the involved clinician, whether the clinician is a psychiatrist, a family practitioner, or another specialist.

Psychotherapy

The major psychotherapeutic approaches to generalized anxiety disorder are cognitive-behavioral, supportive, and insight oriented. Data are still limited on the relative merits of those approaches, although the most sophisticated studies have examined cognitive–behavioral techniques, which seem to have both short-term and long-term efficacy. Cognitive approaches address patients' hypothesized cognitive distortions directly, and behavioral approaches address somatic symptoms directly. The major techniques used in behavioral approaches are relaxation and biofeedback. Some preliminary data indicate that the combination of cognitive and behavioral approaches is more effective than either technique used alone. Supportive therapy offers patients reassurance and comfort, although its long-term efficacy is doubtful. Insight-oriented psychotherapy focuses on uncovering unconscious conflicts and identifying ego strengths. The efficacy of insight-oriented psychotherapy for generalized anxiety disorder is found in many anecdotal case reports, but large controlled studies are lacking.

Most patients experience a marked lessening of anxiety when given the opportunity to discuss their difficulties with a concerned and sympathetic physician. If clinicians discover external situations that are anxiety provoking, they may be able—alone or with the help of the patients or their families—to change the environment and thus reduce the stressful pressures. A reduction in symptoms often allows patients to function effectively in their daily work and relationships and thus gain new rewards and gratification that are themselves therapeutic.

In the psychoanalytic perspective, anxiety sometimes signals unconscious turmoil that deserves investigation. The anxiety can be normal, adaptive, maladaptive, too intense, or too mild, depending on the circumstances. Anxiety appears in numerous situations over the course of the life cycle; in many cases, symptom relief is not the most appropriate course of action.

For patients who are psychologically minded and motivated to understand the sources of their anxiety, psychotherapy may be the treatment of choice. Psychodynamic therapy proceeds with the assumption that anxiety can increase with effective treatment. The goal of the dynamic approach may be to increase the patient's anxiety tolerance (a capacity to experience anxiety without having to discharge it), rather than to eliminate anxiety. Empirical research indicates that many patients who have successful psychotherapeutic treatment may continue to experience anxiety after termination of the psychotherapy, but their increased ego mastery allows them to use the anxiety symptoms as a signal to reflect on internal struggles and to expand their insight and understanding. A psychodynamic approach to patients with generalized anxiety disorder involves a search for the patient's underlying fears.

Mr. B, a 28-year-old man with a history of a generalized anxiety disorder, was a former adolescent alcohol abuser now involved in Alcoholics Anonymous (AA). Because of sexual side effects, he was unwilling to take SSRI antidepressants, buspirone (BuSpar) had been ineffective, and gabapentin (Neurontin) was too sedating. Clonazepam (Klonopin) was effective, but the patient's continued participation in AA led to pressures from AA peers to give up benzodiazepines. Partly because of these pressures, he sought psychodynamic therapy with a psychiatrist. When the psychiatrist suggested that he begin tapering clonazepam, B balked, worried that he would become more anxious. The therapist suggested that it might be useful to bring his anxiety to sessions if their task really was going to be to learn more about his anxiety.

On a tapering dose of clonazepam B's anxiety increased. He complained that his male therapist was unempathic, making him suffer with anxiety while the therapist watched and did nothing. As the treatment unfolded, the therapist learned he had been especially close to his mother, who, with the patient, had been the target of criticism from his often absent, short-tempered, mean-spirited alcoholic father. Patient's mother had surgery and chemotherapy for breast cancer when he was 10 years old. It was shortly after this that his anxiety symptoms began.

When clonazepam was discontinued, there was an outburst of anger at the therapist for making him suffer so much. The therapist quietly accepted patient's anger at him, noting that he had asked the patient to endure more anxiety, while leaving him alone and on his own most of the week. When he suggested that the patient had found in the therapist his absent and sadistic father, he thought this made sense, and he began to trust the therapist more. The patient said he realized that the therapist could endure and understand his anger without needing to retaliate and that he was sticking to a treatment plan they had agreed to from the outset. As the alliance deepened, he struggled to put words to his experience of anxiety. He spoke more of his attachment to his mother and to the way he would cling to her to support her, pressing himself against her ample bosom, while his father would rage at them both while drunk, sometimes suggesting that his clinging to her was unnatural and inspired by lust.

He reported a dream in one session in which he watched passively, frozen with fear and guilt and unable to move, as a man murdered and dismembered a naked woman. His associations to the dream led to painful memories of his mother's disfiguring surgery and to his guilt about not having been able to stop his father from angrily criticizing her both before and after the surgery. He then added there was another part of the dream he had left out because of shame. He had been sexually aroused during the dream. He suddenly reported an intrusive thought that upset him—a thought that the breast cancer had come because he had been unable to protect his mother—and because he had been aroused by her breasts. He wept for the first time in the therapy. Over time the therapist and patient explored the dream and his intrusive thoughts, learning that he felt guilty about having caused his mother's illness and disfiguring surgery not only because he could not protect her from father's rages but also because he felt guilty and ashamed about his attraction to his mother's breasts. He spoke of the way his father's drunken accusation of lust toward his mother was right. He feared, too, that he would be disfigured because of a disease or accident, perhaps by castration, for what he had done to his mother. It was not easy for him to explore these feelings, but as he did, his anxiety diminished. *(Courtesy of Eric M. Plakun, M.D.)*

Pharmacotherapy

The decision to prescribe an anxiolytic to patients with generalized anxiety disorder should rarely be made on the first visit. Because of the long-term nature of the disorder, a treatment plan must be carefully thought out. The major drugs to be considered for the treatment of generalized anxiety disorder are benzodiazepines, the SSRIs, buspirone (BuSpar), and venlafaxine (Effexor). Other drugs that may be useful are the tricyclic drugs (e.g., imipramine [Tofranil]), antihistamines, and the β-adrenergic antagonists (e.g., propranolol [Inderal]) (Table 6.6–3).

Although drug treatment of generalized anxiety disorder is sometimes seen as a 6- to 12-month treatment, some evidence indicates that treatment should be long term, perhaps lifelong. About 25 percent of patients relapse in the first month after the

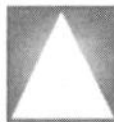

Table 6.6–3
Common Medications for the Treatment of Recurrent Anxiety

Medication	Brand Name	Recommended Initial Dose	Daily Dose (mg)[a]
Antidepressants[b]			
Fluoxetine	Prozac	5 mg/day	20–80
Fluvoxamine	Luvox	50 mg/day	100–300
Paroxetine	Paxil	10 mg/day	20–50
	Paxil CR	12.5 mg/day	25–75
Sertraline	Zoloft	25–50 mg/day	50–200
Citalopram	Celexa	10 mg/day	20–60
Escitalopram	Lexapro	5 mg/day	10–30
Venlafaxine	Effexor XR	37.5 mg/day	75–225
Phenelzine	Nardil	15 mg/day	45–90
Benzodiazepines[c]			
Alprazolam	Xanax	0.25 mg tid	1–4[e]
Clonazepam	Klonopin	0.25 mg bid	1–3
Lorazepam	Ativan	0.5 mg tid	2–6[e]
Azapirone[d]			
Buspirone	BuSpar	7.5 mg bid	30–60

bid, twice daily; tid, three times daily.
All except phenelzine are useful as a primary treatment for obsessive-compulsive disorder.
[a]Some individuals will require higher or lower doses than those listed here.
[b]Useful as a primary treatment for panic disorder (in which lower starting doses are usually used) with or without agoraphobia, generalized anxiety disorder, generalized social anxiety disorder, and posttraumatic stress disorder.
[c]Useful as a primary treatment for panic disorder with or without agoraphobia, generalized anxiety disorder, and generalized social anxiety disorder. May be a useful adjunct to antidepressants in the treatment of posttraumatic stress disorder or obsessive-compulsive disorder.
[d]Useful as a primary treatment for generalized anxiety disorder.
[e]Total daily dose is divided across two to four doses per day.

discontinuation of therapy, and 60 to 80 percent relapse over the course of the next year. Although some patients become dependent on the benzodiazepines, tolerance rarely develops to the therapeutic effects of the benzodiazepines, buspirone, venlafaxine, or the SSRIs.

Benzodiazepines. Benzodiazepines have been the drugs of choice for generalized anxiety disorder. They can be prescribed on an as-needed basis, so that patients take a rapidly acting benzodiazepine when they feel particularly anxious. The alternative approach is to prescribe benzodiazepines for a limited period, during which psychosocial therapeutic approaches are implemented.

Several problems are associated with the use of benzodiazepines in generalized anxiety disorder. About 25 to 30 percent of all patients fail to respond, and tolerance and dependence can occur. Some patients also experience impaired alertness while taking the drugs and therefore are at risk for accidents involving automobiles and machinery.

The clinical decision to initiate treatment with a benzodiazepine should be considered and specific. The patient's diagnosis, the specific target symptoms, and the duration of treatment should all be defined, and the information should be shared with the patient. Treatment for most anxiety conditions lasts for 2 to 6 weeks followed by 1 or 2 weeks of tapering drug use before it is discontinued. The most common clinical mistake with benzodiazepine treatment is to continue treatment indefinitely.

For the treatment of anxiety, it is usual to begin giving a drug at the low end of its therapeutic range and to increase the dosage to achieve a therapeutic response. The use of a benzodiazepine with an intermediate half-life (8 to 15 hours) will likely avoid some of the adverse effects associated with the use of benzodiazepines with long half-lives, and the use of divided doses prevents the development of adverse effects associated with high peak plasma levels. The improvement produced by benzodiazepines may go beyond a simple antianxiety effect. For example, the drugs may cause patients to regard various occurrences in a positive light. The drugs can also have a mild disinhibiting action, similar to that observed after ingesting modest amounts of alcohol.

Buspirone. Buspirone is a 5-HT_{1A} receptor partial agonist and is most likely effective in 60 to 80 percent of patients with generalized anxiety disorder. Data indicate that buspirone is more effective in reducing the cognitive symptoms of generalized anxiety disorder than in reducing the somatic symptoms. Evidence also indicates that patients who have previously had treatment with benzodiazepines are not likely to respond to treatment with buspirone. The lack of response may be caused by the absence, with buspirone treatment, of some of the nonanxiolytic effects of benzodiazepines (e.g., muscle relaxation and the additional sense of well-being). The major disadvantage of buspirone is that its effects take 2 to 3 weeks to become evident, in contrast to the almost immediate anxiolytic effects of the benzodiazepines. One approach is to initiate benzodiazepine and buspirone use simultaneously and then taper off the benzodiazepine use after 2 to 3 weeks, at which point the buspirone should have reached its maximal effects. Some studies have also reported that long-term combined treatment with benzodiazepine and buspirone may be more effective than either drug alone. Buspirone is not an effective treatment for benzodiazepine withdrawal.

Venlafaxine. Venlafaxine is effective in treating the insomnia, poor concentration, restlessness, irritability, and excessive muscle tension associated with generalized anxiety disorder. Venlafaxine is a nonselective inhibitor of the reuptake of three biogenic amines—serotonin, norepinephrine, and, to a lesser extent, dopamine.

Selective Serotonin Reuptake Inhibitors. SSRIs may be effective, especially for patients with comorbid depression. The prominent disadvantage of SSRIs, especially fluoxetine (Prozac), is that they can transiently increase anxiety and cause agitated states. For this reason, the SSRIs sertraline (Zoloft), citalopram (Celexa), or paroxetine (Paxil) are better choices in patients with high anxiety disorder. It is reasonable to begin treatment with sertraline, citalopram, or paroxetine plus a benzodiazepine and then to taper benzodiazepine use after 2 to 3 weeks. Further studies are needed to determine whether SSRIs are as effective for generalized anxiety disorder as they are for panic disorder and OCD.

Other Drugs. If conventional pharmacological treatment (e.g., with buspirone or a benzodiazepine) is ineffective or not completely effective, then a clinical reassessment is indicated to rule out comorbid conditions, such as depression, or to better understand the patient's environmental stresses. Other drugs that have proved useful for generalized anxiety disorder include the tricyclic and tetracyclic drugs. The β-adrenergic receptor antagonists may reduce the somatic manifestations of anxiety but not the underlying condition, and their use is usually limited to situational anxieties, such as performance anxiety.

▲ 6.7 Other Anxiety Disorders

ANXIETY DISORDER ATTRIBUTABLE TO ANOTHER MEDICAL CONDITION

Many medical disorders are associated with anxiety. Symptoms can include panic attacks, generalized anxiety, and other signs of distress. In all cases, the signs and symptoms will be due to the direct physiological effects of the medical condition.

Epidemiology

The occurrence of anxiety symptoms related to general medical conditions is common, although the incidence of the disorder varies for each specific general medical condition.

Etiology

A wide range of medical conditions can cause symptoms similar to those of anxiety disorders (Table 6.7–1). Hyperthyroidism, hypothyroidism, hypoparathyroidism, and vitamin B_{12} deficiency are frequently associated with anxiety symptoms. A pheochromocytoma produces epinephrine, which can cause paroxysmal episodes of anxiety symptoms. Other medical conditions, such as cardiac arrhythmia, can produce physiological symptoms of panic disorder. Hypoglycemia can also mimic the symptoms of an anxiety disorder. The diverse medical conditions that can cause symptoms of anxiety disorder may do so

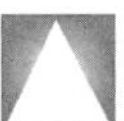

Table 6.7–1
Disorders Associated with Anxiety

Neurological disorders
Cerebral neoplasms
Cerebral trauma and postconcussion syndromes
Cerebrovascular disease
Subarachnoid hemorrhage
Migraine
Encephalitis
Cerebral syphilis
Multiple sclerosis
Wilson's disease
Huntington's disease
Epilepsy
Systemic conditions
Hypoxia
Cardiovascular disease
Cardiac arrhythmias
Pulmonary insufficiency
Anemia
Endocrine disturbances
Pituitary dysfunction
Thyroid dysfunction
Parathyroid dysfunction
Adrenal dysfunction
Pheochromocytoma
Virilization disorders of females
Inflammatory disorders
Lupus erythematosus
Rheumatoid arthritis
Polyarteritis nodosa
Temporal arteritis
Deficiency states
Vitamin B_{12} deficiency
Pellagra
Miscellaneous conditions
Hypoglycemia
Carcinoid syndrome
Systemic malignancies
Premenstrual syndrome
Febrile illnesses and chronic infections
Porphyria
Infectious mononucleosis
Posthepatitic syndrome
Uremia
Toxic conditions
Alcohol and drug withdrawal
Amphetamines
Sympathomimetic agents
Vasopressor agents
Caffeine and caffeine withdrawal
Penicillin
Sulfonamides
Cannabis
Mercury
Arsenic
Phosphorus
Organophosphates
Carbon disulfide
Benzene
Aspirin intolerance

(Adapted from Cumming JL. *Clinical Neuropsychiatry*. Orlando, FL: Grune & Stratton; 1985:214.)

through a common mechanism that involves both the noradrenergic system and the serotonergic system. Each of these conditions is characterized by prominent anxiety that arises as the direct result of some underlying physiological perturbation.

Diagnosis

The diagnosis of anxiety disorder attributable to another medical condition requires the presence of symptoms of an anxiety disorder caused by one or more medical illnesses. The DSM-5 suggests that clinicians to specify whether the disorder is characterized by symptoms of generalized anxiety or panic attacks.

Clinicians should have an increased level of suspicion for the diagnosis when chronic or paroxysmal anxiety is associated with a physical disease known to cause such symptoms in some patients. Paroxysmal bouts of hypertension in an anxious patient may indicate that a workup for a pheochromocytoma is appropriate. A general medical workup may reveal diabetes, an adrenal tumor, thyroid disease, or a neurological condition. For example, some patients with complex partial epilepsy have extreme episodes of anxiety or fear as their only manifestation of the epileptic activity.

Clinical Features

The symptoms of anxiety disorder due to a general medical condition can be identical to those of the primary anxiety disorders. A syndrome similar to panic disorder is the most common clinical picture, and a syndrome similar to a phobia is the least common.

Panic Attacks. Patients who have cardiomyopathy may have the highest incidence of panic disorder secondary to a general medical condition. One study reported that 83 percent of patients with cardiomyopathy awaiting cardiac transplantation had panic disorder symptoms. Increased noradrenergic tone in these patients may be the provoking stimulus for the panic attacks. In some studies, about 25 percent of patients with Parkinson's disease and chronic obstructive pulmonary disease have symptoms of panic disorder. Other medical disorders associated with panic disorder include chronic pain, primary biliary cirrhosis, and epilepsy, particularly when the focus is in the right parahippocampal gyrus.

Generalized Anxiety. A high prevalence of generalized anxiety disorder symptoms has been reported in patients with Sjögren's syndrome, and this rate may be related to the effects of Sjögren's syndrome on cortical and subcortical functions and thyroid function. The highest prevalence of generalized anxiety disorder symptoms in a medical disorder seems to be in Graves' disease (hyperthyroidism), in which as many as two-thirds of all patients meet the criteria for generalized anxiety disorder.

An 86-year-old retired chemical engineer sought help for the onset of a series of attacks over the preceding 4 months in which he experienced marked apprehension, restlessness, a sense that the "walls were caving in," and the need to "get air" to relieve his sense of discomfort. These events typically occurred during the night and awakened him from sound sleep. To feel better, he would need to stick his head out of an open window, regardless of how cold it was outside. His symptoms would gradually improve over 15 to 20 minutes, but complete resolution of these symptoms took a full day. In response to pointed questioning, the patient reported sweating, dizziness, and shortness of breath during these episodes. He imagined that he would die if he could not open the window. He denied palpitations, choking sensations, paresthesia, and nausea. The patient recalled a similar series of attacks almost 30 years earlier during a period of time in which he frequently needed to travel and hence was away from home because of work obligations. The patient denied depressed mood, anhedonia, recent sleep dysfunctions, change in appetite or weight, decreased energy, and feelings of worthlessness. His medical history was notable for a right basal ganglia stroke 6 months earlier. He had a history of hypertension, borderline diabetes, and benign prostatic hypertrophy. Laboratory study results were unremarkable.

A diagnosis of anxiety disorder due to stroke, with panic attacks, was made. The patient was prescribed alprazolam (Xanax), 0.5 mg orally twice a day as needed for panic attacks, and started on escitalopram (Lexapro), 10 mg per day. At a follow-up visit, the patient reported complete resolution of his anxiety symptoms. He remained taking the escitalopram but no longer required the alprazolam. *(Courtesy of LL Lavery, M.D. and EM Whyte, M.D.)*

Phobias. Symptoms of phobias appear to be uncommon, although one study reported a 17 percent prevalence of symptoms of social phobia in patients with Parkinson's disease. Older persons with balance difficulties often complain of a fear of falling, which may express itself by their being unwilling or fearful of walking.

Laboratory Examination

A targeted work-up is required when an anxiety disorder due to another medical condition is being considered as part of the differential diagnosis. If possible, tests should be selected to rule in specific diagnoses suggested by the patient's somatic symptoms (if present).

Test to consider include complete book count, electrolytes, glucose, blood urea nitrogen, creatinine, liver function tests, calcium, magnesium, phosphorus, thyroid function tests, and urine toxicology. Occasionally, additional studies may be indicated to rule out a pheochromocytoma (e.g., urinary catecholamines), a seizure disorder (e.g., EEG), cardiac arrhythmia (e.g., Holter monitoring), and pulmonary disease (pulse oximetry, arterial blood gases). Brain imaging may be useful in ruling out demyelinating disorder, tumor, stroke, or hydrocephalus and is especially important if the anxious individual reports neurological symptoms (e.g., headache, motor or sensory changes, and dizziness), although such complaints may represent somatic manifestations of primary anxiety disorders. Lumbar puncture may be appropriate if an inflammatory or infectious cause is suspected.

Differential Diagnosis

Anxiety, as a symptom, can be associated with many psychiatric disorders in addition to the anxiety disorders themselves. A mental status examination is necessary to determine the presence of mood symptoms or psychotic symptoms that may suggest another psychiatric diagnosis. For a clinician to conclude that a patient has an anxiety disorder caused by a general medical condition, the patient should clearly have anxiety as the predominant symptom and should have a specific causative nonpsychiatric medical disorder. To ascertain the degree to which a general medical condition is causative for the anxiety, the clinician should evaluate the timeline between the medical condition and the anxiety symptoms, the age of onset (primary anxiety disorders usually have their onset before age 35 years), and the patient's family history of both anxiety disorders and relevant general medical conditions (e.g., hyperthyroidism). A diagnosis of adjustment disorder with anxiety must also be considered in the differential diagnosis.

Course and Prognosis

The unremitting experience of anxiety can be disabling and can interfere with every aspect of life, including social, occupational, and psychological functioning. A sudden increase in anxiety level may prompt an affected person to seek medical or psychiatric help more quickly than when the onset is insidious. The treatment or the removal of the primary medical cause of the anxiety usually initiates a clear course of improvement in the anxiety disorder symptoms. In some cases, however, the anxiety disorder symptoms continue even after the primary medical condition is treated (e.g., after an episode of encephalitis). Some symptoms linger for a longer time than other anxiety disorder symptoms. When anxiety disorder symptoms are present for a significant period after the medical disorder has been treated, the remaining symptoms should probably be treated as if they were primary—that is, with psychotherapy, pharmacotherapy, or both.

Treatment

The primary treatment for anxiety disorder due to a general medical condition is to treat the underlying medical condition. If a patient also has an alcohol or other substance use disorder, this disorder must also be addressed therapeutically to gain control of the anxiety disorder symptoms. If the removal of the primary medical condition does not reverse the anxiety disorder symptoms, treatment of these symptoms should follow the treatment guidelines for the specific mental disorder. In general, behavioral modification techniques, anxiolytic agents, and serotonergic antidepressants have been the most effective treatment modalities.

SUBSTANCE-INDUCED ANXIETY DISORDER

Substance-induced disorder is the direct result of a toxic substance, including drugs of abuse, medication, poison, and alcohol, among others.

Epidemiology

Substance-induced anxiety disorder is common, both as the result of the ingestion of so-called recreational drugs and as the result of prescription drug use.

Etiology

A wide range of substances can cause symptoms of anxiety that can mimic any of the DSM-5 anxiety disorders. Although sympathomimetics, such as amphetamine, cocaine, and caffeine, have been most associated with the production of anxiety disorder symptoms, many serotonergic drugs (e.g., LSD and MDMA) can also cause both acute and chronic anxiety syndromes in users. A wide range of prescription medications is also associated with the production of anxiety disorder symptoms in susceptible persons.

Diagnosis

The diagnostic criteria for substance-induced anxiety disorder require the presence of prominent anxiety or panic attacks. The DSM-5 guidelines state that the symptoms should have developed during the use of the substance or within 1 month of the cessation of substance use; however, clinicians may have difficulty determining the relation between substance exposure and anxiety symptoms. The structure of the diagnosis includes specification of (1) the substance (e.g., cocaine), (2) the appropriate state during the onset (e.g., intoxication), and (3) the specific symptom pattern (e.g., panic attacks).

Clinical Features

The associated clinical features of substance-induced anxiety disorder vary with the particular substance involved. Even infrequent use of psychostimulants can result in anxiety disorder symptoms in some persons. Cognitive impairments in comprehension, calculation, and memory can be associated with anxiety disorder symptoms. These cognitive deficits are usually reversible when the substance use is stopped.

Virtually everyone who drinks alcohol, on at least a few occasions, has used it to reduce anxiety, most often social anxiety. In contrast, carefully controlled studies have found that the effects of alcohol on anxiety are variable and can be significantly affected by gender, the amount of alcohol ingested, and cultural attitudes. Nevertheless, alcohol use disorders and other substance-related disorders are commonly associated with anxiety disorders. Alcohol use disorders are about four times more common among patients with panic disorder than among the general population and about two and a half times more common among patients with phobias. Several studies have reported data indicating that genetic diatheses for both anxiety disorders and alcohol use disorders can exist in some families.

Differential Diagnosis

The differential diagnosis for substance-induced anxiety disorder includes the primary anxiety disorders; anxiety disorder due to a general medical condition (for which the patient may be receiving an implicated drug); and mood disorders, which are frequently accompanied by symptoms of anxiety disorders. Personality disorders and malingering must be considered in the differential diagnosis, particularly in some urban emergency departments.

Course and Prognosis

The course and prognosis generally depend on removal of the causally involved substance and the long-term ability of the affected person to limit use of the substance. The anxiogenic effects of most drugs are reversible. When the anxiety does not reverse with cessation of the drug, clinicians should reconsider the diagnosis of substance-induced anxiety disorder or consider the possibility that the substance caused irreversible brain damage.

Treatment

The primary treatment for substance-induced anxiety disorder is the removal of the causally involved substance. Treatment then must focus on finding an alternative treatment if the substance was a medically indicated drug, on limiting the patient's exposure if the substance was introduced through environmental exposure, or on treating the underlying substance-related disorder. If anxiety disorder symptoms continue even after stopping substance use, treatment of the anxiety disorder symptoms with appropriate psychotherapeutic or pharmacotherapeutic modalities may be appropriate.

MIXED ANXIETY-DEPRESSIVE DISORDER

Mixed anxiety-depressive disorder describes patients with both anxiety and depressive symptoms who do not meet the diagnostic criteria for either an anxiety disorder or a mood disorder. The combination of depressive and anxiety symptoms results in significant functional impairment for the affected person. The condition may be particularly prevalent in primary care practices and outpatient mental health clinics. Opponents have argued that the availability of the diagnosis may discourage clinicians from taking the necessary time to obtain a complete psychiatric history to differentiate true depressive disorders from true anxiety disorders. In Europe and especially in China, many of these patients are given a diagnosis of neurasthenia.

Epidemiology

The coexistence of major depressive disorder and panic disorder is common. As many as two-thirds of all patients with depressive symptoms have prominent anxiety symptoms and one-third may meet the diagnostic criteria for panic disorder. Researchers have reported that 20 to 90 percent of all patients with panic disorder have episodes of major depressive disorder. These data suggest that the coexistence of depressive and anxiety symptoms, neither of which meets the diagnostic criteria for other depressive or anxiety disorders, may be common. Presently, however, formal epidemiological data on mixed anxiety-depressive disorder are not available. Nevertheless, some clinicians and researchers have estimated that the prevalence of the disorder in the general population is as high as 10 percent and as high as 50 percent in primary care clinics, although conservative estimates suggest a prevalence of about 1 percent in the general population.

Etiology

Four principal lines of evidence suggest that anxiety symptoms and depressive symptoms are causally linked in some affected patients. First, several investigators have reported similar neuroendocrine findings in depressive disorders and anxiety disorders, particularly panic disorder, including blunted cortisol response to adrenocorticotropic hormone, blunted growth hormone response to clonidine (Catapres), and blunted thyroid-stimulating hormone and prolactin responses to thyrotropin-releasing hormone. Second, several investigators have reported data indicating that hyperactivity of the noradrenergic system is causally relevant to some patients with depressive disorders and with panic disorder. Specifically, these studies have found elevated concentrations of the norepinephrine metabolite (MHPG) in the urine, the plasma, or the CSF of depressed patients and patients with panic disorder who were actively experiencing a panic attack. As with other anxiety and depressive disorders, serotonin and GABA may also be causally involved in mixed anxiety-depressive disorder. Third, many studies have found that serotonergic drugs, such as fluoxetine (Prozac) and clomipramine (Anafranil), are useful in treating both depressive and anxiety disorders. Fourth, a number of family studies have reported data indicating that anxiety and depressive symptoms are genetically linked in at least some families.

Diagnosis

The diagnostic criteria for mixed anxiety-depressive disorder require the presence of subsyndromal symptoms of both anxiety and depression and the presence of some autonomic symptoms, such as tremor, palpitations, dry mouth, and the sensation of a churning stomach. Some preliminary studies have indicated that the sensitivity of general practitioners to a syndrome of mixed anxiety-depressive disorder is low, although this lack of recognition may reflect the lack of an appropriate diagnostic label for the patients.

Clinical Features

The clinical features of mixed anxiety-depressive disorder combine symptoms of anxiety disorders and some symptoms of depressive disorders. In addition, symptoms of autonomic nervous system hyperactivity, such as gastrointestinal complaints, are common and contribute to the high frequency with which the patients are seen in outpatient medical clinics.

Differential Diagnosis

The differential diagnosis includes other anxiety and depressive disorders and personality disorders. Among the anxiety disorders, generalized anxiety disorder is most likely to overlap with mixed anxiety-depressive disorder. Among the mood disorders, dysthymic disorder and minor depressive disorder are most likely to overlap with mixed anxiety-depressive disorder. Among the personality disorders, avoidant, dependent, and obsessive-compulsive personality disorders may have symptoms that resemble those of mixed anxiety-depressive disorder. A diagnosis of a somatoform disorder should also be considered. Only a psychiatric history, a mental status examination, and a working knowledge of the specific criteria can help clinicians differentiate among these conditions. The prodromal signs of schizophrenia may show itself as a mixed picture of mounting anxiety and depression with eventual onset of psychotic symptoms.

Course and Prognosis

On the basis of clinical data to date, patients seem to be equally likely to have prominent anxiety symptoms, prominent depressive symptoms, or an equal mixture of the two symptoms at onset. During the course of the illness, anxiety or depressive symptoms may alternate in their predominance. The prognosis is not known.

Treatment

Because adequate studies comparing treatment modalities for mixed anxiety-depressive disorder are not available, clinicians are probably most likely to provide treatment based on the symptoms present, their severity, and the clinician's own level of experience with various treatment modalities. Psychotherapeutic approaches may involve time-limited approaches, such as cognitive therapy or behavior modification, although some clinicians use a less structured psychotherapeutic approach, such as insight-oriented psychotherapy. Pharmacotherapy for mixed anxiety-depressive disorder can include antianxiety drugs, antidepressant drugs, or both. Among the anxiolytic drugs, some data indicate that the use of triazolobenzodiazepines (e.g., alprazolam [Xanax]) may be indicated because of their effectiveness in treating depression associated with anxiety. A drug that affects the serotonin 5-HT_{1A} receptor, such as buspirone (BuSpar), may also be indicated. Among the antidepressants, despite the noradrenergic theories linking anxiety disorders and depressive disorders, the serotonergic antidepressants may be most effective in treating mixed anxiety-depressive disorder. Venlafaxine (Effexor) is an effective antidepressant that has been approved by the FDA for the treatment of depression as well as generalized anxiety disorder.

7 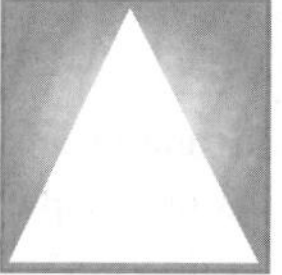

Obsessive-Compulsive and Related Disorders

▲ 7.1 Obsessive-Compulsive Disorder

Obsessive-compulsive disorder (OCD) is represented by a diverse group of symptoms that include intrusive thoughts, rituals, preoccupations, and compulsions. These recurrent obsessions or compulsions cause severe distress to the person. The obsessions or compulsions are time-consuming and interfere significantly with the person's normal routine, occupational functioning, usual social activities, or relationships. A patient with OCD may have an obsession, a compulsion, or both.

An obsession is a recurrent and intrusive thought, feeling, idea, or sensation. In contrast to an obsession, which is a mental event, a compulsion is a behavior. Specifically, a compulsion is a conscious, standardized, recurrent behavior, such as counting, checking, or avoiding. A patient with OCD realizes the irrationality of the obsession and experiences both the obsession and the compulsion as ego-dystonic (i.e., unwanted behavior).

Although the compulsive act may be carried out in an attempt to reduce the anxiety associated with the obsession, it does not always succeed in doing so. The completion of the compulsive act may not affect the anxiety, and it may even increase the anxiety. Anxiety is also increased when a person resists carrying out a compulsion. A variety of OCD conditions are described in this section and those that follow (Sections 7.2 to 7.5).

EPIDEMIOLOGY

The rates of OCD are fairly consistent, with a lifetime prevalence in the general population estimated at 1 to 3 percent. Some researchers have estimated that the disorder is found in as many as 10 percent of outpatients in psychiatric clinics. These figures make OCD the fourth most common psychiatric diagnosis after phobias, substance-related disorders, and major depressive disorder. Epidemiological studies in Europe, Asia, and Africa have confirmed these rates across cultural boundaries.

Among adults, men and women are equally affected with a slight trend toward women in some studies, but among adolescents, boys are more commonly affected than girls. The mean age of onset is about 20 years, although men have a slightly earlier age of onset (mean about 19 years) than women (mean about 22 years). Overall, the symptoms of about two-thirds of affected persons have an onset before age 25, and the symptoms of fewer than 15 percent have an onset after age 35. The onset of the disorder can occur in adolescence or childhood, in some cases as early as 2 years of age. Single persons are more frequently affected with OCD than are married persons, although this finding probably reflects the difficulty that persons with the disorder have maintaining a relationship. OCD occurs less often among blacks than among whites, although access to health care rather than differences in prevalence may explain the variation.

COMORBIDITY

Persons with OCD are commonly affected by other mental disorders. The lifetime prevalence for major depressive disorder in persons with OCD is about 67 percent and for social phobia about 25 percent. Other common comorbid psychiatric diagnoses in patients with OCD include alcohol use disorders, generalized anxiety disorder, specific phobia, panic disorder, eating disorders, and personality disorders. OCD exhibits a superficial resemblance to obsessive-compulsive personality disorder, which is associated with an obsessive concern for details, perfectionism, and other similar personality traits. The incidence of Tourette's disorder in patients with OCD is 5 to 7 percent, and 20 to 30 percent of patients with OCD have a history of tics.

ETIOLOGY

Biological Factors

Neurotransmitters

SEROTONERGIC SYSTEM. Many clinical drug trials that have been conducted support the hypothesis that dysregulation of serotonin is involved in the symptom formation of obsessions and compulsions in the disorder. Data show that serotonergic drugs are more effective in treating OCD than drugs that affect other neurotransmitter systems, but whether serotonin is involved in the cause of OCD is not clear. Clinical studies have assayed cerebrospinal fluid (CSF) concentrations of serotonin metabolites (e.g., 5-hydroxyindoleacetic acid [5-HIAA]) and affinities and numbers of platelet-binding sites of tritiated imipramine (Tofranil), which binds to serotonin reuptake sites, and have reported variable findings of these measures in patients with OCD. In one study, the CSF concentration of 5-HIAA decreased after treatment with clomipramine (Anafranil), focusing attention on the serotonergic system.

NORADRENERGIC SYSTEM. Currently, less evidence exists for dysfunction in the noradrenergic system in OCD. Anecdotal reports show some improvement in OCD symptoms with use of oral clonidine (Catapres), a drug that lowers the amount of norepinephrine released from the presynaptic nerve terminals.

NEUROIMMUNOLOGY. Some interest exists in a positive link between streptococcal infection and OCD. Group A β-hemolytic streptococcal infection can cause rheumatic fever, and approximately 10 to 30 percent of the patients develop Sydenham's chorea and show obsessive-compulsive symptoms.

Brain-Imaging Studies. Neuroimaging in patients with OCD has produced converging data implicating altered function in the neurocircuitry between orbitofrontal cortex, caudate, and thalamus. Various functional brain-imaging studies—for example, positron emission tomography (PET)—have shown increased activity (e.g., metabolism and blood flow) in the frontal lobes, the basal ganglia (especially the caudate), and the cingulum of patients with OCD. The involvement of these areas in the pathology of OCD appears more associated with corticostriatal pathways than with the amygdala pathways, which are the current focus of much anxiety disorder research. Pharmacological and behavioral treatments reportedly reverse these abnormalities. Data from functional brain-imaging studies are consistent with data from structural brain-imaging studies. Both computed tomographic (CT) and magnetic resonance imaging (MRI) studies have found bilaterally smaller caudates in patients with OCD. Both functional and structural brain-imaging study results are also compatible with the observation that neurological procedures involving the cingulum are sometimes effective in the treatment of OCD. One recent MRI study reported increased T1 relaxation times in the frontal cortex, a finding consistent with the location of abnormalities discovered in PET studies.

Genetics. Available genetic data on OCD support the hypothesis that the disorder has a significant genetic component. Relatives of probands with OCD consistently have a threefold to fivefold higher probability of having OCD or obsessive-compulsive features than families of control probands. The data, however, do not yet distinguish the heritable factors from the influence of cultural and behavioral effects on the transmission of the disorder. Studies of concordance for the disorder in twins have consistently found a significantly higher concordance rate for monozygotic twins than for dizygotic twins. Some studies also demonstrate increased rates of a variety of conditions among relatives of OCD probands, including generalized anxiety disorder, tic disorders, body dysmorphic disorder, hypochondriasis, eating disorders, and habits such as nail-biting.

Other Biological Data. Electrophysiological studies, sleep electroencephalogram (EEG) studies, and neuroendocrine studies have contributed data that indicate some commonalities between depressive disorders and OCD. A higher than usual incidence of nonspecific EEG abnormalities occurs in patients with OCD. Sleep EEG studies have found abnormalities similar to those in depressive disorders, such as decreased rapid eye movement latency. Neuroendocrine studies have also produced some analogies to depressive disorders, such as nonsuppression on the dexamethasone-suppression test in about one-third of patients and decreased growth hormone secretion with clonidine infusions.

As mentioned, studies have suggested a possible link between a subset of OCD cases and certain types of motor tic syndromes (i.e., Tourette's disorder and chronic motor tics). A higher rate of OCD, Tourette's disorder, and chronic motor tics are found in relatives of patients with Tourette's disorder than in relatives of controls, whether or not they had OCD. Most family studies of probands with OCD have found increased rates of Tourette's disorder and chronic motor tics only among the relatives of probands with OCD who also have some form of tic disorder. Evidence also suggests cotransmission of Tourette's disorder, OCD, and chronic motor tics within families.

Behavioral Factors

According to learning theorists, obsessions are conditioned stimuli. A relatively neutral stimulus becomes associated with fear or anxiety through a process of respondent conditioning by being paired with events that are noxious or anxiety producing. Thus, previously neutral objects and thoughts become conditioned stimuli capable of provoking anxiety or discomfort.

Compulsions are established in a different way. When a person discovers that a certain action reduces anxiety attached to an obsessional thought, he or she develops active avoidance strategies in the form of compulsions or ritualistic behaviors to control the anxiety. Gradually, because of their efficacy in reducing a painful secondary drive (anxiety), the avoidance strategies become fixed as learned patterns of compulsive behaviors. Learning theory provides useful concepts for explaining certain aspects of obsessive-compulsive phenomena—for example, the anxiety-provoking capacity of ideas not necessarily frightening in themselves and the establishment of compulsive patterns of behavior.

Psychosocial Factors

Personality Factors. OCD differs from obsessive-compulsive personality disorder, which is associated with an obsessive concern for details, perfectionism, and other similar personality traits. Most persons with OCD do not have premorbid compulsive symptoms, and such personality traits are neither necessary nor sufficient for the development of OCD. Only about 15 to 35 percent of patients with OCD have had premorbid obsessional traits.

Psychodynamic Factors. Psychodynamic insight may be of great help in understanding problems with treatment compliance, interpersonal difficulties, and personality problems accompanying the Axis I disorder. Many patients with OCD may refuse to cooperate with effective treatments such as selective serotonin reuptake inhibitors (SSRIs) and behavior therapy. Even though the symptoms of OCD may be biologically driven, psychodynamic meanings may be attached to them. Patients may become invested in maintaining the symptomatology because of secondary gains. For example, a male patient, whose mother stays home to take care of him, may unconsciously wish to hang on to his OCD symptoms because they keep the attention of his mother.

Another contribution of psychodynamic understanding involves the interpersonal dimensions. Studies have shown that relatives will accommodate the patient through active participation in rituals or significant modifications of their daily routines. This form of family accommodation is correlated with stress in the family, rejecting attitudes toward the patient, and poor family functioning. Often, the family members are involved in an effort to reduce the patient's anxiety or to control the patient's expressions of anger. This pattern of relatedness may become internalized and be recreated when the patient enters a treatment setting. By looking at recurring patterns of interpersonal relationships from a psychodynamic perspective, patients may learn how their illness affects others.

Finally, one other contribution of psychodynamic thinking is recognition of the precipitants that initiate or exacerbate symptoms. Often, interpersonal difficulties increase the patient's anxiety and, thus, increase the patient's symptomatology as well. Research suggests that OCD may be precipitated by a number of environmental stressors, especially those involving pregnancy, childbirth, or parental care of children. An understanding of the stressors may assist the clinician in an overall treatment plan that reduces the stressful events themselves or their meaning to the patient.

SIGMUND FREUD. In classic psychoanalytic theory, OCD was termed as *obsessive-compulsive neurosis* and was considered a regression from the oedipal phase to the anal psychosexual phase of development. When patients with OCD feel threatened by anxiety about retaliation for unconscious impulses or by the loss of a significant object's love, they retreat from the oedipal position and regress to an intensely ambivalent emotional stage associated with the anal phase. The ambivalence is connected to the unraveling of the smooth fusion between sexual and aggressive drives characteristic of the oedipal phase. The coexistence of hatred and love toward the same person leaves patients paralyzed with doubt and indecision.

An example of how Freud viewed OCD symptoms is described by Otto Fenichel in the case study presented here.

A patient, who was not analyzed, complained in the first interview that he suffered from the compulsion to look backward constantly, from fear that he might have overlooked something important behind him. These ideas were predominant; he might overlook a coin lying on the ground; he might have injured an insect by stepping on it; or an insect might have fallen on its back and need his help. The patient was also afraid of touching anything, and whenever he had touched an object he had to convince himself that he had not destroyed it. He had no vocation because the severe compulsions disturbed all his working activity; however, he had one passion: housecleaning. He liked to visit his neighbors and clean their houses, just for fun. Another symptom was described by the patient as his "clothes consciousness"; he was constantly preoccupied with the question whether or not his suit fitted. He also stated that sexuality did not play an important part in his life. He had sexual intercourse two or three times a year only, and exclusively with girls in whom he had no personal interest. Later on, he mentioned another symptom. As a child, he had felt his mother to be disgusting and had been terribly afraid of touching her. There was no real reason whatsoever for such a disgust, for the mother had been a nice person.

In the clinical picture for this case study, Freud believed the need to be clean and not to touch is related to anal sexuality, and the disgust for the mother is a reaction against incestuous fears.

One of the striking features of patients with OCD is the degree to which they are preoccupied with aggression or cleanliness, either overtly in the content of their symptoms or in the associations that lie behind them. The psychogenesis of OCD, therefore, may lie in disturbances in normal growth and development related to the anal-sadistic phase of development.

AMBIVALENCE. Ambivalence is an important feature of normal children during the anal-sadistic developmental phase; children feel both love and murderous hate toward the same object, sometimes simultaneously. Patients with OCD often consciously experience both love and hate toward an object. This conflict of opposing emotions is evident in a patient's doing and undoing patterns of behavior and in paralyzing doubt in the face of choices.

MAGICAL THINKING. In magical thinking, regression uncovers early modes of thought rather than impulses; that is, ego functions as well as id functions are affected by regression. Inherent in magical thinking is omnipotence of thought. Persons believe that merely by thinking about an event in the external world they can cause the event to occur without intermediate physical actions. This feeling causes them to fear having an aggressive thought.

DIAGNOSIS AND CLINICAL FEATURES

The diagnostic criteria for OCD in the fifth edition of the *Diagnostic and Statistical Manual of Mental Disorders* (DSM-5) describes the disorder as one in which there are recurrent and persistent thoughts (obsessions) or repetitive behaviors (compulsions). In addition, clinicians can indicate whether the patient's OCD is characterized by good or fair insight, poor insight, or absent insight. Patients with good or fair insight recognize that their OCD beliefs are definitely or probably not true or may or may not be true. Patients with poor insight believe their OCD beliefs are probably true, and patients with absent insight are convinced that their beliefs are true.

Patients with OCD often take their complaints to physicians rather than psychiatrists (Table 7.1–1). Most patients with OCD have both obsessions and compulsions—up to 75 percent in some surveys. Some researchers and clinicians believe that the number may be much closer to 100 percent if patients are carefully assessed for the presence of mental compulsions in addition to behavioral compulsions. For example, an obsession about hurting a child may be followed by a mental compulsion to repeat a specific prayer a specific number of times. Other researchers and clinicians, however, believe that some patients do have only obsessive thoughts without compulsions. Such patients are likely to have repetitious thoughts of a sexual or aggressive act that is reprehensible to them. For clarity, it is best to conceptualize obsessions as thoughts and compulsions as behavior.

Obsessions and compulsions are the essential features of OCD. An idea or an impulse intrudes itself insistently and persistently into a person's conscious awareness. Typical obsessions associated with OCD include thoughts about contamination ("My hands are dirty") or doubts ("I forgot to turn off the stove").

A feeling of anxious dread accompanies the central manifestation, and the key characteristic of a compulsion is that it

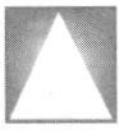

Table 7.1–1
Nonpsychiatric Clinical Specialists Likely to See Obsessive-Compulsive Disorder Patients

Specialist	Presenting Problem
Dermatologist	Chapped hands, eczematoid appearance
Family practitioner	Family member washing excessively, may mention counting or checking compulsions
Oncologist, infectious disease internist	Insistent belief that person has acquired immune deficiency syndrome
Neurologist	Obsessive-compulsive disorder associated with Tourette's disorder, head injury, epilepsy, choreas, other basal ganglia lesions or disorders
Neurosurgeon	Severe, intractable obsessive-compulsive disorder
Obstetrician	Postpartum obsessive-compulsive disorder
Pediatrician	Parent's concern about child's behavior, usually excessive washing
Pediatric cardiologist	Obsessive-compulsive disorder secondary to Sydenham's chorea
Plastic surgeon	Repeated consultations for "abnormal" features
Dentist	Gum lesions from excessive teeth cleaning

From Rapoport JL. The neurobiology of obsessive-compulsive disorder. *JAMA*. 1988;260:2889.

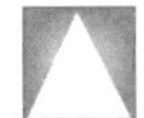

Table 7.1–2
Obsessive-Compulsive Symptoms in Adults

Variable	%
Obsessions (N = 200)	
Contamination	45
Pathological doubt	42
Somatic	36
Need for symmetry	31
Aggressive	28
Sexual	26
Other	13
Multiple obsessions	60
Compulsions (N = 200)	
Checking	63
Washing	50
Counting	36
Need to ask or confess	31
Symmetry and precision	28
Hoarding	18
Multiple comparisons	48
Course of illness (N = 100)[a]	
Type	
Continuous	85
Deteriorative	10
Episodic	2
Not present	71
Present	29

[a]Age at onset: men, 17.5 ± 6.8 years; women, 20.8 ± 8.5 years.
From Rasmussen SA, Eiser JL. The epidemiology and differential diagnosis of obsessive compulsive disorder. *J Clin Psychiatry*. 1992;53(4 Suppl):6.

reduces the anxiety associated with the obsession. The obsession or the compulsion is ego-alien; that is, it is experienced as foreign to the person's experience of himself or herself as a psychological being. No matter how vivid and compelling the obsession or compulsion, the person usually recognizes it as absurd and irrational. The person suffering from obsessions and compulsions usually feels a strong desire to resist them. Nevertheless, about half of all patients offer little resistance to compulsions, although about 80 percent of all patients believe that the compulsion is irrational. Sometimes, patients overvalue obsessions and compulsions—for example, they may insist that compulsive cleanliness is morally correct, even though they have lost their jobs because of time they spent in cleaning.

Symptom Patterns

The presentation of obsessions and compulsions is heterogeneous in adults (Table 7.1–2) and in children and adolescents (Table 7.1–3). The symptoms of an individual patient can overlap and change with time.

Contamination. The most common pattern is an obsession of contamination, followed by washing or accompanied by compulsive avoidance of the presumably contaminated object. The feared object is often hard to avoid (e.g., feces, urine, dust, or germs). Patients may literally rub the skin off their hands by excessive hand washing or may be unable to leave their homes because of fear of germs. Although anxiety is the most common emotional response to the feared object, obsessive shame and disgust are also common. Patients with contamination obsessions usually believe that the contamination is spread from object to object or person to person by the slightest contact.

Pathological Doubt. The second most common pattern is an obsession of doubt, followed by a compulsion of checking. The obsession often implies some danger of violence (e.g., forgetting to turn off the stove or not locking a door). The checking may involve multiple trips back into the house to check the stove, for example. These patients have an obsessional self-doubt and always feel guilty about having forgotten or committed something.

Intrusive Thoughts. In the third most common pattern, there are intrusive obsessional thoughts without a compulsion. Such obsessions are usually repetitious thoughts of a sexual or aggressive act that is reprehensible to the patient. Patients obsessed with thoughts of aggressive or sexual acts may report themselves to police or confess to a priest. Suicidal ideation may also be obsessive; but a careful suicidal assessment of actual risk must always be done.

Symmetry. The fourth most common pattern is the need for symmetry or precision, which can lead to a compulsion of slowness. Patients can literally take hours to eat a meal or shave their faces.

Other Symptom Patterns. Religious obsessions and compulsive hoarding are common in patients with OCD. Compulsive hair pulling and nail biting are behavioral patterns related to OCD. Masturbation may also be compulsive.

Mental Status Examination

On mental status examinations, patients with OCD may show symptoms of depressive disorders. Such symptoms are present

Table 7.1–3
Reported Obsessions and Compulsions for 70 Consecutive Child and Adolescent Patients

Major Presenting Symptom	No. (%) of Reporting Symptoms at Initial Interview[a]
Obsession	
Concern or disgust with bodily wastes or secretions (urine, stool, saliva), dirt, germs, environmental toxins	30 (43)
Fear something terrible may happen (fire, death or illness of loved one, self, or others)	18 (24)
Concern or need for symmetry, order, or exactness	12 (17)
Scrupulosity (excessive praying or religious concerns out of keeping with patient's background)	9 (13)
Lucky and unlucky numbers	6 (8)
Forbidden or perverse sexual thoughts, images, or impulses	3 (4)
Intrusive nonsense sounds, words, or music	1 (1)
Compulsion	
Excessive or ritualized hand washing, showering, bathing, tooth brushing, or grooming	60 (85)
Repeating rituals (e.g., going in and out of door, up and down from chair)	36 (51)
Checking doors, locks, stove, appliances, car brakes	32 (46)
Cleaning and other rituals to remove contact with contaminants	16 (23)
Touching	14 (20)
Ordering and arranging	12 (17)
Measures to prevent harm to self or others (e.g., hanging clothes a certain way)	11 (16)
Counting	13 (18)
Hoarding and collecting	8 (11)
Miscellaneous rituals (e.g., licking, spitting, special dress pattern)	18 (26)

[a]Multiple symptoms recorded, so total exceeds 70.
From Rapoport JL. The neurobiology of obsessive-compulsive disorder. *JAMA*. 1988;260:2889.

in about 50 percent of all patients. Some patients with OCD have character traits suggesting obsessive-compulsive personality disorder (e.g., excessive need for preciseness and neatness), but most do not. Patients with OCD, especially men, have a higher than average celibacy rate. Married patients have a greater than usual amount of marital discord.

Ms. K was referred for psychiatric evaluation by her general practitioner. On interview, Ms. K described a long history of checking rituals that had caused her to lose several jobs and had damaged numerous relationships. She reported, for example, that because she often had the thought that she had not locked the door to the car, it was difficult for her to leave that car until she had checked repeatedly that it was secure. She had broken several car door handles with the vigor of her checking and had been up to an hour late to work because she spent so much time checking her car door. Similarly, she had recurrent thoughts that she had left the door to her apartment unlocked, and she returned several times daily to check her door before she left for work. She reported that checking doors decreased her anxiety about security. Although Ms. K reported that she had occasionally tried to leave her car or apartment without checking the door (e.g., when she was already late for work), she found that she became so worried about her car being stolen or her apartment being broken into that she had difficulty going anywhere. Ms. K reported that her obsessions about security had become so extreme over the past 3 months that she had lost her job due to recurrent tardiness. She recognized the irrational nature of her obsessive concerns but could not bring herself to ignore them. *(Courtesy of Erin B. McClure-Tone, Ph.D. and Daniel S. Pine, M.D.)*

DIFFERENTIAL DIAGNOSIS

Medical Conditions

A number of primary medical disorders can produce syndromes bearing a striking resemblance to OCD. The current conceptualization of OCD as a disorder of the basal ganglia derives from the phenomenological similarity between idiopathic OCD and OCD-like disorders that are associated with basal ganglia diseases, such as Sydenham's chorea and Huntington's disease. Neurological signs of such basal ganglia pathology must be assessed when considering the diagnosis of OCD in a patient presenting for psychiatric treatment. It should also be noted that OCD frequently develops before the age of 30 years, and new-onset OCD in an older individual should raise questions about potential neurological contributions to the disorder.

Tourette's Disorder

OCD is closely related to Tourette's disorder, as the two conditions frequently co-occur, both in individuals over time and within families. About 90 percent of persons with Tourette's disorder have compulsive symptoms, and as many as two-thirds meet the diagnostic criteria for OCD.

In its classic form, Tourette's disorder is associated with a pattern of recurrent vocal and motor tics that bears only a slight resemblance to OCD. The premonitory urges that precede tics often strikingly resemble obsessions, however, and many of the more complicated motor tics are very similar to compulsions.

Other Psychiatric Conditions

Obsessive-compulsive behavior is found in a host of other psychiatric disorders, and the clinician must also rule out these conditions when diagnosing OCD. OCD exhibits a superficial resemblance to obsessive-compulsive personality disorder, which is associated with an obsessive concern for details, perfectionism, and other similar personality traits. The conditions are easily distinguished in that only OCD is associated with a true syndrome of obsessions and compulsions.

Psychotic symptoms often lead to obsessive thoughts and compulsive behaviors that can be difficult to distinguish from OCD with poor insight, in which obsessions border on psychosis. The keys to distinguishing OCD from psychosis are (1) patients with OCD can almost always acknowledge the unreasonable nature of their symptoms, and (2) psychotic illnesses are typically associated with a host of other features that are not characteristic of OCD. Similarly, OCD can be difficult to differentiate from depression because the two disorders often occur comorbidly, and major depression is often associated with obsessive thoughts that, at times, border on true obsessions such as those that characterize OCD. The two conditions are best distinguished by their courses. Obsessive symptoms associated with depression are only found in the presence of a depressive episode, whereas true OCD persists despite remission of depression.

COURSE AND PROGNOSIS

More than half of patients with OCD have a sudden onset of symptoms. The onset of symptoms for about 50 to 70 percent of patients occurs after a stressful event, such as a pregnancy, a sexual problem, or the death of a relative. Because many persons manage to keep their symptoms secret, they often delay 5 to 10 years before coming to psychiatric attention, although the delay is probably shortening with increased awareness of the disorder. The course is usually long but variable; some patients experience a fluctuating course, and others experience a constant one.

About 20 to 30 percent of patients have significant improvement in their symptoms, and 40 to 50 percent have moderate improvement. The remaining 20 to 40 percent of patients either remain ill or their symptoms worsen.

About one-third of patients with OCD have major depressive disorder, and suicide is a risk for all patients with OCD. A poor prognosis is indicated by yielding to (rather than resisting) compulsions, childhood onset, bizarre compulsions, the need for hospitalization, a coexisting major depressive disorder, delusional beliefs, the presence of overvalued ideas (i.e., some acceptance of obsessions and compulsions), and the presence of a personality disorder (especially schizotypal personality disorder). A good prognosis is indicated by good social and occupational adjustment, the presence of a precipitating event, and an episodic nature of the symptoms. The obsessional content does not seem to be related to the prognosis.

TREATMENT

With mounting evidence that OCD is largely determined by biological factors, classic psychoanalytic theory has fallen out of favor. Moreover, because OCD symptoms appear to be largely refractory to psychodynamic psychotherapy and psychoanalysis, pharmacological and behavioral treatments have become common. But psychodynamic factors may be of considerable benefit in understanding what precipitates exacerbations of the disorder and in treating various forms of resistance to treatment, such as noncompliance with medication.

Many patients with OCD tenaciously resist treatment efforts. They may refuse to take medication and may resist carrying out therapeutic homework assignments and other activities prescribed by behavior therapists. The obsessive-compulsive symptoms themselves, no matter how biologically based, may have important psychological meanings that make patients reluctant to give them up. Psychodynamic exploration of a patient's resistance to treatment may improve compliance.

Well-controlled studies have found that pharmacotherapy, behavior therapy, or a combination of both is effective in significantly reducing the symptoms of patients with OCD. The decision about which therapy to use is based on the clinician's judgment and experience and the patient's acceptance of the various modalities.

Pharmacotherapy

The efficacy of pharmacotherapy in OCD has been proved in many clinical trials and is enhanced by the observation that the studies find a placebo response rate of only about 5 percent.

The drugs, some of which are used to treat depressive disorders or other mental disorders, can be given in their usual dosage ranges. Initial effects are generally seen after 4 to 6 weeks of treatment, although 8 to 16 weeks are usually needed to obtain maximal therapeutic benefit. Treatment with antidepressant drugs is still controversial, and a significant proportion of patients with OCD who respond to treatment with antidepressant drugs seem to relapse if the drug therapy is discontinued.

The standard approach is to start treatment with an SSRI or clomipramine and then move to other pharmacological strategies if the serotonin-specific drugs are not effective. The serotonergic drugs have increased the percentage of patients with OCD who are likely to respond to treatment to the range of 50 to 70 percent.

Selective Serotonin Reuptake Inhibitors. Each of the SSRIs available in the United States—fluoxetine (Prozac), fluvoxamine (Luvox), paroxetine (Paxil), sertraline (Zoloft), citalopram (Celexa)—has been approved by the U.S. Food and Drug Administration (FDA) for the treatment of OCD. Higher dosages have often been necessary for a beneficial effect, such as 80 mg a day of fluoxetine. Although the SSRIs can cause sleep disturbance, nausea and diarrhea, headache, anxiety, and restlessness, these adverse effects are often transient and are generally less troubling than the adverse effects associated with tricyclic drugs, such as clomipramine. The best clinical outcomes occur when SSRIs are used in combination with behavioral therapy.

Clomipramine. Of all the tricyclic and tetracyclic drugs, clomipramine is the most selective for serotonin reuptake versus norepinephrine reuptake and is exceeded in this respect only by the SSRIs. The potency of serotonin reuptake of clomipramine is exceeded only by sertraline and paroxetine. Clomipramine was the first drug to be FDA approved for the treatment of OCD. Its dosing must be titrated upward over 2 to 3 weeks to avoid gastrointestinal adverse effects and orthostatic hypotension, and as with other tricyclic drugs, it causes significant sedation and anticholinergic effects, including dry mouth and constipation. As with SSRIs, the best outcomes result from a combination of drug and behavioral therapy.

Other Drugs. If treatment with clomipramine or an SSRI is unsuccessful, many therapists augment the first drug by the addition of valproate (Depakene), lithium (Eskalith), or carbamazepine (Tegretol). Other drugs that can be tried in the treatment of OCD are venlafaxine (Effexor), pindolol (Visken), and the monoamine oxidase inhibitors (MAOIs), especially phenelzine (Nardil). Other pharmacological agents for the treatment of unresponsive patients include buspirone (BuSpar), 5-hydroxytryptamine (5-HT), L-tryptophan, and clonazepam (Klonopin). Adding an atypical antipsychotic such as risperidone (Risperdal) has helped in some cases.

Behavior Therapy

Although few head-to-head comparisons have been made, behavior therapy is as effective as pharmacotherapies in OCD, and some data indicate that the beneficial effects are long lasting with behavior therapy. Many clinicians, therefore, consider behavior therapy the treatment of choice for OCD. Behavior therapy can be conducted in both outpatient and inpatient settings. The principal behavioral approaches in OCD are exposure and response prevention. Desensitization, thought stopping, flooding, implosion therapy, and aversive conditioning have also been used in patients with OCD. In behavior therapy, patients must be truly committed to improvement.

Psychotherapy

In the absence of adequate studies of insight-oriented psychotherapy for OCD, any valid generalizations about its effectiveness are hard to make, although there are anecdotal reports of successes. Individual analysts have seen striking and lasting changes for the better in patients with obsessive-compulsive personality disorder, especially when they are able to come to terms with the aggressive impulses underlying their character traits. Likewise, analysts and dynamically oriented psychiatrists have observed marked symptomatic improvement in patients with OCD in the course of analysis or prolonged insight psychotherapy.

Mr. P, a passive, emotionally vacant, exceedingly polite and quiet man in his 30s, had obsessive-compulsive disorder and sought psychodynamic psychotherapy because he was having difficulty functioning at work or in relationships. Mr. P had counting rituals and a compulsion to keep checking that there were no sharp knives left with their blades exposed and no shoes not properly hung on shoetrees or aligned in closets. In sessions he often spoke endlessly about seemingly empty details of his work life. The therapist became drowsy at one point as he listened to Mr. P, who noticed this and, with uncharacteristic affect in his voice, asked, "Doctor, excuse me, but are you listening?" To this the therapist replied, "No, I guess not. Are you?" Mr. P apologized for having been boring.

This incident led to a direct discussion between them about the way Mr. P's obsessive, circumstantial, and emotionally empty recounting of details was a form of resistance and one in which his therapist had joined him by becoming drowsy in the session. Were they going to do the work of therapy together or not?

In subsequent sessions Mr. P made efforts to speak more about the origin of his symptoms, which began with a ritual of kissing his parents each goodnight nine times lest he be unable to sleep. On one occasion, while explaining this, Mr. P made a slip of speech about having to kiss his father nine times, instead substituting the word "kick" for "kiss." When he heard this, the therapist asked Mr. P if he had noticed the slip. Mr. P insisted he could not have made such a mistake, escalated his protests about this for a minute or two as he became sadder, then burst into sobs. While weeping Mr. P accused the therapist of pretending there had been a slip of speech to make him look bad, and then, with an outburst of anger, recalled the hurt and injury he had felt when the therapist had become drowsy in the session.

Surprised at the intensity of his feelings, Mr. P recalled when his need to kiss his parents goodnight in a ritualized way had begun. It was after he had gotten a new puppy. His controlling and intrusive father had kicked Mr. P's beloved new puppy after the latter had a series of toileting accidents in the house. Mr. P wept as he recalled his revulsion and rage at his father and the way he had later comforted his dog when alone. Mr. P recalled having repeatedly unfolded and refolded the blade of his jackknife to show his dog his weapon and swore to his dog that he would use it on his father if the latter ever tried to hurt him again. Soon after the kicking incident Mr. P's father decided he had had enough of this messy puppy and sent the dog away while Mr. P was at school. Mr. P was bereft for a while, but soon settled into an affectless, timid, and passive way of being.

Mr. P responded to what he had learned about his compulsions by actively trying to suppress them and became more anxious. As his anxiety was explored, memories emerged of Mr. P's earlier struggle with his parents around toileting before the puppy came into his life, when he had received regular enemas from his father to control the frequency of bowel movements. Despite loving his father, Mr. P was also enraged at him for taking his dog away without a chance to say goodbye and for the intrusive and terrifying experience of the enemas, while he was also furious at his mother for not stopping his father. Mr. P also felt humiliated that he had experienced this kind of intrusion into his body and that he had let his dog be given away by his father after swearing that he would protect the puppy from his father.

The meaning of Mr. P's specific rituals about knives and shoes became apparent in the course of his therapy as a result of his reaction to his therapist's lapse in becoming drowsy and a slip of speech that revealed aggression hidden beneath passivity and compliance. Mr. P needed to be sure that no knife blades were exposed because such blades represented the threat of a terrifying assault on his father or an equally terrifying failure to protect the puppy that he loved but lost. Similarly, Mr. P's compulsive need to put shoes properly and safely on shoetrees was linked to an effort to put away the memory of and prevent any recurrence of his beloved puppy being kicked and injured by a shod foot. After these were clarified and Mr. P tried to control his rituals, signal anxiety emerged, and with it the recovery of memories of an earlier struggle with his parents about intrusive control of his toileting behavior. *(Courtesy of E. M. Plakun, M.D.)*

Supportive psychotherapy undoubtedly has its place, especially for those patients with OCD who, despite symptoms of varying degrees of severity, are able to work and make social adjustments. With continuous and regular contact with an interested, sympathetic, and encouraging professional person, patients may be able to function by virtue of this help, without which their symptoms would incapacitate them. Occasionally, when obsessional rituals and anxiety reach an intolerable intensity, it is necessary to hospitalize patients until the shelter of an institution and the removal from external environmental stresses diminish symptoms to a tolerable level.

A patient's family members are often driven to the verge of despair by the patient's behavior. Any psychotherapeutic endeavors must include attention to the family members through provision of emotional support, reassurance, explanation, and advice on how to manage and respond to the patient.

Other Therapies

Family therapy is often useful in supporting the family, helping reduce marital discord resulting from the disorder, and building a treatment alliance with the family members for the good of the patient. Group therapy is useful as a support system for some patients.

For extreme cases that are treatment resistant and chronically debilitating, electroconvulsive therapy (ECT) and psychosurgery should be considered. ECT should be tried before surgery. A psychosurgical procedure for OCD is cingulotomy, which may be successful in treating otherwise severe and treatment-unresponsive patients. Other surgical procedures (e.g., subcaudate tractotomy, also known as *capsulotomy*) have also been used for this purpose.

Deep Brain Stimulation

Nonablative surgical techniques involving indwelling electrodes in various basal ganglia nuclei are under investigation to treat both OCD and Tourette's disorder. Deep brain stimulation (DBS) is performed using MRI-guided stereotactic techniques in which electrodes are implanted in the brain. Complications of DBS include infection, bleeding, or the development of seizures, which are almost always controlled by treatment with phenytoin (Dilantin). Some patients who do not respond to psychosurgery alone and who do not respond to pharmacotherapy or behavior therapy before the operation do respond to pharmacotherapy or behavior therapy after psychosurgery.

OBSESSIVE-COMPULSIVE OR RELATED DISORDER DUE TO ANOTHER MEDICAL CONDITION

Many medical conditions can result in obsessive-compulsive symptoms (i.e., hair pulling, skin picking). The diagnosis of obsessive-compulsive or related disorder attributable to another medical condition is used when obsessive-compulsive symptoms develop in the context of an identifiable medical condition.

OCD-like symptoms have been reported in children following group A β-hemolytic streptococcal infection and have been called *pediatric autoimmune neuropsychiatric disorders associated with streptococcus* (PANDAS). They are believed to result from an autoimmune process that leads to inflammation of the basal ganglia that disrupts cortical–striatal–thalamic axis functioning. For more information, see Section 31.14 OCD in childhood and adolescence.

SUBSTANCE-INDUCED OBSESSIVE-COMPULSIVE OR RELATED DISORDER

Substance-induced obsessive-compulsive or related disorder is characterized by the emergence of obsessive-compulsive or related symptoms as a result of a substance abuse, including drugs, medications, and alcohol. Symptoms present either during use or within a month after substance use, intoxication, or withdrawal. The symptoms cannot be better accounted for by a specific obsessive-compulsive or related disorder or another medical condition. The disturbance cannot occur exclusively during the course of delirium.

OTHER SPECIFIED OBSESSIVE-COMPULSIVE OR RELATED DISORDER

This category is for patients who have symptoms characteristic of obsessive-compulsive and related disorder but do not meet the full criteria for any specific obsessive-compulsive or related disorder. This diagnosis is appropriate under three situations: (1) an atypical presentation, (2) another specific syndrome not listed in DSM-5, and (3) the information presented is insufficient to make a full diagnosis of an obsessive-compulsive or related disorder.

Olfactory Reference Syndrome

Olfactory reference syndrome is characterized by a false belief by the patient that he or she has a foul body odor that is not perceived by others. The preoccupation leads to repetitive behaviors such as washing the body or changing clothes. The patient may have good, fair, poor, or absent insight into the behavior. The syndrome is predominant in males and single status. The mean age of onset is 25 years of age. The belief of a subjective sense of smell that does not exist externally may rise to the level of a somatic delusion, in which case a diagnosis of delusional disorder should be considered. The syndrome has been well-documented in the psychiatric literature, usually classified as a delusion of perception.

In assessing a patient with olfactory reference syndrome, it is important to exclude somatic causes. Some patients with temporal lobe epilepsy may complain of smelling foul odors. Local irritations of the hippocampus from pituitary tumors may also cause olfactory sensations. Patients with inflammation of the frontal, ethmoidal, or sphenoidal sinuses may also have a subjective sense of offensive odors. Olfactory reference syndrome is included in the "other specified" designation for obsessive-compulsive and related disorder of DSM-5.

▲ 7.2 Body Dysmorphic Disorder

Body dysmorphic disorder is characterized by a preoccupation with an imagined defect in appearance that causes clinically significant distress or impairment in important areas of functioning. If a slight physical anomaly is actually present, the person's concern with the anomaly is excessive and bothersome.

The disorder was recognized and named *dysmorphophobia* more than 100 years ago by Emil Kraepelin, who considered it a compulsive neurosis; Pierre Janet called it *obsession de la honte du corps* (obsession with shame of the body). Freud wrote about the condition in his description of the Wolf-Man, who was excessively concerned about his nose. Although dysmorphophobia was widely recognized and studied in Europe, it was not until the publication of the third edition of the

Diagnostic and Statistical Manual of Mental Disorders (DSM-III) in 1980 that dysmorphophobia, as an example of a typical somatoform disorder, was specifically mentioned in the US diagnostic criteria. In the fourth text revision of DSM (DSM-IV-TR), the condition was known as body dysmorphic disorder, because the DSM editors believed that the term *dysmorphophobia* inaccurately implied the presence of a behavioral pattern of phobic avoidance. In the fifth edition of DSM (DSM-5), body dysmorphic disorder is included in the obsessive-compulsive spectrum disorders due to its similarities to obsessive-compulsive disorder (OCD).

EPIDEMIOLOGY

Body dysmorphic disorder is a poorly studied condition, partly because patients are more likely to go to dermatologists, internists, or plastic surgeons than to psychiatrists for this condition. One study of a group of college students found that more than 50 percent had at least some preoccupation with a particular aspect of their appearance, and in about 25 percent of the students, the concern had at least some significant effect on their feelings and functioning. DSM-5 reports a point prevalence in the United States of 2.4 percent.

Available data indicate that the most common age of onset is between 15 and 30 years and women are affected somewhat more often than men. Affected patients are also likely to be unmarried. Body dysmorphic disorder commonly coexists with other mental disorders. One study found that more than 90 percent of patients with body dysmorphic disorder had experienced a major depressive episode in their lifetimes; about 70 percent had experienced an anxiety disorder; and about 30 percent had experienced a psychotic disorder.

ETIOLOGY

The cause of body dysmorphic disorder is unknown. The high comorbidity with depressive disorders, a higher-than-expected family history of mood disorders and OCD, and the reported responsiveness of the condition to serotonin-specific drugs indicate that, in at least some patients, the pathophysiology of the disorder may involve serotonin and may be related to other mental disorders. Stereotyped concepts of beauty emphasized in certain families and within the culture at large may significantly affect patients with body dysmorphic disorder. In psychodynamic models, body dysmorphic disorder is seen as reflecting the displacement of a sexual or emotional conflict onto a nonrelated body part. Such an association occurs through the defense mechanisms of repression, dissociation, distortion, symbolization, and projection.

DIAGNOSIS

The DSM-5 diagnostic criteria for body dysmorphic disorder stipulate preoccupation with a perceived defect in appearance or overemphasis of a slight defect. It also stipulates that at some point during the course of the disorder, the patient performs compulsive behaviors (i.e., mirror checking, excessive grooming) or mental acts (e.g., comparing their appearance to that of others). The preoccupation causes patients significant emotional distress or markedly impairs their ability to function in important areas.

CLINICAL FEATURES

The most common concerns involve facial flaws, particularly those involving specific parts (e.g., the nose). Sometimes the concern is vague and difficult to understand, such as extreme concern over a "scrunchy" chin. One study found that, on average, patients had concerns about four body regions during the course of the disorder. Other body parts of concern are hair, breasts, and genitalia. A proposed variant of dysmorphic disorder among men is the desire to "bulk up" and develop large muscle mass, which can interfere with ordinary living, holding a job, or staying healthy. The specific body part may change during the time a patient is affected with the disorder. Common associated symptoms include ideas or frank delusions of reference (usually about persons' noticing the alleged body flaw), either excessive mirror checking or avoidance of reflective surfaces, and attempts to hide the presumed deformity (with makeup or clothing). The effects on a person's life can be significant; almost all affected patients avoid social and occupational exposure. As many as one-third of patients may be housebound because of worry about being ridiculed for the alleged deformities; and approximately one-fifth of patients attempt suicide. As discussed, comorbid diagnoses of depressive disorders and anxiety disorders are common, and patients may also have traits of OCD, schizoid, and narcissistic personality disorders.

Ms. R, a 28-year-old single woman, presented with the complaint that she is "ugly" and that she feels others are laughing at her because of her ugliness. In reality, Ms. R was an attractive woman. She first became preoccupied with her appearance when she was 13, when she became obsessed with her "facial defects" (e.g., her nose was too fat, her eyes were too far apart). Up until this point, Ms. R was confident, a good student, and socially active. However, her fixation on her face caused her to socially withdraw and have difficulty concentrating in school, which in turn had a negative effect on her grades.

Ms. R dropped out of high school and went for her GED due to her preoccupation. She began to frequently pick at "blemishes" and hairs on her face. She frequently checked herself in mirrors and other reflectively surfaces (e.g., spoons, windows). She found herself thinking about her defects almost all day every day. Despite reassuring comments from family and others, Ms. R could not be convinced that there was nothing wrong with her appearance.

DIFFERENTIAL DIAGNOSIS

The diagnosis of body dysmorphic disorder should not be made if the excessive bodily preoccupation is better accounted for by another psychiatric disorder. Excessive bodily preoccupation is generally restricted to concerns about being fat in anorexia nervosa; to discomfort with, or a sense of wrongness about, his or her primary and secondary sex characteristics occurring in gender identity disorder; and to mood-congruent cognitions involving appearance that occur exclusively during a major depressive episode. Individuals with avoidant personality disorder or social phobia may worry about being embarrassed by imagined or real defects in appearance, but this concern is usually not prominent, persistent, distressing, or impairing. Taijin kyofusho, a diagnosis in Japan, is similar to social phobia but has some features that are more consistent with body dysmorphic disorder, such as the belief that the person has an offensive odor or body parts that are offensive to others. Although individuals with body dysmorphic disorder have obsessional preoccupations about their appearance and may have associated compulsive behaviors (e.g., mirror checking), a separate or additional diagnosis of OCD is made only when the obsessions or compulsions are not restricted to concerns about appearance and are ego-dystonic. An additional diagnosis of delusional disorder, somatic type, can be made in people with body dysmorphic disorder only if their preoccupation with the imagined defect in appearance is held with a delusional intensity. Unlike normal concerns about appearance, the preoccupation with appearance and specific imagined defects in body dysmorphic disorder and the changed behavior because of the preoccupation are excessively time-consuming and are associated with significant distress or impairment.

COURSE AND PROGNOSIS

Body dysmorphic disorder usually begins during adolescence, although it may begin later after a protracted dissatisfaction with the body. Age of onset is not well-understood because variably a long delay occurs between symptom onset and treatment seeking. The onset can be gradual or abrupt. The disorder usually has a long and undulating course with few symptom-free intervals. The part of the body on which concern is focused may remain the same or may change over time.

TREATMENT

Treatment of patients with body dysmorphic disorder with surgical, dermatological, dental, and other medical procedures to address the alleged defects is almost invariably unsuccessful. Although tricyclic drugs, MAOIs, and pimozide (Oral) have reportedly been useful in individual cases, other data indicate that serotonin-specific drugs—for example, clomipramine (Anafranil) and fluoxetine (Prozac)—reduce symptoms in at least 50 percent of patients. In any patient with a coexisting mental disorder, such as a depressive disorder or an anxiety disorder, the coexisting disorder should be treated with the appropriate pharmacotherapy and psychotherapy. How long treatment should be continued after the symptoms of body dysmorphic disorder have remitted is unknown. Augmentation of the SSRI with clomipramine (Anafranil), buspirone (BuSpar), lithium (Eskalith), methylphenidate (Ritalin), or antipsychotics may improve the response rate.

RELATION TO PLASTIC SURGERY

Few data exist about the number of patients seeking plastic surgery who have body dysmorphic disorder. One study found that only 2 percent of the patients in a plastic surgery clinic had the diagnosis, but DSM-5 reports the figure to be 7 to 8 percent. The overall percentage may be much higher, however. Surgical requests are varied: removal of facial sags, jowls, wrinkles, or puffiness; rhinoplasty; breast reduction or enhancement; and penile enlargement. Men who request penile enlargements and women who request cosmetic surgery of the labia of the vagina or the lips of the mouth often are suffering from this disorder. Commonly associated with the belief about appearance is an unrealistic expectation of how much surgery will correct the defect. As reality sets in, the person realizes that life's problems are not solved by altering the perceived cosmetic defect. Ideally, such patients will seek out psychotherapy to understand the true nature of their neurotic feelings of inadequacy. Absent that, patients may take out their unfulfilled expectations and anger by suing their plastic surgeons—who have one of highest malpractice-suit rates of any specialty—or by developing a clinical depression.

▲ 7.3 Hoarding Disorder

Compulsive hoarding is a common and often disabling phenomenon associated with impairment in functions such as eating, sleeping, and grooming. Hoarding may result in health problems and poor sanitation, particularly when hoarding of animals is involved, and may lead to death from fire or falling.

The disorder is characterized by acquiring and not discarding things that are deemed to be of little or no value resulting in excessive clutter of living spaces. Hoarding was originally considered a subtype of OCD, but is now considered to be a separate diagnostic entity. It is commonly driven by an obsessive fear of losing important items that the person believes may be of use at some point in the future, by distorted beliefs about the importance of possessions, and by extreme emotional attachment to possessions.

EPIDEMIOLOGY

Hoarding is believed to occur in approximately 2 to 5 percent of the population, although some studies have found lifetime prevalence as high as 14 percent. It occurs equally among men and women, is more common in single persons and is associated with social anxiety, withdrawal, and dependent personality traits. Hoarding usually begins in early adolescence and persists throughout the life span.

COMORBIDITY

The most significant comorbidity is found between hoarding disorder and OCD with as many as 30 percent of OCD patients showing hoarding behavior.

Studies have found an association between hoarding and compulsive buying. Buying or acquiring needless things (including receiving gifts) may be a source of comfort for hoarders, many of whom find themselves with extra items for a perceived but irrational future need. Approximately half of compulsive buyers display a high level of hoarding; however, up to 20 percent of hoarders do not show signs of excessive buying.

Hoarding is associated with high rates of personality disorders in addition to OCD. These include dependent, avoidant, schizotypal, and paranoid types.

Deficits in attention and executive function that occur in hoarding may resemble those seen in attention-deficit/hyperactivity disorder (ADHD). In one study, 20 percent of hoarding patients met the criteria for ADHD. This finding correlates with the fact that OCD patients with hoarding symptoms had a 10 times higher rate of developing ADHD than those without.

Hoarding behaviors are relatively common among schizophrenic patients and have been noted in dementia and other neurocognitive disorders. One study found hoarding in 20 percent of dementia patients and 14 percent of brain injury patients. Onset of hoarding has been reported in cases of frontotemporal dementia and may follow surgery resulting in structural defects in prefrontal and orbitofrontal cortex. In a study of patients with focal lesions of the telencephalon, 15 percent exhibited a sudden onset of severe and persistent collecting and saving behavior.

Other disorders associated with hoarding include eating disorders, depression, anxiety disorders, substance use disorders (particularly alcohol dependence), kleptomania, and compulsive gambling. Among anxiety disorders, hoarding is most associated with generalized anxiety disorder (27 percent) and social anxiety disorder (14 percent).

ETIOLOGY

Little is known about the etiology of hoarding disorder. Research has shown a familial aspect to hoarding disorder with about 80 percent of hoarders reporting at least one first-degree relative with hoarding behavior. Biological research has shown a lower metabolism in the posterior cingulate cortex and the occipital cortex of hoarders, which may also account for various cognitive impairments within hoarders such as attention and decision-making deficits. One study of the molecular genetics for hoarding found a link between hoarding behavior and markers on chromosomes 4q, 5q, and 17q. Another study found that the catecholamine-O-methyltransferase (COMT) gene on chromosome 22q11.21 might contribute to the genetic susceptibility to hoarding.

DIAGNOSIS

Hoarding disorder is characterized by (1) the acquiring of and failure to discard a large amount of possessions that are deemed useless or of little value; (2) greatly cluttered living areas precluding normal activities; and (3) significant distress and impairment in functioning due to hoarding. DSM-5 includes diagnostic specifiers relate to insight which may be poor, fair, or good. Some patients are completely unaware of the full extent of the problem and totally resistant to treatment. At times delusional beliefs about hoarded items are present.

CLINICAL FEATURES

Hoarding is driven by the fear of losing items that the patient believes will be needed later and a distorted belief about or an emotional attachment to possessions. Most hoarders do not perceive their behavior to be a problem. In fact, many perceive their behavior to be reasonable and part of their identity. Most hoarding patients accumulate possessions passively rather than intentionally, thus clutter accumulates gradually over time. Common hoarded items include newspapers, mail, magazines, old clothes, bags, books, lists, and notes. Hoarding poses risks to not only the patient, but to those around them. Clutter accumulated from hoarding has been attributed to deaths from fire or patients being crushed by their possessions. It can also attract pest infestations that can pose a health risk both to the patient and residents around them. Many sufferers have been evicted from their home or threatened with eviction as a result of their hoarding. In severe cases, hoarding can interfere with work, social interaction, and basic activities such as eating or sleeping.

The pathological nature of hoarding comes from the inability to organize possessions and keep them organized. Many hoard to avoid making decisions about discarding items. Patients with hoarding disorder also overemphasize the importance of recalling information and possessions. For example, a hoarder will keep old newspapers and magazines because they believe that if discarded the information will be forgotten and will never be retrieved again. In addition, patients believe that forgetting information will lead to serious consequences and prefer to keep possessions in sight so as not to forget them.

Ms. T, a 55-year-old single woman, presented to a therapist accompanied by her adult son, who expressed concern about Ms. T's inability to "throw things away." He reported that Ms. T's home was extremely cluttered with "needless things." Whenever he attempted to help her "organize things," however, Ms. T would become agitated and argumentative. Ms. T confirmed her son's complaint and reported having this difficulty for as long as she could remember, but never really viewed it as a problem.

Over the past 5 years, Ms. T's home had become increasingly cluttered to the point that it became more and more difficult to move around within it. She was able to keep the kitchen and bathroom relatively clutter free, but the rest of her home was filled with boxes and bags filled with papers, magazines, clothes, and miscellaneous gifts and trinkets. Her living room was the most affected. Her son reported no longer being able to visit his mother because it was so difficult to move around and there were very few places for them to sit comfortably. This, Ms. T admits, has been a major source of depression for her. Ms. T used to enjoy entertaining family and friends, especially on holidays, but has not had any guests over in years because she felt that her home was no longer "suitable for company." She had made a few attempts to clean out her home, but was unable to discard most items. When asked why she was keeping them, she replied "I may need them later."

DIFFERENTIAL DIAGNOSIS

The diagnosis of hoarding disorder should not be made if the excessive acquisition and inability to discard of possessions is better accounted for by another medical or psychiatric condition. Until recently, hoarding was considered to be a symptom of OCD and obsessive-compulsive personality disorder. However, there are some major differences. Hoarding disorder patients do not display some of the classic symptoms of OCD such as recurring intrusive thoughts or compulsive rituals. Unlike symptoms of OCD, symptoms of hoarding worsen with time, rituals are not fixed, and obsessions about dirt or contamination are absent. OCD patients have better insight into their condition. Symptoms are usually ego-dystonic whereas in hoarding disorder they are ego-syntonic. Hoarding behavior is seldom repetitive and is not viewed as intrusive or distressing to the hoarder. Distress mainly comes at the prospect of discarding items and it manifests more as guilt and anger than anxiety. Hoarding disorder also tends to be less responsive to classic treatments for OCD such as exposure therapy, cognitive–behavioral therapy (CBT), and SSRIs.

Some case reports show the onset of this behavior in patients after suffering brain lesions. Hoarding associated with brain lesions is more purposeless than hoarding which is motivated by emotional attachment or high intrinsic value of possessions. It is a common symptom in moderate to severe dementia. In cases of dementia, hoarding is often associated with a higher prevalence of hiding, rummaging, repetitive behavior, pilfering, and hyperphagia. Onset of the behavior usually coincides with onset of the dementia, starting in an organized manner, and becomes more disorganized as the disease progresses. The onset of dementia in a patient who has hoarded throughout their lifetime can aggravate the hoarding behavior.

Hoarding behavior can be associated with schizophrenia. It is mostly associated with severe cases and is seen as a repetitive behavior associated with delusions, self-neglect and squalor. Bipolar disorder is ruled out by the absence of severe mood swings.

COURSE AND PROGNOSIS

The disorder is a chronic condition with a treatment-resistant course. Treatment seeking does not usually occur until patients are in their 40s or 50s even if the hoarding began during adolescence. Symptoms may fluctuate throughout the course of the disorder, but full remission is rare. Patients have very little insight into their behavior and usually seek treatment under pressure from others. Some patients begin hoarding in response to a stressful event, while others report a slow and steady progression throughout life. Those who report onset due to a stressful event have a later age of onset than those who do not. Those with an earlier age of onset run a longer and more chronic course.

TREATMENT

Hoarding disorder is difficult to treat. Although it shows similarities to OCD, effective treatments for OCD have shown little benefit for patients with hoarding disorder. In one study, only 18 percent of patients responded to medication and CBT. The challenges posed by hoarding patients to typical CBT treatment include poor insight to the behavior and low motivation and resistance to treatment.

The most effective treatment for the disorder is a cognitive–behavioral model that includes training in decision-making and categorizing; exposure and habituation to discarding; and cognitive restructuring. This includes both office and in-home sessions. The role of the therapist in this model is to assist in the development of decision-making skills, to provide feedback about normal saving behavior and to identify and challenge the patient's erroneous beliefs about possessions. The goal in treatment is to get rid of a significant amount of possessions, thereby making the living space livable, and to provide the patient with the skills to maintain a positive balance between the amount of possessions and livable space. Studies have shown a 25 to 34 percent reduction in hoarding behaviors using this method. Restructuring of this method for group and web-based interventions are currently under study and show promise.

Pharmacological treatment studies using SSRIs have shown mixed results. Some studies have shown negative response to SSRI treatment in hoarding patients compared to nonhoarders, while others have found no significant difference between the two groups.

▲ 7.4 Hair-Pulling Disorder (Trichotillomania)

Hair-pulling disorder is a chronic disorder characterized by repetitive hair pulling that leads to variable hair loss that may be visible to others. It is also known as trichotillomania, a term coined by a French dermatologist, Francois Hallopeau in 1889. The disorder was once deemed rare and little about it was described beyond phenomenology. It is now regarded as more common. The disorder is similar to OCD and impulse control in that there is increased tension prior to the hair pulling and a relief of tension or gratification after the hair pulling.

EPIDEMIOLOGY

The prevalence of hair-pulling disorder may be underestimated because of accompanying shame and secretiveness. The diagnosis encompasses at least two categories of hair pulling that differ in incidence, severity, age of presentation, and gender ratio. Other subsets may exist.

The most serious, chronic form of the disorder usually begins in early to mid-adolescence, with a lifetime prevalence ranging from 0.6 percent to as high as 3.4 percent in general populations and with female to male ratio as high as 10 to 1. The number of men may actually be higher, because men are even more likely than women to conceal hair pulling. A patient with chronic hair-pulling disorder is likely to be the only or oldest child in the family.

A childhood type of hair-pulling disorder occurs approximately equally in girls and boys. It is said to be more common than the adolescent or young adult syndrome and is generally far less serious dermatologically and psychologically.

An estimated 35 to 40 percent of patients with hair-pulling disorder chew or swallow the hair that they pull out at one time or another. Of this group, approximately one-third develop potentially hazardous bezoars—hairballs accumulating in the alimentary tract.

COMORBIDITY

Significant comorbidity is found between hair-pulling disorder and OCD; anxiety disorders; Tourette's syndrome; depressive disorders; eating disorders; and various personality disorders—particularly obsessive-compulsive, borderline, and narcissistic personality disorders. Comorbid substance abuse disorder is not encountered as frequently as it is in pathological gambling, kleptomania, and other impulse disorders.

ETIOLOGY

Although hair-pulling disorder is regarded as multidetermined, its onset has been linked to stressful situations in more than one-fourth of all cases. Disturbances in mother-child relationships, fear of being left alone, and recent object loss are often cited as critical factors contributing to the condition. Substance abuse may encourage development of the disorder. Depressive dynamics are often cited as predisposing factors, but no particular personality trait or disorder characterizes patients. Some see self-stimulation as the primary goal of hair pulling.

Family members of hair-pulling disorder patients often have a history of tics, impulse-control disorders, and obsessive-compulsive symptoms, further supporting a possible genetic predisposition.

One study looked at the neurobiology of hair-pulling disorder and found smaller volume of the left putamen and left lenticulate areas. More recently, a study of the genetics of trichotillomania reported a relationship between a serotonin 2A (5-HT_{2A}) receptor gene polymorphism (T102C) and trichotillomania. However, because these studies examined relatively few subjects, these findings need to be replicated in a larger sample to be able to determine the role of basal ganglia abnormalities and serotonin in the etiology of trichotillomania.

DIAGNOSIS AND CLINICAL FEATURES

The fifth edition of the *Diagnostic and Statistical Manual of Mental Disorders* (DSM-V) diagnostic criteria from hair-pulling disorder requires that hair pulling result in hair loss. Before engaging in the behavior, patients with hair-pulling disorder may experience an increasing sense of tension and achieve a sense of relief or gratification from pulling out their hair. All areas of the body may be affected, most commonly the scalp. Other areas involved are eyebrows, eyelashes, and beard; trunk, armpits, and pubic area are less commonly involved.

Two types of hair pulling have been described. *Focused pulling* is the use of an intentional act to control unpleasant personal experiences, such as an urge, bodily sensation (e.g., itching or burning), or thought. In contrast, *automatic pulling* occurs outside the person's awareness and most often during sedentary activities. Most patients have a combination of these types of hair pulling.

Hair loss is characterized by short, broken strands appearing together with long, normal hairs in the affected areas. No abnormalities of the skin or scalp are present. Hair pulling is not reported as being painful, although pruritus and tingling may occur in the involved area. Trichophagy, mouthing of the hair, may follow the hair plucking. Complications of trichophagy include trichobezoars, malnutrition, and intestinal obstruction. Patients usually deny the behavior and often try to hide the resultant alopecia. Head banging, nail biting, scratching, gnawing, excoriation, and other acts of self-mutilation may be present.

> Ms. C, a 27-year-old single woman, came to a local clinic complaining of persistent hair pulling. She first started at age 11, when she began to pick the hairs at the nape of her neck. She would persistently pick at the hair until there was almost none left. Fortunately, her hair was long, so no one noticed the lack of hair at the back of her neck. Over the years, her hair picking progressed until she began picking hair from her entire head, leaving noticeable small bald patches. She strategically hid the bald patches by brushing over the remainder of her hair or with carefully placed scarves and hats. Despite her habit, Ms. C was pretty normal. She got good grades in school and was a year away from getting her Master's degree.
>
> Ms. C's habit was constant, occurring every day, often without her noticing it. She could simply be reading an assignment for school and eventually her hand would find its way into her hair to find a hair to pull. Soon she would notice a small pile of hairs in her book or on her lap, indicating that she had been pulling her hair out for a while. Whenever she tried to stop herself from pulling her hair, she would become increasingly nervous and anxious until she resumed the hair pulling. Her hair pulling sessions lasted anywhere from 10 minutes to an hour.

PATHOLOGY AND LABORATORY EXAMINATION

If necessary, the clinical diagnosis of hair-pulling disorder can be confirmed by punch biopsy of the scalp. In patients with a trichobezoar, blood count may reveal a mild leukocytosis and hypochromic anemia due to blood loss. Appropriate chemistries and radiological studies should also be performed, depending on the bezoar's suspected location and impact on the gastrointestinal (GI) tract.

DIFFERENTIAL DIAGNOSIS

Hair pulling may be a wholly benign condition or it may occur in the context of several mental disorders. The phenomenology of hair-pulling disorder and OCD overlap. As with OCD, hair-pulling disorder is often chronic and recognized by patients as undesirable. Unlike those with OCD, patients with hair-pulling disorder do not experience obsessive thoughts, and the compulsive activity is limited to one act, hair pulling. Patients with factitious disorder actively seek medical attention and the patient role and deliberately simulate illness toward these ends. Patients who malinger or who have factitious disorder may mutilate themselves to get medical attention, but they do not acknowledge the self-inflicted nature of the lesions. Patients with stereotypic movement disorder have stereotypical and rhythmic movements, and they usually do not seem distressed by their behavior. A biopsy may be necessary to distinguish hair-pulling disorder from alopecia areata and tinea capitis.

COURSE AND PROGNOSIS

The mean age at onset of hair-pulling disorder is in the early teens, most frequently before age 17, but onset has also been reported much later in life. The course of the disorder is not well-known; both chronic and remitting forms occur. An early onset (before age 6) tends to remit more readily and responds to suggestions, support, and behavioral strategies. Late onset (after age 13) is associated with an increased likelihood of chronicity and poorer prognosis than the early-onset form. About a third of persons presenting for treatment report a duration of 1 year or less, whereas in some cases, the disorder has persisted for more than two decades.

TREATMENT

No consensus exists on the best treatment modality for hair-pulling disorder. Treatment usually involves psychiatrists and dermatologists in a joint endeavor. Psychopharmacological methods that have been used to treat psychodermatological disorder include topical steroids and hydroxyzine hydrochloride (Vistaril), an anxiolytic with antihistamine properties; antidepressants; and antipsychotics. Initial case reports showed efficacy of SSRIs for hair-pulling disorder. Patients who respond poorly to SSRIs may improve with augmentation with pimozide (Orap), a dopamine receptor antagonist. Other medications that have been reported to have some efficacy for hair-pulling disorder include fluvoxamine (Luvox), citalopram (Celexa), venlafaxine (Effexor), naltrexone (ReVia), and lithium. A report of successful lithium treatment cited the possible effect of the drug on aggression, impulsivity, and mood instability as an explanation. In one study, patients taking naltrexone had a reduction in symptom severity. Case reports also indicate successful treatment with buspirone, clonazepam, and trazodone.

Successful behavioral treatments, such as biofeedback, self-monitoring, desensitization, and habit reversal, have been reported, but most studies have been based on individual cases or a small series of cases with relatively short follow-up periods. Chronic hair-pulling disorder has been treated successfully with insight-oriented psychotherapy. Hypnotherapy has been mentioned as potentially effective in the treatment of dermatological disorders in which psychological factors may be involved; the skin having been shown to be susceptible to hypnotic suggestion.

▲ 7.5 Excoriation (Skin-Picking) Disorder

Excoriation or skin-picking disorder is characterized by the compulsive and repetitive picking of the skin. It can lead to severe tissue damage and result in the need for various dermatological treatments. Throughout history, skin-picking disorder has had many names. In the last edition of the *Diagnostic and Statistical Manual of Mental Disorders* (DSM), it was called trichotillomania. It was also known as skin-picking syndrome, emotional excoriation, nervous scratching artifact, and para-artificial excoriation.

EPIDEMIOLOGY

Skin-picking disorder has lifetime prevalence between 1 and 5 percent in the general population, about 12 percent in the adolescent psychiatric population, and occurs in 2 percent of patients with other dermatologic disorders. It is more prevalent in women than in men.

COMORBIDITY

The repetitive nature of skin-picking behavior is similar to the repetitive compulsive rituals found in OCD and skin-picking disorder is associated with high rates of OCD. In addition, patients with OCD may have obsessions about contamination and skin abnormalities or may be preoccupied with having smooth skin, flawless complexion, and cleanliness. Other comorbid conditions include hair-pulling disorder (trichotillomania, 38 percent), substance dependence (38 percent), major depressive disorder (32 to 58 percent), anxiety disorders (23 to 56 percent), and body dysmorphic disorder (27 to 45 percent). One study reported an association of both borderline and obsessive-compulsive personality disorder (71 percent) in patients with skin-picking disorder.

ETIOLOGY

The cause of skin picking is unknown, however several theories have been postulated. Some theorists speculate that skin-picking behavior is a manifestation of repressed rage at authoritarian parents. These patients pick at their skin and perform other self-destructive acts to assert themselves. Patients may pick as a means to relieve stress. For example, skin picking has been associated with marital conflicts, passing of loved ones, and unwanted pregnancies. According to psychoanalytic theory, the skin is an erotic organ and picking at the skin or scratching the skin leading to excoriations may be a source of erotic pleasure. In that sense it has been considered a masturbatory equivalent. Patients may be unaware of these affects presumed to be in the unconscious. Many patients begin picking at the onset of dermatological conditions such as acne and continue to pick after the condition has cleared.

Abnormalities in serotonin, dopamine, and glutamate metabolism have been theorized to be an underlying neurochemical cause of the disorder, but further research is needed.

DIAGNOSIS

The fifth edition of the *Diagnostic and Statistical Manual of Mental Disorders* (DSM-5) diagnostic criteria for skin-picking disorder requires recurrent skin picking resulting in skin lesions and repeated attempts to decrease or stop picking. The skin picking must cause clinically relevant distress or impairment in functioning. The skin-picking behavior cannot be attributed to another medical or mental condition and cannot be a result of a substance use disorder (e.g., cocaine or methamphetamine use).

CLINICAL FEATURES

The face is the most common site of skin picking. Other common sites are legs, arms, torso, hands, cuticles, fingers, and scalp. While most patients report having a primary picking area, many times they pick other areas of the body in order for the primary area to heal. In severe cases, skin picking can result in physical disfigurement and medical consequences that require medical or surgical interventions (e.g., skin grafts or radiosurgery).

Patients may experience tension prior to picking and a relief and gratification after picking. Many report picking as a means to relieve stress, tension, and other negative feelings. In spite of the relief felt from picking, patients often feel guilty or embarrassed at their behavior. Up to 87 percent of patients report feeling embarrassed by the picking and 58 percent report avoiding social situations. Many patients use bandages, makeup, or clothing to hide their picking. Of skin picking patients, 15 percent report suicidal ideation due to their behavior and about 12 percent have attempted suicide.

Ms. J, a 22-year-old single woman, presented to a psychiatrist at the urging of her dermatologist because of compulsive picking at the skin on her face. She picked at it every day up to 3 times a day in sessions lasting from 20 minutes to over an hour. She had massive scarring and lesions on her face. She went to a physician 6 months prior when one of the lesions had become infected.

Ms. J began picking her face at age 11 at the onset of puberty. At first, she only picked at acne that formed on her face, but as the urge to pick became greater, she started picking at clear patches of skin as well. Due to the scaring and lesions, Ms. J became increasingly withdrawn and avoided all social engagements. She reported feeling great tension prior to picking and only after she began picking did she feel relief.

DIFFERENTIAL DIAGNOSIS

The diagnosis of skin-picking disorder cannot be made if the behavior can be better accounted for by another medical or psychological condition. Many medical and dermatological conditions may result in urges to itch and pick at the skin. Conditions include eczema, psoriasis, diabetes, liver or kidney disease, Hodgkin's disease, polycythemia vera, or systemic lupus. Skin picking can also be seen in Prader–Willi syndrome (97 percent). A thorough physical examination is crucial prior to psychiatric diagnosis.

Skin-picking disorder is similar to OCD and it is associated with high rates of comorbid OCD. The disorders differ in a few ways. Skin-picking disorder is prevalent in females while OCD is equal between genders. The compulsions associated with OCD are usually driven by intrusive thoughts while the compulsion to pick the skin is usually not. Although skin picking generally decreases anxiety, it can also entice pleasure in the patient, which is rarely the case in OCD. Skin picking in OCD patients is usually the result of obsessions about contamination or skin abnormalities.

Skin picking is commonly seen in body dysmorphic disorder. In one study, 45 percent of body dysmorphic patients report lifetime skin-picking disorder and 37 percent report having skin-picking disorder secondary to body dysmorphic disorder. The skin picking in body dysmorphic disorder is primarily centered on removing or minimizing believed imperfection in the patient's appearance.

Substance use disorders often co-occur with skin-picking disorder. Methamphetamine and cocaine use may result in the sensation something crawling on the body or under skin (formication) which can result in skin picking. In order to make the diagnosis of skin-picking disorder, however, skin picking cannot be a physiological effect of substance use.

Factitious Dermatitis

Factitious dermatitis or *dermatitis artefacta* is a disorder in which skin picking is the target of self-inflicted injury and the patient uses more elaborate methods than simple excoriation to self-induce skin lesions. It is seen in 0.3 percent of dermatology patients and has a female to male ratio of 8:1. It can present at any age, but occurs most frequently in adolescents and young adults. It can present as an aggravation of dermatosis, targeting a variety of skin lesions including blisters, ulcers, erythema, edema, purpura, and sinuses. The morphology of factitious dermatitis lesions is often bizarre and linear, with clear-cut, angulated, or geometric edges. Presence of completely normal, unaffected skin adjacent to the horrific looking lesions is a clue to the diagnosis of factitious dermatitis. In addition, the patient's description of history of the skin lesions is usually vague and lacks detail about the appearance and evolution of the lesions.

COURSE AND PROGNOSIS

The onset of skin-picking disorder is either in early adulthood or between 30 and 45 years of age. Onset in children before the age of 10 years has also been seen. The mean age of onset is between 12 and 16 years of age. There may be a lag of time between onset and actual diagnosis. Since little is known about the disorder, many are unaware that it can be treated. Many times patients do not seek treatment until a severe dermatological or medical condition has developed.

Typically, symptoms wax and wane over the course of the patient's life. Approximately 44 percent of women report that amount of picking coincides with their menstrual cycle.

TREATMENT

Skin-picking disorder is difficult to treat and there is little data on effective treatments. Most patients do not actively seek treatment due to embarrassment or because they believe their condition is untreatable. There is support for the use of SSRIs. Studies comparing fluoxetine (Prozac) against placebo has shown to fluoxetine to be superior in reducing skin picking. The opioid antagonist naltrexone has proven to reduce the urge to pick, particularly in patients who experience pleasure from the behavior. Glutamanergic agents and lamotrigine (Lamictal) have also shown efficacy. Nonpharmacological treatments include habit reversal and brief CBT.

Effective therapy requires both psychological and somatic treatment. In some cases mechanical prevention of skin picking by different protective measures may be of use in an effort to break the cycle. Psychotherapy at the same time deals with the underlying emotional factors.

8 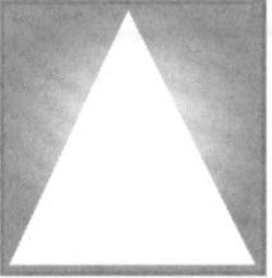

Trauma- and Stressor-Related Disorder

▲ 8.1 Posttraumatic Stress Disorder and Acute Stress Disorder

Both posttraumatic stress disorder (PTSD) and acute stress disorder are marked by increased stress and anxiety following exposure to a traumatic or stressful event. Traumatic or stressful events may include being a witness to or being involved in a violent accident or crime, military combat, or assault, being kidnapped, being involved in a natural disaster, being diagnosed with a life-threatening illness, or experiencing systematic physical or sexual abuse. The person reacts to the experience with fear and helplessness, persistently relives the event, and tries to avoid being reminded of it. The event may be relived in dreams and waking thoughts (flashbacks).

The stressors causing both acute stress disorder and PTSD are sufficiently overwhelming to affect almost everyone. They can arise from experiences in war, torture (discussed in detail below), natural catastrophes, assault, rape, and serious accidents, for example, in cars and in burning buildings. Persons re-experience the traumatic event in their dreams and their daily thoughts; they are determined to avoid anything that brings the event to mind and they undergo a numbing of responsiveness along with a state of hyperarousal. Other symptoms are depression, anxiety, and cognitive difficulties such as poor concentration.

A link between acute mental syndromes and traumatic events has been recognized for more than 200 years. Observations of trauma-related syndromes were documented following the Civil War, and early psychoanalytic writers, including Sigmund Freud, noted a relation between neurosis and trauma. Considerable interest in posttraumatic mental disorders was stimulated by observations of "battle fatigue," "shell shock," and "soldier's heart" in both World Wars I and II. Moreover, increasing documentation of mental reactions to the Holocaust, to a series of natural disasters, and to assault contributed to the growing recognition of a close relation between trauma and psychopathology.

EPIDEMIOLOGY

The lifetime incidence of PTSD is estimated to be 9 to 15 percent and the lifetime prevalence of PTSD is estimated to be about 8 percent of the general population, although an additional 5 to 15 percent may experience subclinical forms of the disorder. The lifetime prevalence rate is 10 percent in women and 4 percent in men. According to the National Vietnam Veterans Readjustment Study (NVVRS), 30 percent of men develop full-blown PTSD after having served in the war and an additional 22.5 percent develop partial PTSD, falling just short of qualifying for the disorder. Among veterans of the Iraq and Afghanistan wars, 13 percent received the diagnosis of PTSD.

Although PTSD can appear at any age, it is most prevalent in young adults, because they tend to be more exposed to precipitating situations. Children can also have the disorder. Men and women differ in the types of traumas to which they are exposed. Historically, men's trauma was usually combat experience, and women's trauma was most commonly assault or rape. The disorder is most likely to occur in those who are single, divorced, widowed, socially withdrawn, or of low socioeconomic level, but anyone can be effected, no one is immune. The most important risk factors, however, for this disorder are the severity, duration, and proximity of a person's exposure to the actual trauma. A familial pattern seems to exist for this disorder, and first-degree biological relatives of persons with a history of depression have an increased risk for developing PTSD following a traumatic event.

COMORBIDITY

Comorbidity rates are high among patients with PTSD, with about two-thirds having at least two other disorders. Common comorbid conditions include depressive disorders, substance-related disorders, anxiety disorders, and bipolar disorders. Comorbid disorders make persons more vulnerable to develop PTSD.

ETIOLOGY

Stressor

By definition, a stressor is the prime causative factor in the development of PTSD. Not everyone experiences the disorder after a traumatic event, however. The stressor alone does not suffice to cause the disorder. Clinicians must also consider individual's preexisting biological and psychosocial factors and events that happened before and after the trauma. For example, a member of a group who lived through a disaster can sometimes better deal with trauma because others have also shared the experience. The stressor's subjective meaning to a person is also important. For example, survivors of a catastrophe may experience guilt feelings (survivor guilt) that can predispose to, or exacerbate, PTSD.

Three weeks after a train derailment, a 42-year-old budget analyst presented to the mental health clinic. He noted that he was embarrassed to seek care, as he was previously a firefighter, but he felt he needed "some reassurance that what I'm experiencing is normal." He reported that, since the wreck, he had been feeling nervous and on edge. He experienced some difficulty focusing his attention at work, and he had occasional intrusive recollections of "the way the ground just shook; the tremendous 'bang' and then the screaming when the train rolled over." He noted that he had spoken with five business colleagues who were also on the train, and three acknowledged similar symptoms. However, they said that they were improving. He was more concerned about the frequency of tearful episodes, sometimes brought on by hearing the name of a severely injured friend, but, at other times, occurring "for no particular reason." In addition, he noted that, when he evacuated the train, rescue workers gave him explicit directions about where to report, and, although he complied, he now felt extremely guilty about not returning to the train to assist in the rescue of others. He reported a modest decrease in appetite and denied weight loss but noted that he had stopped jogging during his lunch break. He had difficulty initiating sleep, so he had begun consuming a "glass or two" of wine before bed to help with this. He did not feel rested on awakening. He denied suicidal ideation or any psychotic symptoms. His sister had taken an antidepressant several years ago, but he did not desire medication. He feared that side effects could further diminish his ability to function at the workplace and could cause him to gain weight. *(Courtesy of D. M. Benedek, M.D., R. J. Ursano, M.D., and H. C. Holloway, M.D.)*

Risk Factors

Even when faced with overwhelming trauma, most persons do not experience PTSD symptoms. The National Comorbidity Study found that 60 percent of males and 50 percent of females had experienced some significant trauma, whereas the reported lifetime prevalence of PTSD, as mentioned earlier, was only about 8 percent. Similarly, events that may appear mundane or less than catastrophic to most persons can produce PTSD in some. Evidence indicates of a dose–response relationship between the degree of trauma and the likelihood of symptoms. Table 8.1–1 summarizes vulnerability factors that appear to play etiological roles in the disorder.

Psychodynamic Factors

The psychoanalytic model of the PTSD hypothesizes that the trauma has reactivated a previously quiescent, yet unresolved psychological conflict. The revival of the childhood trauma results in regression and the use of the defense mechanisms of repression, denial, reaction formation, and undoing. According to Freud, a splitting of consciousness occurs in patients who reported a history of childhood sexual trauma. A preexisting conflict might be symbolically reawakened by the new traumatic event. The ego relives and thereby tries to master and reduce the anxiety. Psychodynamic themes in PTSD are summarized in Table 8.1–2. Persons who suffer from alexithymia, the inability to identify or verbalize feeling states, are incapable of soothing themselves when under stress.

Table 8.1–1
Predisposing Vulnerability Factors in Posttraumatic Stress Disorder

- Presence of childhood trauma
- Borderline, paranoid, dependent, or antisocial personality disorder traits
- Inadequate family or peer support system
- Being female
- Genetic vulnerability to psychiatric illness
- Recent stressful life changes
- Perception of an external locus of control (natural cause) rather than an internal one (human cause)
- Recent excessive alcohol intake

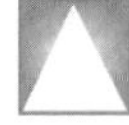

Table 8.1–2
Psychodynamic Themes in Posttraumatic Stress Disorder

- ▲ The subjective meaning of a stressor may determine its traumatogenicity.
- ▲ Traumatic events can resonate with childhood traumas.
- ▲ Somatization and alexithymia may be among the after effects of trauma.
- ▲ Common defenses used include denial, minimization, splitting, projective disavowal, dissociation, and guilt (as a defense against underlying helplessness).
- ▲ Mode of object relatedness involves projection and introjection of the following roles: omnipotent rescuer, abuser, and victim.

Cognitive–Behavioral Factors

The cognitive model of PTSD posits that affected persons cannot process or rationalize the trauma that precipitated the disorder. They continue to experience the stress and attempt to avoid experiencing it by avoidance techniques. Consistent with their partial ability to cope cognitively with the event, persons experience alternating periods of acknowledging and blocking the event. The attempt of the brain to process the massive amount of information provoked by the trauma is thought to produce these alternating periods. The behavioral model of PTSD emphasizes two phases in its development. First, the trauma (the unconditioned stimulus) that produces a fear response is paired, through classic conditioning, with a conditioned stimulus (physical or mental reminders of the trauma, such as sights, smells, or sounds). Second, through instrumental learning, the conditioned stimuli elicit the fear response independent of the original unconditioned stimulus, and persons develop a pattern of avoiding both the conditioned stimulus and the unconditioned stimulus. Some persons also receive secondary gains from the external world, commonly monetary compensation, increased attention or sympathy, and the satisfaction of dependency needs. These gains reinforce the disorder and its persistence.

Biological Factors

The biological theories of PTSD have developed both from preclinical studies of animal models of stress and from measures of biological variables in clinical populations with the disorder. Many neurotransmitter systems have been implicated by both sets of data. Preclinical models of learned helplessness, kindling, and sensitization in animals have led to theories about norepinephrine, dopamine, endogenous opioids, and benzodiazepine receptors and the hypothalamic–pituitary–adrenal (HPA) axis. In clinical populations, data have supported hypotheses that the noradrenergic and endogenous opiate systems, as well as the HPA axis, are hyperactive in at least some patients with PTSD. Other major biological findings are increased activity and responsiveness of the autonomic nervous system, as evidenced by elevated heart rates and blood pressure readings and by abnormal sleep architecture (e.g., sleep fragmentation and increased sleep latency). Some researchers have suggested a similarity between PTSD and two other psychiatric disorders: major depressive disorder and panic disorder.

Noradrenergic System. Soldiers with PTSD-like symptoms exhibit nervousness, increased blood pressure and heart rate, palpitations, sweating, flushing, and tremors—symptoms associated with adrenergic drugs. Studies found increased 24-hour urine epinephrine concentrations in veterans with PTSD and increased urine catecholamine concentrations in sexually abused girls. Further, platelet α_2- and lymphocyte β-adrenergic receptors are downregulated in PTSD, possibly in response to chronically elevated catecholamine concentrations. About 30 to 40 percent of patients with PTSD report flashbacks after yohimbine administration. Such findings are strong evidence for altered function in the noradrenergic system in PTSD.

Opioid System. Abnormality in the opioid system is suggested by low plasma β-endorphin concentrations in PTSD. Combat veterans with PTSD demonstrate a naloxone (Narcan)-reversible analgesic response to combat-related stimuli, raising the possibility of opioid system hyperregulation similar to that in the HPA axis. One study showed that nalmefene (Revex), an opioid receptor antagonist, was of use in reducing symptoms of PTSD in combat veterans.

Corticotropin-Releasing Factor and the HPA Axis. Several factors point to dysfunction of the HPA axis. Studies have demonstrated low plasma and urinary free cortisol concentrations in PTSD. More glucocorticoid receptors are found on lymphocytes, and challenge with exogenous corticotropin-releasing factor (CRF) yields a blunted corticotropin (ACTH) response. Further, suppression of cortisol by challenge with low-dose dexamethasone (Decadron) is enhanced in PTSD. This indicates hyperregulation of the HPA axis in PTSD. Also, some studies have revealed cortisol hypersuppression in trauma-exposed patients who develop PTSD, compared with patients exposed to trauma who do not develop PTSD, indicating that it might be specifically associated with PTSD and not just trauma. Overall, this hyperregulation of the HPA axis differs from the neuroendocrine activity usually seen during stress and in other disorders such as depression. Recently, the role of the hippocampus in PTSD has received increased attention, although the issue remains controversial. Animal studies have shown that stress is associated with structural changes in the hippocampus, and studies of combat veterans with PTSD have revealed a lower average volume in the hippocampal region of the brain. Structural changes in the amygdala, an area of the brain associated with fear, have also been demonstrated.

DIAGNOSIS

The fifth edition of the *Diagnostic and Statistical Manual of Mental Disorders* (DSM-5) criteria for PTSD includes symptoms of intrusion, avoidance, alternations of mood, cognitive difficulties and hyperarousal (see Clinical Features below). In addition, symptoms must be present for at least 1 month. The DSM-5 diagnosis of PTSD allows the physician to specify if the symptoms occur in preschool-aged children or with dissociative (depersonalization/derealization) symptoms. For patients whose symptoms have been present less than 1 month, the appropriate diagnosis may be acute stress disorder.

> Mrs. M sought treatment for symptoms that she developed in the wake of an assault that had occurred about 6 weeks prior to her psychiatric evaluation. While leaving work late one evening, Mrs. M was attacked in a parking lot next to the hospital in which she worked. She was raped and badly beaten but was able to escape and call for help. On referral, Mrs. M reported frequent intrusive thoughts about the assault, including nightmares about the event and recurrent intrusive visions of her assailant. She reported that she now took the bus to work to avoid the scene of the attack and that she had to change her work hours so that she did not have to leave the building after dark. In addition, she reported that she had difficulty interacting with men, particularly those who resembled her attacker, and that she consequently avoided such interactions whenever possible. Mrs. M described increased irritability, difficulty staying asleep at night, poor concentration, and an increased focus on her environment, particularly after dark. *(Courtesy of Erin B. McClure-Tone, Ph.D. and Daniel S. Pine, M.D.)*

CLINICAL FEATURES

Individuals with PTSD show symptoms in three domains: intrusion symptoms following the trauma, avoiding stimuli associated with the trauma, and experiencing symptoms of increased automatic arousal, such as an enhanced startle. Flashbacks, in which the individual may act and feel as if the trauma were reoccurring, represent a classic intrusion symptom. Other intrusion symptoms include distressing recollections or dreams and either physiological or psychological stress reactions to exposure to stimuli that are linked to the trauma. An individual must exhibit at least one intrusion symptom to meet the criteria for PTSD. Symptoms of avoidance associated with PTSD include efforts to avoid thoughts or activities related to the trauma, anhedonia, reduced capacity to remember events related to the trauma, blunted affect, feelings of detachment or derealization, and a sense of a foreshortened future. Symptoms of increased arousal include insomnia, irritability, hypervigilance, and exaggerated startle (see Table 8.1–3).

> A 40-year-old man watched the September 11, 2001, terrorist attack on the World Trade Center on television. Immediately thereafter he developed feelings of panic associated with thoughts that he was going to die. The panic disappeared within a few hours; however, for the next few nights he had nightmares with obsessive thoughts about dying. He sought consultation and reported to the psychiatrist that his wife had been killed in a plane crash 20 years earlier. He described having adapted to the loss "normally" and

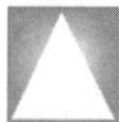

Table 8.1–3
Common Signs and Symptoms of PTSD

Intrusive memories of the event (flash backs)
Frightening dreams
Fear and avoidance of cues that relate to the event
Acute episodes of anxiety, fear, panic, or aggression triggered by cues
Insomnia
Startle reactions
Insomnia
Tendency toward substance abuse (e.g., alcohol)
Detachment from others
Emotional blunting
Anhedonia
Sudden recollection or reliving of traumatic event

was aware that his current symptoms were probably related to that traumatic event. On further exploration in brief psychotherapy, he realized that his reactions to his wife's death were muted and that his relationship with her was ambivalent. At the time of her death, he was contemplating divorce and frequently had wished her dead. He had never fully worked through the mourning process for his wife, and his catastrophic reaction to the terrorist attack was related, in part, to those suppressed feelings. He was able to recognize his feelings of guilt related to his wife and his need for punishment manifested by thinking he was going to die.

Gulf War Syndrome

In the Persian Gulf War against Iraq, which began in 1990 and ended in 1991, approximately 700,000 American soldiers served in the coalition forces. Upon their return, more than 100,000 US veterans reported a vast array of health problems, including irritability, chronic fatigue, shortness of breath, muscle and joint pain, migraine headaches, digestive disturbances, rash, hair loss, forgetfulness, and difficulty concentrating. Collectively, these symptoms were called the *Gulf War syndrome.* The US Department of Defense acknowledged that up to 20,000 troops serving in the combat area may have been exposed to chemical weapons, and the condition is a disorder that in some cases may have been precipitated by exposure to an unidentified toxin (Table 8.1–4). One study of loss of memory found structural change in the right parietal lobe and damage to the basal ganglia with associated neurotransmitter dysfunction. A significant number of veterans have developed amyotrophic lateral sclerosis (ALS), thought to be the result of genetic mutations.

In a 1997 editorial in the *Journal of the American Medical Association,* the relationship of the Persian Gulf War syndrome and stress was stated as follows:

Physicians need to acknowledge that many Gulf War veterans are experiencing stress-related disorders and the physical consequences of stress. These conditions should not be hidden or denied, but rather are well-recognized entities that have been studied extensively in survivors of past wars, most notably the Vietnam conflict. As physicians, we should not accept a diagnosis of stress-related disorder in veterans prior to excluding treatable physical factors, but at the same time, we need to recognize the pervasive presence of stress-related illness such as hypertension, fibromyalgia, and chronic fatigue among Persian Gulf War veterans and manage these illnesses appropriately. As a nation, we need to get beyond the fallacious idea that diseases of the mind either are not real or are shameful and to better recognize that the mind and the body are inextricably linked.

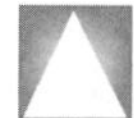

Table 8.1–4
Syndromes Associated with Toxic Exposure[a]

Syndrome	Characteristics	Possible Toxins
1	Impaired cognition	Insect repellant containing N,N′-diethyl-m-toluamide (DEET[b]) absorbed through skin
2	Confusion-ataxia	Exposure to chemical weapons (e.g., sarin)
3	Arthromyoneuropathy	Insect repellant containing DEET in combination with oral pyridostigmine[c]

[a]The three syndromes involved a relatively small group ($N = 249$) of veterans and are based on self-reported descriptions and selection. (Data are from R. W. Haley and T. L. Kurt.)
[b]DEET is a carbonate compound used as an insect repellant. Concentrations above 30% DEET are neurotoxic in children. The military repellant contains 75%. (DEET is available in 100% concentrations as an unregulated over-the-counter preparation usually sold in sport stores.)
[c]Most US troops took low-dose pyridostigmine (Mestinon, 30 mg every 8 hours) for about 5 days in 1991 to protect against exposure to the nerve agent soman.

In addition, thousands of Gulf War veterans developed PTSD and the differentiation between the two disorders has proved difficult. PTSD is caused by psychological stress, and Gulf War syndrome is presumed to be caused by environmental biological stressors. Signs and symptoms often overlap and both conditions may exist at the same time.

9/11/01

On September 11, 2001, terrorist activity destroyed the World Trade Center in New York City and damaged the Pentagon in Washington. It resulted in more than 3,500 deaths and injuries and left many citizens in need of therapeutic intervention. One survey found a prevalence rate of 11.4 percent for PTSD and 9.7 percent for depression in US citizens 1 month after 9/11. It is estimated that more than 25,000 people suffer symptoms of PTSD related to the 9/11 attacks beyond the 1-year mark.

Iraq and Afghanistan

In October 2001, the United States, along with Australia, Canada, and the United Kingdom, invaded Afghanistan in the wake of the September 11, 2001, attacks. On March 20, 2003, US forces, along with their allies, invaded Iraq, marking the beginning of the Iraq War, which officially ended on December 15, 2011.

Both wars caused an estimated 17 percent of returning soldiers to develop PTSD. The rate of PTSD is higher in women soldiers. Women account for 11 percent of those who served in Iraq and Afghanistan and for 14 percent of patients at Veterans Administration (VA) hospitals and clinics. Women soldiers are more likely to seek help than men soldiers. The rate of suicide for active duty personnel in both of these wars have assumed epidemic proportions, with the likelihood of suicide being double that of the general population.

Traumatic brain injury (TBI), the result of direct or indirect trauma to the brain, causes changes in either the gross or microscopic structure of the brain with associated signs and symptoms depending on the location of the lesion. In most cases of TBI there will be signs and symptoms of PTSD as well, complicating the picture. According to the Department of Veterans Affairs, 19 percent of veterans may have TBI.

Natural Disasters

Tsunami. On December 26, 2004, a massive tsunami struck the shores of Indonesia, Sri Lanka, South India, and Thailand and caused serious damage and deaths as far west as the coast of Africa and South Africa. The tsunami caused nearly 300,000 deaths and left more than 1 million people without homes. Many survivors continue to live in fear and show signs of PTSD; fishermen fear venturing out to sea, children fear playing at beaches they once enjoyed, and many families have trouble sleeping for fear of another tsunami.

Hurricane. In August 2005, a category 5 hurricane, Hurricane Katrina, ravaged the Gulf of Mexico, the Bahamas, South Florida, Louisiana, Mississippi, and Alabama. Its high winds and torrential rainfall breached the levee system that protected New Orleans, Louisiana, causing major flooding. More than 1,300 people were killed and tens of thousands were left stranded. In October 2012, Hurricane Sandy landed on the eastern coast of the United States and in the New York–New Jersey metropolitan area caused almost 150 deaths with an estimated 650,000 homes damaged or destroyed. Over 50,000 persons were believed to have developed full blown PTSD as a result.

Earthquake. On January 12, 2010, a 7.0 magnitude earthquake hit Port-au-Prince, the capital of the Republic of Haiti, which had a population of approximately 3 million people. Approximately 316,000 people died, 300,000 were injured, and 1 million were made homeless. The government of Haiti also estimated that 250,000 residences and 30,000 commercial buildings had collapsed or were severely damaged, leaving 10 million cubic meters of rubble.

On March 11, 2011, a 9.0 magnitude earthquake hit northeastern Japan, causing a 10-m tsunami that reached as far as the western coast of the United States, making it the fifth largest earthquake since 1900. Approximately 15,700 people were killed, 4,700 were missing, and 5,700 were injured. It also brought Japan into its second recession in 3 years and triggered the world's biggest nuclear disaster since Chernobyl in 1986.

PTSD developed among those who experienced these disasters, the full extent of which remains to be determined. Some estimates range from 50 to 75 percent of survivors experienced some or all of the signs and symptoms of PTSD.

Torture

The intentional physical and psychological torture of one human by another can have emotionally damaging effects comparable to, and possibly worse than, those seen with combat and other types of trauma. As defined by the United Nations, torture is any deliberate infliction of severe mental pain or suffering, usually through cruel, inhuman, or degrading treatment or punishment. This broad definition includes various forms of interpersonal violence, from chronic domestic abuse to broad-scale genocide. According to Amnesty International, torture is common and widespread in most of the 150 countries worldwide where human rights violations have been documented. Recent figures estimate that between 5 and 35 percent of the world's 14 million refugees have had at least one torture experience, and these numbers do not even account for the consequences of the current political, regional, and religious disputes in various parts of the world where torture is still practiced.

DIFFERENTIAL DIAGNOSIS

Because patients often exhibit complex reactions to trauma, the clinician must be careful to exclude other syndromes as well when evaluating patients presenting in the wake of trauma. It is particularly important to recognize potentially treatable medical contributors to posttraumatic symptomatology, especially head injury during the trauma. Medical contributors can usually be detected through a careful history and physical examination. Other organic considerations that can both cause and exacerbate the symptoms are epilepsy, alcohol-use disorders, and other substance-related disorders. Acute intoxication or withdrawal from some substances may also present a clinical picture that is difficult to distinguish from the disorder until the effects of the substance have worn off.

Symptoms of PTSD can be difficult to distinguish from both panic disorder and generalized anxiety disorder, because all three syndromes are associated with prominent anxiety and autonomic arousal. Keys to correctly diagnosing PTSD involve a careful review of the time course relating the symptoms to a traumatic event. PTSD is also associated with reexperiencing and avoidance of a trauma, features typically not present in panic or generalized anxiety disorder. Major depression is also a frequent concomitant of PTSD. Although the two syndromes are not usually difficult to distinguish phenomenologically, it is important to note the presence of comorbid depression, because this can influence treatment of PTSD. PTSD must be differentiated from a series of related disorders that can exhibit phenomenological similarities, including borderline personality disorder, dissociative disorders, and factitious disorders. Borderline personality disorder can be difficult to distinguish from PTSD. The two disorders can coexist or even be causally related. Patients with dissociative disorders do not usually have the degree of avoidance behavior, the autonomic hyperarousal, or the history of trauma that patients with PTSD report.

COURSE AND PROGNOSIS

PTSD usually develops sometime after the trauma. The delay can be as short as 1 week or as long as 30 years. Symptoms can fluctuate over time and may be most intense during periods of stress. Untreated, about 30 percent of patients recover completely, 40 percent continue to have mild symptoms, 20 percent continue to have moderate symptoms, and 10 percent remain unchanged or become worse. After 1 year, about 50 percent of patients will recover. A good prognosis is predicted by rapid onset of the symptoms, short duration of the symptoms (less than 6 months), good premorbid functioning, strong social supports, and the absence of other psychiatric, medical, or substance-related disorders or other risk factors.

In general, the very young and the very old have more difficulty with traumatic events than do those in midlife. For example, about 80 percent of young children who sustain a burn injury show symptoms of PTSD 1 or 2 years after the initial injury; only 30 percent of adults who suffer such an injury have symptoms of PTSD after 1 year. Presumably, young children do not yet have adequate coping mechanisms to deal with the physical and emotional insults of the trauma. Likewise, older persons are likely to have more rigid coping mechanisms than younger adults and to be less able to muster a flexible approach to dealing with the effects of trauma. Furthermore, the traumatic effects can be exacerbated by physical disabilities characteristic of late life, particularly disabilities of the nervous system and the cardiovascular system, such as reduced cerebral blood flow, failing vision, palpitations, and arrhythmias. Preexisting psychiatric disability, whether a personality disorder or a more serious condition, also increases the effects of particular stressors. PTSD that is comorbid with other disorders is often more severe and perhaps more chronic and may be difficult to treat. The availability of social supports may also influence the development, severity, and duration of PTSD. In general, patients who have a good network of social support are less likely to have the disorder and to experience it in its severe forms and are more likely to recover faster.

TREATMENT

When a clinician is faced with a patient who has experienced a significant trauma, the major approaches are support, encouragement to discuss the event, and education about a variety of coping mechanisms (e.g., relaxation). In encouraging persons to talk about the event it is imperative that the clinician allow the person to proceed at his or her own pace. Some patients will not be willing to talk until well after the event has passed, and those wishes should be respected. To press a person who is reluctant to talk about a trauma into doing so is likely to increase rather than decrease the risk of developing PTSD. The use of sedatives and hypnotics can also be helpful in some cases. When a patient has experienced a traumatic event in the past and has now developed PTSD, the emphasis should be on education about the disorder and its treatment, both pharmacological and psychotherapeutic. The clinician should also work to destigmatize the notion of mental illness and PTSD. Additional support for the patient and the family can be obtained through local and national support groups for patients with PTSD.

Pharmacotherapy

Selective serotonin reuptake inhibitors (SSRIs), such as sertraline (Zoloft) and paroxetine (Paxil), are considered first-line treatments for PTSD, owing to their efficacy, tolerability, and safety ratings. SSRIs reduce symptoms from all PTSD symptom clusters and are effective in improving symptoms unique to PTSD, not just symptoms similar to those of depression or other anxiety disorders. Buspirone (BuSpar) is serotonergic and may also be of use.

The efficacy of imipramine (Tofranil) and amitriptyline (Elavil), two tricyclic drugs, in the treatment of PTSD is supported by a number of well-controlled clinical trials. Although some trials of the two drugs have had negative findings, most of these trials had serious design flaws, including too short a duration. Dosages of imipramine and amitriptyline should be the same as those used to treat depressive disorders, and an adequate trial should last at least 8 weeks. Patients who respond well should probably continue the pharmacotherapy for at least 1 year before an attempt is made to withdraw the drug. Some studies indicate that pharmacotherapy is more effective in treating the depression, anxiety, and hyperarousal than in treating the avoidance, denial, and emotional numbing.

Other drugs that may be useful in the treatment of PTSD include the monoamine oxidase inhibitors (MAOIs) (e.g., phenelzine [Nardil]), trazodone (Desyrel), and the anticonvulsants (e.g., carbamazepine [Tegretol], valproate [Depakene]). Some studies have also revealed improvement in PTSD in patients treated with reversible monoamine oxidase inhibitors (RIMAs). Use of clonidine (Catapres) and propranolol (Inderal), which are antiadrenergic agents, is suggested by the theories about noradrenergic hyperactivity in the disorder. There are almost no positive data concerning the use of antipsychotic drugs in the disorder, so the use of drugs such as haloperidol (Haldol) should be reserved for the short-term control of severe aggression and agitation. Research is ongoing about the use of opioid receptor agonists during traumatic events as a preventative against developing PTSD.

Psychotherapy

Psychodynamic psychotherapy may be useful in the treatment of many patients with PTSD. In some cases, reconstruction of the traumatic events with associated abreaction and catharsis may be therapeutic, but psychotherapy must be individualized because re-experiencing the trauma overwhelms some patients.

Psychotherapeutic interventions for PTSD include behavior therapy, cognitive therapy, and hypnosis. Many clinicians advocate time-limited psychotherapy for the victims of trauma. Such therapy usually takes a cognitive approach and also provides support and security. The short-term nature of psychotherapy minimizes the risk of dependence and chronicity, but issues of suspicion, paranoia, and trust often adversely affect compliance. Therapists should overcome patients' denial of the traumatic event, encourage them to relax, and remove them from the source of the stress. Patients should be encouraged to sleep, using medication if necessary. Support from persons in their environment (e.g., friends and relatives) should be provided. Patients should be encouraged to review and abreact emotional feelings associated with the traumatic event and to plan for future recovery. Abreaction—experiencing the emotions associated with the event—may be helpful for some patients. The amobarbital (Amytal) interview has been used to facilitate this process.

Psychotherapy after a traumatic event should follow a model of crisis intervention with support, education, and the development of coping mechanisms and acceptance of the event. When

PTSD has developed, two major psychotherapeutic approaches can be taken. The first is exposure therapy, in which the patient re-experiences the traumatic event through imaging techniques or in vivo exposure. The exposures can be intense, as in implosive therapy, or graded, as in systematic desensitization. The second approach is to teach the patient methods of stress management, including relaxation techniques and cognitive approaches, to coping with stress. Some preliminary data indicate that, although stress management techniques are effective more rapidly than exposure techniques, the results of exposure techniques last longer.

Another psychotherapeutic technique that is relatively novel and somewhat controversial is eye movement desensitization and reprocessing (EMDR), in which the patient focuses on the lateral movement of the clinician's finger while maintaining a mental image of the trauma experience. The general belief is that symptoms can be relieved as patients work through the traumatic event while in a state of deep relaxation. Proponents of this treatment state it is as effective, and possibly more effective, than other treatments for PTSD and that it is preferred by both clinicians and patients who have tried it.

In addition to individual therapy techniques, group therapy and family therapy have been reported to be effective in cases of PTSD. The advantages of group therapy include sharing of traumatic experiences and support from other group members. Group therapy has been particularly successful with Vietnam veterans and survivors of catastrophic disasters such as earthquakes. Family therapy often helps sustain a marriage through periods of exacerbated symptoms. Hospitalization may be necessary when symptoms are particularly severe or when a risk of suicide or other violence exists.

TRAUMA- OR STRESSOR-RELATED DISORDER UNSPECIFIED

In DSM-5, the category of "unspecified trauma- or stressor-related disorder" is used for patients who develop emotional or behavioral symptoms in response to an identifiable stressor but do not meet the full criteria of any other specified trauma- or stressor-related disorder (e.g., acute stress disorder, PTSD, or adjustment disorder). The symptoms cannot meet the criteria for another mental, medical disorder and is not an exacerbation of a preexisting mental disorder. The symptoms also cannot be attributed to the direct physiological effects of a substance. See Section 8.2 for a discussion of adjustment disorders.

▲ 8.2 Adjustment Disorders

The diagnostic category of adjustment disorders is widely used among clinicians in practice. Adjustment disorders are characterized by an emotional response to a stressful event. It is one of the few diagnostic entities in which an external stressful event is linked to the development of symptoms. Typically, the stressor involves financial issues, a medical illness, or relationship problem. The symptom complex that develops may involve anxious or depressive affect or may present with a disturbance of conduct. By definition, the symptoms must begin within 3 months of the stressor. A variety of subtypes of adjustment disorder are identified in the fifth edition of the *Diagnostic and Statistical Manual of Mental Disorders* (DSM-5). These include adjustment disorder with depressed mood, mixed anxiety and depressed mood, disturbance of conduct, mixed disturbance of emotions and conduct, acute stress disorder, bereavement, and unspecified type.

EPIDEMIOLOGY

The prevalence of the disorder is estimated to be from 2 to 8 percent of the general population. Women are diagnosed with the disorder twice as often as men, and single women are generally overly represented as most at risk. In children and adolescents, boys and girls are equally diagnosed with adjustment disorders. The disorders can occur at any age but are most frequently diagnosed in adolescents. Among adolescents of either sex, common precipitating stresses are school problems, parental rejection and divorce, and substance abuse. Among adults, common precipitating stresses are marital problems, divorce, moving to a new environment, and financial problems.

Adjustment disorders are one of the most common psychiatric diagnoses for disorders of patients hospitalized for medical and surgical problems. In one study, 5 percent of persons admitted to a hospital over a 3-year period were classified as having an adjustment disorder. Up to 50 percent of persons with specific medical problems or stressors have been diagnosed with adjustment disorders. Furthermore, 10 to 30 percent of mental health outpatients and up to 50 percent of general hospital inpatients referred for mental health consultations have been diagnosed with adjustment disorders.

ETIOLOGY

By definition, an adjustment disorder is precipitated by one or more stressors. The severity of the stressor or stressors does not always predict the severity of the disorder; the stressor severity is a complex function of degree, quantity, duration, reversibility, environment, and personal context. For example, the loss of a parent is different for a child 10 years of age than for a person 40 years of age. Personality organization and cultural or group norms and values also contribute to the disproportionate responses to stressors.

Stressors may be single, such as a divorce or the loss of a job, or multiple, such as the death of a person important to a patient, which coincides with the patient's own physical illness and loss of a job. Stressors may be recurrent, such as seasonal business difficulties, or continuous, such as chronic illness or poverty. A discordant intrafamilial relationship can produce an adjustment disorder that affects the entire family system, or the disorder may be limited to a patient who was perhaps the victim of a crime or who has a physical illness. Sometimes, adjustment disorders occur in a group or community setting, and the stressors affect several persons, as in a natural disaster or in racial, social, or religious persecution. Specific developmental stages, such as beginning school, leaving home, getting married, becoming a parent, failing to achieve occupational goals, having the last child leave home, and retiring, are often associated with adjustment disorders.

Psychodynamic Factors

Pivotal to understanding adjustment disorders is an understanding of three factors: the nature of the stressor, the conscious and unconscious meanings of the stressor, and the patient's preexisting vulnerability. A concurrent personality disorder or organic impairment may make a person vulnerable to adjustment disorders. Vulnerability is also associated with the loss of a parent during infancy or being reared in a dysfunctional family. Actual or perceived support from key relationships can affect behavioral and emotional responses to stressors.

Several psychoanalytic researchers have pointed out that the same stress can produce a range of responses in various persons. Throughout his life, Sigmund Freud remained interested in why the stresses of ordinary life produce illness in some and not in others, why an illness takes a particular form, and why some experiences and not others predispose a person to psychopathology. He gave considerable weight to constitutional factors and viewed them as interacting with a person's life experiences to produce fixation.

Psychoanalytic research has emphasized the role of the mother and the rearing environment in a person's later capacity to respond to stress. Particularly important was Donald Winnicott's concept of the good-enough mother, a person who adapts to the infant's needs and provides sufficient support to enable the growing child to tolerate the frustrations in life.

Clinicians must undertake a detailed exploration of a patient's experience of the stressor. Certain patients commonly place all the blame on a particular event when a less obvious event may have had more significant psychological meaning for the patient. Current events may reawaken past traumas or disappointments from childhood, so patients should be encouraged to think about how the current situation relates to similar past events.

Throughout early development, each child develops a unique set of defense mechanisms to deal with stressful events. Because of greater amounts of trauma or greater constitutional vulnerability, some children have less mature defensive constellations than other children. This disadvantage may cause them as adults to react with substantially impaired functioning when they are faced with a loss, a divorce, or a financial setback; those who have developed mature defense mechanisms are less vulnerable and bounce back more quickly from the stressor. Resilience is also crucially determined by the nature of children's early relationships with their parents. Studies of trauma repeatedly indicate that supportive, nurturing relationships prevent traumatic incidents from causing permanent psychological damage.

Psychodynamic clinicians must consider the relation between a stressor and the human developmental life cycle. When adolescents leave home for college, for example, they are at high developmental risk for reacting with a temporary symptomatic picture. Similarly, if the young person who leaves home is the last child in the family, the parents may be particularly vulnerable to a reaction of adjustment disorder. Moreover, middle-aged persons who are confronting their own mortality may be especially sensitive to the effects of loss or death.

Family and Genetic Factors

Some studies suggest that certain persons appear to be at increased risk both for the occurrence of these adverse life events and for the development of pathology once they occur. Findings from a study of more than 2,000 twin pairs indicate that life events and stressors are modestly correlated in twin pairs, with monozygotic twins showing greater concordance than dizygotic twins. Family environmental and genetic factors each accounted for approximately 20 percent of the variance in that study. Another twin study that examined genetic contributions to the development of PTSD symptoms (not necessarily at the level of full disorder and, therefore, relevant to adjustment disorders) also concluded that the likelihood of developing symptoms in response to traumatic life events is partially under genetic control.

DIAGNOSIS AND CLINICAL FEATURES

Although by definition adjustment disorders follow a stressor, the symptoms do not necessarily begin immediately. Up to 3 months may elapse between a stressor and the development of symptoms. Symptoms do not always subside as soon as the stressor ceases; if the stressor continues, the disorder may be chronic. The disorder can occur at any age, and its symptoms vary considerably, with depressive, anxious, and mixed features most common in adults. Physical symptoms, which are most common in children and the elderly, can occur in any age group. Manifestations may also include assaultive behavior and reckless driving, excessive drinking, defaulting on legal responsibilities, withdrawal, vegetative signs, insomnia, and suicidal behavior.

The clinical presentations of adjustment disorder can vary widely. DSM-5 lists six adjustment disorders: with depressed mood; with anxiety; with mixed anxiety and depression; with conduct disturbance; with conduct disturbance and disturbance of emotion; and an unspecified category.

Adjustment Disorder with Depressed Mood

In adjustment disorder with depressed mood, the predominant manifestations are depressed mood, tearfulness, and hopelessness. This type must be distinguished from major depressive disorder and uncomplicated bereavement. Adolescents with this type of adjustment disorder are at increased risk for major depressive disorder in young adulthood.

Adjustment Disorder with Anxiety

Symptoms of anxiety, such as palpitations, jitteriness, and agitation, are present in adjustment disorder with anxiety, which must be differentiated from anxiety disorders.

Adjustment Disorder with Mixed Anxiety and Depressed Mood

In adjustment disorder with mixed anxiety and depressed mood, patients exhibit features of both anxiety and depression that do not meet the criteria for an already established anxiety disorder or depressive disorder.

A 48-year-old married woman, in good health, with no previous psychiatric difficulties, presented to the emergency room reporting that she had overdosed on a handful of antihistamines shortly before she arrived. She described her problems as having started 2 months earlier, soon after her husband unexpectedly requested a divorce. She felt betrayed after having devoted much of her 20-year marriage to being a wife, mother, and homemaker. She was sad and tearful at times, and she occasionally had difficulty sleeping. Otherwise, she had no vegetative symptoms and enjoyed time with family and friends. She felt desperate and suicidal after she realized that "he no longer loved me." After crisis intervention in the emergency setting, she responded well to individual psychotherapy over a 3-month period. She occasionally required benzodiazepines for anxiety during the period of treatment. By the time of discharge, she had returned to her baseline function. She came to terms with the possibility of life after divorce and was exploring her best options under the circumstances. *(Courtesy of Jeffrey W. Katzman, M.D. and Cynthia M. A. Geppert, M.D., Ph.D., M.P.H.)*

Adjustment Disorder with Disturbance of Conduct

In adjustment disorder with disturbance of conduct, the predominant manifestation involves conduct in which the rights of others are violated or age-appropriate societal norms and rules are disregarded. Examples of behavior in this category are truancy, vandalism, reckless driving, and fighting. The category must be differentiated from conduct disorder and antisocial personality disorder.

Adjustment Disorder with Mixed Disturbance of Emotions and Conduct

A combination of disturbances of emotions and of conduct sometimes occurs. Clinicians are encouraged to try to make one or the other diagnosis in the interest of clarity.

Adjustment Disorder Unspecified

Adjustment disorder unspecified is a residual category for atypical maladaptive reactions to stress. Examples include inappropriate responses to the diagnosis of physical illness, such as massive denial, severe noncompliance with treatment, and social withdrawal, without significant depressed or anxious mood.

DIFFERENTIAL DIAGNOSIS

Although uncomplicated bereavement often produces temporarily impaired social and occupational functioning, the person's dysfunction remains within the expectable bounds of a reaction to the loss of a loved one and, thus, is not considered adjustment disorder. Other disorders from which adjustment disorder must be differentiated include major depressive disorder, brief psychotic disorder, generalized anxiety disorder, somatic symptom disorder, substance-related disorder, conduct disorder, and PTSD. These diagnoses should be given precedence in all cases that meet their criteria, even in the presence of a stressor or group of stressors that served as a precipitant. Patients with an adjustment disorder are impaired in social or occupational functioning and show symptoms beyond the normal and expectable reaction to the stressor. Because no absolute criteria help to distinguish an adjustment disorder from another condition, clinical judgment is necessary. Some patients may meet the criteria for both an adjustment disorder and a personality disorder. If the adjustment disorder follows a physical illness, the clinician must make sure that the symptoms are not a continuation or another manifestation of the illness or its treatment.

Acute and Posttraumatic Stress Disorders

The presence of a stressor is a requirement in the diagnosis of adjustment disorder, PTSD, and acute stress disorder. PTSD and acute stress disorder have the nature of the stressor better characterized and are accompanied by a defined constellation of affective and autonomic symptoms. In contrast, the stressor in adjustment disorder can be of any severity, with a wide range of possible symptoms. When the response to an extreme stressor does not meet the acute stress or posttraumatic disorder threshold, the adjustment disorder diagnosis would be appropriate. PTSD is discussed fully in Section 8.1.

COURSE AND PROGNOSIS

With appropriate treatment, the overall prognosis of an adjustment disorder is generally favorable. Most patients return to their previous level of functioning within 3 months. Some persons (particularly adolescents) who receive a diagnosis of an adjustment disorder later have mood disorders or substance-related disorders. Adolescents usually require a longer time to recover than adults.

There is a risk of suicide in patients with adjustment disorder, especially in adolescent patients with adjustment disorder, that has not been fully appreciated. One study of 119 patients with adjustment disorder indicated that 60 percent had documented suicide attempts in the hospital. Fifty percent had attempted suicide immediately prior to their hospital admission. Comorbid diagnoses of substance abuse and personality disorder contributed to the suicide risk profile. A study of the background, pathology, and treatment-related factors of suicidal adolescents found that those with adjustment disorder and suicidality were more likely to have made attempts (up to 25 percent), to exhibit psychomotor restlessness and dysphoric mood, to have experienced a suicide of another person as a stressor, to have poor psychosocial functioning upon treatment entry, and to have received prior psychiatric care.

A 16-year-old high school senior experienced rejection in his first serious relationship. In the weeks after the end of the relationship, he began to exhibit dysphoric mood accompanied by anxiety and psychomotor agitation. He had received counseling in junior high school when his parents divorced and he began using alcohol and marijuana and had been suspended during his freshman year for fighting. A month after the breakup, he began to tell his parents that life was no longer worth living without his former girlfriend. Two months later his parents came home from work and found him hanging in the garage with a note stating he could not go on alone. *(Courtesy of J. W. Katzman, M.D. and C. M. A. Geppert, M.D., Ph.D., M.P.H.)*

TREATMENT

Psychotherapy

Psychotherapy remains the treatment of choice for adjustment disorders. Group therapy can be particularly useful for patients who have had similar stresses—for example, a group of retired persons or patients having renal dialysis. Individual psychotherapy offers the opportunity to explore the meaning of the stressor to the patient so that earlier traumas can be worked through. After successful therapy, patients sometimes emerge from an adjustment disorder stronger than in the premorbid period, although no pathology was evident during that period. Because a stressor can be clearly delineated in adjustment disorders, it is often believed that psychotherapy is not indicated and that the disorder will remit spontaneously. This viewpoint, however, ignores the fact that many persons exposed to the same stressor experience different symptoms, and in adjustment disorders, the response is pathological. Psychotherapy can help persons adapt to stressors that are not reversible or time limited and can serve as a preventive intervention if the stressor does remit.

Psychiatrists treating adjustment disorders must be particularly aware of problems of secondary gain. The illness role may be rewarding to some normally healthy persons who have had little experience with illness's capacity to free them from responsibility. Thus, patients can find therapists' attention, empathy, and understanding, which are necessary for success, rewarding in their own right, and therapists may thereby reinforce patients' symptoms. Such considerations must be weighed before intensive psychotherapy is begun; when a secondary gain has already been established, therapy is difficult. Patients with an adjustment disorder that includes a conduct disturbance may have difficulties with the law, authorities, or school. Psychiatrists should not attempt to rescue such patients from the consequences of their actions. Too often, such kindness only reinforces socially unacceptable means of tension reduction and hinders the acquisition of insight and subsequent emotional growth. In these cases, family therapy can help.

Crisis Intervention

Crisis intervention and case management are short-term treatments aimed at helping persons with adjustment disorders resolve their situations quickly by supportive techniques, suggestion, reassurance, environmental modification, and even hospitalization, if necessary. The frequency and length of visits for crisis support vary according to patients' needs; daily sessions may be necessary, sometimes two or three times each day. Flexibility is essential in this approach.

Pharmacotherapy

No studies have assessed the efficacy of pharmacological interventions in individuals with adjustment disorder, but it may be reasonable to use medication to treat specific symptoms for a brief time. The judicious use of medications can help patients with adjustment disorders, but they should be prescribed for brief periods. Depending on the type of adjustment disorder, a patient may respond to an antianxiety agent or to an antidepressant. Patients with severe anxiety bordering on panic can benefit from anxiolytics such as diazepam (Valium), and those in withdrawn or inhibited states may be helped by a short course of psychostimulant medication. Antipsychotic drugs may be used if there are signs of decompensation or impending psychosis. SSRIs have been found useful in treating symptoms of traumatic grief. Recently, there has been an increase in antidepressant use to augment psychotherapy in patients with adjustment disorders. Pharmacological intervention in this population is most often used, however, to augment psychosocial strategies rather than serving as the primary modality.

9

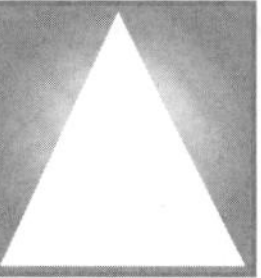

Dissociative Disorders

INTRODUCTION

In psychiatry, *dissociation* is defined as an unconscious defense mechanism involving the segregation of any group of mental or behavioral processes from the rest of the person's psychic activity. Dissociative disorders involve this mechanism so that there is a disruption in one or more mental functions, such as memory, identity, perception, consciousness, or motor behavior. The disturbance may be sudden or gradual, transient or chronic, and the signs and symptoms of the disorder are often caused by psychological trauma.

Amnesia brought on by intrapsychic conflict is coded differently from amnesia brought on by a medical condition such as encephalitis. In the latter case, according to the fifth edition of the *Diagnostic and Statistical Manual of Mental Disorders* (DSM-5), a diagnosis of neurocognitive disorder due to a medical condition would be made; whereas in the former condition, a diagnosis of dissociative amnesia would be made.

DISSOCIATIVE AMNESIA

The main DSM-5 feature of dissociative amnesia is an inability to recall important personal information, usually of a traumatic or stressful nature, that is too extensive to be explained by normal forgetfulness. And, as mentioned above, the disorder does not result from the direct physiological effects of a substance or a neurological or other general medical condition. The different types of dissociative amnesia are listed in Table 9–1.

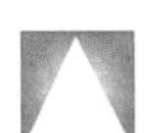

Table 9–1
Types of Dissociative Amnesia

Localized amnesia: Inability to recall events related to a circumscribed period of time
Selective amnesia: Ability to remember some, but not all, of the events occurring during a circumscribed period of time
Generalized amnesia: Failure to recall one's entire life
Continuous amnesia: Failure to recall successive events as they occur
Systematized amnesia: Failure to remember a category of information, such as all memories relating to one's family or to a particular person

A 45-year-old, divorced, left-handed, male bus dispatcher was seen in psychiatric consultation on a medical unit. He had been admitted with an episode of chest discomfort, light-headedness, and left-arm weakness. He had a history of hypertension and had a medical admission in the past year for ischemic chest pain, although he had not suffered a myocardial infarction. Psychiatric consultation was called, because the patient complained of memory loss for the previous 12 years, behaving and responding to the environment as if it were 12 years previously (e.g., he did not recognize his 8-year-old son, insisted that he was unmarried, and denied recollection of current events, such as the name of the current president). Physical and laboratory findings were unchanged from the patient's usual baseline. Brain computed tomography (CT) scan was normal.

On mental status examination, the patient displayed intact intellectual function but insisted that the date was 12 years earlier, denying recall of his entire subsequent personal history and of current events for the past 12 years. He was perplexed by the contradiction between his memory and current circumstances. The patient described a family history of brutal beatings and physical discipline. He was a decorated combat veteran, although he described amnestic episodes for some of his combat experiences. In the military, he had been a champion golden glove boxer noted for his powerful left hand.

He was educated about his disorder and given the suggestion that his memory could return as he could tolerate it, perhaps overnight during sleep or perhaps over a longer time. If this strategy was unsuccessful, hypnosis or an amobarbital (Amytal) interview was proposed. *(Adapted from a case of Richard J. Loewenstein, M.D. and Frank W. Putnam, M.D.)*

Epidemiology

Dissociative amnesia has been reported in a range of approximately 2 to 6 percent of the general population. There may be a slightly higher incidence in women. Cases generally begin to be reported in late adolescence and adulthood. Dissociative amnesia can be especially difficult to assess in preadolescent children because of their more limited ability to describe subjective experience.

Etiology

In many cases of acute dissociative amnesia, the psychosocial environment out of which the amnesia develops is massively conflictual, with the patient experiencing intolerable emotions of shame, guilt, despair, rage, and desperation. These usually result from conflicts over unacceptable urges or impulses, such as intense sexual, suicidal, or violent compulsions. Traumatic experiences such as physical or sexual abuse can induce the disorder. In some cases, the trauma is caused by a betrayal by a trusted, needed other (betrayal trauma). This betrayal is thought to influence the way in which the event is processed and remembered.

Diagnosis and Clinical Features

Classic Presentation. The classic disorder is an overt, florid, dramatic clinical disturbance that frequently results in the patient being brought quickly to medical attention, specifically for symptoms related to the dissociative disorder. It is frequently found in those who have experienced extreme acute trauma. It also commonly develops, however, in the context of profound intrapsychic conflict or emotional stress. Patients may present with intercurrent somatoform or conversion symptoms, alterations in consciousness, depersonalization, derealization, trance states, spontaneous age regression, and even ongoing anterograde dissociative amnesia. Depression and suicidal ideation are reported in many cases. No single personality profile or antecedent history is consistently reported in these patients, although a prior personal or family history of somatoform or dissociative symptoms has been shown to predispose individuals to develop acute amnesia during traumatic circumstances. Many of these patients have histories of prior adult or childhood abuse or trauma. In wartime cases, as in other forms of combat-related posttraumatic disorders, the most important variable in the development of dissociative symptoms, however, appears to be the intensity of combat. Table 9–2 presents the mental status evaluation of dissociative amnesia.

Table 9–2
Mental Status Examination Questions for Dissociative Amnesia

If answers are positive, ask the patient to describe the event. Make sure to specify that the symptom does not occur during an episode of intoxication.

1. Do you ever have blackouts? Blank spells? Memory lapses?
2. Do you lose time? Have gaps in your experience of time?
3. Have you ever traveled a considerable distance without recollection of how you did this or where you went exactly?
4. Do people tell you of things you have said and done that you do not recall?
5. Do you find objects in your possession (such as clothes, personal items, groceries in your grocery cart, books, tools, equipment, jewelry, vehicles, weapons, and so on) that you do not remember acquiring? Out-of-character items? Items that a child might have? Toys? Stuffed animals?
6. Have you ever been told or found evidence that you have talents and abilities that you did not know that you had? For example, musical, artistic, mechanical, literary, athletic, or other talents? Do your tastes seem to fluctuate a lot? For example, food preference, personal habits, taste in music or clothes?
7. Do you have gaps in your memory of your life? Are you missing parts of your memory for your life history? Are you missing memories of some important events in your life? For example, weddings, birthdays, graduations, pregnancies, birth of children?
8. Do you lose track of or tune out conversations or therapy sessions as they are occurring? Do you find that, while you are listening to someone talk, you did not hear all or part of what was just said?
9. What is the longest period of time that you have lost? Minutes? Hours? Days? Weeks? Months? Years? Describe.

Adapted from Loewenstein RJ. An office mental status examination for chronic complex dissociative symptoms and multiple personality disorder. *Psychiatr Clin North Am*. 1991;14:567–604, with permission.

Nonclassic Presentation. These patients frequently come to treatment for a variety of symptoms, such as depression or mood swings, substance abuse, sleep disturbances, somatoform symptoms, anxiety and panic, suicidal or self-mutilating impulses and acts, violent outbursts, eating problems, and interpersonal problems. Self-mutilation and violent behavior in these patients may also be accompanied by amnesia. Amnesia may also occur for flashbacks or behavioral re-experiencing episodes related to trauma.

Differential Diagnosis

The differential diagnosis of dissociative amnesia is listed in Table 9–3.

Ordinary Forgetfulness and Nonpathological Amnesia. Ordinary forgetfulness is a phenomenon that is benign and unrelated to stressful events. In dissociative amnesia, the memory loss is more extensive than in nonpathological amnesia. Other nonpathological forms of amnesia have been described, such as infantile and childhood amnesia, amnesia for sleep and dreaming, and hypnotic amnesia.

Dementia, Delirium, and Amnestic Disorders due to Medical Conditions. In patients with dementia, delirium, and amnestic disorders due to medical conditions, the memory loss for personal information is embedded in a far more extensive set of cognitive, language, attentional, behavioral, and memory problems. Loss of memory for personal identity is usually not found without evidence of a marked disturbance in many domains of cognitive function. Causes of organic amnestic disorders include Korsakoff's psychosis, cerebral vascular accident (CVA), postoperative amnesia, postinfectious amnesia, anoxic amnesia, and transient global amnesia. Electroconvulsive therapy (ECT) may also cause a marked temporary amnesia, as well as persistent memory problems in some cases. Here, however, memory loss for autobiographical experience is unrelated to traumatic or overwhelming experiences and seems to involve many different types of personal experiences, most commonly those occurring just before or during the ECT treatments.

Posttraumatic Amnesia. In posttraumatic amnesia caused by brain injury, a history of a clear-cut physical trauma, a period of unconsciousness or amnesia, or both is usually seen, and there is objective clinical evidence of brain injury.

Seizure Disorders. In most seizure cases, the clinical presentation differs significantly from that of dissociative amnesia, with clear-cut ictal events and sequelae. Patients with pseudoepileptic seizures may also have dissociative symptoms, such as amnesia and an antecedent history of psychological trauma. Rarely, patients with recurrent, complex partial seizures present with ongoing bizarre behavior, memory problems, irritability, or violence, leading to a differential diagnostic puzzle. In some of

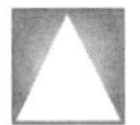

Table 9–3
Differential Diagnosis of Dissociative Amnesia

- Ordinary forgetfulness
  - Age-related cognitive decline
- Nonpathological forms of amnesia
  - Infantile and childhood amnesia
  - Amnesia for sleep and dreaming
  - Hypnotic amnesia
- Dementia
- Delirium
- Amnestic disorders
- Neurological disorders with discrete memory loss episodes
  - Posttraumatic amnesia
  - Transient global amnesia
  - Amnesia related to seizure disorders
- Substance-related amnesia
  - Alcohol
  - Sedative-hypnotics
  - Anticholinergic agents
  - Steroids
  - Marijuana
  - Narcotic analgesics
  - Psychedelics
  - Phencyclidine
  - Methyldopa (Aldomet)
  - Pentazocine (Talwin)
  - Hypoglycemic agents
  - β-blockers
  - Lithium carbonate
  - Many others
- Other dissociative disorders
  - Dissociative fugue
  - Dissociative identity disorder
  - Dissociative disorder not otherwise specified
- Acute stress disorder
- Posttraumatic stress disorder
- Somatization disorder
- Psychotic episode
  - Lack of memory for psychotic episode when returns to nonpsychotic state
- Mood disorder episode
  - Lack of memory for aspects of episode of mania when depressed and vice versa or when euthymic
- Factitious disorder
- Malingering
- Psychophysiological symptoms or disorders
  - Asthma and breathing problems
  - Perimenstrual disorders
  - Irritable bowel syndrome
  - Gastroesophageal reflux disease
  - Somatic memory
- Affective symptoms
  - Depressed mood, dysphoria, or anhedonia
  - Brief mood swings or mood lability
  - Suicidal thoughts and attempts or self-mutilation
  - Guilt and survivor guilt
  - Helpless and hopeless feelings
- Obsessive-compulsive symptoms
  - Ruminations about trauma
  - Obsessive counting, singing
  - Arranging
  - Washing
  - Checking

these cases, the diagnosis can be clarified only by telemetry or ambulatory electroencephalographic (EEG) monitoring.

Substance-Related Amnesia. A variety of substances and intoxicants have been implicated in the production of amnesia. Common offending agents include alcohol, benzodiazepines, ketamine, and hallucinogenic drugs among others.

Transient Global Amnesia. Transient global amnesia can be mistaken for a dissociative amnesia, especially because stressful life events may precede either disorder. In transient global amnesia, however, there is the sudden onset of complete anterograde amnesia and learning abilities; pronounced retrograde amnesia; preservation of memory for personal identity; anxious awareness of memory loss with repeated, often perseverative, questioning; overall normal behavior; lack of gross neurological abnormalities in most cases; and rapid return of baseline cognitive function, with a persistent short retrograde amnesia. The patient usually is older than 50 years of age and shows risk factors for cerebrovascular disease, although epilepsy and migraine have been etiologically implicated in some cases.

Dissociative Identity Disorders. Patients with dissociative identity disorder can present with acute forms of amnesia and fugue episodes. These patients, however, are characterized by a plethora of symptoms, only some of which are usually found in patients with dissociative amnesia. With respect to amnesia, most patients with dissociative identity disorder and those with dissociative disorder not otherwise specified with dissociative identity disorder features report multiple forms of complex amnesia, including recurrent blackouts, fugues, unexplained possessions, and fluctuations in skills, habits, and knowledge.

Acute Stress Disorder, Posttraumatic Stress Disorder, and Somatic Symptom Disorder. Most forms of dissociative amnesia are best conceptualized as part of a group of trauma spectrum disorders that includes acute stress disorder, posttraumatic stress disorder (PTSD), and somatic symptom disorder. Many patients with dissociative amnesia meet full or partial diagnostic criteria for those acute stress disorders or a combination of the three. Amnesia is a criterion symptom of each of the latter disorders.

Malingering and Factitious Amnesia. No absolute way exists to differentiate dissociative amnesia from factitious or malingered amnesia. Malingerers have been noted to continue their deception even during hypnotically or barbiturate-facilitated interviews. A patient who presents to psychiatric attention seeking to recover repressed memories as a chief complaint most likely has a factitious disorder or has been subject to suggestive influences. Most of these individuals actually do not describe bona fide amnesia when carefully questioned, but are often insistent that they must have been abused in childhood to explain their unhappiness or life dysfunction.

Course and Prognosis

Little is known about the clinical course of dissociative amnesia. Acute dissociative amnesia frequently spontaneously resolves once the person is removed to safety from traumatic or overwhelming circumstances. At the other extreme, some patients do develop chronic forms of generalized, continuous, or severe localized amnesia and are profoundly disabled and require high levels of social support, such as nursing home placement or intensive family caretaking. Clinicians should try to restore patients' lost memories to consciousness as soon as possible; otherwise, the repressed memory may form a nucleus in the unconscious mind around which future amnestic episodes may develop.

Treatment

Cognitive Therapy. Cognitive therapy may have specific benefits for individuals with trauma disorders. Identifying the specific cognitive distortions that are based in the trauma may provide an entrée into autobiographical memory for which the patient experiences amnesia. As the patient becomes able to correct cognitive distortions, particularly about the meaning of prior trauma, more detailed recall of traumatic events may occur.

Hypnosis. Hypnosis can be used in a number of different ways in the treatment of dissociative amnesia. In particular, hypnotic interventions can be used to contain, modulate, and titrate the intensity of symptoms; to facilitate controlled recall of dissociated memories; to provide support and ego strengthening for the patient; and, finally, to promote working through and integration of dissociated material.

In addition, the patient can be taught self-hypnosis to apply containment and calming techniques in his or her everyday life. Successful use of containment techniques, whether hypnotically facilitated or not, also increases the patient's sense that he or she can more effectively be in control of alternations between intrusive symptoms and amnesia.

Somatic Therapies. No known pharmacotherapy exists for dissociative amnesia other than pharmacologically facilitated interviews. A variety of agents have been used for this purpose, including sodium amobarbital, thiopental (Pentothal), oral benzodiazepines, and amphetamines.

Pharmacologically facilitated interviews using intravenous amobarbital or diazepam (Valium) are used primarily in working with acute amnesias and conversion reactions, among other indications, in general hospital medical and psychiatric services. This procedure is also occasionally useful in refractory cases of chronic dissociative amnesia when patients are unresponsive to other interventions. The material uncovered in a pharmacologically facilitated interview needs to be processed by the patient in his or her usual conscious state.

Group Psychotherapy. Time-limited and longer-term group psychotherapies have been reported to be helpful for combat veterans with PTSD and for survivors of childhood abuse. During group sessions, patients may recover memories for which they have had amnesia. Supportive interventions by the group members or the group therapist, or both, may facilitate integration and mastery of the dissociated material.

DEPERSONALIZATION/DEREALIZATION DISORDER

Depersonalization is defined as the persistent or recurrent feeling of detachment or estrangement from one's self. The individual may report feeling like an automaton or watching himself or herself in a movie. Derealization is somewhat related and refers to feelings of unreality or of being detached from one's environment. The patient may describe his or her perception of the outside world as lacking lucidity and emotional coloring, as though dreaming or dead. DSM-5 requires the presence of depersonalization, derealization or both in order to make the diagnosis.

Epidemiology

Transient experiences of depersonalization and derealization are extremely common in normal and clinical populations. They are the third most commonly reported psychiatric symptoms, after depression and anxiety. One survey found a 1-year prevalence of 19 percent in the general population. It is common in seizure patients and migraine sufferers; they can also occur with use of psychedelic drugs, especially marijuana, lysergic acid diethylamide (LSD), and mescaline, and less frequently as a side effect of some medications, such as anticholinergic agents. They have been described after certain types of meditation, deep hypnosis, extended mirror or crystal gazing, and sensory deprivation experiences. They are also common after mild to moderate head injury, wherein little or no loss of consciousness occurs, but they are significantly less likely if unconsciousness lasts for more than 30 minutes. They are also common after life-threatening experiences, with or without serious bodily injury. Depersonalization is found two to four times more in women than in men, although some surveys found the disorder to be equal between men and women.

Etiology

Psychodynamic. Traditional psychodynamic formulations have emphasized the disintegration of the ego or have viewed depersonalization as an affective response in defense of the ego. These explanations stress the role of overwhelming painful experiences or conflictual impulses as triggering events.

Traumatic Stress. A substantial proportion, typically one-third to one-half, of patients in clinical depersonalization case series report histories of significant trauma. Several studies of accident victims find as many as 60 percent of those with a life-threatening experience report at least transient depersonalization during the event or immediately thereafter. Military training studies find that symptoms of depersonalization and derealization are commonly evoked by stress and fatigue and are inversely related to performance.

Neurobiological Theories. The association of depersonalization with migraines and marijuana, its generally favorable response to selective serotonin reuptake inhibitors (SSRIs), and the increase in depersonalization symptoms seen with the depletion of L-tryptophan, a serotonin precursor, point to serotonergic involvement. Depersonalization is the primary dissociative symptom elicited by the drug-challenge studies described in the section on neurobiological theories of dissociation. These studies strongly implicate the N-methyl-D-aspartate (NMDA) subtype of the glutamate receptor as central to the genesis of depersonalization symptoms.

Diagnosis and Clinical Features

A number of distinct components comprise the experience of depersonalization, including a sense of (1) bodily changes, (2) duality of self as observer and actor, (3) being cut off from others, and (4) being cut off from one's own emotions. Patients experiencing depersonalization often have great difficulty expressing what they are feeling. Trying to express their subjective suffering with banal phrases, such as "I feel dead," "Nothing seems real," or "I'm standing outside of myself," depersonalized patients may not adequately convey to the examiner the distress they experience. While complaining bitterly about how this is ruining their life, they may nonetheless appear remarkably undistressed.

Ms. R was a 27-year-old, unmarried, graduate student with a master's degree in biology. She complained about intermittent episodes of "standing back," usually associated with anxiety-provoking social situations. When asked about a recent episode, she described presenting in a seminar course. "All of a sudden, I was talking, but it didn't feel like it was me talking. It was very disconcerting. I had this feeling, 'who's doing the talking?' I felt like I was just watching someone else talk. Listening to words come out of my mouth, but I wasn't saying them. It wasn't me. It went on for a while. I was calm, even sort of peaceful. It was as if I was very far away. In the back of the room somewhere—just watching myself. But the person talking didn't even seem like me really. It was like I was watching someone else." The feeling lasted the rest of that day and persisted into the next, during which time it gradually dissipated. She thought that she remembered having similar experiences during high school, but was certain that they occurred at least once a year during college and graduate school.

As a child, Ms. R reported frequent intense anxiety from overhearing or witnessing the frequent violent arguments and periodic physical fights between her parents. In addition, the family was subject to many unpredictable dislocations and moves owing to the patient's father's intermittent difficulties with finances and employment. The patient's anxieties did not abate when the parents divorced when she was a late adolescent. Her father moved away and had little further contact with her. Her relationship with her mother became increasingly angry, critical, and contentious. She was unsure if she experienced depersonalization during childhood while listening to her parents' fights. *(Adapted from a case of Richard J. Loewenstein, M.D. and Frank W. Putnam, M.D.)*

Differential Diagnosis

The variety of conditions associated with depersonalization complicate the differential diagnosis of depersonalization disorder. Depersonalization can result from a medical condition or neurological condition, intoxication or withdrawal from illicit drugs, as a side effect of medications, or can be associated with panic attacks, phobias, PTSD, or acute stress disorder, schizophrenia, or another dissociative disorder. A thorough medical and neurological evaluation is essential, including standard laboratory studies, an EEG, and any indicated drug screens. Drug-related depersonalization is typically transient, but persistent depersonalization can follow an episode of intoxication with a variety of substances, including marijuana, cocaine, and other psychostimulants. A range of neurological conditions, including seizure disorders, brain tumors, postconcussive syndrome, metabolic abnormalities, migraine, vertigo, and Ménière's disease, have been reported as causes. Depersonalization caused by organic conditions tends to be primarily sensory without the elaborated descriptions and personalized meanings common to psychiatric etiologies.

Course and Prognosis

Depersonalization after traumatic experiences or intoxication commonly remits spontaneously after removal from the traumatic circumstances or ending of the episode of intoxication. Depersonalization accompanying mood, psychotic, or other anxiety disorders commonly remits with definitive treatment of these conditions.

Depersonalization disorder itself may have an episodic, relapsing and remitting, or chronic course. Many patients with chronic depersonalization may have a course characterized by severe impairment in occupational, social, and personal functioning. Mean age of onset is thought to be in late adolescence or early adulthood in most cases.

Treatment

Clinicians working with patients with depersonalization/derealization disorder often find them to be a singularly clinically refractory group. Some systematic evidence indicate that SSRI antidepressants, such as fluoxetine (Prozac), may be helpful to patients with depersonalization disorder. Two recent, double-blind, placebo-controlled studies, however, found no efficacy for fluvoxamine (Luvox) and lamotrigine (Lamictal), respectively, for depersonalization disorder. Some patients with depersonalization disorder respond at best sporadically and partially to the usual groups of psychiatric medications, singly or in combination: antidepressants, mood stabilizers, typical and atypical neuroleptics, anticonvulsants, and so forth.

Many different types of psychotherapy have been used to treat depersonalization disorder: psychodynamic, cognitive, cognitive–behavioral, hypnotherapeutic, and supportive. Many such patients do not have a robust response to these specific types of standard psychotherapy. Stress management strategies, distraction techniques, reduction of sensory stimulation, relaxation training, and physical exercise may be somewhat helpful in some patients.

DISSOCIATIVE FUGUE

Dissociative fugue was deleted as a major diagnostic category in DSM-5 and is now diagnosed as a subtype (specifier) of dissociative amnesia. Dissociative fugue can be seen in patients with both dissociative amnesia and dissociative identity disorder. The disorder remains a distinct diagnosis in the *International Statistical Classification of Diseases and Related Health Problems*, 10th edition (ICD-10) and is discussed as a discrete entity in *Synopsis* because of its clinical relevance.

Dissociative fugue is described as sudden, unexpected travel away from home or one's customary place of daily activities, with inability to recall some or all of one's past. This is accompanied by confusion about personal identity or even the assumption of a new identity. The disturbance is not due to the direct physiological effects of a substance or a general medical condition. The symptoms must cause clinically significant distress or impairment in social, occupational, or other important areas of functioning.

Etiology

Traumatic circumstances (i.e., combat, rape, recurrent childhood sexual abuse, massive social dislocations, natural disasters), leading to an altered state of consciousness dominated by a wish to flee, are the underlying causes of most fugue episodes. In some cases, a similar antecedent history is seen, although a psychological trauma is not present at the onset of the fugue episode. In these cases, instead of, or in addition to, external dangers or traumas, the patients are usually struggling with extreme emotions or impulses (i.e., overwhelming fear, guilt, shame, or intense incestuous, sexual, suicidal, or violent urges) that are in conflict with the patient's conscience or ego ideals.

Epidemiology

The disorder is thought to be more common during natural disasters, wartime, or times of major social dislocation and violence, although no systematic data exist on this point. No adequate data exist to demonstrate a gender bias to this disorder; however, most cases describe men, primarily in the military. Dissociative fugue is usually described in adults.

Diagnosis and Clinical Features

Dissociative fugues have been described to last from minutes to months. Some patients report multiple fugues. In most cases in which this was described, a more chronic dissociative disorder, such as dissociative identity disorder, was not ruled out.

In some extremely severe cases of PTSD, nightmares may be terminated by a waking fugue in which the patient runs to another part of the house or runs outside. Children or adolescents may be more limited than adults in their ability to travel. Thus, fugues in this population may be brief and involve only short distances.

A teenage girl was continually sexually abused by her alcoholic father and another family friend. She was threatened with perpetration of sexual abuse on her younger siblings if she told anyone about the abuse. The girl became suicidal but felt that she had to stay alive to protect her siblings. She precipitously ran away from home after being raped by her father and several of his friends as a "birthday present" for one of them. She traveled to a part of the city where she had lived previously with the idea that she would find her grandmother with whom she had lived before the abuse began. She traveled by public transportation and walked the streets, apparently without attracting attention. After approximately 8 hours, she was stopped by the police in a curfew check. When questioned, she could not recall recent events or give her current address, insisting that she lived with her grandmother. On initial psychiatric examination, she was aware of her identity, but she believed that it was 2 years earlier, giving her age as 2 years younger and insisting that none of the events of recent years had occurred. *(Courtesy of Richard J. Loewenstein, M.D. and Frank W. Putnam, M.D.)*

After the termination of a fugue, the patient may experience perplexity, confusion, trance-like behaviors, depersonalization, derealization, and conversion symptoms, in addition to amnesia. Some patients may terminate a fugue with an episode of generalized dissociative amnesia.

As the patient with dissociative fugue begins to become less dissociated, he or she may display mood disorder symptoms, intense suicidal ideation, and PTSD or anxiety disorder symptoms. In the classic cases, an alter identity is created under whose auspices the patient lives for a period of time. Many of these latter cases are better classified as dissociative identity disorder or, if using DSM-5, as other specified dissociative disorder with features of dissociative identity disorder.

Differential Diagnosis

Individuals with dissociative amnesia may engage in confused wandering during an amnesia episode. In dissociative fugue, however, there is *purposeful* travel away from the individual's home or customary place of daily activities, usually with the individual preoccupied by a single idea that is accompanied by a wish to run away.

Patients with dissociative identity disorder may have symptoms of dissociative fugue, usually recurrently throughout their lives. Patients with dissociative identity disorder have multiple forms of complex amnesias and, usually, multiple alter identities that develop, starting in childhood.

In complex partial seizures, patients have been noted to exhibit wandering or semipurposeful behavior, or both, during seizures or in postictal states, for which subsequent amnesia occurs. Seizure patients in an epileptic fugue often exhibit abnormal behavior, however, including confusion, perseveration, and abnormal or repetitive movements. Other features of seizures are typically reported in the clinical history, such as an aura, motor abnormalities, stereotyped behavior, perceptual alterations, incontinence, and a postictal state. Serial or telemetric EEGs, or both, usually show abnormalities associated with behavioral pathology.

Wandering behavior during a variety of general medical conditions, toxic and substance-related disorders, delirium, dementia, and organic amnestic syndromes could theoretically be confused with dissociative fugue. In most cases, however, the somatic, toxic, neurological, or substance-related disorder can be ruled in by the history, physical examination, laboratory tests, or toxicological and drug screening. Use of alcohol or substances may be involved in precipitating an episode of dissociative fugue.

Wandering and purposeful travel can occur during the manic phase of bipolar disorder or schizoaffective disorder. Patients who are manic may not recall behavior that occurred in the euthymic or depressed state and vice versa. In purposeful travel owing to mania, however, the patient is usually preoccupied with grandiose ideas and often calls attention to him or herself because of inappropriate behavior. Assumption of an alternate identity does not occur.

Similarly, peripatetic behavior can occur in some patients with schizophrenia. Memory for events during wandering episodes in such patients may be difficult to ascertain owing to the patient's thought disorder. Patients with dissociative fugue, however, do not demonstrate a psychotic thought disorder or other symptoms of psychosis.

Malingering of dissociative fugue can occur in individuals who are attempting to flee a situation involving legal, financial, or personal difficulties, as well as in soldiers who are attempting to avoid combat or unpleasant military duties. No test, battery of tests, or set of procedures exist that invariably distinguish true dissociative symptoms from those that are malingered. Malingering of dissociative symptoms, such as reports of amnesia for purposeful travel during an episode of antisocial behavior, can be maintained even during hypnotic or pharmacologically facilitated interviews. Many malingerers confess spontaneously or when confronted. In the forensic context, the examiner should always carefully consider the diagnosis of malingering when fugue is claimed.

Course and Prognosis

Most fugues are relatively brief, lasting from hours to days. Most individuals appear to recover, although refractory dissociative amnesia may persist in rare cases. Some studies have described recurrent fugues in most individuals presenting with an episode of dissociative fugue. No systematic modern data exist that attempt to differentiate dissociative fugue from dissociative identity disorder with recurrent fugues.

Treatment

Dissociative fugue is usually treated with an eclectic, psychodynamically oriented psychotherapy that focuses on helping the patient recover memory for identity and recent experience. Hypnotherapy and pharmacologically facilitated interviews are frequently necessary adjunctive techniques to assist with memory recovery. Patients may need medical treatment for injuries sustained during the fugue as well as food and sleep.

Clinicians should be prepared for the emergence of suicidal ideation or self-destructive ideas and impulses as the traumatic or stressful prefugue circumstances are revealed. Psychiatric hospitalization may be indicated if the patient is an outpatient.

Family, sexual, occupational, or legal problems that were part of the original matrix that generated the fugue episode may be substantially exacerbated by the time the patient's original identity and life situation are detected. Thus, family treatment and social service interventions may be necessary to help resolve such complex difficulties.

When dissociative fugue involves assumption of a new identity, it is useful to conceptualize this entity as psychologically vital to protecting the person. Traumatic experiences, memories, cognitions, identifications, emotions, strivings, self-perceptions, or a combination of these have become so conflicting and, yet, so peremptory that the person can resolve them only by embodying them in an alter identity. The therapeutic goal in such cases is neither suppression of the new identity nor fascinated explication of all its attributes. As in dissociative identity disorder, the clinician should appreciate the importance of the psychodynamic information contained within the alter personality state and the intensity of the psychological forces that necessitated its creation. In these cases, the most desirable therapeutic outcome is fusion of the identities, with the person working through and integrating the memories of the experiences that precipitated the fugue.

DISSOCIATIVE IDENTITY DISORDER

Dissociative identity disorder, previously called multiple personality disorder, has been the most extensively researched of all the dissociative disorders. It is characterized by the presence of two or more distinct identities or personality states. The identities or personality states, sometimes called *alters, self-states, alter identities,* or *parts,* among other terms, differ from one another in that each presents as having its own pattern of perceiving, relating to, and thinking about the environment and self, in short, its own personality. It is the paradigmatic dissociative psychopathology in that the symptoms of all the other dissociative disorders are commonly found in patients with dissociative identity disorder: amnesia, fugue, depersonalization, derealization, and similar symptoms.

Until about 1800, patients with dissociative identity disorder were mainly seen as suffering from various states of possession. In the early 1800s, Benjamin Rush built on the clinical reports of others and provided a clinical description of the phenomenology of dissociative identity disorder. Subsequently, both Jean-Martin Charcot and Pierre Janet described the symptoms of the disorder and recognized the dissociative nature of the symptoms. Both Sigmund Freud and Eugen Bleuler recognized the symptoms, although Freud attributed psychodynamic mechanisms to the symptoms and Bleuler considered the symptoms to be reflective of schizophrenia. Perhaps because of an increased appreciation of the problem of child sexual and physical abuse and perhaps because of the cases described in the popular media (*The Three Faces of Eve, Sybil*), awareness of dissociative identity disorder has increased.

Epidemiology

Few systematic epidemiological data exist for dissociative identity disorder. DSM-5 reports a prevalence of about 2 percent in both men and women. Clinical studies report female to male ratios between 5 to 1 and 9 to 1 for diagnosed cases.

Etiology

Dissociative identity disorder is strongly linked to severe experiences of early childhood trauma, usually maltreatment. The rates of reported severe childhood trauma for child and adult patients with dissociative identity disorder range from 85 to 97 percent of cases. Physical and sexual abuses are the most frequently reported sources of childhood trauma. The contribution of genetic factors is only now being systematically assessed, but preliminary studies have not found evidence of a significant genetic contribution.

Diagnosis and Clinical Features

The key feature in diagnosing this disorder is the presence of two or more distinct personality states. There are many other signs and symptoms, however, that define the disorder, and because of great diversity, the diagnosis becomes difficult. These signs and symptoms are listed in Table 9–4, which describes many other associated symptoms commonly found in patients with dissociative personality disorder.

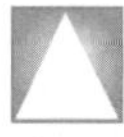

Table 9–4
Dissociative Identity Disorder-Associated Symptoms Commonly Found in Dissociative Identity Disorder

Posttraumatic stress disorder symptoms
- Intrusive symptoms
- Hyperarousal
- Avoidance and numbing symptoms

Somatic symptoms
- Conversion and pseudoneurological symptoms
- Seizure-like episodes
- Pain symptoms
- Headache, abdominal, musculoskeletal, pelvic pain
- Psychophysiological symptoms or disorders
- Asthma and breathing problems
- Perimenstrual disorders
- Irritable bowel syndrome
- Gastroesophageal reflux disease
- Somatic memory

Affective symptoms
- Depressed mood, dysphoria, or anhedonia
- Brief mood swings or mood lability
- Suicidal thoughts and attempts of self-mutilation
- Helpless and hopeless feelings

Obsessive-compulsive symptoms
- Ruminations about trauma
- Obsessive counting, singing
- Arranging
- Washing
- Checking

Mental Status. A careful and detailed mental status is essential in making the diagnosis. It is easy to mistake patients with this disorder as suffering from schizophrenia, borderline personality disorder, or of outright malingering. Table 9–5 lists the questions clinicians should ask in order to make the proper diagnosis.

Memory and Amnesia Symptoms. Dissociative disturbances of memory are manifest in several basic ways and are frequently observable in clinical settings. As part of the general mental status examination, clinicians should routinely inquire about experiences of losing time, blackout spells, and major gaps in the continuity of recall for personal information. Dissociative time loss experiences are too extensive to be explained by normal forgetting and typically have sharply demarcated onsets and offsets.

Patients with dissociative disorder often report significant gaps in autobiographical memory, especially for childhood events. Dissociative gaps in autobiographical recall are usually sharply demarcated and do not fit the normal decline in autobiographical recall for younger ages.

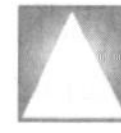

Table 9–5
Mental Status Examination Questions for Dissociative Identity Disorder Process Symptoms

If answers are positive, ask the patient to describe the event. Make sure to specify that the symptom does not occur during an episode of intoxication.

1. Do you act so differently in one situation compared to another situation that you feel almost like you were two different people?
2. Do you feel that there is more than one of you? More than one part of you? Side of you? Do they seem to be in conflict or in a struggle?
3. Does that part (those parts) of you have its (their) own independent way(s) of thinking, perceiving, and relating to the world and the self? Have its (their) own memories, thoughts, and feelings?
4. Does more than one of these entities take control of your behavior?
5. Do you ever have thoughts or feelings, or both, that come from inside you (outside you) that you cannot explain? That do not feel like thoughts or feelings that you would have? That seem like thoughts or feelings that are not under your control (passive influence)?
6. Have you ever felt that your body was engaged in behavior that did not seem to be under your control? For example, saying things, going places, buying things, writing things, drawing or creating things, hurting yourself or others, and so forth? That your body does not seem to belong to you?
7. Do you ever feel that you have to struggle against another part of you that seems to want to do or to say something that you do not wish to do or to say?
8. Do you ever feel that there is a force (pressure, part) inside you that tries to stop you from doing or saying something?
9. Do you ever hear voices, sounds, or conversations in your mind? That seem to be discussing you? Commenting on what you do? Telling you to do or not do certain things? To hurt yourself or others? That seem to be warning you or trying to protect you? That try to comfort, support, or soothe you? That provide important information about things to you? That argue or say things that have nothing to do with you? That have names? Men? Women? Children?
10. I would like to talk with that part (side, aspect, facet) of you (of the mind) that is called the "angry one" (the Little Girl, Janie, that went to Atlantic City last weekend and spend lots of money, etc.). Can that part come forward now, please?
11. Do you frequently have the experience of feeling like you are outside yourself? Inside yourself? Beside yourself, watching yourself as if you were another person?
12. Do you ever feel disconnected from yourself or your body as if you (your body) were not real?
13. Do you frequently experience the world around you as unreal? As if you are in a fog or daze? As if it were painted? Two-dimensional?
14. Do you ever looking in the mirror and not recognize who you see? See someone else there?

Adapted from Loewenstein RJ. An office mental status examination for a chronic complex dissociative symptoms and multiple personality disorder. *Psychiatr Clin North Am*. 1991;14:567, with permission.

Ms. A, a 33-year-old married woman, employed as a librarian in a school for disturbed children, presented to psychiatric attention after discovering her 5-year-old daughter "playing doctor" with several neighborhood children. Although this event was of little consequence, the patient began to become fearful that her daughter would be molested. The patient was seen by her internist and was treated with antianxiety agents and antidepressants, but with little improvement. She sought psychiatric consultation from several clinicians, but repeated, good trials of antidepressants, antianxiety agents, and supportive psychotherapy resulted in limited improvement. After the death of her father from complications of alcoholism, the patient became more symptomatic. He had been estranged from the family since the patient was approximately 12 years of age, owing to his drinking and associated antisocial behavior.

Psychiatric hospitalization was precipitated by the patient's arrest for disorderly conduct in a nearby city. She was found in a hotel, in revealing clothing, engaged in an altercation with a man. She denied knowledge of how she had come to the hotel, although the man insisted that she had come there under a different name for a voluntary sexual encounter.

On psychiatric examination, the patient described dense amnesia for the first 12 years of her life, with the feeling that her "life started at 12 years old." She reported that, for as long as she could remember, she had an imaginary companion, an elderly black woman, who advised her and kept her company. She reported hearing other voices in her head: several women and children, as well as her father's voice repeatedly speaking to her in a derogatory way. She reported that much of her life since 12 years of age was also punctuated by episodes of amnesia: for work, for her marriage, for the birth of her children, and for her sex life with her husband. She reported perplexing changes in skills; for example, she was often told that she played the piano well but had no conscious awareness that she could do so. Her husband reported that she had always been "forgetful" of conversations and family activities. He also noted that, at times, she would speak like a child; at times, she would adopt a southern accent; and, at other times, she would be angry and provocative. She frequently had little recall of these episodes.

Questioned more closely about her early life, the patient appeared to enter a trance and stated, "I just don't want to be locked in the closet" in a child-like voice. Inquiry about this produced rapid shifts in state between alter identities who differed in manifested age, facial expression, voice tone, and knowledge of the patient's history. One spoke in an angry, expletive-filled manner and appeared irritable and preoccupied with sexuality. She discussed the episode with the man in the hotel and stated that it was she who had arranged it. Gradually, the alters described a history of family chaos, brutality, and neglect during the first 12 years of the patient's life, until her mother, also alcoholic, achieved sobriety and fled her husband, taking her children with her. The patient, in the alter identities, described episodes of physical abuse, sexual abuse, and emotional torment by the father, her siblings, and her mother.

After assessment of family members, the patient's mother also met diagnostic criteria for dissociative identity disorder, as did her older sister, who also had been molested. A brother met diagnostic criteria for PTSD, major depression, and alcohol dependence. *(Adapted from a case of Richard J. Loewenstein, M.D. and Frank W. Putnam, M.D.)*

Dissociative Alterations in Identity. Clinically, dissociative alterations in identity may first be manifested by odd first-person plural or third-person singular or plural self-references. In addition, patients may refer to themselves using their own first names or make depersonalized self-references, such as "the body," when describing themselves and others. Patients often describe a profound sense of concretized internal division or personified internal conflicts between parts of themselves. In some instances, these parts may have proper names or may be designated by their predominate affect or function, for example, "the angry one" or "the wife." Patients may suddenly change the way in which they refer to others, for example, "the son" instead of "my son."

Other Associated Symptoms. Most patients with dissociative identity disorder meet criteria for a mood disorder, usually one of the depression spectrum disorders. Frequent, rapid mood swings are common, but these are usually caused by posttraumatic and dissociative phenomena, not a true cyclic mood disorder. Considerable overlap may exist between PTSD symptoms of anxiety, disturbed sleep, and dysphoria and mood disorder symptoms.

Obsessive-compulsive personality traits are common in dissociative identity disorder, and intercurrent obsessive-compulsive disorder (OCD) symptoms are regularly found in patients with dissociative identity disorder, with a subgroup manifesting severe OCD symptoms. OCD symptoms commonly have a posttraumatic quality: checking repeatedly to be sure that no one can enter the house or the bedroom, compulsive washing to relieve a feeling of being dirty because of abuse, and repetitive counting or singing in the mind to distract from anxiety over being abused, for example.

Child and Adolescent Presentations. Children and adolescents manifest the same core dissociative symptoms and secondary clinical phenomena as adults. Age-related differences in autonomy and lifestyle, however, may significantly influence the clinical expression of dissociative symptoms in youth. Younger children, in particular, have a less linear and less continuous sense of time and often are not able to self-identify dissociative discontinuities in their behavior. Often additional informants, such as teachers and relatives, are available to help document dissociative behaviors.

A number of normal childhood phenomena, such as imaginary companionship and elaborated daydreams, must be carefully differentiated from pathological dissociation in younger children. The clinical presentation may be that of an elaborated or autonomous imaginary companionship, with the imaginary companions taking control of the child's behavior, often experienced through passive influence experiences or auditory pseudohallucinations, or both, that command the child to behave in certain ways.

Differential Diagnosis

Table 9–6 lists the most common disorders that must be differentiated from dissociative identity disorder.

Factitious, Imitative, and Malingered Dissociative Identity Disorder. Indicators of falsified or *imitative dissociative identity disorder* are reported to include those typical of other factitious or malingering presentations. These include symptom exaggeration, lies, use of symptoms to excuse antisocial behavior (e.g., amnesia only for bad behavior), amplification of symptoms when under observation, refusal to allow collateral contacts, legal problems, and pseudologia fantastica.

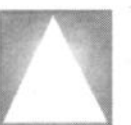

Table 9–6
Differential Diagnosis of Dissociative Identity Disorder

Comorbidity versus differential diagnosis
Affective disorders
Psychotic disorders
Anxiety disorders
Posttraumatic stress disorder
Personality disorders
Neurocognitive disorders
Neurological and seizure disorders
Somatic symptom disorders
Factitious disorders
Malingering
Other dissociative disorders
Deep-trance phenomena

Patients with genuine dissociative identity disorder are usually confused, conflicted, ashamed, and distressed by their symptoms and trauma history. Those with nongenuine disorder frequently show little dysphoria about their disorder.

Course and Prognosis

Little is known about the natural history of untreated dissociative identity disorder. Some individuals with untreated dissociative identity disorder are thought to continue involvement in abusive relationships or violent subcultures, or both, that may result in the traumatization of their children, with the potential for additional family transmission of the disorder. Many authorities believe that some percentage of patients with undiagnosed or untreated dissociative identity disorder die by suicide or as a result of their risk-taking behaviors.

Prognosis is poorer in patients with comorbid organic mental disorders, psychotic disorders (*not* dissociative identity disorder pseudopsychosis), and severe medical illnesses. Refractory substance abuse and eating disorders also suggest a poorer prognosis. Other factors that usually indicate a poorer outcome include significant antisocial personality features, current criminal activity, ongoing perpetration of abuse, and current victimization, with refusal to leave abusive relationships. Repeated adult traumas with recurrent episodes of acute stress disorder may severely complicate the clinical course.

Treatment

Psychotherapy. Successful psychotherapy for the patient with dissociative identity disorder requires the clinician to be comfortable with a range of psychotherapeutic interventions and be willing to actively work to structure the treatment. These modalities include psychoanalytic psychotherapy, cognitive therapy, behavioral therapy, hypnotherapy, and a familiarity with the psychotherapy and psychopharmacological management of the traumatized patient. Comfort with family treatment and systems theory is helpful in working with a patient who subjectively experiences himself or herself as a complex system of selves with alliances, family-like relationships, and intragroup conflict. A grounding in work with patients with somatoform disorders may also be helpful in sorting through the plethora of somatic symptoms with which these patients commonly present.

Cognitive Therapy. Many cognitive distortions associated with dissociative identity disorder are only slowly responsive to cognitive therapy techniques, and successful cognitive interventions may lead to additional dysphoria. A subgroup of patients with dissociative identity disorder does not progress beyond a long-term supportive treatment entirely directed toward stabilization of their multiple multiaxial difficulties. To the extent that they can be engaged in treatment at all, these patients require a long-term treatment focus on symptom containment and management of their overall life dysfunction, as would be the case with any other severely and persistently ill psychiatric patient.

Hypnosis. Hypnotherapeutic interventions can often alleviate self-destructive impulses or reduce symptoms, such as flashbacks, dissociative hallucinations, and passive-influence experiences. Teaching the patient self-hypnosis may help with crises outside of sessions. Hypnosis can be useful for accessing specific alter personality states and their sequestered affects and memories. Hypnosis is also used to create relaxed mental states in which negative life events can be examined without overwhelming anxiety. Clinicians using hypnosis should be trained in its use in general and in trauma populations. Clinicians should be aware of current controversies over the impact of hypnosis on accurate reporting of recollections and should use appropriate informed consent for its use.

Psychopharmacological Interventions. Antidepressant medications are often important in the reduction of depression and stabilization of mood. A variety of PTSD symptoms, especially intrusive and hyperarousal symptoms, are partially medication responsive. Clinicians report some success with SSRI, tricyclic, and monoamine oxidase (MAO) antidepressants, β-blockers, clonidine (Catapres), anticonvulsants, and benzodiazepines in reducing intrusive symptoms, hyperarousal, and anxiety in patients with dissociative identity disorder. Recent research suggests that the α_1-adrenergic antagonist prazosin (Minipress) may be helpful for PTSD nightmares. Case reports suggest that aggression may respond to carbamazepine (Tegretol) in some individuals if EEG abnormalities are present. Patients with obsessive-compulsive symptoms may respond to antidepressants with antiobsessive efficacy. Open-label studies suggest that naltrexone (ReVia) may be helpful for amelioration of recurrent self-injurious behaviors in a subset of traumatized patients.

The atypical neuroleptics, such as risperidone (Risperdal), quetiapine (Seroquel), ziprasidone (Geodon), and olanzapine (Zyprexa), may be more effective and better tolerated than typical neuroleptics for overwhelming anxiety and intrusive PTSD symptoms in patients with dissociative identity disorder. Occasionally, an extremely disorganized, overwhelmed, chronically ill patient with dissociative identity disorder, who has not responded to trials of other neuroleptics, responds favorably to a trial of clozapine (Clozaril).

Electroconvulsive Therapy. For some patients, ECT is helpful in ameliorating refractory mood disorders and does not worsen dissociative memory problems. Clinical experience in tertiary care settings for severely ill patients with dissociative identity disorder suggests that a clinical picture of major depression with persistent, refractory melancholic features across all alter states may predict a positive response to ECT. This response is usually only partial, however, as is typical for most successful somatic treatments in the dissociative identity disorder population.

Target symptoms and somatic treatments for dissociative identity disorder are listed in Table 9–7.

Adjunctive Treatments

Group Therapy. In therapy groups including general psychiatric patients, the emergence of alter personalities can be disruptive to the group process by eliciting excess fascination or by frightening other patients. Therapy groups composed only of patients with dissociative identity disorder are reported to be more successful, although the groups must be carefully structured, must provide firm limits, and should generally focus only on here-and-now issues of coping and adaptation.

Table 9–7
Medications for Associated Symptoms in Dissociative Identity Disorder

Medications and somatic treatments for posttraumatic stress disorder (PTSD), affective disorders, anxiety disorders, and obsessive-compulsive disorder (OCD)
Selective serotonin reuptake inhibitors (no preferred agent, except for OCD symptoms)
Fluvoxamine (Luvox) (for OCD presentations)
Clomipramine (Anafranil) (for OCD presentations)
Tricyclic antidepressants
Monoamine oxidase inhibitors (if patient can reliably maintain diet safely)
Electroconvulsive therapy (for refractory depression with persistent melancholic features across all dissociative identity disorder alters)
Mood stabilizers (more useful for PTSD and anxiety than mood swings)
Divalproex (Depakote)
Lamotrigine (Lamictal)
Oral or intramuscular benzodiazepines
Medications for sleep problems
Low-dose trazodone (Desyrel)
Low-dose mirtazapine (Remeron)
Low-dose tricyclic antidepressants
Low-dose neuroleptics
Benzodiazepines (often less helpful for sleep problems in this population)
Zolpidem (Ambien)
Anticholinergic agents (diphenhydramine [Benadryl], hydroxyzine [Vistaril])
Medications for self-injury, addictions
Naltrexone (ReVia)

Family Therapy. Family or couples therapy is often important for long-term stabilization and to address pathological family and marital processes that are common in patients with dissociative identity disorder and their family members. Education of family and concerned others about dissociative identity disorder and its treatment may help family members cope more effectively with dissociative identity disorder and PTSD symptoms in their loved ones. Group interventions for education and support of family members have also been found helpful. Sex therapy may be an important part of couples' treatment, because patients with dissociative identity disorder may become intensely phobic of intimate contact for periods of time, and spouses may have little idea how to deal with this in a helpful way.

Self-Help Groups. Patients with dissociative identity disorder usually have a negative outcome to self-help groups or 12-step groups for incest survivors. A variety of problematic issues occur in these settings, including intensification of PTSD symptoms because of discussion of trauma material without clinical safeguards, exploitation of the patient with dissociative identity disorder by predatory group members, contamination of that patient's recall by group discussions of trauma, and a feeling of alienation even from these other reputed sufferers of trauma and dissociation.

Expressive and Occupational Therapies. Expressive and occupational therapies, such as art and movement therapy, have proved particularly helpful in treatment of patients with dissociative identity disorder. Art therapy may be used to help with containment and structuring of severe dissociative identity disorder and PTSD symptoms, as well as to permit these patients safer expression of thoughts, feelings, mental images, and conflicts that they have difficulty verbalizing. Movement therapy may facilitate normalization of body sense and body image for these severely traumatized patients. Occupational therapy may help the patient with focused, structured activities that can be completed successfully and may help with grounding and symptom management.

Eye Movement Desensitization and Reprocessing. Eye movement desensitization and reprocessing (EMDR) is a treatment that has recently been advocated for adjunctive treatment of PTSD. There are disagreements in the literature about the usefulness and efficacy of this modality of treatment, and published efficacy studies are discrepant. No systematic studies have been done in dissociative identity disorder patients using EMDR. Case reports suggest that some dissociative identity disorder patients may be destabilized by EMDR procedures, especially those with acutely increased PTSD and dissociative symptoms. Some authorities believe that EMDR can be used as a helpful adjunct for later phases of treatment in well-stabilized dissociative identity disorder outpatients. The International Society for the Study of Trauma and Dissociation dissociative identity disorder treatment guidelines suggest that EMDR only be used in this patient population by clinicians who have taken advanced EMDR training, are knowledgeable and skilled in phasic trauma treatment for dissociative disorders, and have received supervision in the use of EMDR in dissociative identity disorder.

OTHER SPECIFIED OR UNSPECIFIED DISSOCIATIVE DISORDER

The category of dissociative disorder covers all of the conditions characterized by a primary dissociative response that do not meet diagnostic criteria for one of the other DSM-5 dissociative disorders.

Dissociative Trance Disorder

Dissociative trance disorder is manifest by a temporary, marked alteration in the state of consciousness or by loss of the customary sense of personal identity without the replacement by an alternate sense of identity. A variant of this, possession trance, involves single or episodic alternations in the state of consciousness, characterized by the exchange of the person's customary identity with a new identity usually attributed to a spirit, divine power, deity, or another person. In this possessed state, the individual exhibits stereotypical and culturally determined behaviors or experiences being controlled by the possessing entity. There must be partial or full amnesia for the event. The trance or possession state must not be a normally accepted part of a cultural or religious practice and must cause significant distress or functional impairment in one or more of the usual domains. Finally, the dissociative trance state must not occur exclusively during the course of a psychotic disorder and is not the result of any substance use or general medical condition.

Brainwashing

DSM-5 describes this dissociative disorder as "identity disturbance due to prolonged and intense coercive persuasion." Brainwashing occurs largely in the setting of political reform, as has been described at length with the Cultural Revolution in communist China, war imprisonment, torture of political dissidents, terrorist hostages, and, more familiarly in Western culture, totalitarian cult indoctrination. It implies that under conditions of adequate stress and duress, individuals can be made to comply with the demands of those in power, thereby undergoing major changes in their personality, beliefs, and behaviors. Persons subjected to such conditions can undergo considerable harm, including loss of health and life, and they typically manifest a variety of posttraumatic and dissociative symptoms.

The first stage in coercive processes has been likened to the artificial creation of an identity crisis, with the emergence of a new pseudoidentity that manifests characteristics of a dissociative state. Under circumstances of extreme and malignant dependency, overwhelming vulnerability, and danger to one's existence, individuals develop a state characterized by extreme idealization of their captors, with ensuing identification with the aggressor and externalization of their superego, regressive adaptation known as *traumatic infantilism,* paralysis of will, and a state of frozen fright. The coercive techniques that are typically used to induce such a state in the victim have been amply described and include isolation of the subject, degradation, control over all communications and basic daily functions, induction of fear and confusion, peer pressure, assignment of repetitive and monotonous routines, unpredictability of environmental supplies, renunciation of past relationships and values, and various deprivations. Even though physical or sexual abuse, torture, and extreme sensory deprivation and physical neglect can be part of this process, they are not required to define a coercive process. As a result, victims manifest extensive posttraumatic and dissociative symptomatology, including drastic alteration of their identity, values, and beliefs; reduction of cognitive flexibility with regression to simplistic perceptions of good versus evil and dominance versus submission; numbing of experience and blunting of affect; trance-like states and diminished environmental responsiveness; and, in some cases, more severe dissociative symptoms such as amnesia, depersonalization, and shifts in identity.

The treatment of victims of coercion can vary considerably, depending on their particular background, the circumstances involved, and the setting in which help is sought. Although no systematic studies exist in this domain, basic principles involve validation of the traumatic experience and coercive techniques used, cognitive reframing of the events that transpired, exploration of preexisting psychopathology and vulnerabilities (when applicable), and general techniques used in treating posttraumatic and dissociative states. In addition, family interventions and therapy may be required, at least in cases of cult indoctrination, because significant family duress and disruption commonly occur.

Recovered Memory Syndrome

Under hypnosis or during psychotherapy, a patient may recover a memory of a painful experience or conflict—particularly of sexual or physical abuse—that is etiologically significant. When the repressed material is brought back to consciousness, the person not only may recall the experience but may relive it, accompanied by the appropriate affective response (a process called *abreaction*). If the event recalled never really happened but the person believes it to be true and reacts accordingly, it is known as *false memory syndrome.*

The syndrome has led to lawsuits involving accusations of child abuse. However, Thomas E. Gutheil describes memory as a "slender reed—insufficiently strong to bear the weight of a court case." Even if the memory of abuse is real, the perpetrator is not the present person, but the person of the past. Gutheil does not believe that litigation usually serves the patient's psychological goals. Clinical attention should probably be directed toward helping patients cast aside the limiting restrictive role of victim and transcend their past traumas, work through them, and try to get on with their lives.

Ganser Syndrome

Ganser syndrome is a poorly understood condition characterized by the giving of approximate answers (paralogia) together with a clouding of consciousness and is frequently accompanied by hallucinations and other dissociative, somatoform, or conversion symptoms.

Epidemiology. Cases have been reported in a variety of cultures, but the overall frequency of such reports has declined with time. Men outnumber women by approximately 2 to 1. Three of Ganser's first four cases were convicts, leading some authors to consider it to be a disorder of penal populations and, thus, an indicator of potential malingering.

Etiology. Some case reports identify precipitating stressors, such as personal conflicts and financial reverses, whereas others note organic brain syndromes, head injuries, seizures, and medical or psychiatric illness. Psychodynamic explanations are common in the older literature, but organic etiologies are stressed in more recent case studies. It is speculated that the organic insults may act as acute stressors, precipitating the syndrome in vulnerable individuals. Some patients have reported significant histories of childhood maltreatment and adversity.

Diagnosis and Clinical Features. The symptom of *passing over* (*vorbeigehen*) the correct answer for a related, but incorrect one, is the hallmark of Ganser syndrome. The approximate answers often just miss the mark but bear an obvious relation to the question, indicating that it has been understood. When asked how old she was, a 25-year-old woman answered, "I'm not five." If asked to do simple calculations (e.g., 2 + 2 = 5); for general information (the capital of the United States is New York); to identify simple objects (a pencil is a key); or to name colors (green is gray), the patient with Ganser syndrome gives erroneous but comprehensible answers.

A clouding of consciousness also occurs, usually manifest by disorientation, amnesias, loss of personal information, and some impairment of reality testing. Visual and auditory hallucinations occur in roughly one-half of the cases. Neurological examination may reveal what Ganser called *hysterical stigmata,* for example, a nonneurological analgesia or shifting hyperalgesia. It must be accompanied by other dissociative symptoms, such as amnesias, conversion symptoms, or trance-like behaviors.

Differential Diagnosis. Given the reported frequent history of organic brain syndromes, seizures, head trauma, and psychosis in Ganser syndrome, a thorough neurological and medical evaluation is warranted. Differential diagnoses include organic dementia, depressive pseudodementia, confabulation of Korsakoff's syndrome, organic dysphasias, and reactive psychoses. Patients with dissociative identity disorder occasionally may also exhibit Ganser-like symptoms.

Treatment. No systematic treatment studies have been conducted, given the rarity of this condition. In most case reports, the patient has been hospitalized and has been provided with a protective and supportive environment. In some instances, low doses of antipsychotic medications have been reported to be beneficial. Confrontation or interpretations of the patient's approximate answers are not productive, but exploration of possible stressors may be helpful. Hypnosis and amobarbital narcosynthesis have also been used successfully to help patients reveal the underlying stressors that preceded the development of the syndrome, with concomitant cessation of the Ganser symptoms. Usually, a relatively rapid return to normal function occurs within days, although some cases may take a month or more to resolve. The individual is typically amnesic for the period of the syndrome.

10 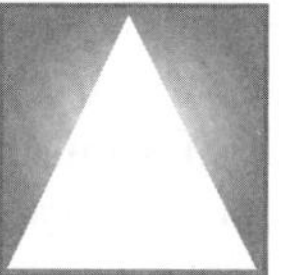

Somatic Symptom and Related Disorders

▲ 10.1 Somatic Symptom Disorder

Somatic symptom disorder, also known as hypochondriasis, is characterized by 6 or more months of a general and nondelusional preoccupation with fears of having, or the idea that one has, a serious disease based on the person's misinterpretation of bodily symptoms. This preoccupation causes significant distress and impairment in one's life; it is not accounted for by another psychiatric or medical disorder; and a subset of individuals with somatic symptom disorder has poor insight about the presence of this disorder.

EPIDEMIOLOGY

In general medical clinic populations, the reported 6-month prevalence of this disorder is 4 to 6 percent, but it may be as high as 15 percent. Men and women are equally affected by this disorder. There are some reports of women having more somatic complaints than men, however. Although the onset of symptoms can occur at any age, the disorder most commonly appears in persons 20 to 30 years of age. Some evidence indicates that this diagnosis is more common among blacks than among whites, but social position, education level, gender, and marital status do not appear to affect the diagnosis. This disorder's complaints reportedly occur in about 3 percent of medical students, usually in the first 2 years, but they are generally transient.

ETIOLOGY

Persons with this disorder augment and amplify their somatic sensations; they have low thresholds for, and low tolerance of, physical discomfort. For example, what persons normally perceive as abdominal pressure, persons with somatic symptom disorder experience as abdominal pain. They may focus on bodily sensations, misinterpret them, and become alarmed by them because of a faulty cognitive scheme.

Somatic symptom disorder can also be understood in terms of a social learning model. The symptoms of this disorder are viewed as a request for admission to the sick role made by a person facing seemingly insurmountable and insolvable problems. The sick role offers an escape that allows a patient to avoid noxious obligations, to postpone unwelcome challenges, and to be excused from usual duties and obligations.

Somatic symptom disorder is sometimes a variant form of other mental disorders, among which depressive disorders and anxiety disorders are most frequently included. An estimated 80 percent of patients with this disorder may have coexisting depressive or anxiety disorders. Patients who meet the diagnostic criteria for somatic symptom disorder may be somatizing subtypes of these other disorders.

The psychodynamic school of thought holds that aggressive and hostile wishes toward others are transferred (through repression and displacement) into physical complaints. The anger of patients with this disorder originates in past disappointments, rejections, and losses, but the patients express their anger in the present by soliciting the help and concern of other persons and then rejecting them as ineffective.

This disorder is also viewed as a defense against guilt, a sense of innate badness, an expression of low self-esteem, and a sign of excessive self-concern. Pain and somatic suffering thus become means of atonement and expiation (undoing) and can be experienced as deserved punishment for past wrongdoing (either real or imaginary) and for a person's sense of wickedness and sinfulness.

DIAGNOSIS

According to the fifth edition of *Diagnostic and Statistical Manual of Mental Disorders* (DSM-5), the diagnostic criteria for somatic symptom disorder require that patients be preoccupied with the false belief that they have a serious disease, based on their misinterpretation of physical signs or sensations the belief must last at least 6 months, despite the absence of pathological findings on medical and neurological examinations. The diagnostic criteria also require that the belief cannot have the intensity of a delusion (more appropriately diagnosed as delusional disorder) and cannot be restricted to distress about appearance (more appropriately diagnosed as body dysmorphic disorder). The symptoms of somatic symptom disorder must be sufficiently intense to cause emotional distress or impair the patient's ability to function in important areas of life. Clinicians may specify the presence of poor insight; patients do not consistently recognize that their concerns about disease are excessive.

CLINICAL FEATURES

Patients with somatic symptom disorder believe that they have a serious disease that has not yet been detected and they cannot be persuaded to the contrary. They may maintain a belief that they have a particular disease or, as time progresses, they may transfer their belief to another disease. Their convictions persist despite negative laboratory results, the benign course of the alleged disease over time, and appropriate reassurances from physicians. Yet, their beliefs are not sufficiently fixed to be delusions. Somatic symptom disorder is often accompanied by symptoms of depression and anxiety and commonly coexists with a depressive or anxiety disorder.

A severe case of somatic symptom disorder that highlights diagnostic, prognostic, and management issues is described in the case study.

Mr. K, a white man in his mid-30s, consulted a general medicine clinic complaining of gastrointestinal problems. Major presenting symptoms were a long list of physical symptoms and concerns mostly related to the gastrointestinal system. These included abdominal pain, left lower quadrant cramps, bloating, persistent sense of fullness in stomach hours after eating, intolerance to foods, constipation, decrease in physical stamina, heart palpitations, and feelings that "skin is getting yellow" and "not getting enough oxygen." A review of systems disclosed disturbances from virtually every organ system, including tired eyes with blurred vision, sore throat and "lump" in throat, heart palpitations, irregular heartbeat, dizziness, trouble breathing, and general weakness.

The patient reported that symptoms started prior to the age of 30 years. For more than a decade, he had been seen by psychiatrists, general practitioners, and all kinds of medical specialists, including surgeons. He used the Internet constantly and traveled extensively in search of expert evaluations, seeking new procedures and diagnostic assessments. He had undergone repeated colonoscopies, sigmoidoscopies, and computed tomographic (CT) scans, magnetic resonance imaging (MRI) studies, and ultrasound examinations of the abdomen that had failed to disclose any pathology. He was on disability and had been unable to work for more than 2 years due to his condition.

About 3 years before his visit to the medicine clinic, his abdominal complaints and his fixed belief that he had an intestinal obstruction led to an exploratory surgical intervention for the first time, apparently with negative findings. However, according to the patient, the surgery "got things even worse," and since then he had been operated on at least five other occasions. During these surgeries he has undergone subtotal colectomies and ileostomies due to possible "adhesions" to rule out "mechanical" obstruction. However, available records from some of the surgeries do not disclose any specific pathology other than "intractable constipation." Pathological specimens were also inconclusive.

The physical examination showed a well-developed, well-nourished male, who was afebrile. A complete physical and neurological examination was normal except for examination of the abdomen, which revealed multiple abdominal scars. Right ileostomy was present, with soft stool in the bag and active bowel sounds. There was no point tenderness and no abdominal distension. During the examination, the patient kept pointing to an area of "hardness" in the left lower quadrant that he thought was a "tight muscle strangling his bowels." However, the examination did not disclose any palpable mass. Skin and extremities were all within normal limits, and all joints had full range of motion and no swelling. Musculature was well-developed. Neurological examination was within normal limits. The patient was scheduled for brief monthly visits by the primary care physician, during which the doctor performed brief physicals, reassured the patient, and allowed the patient to talk about "stressors." The physician avoided invasive tests or diagnostic procedures, did not prescribe any medications, and avoided telling the patient that the symptoms were mental or "all in his head." The primary care physician then referred the patient back to psychiatry.

The psychiatrist confirmed a long list of physical symptoms that started before the age of 30 years, most of which remained medically unexplained. The psychiatric examination revealed some anxiety symptoms, including apprehension, tension, uneasiness, and somatic components such as blushing and palpitations that seemed particularly prominent in front of social situations. Possible symptoms of depression included mild dysphoria, low energy, and sleep disturbance, all of which the patient blamed on his "medical" problems. The mental status examination showed that Mr. K's mood was rather somber and pessimistic, although he denied feeling sad or depressed. Affect was irritable. He was somatically focused and had little if any psychological insight. The examination revealed the presence of a few life stressors (unemployment, financial problems, and family issues) that the patient quickly discounted as unimportant. Although the patient continued to deny having any psychiatric problems or any need for psychiatric intervention or treatment, he agreed to a few regular visits to continue to assess his situation. He refused to engage anyone from his family in this process. Efforts to engage the patient with formal therapy such as cognitive–behavioral therapy (CBT) or a medication trial were all futile, so he was seen only for "supportive psychotherapy," with the hope of developing rapport and preventing additional iatrogenic complications.

During the follow-up period, the patient was operated on at least one more time and continued to complain of abdominal bloating and constipation and to rely on laxatives. The belief that there was a mechanical obstruction of the intestines continued to be firmly held by the patient and bordered on the delusional. However, he continued to refuse pharmacological treatment. The only medication he accepted was a low-dose benzodiazepine for anxiety. He continued to monitor his intestinal function 24 hours per day and to seek evaluation by prominent specialists, traveling to high-profile specialty centers far from home in search of solutions. *(Courtesy of J. I. Escobar, M.D.)*

Although DSM-5 specifies that the symptoms must be present for at least 6 months, transient manifestations can occur after major stresses, most commonly the death or serious illness of someone important to the patient or a serious (perhaps life-threatening) illness that has been resolved but that leaves the patient temporarily affected in its wake. Such states that last fewer than 6 months are diagnosed as "Other Specified Somatic Symptom and Related Disorders" in DSM-5. Transient somatic symptom disorder responses to external stress generally remit when the stress is resolved, but they can become chronic if reinforced by persons in the patient's social system or by health professionals.

DIFFERENTIAL DIAGNOSIS

Somatic symptom disorder must be differentiated from nonpsychiatric medical conditions, especially disorders that show symptoms that are not necessarily easily diagnosed. Such diseases include acquired immunodeficiency syndrome (AIDS), endocrinopathies, myasthenia gravis, multiple sclerosis, degenerative diseases of the nervous system, systemic lupus erythematosus, and occult neoplastic disorders.

Somatic symptom disorder is differentiated from illness anxiety disorder by the emphasis in illness anxiety disorder on fear of having a disease rather than a concern about many symptoms. Patients with illness anxiety disorder usually complain about fewer symptoms than patients with somatic symptom disorder; they are primarily concerned about being sick.

Conversion disorder is acute and generally transient and usually involves a symptom rather than a particular disease. The presence or absence of *la belle indifférence* is an unreliable feature with which to differentiate the two conditions. Patients with body dysmorphic disorder wish to appear normal, but believe that others notice that they are not, whereas those with somatic symptom disorder seek out attention for their presumed diseases.

Somatic symptom disorder can also occur in patients with depressive disorders and anxiety disorders. Patients with panic disorder may initially complain that they are affected by a disease (e.g., heart trouble), but careful questioning during the medical history usually uncovers the classic symptoms of a panic attack. Delusional disorder beliefs occur in schizophrenia and other psychotic disorders, but can be differentiated from somatic symptom disorder by their delusional intensity and by the presence of other psychotic symptoms. In addition, schizophrenic patients' somatic delusions tend to be bizarre, idiosyncratic, and out of keeping with their cultural milieus, as illustrated in the case below.

A 52-year-old man complained "my guts are rotting away." Even after an extensive medical workup, he could not be reassured that he was not ill.

Somatic symptom disorder is distinguished from factitious disorder with physical symptoms and from malingering in that patients with somatic symptom disorder actually experience and do not simulate the symptoms they report.

COURSE AND PROGNOSIS

The course of the disorder is usually episodic; the episodes last from months to years and are separated by equally long quiescent periods. There may be an obvious association between exacerbations of somatic symptoms and psychosocial stressors. Although no well-conducted large outcome studies have been reported, an estimated one-third to one-half of all patients with somatic symptom disorder eventually improve significantly. A good prognosis is associated with high socioeconomic status, treatment-responsive anxiety or depression, sudden onset of symptoms, the absence of a personality disorder, and the absence of a related nonpsychiatric medical condition. Most children with the disorder recover by late adolescence or early adulthood.

TREATMENT

Patients with somatic symptom disorder usually resist psychiatric treatment, although some accept this treatment if it takes place in a medical setting and focuses on stress reduction and education in coping with chronic illness. Group psychotherapy often benefits such patients, in part because it provides the social support and social interaction that seem to reduce their anxiety. Other forms of psychotherapy, such as individual insight-oriented psychotherapy, behavior therapy, cognitive therapy, and hypnosis, may be useful.

Frequent, regularly scheduled physical examinations help to reassure patients that their physicians are not abandoning them and that their complaints are being taken seriously. Invasive diagnostic and therapeutic procedures should only be undertaken, however, when objective evidence calls for them. When possible, the clinician should refrain from treating equivocal or incidental physical examination findings.

Pharmacotherapy alleviates somatic symptom disorder only when a patient has an underlying drug-responsive condition, such as an anxiety disorder or depressive disorder. When somatic symptom disorder is secondary to another primary mental disorder, that disorder must be treated in its own right. When the disorder is a transient situational reaction, clinicians must help patients cope with the stress without reinforcing their illness behavior and their use of the sick role as a solution to their problems.

▲ 10.2 Illness Anxiety Disorder

Illness anxiety disorder is a new diagnosis in the fifth edition of *Diagnostic and Statistical Manual of Mental Disorders* (DSM-5) that applies to those persons who are preoccupied with being sick or with developing a disease of some kind. It is a variant of somatic symptom disorder (hypochondriasis). As stated in DSM-5: Most individuals with hypochondriasis are now classified as having somatic symptom disorder; however, in a minority of cases, the diagnosis of illness anxiety disorder applies instead. In describing the differential diagnosis between the two, according to DSM-5, somatic symptom disorder is diagnosed when somatic symptoms are present, whereas in illness anxiety disorder, there are few or no somatic symptoms and persons are "primarily concerned with the idea they are ill." The diagnosis may also be used for persons who do, in fact, have a medical illness but whose anxiety is out of proportion to their diagnosis and who assume the worst possible outcome imaginable.

EPIDEMIOLOGY

The prevalence of this disorder is unknown aside from using data that relate to hypochondriasis, which gives a prevalence of 4 to 6 percent in a general medical clinic population. In other surveys, up to 15 percent of persons in the general population worry about becoming sick and incapacitated as a result. One might expect the disorder to be diagnosed more frequently in older rather than younger persons. There is no evidence to date that the diagnosis is more common among different races or that gender, social position, education level, and marital status affect the diagnosis.

ETIOLOGY

The etiology is unknown. The social learning model described for somatic symptom disorder may apply to this disorder as well. In that construct, the fear of illness is viewed as a request to play the sick role made by someone facing seemingly insurmountable and insolvable problems. The sick role offers an escape that allows a patient to be excused from usual duties and obligations.

The psychodynamic school of thought is also similar to somatic symptom disorder. Aggressive and hostile wishes toward others are transferred into minor physical complaints or the fear of physical illness. The anger of patients with illness anxiety disorder, as in those with hypochondriasis, originates in past disappointments, rejections, and losses. Similarly, the fear of illness is also viewed as a defense against guilt, a sense of innate badness, an expression of low self-esteem, and a sign of excessive self-concern. The feared illness may also be seen as punishment for past either real or imaginary wrongdoing. The nature of the person's relationships to significant others in his or her past life may also be significant. A parent who died from a specific illness, for example, might be the stimulus for the fear of developing that illness in the offspring of that parent. The type of the fear may also be symbolic of unconscious conflicts that are reflected in the type of illness of which the person is afraid or the organ system selected (e.g., heart, kidney).

DIAGNOSIS

The major DSM-5 diagnostic criteria for illness anxiety disorder are that patients be preoccupied with the false belief that they have or will develop a serious disease and there are few if any physical signs or symptoms. The belief must last at least 6 months, and there are no pathological findings in medical or neurological examinations. The belief cannot have the fixity of a delusion (more appropriately diagnosed as delusional disorder) and cannot be distress about appearance (more appropriately diagnosed as body dysmorphic disorder). The anxiety about illness must be incapacitating and cause emotional distress or impair the patient's ability to function in important areas of life. Some persons with the disorder may visit physicians (care-seeking type) while others may not (care-avoidant type). The majority of patients, however, make repeated visits to physicians and other health care providers.

CLINICAL FEATURES

Patients with illness anxiety disorder, like those with somatic symptom disorder, believe that they have a serious disease that has not yet been diagnosed, and they cannot be persuaded to the contrary. They may maintain a belief that they have a particular disease or, as time progresses, they may transfer their belief to another disease. Their convictions persist despite negative laboratory results, the benign course of the alleged disease over time, and appropriate reassurances from physicians. Their preoccupation with illness interferes with their interaction with family, friends, and coworkers. They are often addicted to Internet searches about their feared illness, inferring the worst from information (or misinformation) they find there.

DIFFERENTIAL DIAGNOSIS

Illness anxiety disorder must be differentiated from other medical conditions. Too often these patients are dismissed as "chronic complainers" and careful medical examinations are not performed. Patients with illness anxiety disorder are differentiated from those with somatic symptom disorder by the emphasis in illness anxiety disorder on fear of having a disease versus the emphasis in somatic symptom disorder on concern about many symptoms; but both may exist to varying degrees in each disorder. Patients with illness anxiety disorder usually complain about fewer symptoms than patients with somatic symptom disorder. Somatic symptom disorder usually has an onset before age 30, whereas illness anxiety disorder has a less specific age of onset. Conversion disorder is acute, generally transient, and usually involves a symptom rather than a particular disease. Pain disorder is chronic, as is hypochondriasis, but the symptoms are limited to complaints of pain. The fear of illness can also occur in patients with depressive and anxiety disorders. If a patient meets the full diagnostic criteria for both illness anxiety disorder and another major mental disorder, such as major depressive disorder or generalized anxiety disorder, the patient should receive both diagnoses. Patients with panic disorder may initially complain that they are affected by a disease (e.g., heart trouble), but careful questioning during the medical history usually uncovers the classic symptoms of a panic attack. Delusional beliefs occur in schizophrenia and other psychotic disorders but can be differentiated from illness anxiety disorder by their delusional intensity and by the presence of other psychotic symptoms. In addition, schizophrenic patients' somatic delusions tend to be bizarre, idiosyncratic, and out of keeping with their cultural milieus.

Illness anxiety disorder can be differentiated from obsessive-compulsive disorder by the singularity of their beliefs and by the absence of compulsive behavioral traits; but there is often an obsessive quality to the patients fear.

COURSE AND PROGNOSIS

Because the disorder is only recently described, there are no reliable data about the prognosis. One may extrapolate from the course of somatic symptom disorder, which is usually episodic; the episodes last from months to years and are separated by equally long quiescent periods. As with hypochondriasis, a good prognosis is associated with high socioeconomic status, treatment-responsive anxiety or depression, sudden onset of symptoms, the absence of a personality disorder, and the absence of a related nonpsychiatric medical condition.

TREATMENT

As with somatic symptom disorder, patients with illness anxiety disorder usually resist psychiatric treatment, although some accept this treatment if it takes place in a medical setting and focuses on stress reduction and education in coping with chronic illness. Group psychotherapy may be of help especially if the group is homogeneous with patients suffering from the same disorder. Other forms of psychotherapy, such as individual insight-oriented psychotherapy, behavior therapy, cognitive therapy, and hypnosis, may be useful.

The role of frequent, regularly scheduled physical examinations is controversial. Some patients may benefit from being reassured that their complaints are being taken seriously and that they do not have the illness of which they are afraid. Others, however, are resistant to seeing a doctor in the first place, or, if having done so, of accepting the fact that there is nothing to worry about. Invasive diagnostic and therapeutic procedures should only be undertaken when objective evidence calls for them. When possible, the clinician should refrain from treating equivocal or incidental physical examination findings.

Pharmacotherapy may be of help in alleviating the anxiety generated by the fear that the patient has about illness, especially if it is one that is life-threatening; but it is only ameliorative and cannot provide lasting relief. That can only come from an effective psychotherapeutic program that is acceptable to the patient and in which he or she is willing and able to participate.

▲ 10.3 Functional Neurological Symptom Disorder (Conversion Disorder)

Conversion disorder, also called functional neurological symptom disorder in the *Diagnostic and Statistical Manual of Mental Disorders,* fifth edition (DSM-5), is an illness of symptoms or deficits that affect voluntary motor or sensory functions, which suggest another medical condition, but that is judged to be caused by psychological factors because the illness is preceded by conflicts or other stressors. The symptoms or deficits of conversion disorder are not intentionally produced, are not caused by substance use, are not limited to pain or sexual symptoms, and the gain is primarily psychological and not social, monetary, or legal.

The syndrome currently known as *conversion disorder* was originally combined with the syndrome known as *somatization disorder* and was referred to as hysteria, conversion reaction, or dissociative reaction. Paul Briquet and Jean-Martin Charcot contributed to the development of the concept of conversion disorder by noting the influence of heredity on the symptom and the common association with a traumatic event. The term conversion was introduced by Sigmund Freud, who, based on his work with Anna O, hypothesized that the symptoms of conversion disorder reflect unconscious conflicts.

EPIDEMIOLOGY

Some symptoms of conversion disorder that are not sufficiently severe to warrant the diagnosis may occur in up to one-third of the general population sometime during their lives. Reported rates of conversion disorder vary from 11 of 100,000 to 300 of 100,000 in general population samples. Among specific populations, the occurrence of conversion disorder may be even higher than that, perhaps making conversion disorder the most common somatoform disorder in some populations. Several studies have reported that 5 to 15 percent of psychiatric consultations in a general hospital and 25 to 30 percent of admissions to a Veterans Administration hospital involve patients with conversion disorder diagnoses.

The ratio of women to men among adult patients is at least 2 to 1 and as much as 10 to 1; among children, an even higher predominance is seen in girls. Symptoms are more common on the left than on the right side of the body in women. Women who present with conversion symptoms are more likely subsequently to develop somatization disorder than women who have not had conversion symptoms. An association exists between conversion disorder and antisocial personality disorder in men. Men with conversion disorder have often been involved in occupational or military accidents. The onset of conversion disorder is generally from late childhood to early adulthood and is rare before 10 years of age or after 35 years of age, but onset as late as the ninth decade of life has been reported. When symptoms suggest a conversion disorder onset in middle or old age, the probability of an occult neurological or other medical condition is high. Conversion symptoms in children younger than 10 years of age are usually limited to gait problems or seizures.

Data indicate that conversion disorder is most common among rural populations, persons with little education, those with low intelligence quotients, those in low socioeconomic groups, and military personnel who have been exposed to combat situations. Conversion disorder is commonly associated with comorbid diagnoses of major depressive disorder, anxiety disorders, and schizophrenia and shows an increased frequency in relatives of probands with conversion disorder. Limited data suggest that conversion symptoms are more frequent in relatives of people with conversion disorder. An increased risk of conversion disorder in monozygotic, but not dizygotic, twin pairs has been reported.

COMORBIDITY

Medical and, especially, neurological disorders occur frequently among patients with conversion disorders. What is typically seen in these comorbid neurological or medical conditions is an elaboration of symptoms stemming from the original organic lesion.

Depressive disorders, anxiety disorders, and somatization disorders are especially noted for their association with conversion disorder. Conversion disorder in schizophrenia is reported, but it is uncommon. Studies of patients admitted to a psychiatric hospital for conversion disorder reveal, on further study, that one-quarter to one-half have a clinically significant mood disorder or schizophrenia.

Personality disorders also frequently accompany conversion disorder, especially the histrionic type (in 5 to 21 percent of cases) and the passive-dependent type (9 to 40 percent of cases). Conversion disorders can occur, however, in persons with no predisposing medical, neurological, or psychiatric disorder.

ETIOLOGY

Psychoanalytic Factors

According to psychoanalytic theory, conversion disorder is caused by repression of unconscious intrapsychic conflict and conversion of anxiety into a physical symptom. The conflict is between an instinctual impulse (e.g., aggression or sexuality) and the prohibitions against its expression. The symptoms allow partial expression of the forbidden wish or urge but disguise it, so that patients can avoid consciously confronting their unacceptable impulses; that is, the conversion disorder symptom has a symbolic relation to the unconscious conflict—for example, vaginismus protects the patient from expressing unacceptable sexual wishes. Conversion disorder symptoms also allow patients to communicate that they need special consideration and special treatment. Such symptoms may function as nonverbal means of controlling or manipulating others.

Learning Theory

In terms of conditioned learning theory, a conversion symptom can be seen as a piece of classically conditioned learned behavior; symptoms of illness, learned in childhood, are called forth as a means of coping with an otherwise impossible situation.

Biological Factors

Increasing data implicate biological and neuropsychological factors in the development of conversion disorder symptoms. Preliminary brain-imaging studies have found hypometabolism of the dominant hemisphere and hypermetabolism of the nondominant hemisphere and have implicated impaired hemispheric communication in the cause of conversion disorder. The symptoms may be caused by an excessive cortical arousal that sets off negative feedback loops between the cerebral cortex and the brainstem reticular formation. Elevated levels of corticofugal output, in turn, inhibit the patient's awareness of bodily sensation, which may explain the observed sensory deficits in some patients with conversion disorder. Neuropsychological tests sometimes reveal subtle cerebral impairments in verbal communication, memory, vigilance, affective incongruity, and attention in these patients.

DIAGNOSIS

The DSM-5 limits the diagnosis of conversion disorder to those symptoms that affect a voluntary motor or sensory function, that is, neurological symptoms. Physicians cannot explain the neurological symptoms solely on the basis of any known neurological condition.

The diagnosis of conversion disorder requires that clinicians find a necessary and critical association between the cause of the neurological symptoms and psychological factors, although the symptoms cannot result from malingering or factitious disorder. The diagnosis of conversion disorder also excludes symptoms of pain and sexual dysfunction and symptoms that occur only in somatization disorder.

DSM-5 describes several types of symptoms or deficits seen in conversion disorder. These include weakness or paralysis; abnormal movements; attacks or seizures; swallowing or speech difficulties such as slurred speech; sensory symptoms and mixed symptoms. These are discussed below.

CLINICAL FEATURES

Paralysis, blindness, and mutism are the most common conversion disorder symptoms. Conversion disorder may be most commonly associated with passive-aggressive, dependent, antisocial, and histrionic personality disorders. Depressive and anxiety disorder symptoms often accompany the symptoms of conversion disorder, and affected patients are at risk for suicide.

Mr. J is a 28-year-old single man who is employed in a factory. He was brought to an emergency department by his father, complaining that he had lost his vision while sitting in the back seat on the way home from a family gathering. He had been playing volleyball at the gathering but had sustained no significant injury except for the volleyball hitting him in the head a few times. As was usual for this man, he had been reluctant to play volleyball because of the lack of his athletic skills and was placed on a team at the last moment. He recalls having some problems with seeing during the game, but his vision did not become ablated until he was in the car on the way home. By the time he got to the emergency department, his vision was improving, although he still complained of blurriness and mild diplopia. The double vision could be attenuated by having him focus on items at different distances.

On examination, Mr. J was fully cooperative, somewhat uncertain about why this would have occurred, and rather nonchalant. Pupillary, oculomotor, and general sensorimotor examinations were normal. After being cleared medically, the patient was sent to a mental health center for further evaluation.

At the mental health center, the patient recounts the same story as he did in the emergency department, and he was still accompanied by his father. He began to recount how his vision started to return to normal when his father pulled over on the side of the road and began to talk to him about the events of the day. He spoke with his father about how he had felt embarrassed and somewhat conflicted about playing volleyball and how he had felt that he really should play because of external pressures. Further history from the patient and his father revealed that this young man had been shy as an adolescent, particularly around athletic participation. He had never had another episode of visual loss. He did recount feeling anxious and sometimes not feeling well in his body during athletic activities.

Discussion with the patient at the mental health center focused on the potential role of psychological and social factors in acute vision loss. The patient was somewhat perplexed by this but was also amenable to discussion. He stated that he clearly recognized that he began seeing and feeling better when his father pulled off to the side of the road and discussed things with him. Doctors admitted that they did not know the cause of the vision loss and that it would likely not return. The patient and his father were satisfied with the medical and psychiatric evaluation and agreed to return for care if there were any further symptoms. The patient was appointed a follow-up time at the outpatient psychiatric clinic. *(Courtesy of Michael A. Hollifield, M.D.)*

Sensory Symptoms

In conversion disorder, anesthesia and paresthesia are common, especially of the extremities. All sensory modalities can be involved, and the distribution of the disturbance is usually inconsistent with either central or peripheral neurological disease. Thus, clinicians may see the characteristic stocking-and-glove anesthesia of the hands or feet or the hemianesthesia of the body beginning precisely along the midline.

Conversion disorder symptoms may involve the organs of special sense and can produce deafness, blindness, and tunnel vision. These symptoms can be unilateral or bilateral, but neurological evaluation reveals intact sensory pathways. In conversion disorder blindness, for example, patients walk around without collisions or self-injury, their pupils react to light, and their cortical-evoked potentials are normal.

Motor Symptoms

The motor symptoms of conversion disorder include abnormal movements, gait disturbance, weakness, and paralysis. Gross rhythmical tremors, choreiform movements, tics, and jerks may be present. The movements generally worsen when attention is called to them. One gait disturbance seen in conversion disorder is *astasia-abasia,* which is a wildly ataxic, staggering gait accompanied by gross, irregular, jerky truncal movements and thrashing and waving arm movements. Patients with the symptoms rarely fall; if they do, they are generally not injured.

Other common motor disturbances are paralysis and paresis involving one, two, or all four limbs, although the distribution of the involved muscles does not conform to the neural pathways. Reflexes remain normal; the patients have no fasciculations or muscle atrophy (except after long-standing conversion paralysis); electromyography findings are normal.

Seizure Symptoms

Pseudoseizures are another symptom in conversion disorder. Clinicians may find it difficult to differentiate a pseudoseizure from an actual seizure by clinical observation alone. Moreover, about one-third of the patient's pseudoseizures also have a coexisting epileptic disorder. Tongue-biting, urinary incontinence and injuries after falling can occur in pseudoseizures, although these symptoms are generally not present. Pupillary and gag reflexes are retained after pseudoseizure, and patients have no postseizure increase in prolactin concentrations.

Other Associated Features

Several psychological symptoms have also been associated with conversion disorder.

Primary Gain. Patients achieve primary gain by keeping internal conflicts outside their awareness. Symptoms have symbolic value; they represent an unconscious psychological conflict.

Secondary Gain. Patients accrue tangible advantages and benefits as a result of being sick; for example, being excused from obligations and difficult life situations, receiving support and assistance that might not otherwise be forthcoming, and controlling other persons' behavior.

La Belle Indifférence. *La belle indifférence* is a patient's inappropriately cavalier attitude toward serious symptoms; that is, the patient seems to be unconcerned about what appears to be a major impairment. That bland indifference is also seen in some seriously ill medical patients who develop a stoic attitude. The presence or absence of *la belle indifférence* is not pathognomonic of conversion disorder, but it is often associated with the condition.

Identification. Patients with conversion disorder may unconsciously model their symptoms on those of someone important to them. For example, a parent or a person who has recently died may serve as a model for conversion disorder. During pathological grief reaction, bereaved persons commonly have symptoms of the deceased.

DIFFERENTIAL DIAGNOSIS

One of the major problems in diagnosing conversion disorder is the difficulty of definitively ruling out a medical disorder. Concomitant nonpsychiatric medical disorders are common in hospitalized patients with conversion disorder, and evidence of a current or previous neurological disorder or a systemic disease affecting the brain has been reported in 18 to 64 percent of such patients. An estimated 25 to 50 percent of patients classified as having conversion disorder eventually receive diagnoses of neurological or nonpsychiatric medical disorders that could have caused their earlier symptoms. Thus, a thorough medical and neurological workup is essential in all cases. If the symptoms can be resolved by suggestion, hypnosis, or parenteral amobartital (Amytal) or lorazepam (Ativan), they are probably the result of conversion disorder.

Neurological disorders (e.g., dementia and other degenerative diseases), brain tumors, and basal ganglia disease must be considered in the differential diagnosis. For example, weakness may be confused with myasthenia gravis, polymyositis, acquired myopathies, or multiple sclerosis. Optic neuritis may be misdiagnosed as conversion disorder blindness. Other diseases that can cause confusing symptoms are Guillain–Barré syndrome, Creutzfeldt–Jakob disease, periodic paralysis, and early neurological manifestations of acquired immunodeficiency syndrome (AIDS). Conversion disorder symptoms occur in schizophrenia, depressive disorders, and anxiety disorders, but these other disorders are associated with their own distinct symptoms that eventually make differential diagnosis possible.

Sensorimotor symptoms also occur in somatization disorder. But somatization disorder is a chronic illness that begins early in life and includes symptoms in many other organ systems. In hypochondriasis, patients have no actual loss or distortion of function; the somatic complaints are chronic and are not limited to neurological symptoms, and the characteristic hypochondriacal attitudes and beliefs are present. If the patient's symptoms are limited to pain, pain disorder can be diagnosed. Patients whose complaints are limited to sexual function are classified as having a sexual dysfunction, rather than conversion disorder.

In both malingering and factitious disorder, the symptoms are under conscious, voluntary control. A malingerer's history is usually more inconsistent and contradictory than that of a patient with conversion disorder, and a malingerer's fraudulent behavior is clearly goal directed.

Table 10.3–1 lists examples of important tests that are relevant to conversion disorder symptoms.

COURSE AND PROGNOSIS

The onset of conversion disorder is usually acute, but a crescendo of symptomatology may also occur. Symptoms or deficits are usually of short duration, and approximately 95 percent of acute cases remit spontaneously, usually within 2 weeks in hospitalized patients. If symptoms have been present for 6 months or longer, the prognosis for symptom resolution is less than 50 percent and diminishes further the longer that conversion is present. Recurrence occurs in one-fifth to one-fourth of people within 1 year of the first episode. Thus, one episode is a predictor for future episodes. A good prognosis is heralded by acute onset, presence of clearly identifiable stressors at the time

Table 10.3–1
Common Symptoms of Conversion Disorder

Motor Symptoms	Sensory Deficits
Involuntary movements	Anesthesia, especially of extremities
Tics	Midline anesthesia
Blepharospasm	Blindness
Torticollis	Tunnel vision
Opisthotonos	Deafness
Seizures	**Visceral Symptoms**
Abnormal gait	Psychogenic vomiting
Falling	Pseudocyesis
Astasia-abasia	Globus hystericus
Paralysis	Swooning or syncope
Weakness	Urinary retention
Aphonia	Diarrhea

Courtesy of Frederick G. Guggenheim, M.D.

of onset, a short interval between onset and the institution of treatment, and above average intelligence. Paralysis, aphonia, and blindness are associated with a good prognosis, whereas tremor and seizures are poor prognostic factors.

TREATMENT

Resolution of the conversion disorder symptom is usually spontaneous, although it is probably facilitated by insight-oriented supportive or behavior therapy. The most important feature of the therapy is a relationship with a caring and confident therapist. With patients who are resistant to the idea of psychotherapy, physicians can suggest that the psychotherapy will focus on issues of stress and coping. Telling such patients that their symptoms are imaginary often makes them worse. Hypnosis, anxiolytics, and behavioral relaxation exercises are effective in some cases. Parenteral amobarbital or lorazepam may be helpful in obtaining additional historic information, especially when a patient has recently experienced a traumatic event. Psychodynamic approaches include psychoanalysis and insight-oriented psychotherapy, in which patients explore intrapsychic conflicts and the symbolism of the conversion disorder symptoms. Brief and direct forms of short-term psychotherapy have also been used to treat conversion disorder. The longer the duration of these patients' sick role and the more they have regressed, the more difficult the treatment.

▲ 10.4 Factitious Disorder

Patients with factitious disorder simulate, induce, or aggravate illness to receive medical attention, regardless of whether or not they are ill. Thus, they may inflict painful, deforming, or even life-threatening injury on themselves, their children, or other dependents. The primary motivation is not avoidance of duties, financial gain, or anything concrete. The motivation is simply to receive medical care and partake in the medical system.

Factitious disorders can lead to significant morbidity or even mortality. Therefore, even though presenting complaints are falsified, the medical and psychiatric needs of these patients must be taken seriously. For example, an operating room technician, the daughter of a physician, repetitively injected herself with *Pseudomonas,* which caused multiple bouts of sepsis and bilateral renal failure that led to her death. Such deaths are not uncommon. In a 1951 article in *Lancet,* Richard Asher coined the term "Munchausen syndrome" to refer to a syndrome in which patients embellish their personal history, chronically fabricate symptoms to gain hospital admission, and move from hospital to hospital. The syndrome was named after Baron Hieronymus Friedrich Freiherr von Munchausen (1720–1797), a German cavalry officer who became a minor celebrity for telling outrageous tall tales—such as travelling on a cannon ball to the moon—based on his military service in the Russo-Turkish War.

EPIDEMIOLOGY

No comprehensive epidemiological data on factitious disorder exist. Limited studies indicate that patients with factitious disorder may comprise approximately 0.8 to 1.0 percent of psychiatry consultation patients. Cases of feigned psychological signs and symptoms are reported much less commonly than those of physical signs and symptoms. A data bank of persons who feign illness has been established to alert hospitals about such patients, many of whom travel from place to place, seek admission under different names, or simulate different illnesses.

Approximately two-thirds of patients with Munchausen syndrome are male. They tend to be white, middle-aged, unemployed, unmarried, and without significant social or family attachments. Patients diagnosed with factitious disorders with physical signs and symptoms are mostly women, who outnumber men 3 to 1. They are usually 20 to 40 years of age with a history of employment or education in nursing or a health care occupation. Factitious physical disorders usually begin for patients in their 20s or 30s, although the literature contains cases ranging from 4 to 79 years of age.

Factitious disorder by proxy (called Factitious Disorder Imposed on Another in the fifth edition of *Diagnostic and Statistical Manual of Mental Disorders* [DSM-5]) is most commonly perpetrated by mothers against infants or young children. Rare or under recognized, it accounts for less than 0.04 percent, or 1,000 of 3 million cases of child abuse reported in the United States each year. Good epidemiological data are lacking, however. This disorder is discussed below.

COMORBIDITY

Many persons diagnosed with factitious disorder have comorbid psychiatric diagnoses (e.g., mood disorders, personality disorders, or substance-related disorders).

ETIOLOGY

Psychosocial Factors

The psychodynamic underpinnings of factitious disorders are poorly understood because the patients are difficult to engage in an exploratory psychotherapy process. They may insist that their symptoms are physical and that psychologically oriented treatment is therefore useless. Anecdotal case reports indicate that many of the patients suffered childhood abuse or deprivation, resulting in frequent hospitalizations during early development. In such circumstances, an inpatient stay may have been regarded as an escape from a traumatic home situation, and the patient may have found a series of caretakers (e.g., doctors, nurses, and hospital workers) to be loving and caring. In contrast, the patients' families of origin included a rejecting mother or an absent father. The usual history reveals that the patient perceives one or both parents as rejecting figures who are unable to form close relationships. The facsimile of genuine illness, therefore, is used to recreate the desired positive parent–child bond. The disorders are a form of repetitional compulsion, repeating the basic conflict of needing and seeking acceptance and love while expecting that they will not be forthcoming. Hence, the patient transforms the physicians and staff members into rejecting parents.

Patients who seek out painful procedures, such as surgical operations and invasive diagnostic tests, may have a masochistic personality makeup in which pain serves as punishment for past sins, imagined or real. Some patients may attempt to master the past and the early trauma of serious medical illness or hospitalization by assuming the role of the patient and reliving the painful and frightening experience over and over again through multiple hospitalizations. Patients who feign psychiatric illness may have had a relative who was hospitalized with the illness they are simulating. Through identification, patients hope to reunite with the relative in a magical way.

Many patients have the poor identity formation and disturbed self-image that is characteristic of someone with borderline personality disorder. Some patients are *as-if personalities* who have assumed the identities of those around them. If these patients are health professionals, they are often unable to differentiate themselves from the patients with whom they come in contact. The cooperation or encouragement of other persons in simulating a factitious illness occurs in a rare variant of the disorder. Although most patients act alone, friends or relatives participate in fabricating the illness in some instances.

Significant defense mechanisms are repression, identification with the aggressor, regression, and symbolization.

Biological Factors

Some researchers have proposed that brain dysfunction may be a factor in factitious disorders. It has been hypothesized that impaired information processing contributes to the *pseudologia fantastica* and aberrant behavior of patients with Munchausen disorder; however, no genetic patterns have been established, and electroencephalographic (EEG) studies noted no specific abnormalities in patients with factitious disorders.

DIAGNOSIS AND CLINICAL FEATURES

Factitious disorder is the faking of physical or psychological signs and symptoms. Clues that should trigger suspicion of the disorder are given in Table 10.4–1. The psychiatric examination should emphasize securing information from any available friends, relatives, or other informants, because interviews with reliable outside sources often reveal the false nature of the patient's illness. Although time-consuming and tedious, verifying all the facts presented by the patient about previous hospitalizations and medical care is essential.

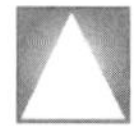

Table 10.4–1
Clues That Should Trigger Suspicion of Factitious Disorder

Unusual, dramatic presentation of symptoms that defy conventional medical or psychiatric understanding
Symptoms do not respond appropriately to usual treatment or medications
Emergence of new, unusual symptoms when other symptoms resolve
Eagerness to undergo procedures or testing or to recount symptoms
Reluctance to give access to collateral sources of information (i.e., refusing to sign releases of information or to give contact information for family and friends)
Extensive medical history or evidence of multiple surgeries
Multiple drug allergies
Medical profession
Few visitors
Ability to forecast unusual progression of symptoms or unusual response to treatment

Table by Dora L. Wang, M.D., Seth Powsner, M.D., and Stuart J. Eisendrath, M.D.

Psychiatric evaluation is requested on a consultation basis in about 50 percent of cases, usually after a simulated illness is suspected. The psychiatrist is often asked to confirm the diagnosis of factitious disorder. Under these circumstances, it is necessary to avoid pointed or accusatory questioning that may provoke truculence, evasion, or flight from the hospital. A danger may exist of provoking frank psychosis if vigorous confrontation is used; in some instances, the feigned illness serves an adaptive function and is a desperate attempt to ward off further disintegration.

Factitious disorder has been divided into two groups depending on the types of signs or symptoms feigned. There is one disorder marked by psychological symptoms and another marked by physical symptoms. Both may occur together. In DSM-5, no distinction is made between the two and the disorder is divided into that "imposed on self" and that "imposed on another" (factitious disorder by proxy). In the discussion that follows, the clinical picture of either psychological symptoms or physical symptoms is considered separately.

Factitious Disorder with Predominantly Psychological Signs and Symptoms

Some patients show psychiatric symptoms judged to be feigned. This determination can be difficult and is often made only after a prolonged investigation. The feigned symptoms frequently include depression, hallucinations, dissociative and conversion symptoms, and bizarre behavior. Because the patient's condition does not improve after routine therapeutic measures are administered, he or she may receive large doses of psychoactive drugs and may undergo electroconvulsive therapy.

Factitious psychological symptoms resemble the phenomenon of pseudomalingering, conceptualized as satisfying the need to maintain an intact self-image, which would be marred by admitting psychological problems that are beyond the person's capacity to master through conscious effort. In this case, deception is a transient ego-supporting device.

Recent findings indicate that factitious psychotic symptoms are more common than had previously been suspected. The

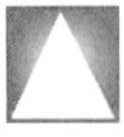

Table 10.4–2
Presentations in Factitious Disorder with Predominantly Psychological Signs and Symptoms

Bereavement	Eating disorder
Depression	Amnesia
Posttraumatic stress disorder	Substance-related disorder
Pain disorder	Paraphilias
Psychosis	Hypersomnia
Bipolar I disorder	Transsexualism
Dissociative identity disorder	

Adapted from Feldman M.D., Eisendrath S.J. *The Spectrum of Factitious Disorders*. Washington, DC: American Psychiatric Press; 1996.

presence of simulated psychosis as a feature of other disorders, such as mood disorders, indicates a poor overall prognosis.

Inpatients who are psychotic and found to have factitious disorder with predominantly psychological signs and symptoms—that is, exclusively simulated psychotic symptoms—generally have a concurrent diagnosis of borderline personality disorder. In these cases, the outcome appears to be worse than that of bipolar I disorder or schizoaffective disorder.

Patients may appear depressed and may explain their depression by offering a false history of the recent death of a significant friend or relative. Elements of the history that may suggest factitious bereavement include a violent or bloody death, a death under dramatic circumstances, and the dead person being a child or a young adult. Other patients may describe either recent and remote memory loss or both auditory and visual hallucinations.

Some patients may use psychoactive substances for the purpose of producing symptoms, such as stimulants to produce restlessness or insomnia, or hallucinogens to produce distortions of reality. Combinations of psychoactive substances can produce very unusual presentations.

Other symptoms, which also appear in the physical type of factitious disorder, include pseudologia fantastica and impostorship. In pseudologia fantastica, limited factual material is mixed with extensive and colorful fantasies. The listener's interest pleases the patient and, thus, reinforces the symptom. The history or the symptoms are not the only distortions of truth. Patients often give false and conflicting accounts about other areas of their lives (e.g., they may claim the death of a parent to play on the sympathy of others). Imposture is commonly related to lying in these cases. Many patients assume the identity of a prestigious person. Men, for example, report being war heroes and attribute their surgical scars to wounds received during battle or in other dramatic and dangerous exploits. Similarly, they may say that they have ties to accomplished or renowned figures.

Table 10.4–2 lists various syndromes feigned by patients who want to be seen as having a mental illness.

Ms. MA was 24 years of age when she first presented in 1973 after an overdose. She gave a history of recurrent overdoses and wrist-slashing attempts since 1969, and, on admission, she stated that she was controlled by her dead sister who kept telling her to take her own life. Her family history was negative.

She was found to be carrying a list of Schneiderian first-rank symptoms in her handbag; she behaved bizarrely, picking imaginary objects out of the wastepaper basket, and opening imaginary doors in the waiting room. She admitted to visual hallucinations and offered four of the first-rank symptoms on her list, but her mental state reverted to normal after 2 days. When she was presented at a case conference, the consensus view was that she had been simulating schizophrenia but had a gross personality disorder; however, the consultant in charge dissented from that general view, feeling that she was genuinely psychotic.

On follow-up, this turned out to be the case. She was readmitted in 1975 and was mute, catatonic, grossly thought disordered, and the diagnosis was changed to that of a schizophrenic illness. She has been followed up regularly since and now presents the picture of a mild schizophrenic defect state; she takes regular depot medication but still complains of auditory hallucinations, hearing her dead sister's voice. She is a day patient. *(Courtesy of Dora Wang, M.D., Deepa N. Nadiga, M.D., and James J. Jenson, M.D.)*

Chronic Factitious Disorder with Predominantly Physical Signs and Symptoms

Factitious disorder with predominantly physical signs and symptoms is the best-known type of Munchausen syndrome. The disorder has also been called hospital addiction, polysurgical addiction—producing the so-called washboard abdomen—and professional patient syndrome, among other names.

The essential feature of patients with the disorder is their ability to present physical symptoms so well that they can gain admission to, and stay in, a hospital. To support their history, these patients may feign symptoms suggesting a disorder involving any organ system. They are familiar with the diagnoses of most disorders that usually require hospital admission or medication and can give excellent histories capable of deceiving even experienced clinicians. Clinical presentations are myriad and include hematoma, hemoptysis, abdominal pain, fever, hypoglycemia, lupus-like syndromes, nausea, vomiting, dizziness, and seizures. Urine is contaminated with blood or feces; anticoagulants are taken to simulate bleeding disorders; insulin is used to produce hypoglycemia; and so on. Such patients often insist on surgery and claim adhesions from previous surgical procedures. They may acquire a "gridiron" or washboard-like abdomen from multiple procedures. Complaints of pain, especially that simulating renal colic, are common, with the patients wanting narcotics. In about half the reported cases, these patients demand treatment with specific medications, usually analgesics. Once in the hospital, they continue to be demanding and difficult. As each test is returned with a negative result, they may accuse doctors of incompetence, threaten litigation, and become generally abusive. Some may sign out abruptly shortly before they believe they are going to be confronted with their factitious behavior. They then go to another hospital in the same or another city and begin the cycle again. Specific predisposing factors are true physical disorders during childhood leading to extensive medical treatment, a grudge against the medical profession, employment as a medical paraprofessional, and an important relationship with a physician in the past.

Factitious Disorder with Combined Psychological and Physical Signs and Symptoms

In combined forms of factitious disorder, both psychological and physical signs and symptoms are present. In one representative report, a patient alternated between feigned dementia, bereavement, rape, and seizures.

Table 10.4–3 provides a comprehensive overview of a variety of signs and symptoms that may be faked and mistaken for genuine illness. The table also includes the means of simulation and possible methods of detection.

Factitious Disorder by Proxy

In this diagnosis, a person intentionally produces physical signs or symptoms in another person who is under the first person's care, hence the DSM-5 diagnosis of "Factitious Disorder Imposed on Another." One apparent purpose of the behavior is for the caretaker to indirectly assume the sick role; another is to be relieved of the caretaking role by having the child hospitalized. The most common case of factitious disorder by proxy involves a mother who deceives medical personnel into believing that her child is ill. The deception may involve a false medical history, contamination of laboratory samples, alteration of records, or induction of injury and illness in the child.

BC, a 1-month-old girl, was admitted for the evaluation of fever. Psychiatric consultation was requested due to inconsistencies in the mother's reporting of medical information despite her presentation as a knowledgeable and caring mother who worked as an emergency medical technician. BC's mother reported her own diagnosis of ovarian cancer when she was 3 months pregnant with BC. She reported undergoing a hysterectomy during her cesarean section, and that she had been getting radiation therapy at a local hospital since BC's birth. The pediatrician called the local hospital with the mother's permission and learned that she had a corpus luteum cyst removed at 3 months' gestation and mild hydronephrosis but no cancer or hysterectomy. BC's mother, when confronted with this, stated only that she might need a kidney transplant for the hydronephrosis.

On further exploration, it was discovered that the mother had brought her children to multiple emergency rooms, giving inaccurate histories that prompted excessive testing. At one visit, she told clinicians that her 2-year-old son had lupus and hypergammaglobulinemia, and at another visit, that he had asthma and seizures. She also pursued a minor cosmetic surgical procedure for him against his pediatrician's recommendation.

Clinicians suspected that BC's mother intentionally fabricated symptoms, such as by warming BC's thermometer, and that she did not actively induce symptoms in her children. She was faithful in keeping medical appointments, and her children appeared healthy and well cared for, despite her factitious behavior. The mother denied a psychiatric history but gave permission for clinicians to contact the local psychiatric hospital, which revealed her history of depression, anorexia, panic disorder, and a suicide attempt resulting in a psychiatric hospitalization. Subsequently, she received psychotherapy and psychopharmacotherapy, which she stopped a few months prior to this presentation. During BC's admission for fever, her mother agreed to resume psychiatric treatment. A social services referral was made, and the pediatrician decided to schedule regular follow-up visits for the children.

PATHOLOGY AND LABORATORY EXAMINATION

Psychological testing may reveal underlying pathology in individual patients. Features that are overrepresented in patients with factitious disorder include normal or above-average intelligence quotient, absence of a formal thought disorder, poor sense of identity, including confusion over sexual identify, poor sexual adjustment, poor frustration tolerance, strong dependence needs, and narcissism. An invalid test profile and elevations of all clinical scales on the Minnesota Multiphasic Personality Inventory-2 (MMPI-2) indicate an attempt to appear more disturbed than is the case ("fake bad").

No laboratory or pathology tests are diagnostic of factitious disorders, although they may help to confirm the diagnosis by demonstrating deception. Certain tests (e.g., drug screening), however, may help confirm or rule out specific mental or medical disorders.

DIFFERENTIAL DIAGNOSIS

Any disorder in which physical signs and symptoms are prominent should be considered in the differential diagnosis, and the possibility of authentic or concomitant physical illness must always be explored. Additionally, a history of many surgeries in patients with factitious disorder may predispose such patients to complications or actual diseases, necessitating even further surgery. Factitious disorder is on a continuum between somatoform disorders and malingering, the goal being to assume the sick role. On the one hand, it is unconscious and nonvolitional, and on the other hand, it is conscious and willful (malingering).

Conversion Disorders

A factitious disorder is differentiated from conversion disorder by the voluntary production of factitious symptoms, the extreme course of multiple hospitalizations, and the seeming willingness of patients with a factitious disorder to undergo an extraordinary number of mutilating procedures. Patients with conversion disorder are not usually conversant with medical terminology and hospital routines, and their symptoms have a direct temporal relation or symbolic reference to specific emotional conflicts.

Hypochondriasis or illness anxiety disorder differs from factitious disorder in that the hypochondriacal patient does not voluntarily initiate the production of symptoms, and hypochondriasis typically has a later age of onset. As with conversion disorder, patients with hypochondriasis do not usually submit to potentially mutilating procedures.

Personality Disorders

Because of their pathological lying, lack of close relationships with others, hostile and manipulative manner, and associated substance abuse and criminal history, patients with factitious disorder are often classified as having antisocial personality disorder. Antisocial persons, however, do not usually volunteer for invasive procedures or resort to a way of life marked by repeated or long-term hospitalization.

Because of attention seeking and an occasional flair for the dramatic, patients with factitious disorder may be classified as

Table 10.4–3
Presentations of Factitious Disorder with Predominantly Physical Signs and Symptoms with Means of Simulation and Possible Methods of Detection

Presentation	Means of Simulation That Have Been Reported	Possible Methods of Detection
Autoimmune		
Goodpasture's syndrome	False history, adding blood to urine	Bronchoalveolar lavage negative for hemosiderin-laden cells
Systemic lupus erythematosus	Malar rash simulated through cosmetics, feigning joint pain	Negative antinuclear antibody test, removability of rash
Dermatological		
Burns	Chemical agents such as oven cleaner	Unnatural shape of lesions, streaks left by chemicals, minor injury to fingers
Excoriations	Self-infliction	Found on accessible parts of the body, or a preponderance of left-sided lesions in a right-handed person
Lesions	Injection of exogenous material such as talc, milk, or gasoline	Puncture marks left by needles, discovery of syringes
Endocrine		
Cushing's syndrome	Steroid ingestion	Evidence of exogenous steroid use
Hyperthyroidism	Thyroxine or L-iodothyronine ingestion	The 24-hour I-131 uptake is suppressed in factitious disease and increased in Graves' disease
Hypoglycemia or insulinoma	1. Insulin injection 2. Ingestion of oral hypoglycemics	1. Insulin to C-peptide ratio greater than 1, detection of serum insulin antibodies 2. Serum levels of hypoglycemic medication
Pheochromocytoma	Epinephrine or metaraminol injection	Analysis of urinary catecholamines may reveal epinephrine only or other suspicious findings
Gastrointestinal		
Diarrhea	Phenolphthalein or castor oil ingestion	Testing of stool for laxatives, increased stool weight
Hemoptysis	Contamination of sputum sample, self-induced trauma such as cuts to tongue	Collect specimen under observation, examine mouth
Ulcerative colitis	Laceration of colon with knitting needle	
Hematological		
Aplastic anemia	Self-administration of chemotherapeutic agents to suppress bone marrow	Hematology/oncology consultation
Anemia	Self-induced phlebotomy	Blood studies
Coagulopathy	Ingestion of warfarin or other anticoagulants	
Infectious disease		
Abdominal abscess	Injection of feces into abdominal wall	Unusual pathogens in microbiology tests
Acquired immunodeficiency syndrome (AIDS)	False history	Collateral information
Neoplastic		
Cancer	False medical and family history, shaving head to simulate chemotherapy	Collateral information, examination
Neurologic		
Paraplegia or quadriplegia	Feigning, fictitious history	Imaging studies, electromyography
Seizures	Feigning, fictitious history	Video electroencephalogram
Obstetrics/gynecology		
Antepartum hemorrhage	Vaginal puncture wounds, use of fake blood	Examination, test blood
Ectopic pregnancy	Feigning abdominal pain while self-injecting human chorionic gonadotropin	Ultrasound
Menorrhagia	Using stolen blood	Type blood
Placenta previa	Intravaginal use of hat pin	Examination
Premature labor	Feigned uterine contractions, manipulation of tocodynamometer	Examination
Premature rupture of membranes	Voiding urine into vagina	Examine fluid
Trophoblastic disease	Addition of human chorionic gonadotropin to urine	
Vaginal bleeding	Self-mutilation with fingernails, nail files, bleach, knives, tweezers, nutpicks, glass, pencils	Examination
Vaginal discharge	Applying cigarette ash to underwear	Examination

(continued)

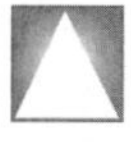

Table 10.4–3
Presentations of Factitious Disorder with Predominantly Physical Signs and Symptoms with Means of Simulation and Possible Methods of Detection (Continued)

Presentation	Means of Simulation That Have Been Reported	Possible Methods of Detection
Systemic		
Fever	Warming thermometer against a lightbulb or other heat source, drinking hot fluids, friction from mouth or anal sphincter, false recordings, injection of pyrogens such as feces, vaccines, thyroid hormone, or tetanus toxoid	Simultaneous taking of temperature from two different locals (orally and rectally), recording the temperature of freshly voided urine, the appearance of cool skin despite high thermometer readings, normal white blood cell count, unusually high or inconsistent temperatures
Urinary		
Bacteriuria	Contamination of urethra or specimen	Unusual pathogen
Hematuria	Contamination of specimen with blood or meat, warfarin ingestion, foreign bodies in bladder (pins)	Collect specimen under observation
Proteinuria	Inserting egg protein into urethra	
Stones	Feigning of renal colic pain, bringing in stones made of exogenous materials or inserting them into urethra	Pathology report

Table by Dora L. Wang, M.D., Seth Powsner, M.D., and Stuart J. Eisendrath, M.D.

having histrionic personality disorder. But not all such patients have a dramatic flair; many are withdrawn and bland.

Consideration of the patient's chaotic lifestyle, history of disturbed interpersonal relationships, identity crisis, substance abuse, self-damaging acts, and manipulative tactics may lead to the diagnosis of borderline personality disorder. Persons with factitious disorder usually do not have the eccentricities of dress, thought, or communication that characterize schizotypal personality disorder patients.

Schizophrenia

The diagnosis of schizophrenia is often based on patients' admittedly bizarre lifestyles, but patients with factitious disorder do not usually meet the diagnostic criteria for schizophrenia unless they have the fixed delusion that they are actually ill and act on this belief by seeking hospitalization. Such a practice seems to be the exception; few patients with factitious disorder show evidence of a severe thought disorder or bizarre delusions.

Malingering

Factitious disorders must be distinguished from malingering. Malingerers have an obvious, recognizable environmental goal in producing signs and symptoms. They may seek hospitalization to secure financial compensation, evade the police, avoid work, or merely obtain free bed and board for the night, but they always have some apparent end for their behavior. Moreover, these patients can usually stop producing their signs and symptoms when they are no longer considered profitable or when the risk becomes too great.

Substance Abuse

Although patients with factitious disorders may have a complicating history of substance abuse, they should be considered not merely as substance abusers but as having coexisting diagnoses.

Ganser's Syndrome

Ganser's syndrome, a controversial condition most typically associated with prison inmates, is characterized by the use of approximate answers. Persons with the syndrome respond to simple questions with astonishingly incorrect answers. For example, when asked about the color of a blue car, the person answers "red" or answers "2 plus 2 equals 5." Ganser's syndrome may be a variant of malingering, in that the patients avoid punishment or responsibility for their actions. Ganser's syndrome can be classified in DSM-5 as a type of dissociative disorder and in *International Statistical Classification of Diseases and Related Health Problems,* 10th edition (ICD-10), it is classified under other dissociative or conversion disorders. In contrast, patients with factitious disorder with predominantly psychological signs and symptoms may *intentionally* give approximate answers.

COURSE AND PROGNOSIS

Factitious disorders typically begin in early adulthood, although they can appear during childhood or adolescence. The onset of the disorder or of discrete episodes of seeking treatment may follow real illness, loss, rejection, or abandonment. Usually, the patient or a close relative had a hospitalization in childhood or early adolescence for a genuine physical illness. Thereafter, a long pattern of successive hospitalizations begins insidiously and evolves. As the disorder progresses, the patient becomes knowledgeable about medicine and hospitals. The onset of the disorder in patients who had early hospitalizations for actual illness is earlier than generally reported.

Factitious disorders are incapacitating to the patient and often produce severe trauma or untoward reactions related to treatment. A course of repeated or long-term hospitalization is obviously incompatible with meaningful vocational work and sustained interpersonal relationships. The prognosis in most cases is poor. A few patients occasionally spend time in jail, usually for minor crimes, such as burglary, vagrancy, and disorderly conduct. Patients may also have a history of intermittent psychiatric hospitalization.

Although no adequate data are available about the ultimate outcome for the patients, a few of them probably die as a result of needless medication, instrumentation, or surgery. In view of the patients' often expert simulation and the risks that they take, some may die without the disorder being suspected. Possible features that indicate a favorable prognosis are (1) the presence of a depressive-masochistic personality; (2) functioning at a borderline, not a continuously psychotic, level; and (3) the attributes of an antisocial personality disorder with minimal symptoms.

TREATMENT

No specific psychiatric therapy has been effective in treating factitious disorders. It is a clinical paradox that patients with the disorders simulate serious illness and seek and submit to unnecessary treatment while they deny to themselves and others their true illness and thus avoid possible treatment for it. Ultimately, the patients elude meaningful therapy by abruptly leaving the hospital or failing to keep follow-up appointments.

Treatment, thus, is best focused on management rather than on cure. Guidelines for the treatment and management of factitious disorder are given in Table 10.4–4. The three major goals in the treatment and management of factitious disorders are to (1) reduce the risk of morbidity and mortality, (2) address the underlying emotional needs or psychiatric diagnosis underlying

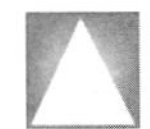

Table 10.4–4
Guidelines for Management and Treatment of Factitious Disorder

- Active pursuit of a prompt diagnosis can minimize the risk of morbidity and mortality.
- Minimize harm. Avoid unnecessary tests and procedures, especially if invasive. Treat according to clinical judgment, keeping in mind that subjective complaints may be deceptive.
- Regular interdisciplinary meetings to reduce conflict and splitting among staff. Manage staff countertransference.
- Consider facilitating healing by using the double-bind technique or face-saving behavioral strategies, such as self-hypnosis or biofeedback.
- Steer the patient toward psychiatric treatment in an empathic, nonconfrontational, face-saving manner. Avoid aggressive direct confrontation.
- Treat underlying psychiatric disturbances, such as Axis I disorders and Axis II disorders. In psychotherapy, address coping strategies and emotional conflicts.
- Appoint a primary care provider as a gatekeeper for all medical and psychiatric treatment.
- Consider involving risk management professionals and bioethicists from an early point.
- Consider appointing a guardian for medical and psychiatric decisions.
- Consider prosecution for fraud, as a behavioral disincentive.

factitious illness behavior, and (3) be mindful of legal and ethical issues. Perhaps the single most important factor in successful management is a physician's early recognition of the disorder. In this way, physicians can forestall a multitude of painful and potentially dangerous diagnostic procedures for these patients. Good liaison between psychiatrists and the medical or surgical staff is strongly advised. Although a few cases of individual psychotherapy have been reported in the literature, no consensus exists about the best approach. In general, working in concert with the patient's primary care physician is more effective than working with the patient in isolation.

The personal reactions of physicians and staff members are of great significance in treating and establishing a working alliance with these patients, who invariably evoke feelings of futility, bewilderment, betrayal, hostility, and even contempt. In essence, staff members are forced to abandon a basic element of their relationship with patients—accepting the truthfulness of the patients' statements. One appropriate psychiatric intervention is to suggest to the staff ways of remaining aware that even though the patient's illness is factitious, the patient is ill.

Physicians should try not to feel resentment when patients humiliate their diagnostic prowess, and they should avoid any unmasking ceremony that sets up the patients as adversaries and precipitates their flight from the hospital. The staff should not perform unnecessary procedures or discharge patients abruptly, both of which are manifestations of anger.

Clinicians who find themselves involved with patients with factitious disorders may become angry at the patients for lying and deceiving them. Hence, therapists must be mindful of countertransference whenever they suspect factitious disorder. Often, the diagnosis is unclear because a definitive physical cause cannot be entirely ruled out. Although the use of confrontation is controversial, at some point in the treatment, patients must be made to face reality. Most patients simply leave treatment when their methods of gaining attention are identified and exposed. In some cases, clinicians should reframe the factitious disorder as a cry for help, so that patients do not view the clinicians' responses as punitive. A major role for psychiatrists working with patients with factitious disorder is to help other staff members in the hospital deal with their own sense of outrage at having been duped. Education about the disorder and some attempt to understand the patient's motivations may help staff members maintain their professional conduct in the face of extreme frustration.

In cases of factitious disorder by proxy, legal intervention has been obtained in several instances, particularly with children. The senselessness of the disorder and the denial of false action by parents are obstacles to successful court action and often make conclusive proof unobtainable. In such cases, the child welfare services should be notified, and arrangements made for ongoing monitoring of the children's health (see Table 10.4–5 for interventions for pediatric factitious disorder by proxy).

Pharmacotherapy of factitious disorders is of limited use. Major mental disorders such as schizophrenia will respond to antipsychotic medication; however, in all cases, medication should be administered carefully because of the potential for abuse. Selective serotonin reuptake inhibitors (SSRIs) may be useful in decreasing impulsive behavior when that is a major component in acting-out factitious behavior.

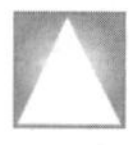

Table 10.4–5
Interventions for Pediatric Factitious Disorder by Proxy

A pediatrician should serve as "gatekeeper" for medical care utilization. All other physicians should coordinate care with the gatekeeper.
Child protective services should be informed whenever a child is harmed.
Family psychotherapy and/or individual psychotherapy should be instituted for the perpetrating parent and the child.
Health insurance companies, school officials, and other non-medical sources should be asked to report possible medical use to the physician gatekeeper. Permission of a parent or of child protective services must first be obtained.
The possibility should be considered of admitting the child to an inpatient or partial hospital setting to facilitate diagnostic monitoring of symptoms and to institute a treatment plan.
The child may require placement in another family. The perpetrating parent may need to be removed from the child through criminal prosecution and incarceration.

Table by Dora L. Wang, M.D., Seth Powsner, M.D., and Stuart J. Eisendrath, M.D.

▲ 10.5 Pain Disorder

In the fourth edition of the *Diagnostic and Statistical Manual of Mental Disorders* (DSM-IV), pain disorder warranted its own diagnostic category; but in the current fifth edition (DSM-5), it is diagnosed as a variant of somatic symptom disorder. Its importance is such, however, that it warrants a separate discussion in this textbook.

A pain disorder is characterized by the presence of, and focus on, pain in one or more body sites and is sufficiently severe to come to clinical attention. Psychological factors are necessary in the genesis, severity, or maintenance of the pain, which causes significant distress, impairment, or both. The physician does not have to judge the pain to be "inappropriate" or "in excess of what would be expected." Rather, the phenomenological and diagnostic focus is on the importance of psychological factors and the degree of impairment caused by the pain. The disorder has been called somatoform pain disorder, psychogenic pain disorder, idiopathic pain disorder, and atypical pain disorder. Pain disorder is diagnosed as "Unspecified Somatic Symptom Disorder" in DSM-5 or it may be designated as a "specifier" under that heading.

EPIDEMIOLOGY

The prevalence of pain disorder appears to be common. Recent work indicates that the 6-month and lifetime prevalence is approximately 5 and 12 percent, respectively. It has been estimated that 10 to 15 percent of adults in the United States have some form of work disability because of back pain alone in any year. Approximately 3 percent of people in a general practice have persistent pain, with at least 1 day per month of activity restriction because of the pain.

Pain disorder can begin at any age. The gender ratio is unknown. Pain disorder is associated with other psychiatric disorders, especially affective and anxiety disorders. Chronic pain appears to be most frequently associated with depressive disorders, and acute pain appears to be more commonly associated with anxiety disorders. The associated psychiatric disorders may precede the pain disorder, may co-occur with it, or may result from it. Depressive disorders, alcohol dependence, and chronic pain may be more common in relatives of individuals with chronic pain disorder. Individuals whose pain is associated with severe depression and those whose pain is related to a terminal illness, such as cancer, are at increased risk for suicide. Differences may exist in how various ethnic and cultural groups respond to pain, but the usefulness of cultural factors for the clinician remains obscure to the treatment of individuals with pain disorder because of a lack of good data and because of high individual variability.

ETIOLOGY

Psychodynamic Factors

Patients who experience bodily aches and pains without identifiable and adequate physical causes may be symbolically expressing an intrapsychic conflict through the body. Patients suffering from alexithymia, who are unable to articulate their internal feeling states in words, express their feelings with their bodies. Other patients may unconsciously regard emotional pain as weak and somehow lacking legitimacy. By displacing the problem to the body, they may feel they have a legitimate claim to the fulfillment of their dependency needs. The symbolic meaning of body disturbances may also relate to atonement for perceived sin, to expiation of guilt, or to suppressed aggression. Many patients have intractable and unresponsive pain because they are convinced they deserve to suffer.

Pain can function as a method of obtaining love, a punishment for wrongdoing, and a way of expiating guilt and atoning for an innate sense of badness. Among the defense mechanisms used by patients with pain disorder are displacement, substitution, and repression. Identification plays a part when a patient takes on the role of an ambivalent love object who also has pain, such as a parent.

Behavioral Factors

Pain behaviors are reinforced when rewarded and are inhibited when ignored or punished. For example, moderate pain symptoms may become intense when followed by the solicitous and attentive behavior of others, by monetary gain, or by the successful avoidance of distasteful activities.

Interpersonal Factors

Intractable pain has been conceptualized as a means for manipulation and gaining advantage in interpersonal relationships, for example, to ensure the devotion of a family member or to stabilize a fragile marriage. Such secondary gain is most important to patients with pain disorder.

Biological Factors

The cerebral cortex can inhibit the firing of afferent pain fibers. Serotonin is probably the main neurotransmitter in the descending inhibitory pathways, and endorphins also play a role in the central nervous system modulation of pain. Endorphin deficiency seems to correlate with augmentation of incoming sensory stimuli. Some patients may have pain disorder, rather than another mental disorder, because of sensory and limbic structural or chemical abnormalities that predispose them to experience pain.

DIAGNOSIS AND CLINICAL FEATURES

Patients with pain disorder are not a uniform group, but a heterogeneous collection of persons with low back pain, headache, atypical facial pain, chronic pelvic pain, and other kinds of pain. A patient's pain may be posttraumatic, neuropathic, neurological, iatrogenic, or musculoskeletal; to meet a diagnosis of pain disorder, however, the disorder must have a psychological factor judged to be significantly involved in the pain symptoms and their ramifications.

Patients with pain disorder often have long histories of medical and surgical care. They visit many physicians, request many medications, and may be especially insistent in their desire for surgery. Indeed, they can be completely preoccupied with their pain and cite it as the source of all their misery. Such patients often deny any other sources of emotional dysphoria and insist that their lives are blissful except for their pain. Their clinical picture can be complicated by substance-related disorders, because these patients attempt to reduce the pain through the use of alcohol and other substances.

At least one study has correlated the number of pain symptoms to the likelihood and severity of symptoms of somatic symptom disorder, depressive disorder, and anxiety disorder. Major depressive disorder is present in about 25 to 50 percent of patients with pain disorder, and dysthymic disorder or depressive disorder symptoms are reported in 60 to 100 percent of the patients. Some investigators believe that chronic pain is almost always a variant of a depressive disorder, a masked or somatized form of depression. The most prominent depressive symptoms in patients with pain disorder are anergia, anhedonia, decreased libido, insomnia, and irritability; diurnal variation, weight loss, and psychomotor retardation appear to be less common.

A 54-year-old accountant sought out his family physician with complaints of severe back pain that came on suddenly while trying to lift a piece of heavy furniture at home. On examination he showed no focal neurological signs but was unable to straighten up into an upright position.

The patient was referred for MRI, which revealed no structural abnormalities. He was advised to have several sessions with a physical therapist to treat what was diagnosed as "back strain," but as the therapy progressed, his pain became more severe, and he complained of muscle tension in his neck in addition to his back and spent most of his days sitting in a chair or lying on a bed board on his bed.

He was eventually referred to a psychiatrist and talked about the stress he was experiencing at work since an assistant that he relied on was fired because of his firm's need to downsize. His work load had increased tremendously as a result. The formulation by the psychiatrist was that the patient was "somatizing" his anger, transforming the strong affect into pain that enabled him to escape from the stressful situation. A course of psychoeducation was begun in which these dynamics were explored. Equally important was his asserting himself at work, explaining that the load he was expected to carry was too much and that help was required. When this was accomplished, the patient's back pain disappeared within a matter of days.

DIFFERENTIAL DIAGNOSIS

Purely physical pain can be difficult to distinguish from purely psychogenic pain, especially because the two are not mutually exclusive. Physical pain fluctuates in intensity and is highly sensitive to emotional, cognitive, attentional, and situational influences. Pain that does not vary and is insensitive to any of these factors is likely to be psychogenic. When pain does not wax and wane and is not even temporarily relieved by distraction or analgesics, clinicians can suspect an important psychogenic component.

Pain disorder must be distinguished from other somatic symptom disorders, although there may be overlap. Patients with hypochondriacal preoccupations may complain of pain, and aspects of the clinical presentation of hypochondriasis, such as bodily preoccupation and disease conviction, can also be present in patients with pain disorder. Patients with hypochondriasis tend to have many more symptoms than patients with pain disorder, and their symptoms tend to fluctuate more than those of patients with pain disorder. Conversion disorder is generally short-lived, whereas pain disorder is chronic. In addition, pain is, by definition, not a symptom in conversion disorder. Malingering patients consciously provide false reports, and their complaints are usually connected to clearly recognizable goals.

The differential diagnosis can be difficult because patients with pain disorder often receive disability compensation or a litigation award. Muscle contraction (tension) headaches, for example, have a pathophysiological mechanism to account for the pain and so are not diagnosed as pain disorder. Patients with pain disorder are not pretending to be in pain, however. As in all of these disorders, symptoms are not imaginary.

COURSE AND PROGNOSIS

The pain in pain disorder generally begins abruptly and increases in severity for a few weeks or months. The prognosis varies, although pain disorder can often be chronic, distressful, and completely disabling. Acute pain disorders have a more favorable prognosis than chronic pain disorders. A wide range of variability is seen in the onset and course of chronic pain disorder. In many cases, the pain has been present for many years by the time the individual comes to psychiatric care, owing to the reluctance of the patient and the physician's tendency to see pain as a psychiatric disorder. People with pain disorder who resume participation in regularly scheduled activities, despite the pain, have a more favorable prognosis than people who allow the pain to become the determining factor in their lifestyle.

TREATMENT

Because it may not be possible to reduce the pain, the treatment approach must address rehabilitation. Clinicians should discuss the issue of psychological factors early in treatment and should frankly tell patients that such factors are important in the cause and consequences of both physical and psychogenic pain. Therapists should also explain how various brain circuits that are involved with emotions (e.g., the limbic system) can influence the sensory pain pathways. For example, persons who hit their head while happy at a party can seem to experience less pain than when they hit their head while angry and at work.

Nevertheless, therapists must fully understand that the patient's experiences of pain are real.

Pharmacotherapy

Analgesic medications do not generally benefit most patients with pain disorder. In addition, substance abuse and dependence are often major problems for such patients who receive long-term analgesic treatment. Sedatives and antianxiety agents are not especially beneficial and are also subject to abuse, misuse, and adverse effects.

Antidepressants, such as tricyclics and SSRIs, are the most effective pharmacological agents. Whether antidepressants reduce pain through their antidepressant action or exert an independent, direct analgesic effect (possibly by stimulating efferent inhibitory pain pathways) remains controversial. The success of SSRIs supports the hypothesis that serotonin is important in the pathophysiology of the disorder. Amphetamines, which have analgesic effects, may benefit some patients, especially when used as an adjunct to SSRIs, but dosages must be monitored carefully.

Psychotherapy

Some outcome data indicate that psychodynamic psychotherapy can benefit patients with pain disorder. The first step in psychotherapy is to develop a solid therapeutic alliance by empathizing with the patient's suffering. Clinicians should not confront somatizing patients with comments such as "*This is all in your head.*" For the patient, the pain is real, and clinicians must acknowledge the reality of the pain, even as they understand that it is largely intrapsychic in origin. A useful entry point into the emotional aspects of the pain is to examine its interpersonal ramifications in the patient's life. In marital therapy, for example, the psychotherapist may soon get to the source of the patient's psychological pain and the function of the physical complaints in significant relationships. Cognitive therapy has been used to alter negative thoughts and to foster a positive attitude.

Other Therapies

Biofeedback can be helpful in the treatment of pain disorder, particularly with migraine pain, myofascial pain, and muscle tension states, such as tension headaches. Hypnosis, transcutaneous nerve stimulation, and dorsal column stimulation have also been used. Nerve blocks and surgical ablative procedures are effective for some patients with pain disorder; but these procedures must be repeated, because the pain returns after 6 to 18 months.

Pain Control Programs

Sometimes it may be necessary to remove patients from their usual settings and place them in a comprehensive inpatient or outpatient pain control program or clinic. Multidisciplinary pain units use many modalities, such as cognitive, behavior, and group therapies. They provide extensive physical conditioning through physical therapy and exercise and offer vocational evaluation and rehabilitation. Concurrent mental disorders are diagnosed and treated, and patients who are dependent on analgesics and hypnotics are detoxified. Inpatient multimodal treatment programs generally report encouraging results.

▲ 10.6 Other Specified or Unspecified Somatic Symptom Disorder

This DSM-5 category is used to describe conditions characterized by one or more unexplained physical symptoms of at least 6 months' duration, which are below the threshold for a diagnosis of somatic symptom disorder. The symptoms are not caused, or fully explained, by another medical, psychiatric, or substance abuse disorder, and they cause clinical significant distress or impairment.

Two types of symptom patterns may be seen in patients with other specified or unspecified somatic symptom disorder: those involving the autonomic nervous system and those involving sensations of fatigue or weakness. In what is sometimes referred to as *autonomic arousal disorder,* some patients are affected with symptoms that are limited to bodily functions innervated by the autonomic nervous system. Such patients have complaints involving the cardiovascular, respiratory, gastrointestinal, urogenital, and dermatological systems. Other patients complain of mental and physical fatigue, physical weakness and exhaustion, and inability to perform many everyday activities because of their symptoms. Some clinicians believe this syndrome is neurasthenia, a diagnosis used primarily in Europe and Asia. The syndrome may overlap with chronic fatigue syndrome, which various research reports have hypothesized to involved psychiatric, virological, and immunological factors. Other conditions included in this unspecified category of somatic symptom disorder are pseudocyesis (discussed in Chapter 23) and conditions that may not have met the 6-month criterion of the other somatic symptom disorders.

11 Feeding and Eating Disorders

▲ 11.1 Anorexia Nervosa

The term "anorexia nervosa" is derived from the Greek term for "loss of appetite" and a Latin word implying nervous origin. Anorexia nervosa is a syndrome characterized by three essential criteria. The first is a self-induced starvation to a significant degree—a behavior. The second is a relentless drive for thinness or a morbid fear of fatness—a psychopathology. The third criterion is the presence of medical signs and symptoms resulting from starvation—a physiological symptomatology. Anorexia nervosa is often, but not always, associated with disturbances of body image, the perception that one is distressingly large despite obvious medical starvation. The distortion of body image is disturbing when present, but not pathognomic, invariable, or required for diagnosis. Two subtypes of anorexia nervosa exist: restricting and binge/purge. The theme in all anorexia nervosa subtypes is the highly disproportionate emphasis placed on thinness as a vital source, sometimes the only source, of self-esteem, with weight, and to a lesser degree, shape, becoming the overriding and consuming daylong preoccupation of thoughts, mood, and behaviors.

Approximately half of anorexic persons will lose weight by drastically reducing their total food intake. The other half of these patients will not only diet but will also regularly engage in binge eating followed by purging behaviors. Some patients routinely purge after eating small amounts of food. Anorexia nervosa is much more prevalent in females than in males and usually has its onset in adolescence. Hypotheses of an underlying psychological disturbance in young women with the disorder include conflicts surrounding the transition from girlhood to womanhood. Psychological issues related to feelings of helplessness and difficulty establishing autonomy have also been suggested as contributing to the development of the disorder. Bulimic symptoms can occur as a separate disorder (bulimia nervosa, which is discussed in Section 11.2) or as part of anorexia nervosa. Persons with either disorder are excessively preoccupied with weight, food, and body shape. The outcome of anorexia nervosa varies from spontaneous recovery to a waxing and waning course to death.

EPIDEMIOLOGY

Anorexia nervosa has been reported more frequently over the past several decades, with increasing reports of the disorder in prepubertal girls and in boys. The most common ages of onset of anorexia nervosa are the midteens, but up to 5 percent of anorectic patients have the onset of the disorder in their early 20s. The most common age of onset is between 14 and 18 years. Anorexia nervosa is estimated to occur in about 0.5 to 1 percent of adolescent girls. It occurs 10 to 20 times more often in females than in males. The prevalence of young women with some symptoms of anorexia nervosa who do not meet the diagnostic criteria is estimated to be close to 5 percent. Although the disorder was initially reported most often among the upper classes, recent epidemiological surveys do not show that distribution. It seems to be most frequent in developed countries, and it may be seen with greatest frequency among young women in professions that require thinness, such as modeling and ballet.

COMORBIDITY

Table 11.1–1 lists comorbid psychiatric conditions associated with anorexia nervosa. Overall, anorexia nervosa is associated with depression in 65 percent of cases, social phobia in 35 percent of cases, and obsessive-compulsive disorder in 25 percent of cases.

ETIOLOGY

Biological, social, and psychological factors are implicated in the causes of anorexia nervosa. Some evidence point to higher concordance rates in monozygotic twins than in dizygotic twins. Sisters of patients with anorexia nervosa are likely to be afflicted, but this association may reflect social influences more than genetic factors. Major mood disorders are more common in family members than in the general population. Neurochemically, diminished norepinephrine turnover and activity are suggested by reduced 3-methoxy-4-hydroxyphenylglycol (MHPG) levels in the urine and the cerebrospinal fluid (CSF) of some patients with anorexia nervosa. An inverse relation is seen between MHPG and depression in these patients; an increase in MHPG is associated with a decrease in depression.

Biological Factors

Endogenous opioids may contribute to the denial of hunger in patients with anorexia nervosa. Preliminary studies show dramatic weight gains in some patients who are given opiate antagonists. Starvation results in many biochemical changes, some of which are also present in depression, such as hypercortisolemia

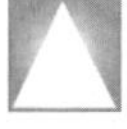

Table 11.1–1
Comorbid Psychiatric Conditions Associated with Anorexia Nervosa

Diagnosis	Restricting-Type Anorexia Nervosa (%)	Binge Eating and Purging Type Anorexia Nervosa (%)
Any affective disorder	57	100
Intermittent depressive disorder	29	44
Major depression	57	66
Minor depression	0	11
Mania/hypomania	0	33
Any anxiety disorder	57	67
Phobic disorder	43	11
Panic disorder	29	22
Generalized anxiety disorder	14	11
Obsessive-compulsive disorder	14	56
Any substance abuse/ dependence	14	33
Drug	14	22
Alcohol	0	33
Schizophrenia	0	0
Any codiagnoses	71	100
Three or more codiagnoses	71	100
Female	100	89
Single	71	89
Age ($x \pm$ SD)	23.6 ± 10.8	25.0 ± 6.4
No. of codiagnoses ($x \pm$ SD)	2.3 ± 2.5	3.8 ± 1.4

SD, standard deviation.

and nonsuppression by dexamethasone. Thyroid function is suppressed as well. These abnormalities are corrected by realimentation. Starvation may produce amenorrhea, which reflects lowered hormonal levels (luteinizing, follicle-stimulating, and gonadotropin-releasing hormones). Some patients with anorexia nervosa, however, may become amenorrheic before significant weight loss. Several computed tomographic (CT) studies reveal enlarged CSF spaces (enlarged sulci and ventricles) in anorectic patients during starvation, a finding that is reversed by weight gain. In one positron emission tomographic (PET) scan study, caudate nucleus metabolism was higher in the anorectic state than after realimentation.

Some authors have proposed a hypothalamic-pituitary axis (neuroendocrine) dysfunction. Some studies have shown evidence for dysfunction in serotonin, dopamine, and norepinephrine, three neurotransmitters involved in regulating eating behavior in the paraventricular nucleus of the hypothalamus. Other humoral factors that may be involved include corticotropin-releasing factor (CRF), neuropeptide Y, gonadotropin-releasing hormone, and thyroid-stimulating hormone. Table 11.1–2 lists the neuroendocrine changes associated with anorexia nervosa.

Social Factors

Patients with anorexia nervosa find support for their practices in society's emphasis on thinness and exercise. No family constellations are specific to anorexia nervosa, but some evidence indicate that these patients have close, but troubled, relationships with their parents. Families of children who present with eating disorders, especially binge eating or purging subtypes, may exhibit high levels of hostility, chaos, and isolation and low levels of nurturance and empathy. An adolescent with a severe eating disorder may tend to draw attention away from strained marital relationships.

Vocational and avocational interests interact with other vulnerability factors to increase the probability of developing eating disorders. In young women, participation in strict ballet schools increases the probability of developing anorexia nervosa at least sevenfold. In high school boys, wrestling is associated with a prevalence of full or partial eating-disorder syndromes during wrestling season of approximately 17 percent, with a minority

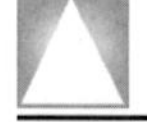

Table 11.1–2
Neuroendocrine Changes in Anorexia Nervosa and Experimental Starvation

Hormone	Anorexia Nervosa	Weight Loss
Corticotropin-releasing hormone (CRH)	Increased	Increased
Plasma cortisol levels	Mildly increased	Mildly increased
Diurnal cortisol difference	Blunted	Blunted
Luteinizing hormone (LH)	Decreased, prepubertal pattern	Decreased
Follicle-stimulating hormone (FSH)	Decreased, prepubertal pattern	Decreased
Growth hormone (GH)	Impaired regulation Increased basal levels and limited response to pharmacological probes	Same
Somatomedin C	Decreased	Decreased
Thyroxine (T_4)	Normal or slightly decreased	Normal or slightly decreased
Triiodothyronine (T_3)	Mildly decreased	Mildly decreased
Reverse T_3	Mildly increased	Mildly increased
Thyrotropin-stimulating hormone (TSH)	Normal	Normal
TSH response to thyrotropin-releasing hormone (TRH)	Delayed or blunted	Delayed or blunted
Insulin	Delayed release	–
C-peptide	Decreased	–
Vasopressin	Secretion uncoupled from osmotic challenge	–
Serotonin	Increased function with weight restoration	
Norepinephrine	Reduced turnover	Reduced turnover
Dopamine	Blunted response to pharmacological probes	–

developing an eating disorder and not improving spontaneously at the end of training. Although these athletic activities probably select for perfectionistic and persevering youth in the first place, pressures regarding weight and shape generated in these social milieus reinforce the likelihood that these predisposing factors will be channeled toward eating disorders.

A gay orientation in men is a proved predisposing factor, not because of sexual orientation or sexual behavior per se, but because norms for slimness, albeit muscular slimness, are very strong in the gay community, only slightly lower than for heterosexual women. In contrast, a lesbian orientation may be slightly protective, because lesbian communities may be more tolerant of higher weights and a more normative natural distribution of body shapes than their heterosexual female counterparts.

Psychological and Psychodynamic Factors

Anorexia nervosa appears to be a reaction to the demand that adolescents behave more independently and increase their social and sexual functioning. Patients with the disorder substitute their preoccupations, which are similar to obsessions, with eating and weight gain for other, normal adolescent pursuits. These patients typically lack a sense of autonomy and selfhood. Many experience their bodies as somehow under the control of their parents, so that self-starvation may be an effort to gain validation as a unique and special person. Only through acts of extraordinary self-discipline can an anorectic patient develop a sense of autonomy and selfhood.

Psychoanalytic clinicians who treat patients with anorexia nervosa generally agree that these young patients have been unable to separate psychologically from their mothers. The body may be perceived as though it were inhabited by the introject of an intrusive and unempathic mother. Starvation may unconsciously mean arresting the growth of this intrusive internal object and thereby destroying it. Often, a projective identification process is involved in the interactions between the patient and the patient's family. Many anorectic patients feel that oral desires are greedy and unacceptable; therefore, these desires are projectively disavowed. Other theories have focused on fantasies of oral impregnation. Parents respond to the refusal to eat by becoming frantic about whether the patient is actually eating. The patient can then view the parents as the ones who have unacceptable desires and can projectively disavow them; that is, others may be voracious and ruled by desire but not the patient.

DIAGNOSIS AND CLINICAL FEATURES

The onset of anorexia nervosa usually occurs between the ages of 10 and 30 years. It is present when (1) an individual voluntarily reduces and maintains an unhealthy degree of weight loss or fails to gain weight proportional to growth; (2) an individual experiences an intense fear of becoming fat, has a relentless drive for thinness despite obvious medical starvation, or both; (3) an individual experiences significant starvation-related medical symptomatology, often, but not exclusively, abnormal reproductive hormone functioning, but also hypothermia, bradycardia, orthostatic, and severely reduced body fat stores; and (4) the behaviors and psychopathology are present for at least 3 months.

The fifth edition of the *Diagnostic and Statistical Manual of Mental Disorders* (DSM-5) requires that patients have a significantly less than minimally normal weight and a marked fear of gaining weight. In spite of being thin, they believe themselves to be fat and restrict their food intake accordingly. They also have little or no insight into the seriousness of their condition nor that their body image is distorted.

There are two subtypes described in DSM-5: (1) the restricting type in which the person loses weight mainly by fasting, dieting, and excessive exercising; and (2) the binge-eating/purging type in which the person has repeated episodes of self-induced vomiting and the use of laxatives, enemas, or diuretics to lose weight. DSM-5 has specific degrees of severity based on body mass index (BMI): Mild: BMI ≥ 17 kg/m^2; Moderate: BMI 16 to 16.99 kg/m^2; Severe: BMI 15 to 15.99 kg/m^2; and Extreme: BMI <15 kg/m^2.

An intense fear of gaining weight and becoming obese is present in all patients with the disorder and undoubtedly contributes to their lack of interest in, and even resistance to, therapy. Most aberrant behavior directed toward losing weight occurs in secret. Patients with anorexia nervosa usually refuse to eat with their families or in public places. They lose weight by drastically reducing their total food intake, with a disproportionate decrease in high-carbohydrate and fatty foods.

As mentioned, the term "anorexia" is a misnomer, because loss of appetite is usually rare until late in the disorder. Evidence that patients are constantly thinking about food is their passion for collecting recipes and for preparing elaborate meals for others. Some patients cannot continuously control their voluntary restriction of food intake and so have eating binges. These binges usually occur secretly and often at night and are frequently followed by self-induced vomiting. Patients abuse laxatives and even diuretics to lose weight, and ritualistic exercising, extensive cycling, walking, jogging, and running are common activities.

Patients with the disorder exhibit peculiar behavior about food. They hide food all over the house and frequently carry large quantities of candies in their pockets and purses. While eating meals, they try to dispose of food in their napkins or hide it in their pockets. They cut their meat into very small pieces and spend a great deal of time rearranging the pieces on their plates. If the patients are confronted with their peculiar behavior, they often deny that their behavior is unusual or flatly refuse to discuss it.

Obsessive-compulsive behavior, depression, and anxiety are other psychiatric symptoms of anorexia nervosa most frequently noted clinically. Patients tend to be rigid and perfectionist, and somatic complaints, especially epigastric discomfort, are usual. Compulsive stealing, usually of candies and laxatives but occasionally of clothes and other items, may occur.

Poor sexual adjustment is frequently described in patients with the disorder. Many adolescent patients with anorexia nervosa have delayed psychosocial sexual development; in adults, a markedly decreased interest in sex often accompanies onset of the disorder. A minority of anorexic patients has a premorbid history of promiscuity, substance abuse, or both but during the disorder show a decreased interest in sex.

Patients usually come to medical attention when their weight loss becomes apparent. As the weight loss grows profound, physical signs such as hypothermia (as low as 35°C), dependent edema, bradycardia, hypotension, and lanugo (the appearance of neonatal-like hair) appear, and patients show a variety of metabolic changes. Some female patients with anorexia nervosa come to medical attention because of amenorrhea, which often appears before their weight loss is noticeable. Some patients induce vomiting or abuse purgatives and diuretics; such behavior causes concern about hypokalemic alkalosis. Impaired water diuresis may be noted.

Electrocardiographic (ECG) changes, such as T wave flattening or inversion, ST segment depression, and lengthening of the QT interval, have been noted in the emaciated stage of anorexia nervosa. ECG changes may also result from potassium loss, which can lead to death. Gastric dilation is a rare complication of anorexia nervosa. In some patients, aortography has shown a superior mesenteric artery syndrome. Other medical complications of eating disorders are listed in Table 11.1–3.

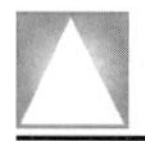

Table 11.1–3
Medical Complications of Eating Disorders

Disorder and System Affected	Consequence
Anorexia nervosa	
Vital signs	Bradycardia, hypotension with marked orthostatic changes, hypothermia, poikilothermia
General	Muscle atrophy, loss of body fat
Central nervous system	Generalized brain atrophy with enlarged ventricles, decreased cortical mass, seizures, abnormal electroencephalogram
Cardiovascular	Peripheral (starvation) edema, decreased cardiac diameter, narrowed left ventricular wall, decreased response to exercise demand, superior mesenteric artery syndrome
Renal	Prerenal azotemia
Hematologic	Anemia of starvation, leukopenia, hypocellular bone marrow
Gastrointestinal	Delayed gastric emptying, gastric dilatation, decreased intestinal lipase and lactase
Metabolic	Hypercholesterolemia, nonsymptomatic hypoglycemia, elevated liver enzymes, decreased bone mineral density
Endocrine	Low luteinizing hormone, low follicle-stimulating hormone, low estrogen or testosterone, low/normal thyroxine, low triiodothyronine, increased reverse triiodothyronine, elevated cortisol, elevated growth hormone, partial diabetes insipidus, increased prolactin
Bulimia Nervosa and Binge Eating and Purging Type Anorexia Nervosa	
Metabolic	Hypokalemic alkalosis or acidosis, hypochloremia, dehydration
Renal	Prerenal azotemia, acute and chronic renal failure
Cardiovascular	Arrhythmias, myocardial toxicity from emetine (ipecac)
Dental	Lingual surface enamel loss, multiple caries
Gastrointestinal	Swollen parotid glands, elevated serum amylase levels, gastric distention, irritable bowel syndrome, melanosis coli from laxative abuse
Musculoskeletal	Cramps, tetany

Subtypes

As mentioned above, Anorexia nervosa has been divided into two clinical subtypes: the food-restricting category and the binge-purging category. In the food-restricting category, present in approximately 50 percent of cases, food intake is highly restricted (usually with attempts to consume fewer than 300 to 500 calories per day and no fat grams), and the patient may be relentlessly and compulsively overactive, with overuse athletic injuries. In the binge-purging subtype, patients alternate attempts at rigorous dieting with intermittent binge or purge episodes. Purging represents a secondary compensation for the unwanted calories, most often accomplished by self-induced vomiting, frequently by laxative abuse, less frequently by diuretics, and occasionally with emetics. Sometimes, repetitive purging occurs without prior binge eating, after ingesting only relatively few calories. Both types may be socially isolated and have depressive disorder symptoms and diminished sexual interest. Over exercising and perfectionistic traits are also common in both types.

A new diagnostic category in DSM-5 is binge eating disorder (see Section 11-3) characterized by episodic bouts of the intake of excessive amounts of food but without purging or similar compensatory behavior.

Those who practice binge eating and purging share many features with persons who have bulimia nervosa without anorexia nervosa. Those who binge eat and purge tend to have families in which some members are obese, and they themselves have histories of heavier body weights before the disorder than do persons with the restricting type. Binge eating–purging persons are likely to be associated with substance abuse, impulse control disorders, and personality disorders. Persons with restricting anorexia nervosa often have obsessive-compulsive traits with respect to food and other matters. Some persons with anorexia nervosa may purge but not binge.

Persons with anorexia nervosa have high rates of comorbid major depressive disorders; major depressive disorder or dysthymic disorder has been reported in up to 50 percent of patients with anorexia nervosa. The suicide rate is higher in persons with the binge eating–purging type of anorexia nervosa than in those with the restricting type.

Patients with anorexia nervosa are often secretive, deny their symptoms, and resist treatment. In almost all cases, relatives or intimate acquaintances must confirm a patient's history. The mental status examination usually shows a patient who is alert and knowledgeable on the subject of nutrition and who is preoccupied with food and weight.

A patient must have a thorough general physical and neurological examination. If the patient is vomiting, a hypokalemic alkalosis may be present. Because most patients are dehydrated, serum electrolyte levels must be determined initially and periodically. Hospitalization may be necessary to deal with medical complications.

A young woman who weighed 10 percent above the average weight but was otherwise healthy, functioning well, and working hard as a university student joined a track team, started training for hours a day, more than her teammates, began to perceive herself as fat and thought that her performance would be enhanced if she lost weight. She started to diet and reduced her weight to 87 percent of the "ideal weight" for her age according to standard tables. At her point of maximum weight loss, her performance actually declined, and she pushed herself even harder in her training regimen. She started to feel apathetic and morbidly afraid of becoming fat. Her food intake became restricted and she stopped eating anything containing fat. Her menstrual periods became skimpy and infrequent but did not cease. *(Courtesy of Arnold E. Andersen, M.D. and Joel Yager, M.D.)*

PATHOLOGY AND LABORATORY EXAMINATION

A complete blood count often reveals leukopenia with a relative lymphocytosis in emaciated patients with anorexia nervosa. If binge eating and purging are present, serum electrolyte determination reveals hypokalemic alkalosis. Fasting serum glucose concentrations are often low during the emaciated phase, and serum salivary amylase concentrations are often elevated if the patient is vomiting. The ECG may show ST segment and T wave changes, which are usually secondary to electrolyte disturbances; emaciated patients have hypotension and bradycardia. Young girls may have a high serum cholesterol level. All these values revert to normal with nutritional rehabilitation and cessation of purging behaviors. Endocrine changes that may occur, such as amenorrhea, mild hypothyroidism, and hypersecretion of corticotrophin-releasing hormone, are caused by the underweight condition and revert to normal with weight gain.

DIFFERENTIAL DIAGNOSIS

The differential diagnosis of anorexia nervosa is complicated by patients' denial of the symptoms, the secrecy surrounding their bizarre eating rituals, and their resistance to seeking treatment. Thus, it may be difficult to identify the mechanism of weight loss and the patient's associated ruminative thoughts about distortions of body image.

Clinicians must ascertain that a patient does not have a medical illness that can account for the weight loss (e.g., a brain tumor or cancer). Weight loss, peculiar eating behaviors, and vomiting can occur in several mental disorders. Depressive disorders and anorexia nervosa have several features in common, such as depressed feelings, crying spells, sleep disturbance, obsessive ruminations, and occasional suicidal thoughts. The two disorders, however, have several distinguishing features. Generally, a patient with a depressive disorder has decreased appetite, whereas a patient with anorexia nervosa claims to have normal appetite and to feel hungry; only in the severe stages of anorexia nervosa do patients actually have decreased appetite. In contrast to depressive agitation, the hyperactivity seen in anorexia nervosa is planned and ritualistic. The preoccupation with recipes, the caloric content of foods, and the preparation of gourmet feasts is typical of patients with anorexia nervosa but is absent in patients with a depressive disorder. In depressive disorders, patients have no intense fear of obesity or disturbance of body image.

Weight fluctuations, vomiting, and peculiar food handling may occur in somatization disorder. On rare occasions, a patient fulfills the diagnostic criteria for both somatization disorder and anorexia nervosa; in such a case, both diagnoses should be made. Generally, the weight loss in somatization disorder is not as severe as that in anorexia nervosa, nor does a patient with somatization disorder express a morbid fear of becoming overweight, as is common in those with anorexia nervosa. Amenorrhea for 3 months or longer is unusual in somatization disorder.

In patients with schizophrenia, delusions about food are seldom concerned with caloric content. More likely, they believe the food to be poisoned. Patients with schizophrenia are rarely preoccupied with a fear of becoming obese and do not have the hyperactivity that is seen in patients with anorexia nervosa. Patients with schizophrenia have bizarre eating habits but not the entire syndrome of anorexia nervosa.

Anorexia nervosa must be differentiated from bulimia nervosa, a disorder in which episodic binge eating, followed by depressive moods, self-deprecating thoughts, and self-induced vomiting occur while patients maintain their weight within a normal range. Patients with bulimia nervosa seldom lose 15 percent of their weight, but the two conditions frequently coexist.

Rare conditions of unknown etiology are seen in which hyperactivity of the vagus nerve causes changes in eating patterns that are associated with weight loss, sometimes of severe degree. In such cases bradycardia, hypotension, and other parasympathomimetic signs and symptoms are seen. Because the vagus nerve relates to the enteric nervous system, eating may be associated with gastric distress such as nausea or bloating. Patients do not generally lose their appetite. Treatment is symptomatic and anticholinergic drugs can reverse hypotension and bradycardia, which may be life-threatening.

COURSE AND PROGNOSIS

The course of anorexia nervosa varies greatly—spontaneous recovery without treatment, recovery after a variety of treatments, a fluctuating course of weight gains followed by relapses, and a gradually deteriorating course resulting in death caused by complications of starvation. One study reviewing subtypes of anorectic patients found that restricting-type anorectic patients seemed less likely to recover than those of the binge eating–purging type. The short-term response of patients to almost all hospital treatment programs is good. Those who have regained sufficient weight, however, often continue their preoccupation with food and body weight, have poor social relationships, and exhibit depression. In general, the prognosis is not good. Studies have shown a range of mortality rates from 5 to 18 percent.

Indicators of a favorable outcome are admission of hunger, lessening of denial and immaturity, and improved self-esteem. Such factors as childhood neuroticism, parental conflict, bulimia nervosa, vomiting, laxative abuse, and various behavioral manifestations (e.g., obsessive-compulsive, hysterical, depressive, psychosomatic, neurotic, and denial symptoms) have been related to poor outcome in some studies, but not in others.

Ten-year outcome studies in the United States have shown that about one-fourth of patients recover completely and another one-half are markedly improved and functioning fairly well. The other one-fourth includes an overall 7 percent mortality rate and those who are functioning poorly with a chronic underweight condition. Swedish and English studies over a 20- and 30-year period show a mortality rate of 18 percent. About half of patients with anorexia nervosa eventually will have the symptoms of bulimia, usually within the first year after the onset of anorexia nervosa.

TREATMENT

In view of the complicated psychological and medical implications of anorexia nervosa, a comprehensive treatment plan, including hospitalization when necessary and both individual and family therapy, is recommended. Behavioral, interpersonal, and cognitive approaches are used and, in many cases, medication may be indicated.

Hospitalization

The first consideration in the treatment of anorexia nervosa is to restore patients' nutritional state; dehydration, starvation, and electrolyte imbalances can seriously compromise health and, in some cases, lead to death. The decision to hospitalize a patient is based on the patient's medical condition and the amount of structure needed to ensure patient cooperation. In general, patients with anorexia nervosa who are 20 percent below the expected weight for their height are recommended for inpatient programs, and patients who are 30 percent below their expected weight require psychiatric hospitalization for 2 to 6 months.

Inpatient psychiatric programs for patients with anorexia nervosa generally use a combination of a behavioral management approach, individual psychotherapy, family education and therapy, and, in some cases, psychotropic medications. Successful treatment is promoted by the ability of staff members to maintain a firm yet supportive approach to patients, often through a combination of positive reinforcers (praise) and negative reinforcers (restriction of exercise). The program must have some flexibility for individualizing treatment to meet patients' needs and cognitive abilities. Patients must become willing participants for treatment to succeed in the long run.

Most patients are uninterested in psychiatric treatment and even resist it; they are brought to a doctor's office unwillingly by agonizing relatives or friends. The patients rarely accept the recommendation of hospitalization without arguing and criticizing the proposed program. Emphasizing the benefits, such as relief of insomnia and depressive signs and symptoms, may help persuade the patients to admit themselves willingly to the hospital. Relatives' support and confidence in the physicians and treatment team are essential when firm recommendations must be carried out. Patients' families should be warned that the patients will resist admission and, for the first several weeks of treatment, will make many dramatic pleas for their families' support to obtain release from the hospital program. Compulsory admission or commitment should be obtained only when the risk of death from the complications of malnutrition is likely. On rare occasions, patients prove that the doctor's statements about the probable failure of outpatient treatment are wrong. They may gain a specified amount of weight by the time of each outpatient visit, but such behavior is uncommon, and a period of inpatient care is usually necessary.

Hospital Management

The following considerations apply to the general management of patients with anorexia nervosa during a hospitalized treatment program. Patients should be weighed daily, early in the morning after emptying the bladder. The daily fluid intake and urine output should be recorded. If vomiting is occurring, hospital staff members must monitor serum electrolyte levels regularly and watch for the development of hypokalemia. Because food is often regurgitated after meals, the staff may be able to control vomiting by making the bathroom inaccessible for at least 2 hours after meals or by having an attendant in the bathroom to prevent the opportunity for vomiting. Constipation in these patients is relieved when they begin to eat normally. Stool softeners may occasionally be given, but never laxatives. If diarrhea occurs, it usually means that patients are surreptitiously taking laxatives. Because of the rare complication of stomach dilation and the possibility of circulatory overload when patients immediately start eating an enormous number of calories, the hospital staff should give patients about 500 calories over the amount required to maintain their present weight (usually 1,500 to 2,000 calories a day). It is wise to give these calories in six equal feedings throughout the day, so that patients need not eat a large amount of food at one sitting. Giving patients a liquid food supplement such as Sustagen may be advisable, because they may be less apprehensive about gaining weight slowly with the formula than by eating food. After patients are discharged from the hospital, clinicians usually find it necessary to continue outpatient supervision of the problems identified in the patients and their families.

Psychotherapy

Cognitive–Behavioral Therapy. Cognitive and behavioral therapy principles can be applied in both inpatient and outpatient settings and have been found effective for inducing weight gain. Monitoring is an essential component of cognitive–behavioral therapy. Patients are taught to monitor their food intake, their feelings and emotions, their binging and purging behaviors, and their problems in interpersonal relationships. Patients are taught cognitive restructuring to identify automatic thoughts and challenge their core beliefs. Problem solving is a specific method whereby patients learn how to think through and devise strategies to cope with their food-related and interpersonal problems. Patients' vulnerability to rely on anorectic behavior as a means of coping can be addressed if they can learn to use these techniques effectively.

Dynamic Psychotherapy. Dynamic expressive–supportive psychotherapy is sometimes used in the treatment of patients with anorexia nervosa, but their resistance may make the process difficult and painstaking. Because patients view their symptoms as constituting the core of their specialness, therapists must avoid excessive investment in trying to change their eating behavior. The opening phase of the psychotherapy process must be geared toward building a therapeutic alliance. Patients may experience early interpretations as though someone else were telling them what they really feel and thereby minimizing and invalidating their own experiences. Therapists who empathize with patients' points of view and take an active interest in what their patients think and feel, however, convey to patients that their autonomy is respected. Above all, psychotherapists must be flexible, persistent, and durable in the face of patients' tendencies to defeat any effort to help them.

Family Therapy. A family analysis should be done for all patients with anorexia nervosa who are living with their families, which is used as a basis for a clinical judgment on what type of family therapy or counseling is advisable. In some cases, family therapy is not possible; however, issues of family relationships can then be addressed in individual therapy. Sometimes, brief counseling sessions with immediate family members is the extent of family therapy required. In one controlled family therapy study in London, anorectic patients under the age of 18 benefited from family therapy, whereas patients over the age of 18 did worse in family therapy than with the control therapy. No controlled studies have been reported on the combination of individual and family therapy; however, in actual practice, most clinicians provide individual therapy and some form of family counseling in managing patients with anorexia nervosa.

Pharmacotherapy

Pharmacological studies have not yet identified any medication that yields definitive improvement of the core symptoms of anorexia nervosa. Some reports support the use of cyproheptadine (Periactin), a drug with antihistaminic and antiserotonergic properties, for patients with the restricting type of anorexia nervosa. Amitriptyline (Elavil) has also been reported to have some benefit. Other medications that have been tried by patients with anorexia nervosa with variable results include clomipramine (Anafranil), pimozide (Orap), and chlorpromazine (Thorazine). Trials of fluoxetine (Prozac) have resulted in some reports of weight gain, and serotonergic agents may yield positive responses in some cases. In patients with anorexia nervosa and coexisting depressive disorders, the depressive condition should be treated. Concern exists about the use of tricyclic drugs in low-weight, depressed patients with anorexia nervosa, who may be vulnerable to hypotension, cardiac arrhythmia, and dehydration. Once an adequate nutritional status has been attained, the risk of serious adverse effects from the tricyclic drugs may decrease; in some patients, the depression improves with weight gain and normalized nutritional status.

▲ 11.2 Bulimia Nervosa

Bulimia nervosa is characterized by episodes of binge eating combined with inappropriate ways of stopping weight gain. Physical discomfort—for example, abdominal pain or nausea—terminates the binge eating, which is often followed by feelings of guilt, depression, or self-disgust. Unlike patients with anorexia nervosa, those with bulimia nervosa typically maintain a normal body weight.

The term *bulimia nervosa* derives from the terms for "ox-hunger" in Greek and "nervous involvement" in Latin. For some patients, bulimia nervosa may represent a failed attempt at anorexia nervosa, sharing the goal of becoming very thin, but occurring in an individual less able to sustain prolonged semi starvation or severe hunger as consistently as classic restricting anorexia nervosa patients. For others, eating binges represent "breakthrough eating" episodes of giving in to hunger pangs generated by efforts to restrict eating so as to maintain a socially desirable level of thinness. Still others use binge eating as a means to self-medicate during times of emotional distress. Regardless of the reason, eating binges provoke panic as individuals feel that their eating has been out of control. The unwanted binges lead to secondary attempts to avoid the feared weight gain by a variety of compensatory behaviors, such as purging or excessive exercise.

EPIDEMIOLOGY

Bulimia nervosa is more prevalent than anorexia nervosa. Estimates of bulimia nervosa range from 1 to 4 percent in young women. As with anorexia nervosa, bulimia nervosa is more common in women than in men, but its onset is often later in adolescence than that of anorexia nervosa. The onset may also occur in early adulthood. Approximately 20 percent of college women experience transient bulimic symptoms at some point during their college years. Although bulimia nervosa is often present in normal-weight young women, they sometimes have a history of obesity. In industrialized countries, the prevalence is about 1 percent of the general population. In the United States, bulimia nervosa may be more prevalent among Hispanics and blacks than non-Hispanic whites.

ETIOLOGY

Biological Factors

Some investigators have attempted to associate cycles of binging and purging with various neurotransmitters. Because antidepressants often benefit patients with bulimia nervosa and because serotonin has been linked to satiety, serotonin and norepinephrine have been implicated. Because plasma endorphin levels are raised in some bulimia nervosa patients who vomit, the feeling of well-being after vomiting that some of these patients experience may be mediated by raised endorphin levels. Increased frequency of bulimia nervosa is found in first-degree relatives of persons with the disorder.

Recent research using functional magnetic resonance imaging (MRI) suggests that overeating in bulimia nervosa may result from an exaggerated perception of hunger signals related to sweet taste mediated by the right anterior insula area of the brain.

Social Factors

Patients with bulimia nervosa, as with those with anorexia nervosa, tend to be high achievers and to respond to societal pressures to be slender. As with anorexia nervosa patients, many patients with bulimia nervosa are depressed and have increased familial depression, but the families of patients with bulimia nervosa are generally less close and more conflictual than the families of those with anorexia nervosa. Patients with bulimia nervosa describe their parents as neglectful and rejecting.

Psychological Factors

Patients with bulimia nervosa, as with those with anorexia nervosa, have difficulties with adolescent demands, but patients with bulimia nervosa are more outgoing, angry, and impulsive than those with anorexia nervosa. Alcohol dependence, shoplifting, and emotional lability (including suicide attempts) are associated with bulimia nervosa. These patients generally experience their uncontrolled eating as more ego-dystonic than do patients with anorexia nervosa and so seek help more readily.

Patients with bulimia nervosa lack superego control and the ego strength of their counterparts with anorexia nervosa. Their difficulties in controlling their impulses are often manifested by substance dependence and self-destructive sexual relationships in addition to the binge eating and purging that characterize the disorder. Many patients with bulimia nervosa have histories of difficulties separating from caretakers, as manifested by the absence of transitional objects during their early childhood years. Some clinicians have observed that patients with bulimia nervosa use their own bodies as transitional objects. The struggle for separation from a maternal figure is played out in the ambivalence toward food; eating may represent a wish to fuse with the caretaker, and regurgitating may unconsciously express a wish for separation.

DIAGNOSIS AND CLINICAL FEATURES

Bulimia nervosa is present when (1) episodes of binge eating occurs relatively frequently (once a week or more) for at least 3 months; (2) compensatory behaviors are practiced after binge eating to prevent weight gain, primarily self-induced vomiting, laxative abuse, diuretics, enemas, abuse of emetics (80 percent of cases), and, less commonly, severe dieting and strenuous exercise (20 percent of cases); (3) weight is not severely lowered as in anorexia nervosa; and (4) the patient has a morbid fear of fatness, a relentless drive for thinness, or both and a disproportionate amount of self-evaluation that depends on body weight and shape. When making a diagnosis of bulimia nervosa, clinicians should explore the possibility that the patient has experienced a brief or prolonged prior bout of anorexia nervosa, which is present in approximately half of those with bulimia nervosa. Binging usually precedes vomiting by about 1 year. DSM-5 also suggests that the person have no concept of how much they do or should eat at any one sitting. The disorder can be classified as mild (1 to 3 episodes per week); moderate (4 to 7 episodes); severe (8 to 13 episodes); and extreme (more than 14 episodes).

Vomiting is common and is usually induced by sticking a finger down the throat, although some patients are able to vomit at will. Vomiting decreases the abdominal pain and the feeling of being bloated and allows patients to continue eating without fear of gaining weight. The acid content of vomitus can damage tooth enamel, a not uncommon finding in patients with the disorder. Depression, sometimes called *postbinge anguish,* often follows the episode. During binges, patients eat food that is sweet, high in calories, and generally soft or smooth textured, such as cakes and pastry. Some patients prefer bulky foods without regard to taste. The food is eaten secretly and rapidly and is sometimes not even chewed. The food ingested is sometimes unusual such as entire loaves of bread or raw or undercooked chicken. Observers of binge eaters often report a feeling of revulsion as they watch the person gorging themselves on such foods.

Annie is a 26-year-old Dutch woman. She works as a nurse in a city hospital and lives alone. Annie would wake up at night, go to her kitchen, and start eating whatever food she could lay her hands on. She stopped only after an hour or two when she could find no more food. The bouts of overeating went on for 5 years until she consulted her general practitioner, who referred her to outpatient psychiatric treatment for a depression related to the eating spells. Annie's spells of uncontrollable overeating were preceded by a feeling of severe tension and were followed by relaxation, although this was coupled with shame and despair. During the year before her referral, the frequency of the overeating spells had increased to two or three times a week. They usually appeared at night after just a few hours of sleep. After eating her way through whatever she could find, she would feel bloated but would not vomit. She tried to get rid of the food by taking large quantities of laxatives. Her weight was unstable, but she managed to keep it within normal limits simply by fasting between the overeating spells. Annie despised obesity but had never really been slim. Her bouts of overeating made her feel increasingly low-spirited and despairing. She had even considered committing suicide by taking an overdose of the sleeping tablets that her general practitioner had prescribed because of her interrupted sleep. Annie managed to do her job adequately and had taken only a few days of sick leave.

Annie was brought up in a village, where her father was a schoolteacher. After secondary school she trained as a nurse and had various jobs on geriatric wards. Annie had always been very sensitive and fearful of criticism and had low self-esteem. She tried hard to live up to expectations and felt frustrated by minor criticisms. She had been in love more than once, but never dared to become engaged because she feared rejection and possibly also because she feared a sexual relationship. She had only a few close friends because she had difficulty engaging in close relationships. She often felt tense and diffident in company. She avoided going to meetings or parties because she feared being criticized or rejected.

On examination Annie appeared quiet and reticent. Her mood was mildly depressed, and she cried silently as she described her difficulties. No psychotic features were suspected. She was otherwise healthy and of average weight. She perceived her own weight to be slightly higher than the weight she would prefer. She said she was afraid of becoming obese. *(Courtesy of International Statistical Classification of Diseases and Related Health Problems, 10th ed. Casebook)*

Most patients with bulimia nervosa are within their normal weight range, but some may be underweight or overweight. These patients are concerned about their body image and their appearance, worried about how others see them, and concerned about their sexual attractiveness. Most are sexually active, compared with anorexia nervosa patients, who are not interested in sex. Pica and struggles during meals are sometimes revealed in the histories of patients with bulimia nervosa.

Bulimia nervosa occurs in persons with high rates of mood disorders and impulse control disorders. Bulimia nervosa is also reported to occur in those at risk for substance-related disorders and a variety of personality disorders. Patients with bulimia nervosa also have increased rates of anxiety disorders, bipolar I disorder, dissociative disorders, and histories of sexual abuse.

Subtypes

Evidence indicates that bulimic persons who purge differ from binge eaters who do not purge in that the latter tend to have less body-image disturbance and less anxiety concerning eating. Those with bulimia nervosa who do not purge tend to be obese. Distinct physiological differences also exist between patients with bulimia who purge and those who do not. Because of all these differences, the diagnosis of bulimia nervous is sometimes subtyped into a purging type, for those who regularly engage in self-induced vomiting or the use of laxatives or diuretics, and a nonpurging type, for those who use strict dieting, fasting, or vigorous exercise but do not regularly engage in purging. Patients who purge may have a different course from that of patients who binge and then diet or exercise.

Patients with purging type may be at risk for certain medical complications such as hypokalemia from vomiting or laxative abuse and hypochloremic alkalosis. Those who vomit repeatedly are at risk for gastric and esophageal tears, although these complications are rare.

PATHOLOGY AND LABORATORY EXAMINATIONS

Bulimia nervosa can result in electrolyte abnormalities and various degrees of starvation, although it may not be as obvious as in low-weight patients with anorexia nervosa. Thus, even normal-weight patients with bulimia nervosa should have laboratory studies of electrolytes and metabolism. In general, thyroid function remains intact in bulimia nervosa, but patients may show nonsuppression on a dexamethasone-suppression test. Dehydration and electrolyte disturbances are likely to occur in patients with bulimia nervosa who purge regularly. These patients commonly exhibit hypomagnesemia and hyperamylasemia. Although not a core diagnostic feature, many patients with bulimia nervosa have menstrual disturbances. Hypotension and bradycardia occur in some patients.

DIFFERENTIAL DIAGNOSIS

The diagnosis of bulimia nervosa cannot be made if the binge-eating and purging behaviors occur exclusively during episodes of anorexia nervosa. In such cases, the diagnosis is anorexia nervosa, binge eating-purging type.

Clinicians must ascertain that patients have no neurological disease, such as epileptic-equivalent seizures, central nervous system tumors, Klüver–Bucy syndrome, or Kleine–Levin syndrome. The pathological features manifested by Klüver–Bucy syndrome are visual agnosia, compulsive licking and biting, examination of objects by the mouth, inability to ignore any stimulus, placidity, altered sexual behavior (hypersexuality), and altered dietary habits, especially hyperphagia. The syndrome is exceedingly rare and is unlikely to cause a problem in differential diagnosis. Kleine–Levin syndrome consists of periodic hypersomnia lasting for 2 to 3 weeks and hyperphagia. As in bulimia nervosa, the onset is usually during adolescence, but the syndrome is more common in men than in women.

Patients with bulimia nervosa who have concurrent seasonal affective disorder and patterns of atypical depression (with overeating and oversleeping in low-light months) may manifest seasonal worsening of both bulimia nervosa and depressive features. In these cases, binges are typically much more severe during winter months. Bright light therapy (10,000 lux for 30 minutes, in early morning, at 18 to 22 in from the eyes) may be a useful component of comprehensive treatment of an eating disorder with seasonal affective disorder.

Some patients with bulimia nervosa—perhaps 15 percent—have multiple comorbid impulsive behaviors, including substance abuse, and lack of ability to control themselves in such diverse areas as money management (resulting in impulse buying and compulsive shopping) and sexual relationships (often resulting in brief, passionate attachments and promiscuity). They exhibit self-mutilation, chaotic emotions, and chaotic sleeping patterns. They often meet criteria for borderline personality disorder and other mixed personality disorders and, not infrequently, bipolar II disorder.

COURSE AND PROGNOSIS

Bulimia nervosa is characterized by higher rates of partial and full recovery compared with anorexia nervosa. As noted in the treatment section, those treated fare much better than those who are untreated. Patients who are untreated tend to remain chronic or may show small, but generally unimpressive, degrees of improvement with time. In a 10-year follow-up study of patients who had previously participated in treatment programs, the number of women who continued to meet the full criteria for bulimia nervosa declined as the duration of follow-up increased. Approximately 30 percent continued to engage in recurrent binge-eating or purging behaviors. A history of substance use problems and a longer duration of the disorder at presentation predicted worse outcome. Approximately 40 percent of women were fully recovered at follow-up. The mortality rate for bulimia nervosa has been estimated at 2 percent per decade according to DSM-5.

TREATMENT

Most patients with uncomplicated bulimia nervosa do not require hospitalization. In general, patients with bulimia nervosa are not as secretive about their symptoms as patients with anorexia nervosa. Therefore, outpatient treatment is usually not difficult, but psychotherapy is frequently stormy and may be prolonged. Some obese patients with bulimia nervosa who have had prolonged psychotherapy do surprisingly well. In some cases—when eating binges are out of control, outpatient treatment does not work, or a patient exhibits such additional psychiatric symptoms as suicidality and substance abuse—hospitalization may become necessary. In addition, electrolyte and metabolic disturbances resulting from severe purging may necessitate hospitalization.

Psychotherapy

Cognitive–Behavioral Therapy. Cognitive–behavioral therapy (CBT) should be considered the benchmark, first-line treatment for bulimia nervosa. The data supporting the efficacy of CBT are based on strict adherence to rigorously implemented, highly detailed, manual-guided treatments that include about 18 to 20 sessions over 5 to 6 months. CBT implements a number of cognitive and behavioral procedures to (1) interrupt the self-maintaining behavioral cycle of binging and dieting and (2) alter the individual's dysfunctional cognitions; beliefs about food, weight, body image; and overall self-concept.

Dynamic Psychotherapy. Psychodynamic treatment of patients with bulimia nervosa has been of limited success. Psychodynamic formulations revealed a tendency to concretize introjective and projective defense mechanisms. In a manner analogous to splitting, patients divide food into two categories: items that are nutritious and those that are unhealthy. Food that is designated nutritious may be ingested and retained because it unconsciously symbolizes good introjects. But junk food is unconsciously associated with bad introjects and, therefore, is expelled by vomiting, with the unconscious fantasy that all destructiveness, hate, and badness are being evacuated. Patients can temporarily feel good after vomiting because of the fantasized evacuation, but the associated feeling of "being all good" is short-lived because it is based on an unstable combination of splitting and projection.

Other Modalities. Controlled trials have shown that a variety of novel ways of administering and facilitating cognitive–behavioral therapy are effective for bulimia nervosa. Some have been incorporated in "stepped-care" programs and including internet-based platforms, computer facilitated programs, email enhanced programs, and administration of cognitive–behavioral therapy via telemedicine to remote areas.

Pharmacotherapy

Antidepressant medications have been shown to be helpful in treating bulimia. This includes the selective serotonin reuptake inhibitors (SSRIs), such as fluoxetine (Prozac). This may be based on elevating central 5-hydroxytryptamine levels. Antidepressant medications can reduce binge eating and purging independent of the presence of a mood disorder. Thus, antidepressants have been used successfully for particularly difficult binge–purge cycles that do not respond to psychotherapy alone. Imipramine (Tofranil), desipramine (Norpramin), trazodone (Desyrel), and monoamine oxidase inhibitors (MAOIs) have been helpful. In general, most of the antidepressants have been effective at dosages usually given in the treatment of depressive disorders. Dosages of fluoxetine that are effective in decreasing binge eating, however, may be higher (60 to 80 mg a day) than those used for depressive disorders. Medication is helpful in patients with comorbid depressive disorders and bulimia nervosa. Carbamazepine (Tegretol) and lithium (Eskalith) have not shown impressive results as treatments for binge eating, but they have been used in the treatment of patients with bulimia nervosa with comorbid mood disorders, such as bipolar I disorder. Evidence indicates that the use of antidepressants alone results in a 22 percent rate of abstinence from binging and purging; other studies show that CBT and medications are the most effective combinations.

▲ 11.3 Binge Eating Disorder and Other Eating Disorders

BINGE EATING DISORDER

Individuals with binge eating disorder engage in recurrent binge eating during which they eat an abnormally large amount of food over a short time. Unlike bulimia nervosa, patients with binge eating disorder do not compensate in any way after a binge episode (e.g., laxative use). Binge episodes often occur in private, generally include foods of dense caloric content, and, during the binge, the person feels he or she cannot control his or her eating.

Epidemiology

Binge eating disorder is the most common eating disorder. It appears in approximately 25 percent of patients who seek medical care for obesity and in 50 to 75 percent of those with severe obesity (BMI greater than 40). It is more common in females (4 percent) than in males (2 percent).

Etiology

The cause of binge eating disorder is unknown. Impulsive and extroverted personality styles are linked to the disorder as are persons who place themselves on a very low calorie diet. Binge eating may also occur during periods of stress. It may be used to reduce anxiety or alleviate depressive moods.

Diagnosis and Clinical Features

To be diagnosed with binge eating disorder, the binges must be characterized by four features: (1) eating more rapidly than normal and to the point of being uncomfortably full, (2) eating large amounts of food even when not hungry, (3) eating alone, and (4) feeling guilty or otherwise upset about the episode. Binges must occur at least once a week for at least 3 months.

Approximately half of individuals with binge eating disorder are obese. Additionally, obese individuals with binge eating disorder have an earlier onset of obesity than those without the disorder. Patients with binge eating disorder are also more likely to have an unstable weight history with frequent episodes of weight cycling (the gaining or losing of more than 10 kg). The disorder may be associated with insomnia, early menarche, neck or shoulder and lower back pain, chronic muscle pain, and metabolic disorders.

Differential Diagnosis

Binge eating disorder and bulimia nervosa share the same core feature of recurrent binge eating. Binge eating disorder is distinct from bulimia nervosa, however, in that binge eating disorder patients do not report recurrent compensatory behavior such as vomiting, laxative abuse, or excessive dieting. Binge eating disorder is distinct from anorexia nervosa in that patients do not exhibit an excessive drive for thinness and are of normal weight or are obese.

The prevalence of binge eating disorder is higher in overweight populations (3 percent) than in the general population (approximately 2 percent). However, there are some distinctions. Obese patients with binge eating disorder have a greater caloric intake during binging and nonbinging episodes, greater eating disorder pathology (i.e., more emotional eating, chaotic eating habits), and higher rates of comorbid psychiatric disorders. Binge eating disorder is also more prevalent in families than obesity.

Course and Prognosis

Little is known about the course of binge eating disorder. Severe obesity is a long-term effect in over 3 percent of patients with the disorder. One prospective study of women in the community with binge eating disorder suggested that by 5 years of follow-up fewer than one-fifth of the sample still had clinically significant eating disorder symptoms.

Treatment

Psychotherapy. CBT is the most effective psychological treatment for binge eating disorder. CBT has been shown to lead to decreases in binge eating and associated problems (e.g., depression); however, studies have not shown marked weight loss as a result of CBT, and CBT combined with psychopharmacological treatments such as SSRIs show better results than CBT alone. Exercise has also shown a reduction in binge eating when combined with CBT. Interpersonal psychotherapy (IPT) has also shown to be effective in the treatment of binge eating disorder; however, therapy focuses more on the interpersonal problems that contribute to the disorder rather than disturbances in eating behavior.

Self-Help Groups. Self-help groups such as Overeaters Anonymous (OA) have proven to be helpful in patients with binge eating disorder. For the treatment of moderate obesity, organizations such as Weight Watchers can be extremely helpful and do not involve common fads or quick fixes.

Psychopharmacotherapy. Symptoms of binge eating may benefit from medication treatment with several SSRIs, desipramine (Norpramin), imipramine (Tofranil), topiramate (Topamax), and sibutramine (Meridia). SSRI medications that have demonstrated improvement in mood as well as binge eating include fluvoxamine (Luvox), citalopram (Celexa), and sertraline (Zoloft). Some studies showed that high-dose SSRI treatment (e.g., fluoxetine [Paxil] at 60 to 100 mg) often initially resulted in weight loss. However, the weight loss was ordinarily short lived, even when medication was continued, and weight always returned when medication was discontinued. Amphetamine and amphetamine-like drugs may help but are of little use over the long term.

Most, but not all, studies show that medication added to CBT is more effective than medication alone. For example, studies indicate that CBT did better than fluvoxamine or desipramine as a monotherapy for binge eating disorder; however, when CBT was used in combination with these agents, more improvement was seen in terms of weight loss compared with CBT alone.

OTHER SPECIFIED FEEDING OR EATING DISORDER

The diagnostic category of "other specified feeding or eating disorder" can be used for eating conditions that may cause significant distress but do not meet the full criteria for a classified eating disorder. Conditions in this category include night eating syndrome, purging disorder, and subthreshold forms of anorexia nervosa, bulimia nervosa, and binge eating disorder.

Night Eating Syndrome

Night eating syndrome is characterized by the consumption of large amounts of food after the evening meal. Individuals generally have little appetite during the day and suffer from insomnia.

Epidemiology. Night eating syndrome occurs in approximately 2 percent of the general population; however, it has a higher prevalence among patients with insomnia, obesity (10 to 15 percent), eating disorders, and other psychiatric disorders. The disorder usually begins in early adulthood.

Etiology. Little is known about the cause of night eating disorder; however, the hormones melatonin, leptin, ghrelin, and cortisol have been studied in relation to the disorder. Night eating syndrome also appears to run in families; patients with night eating syndrome are five times more likely to have a first-degree relative with night eating syndrome.

Diagnosis and Clinical Features. The diagnosis of night eating disorder includes recurrent episodes of hyperphagia or night eating; the lack of desire for food in the morning; and insomnia. Symptoms must persist for at least 3 months and cannot be secondary to another medical or mental condition.

Patients with night eating syndrome usually consume a large portion of their daily calorie intake after the evening meal. They are also more likely to wake up during the night and to eat upon awakening. Nocturnal eating tends to occur during non–rapid eye movement (REM) sleep and is usually short in duration. Patients are also prone to low sleep efficiency. Patients believe that they can only sleep if they eat. Depressed mood is common among these patients, especially during the evening and night hours.

Differential Diagnosis. Night eating disorder is common among patients with other eating disorders, particularly bulimia nervosa and binge eating disorder. Although night eating can be found in bulimia nervosa and binge eating disorder, it is the characteristic sign of night eating disorder. Also, the amount of food consumed during eating episodes is usually lower in night eating disorder than in bulimia nervosa and binge eating disorder. Unlike other eating disorders, patients with night eating syndrome are not overly concerned about body image and weight. Patients with night eating disorder are also at higher risk for obesity and metabolic syndrome.

Sleep-related eating disorder is characterized by recurrent episodes of involuntary eating during the night. These episodes can lead to serious consequences such as the ingesting of nonedible foods or substances, dangerous behaviors while searching for or preparing food, and sleep-related injury. The eating episodes usually occur after the patient has gone to sleep and may occur while the patient is unconscious or asleep. Sleep-related eating disorder also has a high comorbidity with sleepwalking, restless leg syndrome, and obstructive sleep apnea, conditions that are rarely found among night eating syndrome patients. Episodes of sleep-related eating disorder have been reported after the use certain medications, including zolpidem (Ambien), triazolam (Halcion), olanzapine (Zyprexa), and risperidone (Risperdal).

Course and Prognosis. The age of onset for night eating syndrome ranges from the late teens to late 20s and has a long-lasting course with periods of remission with treatment. Patients who experience poor sleep quality are more likely to develop diabetes, obesity, hypertension, and cardiovascular disease.

Treatment. Various studies have shown positive results in patients treated with SSRIs who showed improvement in nighttime awakenings, nocturnal eating, and postevening caloric intake. Weight loss and a reduction in nocturnal eating have been associated with an addition of topiramate to medication regimens.

In patients with comorbid major depression and night eating syndrome, bright light therapy has shown to decrease depressed mood. CBT has also been helpful.

Purging Disorder

Purging disorder is characterized by recurrent purging behavior after consuming a small amount of food in persons of normal weight who have a distorted view of their weight or body image. Purging behavior includes self-induced vomiting, laxative abuse, enemas, and diuretics. To make the diagnosis, the behavior must not be associated with anorexia nervosa. Purging disorder is differentiated from bulimia nervosa because purging behavior occurs after eating small quantities of food or drink and does not occur as a result of a binge episode. Purging episodes should occur at least once a week over a 3-month period before the diagnosis is made.

▲ 11.4 Obesity and the Metabolic Syndrome

Obesity is a chronic illness manifested by an excess of body fat. It is generally measured by the BMI, but a more accurate method is to use body composition analysis also known as *biometric impedance analysis* (BIA). Excess body fat generally results from a greater amount of calories consumed than are burnt off. In healthy individuals, body fat—which is different from the BMI—varies by gender. It ranges from 10 to 13 percent of essential fat to 25 to 31 percent on average of body weight in healthy women. In men, it ranges from 2 to 5 percent of essential fat to 18 to 24 percent on average. The global epidemic of obesity has resulted in an alarming increase in associated morbidity and mortality. Although manifestation of obesity and its comorbid states are largely physical, it has overwhelming psychological ramifications. The diagnosis of obesity using the BMI is discussed below.

COMORBIDITY

Evidence shows a correlation between obesity and psychiatric disorders. In fact, among treatment-seeking obese patients, there is a higher prevalence of morbid psychiatric illness by 40 to 60 percent. Disorders associated with obesity include eating disorders (particularly binge eating disorder), substance use disorders, psychotic disorders (schizophrenia), mood disorders, anxiety disorders, personality disorders, attention-deficit/hyperactivity disorder (ADHD), and posttraumatic stress disorder (PTSD).

There are two eating disorders that can be associated with obesity: bulimia nervosa and binge eating disorder. Both of these disorders are distinct in their clinical characteristics and have some similarities. They both are associated with significant psychopathology and need to be addressed multimodally to ensure success. It is important to note that not all patients with bulimia nervosa are obese; they may be overweight or of normal weight. See Sections 11.2 and 11.3 for further discussions on bulimia nervosa and binge eating disorder, respectively.

EPIDEMIOLOGY

Obesity rates continue to grow at epidemic proportions in the United States and other industrialized nations, representing a serious public health threat to millions of people. In the United States, approximately 36 percent of adults are obese. The prevalence of obesity is highest in minority populations, particularly among non-Hispanic black women. More than one-half of these individuals, 40 years of age or older, are obese and more than 80 percent are overweight. The prevalence of obesity in adolescents in the United States has also increased from about 15 percent in 2000 to about 35 percent in 2012, while the prevalence rates for overweight children ages 6 to 11 range from 14 to 25 percent; however, there has been a slight decrease in recent years.

Obesity also has economic effects. On an individual level, medical spending is approximately 42 percent higher for an obese person compared with that for a person of normal weight. On a national level, costs attributed to both overweight (BMI 25 to 29.9) and obesity (BMI greater than 30) account for 9.1 percent of US health care costs, and if the current trend continues, obesity will account for 16 percent of US health care costs by 2030.

ETIOLOGY

Persons with no medical etiology accumulate fat by eating more calories than are expended as energy; thus intake of energy exceeds its dissipation. To reduce body fat, fewer calories must be consumed or more calories must be burnt. An error of no more than 10 percent in either intake or output would lead to a 30-lb change in body weight in 1 year.

Satiety

Satiety is the feeling that results when hunger is satisfied. Persons stop eating at the end of a meal because they have replenished nutrients that had been depleted. Persons become hungry again when nutrients restored by earlier meals are once again depleted. It seems reasonable that a metabolic signal, derived from food that has been absorbed, is carried by the blood to the brain, where the signal activates receptor cells, probably in the hypothalamus, to produce satiety. Some studies have shown evidence for dysfunction in serotonin, dopamine, and norepinephrine involvement in regulating eating behavior through the hypothalamus. Other hormonal factors that may be involved include CRF, neuropeptide Y, gonadotropin-releasing hormone, and thyroid-stimulating hormone. A newly found substance, obestatin, which is made in the stomach, is a hormone that in animal experiments produces satiety and may have potential use as a weight-loss agent in humans. Hunger results from a decrease in the strength of metabolic signals, secondary to the depletion of critical nutrients.

Cannabinoid receptors are related to appetite and are stimulated with cannabis (marijuana) use. A cannabinoid inverse antagonist has been developed that blocks appetite.

Satiety occurs soon after the beginning of a meal and before the total caloric content of the meal has been absorbed;

therefore, satiety is only one regulatory mechanism controlling food intake. Appetite, defined as the desire for food, is also involved. A hungry person may eat to full satisfaction when food is available, but appetite can also induce a person to overeat past the point of satiety. Appetite may be increased by psychological factors such as thoughts or feelings, and an abnormal appetite may result in an abnormal increase in food intake. Eating is also affected by cannabinoid receptors, which, when stimulated, increase appetite. Marijuana acts on that receptor that accounts for the "munchies" associated with marijuana use. A drug called rimonabant (Acomplia) is an inverse agonist to the cannabidiol receptor, meaning that it blocks appetite. It was withdrawn from the market because of adverse effects; however, in theory, inverse cannabinoid receptor agonists may have clinical use.

The olfactory system may play a role in satiety. Experiments have shown that strong stimulation of the olfactory bulbs in the nose with food odors by use of an inhaler saturated with a particular smell produces satiety for that food. This may have implications for therapy of obesity.

Genetic Factors

The existence of numerous forms of inherited obesity in animals and the ease with which adiposity can be produced by selective breeding make it clear that genetic factors can play a role in obesity. These factors must also be presumed to be important in human obesity.

About 80 percent of patients who are obese have a family history of obesity. This fact can be accounted for not only by genetic factors but also in part by identification with fat parents and by learned oral methods for coping with anxiety. Nonetheless, studies show that identical twins raised apart can both be obese, an observation that suggests a hereditary role. To date, no specific genetic marker of obesity has been found. Table 11.4–1 lists the genetic factors affecting body weight.

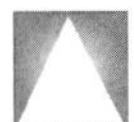

Table 11.4–1
Genetic Factors Affecting Body Weight

	Genetic Factor Description
Leptin	Highly expressed in areas of the hypothalamus that control feeding behavior, hunger, body temperature, and energy expenditure. The mechanisms by which leptin suppresses feeding and exerts its effects on metabolism are largely unknown.
Neuropeptide Y	Synthesized in many areas of the brain; it is a potent stimulator of feeding. Leptin appears to suppress feeding in part by inhibiting expression of neuropeptide Y.
Ghrelin	An acylated, 28-amino acid peptide secreted primarily by the stomach. Ghrelin circulates in the blood and activates neuropeptide Y neurons in the hypothalamic arcuate nucleus, thereby stimulating food intake.
Melanocortin	Acts on certain hypothalamic neurons that inhibit feeding. Targeted disruptions of the melanocortin-4 receptor in mice are associated with development of obesity.
Carboxypeptidase E	The enzyme necessary for processing proinsulin and perhaps other hormones, such as neuropeptide Y. Mice with mutations in this gene gradually become obese as they age and develop hyperglycemia that can be suppressed by treatment with insulin.
Mitochondrial uncoupling proteins	First discovered in brown fat and subsequently identified in white fat and muscle cells. May play an important role in energy expenditure and body weight regulation.
Tubby protein	Highly expressed in the paraventricular nucleus of the hypothalamus and other regions of the brain. Mice with naturally occurring or engineered mutations in the tubby gene show adult onset of obesity, but the mechanisms involved are not known.

Adapted from Comuzzie AG, Williams JT, Martin LJ, Blanger J. Searching for genes underlying normal variation in human adiposity. *J Mol Med.* 2001;79:57.

Developmental Factors

Early in life, adipose tissue grows by increases in both cell number and cell size. Once the number of adipocytes has been established, it does not seem to be susceptible to change. Obesity that begins early in life is characterized by adipose tissue with an increased number of adipocytes of increased size. Obesity that begins in adult life, on the other hand, results solely from an increase in the size of the adipocytes. In both instances, weight reduction produces a decrease in cell size. The greater number and size of adipocytes in patients with juvenile-onset diabetes may be a factor in their widely recognized difficulties with weight reduction and the persistence of their obesity.

The distribution and amount of fat vary in individuals, and fat in different body areas has different characteristics. Fat cells around the waist, flanks, and abdomen (the so-called potbelly) are more active metabolically than those in the thighs and buttocks. The former pattern is more common in men and has a higher correlation with cardiovascular disease than does the latter pattern. Women, whose fat distribution is in the thighs and buttocks, may become obsessed with nostrums that are advertised to reduce fat in these areas (so-called cellulite, which is not a medical term), but no externally applied preparation to reduce this fat pattern exists. Men with abdominal fat may attempt to reduce their girth with machines that exercise the abdominal muscles, but exercise has no effect on loss of this type of fat.

A hormone called leptin, which is made by fat cells, acts as a fat thermostat. When the blood level of leptin is low, more fat is consumed; when high, less fat is consumed. Further research is needed to determine whether this might lead to new ways of managing obesity.

Physical Activity Factors

The marked decrease in physical activity in affluent societies seems to be the major factor in the rise of obesity as a public health problem. Physical inactivity restricts energy expenditure and may contribute to increased food intake. Although food intake increases with increasing energy expenditure over a wide range of energy demands, intake does not decrease proportionately when physical activity falls below a certain minimum level.

Brain-Damage Factors

Destruction of the ventromedial hypothalamus can produce obesity in animals, but this is probably a very rare cause of obesity in humans. There is evidence that the central nervous system, particularly in the lateral and ventromedial hypothalamic areas, adjusts to food intake in response to changing energy requirements so as to maintain fat stores at a baseline determined by a specific set point. This set point varies from one person to another and depends on height and body build.

Health Factors

In only a small number of cases is obesity the consequence of identifiable illness. Such cases include a variety of rare genetic disorders, such as Prader–Willi syndrome, as well as neuroendocrine abnormalities (Table 11.4–2). Hypothalamic obesity results from damage to the ventromedial region of the hypothalamus (VMH), which has been studied extensively in laboratory animals and is a known center of appetite and weight regulation. In humans, damage to the VMH may result from trauma, surgery, malignancy, or inflammatory disease.

Some forms of depression, particularly seasonal affective disorder, are associated with weight gain. Most persons who live in seasonal climates report increases in appetite and weight during the fall and winter months, with decreases in the spring and summer. Depressed patients usually lose weight, but some will gain weight.

Other Clinical Factors

A variety of clinical disorders are associated with obesity. Cushing's disease is associated with a characteristic fat distribution and moon-like face. Myxedema is associated with weight gain, although not invariably. Other neuroendocrine disorders include adiposogenital dystrophy (Fröhlich's syndrome), which is characterized by obesity and sexual and skeletal abnormalities.

Table 11.4–2
Illnesses That Can Explain Some Cases of Obesity

Genetic (dysmorphic) obesities
Autosomal recessive
X-linked
Chromosomal (e.g., Prader–Willi syndrome)

Neuroendocrine obesities
Hypothalamic syndromes
Cushing's syndrome
Hypothyroidism
Polycystic ovarian syndrome (Stein–Leventhal syndrome)
Pseudohypoparathyroidism
Hypogonadism
Growth hormone deficiency
Insulinoma and hyperinsulinism
Iatrogenic obesities

Drugs (psychiatric)
Hypothalamic surgery (neuroendocrine)

Adapted from Bray GA. An approach to the classification and evaluation of obesity. In: Bjorntorp P, Brodoff BN, eds. *Obesity*. Philadelphia: Lippincott Williams & Wilkins; 1992.

Psychotropic Drugs

Long-term use of steroid medications is associated with significant weight gain, as is the use of several psychotropic agents. Patients treated for major depression, psychotic disturbances, and bipolar disorder typically gain 3 to 10 kg, with even larger gains with chronic use. This can produce the so-called metabolic syndrome discussed below.

Psychological Factors

Although psychological factors are evidently crucial to the development of obesity, how such psychological factors result in obesity is not known. The food-regulating mechanism is susceptible to environmental influence, and cultural, family, and psychodynamic factors have all been shown to contribute to the development of obesity. Although many investigators have proposed that specific family histories, precipitating factors, personality structures, or unconscious conflicts cause obesity, overweight persons may suffer from every conceivable psychiatric disorder and come from a variety of disturbed backgrounds. Many obese patients are emotionally disturbed persons who, because of the availability of the overeating mechanism in their environments, have learned to use hyperphagia as a means of coping with psychological problems. Some patients may show signs of serious mental disorder when they attain normal weight because they no longer have that coping mechanism.

DIAGNOSIS AND CLINICAL FEATURES

The diagnosis of obesity, if done in a sophisticated way, involves the assessment of body fat. As this is rarely practical, the use of height and weight to calculate BMI is recommended.

In most cases of obesity, it is not possible to identify the precise etiology, given the multitude of possible causes and their interactions. Instances of secondary obesity (described in Table 11.4–3) are rare but should not be overlooked.

The habitual eating patterns of many obese persons often seem similar to patterns found in experimental obesity. Impaired satiety is a particularly important problem. Obese persons seem inordinately susceptible to food cues in their environment, to the palatability of foods, and to the inability to stop eating if food is available. Obese persons are usually susceptible to all kinds of external stimuli to eating, but they remain relatively unresponsive to the usual internal signals of hunger. Some are unable to distinguish between hunger and other kinds of dysphoria.

DIFFERENTIAL DIAGNOSIS

Other Syndromes

The night eating syndrome, in which persons eat excessively after they have had their evening meal, seems to be precipitated by stressful life circumstances and, once present, tends to recur daily until the stress is alleviated. Night eating may also occur as a result of using sedatives to sleep, which may produce sleepwalking and eating. This has been reported with the use of zolpidem (Ambien) in patients. (See Section 11.3 for further discussion on night eating syndrome.)

Table 11.4–3
Psychiatric Medications and Changes in Body Weight

Tendency to Increase Appetite and Body Weight		
Greatest	**Intermediate**	**Least**
Antidepressant drugs		
Amitriptyline (Elavil)	Doxepin (Adapin, Sinequan)	Amoxapine (Asendin)
	Imipramine (Tofranil)	Desipramine (Norpramin)
	Mirtazapine (Remeron)	Trazodone (Desyrel)
	Nortriptyline (Pamelor)	Tranylcypromine (Parnate)
		Fluoxetine (Prozac)[a]
	Phenelzine (Nardil)	Sertraline (Zoloft)[a]
		Bupropion (Wellbutrin)[a]
	Trimipramine (Surmontil)	Venlafaxine (Effexor)[a]
Mood stabilizers		
Lithium (Eskalith)	Carbamazepine (Tegretol)	Topiramate (Topamax)
Valproic acid (Depakene)		
Antipsychotic drugs		
Chlorpromazine (Thorazine)	Haloperidol (Haldol)	Ziprasidone (Geodon)
		Aripiprazole (Abilify)
Clozapine (Clozaril)	Trifluoperazine (Stelazine)	Molindone (Moban)[a]
Thioridazine (Mellaril)	Perphenazine (Trilafon)	
Mesoridazine (Serentil)	Thiothixene (Navane)	
Olanzapine (Zyprexa)	Fluphenazine (Permitil, Prolixin)	
Sertindole (Serdolect)		
Risperidone (Risperdal)		

[a]May decrease appetite and facilitate weight loss.
Adapted from Allison DB, Mentore JL, Heo M, Chandler LP, Capeller JC, Infante MC, Weiden PJ. Antipsychotic-induced weight gain: A comprehensive research synthesis. *Am J Psychiatry*. 1999;156:1686; and Bernstein JG. Management of psychotropic drug-induced obesity. In: Bjorntorp P, Brodoff BN, eds. *Obesity*. Philadelphia: Lippincott Williams & Wilkins; 1992.

Binge eating disorder is characterized by sudden, compulsive ingestion of very large amounts of food in a short time, usually with great subsequent agitation and self-condemnation. Binge eating also appears to represent a reaction to stress. In contrast to night eating syndrome, however, these bouts of overeating are not periodic, and they are far more often linked to specific precipitating circumstances. Pickwickian syndrome is said to exist when a person is 100 percent over desirable weight and has associated respiratory and cardiovascular pathology.

Body Dysmorphic Disorder (Dysmorphophobia)

Some obese persons feel that their bodies are grotesque and loathsome and that others view them with hostility and contempt. This feeling is closely associated with self-consciousness and impaired social functioning. Emotionally healthy obese persons have no body image disturbances, and only a minority of neurotic obese persons have such disturbances. The disorder is confined mainly to persons who have been obese since childhood; even among them, less than half suffer from it.

COURSE AND PROGNOSIS

Effects on Health

Obesity has adverse effects on health and is associated with a broad range of illnesses (Table 11.4–4). There is a strong correlation between obesity and cardiovascular disorders. Hypertension (blood pressure higher than 140/90 mm Hg) is three times higher for persons who are overweight, and hypercholesterolemia (blood cholesterol over 240 mg/dL) is twice as common. Studies show that blood pressure and cholesterol levels can be reduced by weight reduction. Diabetes, which has clear genetic determinations, can often be reversed with weight reduction, especially type 2 diabetes (mature-onset or noninsulin-dependent diabetes mellitus).

According to the National Institutes of Health data, obese men, regardless of smoking habits, have a higher mortality from colon, rectal, and prostate cancer than men of normal weight. Obese women have a higher mortality from cancer of the gallbladder, biliary passages, breast (postmenopause), uterus (including cervix and endometrium), and ovaries than women of normal weight.

Longevity

Reliable studies indicate that the more overweight a person is, the higher is that person's risk for death. A person who reduces weight to acceptable levels has a mortality decline to normal rates. Weight reduction may be lifesaving for patients with extreme obesity, defined as weight that is twice the desirable weight. Such patients may have cardiorespiratory failure, especially when asleep (sleep apnea).

A number of studies have demonstrated that decreasing caloric intake by 30 percent or more in young or middle-aged laboratory animals prevents or retards age-related chronic

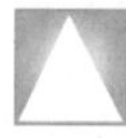

Table 11.4–4
Health Disorders Thought to Be Caused or Exacerbated by Obesity

Heart
Premature coronary heart disease
Left ventricular hypertrophy
Angina pectoris
Sudden death (ventricular arrhythmia)
Congestive heart failure
Vascular system
Hypertension
Cerebrovascular disorder (cerebral infarction or hemorrhage)
Venous stasis (with lower-extremity edema, varicose veins)
Respiratory system
Obstructive sleep apnea
Pickwickian syndrome (alveolar hypoventilation)
Secondary polycythemia
Right ventricular hypertrophy (sometimes leading to failure)
Hepatobiliary system
Cholelithiasis and cholecystitis
Hepatic steatosis
Hormonal and metabolic functions
Diabetes mellitus (insulin independent)
Gout (hyperuricemia)
Hyperlipidemias (hypertriglyceridemia and hypercholesterolemia)
Kidney
Proteinuria and, in very severe obesity, nephrosis
Renal vein thrombosis
Joints, muscles, and connective tissue
Osteoarthritis of knees
Bone spurs of the heel
Osteoarthrosis of spine (in women)
Aggravation of preexisting postural faults
Neoplasia
In women: increased risk of cancer of endometrium, breast, cervix, ovary, gallbladder, and biliary passages
In men: increased risk of cancer of colon, rectum, and prostate

From Vanitallie TB. Obesity: Adverse effects on health and longevity. *Am J Clin Nutr.* 1979;32:2723.

diseases and significantly prolongs the maximal lifespan. The mechanisms through which this effect is mediated are not known, but they may include reductions in metabolic rate, oxidative stress, and inflammation; improved insulin sensitivity; and changes in neuroendocrine and sympathetic nervous system function. Whether long-term calorie restriction with adequate nutrition slows aging in humans is not yet known.

Prognosis

The prognosis for weight reduction is poor, and the course of obesity tends toward inexorable progression. Of patients who lose significant amounts of weight, 90 percent regain it eventually. The prognosis is particularly poor for those who become obese in childhood. Juvenile-onset obesity tends to be more severe, more resistant to treatment, and more likely to be associated with emotional disturbance than is adult obesity.

Discrimination Toward the Obese

Overweight and obese individuals are subject to significant prejudice and discrimination in the United States and other industrialized nations. In a culture in which beauty ideals are thin and highly unrealistic, overweight people are blamed for their condition and are the subject of teasing, bias, and discrimination (sometimes called "fatism"). Income and earning power are suppressed in overweight people, and untoward social conditions, such as absence of romantic relationships, are more common. Furthermore, obese individuals face limited access to health care and may receive biased diagnoses and treatment from medical and mental health providers.

TREATMENT

As mentioned above, many patients routinely treated for obesity may develop anxiety or depression. A high incidence of emotional disturbances has been reported among obese persons undergoing long-term, in-hospital treatment by fasting or severe calorie restriction. Obese persons with extensive psychopathology, those with a history of emotional disturbance during dieting, and those in the midst of a life crisis should attempt weight reduction cautiously and under careful supervision.

Diet

The basis of weight reduction is simple—establish a caloric deficit by bringing intake below output. The simplest way to reduce caloric intake is by means of a low-calorie diet. This strategy requires an adequate amount of protein intake with balanced carbohydrate and fat intake and should be done under medical supervision. The best long-term effects are achieved with a balanced diet that contains readily available foods. For most persons, the most satisfactory reducing diet consists of their usual foods in amounts determined with the aid of tables of food values, which are available in standard books on dieting. Such a diet gives the best chance of long-term maintenance of weight loss. Total unmodified fasts are used for short-term weight loss, but they have associated morbidity including orthostatic hypotension, sodium diuresis, and impaired nitrogen balance.

Ketogenic diets are high-protein, high-fat diets used to promote weight loss. They have high cholesterol content and produce ketosis, which is associated with nausea, hypotension, and lethargy. Many obese persons find it tempting to use a novel or even bizarre diet. Table 11.4–5 contains details and comparisons of various types of diets. Whatever effectiveness these diets may have in large part results from their monotony. When a dieter stops the diet and returns to the usual fare, the incentives to overeat are multiplied.

In general, the best method of weight loss is a balanced diet of 1,100 to 1,200 calories. Such a diet can be followed for long periods but should be supplemented with vitamins, particularly iron, folic acid, zinc, and vitamin B_6.

Exercise

Increased physical activity is an important part of a weight-reduction regimen. Because caloric expenditure in most forms of physical activity is directly proportional to body weight, obese persons expend more calories than persons of normal weight with the same amount of activity. Furthermore, increased physical activity may actually decrease food intake by formerly

Table 11.4–5
Types of Diets

Type of Diet	Calorie Deficit	Weight Loss	Important Supplementary Measures	Content
Low Calorie Diet (LCD)	500–1,000 kcal/day	0.5–1 kg/wk	Diet record very important for success	Carbs 55% Protein 15% Fat <30%
Very Low Calorie Diet (VLCD)	800 kcal/day	15–25% in 8–12 weeks	Support and electrolyte monitoring	Protein 70–100 g/day full replacement of vitamin/mineral/electrolytes
Fasting	<200 kcal/day	50% of weight loss is water weight	Dangerous and not done anymore	Liquids
Popular diets				
1. South Beach diet/New Diet Revolution/Zone diet	<30 g of carb/day	20 lb in 6 months	Difficult to follow over a long period. Cardiac or renal effects need to be evaluated	High fat, low carb
2. Weight Watchers/Jenny Craig/Nutrisystem	Goal is to provide great range of food choice while maintaining a negative energy balance	1–2 lb/wk	Has been shown to reduce cholesterol and blood pressure	Mod fat, balanced nutrient reduction, 20–30% fat, 15–20% protein, 55–60% carbs
3. Ornish program/Pritikin program	Mostly vegetarian diet, no caffeine, no caloric restriction, just one type of food	—	Combines meditation, stress reduction, and smoking cessation	Very low fat, <10–19% cal from fat, 20% protein, and 70% complex carbs like fruit and grain

sedentary persons. This combination of increased caloric expenditure and decreased food intake makes an increase in physical activity a highly desirable feature of any weight-reduction program. Exercise also helps maintain weight loss. It is essential in the treatment of the metabolic syndrome.

Lifestyle Change

A lifestyle change empowers the patient to set goals of weight management. Simple lifestyle modification strategies that patients should be encouraged to follow include:

Personal behavior during a meal:

- ▲ Eat slowly and savor each mouthful
- ▲ Chew each bite 30 times before swallowing
- ▲ Put the fork down between bites
- ▲ Delay eating for 2 to 3 minutes and converse
- ▲ Postpone a snack for 10 minutes
- ▲ Serve food on a smaller plate
- ▲ Divide portions in half so another portion may be permitted

Reduce eating cues:

- ▲ Eat only at one designated place
- ▲ Leave the table as soon as eating is done
- ▲ Do not combine eating with other activities (e.g., reading or watching television)
- ▲ Do not put bowls of food on the table
- ▲ Stock home with healthier food choices
- ▲ Shop for groceries from a list after a full meal
- ▲ Plan meals
- ▲ Keep a food diary to link eating with hunger and nonhunger episodes
- ▲ Substitute other activities for snacking

Pharmacotherapy

Various drugs, some more effective than others, are used to treat obesity. Table 11.4–6 lists the drugs currently available for this use. Drug treatment is effective because it suppresses appetite, but tolerance to this effect may develop after several weeks of use. An initial trial period of 4 weeks with a specific drug can be used; then, if the patient responds with weight loss, the drug can be continued to see whether tolerance develops. If a drug remains effective, it can be dispensed for a longer time until the desired weight is achieved.

Orlistat. One weight-loss medication approved by the Food and Drug Administration (FDA) for long-term use is orlistat (Xenical), which is a selective gastric and pancreatic lipase inhibitor that reduces the absorption of dietary fat (which is then excreted in stool). In clinical trials, orlistat (120 mg, three times a day), in combination with a low-calorie diet, induced losses of approximately 10 percent of initial weight in the first 6 months, which were generally well maintained for periods up to 24 months. Because of its peripheral mechanism of action, orlistat is generally free of the central nervous system effects (i.e., increased pulse, dry mouth, insomnia) that are associated with most weight-loss medications. The principal adverse effects of orlistat are gastrointestinal; patients must consume 30 percent or fewer calories from fat to prevent adverse events that include oily stool, flatulence with discharge, and fecal urgency. A lower dosed over-the-counter formulation of orlistat (Alli) was approved by the FDA in 2007.

Sibutramine. Sibutramine (Meridia) is a β-phenylethylamine that inhibits the reuptake of serotonin and norepinephrine (and dopamine to a limited extent). It was approved by the FDA in

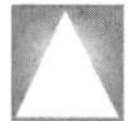

Table 11.4–6
Common Drugs for the Treatment of Obesity

Generic Name	Trade Name(s)	Usual Dosage Range (mg/day)
Amphetamine and dextroamphetamine	Biphetamine	12.5–20
Methamphetamine	Desoxyn	10–15
Benzphetamine	Didrex	75–150
Phendimetrazine	Bontril, Plegine, Prelu-2, X-Trozine	105
Phentermine hydrochloride	Adipex-P, Fastin, Oby-trim	18.75–37.5
Resin	Ionamin	15–30
Diethylpropion hydrochloride	Tenuate	75
Mazindol	Sanorex, Mazanor	3–9
Sibutramine	Meridia	10–15
Orlistat	Xenical	360
Lorcaserin	Belviq	10 twice a day
Phentermine-topiramate	Qsymia	3.75–15 phentermine 23–92 topiramate

1997 for weight loss and the maintenance of weight loss (i.e., long-term use).

Lorcaserin. Lorcaserin (Belviq) has been approved by the FDA for the treatment of obesity in adults. Lorcaserin is a selective serotonin agonist that suppresses appetite and reduces food intake. One double-blind, placebo-controlled trial showed that obese patients lost about 4 percent more of their body weight in 1 year while on lorcaserin compared with controls. Additionally, weight loss was maintained in 70 percent of patients who took lorcaserin for 2 years. Another trial showed that obese patients who took lorcaserin 10 mg, one to two times per day in conjunction with nutritional and exercise programs lost 6 percent of their body weight after 1 year. The recommended dosage is 10 mg twice a day. If the patient does not see a 5 percent reduction of their body weight within 12 weeks of treatment, lorcaserin treatment should be discontinued. Side effects of lorcaserin include headaches, dizziness, fatigue, nausea, dry mouth, and constipation. Rare but serious side effects include a chemical imbalance (serotonin syndrome), suicidal thoughts, psychiatric problems, and problems with memory or comprehension. Pregnant women should not take lorcaserin.

Phentermine-topiramate. Phentermine-topiramate (Qsymia) has been approved by the FDA for weight management treatment in conjunction with diet and exercise. It combines lower doses of immediate-release phentermine, a weight-loss drug prescribed for short-term use, and controlled-release topiramate, an anticonvulsant. Patients should start at the lowest dose (3.75 mg phentermine/23 mg topiramate extended release), then increase to the recommended dose (7.5 mg/46 mg). In some circumstances, patients may have their dose increased to the highest dose (15 mg/92 mg). In clinical trials, patients have shown an average weight loss ranging from 7 percent (lowest dose) to 9 percent (recommended dose) over those taking a placebo. Side effects include paraesthesia, dry mouth, altered taste, increased heart rate, possible birth defects, and psychiatric problems (depression, suicidal thoughts, impaired memory, and concentration). If the patients do not see a 3 percent reduction in their body weight after 12 weeks on the recommended dose, the dosage may be increased to the highest dose. If patients do not see a 5 percent reduction in their body weight after 12 weeks on the highest dose, treatment with Qsymia should be discontinued.

Surgery

Gastroplasty. Vertical banded gastroplasty (VBG) is a restrictive-only operation that involves creating a small gastric reservoir or pouch measuring 15 to 20 mL in volume, which then empties into the residual stomach through a calibrated or banded outlet. On average, patients lose 40 to 50 lb of excess body weight over the first 1 to 2 years postoperatively. Vomiting, electrolyte imbalance, and obstruction may occur. A syndrome called *dumping*, which consists of palpitations, weakness, and sweating, may follow surgical procedures in some patients if they ingest large amounts of carbohydrates in a single meal. Due to such complications, VBG is now only performed in a few centers in the United States.

Gastric Bypass. Since the early 1990s, gastric bypass has greatly replaced VBG as the operation of choice. The procedure involves dividing the stomach into two pouches—a small upper pouch and a larger lower "remnant" pouch—and then rearranging the small intestine to connect to both. The expected weight loss averages 70 percent of excess body weight with the maximum weight loss occurring by 3 years postoperatively. The main complications of gastric bypass surgery are primarily seen during the perioperative period. Mortality is less than 0.5 percent and is mainly due to pulmonary emboli or sepsis secondary to anastomotic leakage. Vitamin B_{12} and iron deficiencies may present and may require oral supplementation. All patients need to take multivitamins postoperatively and need to be followed at regular intervals for nutritional assessment. About 10 to 15 percent of patients will either fail to achieve significant weight loss or regain a significant amount of their loss after 2 or 3 years. This is usually due to consumption of carbohydrates, such as potato chips or other snack foods. Psychological treatment of abnormal eating behaviors is essential to prevent weight gain.

Gastric Banding. Laparoscopic adjustable gastric band was approved by the FDA in 2002 and is one of the least invasive operations for obesity because it does not involve cutting the stomach or the intestine. It involves placing a band around the upper part of the stomach, creating a smaller stomach above the band and a larger stomach below the band. The smaller stomach allows the patient to feel fuller quicker, thus reducing the amount of food intake. Average weight loss is approximately

37 to 50 percent of excess body weight. Complications involve band movement, erosion, malfunction, and slippage (stomach herniating through the band). Improvements in the design of the band and newer placement techniques appear to be reducing complications.

Other Methods. The surgical removal of fat (lipectomy) has no effect on weight loss in the long run nor does liposuction, which has value only for cosmetic reasons. Bariatric surgery is now recommended in individuals who have serious obesity-related health complications and a BMI of greater than 35 kg/m^2 (or a BMI greater than 40 kg/m^2 in the absence of major health complications). Before surgery, candidates should have tried to lose weight using the safer, more traditional options of diet, exercise, and weight loss medication.

Psychotherapy

The psychological problems of obese persons vary, and there is no particular personality type that is more prone to obesity. Some patients may respond to insight-oriented psychodynamic therapy with weight loss, but this treatment has not had much success. Uncovering the unconscious causes of overeating may not alter the behavior of persons who overeat in response to stress, although it may serve to augment other treatment methods. Years after successful psychotherapy many persons who overeat under stress continue to do so. Obese persons seem particularly vulnerable to over dependency on a therapist, and the inordinate regression that may occur during the uncovering psychotherapies should be carefully monitored.

Behavior modification has been the most successful of the therapeutic approaches for obesity and is considered the method of choice. Patients are taught to recognize external cues that are associated with eating and to keep diaries of foods consumed in particular circumstances, such as at the movies or while watching television, or during certain emotional states, such as anxiety or depression. Patients are also taught to develop new eating patterns, such as eating slowly, chewing food well, not reading while eating, and not eating between meals or when not seated. Operant conditioning therapies that use rewards such as praise or new clothes to reinforce weight loss have also been successful. Group therapy helps to maintain motivation, to promote identification among members who have lost weight, and to provide education about nutrition.

Comprehensive Approach

The National Heart, Lung, and Blood Institute formulated key recommendations for patients and the public regarding weight loss. These are listed in Table 11.4–7.

Table 11.4–7
Key Recommendations for Healthy Weight

- ▲ Weight loss to lower elevated blood pressure in overweight and obese persons with high blood pressure.
- ▲ Weight loss to lower elevated levels of total cholesterol, low-density lipoprotein (LDL)-cholesterol, and triglycerides, and to raise low levels of high-density lipoprotein (HDL)-cholesterol in overweight and obese persons with dyslipidemia.
- ▲ Weight loss to lower elevated blood glucose levels in overweight and obese persons with type 2 diabetes.
- ▲ Use the body mass index (BMI) to classify overweight and obesity and to estimate relative risk of disease compared to normal weight.
- ▲ The waist circumference should be used to assess abdominal fat content.
- ▲ The initial goal of weight loss therapy should be to reduce body weight by about 10 percent from baseline. With success, and if warranted, further weight loss can be attempted.
- ▲ Weight loss should be about 1 to 2 lb/wk for a period of 6 months, with the subsequent strategy based on the amount of weight lost.
- ▲ Low calorie diets (LCD) for weight loss in overweight and obese persons. Reducing fat as part of an LCD is a practical way to reduce calories.
- ▲ Reducing dietary fat alone without reducing calories is not sufficient for weight loss. However, reducing dietary fat, along with reducing dietary carbohydrates, can help reduce calories.
- ▲ A diet that is individually planned to help create a deficit of 500 to 1,000 kcal/day should be an integral part of any program aimed at achieving a weight loss of 1 to 2 lb/wk.
- ▲ Physical activity should be part of a comprehensive weight loss therapy and weight control program because it (1) modestly contributes to weight loss in overweight and obese adults, (2) may decrease abdominal fat, (3) increases cardiorespiratory fitness, and (4) may help with maintenance of weight loss.
- ▲ Physical activity should be an integral part of weight loss therapy and weight maintenance. Initially, moderate levels of physical activity for 30 to 45 minutes, 3 to 5 days a week, should be encouraged. All adults should set a long-term goal to accumulate at least 30 minutes or more of moderate-intensity physical activity on most, and preferably all, days of the week.
- ▲ The combination of a reduced calorie diet and increased physical activity is recommended because it produces weight loss that may also result in decreases in abdominal fat and increases in cardiorespiratory fitness.
- ▲ Behavior therapy is a useful adjunct when incorporated into treatment for weight loss and weight maintenance.
- ▲ Weight loss and weight maintenance therapy should employ the combination of LCDs, increased physical activity, and behavior therapy.
- ▲ After successful weight loss, the likelihood of weight loss maintenance is enhanced by a program consisting of dietary therapy, physical activity, and behavior therapy, which should be continued indefinitely. Drug therapy can also be used. However, drug safety and efficacy beyond 1 year of total treatment have not been established.
- ▲ A weight maintenance program should be a priority after the initial 6 months of weight loss therapy.

Formulated from the Obesity Education Institute, National Institute of Health.

METABOLIC SYNDROME

The metabolic syndrome consists of a cluster of metabolic abnormalities associated with obesity and that contribute to an increased risk of cardiovascular disease and type 2 diabetes. The syndrome is diagnosed when a patient has three or more of the following five risk factors: (1) abdominal obesity, (2) high triglyceride level, (3) low HDL cholesterol level, (4) hypertension, and (5) an elevated fasting blood glucose level. Table 11.4–8 lists the criteria as set forth by the World Health Organization (WHO). The syndrome is believed to occur in about 30 percent of the American population, but is also well known in other industrialized countries around the world.

Table 11.4–8
World Health Organization Clinical Criteria for Metabolic Syndrome

Insulin resistance, identified by 1 of the following:
- ▲ Type 2 diabetes
- ▲ Impaired fasting glucose
- ▲ Impaired glucose tolerance
- ▲ Or for those with normal fasting glucose levels (<100 mg/dL), glucose uptake below the lowest quartile for background population under investigation under hyperinsulinemic, euglycemic conditions

Plus any 2 of the following:
- ▲ Antihypertensive medication and/or high blood pressure (≥140 mm Hg systolic or ≥90 mm Hg diastolic)
- ▲ Plasma triglycerides ≥150 mg/dL (≥1.7 mmol/L)
- ▲ BMI >30 kg/m^2 and/or waist:hip ratio >0.9 in men, >0.85 in women
- ▲ Urinary albumin excretion rate ≥20 μg/min or albumin:creatinine ratio ≥30 mg/g

The cause of the syndrome is unknown, but obesity, insulin resistance, and a genetic vulnerability are involved. Treatment involves weight loss, exercise, and the use of statins and antihypertensives as needed to lower lipid levels and blood pressure, respectively. Because of the increased risk of mortality, it is important that the syndrome be recognized early and treated.

Second-generation (atypical) antipsychotic medications have been implicated as a cause of metabolic syndrome. In patients with schizophrenia, treatment with these medications can cause a rapid increase in body weight in the first few months of therapy, which may continue on for more than a year. In addition, insulin resistance leading to type 2 diabetes has been associated with an atherogenic lipid profile.

Clozapine (Clozaril) and olanzapine (Zyprexa) are the two drugs most implicated, but other atypical antipsychotics may also be involved.

Patients prescribed second-generation antipsychotic medications should be monitored periodically with hemoglobin A1c, fasting blood glucose levels at the beginning of treatment and during its course. Lipid profiles should also be obtained. Table 11.4–9 lists screening procedures for patients taking these medications.

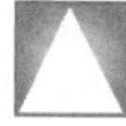

Table 11.4–9
Screen Patients before Prescribing Antipsychotics

- ▲ Personal history of obesity
- ▲ Family history of obesity
- ▲ Diabetes
- ▲ Dyslipidemias
- ▲ Hypertension
- ▲ Cardiovascular disease
- ▲ Body mass index
- ▲ Waist circumference at level of umbilicus
- ▲ Blood pressure
- ▲ Fasting plasma glucose
- ▲ Fasting lipid profile

Data from American Diabetes Association; 2004.

Psychological reactions to the metabolic syndrome depend on the signs and symptoms experienced by the patient. Those who suffer primarily from obesity must deal with self-esteem issues from being overweight as well as the stress of participating in weight loss programs. In many cases of obesity, eating is a way of satisfying deep-seated dependency needs. As weight is lost, some patients become depressed or anxious. Cases of psychosis have been reported in a few markedly obese patients during or after the process of losing a vast amount of weight. Other metabolic discrepancies, particularly variations in blood sugar, may be accompanied by irritability or other mood changes. Finally, fatigue is a common occurrence in patients with this syndrome. As the condition improves, especially if exercise is part of the regimen, fatigue eventually diminishes; but patients may be misdiagnosed as having a dysthymic disorder or chronic fatigue syndrome if metabolic causes of fatigue are not considered.

12

Normal Sleep and Sleep–Wake Disorders

▲ 12.1 Normal Sleep

Sleep is one of the most significant of human behaviors, occupying roughly one-third of human life. It is a universal behavior that has been demonstrated in every animal species studied, from insects to mammals. Sleep is a process the brain requires for proper functioning. Prolonged sleep deprivation leads to severe physical and cognitive impairment and, eventually, death. Sleep may appear to be a passive process but in fact can be associated with a high degree of brain activation. There are several distinct types of sleep that differ both qualitatively and quantitatively. Each type of sleep has unique characteristics, functional importance, and regulatory mechanisms. Selectively depriving a person of one particular type of sleep produces compensatory rebound when the individual is allowed to sleep ad lib. Sleep is particularly relevant to psychiatry since sleep disturbances can occur in virtually all psychiatric illnesses and are frequently part of the diagnostic criteria for specific disorders.

The ancient Greeks ascribed the need for sleep to the god Hypnos (sleep) and his son Morpheus, also a creature of the night, who brought dreams in human forms. Dreams have played an important role in psychoanalysis. Freud believed dreams to be the "royal road to the unconscious." They have figured prominently in art and literature from ancient times to the present.

ELECTROPHYSIOLOGY OF SLEEP

Sleep is made up of two physiological states: non–rapid eye movement (NREM) sleep and rapid eye movement (REM) sleep. In NREM sleep, which is composed of stages 1 through 4, most physiological functions are markedly lower than in wakefulness. REM sleep is a qualitatively different kind of sleep, characterized by a high level of brain activity and physiological activity levels similar to those in wakefulness. About 90 minutes after sleep onset, NREM yields to the first REM episode of the night. This REM latency of 90 minutes is a consistent finding in normal adults; shortening of REM latency frequently occurs with such disorders as narcolepsy and depressive disorders.

For clinical and research applications, sleep is typically scored in epochs of 30 seconds, with stages of sleep defined by the visual scoring of three parameters: electroencephalogram (EEG), electrooculogram (EOG), and electromyogram (EMG) recorded beneath the chin. The EEG records the rapid conjugate eye movements that are the identifying feature of the sleep state (no or few rapid eye movements occur in NREM sleep); the EEG pattern consists of low-voltage, random, fast activity with sawtooth waves; the EMG shows a marked reduction in muscle tone. The criteria defined by Allan Rechtschaffen and Anthony Kales in 1968 are accepted in clinical practice and for research around the world (Table 12.1–1).

In normal persons, NREM sleep is a peaceful state relative to waking. The pulse rate is typically slowed five to ten beats a minute below the level of restful waking and is very regular. Respiration is similarly affected, and blood pressure also tends to be low, with few minute-to-minute variations. The body musculature resting muscle potential is lower in REM sleep than in a waking state. Episodic, involuntary body movements are present in NREM sleep. There are few, if any, REMs and seldom do any penile erections occur in men. Blood flow through most tissues, including cerebral blood flow, is slightly reduced.

The deepest portions of NREM sleep—stages 3 and 4—are sometimes associated with unusual arousal characteristics. When persons are aroused 30 minutes to 1 hour after sleep onset—usually in slow-wave sleep—they are disoriented, and their thinking is disorganized. Brief arousals from slow-wave sleep are also associated with amnesia for events that occur during the arousal. The disorganization during arousal from stage 3 or stage 4 may result in specific problems, including enuresis, somnambulism, and stage 4 nightmares or night terrors.

Polygraphic measures during REM sleep show irregular patterns, sometimes close to aroused waking patterns. Otherwise, if researchers were unaware of the behavioral stage and happened to be recording a variety of physiological measures (aside from muscle tone) during REM periods, they undoubtedly would conclude that the person or animal they were studying was in an active waking state. Because of this observation, REM sleep has also been termed *paradoxical sleep*. Pulse, respiration, and blood pressure in humans are all high during REM sleep—much higher than during NREM sleep and often higher than during waking. Even more striking than the level or rate is the variability from minute to minute. Brain oxygen use increases during REM sleep. The ventilatory response to increased levels of carbon dioxide (CO_2) is depressed during REM sleep, so that no increase in tidal volume occurs as the partial pressure of carbon dioxide (PCO_2) increases. Thermoregulation is altered during REM sleep. In

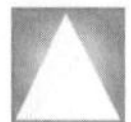

Table 12.1–1
Stages of Sleep—Electrophysiological Criteria

	Electroencephalogram	Electrooculogram	Electromyogram
Wakefulness	Low-voltage, mixed frequency activity Alpha (8–13 cps) activity with eyes closed	Eye movements and eye blinks	High tonic activity and voluntary movements
Nonrapid eye movement sleep			
Stage I	Low-voltage, mixed frequency activity Theta (3–7 cps) activity, vertex sharp waves	Slow eye movements	Tonic activity slightly decreased from wakefulness
Stage II	Low-voltage, mixed frequency background with sleep spindles (12–14 cps bursts) and K complexes (negative sharp wave followed by positive slow wave)	None	Low tonic activity
Stage III	High-amplitude (≥75 μV) slow waves (≤2 cps) occupying 20–50% of epoch	None	Low tonic activity
Stage IV	High-amplitude slow waves occupy >50% of epoch	None	Low tonic activity
REM sleep	Low-voltage, mixed frequency activity Saw-tooth waves, theta activity, and slow alpha activity	REMs	Tonic atonia with phasic twitches

REM, rapid eye movement.
Criteria from Rechtchaffen A, Kales A. *A Manual of Standardized Terminology, Techniques, and Scoring System for Sleep Stages of Human Subjects.* UCLA, Los Angeles: Brain Information Service/Brain Research Institute; 1968.

contrast to the homoeothermic condition of temperature regulation during wakefulness or NREM sleep, a poikilothermic condition (a state in which animal temperature varies with the changes in the temperature of the surrounding medium) prevails during REM sleep. Poikilothermia, which is characteristic of reptiles, results in a failure to respond to changes in ambient temperature with shivering or sweating, whichever is appropriate to maintaining body temperature. Almost every REM period in men is accompanied by a partial or full penile erection. This finding is clinically significant in evaluating the cause of impotence; the nocturnal penile tumescence study is one of the most commonly requested sleep laboratory tests. Another physiological change that occurs during REM sleep is the near-total paralysis of the skeletal (postural) muscles. Because of this motor inhibition, body movement is absent during REM sleep. Probably the most distinctive feature of REM sleep is dreaming. Persons awakened during REM sleep frequently (60 to 90 percent of the time) report that they had been dreaming. Dreams during REM sleep are typically abstract and surreal. Dreaming does occur during NREM sleep, but it is typically lucid and purposeful.

The cyclical nature of sleep is regular and reliable; a REM period occurs about every 90 to 100 minutes during the night (Fig. 12.1–1). The first REM period tends to be the shortest, usually lasting less than 10 minutes; later REM periods may last 15 to 40 minutes each. Most REM periods occur in the last third of the night, whereas most stage 4 sleep occurs in the first third of the night.

These sleep patterns change over a person's life span. In the neonatal period, REM sleep represents more than 50 percent of total sleep time, and the EEG pattern moves from the alert state directly to the REM state without going through stages 1 through 4. Newborns sleep about 16 hours a day, with brief periods of wakefulness. By 4 months of age, the pattern shifts so that the total percentage of REM sleep drops to less than 40 percent, and entry into sleep occurs with an initial period of NREM sleep. By young adulthood, the distribution of sleep stages is as follows:

- ▲ NREM (75 percent)
- ▲ Stage 1: 5 percent
- ▲ Stage 2: 45 percent
- ▲ Stage 3: 12 percent
- ▲ Stage 4: 13 percent
- ▲ REM (25 percent)

This distribution remains relatively constant into old age, although a reduction occurs in both slow-wave sleep and REM sleep in older persons.

SLEEP REGULATION

Most researchers think that there is not one simple sleep control center but a small number of interconnecting systems or centers that are located chiefly in the brainstem and that mutually activate and inhibit one another. Many studies also support the role of serotonin in sleep regulation. Prevention of serotonin synthesis or destruction of the dorsal raphe nucleus of the brainstem, which contains nearly all the brain's serotonergic cell bodies, reduces sleep for a considerable time. Synthesis and release of serotonin by serotonergic neurons are influenced by the availability of amino acid precursors of this neurotransmitter, such as L-tryptophan. Ingestion of large amounts of L-tryptophan (1 to 15 g) reduces sleep latency and nocturnal awakenings. Conversely, L-tryptophan deficiency is associated with less time spent in REM sleep. Norepinephrine-containing neurons with cell bodies located in the locus ceruleus play an important role in controlling normal sleep patterns. Drugs and manipulations that increase the firing of these noradrenergic neurons markedly reduce REM sleep (REM-off neurons) and increase wakefulness. In humans with implanted electrodes (for the control of spasticity), electrical stimulation of the locus ceruleus profoundly disrupts all sleep parameters.

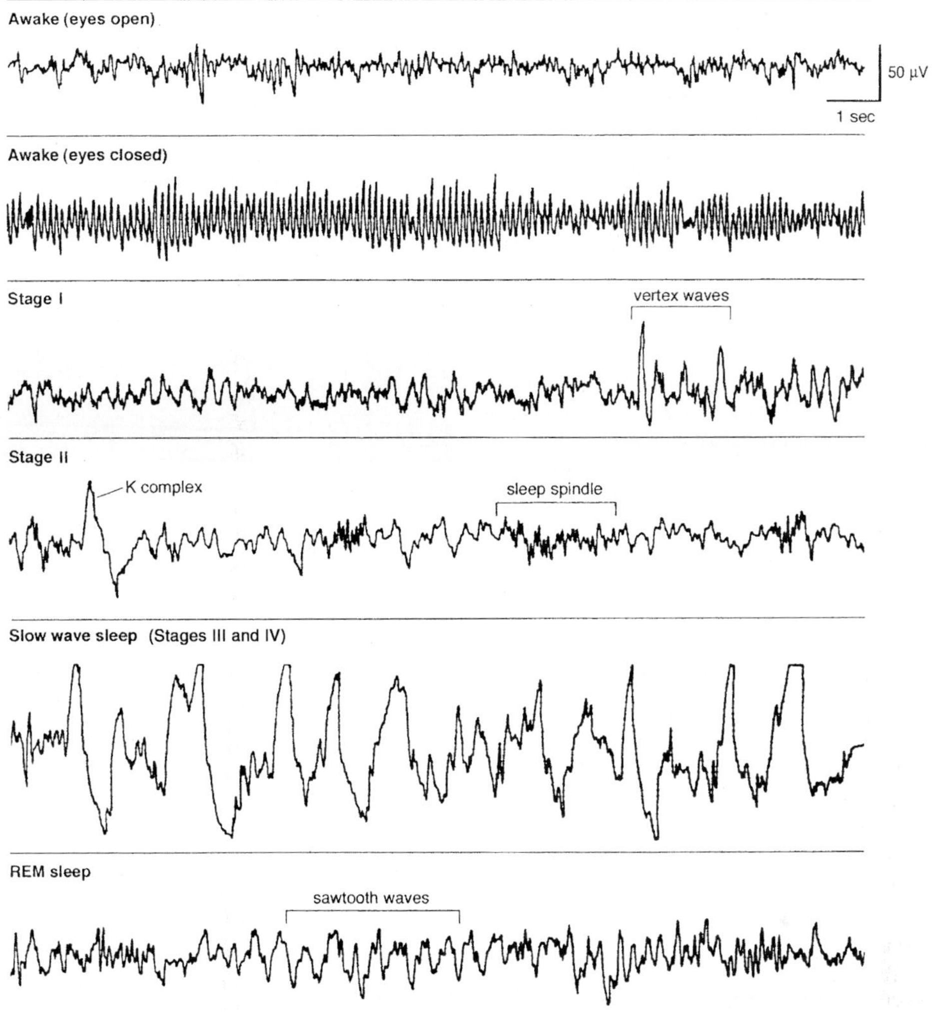

FIGURE 12.1–1

Sleep pattern in a young, healthy subject. REM, rapid eye movement. (From Gillian JC, Seifritz E, Zoltoltoski RK, Salin-Pascual RJ. Basic science of sleep. In: Sadock BJ, Sadock VA, eds. *Kaplan & Sadock's Comprehensive Textbook of Psychiatry.* Vol 1. 7th ed. Philadelphia, PA: Lippincott Williams & Wilkins; 2000:199.)

Brain acetylcholine is also involved in sleep, particularly in the production of REM sleep. In animal studies, the injection of cholinergic-muscarinic agonists into pontine reticular formation neurons (REM-on neurons) results in a shift from wakefulness to REM sleep. Disturbances in central cholinergic activity are associated with the sleep changes observed in major depressive disorder. Compared with healthy persons and nondepressed psychiatric controls, patients who are depressed have marked disruptions of REM sleep patterns. These disruptions include shortened REM latency (60 minutes or less), an increased percentage of REM sleep, and a shift in REM distribution from the last half to the first half of the night. Administration of a muscarinic agonist, such as arecoline, to depressed patients during the first or second NREM period results in a rapid onset of REM sleep. Depression can be associated with an underlying supersensitivity to acetylcholine. Drugs that reduce REM sleep, such as antidepressants, produce beneficial effects in depression. Indeed, about half the patients with major depressive disorder experience temporary improvement when they are deprived of sleep or when sleep is restricted. Conversely, reserpine (Serpasil), one of the few drugs that increase REM sleep, also produces depression. Patients with dementia of the Alzheimer's type have sleep disturbances characterized by reduced REM and slow-wave sleep. The loss of cholinergic neurons in the basal forebrain has been implicated as the cause of these changes.

Melatonin secretion from the pineal gland is inhibited by bright light, so the lowest serum melatonin concentrations occur during the day. The suprachiasmatic nucleus of the hypothalamus may act as the anatomical site of a circadian pacemaker that regulates melatonin secretion and the entrainment of the brain to a 24-hour sleep–wake cycle. Evidence shows that dopamine has an alerting effect. Drugs that increase dopamine concentrations in the brain tend to produce arousal and wakefulness. In contrast, dopamine blockers, such as pimozide (Orap) and the phenothiazines, tend to increase sleep time. A hypothesized homeostatic drive to sleep, perhaps in the form of an endogenous substance—process S—may accumulate during wakefulness and act to induce sleep. Another compound—process C—may act as a regulator of body temperature and sleep duration.

FUNCTIONS OF SLEEP

The functions of sleep have been examined in a variety of ways. Most investigators conclude that sleep serves a restorative, homeostatic function and appears to be crucial for normal thermoregulation and energy conservation. As NREM sleep increases after exercise and starvation, this stage may be associated with satisfying metabolic needs.

Sleep Deprivation

Prolonged periods of sleep deprivation sometimes lead to ego disorganization, hallucinations, and delusions. Depriving persons of REM sleep by awakening them at the beginning of REM cycles increases the number of REM periods and the amount of REM sleep (rebound increase) when they are allowed to sleep without interruption. REM-deprived patients may exhibit irritability and lethargy. In studies with rats, sleep deprivation produces a syndrome that includes a debilitated appearance, skin lesions, increased food intake, weight loss, increased energy expenditure, decreased body temperature, and death. The neuroendocrine changes include increased plasma norepinephrine and decreased plasma thyroxine levels.

Sleep Requirements

Some persons are normally short sleepers who require fewer than 6 hours of sleep each night to function adequately. Long sleepers are those who sleep more than 9 hours each night to function adequately. Long sleepers have more REM periods and more rapid eye movements within each period (known as *REM density*) than short sleepers. These movements are sometimes considered a measure of the intensity of REM sleep and are related to the vividness of dreaming. Short sleepers are generally efficient, ambitious, socially adept, and content. Long sleepers tend to be mildly depressed, anxious, and socially withdrawn. Sleep needs increase with physical work, exercise, illness, pregnancy, general mental stress, and increased mental activity. REM periods increase after strong psychological stimuli, such as difficult learning situations and stress, and after the use of chemicals or drugs that decrease brain catecholamines.

Sleep–Wake Rhythm

Without external clues, the natural body clock follows a 25-hour cycle. The influence of external factors—such as the light–dark cycle, daily routines, meal periods, and other external synchronizers—entrain persons to the 24-hour clock. Sleep is also influenced by biological rhythms. Within a 24-hour period, adults sleep once, sometimes twice. This rhythm is not present at birth but develops over the first 2 years of life. Some women exhibit sleep pattern changes during the phases of the menstrual cycle. Naps taken at different times of the day differ greatly in their proportions of REM and NREM sleep. In a normal nighttime sleeper, a nap taken in the morning or at noon includes a great deal of REM sleep, whereas a nap taken in the afternoon or the early evening has much less REM sleep. A circadian cycle apparently affects the tendency to have REM sleep. Sleep patterns are not physiologically the same when persons sleep in the daytime or during the time when they are accustomed to being awake; the psychological and behavioral effects of sleep differ as well. In a world of industry and communications that often functions 24 hours a day, these interactions are becoming increasingly significant. Even in persons who work at night, interference with the various rhythms can produce problems. The best-known example is jet lag, in which, after flying east to west, persons try to convince their bodies to go to sleep at a time that is out of phase with some body cycles. Most persons adapt within a few days, but some require more time. Conditions in these persons' bodies apparently involve long-term cycle disruption and interference.

▲ 12.2 Sleep–Wake Disorders

Sleep is regulated by several basic mechanisms, and when these systems go awry, sleep disorders occur. Interest in sleep disorders was initially found among psychiatrists, psychologists, and neurologists. The past three decades have witnessed discoveries that make sleep medicine truly multidisciplinary. Research illustrating the medical consequences of sleep-disordered breathing attracted many pulmonary and internal medicine specialists to the field. Sleep–wake disorder-related endocrinology and circadian rhythm research has migrated from the laboratory bench to the bedside. Nonetheless, the seriousness of sleep disorders remains poorly recognized by the general public and the vast majority of clinical practitioners.

Sleep disorders are both dangerous and expensive to treat. Obstructive sleep apnea research verifies its contribution to hypertension, heart failure, and stroke. Investigations link many major industrial catastrophes to sleepiness. Sleepiness is a serious, potentially life-threatening condition that affects not only the sleepy individual but also his or her family, coworkers, and society in general. In fact, sleep-related motor vehicle accidents represent a major public safety concern, and some states have enacted criminal statues to deter sleepy driving. Sleep disorders' direct cost per annum in the United States is estimated at $16 billion, with indirect costs ranging upward to more than $100 billion. Table 12.2–1 lists the terms used in this section to diagnose and describe sleep disorders.

Table 12.2–1
Common Polysomnographic Measures

Sleep latency: Period of time from turning out the lights until the appearance of stage 2 sleep
Early morning awakening: Time of being continuously awake from the last stage of the sleep until the end of the sleep record (usually at 7 AM)
Sleep efficiency: Total sleep time or total time of the sleep record × 100
Apnea index: Number of apneas longer than 10 seconds per hour of sleep
Nocturnal myoclonus index: Number of periodic leg movements per hour
Rapid eye movement (REM) latency: Period of time from the onset of sleep until the first REM period of the night
Sleep-onset REM period: REM sleep within the first 10 minutes of sleep.

SLEEP DISORDER CLASSIFICATION

DSM-5

The fifth edition of the *Diagnostic and Statistical Manual of Mental Disorders* (DSM-5) of the American Psychiatric Association (APA) lists 10 disorders or disorder groups as sleep–wake disorders. The DSM-5 classifies sleep disorders on the basis of clinical diagnostic criteria and presumed etiology. The disorders described in DSM-5 are only a fraction of the known sleep disorders; they provide a framework for clinical assessment. The sleep–wake disorders' current classifications in accordance with the DSM-5 include the following:

1. Insomnia disorder
2. Hypersomnolence disorder
3. Narcolepsy
4. Breathing-related sleep disorders:
   a. Obstructive sleep apnea hypopnea
   b. Central sleep apnea
      i. Idiopathic central sleep apnea
      ii. Cheyne–Stokes breathing
      iii. Central sleep apnea comorbid with opioid use
   c. Sleep-related hypoventilation
5. Circadian rhythm sleep–wake disorders:
   a. Delayed sleep phase type
   b. Advanced sleep phase type
   c. Irregular sleep–wake type
   d. Non–24-hour sleep–wake type
   e. Shift work type
   f. Unspecified type
6. Parasomnias
7. Non-rapid eye movement sleep arousal disorders:
   a. Sleepwalking type
   b. Sleep terror type
8. Nightmare disorder
9. Rapid eye movement sleep behavior disorder
10. Restless legs syndrome
11. Substance/medication-induced sleep disorder

INSOMNIA DISORDER

Insomnia is defined as difficulty initiating or maintaining sleep. It is the most common sleep complaint and may be transient or persistent. Population surveys show a 1-year prevalence rate of 30 to 45 percent in adults.

DSM-5 defines insomnia disorder as dissatisfaction with sleep quantity or quality associated with one or more of the following symptoms: difficulty in initiating sleep, difficulty in maintaining sleep with frequent awakenings or problems returning to sleep, and early morning awakening with inability to return to sleep.

It is now recognized that insomnia can be an independent condition. In the past, practitioners were admonished to treat insomnia's cause rather than the symptoms. There was an implicit notion that by doing so, the sleep problems would improve. Clinical experience suggested otherwise. Consequently, current therapeutics favor providing relief and managing symptoms. In the past it was argued that if insomnia was related to depression, treating the insomnia would mask the depression and thereby interfere with antidepressant treatment regimens. This does not appear to happen.

Descriptively, insomnia can be categorized in terms of how it affects sleep (e.g., sleep-onset insomnia, sleep-maintenance insomnia, or early-morning awakening). Insomnia can also be classified according to its duration (e.g., transient, short term, and long term). According to the Gallup Survey, approximately one-third of US population has several serious bouts of insomnia yearly; however, in 9 percent of the general population, insomnia is a chronic condition. Individuals with chronic insomnia have more than twice as many motor vehicle accidents as the general population, but only 5 percent of those with chronic insomnia see a health care provider to seek help for sleeplessness. Nonetheless, 40 percent or more of those individuals with chronic insomnia self-medicate with over-the-counter drugs, alcohol, or both.

A brief period of insomnia is most often associated with anxiety, either as a sequela to an anxious experience or in anticipation of an anxiety-provoking experience (e.g., an examination or an impending job interview). In some persons, transient insomnia of this kind may be related to grief, loss, or almost any life change or stress. The condition is not likely to be serious, although a psychotic episode or a severe depression sometimes begins with acute insomnia. Specific treatment for the condition is usually not required. When treatment with hypnotic medication is indicated, both the physician and the patient should be clear that the treatment is of short duration and that some symptoms, including a brief recurrence of the insomnia, may be expected when the medication is discontinued.

Persistent insomnia is composed of a fairly common group of conditions in which the problem is difficulty falling asleep or remaining asleep. This insomnia involves two sometimes separable, but often intertwined, problems: somatized tension and anxiety and a conditioned associative response. Patients often have no clear complaint other than insomnia. They may not experience anxiety per se but discharge the anxiety through physiological channels; they may complain chiefly of apprehensive feelings or ruminative thoughts that appear to keep them from falling asleep. Sometimes (but not always) a patient describes the condition's exacerbation at times of stress at work or at home and its remission during vacations.

Sleep state misperception (also known as *subjective insomnia*) is characterized by a dissociation between the patient's experience of sleeping and the objective polygraphic measures of sleep. The ultimate cause of this dissociation is not yet understood, although it appears to be a specific case of a general phenomenon seen in many areas of medicine. Sleep state misperception is diagnosed when a patient complains of difficulty initiating or maintaining sleep and no objective evidence of sleep disruption is found. For example, a patient sleeping in the laboratory reports taking more than an hour to fall asleep, awakening more than 30 times, and sleeping less than 2 hours the entire night. By contrast, the polysomnogram shows sleep onset occurring within 15 minutes, few awakenings, a 90 percent sleep efficiency, and total sleep time exceeding 7 hours. Sleep state misperception can occur in individuals who are apparently free from psychopathology or it can represent a somatic delusion or hypochondriasis. Some patients with sleep state misperception have obsessional features concerning somatic functions. Short-term sleep state misperception can occur during periods of stress, and some clinicians believe it can result from latent or ineffectively treated anxiety or depressive disorders. Cognitive relabeling, diffusing the worry about being unable to sleep, or both can help. Interestingly, anxiolytics can profoundly reduce the perception of sleeplessness without markedly changing sleep physiologically.

Psychophysiological insomnia typically presents as a primary complaint of difficulty in going to sleep. A patient may describe this as having gone on for years and usually denies that it is associated with stressful periods in his or her life. Objects associated with sleep (e.g., the bed, the bedroom) likewise become conditioned stimuli that evoke insomnia. Thus, psychophysiological insomnia is sometimes called *conditioned insomnia.* Psychophysiological insomnia often occurs in combination with other causes of insomnia, including episodes of stress and anxiety disorders, delayed sleep phase syndrome, and hypnotic drug use and withdrawal. In contrast to the insomnia in patients with psychiatric disorders, daytime adaptation is generally good. Work and relationships are satisfying; however, extreme tiredness can exist. Other features include (1) excessive worry about not being able to sleep; (2) trying too hard to sleep; (3) rumination, inability to clear one's mind while trying to sleep; (4) increased muscle tension when attempting to sleep; (5) other somatic manifestations of anxiety; (6) being able to sleep better away from one's own bedroom; and (7) being able to fall asleep when not trying (e.g., watching television). The sleep complaint becomes fixed over time. Interestingly, many patients with psychophysiological insomnia sleep well in the laboratory.

Ms. W, a 41-year-old divorced white woman, presented with a 2.5-year complaint of sleeplessness. She had some difficulty falling asleep (30 to 45 minutes sleep onset latency) and awakened every hour or two after sleep onset. These awakenings could last 15 minutes to several hours, and she estimated approximately 4.5 hours of sleep on an average night. She rarely took daytime naps notwithstanding feeling tired and edgy. She described her sleep problem as follows: "It seems like I never get into a deep sleep. I have never been a heavy sleeper, but now the slightest noise wakes me up. Sometimes I have a hard time getting my mind to shut down." She viewed the bedroom as an unpleasant place of sleeplessness and stated, "I tried staying at a friend's house where it is quiet, but then I couldn't sleep because of the silence."

At times, Ms. W would be unsure whether she was asleep or awake. She had a history of clock watching (to time her wakefulness) but stopped doing this when she realized it was contributing to the problem. Reportedly the insomnia is unrelated to seasonal changes, menstrual cycle, or time-zone translocation. Her basic sleep hygiene was good. Appetite and libido were unchanged. She denied mood disturbance, except that she was quite frustrated and concerned about sleeplessness and its effect on her work. Her work involved sitting at a microscope for 6 hours of a 9-hour working day and meticulously documenting her findings. Her final output had not suffered, but she now had to "double check" for accuracy.

She described herself as a worrier and a Type A personality. She did not know how to relax. For example, on vacation she continually worried about things that could go wrong. She could not even begin to unwind until she had arrived at the destination, checked in, and unpacked. Even then, she was unable to relax.

Medical history was unremarkable except for tonsillectomy (age 16 years), migraine headaches (current), and diet-controlled hypercholesterolemia. She took naproxen (Aleve) as needed for headache. She did not drink caffeinated beverages, smoke tobacco, or drink alcoholic beverages. She did not use recreational drugs.

The problem with insomnia began after relocation to a new city and place of employment. She attributed her insomnia to the noisy neighborhood in which she lived. She first sought treatment 18 months previously. Her family practice physician diagnosed depression and she was started on fluoxetine (Prozac), which made her "climb the walls." Antihistamines were tried next with similar results. She was then switched to low-dose trazodone (Desyrel; for sleep) and developed nausea. After these medical interventions, she sought medical care elsewhere. Zolpidem (Ambien), 5 mg, was prescribed, but it made her feel drugged, and on discontinuation she had withdrawal effects. Another family practice physician diagnosed "nonspecific anxiety disorder" and began buspirone (BuSpar), an experience she described as "having an alien try to climb out of my skin." Buspirone was discontinued. Paroxetine (Paxil) was tried for 8 weeks with no effect. Finally, a psychiatrist was consulted, who diagnosed adult attention-deficit disorder (without hyperactivity) and suggested treatment with methylphenidate (Ritalin). At this point, the patient was convinced that a stimulant would not help her insomnia and demanded referral to a sleep disorders center.

Ms. W's symptoms fell into the broad category of insomnia, and the symptoms had begun after she had moved from one city to another. Environmental sleep disorder (noise) and adjustment sleep disorder (new job, city, and apartment) were likely initial diagnoses. However, a more chronic, endogenous problem had become operative. Ms. W was a "worrier" and meticulous, but she did not reach diagnostic criteria for personality or anxiety disorders. Dyssomnia associated with mood disorder should be considered in any patient with sleep maintenance problems and early-morning awakening insomnia. However, this patient did not have other significant signs of depression. Unfortunately, many patients are misdiagnosed with depression or "masked depression" on the sole basis of an insomnia complaint and unsuccessfully treated with antidepressant medication. Ms. W's job demanded long hours with focused concentration. Her job performance had been superior for many years notwithstanding insomnia. Thus, a diagnosis of attention-deficit disorder was unlikely. Idiopathic insomnia implies a childhood complaint, which Ms. W denied.

The likely working diagnosis was psychophysiological insomnia (PPI). There may have been some sleep state misperception (she was sometimes unclear on whether she was awake or asleep), but this could not adequately account for the constellation of symptoms. An initial treatment plan should include further documentation of the sleep pattern using a sleep log. Behavioral treatments would likely benefit this patient. Medications with sedative effects are sometimes useful during the initial treatment of PPI. However, thus far in this patient they had done more harm than good. She would likely be a challenging patient to treat. *(Courtesy of Max Hirshkowitz, Ph.D., Rhoda G. Seplowitz-Hafkin, M.D., and Amir Sharafkhaneh, M.D., Ph.D.)*

Idiopathic insomnia typically starts early in life, sometimes at birth, and continues throughout life. As the name implies, its cause is unknown; suspected causes include neurochemical imbalance in brainstem reticular formation, impaired regulation of brainstem sleep generators (e.g., raphe nuclei, locus ceruleus), or basal forebrain dysfunction. Treatment is difficult, but improved sleep hygiene, relaxation therapy, and judicious use of hypnotic medicines are reportedly helpful.

Primary insomnia is diagnosed when the chief complaint is nonrestorative sleep or difficulty in initiating or maintaining sleep, and the complaint continues for at least a month (according to ICD-10, the disturbance must occur at least three times a week for a month). The term *primary* indicates that the insomnia is independent of any known physical or mental condition. Primary insomnia is often characterized both by difficulty falling asleep and by repeated awakening. Increased nighttime physiological or psychological arousal and negative conditioning for sleep are frequently evident. Patients with primary insomnia are generally preoccupied with getting enough sleep. The more they try to sleep, the greater the sense of frustration and distress and the more elusive sleep becomes.

Treating Insomnia

Pharmacological Treatment. Primary insomnia is commonly treated with benzodiazepines, zolpidem, eszopiclone (Lunesta), zaleplon (Sonata), and other hypnotics. Hypnotic drugs should be used with care. In general, sleep medications should not be prescribed for more than 2 weeks because tolerance and withdrawal may result. For many years, benzodiazepines were the most commonly prescribed sedative–hypnotic medications for treating insomnia. Benzodiazepine-receptor agonists represent the current standard for sedative–hypnotic medications used to treat insomnia. Long-acting sleep medications (e.g., flurazepam [Dalmane], quazepam [Doral]) are best for middle-of-the-night insomnia; short-acting drugs (e.g., zolpidem, triazolam [Halcion]) are useful for persons who have difficulty falling asleep. The melatonin-receptor agonist ramelteon (Rozerem) has also been approved for treating sleep-onset insomnia. Sedating antidepressants, such as trazodone, are also frequently prescribed as sleep aids.

A variety of over-the-counter (OTC) sleep aids are also available. Nonprescription formulas include sedating antihistamines, protein precursors, and other substances. L-tryptophan was popular and readily available at health food stores until an outbreak of eosinophilia led to its being pulled off the shelves. Melatonin is a leader among self-administered food additives believed by some to alleviate sleeplessness. Melatonin is an endogenous hormone produced by the pineal gland, which is linked to the regulation of sleep. Administration of exogenous melatonin has yielded mixed results, however, in clinical research.

Prescription medicines are rigorously tested in clinical trials; therefore, they hold an advantage over the virtually untested OTCs. To attain U.S. Food and Drug Administration (FDA) approval as a hypnotic, a medication must be safe and effective. Most hypnotic medications are approved for short-term, not long-term, use. Exceptions include zolpidem modified release, eszopiclone, and ramelteon, all of which are approved for long-term therapy. When properly used, hypnotics can provide immediate and adequate relief from sleeplessness. Insomnia, however, usually returns on discontinuation of dosing.

Cognitive–Behavioral Therapy. Cognitive–behavioral therapy (CBT) as a treatment modality uses a combination of behavioral and cognitive techniques to overcome dysfunctional sleep behaviors, misperceptions, and distorted, disruptive thoughts about sleep. Behavioral techniques include universal sleep hygiene, stimulus control therapy, sleep restriction therapy, relaxation therapies, and biofeedback.

Studies repeatedly show significant, sustained improvement in sleep symptoms, including number and duration of awakenings and sleep latency from CBT. Short-term benefits are similar to that of medication, but CBT tends to have lasting benefits even 36 months after treatment. With cessation of the medication, insomnia frequently returns and is sometimes accompanied by rebound insomnia. CBT has not been shown to produce any adverse effects. There are no established "best practice" guidelines for length or quantity of sessions.

CBT, however, is not without limitations. Most data do not compare the efficacy of the individual components of CBT. However, sleep hygiene education alone produces an insignificant effect on sleep. In addition, there are no studies demonstrating evidence for improved efficacy with the combination of the aforementioned components or what cognitive therapy adds to the behavioral component. Intuitively, it would seem that the multicomponent approach addresses many of the variables contributing to insomnia.

The effects of CBT take longer to emerge than effects of medications. Usually when patients finally come for treatment of their insomnia, they are desperate. This makes it difficult to convince them to try a therapy that may take several weeks before it will provide relief. Furthermore, patients do not assume a passive role in this type of therapy; they must be active participants. Many individuals not only want a "quick fix," but they also want to undergo a procedure or have something administered rather than be involved in the therapeutic process. For CBT to be effective, patients must commit to come to multiple sessions and also be open to the idea that modifying thoughts and behaviors about sleep can improve the symptoms of insomnia. The "quick fix" model is more familiar to primary care providers, whereas psychiatrists are used to the delayed response of antidepressants and other psychotropics. Therefore, psychiatrists may be more amenable to recommending CBT. Another barrier for physicians using CBT in clinical practice is that providing CBT for insomnia requires a greater time commitment than prescribing a sleep aid.

Although firmly focused on cognitive and behavioral issues, it helps to extend CBT just slightly into the psychodynamic sphere. For some patients with long-standing difficulty sleeping, being an insomniac becomes an important part of their identity. There may be primary or secondary gain to such identification. It is the negative emotional response (i.e., anger at the inability to control one's sleep, feeling like a failure because one cannot sleep) to insomnia that contributes to its chronicity. In general, these individuals tend to internalize rather than express emotion, feel a heightened need for control, experience interpersonal difficulties, and have significant discontent with past events. For this subset of people, if the emotional response is not addressed, there is more likely to be a limited response to CBT or a relapse of insomnia over time. The clinician who is attuned to a patient's tendency to view something as a failure rather than a challenge will be better able to intercept barriers to treatment.

Universal Sleep Hygiene. A common finding is that a patient's lifestyle leads to sleep disturbance. This is usually phrased as *inadequate sleep hygiene,* referring to a problem in following generally accepted practices to aid sleep. These include, for instance, keeping regular hours of bedtime and arousal, avoiding excessive caffeine, not eating heavy meals before bedtime, and getting adequate exercise. Many behaviors can interfere with sleep and may do so by increasing nervous system arousal near bedtime or by altering circadian rhythms.

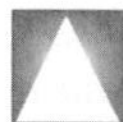

Table 12.2–2
Dos and Don'ts for Good Sleep Hygiene

	DO	DON'T
Maintain regular hours of bedtime and arising	✓	
If you are hungry, have a light snack before bedtime	✓	
Maintain a regular exercise schedule	✓	
Give yourself approximately an hour to wind down before going to bed	✓	
If you are preoccupied or worried about something at bedtime, write it down and deal with it in the morning	✓	
Keep the bedroom cool	✓	
Keep the bedroom dark	✓	
Keep the bedroom quiet	✓	
Take naps		✓
Watch the clock so you know how bad your insomnia actually is		✓
Exercise right before going to bed in order wear yourself out		✓
Watch television in bed when you cannot sleep		✓
Eat a heavy meal before bedtime to help you sleep		✓
Drink coffee in the afternoon and evening		✓
If you cannot sleep, smoke a cigarette		✓
Use alcohol to help in going to sleep		✓
Read in bed when you cannot sleep		✓
Eat in bed		✓
Exercise in bed		✓
Talk on the phone in bed		✓

The focus of universal sleep hygiene is on modifiable environmental and lifestyle components that may interfere with sleep, as well as behaviors that may improve sleep. Treatment should focus on one to three problem areas at a time. Especially because some of these behaviors are difficult to change, only one or two items that are collaboratively chosen by the patient and clinician should be addressed. This gives the patient the best chance at a successful intervention. Overwhelming the patient with too many lifestyle changes or a complex regimen seldom succeeds. Some general "dos and don'ts" are instructive. Sleep-enhancing directives are enumerated in Table 12.2–2. Often a few simple alterations in a patient's habits or sleep environment can be effective. The clinician, however, needs to spend time reviewing both the patient's routine and its irregularity. In some respects, the essence of insomnia is its variability. The day-to-day changes in behavior and the changing severity of sleeplessness can obscure the factors responsible for the problem. A carefully explained program of sleep hygiene, with follow-up, represents a fairly inexpensive but effective intervention. Furthermore, improving sleep habits can enhance sleep even when the major cause of insomnia is physical.

Stimulus Control Therapy. Stimulus control therapy is a deconditioning paradigm developed by Richard Bootzin and colleagues at the University of Arizona. This treatment aims to break the cycle of problems commonly associated with difficulty initiating sleep. By attempting to undo conditioning that undermines sleep, stimulus control therapy helps reduce both primary and reactive factors involved in insomnia. The rules attempt to enhance stimulus cues for sleeping and diminish associations with sleeplessness. The instructions are simple; however, they must be followed consistently. The *first* rule is, go to bed only when sleepy to maximize success. *Second,* use the bed only for sleeping. Do not watch television in bed, do not read, do not eat, and do not talk on the telephone while in bed. *Third,* do not lie in bed and become frustrated if unable to sleep. After a few minutes (do not watch the clock), get up, go to another room, and do something nonarousing until sleepiness returns. The goal is to associate the bed with rapid sleep onset. Rule three should be repeated as often as needed. The *fourth and final* instruction attempts to enhance the mechanisms underlying the circadian and sleep–wake cycles—that is, awaken at the same time every morning (regardless of bedtime, total sleep time, or day of week) and totally avoid napping. Stimulus control therapy does work; however, results might not be seen during the first few weeks or month. If continually practiced, the bouts of insomnia lessen in both frequency and severity.

Sleep Restriction Therapy. Sleep restriction therapy is a strategy designed to increase sleep efficiency by decreasing the amount of time spent awake while lying in bed. Developed by Arthur Spielman, this therapy specifically targets those patients who lie awake in bed unable to sleep. Restricting time in bed can help to consolidate sleep. If the patient reports sleeping only 5 hours of a scheduled 8-hour time in bed, reduce the time in bed. It is advised, however, not to reduce bedtime to less than 4 hours per night and to warn the patient about the hazards of daytime sleepiness. Sleep at other times during the day must be avoided, except in the elderly, who may take a 30-minute nap. The clinician then monitors sleep efficiency (time asleep as a percentage of the time in bed). When sleep efficiency reaches 85 percent (averaged over five nights), time in bed is increased by 15 minutes. Sleep restriction therapy produces a gradual and steady decline in nocturnal wakefulness.

Relaxation Therapy and Biofeedback. The most important aspects of relaxation therapy are that it be performed properly. Self-hypnosis, progressive relaxation, guided imagery, and deep breathing exercises are all effective if they produce relaxation. The goal is to find the optimal technique for each patient, but not all patients need help in relaxing. *Progressive muscle relaxation* is especially useful for patients who experience muscle tension. The patients should purposefully tense (5 to 6 seconds) and then relax (20 to 30 seconds) muscle groups, beginning at the head and ending at the feet. The patient should appreciate the difference between tension and relaxation. *Guided imagery* has the patient visualize a pleasant, restful scene, engaging all of his or her senses. *Breathing exercises* are practiced for at least 20 minutes per day for 2 weeks. Once mastered, the technique should be used once at bedtime for 30 minutes. If it does not work, the patient should try again another night. It is important that the technique not become associated with failure to fall asleep.

The patient is instructed to perform *abdominal breathing* as follows. The patient must become comfortable with each step before moving on to the next:

First, in the supine position, the patient should breathe normally through his or her mouth or nose, whichever is more comfortable, and attend to his or her breathing pattern.

Second, while maintaining that rhythm, the patient should begin to breathe more with his or her abdomen and less with his or her chest.

Third, the patient should pause for a half second after each breath cycle (in and out) and evaluate the breath. How did it feel? Was it smooth? Eventually each breath will become uniform and smooth.

Fourth, the patient should find a place where he or she can best feel the air move in and out. Concentrate on that spot and on the air moving in and out.

Fifth, the patient should visualize intrusive thoughts as floating away; if there are too many thoughts, stop practicing and try again later.

Biofeedback provides stimulus cues for physiological markers of relaxation and can increase self-awareness. A machine is used to measure muscle tension in the forehead or finger temperature. Finger temperature rises when a person becomes more relaxed. Patients require careful and adequate training; simply giving them an instruction tape is not especially helpful. Techniques are ideally mastered during the day for several weeks before application to the sleep problem; this is best achieved outside of the bed. By the time the techniques are applied in bed, the skill should be automatic. Relaxation techniques readily lend themselves to being combined with sleep hygiene and stimulus control therapies. Sometimes, they make for good distractions from thinking about the inability to sleep. The ruminations fuel the insomnia, and if the ruminator can be distracted, then the person may sleep better.

Cognitive Training. This effective, validated treatment for a variety of psychiatric conditions, including major depression and generalized anxiety, has been adapted for use with insomnia. The cognitive aspect of insomnia treatment targets the negative emotional response to an appraisal of a sleep-related situation. The negative emotional response is thought to produce emotional arousal, which in turn contributes to or perpetuates insomnia. People who have maladaptive cognitions tend to exaggerate the negative consequences of insomnia: "There must be something really wrong with me if I can't fall asleep in 40 minutes." They also tend to have unrealistic expectations about their sleep requirements: "If I don't sleep 8 hours a night then my whole day will be ruined." The first step is to identify these cognitions, then challenge their validity, and finally substitute them with more adaptive cognitions.

DH was a 42-year-old man with a 5-year history of insomnia. He identified being fired from his job and the birth of a colicky baby as precipitating factors in his inability to sleep. However, even after he found a new position with better hours and pay and with the child sleeping through the night, DH continued to experience difficulty falling and staying asleep. Perpetuating factors included low back pain and a spouse with periodic limb movement disorder. He reported spending 8 to 9 hours in bed each night and sleeping only 4 to 5 hours intermittently. He watched 1 hour of television in bed before turning out the light for bedtime. He spent hours watching his minutes tick away. He did not awake feeling rested, and when his alarm went off he was frequently already awake and had thoughts such as, "I hardly slept at all last night. I should be able to get more sleep. There must be something wrong with me. Great, I'll be too tired to concentrate on anything today."

Examples of maladaptive thoughts: "I should be able to get more sleep." This is a faulty appraisal of sleeping ability and may relate to a need for control over sleep. This need for control interferes with having a more laissez-faire attitude about a few missed hours of rest. Such thoughts can also lead to feelings of frustration and anger. "Great, I'll be too tired to concentrate on anything today." This is a misattribution of daytime impairment due to poor sleep. DH was also magnifying the negative and discounting the positive with his black-and-white or all-or-nothing thinking. Could DH be too tired to concentrate on some things but not all things? Might his inability to concentrate be due to a myriad of other factors? "There must be something wrong with me (if I can't get enough sleep)." This is catastrophizing and emotional reasoning: Just because a person had a feeling does not mean that the thought or feeling is true. A strongly held belief that sleeplessness negatively affects physical and mental health can set off catastrophizing. *(Courtesy of Max Hirshkowitz, Ph.D., Rhoda G. Seplowitz-Hafkin, M.D., and Amir Sharafkhaneh, M.D., Ph.D.)*

Paradoxical Intention. This is a cognitive technique with conflicting evidence regarding its efficacy. In clinical practice compliance is often a barrier, but it does work for a limited number of patients. The theory is that performance anxiety interferes with sleep onset. Thus, when the patient tries to stay awake for as long as possible rather than trying to fall asleep, performance anxiety will be reduced and sleep latency will improve.

HYPERSOMNOLENCE DISORDER

Excessive sleepiness (hypersomnolence) is a serious, debilitating, potentially life-threatening noncommunicable condition. It affects not only the afflicted individual but also his or her family, coworkers, and the public at large. Sleepiness can be a consequence of (1) insufficient sleep, (2) basic neurologic dysfunction in brain systems regulating sleep, (3) disrupted sleep, or (4) the phase of an individual's circadian rhythm. A sleep history questionnaire is often helpful in diagnosing a patient's sleep disorder (Table 12.2–3). The sleep debt produced by insufficient sleep is cumulative. If one reduces sleep duration by 1 to 2 hours per night and continues this regimen for a week, sleepiness will reach pathological levels. When sleep debt is added to sleep disruption or a basic neurologic dysfunction in sleep mechanisms, there is increasing risk that an individual will lapse unexpectedly into sleep. Sleep onset in such circumstances characteristically occurs without warning. Sleepiness can be episodic and occur as irresistible sleep attacks, occur in the morning as sleep drunkenness, or be chronic. Fatigue, tiredness, and sleepiness are terms that are used by most people synonymously; however, one can be tired but not sleepy, sleepy but not tired, or sleepy and tired. In this section, the term *sleepiness* will refer to drowsiness, a propensity to lapse into sleep, and when extreme, an inability to maintain wakefulness.

Sleepiness adversely affects attention, concentration, memory, and higher-order cognitive processes. Serious results of sleepiness include failure at school, loss of employment, motor vehicle accidents, and industrial disasters. The transportation industry, including trucking, railroad, marine, and aviation, is particularly prone to sleep-related accidents. There are many sleep disorders associated with excessive daytime sleepiness; however, sleep-disordered breathing is by far the most common dyssomnia seen in sleep disorder centers.

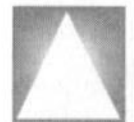

Table 12.2–3
Sleep History Questionnaire

Patient name
Date
Please check the appropriate box or give short answers for the following:

	Yes	No
1. Do you feel sleepy or have sleep attacks during the day?	☐	☐
2. Do you nap during the day?	☐	☐
3. Do you have trouble concentrating during the day?	☐	☐
4. Do you have trouble falling asleep when you first go to bed?	☐	☐
5. Do you awaken during the night?	☐	☐
6. Do you awaken more than once?	☐	☐
7. Do you awaken too early in the morning?	☐	☐
8. How long have you had trouble sleeping?	☐	☐

What do you think precipitated the problem?

____
____
____

9. How would you describe your usual night's sleep (hours of sleep, quality of sleep, etc.)?

____
____
____

	Yes	No
10. Does your schedule for sleep and rising on the weekend differ from what it is during the week?	☐	☐
11. Do others live at home who interrupt your sleep?	☐	☐
12. Are you regularly awakened at night by pain or the need to use the bathroom?	☐	☐
13. Does your job require shift changes or travel?	☐	☐
14. Do you drink caffeinated beverages (coffee, tea, or soft drinks)?	☐	☐

15. Apart from difficulty in sleeping, what, if any, other medical problems do you have?

____
____
____

16. What sleep medications, prescription or nonprescription, do you take? (Please include the dosage, how often you take it, and for how many months or years you have taken it.)

____
____
____

17. What other prescription and over-the-counter medications do you regularly use? (Again, please include the dosage, the frequency, and the duration.)

____
____
____

	Yes	No
18. Have you ever suffered from depression, anxiety, or similar problems?	☐	☐
19. Do you snore?	☐	☐
Questions for the Sleep Partner		
1. Does your sleep partner snore?	☐	☐
2. Does your sleep partner seem to stop breathing repeatedly during the night?	☐	☐
3. Does your sleep partner jerk his or her legs or kick you while he or she is sleeping?	☐	☐
4. Have you ever experienced trouble sleeping? Please explain.	☐	☐

____
____
____
____
____

Primary hypersomnia is diagnosed when no other cause can be found for excessive somnolence occurring for at least 1 month. Some persons are long sleepers who, as with short sleepers, show a normal variation. Their sleep, although long, is normal in architecture and physiology. Sleep efficiency and the sleep–wake schedule are normal. This pattern is without complaints about the quality of sleep, daytime sleepiness, or difficulties with the awake mood, motivation, and performance. Long sleep may be a lifetime pattern, and it appears to have a familial incidence. Many persons are variable sleepers and may become long sleepers at certain times in their lives.

Some persons have subjective complaints of feeling sleepy without objective findings. They do not have a tendency to fall asleep more often than is normal and do not have any objective signs. Clinicians should try to rule out clear-cut causes of excessive somnolence.

Types of Hypersomnia

Kleine–Levin Syndrome. Kleine–Levin syndrome is a relatively rare condition consisting of recurrent periods of prolonged sleep (from which patients may be aroused) with intervening periods of normal sleep and alert waking. During the hypersomniac episodes, wakeful periods are usually marked by withdrawal from social contacts and return to bed at the first opportunity. Kleine–Levin syndrome is the best-recognized recurrent hypersomnia though it is uncommon. It predominantly afflicts males in early adolescence; however, it can occur later in life and in females. With few exceptions, the first attack occurs between the ages of 10 and 21 years. Rare instances of onset in the fourth and fifth decades of life have been reported. In its classic form, the recurrent episodes are associated with extreme sleepiness (18-hour to 20-hour sleep periods), voracious eating, hypersexuality, and disinhibition (e.g., aggression). Episodes typically last for a few days up to several weeks and appear once to ten times per year. A monosymptomatic hypersomnolent form can occur. The frequency of the human leukocyte antigen (HLA) is increased in patients with this syndrome.

Menstrual-Related Hypersomnia. In some women, recurrent episodes of hypersomnia are related to the menstrual cycle, experiencing intermittent episodes of marked hypersomnia at, or shortly before, the onset of their menses. The symptoms typically last for 1 week and resolve with menstruation. Nonspecific EEG abnormalities similar to those associated with Kleine–Levin syndrome have been documented in several instances. Endocrine factors are probably involved, but no specific abnormalities in laboratory endocrine measures have been reported. Treatment with oral contraceptives is effective, and therefore the disorder is believed to be secondary to a hormone imbalance.

Idiopathic Hypersomnia. Idiopathic hypersomnia (IH) presents in several forms. It may be associated with very long sleep periods, after which the individual remains sleepy. IH can also occur without long sleep periods. IH is a disorder of excessive sleepiness in which patients do not have the ancillary symptoms associated with narcolepsy. Unlike narcolepsy, sleep is usually well preserved, and sleep efficiency remains high even in forms associated with very extended sleep schedules (12 hours or more). Furthermore, the patient readily falls asleep if given an opportunity to nap the following day. There is often elevated slow wave sleep; however, the EEG sleep pattern is essentially the same as that found in normal individuals who are sleep deprived. Unlike a sleep-deprived individual, the sleep pattern continues in this profile even after several nights of extended sleep. As the name indicates, the etiology of idiopathic hypersomnia is not known; however, a central nervous system cause is presumed. Three general categories have been developed. Subgroup 1 includes individuals who are HLA-Cw2 positive, have autonomic nervous system dysfunctions, and have other affected family members. Subgroup 2 includes status postviral infection patients (e.g., Guillain–Barré syndrome [ascending polyneuropathy], mononucleosis, and atypical viral pneumonia). Subgroup 3 idiopathic hypersomnia patients are nonfamilial and are not postviral (i.e., truly idiopathic).

Age of onset is characteristically between 15 and 30 years, and the hypersomnia becomes a lifelong problem. In addition to the prolonged, undisturbed, and unrefreshing nocturnal sleep, IH is associated with long nonrefreshing naps, difficulty awakening, sleep drunkenness, and automatic behaviors with amnesia. Other symptoms suggesting autonomic nervous system dysfunction are typical, including migraine-like headaches, fainting spells, syncope, orthostatic hypotension, and Raynaud-type phenomena with cold hands and feet.

Some patients with IH sleep less than 10 hours per night, have difficulty awakening, awake unrefreshed and even confused, and may take unintentional, unrefreshing daytime naps provoked by their daytime somnolence. Onset is typically before 25 years of age, and the course of the disorder is persistent and unremitting.

> A 60-year-old accountant complained of excessive sleepiness and reported that he had to take about five half-hour naps throughout the day. He awakened feeling refreshed but unless he napped he could not function at work. He did not abuse substances and narcolepsy was ruled out; but on history he reported that both his father and paternal grandfather had the same sleep pattern. He was examined in a sleep laboratory and had a normal polysomnograph with 10 hours of uninterrupted sleep. A genetic predisposition for hypersomnolence was presumed to be the cause of his symptoms. He obtained some relief from small doses of amphetamine (2.5 mg) which he would use when he could not take his normal naps because of specific work obligations.

Behaviorally Induced Insufficient Sleep Syndrome. Insufficient sleep syndrome stems from an individual's disregard for the sleep–wake schedule. It is usually subclinical and occurs in a great proportion of the population. Medical help is generally not sought because the individual is aware of the cause of his or her sleepiness. Insufficient sleep, however, is an insidious killer and is related to many vehicular and industrial accidents. When an individual becomes progressively more and more sleep deprived, eventually payment for the sleep debt will be exacted. Excessive sleepiness associated with insufficient sleep can be unmasked by a heavy meal, low-dose alcohol ingestion, a warm room, and sedentary activity. Insufficient sleep syndrome is diagnosed when an individual does not schedule an adequate amount of time for sleep and as a result suffers from daytime sleepiness, fatigue, loss of concentration, memory impairment, irritability, and moodiness. Often the individual will fast and binge on sleep, nap, and extend the sleep period on weekends. Although caffeinated beverages are commonly self-administered, appropriate treatment involves increasing the duration and regularity of sleep. Recent studies indicate that metabolic disorders and insulin resistance may result from chronic insufficient sleep.

Hypersomnia due to a Medical Condition. Medical conditions known to cause hypersomnia include head trauma, stroke, encephalitis, Parkinson's disease, inflammatory conditions, tumors, genetic diseases, and neurodegenerative diseases.

Hypersomnia due to Drug or Substance Use. Sleepiness can be caused by use or abuse of sedative hypnotics, sedating antihistamines, sedating antidepressants, antiepileptics, neuroleptics, and opioid analgesics. Hypersomnia may also be provoked by withdrawal from traditional stimulants (cocaine, amphetamines), caffeine, or nicotine.

Treating Hypersomnia

Hypersomnia caused by insufficient sleep is treated by extending and regularizing the sleep period. If, however, the sleepiness arises from narcolepsy, medical conditions, or idiopathic hypersomnia, it is usually managed pharmacologically. There is no cure for these conditions, but symptoms are managed with either the wake-promoting substance modafinil (Provigil; first-line treatment) or traditional psychostimulants such as amphetamines and their derivatives (if modafinil fails). For narcolepsy (discussed below), REM sleep–suppressing drugs (e.g., many antidepressants) are used to treat the cataplexy. This approach capitalizes on the anticholinergic REM sleep–suppressant properties of these drugs. Because cataplexy is presumably an intrusion of REM sleep phenomena into the awake state, the rationale is clear. Many reports indicate that imipramine (Tofranil) and protriptyline (Vivactil) are quite effective for reducing or eliminating cataplexy. Selective serotonin reuptake inhibitors (SSRIs) have gained popularity because they are associated with fewer side effects than the tricyclic antidepressants. More recently, sodium oxybate (Xyrem) has proven to be extremely effective for reducing cataplexy, even in cases in which the cataplexy was thought to be intractable. Studies also suggest that sodium oxybate helps to improve sleep and relieves some of the sleepiness associated with narcolepsy. Although drug therapies are the treatment of choice, the overall therapeutic approach should include scheduled naps, lifestyle adjustment, psychological counseling, drug holidays to reduce tolerance (if stimulants are used), and careful monitoring of refills, general health, and cardiac status.

NARCOLEPSY

Narcolepsy is a condition characterized by excessive sleepiness, as well as auxiliary symptoms that represent the intrusion of aspects of REM sleep into the waking state. The sleep attacks of narcolepsy represent episodes of irresistible sleepiness, leading to perhaps 10 to 20 minutes of sleep, after which the patient feels refreshed, at least briefly. They can occur at inappropriate times (e.g., while eating, talking, or driving and during sex). The REM sleep includes hypnagogic and hypnopompic hallucinations, cataplexy, and sleep paralysis. The appearance of REM sleep within 10 minutes of sleep onset (sleep-onset REM periods) is also considered evidence of narcolepsy. The disorder can be dangerous because it can lead to automobile and industrial accidents.

Narcolepsy is the prototypical example of sleepiness produced by a basic central nervous system dysfunction of sleep mechanisms. The etiology stems from a genetically triggered hypocretin dysfunction and deficit. It has become apparent that the hypocretin system plays a critical role in narcolepsy. In a canine model of narcolepsy, mutations of hypocretin receptor-2 were identified that result in malfunctioning of this receptor. In human narcolepsy with HLA-DQB1*0602–positive individuals, levels of hypocretin receptor-1 are undetectable in cerebrospinal fluid (CSF). A strong association between narcolepsy and specific HLA suggests an autoimmune process that damages hypocretin-containing cells in the central nervous system (CNS).

Narcolepsy is not as rare as was once thought. It is estimated to occur in 0.02 to 0.16 percent of adults and shows some familial incidence. Narcolepsy is neither a type of epilepsy nor a psychogenic disturbance. It is an abnormality of the sleep mechanisms—specifically, REM-inhibiting mechanisms—and it has been studied in dogs, sheep, and humans. Narcolepsy can occur at any age, but it most frequently begins in adolescence or young adulthood, generally before the age of 30. The disorder either progresses slowly or reaches a plateau that is maintained throughout life.

The most common symptom is sleep attacks: Patients cannot avoid falling asleep. Often associated with the problem (close to 50 percent of long-standing cases) is cataplexy, a sudden loss of muscle tone, such as jaw drop, head drop, weakness of the knees, or paralysis of all skeletal muscles with collapse. Patients often remain awake during brief cataplectic episodes; the long episodes usually merge with sleep and show the electroencephalographic signs of REM sleep.

Other symptoms include hypnagogic or hypnopompic hallucinations, which are vivid perceptual experiences, either auditory or visual, occurring at sleep onset or on awakening. Patients are often momentarily frightened, but within 1 or 2 minutes they return to an entirely normal frame of mind and are aware that nothing was actually there.

Another uncommon symptom is sleep paralysis, most often occurring on awakening in the morning; during the episode, patients are apparently awake and conscious but unable to move a muscle. If the symptom persists for more than a few seconds, as it often does in narcolepsy, it can become extremely uncomfortable. (Isolated brief episodes of sleep paralysis occur in many nonnarcoleptic persons.) Patients with narcolepsy report falling asleep quickly at night but often experience broken sleep.

When the diagnosis is not clinically clear, a nighttime polysomnographic recording reveals a characteristic sleep-onset REM period. A test of daytime multiple sleep latency (several recorded naps at 2-hour intervals) shows rapid sleep onset and usually one or more sleep-onset REM periods. A type of human leukocyte antigen, HLA-DR2, is found in 90 to 100 percent of patients with narcolepsy and only 10 to 35 percent of unaffected persons. One recent study showed that patients with narcolepsy are deficient in the neurotransmitter hypocretin, which stimulates appetite and alertness. Another study found that the number of hypocretin neurons (Hrct cells) in narcoleptics is 85 to 95 percent lower than in nonnarcoleptic brains.

Hypocretin

There is strong evidence that narcolepsy is associated with abnormalities of the hypocretin neurotransmitter system. Low or undetectable levels of hypocretin are found in most patients but some have normal or raised levels. Thus DSM-5 describes two variants of narcolepsy: (1) with hypocretin deficiency and (2) without hypocretin deficiency. DSM-5 also describes narcolepsy with or without cataplexy.

The classic form of narcolepsy (*narcolepsy with cataplexy*) is characterized by a tetrad of symptoms: (1) excessive daytime sleepiness, (2) cataplexy, (3) sleep paralysis, and (4) hypnagogic hallucinations. Patients with narcolepsy often have an abnormal sleep architecture in which REM sleep occurs soon after sleep onset both at night and during daytime naps. This, in connection with the symptom tetrad, makes narcolepsy appear to be a REM sleep intrusion syndrome presumably resultant from dysfunction of REM sleep generator gating mechanisms.

The features of the tetrad match REM sleep characteristics. The sleep paralysis is similar to the muscle atonia that occurs during REM sleep. The hypnagogic hallucinations are vivid "dreams" that occur while the patient is still conscious or partially conscious. However, not all patients have the full constellation of symptoms. Narcolepsy is estimated to afflict 10 to 60 individuals per 10,000. Symptoms commonly appear in the second decade of life. Strong emotions usually act as the "trigger" for cataplexy. Common emotional triggers include laughter and anger. The severity of cataplexy ranges widely from transient weakness in the knees to total paralysis while the patient is fully conscious. Episodes may last from several seconds to minutes. Usually, the patient is unable to speak and may fall to the floor. Nocturnal sleep is often fragmented, and there can be considerable sleep disturbance. Patients may experience depression in relation to the narcolepsy, especially when it is not treated. Social isolation, difficulty with academics and employment, and fear of driving contribute to a sense of loss experienced by patients with narcolepsy.

Treating Narcolepsy

No cure exists for narcolepsy, but symptom management is possible. A regimen of forced naps at a regular time of day occasionally helps patients with narcolepsy and, in some cases, the regimen alone, without medication, can almost cure the condition. When medication is required, stimulants are most commonly used.

Modafinil, an α_1-adrenergic receptor agonist, has been approved by the FDA to reduce the number of sleep attacks and to improve psychomotor performance in narcolepsy. This observation suggests the involvement of noradrenergic mechanisms in the disorder. Modafinil lacks some of the adverse effects of traditional psychostimulants. Nonetheless, the clinician must monitor its use and be sensitive to the patient developing a tolerance.

Sleep specialists often prescribe tricyclic drugs or SSRIs to reduce cataplexy. This approach capitalizes on the REM sleep-suppressant properties of these drugs. Because cataplexy is presumably an intrusion of REM sleep phenomena into the awake state, the rationale is clear. Many reports indicate that imipramine, modafinil, and fluoxetine are effective in reducing or eliminating cataplexy. Although drug therapy is the treatment of choice, the overall therapeutic approach should include scheduled naps, lifestyle adjustment, psychological counseling, drug holidays to reduce tolerance, and careful monitoring of drug refills, general health, and cardiac status.

BREATHING-RELATED SLEEP DISORDERS

Sleep-disordered breathing includes conditions ranging from upper airway resistance syndrome to severe obstructive sleep apnea. Sleep-related breathing impairments such as apnea (absence of airflow) and hypopnea (reduction in airflow) are most often caused by airway obstruction; however, sometimes respiratory reduction results from central (brainstem) changes in ventilatory control, metabolic factors, or heart failure. Each sleep-disordered breathing event can be classified as central, obstructive, or mixed. Central apnea refers to decreased or absent respiratory effort. In DSM-5, three disorders are included under the category of breathing-related sleep disorders: obstructive sleep apnea hypopnea, central sleep apnea, and sleep-related hypoventilation.

Obstructive Sleep Apnea Hypopnea

Obstructive sleep apnea hypopnea, also referred to as obstructive sleep apnea (OSA), is characterized by repetitive collapse or partial collapse of the upper airway during sleep. As a person falls asleep, airway resistance increases. In some individuals this leads to increased respiratory effort or airway occlusion. These periods of functional obstruction of the upper airway result in decreases in arterial oxygen saturation and a transient arousal, after which respiration (at least briefly) resumes normally. An episode of sleep *apnea* is defined as a cessation of breathing for 10 seconds or more during sleep. During an obstructive apnea episode, respiratory effort continues but airflow ceases due to loss of airway patency. A reduction in breathing for at least 10 seconds is termed *hypopnea.* Partial obstructions (hypopnea) can lead to arousals and sleep fragmentation. The consequent reduction in ventilation can decrease oxyhemoglobin concentrations. Predisposing factors for OSA include being male, reaching middle age, being obese, and having micrognathia, retrognathia, nasopharyngeal abnormalities, hypothyroidism, and acromegaly.

A review of more than four million records from the Veterans Health Administration (VHA) found a 2.91 percent prevalence of sleep apnea in that population. Comorbid diagnoses included hypertension (60.1 percent), obesity (30.5 percent), diabetes mellitus (32.9 percent), and cardiovascular disease, including angina and myocardial infarction (27.6 percent), heart failure (13.5 percent), and stroke, including transient ischemic attacks (5.7 percent). Psychiatric comorbidity in the sleep apnea group was significantly higher (P <0.0001) than in the non–sleep apnea group for the diagnoses of mood disorders, anxiety and posttraumatic stress disorder, psychosis, and dementia. There are several theories about the reasons for this association. Psychiatric disorders may be a consequence of sleep apnea (and disturbed sleep and hypoxia). Conversely, psychiatric disorders may predispose people to developing sleep disturbances such as sleep apnea.

Diagnosis. Clinical features associated with OSA hypopnea include excessive sleepiness, snoring, obesity, restless sleep, nocturnal awakenings with choking or gasping for breath, morning dry mouth, morning headaches, and heavy nocturnal sweating. Patients may also have hypertension, erectile failure in men, depression, heart failure, nocturia, polycythemia, and memory impairment as a result of obstructive sleep apnea hypopnea. Obstructive apnea and hypopnea episodes can occur in any state of sleep but are more typical during REM sleep, NREM stage 1, and NREM stage 2 sleep.

On the polysomnogram, episodes of OSA in adults are characterized by multiple periods of at least 10 seconds in duration in which nasal and oral airflow ceases completely (an apnea) or partially (a hypopnea), while the abdominal and chest expansion leads indicate continuing efforts of the diaphragm and accessory muscles of respiration to move air through the obstruction. The arterial oxygen saturation drops and often a bradycardia is seen that may be accompanied by other arrhythmias, such as premature ventricular contractions. At the end, an arousal reflex takes place, seen as a waking signal and possibly as a motor artifact on the EEG channels. At this moment, sometimes called the *breakthrough,* the patient can be observed making brief restless movements in bed.

According to the American Academy of Sleep Medicine scoring manual, polysomnographic recordings are scored for events according to the following rules: Airway obstruction producing complete cessations of breathing for 10 or more seconds is scored as apnea. Partial obstructions with consequent drops in oxygen saturation are designated as hypopnea (4 percent or more required according to Medicare rules), and partial obstructions without significant oxygen saturation but terminated by an arousal are scored as respiratory effort–related arousal (RERA) episodes. The number of apnea episodes per hour of sleep is termed the *apnea index* (AI), the number of apnea plus hypopnea episodes per hour is called the *apnea plus hypopnea index* (AHI), and the number of apnea plus hypopnea plus RERA episodes is designated the *respiratory disturbance index* (RDI).

Treatment. A number of treatments are available for obstructive sleep apnea hypopnea, including weight loss, surgical intervention, positive airway pressure, and oral appliances. Weight loss is known to help many patients. However, because losing weight and keeping it off is difficult and unreliably achieved, the prudent clinician should recommend weight loss but also rely on other therapies.

Aggressive surgical treatments evolved soon after OSA's pathophysiological and potentially life-threatening consequences were recognized. The earliest surgical intervention was designed to create a patent airway; thus, in the late 1970s tracheostomies were performed on individuals with severe apnea. There is little doubt that tracheostomy succeeds in creating an airway. Although no longer the preferred treatment, it remains a standard against which newer, more refined therapies are judged. Second-generation surgical approaches attempt to correct airway obstructions and malformations. Early studies of uvulopalatopharyngoplasty (UPPP) suggested that modification of the soft palate effectively relieved most sleep apnea. Later follow-up results were less impressive. Approximately 30 to 50 percent of patients with sleep apnea benefit from UPPP. These patients are likely those with oropharyngeal obstruction; thus, careful attention to selection criteria presumably improves outcome. However, if obstruction occurs in the posterior airway space (PAS), maxillomandibular surgery may be appropriate. In retrognathic patients or in patients with cephalometrics revealing compromised PAS, moving the jaw forward can achieve impressive normalization of breathing during sleep.

Positive airway pressure (PAP) is the preferred treatment for sleep-disordered breathing. The PAP apparatus consists of a fan-driven blower, a nasal or oronasal mask, and tubing connecting the two. The airflow through the mask provides a positive pressure that offsets oropharyngeal collapse produced by inspiratory negative thoracic pressure. In this manner it acts as a pneumatic splint, thereby maintaining the airway. When the pressure is properly titrated, even the most severe sleep apnea can be alleviated. Results are usually dramatic. PAP devices come in several varieties. The most common are systems that provide a single set continuous positive airway pressure (CPAP). For individuals who find it difficult to exhale against a continuous pressure, bilevel positive airway pressure (BPAP) may provide a solution. BPAP devices have different inspiratory and expiratory pressure settings. More recently, systems that sense the patient's changes in airway resistance and automatically adjust the positive airway pressure (APAP) have been gaining popularity. Such APAP systems should theoretically be able to adapt to changes in pressure requirements produced by sleep deprivation, medications, weight change, sleep stage, illness, and aging. Finally, timed bilevel and servo ventilation systems have also been developed but fall into the category of noninvasive positive pressure ventilation (NIPPV) systems, which are more appropriate for treating other pulmonary diseases and breathing problems in neuromuscular diseases. The tremendous efficacy and remarkable safety of PAP therapies has made them the standard of care for patients who can tolerate sleeping with the machine. The major therapeutic challenge is utilization. Patient education and systematic follow-up are crucial. When problems with the mask, the pressure, nasal stuffiness, and other barriers to routine, nightly use arise, they must be remedied quickly to ensure therapeutic adherence. When used properly, the success of PAP therapy has rendered surgical intervention a secondary option, resorted to mainly after PAP failure, rejection, or nonadherence.

Oral appliances represent another therapeutic option that is gaining popularity. A variety of oral appliances have also been developed to treat snoring, and they appear to be beneficial for mild to moderate OSA cases. The general approach is to manipulate the position of the mandible, lift the palate, or retain the tongue. Randomized trials indicate that some oral appliances improve airway patency sufficiently to treat patients with sleep apnea. However, in patients with severe OSA, improvement does not always reach satisfactory levels; therefore, follow-up evaluations are needed.

In some patients, sleep-disordered breathing occurs only in the supine position. In such situations, preventing patients from sleeping on their backs may produce beneficial results. Tennis balls sewn onto or placed into pockets on the back of the nightshirt or foam wedges may accomplish this goal. Although such interventions are found to be useful in clinical practice, large-scale systematic clinical trials of this approach have not been performed.

Finally, drug therapies have been tried for OSA but without success. Medroxyprogesterone acetate (Provera) was originally thought to be helpful but is seldom used now. Similarly, tricyclic antidepressants sometimes decrease apnea severity by reducing REM sleep, the stage of sleep in which obstructive apnea is usually more frequent. Theophylline was reported to reduce apnea, but further study is needed. There were also animal studies suggesting that mirtazapine (Remeron) and similar serotonin presynaptic–affecting compounds improved breathing; however, studies in humans were disappointing. The only drug therapy approved for use in patients with OSA is the wake-promoting substance modafinil. Modafinil, however, does nothing to treat the pathophysiology of airway occlusion, but rather is used as an adjunct for treating the residual sleepiness that persists in about 8 to 12 percent of patients who are otherwise well treated with and adequately use PAP therapy.

Central Sleep Apnea

Central sleep apnea (CSA), which tends to occur in the elderly, results from periodic failure of CNS mechanisms that stimulate breathing. CSA is defined as the absence of breathing due to lack of respiratory effort. It is a disorder of ventilatory control in which repeated episodes of apneas and hypopneas occur in a periodic or intermittent pattern during sleep caused by variability in respiratory effort. The original teaching was that OSA results in a complaint of excessive sleepiness, whereas CSA is manifest as insomnia, but later case series have emphasized that either symptom may appear in either disorder. The polysomnogramic features of CSA are similar to those of OSA, except that, during the periods of apnea, a cessation of respiratory effort is seen in the abdominal and chest expansion leads. DSM-5 specifies three subtypes of CSA: idiopathic CSA, Cheyne–Stokes breathing pattern, and CSA comorbid with opioid use. However, there are several different etiologies that can result in diminished effort to breathe, including the three subtypes above, as well as high altitude, brainstem lesions, specific medical conditions, specific drugs or substances, and congenital abnormalities.

Idiopathic CSA. There is an idiopathic form of CSA. Patients typically have low normal arterial carbon dioxide tension ($PaCO_2$) while awake and have a high ventilatory response to CO_2. They present with daytime sleepiness, insomnia, or awakening with shortness of breath. Respiratory cessations during sleep occur independent of ventilatory effort. Polysomnography reveals five or more central apneas per hour of sleep.

Cheyne–Stokes Breathing. Cheyne–Stokes breathing is a unique breathing pattern consisting of prolonged hyperpneas during which tidal volume gradually waxes and wanes in a crescendo–decrescendo fashion. The hyperpneas alternate with apnea and hypopnea episodes that are associated with reduced ventilatory effort. This pattern is most common in older men with congestive heart failure or stroke. As with primary CSA, the patient presents with daytime sleepiness, insomnia, and awakening short of breath. Polysomnography reveals ten or more central apnea and hypopnea episodes per hour of sleep.

CSA Comorbid with Opioid Use. This is a third subtype of CSA in DSM-5, specified if opioid use disorder is present. There is an association with chronic use of long-acting opioid medications and impairment of neuromuscular respiratory control leading to CSA.

CSA due to High Altitude. Central apnea at sleep onset is universal at elevations above 7,600 m but can occur at 5,000 m (especially with a rapid ascent). This subtype is no longer included in DSM-5 but may still have clinical significance. Periods of central apnea alternate with periods of hyperpnea in a 12-second to 34-second cycle. This is an extension of normal respiratory control at sleep onset where medullary pH receptors raise their set-point and require lower pH to respond. At high altitudes, hyperventilation causes a hypocapnic alkalosis that reduces ventilation during sleep. Sleep architecture may suffer, with increased duration in stages 1 and 2 and less slow wave sleep. REM sleep may not be affected. This condition can be treated with acetazolamide, which lowers serum pH and increases the respiratory drive. Acetazolamide side effects include metabolic acidosis, electrolyte imbalance, anaphylaxis, Stevens-Johnson syndrome, toxic epidermal necrolysis, and agranulocytosis. Common reactions include but are not limited to fatigue, anorexia, taste changes, polyuria, diarrhea, melena, tinnitus, and photosensitivity.

CSA due to Medical Condition That Is Not Cheyne–Stokes. This form of CSA is usually caused by a brainstem lesion associated with a wide range of variable etiologies. Cardiac and renal disorders can also cause central apnea. Diagnostic criteria requires polysomnographically verified rate of 10 or more central apneas and hypopneas per hour of sleep with a crescendo–decrescendo breathing pattern accompanied by arousals and fragmented sleep.

CSA due to Drug or Substance Use. Central apnea episodes can be provoked by a variety of drugs or drug combinations, most notably long-acting opiates. However, other substances or medications have also been associated with alterations in neuromuscular control leading to CSA. Diagnostic criteria are a central apnea index (number of episodes per hour) of 5 or more and the patient taking a drug(s) for at least 2 months.

Primary Sleep Apnea of Infancy. This form of CSA involves prolonged apneas or hypopneas with concomitant hypoxemia, bradycardia, or both. This condition afflicts preterm neonates, presumably because their brainstems are not fully developed. The condition may be exacerbated by other medical problems that further compromise the infant's physiological and developmental status.

Sleep-Related Hypoventilation

Idiopathic Hypoventilation. Patients with idiopathic hypoventilation have normal lungs and a decrease in alveolar ventilation resulting in sleep-related arterial oxygen desaturation likely due to blunted chemoresponsiveness. They do not have lung disease, obesity, kyphoscoliosis, or other structural conditions that might cause hypoventilation. Polysomnography shows episodes of shallow breathing longer than 10 seconds in duration associated with arterial oxygen desaturation and frequent arousals from sleep associated with the breathing disturbances or bradytachycardia. Patients often complain of excessive daytime sleepiness, frequent arousals during sleep, or insomnia.

Congenital Central Alveolar Hypoventilation. Sometimes called Ondine's curse, congenital central alveolar hypoventilation parasomnia cannot be explained by primary pulmonary disease or ventilatory muscle weakness. The sleep-related hypoventilation results from a failure in automatic control of breathing. Although present at birth, congenital central hypoventilation syndrome may initially be unrecognized. In severe forms, treatment requires continual ventilatory support.

Comorbid Sleep-Related Hypoventilation. Comorbid sleep-related hypoventilation occurs when hypoventilation is a consequence of a medical condition, for example, pulmonary parenchymal or vascular pathology, lower airway obstruction, or neuromuscular or chest wall disorders.

SLEEP-RELATED HYPOVENTILATION DUE TO PULMONARY PARENCHYMAL OR VASCULAR PATHOLOGY. Parenchymal lung disease or vascular disease is the primary cause of the hypoxemia. These diseases include interstitial lung diseases, idiopathic and secondary forms of pulmonary hypertension, cystic fibrosis (which affects lung parenchyma and lower airway), and hemoglobinopathies such as sickle cell anemia. Nocturnal hypoxemia can lead to pulmonary artery hypertension, cor pulmonale, and neurocognitive dysfunction. Sleep studies reveal sustained oxyhemoglobin desaturation during sleep occurring in the absence of detectable apnea or hypopnea episodes.

SLEEP-RELATED HYPOVENTILATION DUE TO LOWER AIRWAY OBSTRUCTION. This is diagnosed by a forced expiratory volume in 1 second (FEV1)/forced vital capacity (FVC) ratio that is less than 70 percent of predicted value on pulmonary function tests (PFTs). Chronic obstructive pulmonary disease (COPD) including emphysema and chronic bronchitis, α-1-antitrypsin deficiency, bronchiectasis, and cystic fibrosis form the majority of disorders that cause this sleep disturbance. Nocturnal hypoxemia can potentially lead to pulmonary artery hypertension and cor pulmonale. Sustained hypoxemia can also cause brain damage. Sleep studies reveal sustained oxyhemoglobin desaturation during sleep occurring in the absence of detectable apnea or hypopnea episodes.

SLEEP-RELATED HYPOVENTILATION DUE TO NEUROMUSCULAR AND CHEST WALL DISORDERS. Myasthenia gravis and amyotrophic lateral sclerosis (ALS) occurring together with OSA can exacerbate the hypoxemia produced by the neuromuscular and chest wall disorders.

CIRCADIAN RHYTHM SLEEP DISORDERS

Circadian rhythm sleep disorders include a wide range of conditions involving a misalignment between desired and actual sleep periods. This collection of sleep disorders shares the same basic underlying etiology—a desynchrony between an individual's internal circadian biological clock and the desired or conventional sleep–wake cycle. The circadian (*circa* plus *dias,* "approximately 1 day") pacemaker is located in the suprachiasmatic nucleus (SCN). SCN firing oscillates with an almost sinusoidal pattern, the period of which is 24 hours, and the output correlates with the daily fluctuations in core body temperature. SCN firing patterns persists even in cerveau isolé preparations (an animal with its mesencephalon transected). Mismatched circadian clock and desired schedules can arise from improper phase relationships between the two, travel across time zones, or dysfunctions in the basic biological rhythm.

Under normal circumstances the internal circadian pacemaker is reset each day by bright light, social cues, stimulants, and activity. In cases in which these factors fail to reentrain the circadian rhythm, the circadian sleep disorders occur. DSM-5 lists six types of circadian rhythm sleep disorders: delayed sleep phase type, advanced sleep phase type, irregular sleep–wake type, non–24-hour sleep–wake type, shift work type, and unspecified type. Jet lag type and "due to a medical condition" are not included in DSM-5 but are included in other classification systems such as ICSD-2.

Delayed Sleep Phase Type

The delayed sleep phase circadian disorder occurs when the biological clock runs slower than 24 hours or is shifted later than the desired schedule. This produces a phase delay in the sleepiness–alertness cycle. Individuals with delayed sleep phase are more alert in the evening and early nighttime, stay up later, and are more tired in the morning. These individuals are commonly referred to as *night owls.*

Advanced Sleep Phase Type

Advanced sleep phase occurs when the circadian rhythm cycle is shifted earlier. Therefore, the sleepiness cycle is advanced with respect to clock time. Individuals with advanced sleep phase are drowsy in the evening, want to retire to bed earlier, awaken earlier, and are more alert in the early morning. Individuals with this pattern of advanced sleep phase are sometimes called *early birds* or *larks.*

Irregular Sleep–Wake Type

The irregular sleep–wake pattern occurs when the circadian sleep–wake rhythm is absent or pathologically diminished. The sleep–wake pattern is temporally disorganized, and the timing of sleep and wakefulness is unpredictable. Individuals with this condition have a normal amount of sleep during a 24-hour period; however, it is fragmented into three or more episodes that occur irregularly. There are symptoms of insomnia at night and excessive sleepiness during the day. Long daytime naps and inappropriate nocturnal wakefulness occur. Except in unusual circumstances, activities of daily life are significantly impaired. A history of reclusion or isolation may be associated with this disorder because decreased exposure to external stimuli can contribute to symptoms. Irregular sleep–wake type is typically associated with neurodegenerative disorders, such as Alzheimer's disease and some neurodevelopmental disorders in children.

Non–24-Hour Sleep–Wake Type (Free Running)

When the circadian sleep–wake pacemaker has a cycle length greater or less than 24 hours and is not reset each morning, a person may develop this type of circadian rhythm disorder, such as in blind or visually impaired persons. Under normal circumstances, resynchronization of the circadian rhythm occurs daily in response to the light–dark cycle. Problems occur incrementally when internal and environmental clocks become more and more out of phase. If the circadian clock's period is longer than 24 hours and does not reset each day, the patient experiences progressively worsening sleep-onset insomnia and daytime sleepiness. Sleep problems peak when circadian and environmental clocks are 12 hours out of phase and then begin to lessen, emulating progressively resolving advanced sleep phase. Eventually the clocks correlate, and the sleep–wake cycle is normal for a few days, after which the insomnia–hypersomnia cycle begins again. For this reason, non–24-hour sleep–wake disorder has been called *periodic insomnia* and *periodic excessive sleepiness.* Traumatic brain injury (TBI) has been associated with non–24-hour sleep–wake type. Blindness is a known risk factor. In both sighted and blind individuals, sequential measurement of phase markers such as melatonin may help in determining circadian phase. Both phototherapy and melatonin are being tried as treatments for this disorder.

Shift Work Type

Many service industries require 24-hour operation (e.g., transportation, health care). Similarly, as Western cultures became more capital intensive, mining and manufacturing became around-the-clock enterprises. The number of individuals doing shift work has been increasing steadily for decades. Shift workers commonly suffer from insomnia, excessive sleepiness, or both. Some individuals require only a short time to adjust to a shift change, whereas others have great difficulty. Frequent shift rotation adds to the problem. Furthermore, to meet social demands, shift workers often adopt a nonshifted sleep–wake schedule on weekends and holidays. Even those individuals who try to stay shifted usually retain an unshifted circadian rhythm. The result can be severe insomnia when attempting to sleep and excessive sleepiness when attempting to remain awake. The result is profound sleep deprivation as circadian rhythm continues to be poorly entrained to the sleep–wake schedule. The natural low point in the normal sleep–wake rhythm occurs at approximately 3:00 to 5:00 AM. Of interest, this is precisely the time frame during which transportation and industrial accidents commonly occur as a direct consequence of sleepiness. Though unclear, DSM-5 seems to indicate that individuals experiencing jet lag are included under this subtype, noting that, despite different etiologies, individuals who travel across many time zones frequently may experience effects similar to those of shift work disorder.

Jet Lag Type

Removed from DSM-5, jet lag is still recognized as a circadian rhythm sleep disorder by the ICSD-2. With the advent of high-speed air travel, an induced desynchrony between circadian and environmental clocks became possible. Thus, the term *jet lag* came into use. When an individual rapidly travels across many time zones, either a circadian phase advance or a phase delay is induced, depending on the direction of travel. Typically, translocation of one or two time zones will not produce a sustained problem; however, overseas travel can be marked by great difficulty in adjusting one's sleep–wake routine. Individuals who frequently travel for business can find themselves quite impaired at the time they need to make important decisions. Furthermore, "night owls" will experience greater difficulty adjusting to eastward travel because resynchronization requires phase advance. Similarly, "larks" theoretically will have more difficulty with westward travel. The number of time zones crossed is a critical factor. Normally, healthy individuals can easily adapt to one to two time zone changes per day; therefore, natural adjustment to an 8-hour translocation may take 4 or more days.

Due to Medical Condition

During illnesses that keep patients bedridden, during hospitalizations, and in some forms of dementia, individuals often sleep ad lib. The resulting chaotic sleep–wake pattern adversely affects the circadian rhythm. The breakdown in the sleep–wake cycle may be further exacerbated by medication with sedative properties. Sleep in patients in the intensive care unit is disturbed by noise, light, and the therapeutic and monitoring procedures being performed. The resulting disorganized sleep–wake pattern can produce a significant sleep disorder. In addition, abuse of recreational street drugs (e.g., methamphetamine and 3,4-methylenedioxymethamphetamine ["ecstasy"]) is associated with individuals remaining awake overnight or continuously for several days at a time. These episodes of prolonged wakefulness ultimately produce periods of profound hypersomnia (commonly called *crashing*).

Treatment of Circadian Rhythm Sleep Disorders

Chronotherapy is one technique used to reset the biological clock. It involves progressively phase delaying a person until the circadian oscillator is synchronized with the desired sleep–wake schedule. When individuals are deprived of environmental time cues and told to sleep when they feel sleepy, the typical "day" lasts 25 to 26 hours. This suggests that young and middle-aged adults have a propensity to phase delay. Thus, phase delaying each night by 2 to 3 hours is thought to be easier than phase advancing because it capitalizes on a natural tendency. Halting the phase delay at the appropriate moment and maintaining the desired synchrony can be a challenge. The patient also has to cope with an odd sleep–wake schedule for the better part of a week during therapy (which can interfere with school or work). For these reasons, the development of light therapy has in the past few years superseded chronotherapy.

Light or Phototherapy. Sleep disorders' research indicates that exposing an individual to bright lights (greater than 10,000 lux) can alter the endogenous biological rhythm. With precise timing of bright light exposure, the biological clock can be stopped and reset. Exposure to light modifies the set-point of the biological clock. Using core body temperature as a physiological marker, one can use bright lights to produce phase delay when presented before the temperature nadir. By contrast, light exposure after the temperature nadir evokes phase advance. The closer one presents light to the point of inflection (temperature nadir), the more robust is the response in altering the cycle. Thus, early morning bright-light therapy can be used to phase advance individuals with delayed sleep phase syndrome. Similarly, exposure to bright light in the evening can help patients with advanced sleep phase syndrome. More recently, it was discovered that the blue part of the light spectrum is the crucial ingredient in phase setting and shifting. Light therapy is being applied to reset the circadian rhythm of shift workers, astronauts, and individuals experiencing jet lag.

Melatonin. Experimental use of melatonin to treat circadian rhythm disorders in the blind, e.g. non–24-hour sleep–wake disorder (see above), has proven successful. Researchers posit that melatonin secretion acts as the biological substrate for the internal circadian oscillator. Under normal circumstances, melatonin levels begin to rise at dusk and remain elevated until dawn. Bright light suppresses the release of melatonin. Melatonin, in a sense, is the signal of darkness in the brain. As such, it can be used clinically to manage sighted patients with disturbed sleep–wake cycles. Melatonin is available over the counter. A prescription form of melatonin (Circadin) is available in Europe, and a synthetic melatonin agonist (ramelteon [Rozerem]) is available in the United States. Ramelteon is FDA approved for treating patients with sleep-onset insomnia but is used off label for the entire spectrum of circadian rhythm sleep disorders. Of interest, the only medication approved for shift work sleep disorder is the wake-promoting compound modafinil. Modafinil is approved for treating sleepiness occurring during night shift work.

PARASOMNIAS

Parasomnias are sometimes referred to as disorders of partial arousal. In general, the parasomnias are a diverse collection of sleep disorders characterized by physiological or behavioral phenomena that occur during or are potentiated by sleep. One conceptual framework posits many parasomnias as overlaps or intrusions of one basic sleep–wake state into another. Wakefulness, NREM sleep, and REM sleep can be characterized as three basic states that differ in their neurological organization. During wakefulness, both the body and brain are active. In NREM sleep, both the body and brain are much less active. REM sleep, however, pairs an atonic body with an active brain (capable of creating elaborate dream fantasies). Regional cerebral blood flow, magnetic resonance imaging (MRI), and other imaging studies confirm increased brain activation during REM sleep. It certainly appears that in some parasomnias there are state boundary violations. For example, sleepwalking and sleep terrors involve momentary or partial wakeful behaviors suddenly occurring in NREM (slow wave) sleep. Similarly, isolated sleep paralysis is the persistence of REM sleep atonia into the wakefulness transition, whereas REM sleep behavior disorder is the failure of the mechanism, creating paralytic atonia such that individuals literally act out their dreams.

The frequency of significant parasomnias is variable, and the clinical significance often has more to do with the medical consequences or the evoked level of distress than with how often the abnormal events occur. For example, biannual REM sleep behavior disorder, in which the patient is seriously injured while enacting a dream, is more clinically urgent than weekly bruxism. Similarly, monthly recurrent nightmares that provoke severe insomnia and fear of sleeping can be more distressing than night terrors of the same frequency (at least to the patient). The irregularities of occurrence of most parasomnias make them difficult to document in the sleep laboratory. Sleep studies, however, are often conducted to make a differential diagnosis and rule out that the unusual behavior is secondary to seizure, sleep-disordered breathing, or another sleep disorder.

NREM Sleep Arousal Disorders

Sleepwalking. Sleepwalking in its classic form, as the name implies, is a condition in which an individual arises from bed and ambulates without fully awakening. It is sometimes called somnambulism, and individuals can engage in a variety of complex behaviors while unconscious. Sleepwalking usually occurs during slow wave sleep and lies in the middle of a parasomnia continuum that ranges from "confused arousal" to "sleep terror." Sleepwalks characteristically begin toward the end of the first or second slow wave sleep episodes. Sleep deprivation and interruption of slow wave sleep appear to exacerbate, or even provoke, sleepwalking in susceptible individuals. Sleepwalking episodes may range from sitting up and attempting to walk to conducting an involved sequence of semipurposeful actions. The sleepwalker often can successfully interact with the environment (e.g., avoiding tripping over objects). However, the sleepwalker may interact with the environment inappropriately, which sometimes results in injury (e.g., stepping out of an upstairs window or walking into the roadway). There are cases in which sleepwalkers have committed acts of violence. An individual who is sleepwalking is difficult to awaken. Once awake, the sleepwalker will usually appear confused. It is best to gently attempt to lead sleepwalkers back to bed rather than to attempt to awaken them by grabbing, shaking, or shouting. In their confused state, sleepwalkers may think they are being attacked and may react violently to defend themselves. Sleepwalking in adults is rare, has a familial pattern, and may occur as a primary parasomnia or secondary to another sleep disorder (e.g., sleep apnea). By contrast, sleepwalking is very common in children and has peak prevalence between ages 4 and 8 years. After adolescence, it usually disappears spontaneously. Nightly to weekly sleepwalking episodes associated with physical injury to the patient and others are considered severe. There are "specialized" forms of sleepwalking, most notably sleep-related eating behavior and sexsomnia.

SLEEP-RELATED EATING. This occurs when an individual experiences episodes of ingesting food during sleep with varying degrees of amnesia. Individuals may find evidence of these episodes the next morning with little to no memory of their eating.

SEXSOMNIA. Sleep-related sexual behavior, or sexsomnia, is when a person engages in sexual activities (e.g., masturbation, fondling, sexual intercourse) during sleep without conscious awareness.

Sleep Terrors. Sleep terror disorder is an arousal in the first third of the night during deep NREM (stages 3 and 4) sleep. It is characterized by a sudden arousal with intense fearfulness. They usually begin with a piercing scream or cry and are accompanied by behavioral manifestations of intense anxiety bordering on panic. Autonomic and behavioral correlates of fright typically mark the experience. In a typical case of night terrors, no signs of temporal lobe epilepsy or other seizure disorders are seen, either clinically or on EEG recordings. An individual experiencing a sleep terror usually sits up in bed, is unresponsive to stimuli, and, if awakened, is confused or disoriented. Vocalizations may occur, but they usually are incoherent. Notwithstanding the intensity of these events, amnesia for the episodes usually occurs. Like sleepwalking, these episodes usually arise from slow wave sleep. Fever and CNS depressant withdrawal potentiate sleep terror episodes. Unlike nightmares, in which an elaborate dream sequence unfolds, sleep terrors may be devoid of images or contain only fragments of very brief but frighteningly vivid but sometimes static images. It is sometimes called *pavor nocturnus,* incubus, or night terror, and a familial pattern has been reported. As with other slow wave sleep parasomnias, sleep deprivation can provoke or exacerbate sleep terrors. Psychopathology is seldom associated with sleep terrors in children; however, a history of traumatic experience or frank psychiatric problems is often comorbid in adults with this disorder. Severity ranges from less than once per month to almost nightly occurrence (with injury to the patient or others).

Parasomnias Usually Associated with REM Sleep

REM Sleep Behavior Disorder (Including Parasomnia Overlap Disorder and Status Dissociatus). REM behavior disorder (RBD) involves a failure of the patient to have atonia (sleep paralysis) during the REM stage sleep. The result is that the patient literally enacts his or her dreams. Under normal circumstances, the dreamer is immobilized by REM-related hypopolarization of α and γ motor neurons. Without this paralysis or with intermittent atonia, punching, kicking, leaping, and running from bed during attempted dream enactment occur. The activity has been correlated with dream imagery, and, unlike during sleepwalking, the individual seems unaware of the actual environment but rather is acting on the dream sensorium. Thus, a sleepwalker may calmly go to a bedroom window, open it, and step out. By contrast, a person with REM sleep behavior disorder would more likely dive through the window thinking it is a dream-visualized lake. Patients and bed partners frequently sustain injury, which is sometimes serious (e.g., lacerations, fractures). A wide variety of drugs and comorbid conditions can precipitate or worsen RBD. In animals, presumed RBD can be produced with bilateral peri–locus coeruleus lesions. In humans, there is a suggestion that RBD may result from diffuse hemispheric lesions, bilateral thalamic abnormalities, or brainstem lesions. Clonazepam (Klonopin) has been used successfully to treat RBD.

Recurrent Isolated Sleep Paralysis. Sleep paralysis is, as the name implies, an inability to make voluntary movements during sleep. It becomes a parasomnia when it occurs at sleep onset or on awakening, a time when the individual is partially conscious and aware of the surroundings. This inability to move can be extremely distressing, especially when it is coupled with the feeling that there is an intruder in the house or when hypnagogic hallucinations are occurring. Sleep paralysis is one of the tetrad of symptoms associated with narcolepsy; however, it is known to occur (with or without hypnagogia) in individuals that have neither cataplexy nor excessive daytime sleepiness. Although it is sometimes frightening, sleep paralysis is a feature of normal REM sleep briefly intruding into wakefulness. The paralysis may last from 1 to several minutes. It is interesting that the occurrence of sleep paralysis with hypnagogia may account for a variety of experiences in which the sleeper is confronted or attacked by some sort of "creature." The common description is that a "presence" was felt to be near, the individual was paralyzed, and the creature talks, attacks, or sits on the sleeper's chest and then vanishes. Whether it is called an incubus, "Old Hag," a vampire, ghost oppression (*kanashibari* in Japanese), witch riding, or an alien encounter, elements common to sleep paralysis are seen. Irregular sleep, sleep deprivation, psychological stress, and shift work are thought to increase the likelihood of sleep paralysis occurring. Occasional sleep paralysis occurs in 7 to 8 percent of young adults. Estimates of at least one experience of sleep paralysis during the lifetime range from 25 to 50 percent. Improved sleep hygiene and assurance of sufficient sleep are first-line therapies. Sometimes, if the individual voluntarily makes very rapid eye movements or is touched by another person, the episode will terminate.

Nightmare Disorder. Nightmares are frightening or terrifying dreams. Sometimes called *dream anxiety attacks,* they produce sympathetic activation and ultimately awaken the dreamer. Nightmares occur in REM sleep and usually evolve from a long, complicated dream that becomes increasingly frightening. The person having been aroused to wakefulness, he or she typically remembers the dream (in contrast to sleep terrors). Some nightmares are recurrent, and reportedly when they occur in association with posttraumatic stress disorder they may be recollections of actual events. Common in children ages 3 to 6 years (prevalence estimates range from 10 to 50 percent), nightmares are rare in adults (1 percent or less). Frequent and distressing nightmares are sometimes responsible for insomnia because the individual is afraid to sleep. In Freudian terms, the nightmare is an example of the failure of the dream process that defuses the emotional content of the dream by disguising it symbolically, thus preserving sleep. Most patients afflicted with nightmares are free from psychiatric conditions. Nonetheless, individuals at risk for nightmares include those with schizotypal, borderline, and schizoid personality disorders, as well as those with schizophrenia. Having thin boundaries makes these individuals more vulnerable; furthermore, they may be at risk for schizophrenia. Traumatic events are known to induce nightmares, sometimes immediately, but at other times delayed. The nightmares can persist for many years. Several medications are known to sometimes provoke nightmares, including L-DOPA and β-adrenergic blockers, as does withdrawal from REM suppressant medications. Finally, drug or alcohol abuse is associated with nightmares.

Frequently occurring nightmares often produce a "fear of sleeping" type of insomnia. In turn, the insomnia may provoke sleep deprivation, which is known to exacerbate nightmares. In this manner, a vicious cycle is created. Treatment using behavioral techniques can be helpful. Universal sleep hygiene, stimulus control therapy, lucid dream therapy, and cognitive therapy reportedly improve sleep and reduce nightmares. In patients with nightmares related to posttraumatic stress disorder, nefazodone (an atypical antidepressant) reportedly provides therapeutic benefit. Benzodiazepines may also be helpful; however, systematic controlled trials are lacking.

Evidence for the use of prazosin (Minipress), a central nervous system α-1–receptor antagonist, in the treatment of posttraumatic stress disorder–related nightmares is growing. Prazosin significantly increased total sleep time and REM sleep time and significantly reduced trauma-related nightmares and distressed awakenings.

Other Parasomnias

Sleep Enuresis. Sleep enuresis is a disorder in which the individual urinates during sleep while in bed. *Bed-wetting,* as it is commonly called, has primary and secondary forms. In children, primary sleep enuresis is the continuance of bed-wetting since infancy. Secondary enuresis refers to relapse after toilet training was complete and there was a period during which the child remained dry. Usually, after toilet training bed-wetting spontaneously resolves before age 6 years. Prevalence progressively declines from 30 percent at age 4 years, to 10 percent at age 6 years, to 5 percent at age 10 years, and to 3 percent at age 12 years.

Parental primary enuresis increases the likelihood that the children will also have enuresis. A single recessive gene is suspected. Secondary enuresis in children may occur with the birth of a sibling and represent a "cry for attention." Secondary enuresis can also be associated with nocturnal seizures, sleep deprivation, and urological anomalies. In adults, sleep enuresis is sometimes seen in patients with sleep-disordered breathing. In most cases, embarrassment, shame, and guilt are the most serious consequences. Nonetheless, if sleep enuresis is not addressed, it may leave psychosocial scars. A variety of medications have been used to treat sleep enuresis, including imipramine, oxybutynin chloride, and synthetic vasopressin. Behavioral treatments, including bladder training, using conditioning devices (bell and pad), and fluid restriction, have reportedly had good success when properly administered. Other treatments include psychotherapy, motivational strategies, and hypnotherapy.

Sleep-Related Groaning (Catathrenia). This disorder is a chronic condition characterized by prolonged, frequently loud groans during sleep. The groaning can occur in any sleep stage. The parasomnia may begin during childhood but often remains occult until the child has to share a room. Catathrenia is not related to any psychiatric or physiologic abnormalities. There is no known treatment, and it reportedly does not improve with CPAP therapy. Polysomnography with respiratory-sound monitoring reveals sounds during exhalation and respiratory dysrhythmia.

Sleep-Related Hallucinations. Sleep-related hallucinations are typically visual images occurring at sleep onset (hypnagogic) or on awakening (hypnopompic) from sleep. Sometimes difficult to differentiate from dreams, they are common in patients with narcolepsy. Complex hallucinations are rare and usually happen with abrupt awakening and without remembrance dreaming. Images tend to be vivid and immobile and persists for several minutes (usually disappearing when a light is turned on). The images can be frightening.

Sleep-Related Eating Disorder. This syndrome involves an inability to get back to sleep after awakening unless the individual has something to eat or drink. After eating or drinking, return to sleep is normal. Nocturnal eating (drinking) syndrome predominantly affects infants and children; however, adult cases have been reported. It is believe that the problem is mainly associated with breastfeeding or bottle feeding. An infant will drink 4 to 8 oz or more at each awakening. Wetting is also excessive. Infants should be able to sleep through the night without feeding after age 6 months; however, in afflicted individuals, this does not happen. The syndrome invariably leads to the caregiver becoming sleep deprived. In adults, nocturnal eating can be conditioned to awakening. Eating may become obsessional, and several small meals may be eaten during the course of a night. The individual may be unaware of the activity, and weight gain can become a problem.

Parasomnia due to Drug or Substance Use and Parasomnia due to Medical Conditions. Many drugs and substances can trigger parasomnias, particularly those agents that lighten sleep; however, alcohol is notorious for producing sleepwalking (even in individuals who have taken sleeping pills). RBD can be provoked or worsened by biperiden (Akineton), tricyclic antidepressants, monoamine oxidase inhibitors (MAOIs), caffeine, venlafaxine (Effexor), selegiline (Eldepryl), and serotonin agonists. RBD may also occur during withdrawal from alcohol, meprobamate (Meprospan), pentazocine (Talwin), and nitrazepam (Nitrazadon). Medications known to provoke nightmares include L-DOPA and β-blockers. Nightmares can also be caused by drug-induced REM sleep rebound (e.g., withdrawal from REM-suppressing drugs such as methamphetamine) and alcohol abuse or withdrawal.

Seizure disorder should always be on the top of a differential diagnosis list for most parasomnias. In fact, the American Academy of Sleep Medicine practice guidelines concerning the indications for polysomnography include using sleep testing to rule out seizures when diagnosing sleep terror, sleepwalking, RBD, nightmares, and other parasomnias. Sleep-related breathing disorders are also known to trigger sleepwalking, enuresis, sleep terror, confusional arousal, and nightmares. RBD is associated with a variety of neurological conditions, including Parkinson's disease, dementia, progressive supranuclear palsy, Shy–Drager syndrome (a movement disorder with autonomic arousal symptoms), narcolepsy, and others.

Ms. R, a 20-year-old white woman, was referred with symptoms of talking, mumbling, and crying out during sleep. At least twice per week she screamed in her sleep. She was bothered with excessive sleepiness and falling asleep inappropriately, such as during a conversation. When inactive, she was tired and sleepy, even after a full 8-hour night of sleep. However, she had energy when motivated and led a vigorous life. Once, she awakened outside of her apartment and her roommate had to let her back in because she had locked herself out. She did not recall the sleepwalking episode or other nocturnal wanderings but sometimes remembered yelling. From the history, crying seemed to occur in light sleep, but she rarely recalled any sleep-related thoughts or dreams. However, there was a history of occasional nightmares and bruxism. The patient used an oral appliance to protect her teeth. Leg kicking and mild snoring without gasping or choking were noted. The patient also complained of leg kicking during sleep. Her sleep–wake schedule was irregular, and she averaged between 5 and 7 hours of sleep per night. She occasionally awakened with a headache in the morning.

Previous health history included a hospitalization for febrile convulsions during infancy, ophthalmologic surgery for strabismus during childhood, and tonsillectomy as a teenager. Her health was otherwise excellent. The patient did not smoke tobacco or drink alcohol.

By history, Ms. R had one or more of the parasomnias. Sleep talking alone does not require a sleep study, but this patient had nocturnal wanderings. Polysomnography with clinical EEG are indicated to rule out unrecognized nocturnal seizure disorder or other organic factors inducing sleepwalking. Sleepwalking is common and not necessarily considered abnormal in young children; however, in the adult it is rare and merits careful evaluation. Ms. R's excessive daytime sleepiness was likely due to insufficient sleep (5 to 7 hours per night) and possibly parasomnia-related disruption. Of interest, many parasomnias are exacerbated by sleep deprivation, as is nocturnal seizure disorder.

Sleep studies were performed using comprehensive, attended, laboratory polysomnography. Prior to the overnight study, a clinical EEG was performed. The clinical EEG study did not reveal any significant abnormal EEG activity during baseline, photic stimulation, or hyperventilation. An extended EEG montage was used during the sleep study. Overall sleep quality was within the normal range. Sleep efficiency was 96 percent, and latency to sleep was 1 minute. REM sleep percentage was elevated (31 percent), and latency to REM sleep was less than normal (57 minutes). Slow wave sleep was normal in percentage, but EEG delta activity was of very high amplitude. The overall macroarchitectural sleep pattern suggested rebound from sleep deprivation.

By contrast, sleep microarchitecture contained many abnormal features. There were high-amplitude paroxysmal EEG bursts. Excessively prolonged sleep spindles were noted, and rhythmic K complexes were observed. There was one arousal out of slow wave sleep, with rhythmic EEG discharges alternating with sharp waves. Sharps and spikes occurred several times; however, the focus was difficult to localize (possibly right temporal lobe). There were frequent body movements and full body jerks, most of which occurred during NREM sleep. There were episodes of moaning during slow wave sleep and laughing during stage 2 sleep that was followed by high-amplitude theta bursts and REM sleep. There were frequent movements and arousals from REM sleep but no REM-related spikes or sharp waves. Seizure-like EEG activity was noted during the night and occurred predominantly during slow wave sleep. However, the patient did not attempt to sleepwalk. Sharp wave-and-spike activity increased during the final 45 minutes of the sleep study.

The patient did not have any sleep-related breathing impairment, and oxygen saturation nadir was 90 percent. She had no periodic limb movements during sleep, and polygraphic features associated with restless legs syndrome were absent. *(Courtesy of Max Hirshkowitz, Ph.D., Rhoda G. Seplowitz-Hafkin, M.D., and Amir Sharafkhaneh, M.D., Ph.D.)*

SLEEP-RELATED MOVEMENT DISORDERS

Restless Legs Syndrome

Restless legs syndrome (RLS) (also known as *Ekbom syndrome*) is an uncomfortable, subjective sensation of the limbs, usually the legs, sometimes described as a "creepy crawly" feeling, and the irresistible urge to move the legs when at rest or while trying to fall asleep. Patients often report the sensation of ants walking on the skin and crawling feelings in their legs. It tends to be worse at night and moving the legs or walking helps to alleviate the discomfort. Thus, as the individual is lying in bed and relaxing, he or she is disturbed by these sensations. Then he or she moves the legs and again tries to fall asleep. This cycle sometimes continues for hours and results in profound insomnia. A National Institutes of Health workshop established criteria for the diagnosis of RLS. Uremia, neuropathies, and iron and folic acid deficiency anemias can produce secondary RLS. RLS is also reported in association with fibromyalgia, rheumatoid arthritis, diabetes, thyroid diseases, and COPD. Detailed history and physical examination are important parts of the RLS workup. In addition, the ferritin level should be checked in every patient with symptoms consistent with RLS. Pharmacologically, the dopaminergic agonists pramipexole (Mirapex) and ropinirole (Requip) are FDA approved and represent the treatments of choice. Other agents used to treat RLS include dopamine precursors (e.g., levodopa), benzodiazepines, opiates, and antiepileptic drugs (e.g., gabapentin [Neurontin]). Nonpharmacological treatments include avoiding alcohol use close to bedtime, massaging the affected parts of the legs, taking hot baths, applying hot or cold to the affected areas, and engaging in moderate exercise.

Periodic Limb Movement Disorder

Periodic limb movement disorder (PLMD), previously called *nocturnal myoclonus,* involves brief, stereotypic, repetitive, nonepileptiform movements of the limbs, usually the legs. It occurs primarily in NREM sleep and involves an extension of the big toe. A partial flexion of the ankle, knee, and hip may also occur. These movements range from 0.5 to 5 seconds in duration and occur every 20 to 40 seconds. The leg movements are frequently associated with brief arousals from sleep and as a result can (but do not always) disturb sleep architecture. The prevalence of PLMD increases with aging and can occur in association with folate deficiency, renal disease, anemia, and the use of antidepressants. Pharmacotherapy for PLMD associated with RLS is the same as for RLS. Clinical trials of pharmacotherapy for other forms of PLMD are lacking. However, benzodiazepines, especially clonazepam, and opiates improve sleep in patients with PLMD.

Sleep-Related Leg Cramps

Nocturnal leg cramps are much like leg cramps that occur during wakefulness. They usually affect the calf and are painful muscle contractions. The pain awakens the sleeper and thereby disrupts sleep. Metabolic disorders, mineral deficiencies, electrolytic imbalances, diabetes, and pregnancy are known precipitators. The reason that some individuals have repeated leg cramps during sleep and not during the day is not known.

Sleep-Related Bruxism

Sleep-related bruxism is diagnosed when an individual grinds or clenches the teeth during sleep. Formerly classified as a parasomnia, sleep bruxism can produce abnormal wear on the teeth, damage teeth, provoke tooth and jaw pain, or make loud unpleasant sounds that disturb the bed partner. Sometimes atypical facial pain and headache also result. More than 85 percent of the population may brux at one time or another; however, it is clinically significant in only about 5 percent. Teeth grinding occurs in any sleep stage but appears to be most common at transition to sleep, in stage 2 sleep, and during REM sleep. Some evidence indicates that teeth grinding during REM sleep is more commonly associated with dental wear or damage. Sleep bruxism does not appear to be exacerbated by dental malocclusion. It worsens during periods of stress. Researchers studying sleep bruxism have found that many patients seem to have less frequent teeth grinding when sleeping in the laboratory; therefore, repeated study may be needed to document the disorder. By contrast, bruxism frequently appears on polysomnographic recordings made for other purposes. Sleep bruxism may occur secondary to sleep-related breathing disorders, the use of psychostimulants (e.g., amphetamine, cocaine), alcohol ingestion, and treatment with SSRIs. Differential diagnosis should rule out nocturnal seizures. Sleep bruxism can occur infrequently (monthly), regularly (weekly), or frequently (nightly). Severity is judged on the basis of sleep disruption, consequent pain, and dental damage. The usual treatment involves having the patient wear an oral appliance to protect the teeth during sleep. There are two basic types of appliances: the soft one (mouth guard) is typical used in the short term, whereas the hard acrylic one (bite splint) is used longer term and requires regular follow-up. Relaxation, biofeedback, hypnosis, physical therapy, and stress management are also used to treat sleep bruxism. A variety of drug therapies have been tried (benzodiazepines, muscle relaxants, dopaminergic agonists, and propranolol [Inderal]), but outcome data are not available.

Sleep-Related Rhythmic Movement Disorder

This sleep disorder is marked by repetitive, rhythmic movements usually involving the head and neck. Usually occurring at the transition from wakefulness to sleep, this movement disorder may also continue during light sleep. Formerly classified as a parasomnia, sleep-related rhythmic movement disorder has many names, including *jactatio capitis nocturna,* head banging, head rolling, body rocking, and *rhythmie du sommeil.* A majority of infants body rock. Some clinicians believe that body rocking develops from the soothing effect of vestibular stimulation. If the rhythmic movement persists into childhood and involves head banging, the risk of injury increases. The male to female ratio is 4 to 1. Severity ranges from less than one episode weekly to nightly episodes producing injury.

Sleep-Related Movement Disorder due to Drug or Substance Use and Sleep-Related Movement Disorder due to Medical Condition

A variety of drugs, substances, and comorbid conditions can produce or exacerbate sleep-related movement disorders. Stimulants can produce rhythmic movement disorders and bruxism. Antidepressants (including most tricyclics and SSRIs), antiemetics, lithium (Eskalith), calcium-channel blockers, antihistamines, and neuroleptics can provoke restless legs symptoms and periodic limb movement disorder. Neurologic diseases that are associated with daytime movement disorders can also be associated with sleep-related movement disorders. Stress, anxiety, and sleep deprivation may contribute to bruxism.

ISOLATED SYMPTOMS, APPARENTLY NORMAL VARIANTS, AND UNRESOLVED ISSUES

Long Sleeper

Some individuals are sleepy when they have what most people consider a normal amount of sleep; however, when given the chance to sleep 10 to 12 hours, they are refreshed. These people are classified as long sleepers. This pattern of requiring more than the average amount of sleep is usually present since childhood. Polysomnography may help to differentiate a long sleeper from someone with idiopathic hypersomnia. There may be associated autonomic nervous system dysfunction or polysomnographic evidence of elevated slow wave sleep percentage in patients with idiopathic hypersomnia.

Short Sleeper

People who fall under the category of short sleeper require less than 5 hours of sleep per 24-hour period in order to maintain normal daytime functioning and mood. This appears to run in families, but the specific genes are unknown.

Snoring

Primary snoring consists of loud snoring in the absence of recurrent apnea or hypopnea episodes. The sound may disturb the bed partner to the extent that the persons sleep in separate rooms. To be classified as primary snoring, the individual must not be suffering from excessive sleepiness. Snoring may become louder when the individual sleeps supine or during REM sleep. A variety of oral appliances have been developed to decrease snoring (see “Treatment” under “Breathing-Related Sleep Disorders”).

Sleep Talking

As the name implies, sleep talking in its classic form involves unconscious speech during sleep. It is seldom recognized in an individual unless it annoys the bed partner. It can be induced by fever, stress, or conversing with the sleeper. Somniloquy may accompany sleep terror, sleepwalking, confusional arousals, OSA, and REM sleep behavior disorder.

Sleep Starts (Hypnic Jerk)

Sleep starts are sudden, brief muscle contractions that occur at the transition between wakefulness and sleep in 60 to 70 percent of adults. The contractions commonly involve the legs; however, sometimes there is movement in the arms and head. This “hypnic jerk,” as it is sometimes called, is usually benign. The sleep start, however, can interfere with the ability to fall asleep and may be accompanied by sensations of falling, a hallucinated flash of light, or a loud crackling sound. In severe cases the sleep start produces profound sleep-onset insomnia.

Benign Sleep Myoclonus of Infancy

Previously called benign neonatal sleep myoclonus, this disorder is characterized by asynchronous jerking of limbs and trunk during quiet sleep in neonates. This benign, apparently rare parasomnia usually begins within the first week of life and may last a few days or several months. No treatment is recommended.

Hypnagogic Foot Tremor and Alternating Leg Muscle Activation during Sleep

Hypnagogic foot tremor (HFT) occurs at sleep onset or during stages 1 and 2 of sleep. It consists in a rhythmic movement of the toes or feet for seconds to minutes. Alternating leg muscle activation (ALMA) consists of brief activation of the anterior tibialis in one leg and then the other.

Propriospinal Myoclonus at Sleep Onset

This is a spinal cord–mediated movement disorder that is sometimes associated with spinal cord lesions. Movements appear during times of wakeful relaxation and then may interfere with sleep onset. They start in the abdominal and truncal muscles and then progress to the neck and proximal muscles of the limbs. Treatment with clonazepam or anticonvulsants may be effective.

Excessive Fragmentary Myoclonus

These small movements or muscle fasciculations of the fingers, toes, or corners of the mouth are involuntary and can occur during wakefulness or sleep. Although no visible movement is present, the patient is typically aware of the twitching. In patients with apnea, twitching may worsen during periods of hypoxemia.

OTHER SLEEP DISORDERS

Other Physiological (Organic) Sleep Disorders

This category is for sleep disorders that do not fit into any other ICSD-2 classification. The disorders in this category are suspected to have a medical or physiological etiology even if the etiology is not known at the time of diagnosis.

Other Sleep Disorder Not due to Substance Use or Known Physiological Conditions

This category is for sleep disorders that do not fit into any other ICSD-2 classification and are believed to be due to psychiatric or behavioral factors.

Environmental Sleep Disorder

This is a sleep disorder secondary to environmental factors that contribute to insomnia or daytime somnolence (from insomnia or poor sleep). Noise, heat, cold, light, bed partner noise, bed partner activity, or perceived danger can induce an environmental sleep disorder. The insomnia or hypersomnia are directly caused by the disturbing environmental factor. An example of an environmental factor is having a neighbor who plays music loudly every night. Onset, course, and termination of the problem are correlated with the introduction, presence, and removal of the specific factor or factors. Thus, treatment involves identifying and removing the environmental irritant.

TOOLS IN SLEEP MEDICINE

Clinical Interview

A careful and thorough clinical interview is one of the most informative parts of a patient workup for sleep disorders. The habitual bedtime and arising times for both weekdays and weekends, the frequency, duration, and refreshingness of naps, and overall level of sleepiness are good places to begin. Specific sleep problems relating to difficulty initiating and maintaining sleep are important, including whether there is rumination at bedtime, fear of not being able to sleep, or excessive worry when attempting to sleep. Leg movement, leg sensations, leg cramps, teeth grinding, dream enactments (with or without injury), and other movements should be queried. Morning headaches, morning dry mouth, nocturnal reflux, hyperhidrosis, nocturia, enuresis, nocturnal tongue biting, nightmares, sleep terrors, and other sleep-related problems should be reviewed. Asking about the presence of family pets and whether they sleep in the bedroom (or bed) can be important in some cases.

Polysomnography

Polysomnography is the continuous, attended, comprehensive recording of the biophysiological changes that occur during sleep. Each 30-second segment of the recording is considered an "epoch." A polysomnogram is typically recorded at night and lasts between 6 and 8 hours. Brain wave activity, eye movements, submental electromyography activity, nasal–oral airflow, respiratory effort, oxyhemoglobin saturation, heart rhythm, and leg movements during sleep are measured. Body position is usually noted, and snoring sounds may be recorded. Brain wave activity, eye movements, and submental electromyogram are important for identifying sleep stages. Muscle tension and movements subside with deeper sleep and can also be useful in the diagnosis of periodic limb movement disorder and restless legs syndrome. Nasal airflow, respiratory effort, and oxyhemoglobin saturation are instrumental in diagnosing sleep apnea and other sleep-related breathing disorders.

Indications for polysomnography include (1) diagnosis of sleep-related breathing disorders, (2) positive airway pressure titration and assessment of treatment efficacy, and (3) evaluation of sleep-related behaviors that are violent or may potentially harm the patient or bed partner. Polysomnography can also be used to diagnose atypical parasomnias, sleep-related problems secondary to neuromuscular disorders, periodic limb movement disorder, and arousals secondary to seizure disorder. In addition, patients with excessive daytime sleepiness or those who wake up gasping or choking should be referred for polysomnography. A sleep study is not needed to diagnose RLS.

Referrals for polysomnography should be considered in cases in which sleeplessness has been present for 6 months or more for a minimum of four nights a week. It should also be considered when insomnia has not responded to pharmacological or behavioral therapy, sleep-promoting medications are contraindicated, or a medical or psychiatric cause has been excluded. Referral should also be made if the treatment of an underlying medical or psychiatric comorbidity has failed to resolve the insomnia.

Polysomnography is also recommended to assess sleep quality and quantity on the night just prior to a multiple sleep latency test being conducted to diagnose narcolepsy.

Multiple Sleep Latency Test

The multiple sleep latency test (MSLT) is indicated for diagnosing narcolepsy. Beginning 2 hours after morning awakening, 20-minute nap opportunities are provided during which the patient is instructed to let himself or herself fall asleep and not resist falling asleep. Electroencephalographic, electrooculographic, and submental electromyography activity is recorded to determine sleep stage. The latency to sleep is used to assess the level of sleepiness, and the appearance of REM sleep on two or more nap opportunities confirms narcolepsy, especially when other ancillary symptoms are present (e.g., cataplexy, sleep paralysis, hypnagogia, and excessive sleepiness). If the patient falls asleep on a given nap opportunity, the nap is terminated 15 minutes after initial sleep onset. If the patient does not fall asleep, the session is terminated after 20 minutes of recording. Five nap opportunities are provided at 2-hour intervals across the day.

Maintenance of Wakefulness Test

Similar procedurally to the MSLT, the maintenance of wakefulness test (MWT) provides 40-minute test sessions at 2-hour intervals across the day, but the patient is instructed to try to remain awake. This technique is used to assess treatment outcomes and is sometimes required as part of "fit for duty" testing. Patients sit in a comfortable chair or on the bed with a bolster pillow in a darkened room while recordings are made. The first epoch of stage 2, 3, or 4 sleep or REM or three consecutive epochs of stage 1 mark unequivocal sleep onset. Falling asleep on MWT indicates some level of sleepiness. Fifty-nine percent of volunteers (presumably normal) remain awake for the entire 40 minutes across all four trials (using unequivocal sleep criteria). Any sleep latency of less than 8 minutes is abnormal. Sleep latency ranging from 8 to 40 minutes is of unknown significance. The mean sleep latency (first sleep epoch) is 30.4 ± 11.2 minutes, and the upper 95 percent confidence interval is 40 minutes.

Actigraphy

An actigraph is a device that measures and records movement. It is usually worn on the wrist (like a watch) and can be used as a rough measure of the sleep–wake cycle. Depending on the model and the settings, it can make continuous recordings for days or weeks. It can be especially useful for assessing insomnia, circadian rhythm disorders, movement disorders, and an assortment of rare events.

Home Sleep Testing

Recently approved by Medicare, home sleep testing involves recording a limited number of cardiopulmonary parameters to assess patients for sleep-related breathing disorders. Home sleep testing is much less expensive than polysomnography. Usually, airflow, respiratory effort, heart rhythm, snoring sounds, and oximetry are recorded. A number of devices are commercially available that are capable of detecting sleep apnea in patients with moderate to severe pathophysiology. Negative studies are problematic because home sleep testing is less sensitive than full laboratory polysomnography. Patients with negative tests notwithstanding obvious symptoms or comorbidity should be scheduled for laboratory sleep study. In addition, home sleep testing does not check for the full spectrum of sleep disorders; therefore, residual symptoms after a breathing disorder is diagnosed in this manner need careful follow-up.

Sleep Apps

A variety of commercial smart phone sleep applications have been developed to deal with sleep disorders. Some provide "white noise" to help induce sleep in those sensitive to noise; others gather data about respiratory rate, body movement and depth of sleep while the phone is on the bed or under the pillow of the person in bed. There is no scientific evidence as to the efficacy of the many different sleep apps on the market although there are anecdotal reports of some persons receiving benefit from their use.

13 Human Sexuality and Sexual Dysfunctions

▲ 13.1 Normal Sexuality

Sexuality is determined by anatomy, physiology, the culture in which a person lives, relationships with others, and developmental experiences throughout the life cycle. It includes the perception of being male or female and private thoughts and fantasies as well as behavior. To the average person, sexual attraction to another person and the passion and love that follow are deeply associated with feelings of intimate happiness.

Normal sexual behavior brings pleasure to oneself and one's partner and involves stimulation of the primary sex organs including coitus; it is devoid of inappropriate feelings of guilt or anxiety and is not compulsive. Societal understanding of what defines normal sexual behavior is inconstant and varies from era to era, reflecting the cultural mores of the time.

Sexuality has always been an area of interest to the medical community. In the classical era, Hippocrates cited the clitoris as the site of female sexual arousal, the first physician historically recorded to have made that assessment. In the middle ages, Islamic physicians recommended coitus interruptus as a form of birth control. At the end of the Renaissance and the beginning of the Reformation, a linen sheath was devised as a condom, not for purposes of birth control, but as protection against syphilis. During the Victorian era, sexologists such as Havelock Ellis and Richard von Krafft-Ebing presented diverging perspectives on sexual behavior. During that same period, Sigmund Freud developed his innovative theories on libido, childhood sexuality, and the effects of the sexual impulse on human behavior. In the modern era, the research of Alfred Kinsey, the work of William Masters and Virginia Johnson, and the development of drugs that prevent contraception, aid erection, and replace hormones that decrease with menopause and aging contributed to the development of an era of sexual liberality. Sex has also been a consistent focus of curiosity and interest to humankind in general. Depictions of sexual behavior have existed from the time of prehistoric cave drawings through Leonardo da Vinci's anatomical illustrations of intercourse to current pornographic sites on the Internet.

TERMS

Sexuality and total personality are so entwined that to speak of sexuality as a separate entity is virtually impossible. The term *psychosexual,* therefore, is used to describe personality development and functioning as these are affected by sexuality. The term *psychosexual* applies to more than sexual feelings and behavior, and it is not synonymous with *libido* in the broad Freudian sense.

Freud's generalization that all pleasurable impulses and activities are originally sexual has given laypersons a somewhat distorted view of sexual concepts and has presented psychiatrists with a confused picture of motivation. For example, some oral activities are directed toward obtaining food, and others are directed toward achieving sexual gratification. Both activities are pleasure seeking and use the same organ, but they are not, as Freud contended, both necessarily sexual. Labeling of all pleasure-seeking behaviors as sexual makes it impossible to specify precise motivations. Persons may also use sexual activities for gratification of nonsexual needs, such as dependency, aggression, power, and status. Although sexual and nonsexual impulses can jointly motivate behavior, the analysis of behavior depends on understanding the underlying individual motivations and their interactions.

CHILDHOOD SEXUALITY

Before Freud described the effects of childhood experiences on personalities of adults, the universality of sexual activity and sexual learning in children was unrecognized. Most sexual learning experiences in childhood occur without the parents' knowledge, but awareness of a child's sex does influence parental behavior. Male infants, for instance, tend to be handled more vigorously and female infants tend to be cuddled more. Fathers spend more time with their infant sons than with their daughters, and they also tend to be more aware of their sons' adolescent concerns than of their daughters' anxieties. Boys are more likely than girls to be physically disciplined. A child's sex affects parental tolerance for aggression and reinforcement or extinction of activity and of intellectual, aesthetic, and athletic interests.

Observation of children reveals that genital play in infants is part of normal development. According to Harry Harlow, interaction with mothers and peers is necessary for the development of effective adult sexual behavior in monkeys, a finding that has relevance to the normal socialization of children. During a critical period in development, infants are especially susceptible to certain stimuli; later, they may be immune to these stimuli. The detailed relation of critical periods to psychosexual development has yet to be established; Freud's stages of psychosexual development—oral, anal, phallic, latent, and genital—presumably provide a broad framework.

PSYCHOSEXUAL FACTORS

Sexuality depends on four interrelated psychosexual factors: sexual identity, gender identity, sexual orientation, and sexual behavior. These factors affect personality, growth, development, and functioning. Sexuality is something more than physical sex, coital or noncoital, and something less than all behaviors directed toward attaining pleasure.

Sexual Identity and Gender Identity

Sexual identity is the pattern of a person's biological sexual characteristics: chromosomes, external genitalia, internal genitalia, hormonal composition, gonads, and secondary sex characteristics. In normal development, these characteristics form a cohesive pattern that leaves a person in no doubt about his or her sex. Gender identity is a person's sense of maleness or femaleness. Sexual identity and gender identity are interactive. Genetic influences and hormones affect behavior, and the environment affects hormonal production and gene expression (Table 13.1–1).

Sexual Identity. Modern embryological studies have shown that all mammalian embryos, whether genetically male (XY genotype) or genetically female (XX genotype), are anatomically female during the early stages of fetal life. Differentiation of the male from the female results from the action of fetal androgens; the action begins about the sixth week of embryonic life and is completed by the end of the third month. Recent research has focused on the possible roles of key genes in fetal sexual development. A testis develops as a result of SRY and SOX9 action, and an ovary develops in the absence of such action. DAX1 plays a part in the fetal development of both sexes and WNT4 action is needed for the development of the mullerian ducts in the female fetus. Other studies have explained the effects of fetal hormones on the masculinization or feminization of the brain. In animals, prenatal hormonal stimulation of the brain is necessary for male and female reproductive and copulatory behavior. The fetus is also vulnerable to exogenously administered androgens during that period. For instance, if a pregnant woman receives sufficient exogenous androgens, her female fetus that possesses ovaries can develop external genitalia resembling those of a male fetus.

In the past, newborns with ambiguous genitalia were assigned their sexual identity at birth. The theory underlying this action was that parents and child would feel less confusion, and that the child would accept the assigned sex and more easily develops a stable sense of being male or female. Although this worked for some children, others developed a gender identity at odds with their assigned sex. For example, an infant designated female at birth could feel itself to be male throughout childhood, and more emphatically at puberty. In some cases, this conflict led to depression and even suicide. Current practice usually allows the child to develop with the ambiguity, which permits a sense of gender identity to evolve as the child grows. The gender identity is then more congruent with the child's emotional sense of maleness or femaleness. Ideally, the family receives support from a medical team composed of a pediatrician, an endocrinologist, and a psychiatrist throughout this developmental process.

Gender Identity. In infants with an unambiguous sexual identity, almost everyone has a firm conviction that "I am male" or "I am female" by 2 to 3 years of age. Yet, even if maleness and femaleness develop normally, persons must still develop a sense of masculinity or femininity.

Gender identity, according to Robert Stoller, "connotes psychological aspects of behavior related to masculinity and femininity." Stoller considers gender social and sex biological: "Most often the two are relatively congruent, that is, males tend to be manly and females womanly." But sex and gender can develop in conflicting or even opposite ways. Gender identity results from an almost infinite series of cues derived from experiences with family members, teachers, friends, and coworkers, and from cultural phenomena. Physical characteristics derived

Table 13.1–1
Classification of Intersexual Disorders[a]

Syndrome	Description
Virilizing adrenal hyperplasia (adrenogenital syndrome)	Results from excess androgens in fetus with XX genotype; most common female intersex disorder; associated with enlarged clitoris, fused labia, hirsutism in adolescence
Turner's syndrome	Results from absence of second female sex chromosome (XO); associated with web neck, dwarfism, cubitus valgus; no sex hormones produced; infertile
Klinefelter's syndrome	Genotype is XXY; male habitus present with small penis and rudimentary testes because of low androgen production; weak libido; usually assigned as male
Androgen insensitivity syndrome (testicular-feminizing syndrome)	Congenital X-linked recessive disorder that results in inability of tissues to respond to androgens; external genitals look female and cryptorchid testes present; in extreme form patient has breasts, normal external genitals, short blind vagina, and absence of pubic and axillary hair
Enzymatic defects in XY genotype (e.g., 5-α-reductase deficiency, 17-hydroxy-steroid deficiency)	Congenital interruption in production of testosterone that produces ambiguous genitals and female habitus
Hermaphroditism	True hermaphrodite is rare and characterized by both testes and ovaries in same person (may be 46 XX or 46 XY)
Pseudohermaphroditism	Usually the result of endocrine or enzymatic defect (e.g., adrenal hyperplasia) in persons with normal chromosomes; female pseudohermaphrodites have masculine-looking genitals but are XX; male pseudohermaphrodites have rudimentary testes and external genitals and are XY

[a]Intersexual disorders include a variety of syndromes that produce persons with gross anatomical or physiological aspects of the opposite sex.

from a person's biological sex—such as physique, body shape, and physical dimensions—interrelate with an intricate system of stimuli, including rewards and punishment and parental gender labels, to establish gender identity.

Thus, formation of gender identity arises from parental and cultural attitudes, the infant's external genitalia, and a genetic influence, which is physiologically active by the sixth week of fetal life. Although family, cultural, and biological influences may complicate establishment of a sense of masculinity or femininity, persons usually develop a relatively secure sense of identification with their biological sex—a stable gender identity.

Gender Role. Related to, and in part derived from, gender identity is gender role behavior. John Money and Anke Ehrhardt described gender role behavior as all those things that a person says or does to disclose himself or herself as having the status of boy or man, girl or woman, respectively. A gender role is not established at birth but is built up cumulatively through (1) experiences encountered and transacted through casual and unplanned learning, (2) explicit instruction and inculcation, and (3) spontaneously putting two and two together to make sometimes four and sometimes five. The usual outcome is a congruence of gender identity and gender role. Although biological attributes are significant, the major factor in achieving the role appropriate to a person's sex is learning.

Research on sex differences in children's behavior reveals more psychological similarities than differences. Girls, however, are found to be less susceptible to tantrums after the age of 18 months than are boys, and boys generally are more physically and verbally aggressive than are girls from age 2 onward. Little girls and little boys are similarly active, but boys are more easily stimulated to sudden bursts of activity when they are in groups. Some researchers speculate that, although aggression is a learned behavior, male hormones may have sensitized boys' neural organizations to absorb these lessons more easily than do girls.

Persons' gender roles can seem to be opposed to their gender identities. Persons may identify with their own sex and yet adopt the dress, hairstyle, or other characteristics of the opposite sex. Or, they may identify with the opposite sex and yet for expediency adopt many behavioral characteristics of their own sex. A further discussion of gender issues appears in Chapter 14.

Sexual Orientation

Sexual orientation describes the object of a person's sexual impulses: heterosexual (opposite sex), homosexual (same sex), or bisexual (both sexes). A group of people have defined themselves as "asexual" and assert this as a positive identity. Some researchers believe this lack of attraction to any object is a manifestation of a desire disorder. Other people wish not to define their sexual orientation at all and avoid labels. Still others describe themselves as polysexual or pansexual.

Sexual Behavior

The Central Nervous System and Sexual Behavior

THE BRAIN

Cortex. The cortex is involved in both controlling sexual impulses and processing sexual stimuli that may lead to sexual activity. In studies of young men, some areas of the brain have been found to be more active during sexual stimulation than others. These include the orbitofrontal cortex, which is involved in emotions; the left anterior cingulate cortex, which is involved in hormone control and sexual arousal; and the right caudate nucleus, whose activity is a factor in whether sexual activity follows arousal.

Limbic System. In all mammals, the limbic system is directly involved with elements of sexual functioning. Chemical or electrical stimulation of the lower part of the septum and the contiguous preoptic area, the fimbria of the hippocampus, the mammillary bodies, and the anterior thalamic nuclei have all elicited penile erections.

Studies of the brain in women have revealed that those areas activated by emotions of fear or anxiety are notably quiescent when the woman experiences an orgasm.

Brainstem. Brainstem sites exert inhibitory and excitatory control over spinal sexual reflexes. The nucleus paragigantocellularis projects directly to pelvic efferent neurons in the lumbosacral spinal cord, apparently causing them to secrete serotonin, which is known to inhibit orgasms. The lumbosacral cord also receives projections from other serotonergic nuclei in the brainstem.

Brain Neurotransmitters. Many neurotransmitters, including dopamine, epinephrine, norepinephrine, and serotonin, are produced in the brain and affect sexual function. For example, an increase in dopamine is presumed to increase libido. Serotonin, produced in the upper pons and midbrain, exerts an inhibitory effect on sexual function. Oxytocin is released with orgasm and is believed to reinforce pleasurable activities.

SPINAL CORD. Sexual arousal and climax are ultimately organized at the spinal level. Sensory stimuli related to sexual function are conveyed via afferents from the pudendal, pelvic, and hypogastric nerves. Several separate experiments suggest that sexual reflexes are mediated by spinal neurons in the central gray region of the lumbosacral segments.

Physiological Responses. Sexual response is a true psychophysiological experience. Arousal is triggered by both psychological and physical stimuli; levels of tension are experienced both physiologically and emotionally; and, with orgasm, normally a subjective perception of a peak of physical reaction and release occurs along with a feeling of well-being. Psychosexual development, psychological attitudes toward sexuality, and attitudes toward one's sexual partner are directly involved with, and affect, the physiology of human sexual response.

Normally, men and women experience a sequence of physiological responses to sexual stimulation. In the first detailed description of these responses, Masters and Johnson observed that the physiological process involves increasing levels of vasocongestion and myotonia (tumescence) and the subsequent release of the vascular activity and muscle tone as a result of orgasm (detumescence). Tables 13.1–2 and 13.1–3 describe the physiologic male and female sexual response cycles. It is important to remember that the sequence of responses can overlap and fluctuate. A sexual fantasy or the desire to have sex frequently precedes the physiological responses of excitement, orgasm, and resolution, particularly in the male. In addition, a person's subjective experiences are as important to sexual satisfaction as the objective physiologic response.

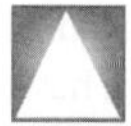

Table 13.1–2
Male Sexual Response Cycle[a]

Organ	Excitement Phase	Orgasmic Phase	Resolution Phase
	Lasts several minutes to several hours; heightened excitement before orgasm, 30 seconds to 3 minutes	3 to 15 seconds	10 to 15 minutes; if no orgasm, ½ to 1 day
Skin	Just before orgasm: sexual flush inconsistently appears; maculopapular rash originates on abdomen and spreads to anterior chest wall, face, and neck and can include shoulders and forearms	Well-developed flush	Flush disappears in reverse order of appearance; inconsistently appearing film of perspiration on soles of feet and palms of hands
Penis	Erection in 10 to 30 seconds caused by vasocongestion of erectile bodies of corpus cavernosa of shaft; loss of erection may occur with introduction of asexual stimulus, loud noise; with heightened excitement, size of glands and diameter of penile shaft increase further	Ejaculation; emission phase marked by three to four 0.8-second contractions of vas, seminal vesicles, prostate; ejaculation proper marked by 0.8-second contractions of urethra and ejaculatory spurt of 12 to 20 in at age 18, decreasing with age to seepage at 70	Erection: partial involution in 5 to 10 seconds with variable refractory period; full detumescence in 5 to 30 minutes
Scrotum and testes	Tightening and lifting of scrotal sac and elevation of testes; with heightened excitement, 50% increase in size of testes over unstimulated state and flattening against perineum, signaling impending ejaculation	No change	Decrease to baseline size because of loss of vasocongestion; testicular and scrotal descent within 5 to 30 minutes after orgasm; involution may take several hours if no orgasmic release takes place
Cowper's glands	2 to 3 drops of mucoid fluid that contain viable sperm are secreted during heightened excitement	No change	No change
Other	Breasts: inconsistent nipple erection with heightened excitement before orgasm Myotonia: semispastic contractions of facial, abdominal, and intercostal muscles Tachycardia: up to 175 beats a minute Blood pressure: rise in systolic 20 to 80 mm Hg; in diastolic 10 to 40 mm Hg Respiration: increased	Loss of voluntary muscular control Rectum: rhythmical contractions of sphincter Heart rate: up to 180 beats a minute Blood pressure: up to 40 to 100 mm Hg systolic; 20 to 50 mm Hg diastolic Respiration: up to 40 respirations a minute	Return to baseline state in 5 to 10 minutes A refractory period follows orgasm, during which time the male cannot be rearoused to erection and is unresponsive to stimulation. The length of the refractory period is age and situation dependent

[a]A desire phase consisting of sex fantasies and desire to have sex precedes excitement phase.
Table by Virginia Sadock, M.D.

HORMONES AND SEXUAL BEHAVIOR

In general, substances that increase dopamine levels in the brain increase desire, whereas substances that augment serotonin decrease desire. Testosterone increases libido in both men and women, although estrogen is a key factor in the lubrication involved in female arousal and may increase sensitivity in the woman to stimulation. Recent studies indicate that estrogen is also a factor in the male sexual response and that a decrease in estrogen in the middle-aged male results in greater fat accumulation just as it does in women. Progesterone mildly depresses desire in men and women as do excessive prolactin and cortisol. Oxytocin is involved in pleasurable sensations during sex and is found in higher levels in men and women following orgasm.

GENDER DIFFERENCES IN DESIRE AND EROTIC STIMULI

Sexual impulses and desire exist in men and women. In measuring desire by the frequency of spontaneous sexual thoughts, interest in participating in sexual activity, and alertness to sexual cues, males generally possess a higher baseline level of desire than do women, which may be biologically determined. Motivations for having sex, other than desire, exist in both men and women, but seem to be more varied and prevalent in women. In women they may include a wish to reinforce the pair bond, the need for a feeling of closeness, a way of preventing the man from straying, or a desire to please the partner.

Although explicit sexual fantasies are common to both sexes, the external stimuli for the fantasies frequently differ for men and women. Many men respond sexually to visual stimuli of nude or barely dressed women. Women report responding sexually to romantic stories such as a demonstrative hero whose passion for the heroine impels him toward a lifetime commitment to her. A complicating factor is that a woman's subjective sense of arousal is not always congruent with her physiological state of arousal. Specifically, her sense of excitement may reflect a readiness to be aroused rather than physiological lubrication. Conversely, she may experience signs of arousal, including vaginal lubrication, without being aware of them. This situation rarely occurs in men.

Table 13.1–3
Female Sexual Response Cycle[a]

Organ	Excitement Phase	Orgasmic Phase	Resolution Phase
	Lasts several minutes to several hours; heightened excitement before orgasm, 30 seconds to 3 minutes	3 to 15 seconds	10 to 15 minutes; if no orgasm, 1/2 to 1 day
Skin	Just before orgasm: sexual flush inconsistently appears; maculopapular rash originates on abdomen and spreads to anterior chest wall, face, and neck; can include shoulders and forearms	Well-developed flush	Flush disappears in reverse order of appearance; inconsistently appearing film of perspiration on soles of feet and palms of hands
Breasts	Nipple erection in two-thirds of women, venous congestion and areolar enlargement; size increases to one-fourth over normal	Breasts may become tremulous	Return to normal in about 30 minutes
Clitoris	Enlargement in diameter of glands and shaft; just before orgasm, shaft retracts into prepuce	No change	Shaft returns to normal position in 5 to 10 seconds; detumescence in 5 to 30 minutes; if no orgasm, detumescence takes several hours
Labia majora	Nullipara: elevate and flatten against perineum Multipara: congestion and edema	No change	Nullipara: decrease to normal size in 1 to 2 minutes Multipara: decrease to normal size in 10 to 15 minutes
Labia minora	Size increased two to three times over normal; change to pink, red, deep red before orgasm	Contractions of proximal labia minora	Return to normal within 5 minutes
Vagina	Color change to dark purple; vaginal transudate appears 10 to 30 seconds after arousal; elongation and ballooning of vagina; lower third of vagina constricts before orgasm	3 to 15 contractions of lower third of vagina at intervals of 0.8 second	Ejaculate forms seminal pool in upper two-thirds of vagina; congestion disappears in seconds or, if no orgasm, in 20 to 30 minutes
Uterus	Ascends into false pelvis; labor-like contractions begin in heightened excitement just before orgasm	Contractions throughout orgasm	Contractions cease, and uterus descends to normal position
Other	Myotonia A few drops of mucoid secretion from Bartholin's glands during heightened excitement Cervix swells slightly and is passively elevated with uterus	Loss of voluntary muscular control Rectum: rhythmical contractions of sphincter Hyperventilation and tachycardia	Return to baseline status in seconds to minutes Cervix color and size return to normal, and cervix descends into seminal pool

[a]A desire phase consisting of sex fantasies and desire to have sex may precede or overlap with the excitement phase.
Table by Virginia Sadock, M.D.

MASTURBATION

Masturbation is usually a normal precursor of object-related sexual behavior. No other form of sexual activity has been more frequently discussed, more roundly condemned, and more universally practiced than masturbation. Research by Kinsey into the prevalence of masturbation indicated that nearly all men and three-fourths of all women masturbate sometime during their lives.

Longitudinal studies of development show that sexual self-stimulation is common in infancy and childhood. Just as infants learn to explore the functions of their fingers and mouths, they learn to do the same with their genitalia. At about 15 to 19 months of age, both sexes begin genital self-stimulation. Pleasurable sensations result from any gentle touch to the genital region. Those sensations, coupled with the ordinary desire for exploration of the body, produce a normal interest in masturbatory pleasure at that time. Children also develop an increased interest in the genitalia of others—parents, children, and even animals. As youngsters acquire playmates, the curiosity about their own and others' genitalia motivates episodes of exhibitionism or genital exploration. Such experiences, unless blocked by guilty fear, contribute to continued pleasure from sexual stimulation.

With the approach of puberty, the upsurge of sex hormones, and the development of secondary sex characteristics, sexual curiosity intensifies, and masturbation increases. Adolescents are physically capable of coitus and orgasm, but are usually inhibited by social restraints. The dual and often conflicting pressures of establishing their sexual identities and controlling their sexual impulses produce a strong physiological sexual tension in teenagers that demands release, and masturbation is a normal way to reduce sexual tensions. In general, males learn to masturbate to orgasm earlier than females and masturbate more frequently. An important emotional difference between the adolescent and the youngster of earlier years is the presence of coital fantasies during masturbation in the adolescent. These fantasies are an important adjunct to the development of sexual identity; in the comparative safety of the imagination, the adolescent learns to perform the adult sex role. This autoerotic activity is usually maintained into the young adult years, when it is normally replaced by coitus.

Couples in a sexual relationship do not abandon masturbation entirely. When coitus is unsatisfactory or is unavailable because of illness or the absence of the partner, self-stimulation often serves an adaptive purpose, combining sensual pleasure and tension release.

Kinsey reported that when women masturbate, most prefer clitoral stimulation. Masters and Johnson stated that women prefer the shaft of the clitoris to the glans because the glans is hypersensitive to intense stimulation. Most men masturbate by vigorously stroking the penile shaft and glans.

Several studies found that in men, orgasm from masturbation raised the serum prostate-specific antigen (PSA) significantly. Male patients scheduled for PSA tests should be advised not to masturbate (or have coitus) for at least 7 days prior to the examination.

Moral taboos against masturbation have generated myths that masturbation causes mental illness or decreased sexual potency. No scientific evidence supports such claims. Masturbation is a psychopathological symptom only when it becomes a compulsion beyond a person's willful control. Then, it is a symptom of emotional disturbance, not because it is sexual but because it is compulsive. Masturbation is probably a universal aspect of psychosexual development and, in most cases, it is adaptive.

COITUS

The first coitus is a rite of passage for both men and women. In the United States, the overwhelming majority of people have experienced coitus by young adulthood, by their early 20s. In a study of persons ages 18 to 59, over 95 percent had included coitus in their last sexual interaction.

The young man experiencing intercourse for the first time is vulnerable in his pride and self-esteem. Cultural myths still perpetuate the idea that he should be able to have an erection with no, or little, stimulation, and that he should have an easy mastery over the situation, even though it is an act that he has never before experienced. Cultural pressure on the woman with her first coitus reflects remaining cultural ambivalence about her loss of virginity, despite the current era of sexual liberality. This is demonstrated in the statistic that only 50 percent of young women use contraception during their first coitus, and of that 50 percent, an even smaller number use it consistently thereafter. Young women with a history of masturbation are more likely to approach intercourse with positive anticipation and confidence.

In the last decade, coitus has also been part of the sexual repertoire of elderly adults, due to the development of sildenafil type drugs, which facilitate erections in men, and hormonally enhanced creams or hormonal pills, which counteract vaginal atrophy in postmenopausal women. Prior to the development of these drugs, many elderly adults enjoyed gratifying sex play, exclusive of coitus.

HOMOSEXUALITY

In 1973 homosexuality was eliminated as a diagnostic category by the American Psychiatric Association, and in 1980, it was removed from the Diagnostic and Statistical Manual of Mental Disorders (DSM). The 10th revision of the *International Statistical Classification of Diseases and Related Health Problems* (ICD-10) states: "Sexual orientation alone is not to be regarded as a disorder." This change reflects a change in the understanding of homosexuality, which is now considered to occur with some regularity as a variant of human sexuality, not as a pathological disorder. As David Hawkins wrote, "The presence of homosexuality does not appear to be a matter of choice; the expression of it is a matter of choice."

Definition

The term *homosexuality* often describes a person's overt behavior, sexual orientation, and sense of personal or social identity. Many persons prefer to identify sexual orientation by using terms such as *lesbians* and *gay men,* rather than *homosexual,* which may imply pathology and etiology based on its origin as a medical term, and refer to sexual behavior with terms such as *same sex* and *male–female.* Hawkins wrote that the terms *gay* and *lesbian* refer to a combination of self-perceived identity and social identity; they reflect a person's sense of belonging to a social group that is similarly labeled. Homophobia is a negative attitude toward, or fear of, homosexuality or homosexuals. Heterosexism is the belief that a heterosexual relationship is preferable to all others; it implies discrimination against those practicing other forms of sexuality.

Prevalence

Recent research reports rates of homosexuality in 2 to 4 percent of the population. In a 2011 Williams Institute report 8.2 percent of Americans reported one or more episodes of same-sex sexual behavior and 11 percent reported some same-sex attraction without ever acting it out. In a 2013 U.S. National Institute of Health Survey, 96.6 percent of adults identified as straight, 1.6 percent identified as gay or lesbian, and 0.7 percent identified as bisexual. The remaining 1.1 percent of adults identified as "something else."

Some lesbians and gay men, particularly the latter, report being aware of same-sex romantic attractions before puberty. According to Kinsey's data, about half of all prepubertal boys have had some genital experience with a male partner. These experiences are often exploratory, particularly when shared with a peer, not an adult, and typically lack a strong affective component. Most gay men recall the onset of romantic and erotic attractions to same-sex partners during early adolescence. For women, the onset of romantic feelings toward same-sex partners may also be in preadolescence, but the clear recognition of a same-sex partner preference typically occurs in middle to late adolescence or in young adulthood. More lesbians than gay men appear to have engaged in heterosexual experiences. In one study, 56 percent of lesbians had experienced heterosexual intercourse before their first genital homosexual experience, compared with 19 percent of gay men who had sampled heterosexual intercourse first. Nearly 40 percent of the lesbians had had heterosexual intercourse during the year preceding the survey.

Theoretical Issues

Psychological Factors

The determinants of homosexual behavior are enigmatic. Freud viewed homosexuality as an arrest of psychosexual development and mentioned castration fears and fears of maternal engulfment in the preoedipal phase of psychosexual development. According to psychodynamic theory, early life situations that can result in male homosexual behavior include a strong fixation on the mother; lack of effective fathering; inhibition of masculine development by the parents; fixation at, or regression to, the narcissistic stage of development; and losses when competing with brothers and sisters. Freud's views on the causes of female homosexuality included a lack of resolution of penis envy in association with unresolved oedipal conflicts.

Freud did not consider homosexuality a mental illness. In "Three Essays on the Theory of Sexuality," he wrote that homosexuality "is found in persons who exhibit no other serious deviations from normal whose efficiency is unimpaired and who are indeed distinguished by especially high intellectual development and ethical culture." In "Letter to an American Mother," Freud wrote, "Homosexuality is assuredly no advantage, but it is nothing to be ashamed of, no vice, no degradation, it cannot be classified as an illness; we consider it to be a variation of the sexual functions produced by a certain arrest of sexual development."

New Concepts of Psychoanalytic Factors

Some psychoanalysts have advanced new psychodynamic formulations that contrast with classic psychoanalytic theory. According to Richard Isay, gay men have described same-sex fantasies that occurred when they were 3 to 5 years of age, at about the same age that heterosexuals have male–female fantasies. Isay wrote that same-sex erotic fantasies in gay men center on the father or the father surrogate.

The child's perception of, and exposure to, these erotic feelings may account for such "atypical" behavior as greater secretiveness than other boys, self-isolation, and excessive emotionality. Some "feminine" traits may also be caused by identification with the mother or a mother surrogate. Such characteristics usually develop as a way of attracting the father's love and attention in a manner similar to the way the heterosexual boy may pattern himself after his father to gain his mother's attention.

The psychodynamics of homosexuality in women may be similar. The little girl does not give up her original fixation on the mother as a love object and continues to seek it in adulthood.

Biological Factors

Recent studies indicate that genetic and biological components may contribute to sexual orientation. Gay men reportedly exhibit lower levels of circulatory androgens than do heterosexual men. Prenatal hormones appear to play a role in the organization of the central nervous system: The effective presence of androgens in prenatal life is purported to contribute to a sexual orientation toward females, and a deficiency of prenatal androgens (or tissue insensitivity to them) may lead to a sexual orientation toward males. Preadolescent girls exposed to large amounts of androgens before birth are uncharacteristically aggressive, and boys exposed to excessive female hormones in utero are less athletic, less assertive, and less aggressive than other boys. Women with hyperadrenocorticalism are lesbian and bisexual in greater proportion than women in the general population.

Genetic studies have shown a higher incidence of homosexual concordance among monozygotic twins than among dizygotic twins; these results suggest a genetic predisposition, but chromosome studies have been unable to differentiate homosexuals from heterosexuals. Gay men show a familial distribution; they have more brothers who are gay than do heterosexual men. One study found that 33 of 40 pairs of gay brothers shared a genetic marker on the bottom half of the X chromosome. Another study found that a group of cells in the hypothalamus was smaller in women and in gay men than in heterosexual men. Neither of these studies has been replicated.

Relationship Patterns. Relationship patterns among gay men and lesbians are not dissimilar to those of heterosexuals. Some same-sex pairs live in a common household in either a monogamous or a primary relationship for decades; others typically have only fleeting sexual contacts. Although many gay men form stable relationships, male–male relationships appear to be less stable and more fleeting than female–female relationships. Opinion polls have found changes in American attitudes toward homosexuality, indicating a greater acceptance of homosexuals than in the past. This change was dramatically illustrated in the 2015 landmark opinion, in which the U.S. Supreme Court ruled that same-sex couples can marry nationwide, establishing a new civil right and handing gay rights advocates a historic victory. In the 5–4 ruling, Justice Anthony Kennedy wrote for the majority with the four liberal justices. Each of the four conservative justices wrote their own dissent.

Psychopathology. The range of psychopathology that may be found among lesbians and gay men parallels that found among heterosexuals; some studies have reported a high suicide rate, however. Distress resulting only from conflict between gay men or lesbians and the societal value structure is not classifiable as a disorder. If the distress is sufficiently severe to warrant a diagnosis, adjustment disorder or a depressive disorder should be considered. Some gay men and lesbians with major depressive disorder may experience guilt and self-hatred that become directed toward their sexual orientation; then the desire for sexual reorientation is only a symptom of the depressive disorder.

Coming Out. According to Rochelle Klinger and Robert Cabaj, coming out is a "process by which an individual acknowledges his or her sexual orientation in the face of societal stigma and with successful resolution accepts himself or herself." The authors wrote:

> Successful coming out involves the individual accepting his or her sexual orientation and integrating it into all spheres (e.g., social, vocational, and familial). Another milestone that individuals and couples must eventually confront is the degree of disclosure of sexual orientation to the external world. Some degree of disclosure is probably necessary for successful coming out.

Difficulty negotiating coming out and disclosure is a common cause of relationship difficulties. For each person, problems resolving the coming out process can contribute to poor self-esteem caused by internalized homophobia and lead to deleterious effects on the person's ability to function in the relationship. Conflict can also arise within a relationship when partners disagree on the degree of disclosure.

LOVE AND INTIMACY

Freud postulated that psychological health could be determined by a person's ability to function well in two spheres, work and love. A person able to give and receive love with a minimum of fear and conflict has the capacity to develop genuinely intimate relationships with others. A desire to maintain closeness to the love object typifies being in love. Mature love is marked by the intimacy that is a special attribute of the relationship between two persons. When involved in an intimate relationship, the person actively strives for the growth and happiness of the loved person. Sex frequently acts as a catalyst in forming and maintaining intimate relationships. The quality of intimacy in a mature sexual relationship is what Rollo May called "active receiving," in which a person, while loving, permits himself or herself to be loved. May describes the value of sexual love as an expansion of self-awareness, the experience of tenderness, an increase of self-affirmation and pride, and sometimes, at the moment of orgasm, loss of feeling of separateness. In that setting, sex and love are reciprocally enhancing and healthily fused.

Some persons experience conflicts that prevent them from fusing tender and passionate impulses. This can inhibit the expression of sexuality in a relationship, interfere with feelings of closeness to another person, and diminish a person's sense of adequacy and self-esteem. When these problems are severe, they may prevent the formation of, or commitment to, an intimate relationship.

SEX AND THE LAW

Medicine and the law both assess the impact of sexuality on the individual and society and determine what is healthy or legal behavior. Appropriateness or legality of sexual behavior, however, is not always viewed the same way by professionals in both disciplines. The issues at the interface of sexual science and the law often are emotionally charged and reflect cultural divisions about acceptable sexual mores. They include abortion, pornography, prostitution, sex education, the treatment of sex offenders, and the right to sexual privacy, among other issues. Laws regarding these issues (e.g., criminalization of oral or anal sex by consenting adults, or the need for parental permission by minors who are requesting an abortion) vary from state to state.

TAKING A SEX HISTORY

A sex history provides important information about patients, regardless of the presence of a sexual disorder or whether that is the patient's chief complaint. The information can be obtained gradually, through open-ended questions. The outline in Table 13.1–4 provides a guide to the topics to be covered and a structure that can be used when time is limited.

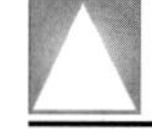

Table 13.1–4
Taking a Sex History

I. Identifying data
  A. Age
  B. Sex
  C. Occupation
  D. Relationship status—single, married, number of times previously married, separated, divorced, cohabiting, serious involvement, casual dating (difficulty forming or keeping relationships should be assessed throughout the interview)
  E. Sexual orientation—heterosexual, homosexual, or bisexual (this may also be ascertained later in the interview)
II. Current functioning
  A. Unsatisfactory to highly satisfactory
  B. If unsatisfactory, why?
  C. Feeling about partner satisfaction
  D. Dysfunctions?—e.g., lack of desire, erectile disorder, inhibited female interest/arousal, anorgasmia, premature ejaculation, retarded ejaculation, pain associated with intercourse (dysfunction discussed below)
    1. Onset—lifelong or acquired
      a. If acquired, when?
      b. Did onset coincide with drug use (medications or illegal recreational drugs), life stresses (e.g., loss of job, birth of child), interpersonal difficulties
    2. Generalized—occurs in most situations or with most partners
    3. Situational
      a. Only with current partner
      b. In any committed relationship
      c. Only with masturbation
      d. In socially proscribed circumstance (e.g., affair)
      e. In definable circumstance (e.g., very late at night, in parental home, when partner initiated sex play)
  E. Frequency—partnered sex (coital and noncoital sex play)
  F. Desire/libido—how often are sexual feelings, thoughts, fantasies, dreams, experienced? (per day, week, etc.)
  G. Description of typical sexual interaction
    1. Manner of initiation or invitation (e.g., verbal or physical? Does same person always initiate?)
    2. Presence, type, and extent of foreplay (e.g., kissing, caressing, manual or oral genital stimulation)
    3. Coitus? positions used?
    4. Verbalization during sex? if so, what kind?
    5. Afterplay? (whether sex act is completed or disrupted by dysfunction); typical activities (e.g., holding, talking, return to daily activities, sleeping)
    6. Feeling after sex: relaxed, tense, angry, loving
  H. Sexual compulsivity?—intrusion of sexual thoughts or participation in sexual activities to a degree that interferes with relationships or work, requires deception and may endanger the patient

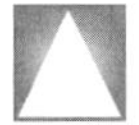

Table 13.1–4
Taking a Sex History (Continued)

III. Past sexual history
  A. Childhood sexuality
    1. Parental attitudes about sex—degree of openness of reserve (assess unusual prudery or seductiveness)
    2. Parents' attitudes about nudity and modesty
    3. Learning about sex
      a. From parents? (initiated by child's questions or parent volunteering information? which parent? what was child's age?) subjects covered (e.g., pregnancy, birth, intercourse, menstruation, nocturnal emission, masturbation)
      b. From books, magazines, or friends at school or through religious group?
      c. Significant misinformation
      d. Feeling about information
    4. Viewing or hearing primal scene—reaction?
    5. Viewing sex play or intercourse of person other than parent
    6. Viewing sex between pets or other animals
  B. Childhood sex activities
    1. Genital self-stimulation before adolescence; age? reaction if apprehended?
    2. Awareness of self as boy or girl; bathroom sensual activities? (regarding urine, feces, odor, enemas)
    3. Sexual play or exploration with another child (playing doctor)—type of activity (e.g., looking, manual touching, genital touching); reactions or consequences if apprehended (by whom?)

IV. Adolescence
  A. Age of onset of puberty—development of secondary sex characteristics, age of menarche for girl, wet dreams or first ejaculation for boy (preparation for and reaction to)
  B. Sense of self as feminine or masculine—body image, acceptance by peers (opposite sex and same sex), sense of sexual desirability, onset of coital fantasies
  C. Sex activities
    1. Masturbation—age begun; ever punished or prohibited? method used, accompanying fantasies, frequency (questions about masturbation and fantasies are among the most sensitive for patients to answer)
    2. Homosexual activities—ongoing or rare and experimental episodes, approached by others? If homosexual, has there been any heterosexual experimentation?
    3. Dating—casual or steady, description of first crush, infatuation, or first love.
    4. Experiences of kissing, necking, petting ("making out" or "fooling around"), age begun, frequency, number of partners, circumstances, type(s) of activity
    5. Orgasm—when first experienced? (may not be experienced during adolescence), with masturbation, during sleep, or with partner? with intercourse or other sex play? frequency?
    6. First coitus—age, circumstances, partner, reactions (may not be experienced during adolescence); contraception and/or safe sex precautions used

V. Adult sexual activities (may be experienced by some adolescents)
  A. Premarital sex
    1. Types of sex play experiences—frequency of sexual interactions, types and number of partners
    2. Contraception and/or safe sex precautions used
    3. First coitus (if not experienced in adolescence) age, circumstances, partner
    4. Cohabitation—age begun, duration, description of partner, sexual fidelity, types of sexual activity, frequency, satisfaction, number of cohabiting relationships, reasons for breakup(s)
    5. Engagement—age, activity during engagement period with fiancé(e), with others; length of engagement
  B. Marriage (if multiple marriages have occurred, explore sexual activity, reasons for marriage, and reasons for divorce in each marriage)
    1. Types and frequency of sexual interaction—describe typical sexual interaction (see above), satisfaction with sex life? view of partner's feeling
    2. First sexual experience with spouse—when? what were the circumstances? was it satisfying? disappointing?
    3. Honeymoon—setting, duration, pleasant or unpleasant, sexually active, frequency? problems? compatibility?
    4. Effect of pregnancies and children on marital sex
    5. Extramarital sex—number of incidents, partner; emotional attachment to extramarital partners? feelings about extramarital sex
    6. Postmarital masturbation—frequency? effect on marital sex?
    7. Extramarital sex by partner—effect on interviewee
    8. Ménage à trois or multiple sex (swinging)
    9. Areas of conflict in marriage (e.g., parenting, finances, division of responsibilities, priorities)

VI. Sex after widowhood, separation, divorce—celibacy, orgasms in sleep, masturbation, noncoital sex play, intercourse (number of and relationship to partners), other

VII. Special issues
  A. History of rape, incest, sexual or physical abuse
  B. Spousal abuse (current)
  C. Chronic illness (physical or psychiatric)
  D. History or presence of sexually transmitted diseases
  E. Fertility problems
  F. Abortions, miscarriages, or unwanted or illegitimate pregnancies
  G. Gender identity conflict (e.g., transsexualism, wearing clothes of opposite sex)
  H. Paraphilias (e.g., fetishes, voyeurism, sadomasochism)

▲ 13.2 Sexual Dysfunctions

The essential features of sexual dysfunctions are an inability to respond to sexual stimulation, or the experience of pain during the sexual act. Dysfunction can be defined by disturbance in the subjective sense of pleasure or desire usually associated with sex, or by the objective performance. In the *Diagnostic and Statistical Manual of Mental Disorders*, fifth edition (DSM-5), the sexual dysfunctions include male hypoactive sexual desire disorder, female sexual interest/arousal disorder, erectile disorder, female orgasmic disorder, delayed ejaculation, premature (early) ejaculation, genito-pelvic pain/penetration disorder, substance/medication induced sexual dysfunction, other specified sexual dysfunction, and unspecified sexual dysfunction. Sexual dysfunctions are diagnosed only when they are a major part of the clinical picture. If more than one dysfunction exists, they should all be diagnosed. Sexual dysfunctions can be lifelong or acquired, generalized or situational, and result from psychological factors, physiological factors, combined factors, and numerous stressors including prohibitive cultural mores, health and partner issues, and relationship conflicts. If the dysfunction is attributable entirely to a general medical condition, substance use, or adverse effects of medication, then sexual dysfunction due to a general medical condition or substance-induced sexual dysfunction is diagnosed. In DSM-5, specification of the severity of the dysfunction is indicated by noting whether the patient's distress is mild, moderate, or severe.

Sexual dysfunctions are frequently associated with other mental disorders, such as depressive disorders, anxiety disorders, personality disorders, and schizophrenia. In many instances, a sexual dysfunction may be diagnosed in conjunction with another psychiatric disorder. If the dysfunction is largely attributable to an underlying psychiatric disorder, only the underlying disorder should be diagnosed. Sexual dysfunctions are usually self-perpetuating, with the patients increasingly subjected to ongoing performance anxiety and a concomitant inability to experience pleasure. In relationships, the sexually functional partner often reacts with distress or anger due to feelings of deprivation or a sense that he or she is an insufficiently attractive or adequate sexual partner. In such cases, the clinician must consider whether the sexual problem preceded or arose from relationship difficulties and weigh whether a diagnosis of sexual dysfunction relevant to relationship issues is more appropriate.

DESIRE, INTEREST, AND AROUSAL DISORDERS

Male Hypoactive Sexual Desire Disorder

This dysfunction is characterized by a deficiency or absence of sexual fantasies and desire for sexual activity for a minimum duration of approximately 6 months. Men for whom this is a lifelong condition have never experienced many spontaneous erotic/sexual thoughts. Minimal spontaneous sexual thinking or minimal desire for sex ahead of sexual experiences is not considered a diagnosable disorder in women, particularly if desire is triggered during the sexual encounter. The reported prevalence of low desire is greatest at the younger and older ends of the age spectrum, with only 2 percent of men ages 16 to 44 affected by this disorder. A reported 6 percent of men ages 18 to 24, and 40 percent of men ages 66 to 74, have problems with sexual desire. Some men may confuse decreased desire with decreased activity. Their erotic thoughts and fantasies are undiminished, but they no longer act on them due to health issues, unavailability of a partner, or another sexual dysfunction such as erectile disorder.

A variety of causative factors are associated with low sexual desire. Patients with desire problems often use inhibition of desire defensively, to protect against unconscious fears about sex. Sigmund Freud conceptualized low sexual desire as the result of inhibition during the phallic psychosexual phase of development and of unresolved oedipal conflicts. Some men, fixated at the phallic state of development, are fearful of the vagina and believe that they will be castrated if they approach it. Freud called this concept *vagina dentata;* he theorized that men avoid contact with the vagina when they unconsciously believe that the vagina has teeth. Lack of desire can also result from chronic stress, anxiety, or depression.

Abstinence from sex for a prolonged period sometimes results in suppression of sexual impulses. Loss of desire may also be an expression of hostility to a partner or the sign of a deteriorating relationship. The presence of desire depends on several factors: biological drive, adequate self-esteem, the ability to accept oneself as a sexual person, the availability of an appropriate partner, and a good relationship in nonsexual areas with a partner. Damage to, or absence of, any of these factors can diminish desire.

In making the diagnosis, clinicians must evaluate a patient's age, general health, any medication regimen, and life stresses. The clinician must attempt to establish a baseline of sexual interest before the disorder began. The need for sexual contact and satisfaction varies among persons and over time in any given person. The diagnosis should not be made unless the lack of desire is a source of distress to a patient.

Female Sexual Interest/Arousal Disorder

The combination of interest (or desire) and arousal into one dysfunction category reflects the recognition that women do not necessarily move stepwise from desire to arousal, but often experience desire synchronously with, or even following, beginning feelings of arousal. This is particularly true for women in long-term relationships. As a corollary, women experiencing sexual dysfunction may experience either/or both inability to feel interest or arousal, and they may often have difficulty achieving orgasm or experience pain in addition. Some may experience dysfunction across the entire range of sexual response/pleasure. Complaints in this dysfunction category present variously as a decrease or paucity of erotic feelings, thoughts, or fantasies; a decreased impulse to initiate sex; a decreased or absent receptivity to partner overtures; or an inability to respond to partner stimulation.

A complicating factor in this diagnosis is that a subjective sense of arousal is often poorly correlated with genital lubrication in both normal and dysfunctional women. Therefore, complaints of lack of pleasure are sufficient for this diagnosis even when vaginal lubrication and congestion are present. A woman complaining of lack of arousal may lubricate vaginally, but may not experience a subjective sense of excitement. Some studies using functional magnetic resonance imaging (fMRI) have revealed a low correlation between brain activation in areas controlling genital response and simultaneous ratings of subjective arousal. Physiological studies of sexual dysfunctions indicate that a hormonal pattern may contribute to responsiveness in women who have arousal dysfunction. William Masters and Virginia Johnson found that women are particularly desirous of sex before the onset of the menses. Other women report feeling the greatest sexual excitement immediately after the menses or at the time of ovulation. Alterations in testosterone, estrogen, prolactin, and thyroxin levels have been implicated in female sexual arousal disorder. In addition, medications with antihistaminic or anticholinergic properties cause a decrease in vaginal lubrication.

Factors such as life stresses, aging, menopause, adequate sexual stimulation, general health, and medication regimen must be evaluated before making this diagnosis. Relationship problems are particularly relevant to acquired interest/arousal disorder. In one study of couples with markedly decreased sexual interaction, the most prevalent etiology was marital discord.

Male Erectile Disorder

Male erectile disorder was historically called *impotence*. The term was dropped for a more medical designation, but also because it was considered derogatory and had negative connotations for the man with the problem. However, it describes with accuracy the feelings of powerlessness, helplessness, and resultant low self-esteem men with this dysfunction frequently suffer. A man with lifelong male erectile disorder has never been able to obtain an erection sufficient for insertion. In acquired male erectile disorder, a man has successfully achieved penetration at some time in his sexual life but is later unable to do so. In situational male erectile disorder, a man is able to have coitus in certain circumstances but not in others; for example, he may function effectively with a prostitute but be unable to have an erection when with his partner.

Acquired male erectile disorder has been reported in 10 to 20 percent of all men. Freud declared it common among his patients. Erectile disorder is the chief complaint of more than 50 percent of all men treated for sexual disorders. Lifelong male erectile disorder is rare; it occurs in about 1 percent of men younger than age 35. The incidence of erectile disorder increases with age. It has been reported variously as 2 to 8 percent of the young adult population. Alfred Kinsey reported that 75 percent of all men were impotent at age 80. There is a reported incidence of 40 to 50 percent in men between ages of 60 and 70. All men older than 40, Masters and Johnson claimed, have a fear of impotence, which the researchers believed reflected the masculine fear of loss of virility with advancing age. Male erectile disorder, however, is not universal in aging men; having an available sex partner is related to continuing potency, as is a history of consistent sexual activity and the absence of vascular, neurologic, or endocrine disease. Twenty percent of men fear erectile dysfunction prior to their first coitus; the reported incidence of actual erectile dysfunction during first coitus is 8 percent. As Stephen Levine has stated, the first sexual encounter "is a horse race between excitement and anxiety."

Male erectile disorder can be organic or psychological, or a combination of both, but in young and middle-aged men the cause is usually psychological. A good history is of primary importance in determining the cause of the dysfunction. If a man reports having spontaneous erections at times when he does not plan to have intercourse, having morning erections, or having good erections with masturbation or with partners other than his usual one, the organic causes of his erectile disorder can be considered negligible, and costly diagnostic procedures can be avoided. Male erectile disorder caused by a general medical condition or a pharmacological substance is discussed later in this section.

Freud ascribed one type of erectile disorder to an inability to reconcile feelings of affection toward a woman with feelings of desire for her. Men with such conflicting feelings can function only with women whom they see as degraded (Madonna–Putana complex). Other factors that have been cited as contributing to impotence include a punitive superego, an inability to trust, and feelings of inadequacy or a sense of being undesirable as a partner. A man may be unable to express a sexual impulse because of fear, anxiety, anger, or moral prohibition. In an ongoing relationship, the disorder may reflect difficulties between the partners, particularly when a man cannot communicate his needs or his anger in a direct and constructive way. In addition, episodes of erectile disorder are reinforcing, with the man becoming increasingly anxious before each sexual encounter.

Mr. Y came for therapy after his wife complained about their lack of sexual interaction. The patient avoided sex because of his frequent erectile dysfunction and the painful feelings of inadequacy he suffered after his "failures." He presented as an articulate, gentle, and self-blaming man.

He was faithful to his wife but masturbated frequently. His fantasies involved explicit sadistic components, including hanging and biting women. The contrast between his angry, aggressive fantasies and his loving, considerate behavior toward his wife symbolized his conflicts about his sexuality, his masculinity, and his mixed feelings about women. He was diagnosed with erectile disorder, situational type.

ORGASM DISORDERS

Female Orgasmic Disorder

Female orgasmic disorder, sometimes called *inhibited female orgasm* or *anorgasmia,* is defined as the recurrent or persistent inhibition of female orgasm, as manifested by the recurrent delay in, or absence of orgasm after a normal sexual excitement phase that a clinician judges to be adequate in focus, intensity, and duration—in short, a woman's inability to achieve orgasm by masturbation or coitus. Women who can achieve orgasm by one of these methods are not necessarily categorized as anorgasmic, although some sexual inhibition may be postulated. The complaint is reported by the woman, herself. However, some anorgasmic women are not distressed by the lack of climax and derive pleasure from sexual activity. In the latter instance, a woman may present with this complaint because her partner is troubled by her lack of orgasm.

Research on the physiology of the female sexual response has shown that orgasms caused by clitoral stimulation and those caused by vaginal stimulation are physiologically identical. Freud's theory that women must give up clitoral sensitivity for vaginal sensitivity to achieve sexual maturity is now considered misleading, but some women report that they gain a special sense of satisfaction from an orgasm precipitated by coitus. Some researchers attribute this satisfaction to the psychological feeling of closeness engendered by the act of coitus, but others maintain that the coital orgasm is a physiologically different experience. Many women achieve orgasm during coitus by a combination of manual clitoral stimulation and penile vaginal stimulation.

A woman with lifelong female orgasmic disorder has never experienced orgasm by any kind of stimulation. A woman with acquired orgasmic disorder has previously experienced at least one orgasm, regardless of the circumstances or means of stimulation, whether by masturbation or while dreaming during sleep. Studies have shown that women achieve orgasm more consistently with masturbation than with partnered sex. Kinsey found that 5 percent of married women older than age 35 years had never achieved orgasm by any means. The incidence of never having experienced orgasm is reported as 10 percent among all women. The incidence of orgasm increases with age. According to Kinsey, the first orgasm occurs during adolescence in about 50 percent of women as a result of masturbation or genital caressing with a partner; the rest usually experience orgasm as they get older. Lifelong female orgasmic disorder is more common among unmarried women than married women. Increased orgasmic potential in women older than 35 years of age has been explained on the basis of less psychological inhibition, greater sexual experience, or both.

Acquired female orgasmic disorder is a common complaint in clinical populations. One clinical treatment facility reported having about four times as many nonorgasmic women in its practice as female patients with all other sexual disorders. In another study, 46 percent of women complained of difficulty reaching orgasm. Inhibition of arousal and orgasmic problems often occur together. The overall prevalence of female orgasmic disorder from all causes is estimated to be 30 percent. A recent twin study suggests that orgasmic dysfunction in some females has a genetic basis and cannot be attributed solely to psychological differences. That study demonstrated an estimated heritability for difficulty reaching orgasm with intercourse of 34 percent and an estimated heritability in women who could not climax with masturbation of 45 percent.

Numerous psychological factors are associated with female orgasmic disorder. They include fears of impregnation, rejection by a sex partner, and damage to the vagina; hostility toward men; poor body image; and feelings of guilt about sexual impulses. Some women equate orgasm with loss of control or with aggressive, destructive, or violent impulses; their fear of these impulses may be expressed through inhibition of arousal or orgasm. Cultural expectations and social restrictions on women are also relevant. Many women have grown up to believe that sexual pleasure is not a natural entitlement for so-called decent women. Nonorgasmic women may be otherwise symptom free or may experience frustration in a variety of ways; they may have such pelvic complaints as lower abdominal pain, itching, and vaginal discharge, as well as increased tension, irritability, and fatigue.

Delayed Ejaculation

In male delayed ejaculation, sometimes called *retarded ejaculation,* a man achieves ejaculation during coitus with great difficulty, if at all. The problem is rarely present with masturbation, but appears as a problem during partnered sex. A man with lifelong delayed ejaculation has never been able to ejaculate during partnered sexual activity. The problem is usually most pronounced during coital activity. The disorder is diagnosed as acquired if it develops after previously normal functioning. Some researchers think that orgasm and ejaculation should be differentiated, especially in the case of men who ejaculate but complain of a decreased or absent subjective sense of pleasure during the orgasmic experience (orgasmic anhedonia).

The incidence of delayed ejaculation is much lower than the incidence of premature ejaculation or erectile disorder. Masters and Johnson reported an incidence of delayed ejaculation of only 3.8 percent in one group of 447 men with sexual dysfunctions. A general prevalence of 5 percent has been reported. However, an increase in the presentation of this disorder in sex therapy programs has been seen in the last decade. This has been attributed to the increasing use of antidepressants, which can have a side effect of delayed ejaculation, as well as a high use of Internet pornography sites. These sites offer a level of stimulation involving such variety of people and acts that they may inure the man to the stimulation of more typical partnered activity. Recent studies of adolescent males who use these sites frequently, prior to live sexual interaction, have reported that these teens do not develop neuronal synapses that will enable them to respond to usual partnered interactions with sufficient pleasure to allow them to achieve climax.

Lifelong delayed ejaculation indicates severe psychopathology. A man may come from a rigid, puritanical background; he may perceive sex as sinful and the genitals as dirty; and he may have conscious or unconscious incest wishes and guilt. He usually has difficulty with closeness in areas beyond those of sexual relations. In a few cases, the condition is aggravated by an attention-deficit/hyperactivity disorder. A man's distractibility prevents sufficient arousal for climax to occur.

In an ongoing relationship, acquired male delayed ejaculation disorder frequently reflects interpersonal difficulties. The disorder may be a man's way of coping with real or fantasized changes in a relationship, such as plans for pregnancy about which the man is ambivalent, the loss of sexual attraction to the partner, or demands by the partner for greater commitment as expressed by sexual performance. In some men, the inability to ejaculate reflects unexpressed hostility toward a woman. The problem is more common among men with obsessive-compulsive disorder (OCD) than among others.

A couple presented with the man as the identified patient; he was unable to ejaculate with intercourse. He had always had difficulty reaching climax, except in rare circumstances. He ejaculated once when he was with two women at the same time and once when he was experimenting with cocaine. He currently was not using any substances except for a moderate use of alcohol. This patient was committed to his marriage, although he had extramarital sexual experiences. He did not ejaculate with coitus in those situations either, although he could climax with oral sex. He stated he was more interested in "the conquest" than in the sex itself. He could climax with masturbation, although he rarely masturbated himself, but went to massage parlors. He had issues with anger at women and considered his wife to be excessively critical.

He had difficulty doing any of the exercises that required him to pleasure his wife. His difficulty giving also made it hard for him to enjoy mutual pleasuring. It was easier for him to be the recipient of stimulation. Because of this patient's problems with impulsiveness, narcissism, and dependency, it was necessary to combine introspective psychotherapy with a regimen of behavioral exercises.

The patient was diagnosed with delayed ejaculation, lifelong type.

Premature (Early) Ejaculation

In premature ejaculation, men persistently or recurrently achieve orgasm and ejaculation before they wish to. The diagnosis is made when a man regularly ejaculates before or within approximately 1 minute after penetration. DSM-5 refers only to "vaginal penetration" in its diagnostic criteria, even though it is entirely possible for the disorder to occur in men who are homosexual and do not engage in vaginal penetration. DSM-5 defines the disorder as mild if ejaculation occurs within approximately 30 seconds to 1 minute of vaginal penetration, moderate if ejaculation occurs within approximately 15 to 30 seconds of vaginal penetration, and severe when ejaculation occurs at the start of sexual activity or within approximately 15 seconds of vaginal penetration. A difficulty with these specifiers involves time distortions, which patients make in both overestimating and underestimating time from penetration to climax and objective time measurements are obviously not possible. Clinicians need to consider factors that affect the duration of the excitement phase of the sexual response, such as age, the novelty of the sex partner, and the frequency of coitus. As with the other sexual dysfunctions, premature ejaculation is not diagnosed when it is caused exclusively by organic factors or when it is symptomatic of another clinical psychiatric syndrome.

Premature ejaculation is more commonly reported among college-educated men than among men with less education. The complaint is thought to be related to their concern for partner satisfaction, but the true cause of this increased frequency has not been determined. Premature ejaculation is the chief complaint of about 35 to 40 percent of men treated for sexual disorders. In DSM-5, the writers state that the disorder, with its newly defined time parameter, would now be an accurate diagnosis for only 1 to 3 percent of men. Some researchers divide men who experience premature ejaculation into two groups: those who are physiologically predisposed to climax quickly because of shorter nerve latency time and those with a psychogenic or behaviorally conditioned cause. Difficulty in ejaculatory control can be associated with anxiety regarding the sex act, with unconscious fears about the vagina, or with negative cultural conditioning. Men whose early sexual contacts occurred largely with prostitutes who demanded that the sex act proceed quickly or whose sexual contacts took place in situations in which discovery would be embarrassing (e.g., in a shared dormitory room or in the parental home) might have been conditioned to achieve orgasm rapidly. With young, inexperienced men, who have the problem, it may resolve in time. In ongoing relationships, the partner has a great influence on a premature ejaculator, and a stressful marriage exacerbates the disorder. The developmental background and the psychodynamics found in premature ejaculation and in erectile disorder are similar.

SEXUAL PAIN DISORDERS

Genito-Pelvic Pain/Penetration Disorder

In DSM-5, this disorder refers to one or more of the following complaints, of which any two or more may occur together: difficulty having intercourse; genito-pelvic pain; fear of pain or penetration; and tension of the pelvic floor muscles. Previously, these pain disorders were diagnosed as *dyspareunia* or *vaginismus*. These former diagnoses could coexist or one could lead to the other and could understandably lead to fear of pain with sex. Thus, it is reasonable to gather these diagnoses into one diagnostic category. For the purposes of clinical discussion, however, the distinct categories of dyspareunia and vaginismus remain clinically useful.

Dyspareunia

Dyspareunia is recurrent or persistent genital pain occurring before, during, or after intercourse. Dyspareunia is related to, and often coincides with, vaginismus. Repeated episodes of vaginismus can lead to dyspareunia and vice versa; in either case, somatic causes must be ruled out. A pain disorder should not be diagnosed when an organic basis for pain is found or when it is caused by a lack of lubrication. DSM-5 cites that 15 percent of women in North America report recurrent pain during intercourse.

In most cases, dynamic factors are considered causative. Chronic pelvic pain is a common complaint in women with a history of rape or childhood sexual abuse. Painful coitus can result from tension and anxiety about the sex act that cause women to involuntarily contract their pelvic floor muscles. The pain is real and makes intercourse unpleasant or unbearable. Anticipation of further pain may cause women to avoid coitus altogether. If a partner proceeds with intercourse regardless of a woman's state of readiness, the condition is aggravated. There is an increase in reported dyspareunia postmenopausally due to hormonally induced physiological changes in the vagina; however, specific complaints of difficulty having intercourse occur more often in premenopausal women. There is some increase in dyspareunia in the immediate postpartum population, but it is usually temporary. Dyspareunia may present as any of the four complaints listed under genito-pelvic pain/penetration disorder and should be diagnosed as genito-pelvic pain/penetration disorder.

Vaginismus

Defined as a constriction of the outer third of the vagina due to involuntary pelvic floor muscle tightening or spasm, vaginismus interferes with penile insertion and intercourse. This response may occur during a gynecological examination when involuntary vaginal constriction prevents the introduction of the speculum into the vagina. The diagnosis is not made when the dysfunction is caused exclusively by organic factors or when it is symptomatic of another mental disorder.

Vaginismus may be complete, that is no penetration of the vagina is possible, whether by the penis, fingers, a speculum during gynecologic exam, or even if the woman tries to use the smallest size tampon. Many women who discover this complaint when they become sexually active have avoided the use of tampons previously. In a less severe form of vaginismus, pelvic floor muscle tightening due to pain or fear of pain makes penetration difficult, but not impossible. Penetration may be achieved with the smallest size speculum or little fingers. In mild cases, the muscles relax after the initial difficulty with penetration and the woman can continue with sexual play, sometimes even with coitus.

Miss B was a 27-year-old single woman who presented for therapy because of an inability to have intercourse. She described episodes with a recent boyfriend in which he had tried vaginal penetration but had been unable to enter. The boyfriend did not have erectile dysfunction. Miss B experienced desire and was able to achieve orgasm through manual or oral stimulation. For almost a year, she and her boyfriend had sex play without intercourse. However, he complained increasingly about his frustration at the lack of coitus, which he had enjoyed in previous relationships. Miss B had a conscious fear of penetration and dreaded going to the gynecologist, although she was able to use tampons when she menstruated. She was diagnosed with genito-pelvic pain/penetration disorder, lifelong type.

Vaginismus is less prevalent than female orgasmic disorder. It most often afflicts highly educated women and those in high socioeconomic groups. Women with vaginismus may consciously wish to have coitus, but unconsciously wish to keep a penis from entering their bodies. A sexual trauma, such as rape, may cause vaginismus. Anticipation of pain at the first coital experience may cause vaginismus. Clinicians have noted that a strict religious upbringing in which sex is associated with sin is frequent in these patients. Other women have problems in dyadic relationships; if women feel emotionally abused by their partners, they may protest in this nonverbal fashion. Some women who have experienced significant pain in childhood due to surgical or dental interventions become guarded about any breach of body integrity and develop vaginismus. Vaginismus may present as any of the four complaints under genito-pelvic pain/penetration disorder and should be diagnosed as genito-pelvic pain/penetration disorder.

Table 13.2–1
Diseases and Other Medical Conditions Implicated in Male Erectile Disorder

Infectious and parasitic diseases	Neurological disorders
Elephantiasis	Multiple sclerosis
Mumps	Transverse myelitis
Cardiovascular disease[a]	Parkinson's disease
Atherosclerotic disease	Temporal lobe epilepsy
Aortic aneurysm	Traumatic and neoplastic spinal cord diseases[a]
Leriche's syndrome	Central nervous system tumor
Cardiac failure	Amyotrophic lateral sclerosis
Renal and urological disorders	Peripheral neuropathy
Peyronie's disease	General paresis
Chronic renal failure	Tabes dorsalis
Hydrocele and varicocele	Pharmacological factors
Hepatic disorders	Alcohol and other dependence-inducing substances (heroin, methadone, morphine, cocaine, amphetamines, and barbiturates)
Cirrhosis (usually associated with alcohol dependence)	Prescribed drugs (psychotropic drugs, antihypertensive drugs, estrogens, and antiandrogens)
Pulmonary disorders	Poisoning
Respiratory failure	Lead (plumbism)
Genetics	Herbicides
Klinefelter's syndrome	Surgical procedures[a]
Congenital penile vascular and structural abnormalities	Perineal prostatectomy
Nutritional disorders	Abdominal-perineal colon resection
Malnutrition	Sympathectomy (frequently interferes with ejaculation)
Vitamin deficiencies	Aortoiliac surgery
Obesity	Radical cystectomy
Endocrine disorders[a]	Retroperitoneal lymphadenectomy
Diabetes mellitus	Miscellaneous
Dysfunction of the pituitary-adrenal-testis axis	Radiation therapy
Acromegaly	Pelvic fracture
Addison's disease	Any severe systemic disease or debilitating condition
Chromophobe adenoma	
Adrenal neoplasia	
Myxedema	
Hyperthyroidism	

[a]In the United States, an estimated 2 million men are impotent because they have diabetes mellitus; an additional 300,000 are impotent because of other endocrine diseases; 1.5 million are impotent as a result of vascular disease; 180,000 because of multiple sclerosis; 400,000 because of traumas and fractures leading to pelvic fractures or spinal cord injuries; and another 650,000 are impotent as a result of radical surgery, including prostatectomies, colostomies, and cystectomies.

SEXUAL DYSFUNCTION DUE TO A GENERAL MEDICAL CONDITION

Male Erectile Disorder due to a General Medical Condition

The incidence of psychological, as opposed to organic, male erectile disorder has been the focus of many studies. Statistics indicate that 20 to 50 percent of men with erectile disorder have an organic basis for the disorder. A physiologic etiology is more likely in men older than 50 and the most likely cause in men older than age 60. The organic causes of male erectile disorder are listed in Table 13.2–1. Side effects of medication can impair male sexual functioning in a variety of ways (Table 13.2–2). Castration (removal of the testes) does not always lead to sexual dysfunction, because erection may still occur. A reflex arc, fired when the inner thigh is stimulated, passes through the sacral cord erectile center to account for the phenomenon.

A number of procedures, benign and invasive, are used to help differentiate organically caused erectile disorder from functional erectile disorder. The procedures include monitoring nocturnal penile tumescence (erections that occur during sleep), normally associated with rapid eye movement; monitoring tumescence with a strain gauge; measuring blood pressure in the penis with a penile plethysmograph or an ultrasound (Doppler) flowmeter, both of which assess blood flow in the internal pudendal artery; and measuring pudendal nerve

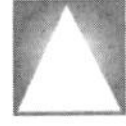

Table 13.2–2
Some Pharmacological Agents Implicated in Male Sexual Dysfunctions

Drug	Impairs Erection	Impairs Ejaculation
Psychiatric drugs		
Cyclic drugs[a]		
Imipramine (Tofranil)	+	+
Protriptyline (Vivactil)	+	+
Desipramine (Pertofrane)	+	+
Clomipramine (Anafranil)	+	+
Amitriptyline (Elavil)	+	+
Trazodone (Desyrel)[b]	–	–
Monoamine oxidase inhibitors		
Tranylcypromine (Parnate)	+	
Phenelzine (Nardil)	+	+
Pargyline (Eutonyl)	–	+
Isocarboxazid (Marplan)	–	+
Other mood-active drugs		
Lithium (Eskalith)	+	
Amphetamines	+	+
Fluoxetine (Prozac)[c]	–	+
Antipsychotics[d]		
Fluphenazine (Prolixin)	+	
Thioridazine (Mellaril)	+	+
Chlorprothixene (Taractan)	–	+
Mesoridazine (Serentil)	–	+
Perphenazine (Trilafon)	–	+
Trifluoperazine (Stelazine)	–	+
Reserpine (Serpasil)	+	+
Haloperidol (Haldol)	–	+
Antianxiety agent[e]		
Chlordiazepoxide (Librium)	–	+
Antihypertensive drugs		
Clonidine (Catapres)	+	
Methyldopa (Aldomet)	+	+
Spironolactone (Aldactone)	+	–
Hydrochlorothiazide	+	–
Guanethidine (Ismelin)	+	+
Commonly abused substances		
Alcohol	+	+
Barbiturates	+	+
Cannabis	+	–
Cocaine	+	+
Heroin	+	+
Methadone	+	–
Morphine	+	+
Miscellaneous drugs		
Antiparkinsonian agents	+	+
Clofibrate (Atromid-S)	+	–
Digoxin (Lanoxin)	+	–
Glutethimide (Doriden)	+	+
Indomethacin (Indocin)	+	–
Phentolamine (Regitine)	–	+
Propranolol (Inderal)	+	–

[a]The incidence of male erectile disorder associated with the use of tricyclic drugs is low.
[b]Trazodone has been causative in some cases of priapism.
[c]All SSRIs can produce sexual dysfunction, more commonly, in men.
[d]Impairment of sexual function is not a common complication of the use of antipsychotics. Priapism has occasionally occurred in association with the use of antipsychotics.
[e]Benzodiazepines have been reported to decrease libido, but in some patients the diminution of anxiety caused by those drugs enhances sexual function.

latency time. Other diagnostic tests that delineate organic bases for impotence include glucose tolerance tests, plasma hormone assays, liver and thyroid function tests, prolactin and follicle-stimulating hormone (FSH) determinations, and cystometric examinations. Invasive diagnostic studies include penile arteriography, infusion cavernosonography, and radioactive xenon penography. Invasive procedures require expert interpretation and are used only for patients who are candidates for vascular reconstructive procedures.

Dyspareunia due to a General Medical Condition

An estimated 30 percent of all surgical procedures on the female genital area result in temporary dyspareunia. In addition, 30 to 40 percent of women with the complaint who are seen in sex therapy clinics have pelvic pathology. Organic abnormalities leading to dyspareunia and vaginismus include irritated or infected hymenal remnants, episiotomy scars, Bartholin's gland infection, various forms of vaginitis and cervicitis, endometriosis, and adenomyosis. Postcoital pain has been reported by women with myomata, endometriosis, and adenomyosis, and is attributed to the uterine contractions during orgasm. Postmenopausal women may have dyspareunia resulting from thinning of the vaginal mucosa and reduced lubrication.

Two conditions not readily apparent on physical examination that produce dyspareunia are vulvar vestibulitis and interstitial cystitis. The former may present with chronic vulvar pain and the latter produces pain most intensely following orgasm. Dyspareunia can also occur in men, but it is uncommon and is usually associated with an organic condition, such as Peyronie's disease, which consists of sclerotic plaques on the penis that cause penile curvature.

Male Hypoactive Sexual Desire Disorder and Female Interest/Arousal Disorder due to a General Medical Condition

Sexual desire commonly decreases after major illness or surgery, particularly when the body image is affected after such procedures as mastectomy, ileostomy, hysterectomy, and prostatectomy. Illnesses that deplete a person's energy, chronic conditions that require physical and psychological adaptation, and serious illnesses that can cause a person to become depressed can all markedly lessen sexual desire.

In some cases, biochemical correlates are associated with hypoactive sexual desire disorder (Table 13.2–3). A recent study found markedly lower levels of serum testosterone in men complaining of low desire than in normal controls in a sleep-laboratory situation. Drugs that depress the central nervous system (CNS) or decrease testosterone production can decrease desire.

Other Male Sexual Dysfunction due to a General Medical Condition

Delayed ejaculation can have physiological causes and can occur after surgery on the genitourinary tract, such as prostatectomy. It may also be associated with Parkinson's disease

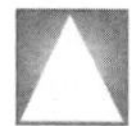

Table 13.2–3
Neurophysiology of Sexual Dysfunction

	DA	5-HT	NE	ACh	Clinical Correlation
Erection	↑	°	α, β ↓↑	M	Antipsychotics may lead to erectile dysfunction (DA block): DA agonists may lead to enhanced erection and libido; priapism with trazodone (α_1, block); β-blockers may lead to impotence
Ejaculation and orgasm	°	± ↓	α_1 ↑	M	α-Blockers (tricyclic drugs, MAOIs, thioridazine) may lead to impaired ejaculation; 5-HT agents may inhibit orgasm

↑, facilities; ↓, inhibits or decreases; ±, some; ACh, acetylcholine; DA, dopamine; 5-HT, serotonin; M, modulates; NE, norepinephrine; °, minimal.
Reprinted from Segraves R. *Psychiatric Times*. 1990.

and other neurological disorders involving the lumbar or sacral sections of the spinal cord. The antihypertensive drug guanethidine monosulfate (Ismelin), methyldopa (Aldomet), the phenothiazines, the tricyclic drugs, and the selective serotonin reuptake inhibitors (SSRIs), among others, have been implicated in retarded ejaculation. In addition, delayed ejaculation must be differentiated from retrograde ejaculation, in which ejaculation occurs but the seminal fluid passes backward into the bladder. Retrograde ejaculation always has an organic cause. It can develop after genitourinary surgery and it is also associated with medications that have anticholinergic adverse effects, such as the phenothiazines.

Other Female Sexual Dysfunction due to a General Medical Condition

Some medical conditions—specifically, endocrine diseases such as hypothyroidism, diabetes mellitus, and primary hyperprolactinemia—can affect a woman's ability to have orgasms. Several drugs also affect some women's capacity to have orgasms (Table 13.2–4). Antihypertensive medications, CNS stimulants, tricyclic drugs, SSRIs, and, frequently, monoamine oxidase inhibitors (MAOIs) have interfered with female orgasmic capacity. One study of women taking MAOIs, however, found that after 16 to 18 weeks of pharmacotherapy, the adverse effect of the medication disappeared and the women were able to re-experience orgasms, although they continued taking an undiminished dose of the drug.

Substance/Medication-Induced Sexual Dysfunction

The diagnosis of substance-induced sexual dysfunction is used when evidence of substance intoxication or withdrawal is apparent from the history, physical examination, or laboratory findings. The disturbance in sexual function must be predominant in the clinical picture. Distressing sexual dysfunction occurs soon after significant substance intoxication or withdrawal, or after exposure to a medication or a change in medication use. Specified substances include alcohol, amphetamines or related substances, cocaine, opioids, sedatives, hypnotics, or anxiolytics, and other or unknown substances.

Abused recreational substances affect sexual function in various ways. In small doses, many substances enhance sexual performance by decreasing inhibition or anxiety or by causing a temporary elevation of mood. With continued use, however, erectile engorgement and orgasmic and ejaculatory capacities become impaired. The abuse of sedatives, anxiolytics, hypnotics, and particularly opiates and opioids nearly always depresses desire. Alcohol may foster the initiation of sexual activity by removing inhibition, but it also impairs performance. Cocaine and amphetamines produce the following similar effects: Although no direct evidence indicates that sexual drive is enhanced, users initially have feelings of increased energy and may become sexually active; ultimately, dysfunction occurs. Men usually go through two stages: an experience of prolonged erection without ejaculation, and then a gradual loss of erectile capability.

Patients recovering from substance dependency may need therapy to regain sexual function, partly because of psychological readjustment to a nondependent state. Many substance abusers have always had difficulty with intimate interactions. Others who spent their crucial developmental years under the influence of a substance have missed the experiences that would have enabled them to learn social and sexual skills.

Table 13.2–4
Some Antipsychotic Drugs Implemented in Inhibited Female Orgasm[a]

Tricyclic antidepressants
Imipramine (Tofranil)
Clomipramine (Anafranil)
Nortriptyline (Aventyl)
Monoamine oxidase inhibitors
Tranylcypromine (Parnate)
Phenelzine (Nardil)
Isocarboxazid (Marplan)
Dopamine receptor antagonists
Thioridazine (Mellaril)
Trifluoperazine (Stelazine)

Selective serotonin reuptake inhibitors
Fluoxetine (Prozac)
Paroxetine (Paxil)
Sertraline (Zoloft)
Fluvoxamine (Luvox)
Citalopram (Celexa)

[a]The interrelation between female sexual dysfunction and pharmacological agents has been less extensively evaluated than male reactions. Oral contraceptives are reported to decrease libido in some women, and some drugs with anticholinergic side effects may impair arousal as well as orgasm. Prolonged use of oral contraceptives may also cause physiologic menopausal-like changes resulting in genito-pelvic pain/penetration disorder. Benzodiazepines have been reported to decrease libido, but in some patients the diminution of anxiety caused by those drugs enhances sexual function. Both increase and decrease in libido have been reported with psychoactive agents. It is difficult to separate those effects from the underlying condition or from improvement of the condition. Sexual dysfunction associated with the use of a drug disappears when use of the drug is discontinued.

Pharmacological Agents Implicated in Sexual Dysfunction

Almost every pharmacological agent, particularly those used in psychiatry, has been associated with an effect on sexuality. In men, these effects include decreased sex drive, erectile failure, decreased volume of ejaculate, and delayed or retrograde ejaculation. In women, decreased sex drive, decreased vaginal lubrication, inhibited or delayed orgasm, and decreased or absent vaginal contractions may occur. Drugs may also enhance the sexual responses and increase the sex drive, but this is less common than adverse effects. The effects of psychoactive drugs are detailed later in this section.

Antipsychotic Drugs. Most antipsychotic drugs are dopamine receptor antagonists that also block adrenergic and cholinergic receptors, thus accounting for the adverse sexual effects (Table 13.2–5). Chlorpromazine (Thorazine) and trifluoperazine (Stelazine) are potent anticholinergics, and they impair erection and ejaculation. With some drugs, the seminal fluid backs up into the bladder rather than being propelled through the penile urethra. Patients still have a pleasurable sensation, but the orgasm is dry. When urinating after orgasm, the urine may be milky white because it contains the ejaculate. The condition is startling but harmless. Paradoxically, some rare cases of priapism have been reported with antipsychotics.

Antidepressant Drugs. The tricyclic and tetracyclic antidepressants have anticholinergic effects that interfere with erection and delay ejaculation. Because the anticholinergic effects vary among the cyclic antidepressants, those with the fewest effects (e.g., desipramine [Norpramin]) produce the fewest sexual adverse effects. The effects of the tricyclics and tetracyclics have not been documented sufficiently in women; however, few women seem to complain of any effects.

Table 13.2–5
Diagnostic Issues with Sex and Some Antipsychotic Drugs

Differential diagnosis of drug-induced sexual dysfunction	Problem after drug therapy started or drug overdose Problem not situation or partner specific Not a lifelong or recurrent problem No obvious nonpharmacological precipitant Dissipates with drug discontinuation
Antipsychotic drugs and ejaculatory problems	Perphenazine Chlorpromazine Trifluoperazine Haloperidol Mesoridazine Chlorprothixene
Antipsychotic drugs and priapism	Perphenazine Mesoridazine Chlorpromazine Thioridazine Fluphenazine Molindone Risperidone Clozapine

Table by R. T. Segraves, M.D.

Some men report increased sensitivity of the glans that is pleasurable and that does not interfere with erection, although it delays ejaculation. In some cases, however, the tricyclic causes painful ejaculation, perhaps as the result of interference with seminal propulsion caused by interference with, in turn, urethral, prostatic, vas, and epididymal smooth muscle contractions. Clomipramine (Anafranil) has been reported to increase sex drive in some persons. Selegiline (Deprenyl), a selective MAO type B (MAO_B) inhibitor, and bupropion (Wellbutrin) have also been reported to increase sex drive, possibly by dopaminergic activity and increased production of norepinephrine.

Venlafaxine (Effexor) and the SSRIs most often have adverse effects because of the rise in serotonin levels. A lowering of the sex drive and difficulty reaching orgasm occur in both sexes. Reversal of those negative effects has been achieved with cyproheptadine (Periactin), an antihistamine with antiserotonergic effects, and with methylphenidate (Ritalin), which has adrenergic effects. Trazodone (Desyrel) is associated with the rare occurrence of priapism, the symptom of prolonged erection in the absence of sexual stimuli. That symptom appears to result from the α_2-adrenergic antagonism of trazodone.

The MAOIs affect biogenic amines broadly. Accordingly, they produce impaired erection, delayed or retrograde ejaculation, vaginal dryness, and inhibited orgasm. Tranylcypromine (Parnate) has a paradoxical sexually stimulating effect in some persons, possibly as a result of its amphetamine-like properties.

Mr. W presented with the complaint of inability to achieve orgasm. His problem dated from the time, 18 months previously, when he had been placed on fluoxetine (Prozac). Before that time, he had been able to achieve orgasm through masturbation and through coitus with his wife.

Mr. W tried several other SSRIs, as well as venlafaxine, but the side effect of delayed ejaculation persisted. None of the usual antidotes to SSRI-induced anorgasmia proved effective, and the patient then was tried on antidepressants of other categories. Mr. W was able to respond to bupropion and clonazepam (Klonopin). This combination treated his depression and anxiety, and his delayed ejaculation resolved.

He was diagnosed with pharmacologically induced delayed ejaculation.

GENERAL EFFECTS. Because depression is associated with a decreased libido, varying levels of sexual dysfunction and anhedonia are part of the disease process. Some patients report improved sexual functioning as their depression improves as a result of antidepressant medication. The phenomenon makes the evaluation of sexual side effects difficult; also, the side effects may disappear with time, perhaps because a biogenic amine homeostatic mechanism comes into play.

Lithium. Lithium (Eskalith) regulates mood and, in the manic state, may reduce hypersexuality, possibly by a dopamine antagonist activity. In some patients, impaired erection has been reported.

Sympathomimetics. Psychostimulants, which are sometimes used in the treatment of depression, include amphetamines, methylphenidate, and pemoline (Cylert), which raise the plasma levels of norepinephrine and dopamine. Libido is increased; however, with prolonged use, men may experience a loss of desire and erections.

α-Adrenergic and β-Adrenergic Receptor Antagonists. α-Adrenergic and β-adrenergic receptor antagonists are used in the treatment of hypertension, angina, and certain cardiac arrhythmias. They diminish tonic sympathetic nerve outflow from vasomotor centers in the brain. As a result, they can cause impotence, decrease the volume of ejaculate, and produce retrograde ejaculation. Changes in libido have been reported in both sexes.

Suggestions have been made to use the side effects of drugs therapeutically. Thus, a drug that delays or interferes with ejaculation (e.g., fluoxetine) might be used to treat premature ejaculation.

Anticholinergics. The anticholinergics block cholinergic receptors and include such drugs as amantadine (Symmetrel) and benztropine (Cogentin). They produce dryness of the mucous membranes (including those of the vagina) and erectile disorder. However, amantadine may reverse SSRI-induced orgasmic dysfunction through its dopaminergic effect.

Antihistamines. Drugs such as diphenhydramine (Benadryl) have anticholinergic activity and are mildly hypnotic. They may inhibit sexual function as a result. Cyproheptadine, although an antihistamine, also has potent activity as a serotonin antagonist. It is used to block the serotonergic sexual adverse effects produced by SSRIs, such as delayed orgasm.

Antianxiety Agents. The major class of anxiolytics is the benzodiazepines (e.g., diazepam [Valium]). They act on the γ-aminobutyric acid (GABA) receptors, which are believed to be involved in cognition, memory, and motor control. Because benzodiazepines decrease plasma epinephrine concentrations, they diminish anxiety, and as a result they improve sexual function in persons inhibited by anxiety.

Alcohol. Alcohol suppresses CNS activity generally and can produce erectile disorders in men as a result. Alcohol has a direct gonadal effect that decreases testosterone levels in men; paradoxically, it can produce a slight rise in testosterone levels in women. The latter finding may account for women who report increased libido after drinking small amounts of alcohol. The long-term use of alcohol reduces the ability of the liver to metabolize estrogenic compounds. In men, that produces signs of feminization (such as gynecomastia as a result of testicular atrophy).

Opioids. Opioids, such as heroin, have adverse sexual effects, such as erectile failure and decreased libido. The alteration of consciousness may enhance the sexual experience in occasional users.

Hallucinogens. The hallucinogens include lysergic acid diethylamide (LSD), phencyclidine (PCP), psilocybin (from some mushrooms), and mescaline (from peyote cactus). In addition to inducing hallucinations, the drugs cause loss of contact with reality and an expanding and heightening of consciousness. Some users report that the sexual experience is similarly enhanced, but others experience anxiety, delirium, or psychosis, which clearly interfere with sexual function.

Cannabis. The altered state of consciousness produced by cannabis may enhance sexual pleasure for some persons. Its prolonged use depresses testosterone levels.

Barbiturates and Similarly Acting Drugs. Barbiturates and similarly acting sedative-hypnotic drugs may enhance sexual responsiveness in persons who are sexually unresponsive as a result of anxiety. They have no direct effect on the sex organs; however, they do produce an alteration in consciousness that some persons find pleasurable. These drugs are subject to abuse, and use can be fatal when combined with alcohol or other CNS depressants.

Methaqualone (Quaalude) acquired a reputation as a sexual enhancer, which had no biological basis in fact. It is no longer marketed in the United States.

TREATMENT

Before 1970, the most common treatment of sexual dysfunctions was individual psychotherapy. After 1970 dual-sex therapy (see below) developed by William Masters and Virginia Johnson became the treatment of choice. Classic psychodynamic theory holds that sexual inadequacy has its roots in early developmental conflicts, and the sexual disorder is treated as part of a pervasive emotional disturbance. Treatment focuses on the exploration of unconscious conflicts, motivation, fantasy, and various interpersonal difficulties. One of the assumptions of therapy is that removal of the conflicts allows the sexual impulse to become structurally acceptable to the ego, and thereby the patient finds appropriate means of satisfaction in the environment. The symptoms of sexual dysfunctions, however, frequently become secondarily autonomous and continue to persist, even when other problems evolving from the patients' pathology have been resolved. The addition of behavioral techniques is often necessary to cure the sexual problem.

Dual-Sex Therapy

The theoretical basis of dual-sex therapy is the concept of the marital unit or dyad as the object of therapy; the approach represented the major advance in the diagnosis and treatment of sexual disorders in the 20th century. In dual-sex therapy, treatment is based on a concept that the couple must be treated when a dysfunctional person is in a relationship. Because both are involved in a sexually distressing situation, both must participate in the therapy program. The sexual problem often reflects other areas of disharmony or misunderstanding in the relationship so that the entire relationship is treated, with emphasis on the sexual functioning of the partners.

The keystone of the program is the roundtable session in which a male and female therapy team clarifies, discusses, and works through problems with the couple. The four-way sessions require active participation by the patients. Therapists and patients discuss the psychological and physiological aspects of sexual functioning, and therapists have an educative attitude. Therapists suggest specific sexual activities for the couple to follow in the privacy of their home. The aim of the therapy is to establish or reestablish communication within the partner unit. Sex is emphasized as a natural function that flourishes in the appropriate domestic climate, and improved communication is encouraged toward that end. In a variation of this therapy that has proved effective, one therapist may treat the couple. Treatment is short term and is behaviorally oriented. The therapists attempt to reflect the situation as they see it, rather than interpret underlying dynamics. An undistorted picture of the relationship presented by the therapists often corrects the myopic, narrow view held by each partner. This new perspective can interrupt the couple's destructive pattern of relating and can encourage improved, more effective communication. Specific exercises are prescribed for the couple to treat their particular problems. Sexual inadequacy often involves lack of information, misinformation, and performance fear. Therefore, the couple is specifically prohibited from any sexual play other than that prescribed by the therapists. Beginning exercises usually focus on heightening sensory awareness to touch, sight, sound, and smell. Initially, intercourse is interdicted, and the couple learn to give and receive bodily pleasure without the pressure of performance or penetration. At the same time, they learn how to communicate nonverbally in a mutually satisfactory way, and they learn that sexual foreplay is an enjoyable alternative to intercourse and orgasm.

During the sensate focus exercises, the couple receives much reinforcement to reduce anxiety. They are urged to use fantasies to distract them from obsessive concerns about performance (spectatoring). The needs of both the dysfunctional partner and the nondysfunctional partner are considered. If either partner becomes sexually excited by the exercises, the other is encouraged to bring him or her to orgasm by manual or oral means. Open communication between the partners is urged, and the expression of mutual needs is encouraged. Resistances, such as claims of fatigue or not enough time to complete the exercises, are common and must be dealt with by the therapists. Issues of body image, fear of being touched, and difficulty touching oneself arise frequently. Genital stimulation is eventually added to general body stimulation. The couple is instructed sequentially to try various positions for intercourse, without necessarily completing the act, and to use varieties of stimulating techniques before they are instructed to proceed with intercourse.

Psychotherapy sessions follow each new exercise period, and problems and satisfactions, both sexual and in other areas of the couple's lives, are discussed. Specific instructions and the introduction of new exercises geared to the individual couple's progress are reviewed in each session. Gradually, the couple gains confidence and learns to communicate, verbally and sexually. Sex therapy is most effective when the sexual dysfunction exists apart from other psychopathology.

Over the past few years, it has been shown that similar results can be obtained with one therapist providing sex therapy and dual sex therapy is conducted to a much lesser degree than previously. Some couples prefer to be treated by a man, others by a woman and while these wishes should be accommodated, it is not always possible to do so. In such instances, the objections should be explored and the couple reassured that whatever embarrassment one or the other may anticipate will quickly diminish as therapy proceeds.

Specific Techniques and Exercises

Various techniques are used to treat the various sexual dysfunctions. In cases of vaginismus, a woman is advised to dilate her vaginal opening with her fingers or with size-graduated dilators. Dilators are also used to treat cases of dyspareunia. Sometimes, treatment is coordinated with specially trained physiotherapists who work with the patients to help them relax their perineal muscles.

In cases of premature ejaculation, an exercise known as the squeeze technique is used to raise the threshold of penile excitability. In this exercise, the man or the woman stimulates the erect penis until the earliest sensations of impending ejaculation are felt. At this point, the woman forcefully squeezes the coronal ridge of the glans, the erection is diminished, and ejaculation is inhibited. The exercise program eventually raises the threshold of the sensation of ejaculatory inevitability and allows the man to focus on sensations of arousal without anxiety and develop confidence in his sexual performance. A variant of the exercise is the stop–start technique developed by James H. Semans, in which the woman stops all stimulation of the penis when the man first senses an impending ejaculation. No squeeze is used. Research has shown that the presence or absence of circumcision has no bearing on a man's ejaculatory control; the glans is equally sensitive in the two states. Sex therapy has been most successful in the treatment of premature ejaculation.

A man with a sexual desire disorder or male erectile disorder is sometimes told to masturbate to prove that full erection and ejaculation are possible. Delayed ejaculation is managed initially by extravaginal ejaculation and then by gradual vaginal entry after stimulation to a point near ejaculation. Most importantly, the early exercises forbid ejaculation to remove the pressure to climax and allow the man to immerse himself in sexual pleasuring.

In cases of lifelong female orgasmic disorder, the woman is directed to masturbate, sometimes using a vibrator. The shaft of the clitoris is the masturbatory site most preferred by women, and orgasm depends on adequate clitoral stimulation. An area on the anterior wall of the vagina has been identified in some women as a site of sexual excitation, known as the *G-spot;* but reports of an ejaculatory phenomenon at orgasm in women following the stimulation of the G-spot have not been satisfactorily verified.

Hypnotherapy

Hypnotherapists focus specifically on the anxiety-producing situation—that is, the sexual interaction that results in dysfunction. The successful use of hypnosis enables patients to gain control over the symptom that has been lowering self-esteem and disrupting psychological homeostasis. The patient's cooperation is first obtained and encouraged during a series of nonhypnotic sessions with the therapist. Those discussions permit the development of a secure doctor–patient relationship, a sense of physical and psychological comfort on the part of the patient, and the establishment of mutually desired treatment goals. During this time, the therapist assesses the patient's capacity for the trance experience. The nonhypnotic sessions also permit the clinician to take a psychiatric history and perform a mental status examination before beginning hypnotherapy. The focus of treatment is on symptom removal and attitude alteration. The patient is instructed in developing alternative means of dealing with the anxiety-provoking situation, the sexual encounter.

In addition, patients are taught relaxation techniques to use on themselves before sexual relations. With these methods to alleviate anxiety, the physiological responses to sexual stimulation can more readily result in pleasurable excitation and discharge. Psychological impediments to vaginal lubrication, erection, and orgasms are removed, and normal sexual functioning ensues. Hypnosis may be added to a basic individual psychotherapy program to accelerate the effects of psychotherapeutic intervention.

Behavior Therapy

Behavioral approaches were initially designed for the treatment of phobias but are now used to treat other problems as well. Behavior therapists assume that sexual dysfunction is learned maladaptive behavior, which causes patients to be fearful of sexual interaction. Using traditional techniques, therapists set up a hierarchy of anxiety-provoking situations, ranging from least threatening (e.g., the thought of kissing) to most threatening (e.g., the thought of penile penetration). The behavior therapist enables the patient to master the anxiety through a standard program of systematic desensitization, which is designed to inhibit the learned anxious response by encouraging behaviors antithetical to anxiety. The patient first deals with the least anxiety-producing situation in fantasy and progresses by steps to the most anxiety-producing situation. Medication, hypnosis, and special training in deep muscle relaxation are sometimes used to help with the initial mastery of anxiety.

Assertiveness training is helpful in teaching patients to express sexual needs openly and without fear. Exercises in assertiveness are given in conjunction with sex therapy; patients are encouraged to make sexual requests and to refuse to comply with requests perceived as unreasonable. Sexual exercises may be prescribed for patients to perform at home, and a hierarchy may be established, starting with those activities that have proved most pleasurable and successful in the past.

One treatment variation involves the participation of the patient's sexual partner in the desensitization program. The partner, rather than the therapist, presents items of increasing stimulation value to the patient. A cooperative partner is necessary to help the patient carry gains made during treatment sessions to sexual activity at home.

Mindfulness

Mindfulness is a cognitive technique that has been helpful in the treatment of sexual dysfunction. The patient is directed to focus on the moment and maintain an awareness of sensations—visual, tactile, auditory, and olfactory—that he or she experiences in the moment. The aim is to distract the patient from spectatoring (watching him or herself) and center the person on the sensations that lead to arousal and/or orgasm. Hopefully, this shift in focus allows patients to become immersed in the pleasure of the experience and remove themselves from self-judgment and performance anxiety.

Group Therapy

Group therapy has been used to examine both intrapsychic and interpersonal problems in patients with sexual disorders. A therapy group provides a strong support system for a patient who feels ashamed, anxious, or guilty about a particular sexual problem. It is a useful forum in which to counteract sexual myths, correct misconceptions, and provide accurate information about sexual anatomy, physiology, and varieties of behavior.

Groups for the treatment of sexual disorders can be organized in several ways. Members may all share the same problem, such as premature ejaculation; members may all be of the same sex with different sexual problems; or groups may be composed of both men and women who are experiencing a variety of sexual problems. Group therapy can be an adjunct to other forms of therapy or the prime mode of treatment. Groups organized to treat a particular dysfunction are usually behavioral in approach.

Groups composed of married couples with sexual dysfunctions have also been effective. A group provides the opportunity to gather accurate information, offers consensual validation of individual preferences, and enhances self-esteem and self-acceptance. Techniques, such as role playing and psychodrama, may be used in treatment. Such groups are not indicated for couples when one partner is uncooperative, when a patient has a severe depressive disorder or psychosis, when a patient finds explicit sexual audiovisual material repugnant, or when a patient fears or dislikes groups.

Analytically Oriented Sex Therapy

One of the most effective treatment modalities is the use of sex therapy integrated with psychodynamic and psychoanalytically oriented psychotherapy. The sex therapy is conducted over a longer period than usual, which allows learning or relearning of sexual satisfaction under the realities of patients' day-to-day lives. The addition of psychodynamic conceptualizations to behavioral techniques used to treat sexual dysfunctions allows the treatment of patients with sexual disorders associated with other psychopathology.

The material and dynamics that emerge in patients in analytically oriented sex therapy are the same as those in psychoanalytic therapy, such as dreams, fear of punishment, aggressive feelings, difficulty in trusting a partner, fear of intimacy, oedipal feelings, and fear of genital mutilation. The combined approach of analytically oriented sex therapy is used by the general psychiatrist who carefully judges the optimal timing of sex therapy and the ability of patients to tolerate the directive approach that focuses on their sexual difficulties.

Biological Treatments

Biological treatments, including pharmacotherapy, surgery, and mechanical devices, are used to treat specific cases of sexual disorder. Most of the recent advances involve male sexual dysfunction. Current studies are under way to test biological treatment of sexual dysfunction in women.

Pharmacotherapy. The major new medications to treat sexual dysfunction are sildenafil (Viagra) and its congeners (Table 13.2–6); oral phentolamine (Vasomax); alprostadil (Caverject, Idex), and injectable medications; papaverine, prostaglandin E1, phentolamine, or some combination of these (Edex); and a transurethral alprostadil (MUSE), all used to treat erectile disorder.

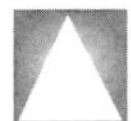

Table 13.2–6
Pharmacokinetics of the PDE-5 Inhibitors

	Sildenafil 100 mg	Vardenafil 20 mg	Tadalafil 20 mg
Maximum concentration	450 ng/mL	20.9 ng/mL	378 ng/mL
Time to maximum concentration	1.0 hours	0.7 hours	2.0 hours
Half-life	4 hours	3.9 hours	17.5 hours

From Arnold LM. Vardenafil & Tadalafil: Options for erectile dysfunction. *Curr Psychiatr.* 2004;3(2):46.

Sildenafil is a nitric oxide enhancer that facilitates the inflow of blood to the penis necessary for an erection. The drug takes effect about 1 hour after ingestion, and its effect can last up to 4 hours. Sildenafil is not effective in the absence of sexual stimulation. The most common adverse events associated with its use are headaches, flushing, and dyspepsia. The use of sildenafil is contraindicated for persons taking organic nitrates. The concomitant action of the two drugs can result in large, sudden, and sometimes fatal drops in systemic blood pressure. Sildenafil is not effective in all cases of erectile dysfunction. It fails to produce an erection that is sufficiently rigid for penetration in about 50 percent of men who have had radical prostate surgery or in those with long-standing insulin-dependent diabetes. It is also ineffective in certain cases of nerve damage.

A small number of patients developed nonarteritic ischemic optic neuropathy (NAION) soon after use of sildenafil. Six patients had vision loss within 24 hours after use of the agent. Both eyes were affected in one individual. All affected individuals had preexisting hypertension, diabetes, elevated cholesterol, or hyperlipidemia. Although very rare, sildenafil may provoke NAION in individuals with an arteriosclerotic risk profile. Very rare cases of hearing loss have also been reported.

Sildenafil use in women results in vaginal lubrication, but not in increased desire. Anecdotal reports, however, describe individual women who have experienced intensified excitement with sildenafil.

Oral phentolamine and apomorphine are not U.S. Food and Drug Administration (FDA) approved at present, but have proved effective as potency enhancers in men with minimal erectile dysfunction. Phentolamine reduces sympathetic tone and relaxes corporeal smooth muscle. Adverse events include hypotension, tachycardia, and dizziness. Apomorphine effects are mediated by the autonomic nervous system and result in vasodilation that facilitates the inflow of blood to the penis. Adverse events include nausea and sweating.

In contrast to the oral medications, injectable and transurethral forms of alprostadil act locally on the penis and can produce erections in the absence of sexual stimulation. Alprostadil contains a naturally occurring form of prostaglandin E, a vasodilating agent. Alprostadil may be administered by direct injection into the corpora cavernosa or by intraurethral insertion of a pellet through a canula. The firm erection produced within 2 to 3 minutes after administration of the drug may last as long as 1 hour. Infrequent and reversible adverse effects of injections include penile bruising and changes in liver function test results. Possible hazardous sequelae exist, including priapism and sclerosis of the small veins of the penis. Users of transurethral alprostadil sometimes complain of burning sensations in the penis.

Two small trials found different topical agents effective in alleviating erectile dysfunction. One cream consists of three vasoactive substances known to be absorbed through the skin: aminophylline, isosorbide dinitrate, and co-dergocrine mesylate, which is a mixture of ergot alkaloids. The other is a gel containing alprostadil and an additional ingredient, which temporarily makes the outer layer of the skin more permeable.

In addition, a cream incorporating alprostadil has been developed to treat female sexual arousal disorder; the initial results are promising. In a trial of postmenopausal women with arousal problems who were already on hormonal therapy, vaginally applied phentolamine mesylate, an α-receptor antagonist, significantly increased vasocongestion and a subjective sense of arousal

A drug to increase desire in women, flibanserin, which had previously been denied approval by the FDA was approved for use in 2015 largely as a result of pressure from the pharmaceutical company with the patent on the drug and from some women groups who felt that sexism trumped scientific data in that first disapproval. Flibanserin sold under the trade name Addyi, is used for the treatment of premenopausal women with hypoactive sexual desire disorder. The medication was found to increase the number of satisfying sexual events from about two to three times per month to about four times per month which was almost equal to results from placebo. Flibanserin is presumed to work by increasing dopamine and norepinephrine levels and decreasing serotonin levels in the brain, actions believed to be mediated by activation of the 5-HT_{1A} receptor; but its exact mechanism of action is unknown. Adverse events include dizziness, nausea, fatigue, day-time sleepiness, and interrupted night-time sleep. Drinking alcohol while on flibanserin was associated with a severe drop in blood pressure in close to 20 percent of women. Because of limited postmarketing data, clinicians should be extremely cautious about prescribing the drug.

Numerous other pharmacological agents have been used to treat the various sexual disorders. Intravenous methohexital sodium (Brevital) has been used in desensitization therapy. Antianxiety agents may have some application in tense patients, although these drugs can interfere with the sexual response. The side effects of antidepressants, in particular the SSRIs and tricyclic drugs, have been used to prolong the sexual response in patients with premature ejaculation. This approach is particularly useful in patients who are refractory to behavioral techniques who may fall into the category of physiologically disposed premature ejaculators. Topical anesthetic creams are also reported to be helpful in decreasing the intravaginal ejaculation latency time (IELT) in cases of premature ejaculation. Antidepressants are advocated in treatment of patients who are phobic of sex and in those with posttraumatic stress disorder following rape. Trazodone is an antidepressant that improves nocturnal erections. The risks of taking such medications must be carefully weighed against their possible benefits. Bromocriptine (Parlodel) is used in the treatment of hyperprolactinemia, which is frequently associated with hypogonadism. In such patients, it is necessary to rule out pituitary tumors. Bromocriptine, a dopamine agonist, may improve sexual function impaired by hyperprolactinemia.

A number of substances have popular standing as aphrodisiacs; for example, ginseng root and yohimbine (Yocon). Studies, however, have not confirmed any aphrodisiac properties. Yohimbine, an α-receptor antagonist, may cause dilation of the penile artery; however, the American Urologic Association does not recommend its use to treat organic erectile dysfunction. Many recreational drugs, including cocaine, amphetamines, alcohol, and cannabis, are considered enhancers of sexual performance. Although they may provide the user with an initial benefit because of their tranquilizing, disinhibiting, or mood-elevating effects, consistent or prolonged use of any of these substances impairs sexual functioning.

Dopaminergic agents have been reported to increase libido and improve sex function. Those drugs include L-dopa, a dopamine precursor, and bromocriptine, a dopamine agonist. The antidepressant bupropion has dopaminergic effects and has increased sex drive in some patients. Selegiline, an MAOI, is selective for MAO_B and is dopaminergic. It improves sexual functioning in older persons.

HORMONE THERAPY. Androgens increase the sex drive in women and in men with low testosterone concentrations. Women may experience virilizing effects, some of which are irreversible (e.g., deepening of the voice). In men, prolonged use of androgens produces hypertension and prostatic enlargement. Testosterone is most effective when given parenterally; however, effective oral and transdermal preparations are available.

Women who use estrogens for replacement therapy or for contraception may report decreased libido; in such cases, a combined preparation of estrogen and testosterone has been used effectively. Estrogen itself prevents thinning of the vaginal mucous membrane and facilitates lubrication. Several forms of locally delivered estrogen—vaginal rings, vaginal creams, and vaginal tablets—provide alternate administration routes to treat women with arousal problems or genital atrophy. Because tablets, creams, and rings do not significantly increase circulating estrogen levels, these devices may be considered for patients with breast cancer with arousal problems.

ANTIANDROGENS AND ANTIESTROGENS. Estrogens and progesterone are antiandrogens that have been used to treat compulsive sexual behavior in men, usually in sex offenders. Clomiphene (Clomid) and tamoxifen (Nolvadex) are both antiestrogens, and both stimulate gonadotropin-releasing hormone (GnRH) secretion and increase testosterone concentrations, thereby increasing libido. Women being treated for breast cancer with tamoxifen report an increased libido. However, tamoxifen may cause uterine cancer.

Mechanical Treatment Approaches. In male patients with arteriosclerosis (especially of the distal aorta, known as Leriche's syndrome), the erection may be lost during active pelvic thrusting. The need for increased blood in the gluteal muscles and others served by the ilial or hypogastric arteries takes blood away (steals) from the pudendal artery and, thus, interferes with penile blood flow. Relief may be obtained by decreasing pelvic thrusting, which is also aided by the woman's superior coital position.

Vacuum Pump. Vacuum pumps are mechanical devices that patients without vascular disease can use to obtain erections. The blood drawn into the penis following the creation of the vacuum is kept there by a ring placed around the base of the penis. This device has no adverse effects, but it is cumbersome, and partners must be willing to accept its use. Some women complain that the penis is redder and cooler than when erection is produced by natural circumstances, and they find the process and the result objectionable. Some men describe the process as painful.

A similar device, called EROS, has been developed to create clitoral erections in women. EROS is a small suction cup that fits over the clitoral region and draws blood into the clitoris. Studies have reported its success in treating female sexual arousal disorder. Vibrators used to stimulate the clitoral area have been successful in treating anorgasmic women.

Surgical Treatment

MALE PROSTHESES. Surgical treatment is infrequently advocated, but penile prosthetic devices are available for men with inadequate erectile responses who are resistant to other treatment methods or who have medically caused deficiencies. The two main types of prostheses are (1) a semirigid rod prosthesis that produces a permanent erection that can be positioned close to the body for concealment and (2) an inflatable type that is implanted with its own reservoir and pump for inflation and deflation. The latter type is designed to mimic normal physiological functioning.

VASCULAR SURGERY. When vascular insufficiency is present due to atherosclerosis or other blockage, bypass surgery of penile arteries has been attempted in selected cases with some success.

Outcome

Demonstrating the effectiveness of traditional outpatient psychotherapy is just as difficult when therapy is oriented to sexual problems as it is in general. The more severe the psychopathology associated with a problem of long duration, the more adverse the outcome is likely to be. The results of different treatment methods have varied considerably since Masters and Johnson first reported positive results for their treatment approach in 1970. Masters and Johnson studied the failure rates of their patients (defined as the failure to initiate reversal of the basic symptom of the presenting dysfunction). They compared initial failure rates with 5-year follow-up findings for the same couples. Although some have criticized their definition of the percentage of presumed successes, other studies have confirmed the effectiveness of their approach.

The more difficult treatment cases involve couples with severe marital discord. Desire disorders are particularly difficult to treat. They require longer, more intensive therapy than some other disorders, and their outcomes vary greatly.

When behavioral approaches are used, empirical criteria that predict outcome are more easily isolated. Using these criteria, for instance, couples who regularly practice assigned exercises appear to have a much greater likelihood of success than do more resistant couples or those whose interaction involves sadomasochistic or depressive features or mechanisms of blame and projection. Attitude flexibility is also a positive prognostic factor. Overall, younger couples tend to complete sex therapy more often than older couples. Couples whose interactional difficulties center on their sex problems, such as inhibition, frustration, or fear of performance failure, are also likely to respond well to therapy.

Although most therapists prefer to treat a couple for sexual dysfunction, treatment of individual persons has also been successful. In general, methods that have proved effective singly or in combination include training in behavioral sexual skills, systematic desensitization, directive marital counseling, traditional psychodynamic approaches, group therapy, and pharmacotherapy.

OTHER SPECIFIED SEXUAL DYSFUNCTIONS

Many sexual disorders are not classifiable as sexual dysfunctions or as paraphilias. These unclassified disorders are rare, poorly documented, not easily classified, or not specifically described in DSM-5. Nevertheless, they are syndromes that therapists have seen clinically.

Postcoital Dysphoria

Postcoital dysphoria occurs during the resolution phase of sexual activity, when persons normally experience a sense of general well-being and muscular and psychological relaxation. Some persons, however, undergo postcoital dysphoria at this time and, after an otherwise satisfactory sexual experience, become depressed, tense, anxious, and irritable, and show psychomotor agitation. They often want to get away from their partners and may become verbally or even physically abusive. The incidence of the disorder is unknown, but it is more common in men than in women. The causes relate to the person's attitude toward sex in general and toward the partner in particular. The disorder may occur in adulterous sex and in contacts with prostitutes. The fear of acquired immunodeficiency syndrome (AIDS) causes some persons to experience postcoital dysphoria. Treatment requires insight-oriented psychotherapy to help patients understand the unconscious antecedents to their behavior and attitudes.

Couple Problems

At times, a complaint arises from the spousal unit or the couple, rather than from an individual dysfunction. For example, one partner may prefer morning sex, but the other functions more readily at night, or the partners have unequal frequencies of desire.

Unconsummated Marriage

A couple involved in an unconsummated marriage has never had coitus and is typically uninformed and inhibited about sexuality. The partners' feelings of guilt, shame, or inadequacy are increased by their problem, and they experience conflict between their need to seek help and their need to conceal their difficulty. Couples may seek help for the problem after having been married several months or several years. Masters and Johnson reported one unconsummated marriage of 17 years' duration.

Frequently, the couple does not seek help directly; the woman may reveal the problem to her gynecologist on a visit ostensibly concerned with vague vaginal or other somatic complaints. On examining her, the gynecologist may find an intact hymen. In some cases, however, the wife may have undergone a hymenectomy to resolve the problem, but the surgery may aggravate the situation without solving the basic problem. The surgical procedure is another stress and often increases the couple's feelings of inadequacy. The wife may feel put upon, abused, or mutilated, and the husband's concern about his manliness may increase. An inquiry by a physician who is comfortable dealing with sexual problems may be the first opening to a frank discussion of the couple's distress. Often, the pretext of the medical visit is a discussion of contraceptive methods or—even more ironically—a request for an infertility workup. Once presented, the complaint can often be treated successfully. The duration of the problem does not significantly affect the prognosis or the outcome of the case.

The causes of unconsummated marriage are varied: lack of sex education, sexual prohibitions overly stressed by parents or society, problems of an oedipal nature, immaturity in both partners, overdependence on primary families, and problems in sexual identification. Religious orthodoxy, with severe control of sexual and social development, and equating sexuality with sin or uncleanliness has also been cited as a dominant cause. Many women involved in an unconsummated marriage have distorted concepts about their vaginas. They may fear that it is too small or too soft, or they may confuse the vagina with the rectum and thus feel unclean. Men may share these distortions about the vagina and perceive it as dangerous to themselves. Similarly, both partners may have distortions about the man's penis and perceive it as a weapon, as too large, or as too small. Many patients can be helped by simple education about genital anatomy and physiology, by suggestions for self-exploration, and by correct information from a physician. The problem of unconsummated marriage is best treated by seeing both members of the couple. Dual-sex therapy involving a male–female cotherapist team has been markedly effective. Other forms of conjoint therapy, marital counseling, traditional psychotherapy on a one-to-one basis, and counseling from a sensitive family physician, gynecologist, or urologist are also helpful.

Body Image Problems

Some persons are ashamed of their bodies and experience feelings of inadequacy related to self-imposed standards of masculinity or femininity. They may insist on sex only during total darkness, not allow certain body parts to be seen or touched, or seek unnecessary operative procedures to deal with their imagined inadequacies. Body dysmorphic disorder should be ruled out.

Sex Addiction and Compulsivity

The concept of sex addiction developed over the last two decades to refer to persons who compulsively seek out sexual experiences and whose behavior becomes impaired if they are unable to gratify their sexual impulses. The concept of sex addiction derived from the model of addiction to such drugs as heroin or addiction to behavioral patterns, such as gambling. Addiction implies psychological dependence, physical dependence, and the presence of a withdrawal syndrome if the substance (e.g., the drug) is unavailable or the behavior (e.g., gambling) is frustrated.

In DSM-5, the terms *sex addiction* or *compulsive sexuality* are not used, nor is it a disorder that is universally recognized or accepted. Nevertheless, the phenomenon of a person whose life revolves around sex-seeking behavior and activities, who spends an excessive amount of time in such behavior, and who often tries to stop such behavior but is unable to do so is well known to clinicians. Such persons show repeated and increasingly frequent attempts to have a sexual experience, deprivation of which gives rise to symptoms of distress. Sex addiction is a useful concept heuristically, in that it can alert the clinician to seek an underlying cause for the manifest behavior. There is interest in making it a new official diagnostic category, which the authors support.

Diagnosis. Sex addicts are unable to control their sexual impulses, which can involve the entire spectrum of sexual fantasy or behavior. Eventually, the need for sexual activity increases, and the person's behavior is motivated largely by the persistent desire to experience the sex act. The history usually reveals a long-standing pattern of such behavior, which the person repeatedly has tried to stop, but without success. Although a patient may have feelings of guilt and remorse after the act, these feelings do not suffice to prevent its recurrence. The patient may report that the need to act out is most severe during stressful periods or when angry, depressed, anxious, or otherwise dysphoric. Most acts culminate in a sexual orgasm. Eventually, the sexual activity interferes with the person's social, vocational, or marital life, which begins to deteriorate. The signs of sexual addiction are listed in Table 13.2–7.

Types of Behavioral Patterns. The paraphilias constitute the behavioral patterns most often found in the sex addict. The essential features of a paraphilia are recurrent, intense sexual urges or behaviors, including exhibitionism, fetishism, frotteurism, sadomasochism, cross-dressing, voyeurism, and pedophilia. Paraphilias are associated with clinically significant distress and almost invariably interfere with interpersonal relationships, and they often lead to legal complications. In addition to the paraphilias, however, sex addiction can also include behavior that is considered normal, such as coitus and masturbation, except that it is promiscuous and uncontrolled.

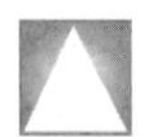

Table 13.2–7
Signs of Sexual Addiction

1. Out-of-control behavior
2. Severe adverse consequences (medical, legal, interpersonal) due to sexual behavior
3. Persistent pursuit of self-destructive or high-risk sexual behavior
4. Repeated attempts to limit or stop sexual behavior
5. Sexual obsession and fantasy as a primary coping mechanism
6. The need for increasing amounts of sexual activity
7. Severe mood changes related to sexual activity (e.g., depression, euphoria)
8. Inordinate amount of time spent in obtaining sex, being sexual, or recovering from sexual experience
9. Interference of sexual behavior in social, occupational, or recreational activities

Data from Carnes P. *Don't Call It Love*. New York: Bantam Books; 1991.

In the 19th century, Krafft-Ebing reported on several cases of abnormally increased sexual desire. One involved a 36-year-old married teacher, the father of seven children, who masturbated repeatedly while sitting at his desk in front of his pupils, after which he was "penitent and filled with shame." He indulged in coitus three or four times a day in addition to his repeated masturbatory act. In another case, a young woman masturbated almost incessantly and was unable to control her impulses. She had frequent coitus with many men, but neither coitus nor masturbation sufficed, and she eventually was placed in an institution. Krafft-Ebing referred to the condition as "sexual hyperaesthesia," which he believed could occur in otherwise normal persons. In this case, the clinician would have to differentiate between a diagnosis of sex addiction or persistent genital arousal disorder (PGAD). This is not a diagnostic category in DSM-5, but has received attention by sex therapists. Women with PGAD complain that their sense of arousal is not satisfied by orgasm or multiple orgasms. The ongoing sense of arousal is distressing, intensely uncomfortable, and has led to one reported case of suicide. In contrast to sex addicts, women with PGAD are not even temporarily satisfied, physically or emotionally, by orgasm. Some theorists suspect a neurologic etiology.

In many cases, sex addiction is the final common pathway of a variety of other disorders. In addition to the paraphilias that are often present, the patient may have an associated major mood disorder or schizophrenia. Antisocial personality disorder and borderline personality disorder are common.

DON JUANISM. Some men who appear to be hypersexual, as manifested by their need to have many sexual encounters or conquests, use their sexual activities to mask deep feelings of inferiority. Some have unconscious homosexual impulses, which they deny by compulsive sexual contacts with women. After having sex, most Don Juans are no longer interested in the woman. The condition is sometimes referred to as *satyriasis* or *sex addiction*.

NYMPHOMANIA. Nymphomania signifies a woman's excessive or pathological desire for coitus. Of the few scientific studies of the condition, those patients who were studied usually have had one or more sexual disorders, often including female orgasmic disorder. The woman often has an intense fear of losing love and, through her actions, attempts to satisfy her dependence needs rather than gratify her sexual impulses. This disorder is a form of sex addiction.

Comorbidity. Comorbidity (dual diagnosis) refers to the presence of an addiction that coexists with another psychiatric disorder. For example, about 50 percent of patients with substance-use disorder also have an additional psychiatric disorder. Similarly, many sex addicts have an associated psychiatric disorder. Dual diagnosis implies that the psychiatric illness and the addiction are separate disorders; one does not cause the other. The diagnosis of comorbidity is often difficult to make because addictive behavior (of all types) can produce extreme anxiety and severe disturbances in mood and affect, especially while the addictive behavior is treated. If, after a period of abstinence, symptoms of a psychiatric disorder remain, the comorbid condition is more easily recognized and diagnosed than during the addictive period. Finally, a high correlation is found between sex addiction and substance-use disorders (up to 80 percent in some studies), which not only complicates the task of diagnosis, but also complicates treatment.

Treatment. Self-help groups based on the 12-step concept used in Alcoholics Anonymous (AA) have been used successfully with many sex addicts. They include such groups as Sexaholics Anonymous (SA), Sex and Love Addicts Anonymous (SLAA), and Sex Addicts Anonymous (SAA). The groups differ in that some are for men or women, or for married persons or couples. All advocate some abstinence from either the addictive behavior or sex in general. Should a substance-use disorder also be present, the patient often requires referral to AA or Narcotics Anonymous (NA) as well. Patients may enter an inpatient treatment unit when they lack sufficient motivation to control their behavior on an outpatient basis or may be a danger to themselves or others. In addition, severe medical or psychiatric symptoms may require careful supervision and treatment best carried out in a hospital.

A 42-year-old married businessman with two children was considered a model of virtue in his community. He was active in his church and on the boards of several charitable organizations. He was living a secret life, however, and would lie to his wife, telling her that he was at a board meeting when he was actually visiting massage parlors for paid sex. He eventually was engaging in the behavior four to five times a day, and although he tried to quit many times, he was unable to do so. He knew that he was harming himself by putting his reputation and marriage at risk.

The patient presented himself to the psychiatric emergency room, stating that he would prefer to be dead rather than continue the behavior described. He was admitted with a diagnosis of major depressive disorder and started on a daily dose of 20 mg of fluoxetine. In addition, he received 100 mg of medroxyprogesterone intramuscularly once a day. His need to masturbate diminished markedly and ceased entirely on the third hospital day, as did his mental preoccupation with sex. The medroxyprogesterone was discontinued on the sixth day, when he was discharged. He continued to take fluoxetine, enrolled in a local SA group, and entered individual and couples psychotherapy. His addictive behavior eventually stopped, he was having satisfactory sexual relations with his wife, and he was no longer suicidal or depressed.

Psychotherapy. Insight-oriented psychotherapy may help patients understand the dynamics of their behavioral patterns. Supportive psychotherapy can help repair the interpersonal, social, or occupational damage that occurs. Cognitive behavioral therapy helps the patient recognize dysphoric states that precipitate sexual acting out. Marital therapy or couples therapy can help the patient regain self-esteem, which is severely impaired by the time a treatment program is begun. It is also helpful to the partners who need assistance in understanding the disease and dealing with their own complex reactions to the situation. Finally, psychotherapy may be of help in the treatment of any associated psychiatric disorder.

Pharmacotherapy. Most specialists in general addiction avoid the use of psychotropic agents, especially in the early stages of treatment. Substance-dependent persons have a tendency to abuse those agents, especially agents with a high abuse potential, such as the benzodiazepines. Pharmacotherapy is of use in the treatment of associated psychiatric disorders, such as major depressive disorders and schizophrenia.

Certain medications may be of use in treating sex addiction, however, because of their specific effects on reducing the sex drive. SSRIs reduce libido in some persons, a side effect that is used therapeutically. Compulsive masturbation is an example of a behavioral pattern that may benefit from such medication. Medroxyprogesterone acetate diminishes libido in men and, thus, makes it easier to control sexually addictive behavior.

The use of antiandrogens in women to control hypersexuality has not been tested sufficiently, but because androgenic compounds contribute to the sex drive in women, antiandrogens could be of benefit. Antiandrogenic agents (cyproterone acetate) are not available in the United States but are used in Europe with varying success. Use of the antiandrogenic medications is controversial, and objected by clinicians who see it a chemical castration and believe that it is an inappropriate treatment approach.

Distress about Sexual Orientation

Distress about sexual orientation is characterized by dissatisfaction with sexual arousal patterns, and it is usually applied to dissatisfaction with homosexual arousal patterns, a desire to increase heterosexual arousal, and strong negative feelings about being homosexual. Occasional statements to the effect that life would be easier if the person were not homosexual do not constitute persistent and marked distress about sexual orientation.

Treatment of sexual orientation distress also known as conversion or reparative therapy is controversial. One study reported that with a minimum of 350 hours of psychoanalytic therapy, about a third of 100 bisexual and gay men who wanted to change their sexual orientation achieved a heterosexual reorientation at a 5-year follow-up; this study has been challenged, however, and never replicated. Behavior therapy and avoidance conditioning techniques have also been used, but these techniques may change behavior only in the laboratory setting. Prognostic factors weighing in favor of heterosexual reorientation for men include being younger than 35 years of age, having some experience of heterosexual arousal, and being highly motivated to reorient.

Another and more prevalent style of intervention is directed at enabling persons with persistent and marked distress about sexual orientation to live comfortably with homosexuality without shame, guilt, anxiety, or depression. Gay counseling centers are engaged with patients in such treatment programs. At present, outcome studies of such centers have not been reported in detail. Few data are available about the treatment of women with persistent and marked distress about sexual orientation, and these are primarily from single-case studies with variable outcomes. The American Psychiatric Association opposes conversion therapy on two grounds: it is based on the assumption that homosexuality is a disease and that it has not been proved to work. Opponents of conversion therapy consider it to be not only unethical but illegal and some groups advocate laws that prohibit therapists from engaging in or advocating such approaches. Overall, conversion therapy has been discredited.

Persistent Genital Arousal Disorder

PGAD has previously been called persistent sexual arousal syndrome. It has been diagnosed in women who complain of a continual feeling of sexual arousal, which is uncomfortable, demands release, and interferes with life pleasures and activities. These women masturbate frequently, sometimes incessantly, because climax provides relief. However, the relief is temporary and the sense of arousal returns rapidly and remains. The sense of arousal in these cases is neither pleasurable nor exciting, and the women are not interested in a sexual experience but in relief from their symptoms. Some women have reported masturbating so frequently to alleviate the arousal that they have irritated their genitalia severely. One case of attempted suicide has been reported with this syndrome, with the woman stating that she could no longer tolerate the sensations and that she had masturbated so often that her vulva was raw.

Female Premature Orgasm

Data on female premature orgasm are lacking. A case of multiple spontaneous orgasms without sexual stimulation was seen in a woman; the cause was an epileptogenic focus in the temporal lobe. Instances have been reported of women taking antidepressants (e.g., fluoxetine and clomipramine) who experience spontaneous orgasm associated with yawning.

Postcoital Headache

Postcoital headache, characterized by headache immediately after coitus, may last for several hours. It is usually described as throbbing and is localized in the occipital or frontal area. The cause is unknown. There may be vascular, muscle-contraction (tension), or psychogenic causes. Coitus may precipitate migraine or cluster headaches in predisposed persons.

Orgasmic Anhedonia

Orgasmic anhedonia is a condition in which a person has no physical sensation of orgasm, even though the physiological component (e.g., ejaculation) remains intact. Organic causes, such as sacral and cephalic lesions that interfere with afferent pathways from the genitalia to the cortex, must be ruled out. Psychiatric causes usually relate to extreme guilt about experiencing sexual pleasure. These feelings produce a dissociative response that isolates the affective component of the orgasmic experience from consciousness.

Masturbatory Pain

Persons may experience pain during masturbation. Organic causes should always be ruled out; a small vaginal tear or early Peyronie's disease can produce a painful sensation. The condition should be differentiated from compulsive masturbation. Persons may masturbate to the extent that they do physical damage to their genitals and eventually experience pain during subsequent masturbatory acts. Such cases constitute a separate sexual disorder and should be so classified.

Certain masturbatory practices have resulted in what has been called autoerotic asphyxiation. The practices involve persons masturbating while hanging by the neck to heighten the erotic sensations and the orgasm's intensity through the mechanism of mild hypoxia. Although the persons intend to release themselves from the noose after orgasm, an estimated 500 to 1,000 persons a year accidentally kill themselves by hanging. Most who indulge in the practice are male; transvestism is often associated with the habit, and most deaths occur among adolescents. Such masochistic practices are usually associated with severe mental disorders, such as schizophrenia and major mood disorders.

▲ 13.3 Paraphilic Disorders

Paraphilias or perversions are sexual stimuli or acts that are deviations from normal sexual behaviors, but are necessary for some persons to experience arousal and orgasm. According to the *Diagnostic and Statistical Manual of Mental Disorders*, fifth edition (DSM-5), the term paraphilic disorder is reserved for those cases in which a sexually deviant fantasy or impulse has been expressed behaviorally. Individuals with paraphilic interests can experience sexual pleasure, but they are inhibited from responding to stimuli that are normally considered erotic. The paraphiliac person's sexuality is mainly restricted to specific deviant stimuli or acts. Persons that occasionally experiment with paraphilic behavior (e.g., infrequent episode of bondage or dressing in costumes), but are capable of responding to more typical erotic stimuli, are not seen as having paraphilic disorders.

Paraphilic disorders can range from nearly normal behavior to behavior that is destructive or hurtful only to a person's self or to a person's self and partner, and finally to behavior that is deemed destructive or threatening to the community at large. DSM-5 lists pedophilia, frotteurism, voyeurism, exhibitionism, sexual sadism, sexual masochism, fetishism, and transvestism with explicit diagnostic criteria because of their threat to others and/or because they are relatively common paraphilias. There are many other paraphilias that may be diagnosed. A paraphilia is clinically significant if the person has acted on these fantasies or if these fantasies cause marked distress or interpersonal difficulty or job-related difficulty. However, when the fantasy has not been acted upon, the term paraphilic disorder should not be applied. In the paraphilias listed earlier, with the exception of pedophilia, the specifiers, "in a controlled environment" (where the fantasy cannot easily be acted upon due to circumstances, such as being in an institution) and "in full remission" (when the patient has not acted on the fantasies for 5 years and there has been no impairment in interpersonal or occupational functioning in an uncontrolled environment for 5 years) are added.

A special fantasy with its unconscious and conscious components is the pathognomonic element of the paraphilia, with sexual arousal and orgasm being associated phenomena that *reinforce the fantasy or impulse.* The influence of these fantasies and their behavioral manifestations often extend beyond the sexual sphere to pervade people's lives.

The major functions of human sexual behavior are to assist in bonding, to create mutual pleasure in cooperation with a partner, to express and enhance love between two persons, and to procreate. Paraphilic disorders entail divergent behaviors in that those acts involve aggression, victimization, and extreme one-sidedness. The behaviors exclude or harm others and disrupt the potential for bonding between persons. Moreover, paraphilic sexual scripts often serve other vital psychic functions. They may assuage anxiety, bind aggression, or stabilize identity.

EPIDEMIOLOGY

Paraphilias are practiced by only a small percentage of the population, but the insistent, repetitive nature of the disorders results in a high frequency of such acts. Thus, a large proportion of the population has been victimized by persons with paraphilic disorders. It has been suggested that the prevalence of paraphilias is significantly higher than the number of cases diagnosed in general clinical facilities, based on the large commercial market in paraphilic pornography and paraphernalia. It is not known how many of the consumers of this material act on paraphilic fantasies or cannot respond to typical erotic stimuli.

Among legally identified cases of paraphilic disorders, pedophilia is most common. Of all children, 10 to 20 percent have been molested by age 18. Because a child is the object, the act is taken more seriously, and greater effort is spent tracking down the culprit than in other paraphilic disorders. Persons with exhibitionism who publicly display themselves to young children are also commonly apprehended. Those with voyeurism may be apprehended, but their risk is not great. Of adult females, 20 percent have been the targets of persons with exhibitionism and voyeurism. Sexual masochism and sexual sadism are underrepresented in any prevalence estimates. Sexual sadism usually comes to attention only in sensational cases of rape, brutality, and lust murder. The excretory paraphilic disorders are scarcely reported, because activity usually takes place between consenting adults or between prostitute and client. Persons with fetishism rarely become entangled in the legal system. Those with transvestism may be arrested occasionally for disturbing the peace or on other misdemeanor charges if they are obviously men dressed in women's clothes, but arrest is more common among those with gender identity disorders. Zoophilia as a true paraphilic disorder is rare (Table 13.3–1).

As usually defined, the paraphilias seem to be largely male conditions. Fetishism almost always occurs in men. More than 50 percent of all paraphilias have their onset before age 18. Patients with paraphilia frequently have three to five paraphilias, either concurrently or at different times in their lives. This pattern of occurrence is especially the case with exhibitionism, fetishism, sexual masochism, sexual sadism, transvestic fetishism, voyeurism, and zoophilia (see Table 13.3–1). The occurrence of paraphilic behavior peaks between ages 15 and 25 and gradually declines. DSM-5 suggests the paraphilia designation be reserved for those ages 18 and older to avoid pathologizing normal sexual curiosity and occasional experimentation in adolescence. In men older than 50, criminal paraphilic acts are rare.

Table 13.3–1
Frequency of Paraphilic Acts Committed by Patients with Paraphilia Seeking Outpatient Treatment

Diagnostic Category	Patients with Paraphilia Seeking Outpatient Treatment (%)	Paraphilic Acts per Patient with Paraphilia[a]
Pedophilia	45	5
Exhibitionism	25	50
Voyeurism	12	17
Frotteurism	6	30
Sexual masochism	3	36
Transvestic fetishism	3	25
Sexual sadism	3	3
Fetishism	2	3
Zoophilia	1	2

[a]Median number.
(Courtesy of Gene G. Abel, M.D.)

Those that occur are practiced in isolation or with a cooperative partner.

ETIOLOGY

Psychosocial Factors

In the classic psychoanalytic model, persons with a paraphilia have failed to complete the normal developmental process toward sexual adjustment, but the model has been modified by new psychoanalytic approaches. What distinguishes one paraphilia from another is the method chosen by a person (usually male) to cope with the anxiety caused by the threat of castration by the father and separation from the mother. However bizarre its manifestation, the resulting behavior provides an outlet for the sexual and aggressive drives that would otherwise have been channeled into normal sexual behavior.

Failure to resolve the oedipal crisis by identifying with the father-aggressor (for boys) or mother-aggressor (for girls) results in either improper identification with the opposite-sex parent or an improper choice of object for libido cathexis. Classic psychoanalytic theory holds that transsexualism and transvestic fetishism are disorders because each involves identification with the opposite-sex parent instead of the same-sex parent; for instance, a man dressing in women's clothes is believed to identify with his mother. Exhibitionism and voyeurism may be attempts to calm anxiety about castration because the reaction of the victim or the arousal of the voyeur reassures the paraphilic person that the penis is intact. Fetishism is an attempt to avoid anxiety by displacing libidinal impulses to inappropriate objects. A person with a shoe fetish unconsciously denies that women have lost their penises through castration by attaching libido to a phallic object, the shoe, which symbolizes the female penis. Persons with pedophilia and sexual sadism have a need to dominate and control their victims to compensate for their feelings of powerlessness during the oedipal crisis. Some theorists believe that choosing a child as a love object is a narcissistic act. Persons with sexual masochism overcome their fear of injury and their sense of powerlessness by showing that they are impervious to harm. Another theory proposes that the masochist directs the aggression inherent in all paraphilias toward herself or himself. Although recent developments in psychoanalysis place more emphasis on treating defense mechanisms than on oedipal traumas, psychoanalytic therapy for patients with a paraphilia remains consistent with Sigmund Freud's theory.

Other theories attribute the development of a paraphilia to early experiences that condition or socialize children into committing a paraphilic act. The first shared sexual experience can be important in that regard. Molestation as a child can predispose a person to accept continued abuse as an adult or, conversely, to become an abuser of others. Also, early experiences of abuse that are not specifically sexual, such as spanking, enemas, or verbal humiliation, can be sexualized by a child and can form the basis for a paraphilia. Such experiences can result in the development of an *eroticized child.*

A 34-year-old man presented for treatment with a chief complaint of erectile disorder. He was frequently unable to obtain an erection sufficient for coitus with his wife. The problem disappeared whenever she was willing to act out his bondage fantasy and tie him up with ropes, a scenario he intensely desired. He explained that he felt free to be sexual when he was tied up because it reassured him that he could move vigorously and not hurt the woman. In addition, he gave a history of being tied up "in fun" when he was a child by a babysitter who would then tickle him until he begged her to stop.

The onset of paraphilic acts can result from persons' modeling their behavior on the behavior of others who have carried out paraphilic acts, mimicking sexual behavior depicted in the media, or recalling emotionally laden events from the past, such as their own molestation. Learning theory indicates that because the fantasizing of paraphilic interests begins at an early age and because personal fantasies and thoughts are not shared with others (who could block or discourage them), the use and misuse of paraphilic fantasies and urges continue uninhibited until late in life. Only then do persons begin to realize that such paraphilic interests and urges are inconsistent with societal norms. By that time, however, the repetitive use of such fantasies has become ingrained, and the sexual thoughts and behaviors have become associated with, or conditioned to, paraphilic fantasies.

Biological Factors

Several studies have identified abnormal organic findings in persons with paraphilias. None has used random samples of such persons; instead, they have extensively investigated patients with paraphilia who were referred to large medical centers. Among these patients, those with positive organic findings included 74 percent with abnormal hormone levels, 27 percent with hard or soft neurological signs, 24 percent with chromosomal abnormalities, 9 percent with seizures, 9 percent with dyslexia, 4 percent with abnormal electroencephalography (EEG) studies, 4 percent with major mental disorders, and 4 percent with mental handicaps. The question is whether these abnormalities are causally related to paraphilic interests or are incidental findings that bear no relevance to the development of paraphilia.

Psychophysiological tests have been developed to measure penile volumetric size in response to paraphilic and nonparaphilic stimuli. The procedures may be of use in diagnosis and treatment, but are of questionable diagnostic validity because some men are able to suppress their erectile responses.

DIAGNOSIS AND CLINICAL FEATURES

In DSM-5, the criteria for paraphilic disorder requires the patient to have experienced intense and recurrent arousal from their deviant fantasy for at least 6 months and to have acted on the paraphilic impulse. The presence of a paraphilic fantasy, however, may still distress a patient even if there has been no behavioral elaboration. The fantasy distressing the patient contains unusual sexual material that is relatively fixed and shows only minor variations. Arousal and orgasm depend on the mental elaboration, if not the behavioral playing out of the fantasy. Sexual activity is ritualized or stereotyped and makes use of degraded, reduced, or dehumanized objects.

Exhibitionism

Exhibitionism is the recurrent urge to expose the genitals to a stranger or to an unsuspecting person. Sexual excitement occurs in anticipation of the exposure, and orgasm is brought about by masturbation during or after the event. In almost 100 percent of cases, those with exhibitionism are men exposing themselves to women. The dynamic of men with exhibitionism is to assert their masculinity by showing their penises and by watching the victims' reactions—fright, surprise, and disgust. In this paraphilic disorder, men unconsciously feel castrated and impotent. Wives of men with exhibitionism often substitute for the mothers to whom the men were excessively attached during childhood, or conversely, by whom they were rejected. In other related paraphilias, the central themes involve derivatives of looking or showing.

A substance-abusing professional was finally able to attain sobriety at age 33 years. With this accomplishment, he met a woman and got married, began to work steadily for the first time in his life, and was able to impregnate his new wife. His preferred sexual activity had been masturbation in semi-public places. The patient had a strong sense that his mother had always thought him to be inadequate, did not like to spend time with him, and constantly made negative comparisons between him and his "all-boy" younger brother. He recalled several times when his father had tried to explain his mother's antipathy: "It is just one of those things son: your mother does not seem to like you." Without substance abuse, he gave up his exhibitionism, but he quickly developed sexual incapacity with his wife and became "addicted" to phone sex. *(Courtesy of Stephen B. Levine, M.D.)*

Specifiers added to exhibitionistic disorder by DSM-5 differentiate arousal from exposing genitals to prepubertal children, to physically mature individuals, or to both prepubertal children and physically mature individuals.

Fetishism

In fetishism the sexual focus is on objects (e.g., shoes, gloves, pantyhose, and stockings) that are intimately associated with the human body, or on nongenital body parts. The latter focus is sometimes called partialism and is discussed later. DSM-5 applies the diagnosis fetishistic disorder to partialism and attaches the following specifiers to fetishistic disorder: body part(s); nonliving parts; other. The particular fetish used is linked to someone closely involved with a patient during childhood and has a quality associated with this loved, needed, or even traumatizing person. Usually, the disorder begins by adolescence, although the fetish may have been established in childhood. Once established, the disorder tends to be chronic.

Sexual activity may be directed toward the fetish itself (e.g., masturbation with or into a shoe), or the fetish may be incorporated into sexual intercourse (e.g., the demand that high-heeled shoes be worn). The disorder is almost exclusively found in men. According to Freud, the fetish serves as a symbol of the phallus to persons with unconscious castration fears. Learning theorists believe that the object was associated with sexual stimulation at an early age.

A 50-year-old man entered treatment with a chief complaint of erectile disorder experienced primarily with his wife. He was suffering from a moderate depression that related to both his marital issues and business problems. He had no erectile problems with women he picked up in bars or knew and arranged to meet in bars. Bars were his chosen venue in part because smoking had been prohibited in other public areas in his city and a woman's act of smoking a cigarette was necessary to his sexual arousal. His family history included an alcoholic mother and an emotionally abusive father who was a chain smoker. On family car trips the father would smoke, with all the car windows up. If the patient complained of feeling nauseous the father would tell him to "shut up." He recalled being very attracted to a Sunday school teacher who smoked when he was 6 years old. He first smoked when he was 13, sneaking and hiding behind his house. His first cigarette was one he stole from a pack on his mother's night table.

Frotteurism

Frotteurism is usually characterized by a man's rubbing his penis against the buttocks or other body parts of a fully clothed woman to achieve orgasm. At other times, he may use his hands to rub an unsuspecting victim. The acts usually occur in crowded places, particularly in subways and buses. Those with frotteurism are extremely passive and isolated, and frottage is often their only source of sexual gratification. The expression of aggression in this paraphilia is readily apparent.

Pedophilia

Pedophilia involves recurrent intense sexual urges toward, or arousal by, children 13 years of age or younger, over a period of at least 6 months. In legal terms, persons with pedophilia are at least 16 years of age and at least 5 years older than the victims. When a perpetrator is a late adolescent involved in an ongoing sexual relationship with a 12- or 13-year-old, the diagnosis is not warranted.

Most child molestations involve genital fondling or oral sex. Vaginal or anal penetration of children occurs infrequently, except in cases of incest. Although most child victims coming to public attention are girls, this finding appears to be a product of the referral process. Offenders report that when they touch a child, most (60 percent) of the victims are boys. This figure is in sharp contrast to the figure for nontouching victimization of children, such as window peeping and exhibitionism; 99 percent of all such cases are perpetrated against girls. DSM-5 adds the following specifiers to a diagnosis of pedophilic disorder: sexually attracted to males; sexually attracted to females; or sexually attracted to both. Of persons with pedophilia, 95 percent are heterosexual, and 50 percent have consumed alcohol to excess at the time of the incident. In addition to their pedophilia, a significant number of the perpetrators are concomitantly or have previously been involved in exhibitionism, voyeurism, or rape.

Incest is related to pedophilia by the frequent selection of an immature child as a sex object, the subtle or overt element of coercion, and occasionally the preferential nature of the adult–child liaison.

A 62-year-old married janitor who worked as a fourth-grade school teacher for 26 years was referred for help after his family discovered that he had repeatedly fondled the genitals of his 4- and 6-year-old granddaughters. A father of five, he had not had sex with his wife for 30 years. He was generous, helpful, and cooperative with his children and grandchildren. Intellectually slow, he preferred comic books and had a charming manner of playing with young children "like he was one himself." By his estimate he had touched the buttocks and genitals of at least 300 girl students, thinking only of how they did not know what he was doing because he was being affectionate and they were too young to realize what was happening. He loved the anticipation and excitement of this behavior. His teaching career ended when parents complained to a principal. The patient had tried to touch his 12-year-old daughter who angrily warned him to stay away from her, but he had also managed to touch her friends and his best friend's daughters as they neared puberty. *(Adapted from a case courtesy of Stephen B. Levine, M.D.)*

Sexual Masochism

Masochism takes its name from the activities of Leopold von Sacher-Masoch, a 19th century Austrian novelist whose characters derived sexual pleasure from being abused and dominated by women. According to the DSM-5, persons with sexual masochism have a recurrent preoccupation with sexual urges and fantasies involving the act of being humiliated, beaten, bound, or otherwise made to suffer. A specifier added to this disorder diagnosis is: with asphyxiophilia; also called autoerotic asphyxiation, this is the practice of achieving or heightening sexual arousal with restriction of breathing. Sexual masochistic practices are more common among men than among women. Freud believed masochism resulted from destructive fantasies turned against the self. In some cases, persons can allow themselves to experience sexual feelings only when punishment for the feelings follows. Persons with sexual masochism may have had childhood experiences that convinced them that pain is a prerequisite for sexual pleasure. About 30 percent of those with sexual masochism also have sadistic fantasies. Moral masochism involves a need to suffer, but is not accompanied by sexual fantasies.

A 27-year-old woman presented for an interview with the director of a course to which she had applied and which she was eager to take. She appeared at the interview in the company of a man whom she introduced to the director, saying, "This is my lover." When asked about this unusual behavior during the interview, the applicant stated that her companion had ordered her to bring him and make that introduction. She further explained that she was part of a group that utilized sadomasochistic techniques in their sexual play.

Sexual Sadism

DSM-5 defines sexual sadism as the recurrent and intense sexual arousal from the physical and psychological suffering of another person. A person must have experienced these feelings for at least 6 months, and must have acted on sadistic fantasies to receive a diagnosis of sexual sadism disorder. Persons who deny behavioral elaboration of their paraphilic fantasies and who say they suffer no distress, or interpersonal or social difficulties, as a consequence of their paraphilias are designated as having an ascertained sexual sadism interest.

The onset of the disorder is usually before the age of 18 years, and most persons with sexual sadism are male. According to psychoanalytic theory, sadism is a defense against fears of castration; persons with sexual sadism do to others what they fear will happen to them and derive pleasure from expressing their aggressive instincts. The disorder was named after the Marquis de Sade, an 18th century French author and military officer who was repeatedly imprisoned for his violent sexual acts against women. Sexual sadism is related to rape, although rape is more aptly considered an expression of power. Some sadistic rapists, however, kill their victims after having sex (so-called lust murders). In many cases, these persons have underlying schizophrenia. John Money believes that lust murderers suffer from dissociative disorder and perhaps have a history of head trauma. He lists five contributory causes of sexual sadism: hereditary predisposition, hormonal malfunctioning, pathological relationships, a history of sexual abuse, and the presence of other mental disorders.

Voyeurism

Voyeurism, also known as *scopophilia,* is the recurrent preoccupation with fantasies and acts that involve observing unsuspecting persons who are naked or engaged in grooming or sexual activity. Masturbation to orgasm usually accompanies or follows the event. The first voyeuristic act usually occurs during childhood, and the paraphilia is most common in men. When persons with voyeurism are apprehended, the charge is usually loitering.

Transvestism

Transvestism, formerly called transvestic fetishism, is described as fantasies and sexual urges to dress in opposite gender clothing as a means of arousal and as an adjunct to masturbation or coitus. The diagnosis is given when the transvestic fantasies have been acted upon for at least 6 months. DSM-5 requires specifiers with a diagnosis of transvestic disorder: with fetishism is added if the patient is aroused by fabrics, materials, or garments; with autogynephilia is added if the patient is sexually aroused by thoughts or images of himself as a female.

Transvestism typically begins in childhood or early adolescence. As years pass, some men with transvestism want to dress and live permanently as women. Very rarely, women want to dress and live as men. These persons are classified in DSM-5 as persons with transvestic disorder and gender dysphoria. Usually, a person wears more than one article of opposite sex clothing; frequently, an entire wardrobe is involved. When a man with transvestism is cross-dressed, the appearance of femininity may be striking, although not usually to the degree found in transsexualism. When not dressed in women's clothes, men with transvestism may be hypermasculine in appearance and occupation. Cross-dressing can be graded from solitary, depressed, guilt-ridden dressing to ego-syntonic, social membership in a transvestite subculture.

The overt clinical syndrome of transvestism may begin in latency, but is more often seen around pubescence or in adolescence. Frank dressing in opposite sex clothing usually does not begin until mobility and relative independence from parents are well established.

Other Specified Paraphilic Disorder

This classification includes various paraphilias that cause personal distress and that have been acted upon for 6 months that do not meet the criteria for any of the aforementioned categories. The same definition applies to Unspecified Paraphilic Disorder, with the difference that the clinician does not wish to specify the particular paraphilia for reasons that may include not having sufficient information.

Telephone and Computer Scatologia. Telephone scatologia is characterized by obscene phone calling and involves an unsuspecting partner. Tension and arousal begin in anticipation of phoning; the recipient of the call listens while the telephoner (usually male) verbally exposes his preoccupations or induces her to talk about her sexual activity. The conversation is accompanied by masturbation, which is often completed after the contact is interrupted.

Persons also use interactive computer networks, sometimes compulsively, to send obscene messages by electronic mail and to transmit sexually explicit messages and video images. Because of the anonymity of the users in chat rooms who use aliases, online or computer sex (cybersex) allows some persons to play the role of the opposite sex ("genderbending"), which represents an alternative method of expressing transvestic or transsexual fantasies. A danger of online cybersex is that pedophiles often make contact with children or adolescents who are lured into meeting them and are then molested. Many online contacts develop into offline liaisons. Although some persons report that the offline encounters develop into meaningful relationships, most such meetings are filled with disappointment and disillusionment, as the fantasized person fails to meet unconscious expectations of the ideal partner. In other situations, when adults meet, rape or even homicide may occur.

Necrophilia. Necrophilia is an obsession with obtaining sexual gratification from cadavers. Most persons with this disorder find corpses in morgues, but some have been known to rob graves or even to murder to satisfy their sexual urges. In the few cases studied, those with necrophilia believed that they were inflicting the greatest conceivable humiliation on their lifeless victims. According to Richard von Krafft-Ebing, the diagnosis of psychosis is, under all circumstances, justified.

Partialism. Persons with the disorder of partialism concentrate their sexual activity on one part of the body to the exclusion of all others. Mouth–genital contact—such as cunnilingus (oral contact with a woman's external genitals), fellatio (oral contact with the penis), and anilingus (oral contact with the anus)—is normally associated with foreplay; Freud recognized the mucosal surfaces of the body as erotogenic and capable of producing pleasurable sensation. But when a person uses these activities as the sole source of sexual gratification and cannot have or refuses to have coitus, a paraphilia exists. It is also known as *oralism.*

Zoophilia. In zoophilia, animals—which may be trained to participate—are preferentially incorporated into arousal fantasies or sexual activities, including intercourse, masturbation, and oral–genital contact. Zoophilia as an organized paraphilia is rare. For many persons, animals are the major source of relatedness, so it is not surprising that a broad variety of domestic animals are used sensually or sexually.

Sexual relations with animals may occasionally be an outgrowth of availability or convenience, especially in parts of the world where rigid convention precludes premarital sexuality and in situations of enforced isolation. Because masturbation is also available in such situations, however, a predilection for animal contact is probably present in opportunistic zoophilia.

Coprophilia and Klismaphilia. Coprophilia is sexual pleasure associated with the desire to defecate on a partner, to be defecated on, or to eat feces (coprophagia). A variant is the compulsive utterance of obscene words (coprolalia). These paraphilias are associated with fixation at the anal stage of psychosexual development. Similarly, klismaphilia, the use of enemas as part of sexual stimulation, is related to anal fixation.

Urophilia. Urophilia, a form of urethral eroticism, is interest in sexual pleasure associated with the desire to urinate on a partner or to be urinated on. In both men and women, the disorder may be associated with masturbatory techniques involving the insertion of foreign objects into the urethra for sexual stimulation.

Masturbation. Masturbation is a normal activity that is common in all stages of life from infancy to old age, but this viewpoint was not always accepted. Freud believed that neurasthenia was caused by excessive masturbation. In the early 1900s, *masturbatory insanity* was a common diagnosis in hospitals for the criminally insane in the United States. Masturbation can be defined as a person's achieving sexual pleasure—which usually results in orgasm—by himself or herself (autoeroticism). Alfred Kinsey found it to be more prevalent in males than in females, but this difference may no longer exist. The frequency of masturbation varies from three to four times a week in adolescence to one to two times a week in adulthood. It is common among married persons; Kinsey reported that it occurred on the average of once a month among married couples.

The techniques of masturbation vary in both sexes and among persons. The most common technique is direct stimulation of the clitoris or penis with the hand or the fingers. Indirect stimulation can also be used, such as rubbing against a pillow or squeezing the thighs. Kinsey found that 2 percent of women are capable of achieving orgasm through fantasy alone. Men and women have been known to insert objects in the urethra to achieve orgasm. The hand vibrator is now used as a masturbatory device by both sexes.

Masturbation is abnormal when it is the only type of sexual activity performed in adulthood if a partner is or might be available, when its frequency indicates a compulsion or sexual dysfunction, or when it is consistently preferred to sex with a partner.

Hypoxyphilia. Hypoxyphilia is the desire to achieve an altered state of consciousness secondary to hypoxia while experiencing orgasm. Persons may use a drug (e.g., a volatile nitrite or nitrous oxide) to produce hypoxia. Autoerotic asphyxiation is also associated with hypoxic states, but it should be classified as a form of sexual masochism.

DIFFERENTIAL DIAGNOSIS

Clinicians must differentiate a paraphilia from an experimental act that is not recurrent or compulsive and that is done for its novelty. Paraphilic activity most likely begins during adolescence. Some paraphilias (especially the bizarre types) are associated with other mental disorders, such as schizophrenia. Brain diseases especially those involving the frontal lobes, can also release perverse impulses. There have been a few case reports of temporal lobe seizures being corrected with paraphilic acts.

COURSE AND PROGNOSIS

The difficulty in controlling or curing paraphilic disorders rests in the fact that it is hard for people to give up sexual pleasure with no assurance that new routes to sexual gratification will be secured. A poor prognosis for paraphilic disorder is associated with an early age of onset, a high frequency of acts, no guilt or shame about the act, and substance abuse. The course and the prognosis are better when patients have a history of coitus in addition to the paraphilia, and when they are self-referred rather than referred by a legal agency.

TREATMENT

Five types of psychiatric interventions are used to treat persons with paraphilic disorder and paraphilic interests: external control, reduction of sexual drives, treatment of comorbid conditions (e.g., depression or anxiety), cognitive–behavioral therapy, and dynamic psychotherapy.

Prison is an external control mechanism for sexual crimes that usually does not contain a treatment element. When victimization occurs in a family or work setting, the external control comes from informing supervisors, peers, or other adult family members of the problem and advising them about eliminating opportunities for the perpetrator to act on urges.

Drug therapy, including antipsychotic or antidepressant medication, is indicated for the treatment of schizophrenia or depressive disorders if the paraphilia is associated with these disorders. Antiandrogens, such as cyproterone acetate in Europe and medroxyprogesterone acetate (Depo-Provera) in the United States, may reduce the drive to behave sexually by decreasing serum testosterone levels to subnormal concentrations. Serotonergic agents, such as fluoxetine (Prozac), have been used with limited success in some patients with paraphilia.

Cognitive–behavioral therapy is used to disrupt learned paraphilic patterns and modify behavior to make it socially acceptable. The interventions include social skills training, sex education, cognitive restructuring (confronting and destroying the rationalizations used to support victimization of others), and development of victim empathy. Imaginal desensitization, relaxation technique, and learning what triggers the paraphilic impulse so that such stimuli can be avoided are also taught. In modified aversive behavior rehearsal, perpetrators are videotaped acting out their paraphilia with a mannequin. Then the patient with paraphilic disorder is confronted by a therapist and a group of other offenders who ask questions about feelings, thoughts, motives associated with the act and repeatedly try to correct cognitive distortions and point out lack of victim empathy to the patient.

Insight-oriented psychotherapy is a long-standing treatment approach. Patients have the opportunity to understand their dynamics and the events that caused the paraphilia to develop. In particular, they become aware of the daily events that cause them to act on their impulses (e.g., a real or fantasized rejection). Treatment helps them deal more effectively with life stresses and enhances their capacity to relate to a life partner. In addition, psychotherapy allows patients to regain self-esteem, which in turn allows them to approach a partner in a more normal sexual manner. Sex therapy is an appropriate adjunct to the treatment of patients with specific sexual dysfunctions when they attempt nondeviant sexual activities.

Good prognostic indicators include the presence of only one paraphilia, normal intelligence, the absence of substance abuse, the absence of nonsexual antisocial personality traits, and the presence of a successful adult attachment. Paraphilic disorders, however, remain significant treatment challenges even under these circumstances.

14

Gender Dysphoria

INTRODUCTION

The term *gender dysphoria* appears as a diagnosis for the first time in the fifth edition of the *Diagnostic and Statistical Manual of Mental Disorders* (DSM-5) to refer to those persons with a marked incongruence between their experienced or expressed gender and the one they were assigned at birth. It was known as gender identity disorder in the previous edition of DSM.

The term *gender identity* refers to the sense one has of being male or female, which corresponds most often to the person's anatomical sex. Persons with gender dysphoria express their discontent with their assigned sex as a desire to have the body of the other sex or to be regarded socially as a person of the other sex.

The term *transgender* is a general term used to refer to those who identify with a gender different from the one they were born with (sometimes referred to as their assigned gender). Transgender people are a diverse group: There are those who want to have the body of another sex known as transsexuals; those who feel they are between genders, of both genders, or of neither gender known as genderqueer; and those who wear clothing traditionally associated with another gender, but who maintain a gender identity that is the same as their birth-assigned gender known as cross-dressers. Contrary to popular belief, most transgender people do not have genital surgery. Some do not desire it and others who do may be unable to afford it. Transgender people may be of any sexual orientation. For example, a transgender man, assigned female at birth, may identify as gay (attracted to other men), straight (attracted to women), or bisexual (attracted to both men and women).

In DSM-5, no distinction is made for the overriding diagnostic term *gender dysphoria* as a function of age. However, criteria for diagnosis in children or adolescents are somewhat different. In children, gender dysphoria can manifest as statements of wanting to be the other sex and as a broad range of sex-typed behaviors conventionally shown by children of the other sex. Gender identity crystallizes in most persons by age 2 or 3 years. A specifier is noted if the gender dysphoria is associated with a disorder of sex development.

EPIDEMIOLOGY

Children

Most children with gender dysphoria are referred for clinical evaluation in early grade school years. Parents, however, typically report that the cross-gender behaviors were apparent before 3 years of age. Among a sample of boys younger than age 12 who were referred for a range of clinical problems, the reported desire to be the other sex was 10 percent. For clinically referred girls younger than age 12, the reported desire to be the other sex was 5 percent. The sex ratio of children referred for gender dysphoria is 4 to 5 boys for each girl, which is hypothesized to be due in part to societal stigma directed toward feminine boys. The sex ratio is equal in adolescents referred for gender dysphoria. Researchers have observed that many children considered to have shown gender nonconforming behavior do not grow up to be transgender adults; conversely many people who later come out as transgender adults report that they were not identified as gender nonconforming during childhood.

Adults

The estimates of gender dysphoria in adults emanate from European hormonal/surgical clinics with a prevalence of 1 in 11,000 male-assigned and 1 in 30,000 female-assigned people. DSM-5 reports a prevalence rate ranging from 0.005 to 0.014 percent for male-assigned and 0.002 to 0.003 percent for female-assigned people. Most clinical centers report a sex ratio of three to five male patients for each female patient. Most adults with gender dysphoria report having felt different from other children of their same sex, although, in retrospect, many could not identify the source of that difference. Many report feeling extensively cross-gender identified from the earliest years, with the cross-gender identification becoming more profound in adolescence and young adulthood. Overall the prevalence of male to female dysphoria is higher than female to male dysphoria. An important factor in diagnosis is that there is greater social acceptance of birth-assigned females dressing and behaving as boys (so-called tomboys) than there is of birth-assigned males acting as females (so-called sissies). Some researchers speculate that one in 500 adults may fall somewhere on a transgender spectrum, based on population data rather than clinical data.

ETIOLOGY

Biological Factors

For mammals, the resting state of tissue is initially female; as the fetus develops, a male is produced only if androgen (set off by the Y chromosome, which is responsible for testicular development) is introduced. Without testes and androgen, female external genitalia develop. Thus, maleness and masculinity depend on fetal and perinatal androgens. Sexual behavior in lower animals is governed by sex steroids, but this effect diminishes as the evolutionary tree is scaled. Sex steroids influence the expression of sexual behavior in mature men or women; that is, testosterone can increase libido and aggressiveness in women, and estrogen can decrease libido and aggressiveness in men. But masculinity, femininity, and gender identity may result more from postnatal life events than from prenatal hormonal organization.

Brain organization theory refers to masculinization or feminization of the brain in utero. Testosterone affects brain neurons that contribute to the masculinization of the brain in such areas as the hypothalamus. Whether testosterone contributes to so-called masculine or feminine behavioral patterns remains a controversial issue.

Genetic causes of gender dysphoria are under study but no candidate genes have been identified, and chromosomal variations are uncommon in transgender populations. Case reports of identical twins have shown some pairs that are concordant for transgender issues and others not so affected.

A variety of other approaches to understanding gender dysphoria are underway. These include imaging studies that have shown changes in white matter tracts, cerebral blood flow, and cerebral activation patterns in patients with gender dysphoria; but such studies have not been replicated. An incidental finding is that transgender persons are likely to be left handed, the significance of which in unknown.

Psychosocial Factors

Children usually develop a gender identity consonant with their assigned sex. The formation of gender identity is influenced by the interaction of children's temperament and parents' qualities and attitudes. Culturally acceptable gender roles exist: Boys are not expected to be effeminate, and girls are not expected to be masculine. There are boys' games (e.g., cops and robbers) and girls' toys (e.g., dolls and dollhouses). These roles are learned, although some investigators believe that some boys are temperamentally delicate and sensitive and that some girls are aggressive and energized—traits that are stereotypically known in today's culture as feminine and masculine, respectively. However, greater tolerance for mild cross-gender activity in children has developed in the last few decades.

Sigmund Freud believed that gender identity problems resulted from conflicts experienced by children within the Oedipal triangle. In his view, these conflicts are fueled by both real family events and children's fantasies. Whatever interferes with a child's loving the opposite-sex parent and identifying with the same-sex parent interferes with normal gender identity development.

Since Freud, psychoanalysts have postulated that the quality of the mother–child relationship in the first years of life is paramount in establishing gender identity. During this period, mothers normally facilitate their children's awareness of, and pride in, their gender: Children are valued as little boys and girls. Analysts argue that devaluing, hostile mothering can result in gender problems. At the same time, the separation–individuation process is unfolding. When gender problems become associated with separation–individuation problems, the result can be the use of sexuality to remain in relationships characterized by shifts between a desperate infantile closeness and a hostile, devaluing distance.

Some children are given the message that they would be more valued if they adopted the gender identity of the opposite sex. Rejected or abused children may act on such a belief. Gender identity problems can also be triggered by a mother's death, extended absence, or depression, to which a young boy may react by totally identifying with her—that is, by becoming a mother to replace her.

The father's role is also important in the early years, and his presence normally helps the separation–individuation process. Without a father, mother and child may remain overly close. For a girl, the father is normally the prototype of future love objects; for a boy, the father is a model for male identification.

Learning theory postulates that children may be rewarded or punished by parents and teachers on the basis of gendered behavior, thus influencing the way children express their gender identities. Children also learn how to label people according to gender and eventually learn that gender is not dictated by surface appearance such as clothing or hairstyle.

DIAGNOSIS AND CLINICAL FEATURES

Children

The DSM-5 defines gender dysphoria in children as incongruence between expressed and assigned gender, with the most important criterion being a desire to be another gender or insistence that one is another gender. By emphasizing the importance of the child's self-perception, the creators of the diagnosis attempt to limit its use to those children who clearly state their wishes to be another gender, rather than encompassing a broader group of children who might be considered by adults to be gender nonconforming. However, a child's behavior may also lead to this diagnosis.

Many children with gender dysphoria prefer clothing typical of another gender, preferentially choose playmates of another gender, enjoy games and toys associated with another gender, and take on the roles of another gender during play. For a diagnosis to be made, these social characteristics must be accompanied by other traits less likely to be socially influenced, such as a strong desire to be the other gender, dislike of one's sexual anatomy, or desire for primary or secondary sexual characteristics of the desired gender. Children may express a desire to have different genitals, state that their genitals are going to change, or urinate in the position (standing or sitting) typical of another gender. It is notable that characteristics used to diagnose children with gender dysphoria must be accompanied by clinically significant distress or impairment on the part of the child, and not simply on the part of the adult caregivers, who may be uncomfortable with gender nonconformity.

Differential Diagnosis of Children

Children diagnosed with gender dysphoria, predicted to be more likely than others to identify as transgender as adults, are differentiated from other gender nonconforming children by statements about desired anatomical changes, as well as persistence of the diagnosis over time. Children whose gender dysphoria persists over time may make repeated statements about a desire to be or belief that they are another gender. Other gender nonconforming children may make these statements for short periods but not repeatedly, or may not make these types of statements, and may instead prefer clothing and behaviors associated with another gender, but show contentment with their birth-assigned gender.

The diagnosis of gender dysphoria no longer excludes intersex people, and instead is coded with a specifier in the cases where intersex people are gender dysphoric in relation to their birth-assigned gender. A medical history is important to distinguish between those children with intersex conditions and those without. The standards of care for intersex children have changed dramatically over the last few decades due to activism by intersex adults and supportive medical and mental health professionals. Historically, intersex babies were often subjected to early surgical procedures to create more standard male or female appearances. These procedures had the potential to cause sexual dysfunction, such as inability to orgasm, and permanent sterility. Recently, these practices have changed considerably so that more intersex people are given the chance to make decisions about their bodies later in life.

Adolescents and Adults

Adolescents and adults diagnosed with gender dysphoria must also show an incongruence between expressed and assigned gender. In addition, they must meet at least two of six criteria, half of which are related to their current (or in the cases of early adolescents, future) secondary sex characteristics or desired secondary sex characteristics. Other criteria include a strong desire to be another gender, be treated as another gender, or the belief that one has the typical feelings and reactions of another gender.

In practice, most adults who present to mental health practitioners with reports of gender-related concerns are aware of the concept of transgender identity. They may be interested in therapy to explore gender issues, or may be making contact in order to request a letter recommending hormone treatment or surgery. The cultural trope of being "trapped in the wrong body" does not apply to all, or even most, people who identify as transgender, so clinicians should be aware to use open and affirming approaches, taking language cues from their patients.

The DSM-5 criteria are noticeably open to the idea that some people do not fit into the traditional gender binary, and may desire to be alternative genders, such as genderqueer. Like the diagnosis in childhood, the adolescent and adult diagnosis also requires that those diagnosed be personally distressed or impaired by their feelings, rather than their behaviors or identities being pathologized by others while not upsetting to the people themselves. The adolescent and adult criteria also contain a posttransition specifier, which can be used for those people who live in their affirmed genders. They are required, however, to have undergone or be preparing to undergo at least one medical or surgical procedure in order to qualify for this specifier.

Differential Diagnosis of Adolescents and Adults

Those who meet the criteria for a diagnosis of gender dysphoria must experience clinical distress or impairment related to their gender identity. This excludes from the diagnosis those transgender or gender nonconforming people who are not clinically distressed by their gender identities. There are certain mental illnesses in which transgender identity may be a component of delusional thinking, such as in *schizophrenia.* However, this is extremely rare and can be differentiated from transgender identity or gender dysphoria through the diminishment of transgender feelings with the successful treatment of psychosis versus the persistence of these feelings in periods that are psychosis free. *Body dysmorphic disorder* may be a differential diagnosis for some patients who present with a desire to change gendered body parts. However, those with body dysmorphic disorder generally focus on a body part because of a belief that it is abnormal, rather than due to a desire to change their assigned gender. The *Paraphilic Disorders* chapter of the DSM-5 contains the diagnosis *transvestic disorder,* which is defined as recurrent and intense sexual arousal from cross-dressing that causes clinically significant distress or impairment. This diagnosis is differentiated from gender dysphoria by the patient's gender identity being consistent with their gender assigned at birth, and by sexual excitement linked to cross-dressing coming to interfere with the person's life.

COURSE AND PROGNOSIS

Children

Children typically begin to develop a sense of their gender identity around age 3. At this point they may develop gendered behaviors and interests, and some may begin to express a desire to be another gender. It is often around school age that children are first brought for clinical consultations, as this is when they begin to interact heavily with classmates and to be scrutinized by adults other than their caregivers. Some children who will later identify as transgender as adults do not show behaviors consistent with another gender at this age. Some say later that they worked hard to appear stereotypical to their assigned gender, whereas others deny being able to recall gender identity concerns. Approaching puberty, many children diagnosed with gender dysphoria begin to show increased levels of anxiety related to anticipated changes to their bodies.

Children diagnosed with gender dysphoria do not necessarily grow up to identify as transgender adults. A number of studies have demonstrated that more than half of those diagnosed with gender identity disorder, based on the DSM-IV, later identify with their birth-assigned gender once they reach adulthood. Those children who do identify as transgender as adults have been shown to have more extreme gender dysphoria as children. Many studies show increased rates of gay and bisexual identity among those who were gender nonconforming as children.

Comorbidity in Children

Children diagnosed with gender dysphoria show higher rates than other children of depressive disorders, anxiety disorders, and impulse-control disorders. This is likely related to the stigma faced by these children related to their gendered behaviors and identities. There are also reports that those diagnosed with gender dysphoria are more likely than others to fall on the autism spectrum. Some researchers posit that this may be related to intrauterine hormone exposure.

Adults

Some people diagnosed with gender dysphoria as adults recall the continuous development of transgender identity since childhood. In these cases, some have periods of hiding their gender identity, many entering into stereotypic activities and employment in order to convince themselves and others that they do not have gender nonconforming identities. Others do not recall gender identity issues during childhood. Lesbian and gay communities are often havens for gender nonconforming people, and some people identify as gay, lesbian, or bisexual before coming out as transgender.

Comorbidity in Adults

Adults diagnosed with gender dysphoria show higher rates than other adults of depressive disorders, anxiety disorders, suicidality and self-harming behaviors, and substance abuse. The lifetime rate of suicidal thoughts in transgender people is thought to be about 40 percent. The minority stress model predicts increases in mental illness in groups that are stigmatized, discriminated against, harassed, and abused at higher rates than others. DSM-5 reports that persons with late-onset gender dysphoria may have greater fluctuations in the extent of their distress and more ambivalence about and less satisfaction after sex reassignment surgery.

TREATMENT

Children

Treatment of gender identity issues in children typically consists of individual, family, and group therapy that guides children in exploring their gendered interests and identities. There are some providers who practice reparative, or conversion therapy, which attempts to change a person's gender identity or sexual orientation. This type of therapy is contrary to position statements by the American Psychiatric Association and practice guidelines of the American Academy of Child and Adolescent Psychiatry.

Adolescents

As gender-nonconforming children approach puberty, some show intense fear and preoccupation related to the physical changes they anticipate or are beginning to experience. In addition to providing psychotherapy, many clinicians use these adolescents' reactions to the first signs of puberty as a compass to determine if puberty-blocking medications should be a consideration. Puberty-blocking medications are gonadotropin-releasing hormone (GnRH) agonists that can be used to temporarily block the release of hormones that lead to secondary sex characteristics, giving adolescents and their families time to reflect on the best options moving forward. GnRH agonists have been used for many years in other populations (e.g., children with precocious puberty) and are felt to be safe. However, such steps should be considered carefully.

Adults

Treatment of adults who identify as transgender may include psychotherapy to explore gender issues, hormonal treatment, and surgical treatment. Hormonal and surgical interventions may decrease depression and improve quality of life for such persons.

Mental Health Treatment

The history of poor treatment and medicalization of transgender people by mental health providers has led to a decreased interest on the part of trans-identified people in engaging in mental health care. Many surgeons, and some physicians who prescribe transition-related hormones, require a letter from a mental health provider, so many transgender people are engaged with mental health in a gatekeeping model. Many community clinics are now using informed consent models for hormone treatment, thereby decreasing the need for mental health providers to play the role of gatekeepers. The World Professional Association for Transgender Health (WPATH) Standards of Care (SOC) for the health of transsexual, transgender, and gender-nonconforming people have recently become more flexible and open to informed consent models. Some mental health providers are specializing in working with transgender populations, and this is increasing the rate at which transgender people engage in psychotherapy.

Hormones

Hormone treatment of transgender men is primarily accomplished with testosterone, usually taken by injection every week or every other week. Initial changes with testosterone therapy include increased acne, muscle mass, and libido, as well as cessation of menses, usually within the first few months. Subsequent, and more permanent, changes include deepening of the voice, increased body hair, and enlargement of the clitoris. Monitoring includes hemoglobin/hematocrit levels, as testosterone can rarely cause an increase in red blood cell counts that can lead to stroke. Like all steroid hormones, testosterone is processed in the liver, so routine liver function tests should be obtained. Clinicians also want to monitor cholesterol and screen for diabetes, as testosterone treatment may increase the likelihood of lipid abnormalities and diabetes. Those beginning hormone treatments are routinely counseled on fertility, as future fertility may be affected on testosterone.

Transgender women may take estrogen, testosterone-blockers, or progesterone, often in combination. These hormones can cause softening of the skin and redistribution of fat, as well as breast growth. Breast development varies between people, but does not generally exceed bra cup size B. It is generally recommended to be on hormones for 18 to 24 months before having breast augmentation, allowing the breasts to develop to their final size. Sex drive can decrease, as well as erections and ejaculation. Body hair can decrease somewhat, but often not as much as desired, prompting many women to obtain electrolysis. There is no change in voice, as testosterone has permanently altered the vocal cords, and many women seek out voice coaching. Those on estrogen should avoid cigarette smoking, as the combination can lead to increased risk of blood clots. Blood pressure should be monitored, as well as liver function and cholesterol. In addition, providers routinely test prolactin as this hormone can increase on estrogen therapy, and in rare cases transgender women may develop prolactinomas. Reproductive counseling is very important before beginning estrogen treatment because permanent sterility is almost always the outcome.

Surgery

Many fewer people undergo gender-related surgeries than take hormones. Some people do not desire gender-related surgeries. Others cannot afford them, or are not convinced that they will be satisfied with currently available results.

The most common type of surgery for both trans-men and trans-women is "top surgery," or chest surgery. Transgender men may have surgery to construct a male-contoured chest. Trans-women may have breast augmentation.

"Bottom surgery" is less common. Transgender men may have a metoidioplasty, in which the clitoris is freed from the ligament attaching it to the body, and tissue is added, increasing its length and girth. Scrotoplasty, the placement of testicular implants, is another way to create male-appearing genitalia. Phalloplasty, the creation of a penis, is less commonly performed because it is expensive, involves multiple procedures, requires donor skin from another part of the body, and has limited functionality. Bottom surgery for women is typically vaginoplasty, also commonly known as sex reassignment surgery (SRS). In this procedure, the testicles are removed, the penis is reconstructed to form a clitoris, and a vagina is created. Techniques for vaginoplasty are becoming very good, but the procedure remains expensive. Because of this, some women, especially those with less money, may have orchiectomies, where the testes alone are removed. These can be in-office procedures with local anesthetic, and are effective in substantially decreasing the body's production of androgens like testosterone. Less widely discussed, but important to many women, are facial feminization surgeries that alter the cheeks, forehead, nose, and lips to create a more feminine facial appearance. The face is often used by persons to recognize gender in another person and having facial features that match one's affirmed gender can facilitate social interaction and provide safety from harassment and violence. Transgender men rarely undergo facial surgeries, as testosterone typically causes the face to appear more masculine.

Because surgery is inaccessible to many, there are rare cases of self-surgery and some people have surgeries performed under unsafe conditions. Women may inject industrial grade silicone to produce body curves. Silicone injection that is not done under the supervision of a medical professional can result in body mutilation, infection, and even silicone blood clots that can lead to embolism and death.

Other Specified

The category *other specified gender dysphoria* can be used in cases where the presentation causes clinically significant distress or impairment but does not meet the full criteria for gender dysphoria. If this diagnosis is used, the clinician records the specific reason that the full criteria were not met.

Unspecified

The category *unspecified gender dysphoria* can be applied when full criteria are not met and the clinician chooses not to specify why they are not met.

A 27-year-old assigned female at birth was referred to a gender identity clinic reporting having felt different as a child from other girls, although unable then to identify the source. As a young girl, she enjoyed playing sports with girls and boys, but generally preferred the companionship of boys. She preferred wearing unisex or boyish clothes and resisted wearing a skirt or dress. Everyone referred to her as a tomboy. She tried to hide her breast development by wearing loose fitting tops and stooping forward. Menses were embarrassing and poignantly reminded her of her femaleness, which was becoming increasingly alienating. As sexual attractions evolved, they were directed exclusively to female partners. In her late teens, she had one sexual experience with a man, and it was aversive. She began socializing in lesbian circles, but did not feel comfortable there and did not consider herself lesbian, but more a man. For sexual partners, she wanted heterosexual women and wanted to be considered by the partner as a man. As gender dysphoric feelings became increasingly pronounced, she consulted transsexual sites on the Internet and contacted a female-to-male transsexual community support group. She then set into motion the process of clinical referral. She transitioned to living as a man, had a name change, and was administered androgen injections. The patient's voice deepened, facial and body hair grew, menses stopped, and sex drive increased, along with clitoral hypertrophy. After 2 years, the patient underwent bilateral mastectomy and is on the wait list for phalloplasty and hysterectomy-oopherectomy. Employment as a man continues, as does a 3-year relationship with a female partner. The partner has a child from a previous marriage. *(Adapted from case of Richard Green, M.D.)*

Intersex Conditions

Intersex conditions include a variety of syndromes in which persons are born with anatomies that do not correspond with typical male or female bodies.

Congenital Adrenal Hyperplasia

Congenital adrenal hyperplasia is a condition in which an enzymatic defect in the production of adrenal cortisol, beginning prenatally, leads to overproduction of adrenal androgens and, when the chromosomes are XX, virilization of the female fetus. Postnatally, excessive adrenal androgen can be controlled by steroid administration.

The androgenization can range from mild clitoral enlargement to external genitals that look like a normal scrotal sac, testes, and a penis, but behind these external genitals are a vagina and a uterus. Other parts of the body remain feminized (i.e., there is breast development at puberty). Most people with congenital adrenal hyperplasia are raised female, except in cases of extreme virilization. If the parents are uncertain about the sex of their child, sometimes an intersex identity results. Gender identity usually reflects the rearing practices, but hormones may help determine behavior. Studies showed that sex-disordered children raised as girls had a more intense tomboy quality than that found in a control group. The girls most often had a heterosexual orientation, but higher rates of bisexual or homosexual behavior were reported. In those brought up female, about 5% show severe gender dysphoria, whereas about 12% of those assigned male are gender dysphoric.

Androgen Insensitivity Syndrome

Androgen insensitivity syndrome was formerly called *testicular feminization.* In persons with complete androgen insensitivity and the XY karyotype, tissue cells are unable to use testosterone or other androgens. Therefore, the person appears to be a normal female at birth and is raised as a girl. She is later found to have cryptorchid testes, which produce the testosterone to which the tissues do not respond, and minimal or absent internal sexual organs. Secondary sex characteristics at puberty are female because of the small, but sufficient, amount of estrogens, which results from the conversion of testosterone into estradiol. The patients usually sense themselves as females and are feminine. However, some experience gender conflicts and distress. In partial androgen insensitivity, persons may have a range of anatomical structures and gender identities.

Turner's Syndrome

In Turner's syndrome, one sex chromosome is missing, such that the sex karyotype is simply X. Persons with Turner's syndrome have female genitalia, are short, and sometimes have anomalies such as a shield-shaped chest and a webbed neck. As a consequence of dysfunctional ovaries, they require exogenous estrogen to develop female secondary sex characteristics. Gender identity is typically female.

Klinefelter's Syndrome

An extra X chromosome is present in Klinefelter's syndrome, such that the karyotype is XXY. At birth, persons with Klinefelter's appear to be normal males. Excessive gynecomastia may occur in adolescence. Testes are small, usually without sperm production. They are tall, and body habitus is eunuchoid. Reports suggest a higher rate of gender dysphoria.

5-α-Reductase Deficiency

In 5-α-reductase deficiency, an enzymatic defect prevents the conversion of testosterone to dihydrotestosterone, which is required for prenatal virilization of the genitalia. At birth, the affected person appears to be female, although some variance is visible. In earlier generations, before childhood identification of the disorder was common, these persons, raised as girls, virilized at puberty and usually changed their gender identity to male. Later generations were expected to virilize and, thus, may have been raised with ambiguous gender. Over half of those with 5-α-reductase deficiency identify as male as adults. There are reports of a small number of patients for whom early removal of the testes and socialization as girls have resulted in a female gender identity.

Treatment

Because intersex conditions are present at birth, treatment must be timely. The appearance of the genitalia in diverse conditions is often ambiguous, and a decision must be made about the assigned sex (boy or girl) and how the child should be reared.

Intersex conditions should be addressed as early as possible, so that the entire family can regard the child in a consistent, relaxed manner. This is particularly important because intersex patients may have gender identity problems because of complicated biological influences and familial confusion about their actual sex. When intersex conditions are discovered, a panel of pediatric, urological, and psychiatric experts works with the family to determine the sex of rearing on the basis of clinical examination, urological studies, buccal smears, chromosomal analyses, and assessment of the parental wishes.

Education of parents and presentation of the range of options open to them is essential, because parents respond to the infant's genitalia in ways that promote the formation of gender identity. Although the label of boy or girl may be assigned to the infant on the basis of chromosomal and urological examination, the parents can then react to the child according to sex role assignment with leeway to adjust the sex assignment should the child act definitively as a member of the sex different from the one designated. Some studies have shown that an equal number of persons assigned to be female at birth choose to become male as adults as do those assigned to be male at birth who choose to become female. In general, the sex of rearing is the best predictor of later gender identity.

In the past, many intersex infants underwent surgical procedures at an early age in order to normalize genital appearance. It is easier to surgically assign a child to be female than to assign one to be male, because male-to-female genital surgical procedures are far more advanced than female-to-male procedures. That is an insufficient reason, however, to assign a chromosomal male to be female.

The standards of care related to intersex infants have changed considerably due to work by intersex people and their allies, so that it is no longer recommended that infants have immediate surgical procedures performed. Instead, families are encouraged to choose a sex of rearing that is flexible, and to wait for the intersex person to decide on their own later whether to have surgery. Early surgeries are typically avoided now because they may interfere with later reproductive capacity and sexual functioning.

Transvestic Disorder

Transvestic disorder appears in the DSM-5 section on *Paraphilic Disorders,* and is defined as a period of at least 6 months of recurrent and intense sexual arousal from cross-dressing that causes clinically significant distress or impairment. Those who cross-dress are diverse, and many use cross-dressing as a form of entertainment or pleasure that does not cause distress, and therefore do not meet the criteria for this diagnosis. Cross-dressing does not imply gender dysphoria—many people who cross-dress do so while retaining a gender identity that matches their assigned gender. Cross-dressers do not necessarily have a preoccupation with getting rid of their primary and secondary sex characteristics and acquiring the sex characteristics of the other sex. However, there are those who may be diagnosed with both gender dysphoria and transvestic disorder.

The prevalence of transvestic disorder is unknown. It is more common in males and extremely rarely diagnosed in females, most likely due to comparable societal acceptance of women dressing in male-typical clothing. Those diagnosed with transvestic disorder often remember a fascination with female clothing in childhood. They may have periods of stress-related cross-dressing that produces sexual excitement, but also reduces tension and anxiety. There may be periods where the person buys a number of articles of clothing, wears them for sexual excitement, and then becomes distressed by their behavior and throws them out. Transvestic disorder can coexist with other paraphilic disorders, most commonly *sexual masochism disorder* and *fetishistic disorder.*

Treatment. A combined approach, using psychotherapy and pharmacotherapy, is often useful in the treatment of transvestic disorder. The stress factors that precipitate the behavior are identified in therapy. The goal is to help patients cope with the stressors appropriately and, if possible, eliminate them. Intrapsychic dynamics about attitudes toward men and women are examined, and unconscious conflicts are identified. Medication, such as antianxiety and antidepressant agents, is used to treat the symptoms. Because cross-dressing can occur impulsively, medications that reinforce impulse control may be helpful, such as fluoxetine (Prozac). Behavior therapy and hypnosis are alternative methods that may be of use in selected patients.

15 Disruptive, Impulse-Control, and Conduct Disorders

INTRODUCTION

Five conditions comprise the category of *disruptive, impulse-control, and conduct disorders*. They include two that are associated with childhood: (1) oppositional defiant disorder and (2) conduct disorder, both of which are discussed in the child psychiatry section of this text in Sections 27.12d and 27.12e, respectively. The remaining three disorders are intermittent explosive disorder, kleptomania, and pyromania, which are discussed in subsequent text of this chapter. Each disorder is characterized by the inability to resist an intense impulse, drive, or temptation to perform a particular act that is obviously harmful to self or others, or both. Before the event, the individual usually experiences mounting tension and arousal, sometimes—but not consistently—mingled with conscious anticipatory pleasure. Completing the action brings immediate gratification and relief. Within a variable time afterward, the individual experiences a conflation of remorse, guilt, self-reproach, and dread. These feelings may stem from obscure unconscious conflicts or awareness of the deed's impact on others (including the possibility of serious legal consequences in syndromes such as kleptomania). Shameful secretiveness about the repeated impulsive activity frequently expands to pervade the individual's entire life, often significantly delaying treatment.

ETIOLOGY

Psychodynamic, psychosocial, and biological factors all play an important role in impulse-control disorders; however, the primary causal factor remains unknown. Some impulse-control disorders may have common underlying neurobiological mechanisms. Fatigue, incessant stimulation, and psychic trauma can lower a person's resistance to control impulses.

Psychodynamic Factors

An impulse is a disposition to act to decrease heightened tension caused by the buildup of instinctual drives or by diminished ego defenses against the drives. The impulse disorders have in common an attempt to bypass the experience of disabling symptoms or painful affects by acting on the environment.

In his work with adolescents who were delinquent, August Aichhorn described impulsive behavior as related to a weak superego and weak ego structures associated with psychic trauma produced by childhood deprivation.

Otto Fenichel linked impulsive behavior to attempts to master anxiety, guilt, depression, and other painful affects by means of action. He thought that such actions defend against internal danger and that they produce a distorted aggressive or sexual gratification. To observers, impulsive behaviors may appear irrational and motivated by greed, but they may actually be endeavors to find relief from pain.

Heinz Kohut considered many forms of impulse-control problems, including gambling, kleptomania, and some paraphilic behaviors, to be related to an incomplete sense of self. He observed that when patients do not receive the validating and affirming responses that they seek from persons in significant relationships with them, the self might fragment. As a way of dealing with this fragmentation and regaining a sense of wholeness or cohesion in the self, persons may engage in impulsive behaviors that to others appear self-destructive. Kohut's formulation has some similarities to Donald Winnicott's view that impulsive or deviant behavior in children is a way for them to try to recapture a primitive maternal relationship. Winnicott saw such behavior as hopeful in that the child searches for affirmation and love from the mother rather than abandoning any attempt to win her affection.

Patients attempt to master anxiety, guilt, depression, and other painful affects by means of actions, but such actions aimed at obtaining relief seldom succeed even temporarily.

Psychosocial Factors

Psychosocial factors implicated causally in impulse-control disorders are related to early life events. The growing child may have had improper models for identification, such as parents who had difficulty controlling impulses. Other psychosocial factors associated with the disorders include exposure to violence in the home, alcohol abuse, promiscuity, and antisocial behavior.

Biological Factors

Many investigators have focused on possible organic factors in the impulse-control disorders, especially for patients with overtly violent behavior. Experiments have shown that impulsive and violent activity is associated with specific brain regions, such as the limbic system, and that the inhibition of such behaviors is associated with other brain regions. A relation has been found between low cerebrospinal fluid (CSF) levels of 5-hydroxyindoleacetic acid (5-HIAA) and impulsive aggression. Certain hormones, especially testosterone, have also been associated with violent and aggressive behavior. Some reports have described a relation between temporal lobe epilepsy and certain impulsive violent behaviors, as well as an association of aggressive behavior in patients who have histories of head trauma with increased numbers of emergency room visits and other potential organic antecedents. A high incidence of mixed cerebral dominance may be found in some violent populations.

Considerable evidence indicates that the serotonin neurotransmitter system mediates symptoms evident in impulse-control disorders. Brainstem and CSF levels of 5-HIAA are decreased, and serotonin-binding sites are increased in persons who have committed suicide. The dopaminergic and noradrenergic systems have also been implicated in impulsivity.

Impulse-control disorder symptoms can continue into adulthood in persons whose disorder has been diagnosed as childhood attention-deficit/hyperactivity disorder (ADHD). Lifelong or acquired mental deficiency, epilepsy, and even reversible brain syndromes have long been implicated in lapses in impulse control.

INTERMITTENT EXPLOSIVE DISORDER

Intermittent explosive disorder manifests as discrete episodes of losing control of aggressive impulses; these episodes can result in serious assault or the destruction of property. The aggressiveness expressed is grossly out of proportion to any stressors that may have helped elicit the episodes. The symptoms, which patients may describe as spells or attacks, appear within minutes or hours and, regardless of duration, remit spontaneously and quickly. After each episode, patients usually show genuine regret or self-reproach, and signs of generalized impulsivity or aggressiveness are absent between episodes. The diagnosis of intermittent explosive disorder should not be made if the loss of control can be accounted for by schizophrenia, antisocial or borderline personality disorder, ADHD, conduct disorder, or substance intoxication.

The term *epileptoid personality* has been used to convey the seizure-like quality of the characteristic outbursts, which are not typical of the patient's usual behavior, and to convey the suspicion of an organic disease process, for example, damage to the central nervous system. Several associated features suggest the possibility of an epileptoid state: the presence of auras; postictal-like changes in the sensorium, including partial or spotty amnesia; and hypersensitivity to photic, aural, or auditory stimuli.

Epidemiology

Intermittent explosive disorder is underreported. The disorder appears to be more common in men than in women. The men are likely to be found in correctional institutions and the women in psychiatric facilities. In one study, about 2 percent of all persons admitted to a university hospital psychiatric service had disorders that were diagnosed as intermittent explosive disorder; 80 percent were men.

Evidence indicates that intermittent explosive disorder is more common in first-degree biological relatives of persons with the disorder than in the general population. Many factors other than a simple genetic explanation may be responsible.

Comorbidity

High rates of fire setting in patients with intermittent explosive disorder have been reported. Other disorders of impulse control and substance use and mood, anxiety, and eating disorders have also been associated with intermittent explosive disorder.

Etiology

Psychodynamic Factors. Psychoanalysts have suggested that explosive outbursts occur as a defense against narcissistic injurious events. Rage outbursts serve as interpersonal distance and protect against any further narcissistic injury.

Psychosocial Factors. Typical patients have been described as physically large, but dependent, men whose sense of masculine identity is poor. A sense of being useless and impotent or of being unable to change the environment often precedes an episode of physical violence, and a high level of anxiety, guilt, and depression usually follows an episode.

An unfavorable childhood environment often filled with alcohol dependence, beatings, and threats to life is usual in these patients. Predisposing factors in infancy and childhood include perinatal trauma, infantile seizures, head trauma, encephalitis, minimal brain dysfunction, and hyperactivity. Investigators who have concentrated on psychogenesis as causing episodic explosiveness have stressed identification with assaultive parental figures as symbols of the target for violence. Early frustration, oppression, and hostility have been noted as predisposing factors. Situations that are directly or symbolically reminiscent of early deprivations (e.g., persons who directly or indirectly evoke the image of the frustrating parent) become targets for destructive hostility.

Biological Factors. Some investigators suggest that disordered brain physiology, particularly in the limbic system, is involved in most cases of episodic violence. Compelling evidence indicates that serotonergic neurons mediate behavioral inhibition. Decreased serotonergic transmission, which can be induced by inhibiting serotonin synthesis or by antagonizing its effects, decreases the effect of punishment as a deterrent to behavior. The restoration of serotonin activity, by administering serotonin precursors such as L-tryptophan or drugs that increase synaptic serotonin levels, restores the behavioral effect of punishment. Restoring serotonergic activity by administration of L-tryptophan or drugs that increase synaptic serotonergic levels appears to restore control of episodic violent tendencies. Low levels of CSF 5-HIAA have been correlated with impulsive aggression. High CSF testosterone concentrations are correlated with aggressiveness and interpersonal violence in men. Antiandrogenic agents have been shown to decrease aggression.

Familial and Genetic Factors. First-degree relatives of patients with intermittent explosive disorder have higher rates of impulse-control disorders, depressive disorders, and substance use disorders. Biological relatives of patients with the disorder were more likely to have histories of temper or explosive outbursts than the general population.

Diagnosis and Clinical Features

The diagnosis of intermittent explosive disorder should be the result of history-taking that reveals several episodes of loss of control associated with aggressive outbursts. One discrete episode does not justify the diagnosis. The histories typically describe a childhood in an atmosphere of alcohol dependence, violence, and emotional instability. Patients' work histories are poor; they report job losses, marital difficulties, and trouble with the law. Most patients have sought psychiatric help in the past but to no avail. Anxiety, guilt, and depression usually follow an outburst, but this is not a constant finding. Neurological examination sometimes reveals soft neurological signs, such as left–right ambivalence and perceptual reversal. Electroencephalography (EEG) findings are frequently normal or show nonspecific changes.

A 36-year-old real estate agent sought assistance for difficulty with his anger. He was quite competent at his job, although he frequently lost clients when he became enraged over their indecisiveness. On a number of occasions, he became verbally abusive, leading clients to find ways out of escrow closings. The impulsive aggression also led to termination of multiple relationships because sudden angry outbursts contained demeaning accusations toward his girlfriends. This occurred frequently in the absence of any clear conflict. On multiple occasions, the patient became so uncontrollably enraged that he threw things across the room, including books, his desk, and the contents of the refrigerator. Between episodes, he was a kind and likable individual with many friends. He enjoyed drinking on the weekends and had a history of two arrests for driving while intoxicated. On one of these occasions, he became involved in a verbal altercation with a police officer. He had a history of drug experimentation in college that included cocaine and marijuana.

Mental status examination revealed a generally cooperative patient. However, he became quite defensive when questioned about his anger and easily felt accused and blamed by the interviewer for his past behaviors. He had no significant medical history and no signs of neurological problems. He had never been in psychiatric treatment prior to this evaluation. He was on no medications. He denied any symptoms of a mood disorder or any other antisocial activity.

Treatment included the use of carbamazepine (Tegretol) and a combination of supportive and cognitive-behavioral psychotherapy. The patient's angry outbursts improved as he became aware of early signs that he was about to lose control. He learned techniques to avoid confrontation when he was faced with these warning signs. *(Courtesy of Vivien K. Burt, M.D., Ph.D., and Jeffrey William Katzman, M.D.)*

Physical Findings and Laboratory Examination

Persons with the disorder have a high incidence of soft neurological signs (e.g., reflex asymmetries), nonspecific EEG findings, abnormal neuropsychological testing results (e.g., letter reversal difficulties), and accident susceptibility. Blood chemistry (liver and thyroid function tests, fasting blood glucose, electrolytes), urinalysis (including drug toxicology), and syphilis serology may help rule out other causes of aggression. Magnetic resonance imaging (MRI) may reveal changes in the prefrontal cortex, which is associated with loss of impulse control.

Differential Diagnosis

The diagnosis of intermittent explosive disorder can be made only after disorders associated with the occasional loss of control of aggressive impulses have been ruled out as the primary cause. These other disorders include psychotic disorders, personality change because of a general medical condition, antisocial or borderline personality disorder, and substance intoxication (e.g., alcohol, barbiturates, hallucinogens, and amphetamines), epilepsy, brain tumors, degenerative diseases, and endocrine disorders.

Conduct disorder is distinguished from intermittent explosive disorder by its repetitive and resistant pattern of behavior, as opposed to an episodic pattern. Intermittent explosive disorder differs from the antisocial and borderline personality disorders because, in the personality disorders, aggressiveness and impulsivity are part of patients' characters and, thus, are present between outbursts. In paranoid and catatonic schizophrenia, patients may display violent behavior in response to delusions and hallucinations, and they show gross impairments in reality testing. Hostile patients with mania may be impulsively aggressive, but the underlying diagnosis is generally apparent from their mental status examinations and clinical presentations.

Amok is an episode of acute violent behavior for which the person claims amnesia. Amok is usually seen in southeastern Asia, but it has been reported in North America. Amok is distinguished from intermittent explosive disorder by a single episode and prominent dissociative features.

Course and Prognosis

Intermittent explosive disorder may begin at any stage of life, but usually appears between late adolescence and early adulthood. The onset can be sudden or insidious, and the course can be episodic or chronic. In most cases, the disorder decreases in severity with the onset of middle age, but heightened organic impairment can lead to frequent and severe episodes.

Treatment

A combined pharmacological and psychotherapeutic approach has the best chance of success. Psychotherapy with patients who have intermittent explosive disorder is difficult, however, because of their angry outbursts. Therapists may have problems with countertransference and limit-setting. Group psychotherapy may be helpful, and family therapy is useful, particularly when the explosive patient is an adolescent or a young adult. A goal of therapy is to have the patient recognize and verbalize the thoughts or feelings that precede the explosive outbursts instead of acting them out.

Anticonvulsants have long been used, with mixed results, in treating explosive patients. Lithium (Eskalith) has been reported useful in generally lessening aggressive behavior, and carbamazepine, valproate (Depakene) or divalproex (Depakote), and phenytoin (Dilantin) have been reported helpful. Some clinicians have also used other anticonvulsants (e.g., gabapentin [Neurontin]). Benzodiazepines are sometimes used but have been reported to produce a paradoxical reaction of dyscontrol in some cases.

Antipsychotics (e.g., phenothiazines and serotonin–dopamine antagonists) and tricyclic drugs have been effective in some cases, but clinicians must then question whether schizophrenia or a mood disorder is the true diagnosis. With a likelihood of subcortical seizure-like activity, medications that lower the seizure threshold can aggravate the situation. Selective serotonin reuptake inhibitors (SSRIs), trazodone (Desyrel), and buspirone (BuSpar) are useful in reducing impulsivity and aggression.

Propranolol (Inderal) and other β-adrenergic receptor antagonists and calcium channel inhibitors have also been effective in some cases. Some neurosurgeons have performed operative treatments for intractable violence and aggression. No evidence indicates that such treatment is effective.

KLEPTOMANIA

The essential feature of kleptomania is a recurrent failure to resist impulses to steal objects not needed for personal use or for monetary value. The objects taken are often given away, returned surreptitiously, or kept and hidden. Persons with kleptomania usually have the money to pay for the objects they impulsively steal.

As with other impulse-control disorders, kleptomania is characterized by mounting tension before the act, followed by gratification and lessening of tension with or without guilt, remorse, or depression after the act. The stealing is not planned and does not involve others. Although the thefts do not occur when immediate arrest is probable, persons with kleptomania do not always consider their chances of being apprehended, although repeated arrests lead to pain and humiliation. These persons may feel guilt and anxiety after the theft, but they do not feel anger or vengeance. Furthermore, when the object stolen is the goal, the diagnosis is not kleptomania; in kleptomania, the act of stealing is itself the goal.

Epidemiology

The prevalence of kleptomania is not known, but it is estimated to be about 0.6 percent. The range varies from 3.8 to 24 percent of those arrested for shoplifting. There are reports that it occurs in fewer than 5 percent of identified shoplifters. The male-to-female ratio is 1:3 in clinical samples.

Comorbidity

Patients with kleptomania are said to have a high lifetime comorbidity of major mood disorders (usually, but not exclusively, depressive) and various anxiety disorders. Associated conditions also include other disorders such as pathological gambling and compulsive shopping, eating disorders, and substance use disorders, alcoholism in particular.

Etiology

Psychosocial Factors. The symptoms of kleptomania tend to appear in times of significant stress, for example, losses, separations, and endings of important relationships. Some psychoanalytic writers have stressed the expression of aggressive impulses in kleptomania; others have discerned a libidinal aspect. Those who focus on symbolism see meaning in the act itself, the object stolen, and the victim of the theft.

Analytic writers have focused on stealing by children and adolescents. Anna Freud pointed out that the first thefts from mother's purse indicate the degree to which all stealing is rooted in the oneness between mother and child. Karl Abraham wrote of the central feeling of being neglected, injured, or unwanted. One theoretician established seven categories of stealing in chronically acting-out children:

1. As a means of restoring the lost mother–child relationship
2. As an aggressive act
3. As a defense against fears of being damaged (perhaps a search by girls for a penis or a protection against castration anxiety in boys)
4. As a means of seeking punishment
5. As a means of restoring or adding to self-esteem
6. In connection with, and as a reaction to, a family secret
7. As excitement (*lust angst*) and a substitute for a sexual act

One or more of these categories can also apply to adult kleptomania.

Biological Factors. Brain diseases and mental retardation have been associated with kleptomania, as they have with other disorders of impulse control. Focal neurological signs, cortical atrophy, and enlarged lateral ventricles have been found in some patients. Disturbances in monoamine metabolism, particularly of serotonin, have been postulated.

Family and Genetic Factors. In one study, 7 percent of first-degree relatives had obsessive-compulsive disorder (OCD). In addition, a higher rate of mood disorders has been reported in family members.

Diagnosis and Clinical Features

The essential feature of kleptomania is recurrent, intrusive, and irresistible urges or impulses to steal unneeded objects. Patients with kleptomania may also be distressed about the possibility or actuality of being apprehended and may manifest signs of depression and anxiety. Patients feel guilty, ashamed, and embarrassed about their behavior. They often have serious problems with interpersonal relationships and often show signs of personality disturbance. In one study of patients with kleptomania, the frequency of stealing ranged from less than 1 to 120 episodes a month. Most patients with kleptomania steal from retail stores, but they may also steal from family members in their own households.

Jane was a 42-year-old, highly successful, single executive from a wealthy background. She called herself a "shop-'til-you-drop type" and had always been able to afford the expensive designer clothing that she loved. Since college, her "legit" shopping had been paralleled by "boosting" cheap panties and brassieres from discount stores. She did not wear the stolen items; indeed, she considered them "sleazy." She could never bring herself to get rid of them either and kept boxes filled with pilfered lingerie in a storage facility.

Jane talked or bought her way out of trouble until her 30s, when she was arrested while stealing pantyhose from the same K-Mart for the third time in as many months. As a condition of probation, she was ordered to see a psychiatrist. Her attendance was sporadic, and several more thefts occurred over the next 2 years. She also experienced substantial depression, which she tried to alleviate by heavy drinking.

Jane finally began taking her problem seriously after yet another arrest precipitated a suicidal gesture. She began keeping appointments regularly and consented to taking citalopram (Celexa) and naltrexone (ReVia). She believes that her participation in an Alcoholics Anonymous (AA) group for high-pressured executives has been at least as effective—if not more so—in controlling her stealing. *(Courtesy of Harvey Roy Greenberg, M.D.)*

Differential Diagnosis

Episodes of theft occasionally occur during psychotic illness, for example, acute mania, major depression with psychotic features, or schizophrenia. Psychotic stealing is obviously a product of pathological elevation or depression of mood or command hallucinations or delusions. Theft in individuals with antisocial personality disorder is deliberately undertaken for personal gain, with some degree of premeditation and planning, often executed with others. Antisocial stealing regularly involves the threat of harm or actual violence, particularly to elude capture. Guilt and remorse are distinctively lacking, or patients are patently insincere. Shoplifting has become a national epidemic. Few shoplifters have true kleptomania; most are teenagers and young adults who "boost" in pairs or small groups for "kicks," as well as goods, and do not have a major psychiatric disorder. Acute intoxication with drugs or alcohol may precipitate theft in an individual with another psychiatric disorder or without significant psychopathology. Patients with Alzheimer's disease or other dementing organic illness may leave a store without paying, owing to forgetfulness rather than larcenous intent. Malingering kleptomania is common in apprehended antisocial types, as well as nonantisocial youthful shoplifters. Given a sufficiently intelligent perpetrator, the fictive version can be difficult to distinguish from the genuine disorder.

Course and Prognosis

Kleptomania may begin in childhood, although most children and adolescents who steal do not become kleptomaniac adults. The onset of the disorder generally is late adolescence. Women are more likely than men to present for psychiatric evaluation or treatment. Men are more likely to be sent to prison. Men tend to present with the disorder at about 50 years of age; women present at about 35 years of age. In quiescent cases, new bouts of the disorder may be precipitated by loss or disappointment.

The course of the disorder waxes and wanes, but tends to be chronic. Persons sometimes have bouts of being unable to resist the impulse to steal, followed by free periods that last for weeks or months. The spontaneous recovery rate of kleptomania is unknown.

Serious impairment and complications are usually secondary to being caught, particularly to being arrested. Many persons seem never to have consciously considered the possibility of facing the consequences of their acts, a feature that agrees with some descriptions of patients with kleptomania (sometimes, as persons who feel wronged and therefore entitled to steal). Often, the disorder in no way impairs a person's social or work functioning.

The prognosis with treatment can be good, but few patients come for help of their own accord.

Treatment

Because true kleptomania is rare, reports of treatment tend to be individual case descriptions or a short series of cases. Insight-oriented psychotherapy and psychoanalysis have been successful, but depend on patients' motivations. Those who feel guilt and shame may be helped by insight-oriented psychotherapy because of their increased motivation to change their behavior.

Behavior therapy, including systematic desensitization, aversive conditioning, and a combination of aversive conditioning and altered social contingencies, has been reported successful, even when motivation was lacking. The reports cite follow-up studies of up to 2 years. SSRIs, such as fluoxetine (Prozac) and fluvoxamine (Luvox), appear to be effective in some patients with kleptomania. Case reports indicated successful treatment with tricyclic drugs, trazodone, lithium, valproate, naltrexone, and electroconvulsive therapy.

PYROMANIA

Pyromania is the recurrent, deliberate, and purposeful setting of fires. Associated features include tension or affective arousal before setting the fires; fascination with, interest in, curiosity about, or attraction to fire and the activities and equipment associated with firefighting; and pleasure, gratification, or relief when setting fires or when witnessing or participating in their aftermath. Patients may make considerable advance preparations before starting a fire. Pyromania differs from arson in that the latter is done for financial gain, revenge, or other reasons and is planned beforehand.

Epidemiology

No information is available on the prevalence of pyromania, but only a small percentage of adults who set fires can be classified as having pyromania. The disorder is found far more often in men than in women, with a male-to-female ratio of approximately 8:1. More than 40 percent of arrested arsonists are younger than 18 years of age.

Comorbidity

Pyromania is significantly associated with substance abuse disorder (especially alcoholism); affective disorders, depressive or bipolar; other impulse-control disorders, such as kleptomania in female fire setters; and various personality disturbances, such as inadequate and borderline personality disorders. Attention-deficit/hyperactivity disorder and learning disabilities may be conspicuously associated with childhood pyromania; this constellation frequently persists into adulthood. Persons who set fires are more likely to be mildly retarded than are those in the general population. Some studies have noted an increased incidence of alcohol use disorders in persons who set fires. Fire setters also tend to have a history of antisocial traits, such as truancy, running away from home, and delinquency. Enuresis has been considered a common finding in the history of fire setters, although controlled studies have failed to confirm this. Studies, however, have found an association between cruelty to animals and fire setting. Childhood and adolescent fire setting is often associated with ADHD or adjustment disorders.

Etiology

Psychosocial. Freud saw fire as a symbol of sexuality. He believed the warmth radiated by fire evokes the same sensation that accompanies a state of sexual excitation, and a flame's shape and movements suggest a phallus in activity. Other psychoanalysts have associated pyromania with an abnormal craving for power and social prestige. Some patients with pyromania are volunteer firefighters who set fires to prove themselves brave, to force other firefighters into action, or to demonstrate their power to extinguish a blaze. The incendiary act is a way to vent accumulated rage over frustration caused by a sense of social, physical, or sexual inferiority. Several studies have noted that the fathers of patients with pyromania were absent from the home. Thus, one explanation of fire setting is that it represents a wish for the absent father to return home as a rescuer, to put out the fire, and to save the child from a difficult existence.

Female fire setters, in addition to being much fewer in number than male fire setters, do not start fires to put firefighters into action as men frequently do. Frequently noted delinquent trends in female fire setters include promiscuity without pleasure and petty stealing, often approaching kleptomania.

Biological Factors. Significantly low CSF levels of 5-HIAA and 3-methoxy-4-hydroxyphenylglycol (MHPG) have been found in fire setters, which suggests possible serotonergic or adrenergic involvement. The presence of reactive hypoglycemia, based on blood glucose concentrations on glucose tolerance tests, has been put forward as a cause of pyromania. Further studies are needed, however.

Diagnosis and Clinical Features

Persons with pyromania often regularly watch fires in their neighborhoods, frequently set off false alarms, and show interest in firefighting paraphernalia. Their curiosity is evident, but they show no remorse and may be indifferent to the consequences for life or property. Fire setters may gain satisfaction from the resulting destruction; frequently, they leave obvious clues. Commonly associated features include alcohol intoxication, sexual dysfunctions, below-average intelligence quotient (IQ), chronic personal frustration, and resentment toward authority figures. Some fire setters become sexually aroused by the fire.

Differential Diagnosis

Clinicians should have little trouble distinguishing between pyromania and the fascination of many young children with matches, lighters, and fire as part of the normal investigation of their environments. Pyromania must also be separated from incendiary acts of sabotage carried out by dissident political extremists or by "paid torchers," termed arsonists in the legal system.

When fire setting occurs in conduct disorder and antisocial personality disorder, it is a deliberate act, not a failure to resist an impulse. Fires may be set for profit, sabotage, or retaliation. Patients with schizophrenia or mania may set fires in response to delusions or hallucinations. Patients with brain dysfunction (e.g., dementia), mental retardation, or substance intoxication may set fires because of a failure to appreciate the consequences of the act.

Course and Prognosis

Although fire setting often begins in childhood, the typical age of onset of pyromania is unknown. When the onset is in adolescence or adulthood, the fire setting tends to be deliberately destructive. Fire setting in pyromania is episodic and may wax and wane in frequency. The prognosis for treated children is good, and complete remission is a realistic goal. The prognosis for adults is guarded, because they frequently deny their actions, refuse to take responsibility, are dependent on alcohol, and lack insight.

Treatment

Little has been written about the treatment of pyromania, and treating fire setters has been difficult because of their lack of motivation. No single treatment has been proved effective; thus a number of modalities, including behavioral approaches, should be tried. Because of the recurrent nature of pyromania, any treatment program should include supervision of patients to prevent a repeated episode of fire setting. Incarceration may be the only method of preventing a recurrence. Behavior therapy can then be administered in the institution.

Fire setting by children must be treated with the utmost seriousness. Intensive interventions should be undertaken when possible, but as therapeutic and preventive measures, not as punishment. In the case of children and adolescents, treatment of pyromania or fire setting should include family therapy.

OTHER SPECIFIED OR UNSPECIFIED DISORDERS

This DSM-5 diagnostic category is a residual category for disorders that do not meet the criteria for the disorders described earlier. Some of the disorders listed below stand at the borderline between impulsive and compulsive disorders. Important, although subtle, distinctions exist between the two terms. An *impulse* is a tension state that can exist without an action; a *compulsion* is a tension state that always has an action component. The disorders are classified here as compulsions because the patients feel "compelled" to act out their pathological behavior; they cannot resist the impulse to do so. Impulses are acted on with the expectation of receiving pleasure; compulsions are usually ego-dystonic; for example, the patient does not like having to perform the act even though compelled to do so. An exception to the rule that impulses are associated with pleasure involves those cases in which feelings of guilt follow the act and disturb the sense of pleasure. Similarly, not all compulsions are ego-dystonic; for example, certain compulsive video game playing may have a pleasurable component. Both impulsive and compulsive behaviors are characterized by their repetitive nature; however, the repeated acting out of impulses leads to psychosocial impairment, whereas compulsive behavior does not always carry that risk. Because of the repetitive and pleasurable nature of many of the behavioral patterns in this group of disorders, they are often referred to as addictions.

Internet Compulsion

Also called *Internet Addiction,* such persons spend almost all their waking hours at the computer terminal. Their patterns of use are repetitive and constant, and they are unable to resist strong urges to use the computer or to "surf the Web." Internet addicts may gravitate to certain sites that meet specific needs (e.g., shopping, sex, and interactive games, among others). In DSM-5 there is a condition proposed for further study called "Internet gaming disorder," which refers to persons who continually use the Internet to play games to the extent that it interferes with social relations and work performance. But as mentioned earlier, the disorder need not be limited to games. Other activities may be involved.

Internet Use and Abuse. Web sites and organizations offer opportunities for people with similar interests to find one another and begin relationships. The Internet has been useful as a matchmaker, with millions of subscribers to dating services. People meet on the Internet, fall in love, and may even marry. During this process some fact fudging is not uncommon. In Second Life and similar alternate universe games, creative identity deception is expected. This use can become problematic and thus can be termed "abuse" in various ways.

VICTIMS. Deception can take a malignant turn as sexual predators deceive their victims with false identities only to exploit and harm them when they meet. These contacts are unregulated and difficult to detect except by monitoring and checking the computers used. There are weekly reports of minors having been lured into sometimes lethal situations by sexual predators. Occasionally there is a report of a couple that met to marry only to discover they had missed verifying crucial details, such as each other's sex.

Some people who make little use of the Internet nonetheless become victims and enter treatment. The suicide of one teenager after reading untruths entered by a peer's malicious mother ("cyberbullying") has inspired laws to criminalize such behavior. Internet identity theft is also rampant. An underreported and growing problem, medical identity theft, is harder to detect and remedy, often requiring painstaking record correction.

The combination of anonymity, convenience, and escape (the ACE model) promotes the Internet as a focus of psychopathology. Internet addiction is mentioned on 385,000 Web pages, a 180-fold increase in 4 years, with those at risk suffering from depression, bipolar disorder, anxiety, low self-esteem, or addiction to substances, at least previously. Online surveys find that 4 to 10 percent of users meet criteria for "Internet addiction," defined as having at least five of the following signs and symptoms: (1) preoccupation with the Internet; (2) increasing amount of time spent online; (3) failure to cut back use with concomitant restlessness; (4) moodiness or depression; (5) staying online longer than originally intended; (6) running the risk of losing a job, relationship, or other opportunity because of Internet use; and (7) lying to conceal the extent of Internet use and/or using the Internet to escape negative feelings. General population surveys show a prevalence of 0.3 to 0.7 percent, with higher rates when family members are queried. The "addicted" averaged 38.5 hours per week on a computer, whereas others averaged 4.9 hours per week. Forty percent got less than 4 hours of sleep per night because of Internet use. Impairment was evident in increased divorce rates, vocational impairment, legal problems, and personal distress. Subgroups on Internet use include (1) cybersex addiction (viewing pornography); (2) cyber-relational addiction (online relationships become more important than those in one's physical world); online gaming (gambling, stock trading), compulsive, debt-inducing shopping, and others; (3) information overload; (4) net compulsivity; and (5) computer (non-Internet) addiction (e.g., computer games). About 30 percent of those "addicted" reported using the Internet to escape negative feelings and because it was always available at low cost. It is possible to lose real money on the Internet, gambling constantly and continually without being seen to do so. More money is made on sex via the Internet than through the sale of anything else. Combinations abound, as in the 873,000 sites mentioning both "cybersex" and "casino."

Treatment for Internet Addicts. A subset of Web pages offer a chance to evaluate one's Internet use as possibly pathological and offer both education and online counseling, with some urging face-to-face counseling as a way of becoming less involved with the Internet. A rough idea of the ratio of what is offered as possible sources of help online is the number of sites mentioning "cybersex" (close 4 million) compared to those mentioning "cybersex addiction" (about 20,000). There are many mentions and variants on "Center for Internet Addiction" often represented only by single practitioners with some ancillary staff.

Mobile or Cell Phone Compulsion

Some persons compulsively use mobile phones to call others—friends, acquaintances, or business associates. They justify their need to contact others by giving plausible reasons for calling; but underlying conflicts may be expressed in the behavior, such as fear of being alone, the need to satisfy unconscious dependency needs, or undoing a hostile wish toward a loved one, among others (e.g., "I just want to make sure you are OK.").

Repetitive Self-Mutilation

Persons who repeatedly cut themselves or do damage to their bodies may do so in a compulsive manner. In all cases, another disorder will be found. Parasuicidal behavior is common in borderline personality disorder. Compulsive body piercing or tattooing may be a symptom of a paraphilia or a depressive equivalent.

In DSM-5 there is a proposed diagnosis called "nonsuicidal self-injury" to refer to persons who repeatedly damage their bodies, who, however, do not wish to die, contrasted with those persons who harm themselves with true suicidal intent. There is secondary gain to this self-injurious behavior such as getting the attention of others, the so-called "cry for help," or obtaining relief from dysphoric states. It has been postulated that cutting the skin or inflicting bodily pain may release endorphins or raise dopamine levels in the brain, both of which contribute to a euthymic or elated mood, thus alleviating depressed states of mind in those who practice self-mutilation.

Compulsive Sexual Behavior

Some persons repeatedly seek out sexual gratification, often in perverse ways (e.g., exhibitionism). They are unable to control their behavior and may not experience feelings of guilt after an episode of acting-out behavior. Sometimes called *sexual addiction,* this condition is discussed extensively in Section 13.2.

16 Substance Related and Addictive Disorders

▲ 16.1 Introduction and Overview

The most commonly abused drugs have been part of human existence for thousands of years. For example, opium has been used for medicinal purposes for at least 3,500 years, references to cannabis (marijuana) as a medicinal can be found in ancient Chinese herbals, wine is mentioned frequently in the Bible, and the natives of the Western Hemisphere smoked tobacco and chewed coca leaves. As new drugs were discovered and new routes of administration developed, new problems related to their use emerged. Substance use disorders are complicated psychiatric conditions and like other psychiatric disorders, both biological factors and environmental circumstances are etiologically significant.

This chapter covers substance dependence and substance abuse with descriptions of the clinical phenomena associated with the use of 11 designated classes of pharmacological agents: alcohol, amphetamines or similarly acting agents, caffeine, cannabis, cocaine, hallucinogens, inhalants, nicotine, opioids, phencyclidine (PCP) or similar agents, and a group that includes sedatives, hypnotics, and anxiolytics. A residual 12th category includes a variety of agents not in the 11 designated classes, such as anabolic steroids and nitrous oxide.

TERMINOLOGY

Various terms have been used over the years to refer to drug abuse. For example, the term *dependence* has been and is used in one of two ways when discussing substance use disorders. In *behavioral dependence,* substance-seeking activities and related evidence of pathological use patterns are emphasized, whereas *physical dependence* refers to the physical (physiological) effects of multiple episodes of substance use. Psychological dependence, also referred to as habituation, is characterized by a continuous or intermittent craving (i.e., intense desire) for the substance to avoid a dysphoric state. Behavioral, physical, and psychological dependences are the hallmark of substance use disorders.

Somewhat related to dependence are the related words *addiction* and *addict*. The word *addict* has acquired a pejorative connotation that ignores the concept of substance abuse as a medical disorder. *Addiction* has also been trivialized in popular usage, as in the terms *TV addiction* and *money addiction;* however, the term still has value. There are common neurochemical and neuroanatomical substrates found among all addictions, whether it is to substances or to gambling, sex, stealing, or eating. These various addictions may have similar effects on the activities of specific reward areas of the brain, such as the ventral tegmental area, the locus ceruleus, and the nucleus accumbens.

Codependence

The terms *coaddiction* and, more commonly, *codependency* or *codependence* are used to designate the behavioral patterns of family members who have been significantly affected by another family member's substance use or addiction. The terms have been used in various ways and no established criteria for codependence exist.

Enabling

Enabling was one of the first, and more agreed on, characteristics of codependence or coaddiction. Sometimes, family members feel that they have little or no control over the enabling acts. Either because of the social pressures for protecting and supporting family members or because of pathological interdependencies, or both, enabling behavior often resists modification. Other characteristics of codependence include unwillingness to accept the notion of addiction as a disease. The family members continue to behave as if the substance-using behavior were voluntary and willful (if not actually spiteful), and the user cares more for alcohol and drugs than for family members. This results in feelings of anger, rejection, and failure. In addition to those feelings, family members may feel guilty and depressed because addicts, in an effort to deny loss of control over drugs and to shift the focus of concern away from their use, often try to place the responsibility for such use on other family members, who often seem willing to accept some or all of it.

Denial

Family members, as with the substance users themselves, often behave as if the substance use that is causing obvious problems were not really a problem; that is, they engage in denial. The reasons for the unwillingness to accept the obvious vary. Sometimes denial is self-protecting, in that the family members

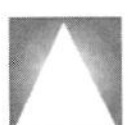

Table 16.1–1
Terms Used in Substance-Related Disorders

Dependence The repeated use of a drug or chemical substance, with or without physical dependence. Physical dependence indicates an altered physiologic state caused by repeated administration of a drug, the cessation of which results in a specific syndrome.

Abuse Use of any drug, usually by self-administration, in a manner that deviates from approved social or medical patterns.

Misuse Similar to abuse, but usually applies to drugs prescribed by physicians that are not used properly.

Addiction The repeated and increased use of a substance, the deprivation of which gives rise to symptoms of distress and an irresistible urge to use the agent again and which leads also to physical and mental deterioration.

Intoxication A reversible syndrome caused by a specific substance (e.g., alcohol) that affects one or more of the following mental functions: memory, orientation, mood, judgment, and behavioral, social, or occupational functioning.

Withdrawal A substance-specific syndrome that occurs after stopping or reducing the amount of the drug or substance that has been used regularly over a prolonged period of time. The syndrome is characterized by physiologic signs and symptoms in addition to psychological changes, such as disturbances in thinking, feeling, and behavior. Also called *abstinence syndrome* or *discontinuation syndrome.*

Tolerance Phenomenon in which, after repeated administration, a given dose of drug produces a decreased effect or increasingly larger doses must be administered to obtain the effect observed with the original dose. *Behavioral tolerance* reflects the ability of the person to perform tasks despite the effects of the drug.

Cross-tolerance Refers to the ability of one drug to be substituted for another, each usually producing the same physiologic and psychological effect (e.g., diazepam and barbiturates). Also known as *cross-dependence.*

Neuroadaptation Neurochemical or neurophysiologic changes in the body that result from the repeated administration of a drug. Neuroadaptation accounts for the phenomenon of tolerance. *Pharmacokinetic adaptation* refers to adaptation of the metabolizing system in the body. *Cellular or pharmacodynamic adaptation* refers to the ability of the nervous system to function despite high blood levels of the offending substance.

Codependence Term used to refer to family members affected by or influencing the behavior of the substance abuser. Related to the term *enabler,* which is a person who facilitates the abuser's addictive behavior (e.g., providing drugs directly or money to buy drugs). Enabling also includes the unwillingness of a family member to accept addiction as a medical-psychiatric disorder or to deny that person is abusing a substance.

believe that if a drug or alcohol problem exists, then they are responsible.

As with the addicts themselves, codependent family members seem unwilling to accept the notion that outside intervention is needed and, despite repeated failures, continue to believe that greater willpower and greater efforts at control can restore tranquility. When additional efforts at control fail, they often attribute the failure to themselves rather than to the addict or the disease process, and along with failure come feelings of anger, lowered self-esteem, and depression. A summary of some key terms related to substance use disorders is given in Table 16.1–1.

EPIDEMIOLOGY

The National Institute of Drug Abuse (NIDA) and other agencies, such as the National Survey of Drug Use and Health (NSDUH), conduct periodic surveys of the use of illicit drugs in the United States. It is estimated that more than 22 million persons older than the age of 12 years (about 10 percent of the total US population) are classified as having a substance-related disorder. Of this group, almost 15 million are dependent on, or abuse, alcohol.

In 2012, 669,000 persons were dependent on, or abused, heroin; 1.7 percent (4.3 million) abused marijuana; 0.4 percent (1 million) abused cocaine; and 2 million were classified as dependent on, or abuse of, pain relievers.

With regard to age at first use, those who started using drugs at an earlier age (14 years or younger) were more likely to become addicted than those who started at a later age. This applied to all substances of abuse, but particularly to alcohol. Among adults aged 21 or older who first tried alcohol at age 14 or younger, 15 percent were classified as alcoholics compared with only 3 percent who first used alcohol at age 21 or older.

Rates of abuse also varied according to age. The rate for dependence or abuse is highest among adults age 18 to 25 (19 percent) compared to youths age 12 to 17 (6 percent) and adults age 26 or older (7 percent). After age 21, a general decline occurred with age. By age 65, only about 1 percent of persons have used an illicit substance within the past year, which lends credence to the clinical observation that addicts tend to "burn out" as they age.

More men than women use drugs; the highest lifetime rate is among American Indian or Alaska natives; whites are more affected than blacks or African Americans; those with some college education use more substances than those with less education; and the unemployed have higher rates that those with either part-time or full-time employment.

Rates of substance dependence or abuse varied by region in the United States. Rates were slightly higher in the West (9 percent) and Midwest (9 percent) than in the Northeast (8 percent) and South (8 percent). Rates were similar in small metropolitan counties and large metropolitan counties (both at 9 percent) and were lowest in completely rural counties (7 percent). Rates are also higher among persons on parole or on supervised release from jail (34 percent vs. 9 percent). The number of persons driving while under the influence of drugs or alcohol is on a decline. The percentage driving under the influence of alcohol decreased from 14 percent in 2002 to 11 percent in 2010, and those driving under the influence of drugs decreased from 5 percent to 4 percent during the same period. A comprehensive survey of drug use and trends in the United States is available at www.samhsa.gov.

ETIOLOGY

The model of substance use disorders is the result of a process in which multiple interacting factors influence drug-using behavior and the loss of judgment with respect to decisions about using a given drug. Although the actions of a given drug are critical in the process, it is not assumed that all people who become dependent on the same drug experience its effects in the same way or are motivated by the same set of factors. Furthermore, it is postulated that different factors may be more or less important at different stages of the process. Thus, drug availability, social acceptability, and peer pressures may be the major determinants of initial experimentation with a drug, but other factors, such as personality and individual biology, probably are more important in how the effects of a given drug are perceived and the degree to which repeated drug use produces changes in the central nervous system (CNS). Still other factors, including the particular actions of the drug, may be primary determinants of whether drug use progresses to drug dependence, whereas still others may be important influences on the likelihood that drug use (1) leads to adverse effects or (2) to successful recovery from dependence.

It has been asserted that addiction is a "brain disease," that the critical processes that transform voluntary drug-using behavior to compulsive drug use are changes in the structure and neurochemistry of the brain of the drug user. Sufficient evidence now indicates that such changes in relevant parts of the brain do occur. The perplexing and unanswered question is whether these changes are both necessary and sufficient to account for the drug-using behavior. Many argue that they are not, that the capacity of drug-dependent individuals to modify their drug-using behavior in response to positive reinforcers or aversive contingencies indicates that the nature of addiction is more complex and requires the interaction of multiple factors.

The central element is the drug-using behavior itself. The decision to use a drug is influenced by immediate social and psychological situations as well as by the person's more remote history. Use of the drug initiates a sequence of consequences that can be rewarding or aversive and which, through a process of learning, can result in a greater or lesser likelihood that the drug-using behavior will be repeated. For some drugs, use also initiates the biological processes associated with tolerance, physical dependence, and sensitization. In turn, tolerance can reduce some of the adverse effects of the drug, permitting or requiring the use of larger doses, which then can accelerate or intensify the development of physical dependence. Above a certain threshold, the aversive qualities of a withdrawal syndrome provide a distinct recurrent motive for further drug use. Sensitization of motivational systems can increase the salience of drug-related stimuli.

Psychodynamic Factors

The range of psychodynamic theories about substance abuse reflects the various popular theories during the last 100 years. According to classic theories, substance abuse is a masturbatory equivalent (some heroin users describe the initial "rush" as similar to a prolonged sexual orgasm), a defense against anxious impulses, or a manifestation of oral regression (i.e., dependency). Recent psychodynamic formulations relate substance use as a reflection of disturbed ego functions (i.e., the inability to deal with reality). As a form of self-medication, alcohol may be used to control panic, opioids to diminish anger, and amphetamines to alleviate depression. Some addicts have great difficulty recognizing their inner emotional states, a condition called *alexithymia* (i.e., being unable to find words to describe their feelings).

Learning and Conditioning. Drug use, whether occasional or compulsive, can be viewed as behavior maintained by its consequences. Drugs can reinforce antecedent behaviors by terminating some noxious or aversive state such as pain, anxiety, or depression. In some social situations, the drug use, apart from its pharmacological effects, can be reinforcing if it results in special status or the approval of friends. Each use of the drug evokes rapid positive reinforcement, either as a result of the rush (the drug-induced euphoria), alleviation of disturbed affects, alleviation of withdrawal symptoms, or any combination of these effects. In addition, some drugs may sensitize neural systems to the reinforcing effects of the drug. Eventually, the paraphernalia (needles, bottles, cigarette packs) and behaviors associated with substance use can become secondary reinforcers, as well as cues signaling availability of the substance, and in their presence, craving or a desire to experience the effects increases.

Drug users respond to the drug-related stimuli with increased activity in limbic regions, including the amygdala and the anterior cingulate. Such drug-related activation of limbic areas has been demonstrated with a variety of drugs, including cocaine, opioids, and cigarettes (nicotine). Of interest, the same regions activated by cocaine-related stimuli in cocaine users are activated by sexual stimuli in both normal controls and cocaine users.

In addition to the operant reinforcement of drug-using and drug-seeking behaviors, other learning mechanisms probably play a role in dependence and relapse. Opioid and alcohol withdrawal phenomena can be conditioned (in the pavlovian or classic sense) to environmental or interoceptive stimuli. For a long time after withdrawal (from opioids, nicotine, or alcohol), the addict exposed to environmental stimuli previously linked with substance use or withdrawal may experience conditioned withdrawal, conditioned craving, or both. The increased feelings of craving are not necessarily accompanied by symptoms of withdrawal. The most intense craving is elicited by conditions associated with the availability or use of the substance, such as watching someone else use heroin or light a cigarette or being offered some drug by a friend. Those learning and conditioning phenomena can be superimposed on any preexisting psychopathology, but preexisting difficulties are not required for the development of powerfully reinforced substance-seeking behavior.

Genetic Factors

Strong evidence from studies of twins, adoptees, and siblings brought up separately indicates that the cause of alcohol abuse has a genetic component. Many less conclusive data show that other types of substance abuse or substance dependence have a genetic pattern in their development. Researchers recently have used restriction fragment length polymorphism (RFLP) in the study of substance abuse and substance dependence, and associations to genes that affect dopamine production have been postulated.

Neurochemical Factors

Receptors and Receptor Systems. With the exception of alcohol, researchers have identified particular neurotransmitters or neurotransmitter receptors involved with most substances of abuse. Some researchers base their studies on such hypotheses.

The opioids, for example, act on opioid receptors. A person with too little endogenous opioid activity (e.g., low concentrations of endorphins) or with too much activity of an endogenous opioid antagonist may be at risk for developing opioid dependence. Even in a person with completely normal endogenous receptor function and neurotransmitter concentration, the long-term use of a particular substance of abuse may eventually modulate receptor systems in the brain so that the presence of the exogenous substance is needed to maintain homeostasis. Such a receptor-level process may be the mechanism for developing tolerance within the CNS. Demonstrating modulation of neurotransmitter release and neurotransmitter receptor function has proved difficult, however, and recent research focuses on the effects of substances on the second-messenger system and on gene regulation.

Pathways and Neurotransmitters. The major neurotransmitters possibly involved in developing substance abuse and substance dependence are the opioid, catecholamine (particularly dopamine), and γ-aminobutyric acid (GABA) systems. The dopaminergic neurons in the ventral tegmental area are particularly important. These neurons project to the cortical and limbic regions, especially the nucleus accumbens. This pathway is probably involved in the sensation of reward and may be the major mediator of the effects of such substances as amphetamine and cocaine. The locus ceruleus, the largest group of adrenergic neurons, probably mediates the effects of the opiates and the opioids. These pathways have collectively been called the *brain-reward circuitry.*

COMORBIDITY

Comorbidity is the occurrence of two or more psychiatric disorders in a single patient at the same time. A high prevalence of additional psychiatric disorders is found among persons seeking treatment for alcohol, cocaine, or opioid dependence; some studies have shown that up to 50 percent of addicts have a comorbid psychiatric disorder. Although opioid, cocaine, and alcohol abusers with current psychiatric problems are more likely to seek treatment, those who do not seek treatment are not necessarily free of comorbid psychiatric problems; such persons may have social supports that enable them to deny the impact that drug use is having on their lives. Two large epidemiological studies have shown that even among representative samples of the population, those who meet the criteria for alcohol or drug abuse and dependence (excluding tobacco dependence) are also far more likely to meet the criteria for other psychiatric disorders also.

In various studies, a range of 35 to 60 percent of patients with substance abuse or substance dependence also meets the diagnostic criteria for antisocial personality disorder. The range is even higher when investigators include persons who meet all the antisocial personality disorder diagnostic criteria, except the requirement that the symptoms started at an early age. That is, a high percentage of patients with substance abuse or substance dependence diagnoses have a pattern of antisocial behavior, whether it was present before the substance use started or developed during the course of the substance use. Patients with substance abuse or substance dependence diagnoses who have antisocial personality disorder are likely to use more illegal substances; to have more psychopathology; to be less satisfied with their lives; and to be more impulsive, isolated, and depressed than patients with antisocial personality disorders alone.

Depression and Suicide

Depressive symptoms are common among persons diagnosed with substance abuse or substance dependence. About one-third to one-half of all those with opioid abuse or opioid dependence and about 40 percent of those with alcohol abuse or alcohol dependence meet the criteria for major depressive disorder sometime during their lives. Substance use is also a major precipitating factor for suicide. Persons who abuse substances are about 20 times more likely to die by suicide than the general population. About 15 percent of persons with alcohol abuse or alcohol dependence have been reported to commit suicide. This frequency of suicide is second only to the frequency in patients with major depressive disorder.

DIAGNOSTIC CLASSIFICATION

There are four major diagnostic categories in the *Diagnostic and Statistical Manual of Mental Disorders*, fifth edition (DSM-5): (1) Substance Use Disorder, (2) Substance Intoxication, (3) Substance Withdrawal, and (4) Substance-Induced Mental Disorder.

Substance Use Disorder

Substance use disorder is the diagnostic term applied to the specific substance abused (e.g., alcohol use disorder, opioid use disorder) that results from the prolonged use of the substance. The following points should be considered in making this diagnosis. These criteria apply to all substances of abuse. In the sections that follow on the specific drugs of abuse these criteria should be applied in making the diagnosis of substance use disorder.

A maladaptive pattern of substance use leading to clinically significant impairment or distress, as manifested by two (or more) of the following, occurring within a 12-month period:

1. Recurrent substance use resulting in a failure to fulfill major role obligations at work, school, or home (e.g., repeated absences or poor work performance related to substance use; substance-related absences, suspensions, or expulsions from school; neglect of children or household).
2. Recurrent substance use in situations in which it is physically hazardous (e.g., driving an automobile or operating a machine when impaired by substance use).
3. Continued substance use despite having persistent or recurrent social or interpersonal problems caused or exacerbated by the effects of the substance (e.g., arguments with spouse about consequences of intoxication, physical fights).
4. Tolerance, as defined by either of the following:
   a. A need for markedly increased amounts of the substance to achieve intoxication or desired effect.
   b. Markedly diminished effect with continued use of the same amount of the substance.
5. Withdrawal, as manifested by either of the following:
   a. The characteristic withdrawal syndrome for the substance.
   b. The same (or a closely related) substance is taken to relieve or avoid withdrawal symptoms.

6. The substance is often taken in larger amounts or over a longer period than was intended.
7. There is a persistent desire or unsuccessful efforts to cut down or control substance use.
8. A great deal of time is spent in activities necessary to obtain the substance, use the substance, or recover from its effects.
9. Important social, occupational, or recreational activities are given up or reduced because of substance use.
10. The substance use is continued despite knowledge of having a persistent or recurrent physical or psychological problem that is likely to have been caused or exacerbated by the substance.
11. Craving or a strong desire or urge to use a specific substance.

Substance Intoxication

Substance intoxication is the diagnosis used to describe a syndrome (e.g., alcohol intoxication or simple drunkenness) characterized by specific signs and symptoms resulting from recent ingestion or exposure to the substance. A general description of substance intoxication includes the following points:

1. The development of a reversible substance-specific syndrome due to recent ingestion of (or exposure to) a substance. Note: Different substances may produce similar or identical syndromes.
2. Clinically significant maladaptive behavioral or psychological changes that are due to the effect of the substance on the central nervous system (e.g., belligerence, mood lability, cognitive impairment, impaired judgment, impaired social or occupational functioning) and develop during or shortly after use of the substance.
3. The symptoms are not due to a general medical condition and are not better accounted for by another mental disorder.

Substance Withdrawal

Substance withdrawal is the diagnosis used to describe a substance specific syndrome that results from the abrupt cessation of heavy and prolonged use of a substance (e.g., opioid withdrawal). A general description of substance withdrawal requires the following criteria to be met:

1. The development of a substance-specific syndrome due to the cessation of (or reduction in) substance use that has been heavy and prolonged.
2. The substance-specific syndrome causes clinically significant distress or impairment in social, occupational, or other important areas of functioning.
3. The symptoms are not due to a general medical condition and are not better accounted for by another mental disorder.

In the discussion of each drug in the sections that follow, the criteria listed above, derived from the DSM-5, can be applied. Thus, in place of the word substance, the clinician should indicate the specific substance or drug that is used or that caused intoxication or withdrawal.

TREATMENT AND REHABILITATION

Some persons who develop substance-related problems recover without formal treatment, especially as they age. For patients with less severe disorders, such as nicotine addiction, relatively brief interventions are often as effective as more intensive treatments. Because these brief interventions do not change the environment, alter drug-induced brain changes, or provide new skills, a change in the patient's motivation (cognitive change) probably has the best impact on the drug-using behavior. For those individuals who do not respond or whose dependence is more severe, a variety of interventions described below appear to be effective.

It is useful to distinguish among specific procedures or techniques (e.g., individual therapy, family therapy, group therapy, relapse prevention, and pharmacotherapy) and treatment programs. Most programs use a number of specific procedures and involve several professional disciplines as well as nonprofessionals who have special skills or personal experience with the substance problem being treated. The best treatment programs combine specific procedures and disciplines to meet the needs of the individual patient after a careful assessment.

No classification system is generally accepted for either the specific procedures used in treatment or programs using various combinations of procedures. This lack of standardized terminology for categorizing procedures and programs presents a problem, even when the field of interest is narrowed from substance problems in general to treatment for a single substance, such as alcohol, tobacco, or cocaine. Except in carefully monitored research projects, even the definitions of specific procedures (e.g., individual counseling, group therapy, and methadone maintenance) tend to be so imprecise that usually just what transactions are supposed to occur cannot be inferred. Nevertheless, for descriptive purposes, programs are often broadly grouped on the basis of one or more of their salient characteristics: whether the program is aimed at merely controlling acute withdrawal and consequences of recent drug use (detoxification) or is focused on longer-term behavioral change; whether the program makes extensive use of pharmacological interventions; and the degree to which the program is based on individual psychotherapy, Alcoholics Anonymous (AA) or other 12-step principles, or therapeutic community principles. For example, government agencies recently categorized publicly funded treatment programs for drug dependence as (1) methadone maintenance (mostly outpatient), (2) outpatient drug-free programs, (3) therapeutic communities, or (4) short-term inpatient programs.

Selecting a Treatment

Not all interventions are applicable to all types of substance use or dependence, and some of the more coercive interventions used for illicit drugs are not applicable to substances that are legally available, such as tobacco. Addictive behaviors do not change abruptly, but through a series of stages. Five stages in this gradual process have been proposed: precontemplation, contemplation, preparation, action, and maintenance. For some types of addictions the therapeutic alliance is enhanced when the treatment approach is tailored to the patient's stage of readiness to change. Interventions for some drug use disorders may have a specific pharmacological agent as an important component; for example, disulfiram, naltrexone (ReVia), or acamprosate for alcoholism; methadone (Dolophine), levomethadyl acetate (ORLAAM), or buprenorphine (Buprenex) for heroin addiction; and nicotine delivery devices or bupropion (Zyban) for tobacco dependence. Not all interventions are likely to be useful to healthcare professionals. For example, many youthful offenders with histories of drug use or dependence are now remanded to special facilities (boot camps); other programs for offenders (and sometimes for employees) rely almost exclusively on the deterrent effect of frequent urine testing; and a third group are built around religious conversion or rededication in a specific religious sect or denomination. In contrast to the numerous studies suggesting some value for brief interventions for smoking and for problem drinking, few controlled studies are conducted of brief interventions for those seeking treatment for dependence on illicit drugs.

In general, brief interventions (e.g., a few weeks of detoxification, whether in or out of a hospital) used for persons who are severely dependent on illicit opioids have limited effect on outcome measured a few months later. Substantial reductions in illicit drug use, antisocial behaviors, and psychiatric distress among patients dependent on cocaine or heroin are much more likely following treatment lasting at least 3 months. Such a time-in-treatment effect is seen across very different modalities, from residential therapeutic communities to ambulatory methadone maintenance programs. Although some patients appear to benefit from a few days or weeks of treatment, a substantial percentage of users of illicit drugs drop out (or are dropped) from treatment before they have achieved significant benefits.

Some of the variance in treatment outcomes can be attributed to differences in the characteristics of patients entering treatment and by events and conditions following treatment. Programs based on similar philosophical principles and using what seem to be similar therapeutic procedures vary greatly in effectiveness, however. Some of the differences among programs that seem to be similar reflect the range and intensity of services offered. Programs with professionally trained staffs that provide more comprehensive services to patients with more severe psychiatric difficulties are more likely able to retain those patients in treatment and help them make positive changes. Differences in the skills of individual counselors and professionals can strongly affect outcomes.

Such generalizations concerning programs serving illicit drug users may not hold for programs dealing with those seeking treatment for alcohol, tobacco, or even cannabis problems uncomplicated by heavy use of illicit drugs. In such cases, relatively brief periods of individual or group counseling can produce long-lasting reductions in drug use. The outcomes usually considered in programs dealing with illicit drugs have typically included measures of social functioning, employment, and criminal activity, as well as decreased drug-using behavior.

Treatment of Comorbidity

Treatment of the severely mentally ill (primarily those with schizophrenia and schizoaffective disorders) who are also drug dependent continues to pose problems for clinicians. Although some special facilities have been developed that use both antipsychotic drugs and therapeutic community principles, for the most part, specialized addiction agencies have difficulty treating these patients. Generally, integrated treatment in which the same staff can treat both the psychiatric disorder and the addiction is more effective than either parallel treatment (a mental health and a specialty addiction program providing care concurrently) or sequential treatment (treating either the addiction or the psychiatric disorder first and then dealing with the comorbid condition).

Services and Outcome

The extension of managed care into the public sector has produced a major reduction in the use of hospital-based detoxification and virtual disappearance of residential rehabilitation programs for alcoholics. Managed-care organizations, however, tend to assume that the relatively brief courses of outpatient counseling that are effective with private-sector alcoholic patients are also effective with patients who are dependent on illicit drugs and who have minimal social supports. For the present, the trend is to provide the care that costs the least over the short term and to ignore studies showing that more services can produce better long-term outcomes.

Treatment is often a worthwhile social expenditure. For example, treatment of antisocial illicit drug users in outpatient settings can decrease antisocial behavior and reduce rates of human immunodeficiency virus (HIV) seroconversion that more than offset the treatment cost. Treatment in a prison setting can decrease postrelease costs associated with drug use and rearrests. Despite such evidence, problems exist in maintaining public support for treatment of substance dependence in both the public and private sectors. This lack of support suggests that these problems continue to be viewed, at least in part, as moral failings rather than as medical disorders.

▲ 16.2 Alcohol-Related Disorders

Alcoholism is among the most common psychiatric disorders observed in the Western world. Alcohol-related problems in the United States contribute to 2 million injuries each year, including 22,000 deaths. Recent years have witnessed a blossoming of clinically relevant research regarding alcohol abuse and dependence, including information on specific genetic influences, the clinical course of these conditions, and the development of new and helpful treatments.

Alcohol is a potent drug that causes both acute and chronic changes in almost all neurochemical systems. Thus alcohol abuse can produce serious temporary psychological symptoms including depression, anxiety, and psychoses. Long-term, escalating levels of alcohol consumption can produce tolerance as well as such intense adaptation of the body that cessation of use can precipitate a withdrawal syndrome usually marked by insomnia, evidence of hyperactivity of the autonomic nervous system, and feelings of anxiety. Therefore, in an adequate evaluation of life problems and psychiatric symptoms in a patient, the clinician must consider the possibility that the clinical situation reflects the effects of alcohol.

EPIDEMIOLOGY

Psychiatrists need to be concerned about alcoholism because this condition is common; intoxication and withdrawal mimic many major psychiatric disorders, and the usual person with alcoholism does not fit the stereotype (i.e., so called "nasty knock-down drinkers").

Prevalence of Drinking

At some time during life, 90 percent of the population in the United States drinks, with most people beginning their alcohol intake in the early to middle teens (Table 16.2–1). By the end of high school, 80 percent of students have consumed alcohol, and more than 60 percent have been intoxicated. At any time, two of three men are drinkers, with a ratio of persisting alcohol intake of approximately 1.3 men to 1.0 women, and the highest prevalence of drinking from the middle or late teens to the mid-20s.

Men and women with higher education and income are most likely to imbibe, and, among religious denominations, Jews have the highest proportion who consume alcohol but among the lowest rates of alcohol dependence. Other ethnicities, such as the Irish, have higher rates of severe alcohol problems, but they also have significantly higher rates of abstentions. Some estimates show that more than 60 percent of men and women in some Native American and Inuit tribes have been alcohol dependent at some time. In the United States, the average adult consumes 2.2 gallons of absolute alcohol a year, a decrease from 2.7 gallons per capita in 1981.

Drinking alcohol-containing beverages is generally considered an acceptable habit in the United States. About 90 percent of all US residents have had an alcohol-containing drink at least once in their lives, and about 51 percent of all US adults are current users of alcohol. After heart disease and cancer, alcohol-related disorders constitute the third largest health problem in the United States today. Beer accounts for about one-half of all alcohol consumption, liquor for about one-third, and wine for about one-sixth. About 30 to 45 percent of all adults in the United States have had at least one transient episode of an alcohol-related problem, usually an alcohol-induced amnestic episode (e.g., a blackout), driving a motor vehicle while intoxicated, or missing school or work because of excessive drinking. About 10 percent of women and 20 percent of men have met the diagnostic criteria for alcohol abuse during their lifetimes, and 3 to 5 percent of women and 10 percent of men have met the diagnostic criteria for the more serious diagnosis of alcohol dependence during their lifetimes. About 200,000 deaths each year are directly related to alcohol abuse. The common causes of death among persons with the alcohol-related disorders are suicide, cancer, heart disease, and hepatic disease. Although persons involved in automotive fatalities do not always meet the diagnostic criteria for an alcohol-related disorder, drunk drivers are involved in about 50 percent of all automotive fatalities, and this percentage increases to about 75 percent when only accidents occurring in the late evening are considered. Alcohol use and alcohol-related disorders are associated with about 50 percent of all homicides and 25 percent of all suicides. Alcohol abuse reduces life expectancy by about 10 years, and alcohol leads all other substances in substance-related deaths. Table 16.2–2 lists other epidemiological data about alcohol use.

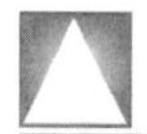

Table 16.2–1
Alcohol Epidemiology

Condition	Population (%)
Ever had a drink	90
Current drinker	60–70
Temporary problems	40+
Abuse[a]	Male: 10+ Female: 5+
Dependence[a]	Male: 10 Female: 3–5

[a]20–30% of psychiatric patients.

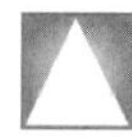

Table 16.2–2
Epidemiological Data for Alcohol-Related Disorders

Race and Ethnicity	Whites have the highest rate of alcohol use. Hispanics and blacks have similar rate of binge use, but is lower among blacks than among whites.
Gender	Men are much more likely than women to be binge drinkers and heavy drinkers.
Region and Urbanicity	Alcohol use is highest in western states and lowest in southern states. North central and northeast regions are about the same. The rate of past month alcohol use was 56% in large metropolitan areas, 52% in small metropolitan areas, and 46% in nonmetropolitan areas. Little variation seen in binge and heavy alcohol use rates by population density.
Education	About 70% of adults with college degrees are current drinkers, compared with only 40% of those with less than a high school education. Binge alcohol use rates are similar across different levels of education.
Socioeconomic Class	Alcohol-related disorders appear among persons of all socioeconomic classes. Persons who are stereotypical skid-row alcoholics constitute less than 5% of those with alcohol-related disorders.

COMORBIDITY

The psychiatric diagnoses most commonly associated with the alcohol-related disorders are other substance-related disorders, antisocial personality disorder, mood disorders, and anxiety disorders. Although the data are somewhat controversial, most suggest that persons with alcohol-related disorders have a markedly higher suicide rate than the general population.

Antisocial Personality Disorder

A relation between antisocial personality disorder and alcohol-related disorders has frequently been reported. Some studies suggest that antisocial personality disorder is particularly common in men with an alcohol-related disorder and can precede the development of the alcohol-related disorder. Other studies, however, suggest that antisocial personality disorder and alcohol-related disorders are completely distinct entities that are not causally related.

Mood Disorders

About 30 to 40 percent of persons with an alcohol-related disorder meet the diagnostic criteria for major depressive disorder sometime during their lifetimes. Depression is more common in women than in men with these disorders. Several studies reported that depression is likely to occur in patients with alcohol-related disorders who have a high daily consumption of alcohol and a family history of alcohol abuse. Persons with alcohol-related disorders and major depressive disorder are at great risk for attempting suicide and are likely to have other substance-related disorder diagnoses. Some clinicians recommend antidepressant drug therapy for depressive symptoms that remain after 2 to 3 weeks of sobriety. Patients with bipolar I disorder are thought to be at risk for developing an alcohol-related disorder; they may use alcohol to self-medicate their manic episodes. Some studies have shown that persons with both alcohol-related disorder and depressive disorder diagnoses have concentrations of dopamine metabolites (homovanillic acid) and GABA in their cerebrospinal fluid (CSF).

Anxiety Disorders

Many persons use alcohol for its efficacy in alleviating anxiety. Although the comorbidity between alcohol-related disorders and mood disorders is fairly widely recognized, it is less well known that perhaps 25 to 50 percent of all persons with alcohol-related disorders also meet the diagnostic criteria for an anxiety disorder. Phobias and panic disorder are particularly frequent comorbid diagnoses in these patients. Some data indicate that alcohol may be used in an attempt to self-medicate symptoms of agoraphobia or social phobia, but an alcohol-related disorder is likely to precede the development of panic disorder or generalized anxiety disorder.

Suicide

Most estimates of the prevalence of suicide among persons with alcohol-related disorders range from 10 to 15 percent, although alcohol use itself may be involved in a much higher percentage of suicides. Some investigators have questioned whether the suicide rate among persons with alcohol-related disorders is as high as the numbers suggest. Factors that have been associated with suicide among persons with alcohol-related disorders include the presence of a major depressive episode, weak psychosocial support systems, a serious coexisting medical condition, unemployment, and living alone.

ETIOLOGY

Many factors affect the decision to drink, the development of temporary alcohol-related difficulties in the teenage years and the 20s, and the development of alcohol dependence. The initiation of alcohol intake probably depends largely on social, religious, and psychological factors, although genetic characteristics might also contribute. The factors that influence the decision to drink or those that contribute to temporary problems might differ, however, from those that add to the risk for the severe, recurring problems of alcohol dependence.

A similar interplay between genetic and environmental influences contributes to many medical and psychiatric conditions, and, thus, a review of these factors in alcoholism offers information about complex genetic disorders overall. Dominant or recessive genes, although important, explain only relatively rare conditions. Most disorders have some level of genetic predisposition that usually relates to a series of different genetically influenced characteristics, each of which increases or decreases the risk for the disorder.

It is likely that a series of genetic influences combine to explain approximately 60 percent of the proportion of risk for alcoholism, with environment responsible for the remaining proportion of the variance. The divisions offered in this section, therefore, are more heuristic than real, because it is the combination of a series of psychological, sociocultural, biological, and other factors that are responsible for the development of severe, repetitive alcohol-related life problems.

Psychological Theories

A variety of theories relate to the use of alcohol to reduce tension, increase feelings of power, and decrease the effects of psychological pain. Perhaps the greatest interest has been paid to the observation that people with alcohol-related problems often report that alcohol decreases their feelings of nervousness and helps them cope with the day-to-day stresses of life. The psychological theories are built, in part, on the observation among nonalcoholic people that the intake of low doses of alcohol in a tense social setting or after a difficult day can be associated with an enhanced feeling of well-being and an improved ease of interactions. In high doses, especially at falling blood alcohol levels, however, most measures of muscle tension and psychological feelings of nervousness and tension are increased. Thus, tension-reducing effects of this drug might have an impact most on light to moderate drinkers or add to the relief of withdrawal symptoms, but play a minor role in causing alcoholism. The theories that focus on alcohol's potential to enhance feelings of being powerful and sexually attractive and to decrease the effects of psychological pain are difficult to evaluate definitively.

Psychodynamic Theories

Perhaps related to the disinhibiting or anxiety-lowering effects of lower doses of alcohol is the hypothesis that some people may use this drug to help them deal with self-punitive harsh superegos and to decrease unconscious stress levels. In addition, classic psychoanalytical theory hypothesizes that at least some alcoholic people may have become fixated at the oral stage of development and use alcohol to relieve their frustrations by taking the substance by mouth. Hypotheses regarding arrested phases of psychosexual development, although heuristically useful, have had little effect on the usual treatment approaches and are not the focus of extensive ongoing research. Similarly, most studies have not been able to document an "addictive personality" present in most alcoholics and associated with a propensity to lack control of intake of a wide range of substances and foods. Although pathological scores on personality tests are often seen during intoxication, withdrawal, and early recovery, many of these characteristics are not found to predate alcoholism, and most disappear with abstinence. Similarly, prospective studies of children of alcoholics who themselves have no co-occurring disorders usually document high risks mostly for alcoholism. As is described later in this text, one partial exception occurs with the extreme levels of impulsivity seen in the 15 to 20 percent of alcoholic men with antisocial personality disorder, because they have high risks for criminality, violence, and multiple substance dependencies.

Behavioral Theories

Expectations about the rewarding effects of drinking, cognitive attitudes toward responsibility for one's behavior, and subsequent reinforcement after alcohol intake all contribute to the decision to drink again after the first experience with alcohol and to continue to imbibe despite problems. These issues are important in efforts to modify drinking behaviors in the general population, and they contribute to some important aspects of alcoholic rehabilitation.

Sociocultural Theories

Sociocultural theories are often based on extrapolations from social groups that have high and low rates of alcoholism. Theorists hypothesize that ethnic groups, such as Jews, who introduce children to modest levels of drinking in a family atmosphere and eschew drunkenness have low rates of alcoholism. Some other groups, such as Irish men or some American Indian tribes with high rates of abstention but a tradition of drinking to the point of drunkenness among drinkers, are believed to have high rates of alcoholism. These theories, however, often depend on stereotypes that tend to be erroneous, and prominent exceptions to these rules exist. For example, some theories based on observations of the Irish and the French have incorrectly predicted high rates of alcoholism among the Italians.

Yet, environmental events, presumably including cultural factors, account for as much as 40 percent of the alcoholism risk. Thus, although these are difficult to study, it is likely that cultural attitudes toward drinking, drunkenness, and personal responsibility for consequences are important contributors to the rates of alcohol-related problems in a society. In the final analysis, social and psychological theories are probably highly relevant, because they outline factors that contribute to the onset of drinking, the development of temporary alcohol-related life difficulties, and even alcoholism. The problem is how to gather relatively definitive data to support or refute the theories.

Childhood History

Researchers have identified several factors in the childhood histories of persons with later alcohol-related disorders and in children at high risk for having an alcohol-related disorder because one or both of their parents are affected. In experimental studies, children at high risk for alcohol-related disorders have been found to possess, on average, a range of deficits on neurocognitive testing, low amplitude of the P300 wave on evoked potential testing, and a variety of abnormalities on electroencephalography (EEG) recordings. Studies of high-risk offspring in their 20s have also shown a generally blunted effect of alcohol compared with that seen in persons whose parents have not been diagnosed with alcohol-related disorder. These findings suggest that a heritable biological brain function may predispose a person to an alcohol-related disorder. A childhood history of attention-deficit/hyperactivity disorder (ADHD), conduct disorder, or both, increases a child's risk for an alcohol-related disorder as an adult. Personality disorders, especially antisocial personality disorder, as noted earlier, also predispose a person to an alcohol-related disorder.

Genetic Theories

Four lines of evidence support the conclusion that alcoholism is genetically influenced. First, a threefold to fourfold increased risk for severe alcohol problems is seen in close relatives of alcoholic people. The rate of alcohol problems increases with the number of alcoholic relatives, the severity of their illness, and the closeness of their genetic relationship to the person under study. The family investigations do little to separate the importance of genetics and environment, and the second approach, twin studies, takes the data a step further. The rate of similarity, or concordance, for severe alcohol-related problems is significantly higher in identical twins of alcoholic individuals than in fraternal twins in most investigations, which estimate that genes explain 60 percent of the variance, with the remainder relating to nonshared, probably adult environmental influences. Third, the adoption-type studies have all revealed a significantly enhanced risk for alcoholism in the offspring of alcoholic parents, even when the children had been separated from their biological parents close to birth and raised without any knowledge of the problems within the biological family. The risk for severe alcohol-related difficulties is not further enhanced by being raised in an alcoholic adoptive family. Finally, studies in animals support the importance of a variety of yet-to-be-identified genes in the free-choice use of alcohol, subsequent levels of intoxication, and some consequences.

EFFECTS OF ALCOHOL

The term *alcohol* refers to a large group of organic molecules that have a hydroxyl group (OH) attached to a saturated carbon atom. Ethyl alcohol, also called *ethanol,* is the common form of alcohol; sometimes referred to as *beverage alcohol,* ethyl alcohol is used for drinking. The chemical formula for ethanol is CH_3CH_2OH.

The characteristic tastes and flavors of alcohol-containing beverages result from their methods of production, which produce various congeners in the final product, including methanol, butanol, aldehydes, phenols, tannins, and trace amounts of various metals. Although the congeners may confer some differential psychoactive effects on the various alcohol-containing beverages, these differences are minimal compared with the effects of ethanol itself. A single drink is usually considered to contain about 12 g of ethanol, which is the content of 12 oz of beer (7.2 proof, 3.6 percent ethanol in the United States), one 4-oz glass of nonfortified wine, or 1 to 1.5 oz of an 80-proof (40 percent ethanol) liquor (e.g., whiskey or gin). In calculating patients' alcohol intake, however, clinicians should be aware that beers vary in their alcohol content, that beers are available in small and large cans and mugs, that glasses of wine range from 2 to 6 oz, and that mixed drinks at some bars and in most homes contain 2 to 3 oz of liquor. Nonetheless, using the moderate sizes of drinks, clinicians can estimate that a single drink increases the blood alcohol level of a 150-lb man by 15 to 20 mg/dL, which is about the concentration of alcohol that an average person can metabolize in 1 hour.

The possible beneficial effects of alcohol have been publicized, especially by the makers and the distributors of alcohol. Most attention has been focused on some epidemiological data that suggest that one or two glasses of red wine each day lower the incidence of cardiovascular disease; these findings, however, are highly controversial.

Absorption

About 10 percent of consumed alcohol is absorbed from the stomach, and the remainder from the small intestine. Peak blood concentration of alcohol is reached in 30 to 90 minutes and usually in 45 to 60 minutes, depending on whether the alcohol was ingested on an empty stomach (which enhances absorption) or with food (which delays absorption). The time to peak blood concentration also depends on the time during which the alcohol was consumed; rapid drinking reduces the time to peak concentration, slower drinking increases it. Absorption is most rapid with beverages containing 15 to 30 percent alcohol (30 to 60 proof). There is some dispute about whether carbonation (e.g., in champagne and in drinks mixed with seltzer) enhances the absorption of alcohol.

The body has protective devices against inundation by alcohol. For example, if the concentration of alcohol in the stomach becomes too high, mucus is secreted and the pyloric valve closes. These actions slow the absorption and keep the alcohol from passing into the small intestine, where there are no significant restraints on absorption. Thus, a large amount of alcohol can remain unabsorbed in the stomach for hours. Furthermore, pylorospasm often results in nausea and vomiting.

Once alcohol is absorbed into the bloodstream, it is distributed to all body tissues. Because alcohol is uniformly dissolved in the body's water, tissues containing a high proportion of water receive a high concentration of alcohol. The intoxicating effects are greater when the blood alcohol concentration is rising than when it is falling (the Mellanby effects). For this reason, the rate of absorption bears directly on the intoxication response.

Metabolism

About 90 percent of absorbed alcohol is metabolized through oxidation in the liver; the remaining 10 percent is excreted unchanged by the kidneys and lungs. The rate of oxidation by the liver is constant and independent of the body's energy requirements. The body can metabolize about 15 mg/dL per hour, with a range of 10 to 34 mg/dL per hour. That is, the average person oxidizes three-fourths of an ounce of 40 percent (80 proof) alcohol in an hour. In persons with a history of excessive alcohol consumption, upregulation of the necessary enzymes results in rapid alcohol metabolism.

Alcohol is metabolized by two enzymes: alcohol dehydrogenase (ADH) and aldehyde dehydrogenase. ADH catalyzes the conversion of alcohol into acetaldehyde, which is a toxic compound; aldehyde dehydrogenase catalyzes the conversion of acetaldehyde into acetic acid. Aldehyde dehydrogenase is inhibited by disulfiram (Antabuse), often used in the treatment of alcohol-related disorders. Some studies have shown that women have a lower ADH blood content than men; this fact may account for woman's tendency to become more intoxicated than men after drinking the same amount of alcohol. The decreased function of alcohol-metabolizing enzymes in some Asian persons can also lead to easy intoxication and toxic symptoms.

Effects on the Brain

Biochemistry. In contrast to most other substances of abuse with identified receptor targets—such as the N-methyl-D-aspartate (NMDA) receptor of PCP—no single molecular target has been identified as the mediator for the effects of alcohol. The longstanding theory about the biochemical effects of alcohol concerns its effects on the membranes of neurons. Data support the hypothesis that alcohol produces its effects by intercalating itself into membranes and, thus, increasing fluidity of the membranes with short-term use. With long-term use, however, the theory hypothesizes that the membranes become rigid or stiff. The fluidity of the membranes is critical to normal functioning of receptors, ion channels, and other membrane-bound functional proteins. In recent studies, researchers have attempted to identify specific molecular targets for the effects of alcohol. Most attention has been focused on the effects of alcohol at ion channels. Specifically, studies have found that alcohol ion channel activities associated with the nicotinic acetylcholine, serotonin 5-hydroxytryptamine 3 (5-HT_3), and GABA type A ($GABA_A$) receptors are enhanced by alcohol, whereas ion channel activities associated with glutamate receptors and voltage-gated calcium channels are inhibited.

Behavioral Effects. As the net result of the molecular activities, alcohol functions as a depressant much like the barbiturates and the benzodiazepines, with which alcohol has some cross-tolerance and cross-dependence. At a level of 0.05 percent alcohol in the blood, thought, judgment, and restraint are loosened and sometimes disrupted. At a concentration of 0.1 percent, voluntary motor actions usually become perceptibly clumsy. In most states, legal intoxication ranges from 0.1 to 0.15 percent blood alcohol level. At 0.2 percent, the function of the entire motor area of the brain is measurably depressed, and the parts of the brain that control emotional behavior are also affected. At 0.3 percent, a person is commonly confused or may become stuporous; at 0.4 to 0.5 percent, the person falls into a coma. At higher levels, the primitive centers of the brain that control breathing and heart rate are affected, and death ensues secondary to direct respiratory depression or the aspiration of vomitus. Persons with long-term histories of alcohol abuse, however, can tolerate much higher concentrations of alcohol than can alcohol-naïve persons; their alcohol tolerance may cause them to falsely appear less intoxicated than they really are.

Sleep Effects. Although alcohol consumed in the evening usually increases the ease of falling asleep (decreased sleep latency), alcohol also has adverse effects on sleep architecture.

Specifically, alcohol use is associated with a decrease in rapid eye movement sleep (REM or dream sleep) and deep sleep (stage 4) and more sleep fragmentation, with more and longer episodes of awakening. Therefore, the idea that drinking alcohol helps persons fall asleep is a myth.

Other Physiological Effects

Liver. The major adverse effects of alcohol use are related to liver damage. Alcohol use, even as short as week-long episodes of increased drinking, can result in an accumulation of fats and proteins, which produce the appearance of a fatty liver, sometimes found on physical examination as an enlarged liver. The association between fatty infiltration of the liver and serious liver damage remains unclear. Alcohol use, however, is associated with the development of alcoholic hepatitis and hepatic cirrhosis.

Gastrointestinal System. Long-term heavy drinking is associated with developing esophagitis, gastritis, achlorhydria, and gastric ulcers. The development of esophageal varices can accompany particularly heavy alcohol abuse; the rupture of the varices is a medical emergency often resulting in death by exsanguination. Disorders of the small intestine occasionally occur, and pancreatitis, pancreatic insufficiency, and pancreatic cancer are also associated with heavy alcohol use. Heavy alcohol intake can interfere with the normal processes of food digestion and absorption; as a result, consumed food is inadequately digested. Alcohol abuse also appears to inhibit the intestine's capacity to absorb various nutrients, such as vitamins and amino acids. This effect, coupled with the often poor dietary habits of those with alcohol-related disorders, can cause serious vitamin deficiencies, particularly of the B vitamins.

Other Bodily Systems. Significant intake of alcohol has been associated with increased blood pressure, dysregulation of lipoprotein and triglyceride metabolism, and increased risk for myocardial infarction and cerebrovascular disease. Alcohol has been shown to affect the hearts of nonalcoholic persons who do not usually drink, increasing the resting cardiac output, the heart rate, and the myocardial oxygen consumption. Evidence indicates that alcohol intake can adversely affect the hematopoietic system and can increase the incidence of cancer, particularly head, neck, esophageal, stomach, hepatic, colonic, and lung cancer. Acute intoxication may also be associated with hypoglycemia, which, when unrecognized, may be responsible for some of the sudden deaths of persons who are intoxicated. Muscle weakness is another side effect of alcoholism. Recent evidence shows that alcohol intake raises the blood concentration of estradiol in women. The increase in estradiol correlates with the blood alcohol level.

Laboratory Tests. The adverse effects of alcohol appear in common laboratory tests, which can be useful diagnostic aids in identifying persons with alcohol-related disorders. The γ-glutamyl transpeptidase levels are high in about 80 percent of those with alcohol-related disorders, and the mean corpuscular volume (MCV) is high in about 60 percent, more so in women than in men. Other laboratory test values that may be high in association with alcohol abuse are those of uric acid, triglycerides, aspartate aminotransferase (AST), and alanine aminotransferase (ALT).

Drug Interactions. The interaction between alcohol and other substances can be dangerous, even fatal. Certain substances, such as alcohol and phenobarbital (Luminal), are metabolized by the liver, and their prolonged use can lead to acceleration of their metabolism. When persons with alcohol-related disorders are sober, this accelerated metabolism makes them unusually tolerant to many drugs such as sedatives and hypnotics; when they are intoxicated, however, these drugs compete with the alcohol for the same detoxification mechanisms, and potentially toxic concentrations of all involved substances can accumulate in the blood.

The effects of alcohol and other CNS depressants are usually synergistic. Sedatives, hypnotics, and drugs that relieve pain, motion sickness, head colds, and allergy symptoms must be used with caution by persons with alcohol-related disorders. Narcotics depress the sensory areas of the cerebral cortex and can produce pain relief, sedation, apathy, drowsiness, and sleep; high doses can result in respiratory failure and death. Increasing the dosages of sedative-hypnotic drugs, such as chloral hydrate (Noctec) and benzodiazepines, especially when they are combined with alcohol, produces a range of effects from sedation to motor and intellectual impairment to stupor, coma, and death. Because sedatives and other psychotropic drugs can potentiate the effects of alcohol, patients should be instructed about the dangers of combining CNS depressants and alcohol, particularly when they are driving or operating machinery.

DISORDERS

Alcohol Use Disorder

Diagnosis and Clinical Features. In the fifth edition of *Diagnostic and Statistical Manual of Mental Disorders* (DSM-5), all substance use disorders use the same general criteria for dependence and abuse (see Section 16.1). A need for daily use of large amounts of alcohol for adequate functioning, a regular pattern of heavy drinking limited to weekends, and long periods of sobriety interspersed with binges of heavy alcohol intake lasting for weeks or months strongly suggest alcohol dependence and alcohol abuse. The drinking patterns are often associated with certain behaviors: the inability to cut down or stop drinking; repeated efforts to control or reduce excessive drinking by "going on the wagon" (periods of temporary abstinence) or by restricting drinking to certain times of the day; binges (remaining intoxicated throughout the day for at least 2 days); occasional consumption of a fifth of spirits (or its equivalent in wine or beer); amnestic periods for events occurring while intoxicated (blackouts); the continuation of drinking despite a serious physical disorder that the person knows is exacerbated by alcohol use; and drinking nonbeverage alcohol, such as fuel and commercial products containing alcohol. In addition, persons with alcohol dependence and alcohol abuse show impaired social or occupational functioning because of alcohol use (e.g., violence while intoxicated, absence from work, job loss), legal difficulties (e.g., arrest for intoxicated behavior and traffic accidents while intoxicated), and arguments or difficulties with family members or friends about excessive alcohol consumption.

Mark, a 45-year-old divorced man, was examined in a hospital emergency room because he had been confused and unable to care for himself of the preceding 3 days. His brother, who brought him to the hospital, reported that the patient has consumed large quantities of beer and wine daily for more than 5 years. His home and job lives were reasonably stable until his divorce 5 years prior. The brother indicated that Mark's drinking pattern since the divorce has been approximately 5 beers and a fourth of wine a day. Mark often experienced blackouts from drinking and missed days of work frequently. As a result, Mark has lost several jobs in the past 5 years. Although he usually provides for himself marginally with small jobs, 3 days earlier he ran out of money and alcohol and resorted to panhandling on the streets for cash to buy food. Mark had been poorly nourished, having one meal per day at best and was evidently relying on beer as his prime source of nourishment.

On examination, Mark alternates between apprehension and chatty, superficial warmth. He is pretty keyed up and talks constantly in a rambling and unfocused manner. His recognition of the physician varies; at times he recognizes him and other times he becomes confused and believes the doctor to be his other brother who lives in another state. On two occasions he referred to the physician by said brother's name and asked when he arrived in town, evidently having lost track of the interview up to that point. He has a gross hand tremor at rest and is disoriented to time. He believes he's in a parking lot rather than a hospital. Efforts at memory and calculation testing fail because Mark's attention shifts so rapidly.

Subtypes of Alcohol Dependence. Various researchers have attempted to divide alcohol dependence into subtypes based primarily on phenomenological characteristics. One recent classification notes that type A alcohol dependence is characterized by late onset, few childhood risk factors, relatively mild dependence, few alcohol-related problems, and little psychopathology. Type B alcohol dependence is characterized by many childhood risk factors, severe dependence, an early onset of alcohol-related problems, much psychopathology, a strong family history of alcohol abuse, frequent polysubstance abuse, a long history of alcohol treatment, and a lot of severe life stresses. Some researchers have found that type A persons who are alcohol dependent may respond to interactional psychotherapies, whereas type B persons who are alcohol dependent may respond to training in coping skills.

Other subtyping schemes of alcohol dependence have received fairly wide recognition in the literature. One group of investigators proposed three subtypes: earlystage problem drinkers, who do not yet have complete alcohol dependence syndromes; affiliative drinkers, who tend to drink daily in moderate amounts in social settings; and schizoid-isolated drinkers, who have severe dependence and tend to drink in binges and often alone.

Another investigator described gamma alcohol dependence, which is thought to be common in the United States and represents the alcohol dependence seen in those who are active in Alcoholics Anonymous (AA). This variant concerns control problems in which persons are unable to stop drinking once they start. When drinking is terminated as a result of ill health or lack of money, these persons can abstain for varying periods. In delta alcohol dependence, perhaps more common in Europe than in the United States, persons who are alcohol dependent must drink a certain amount each day but are unaware of a lack of control. The alcohol use disorder may not be discovered until a person who must stop drinking for some reason exhibits withdrawal symptoms.

Another researcher has suggested a *type I, male-limited* variety of alcohol dependence, characterized by late onset, more evidence of psychological than of physical dependence, and the presence of guilt feelings. *Type II, male-limited* alcohol dependence is characterized by onset at an early age, spontaneous seeking of alcohol for consumption, and a socially disruptive set of behaviors when intoxicated.

Four subtypes of alcoholism were postulated by still another investigator. The first is *antisocial alcoholism,* typically with a predominance in men, a poor prognosis, early onset of alcohol-related problems, and a close association with antisocial personality disorder. The second is *developmentally cumulative alcoholism,* with a primary tendency for alcohol abuse that is exacerbated with time as cultural expectations foster increased opportunities to drink. The third is *negative-affect alcoholism,* which is more common in women than in men; according to this hypothesis, women are likely to use alcohol for mood regulation and to help ease social relationships. The fourth is *developmentally limited alcoholism,* with frequent bouts of consuming large amounts of alcohol; the bouts become less frequent as persons age and respond to the increased expectations of society about their jobs and families.

Alcohol Intoxication

The DSM-5 diagnostic criteria for alcohol intoxication (also called simple drunkenness) are based on evidence of recent ingestion of ethanol, maladaptive behavior, and at least one of several possible physiological correlates of intoxication (Table 16.2–3). As a conservative approach to identifying blood levels that are likely to have major effects on driving abilities, the legal definition of intoxication in most states in the United States requires a blood concentration of 80 or 100 mg ethanol per deciliter of blood (mg/dL), which is the same as 0.08 to 0.10 g/dL. The following is an outline of the rough estimates of the levels of impairment likely to be seen at various blood alcohol concentrations, for most people. Evidence of behavioral changes, a slowing in motor performance, and a decrease in the ability to think clearly occurs at doses as low as 20 to 30 mg/dL, as shown in Table 16.2–4. Blood concentrations between 100 and 200 mg/dL are likely to increase the impairment in coordination and judgment to severe problems with coordination (ataxia), increasing lability of mood, and progressively greater levels of cognitive deterioration. Anyone who does not show significant levels of impairment in motor and mental performance at approximately 150 mg/dL probably has

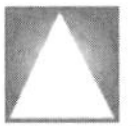

Table 16.2–3
Signs of Alcohol Intoxication

1. Slurred speech
2. Dizziness
3. Incoordination
4. Unsteady gait
5. Nystagmus
6. Impairment in attention or memory
7. Stupor or coma
8. Double vision

Table 16.2–4
Impairment Likely to Be Seen at Different Blood Alcohol Concentrations

Level	Likely Impairment
20–30 mg/dL	Slowed motor performance and decreased thinking ability
30–80 mg/dL	Increase in motor and cognitive problems
80–200 mg/dL	Increase in incoordination and judgment errors Mood lability Deterioration in cognition
200–300 mg/dL	Nystagmus, marked slurring of speech, and alcoholic blackouts
>300 mg/dL	Impaired vital signs and possible death

significant pharmacodynamic tolerance. In that range, most people without significant tolerance also experience relatively severe nausea and vomiting. With blood alcohol concentrations in the 200 to 300 mg/dL range, the slurring of speech is likely to become more intense, and memory impairment (*anterograde amnesia* or *alcoholic blackouts*) becomes pronounced. Further increases in blood alcohol concentration result in the first level of anesthesia, and the nontolerant person who reaches 400 mg/dL or more risks respiratory failure, coma, and death.

Alcohol Withdrawal

Alcohol withdrawal, even without delirium, can be serious; it can include seizures and autonomic hyperactivity. Conditions that may predispose to, or aggravate, withdrawal symptoms include fatigue, malnutrition, physical illness, and depression. The DSM-5 criteria for alcohol withdrawal require the cessation or reduction of alcohol use that was heavy and prolonged as well as the presence of specific physical or neuropsychiatric symptoms. The diagnosis also allows for the specification "with perceptual disturbances." One positron emission tomography (PET) study of blood flow during alcohol withdrawal in otherwise healthy persons with alcohol dependence reported a globally low rate of metabolic activity, although, with further inspection of the data, the authors concluded that activity was especially low in the left parietal and right frontal areas.

The classic sign of alcohol withdrawal is tremulousness, although the spectrum of symptoms can expand to include psychotic and perceptual symptoms (e.g., delusions and hallucinations), seizures, and the symptoms of delirium tremens (DTs), called alcohol delirium in DSM-5. Tremulousness (commonly called the "shakes" or the "jitters") develops 6 to 8 hours after the cessation of drinking, the psychotic and perceptual symptoms begin in 8 to 12 hours, seizures in 12 to 24 hours, and DTs anytime during the first 72 hours, although physicians should watch for the development of DTs for the first week of withdrawal. The syndrome of withdrawal sometimes skips the usual progression and, for example, goes directly to DTs.

The tremor of alcohol withdrawal can be similar to either physiological tremor, with a continuous tremor of great amplitude and of more than 8 Hz, or familial tremor, with bursts of tremor activity slower than 8 Hz. Other symptoms of withdrawal include general irritability, gastrointestinal symptoms (e.g., nausea and vomiting), and sympathetic autonomic hyperactivity, including anxiety, arousal, sweating, facial flushing, mydriasis, tachycardia, and mild hypertension. Patients experiencing alcohol withdrawal are generally alert but may startle easily.

Twenty-nine-year-old Mr. F had been a heavy drinker for 8 years. One evening after work, he started drinking with friends and drank throughout the evening. He fell asleep in the early morning hours and upon awakening had a strong desire to drink and decided not to attend work. He had several Bloody Marys instead of food because food did not appeal to him. He went to a local bar in the afternoon and consumed large quantities of beer. That evening he met with some friends and continued to drink.

This drinking pattern continued for the next week. The beginning of the following week he attempted to have a cup of coffee and found that his hands were shaking so much that he could not get the cup to his mouth to drink. He eventually managed to pour himself some wine in a glass and drank as much as he could. His hands then became less shaky, but he now felt nauseous and began having dry heaves. He tried to drink repeatedly but he could not keep the alcohol down. He felt very ill and anxious so he contacted his physician who recommended he report to a hospital.

Upon evaluation, Mr. F was alert. He had a marked resting and intention tremor of the hands, and his tongue and eyelids were tremulous. He was oriented and had no memory impairment. When inquired about his drinking, Mr. F admits to drinking several drinks each day for the past 8 years, but claims that his drinking never interfered with his work or his relations with colleagues or friends. He denies having any aftereffects from his drinking other than mild hangovers. He denies ever having a binge such as this before and denies ever needing to drink daily in order to function adequately. He admits, however, that he has never tried to reduce or stop drinking.

Withdrawal Seizures. Seizures associated with alcohol withdrawal are stereotyped, generalized, and tonic–clonic in character. Patients often have more than one seizure 3 to 6 hours after the first seizure. Status epilepticus is relatively rare and occurs in less than 3 percent of patients. Although anticonvulsant medications are not required in the management of alcohol withdrawal seizures, the cause of the seizures is difficult to establish when a patient is first assessed in the emergency room; thus, many patients with withdrawal seizures receive anticonvulsant medications, which are then discontinued once the cause of the seizures is recognized. Seizure activity in patients with known alcohol abuse histories should still prompt clinicians to consider other causative factors, such as head injuries, CNS infections, CNS neoplasms, and other cerebrovascular diseases; long-term severe alcohol abuse can result in hypoglycemia, hyponatremia, and hypomagnesemia—all of which can also be associated with seizures.

Treatment. The primary medications to control alcohol withdrawal symptoms are the benzodiazepines (Table 16.2–5). Many studies have found that benzodiazepines help control seizure activity, delirium, anxiety, tachycardia, hypertension, diaphoresis, and tremor associated with alcohol withdrawal. Benzodiazepines can be given either orally or parenterally; neither diazepam (Valium) nor chlordiazepoxide (Librium), however, should be given intramuscularly (IM) because of their erratic absorption by this route. Clinicians must titrate the dosage of the benzodiazepine, starting with a high dosage and lowering the dosage as the

Table 16.2–5
Drug Therapy for Alcohol Intoxication and Withdrawal

Clinical Problem	Drug	Route	Dosage	Comment
Tremulousness and mild to moderate agitation	Chlordiazepoxide	Oral	25–100 mg every 4–6 hr	Initial dose can be repeated every 2 hr until patient is calm; subsequent doses must be individualized and titrated
	Diazepam	Oral	5–20 mg every 4–6 hr	
Hallucinosis	Lorazepam	Oral	2–10 mg every 4–6 hr	
Extreme agitation	Chlordiazepoxide	Intravenous	0.5 mg/kg at 12.5 mg/min	Give until patient is calm; subsequent doses must be individualized and titrated
Withdrawal seizures	Diazepam	Intravenous	0.15 mg/kg at 2.5 mg/min	
Delirium tremens	Lorazepam	Intravenous	0.1 mg/kg at 2.0 mg/min	

Adapted from Koch-Weser J, Sellers EM, Kalant J. Alcohol intoxication and withdrawal. *N Engl J Med.* 1976;294:757.

patient recovers. Sufficient benzodiazepines should be given to keep patients calm and sedated but not so sedated that they cannot be aroused for clinicians to perform appropriate procedures, including neurological examinations.

Although benzodiazepines are the standard treatment for alcohol withdrawal, studies have shown that carbamazepine (Tegretol) in daily doses of 800 mg is as effective as benzodiazepines and has the added benefit of minimal abuse liability. Carbamazepine use is gradually becoming common in the United States and Europe. The β-adrenergic receptor antagonists and clonidine (Catapres) have also been used to block the symptoms of sympathetic hyperactivity, but neither drug is an effective treatment for seizures or delirium.

Delirium

Diagnosis and Clinical Features. Patients with recognized alcohol withdrawal symptoms should be carefully monitored to prevent progression to alcohol withdrawal delirium, the most severe form of the withdrawal syndrome, also known as DTs. Alcohol withdrawal delirium is a medical emergency that can result in significant morbidity and mortality. Patients with delirium are a danger to themselves and to others. Because of the unpredictability of their behavior, patients with delirium may be assaultive or suicidal or may act on hallucinations or delusional thoughts as if they were genuine dangers. Untreated, DTs has a mortality rate of 20 percent, usually as a result of an intercurrent medical illness such as pneumonia, renal disease, hepatic insufficiency, or heart failure. Although withdrawal seizures commonly precede the development of alcohol withdrawal delirium, delirium can also appear unheralded. The essential feature of the syndrome is delirium occurring within 1 week after a person stops drinking or reduces the intake of alcohol. In addition to the symptoms of delirium, the features of alcohol intoxication delirium include autonomic hyperactivity such as tachycardia, diaphoresis, fever, anxiety, insomnia, and hypertension; perceptual distortions, most frequently visual or tactile hallucinations; and fluctuating levels of psychomotor activity, ranging from hyperexcitability to lethargy.

About 5 percent of persons with alcohol-related disorders who are hospitalized have DTs. Because the syndrome usually develops on the third hospital day, a patient admitted for an unrelated condition may unexpectedly have an episode of delirium, the first sign of a previously undiagnosed alcohol-related disorder. Episodes of DTs usually begin in a patient's 30s or 40s after 5 to 15 years of heavy drinking, typically of the binge type. Physical illness (e.g., hepatitis or pancreatitis) predisposes to the syndrome; a person in good physical health rarely has DTs during alcohol withdrawal.

Mr. R, a 40-year-old man, was admitted to the orthopedic department of a general hospital after experiencing a fall down stairs and breaking his leg. On the third day of his hospital stay, he became increasingly nervous and started to tremble. He was unable to sleep at night, talked incoherently, and was obviously very anxious. Mr. R, when asked, denied an alcohol problem other than an occasional glass of wine.

When asked directly, his wife admitted that Mr. R drank large quantities of wine for over 4 years. During the previous year, his drinking would begin every evening when he came home from work and would not end until he fell asleep. On the evening of admittance, the fall occurred before he was able to consume any alcohol.

During the few weeks prior to his admittance, Mr. R had eaten very little. On several occasions, Mrs. R noticed that Mr. R was unable to recall even important events from the previous day. He had a car accident 3 years prior but without major injury. Mr. R had no other major health problems. His relationship with Mrs. R became very difficult after he began drinking and Mrs. R was seriously contemplating divorce. Mr. R had a tense relationship with his four children and he often argued with them. Recently, the children tried to avoid Mr. R as much as possible.

On examination, Mr. R's speech was rambling and incoherent. He believed that he was still at work and that he had a job to finish. At times he thought the physicians and nurses were his co-workers. At times he picked at bugs that he could see on his bed sheets. He was disoriented in time and was startled easily by sounds from outside the room. He sweats profusely and could not hold a glass without spilling some of the contents.

Treatment. The best treatment for DTs is prevention. Patients withdrawing from alcohol who exhibit withdrawal phenomena should receive a benzodiazepine, such as 25 to 50 mg of chlordiazepoxide every 2 to 4 hours until they seem to be out of danger. Once the delirium appears, however, 50 to 100 mg of chlordiazepoxide should be given every 4 hours orally, or lorazepam (Ativan) should be given intravenously (IV) if oral medication is not possible (Table 16.2–5). Antipsychotic medications that may reduce the seizure threshold in patients should be avoided. A high-calorie, high-carbohydrate diet supplemented by multivitamins is also important.

Physically restraining patients with the DTs are risky; they may fight against the restraints to a dangerous level of exhaustion. When patients are disorderly and uncontrollable, a seclusion room can be used. Dehydration, often exacerbated by diaphoresis and fever, can be corrected with fluids given by mouth or IV. Anorexia, vomiting, and diarrhea often occur during withdrawal. Antipsychotic medications should be avoided because they can reduce the seizure threshold in the patient. The emergence of focal neurological symptoms, lateralizing seizures, increased intracranial pressure, or evidence of skull fractures or other indications of CNS pathology should prompt clinicians to examine a patient for additional neurological disease. Nonbenzodiazepine anticonvulsant medication is not useful in preventing or treating alcohol withdrawal convulsions, although benzodiazepines are generally effective.

Warm, supportive psychotherapy in the treatment of DTs is essential. Patients are often bewildered, frightened, and anxious because of their tumultuous symptoms, and skillful verbal support is imperative.

Alcohol-Induced Persisting Dementia

Alcohol-induced persisting dementia is a poorly studied, heterogeneous long-term cognitive problem that can develop in the course of alcoholism. Global decreases in intellectual functioning, cognitive abilities, and memory are observed, but recent memory difficulties are consistent with the global cognitive impairment, an observation that helps to distinguish this from alcohol-induced persisting amnestic disorder. Brain functioning tends to improve with abstinence, but perhaps half of all affected patients have long-term and even permanent disabilities in memory and thinking. Approximately 50 to 70 percent of these patients evidence increased size of the brain ventricles and shrinkage of the cerebral sulci, although these changes appear to be partially or completely reversible during the first year of complete abstinence.

Alcohol-Induced Persisting Amnestic Disorder

Diagnosis and Clinical Features. The essential feature of alcohol-induced persisting amnestic disorder is a disturbance in short-term memory caused by prolonged heavy use of alcohol. Because the disorder usually occurs in persons who have been drinking heavily for many years, the disorder is rare in persons younger than age 35.

Wernicke–Korsakoff Syndrome. The classic names for alcohol-induced persisting amnestic disorder are Wernicke's encephalopathy (a set of acute symptoms) and Korsakoff's syndrome (a chronic condition). Whereas Wernicke's encephalopathy is completely reversible with treatment, only about 20 percent of patients with Korsakoff's syndrome recover. The pathophysiological connection between the two syndromes is thiamine deficiency, caused either by poor nutritional habits or by malabsorption problems. Thiamine is a cofactor for several important enzymes and may also be involved in conduction of the axon potential along the axon and in synaptic transmission. The neuropathological lesions are symmetrical and paraventricular, involving the mammillary bodies, the thalamus, the hypothalamus, the midbrain, the pons, the medulla, the fornix, and the cerebellum.

Wernicke's encephalopathy, also called *alcoholic encephalopathy,* is an acute neurological disorder characterized by ataxia (affecting primarily the gait), vestibular dysfunction, confusion, and a variety of ocular motility abnormalities, including horizontal nystagmus, lateral orbital palsy, and gaze palsy. These eye signs are usually bilateral but not necessarily symmetrical. Other eye signs may include a sluggish reaction to light and anisocoria. Wernicke's encephalopathy may clear spontaneously in a few days or weeks or may progress into Korsakoff's syndrome.

Treatment. In the early stages, Wernicke's encephalopathy responds rapidly to large doses of parenteral thiamine, which is believed to be effective in preventing the progression into Korsakoff's syndrome. The dosage of thiamine is usually initiated at 100 mg by mouth two to three times daily and is continued for 1 to 2 weeks. In patients with alcohol-related disorders who are receiving IV administration of glucose solution, it is good practice to include 100 mg of thiamine in each liter of the glucose solution.

Korsakoff's syndrome is the chronic amnestic syndrome that can follow Wernicke's encephalopathy, and the two syndromes are believed to be pathophysiologically related. The cardinal features of Korsakoff's syndrome are impaired mental syndrome (especially recent memory) and anterograde amnesia in an alert and responsive patient. The patient may or may not have the symptom of confabulation. Treatment of Korsakoff's syndrome is also thiamine given 100 mg by mouth two to three times daily; the treatment regimen should continue for 3 to 12 months. Few patients who progress to Korsakoff's syndrome ever fully recover, although many have some improvement in their cognitive abilities with thiamine and nutritional support.

Blackouts. Blackouts are similar to episodes of transient global amnesia in that they are discrete episodes of anterograde amnesia that occur in association with alcohol intoxication. The periods of amnesia can be particularly distressing when persons fear that they have unknowingly harmed someone or behaved imprudently while intoxicated. During a blackout, persons have relatively intact remote memory but experience a specific short-term memory deficit in which they are unable to recall events that happened in the previous 5 or 10 minutes. Because their other intellectual faculties are well preserved, they can perform complicated tasks and appear normal to casual observers. The neurobiological mechanisms for alcoholic blackouts are now known at the molecular level; alcohol blocks the consolidation of new memories into old memories, a process that is thought to involve the hippocampus and related temporal lobe structures.

Alcohol-Induced Psychotic Disorder

Diagnosis and Clinical Features. Approximately 3 percent of alcoholic persons experience auditory hallucinations or paranoid delusions in the context of heavy drinking or withdrawal. The most common auditory hallucinations are voices, but they are often unstructured. The voices are characteristically maligning, reproachful, or threatening, although some patients report that the voices are pleasant and nondisruptive. The hallucinations usually last less than a week, but during that week impaired reality testing is common. After the episode, most patients realize the hallucinatory nature of the symptoms.

Hallucinations after alcohol withdrawal are considered rare, and the syndrome is distinct from alcohol withdrawal delirium. The hallucinations can occur at any age, but usually appear in persons abusing alcohol for a long time. Although the hallucinations usually resolve within a week, some linger; in these cases, clinicians must consider other psychotic disorders in the differential diagnosis. Alcohol withdrawal-related hallucinations are differentiated from the hallucinations of schizophrenia by the temporal association with alcohol withdrawal, the absence of a classic history of schizophrenia, and their usually short-lived duration. Alcohol withdrawal-related hallucinations are differentiated from the DTs by the presence of a clear sensorium in patients.

Mr. G was a 40-year-old unemployed man living alone in a studio apartment and was brought to the hospital by the police. He contacted them complaining that he heard voices of men on the street below his window talking about him and threatening to kill him. He stated that every time he looked out the window the men had always disappeared.

Mr. G had a 15-year history of almost daily alcohol use. He was intoxicated each day and often experienced shakes upon awakening in the morning. On the previous day, he had only one glass of beer instead of his usual four because of gastrointestinal problems. He was fully alert and oriented.

Treatment. The treatment of alcohol withdrawal-related hallucinations is much like the treatment of DTs—benzodiazepines, adequate nutrition, and fluids, if necessary. If this regimen fails or for long-term cases, antipsychotics may be used.

Alcohol-Induced Mood Disorder

Heavy intake of alcohol over several days results in many of the symptoms observed in major depressive disorder, but the intense sadness markedly improves within several days to 1 month of abstinence. Eighty percent of people with alcoholism report histories of intense depression, including 30 to 40 percent who were depressed for 2 or more weeks at a time. However, only 10 to 15 percent of alcoholic persons have ever had depression that meets the criteria for major depressive disorder when they have not been drinking heavily.

Even severe substance-induced depressions are likely to improve fairly rapidly with abstinence, without medication or intensive psychotherapy aimed at the depressive symptoms. A logical approach for these substance-induced conditions is to teach the patient how to best view and deal with the temporary sadness through education and cognitive-behavioral treatment, and to watch and wait at least 2 to 4 weeks before starting antidepressant medications.

A consultation was requested on a 42-year-old woman with alcohol dependence who complained of persisting severe depressive symptoms despite 5 days of abstinence. In the initial stage of the interview, she noted that she had "always been depressed" and felt that she "drank to cope with the depressive symptoms." Her current complaint included a prominent sadness that had persisted for several weeks, difficulties concentrating, initial and terminal insomnia, and a feeling of hopelessness and guilt. In an effort to distinguish between an alcohol-induced mood disorder and an independent major depressive episode, a time-line–based history was obtained. This focused on the age of onset of alcohol dependence, periods of abstinence that extended for several months or more since the onset of dependence, and the ages of occurrence of clear major depressive episodes lasting several weeks or more at a time. Despite this patient's original complaints, it became clear that there had been no major depressive episodes prior to her mid-20s when alcohol dependence began, and that during a 1-year period of abstinence related to the gestation and neonatal period of her son, her mood had significantly improved. A provisional diagnosis of an alcohol-induced mood disorder was made. The patient was offered education, reassurance, and cognitive therapy to help her to deal with the depressive symptoms, but no antidepressant medications were prescribed. The depressive symptoms remained at their original intensity for several additional days and then began to improve. By approximately 3 weeks abstinent the patient no longer met criteria for a major depressive episode, although she demonstrated mood swings similar to dysphemia for several additional weeks. This case is a fairly typical example of an alcohol-induced mood disorder in an individual with alcohol dependence. *(Courtesy of Marc A. Shuckit, M.D.)*

Alcohol-Induced Anxiety Disorder

Anxiety symptoms fulfilling the diagnostic criteria for alcohol-induced anxiety disorder are also common in the context of acute and protracted alcohol withdrawal. Almost 80 percent of alcoholic persons report panic attacks during at least one acute withdrawal episode; their complaints can be sufficiently intense for the clinician to consider diagnosing panic disorder. Similarly, during the first 4 weeks or so of abstinence, people with severe alcohol problems are likely to avoid some social situations for fear of being overwhelmed by anxiety (i.e., they have symptoms resembling social phobia); their problems can at times be severe enough to resemble agoraphobia. However, when psychological or physiological symptoms of anxiety are observed in alcoholic persons only in the context of heavy drinking or within the first several weeks or month of abstinence, the symptoms are likely to diminish and subsequently disappear with time alone.

A 48-year-old woman was referred for evaluation and treatment of her recent onset of panic attacks. These episodes occurred two to three times per week over the preceding 6 months, with each lasting typically between 10 and 20 minutes. Panic symptoms occurred regardless of levels of life stress and could not be explained by current medications or medical conditions. The workup included an evaluation of her laboratory test values, which revealed a carbohydrate-deficient transferrin (CDT) level of 28 U/L, a uric acid level of 7.1 mg, and a γ-glutamyltransferase value of 47. All other blood tests were within normal limits.

The atypical age of onset of the panic attacks, along with the blood results, encouraged the clinician to probe further regarding the pattern of alcohol-related life problems with both the patient and, separately, her spouse. This step documented a history of alcohol dependence with an onset at approximately 35 years of age, with no evidence of panic disorder before that date. Nor did the patient have repetitive panic attacks beyond 2 weeks of abstinence during her frequent periods of nondrinking, which often lasted for 3 or 4 months. A working diagnosis of alcohol dependence with an alcohol-induced anxiety disorder characterized by panic attacks was made, and the patient was encouraged to abstain and was appropriately treated for possible withdrawal symptoms. Over the subsequent 3 weeks after a taper of benzodiazepines used for the treatment of withdrawal, the panic symptoms diminished in intensity and subsequently disappeared. *(Courtesy of Marc A. Schuckit, M.D.)*

Alcohol-Induced Sexual Dysfunction

The formal diagnosis of symptoms of sexual dysfunction associated with alcohol intoxication is alcohol-induced sexual dysfunction (see Section 13.2).

Alcohol-Induced Sleep Disorder

The diagnostic criteria for alcohol-induced sleep disorders with an onset during either alcohol intoxication or alcohol withdrawal are found in the sleep disorders section (see Section 12.2).

Unspecified Alcohol-Related Disorder

The diagnosis of unspecified alcohol-related disorder is used for alcohol-related disorders that do not meet the diagnostic criteria for any of the other diagnoses.

Idiosyncratic Alcohol Intoxication

Whether there is such a diagnostic entity as idiosyncratic alcohol intoxication is under debate. Several well-controlled studies of persons who supposedly have the disorder have raised questions about the validity of the designation. The condition has been variously called pathologic, complicated, atypical, and paranoid alcohol intoxication; all these terms indicate that a severe behavioral syndrome develops rapidly after a person consumes a small amount of alcohol that would have minimal behavioral effects on most persons. The diagnosis is important in the forensic arena because alcohol intoxication is not generally accepted as a reason for judging persons not responsible for their activities. Idiosyncratic alcohol intoxication, however, can be used in a person's defense if a defense lawyer can argue successfully that the defendant has an unexpected, idiosyncratic, pathological reaction to a minimal amount of alcohol.

In anecdotal reports, persons with idiosyncratic alcohol intoxication have been described as confused and disoriented and as experiencing illusions, transitory delusions, and visual hallucinations. Persons may display greatly increased psychomotor activity and impulsive, aggressive behavior. They can be dangerous to others and they may also exhibit suicidal ideation and make suicide attempts. The disorder, usually described as lasting for a few hours, terminates in prolonged sleep, and those affected cannot recall the episodes on awakening. The cause of the condition is unknown, but it is reported to be most common in persons with high levels of anxiety. According to one hypothesis, alcohol causes sufficient disorganization and loss of control to release aggressive impulses. Another suggestion is that brain damage, particularly encephalitic or traumatic damage, predisposes some persons to an intolerance for alcohol and thus to abnormal behavior after they ingest only small amounts. Other predisposing factors may include advancing age, using sedative-hypnotic drugs, and feeling fatigued. A person's behavior while intoxicated tends to be atypical; after one weak drink, a quiet, shy person becomes belligerent and aggressive.

In treating idiosyncratic alcohol intoxication, clinicians must help protect patients from harming themselves and others. Physical restraint may be necessary, but is difficult because of the abrupt onset of the condition. Once a patient has been restrained, injection of an antipsychotic drug, such as haloperidol (Haldol), is useful for controlling assaultiveness. This condition must be differentiated from other causes of abrupt behavioral change, such as complex partial epilepsy. Some persons with the disorder reportedly showed temporal lobe spiking on an EEG after ingesting small amounts of alcohol.

Other Alcohol-Related Neurological Disorders

Only the major neuropsychiatric syndromes associated with alcohol use have been discussed here. The complete list of neurological syndromes is lengthy (Table 16.2–6). Alcoholic pellagra encephalopathy is one diagnosis of potential interest to psychiatrists presented with a patient who appears to have Wernicke–Korsakoff syndrome but who does not respond to thiamine treatment. The symptoms of alcoholic pellagra encephalopathy include confusion, clouding of consciousness, myoclonus, oppositional hypertonias, fatigue, apathy, irritability, anorexia, insomnia, and sometimes delirium. Patients have a niacin (nicotinic acid) deficiency, and the specific treatment is 50 mg of niacin by mouth four times daily or 25 mg parenterally two to three times daily.

Fetal Alcohol Syndrome

Data indicate that women who are pregnant or are breast-feeding should not drink alcohol. Fetal alcohol syndrome, the leading cause of intellectual disability in the United States, occurs when mothers who drink alcohol expose fetuses to alcohol in utero. The alcohol inhibits intrauterine growth and postnatal development. Microcephaly, craniofacial malformations, and limb and heart defects are common in affected infants. Short adult stature and development of a range of adult maladaptive behaviors have also been associated with fetal alcohol syndrome.

Women with alcohol-related disorders have a 35 percent risk of having a child with defects. Although the precise mechanism of the damage to the fetus is unknown, the damage seems to result from exposure in utero to ethanol or to its metabolites; alcohol may also cause hormone imbalances that increase the risk of abnormalities.

PROGNOSIS

Between 10 and 40 percent of alcoholic persons enter some kind of formal treatment program during the course of their alcohol problems. A number of prognostic signs are favorable. First is the absence of preexisting antisocial personality disorder or

Table 16.2–6
Neurological and Medical Complications of Alcohol Use

Alcohol intoxication
- Acute intoxication
- Pathological intoxication (atypical, complicated, unusual)
- Blackouts

Alcohol withdrawal syndromes
- Tremulousness (the shakes or the jitters)
- Alcoholic hallucinosis (horrors)
- Withdrawal seizures (rum fits)
- Delirium tremens (shakes)

Nutritional diseases of the nervous system secondary to alcohol abuse
- Wernicke–Korsakoff syndrome
- Cerebellar degeneration
- Peripheral neuropathy
- Optic neuropathy (tobacco-alcohol amblyopia)
- Pellagra

Alcoholic diseases of uncertain pathogenesis
- Central pontine myelinolysis
- Marchiafava–Bignami disease
- Fetal alcohol syndrome
- Myopathy
- Alcoholic dementia
- Alcoholic cerebral atrophy

Systemic diseases due to alcohol with secondary neurological complications
- Liver disease
- Hepatic encephalopathy
- Acquired (non-Wilsonian) chronic hepatocerebral degeneration
- Gastrointestinal diseases
- Malabsorption syndromes
- Postgastrectomy syndromes
- Possible pancreatic encephalopathy

Cardiovascular diseases
- Cardiomyopathy with potential cardiogenic emboli and cerebrovascular disease
- Arrhythmias and abnormal blood pressure leading to cerebrovascular disease
- Hematological disorders
- Anemia, leukopenia, thrombocytopenia (could possibly lead to hemorrhagic cerebrovascular disease)

Infectious disease, especially meningitis (especially pneumococcal and meningococcal)

Hypothermia and hyperthermia

Hypotension and hypertension

Respiratory depression and associated hypoxia

Toxic encephalopathies, including alcohol and other substances

Electrolyte imbalances leading to acute confusional states and, rarely, local neurological signs and symptoms
- Hypoglycemia
- Hyperglycemia
- Hyponatremia
- Hypercalcemia
- Hypomagnesemia
- Hypophosphatemia

Increased incidence of trauma
- Epidural, subdural, and intracerebral hematoma
- Spinal cord injury
- Posttraumatic seizure disorders
- Compressive neuropathies and brachial plexus injuries (Saturday night palsies)
- Posttraumatic symptomatic hydrocephalus (normal pressure hydrocephalus)
- Muscle crush injuries and compartmental syndromes

From Rubino FA. Neurologic complications of alcoholism. *Psychiatr Clin North Am*. 1992;15:361.

a diagnosis of other substance abuse or dependence. Second, evidence of general life stability with a job, continuing close family contacts, and the absence of severe legal problems also bodes well for the patient. Third, if the patient stays for the full course of the initial rehabilitation (perhaps 2 to 4 weeks), the chances of maintaining abstinence are good. The combination of these three attributes predicts at least a 60 percent chance for 1 or more years of abstinence. Few studies have documented the long-term course, but researchers agree that 1 year of abstinence is associated with a good chance for continued abstinence over an extended period. Alcoholic persons with severe drug problems (especially intravenous drug use or cocaine or amphetamine dependence) and those who are homeless may have only a 10 to 15 percent chance of achieving 1 year of abstinence, however.

Accurately predicting whether any specific person will achieve or maintain abstinence is impossible, but the prognostic factors listed earlier are associated with an increased likelihood of abstinence. The factors reflecting life stability, however, probably explain only 20 percent or less of the course of alcohol use disorders. Many forces that are difficult to measure affect the clinical course significantly; they are likely to include such intangibles as motivational level and the quality of the patient's social support system.

In general, alcoholic persons with preexisting independent major psychiatric disorders—such as antisocial personality disorder, schizophrenia, and bipolar I disorder—are likely to run the course of their independent psychiatric illness. Thus, for example, clinicians must treat the patient with bipolar I disorder who has secondary alcoholism with appropriate psychotherapy and lithium (Eskalith), use relevant psychological and behavioral techniques for the patient with antisocial personality disorder, and offer appropriate antipsychotic medications on a long-term basis to the patient with schizophrenia. The goal is to minimize the symptoms of the independent psychiatric disorder in the hope that greater life stability will be associated with a better prognosis for the patient's alcohol problems.

TREATMENT AND REHABILITATION

Three general steps are involved in treating the alcoholic person after the disorder has been diagnosed: intervention, detoxification, and rehabilitation. These approaches assume that all possible efforts have been made to optimize medical functioning and to address psychiatric emergencies. Thus, for example, an alcoholic person with symptoms of depression sufficiently severe to be suicidal requires inpatient hospitalization for at least several days until the suicidal ideation disappears. Similarly, a person presenting with cardiomyopathy, liver difficulties, or gastrointestinal bleeding first needs adequate treatment of the medical emergency.

The patient with alcohol abuse or dependence must then be brought face-to-face with the reality of the disorder (intervention), be detoxified if needed, and begin rehabilitation. The essentials of these three steps for an alcoholic person with independent psychiatric syndromes closely resemble the approaches used for the primary alcoholic person without independent psychiatric syndromes. In the former case, however, the treatments are applied after the psychiatric disorder has been stabilized to the extent possible.

Intervention

The goal in the intervention step, which has also been called *confrontation,* is to break through feelings of denial and help the patient recognize the adverse consequences likely to occur if the disorder is not treated. Intervention is a process aimed at maximizing the motivation for treatment and continued abstinence.

This step often involves convincing patients that they are responsible for their own actions while reminding them of how alcohol has created significant life impairments. The psychiatrist often finds it useful to take advantage of the person's chief presenting complaint, whether it is insomnia, difficulties with sexual performance, an inability to cope with life stresses, depression, anxiety, or psychotic symptoms. The psychiatrist can then explain how alcohol has either created or contributed to these problems and can reassure the patient that abstinence can be achieved with a minimum of discomfort.

JP, a 47-year-old physician, was confronted regarding his alcohol-related behaviors by his wife and 21-year-old daughter. They told him about his slurred speech on several recent occasions when the daughter called home, as well as a large number of wine bottles in the trash each week. JP's wife complained of the hours he spent alone in his study and his practice of staying up after she went to bed, retiring later with alcohol on his breath. She also related her concern about his consumption of about 10 or 12 drinks at a recent party, with the resulting tendency to isolate himself from the other guests. She then reminded him of his need to pack liquor when they go on trips where alcohol may not be readily available, and the tremor of his hands some mornings after being drunk the night before. The family shared their concern directly with JP at a time when he was not actively intoxicated, emphasizing specific times and events when his impairment with alcohol occurred. They had also made an appointment with the clinician at an alcohol and drug treatment program so that a next step could be established if the intervention was successful. *(Adapted from Marc A. Schuckit, M.D.)*

A physician intervening with a patient can use the same nonjudgmental but persistent approach each time an alcohol-related impairment is identified. It is the persistence rather than exceptional interpersonal skills that usually gets results. A single intervention is rarely sufficient. Most alcoholic persons need a series of reminders of how alcohol contributed to each developing crisis before they seriously consider abstinence as a long-term option.

Family

The family can be of great help in the intervention. Family members must learn not to protect the patient from the problems caused by alcohol; otherwise, the patient may not be able to gather the energy and the motivation necessary to stop drinking. In addition, during the intervention stage, the family can suggest that the patient meet with persons who are recovering from alcoholism, perhaps through AA, and family members can meet with groups, such as Al-Anon, that reach out to family members. Those support groups for families meet many times a week and help family members and friends see that they are not alone in their fears, worry, and feelings of guilt. Participants share coping strategies and help each other find community resources. The groups can be most useful in helping family members rebuild their lives, even if the alcoholic person refuses to seek help.

Detoxification

Most persons with alcohol dependence have relatively mild symptoms when they stop drinking. If the patient is in relatively good health, is adequately nourished, and has a good social support system, the depressant withdrawal syndrome usually resembles a mild case of the flu. Even intense withdrawal syndromes rarely approach the severity of symptoms described by some early textbooks in the field.

The essential first step in detoxification is a thorough physical examination. In the absence of a serious medical disorder or combined drug abuse, severe alcohol withdrawal is unlikely. The second step is to offer rest, adequate nutrition, and multiple vitamins, especially those containing thiamine.

Mild or Moderate Withdrawal. Withdrawal develops because the brain has physically adapted to the presence of a brain depressant and cannot function adequately in the absence of the drug. Giving sufficient brain depressant on the first day to diminish symptoms and then weaning the patient off the drug over the next 5 days offers most patients optimal relief and minimizes the possibility that severe withdrawal will develop. Any depressant—including alcohol, barbiturates, or any of the benzodiazepines—can work, but most clinicians choose a benzodiazepine for its relative safety. Adequate treatment can be given with either short-acting drugs (e.g., lorazepam), or long-acting substances (e.g., chlordiazepoxide and diazepam).

An example of treatment is the administration of 25 mg of chlordiazepoxide by mouth three or four times a day on the first day, with a notation to skip a dose if the patient is asleep or feeling sleepy. An additional one or two 25-mg doses can be given during the first 24 hours if the patient is jittery or shows signs of increasing tremor or autonomic dysfunction. Whatever benzodiazepine dosage is required on the first day can be decreased by 20 percent each subsequent day, with a resulting need for no further medication after 4 or 5 days. When giving a long-acting agent, such as chlordiazepoxide, the clinician must avoid producing excessive sleepiness through overmedication; if the patient is sleepy, the next scheduled dose should be omitted. When taking a short-acting drug, such as lorazepam, the patient must not miss any dose because rapid changes in benzodiazepine concentrations in the blood can precipitate severe withdrawal.

A social model program of detoxification saves money by avoiding medications while using social supports. This less-expensive regimen can be helpful for mild or moderate withdrawal syndromes. Some clinicians have also recommended β-adrenergic receptor antagonists (e.g., propranolol [Inderal]) or α-adrenergic receptor agonists (e.g., clonidine), although these medications do not appear to be superior to the benzodiazepines. Unlike the brain depressants, these other agents do little to decrease the risk of seizures or delirium.

Severe Withdrawal. For the approximately 1 percent of alcoholic patients with extreme autonomic dysfunction, agitation, and confusion—that is, those with alcoholic withdrawal delirium, or DTs—no optimal treatment has yet been developed.

The first step is to ask why such a severe and relatively uncommon withdrawal syndrome has occurred; the answer often relates to a severe concomitant medical problem that needs immediate treatment. The withdrawal symptoms can then be minimized through the use of either benzodiazepines (in which case high doses are sometimes required) or antipsychotic agents, such as haloperidol. Once again, on the first or second day, doses are used to control behavior, and the patient can be weaned off the medication by about the fifth day.

Another 1 percent of patients may have a single grand mal convulsion; the rare person has multiple fits, with the peak incidence on the second day of withdrawal. Such patients require neurological evaluation, but in the absence of evidence of a seizure disorder, they do not benefit from anticonvulsant drugs.

Protracted Withdrawal. Symptoms of anxiety, insomnia, and mild autonomic overactivity are likely to continue for 2 to 6 months after the acute withdrawal has disappeared. Although no pharmacological treatment for this syndrome appears appropriate, it is possible that some of the medications used for the rehabilitation phase, especially acamprosate (Campral), may work by diminishing some of these symptoms. It is important that the clinician warn the patient that some level of sleep problems or feelings of nervousness might remain after acute withdrawal and discuss cognitive and behavioral approaches that might be appropriate to helping the patient feel more comfortable. These protracted withdrawal symptoms may enhance the probability of relapse.

Rehabilitation

For most patients, rehabilitation includes three major components: (1) continued efforts to increase and maintain high levels of motivation for abstinence; (2) work to help the patient readjust to a lifestyle free of alcohol; and (3) relapse prevention. Because these steps are carried out in the context of acute and protracted withdrawal syndromes and life crises, treatment requires repeated presentations of similar materials that remind the patient how important abstinence is and that help the patient develop new day-to-day support systems and coping styles.

No single major life event, traumatic life period, or identifiable psychiatric disorder is known to be a unique cause of alcoholism. In addition, the effects of any causes of alcoholism are likely to have been diluted by the effects of alcohol on the brain and the years of an altered lifestyle, so that the alcoholism has developed a life of its own. This is true even though many alcoholic persons believe that the cause was depression, anxiety, life stress, or pain syndromes. Research, data from records, and resource persons usually reveal that alcohol contributed to the mood disorder, accident, or life stress, not vice versa.

The same general treatment approach is used in inpatient and outpatient settings. Selection of the more expensive and intensive inpatient mode often depends on evidence of additional severe medical or psychiatric syndromes, the absence of appropriate nearby outpatient groups and facilities, and the patient's history of having failed in outpatient care. The treatment process in either setting involves intervention, optimizing physical and psychological functioning, enhancing motivation, reaching out to family, and using the first 2 to 4 weeks of care as an intensive period of help. Those efforts must be followed by at least 3 to 6 months of less frequent outpatient care. Outpatient care uses a combination of individual and group counseling, judicious avoidance of psychotropic medications unless needed for independent disorders, and involvement in such self-help groups as AA.

Counseling. Counseling efforts in the first several months should focus on day-to-day life issues to help patients maintain a high level of motivation for abstinence and to enhance their functioning. Psychotherapy techniques that provoke anxiety or that require deep insights have not been shown to be of benefit during the early months of recovery and, at least theoretically, may actually impair efforts at maintaining abstinence. Thus, this discussion focuses on the efforts likely to characterize the first 3 to 6 months of care.

Counseling or therapy can be carried out in an individual or group setting; few data indicate that either approach is superior. The technique used is not likely to matter greatly and usually boils down to simple day-to-day counseling or almost any behavioral or psychotherapeutic approach focusing on the here and now. To optimize motivation, treatment sessions should explore the consequences of drinking, the likely future course of alcohol-related life problems, and the marked improvement that can be expected with abstinence. Whether in an inpatient or an outpatient setting, individual or group counseling is usually offered a minimum of three times a week for the first 2 to 4 weeks, followed by less intense efforts, perhaps once a week, for the subsequent 3 to 6 months.

Much time in counseling deals with how to build a lifestyle free of alcohol. Discussions cover the need for a sober peer group, a plan for social and recreational events without drinking, and approaches for reestablishing communication with family members and friends.

The third major component, relapse prevention, first identifies situations in which the risk for relapse is high. The counselor must help the patient develop modes of coping to be used when the craving for alcohol increases or when any event or emotional state makes a return to drinking likely. An important part of relapse prevention is reminding the patient about the appropriate attitude toward slips. Short-term experiences with alcohol can never be used as an excuse for returning to regular drinking. The efforts to achieve and maintain a sober lifestyle are not a game in which all benefits are lost with that first sip. Rather, recovery is a process of trial and error; patients use slips that occur to identify high-risk situations and to develop more appropriate coping techniques.

Most treatment efforts recognize the effects that alcoholism has on the significant persons in the patient's life, and an important aspect of recovery involves helping family members and close friends understand alcoholism and realize that rehabilitation is an ongoing process that lasts for 6 to 12 or more months. Couples and family counseling and support groups for relatives and friends help the persons involved to rebuild relationships, to learn how to avoid protecting the patient from the consequences of any drinking in the future, and to be as supportive as possible of the alcoholic patient's recovery program.

Medications. If detoxification has been completed and the patient is not one of the 10 to 15 percent of alcoholic persons who have an independent mood disorder, schizophrenia, or anxiety disorder, little evidence favors prescribing psychotropic medications for the treatment of alcoholism. Lingering levels of anxiety and insomnia as part of a reaction to life stresses and protracted abstinence should be treated with behavior modification approaches and reassurance. Medications for these symptoms (including benzodiazepines) are likely to lose their effectiveness much faster than the insomnia disappears; thus, the patient may increase the dose and have subsequent problems. Similarly, sadness and mood swings can linger at low levels for several months. Controlled clinical trials, however, indicate no benefit in prescribing antidepressant medications or lithium to treat the average alcoholic person who has no independent or long-lasting psychiatric disorder. The mood disorder will clear before the medications can take effect, and patients who resume drinking while on the medications face significant potential dangers. With little or no evidence that the medications are effective, the dangers significantly outweigh any potential benefits from their routine use.

One possible exception to the proscription against the use of medications is the alcohol-sensitizing agent disulfiram. Disulfiram is given in daily doses of 250 mg before the patient is discharged from the intensive first phase of outpatient rehabilitation or from inpatient care. The goal is to place the patient in a condition in which drinking alcohol precipitates an uncomfortable physical reaction, including nausea, vomiting, and a burning sensation in the face and stomach. Few data prove

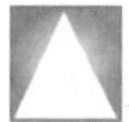

Table 16.2–7
Medications for Treating Alcohol Dependence

	Disulfiram (Antabuse)	Naltrexone (ReVia)	Acamprosate (Campral)
Action	Inhibits intermediate metabolism of alcohol, causing a build-up of acetaldehyde and a reaction of flushing, sweating, nausea, and tachycardia if a patient drinks alcohol	Blocks opioid receptors, resulting in reduced craving and reduced reward in response to drinking	Affects glutamate and GABA neurotransmitter systems, but its alcohol-related action is unclear
Contraindications	Concomitant use of alcohol or alcohol-containing preparations or metronidazole; coronary artery disease; severe myocardial disease	Currently using opioids or in acute opioid withdrawal; anticipated need for opioid analgesics; acute hepatitis or liver failure	Severe renal impairment (CrCl ≤ 30 mL/min)
Precautions	High impulsivity—likely to drink while using it; psychoses (current or history); diabetes mellitus; epilepsy; hepatic dysfunction; hypothyroidism; renal impairment; rubber contact dermatitis	Other hepatic disease; renal impairment; history of suicide attempts. If opioid analgesia is required, larger doses may be required, and respiratory depression may be deeper and more prolonged.	Moderate renal impairment (dose adjustment for CrCl between 30 and 50 mL/min); depression or suicidality
Serious Adverse Reactions	Hepatitis; optic neuritis; peripheral neuropathy; psychotic reactions. Pregnancy Category C.	Will precipitate severe withdrawal if patient is dependent on opioids; hepatoxicity (uncommon at usual doses). Pregnancy Category C.	Anxiety; depression. Rare events include the following: suicide attempt, acute kidney failure, heart failure, mesenteric arterial occlusion, cardiomyopathy, deep thrombophlebitits, and shock. Pregnancy Category C.
Common Side Effects	Metallic after-taste; dermatitis	Nausea; abdominal pain; constipation; dizziness; headache; anxiety; fatigue	Diarrhea; flatulence; nausea; abdominal pain; headache; back pain; infection; flu syndrome; chills; somnolence; decreased libido; amnesia; confusion
Examples of Drug Interactions	Amitryptyline; anticoagulants such as warfarin; diazepam; isoniazid; metronidazole; phenytoin; theophylline; warfarin; any nonprescription drug containing alcohol	Opioid analgesics (blocks action); yohimbine (use with naltrexone increases negative drug effects)	No clinically relevant interactions known
Usual Adult Dosage	*Oral dose:* 250 mg daily (range 125–500 mg) *Before prescribing:* (1) warn that the patient should not take disulfiram for at least 12 hours after drinking and that a disulfiram-alcohol reaction can occur up to 2 weeks after the last dose; and (2) warn about alcohol in the diet (e.g., sauces and vinegars) and in medications and toiletries *Follow up:* Monitor liver function tests periodically	*Oral dose:* 50 mg daily *Before prescribing:* Evaluate for possible current opioid use; consider a urine toxicology screen for opioids, including synthetic opioids. Obtain liver function tests *Follow up:* Monitor liver function tests periodically	*Oral dose:* 666 mg (two 333-mg tablets) three times daily *or,* for patients with moderate renal impairment (CrCl 30–50 mL/min), reduce to 333 mg (one tablet) three times daily *Before prescribing:* Establish abstinence

CrCl, creatinine clearance; GABA, γ-aminobutyric acid.

that disulfiram is more effective than a placebo, however, probably because most persons stop taking the disulfiram when they resume drinking. Many clinicians have stopped routinely prescribing the agent, partly in recognition of the dangers associated with the drug itself: mood swings, rare instances of psychosis, the possibility of increased peripheral neuropathies, the relatively rare occurrence of other significant neuropathies, and potentially fatal hepatitis. Moreover, patients with preexisting heart disease, cerebral thrombosis, diabetes, and a number of other conditions cannot be given disulfiram because an alcohol reaction to the disulfiram could be fatal.

Two additional promising pharmacological interventions have recently been studied. The first involves the opioid antagonist naltrexone (ReVia), which at least theoretically is believed possibly to decrease the craving for alcohol or blunt the rewarding effects of drinking. In any event, two relatively small (approximately 90 patients on the active drug across the studies) and short-term (3 months of active treatment) investigations using 50 mg per day of this drug had potentially promising results. Evaluating the full impact of this medication, however, will require longer-term studies of relatively large groups of more diverse patients.

The second medication of interest, acamprosate (Campral), has been tested in more than 5,000 alcohol-dependent patients in Europe. This drug is not yet available in the United States. Used in dosages of approximately 2,000 mg per day, this medication was associated with approximately 10 to 20 percent more positive outcomes than placebo when used in the context of the usual psychological and behavioral treatment regimens for alcoholism. The mechanism of action of acamprosate is not known, but it may act directly or indirectly at GABA receptors or at NMDA sites, the effects of which alter the development of tolerance or physical dependence on alcohol. A summary of medications used for alcohol dependence is given in Table 16.2–7.

Another medication with potential promise in the treatment of alcoholism is the nonbenzodiazepine antianxiety drug buspirone (BuSpar), although the effect of this drug on alcohol rehabilitation is inconsistent between studies. No evidence exists that antidepressant medications, such as the selective serotonin reuptake inhibitors (SSRIs), lithium, or antipsychotic medications, are significantly effective in the treatment of alcoholism.

Alcoholics Anonymous. Clinicians must recognize the potential importance of self-help groups such as AA. Members of AA have help available 24 hours a day, associate with a sober peer group, learn that it is possible to participate in social functions without drinking, and are given a model of recovery by observing the accomplishments of sober members of the group.

Learning about AA usually begins during inpatient or outpatient rehabilitation. The clinician can play a major role in helping patients understand the differences between specific groups. Some are composed only of men or women, and others are mixed; some meetings are composed mostly of blue collar men and women, whereas others are mostly for professionals; some groups place great emphasis on religion, and others are eclectic. Patients with coexisting psychiatric disorders may need some additional education about AA. The clinician should remind them that some members of AA may not understand their special need for medications and should arm the patients with ways of coping when group members inappropriately suggest that the required medications be stopped. Although difficult to evaluate using double-blind controls, most studies indicate that participation in AA is associated with improved outcomes, and incorporation into treatment programs saves money.

▲ 16.3 Caffeine-Related Disorders

Caffeine is the most widely consumed psychoactive substance in the world. Caffeine is found in more than 60 species of plants and belongs to the methylxanthine class of alkaloids, which also includes theobromine (found in chocolate) and theophylline (often used in the treatment of asthma). In the United States, 87 percent of children and adults consume foods and beverages containing caffeine. Caffeine affects various neurobiological and physiological systems and produces significant psychological effects. Its habitual use can result in psychiatric symptoms and disorders. In rare cases, death related to caffeine overdose has occurred. Its widely accepted integration into daily customs can lead to an underestimation of the role that caffeine may play in one's daily life and can make the recognition of caffeine-associated disorders particularly challenging. Hence, it is important for the clinician to be familiar with caffeine, its effects, and problems that can be associated with its use.

Caffeine use is associated with five disorders: caffeine use disorder, caffeine intoxication, caffeine withdrawal, caffeine-induced anxiety disorder, and caffeine-induced sleep disorder.

EPIDEMIOLOGY

Caffeine is contained in drinks, foods, prescription medicines, and over-the-counter medicines (Table 16.3–1). An adult in the United States consumes about 200 mg of caffeine per day on average, although 20 to 30 percent of all adults consume more than 500 mg per day. The per capita use of coffee in the United States is 10.2 pounds per year. A cup of coffee generally contains 100 to 150 mg of caffeine; tea contains about one-third as much. Many over-the-counter medications contain one-third to one-half as much caffeine as a cup of coffee, and some migraine medications and over-the-counter stimulants contain more caffeine than a cup of coffee. Cocoa, chocolate, and soft drinks contain significant amounts of caffeine, enough to cause some symptoms of caffeine intoxication in small children when they ingest a candy bar and a 12-ounce cola drink.

Caffeine consumption also varies by age. The average daily caffeine consumption of caffeine consumers of all ages is 2.79 mg/kg of body weight in the United States. A substantial amount of caffeine is consumed even by young children (i.e., more than 1 mg/kg for children between the ages of 1 and 5 years). Worldwide, estimates place the average daily per capita caffeine consumption at about 70 mg. Up to 85 percent of adults consume caffeine in any given year.

COMORBIDITY

Persons with caffeine-related disorders are more likely to have additional substance-related disorders than are those without diagnoses of caffeine-related disorders. About two-thirds of

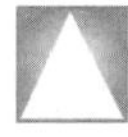

Table 16.3–1
Common Sources of Caffeine and Representative Decaffeinated Products

Source	Caffeine per Unit (mg)
Beverages and foods (5–6 oz)	
Fresh drip coffee, brewed coffee	90–140
Instant coffee	66–100
Tea (leaf or bagged)	30–100
Cocoa	5–50
Decaffeinated coffee	2–4
Chocolate bar or ounce of baking chocolate	25–35
Soft drinks (8–12 oz)	
Pepsi, Coke, Tab, Royal Crown Cola, Dr. Pepper, Mountain Dew	25–50
Canada Dry Ginger Ale, Caffeine-Free Coke, Caffeine-Free Pepsi, 7-Up, Sprite, Squirt, Caffeine-Free Tab	0
Prescription medications (1 tablet or capsule)	
Cafergot, Migralam	100
Anoquan, Aspir-code, BAC, Darvon, Fiorinal	32–50
Over-the-counter analgesics and cold preparations (1 tablet or capsule)	
Excedrin	60
Aspirin compound, Anacin, B-C powder, Capron, Cope, Dolor, Midol, Nilain, Norgesic, PAC, Trigesic, Vanquish	~30
Advil, aspirin, Empirin, Midol 200, Nuprin, Pamprin	0
Over-the-counter stimulants and appetite suppressants (1 tablet or capsule)	
Caffin-TD, Caffedrine	250
Vivarin, Ver	200
Quick-Pep	140–150
Amostant, Anorexin, Appedrine, Nodoz, Wakoz	100

Adapted from table by Jerome H. Jaffe, M.D.

those who consume large amounts of caffeine daily also use sedative and hypnotic drugs.

ETIOLOGY

After exposure to caffeine, continued caffeine consumption can be influenced by several different factors, such as the pharmacological effects of caffeine, caffeine's reinforcing effects, genetic predispositions to caffeine use, and personal attributes of the consumer.

Neuropharmacology

Caffeine, a methylxanthine, is more potent than another commonly used methylxanthine, theophylline (Primatene). The half-life of caffeine in the human body is 3 to 10 hours, and the time of peak concentration is 30 to 60 minutes. Caffeine readily crosses the blood–brain barrier. Caffeine acts primarily as an antagonist of the adenosine receptors. Adenosine receptors activate an inhibitory G protein (Gi) and, thus, inhibit the formation of the second-messenger cyclic adenosine monophosphate (cAMP). Caffeine intake, therefore, results in an increase in intraneuronal cAMP concentrations in neurons with adenosine receptors. Three cups of coffee are estimated to deliver so much caffeine to the brain that about 50 percent of the adenosine receptors are occupied by caffeine. Several experiments indicate that caffeine, especially at high doses or concentrations, can affect dopamine and noradrenergic neurons. Specifically, dopamine activity may be enhanced by caffeine, a hypothesis that could explain clinical reports associating caffeine intake with an exacerbation of psychotic symptoms in patients with schizophrenia. Activation of noradrenergic neurons has been hypothesized to be involved in the mediation of some symptoms of caffeine withdrawal.

Subjective Effects, Benefits, and Reinforcement

Single low to moderate doses of caffeine (i.e., 20 to 200 mg) can produce a profile of subjective effects in humans that is generally identified as pleasurable. Thus, studies have shown that such doses of caffeine result in increased ratings on measures such as well-being, energy and concentration, and motivation to work. Coffee contains hundreds of biologically active compounds in addition to caffeine. For example, one compound contained in coffee called chlorogenic acid has antioxidant and anti-inflammatory properties. Such compounds have been shown to improve glucose metabolism, insulin sensitivity, and decrease insulin resistance. Coffee may also reduce the risk of ischemic stroke and be protective against neurodegenerative disorders such as Alzheimer's and Parkinson's disease. Other purported benefits include improved asthma control, improved liver function in those with chronic liver disease and increased hair growth in balding men and women. Many of these effects on the benefits of coffee are anecdotal with very few controlled studies, however potent doses of caffeine in the range of 300 to 800 mg (the equivalent of several cups of brewed coffee ingested at once) produce effects that are often rated as being unpleasant, such as anxiety and nervousness. Although animal studies have generally found it difficult to demonstrate that caffeine functions as a reinforcer, well-controlled studies in humans have shown that people choose caffeine over placebo when given the choice under controlled experimental conditions. In habitual users, the reinforcing effects of caffeine are potentiated by the ability to suppress low-grade withdrawal symptoms after overnight abstinence. Thus, the profile of caffeine's subjective effects, benefits, and its ability to function as a reinforcer contribute to the regular use of caffeine.

Genetics and Caffeine Use

Some genetic predisposition may exist to continued coffee use after exposure to coffee. Investigations comparing coffee or caffeine use in monozygotic and dizygotic twins have shown higher concordance rates for monozygotic twins for total caffeine consumption, heavy use, caffeine tolerance, caffeine withdrawal, and caffeine intoxication, with heritabilities ranging between 35 and 77 percent. Multivariate structural equation modeling of caffeine use, cigarette smoking, and alcohol use suggests that a common genetic factor—polysubstance use—underlies use of these three substances.

Age, Sex, and Race

The relationship between long-term chronic caffeine use and demographical features, such as age, sex, and race, has not been widely studied. Some evidence suggest that middle-aged people may use more caffeine, although caffeine use in adolescents is not uncommon. No known evidence indicates that caffeine use differs between men and women, and no data specifically address caffeine use for different races. Some evidence suggests that, for both children and adults in the United States, whites consume more caffeine than blacks.

Special Populations

Cigarette smokers consume more caffeine than nonsmokers. This observation may reflect a common genetic vulnerability to caffeine use and cigarette smoking. It may also be related to increased rates of caffeine elimination in cigarette smokers. Preclinical and clinical studies indicate that regular caffeine use can potentiate the reinforcing effects of nicotine.

Heavy use and clinical dependence on alcohol is associated with heavy use and clinical dependence on caffeine as well. Individuals with anxiety disorders tend to report lower levels of caffeine use, although one study showed that a greater proportion of heavy caffeine consumers also use benzodiazepines. Several studies have also shown high daily amounts of caffeine use in psychiatric in-patients. For example, several studies have found that such patients consume the equivalent of an average of five or more cups of brewed coffee each day. Finally, high daily caffeine consumption has also been noted in prisoners.

Personality

Although attempts have been made to link preferential use of caffeine to particular personality types, results from these studies do not suggest that any particular personality type is especially linked to caffeine use.

Effects on Cerebral Blood Flow

Most studies have found that caffeine results in global cerebral vasoconstriction, with a resultant decrease in cerebral blood flow (CBF), although this effect may not occur in persons over 65 years of age. According to one recent study, tolerance does not develop to these vasoconstrictive effects, and the CBF shows a rebound increase after withdrawal from caffeine. Some clinicians believe that caffeine use can cause a similar constriction in the coronary arteries and produce angina in the absence of atherosclerosis.

DIAGNOSIS

The diagnosis of caffeine intoxication or other caffeine-related disorders depends primarily on a comprehensive history of a patient's intake of caffeine-containing products. The history should cover whether a patient has experienced any symptoms of caffeine withdrawal during periods when caffeine consumption was either stopped or severely reduced. The differential diagnosis for caffeine-related disorders should include the following psychiatric diagnoses: generalized anxiety disorder, panic disorder with or without agoraphobia, bipolar II disorder, ADHD, and sleep disorders. The differential diagnosis should include the abuse of caffeine-containing over-the-counter medications, anabolic steroids, and other stimulants, such as amphetamines and cocaine. A urine sample may be needed to screen for these substances. The differential diagnosis should also include hyperthyroidism and pheochromocytoma.

Caffeine Intoxication

The fifth edition of the *Diagnostic and Statistical Manual of Mental Disorders* (DSM-5) diagnostic criteria for caffeine intoxication includes the recent consumption of caffeine, usually in excess of 250 mg. The annual incidence of caffeine intoxication is an estimated 10 percent, although some clinicians and investigators suspect that the actual incidence is much higher. The common symptoms associated with caffeine intoxication include anxiety, psychomotor agitation, restlessness, irritability, and psychophysiological complaints such as muscle twitching, flushed face, nausea, diuresis, gastrointestinal distress, excessive perspiration, tingling in the fingers and toes, and insomnia. Consumption of more than 1 g of caffeine can produce rambling speech, confused thinking, cardiac arrhythmias, inexhaustibleness, marked agitation, tinnitus, and mild visual hallucinations (light flashes). Consumption of more than 10 g of caffeine can cause generalized tonic–clonic seizures, respiratory failure, and death.

> Ms. B, a 30-year-old, went for consultation due to "anxiety attacks." The attacks occurred mid- to late afternoon, when Ms. B became restless, nervous, and easily excited and sometimes was noticed to be flushed, sweating, and, according to coworkers, "talking a mile a minute." In response to questioning, Ms. B admitted to consuming six to seven cups of coffee each day before the time the attacks usually occurred.

Caffeine Withdrawal

The appearance of withdrawal symptoms reflects the tolerance and physiological dependence that develop with continued caffeine use. Several epidemiological studies have reported symptoms of caffeine withdrawal in 50 to 75 percent of all caffeine users studied. The most common symptoms are headache and fatigue; other symptoms include anxiety, irritability, mild depressive symptoms, impaired psychomotor performance, nausea, vomiting, craving for caffeine, and muscle pain and stiffness. The number and severity of the withdrawal symptoms are correlated with the amount of caffeine ingested and the abruptness of the withdrawal. Caffeine withdrawal symptoms have their onset 12 to 24 hours after the last dose; the symptoms peak in 24 to 48 hours and resolve within 1 week.

The induction of caffeine withdrawal can sometimes be iatrogenic. Physicians often ask their patients to discontinue caffeine intake before certain medical procedures, such as endoscopy, colonoscopy, and cardiac catheterization. In addition, physicians often recommend that patients with anxiety symptoms, cardiac arrhythmias, esophagitis, hiatal hernias, fibrocystic disease of the breast, and insomnia to stop caffeine intake. Some persons simply decide that it would be good for them to stop using caffeine-containing products. In all these situations, caffeine users should taper the use of caffeine-containing products over a 7- to 14-day period rather than stop abruptly.

Mr. F was a 43-year-old attorney who was brought for a psychiatric consultation by his wife. Mr. F had been complaining of fatigue, loss of motivation, sleepiness, headache, nausea, and difficulty concentrating. His symptoms occurred mostly over the weekends. He withdrew from weekend social activities due to his symptoms, which worried Mrs. F because he seems fine during the week. Mr. F is in good health with no recent history of medical disorders.

Mr. F worked in a very busy law practice, many times working 60-hour weeks, and barely sees his family during the week. At work he is often anxious, restless, and constantly busy. He worries about his job so much that he has difficulty sleeping on weeknights. He denies any marital or family problems, other than those caused by his not wanting to do anything over the weekend.

At work, Mr. F regularly consumes approximately 4 to 5 cups of coffee per day. He cut out coffee on the weekends because he felt that it may be contributing to his anxiety and sleeplessness.

Caffeine-Induced Anxiety Disorder

The anxiety related to caffeine use can resemble that of generalized anxiety disorder. Patients with the disorder may be perceived as "wired," overly talkative, and irritable; they may complain of not sleeping well and of having energy to burn. Caffeine can induce and exacerbate panic attacks in persons with a panic disorder, and although a causative association between caffeine and a panic disorder has not yet been demonstrated, patients with panic disorder should avoid caffeine.

Mr. B was a 28-year-old single African American male graduate student who was in good health and had no history of previous psychiatric evaluation or treatment. He took no medications, did not smoke or consume alcohol, and had no current or past history of illicit drug use.

His chief complaint was that he had begun feeling mounting "anxiety" when working in the laboratory where he was pursuing his graduate studies. His work had been progressive well, he felt his relationship with his advisor was good and supportive, and he could not identify any problems with staff or peers that might explain his anxiety. He had been working long hours, but found the work interesting and had recently had his first paper accepted for publication.

Despite these successes, he reported feeling a "crescendoing anxiety" as his day would progress. He noted that by the afternoon he would be experiencing palpitations, bursts of his heart racing, tremors in his hands, and an overall feeling of "being on the edge." He also noted a nervous energy in the afternoons. These experiences were occurring daily and seemed confined to the laboratory (although he admitted he was in the laboratory every day of the week).

When reviewing Mr. B's caffeine intake, it was found that he was consuming excessive amounts of coffee. Staff made a large urn of caffeinated coffee each morning, and Mr. B routinely started with a large mug of coffee. Over the course of the morning he would consume three to four mugs of coffee (the equivalent of about six or eight 6-oz cups of coffee), and continued this level of use throughout the afternoon. He occasionally had a single can of a caffeinated soft drink, and used no other forms of caffeine on a regular basis. Mr. B estimated that he drank a total of six to eight or more mugs of coffee per day (which was estimated to be at least 1,200 mg of caffeine per day). Once pointed out to him, he realized that this level of caffeine consumption was considerably higher than at any other time in his life. He admitted he liked the taste of coffee and felt a burst of energy in the morning when he drank coffee that helped him start his day.

Mr. B and his physician developed a plan to decrease his caffeine use by tapering off caffeine. Mr. B was successful in decreasing his caffeine use and had good resolution of his anxiety symptoms once his daily caffeine use had markedly decreased. *(Courtesy of Laura M. Juliano, Ph.D. and Roland R. Griffiths, Ph.D.)*

Caffeine-Induced Sleep Disorder

Caffeine is associated with delay in falling asleep, inability to remain asleep, and early morning awakening.

Caffeine Use Disorder

The DSM has typically excluded caffeine from its diagnostic schema for substance dependence; however it has been included as a research diagnosis within DSM-5 to encourage further study. Proposed diagnostic criteria for caffeine use disorder include failed efforts to reduce or control use, larger amounts consumed over time, experiencing withdrawal symptoms that lead to cravings, and consumption of caffeine for in order to perform social or occupational obligations. Three or more of these features within a 12 month period may be diagnostic of a disorder. No studies have examined the course and prognosis for patients with a diagnosis of caffeine use disorder. Given the wide prevalence and social acceptability of caffeine use, there is an obvious need for diagnostic threshold higher than that used for the other substance use disorders. It is important to examine cases that have sufficient clinical importance to be labeled a mental disorder so as not to pathologize normal, socially acceptable patterns of use.

Ms. G was a 35-year-old married, white homemaker with three children, aged 8, 6, and 2. She took no prescription medications, took a multivitamin and vitamins C and E on a daily basis, did not smoke, and had no history of psychiatric problems. She drank moderate amounts of alcohol on the weekends, had smoked marijuana in college but had not used it since, and had no other history of illicit drug use.

She had started consuming caffeinated beverages while in college, and her current beverage of choice was caffeinated diet cola. Ms. G had her first soft drink early in the morning, shortly after getting out of bed, and she jokingly called it her "morning hit." She spaced out her bottles of soft drinks over the course of the day, with her last bottle at dinnertime. She typically drank four to five 20-oz bottles of caffeinated diet cola each day.

She and her husband had argued about her caffeinated soft drink use in the past, and her husband had believed she should not drink caffeinated soft drinks while pregnant. However, she had continued to do so during each of her pregnancies. Despite a desire to stop drinking caffeinated soft drinks, she was unable to do so. She described having a strong desire to drink caffeinated soft drinks, and if she resisted this desire, she found that she could not think of anything else. She drank caffeinated soft drinks in her car, which had a manual transmission, and noted that she fumbled while shifting and holding the soft drink and spilled it in the car. She also noted that her teeth had become yellowed, and she suspected this was related to her tendency to swish soft drink in her mouth before swallowing it. When asked to describe a time when she stopped using soft drinks, she reported that she had run out of it on the day one of her children was to have a birthday party, and she did not have time to leave her home to buy more. In the early afternoon of that day, a few hours before the scheduled start of the party, she felt extreme lethargy, a severe headache, irritability, and craving for a soft drink. She called her husband and told him she planned to cancel the party. She then went to the grocery store to buy soft drinks, and after drinking two bottles, she felt well enough to host the party.

Although initially expressing interest in decreasing or stopping her caffeinated soft drink use, Ms. G did not attend scheduled follow-up appointments after her first evaluation. When finally contacted at home, she reported she had only sought help initially at her husband's request, and she had decided to try to cut down on her caffeine use on her own. *(Courtesy of Eric Stain, M.D.)*

Caffeine-Related Disorder Not Elsewhere Classified

This category is used for caffeine-related disorders that do not meet the criteria for caffeine use disorder, caffeine intoxication, caffeine withdrawal, caffeine-induced anxiety disorder, or caffeine-induced sleep disorder.

CLINICAL FEATURES

Signs and Symptoms

After the ingestion of 50 to 100 mg of caffeine, common symptoms include increased alertness, a mild sense of well-being, and a sense of improved verbal and motor performance. Caffeine ingestion is also associated with diuresis, cardiac muscle stimulation, increased intestinal peristalsis, increased gastric acid secretion, and (usually mildly) increased blood pressure.

Caffeine Use and Nonpsychiatric Illnesses

Despite numerous studies examining the relationship between caffeine use and physical illness, significant health risk from nonreversible pathological consequences of caffeine use, such as cancer, heart disease, and human reproduction, has not been conclusively demonstrated. Nonetheless, caffeine use is often considered to be contraindicated for various conditions, including generalized anxiety disorder, panic disorder, primary insomnia, gastroesophageal reflux, and pregnancy. In addition, the modest ability of caffeine to increase blood pressure and the documented cholesterol-elevating compounds of unfiltered coffee have raised the issue of the relationship of caffeine and coffee use to cardiovascular disease. Finally, there may be a mild association between higher daily caffeine use in women and delayed conception and slightly lower birth weight. Studies, however, have not found such associations, and effects, when found, are usually with relatively high daily dosages of caffeine (e.g., the equivalent of five cups of brewed coffee per day). For a woman who is considering pregnancy, especially if there is some difficulty in conceiving, it may be useful to counsel the elimination of caffeine use. Similarly, for a woman who becomes pregnant and has moderate to high daily caffeine consumption, a discussion about decreasing her daily caffeine use may be warranted.

Death from Caffeine Overdose

Caffeine overdose can cause death in rare cases. Fatal intoxication (sometimes used as a method of suicide) from ingestion of large doses of caffeine has been reported. In the acute phase, toxic effects cause serious gastric irritation that leads to vomiting and abdominal pain. Significant central nervous system effects including agitation, altered consciousness, rigidity and seizures may also occur. Cardiovascular effects may result in death due to increased circulation of catecholamines leading to cardiac arrhythmia, most often ventricular fibrillation. Oral ingestion of caffeine tablets or other caffeine medications including pure caffeine powder are the most common forms of ingestion that lead to overdose. Toxic levels of caffeine are unlikely through ingestion of caffeinated beverages, as the acute GI upset causes vomiting preventing toxic accumulation. There are no restrictions on the purchase of large quantities of pure caffeine and warning labels about the risk of fatal overdose are lacking. However, in September of 2015, the FDA issued warning to producers of pure powdered caffeine to add warning labels and the amounts of caffeine contained in products sold to consumers.

TREATMENT

Analgesics, such as aspirin, almost always can control the headaches and muscle aches that may accompany caffeine withdrawal. Rarely do patients require benzodiazepines to relieve withdrawal symptoms. If benzodiazepines are used for this purpose, they should be used in small dosages for a brief time, about 7 to 10 days at the longest.

The first step in reducing or eliminating caffeine use is to have patients determine their daily consumption of caffeine. This can best be accomplished by having the patient keep a daily food diary. The patient must recognize all sources of caffeine in the diet, including forms of caffeine (e.g., beverages, medications), and accurately record the amount consumed. After several days of keeping such a diary, the clinician can meet with the patient, review the diary, and determine the average daily caffeine dose in milligrams.

The patient and clinician should then decide on a fading schedule for caffeine consumption. Such a schedule could involve a decrease in increments of 10 percent every few days. Because caffeine is typically consumed in beverage form, the patient can use a substitution procedure in which a decaffeinated beverage is gradually used in place of the caffeinated beverage. The diary should be maintained during this time, so that the patient's progress can be monitored. The fading should be individualized for each patient, so that the rate of decrease in caffeine consumption minimizes withdrawal symptoms. The patient should probably avoid stopping all caffeine use abruptly, because withdrawal symptoms are likely to develop with sudden discontinuation of all caffeine use.

▲ 16.4 Gambling Disorder

Gambling disorder is characterized by persistent and recurrent maladaptive gambling that causes economic problems and significant disturbances in personal, social, or occupational functioning. Aspects of the maladaptive behavior include (1) a preoccupation with gambling; (2) the need to gamble with increasing amounts of money to achieve the desired excitement; (3) repeated unsuccessful efforts to control, cut back, or stop gambling; (4) gambling as a way to escape from problems; (5) gambling to recoup losses; (6) lying to conceal the extent of the involvement with gambling; (7) the commission of illegal acts to finance gambling; (8) jeopardizing or losing personal and vocational relationships because of gambling; and (9) a reliance on others for money to pay off debts.

Previous editions of the *Diagnostic and Statistical Manual of Mental Disorders* (DSM) include pathological gambling disorder in the impulse-control disorder category because of patient's preoccupation or compulsion to gamble. However, the criteria for the disorder are structured more like a substance-related or addiction disorder than an impulse-control disorder, with the need to gamble with increased amounts of money to achieve desired excitement (tolerance) and feelings of irritability and restlessness when attempting to reduce or stop gambling (withdrawal). Substance use is often a common comorbidity with gambling. Thus, in the fifth edition of the DSM (DSM-5), gambling disorder is included in the section on substance use and addictive disorders and is diagnosed as a non–substance-related disorder.

Table 16.4–1
Lifetime Prevalence of Gambling Types

Type of Gambling	Prevalence (%)
A. Sports betting	
Office sports pool	44.3
Sports with bookie or parlay cards	5.8
Betting on horse/dog races/dog or cock fights	25.0
Gambling at a casino	44.7
B. Other types of gambling that involve some aspect of mental or physical skill	
Games involving mental skill (e.g., cards)	35.8
Games involving physical skill (e.g., pool)	22.7
Speculating on high-risk investments	8.4
Internet gambling	1.0
C. Types of gambling that largely involve chance	
Playing lotto/numbers	62.2
Gambling machines (e.g., video poker)	26.1
Slot machines/bingo/pull-tabs	48.9

Adapted from Kessler RC, Hwang I, LaBrie R, Petuhova M, Sampson NA, Winters KC, Shaffer HJ. DSM-IV pathological gambling in the National Comorbidity Survey Replication Psychological Med. 2008;38:1355.

EPIDEMIOLOGY

Although comprehensive worldwide statistics have yet to be compiled, excellent local studies all point to a 3 to 5 percent rate of problem gamblers in the general population and an approximate 1 percent rate of individuals meeting the requirements for gambling disorder. Problem gambling is more common in men and young adults than in women and older adults; however, escalation has been noted in the poor, notably poor minorities; adolescents; elderly retirees; and women. One of three pathological gamblers is now female: it has been suggested that women are gambling more because of an increased presence in the workplace that provides them with more cash. These groups are still underserved with regard to research and treatment. The prevalence of gambling disorder in individuals who have a substance use disorder is higher, with various surveys showing rates of 10 to 18 percent of patients with substance abuse being pathological gamblers.

As every type of gambling has become increasingly accessible over the last few decades, the rate of normal and pathological gambling has risen spectacularly, especially in locales with legalized gambling. The most popular types of gambling are numbers/lotto (62.2 percent), slot machines or bingo (48.9 percent), gambling at a casino (44.7 percent), and office sports pools (44.3 percent) (Table 16.4–1). The least popular are betting on sports with a bookie or parlay card, internet gambling, and speculating on high-risk investments.

Family histories of pathological gamblers show an increased rate of substance abuse (particularly alcoholism) and depressive disorders. A parent or influential relative of the patient often has been a problem or pathological gambler. The family circle is likely to be competitively and materialistically oriented, evincing intense admiration for money and associated symbols of success. In this respect, compulsive gambling has been called the dark side of the American dream.

COMORBIDITY

Significant comorbidity occurs between pathological gambling and mood disorders (especially, major depression and bipolarity) and other substance use and addictive disorders (notably, alcohol and stimulant abuse and caffeine and tobacco dependence). Comorbidity also exists with ADHD (particularly in childhood), various personality disorders (notably, narcissistic, antisocial, and borderline personality disorders), and disruptive, impulse control, and conduct disorders. Although many pathological gamblers have obsessive personality traits, full-blown obsessive-compulsive disorder (OCD) is uncommon in this group.

ETIOLOGY

Psychosocial Factors

Several factors may predispose persons to develop the disorder: loss of a parent by death, separation, divorce, or desertion before a child is 15 years of age; inappropriate parental discipline (absence, inconsistency, or harshness); exposure to, and availability of, gambling activities for adolescents; a family emphasis on material and financial symbols; and a lack of family emphasis on saving, planning, and budgeting.

Psychoanalytic theory has focused on a number of core character difficulties. Sigmund Freud suggested that compulsive gamblers have an unconscious desire to lose, and gamble to relieve unconscious feelings of guilt. Another suggestion is that the gamblers are narcissists, whose grandiose and omnipotent fantasies lead them to believe they can control events and even predict their outcome. Learning theorists view uncontrolled gambling as resulting from erroneous perceptions about control of impulses.

Biological Factors

Several studies have suggested that gamblers' risk-taking behavior may have an underlying neurobiological cause. These theories have centered on both serotonergic and noradrenergic receptor systems. Male pathological gamblers may have subnormal 3-methoxy-4-hydroxyphenyl glycol (MHPG) concentrations in plasma, increased MHPG concentrations in the CSF, and increased urinary output of norepinephrine. Evidence also implicates serotonergic regulatory dysfunction in the pathological gambler. Chronic gamblers have low platelet monoamine oxidase (MAO) activity, a marker of serotonin activity, also linked to difficulties with inhibition. Further studies are needed to confirm these findings.

DIAGNOSIS AND CLINICAL FEATURES

In addition to the features already described, pathological gamblers often appear overconfident, somewhat abrasive, energetic, and free spending. They often show obvious signs of personal stress, anxiety, and depression. They commonly have the attitude that money is both the cause of, and the solution to all their problems. As their gambling increases, they are usually forced to lie to obtain money and to continue gambling while hiding the extent of their gambling. They make no serious attempt to budget or save money. When their borrowing resources are strained, they are likely to engage in antisocial behavior to obtain money for gambling. Their criminal behavior is typically nonviolent, such as forgery, embezzlement, or fraud, and they consciously intend to return or repay the money. Complications include alienation from family members and acquaintances, the loss of life accomplishments, suicide attempts, and association with fringe and illegal groups. Arrest for nonviolent crimes may lead to imprisonment.

Gerry was a 35-year-old former auto dealership owner. Two of his uncles were compulsive gamblers, and his paternal grandfather was hospitalized with major depressive illness. He played poker and had been a racecourse habitué since the age of 15 years. He had dropped out of college after a few months and become a car sales representative. Soon he was promoted to showroom manager and then went out on his own. By age 32 years, he was a multimillionaire owner of a dealership chain, happily married with two children.

Gerry continued to gamble frequently. He was a successful weekend sports bettor, as well as a consistent winner at weekly gin rummy and poker games and occasional jaunts to Las Vegas and Atlantic City.

In the context of his wife giving birth to a stillborn child, Gerry started going to casinos more often, gradually increasing the size of bets at blackjack and craps. His sport wagers also escalated. His games at home gradually became boring—"there was zilch action." He began frequenting an illegal local poker parlor that featured high-stake action.

Over several years, Gerry slipped into a typical gambling spiral. He accumulated several million dollars in debts and lied to family and colleagues about his whereabouts. He raided business and personal accounts, including his children's college funds, maxed out credit cards, and borrowed from loan sharks at exorbitant rates. He grew profoundly depressed and seriously thought of killing himself in a car crash so that his insurance would "take care of my family after I am gone."

Gerry's dire situation was unmasked when his Porsche was repossessed one Sunday morning. Initially his wife threatened to divorce him. However, a wealthy relative intervened and bailed him out. He swore never to gamble again, entered Gamblers Anonymous, and within 2 months resumed his frantic chasing.

Over the next decade, Gerry underwent four more episodes of recovery and relapse. His wife divorced him, he lost his dealerships, and had to declare bankruptcy. Gerry finally enrolled in a pilot dual-diagnostic recovery program, where he was diagnosed with atypical bipolar disorder. His treatment included Gamblers Anonymous meetings, individual and family counseling, and pharmacotherapy with bupropion (Wellbutrin) and lamotrigine (Lamictal).

Gerry eventually reconciled with his wife and family. He returned to selling cars, started living modestly, and continued to attend Gamblers Anonymous meetings regularly. However, he declared emphatically that he always considers himself always one step away from becoming a "degenerate gambler" again. *(Courtesy of Harvey Roy Greenberg, M.D.)*

PSYCHOLOGICAL TESTING AND LABORATORY EXAMINATION

Male patients with gambling disorders have shown abnormalities in platelet MAO activity. Patients with pathological gambling often display high levels of impulsivity on neuropsychological tests. German studies have demonstrated increased cortisol levels in the saliva of gamblers while they gamble, which can account for the euphoria that occurs during the experience and its addictive potential.

DIFFERENTIAL DIAGNOSIS

Social gambling is distinguished from pathological gambling in that the former occurs with friends, on special occasions, and with predetermined acceptable and tolerable losses. Gambling that is symptomatic of a manic episode can usually be distinguished from pathological gambling by the history of a marked mood change and the loss of judgment preceding the gambling.

Manic-like mood changes are common in pathological gambling, but they always follow winning and are usually succeeded by depressive episodes because of subsequent losses. Persons with antisocial personality disorder may have problems with gambling. When both disorders are present, both should be diagnosed.

COURSE AND PROGNOSIS

Pathological gambling usually begins in adolescence for men and late in life for women. The disorder waxes and wanes and tends to be chronic. Four phases are seen in pathological gambling:

1. The winning phase, ending with a big win, equal to about a year's salary, which hooks patients. Women usually do not have a big win, but use gambling as an escape from problems.

2. The progressive-loss phase, in which patients structure their lives around gambling and then move from being excellent gamblers to being stupid ones who take considerable risks, cash in securities, borrow money, miss work, and lose jobs.
3. The desperate phase, with patients frenziedly gambling with large amounts of money, not paying debts, becoming involved with loan sharks, writing bad checks, and possibly embezzling.
4. The hopeless stage of accepting that losses can never be made up, but the gambling continues because of the associated arousal or excitement. The disorder may take up to 15 years to reach the last phase, but then, within a year or two, patients have totally deteriorated.

TREATMENT

Gamblers seldom come forward voluntarily to be treated. Legal difficulties, family pressures, or other psychiatric complaints bring gamblers to treatment. Gamblers Anonymous (GA) was founded in Los Angeles in 1957 and modeled on Alcoholics Anonymous (AA) (Table 16.4–2). It is accessible, at least in large cities, and is an effective treatment for gambling in some patients. GA is a method of inspirational group therapy that involves public confession, peer pressure, and the presence of reformed gamblers (as with sponsors in AA) available to help members resist the impulse to gamble. The dropout rate from GA is high, however. In some cases, hospitalization may help by removing patients from their environments. Insight-oriented psychotherapy should not be sought until patients have been away from gambling for 3 months. At this point, patients who are pathological gamblers may become excellent candidates for this form of psychotherapy. Family therapy is often valuable. Cognitive–behavioral therapy (e.g., relaxation techniques combined with visualization of gambling avoidance) has had some success.

Psychopharmacological treatment, once largely unsuccessful, now plays a significant role in the management of pathological gamblers. Effective agents include antidepressants, notably selective serotonin reuptake inhibitors (SSRIs) and bupropion (Wellbutrin, Zyban); mood stabilizers, including sustained-release lithium (Eskalith) and antiepileptics such as topiramate (Topamax); atypical antipsychotics; and opioid agents such as naltrexone (ReVia). In many patients it is difficult to determine whether an antidepressant or mood stabilizer alleviates gambling cravings directly or via treatment of a comorbid condition, particularly depressive or bipolar disorders.

Table 16.4–2
Twelve Steps of Gambler's Anonymous

1. We admitted we were powerless over gambling—that our lives had become unmanageable.
2. Came to believe that a Power greater than ourselves could restore us to a normal way of thinking and living.
3. Made a decision to turn our will and our lives over to the care of this Power of our own understanding.
4. Made a searching and fearless moral and financial inventory of ourselves.
5. Admitted to ourselves and to another human being the exact nature of our wrongs.
6. Were entirely ready to have these defects of character removed.
7. Humbly asked God (of our understanding) to remove our shortcomings.
8. Made a list of all persons we had harmed and became willing to make amends to them all.
9. Make direct amends to such people wherever possible, except when to do so would injure them or others.
10. Continued to take personal inventory and when we were wrong, promptly admitted it.
11. Sought through prayer and meditation to improve our conscious contact with God as we understood Him, praying only for knowledge of His will for us and the power to carry that out.
12. Having made an effort to practice these principles in all our affairs, we tried to carry this message to other compulsive gamblers.

From Gamblers Anonymous. Available at www.gamblersanonymous.org/ga/content/recovery-program

▲ 16.5 Hallucinogen-Related Disorders

Hallucinogens, by definition, are intoxicants. The use of hallucinogenic drugs is associated with panic attacks, hallucinogen persisting perception disorder (flashbacks), psychosis, delirium, and mood and anxiety disorders. Hallucinogens have been used for thousands of years, and drug-induced hallucinogenic states have been part of social and religious rituals. The discovery of lysergic acid diethylamide (LSD) in 1943 increased the use and misuse of hallucinogens because such synthetic hallucinogens are easily made, easily distributed, sold cheaply, and much more potent than their botanical counterparts. This paved the way to the abuse of synthetic hallucinogens and the development of several associated psychiatric disorders that are now seen in psychiatric practice.

PREPARATIONS

Hallucinogens are natural and synthetic substances that are variously called *psychedelics* or *psychotomimetics* because, in addition to inducing hallucinations, they produce a loss of contact with reality and an experience of expanded and heightened consciousness. The hallucinogens are classified as Schedule I controlled substances; the U.S. Food and Drug Administration (FDA) has decreed that they have no medical use and a high abuse potential.

The classic, naturally occurring hallucinogens are psilocybin (from some mushrooms) and mescaline (from peyote cactus); others are harmine, harmaline, ibogaine, and dimethyltryptamine (DMT). The classic synthetic hallucinogen is LSD, synthesized in 1938 by Albert Hoffman, who later accidentally ingested some of the drug and experienced the first LSD-induced hallucinogenic episode. Some researchers classify the substituted or so-called designer amphetamines, such as 3,4-methylenedioxyamphetamine (MDMA), as hallucinogens. Because these drugs are structurally related to amphetamines, this textbook classifies them as stimulant substances, and they are covered in Section 16.9. Table 16.5–1 lists some representative hallucinogens.

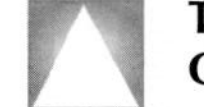

Table 16.5–1
Overview of Representative Hallucinogens

Agent	Locale	Chemical Classification	Biological Sources	Common Route	Typical Dose	Duration of Effects	Adverse Reactions
Lysergic acid diethylamide (LSD)	Globally distributed, semisynthetic	Indolealkylamine	Fungus in rye yields lysergic acid	Oral	100 μg	6–12 hr	Extensive, including pandemic 1965–1975
Mescaline	Southwestern U.S.	Phenethylamine	Peyote cactus, *L. williamsii*	Oral	200–400 mg or 4–6 cactus buttons	10–12 hr	Little or none verified
Methylenedioxyamphetamine (MDA)	U.S., synthetic	Phenethylamine	Synthetic	Oral	80–160 mg	8–12 hr	Documented
Methylenedioxy-methamphetamine (MDMA)	U.S., synthetic	Phenethylamine	Synthetic	Oral	80–150 mg	4–6 hr	Documented
Psilocybin	Southern U.S., Mexico, South America	Phosphorylated hydroxylated DMT	Psilocybin mushrooms	Oral	4–6 mg or 5–10 g of dried mushroom	4–6 hr	Psychosis
Ibogaine	West Central Africa	Indolealkylamine	Tabernanthe iboga	Eating powdered root	200–400 mg	8–48 hr	CNS excitation, death
Ayahuasca	South American tropics	Harmine, other β-carbolines	Bark or leaves of *Banisteriopsis caapi*	As a tea	300–400 mg	4–8 hr	None reported
Dimethyltryptamine	South America, synthetic	Substituted tryptamine	Leaves of *Virola calophylla*	As a snuff, IV	0.2 mg/kg IV	30 min	None reported
Morning glory	American tropics and warm zones	D-lysergic acid alkaloids	Seeds of *Ipomoea violacea, Turbina corymbosa*	Orally as infusion	7–13 seeds	3 hr	Toxic delirium
Nutmeg and mace	Warm zones of Europe, Africa, Asia	Myristicin and aromatic ethers	Fruit of *Myristica fragrans,* commercial species	Orally or as a snuff	1 teaspoon, 5–15 g	Unknown	Similar to atropinism, with seizures, death
Yopo/Cohoba	Northern South America, Argentina	β-Carbolines and tryptamines	Beans of *Anadenanthera peregrina*	Smoked or as a snuff	Unknown	Unknown	Ataxia, hallucinations, seizures
Bufotenin	Northern South America, Argentina	5-OH-dimethyl-tryptamine	Skin glands of toads; seeds of *A. peregrina*	As a snuff or IV	Unknown	15 min	None reported
Phencyclidine (PCP)	U.S., synthetic	1-phenylcyclohexylpiperidine	Synthetic	Oral, smoked, as a snuff, IV	5–10 mg	4–6 hr	Psychotic
Ketamine	U.S., synthetic	(+/-)-2-(2-chlorophenyl)-2-(methylamino)-cyclohexanone	Synthetic	Oral, snorted, IV		1–2 hr	Psychotic

Adapted from Henry David Abraham, M.D.

PCP; 1–1 (phenylcyclohexyl) piperidine, also known as *angel dust,* was first developed as a novel anesthetic in the late 1950s. This drug and the closely related compound ketamine were termed as *dissociative anesthetics,* because they produced a condition in which subjects were awake but apparently insensitive to, or dissociated from, the environment. Phencyclidine and ketamine exert their unique behavioral effects by blocking NMDA-type receptors for the excitatory neurotransmitter glutamate. Their intoxication can present with a variety of symptoms, from anxiety to psychosis. Phencyclidine and ketamine are classified as Schedule II and Schedule III controlled substances, respectively. Although different in pharmacology and clinical effects, the fifth edition of the *Diagnostic and Statistical Manual of Mental Disorders* (DSM-5) includes PCP and ketamine within the hallucinogen category due to their hallucinogenic effects.

EPIDEMIOLOGY

The incidence of hallucinogen use has exhibited two notable periods of increase. Between 1965 and 1969, there was a tenfold increase in the estimated annual number of initiates. This increase was driven primarily by the use of LSD. The second period of increase in first-time hallucinogen use occurred from around 1992 until 2000, fueled mainly by increases in use of ecstasy (i.e., MDMA). Decreases in initiation of both LSD and ecstasy were evident between then and 2013, coinciding with an overall drop in hallucinogen incidence from 1.6 million to 1.1 million.

The NSDUH found that approximately 10 percent of persons age 12 years or older reported lifetime use of hallucinogens. Of this group, 9 percent reported lifetime use of LSD, 6 percent reported lifetime use of ecstasy, and 3 percent reported lifetime use of PCP. The highest rates of current use are among 18 to 25 year olds (2 percent) followed by 12 to 17 year olds (0.9 percent) and adults 25 years or older (0.2 percent). Males (11 percent) are more likely than females (9 percent) to use hallucinogens. Approximately 331,000 persons age 12 years or older were dependent on or abused hallucinogens within the past year.

Hallucinogen use is most common among young (15 to 35 years of age) white men. The ratio of whites to blacks who have used a hallucinogen is 2:1; the white to Hispanic ratio is about 1.5:1. Men represent 62 percent of those who have used a hallucinogen at some time and 75 percent of those who have used a hallucinogen in the preceding month. Persons 26 to 34 years of age show the highest use of hallucinogens, with 16 percent having used a hallucinogen at least once. Persons 18 to 25 years of age have the highest recent use of a hallucinogen.

Cultural factors influence the use of hallucinogens; their use in the western United States is significantly higher than in the southern United States. Hallucinogen use is associated with less morbidity and less mortality than use of some other substances. For example, one study found that only 1 percent of substance-related emergency room visits were related to hallucinogens, compared with 40 percent for cocaine-related problems. Of persons visiting the emergency room for hallucinogen-related reasons, however, more than 50 percent were younger than 20 years of age. Resurgence in the popularity of hallucinogens has been reported.

Phencyclidine

Phencyclidine and some related substances are relatively easy to synthesize in illegal laboratories and relatively inexpensive to buy on the street. The variable quality of the laboratories, however, results in a range of potency and purity. PCP use varies most markedly with geography. Most users of PCP also use other substances, particularly alcohol, but also opiates, opioids, marijuana, amphetamines, and cocaine. PCP is frequently added to marijuana, with severe untoward effects on users. The actual rate of PCP dependence and abuse is not known, but PCP is associated with 3 percent of substance abuse deaths and 32 percent of substance-related emergency room visits nationally.

In the United States, 2.5 percent of those aged 12 and older acknowledged ever using PCP. The highest lifetime prevalence was in those aged 26 to 34 years (4 percent), whereas the highest proportion using PCP in the prior year (0.7 percent) was in those aged 12 to 17 years.

Some areas of some cities have a tenfold higher usage rate of PCP than other areas. The highest PCP use in the United States is in Washington, DC, where PCP accounts for 18 percent of all substance-related deaths and more than 1,000 emergency room visits per year. In Los Angeles, Chicago, and Baltimore, the comparable figure is 6 percent. Overall, most users are between 18 and 25 years of age and they account for 50 percent of cases. Patients are more likely to be male rather than female, especially those who visit emergency rooms. There are twice as many white as black users, although blacks account for more visits to hospitals for PCP-related disorders than do whites. PCP use appears to be rising, with some reports showing a 50 percent increase, particularly in urban areas.

NEUROPHARMACOLOGY

Although most hallucinogenic substances vary in their pharmacological effects, LSD can serve as a hallucinogenic prototype. The pharmacodynamic effect of LSD remains controversial, although it is generally agreed that the drug acts on the serotonergic system, either as an antagonist or as an agonist. Data at this time suggest that LSD acts as a partial agonist at postsynaptic serotonin receptors.

Most hallucinogens are well absorbed after oral ingestion, although some are ingested by inhalation, smoking, or intravenous injection. Tolerance for LSD and other hallucinogens develops rapidly and is virtually complete after 3 or 4 days of continuous use. Tolerance also reverses quickly, usually in 4 to 7 days. Neither physical dependence nor withdrawal symptoms occur with hallucinogens, but a user can develop a psychological dependence on the insight-inducing experiences of episodes of hallucinogen use.

Phencyclidine

Phencyclidine and its related compounds are variously sold as a crystalline powder, paste, liquid, or drug-soaked paper (blotter). PCP is most commonly used as an additive to a cannabis- or parsley-containing cigarette. Experienced users report that the effects of 2 to 3 mg of smoked PCP occur in about 5 minutes and plateau in 30 minutes. The bioavailability of PCP is about 75 percent when taken by intravenous administration and about

30 percent when smoked. The half-life of PCP in humans is about 20 hours, and the half-life of ketamine in humans is about 2 hours.

The primary pharmacodynamic effect of PCP and ketamine is as an antagonist at the NMDA subtype of glutamate receptors. PCP binds to a site within the NMDA-associated calcium channel and prevents the influx of calcium ions. PCP also activates the dopaminergic neurons of the ventral tegmental area, which project to the cerebral cortex and the limbic system. Activation of these neurons is usually involved in mediating the reinforcing qualities of PCP.

Tolerance for the effects of PCP occurs in humans, although physical dependence generally does not occur. In animals that are administered more PCP per pound for longer times than most humans, PCP does induce physical dependence, however, with marked withdrawal symptoms of lethargy, depression, and craving. Physical symptoms of withdrawal in humans are rare, probably as a function of dose and duration of use. Although physical dependence on PCP is rare in humans, psychological dependence on both PCP and ketamine are common, and some users become psychologically dependent on the PCP-induced psychological state.

That PCP is made in illicit laboratories contributes to the increased likelihood of impurities in the final product. One such contaminant is 1-piperidenocyclohexane carbonitrite, which releases hydrogen cyanide in small quantities when ingested. Another contaminant is piperidine, which can be recognized by its strong, fishy odor.

DIAGNOSIS

Hallucinogen Use Disorder

Long-term hallucinogen use is not common. Some long-term users of PCP are said to be "crystallized," a syndrome characterized by dulled thinking, decreased reflexes, loss of memory, loss of impulse control, depression, lethargy, and impaired concentration. Although psychological dependence occurs, it is rare, in part because each LSD experience is different and in part because there is no reliable euphoria.

B, a 16-year-old boy from divorced parents, was admitted to the psychiatric unit of a local hospital. He had slashed his wrists with a knife, severing nerves and tendons in his left hand, and drifted in and out of consciousness during the night. He finally contacted the mother of a friend who lived nearby in the morning who immediately brought him to the hospital.

B had a history of juvenile delinquency from the age of 13 when he began hanging out with some older boys at his junior high school. He and his friends shoplifted, stole, smoked marijuana, and took LSD. B's grades dropped and he got in trouble at school on two occasions for getting into fights with other students.

On admission, B stated that he did not intend on committing suicide when he slashed his wrist. After some questioning, he revealed that he had been "dropping acid" with some friend and after they left he thought he heard the sirens of police cars approaching his home. He did not wish to get arrested, so he slashed his wrist and then lost consciousness. He denies feeling depressed, although he claims his life is pointless and that he felt it made no difference whether he lived or died.

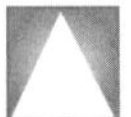

Table 16.5–2
Physiological Changes from Hallucinogens

1. Pupillary dilation
2. Tachycardia
3. Sweating
4. Palpitations
5. Blurring of vision
6. Tremors
7. Incoordination

Hallucinogen Intoxication

Intoxication with hallucinogens is characterized by maladaptive behavioral and perceptual changes and by certain physiological signs (Table 16.5–2). The differential diagnosis for hallucinogen intoxication includes anticholinergic and amphetamine intoxication and alcohol withdrawal. The preferred treatment for hallucinogen intoxication is talking down the patient; during this process, guides can reassure patients that the symptoms are drug induced, that they are not going crazy, and that the symptoms will resolve shortly. In the most severe cases, dopaminergic antagonists—for example, haloperidol (Haldol)—or benzodiazepines—for example, diazepam (Valium)—can be used for a limited time. Hallucinogen intoxication usually lacks a withdrawal syndrome.

Short-term PCP intoxication can have potentially severe complications and must often be considered a psychiatric emergency. Some patients may be brought to psychiatric attention within hours of ingesting PCP, but often 2 to 3 days elapse before psychiatric help is sought. Persons who lose consciousness are brought for help earlier than those who remain conscious. Most patients recover completely within a day or two, but some remain psychotic for as long as 2 weeks. Patients who are first seen in a coma often exhibit disorientation, hallucinations, confusion, and difficulty communicating on regaining consciousness. These symptoms may also be seen in noncomatose patients, but their symptoms appear to be less severe than those of comatose patients. Behavioral disturbances sometimes are severe; they can include public masturbation, stripping off clothes, violence, urinary incontinence, crying, and inappropriate laughing. Patients frequently have amnesia for the entire period of the psychosis.

A 17-year-old male patient was brought to the emergency room by the police, having been found disoriented on the street. As the police attempted to question him, he became increasingly agitated; when they attempted to restrain him, he became assaultive. Attempts to question or to examine him in the emergency department evoked increased agitation.

Initially, it was impossible to determine vital signs or to draw blood. Based on the observation of horizontal, vertical, and rotator nystagmus, a diagnosis of PCP intoxication was entertained. Within a few minutes of being placed in a darkened examination room, his agitation markedly decreased. Blood pressure was 170/100; other vital signs were within normal limits. Blood was drawn for toxicological examination. The patient agreed to take 20 mg of diazepam (Valium) orally. Thirty minutes later, he was less agitated and could be interviewed, although he responded to questions in a fragmented fashion and was slightly dysarthic. He stated that he must have inadvertently taken a larger-than-usual dose of "dust," which he reported having used once or twice a week for several years. He denied use of any other substance and any history of mental disorder. He was disoriented to time and place. The qualitative toxicology screen revealed PCP and no other drugs. Results of neurological examination were within normal limits, but brisk deep tendon reflexes were noted. Some 90 minutes after arrival, his temperature, initially normal, was elevated to 38°C, his blood pressure had increased to 182/110, and he was poorly responsive to stimulation. He was admitted to a medical bed. His blood pressure and level of consciousness continued to fluctuate over the ensuing 18 hours. Results of hematological and biochemical analyses of blood, as well as urinalyses, remained within normal limits. A history obtained from his family revealed that the patient had had multiple emergency room visits for complications from PCP use during the previous several years. He had completed a 30-day residential treatment program and had participated in several outpatient programs but had consistently relapsed. The patient was discharged after vital signs and level of consciousness had been within normal limits for 8 hours. At discharge, nystagmus and dysarthria were no longer present. A referral to an outpatient treatment program was made. *(Courtesy of Daniel C. Javitt, M.D., Ph.D. and Stephen R. Zukin, M.D.)*

Hallucinogen Persisting Perception Disorder

Long after ingesting a hallucinogen, a person can experience a flashback of hallucinogenic symptoms. This syndrome is diagnosed as *hallucinogen persisting perception disorder* in the fifth edition of the *Diagnostic and Statistical Manual of Mental Disorders* (DSM-5). According to studies, from 15 to 80 percent of users of hallucinogens report having experienced flashbacks. The differential diagnosis for flashbacks includes migraine, seizures, visual system abnormalities, and posttraumatic stress disorder. The following can trigger a flashback: emotional stress; sensory deprivation, such as monotonous driving; or use of another psychoactive substance, such as alcohol or marijuana.

Flashbacks are spontaneous, transitory recurrences of the substance-induced experience. Most flashbacks are episodes of visual distortion, geometric hallucinations, hallucinations of sounds or voices, false perceptions of movement in peripheral fields, flashes of color, trails of images from moving objects, positive afterimages and halos, macropsia, micropsia, time expansion, physical symptoms, or relived intense emotion. The episodes usually last a few seconds to a few minutes, but sometimes last longer. Most often, even in the presence of distinct perceptual disturbances, the person has insight into the pathological nature of the disturbance. Suicidal behavior, major depressive disorder, and panic disorders are potential complications.

A 20-year-old undergraduate presented with a chief complaint of seeing the air. The visual disturbance consisted of perception of white pinpoint specks too numerous to count in both the central and peripheral visual fields. They were constantly present and were accompanied by the perception of trails of moving objects left behind as they passed through the patient's visual field. Attending a hockey game was difficult, as the brightly dressed players left streaks of their own images against the white of the ice for seconds at a time. The patient also described the false perception of movement in stable objects, usually in his peripheral visual fields; halos around objects; and positive and negative afterimages. Other symptoms included mild depression, daily bitemporal headache, and a loss of concentration in the last year.

The visual syndrome had gradually emerged over the last 3 months following experimentation with the hallucinogenic drug LCD-25 on three separate occasions. He feared he had sustained some kind of "brain damage" from the drug experience. He denied use of any other agents, including amphetamines, phencyclidine, narcotics, or alcohol, to excess. He had smoked marijuana twice a week for a period of 7 months at age 17.

The patient had consulted two ophthalmologists, both of whom confirmed that the white pinpoint specks were not vitreous floaters (diagnostically insignificant particulate matter floating in the vitreous humor of the eye that can cause the perception of "specks"). A neurologist's examination also proved negative. A therapeutic trial of an anticonvulsant medication resulted in a 50 percent improvement in the patient's visual symptoms and remission of his depression.

Hallucinogen Intoxication Delirium

Hallucinogen intoxication delirium is a relatively rare disorder beginning during intoxication in those who have ingested pure hallucinogens. An estimated 25 percent of all PCP-related emergency room patients may meet the criteria for hallucinogen intoxication delirium. Hallucinogens are often mixed with other substances, however, and the other components or their interactions with the hallucinogens can produce clinical delirium.

Hallucinogen-Induced Psychotic Disorders

If psychotic symptoms are present in the absence of retained reality testing, a diagnosis of hallucinogen-induced psychotic disorder may be warranted. The most common adverse effect of LSD and related substances is a "bad trip," an experience resembling the acute panic reaction to cannabis but sometimes more severe; a bad trip can occasionally produce true psychotic symptoms. The bad trip generally ends when the immediate effects of the hallucinogen wear off, but its course is variable. Occasionally, a protracted psychotic episode is difficult to distinguish from a nonorganic psychotic disorder. Whether a chronic psychosis after drug ingestion is the result of the drug ingestion, is unrelated to the drug ingestion, or is a combination of both the drug ingestion and predisposing factors is currently unanswerable.

Occasionally, the psychotic disorder is prolonged, a reaction thought to be most common in persons with preexisting schizoid personality disorder and prepsychotic personalities, an unstable ego balance, or much anxiety. Such persons cannot cope with the perceptual changes, body-image distortions, and symbolic unconscious material stimulated by the hallucinogen. The rate of previous mental instability in persons hospitalized for LSD reactions is high. Adverse reactions occurred in the late 1960s when LSD was being promoted as a self-prescribed psychotherapy for emotional crises in the lives of seriously disturbed persons. Now that this practice is less frequent, prolonged adverse reactions are less common.

A 22-year-old female photography student presented to the hospital with inappropriate mood and bizarre thinking. She had no prior psychiatric history. Nine days before admission, she ingested one or two psilocybin mushrooms. Following the immediate ingestion, the patient began to giggle. She then described euphoria, which progressed to auditory hallucinations and belief in the ability to broadcast her thoughts on the media. Two days later she repeated the ingestion, and continued to exhibit psychotic symptoms to the day of admission. When examined she heard voices telling her she could be president, and reported the sounds of "lambs crying." She continued to giggle inappropriately, bizarrely turning her head from side to side ritualistically. She continued to describe euphoria, but with an intermittent sense of hopelessness in a context of thought blocking. Her self-description was "feeling lucky." She was given haloperidol, 10 mg twice a day, along with benztropine (Cogentin) 1 mg three times a day and lithium carbonate (Eskalith) 300 mg twice a day. On this regimen her psychosis abated after 5 days.

Hallucinogen-Induced Mood Disorder

Unlike cocaine-induced mood disorder and amphetamine-induced mood disorder, in which the symptoms are somewhat predictable, mood disorder symptoms accompanying hallucinogen abuse can vary. Abusers may experience manic-like symptoms with grandiose delusions or depression-like feelings and ideas or mixed symptoms. As with the hallucinogen-induced psychotic disorder symptoms, the symptoms of hallucinogen-induced mood disorder usually resolve once the drug has been eliminated from the person's body.

Hallucinogen-Induced Anxiety Disorder

Hallucinogen-induced anxiety disorder also varies in its symptom pattern, but few data about symptom patterns are available. Anecdotally, emergency room physicians who treat patients with hallucinogen-related disorders frequently report panic disorder with agoraphobia. Anxiety is probably the most common symptom causing a PCP-intoxicated person to seek help in an emergency room.

Unspecified Hallucinogen-Related Disorder

When a patient with a hallucinogen-related disorder does not meet the diagnostic criteria for any of the standard hallucinogen-related disorders, the patient may be classified as having unspecified hallucinogen-related disorder. DSM-5 does not have a diagnostic category of hallucinogen withdrawal, but some clinicians anecdotally report a syndrome with depression and anxiety after cessation of frequent hallucinogen use. Such a syndrome may best fit the diagnosis of unspecified hallucinogen-related disorder.

CLINICAL FEATURES

Lsysergic Acid Diethylamide

A large class of hallucinogenic compounds with well-studied structure–activity relationships is represented by the prototype LSD. LSD is a synthetic base derived from the lysergic acid nucleus from the ergot alkaloids. That family of compounds was discovered in rye fungus and was responsible for lethal outbreaks of St. Anthony's fire in the Middle Ages. The compounds are also present in morning glory seeds in low concentrations. Many homologs and analogs of LSD have been studied. None of them has potency exceeding that of LSD.

Physiological symptoms from LSD are typically few and relatively mild. Dilated pupils, increased deep tendon motor reflexes and muscle tension, and mild motor incoordination and ataxia are common. Increased heart rate, respiration, and blood pressure are modest in degree and variable, as are nausea, decreased appetite, and salivation.

The usual sequence of changes follows a pattern of somatic symptoms appearing first, then mood and perceptual changes, and, finally, psychological changes, although effects overlap and, depending on the particular hallucinogen, the time of onset and offset varies. The intensity of LSD effects in a nontolerant user generally is proportional to dose, with 25 μg as an approximate threshold dose.

The syndrome produced by LSD resembles that produced by mescaline, psilocybin, and some of the amphetamine analogs. The major difference among LSD, psilocybin, and mescaline is potency. A 1.5 μg/kg dose of LSD is roughly equivalent to 225 μg/kg of psilocybin, which is equivalent to 5 mg/kg of mescaline. With mescaline, onset of symptoms is slower and more nausea and vomiting occurs but in general, the perceptual effects are more similar than different.

Tolerance, particularly to the sensory and other psychological effects, is evident as soon as the second or third day of successive LSD use. Four to 6 days free of LSD are necessary to lose significant tolerance. Tolerance is associated with frequent use of any of the hallucinogens. Cross-tolerance among mescaline, psilocybin, and LSD occurs, but not between amphetamine and LSD, despite the chemical similarity of amphetamine and mescaline.

Previously distributed as tablets, liquid, powder, and gelatin squares, in recent years, LSD has been commonly distributed as "blotter acid." Sheets of paper are soaked with LSD, and dried and perforated into small squares. Popular designs are stamped on the paper. Each sheet contains as many as a few hundred squares; one square containing 30 to 75 μg of LSD is one chewed dose, more or less. Planned massive ingestion is uncommon but massive ingestion happens by accident.

The onset of action of LSD occurs within an hour, peaks in 2 to 4 hours, and lasts 8 to 12 hours. The sympathomimetic effects of LSD include tremors, tachycardia, hypertension, hyperthermia, sweating, blurring of vision, and mydriasis. Death caused by cardiac or cerebrovascular pathology related to hypertension or hyperthermia can occur with hallucinogenic use. A syndrome similar to neuroleptic malignant syndrome has reportedly been associated with LSD. Death can also be caused by a physical injury when LSD use impairs judgment about traffic or a person's ability to fly, for example. The psychological effects are usually well tolerated, but when persons cannot recall experiences or appreciate that the experiences are substance induced, they may fear the onset of insanity.

With hallucinogen use, perceptions become unusually brilliant and intense. Colors and textures seem to be richer, contours sharpened, music more emotionally profound, and smells and tastes heightened. Synesthesia is common; colors may be heard or sounds seen. Changes in body image and alterations of time and space perception also occur. Hallucinations are usually visual, often of geometric forms and figures, but auditory and tactile hallucinations are sometimes experienced. Emotions become unusually intense and may change abruptly and often; two seemingly incompatible feelings may be experienced at the same time. Suggestibility is greatly heightened, and sensitivity or detachment from other persons may arise. Other common features are a seeming awareness of internal organs, the recovery of lost early memories, the release of unconscious material in symbolic form, and regression and the apparent reliving of past events, including birth. Introspective reflection and feelings of religious and philosophical insight are common. The sense of self is greatly changed, sometimes to the point of depersonalization, merging with the external world, separation of self from body, or total dissolution of the ego in mystical ecstasy.

There is no clear evidence of a drastic personality change or chronic psychosis produced by long-term LSD use by moderate users not otherwise predisposed to these conditions. Some heavy users of hallucinogens, however, may experience chronic anxiety or depression and may benefit from a psychological or pharmacological approach that addresses the underlying problem.

Many persons maintain that a single experience with LSD has given them increased creative capacity, new psychological insight, relief from neurotic or psychosomatic symptoms, or a desirable change in personality. In the 1950s and 1960s, psychiatrists showed great interest in LSD and related substances, both as potential models for functional psychosis and as possible pharmacotherapeutic agents. The availability of these compounds to researchers in the basic neurosciences has led to many scientific advances.

Phenethylamines

Phenethylamines are compounds with chemical structures similar to those of the neurotransmitters dopamine and norepinephrine. Mescaline (3,4,5-trimethoxyphenethylamine), a classic hallucinogen in every sense of the term, was the first hallucinogen isolated from the peyote cactus that grows in the southwestern United States and northern Mexico. Mescaline human pharmacology was characterized in 1896 and its structure verified by synthesis 23 years later. Although many psychoactive plants have been recognized dating to before recorded history, mescaline was the only structurally identified hallucinogen until LSD was described in 1943.

Mescaline

Mescaline is usually consumed as peyote "buttons," picked from the small blue-green cacti *Lophophora williamsii* and *Lophophora diffusa.* The buttons are the dried, round, fleshy cacti tops. Mescaline is the active hallucinogenic alkaloid in the buttons. Use of peyote is legal for the Native American Church members in some states. Adverse reactions to peyote are rare during structured religious use. Peyote usually is not consumed casually because of its bitter taste and sometimes severe nausea and vomiting that precede the hallucinogenic effects.

Many structural variations of mescaline have been investigated and structural activity relationships fairly well characterized. One analog, 2,5-dimethoxy-4-methylamphetamine (DOM), also known as STP, an unusually potent amphetamine with hallucinogen properties, had a relatively brief period of illicit popularity and notoriety in the 1960s, but it appears to have disappeared from the illicit market.

Another series of phenethylamine analogs with hallucinogenic properties is the 3,4-methylenedioxyamphetamine (MDA)–related amphetamines. The currently most popular and, to society, most troublesome member of this large family of drugs is MDMA, or ecstasy, more a relatively mild stimulant than hallucinogen. MDMA produces an altered state of consciousness with sensory changes and, most important for some users, a feeling of enhanced personal interactions.

Many plants contain N,N-DMT, which is also found normally in human biofluids at very low concentrations. When DMT is taken parenterally or by sniffing, a brief, intense hallucinogenic episode can result. As with mescaline in the phenethylamine group, DMT is one of the oldest, best documented, but least potent of the tryptamine hallucinogens. Synthesized homologs of DMT have been evaluated in humans and structure activity relationships have been reasonably well described.

Psilocybin Analogs

An unusual collection of tryptamines has its origin in the world of fungi. The natural prototype is psilocybin itself. That and related homologs have been found in as many as 100 species of mushroom, largely of the *Psilocybe* genus.

Psilocybin is usually ingested as mushrooms. Many species of psilocybin-containing mushrooms are found worldwide. In the United States, large *Psilocybe cubensis* (gold caps) grow in Florida and Texas and are easily grown with cultivation kits advertised in drug-oriented magazines and on the Internet. The tiny *Psilocybe semilanceata* (liberty cap) grows in lawns and pastures in the Pacific Northwest. Psilocybin remains active when the mushrooms are dried or cooked into omelets or other foods.

Psilocybin mushrooms are used in religious activities by Mexican Indians. They are valued in Western society by users who prefer to ingest a mushroom rather than a synthetic chemical. Of course, one danger of eating wild mushrooms is misidentification and ingestion of a poisonous variety. At a large American university, 24 percent of students reported using psychedelic mushrooms or mescaline, compared with 17 percent who reported LSD use. Psilocybin sold as pills or capsules usually contains PCP or LSD instead.

Studies are underway in several medical centers in the United States (including New York University) to examine the use of psilocybin in terminally ill patients.

Preliminary reports indicate that the psilocybin is helpful in reducing morbid anxiety about death and dying. It may play an important role in palliative care medicine in the future.

Phencyclidine

The amount of PCP varies greatly from PCP-laced cigarette to cigarette; 1 g may be used to make as few as four or as many as several dozen cigarettes. Less than 5 mg of PCP is considered a low dose, and doses above 10 mg are considered high. Dose variability makes it difficult to predict the effect, although smoking PCP is the easiest and most reliable way for users to titrate the dose.

Persons who have just taken PCP are frequently uncommunicative, appear to be oblivious, and report active fantasy production. They experience speedy feelings, euphoria, bodily warmth, tingling, peaceful floating sensations, and, occasionally, feelings of depersonalization, isolation, and estrangement. Sometimes, they have auditory and visual hallucinations. They often have striking alterations of body image, distortions of space and time perception, and delusions. They may experience intensified dependence feelings, confusion, and disorganization of thought. Users may be sympathetic, sociable, and talkative at one moment but hostile and negative at another. Anxiety is sometimes reported; it is often the most prominent presenting symptom during an adverse reaction. Nystagmus, hypertension, and hyperthermia are common effects of PCP. Head-rolling movements, stroking, grimacing, muscle rigidity on stimulation, repeated episodes of vomiting, and repetitive chanting speech are sometimes observed.

The short-term effects last 3 to 6 hours and sometimes give way to a mild depression in which the user becomes irritable, somewhat paranoid, and occasionally belligerent, irrationally assaultive, suicidal, or homicidal. The effects can last for several days. Users sometimes find that it takes 1 to 2 days to recover completely; laboratory tests show that PCP can remain in the patient's blood and urine for more than a week.

Ketamine

Ketamine is a dissociative anesthetic agent, originally derived from PCP, which is available for use in human and veterinary medicine. It has become a drug of abuse, with sources exclusively from stolen supplies. It is available as a powder or in solution for intranasal, oral, inhalational, or (rarely) intravenous use. Ketamine functions by working at the NMDA receptor and, as with PCP, can cause hallucinations and a dissociated state in which the patient has an altered sense of the body and reality and little concern for the environment.

Ketamine causes cardiovascular stimulation and no respiratory depression. On physical examination, the patient may be hypertensive and tachycardic, have increased salivation and bidirectional or rotary nystagmus, or both. The onset of action is within seconds when used intravenously, and analgesia lasting 40 minutes and dissociative effects lasting for hours have been described. Cardiovascular status should be monitored and supportive care administered. A dystonic reaction has been described, as have flashbacks, but a more common complication is related to a lack of concern for the environment or personal safety.

Ketamine has a briefer duration of effect than PCP. Peak ketamine levels occur approximately 20 minutes after intramuscular injection. After intranasal administration, the duration of effect is approximately 1 hour. Ketamine is N-demethylated by liver microsomal cytochrome P450 (CYP), especially CYP3A, into norketamine. Ketamine, norketamine, and dehydronorketamine can be detected in urine, with half-lives of 3, 4, and 7 hours, respectively. Urinary ketamine and norketamine levels vary widely from individual to individual and can range from 10 to 7,000 ng/mL after intoxication. As of yet, the relationship between serum ketamine levels and clinical symptoms has not been formally studied. Ketamine is often used in combination with other drugs of abuse, especially cocaine. Ketamine does not appear to interfere with, and may enhance, cocaine metabolism.

Ketamine is being studied for use in the treatment of depression. Although not approved by the FDA for the treatment of depression, it has been used effectively in selected cases to relieve depression, especially in patients who are suicidal. The antidepressant effects are short lived however, and patients must be treated on a weekly basis with ketamine infusions. Further study is warranted on its effectiveness over the long term.

ADDITIONAL HALLUCINOGENS

Canthinones

Canthinones are alkaloids similar to amphetamines naturally found in the khat plant and synthetically made and known as "bath salts." They are CNS stimulants that cause a massive release of dopamine, and a single dose can last up to 8 hours. They produce profound toxic effects that can lead to seizures, strokes, and/or death. Hallucinations and delusions are common. They are swallowed, injected, or "snorted" to produce the desired euphoric effect.

Ibogaine

Ibogaine is a complex alkaloid found in the African shrub *Tabernanthe iboga.* Ibogaine is a hallucinogen at the 400 mg dose range. The plant originates in Africa and traditionally is used in sacramental initiation ceremonies. Although it has not been a popular hallucinogen because of its unpleasant somatic effects when taken at hallucinogenic doses, patients exposed to ibogaine may be encountered by a psychiatrist because of the therapeutic claims.

Ayahuasca

Ayahuasca, much discussed on Internet hallucinogen websites, originally referred to a decoction from one or more South American plants. The substance contains the alkaloids harmaline and harmine. Both of those β-carboline alkaloids have hallucinogenic properties, but the resulting visual sensory alterations are accompanied by considerable nausea. Amazon native tribes discovered that adding leaves from plants containing substantial amounts of DMT markedly enhanced the visual and sacramental impact of ayahuasca. Thus, neither component in the ayahuasca plant mixture works well alone but when taken in combination an extremely effective hallucinogenic agent results.

In recent years, the term *ayahuasca* has evolved to a less specific term to refer to any mixture of two things that are hallucinogenic when taken in combination. For example, harmine and harmaline are available as fine chemicals and when taken along with many botanicals containing DMT result in a mixture with hallucinogen properties, initially intense but usually of brief duration.

Salvia Divinorum

American Indians in northern Oaxaca, Mexico, have used *Salvia divinorum* as a medicine and as a sacred sacrament, which is now widely discussed, advertised, and sold on the Internet. When the plant is chewed or dried leaves smoked, it produces hallucinogen effects. Salvinorin-A, an active component in the plant, is parenterally potent, active at 250-μg doses when smoked, and of scientific and potential medical interest because it binds to the opioid κ-receptor.

TREATMENT

Hallucinogen Intoxication

A basic principle in treatment is providing reassurance and supportive care. Patients experiencing intense and unpleasant hallucinogen intoxication can be helped by a quiet environment, verbal reassurance, and the passage of time. More rapid relief of intense anxiety is likely after oral administration of 20 mg of diazepam (Valium) or, if oral administration presents problems, an equivalent parenteral dose of a benzodiazepine. Anxiety and other symptoms generally diminish within 20 minutes of medication administration, compared to hours with only psychological and environmental support; however, perceptual symptoms may persist. Patients may need gentle restraint if they are in danger to themselves or others, but restraints should be avoided if possible. Neuroleptic medications, particularly if given at excessive doses, may worsen symptoms and are best avoided unless the diagnosis remains unclear and behavior cannot otherwise be managed. The marketing of lower doses of LSD and a more sophisticated approach to treatment of casualties by drug users themselves have combined to reduce the appearance of this once-common disorder in psychiatric treatment facilities.

Hallucinogen Persisting Disorder

Treatment for hallucinogen persisting perception disorder is palliative. The first step in the process is correct identification of the disorder; it is not uncommon for the patient to consult a number of specialists before the diagnosis is made. Pharmacological approaches include long-lasting benzodiazepines, such as clonazepam (Klonopin) and, to a lesser extent, anticonvulsants including valproic acid (Depakene) and carbamazepine (Tegretol). Currently, no drug is completely effective in ablating symptoms. Antipsychotic agents should be used only in the treatment of hallucinogen-induced psychoses, because they may have a paradoxical effect and exacerbate symptoms. A second dimension of treatment is behavioral. The patient must be instructed to avoid gratuitous stimulation in the form of over-the-counter drugs, caffeine, and alcohol, and avoidable physical and emotional stressors. Marijuana smoke is a particularly strong intensifier of the disorder, even when passively inhaled. Finally, three comorbid conditions are associated with hallucinogen persisting perception disorder: panic disorder, major depression, and alcohol dependence. All these conditions require primary prevention and early intervention.

Hallucinogen-Induced Psychosis

Treatment of hallucinogen-induced psychosis does not differ from conventional treatment for other psychoses. In addition to antipsychotic medications, a number of agents are reportedly effective, including lithium carbonate, carbamazepine, and electroconvulsive therapy. Antidepressant drugs, benzodiazepines, and anticonvulsant agents may each have a role in treatment as well. One hallmark of this disorder is that, as opposed to schizophrenia, in which negative symptoms and poor interpersonal relatedness may commonly be found, patients with hallucinogen-induced psychosis exhibit the positive symptoms of hallucinations and delusions while retaining the ability to relate to the psychiatrist. Medical therapies are best applied in a context of supportive, educational, and family therapies. The goals of treatment are the control of symptoms, a minimal use of hospitals, daily work, the development and preservation of social relationships, and the management of comorbid illnesses such as alcohol dependence.

Phencyclidine

Treatment of PCP intoxication aims to reduce systemic PCP levels and to address significant medical, behavioral, and psychiatric issues. For intoxication and PCP-induced psychotic disorder, although resolution of current symptoms and signs is paramount, the long-term goal of treatment is to prevent relapse to PCP use. PCP levels can fluctuate over many hours or even days, especially after oral administration. A prolonged period of clinical observation is therefore mandatory before concluding that no serious or life-threatening complications will ensue.

Trapping of ionized PCP in the stomach has led to the suggestion of continuous nasogastric suction as a treatment for PCP intoxication. This strategy, however, can be needlessly intrusive and can induce electrolyte imbalances. Administration of activated charcoal is safer, and it binds PCP and diminishes toxic effects of PCP in animals.

Trapping of ionized PCP in urine has led to the suggestion of urinary acidification as an aid to drug elimination. This strategy, however, may be ineffective and is potentially dangerous. Only a small portion of PCP is excreted in urine, metabolic acidosis itself carries significant risks, and acidic urine can increase the risk of renal failure secondary to rhabdomyolysis. Because of the extremely large volume of distribution of PCP, neither hemodialysis nor hemoperfusion can significantly promote drug clearance.

No drug is known to function as a direct PCP antagonist. Any compound binding to the PCP receptor, which is located within the ion channel of the NMDA receptor, would block NMDA receptor–mediated ion fluxes as does PCP itself. NMDA-receptor mechanisms predict that pharmacological strategies promoting NMDA receptor activation (e.g., administration of a glycine site agonist drug) would promote rapid dissociation of PCP from its binding sites. No clinical trials of NMDA agonists for PCP or ketamine intoxication in humans have been carried out to date. Treatment must therefore be supportive and directed at specific symptoms and signs of toxicity. Classic measures should be used for medical crises, including seizures, hypothermia, and hypertensive crisis.

Because PCP disrupts sensory input, environmental stimuli can cause unpredictable, exaggerated, distorted, or violent reactions. A cornerstone of treatment, therefore, is minimization of sensory inputs to PCP-intoxicated patients. Patients should be evaluated and treated in an environment that is as quiet and isolated as possible. Precautionary physical restraint is recommended by some authorities, with the risk of rhabdomyolysis from struggle against the restraints balanced by the avoidance of violent or disruptive behavior. Pharmacological sedation can be accomplished with oral or IM antipsychotics or benzodiazepines; no convincing evidence indicates that either class of compounds is clinically superior. Because of the anticholinergic actions of PCP at high doses, neuroleptics with potent intrinsic anticholinergic properties should be avoided.

▲ 16.6 Inhalant-Related Disorders

Inhalant drugs (also called *volatile substances* or *solvents*) are volatile hydrocarbons that vaporize to gaseous fumes at room temperature and are inhaled through the nose or mouth to enter the bloodstream via the transpulmonary route. These compounds are commonly found in many household products and are divided into four commercial classes: (1) solvents for glues and adhesives, (2) propellants (e.g., for aerosol paint sprays, hair sprays, and shaving cream), (3) thinners (e.g., for paint products and correction fluids), and (4) fuels (e.g., gasoline, propane). These drugs are believed to share some similar pharmacological properties despite their chemical differences.

Persons, especially adolescents, like to inhale these products for their intoxicating effect. Inhalants are associated with a number of problems including conduct disorder, mood disorders, suicidality, and physical and sexual abuse or neglect. In some cases, an early time-limited use of inhalants may signal a lifelong problem with externalizing behaviors and risk-taking propensity. A smaller subgroup use inhalants chronically and such use has been associated with multiple sequelae, including major behavioral and organ pathology from the drugs' toxicity.

The fifth edition of *Diagnostic and Statistical Manual of Mental Disorders* (DSM-5) excludes anesthetic gases (e.g., nitrous oxide and ether) and short-acting vasodilators (e.g., amyl nitrite) from the inhalant-related disorders, which are classified as other (or unknown) substance-related disorders and are discussed in Section 16.13.

EPIDEMIOLOGY

Inhalant substances are easily available, legal, and inexpensive. These three factors contribute to the high use of inhalants among poor and young persons. Approximately 6 percent of persons in the United States had used inhalants at least once, and about 1 percent of persons are current users. Among young adults 18 to 25 years of age, 11 percent had used inhalants at least once, and 2 percent were current users. Among adolescents 12 to 17 years of age, 7 percent had used inhalants at least once, and 1.1 percent were current users. In one study of high school seniors, 18 percent reported having used inhalants at least once, and 2.7 percent reported having used inhalants within the preceding month. White users of inhalants are more common than either Black or Hispanic users. Most users (up to 80 percent) are male. Some data suggest that inhalant use may be more common in suburban communities in the United States than in urban communities.

Inhalant use accounts for 1 percent of all substance-related deaths and less than 0.5 percent of all substance-related emergency room visits. About 20 percent of the emergency room visits for inhalant use involve persons younger than 18 years of age. Inhalant use among adolescents may be most common in those whose parents or older siblings use illegal substances. Inhalant use among adolescents is also associated with an increased likelihood of conduct disorder or antisocial personality disorder.

NEUROPHARMACOLOGY

Inhalants most used by American adolescents are (in descending order) gasoline, glue (which usually contains toluene), spray paint, solvents, cleaning fluids, and assorted other aerosols. Sniffing vapor through the nose or huffing (taking deep breaths) through the mouth leads to transpulmonary absorption with very rapid drug access to the brain. Breathing through a solvent-soaked cloth, inhaling fumes from a glue-containing bag, huffing vapor sprayed into a plastic bag, or breathing vapor from a gasoline can are common. Approximately 15 to 20 breaths of 1 percent gasoline vapor produce several hours of intoxication. Inhaled toluene concentrations from a glue-containing bag may reach 10,000 ppm, and vapors from several tubes of glue may be inhaled each day. By comparison, one study of just 100 ppm of toluene showed that a 6-hour exposure produced a temporary neuropsychological performance decrement of approximately 10 percent.

Inhalants generally act as a CNS depressant. Tolerance for inhalants can develop, although withdrawal symptoms are usually fairly mild.

Inhalants are rapidly absorbed through the lungs and rapidly delivered to the brain. The effects appear within 5 minutes and can last for 30 minutes to several hours, depending on the inhalant substance and the dose. The concentrations of many inhalant substances in blood are increased when used in combination with alcohol, perhaps because of competition for hepatic enzymes. Although about one-fifth of an inhalant substance is excreted unchanged by the lungs, the remainder is metabolized by the liver. Inhalants are detectable in the blood for 4 to 10 hours after use, and blood samples should be taken in the emergency room when inhalant use is suspected.

Much like alcohol, inhalants have specific pharmacodynamic effects that are not well understood. Because their effects are generally similar and additive to the effects of other CNS depressants (e.g., ethanol, barbiturates, and benzodiazepines), some investigators have suggested that inhalants operate by enhancing the GABA system. Other investigators have suggested that inhalants work through membrane fluidization, which has also been hypothesized to be a pharmacodynamic effect of ethanol.

DIAGNOSIS

Inhalant Use Disorder

Most persons probably use inhalants for a short time without developing a pattern of long-term use resulting in dependence and abuse. Nonetheless, dependence and abuse of inhalants occur and are diagnosed according to the DSM-5 (see page 621).

Inhalant Intoxication

The diagnostic criteria for inhalant intoxication specify the presence of maladaptive behavioral changes and at least two physical symptoms. The intoxicated state is often characterized by apathy, diminished social and occupational functioning, impaired judgment, and impulsive or aggressive behavior, and it can be accompanied by nausea, anorexia, nystagmus, depressed reflexes, and diplopia. With high doses and long exposures, a user's neurological status can progress to stupor and unconsciousness, and a person may later be amnestic for the period of intoxication. Clinicians can sometimes identify a recent user of inhalants by rashes around the patient's nose and mouth; unusual breath odors; the residue of the inhalant substances on the patient's face, hands, or clothing; and irritation of the patient's eyes, throat, lungs, and nose. The disorder can be chronic, as in the following case.

A 16-year-old single Hispanic female was referred to a university substance-treatment program for evaluation. The patient had been convicted for auto theft, menacing with a weapon, and being out of control by her family. By age 15, she had regularly been using inhalants and drinking alcohol heavily. She had tried typewriter-erasing fluid, bleach, tile cleaner, hairspray, nail polish, glue, and gasoline, but preferred spray paint. She had sniffed paint many times each day for about 6 months at age 15, using a maximum of eight paint cans per day. The patient said, "It blacks out everything." Sometimes she had lost consciousness, and she believed that the paint had impaired her memory and made her "dumb." *(Courtesy of Thomas J. Crowley, M.D.)*

Inhalant Intoxication Delirium

Delirium can be induced by the effects of the inhalants themselves, by pharmacodynamic interactions with other substances, and by the hypoxia that may be associated with either the inhalant or its method of inhalation. If the delirium results in severe behavioral disturbances, short-term treatment with a dopamine receptor antagonist, such as haloperidol (Haldol), may be necessary. Benzodiazepines should be avoided because of the possibility of increasing the patient's respiratory depression.

Inhalant-Induced Persisting Dementia

Inhalant-induced persisting dementia, as with delirium, may result from the neurotoxic effects of the inhalants themselves; the neurotoxic effects of the metals (e.g., lead) commonly used in inhalants; or the effects of frequent and prolonged periods of hypoxia. The dementia caused by inhalants is likely to be irreversible in all but the mildest cases.

Inhalant-Induced Psychotic Disorder

Clinicians can specify hallucinations or delusions as the predominant symptoms. Paranoid states are probably the most common psychotic syndromes during inhalant intoxication.

Inhalant-Induced Mood Disorder and Inhalant-Induced Anxiety Disorder

Inhalant-induced mood disorder and inhalant-induced anxiety disorder allow the classification of inhalant-related disorders characterized by prominent mood and anxiety symptoms. Depressive disorders are the most common mood disorders associated with inhalant use, and panic disorders and generalized anxiety disorder are the most common anxiety disorders.

Other Inhalant-Induced Disorders

Other Inhalant-Induced Disorder is the recommended DSM-5 diagnosis for inhalant-related disorders that do not fit into one of the diagnostic categories discussed earlier.

CLINICAL FEATURES

In small initial doses, inhalants can be disinhibiting and produce feelings of euphoria and excitement as well as pleasant floating sensations, the effects for which persons presumably use the drugs. High doses of inhalants can cause psychological symptoms of fearfulness, sensory illusions, auditory and visual hallucinations, and distortions of body size. The neurological symptoms can include slurred speech, decreased speed of talking, and ataxia. Long-term use can be associated with irritability, emotional lability, and impaired memory.

Tolerance for the inhalants does develop for some users; a withdrawal syndrome can accompany the cessation of inhalant use. The withdrawal syndrome does not occur frequently; when it does, it can be characterized by sleep disturbances, irritability, jitteriness, sweating, nausea, vomiting, tachycardia, and (sometimes) delusions and hallucinations.

Organ Pathology and Neurological Effects

Inhalants are associated with many potentially serious adverse effects. The most serious of these is death, which can result from respiratory depression, cardiac arrhythmias, asphyxiation, aspiration of vomitus, or accident or injury (e.g., driving while intoxicated with inhalants). Placing an inhalant-soaked rag and one's head into a plastic bag, a common procedure for inhalant users, can cause coma and suffocation.

Chronic inhalant users may have numerous neurological problems. Computed tomography (CT) and magnetic resonance imaging (MRI) reveal diffuse cerebral, cerebellar, and brainstem atrophy with white matter disease, a leukoencephalopathy. Single photon emission CT (SPECT) of former solvent-abusing adolescents showed both increases and decreases of blood flow in different cerebral areas. Several studies of house painters and factory workers who have been exposed to solvents for long periods also have found evidence of brain atrophy on CT scans, with decreased cerebral blood flow.

Neurological and behavioral signs and symptoms can include hearing loss, peripheral neuropathy, headache, paresthesias, cerebellar signs, persisting motor impairment, parkinsonism, apathy, poor concentration, memory loss, visual–spatial dysfunction, impaired processing of linguistic material, and lead encephalopathy. White matter changes, or pontine atrophy on MRI, have been associated with worse intelligence quotient (IQ) test results. The combination of organic solvents with high concentrations of copper, zinc, and heavy metals has been associated with the development of brain atrophy, temporal lobe epilepsy, decreased IQ, and a variety of EEG changes.

Other serious adverse effects associated with long-term inhalant use include irreversible hepatic disease or renal damage (tubular acidosis) and permanent muscle damage associated with rhabdomyolysis. Additional adverse effects include cardiovascular and pulmonary symptoms (e.g., chest pain and bronchospasm) as well as gastrointestinal (GI) symptoms (e.g., pain, nausea, vomiting, and hematemesis). There are several clinical reports of *toluene embryopathy,* with signs such as those of fetal alcohol syndrome. These include low birth weight, microcephaly, shortened palpebral fissures, small face, low-set ears, and other dysmorphic signs. These babies reportedly develop slowly, show hyperactivity, and have cerebellar dysfunction. No convincing evidence indicates, however, that toluene, the best-studied inhalant, produces genetic damage in somatic cells.

TREATMENT

Inhalant intoxication, as with alcohol intoxication, usually requires no medical attention and resolves spontaneously. However, effects of the intoxication, such as coma, bronchospasm, laryngospasm, cardiac arrhythmias, trauma, or burns, need treatment. Otherwise, care primarily involves reassurance, quiet support, and attention to vital signs and level of consciousness. Sedative drugs, including benzodiazepines, are contraindicated because they worsen inhalant intoxication.

No established treatment exists for the cognitive and memory problems of inhalant-induced persisting dementia. Street outreach and extensive social service support have been offered to severely deteriorated, inhalant-dependent, homeless adults. Patients may require extensive support within their families or in foster or domiciliary care.

The course and treatment of inhalant-induced psychotic disorder are like those of inhalant intoxication. The disorder is brief, lasting a few hours to (at most) a very few weeks beyond the intoxication. Confusion, panic, and psychosis mandate special attention to patient safety. Severe agitation may require cautious control with haloperidol (5 mg intramuscularly per 70 kg body weight). Sedative drugs should be avoided because they may aggravate the psychosis. Inhalant-induced anxiety and mood disorders may precipitate suicidal ideation, and patients should be carefully evaluated for that possibility. Antianxiety medications and antidepressants are not useful in the acute phase of the disorder; they may be of use in cases of a coexisting anxiety or depressive illness.

Day Treatment and Residential Programs

Day treatment and residential programs have been used successfully, especially for adolescent abusers with combined substance dependence and other psychiatric disorders. Treatment addresses the comorbid state which, in most cases, is conduct disorder or, in other instances, may be ADHD, major depressive disorder, dysthymic disorder, and posttraumatic stress disorder (PTSD). Attention is also directed to experiences of abuse or neglect, which is very common in these patients. Both group and individual therapies are used that are behaviorally oriented, with immediate rewards for progress toward objectively defined goals in treatment and punishments for lapses to previous behaviors. Patients attend on-site schools with special education teachers, together with planned recreational activities, and the programs provide birth control consultations. The patients' families, often very chaotic, are engaged in modifications of structural family therapy or multisystemic therapy, both of which have good empirical support. Participation in 12-step programs is required. Treatment interventions are coordinated closely with interventions by community social workers and probation officers. Progress is monitored with urine and breath samples analyzed for alcohol and other drugs at intake and frequently during treatment.

Treatment usually lasts 3 to 12 months. Termination is considered successful if the youth has practiced a plan to stay abstinent; is showing fewer antisocial behaviors; has a plan to continue any needed psychiatric treatment (e.g., treatment for comorbid depression); has a plan to live in a supportive, drug-free environment; is interacting with the family in a more productive way; is working or attending school; and is associating with drug-free, nondelinquent peers.

▲ 16.7 Opioid-Related Disorders

Opioids have been used for analgesic and other medicinal purposes for thousands of years, but they also have a long history of misuse for their psychoactive effects. Continued opioid misuse can result in syndromes of abuse and dependence and cause disturbances in mood, behavior, and cognition that can mimic other psychiatric disorders. In developed countries, the opioid drug most frequently associated with abuse and dependence is heroin; however, there is growing public health concern about prescription opioids, which are widely available, have significant abuse liability, and are used increasingly for purposes. Opioid addiction affects the young and the old, the wealthy and the poor, and the professional and the unemployed. Over the last few decades, there have been significant advances in treatment and understanding of opioid dependence. It is increasingly accepted that opioid dependence is often a chronic, relapsing disorder amenable to medical treatment and intervention. Table 16.7–1 lists various opioids that are used therapeutically in the United States, with the exception of heroin.

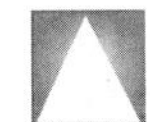

Table 16.7–1
Opioids

Proprietary Name	Trade Name
Morphine	
Heroin (diacetylmorphine)	
Hydromorphone (dihydromorphinone)	Dilaudid
Oxymorphone (dihydro hydroxymorphinone)	Numorphan
Levorphanol	Levo-Dromoran
Methadone	Dolophine
Meperidine (pethidine)	Demerol, Pethadol
Fentanyl	Sublimaze
Codeine	
Hydrocodone (dihydrocodeinone)	Hycodan, others
Drocode (dihydrocodeine)	Synalgos-DC, Compal
Oxycodone (dihydrohydroxycodeinone)	Roxicodone, OxyContin, Percodan, Percocet, Vicodin
Propoxyphene	Darvon, others
Buprenorphine	Buprenex
Pentazocine	Talwin
Nalbuphine	Nubain
Butorphanol	Stadol

Opioid dependence is a cluster of physiological, behavioral, and cognitive symptoms, which together indicate repeated and continuing use of opioid drugs, despite significant problems related to such use. Drug dependence, in general, has been defined by the World Health Organization (WHO) as a syndrome in which the use of a drug or class of drugs takes on a much higher priority for a given person than other behaviors that once had a higher value. These brief definitions each have as their central features an emphasis on the drug-using behavior itself, its maladaptive nature, and how the choice to engage in that behavior shifts and becomes constrained as a result of interaction with the drug over time.

Opioid abuse is a term used to designate a pattern of maladaptive use of an opioid drug leading to clinically significant impairment or distress and occurring within a 12-month period, but one in which the symptoms have never met the criteria for opioid dependence.

The opioid-induced disorders include such common phenomena as opioid use disorder, opioid intoxication, opioid withdrawal, opioid-induced sleep disorder, and opioid-induced sexual dysfunction. Opioid intoxication delirium is occasionally seen in hospitalized patients. Opioid-induced psychotic disorder, opioid-induced mood disorder, and opioid-induced anxiety disorder, by contrast, are quite uncommon with μ-agonist opioids, but have been seen with certain mixed agonist–antagonist opioids acting at other receptors. The diagnosis of opioid-related disorder not elsewhere classified is used for situations that do not meet the criteria for any of the other opioid-related disorders.

In addition to the morbidity and mortality associated directly with the opioid-related disorders, the association between the transmission of the HIV and intravenous opioid and opiate use is now recognized as a leading national health concern. The words *opiate* and *opioid* come from the word opium, the juice of the opium poppy, *Papaver somniferum,* which contains approximately 20 opium alkaloids, including morphine.

Many synthetic opioids have been manufactured, including meperidine (Demerol), methadone (Dolophine), pentazocine (Talwin), and propoxyphene (Darvon). Methadone is the current gold standard in the treatment of opioid dependence. Opioid antagonists have been synthesized to treat opioid overdose and opioid dependence. This class of drugs includes naloxone (Narcan), naltrexone (ReVia), nalorphine, levallorphan, and apomorphine. Compounds with mixed agonist and antagonist activity at opioid receptors have been synthesized and include pentazocine, butorphanol (Stadol), and buprenorphine (Buprenex). Studies have found buprenorphine to be an effective treatment for opioid dependence.

EPIDEMIOLOGY

The use and dependence rates derived from national surveys do not accurately reflect fluctuations in drug use among opioid-dependent and previously opioid-dependent populations. When the supply of illicit heroin increases in purity or decreases in price, use among that vulnerable population tends to increase, with subsequent increases in adverse consequences (emergency room visits) and requests for treatment. The number of current heroin users in the United States has been estimated to be between 600,000 and 800,000. The number of people estimated to have used heroin at any time in their lives (lifetime users) is estimated at approximately 3 million.

In 2010, an estimated 140,000 persons had used heroin for the first time within the past 12 months. The average age of first use among recent initiates was 21.3 years in 2010. Opioid use in the United States experienced a resurgence in the 1990s, with emergency department visits related to heroin abuse doubling between 1990 and 1995. This increase in heroin use was associated with an increase in heroin purity and a decrease in its street price. In the late 1990s, heroin use increased among people who were 18 to 25 years of age, and a brief upsurge was seen in the use of oxycodone (OxyContin). Methods of administration other than injecting, such as smoking and snorting, increased in popularity. In 2010, the number of new nonmedical users of psychiatry of oxycodone was 598,000, with an average age of first use of 22.8 years. Comparable data on past year oxycodone initiation are not available for prior years, but calendar year estimates of oxycodone initiation show a steady increase in the number of initiates from 1995, the year this drug was first available, through 2003. The male-to-female ratio of persons with heroin dependence is approximately 3:1. Users of opioids typically started to use substances in their teens and early 20s; currently, most persons with opioid dependence are in their 30s and 40s. The tendency for dependence to remit generally begins after age 40 years and has been called "maturing out." Many persons, however, have remained opioid dependent for 50 years or longer. In the United States, persons tend to experience their first opioid-induced experience in their early teens or even as young as 10 years of age. Early induction into the drug culture is likely in communities in which substance abuse is rampant and in families in which the parents are substance abusers. A heroin habit can cost a person hundreds of dollars a day; thus, a person with opioid dependence needs to obtain money through criminal activities and prostitution. The involvement of persons with opioid dependence in prostitution accounts for much of the spread of HIV. The lifetime prevalence for heroin use is approximately 1 percent, with 0.2 percent having taken the drug during the prior year.

NEUROPHARMACOLOGY

The primary effects of the opioid drugs are mediated via the opioid receptors, which were discovered in the first half of the 1970s (published in 1973). The μ-opioid receptors are involved in the regulation and mediation of analgesia, respiratory depression, constipation, and drug dependence; the κ-opioid receptors, with analgesia, diuresis, and sedation; and the Δ-opioid receptors, with analgesia.

In 1975, the enkephalins, two endogenous pentapeptides with opioid-like actions, were identified. This discovery led to the identification of three classes of endogenous opioids within the brain, including the endorphins, the dynorphins, and the enkephalins. The term "endorphin" (a contraction of "endogenous" and "morphine") was coined by Dr. Eric Simon, Professor of psychiatry at NYU School of Medicine, one of the scientists who discovered the opioid receptors, to serve as a generic name for all molecules with morphine-like activity found in the brain. Endorphins are involved in neural transmission and pain suppression. They are released naturally in the body when a person is physically hurt or severely stressed and are thought to account for the absence of pain during acute injuries.

The endogenous opioids also have significant interactions with other neuronal systems, such as the dopaminergic and noradrenergic neurotransmitter systems. Several types of data indicate that the addictive rewarding properties of opioids are mediated through activation of the ventral tegmental area dopaminergic neurons that project to the cerebral cortex and the limbic system.

Heroin, the most commonly abused opioid, is more lipid soluble than morphine. This allows it to cross the blood–brain barrier faster and have a more rapid and pleasurable onset than morphine. Heroin was first introduced as a treatment for morphine addiction, but heroin, in fact, is more dependence producing than morphine. Codeine, which occurs naturally as approximately 0.5 percent of the opiate alkaloids in opium, is absorbed easily through the gastrointestinal tract and is subsequently transformed into morphine in the body. Results of at least one study using positron emission tomography (PET) have suggested that one effect of all opioids is decreased cerebral blood flow in selected brain regions in persons with opioid dependence. There is interesting evidence indicating that the endorphins are involved in other addictions, such as alcoholism, cocaine, and cannabinoid addiction. The opioid antagonist, naltrexone, has shown value in mitigating alcohol addiction.

The discovery of this new endorphinergic neuromodulatory system has led to the discovery of an endogenous cannabinoid system and has stimulated many outstanding laboratories to do research toward improved pain management and prevention and treatment of narcotic addiction.

Table 16.7–2
Non–Substance-Related Psychiatric Disorders in Opioid Users

Diagnostic Category[a]	Lifetime Rates % (Current Rates %) Men (N = 378)	Women (N = 338)	Total
Mood disorder	11.4 (2.1)	27.5 (5.3)	19.0 (3.6)
Major depressive disorder	8.7 (1.3)	23.7 (5.3)	15.8 (3.2)
Dysthymic disorder	2.4 (2.4)	4.4 (4.4)	3.4 (3.4)
Bipolar I disorder	0.8 (0.8)	0.0 (0.0)	0.4 (0.4)
Anxiety disorder	6.1 (3.4)	10.7 (6.8)	8.2 (5.0)
Simple phobia	1.9 (1.9)	5.3 (3.6)	3.5 (2.7)
Social phobia	1.9 (0.8)	3.6 (2.7)	2.7 (1.7)
Panic disorder	2.1 (0.3)	1.8 (0.9)	2.0 (0.6)
Agoraphobia	0.0 (0.0)	0.6 (0.3)	0.3 (0.1)
Obsessive-compulsive disorder	0.5 (0.5)	0.0 (0.0)	0.3 (0.3)
General anxiety disorder	0.8 (0.8)	0.0 (0.0)	0.1 (0.1)
Eating disorders	0.0 (0.0)	1.5 (0.0)	0.7 (0.0)
Bulimia nervosa	0.0 (0.0)	0.9 (0.0)	0.4 (0.0)
Anorexia nervosa	0.0 (0.0)	0.6 (0.0)	0.3 (0.0)
Schizophrenia	0.0 (0.0)	0.3 (0.3)	0.1 (0.1)

[a]Multiple disorders possible.

Adapted from Brooner RK, King VL, Kidorf M, Schmidt CW, Bigelow GE. Psychiatric and substance use comorbidity among treatment-seeking opioid abusers. *Arch Gen Psychiatry*. 1997;54:71.

Tolerance and Dependence

Tolerance to all actions of opioid drugs does not develop uniformly. Tolerance to some actions of opioids can be so high that a 100-fold increase in dose is required to produce the original effect. For example, terminally ill cancer patients may need 200 to 300 mg a day of morphine, whereas a dose of 60 mg can easily be fatal to an opioid-naive person. The symptoms of opioid withdrawal do not appear unless a person has been using opioids for a long time or when cessation is particularly abrupt, as occurs functionally when an opioid antagonist is given. The long-term use of opioids results in changes in the number and sensitivity of opioid receptors, which mediate at least some of the effects of tolerance and withdrawal. Although long-term use is associated with increased sensitivity of the dopaminergic, cholinergic, and serotonergic neurons, the effect of opioids on the noradrenergic neurons is probably the primary mediator of the symptoms of opioid withdrawal. Short-term use of opioids apparently decreases the activity of the noradrenergic neurons in the locus ceruleus; long-term use activates a compensatory homeostatic mechanism within the neurons; and opioid withdrawal results in rebound hyperactivity. This hypothesis also provides an explanation for why clonidine (Catapres), an α_2-adrenergic receptor agonist that decreases the release of norepinephrine, is useful in the treatment of opioid withdrawal symptoms.

COMORBIDITY

Approximately 90 percent of persons with opioid dependence have an additional psychiatric disorder. The most common comorbid psychiatric diagnoses are major depressive disorder, alcohol use disorders, antisocial personality disorder, and anxiety disorders. Approximately 15 percent of persons with opioid dependence attempt to commit suicide at least once. The high prevalence of comorbidity with other psychiatric diagnoses (Table 16.7–2) highlights the need to develop a broad-based treatment program that also addresses patients' associated psychiatric disorders.

ETIOLOGY

Psychosocial Factors

Opioid dependence is not limited to low socioeconomic status (SES), although the incidence of opioid dependence is greater in these groups than in higher SES groups. Social factors associated with urban poverty probably contribute to opioid dependence. Approximately 50 percent of urban heroin users are children of single parents or divorced parents and are from families in which at least one other member has a substance-related disorder. Children from such settings are at high risk for opioid dependence, especially if they also evidence behavioral problems in school or other signs of conduct disorder.

Some consistent behavior patterns seem to be especially pronounced in adolescents with opioid dependence. These patterns have been called the *heroin behavior syndrome:* underlying depression, often of an agitated type and frequently accompanied by anxiety symptoms; impulsiveness expressed by a passive-aggressive orientation; fear of failure; use of heroin as an anti-anxiety agent to mask feelings of low self-esteem, hopelessness, and aggression; limited coping strategies and low frustration tolerance, accompanied by the need for immediate gratification; sensitivity to drug contingencies, with a keen awareness of the relation between good feelings and the act of drug taking; feelings of behavioral impotence counteracted by momentary control over the life situation by means of substances; disturbances in social and interpersonal relationships with peers maintained by mutual substance experiences.

Biological and Genetic Factors

Evidence now exists for common and drug-specific, genetically transmitted vulnerability factors that increase the likelihood of developing drug dependence. Individuals who abuse a substance from any category are more likely to abuse substances from other categories. Monozygotic twins are more likely than dizygotic twins to be concordant for opioid dependence. Multivariate modeling techniques have indicated that not only was the genetic contribution high for heroin abuse in this group, but also a higher proportion of the variance because of genetic factors was not shared with the common vulnerability factor—that is, it was specific for opioids.

A person with an opioid-related disorder may have had genetically determined hypoactivity of the opiate system. Researchers are investigating the possibility that such hypoactivity may be caused by too few, or less-sensitive, opioid receptors, by release of too little endogenous opioid, or by overly high concentrations of a hypothesized endogenous opioid antagonist. A biological predisposition to an opioid-related disorder may also be associated with abnormal functioning in either the dopaminergic or the noradrenergic neurotransmitter system.

Psychodynamic Theory

In psychoanalytic literature, the behavior of persons addicted to narcotics has been described in terms of libidinal fixation, with regression to pregenital, oral, or even more archaic levels of psychosexual development. The need to explain the relation of drug abuse, defense mechanisms, impulse control, affective disturbances, and adaptive mechanisms led to the shift from psychosexual formulations to formulations emphasizing ego psychology. Serious ego pathology, often thought to be associated with substance abuse, is considered to indicate profound developmental disturbances. Problems of the relation between the ego and affects emerge as a key area of difficulty.

DIAGNOSIS

Opioid Use Disorder

Opioid use disorder is a pattern of maladaptive use of an opioid drug, leading to clinically significant impairment or distress and occurring within a 12-month period.

> A 42-year-old executive in a public relations firm was referred for psychiatric consultation by his surgeon, who discovered him sneaking large quantities of a codeine-containing cough medicine into the hospital. The patient had been a heavy cigarette smoker for 20 years and had a chronic, hacking cough. He had come into the hospital for a hernia repair and found the pain from the incision unbearable when he coughed.
>
> A back operation 5 years previously had led his doctors to prescribe codeine to help relieve the incisional pain at that time. Over the intervening 5 years, however, the patient had continued to use codeine-containing tablets and had increased his intake to 60 to 90 mg daily. He stated that he often "just took them by the handful—not to feel good, you understand, just to get by." He spent considerable time and effort developing a circle of physicians and pharmacists to whom he would "make the rounds" at least three times a week to obtain new supplies of pills. He had tried several times to stop using codeine, but had failed. During this period he lost two jobs because of lax work habits and was divorced by his wife of 11 years.

Opioid Intoxication

Opioid intoxication includes maladaptive behavioral changes and specific physical symptoms of opioid use. In general, altered mood, psychomotor retardation, drowsiness, slurred speech, and impaired memory and attention in the presence of other indicators of recent opioid use strongly suggest a diagnosis of opioid intoxication.

Opioid Withdrawal

The *Diagnostic and Statistical Manual of Mental Disorders,* fifth edition (DSM-5) diagnostic criteria for opioid withdrawal are described below. The general rule about the onset and duration of withdrawal symptoms is that substances with short durations of action tend to produce short, intense withdrawal syndromes and substances with long durations of action produce prolonged, but mild, withdrawal syndromes. An exception to the rule, narcotic antagonist-precipitated withdrawal after long-acting opioid dependence can be severe.

An abstinence syndrome can be precipitated by administration of an opioid antagonist. The symptoms can begin within seconds of such an intravenous injection and peak in approximately 1 hour. Opioid craving rarely occurs in the context of analgesic administration for pain from physical disorders or surgery. The full withdrawal syndrome, including intense craving for opioids, usually occurs only secondary to abrupt cessation of use in persons with opioid dependence.

Morphine and Heroin. The morphine and heroin withdrawal syndrome begins 6 to 8 hours after the last dose, usually after a 1- to 2-week period of continuous use or after the administration of a narcotic antagonist. The withdrawal syndrome reaches its peak intensity during the second or third day and subsides during the next 7 to 10 days, but some symptoms may persist for 6 months or longer.

Meperidine. The withdrawal syndrome from meperidine begins quickly, reaches a peak in 8 to 12 hours, and ends in 4 to 5 days.

Methadone. Methadone withdrawal usually begins 1 to 3 days after the last dose and ends in 10 to 14 days.

Symptoms. Opioid withdrawal consists of severe muscle cramps and bone aches, profuse diarrhea, abdominal cramps, rhinorrhea, lacrimation, piloerection or gooseflesh (from which comes the term *cold turkey* for the abstinence syndrome), yawning, fever, pupillary dilation, hypertension, tachycardia, and temperature dysregulation, including hypothermia and hyperthermia. Persons with opioid dependence seldom die from opioid withdrawal, unless they have a severe preexisting physical illness such as cardiac disease. Residual symptoms—such as insomnia, bradycardia, temperature dysregulation, and a craving for opioids—can persist for months after withdrawal. Associated features of opioid withdrawal include restlessness, irritability, depression, tremor, weakness, nausea, and vomiting. At any time during the abstinence syndrome, a single injection of morphine or heroin eliminates all the symptoms.

Opioid Intoxication Delirium

Opioid intoxication delirium is most likely to happen when opioids are used in high doses, are mixed with other psychoactive compounds, or are used by a person with preexisting brain damage or a CNS disorder (e.g., epilepsy).

Opioid-Induced Psychotic Disorder

Opioid-induced psychotic disorder can begin during opioid intoxication. Clinicians can specify whether hallucinations or delusions are the predominant symptoms.

Opioid-Induced Mood Disorder

Opioid-induced mood disorder can begin during opioid intoxication. Opioid-induced mood disorder symptoms can have a manic, depressed, or mixed nature, depending on a person's response to opioids. A person coming to psychiatric attention with opioid-induced mood disorder usually has mixed symptoms, combining irritability, expansiveness, and depression.

Opioid-Induced Sleep Disorder and Opioid-Induced Sexual Dysfunction

Hypersomnia is likely to be more common with opioids than insomnia. The most common sexual dysfunction is likely to be impotence.

Unspecified Opioid-Related Disorder

The DSM-5 includes diagnoses for other opioid-related disorders with symptoms of delirium, abnormal mood, psychosis, abnormal sleep, and sexual dysfunction. Clinical situations that do not fit into these categories exemplify appropriate cases for the use of the DSM-5 diagnosis of unspecified opioid-related disorder.

CLINICAL FEATURES

Opioids can be taken orally, snorted intranasally, and injected intravenously or subcutaneously. Opioids are subjectively addictive because of the euphoric high (the rush) that users experience, especially those who take the substances intravenously. The associated symptoms include a feeling of warmth, heaviness of the extremities, dry mouth, itchy face (especially the nose), and facial flushing. The initial euphoria is followed by a period of sedation, known in street parlance as "nodding off." Opioid use can induce dysphoria, nausea, and vomiting in opioid-naive persons.

The physical effects of opioids include respiratory depression, pupillary constriction, smooth muscle contraction (including the ureters and the bile ducts), constipation, and changes in blood pressure, heart rate, and body temperature. The respiratory depressant effects are mediated at the level of the brainstem.

Adverse Effects

The most common and most serious adverse effect associated with the opioid-related disorders is the potential transmission of hepatitis and HIV through the use of contaminated needles by more than one person. Persons can experience idiosyncratic allergic reactions to opioids, which result in anaphylactic shock, pulmonary edema, and death if they do not receive prompt and adequate treatment. Another serious adverse effect is an idiosyncratic drug interaction between meperidine and MAOIs, which can produce gross autonomic instability, severe behavioral agitation, coma, seizures, and death. Opioids and MAOIs should not be given together for this reason.

Opioid Overdose

Death from an overdose of an opioid is usually attributable to respiratory arrest from the respiratory depressant effect of the drug. The symptoms of overdose include marked unresponsiveness, coma, slow respiration, hypothermia, hypotension, and bradycardia. When presented with the clinical triad of coma, pinpoint pupils, and respiratory depression, clinicians should consider opioid overdose as a primary diagnosis. They can also inspect the patient's body for needle tracks in the arms, legs, ankles, groin, and even the dorsal vein of the penis.

MPTP-Induced Parkinsonism

In 1976, after ingesting an opioid contaminated with methyl-phenyltetrahydropyridine (MPTP), several persons developed a syndrome of irreversible parkinsonism. The mechanism for the neurotoxic effect is as follows: MPTP is converted into 1-methyl-4-phenylpyridinium (MPP+) by the enzyme monoamine oxidase and is then taken up by dopaminergic neurons. Because MPP+ binds to melanin in substantia nigra neurons, MPP+ is concentrated in these neurons and eventually kills the cells. PET studies of persons who ingested MPTP but remained asymptomatic have shown a decreased number of dopamine-binding sites in the substantia nigra. This decrease reflects a loss in the number of dopaminergic neurons in that region.

TREATMENT AND REHABILITATION

Overdose Treatment

The first task in overdose treatment is to ensure an adequate airway. Tracheopharyngeal secretions should be aspirated; an airway may be inserted. The patient should be ventilated mechanically until naloxone, a specific opioid antagonist, can be given. Naloxone is administered intravenously at a slow rate—initially approximately 0.8 mg per 70 kg of body weight. Signs of improvement (increased respiratory rate and pupillary dilation) should occur promptly. In opioid-dependent patients, too much naloxone may produce signs of withdrawal as well as reversal of overdosage. If no response to the initial dosage occurs, naloxone administration may be repeated after intervals of a few minutes. Previously, it was thought that if no response was observed after 4 to 5 mg, the CNS depression was probably not caused solely by opioids. The duration of action of naloxone is short compared with that of many opioids, such as methadone and levomethadyl acetate, and repeated administration may be required to prevent recurrence of opioid toxicity.

Medically Supervised Withdrawal and Detoxification

Opioid Agents for Treating Opioid Withdrawal: Methadone. Methadone is a synthetic narcotic (an opioid) that substitutes for heroin and can be taken orally. When given to addicts to replace their usual substance of abuse, the drug suppresses withdrawal symptoms. A daily dose of 20 to 80 mg suffices to stabilize a patient, although daily doses of up to 120 mg have been used. The duration of action for methadone exceeds 24 hours; thus, once-daily dosing is adequate. Methadone maintenance is continued until the patient can be withdrawn from methadone, which itself causes dependence. An abstinence syndrome occurs with methadone withdrawal, but patients are detoxified from methadone more easily than from heroin. Clonidine (0.1 to 0.3 mg three to four times a day) is usually given during the detoxification period.

Methadone maintenance has several advantages. First, it frees persons with opioid dependence from using injectable heroin and, thus, reduces the chance of spreading HIV through contaminated needles. Second, methadone produces minimal euphoria and rarely causes drowsiness or depression when taken for a long time. Third, methadone allows patients to engage in gainful employment instead of criminal activity. The major disadvantage of methadone use is that patients remain dependent on a narcotic.

Other Opioid Substitutes

LEVOMETHADYL (LAAM). LAAM is an opioid agonist that suppresses opioid withdrawal. It is no longer used, however, because some patients developed prolonged QT intervals associated with potentially fatal arrhythmias (*torsades de pointes*).

BUPRENORPHINE. As with methadone and LAAM, buprenorphine is an opioid agonist approved for opioid dependence in 2002. It can be dispensed on an outpatient basis, but prescribing physicians must demonstrate that they have received special training in its use. Buprenorphine in a daily dose of 8 to 10 mg appears to reduce heroin use. Buprenorphine is also effective in thrice-weekly dosing because of its slow dissociation from opioid receptors. After repeated administration, it attenuates or blocks the subjective effects of parenterally administered opioids such as heroin or morphine. A mild opioid withdrawal syndrome occurs if the drug is abruptly discontinued after chronic administrations.

Opioid Antagonists. Opioid antagonists block or antagonize the effects of opioids. Unlike methadone, they do not exert narcotic effects and do not cause dependence. Opioid antagonists include naloxone, which is used in the treatment of opioid overdose because it reverses the effects of narcotics, and naltrexone, the longest-acting (72 hours) antagonist. The theory for using an antagonist for opioid-related disorders is that blocking opioid agonist effects, particularly euphoria, discourages persons with opioid dependence from substance-seeking behavior and, thus, deconditions this behavior. The major weakness of the antagonist treatment model is the lack of any mechanism that compels a person to continue to take the antagonist. In this respect, it resembles the use of Antabuse in the treatment of alcoholism; patients must be motivated to take the drug.

Recently, programs have been developed in which first responders, including police, have been given Naltrexone kits (which include naltrexone nasal spray) to use in persons who have taken an overdose of opioids, usually heroin. A number of deaths have been prevented as a result of these interventions.

Pregnant Women with Opioid Dependence

Neonatal addiction is a significant problem. Approximately three-fourths of all infants born to addicted mothers experience the withdrawal syndrome.

Neonatal Withdrawal. Although opioid withdrawal is rarely fatal for the otherwise healthy adult, it is hazardous to the fetus and can lead to miscarriage or fetal death. Maintaining a pregnant woman with opioid dependence on a low dose of methadone (10 to 40 mg daily) may be the least hazardous course to follow. At this dose, neonatal withdrawal is usually mild and can be managed with low doses of paregoric. If pregnancy begins while a woman is taking high doses of methadone, the dosage should be reduced slowly (e.g., 1 mg every 3 days), and fetal movements should be monitored. If withdrawal is necessary or desired, it is least hazardous during the second trimester.

Fetal AIDS Transmission. Acquired immune deficiency syndrome (AIDS) is the other major risk to the fetus of a woman with opioid dependence. Pregnant women can pass HIV, the causative agent of AIDS, to the fetus through the placental circulation. An HIV-infected mother can also pass HIV to the infant through breast-feeding. The use of zidovudine (Retrovir) alone or in combination with other anti-HIV medication in infected women can decrease the incidence of HIV in newborns.

Psychotherapy

The entire range of psychotherapeutic modalities is appropriate for treating opioid-related disorders. Individual psychotherapy, behavioral therapy, cognitive-behavioral therapy, family therapy, support groups (e.g., Narcotics Anonymous [NA]), and social skills training may all prove effective for specific patients. Social skills training should be particularly emphasized for patients with few social skills. Family therapy is usually indicated when the patient lives with family members.

Therapeutic Communities

Therapeutic communities are residences in which all members have a substance abuse problem. Abstinence is the rule; to be admitted to such a community, a person must show a high level of motivation. The goals are to effect a complete change of lifestyle, including abstinence from substances; to develop personal honesty, responsibility, and useful social skills; and to eliminate antisocial attitudes and criminal behavior.

The staff members of most therapeutic communities are persons with former substance dependence who often put prospective candidates through a rigorous screening process to test their motivation. Self-help through the use of confrontational groups and isolation from the outside world and from friends associated with the drug life are emphasized. The prototypical community for persons with substance dependence is Phoenix House, where the residents live for long periods (usually 12 to 18 months) while receiving treatment. They are allowed to return to their old environments only when they have demonstrated their ability to handle increased responsibility within the therapeutic community. Therapeutic communities can be effective but require large staffs and extensive facilities. Moreover, dropout rates are high; up to 75 percent of those who enter therapeutic communities leave within the first month.

Education and Needle Exchange

Although the essential treatment of opioid use disorders is encouraging persons to abstain from opioids, education about the transmission of HIV must receive equal attention. Persons with opioid dependence who use intravenous or subcutaneous routes of administration must be taught available safe-sex practices. Free needle-exchange programs are often subject to intense political and societal pressures but, where allowed, should be made available to persons with opioid dependence. Several studies have indicated that unsafe needle sharing is common when it is difficult to obtain enough clean needles and is also common in persons with legal difficulties, severe substance problems, and psychiatric symptoms. These are just the persons most likely to be involved in transmitting HIV.

Narcotic Anonymous

Narcotics Anonymous is a self-help group of abstinent drug addicts modeled on the 12-step principles of Alcoholics Anonymous (AA). Such groups now exist in most large cities and can provide useful group support. The outcome for patients treated in 12-step programs is generally good, but the anonymity that is at the core of the 12-step model has made detailed evaluation of its efficacy in treating opioid dependence difficult.

▲ 16.8 Sedative-, Hypnotic-, or Anxiolytic-Related Disorders

The drugs discussed in this section are referred to as *anxiolytic* or *sedative–hypnotic* drugs. Their sedative or calming effects are on a continuum with their hypnotic or sleep-inducing effects. In addition to their psychiatric indications, these drugs are also used as antiepileptics, muscle relaxants, anesthetics, and anesthetic adjuvants. Alcohol and all drugs of this class are cross-tolerant, and their effects are additive. Physical and psychological dependence develops to these drugs, and all are associated with withdrawal symptoms. In the practice of psychiatry and addiction medicine, the drug class that is clinically most important is the benzodiazepines.

The three major groups of drugs associated with this class of substance-related disorders are benzodiazepines, barbiturates, and barbiturate-like substances. Each group is discussed below.

BENZODIAZEPINES

Many benzodiazepines, differing primarily in their half-lives, are available in the United States. Examples of benzodiazepines are diazepam, flurazepam (Dalmane), oxazepam (Serax), and chlordiazepoxide (Librium). Benzodiazepines are used primarily as anxiolytics, hypnotics, antiepileptics, and anesthetics, as well as for alcohol withdrawal. After their introduction in the United States in the 1960s, benzodiazepines rapidly became the most prescribed drugs; approximately 15 percent of all persons in the United States have had a benzodiazepine prescribed by a physician. Increasing awareness of the risks for dependence on benzodiazepines and increased regulatory requirements, however, have decreased the number of benzodiazepine prescriptions. The Drug Enforcement Agency (DEA) classifies all benzodiazepines as Schedule IV controlled substances.

Flunitrazepam (Rohypnol), a benzodiazepine used in Mexico, South America, and Europe but not available in the United States, has become a drug of abuse. When taken with alcohol, it has been associated with promiscuous sexual behavior and rape. It is illegal to bring flunitrazepam into the United States. Although misused in the United States, it remains a standard anxiolytic in many countries.

Non-benzodiazepine sedatives such as zolpidem (Ambien), zaleplon (Sonata), and eszopiclone (Lunesta)—the so-called Z drugs—have clinical effects similar to the benzodiazepines and are also subject to misuse and dependence.

BARBITURATES

Before the introduction of benzodiazepines, barbiturates were frequently prescribed, but because of their high abuse potential, their use is much rarer today. Secobarbital (popularly known as "reds," "red devils," "seggies," and "downers"), pentobarbital (Nembutal) (known as "yellow jackets," "yellows," and "nembies"), and a secobarbital–amobarbital combination (known as "reds and blues," "rainbows," "double-trouble," and "tooies") are easily available on the street from drug dealers. Pentobarbital, secobarbital, and amobarbital (Amytal) are now under the same federal legal controls as morphine.

The first barbiturate, barbital (Veronal), was introduced in the United States in 1903. Barbital and phenobarbital (Solfoton, Luminal), which was introduced shortly thereafter, are long-acting drugs with half-lives of 12 to 24 hours. Amobarbital is an intermediate-acting barbiturate with a half-life of 6 to 12 hours. Pentobarbital and secobarbital are short-acting barbiturates with half-lives of 3 to 6 hours. Although barbiturates are useful and effective sedatives, they are highly lethal with only ten times the normal dose producing coma and death.

BARBITURATE-LIKE SUBSTANCES

The most commonly abused barbiturate-like substance is methaqualone, which is no longer manufactured in the United States. It is often used by young persons who believe that the substance heightens the pleasure of sexual activity. Abusers of methaqualone commonly take one or two standard tablets (usually 300 mg per tablet) to obtain the desired effects. The street names for methaqualone include "mandrakes" (from the United Kingdom preparation Mandrax) and "soapers" (from the brand name Sopor). "Luding out" (from the brand name Quaalude) means getting high on methaqualone, which is often combined with excessive alcohol intake.

Other barbiturate-like substances include meprobamate (Equanil), a carbamate derivative that has weak efficacy as an antianxiety agent but has muscle-relaxant effects and is used for that purpose; chloral hydrate, a hypnotic that is highly toxic to the GI system and, when combined with alcohol, is known as a "mickey finn"; and ethchlorvynol, a rapidly acting sedative agent with anticonvulsant and muscle-relaxant properties. All are subject to abuse.

EPIDEMIOLOGY

Approximately 6 percent of individuals have used either sedatives or tranquilizers illicitly, including 0.3 percent who reported illicit use of sedatives in the prior year and 0.1 percent who reported use of sedatives in the prior month. The age group with the highest lifetime prevalence of sedative (3 percent) or tranquilizer (6 percent) use was 26 to 34 years of age, and those aged 18 to 25 were most likely to have used sedatives or tranquilizers in the prior year. About one-fourth to one-third of all substance-related emergency room visits involve substances of this class. The patients have a female-to-male ratio of 3:1 and a white-to-black ratio of 2:1. Some persons use benzodiazepines alone, but persons who use cocaine often use benzodiazepines to reduce withdrawal symptoms, and opioid abusers use them to enhance the euphoric effects of opioids. Because they are easily obtained, benzodiazepines are also used by abusers of stimulants, hallucinogens, and PCP to help reduce the anxiety that can be caused by those substances.

Whereas barbiturate abuse is common among mature adults who have long histories of abuse of these substances, benzodiazepines are abused by a younger age group, usually those under 40 years of age. This group may have a slight male predominance and has a white-to-black ratio of approximately 2:1. Benzodiazepines are probably not abused as frequently as other substances for the purpose of getting "high," or inducing a euphoric feeling. Rather, they are used when a person wishes to experience a general relaxed feeling.

NEUROPHARMACOLOGY

The benzodiazepines, barbiturates, and barbiturate-like substances all have their primary effects on the GABA type A ($GABA_A$) receptor complex, which contains a chloride ion channel, a binding site for GABA, and a well-defined binding site for benzodiazepines. The barbiturates and barbiturate-like substances are also believed to bind somewhere on the $GABA_A$ receptor complex. When a benzodiazepine, barbiturate, or barbiturate-like substance does bind to the complex, the effect is to increase the affinity of the receptor for its endogenous neurotransmitter, GABA, and to increase the flow of chloride ions through the channel into the neuron. The influx of negatively charged chloride ions into the neuron is inhibitory, and hyperpolarizes the neuron relative to the extracellular space.

Although all the substances in this class induce tolerance and physical dependence, the mechanisms behind these effects are best understood for the benzodiazepines. After long-term benzodiazepine use, the receptor effects caused by the agonist are attenuated. Specifically, GABA stimulation of the $GABA_A$ receptors results in less chloride influx than was caused by GABA stimulation before the benzodiazepine administration. This downregulation of receptor response is not caused by a decrease in receptor number or by decreased affinity of the receptor for GABA. The basis for the downregulation seems to be in the coupling between the GABA binding site and the activation of the chloride ion channel. This decreased efficiency in coupling may be regulated within the $GABA_A$ receptor complex itself or by other neuronal mechanisms.

DIAGNOSIS

Sedative, Hypnotic, or Anxiolytic Use Disorder

Sedative, hypnotic, or anxiolytic use disorder is diagnosed according to the general criteria in the fifth edition of the *Diagnostic and Statistical Manual of Mental Disorders* (DSM-5) for substance use disorder (see Section 16.1).

Sedative, Hypnotic, or Anxiolytic Intoxication

The intoxication syndromes induced by all these drugs are similar, and include incoordination, dysarthria, nystagmus, impaired memory, gait disturbance, and in severe cases stupor, coma, or death. The diagnosis of intoxication by one of this class of substances is best confirmed by obtaining a blood sample for substance screening.

Benzodiazepines. Benzodiazepine intoxication can be associated with behavioral disinhibition, potentially resulting in hostile or aggressive behavior in some persons. The effect is perhaps most common when benzodiazepines are taken in combination with alcohol. Benzodiazepine intoxication is associated with less euphoria than is intoxication by other drugs in this class. This characteristic is the basis for the lower abuse and dependence potential of benzodiazepines than of barbiturates.

Barbiturates and Barbiturate-like Substances. When barbiturates and barbiturate-like substances are taken in relatively low doses, the clinical syndrome of intoxication is indistinguishable from that associated with alcohol intoxication. The symptoms include sluggishness, incoordination, difficulty thinking, poor memory, slow speech and comprehension, faulty judgment, disinhibited sexual aggressive impulses, narrowed range of attention, emotional lability, and exaggerated basic personality traits. The sluggishness usually resolves after a few hours, but depending primarily on the half-life of the abused substance, impaired judgment, distorted mood, and impaired motor skills may remain for 12 to 24 hours. Other potential symptoms are hostility, argumentativeness, moroseness, and, occasionally, paranoid and suicidal ideation. The neurological effects include nystagmus, diplopia, strabismus, ataxic gait, positive Romberg's sign, hypotonia, and decreased superficial reflexes.

Sedative, Hypnotic, or Anxiolytic Withdrawal

Benzodiazepines. The severity of the withdrawal syndrome associated with the benzodiazepines varies significantly depending on the average dose and the duration of use, but a mild withdrawal syndrome can follow even short-term use of relatively low doses of benzodiazepines. A significant withdrawal syndrome is likely to occur at cessation of dosages in the range of 40 mg a day for diazepam, for example, although 10 to 20 mg a day, taken for a month, can also result in a withdrawal syndrome when drug administration is stopped. The onset of withdrawal symptoms usually occurs 2 to 3 days after the cessation of use, but with long-acting drugs, such as diazepam, the latency before onset can be 5 or 6 days. The symptoms include anxiety, dysphoria, intolerance for bright lights and loud noises, nausea, sweating, muscle twitching, and sometimes seizures (generally at dosages of 50 mg a day or more of diazepam). Table 16.8–1 lists the signs and symptoms of benzodiazepine withdrawal.

Barbiturates and Barbiturate-like Substances. The withdrawal syndrome for barbiturate and barbiturate-like substances ranges from mild symptoms (e.g., anxiety, weakness, sweating, and insomnia) to severe symptoms (e.g., seizures, delirium, cardiovascular collapse, and death). Persons who have been abusing phenobarbital in the range of 400 mg a day may experience mild withdrawal symptoms; those who have been abusing the substance in the range of 800 mg a day can experience orthostatic hypotension, weakness, tremor, and severe anxiety. Approximately 75 percent of these persons have withdrawal-related seizures. Users of dosages higher than 800 mg a day may experience anorexia, delirium, hallucinations, and repeated seizures.

Most symptoms appear in the first 3 days of abstinence, and seizures generally occur on the second or third day, when the symptoms are worst. If seizures do occur, they always precede the development of delirium. The symptoms rarely occur more than a week after stopping the substance. A psychotic disorder, if it develops, starts on the third to eighth day. The various associated symptoms generally run their course within 2 to 3 days, but can last as long as 2 weeks. The first episode of the syndrome usually occurs after 5 to 15 years of heavy substance use.

Table 16.8–1
Signs and Symptoms of the Benzodiazepine Discontinuation Syndrome

The following signs and symptoms may be seen when benzodiazepine therapy is discontinued; they reflect the return of the original anxiety symptoms (recurrence), worsening of the original anxiety symptoms (rebound), or emergence of new symptoms (true withdrawal):

Disturbances of mood and cognition
Anxiety, apprehension, dysphoria, pessimism, irritability, obsessive rumination, and paranoid ideation

Disturbances of sleep
Insomnia, altered sleep–wake cycle, and daytime drowsiness

Physical signs and symptoms
Tachycardia, elevated blood pressure, hyperreflexia, muscle tension, agitation/motor restlessness, tremor, myoclonus, muscle and joint pain, nausea, coryza, diaphoresis, ataxia, tinnitus, and grand malseizures

Perceptual disturbances
Hyperacusis, depersonalization, blurred vision, illusions, and hallucinations

Other Sedative-, Hypnotic-, or Anxiolytic-Induced Disorders

Delirium. Delirium that is indistinguishable from delirium tremens associated with alcohol withdrawal is seen more commonly with barbiturate withdrawal than with benzodiazepine withdrawal. Delirium associated with intoxication can be seen with either barbiturates or benzodiazepines if the dosages are sufficiently high.

Persisting Dementia. The existence of the sedative/hypnotic-induced persisting dementia is controversial, because uncertainty exists whether a persisting dementia is caused by the substance use itself or by associated features of the substance use.

Persisting Amnestic Disorder. Amnestic disorders associated with sedatives and hypnotics may be underdiagnosed. One exception is the increased number of reports of amnestic episodes associated with short-term use of benzodiazepines with short half-lives (e.g., triazolam [Halcion]).

Psychotic Disorders. The psychotic symptoms of barbiturate withdrawal can be indistinguishable from those of alcohol-associated delirium tremens. Agitation, delusions, and hallucinations are usually visual, but sometimes tactile or auditory features develop after about 1 week of abstinence. Psychotic symptoms associated with intoxication or withdrawal are more common with barbiturates than with benzodiazepines. They are diagnosed in DSM-5 as sedative, hypnotic, or anxiolytic withdrawal with perceptual disturbances when reality testing is intact (the individual is aware that the drug is causing the psychotic symptoms). If reality testing is not intact (the individual believes the hallucinations are real), a diagnosis of substance/medication-induced psychotic disorder is more appropriate. Clinicians can further specify whether delusions or hallucinations are the predominant symptoms, including the type (e.g., auditory, visual, or tactile).

Other Disorders. Sedative and hypnotic use has also been associated with mood disorders, anxiety disorders, sleep disorders, and sexual dysfunctions.

Unspecified Sedative-, Hypnotic-, or Anxiolytic-Related Disorder. When none of the previously discussed diagnostic categories is appropriate for a person with sedative-, hypnotic-, or anxiolytic-related disorder, and he or she does not meet the diagnostic criteria for any general substance-related disorder, the appropriate diagnosis is unspecified sedative-, hypnotic-, or anxiolytic-related disorder.

CLINICAL FEATURES

Patterns of Abuse

Oral Use. Sedatives and hypnotics can all be taken orally, either occasionally to achieve a time-limited specific effect or regularly to obtain a constant, usually mild, intoxication state. The occasional use pattern is associated with young persons who take the substance to achieve specific effects—relaxation for an evening, intensification of sexual activities, and a short-lived period of mild euphoria. The user's personality and expectations about the substance's effects and the setting in which the substance is taken also affect the substance-induced experience. The regular use pattern is associated with middle-aged, middle-class persons who usually obtain the substance from a family physician as a prescription for insomnia or anxiety. Abusers of this type may have prescriptions from several physicians, and the pattern of abuse may go undetected until obvious signs of abuse or dependence are noticed by the person's family, coworkers, or physicians.

Intravenous Use. A severe form of abuse involves the intravenous use of this class of substances. The users are mainly young adults who are intimately involved with illegal substances. Intravenous barbiturate use is associated with a pleasant, warm, drowsy feeling, and users may be inclined to use barbiturates more than opioids because barbiturates are less costly. The physical dangers of injection include transmission of the HIV, cellulitis, vascular complications from accidental injection into an artery, infections, and allergic reactions to contaminants. Intravenous use is associated with rapid and profound tolerance and dependence and a severe withdrawal syndrome.

Overdose

Benzodiazepines. In contrast to the barbiturates and the barbiturate-like substances, the benzodiazepines have a large margin of safety when taken in overdoses, a feature that has contributed significantly to their rapid acceptance. The ratio of lethal dose to effective dose is approximately 200 to 1 or higher, because of the minimal degree of respiratory depression associated with the benzodiazepines. A list of equivalent therapeutic doses of benzodiazepines is given in Table 16.8–2. Even when grossly excessive amounts (more than 2 g) are taken in suicide attempts, the symptoms include only drowsiness, lethargy, ataxia, some confusion, and mild depression of the user's vital signs. A much more serious condition prevails when benzodiazepines are taken in overdose in combination with other sedative–hypnotic substances, such as alcohol. In such cases, small doses of benzodiazepines can cause death. The availability of flumazenil (Romazicon), a specific benzodiazepine antagonist, has reduced the lethality of the benzodiazepines. Flumazenil can be used in emergency rooms to reverse the effects of the benzodiazepines.

Barbiturates. Barbiturates are lethal when taken in overdose because they induce respiratory depression. In addition to intentional suicide attempts, accidental or unintentional overdoses are common. Barbiturates in home medicine cabinets are a common cause of fatal drug overdoses in children. As with benzodiazepines, the lethal effects of the barbiturates are additive to those of other sedatives or hypnotics, including alcohol and benzodiazepines. Barbiturate overdose is characterized by the induction of coma, respiratory arrest, cardiovascular failure, and death.

The lethal dose varies with the route of administration and the degree of tolerance for the substance after a history of long-term abuse. For the most commonly abused barbiturates, the ratio of lethal dose to effective dose ranges between 3:1 and 30:1. Dependent users often take an average daily dose of 1.5 g of a short-acting barbiturate, and some have been reported to take as much as 2.5 g a day for months.

The lethal dose is not much greater for the long-term abuser than for the neophyte. Tolerance develops quickly, to the point at which withdrawal in a hospital becomes necessary to prevent accidental death from overdose.

Table 16.8–2
Approximate Therapeutic Equivalent Doses of Benzodiazepines

Generic Name	Trade Name	Dose (mg)
Alprazolam	Xanax	1
Chlordiazepoxide	Librium	25
Clonazepam	Klonopin	0.5–1.0
Clorazepate	Tranxene	15
Diazepam	Valium	10
Estazolam	ProSom	1
Flurazepam	Dalmane	30
Lorazepam	Ativan	2
Oxazepam	Serax	30
Temazepam	Restoril	20
Triazolam	Halcion	0.25
Quazepam	Doral	15
Zolpidem	Ambien	10
Zaleplon	Sonata	10

Barbiturate-like Substances. The barbiturate-like substances vary in their lethality and are usually intermediate between the relative safety of the benzodiazepines and the high lethality of the barbiturates. An overdose of methaqualone, for example, can result in restlessness, delirium, hypertonia, muscle spasms, convulsions, and, in very high doses, death. Unlike barbiturates, methaqualone rarely causes severe cardiovascular or respiratory depression, and most fatalities result from combining methaqualone with alcohol.

TREATMENT AND REHABILITATION

Withdrawal

Benzodiazepines. Because some benzodiazepines are eliminated from the body slowly, symptoms of withdrawal can continue to develop for several weeks. To prevent seizures and other withdrawal symptoms, clinicians should gradually reduce the dosage. Several reports indicate that carbamazepine (Tegretol) may be useful in the treatment of benzodiazepine withdrawal. Table 16.8–3 lists guidelines for treating benzodiazepine withdrawal.

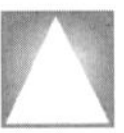

Table 16.8–3
Guidelines for Treatment of Benzodiazepine Withdrawal

1. Evaluate and treat concomitant medical and psychiatric conditions.
2. Obtain drug history and urine and blood sample for drug and ethanol assay.
3. Determine required dose of benzodiazepine or barbiturate for stabilization, guided by history, clinical presentation, drug-ethanol assay, and (in some cases) challenge dose.
4. Detoxification from supratherapeutic dosages:
   a. Hospitalize if there are medical or psychiatric indications, poor social supports, or polysubstance dependence or the patient is unreliable.
   b. Some clinicians recommend switching to longer-acting benzodiazepine for withdrawal (e.g., diazepam, clonazepam); others recommend stabilizing on the drug that patient was taking or on phenobarbital.
   c. After stabilization, reduce dosage by 30% on the second or third day and evaluate the response, keeping in mind that symptoms that occur after decreases in benzodiazepines with short elimination half-lives (e.g., lorazepam) appear sooner than with those with longer elimination half-lives (e.g., diazepam).
   d. Reduce dosage further by 10–25% every few days if tolerated.
   e. Use adjunctive medications if necessary—carbamazepine, β-adrenergic receptor antagonists, valproate, clonidine, and sedative antidepressants have been used but their efficacy in the treatment of the benzodiazepine abstinence syndrome has not been established).
5. Detoxification from therapeutic dosages:
   a. Initiate 10–25% dose reduction and evaluate response.
   b. Dose, duration of therapy, and severity of anxiety influence the rate of taper and need for adjunctive medications.
   c. Most patients taking therapeutic doses have uncomplicated discontinuation.
6. Psychological interventions may assist patients in detoxification from benzodiazepines and in the long-term management of anxiety.

Courtesy of Domenic A. Ciraulo, M.D., and Ofra Sarid-Segal, M.D.

Barbiturates. To avoid sudden death during barbiturate withdrawal, clinicians must follow conservative clinical guidelines. Clinicians should not give barbiturates to a comatose or grossly intoxicated patient. A clinician should attempt to determine a patient's usual daily dose of barbiturates and then verify the dosage clinically. For example, a clinician can give a test dose of 200 mg of pentobarbital every hour until a mild intoxication occurs but withdrawal symptoms are absent (Table 16.8–4). The clinician can then taper the total daily dose at a rate of approximately 10 percent of the total daily dose. Once the correct dosage is determined, a long-acting barbiturate can be used for the detoxification period. During this process, the patient may begin to experience withdrawal symptoms, in which case the clinician should halve the daily decrement.

In the withdrawal procedure, phenobarbital can be substituted for the more commonly abused short-acting barbiturates. The effects of phenobarbital last longer, and because barbiturate blood levels fluctuate less, phenobarbital does not cause observable toxic signs or a serious overdose. An adequate dose is 30 mg of phenobarbital for every 100 mg of the short-acting substance. The user should be maintained for

Table 16.8–4
Pentobarbital Test Dose Procedure for Barbiturate Withdrawal

Symptoms after Test Dose of 200 mg Oral Pentobarbital	Estimated 24-Hour Oral Pentobarbital Dose (mg)	Estimated 24-Hour Oral Phenobarbital Dose (mg)
Level I: Asleep but arousable; withdrawal symptoms not likely	0	0
Level II: Mild sedation; patient may have slurred speech, ataxia, nystagmus	500–600	150–200
Level III: Patient is comfortable: no evidence of sedation; may have nystagmus	800	250
Level IV: No drug effect	1,000–1,200	300–600

at least 2 days at that level before the dose is reduced further. The regimen is analogous to the substitution of methadone for heroin.

After withdrawal is complete, the patient must overcome the desire to start taking the substance again. Although substitution of nonbarbiturate sedatives or hypnotics for barbiturates has been suggested as a preventive therapeutic measure, this often results in replacing one substance dependence with another. If a user is to remain substance-free, follow-up treatment, usually with psychiatric help and community support, is vital. Otherwise, a patient will almost certainly return to barbiturates or a substance with similar hazards.

Overdose

The treatment of overdose of this class of substances involves gastric lavage, activated charcoal, and careful monitoring of vital signs and CNS activity. Patients who overdose and come to medical attention while awake should be kept from slipping into unconsciousness. Vomiting should be induced, and activated charcoal should be administered to delay gastric absorption. If a patient is comatose, the clinician must establish an intravenous fluid line, monitor the patient's vital signs, insert an endotracheal tube to maintain a patent airway, and provide mechanical ventilation, if necessary. Hospitalization of a comatose patient in an intensive care unit is usually required during the early stages of recovery from such overdoses.

EXPERT OPINION

The International Study of Expert Judgment on Therapeutic Use of Benzodiazepines and Other Psychotherapeutic Medications was designed to gather systematic data on the opinions of leading clinicians concerning the benefits and risks of benzodiazepines and alternative treatments of anxiety. This survey study addressed the relative risks of benzodiazepines compared with other agents and comparative risks within the class. The expert panel assessed risk based on a drug's potential to produce tolerance, rebound symptoms, a withdrawal syndrome, and ease of discontinuation.

Two-thirds of the expert panel reported that long-term use of benzodiazepines for the treatment of anxiety disorders does not pose a high risk of dependence and abuse. Although agreement was that the pharmacological properties of the medication may be the most important contributor to development of withdrawal symptoms, no consensus existed on whether benzodiazepines with shorter and longer half-lives have similar dependence potential. A clear consensus was that the differences in withdrawal symptoms are clinically negligible with gradual dose tapering. Because differences in abuse liability among the various benzodiazepines have not been demonstrated in humans, and because the benefits of benzodiazepine treatment clearly outweigh the risks, most physicians on the expert panel opposed increased restrictions on benzodiazepine prescribing.

Despite the expert opinion stated earlier, state and federal agencies have attempted to restrict the distribution of benzodiazepines by requiring special reporting forms. For example, in New York State, through the use of a newly enacted prescription monitoring program (PMP) called I-STOP, effective since August 27, 2013, doctors cannot write a prescription for a benzodiazepine unless they first search a computerized database that contains the names of all persons in the state who were ever prescribed benzodiazepines and other controlled substances. Governments have taken these and other such measures in an attempt to stem the tide of abuse. However most abuse results from the illicit manufacture, sale, and diversion of substances, particularly to cocaine and opioid addicts, not from physicians' prescriptions or legitimate pharmaceutical companies. These programs do not stem the tide of illegal use of valuable medications and interfere in the practice of medicine and in the confidential relationship between doctor and patient.

▲ 16.9 Stimulant-Related Disorders

AMPHETAMINES

Amphetamines and amphetamine-like drugs are among the most widely used illicit substances, second only to cannabis, in the United States, Asia, Great Britain, Australia, and several other Western European countries. Methamphetamine, a congener of amphetamine, has become even more popular in recent years.

The racemic amphetamine sulfate (Benzedrine) was first synthesized in 1887, and it was introduced to clinical practice in 1932 as an over-the-counter inhaler for the treatment of nasal congestion and asthma. In 1937, amphetamine sulfate tablets were introduced for the treatment of narcolepsy, postencephalitic Parkinsonism, depression, and lethargy. In the 1970s, a variety of social and regulatory factors began to curb widespread amphetamine distribution. The current U.S. Food and Drug Administration (FDA)–approved indications for amphetamine are limited to ADHD and narcolepsy; however, amphetamines are also used in the treatment of obesity, depression, dysthymia, chronic fatigue syndrome, AIDS, dementia, multiple sclerosis, fibromyalgia, and neurasthenia.

Preparations

The major amphetamines currently available and used in the United States are dextroamphetamine (Dexedrine), methamphetamine (Desoxyn), a mixed dextroamphetamine-amphetamine salt (Adderall), and the amphetamine-like compound methylphenidate (Ritalin). These drugs go by such street names as ice, crystal, crystal meth, and speed. As a general class, the amphetamines are referred to as analeptics, sympathomimetics, stimulants, and psychostimulants. The typical amphetamines are used to increase performance and to induce a euphoric feeling, for example, by students studying for examinations, by long-distance truck drivers on trips, by business people with important deadlines, by athletes in competition, and by soldiers during wartime. Although not as addictive as cocaine, amphetamines are nonetheless addictive drugs.

Other amphetamine-like substances are ephedrine, pseudoephedrine, and phenylpropanolamine (PPA). These drugs, PPA in particular, can dangerously exacerbate hypertension, precipitate a toxic psychosis, cause intestinal infarction, or result in death. The safety margin for PPA is particularly narrow, and three to four times the normal dose can result in life-threatening hypertension. In 2005, medications containing PPA were recalled by the FDA, and in 2006, the FDA prohibited the sale of over-the-counter medications containing ephedrine and regulated the sale of over-the-counter medications containing pseudoephedrine, which was being used illegally to make methamphetamine.

Amphetamine-type drugs with abuse potential also include phendimetrazine (Preludin), which is included in Schedule II of the Controlled Substance Act (CSA), and diethylpropion (Tenuate), benzphetamine (Didrex), and phentermine (Ionamin), which are included in Schedules III or IV of the CSA. It is presumed that all these drugs are capable of producing all the listed amphetamine-induced disorders. Modafinil (Provigil), used in the treatment of narcolepsy, also has stimulant and euphorigenic effects in humans, but its toxicity and likelihood of producing amphetamine-induced disorders are unknown.

Methamphetamine is a potent form of amphetamine that abusers of the substance inhale, smoke, or inject intravenously. Its psychological effects last for hours and are described as particularly powerful. Unlike cocaine (see discussion later in this section), which must be imported, methamphetamine is a synthetic drug that can be manufactured domestically in illicit laboratories.

Other agents called *substituted* or *designer amphetamines* are discussed separately later in this section.

Epidemiology

Amphetamine-type stimulant abuse represents major public health and law enforcement problems in the United States and abroad, primarily due to the consumption of methamphetamine. According to the Community Epidemiology Work Group, methamphetamine abuse occurs at epidemic levels in Hawaii, on the West Coast, and in some Southern states, and continues to spread eastward. Nationally, treatment admission rates for methamphetamine dependence more than doubled between 1995 and 2012, and in the western United States, treatment admission rates for methamphetamine dependence are higher than those of either cocaine or heroin. According to the National Association of Counties, nearly half (48 percent) of 500 county law enforcement agencies in the United States name methamphetamine as the primary drug problem, more than cocaine (22 percent), marijuana (22 percent), and heroin (2 percent) combined. Similarly, almost 40 percent of state and local law enforcement agencies identify methamphetamine as their greatest drug threat, second only to cocaine, a higher percentage than any other drug.

On a global basis, use of amphetamine-type stimulants, including methamphetamine, is also a major concern, ranking as the second most widely used substance, following marijuana, according to a report from the United Nations Office on Drugs and Crime. According to the 2010 National Survey on Drug Use and Health (NSDUH), 353,000 persons 12 years or older were current users of methamphetamine (0.1 percent).

Neuropharmacology

All the amphetamines are rapidly absorbed orally and have a rapid onset of action, usually within 1 hour when taken orally. The classic amphetamines are also taken intravenously and have an almost immediate effect by this route. Nonprescribed amphetamines and designer amphetamines are also inhaled ("snorting"). Tolerance develops with both classic and designer amphetamines, although amphetamine users often overcome the tolerance by taking more of the drug. Amphetamine is less addictive than cocaine, as evidenced by experiments on rats in which not all animals spontaneously self-administered low doses of amphetamine.

The classic amphetamines (i.e., dextroamphetamine, methamphetamine, and methylphenidate) produce their primary effects by causing the release of catecholamines, particularly dopamine, from presynaptic terminals. The effects are particularly potent for the dopaminergic neurons projecting from the ventral tegmental area to the cerebral cortex and the limbic areas. This pathway has been termed the *reward circuit pathway,* and its activation is probably the major addicting mechanism for the amphetamines. The designer amphetamines cause the release of catecholamines (dopamine and norepinephrine) and of serotonin, the neurotransmitter implicated as the major neurochemical pathway for hallucinogens. Therefore, the clinical effects of designer amphetamines are a blend of the effects of classic amphetamines and those of hallucinogens.

COCAINE

Cocaine has been used in its raw form for more than 15 centuries. In the United States, cycles of widespread stimulant misuse and associated problems have occurred for more than 100 years. Cocaine and cocaine use disorders became a major public health issue in the 1980s when an epidemic of use spread throughout the country. Due to education and intervention, cocaine use has since declined. However, high rates of legal, psychiatric, medical, and social problems related to cocaine use still exist, thus cocaine-related disorders remain an important public health issue.

Cocaine is an alkaloid derived from the shrub *Erythroxylum coca,* which is indigenous to South America, where the leaves of the shrub are chewed by local inhabitants to obtain the stimulating effects. The cocaine alkaloid was first isolated in 1855 and first used as a local anesthetic in 1880. It is still used as a local anesthetic, especially for eye, nose, and throat surgery, for which its vasoconstrictive and analgesic effects are helpful. In 1884, Sigmund Freud made a study of cocaine's general pharmacological effects and, for a period of time, according to his biographers, was addicted to the drug. In the 1880s and 1890s, cocaine was widely touted as a cure for many ills and was listed in the 1899 *Merck Manual.* It was the active ingredient in the beverage Coca-Cola until 1903. In 1914, however, once its addictive and adverse effects had been recognized, cocaine was classified as a narcotic, along with morphine and heroin.

Epidemiology

Cocaine Use. In 2012, 1.5 million (0.6 percent) persons aged 12 years or older used cocaine in the past month. Persons aged 18 to 25 (1.5 percent) had a higher rate of past month cocaine use than persons aged 26 or older (0.5 percent) and youths aged 12 to 17 (0.9 percent). Males (0.8 percent) were twice as likely as females (0.4 percent) to have used cocaine in the past year. Asians had the lowest rate of past year cocaine use (0.5 percent) compared with other racial or ethnic groups.

Cocaine Abuse and Dependence. It is estimated that more than 1.0 million (0.4 percent) persons aged 12 or older meet the criteria for abuse of, or dependence on, cocaine. Persons aged 18 to 25 (0.9 percent) had the highest rate of past year cocaine abuse or dependence, followed by persons aged 26 or older (0.4 percent) and youths aged 12 to 17 (0.2 percent). Males (0.9 percent) were more than twice as likely as females (0.4 percent) to have met the criteria for cocaine abuse or dependence. Blacks (1.1 percent) and Hispanics (0.9 percent) had higher rates of cocaine abuse or dependence than whites (0.5 percent), and the rate for Asians (0.1 percent) was lower than that for blacks, Hispanics, whites, American Indians or Alaskan Natives (1.2 percent), and non-Hispanic persons who identified themselves with two or more races (0.9 percent).

Crack Cocaine. An estimated 1.1 million (0.4 percent) persons aged 12 or older used crack cocaine in the past year, and 492,000 (0.2 percent) persons used crack cocaine in the past month. Persons aged 18 to 25 (0.5 percent) had the highest rate of past year crack use, followed by persons aged 26 or older (0.4 percent) and youths aged 12 to 17 (0.1 percent). Males (0.5 percent) were twice as likely as females (0.3 percent) to have used crack cocaine in the past year. Asians had the lowest rate of past year crack cocaine use (0.1 percent) compared with other racial or ethnic groups. Blacks (0.9 percent), whites (0.4 percent), Hispanics or Latinos (0.3 percent), and persons who identified themselves with two or more non-Hispanic races (0.9 percent) had higher rates of past year crack cocaine use than American Indians or Alaska Natives (0.2 percent) and Native Hawaiians or Other Pacific Islanders (0.1 percent).

Current cocaine use is on the decline, primarily because of increased awareness of cocaine's risks, as well as a comprehensive public campaign about cocaine and its effects. The societal effects of the decrease in cocaine use, however, have been somewhat offset by the frequent use over the past years of crack.

Comorbidity

As with other substance-related disorders, cocaine-related disorders are often accompanied by additional psychiatric disorders. The development of mood disorders and alcohol-related disorders usually follows the onset of cocaine-related disorders, whereas anxiety disorders, antisocial personality disorder, and ADHD are thought to precede the development of cocaine-related disorders. Most studies of comorbidity in patients with cocaine-related disorders have shown that major depressive disorder, bipolar II disorder, cyclothymic disorder, anxiety disorders, and antisocial personality disorder are the most commonly associated psychiatric diagnoses.

Etiology

Genetic Factors. The most convincing evidence to date of a genetic influence on cocaine dependence comes from studies of twins. Monozygotic twins have higher concordance rates for stimulant dependence (cocaine, amphetamines, and amphetamine-like drugs) than dizygotic twins. The analyses indicate that genetic factors and unique (unshared) environmental factors contribute about equally to the development of stimulant dependence.

Sociocultural Factors. Social, cultural, and economic factors are powerful determinants of initial use, continuing use, and relapse. Excessive use is far more likely in countries where cocaine is readily available. Different economic opportunities may influence certain groups more than others to engage in selling illicit drugs, and selling is more likely to be carried out in familiar communities than in communities where the seller runs a high risk of arrest.

Learning and Conditioning. Learning and conditioning are also considered important in perpetuating cocaine use. Each inhalation or injection of cocaine yields a "rush" and a euphoric experience that reinforces the antecedent drug-taking behavior. In addition, the environmental cues associated with substance use become associated with the euphoric state so that long after a period of cessation, such cues (e.g., white powder and paraphernalia) can elicit memories of the euphoric state and reawaken craving for cocaine.

In cocaine abusers (but not in normal controls), cocaine-related stimuli activate brain regions subserving episodic and working memory and produce electroencephalography (EEG) arousal (desynchronization). Increased metabolic activity in the limbic-related regions, such as the amygdala, parahippocampal gyrus, and dorsolateral prefrontal cortex, reportedly correlates with reports of craving for cocaine, but the degree of EEG arousal does not.

Pharmacological Factors. As a result of actions in the CNS, cocaine can produce a sense of alertness, euphoria, and well-being. Users may experience decreased hunger and less need for sleep. Performance impaired by fatigue is usually improved. Some users believe that cocaine enhances sexual performance.

Neuropharmacology

Cocaine's primary pharmacodynamic action related to its behavioral effects is competitive blockade of dopamine reuptake by the dopamine transporter. This blockade increases the concentration of dopamine in the synaptic cleft and results in increased activation of both dopamine type 1 (D_1) and type 2 (D_2) receptors. The effects of cocaine on the activity mediated by D_3, D_4, and D_5 receptors are not yet well understood, but at least one preclinical study has implicated the D_3 receptor. Although the behavioral effects are attributed primarily to the blockade of dopamine reuptake, cocaine also blocks the reuptake of norepinephrine and serotonin. The behavioral effects related to these activities are receiving increased attention in the scientific literature. The effects of cocaine on cerebral blood flow and cerebral glucose use have also been studied. Results in most studies generally showed that cocaine is associated with decreased cerebral blood flow and possibly with the development of patchy areas of decreased glucose use.

The behavioral effects of cocaine are felt almost immediately and last for a relatively brief time (30 to 60 minutes); thus users require repeated doses of the drug to maintain the feelings of intoxication. Despite the short-lived behavioral effects, metabolites of cocaine can be present in the blood and urine for up to 10 days.

Cocaine has powerful addictive qualities. Because of its potency as a positive reinforcer of behavior, psychological dependence on cocaine can develop after a single use. With repeated administration, both tolerance and sensitivity to various effects of cocaine can arise, although the development of tolerance or sensitivity is apparently caused by many factors and is not easily predicted. Physiological dependence on cocaine does occur, although cocaine withdrawal is mild compared with withdrawal from opiates and opioids.

Researchers recently reported that positron emission tomography (PET) scans of the brains of patients being treated for cocaine addiction show high activation in the mesolimbic dopamine system when addicts profoundly crave a drug. Researchers exposed patients to cues that had previously caused them to crave cocaine, and patients described feelings of intense cravings for the drug while PET scans showed activation in areas from the amygdala and the anterior cingulate to the tip of both temporal lobes. Some researchers claim that the mesolimbic dopamine system is also active in patients with nicotine addiction, and the same system has been linked to cravings for heroin, morphine, amphetamines, marijuana, and alcohol.

The D_2 receptors in the mesolimbic dopamine system have been held responsible for the heightened activity during periods of craving. PET scans of patients recovering from cocaine addiction are reported to show a drop in neuronal activity consistent with a lessened ability to receive dopamine, and the reduction in this ability, although it decreases over time, is apparent as long as a year and a half after withdrawal. The pattern of reduced brain activity reflects the course of the craving; between the third and fourth weeks of withdrawal, the activity is at its lowest level, and the risk of patient relapse is highest. After about 1 year, the brains of former addicts are almost back to normal, although whether the dopamine cells ever return to a completely normal state is debatable.

Methods of Use

Because drug dealers often dilute cocaine powder with sugar or procaine, street cocaine varies greatly in purity. Cocaine is sometimes cut with amphetamine. The most common method of using cocaine is inhaling the finely chopped powder into the nose, a practice referred to as "snorting" or "tooting." Other methods of ingesting cocaine are subcutaneous or intravenous injection and smoking (freebasing). Freebasing involves mixing street cocaine with chemically extracted pure cocaine alkaloid (the freebase) to get an increased effect. Smoking is also the method used to ingest crack cocaine. Inhaling is the least dangerous method of cocaine use; intravenous injection and smoking are the most dangerous. The most direct methods of ingestion are often associated with cerebrovascular diseases, cardiac abnormalities, and death. Although cocaine can be taken orally, it is rarely ingested via this, the least effective, route.

Crack. Crack, a freebase form of cocaine, is extremely potent. It is sold in small, ready-to-smoke amounts, often called "rocks." Crack cocaine is highly addictive; even one or two experiences with the drug can cause intense craving for more. Users have been known to resort to extremes of behavior to obtain the money to buy more crack. Reports from urban emergency rooms have also associated extremes of violence with crack abuse.

DIAGNOSIS AND CLINICAL FEATURES

Stimulant Use Disorder

The fifth edition of the *Diagnostic and Statistical Manual of Mental Disorders* (DSM-5) diagnostic criteria for stimulant use disorder are similar to the criteria used for other substance use disorders.

Amphetamine dependence can result in a rapid downward spiral of a person's abilities to cope with work- and family-related obligations and stresses. A person who abuses amphetamines requires increasingly high doses of amphetamine to obtain the usual high, and physical signs of amphetamine abuse (e.g., decreased weight and paranoid ideas) almost always develop with continued abuse.

Mr. H, a 35-year-old married man, was admitted to a psychiatric hospital because he felt persecuted by gang members who were out to kill him. He could not explain why they wished to kill him, but he heard voices from people whom he suspected to be mob drug dealers and they were discussing that they should kill him. He used methamphetamine for several years, so he had dealt with drug dealers before. He began using at age 27 at the persuasion of a friend to try it. After an injection of 20 mg, he felt good and powerful and his sleepiness and fatigue disappeared. After a few tries Mr. H found that he could not stop using it. He constantly thought about how he would obtain the drug and started increasing the dosage he used. During times that he could not get methamphetamine, he felt lethargic and sleepy and became irritable and dysphoric. Mr. H's wife learned of his drug use and attempted to persuade him to stop using it. He lost his job 2 months prior to his admission because he was repeatedly abusive to work colleagues because he felt that they were trying to harm him. With no income, Mr. H had to cut down his use of methamphetamine to only occasional usage. He finally decided to quit when his wife threatened to divorce him. Once he stopped using, he felt very tired, seemed gloomy, and often sat in his favorite chair and did nothing. After a few weeks, Mr. H told his wife that he did not wish to leave the house because he had heard dealers on the street talking about him. He wanted all doors and windows locked, and he refused to eat in fear that the food may be poisoned.

On examination, Mr. H seemed withdrawn, only giving short answers to questions. He was in clear consciousness and fully oriented and showed no marked impairment of cognitive functions. Physical and neurological testing showed no abnormalities except needle scars on his arms from methamphetamine injections. An EEG was normal.

Clinically and practically, cocaine use disorder can be suspected in patients who evidence unexplained changes in personality. Common changes associated with cocaine use are irritability, impaired ability to concentrate, compulsive behavior, severe insomnia, and weight loss. Colleagues at work and family members may notice a person's general and increasing inability to perform the expected tasks associated with work and family life. The patient may show new evidence of increased debt or inability to pay bills on time because of the large sums used to buy cocaine. Cocaine abusers often excuse themselves from work or social situations every 30 to 60 minutes to find a secluded place to inhale more cocaine. Because of the vasoconstricting effects of cocaine, users almost always develop nasal congestion, which they may attempt to self-medicate with decongestant sprays.

Mr. D, a 45-year-old married man, was referred by his therapist to a private outpatient substance abuse treatment program for evaluation and treatment of a possible cocaine problem. According to the therapist, Mr. D's wife expressed concern for a possible substance abuse problem on several occasions. A few days prior, Mr. D admitted to the therapist and his wife that he "occasionally" used cocaine for the past year. His wife insisted that he obtain treatment for his drug problem or else she would file for divorce. Mr. D reluctantly conceded to treatment, but insisted that his cocaine use was not a problem and that he felt capable of stopping without entering a treatment program.

During the initial evaluation interview, Mr. D reported that he currently used cocaine, intranasally, 3 to 5 days a week, and that this pattern has been continuing for a year and a half. On average, he consumes a total of 1 to 2 g of cocaine weekly. He mostly uses cocaine at work, in his office or in the bathroom. He usually started thinking about cocaine during his drive to work in the morning and once at work was unable avoid thinking about the cocaine in his desk drawer. Despites his attempts at distraction and postponing use, he usually takes his first line of cocaine within an hour of arriving at work. On some days he will take another two to three lines over the course of the day, but, on days where he is frustrated and stressed, he may take a line or two every hour from morning until late afternoon. He rarely uses cocaine at home and never uses in front of his wife or his three daughters. He occasionally takes a line or two during a weekday evening or weekends at home when everyone else is out of the house. He denies current use of alcohol or any other illicit drug. He denies any history of alcohol or drug abuse and any history of emotional or marital problems.

Stimulant Intoxication

The diagnostic criteria for stimulant intoxication emphasize behavioral and physical signs and symptoms of stimulant use.

Persons use stimulants for their characteristic effects of elation, euphoria, heightened self-esteem, and perceived improvement on mental and physical tasks. With high doses, symptoms of intoxication include agitation, irritability, impaired judgment, impulsive and potentially dangerous sexual behavior, aggression, a generalized increase in psychomotor activity, and potentially, symptoms of mania. The major associated physical symptoms are tachycardia, hypertension, and mydriasis.

Mrs. T, a 45-year-old married business woman, was admitted to psychiatric service after a 3-month period in which she became increasingly mistrustful of others and suspicious of business associates. She took statements from others out of context, twisting their words, and making inappropriately hostile and accusatory comments. On one occasion, Mrs. T physically attacked a coworker in a bar accusing her of having an affair with her husband and plotting with other coworkers to kill her.

One year previously, Mrs. T was prescribed methylphenidate for narcolepsy due to daily irresistible sleep attacks and episodes of sudden loss of muscle tone when she became emotionally excited. After taking the medication, Mrs. T became asymptomatic and was able to work effectively and have an active social life with family and friends.

In the 5 months before admission, Mrs. T had been using increasingly large doses of methylphenidate to maintain alertness late at night because of an increased amount of work that could not be handled during the day. She reported that during this time she often could feel her heart race and that she had trouble sitting still.

Mr. P, an 18-year-old man, was brought to a hospital emergency room via ambulance in the middle of the night. He was accompanied by a friend who decided to call an ambulance because he felt Mr. P was going to die. Mr. P was agitated and argumentative, his breathing was irregular and rapid, his pulse was rapid, and his pupils were dilated. His friend eventually admitted that they used a lot of cocaine that evening.

When his mother arrived at the hospital, Mr. P's condition had somewhat improved, although his loud singing created a commotion in the emergency room. His mother states Mr. P has some disciplinary problems; he is disobedient, resentful, and violently argumentative. He had been arrested on a few occasions for shoplifting and for driving while intoxicated. His mother suspected that Mr. P was using drugs due to his behavior and because she heard him talk to his friends about drugs; however, she has no direct proof of his use.

Within 24 hours, Mr. P was well and willing to talk. He boastfully stated that he had been using alcohol and various drugs regularly since he was 13. It started with just alcohol and marijuana, but once he entered high school and became acquainted with older youths, he experimented with other drugs such as speed and cocaine. By the time he was 16, he was using combinations of alcohol, speed, marijuana, and cocaine. He settled on just cocaine after a year of mixing drugs.

Mr. P frequently skipped school and when he attended school he was usually intoxicated. To support his habit, he acquired money in various schemes, such as borrowing money from friends that he had no intention of paying back or stealing car radios or stealing from his mother.

Despite his blatant admission of drug use, Mr. P denies having a problem. When asked about his ability to control his drug use, he defensively replies "Of course I can. No problem. I just don't see any damn reason to stop."

Stimulant Withdrawal

After stimulant intoxication, a "crash" occurs with symptoms of anxiety, tremulousness, dysphoric mood, lethargy, fatigue, nightmares (accompanied by rebound rapid eye movement [REM] sleep), headache, profuse sweating, muscle cramps, stomach cramps, and insatiable hunger. The withdrawal symptoms generally peak in 2 to 4 days and are resolved in 1 week. The most serious withdrawal symptom is depression, which can be particularly severe after the sustained use of high doses of stimulants and which can be associated with suicidal ideation or behavior. A person in the state of withdrawal can experience powerful and intense cravings for cocaine, especially because taking cocaine can eliminate the unpleasant withdrawal symptoms. Persons experiencing cocaine withdrawal often attempt to self-medicate with alcohol, sedatives, hypnotics, or antianxiety agents such as diazepam (Valium).

Stimulant Intoxication Delirium

Delirium associated with stimulant use generally results from high doses of a stimulant or from sustained use, and so sleep deprivation affects the clinical presentation. The combination of stimulants with other substances and the use of stimulants by a person with preexisting brain damage can also cause development of delirium. It is not uncommon for university students who are using amphetamines to cram for examinations to exhibit this type of delirium.

Stimulant-Induced Psychotic Disorder

The hallmark of stimulant-induced psychotic disorder is the presence of paranoid delusions and hallucinations, which occurs in up to 50 percent of stimulant users. Auditory hallucinations are also common, but visual and tactile hallucinations are less common than paranoid delusions. The sensation of bugs crawling beneath the skin (formication) has been reported to be associated with cocaine use. The presence of these symptoms depends on the dose, duration of use, and the user's sensitivity to the substance. Cocaine-induced psychotic disorders are most common with intravenous use and crack users, and the psychotic symptoms are more common in men than in women. The treatment of choice for amphetamine-induced psychotic disorder is the short-term use of an antipsychotic medication such as haloperidol (Haldol).

Mr. H is a 20-year-old college student who was functioning well until the weeks of his finals, when he began taking large amounts of cocaine because he felt he was unprepared for his tests. He began having delusional beliefs that he was being followed by the police and a detective at the request of his parents in order to spy on him. He also believed that his roommate would give reports to the detective about his study habits and social life. He was brought to the emergency room after he threatened to harm his roommate if he continued to report on him.

During evaluation, Mr. P reported sleeplessness and auditory hallucinations that told him that his roommate was conspiring against him. He was very agitated and paced continuously. After admission to the hospital, Mr. P was given antipsychotics and sleeping medications and recovered in 3 days.

Stimulant-Induced Mood Disorder

The DSM-5 allows for the diagnoses of stimulant-induced bipolar disorder and stimulant-induced depressive disorder, either of which can begin during either intoxication or withdrawal. In general, intoxication is associated with manic or mixed mood features, whereas withdrawal is associated with depressive mood features.

Stimulant-Induced Anxiety Disorder

The DSM-5 allows for the diagnosis of stimulant-induced anxiety disorder. The onset of stimulant-induced anxiety disorder can also occur during intoxication or withdrawal. Stimulants can induce symptoms similar to those seen in panic disorder, and phobic disorders, in particular.

Stimulant-Induced Obsessive-Compulsive Disorder

The DSM-5 allows for the diagnosis of stimulant-induced obsessive-compulsive disorder. The onset can occur during intoxication or withdrawal. After high doses of stimulants, some individuals develop time-limited stereotyped behaviors or rituals (i.e., picking at clothing, and arranging and rearranging items purposelessly) that share some features with the type of compulsions seen in obsessive-compulsive disorder.

Stimulant-Induced Sexual Dysfunction

The DSM-5 allows for the diagnosis of stimulant-induced sexual dysfunction. Amphetamines may be prescribed as an antidote to the sexual side effects of serotonergic agents such as fluoxetine (Prozac), but stimulants are often misused by persons to enhance sexual experiences. High doses and long-term use are associated with erectile disorder and other sexual dysfunctions.

Stimulant-Induced Sleep Disorder

Stimulant-induced sleep disorder can begin during either intoxication or withdrawal, and sleep dysfunction can vary depending on the onset. Stimulant intoxication can produce insomnia and sleep deprivation, whereas persons undergoing stimulant withdrawal can experience hypersomnolence and nightmares.

ADVERSE EFFECTS

Amphetamines

Physical. Amphetamine abuse can produce adverse effects, the most serious of which include cerebrovascular, cardiac, and gastrointestinal effects. Among the specific life-threatening conditions are myocardial infarction, severe hypertension, cerebrovascular disease, and ischemic colitis. A continuum of neurological symptoms, from twitching to tetany to seizures to coma and death, is associated with increasingly high amphetamine doses. Intravenous use of amphetamines can transmit HIV and hepatitis and further the development of lung abscesses, endocarditis, and necrotizing angiitis. Several studies have shown that abusers of amphetamines knew little—or did not care—about safe-sex practices and the use of condoms. The non–life-threatening adverse effects of amphetamine abuse include flushing, pallor, cyanosis, fever, headache, tachycardia, palpitations, nausea, vomiting, bruxism (teeth grinding), shortness of breath, tremor, and ataxia. Pregnant women who use amphetamines often have babies with low birthweight, small head circumference, early gestational age, and growth retardation.

Psychological. The adverse psychological effects associated with amphetamine use include restlessness, dysphoria, insomnia, irritability, hostility, and confusion. Amphetamine use can also induce symptoms of anxiety disorders, such as generalized anxiety disorder and panic disorder, as well as ideas of reference, paranoid delusions, and hallucinations.

Cocaine

A common adverse effect associated with cocaine use is nasal congestion; serious inflammation, swelling, bleeding, and ulceration of the nasal mucosa can also occur. Long-term use of cocaine can also lead to perforation of the nasal septa. Freebasing and smoking crack can damage the bronchial passages and the lungs. The intravenous use of cocaine can result in infection, embolisms, and the transmission of HIV. Minor neurological complications with cocaine use include the development of acute dystonia, tics, and migraine-like headaches. The major complications of cocaine use, however, are cerebrovascular, epileptic, and cardiac. About two-thirds of these acute toxic effects occur within 1 hour of intoxication, about one-fifth occur in 1 to 3 hours, and the remainder occurs up to several days later.

Cerebrovascular Effects. The most common cerebrovascular diseases associated with cocaine use are nonhemorrhagic cerebral infarctions. When hemorrhagic infarctions do occur, they can include subarachnoid, intraparenchymal, and intraventricular hemorrhages. Transient ischemic attacks have also been associated with cocaine use. Although these vascular disorders usually affect the brain, spinal cord hemorrhages have also been reported. The obvious pathophysiological mechanism for these vascular disorders is vasoconstriction, but other pathophysiological mechanisms have also been proposed.

Seizures. Seizures have been reported to account for 3 to 8 percent of cocaine-related emergency room visits. Cocaine is the substance of abuse most commonly associated with seizures; the second most common substance is amphetamine. Cocaine-induced seizures are usually single events, although multiple seizures and status epilepticus are also possible. A rare and easily misdiagnosed complication of cocaine use is partial complex status epilepticus, which should be considered as a diagnosis in a patient who seems to have cocaine-induced psychotic disorder with an unusually fluctuating course. The risk of having cocaine-induced seizures is highest in patients with a history of epilepsy who use high doses of cocaine as well as crack.

Cardiac Effects. Myocardial infarctions and arrhythmias are perhaps the most common cocaine-induced cardiac abnormalities. Cardiomyopathies can develop with long-term use of cocaine, and cardioembolic cerebral infarctions can be a further complication of cocaine-induced myocardial dysfunction.

Death. High doses of cocaine are associated with seizures, respiratory depression, cerebrovascular diseases, and myocardial infarctions—all of which can lead to death in persons who use cocaine. Users may experience warning signs of syncope or chest pain but may ignore these signs because of the irrepressible desire to take more cocaine. Deaths have also been reported with the ingestion of "speedballs," which are combinations of opioids and cocaine.

Other Agents

Substituted Amphetamines. MDMA is one of a series of substituted amphetamines that also includes MDEA, MDA, DOB (2,5-dimethoxy-4-bromoamphetamine), PMA (paramethoxyamphetamine), and others. These drugs produce subjective effects resembling those of amphetamine and LSD, and in that sense, MDMA and similar analogues may represent a distinct category of drugs.

A methamphetamine derivative that came into use in the 1980s, MDMA was not technically subject to legal regulation at the time. Although it has been labeled a "designer drug" in the belief that it was deliberately synthesized to evade legal regulation, it was actually synthesized and patented in 1914. Several psychiatrists used it as an adjunct to psychotherapy and concluded that it had value. At one time, it was advertised as legal and was used in psychotherapy for its subjective effects. It was never approved by the FDA, however. Its use raised questions of both safety and legality, because the related amphetamine derivatives MDA, DOB, and PMA had caused a number of overdose deaths, and MDA was known to cause extensive destruction of serotonergic nerve terminals in the CNS. Using emergency scheduling authority, the Drug Enforcement Agency made MDMA a Schedule I drug under the CSA, along with LSD, heroin, and marijuana. Despite its illegal status, MDMA continues to be manufactured, distributed, and used in the United States, Europe, and Australia. Its use is common in Australia and Great Britain at extended dances ("raves") popular with adolescents and young adults.

MECHANISMS OF ACTION. The unusual properties of the drugs may be a consequence of the different actions of the optical isomers: the *R*(−) isomers produce LSD-like effects and the amphetamine-like properties are linked to *S*(+) isomers. The LSD-like actions, in turn, may be linked to the capacity to release serotonin. The various derivatives may exhibit significant differences in subjective effects and toxicity. Animals in laboratory experiments will self-administer the drugs, suggesting prominent amphetamine-like effects.

SUBJECTIVE EFFECTS. After taking usual doses (100 to 150 mg), MDMA users experience elevated mood and, according to various reports, increased self-confidence and sensory sensitivity; peaceful feelings coupled with insight, empathy, and closeness to persons; and decreased appetite. Difficulty concentrating and an increased capacity to focus have both been reported. Dysphoric reactions, psychotomimetic effects, and psychosis have also been reported. Higher doses seem more likely to produce psychotomimetic effects. Sympathomimetic effects of tachycardia, palpitation, increased blood pressure, sweating, and bruxism are common. The subjective effects are reported to be prominent for approximately 4 to 8 hours, but they may not last as long or may last longer, depending on the dose and route of administration. The drug is usually taken orally but is also snorted and injected. Both tachyphylaxis and some tolerance are reported by users.

TOXICITY. Although it is not as toxic as MDA, various somatic toxicities have been attributed to MDMA use as well as fatal overdoses. It does not appear to be neurotoxic when injected into the brains of animals, but it is metabolized to MDA in both animals and humans. In animals, MDMA produces selective, long-lasting damage to serotonergic nerve terminals. It is not certain if the levels of the MDA metabolite reached in humans after the usual doses of MDMA suffice to produce lasting damage. Users of MDMA show differences in neuroendocrine responses to serotonergic probes, and studies of former MDMA users show global and regional decreases in serotonin transporter binding, as measured by PET.

Currently, no established clinical uses exist for MDMA, although before its regulation, there were several reports of its beneficial effects as an adjunct to psychotherapy.

Khat. The fresh leaves of *Catha edulis,* a bush native to East Africa, have been used as a stimulant in the Middle East, Africa, and the Arabian Peninsula for at least 1,000 years. Khat is still widely used in Ethiopia, Kenya, Somalia, and Yemen. The amphetamine-like effects of khat have long been recognized, and although efforts to isolate the active ingredient were first undertaken in the nineteenth century, only since the 1970s has cathinone (*S*[−]α-aminopropiophenone or *S*[−]2-amino-1-phenyl-1-propanone) been identified as the substance responsible. Cathinone is a precursor moiety that is normally enzymatically converted in the plant to the less-active entities norephedrine and cathine (norpseudoephedrine), which explains why only the fresh leaves of the plant are valued for their stimulant effects. Cathinone has most of the CNS and peripheral actions of amphetamine and appears to have the same mechanism of action. In humans, it elevates mood, decreases hunger, and alleviates fatigue. At high doses, it can induce an amphetamine-like psychosis in humans. Because it is typically absorbed buccally after chewing the leaf and because the alkaloid is metabolized relatively rapidly, high toxic blood levels are rarely reached. Concern about khat use is linked to its dependence-producing properties rather than to its acute toxicity. It is estimated that five million doses are consumed each day, despite prohibition of its use in a number of African and Arab countries.

In the 1990s, several clandestine laboratories began synthesizing methcathinone, a drug with actions similar to those of cathinone. Known by a number of street names (e.g., bath salts, "CAT," "goob," and "crank"), its popularity is primarily owing to its ease of synthesis from ephedrine or pseudoephedrine, which were readily available until placed under special controls. Methcathinone has been moved to Schedule I of the CSA. The patterns of use, adverse effects, and complications closely resemble those reported for amphetamine.

"Club Drugs." The use of a certain group of substances popularly called *club drugs* is often associated with dance clubs, bars, and all-night dance parties (raves). The group includes LSD, γ-hydroxybutyrate (GHB), ketamine, methamphetamine, MDMA (ecstasy), and Rohypnol or "roofies" (flunitrazepam).

These substances are not all in the same drug class, and they do not produce the same physical or subjective effects. GHB, ketamine, and Rohypnol have been called *date rape drugs* because they produce disorienting and sedating effects, and often users cannot recall what occurred during all or part of an episode under the influence of the drug. Hence, it is alleged that these drugs might be surreptitiously placed in a beverage, or a person might be convinced to take the drug and then not recall clearly what occurred after ingestion.

Emergency department mentions of GHB, ketamine, and Rohypnol are relatively few. Of the club drugs, methamphetamine is the substance that accounts for the largest share of treatment admissions.

TREATMENT AND REHABILITATION

Amphetamines

The treatment of amphetamine-related (or amphetamine-like) disorders shares with cocaine-related disorders the difficulty of helping patients remain abstinent from the drug, which is powerfully reinforcing and induces craving. An inpatient setting and the use of multiple therapeutic methods (individual, family, and group psychotherapy) are usually necessary to achieve lasting abstinence. The treatment of specific amphetamine-induced disorders (e.g., amphetamine-induced psychotic disorder and amphetamine-induced anxiety disorder) with specific drugs (e.g., antipsychotic and anxiolytics) may be necessary on a short-term basis. Antipsychotics may be prescribed for the first few days. In the absence of psychosis, diazepam (Valium) is useful to treat patients' agitation and hyperactivity.

Physicians should establish a therapeutic alliance with patients to deal with the underlying depression, personality disorder, or both. Because many patients are heavily dependent on the drug, however, psychotherapy may be especially difficult.

Comorbid conditions, such as depression, may respond to antidepressant medication. Bupropion (Wellbutrin) may be of use after patients have withdrawn from amphetamine. It has the effect of producing feelings of well-being as these patients cope with the dysphoria that may accompany abstinence.

Cocaine

Detoxification. The cocaine withdrawal syndrome is distinct from that of opioids, alcohol, or sedative–hypnotic agents, because no physiological disturbances necessitate inpatient or residential drug withdrawal. Thus, it is generally possible to engage in a therapeutic trial of outpatient withdrawal before deciding whether a more intensive or controlled setting is required for patients unable to stop without help in limiting their access to cocaine. Patients withdrawing from cocaine typically experience fatigue, dysphoria, disturbed sleep, and some craving; some may experience depression. No pharmacological agents reliably reduce the intensity of withdrawal, but recovery over a week or two is generally uneventful. It may take longer, however, for sleep, mood, and cognitive function to recover fully.

Most cocaine users do not come to treatment voluntarily. Their experience with the substance is too positive, and the negative effects are perceived as too minimal, to warrant seeking treatment. Those who do not seek treatment often have polysubstance-related disorder, fewer negative consequences associated with cocaine use, fewer work- or family-related obligations, and increased contact with the legal system and with illegal activities.

The major hurdle to overcome in the treatment of cocaine-related disorders is the user's intense craving for the drug. Although animal studies have shown that cocaine is a powerful inducer of self-administration, these studies have also shown that animals limit their use of cocaine when negative reinforcers are experimentally linked to the cocaine intake. In humans, negative reinforcers may take the form of work and family-related problems brought on by cocaine use. Therefore, clinicians must take a broad treatment approach and include social, psychological, and perhaps biological strategies in the treatment program.

Attaining abstinence from cocaine in patients may require complete or partial hospitalization to remove them from the usual social settings in which they had obtained or used cocaine. Frequent, unscheduled urine testing is almost always necessary to monitor patients' continued abstinence, especially in the first weeks and months of treatment. Relapse prevention therapy (RPT) relies on cognitive and behavioral techniques in addition to hospitalization and outpatient therapy to achieve the goal of abstinence.

Psychosocial Therapies. Psychological intervention usually involves individual, group, and family modalities. In individual therapy, therapists should focus on the dynamics leading to cocaine use, the perceived positive effects of the cocaine, and other ways to achieve these effects. Group therapy and support groups, such as Narcotics Anonymous, often focus on discussions with other persons who use cocaine and on sharing experiences and effective coping methods. Family therapy is often an essential component of the treatment strategy. Common issues discussed in family therapy are the ways the patient's past behavior has harmed the family and the responses of family members to these behaviors. Therapy should also focus, however, on the future and on changes in the family's activities that may help the patient stay off the drug and direct energies in different directions. This approach can be used on an outpatient basis.

NETWORK THERAPY. Network therapy was developed as a specialized type of combined individual and group therapy to ensure greater success in the office-based treatment of addicted patients. Network therapy uses both psychodynamic and cognitive-behavioral approaches to individual therapy while engaging the patient in a group support network. The group, composed of the patient's family and peers, is used as a therapeutic network joining the patient and therapist at intervals in therapy sessions. The approach promotes group cohesiveness as a vehicle for engaging patients in this treatment. This network is managed by the therapist to provide cohesiveness and support and to promote compliance with treatment. Although network therapy has not received systematic controlled evaluation, it is frequently applied in the psychiatric practice because it is one of the few manualized approaches that has been designed for use by individual practitioners in an office setting.

Pharmacological Adjuncts. Presently, no pharmacological treatments produce decreases in cocaine use comparable to the decreases in opioid use seen when heroin users are treated with methadone, levomethadyl acetate (ORLAAM) (commonly called L-a-acetylmethadol [LAAM]), or buprenorphine (Buprenex). A variety of pharmacological agents, most of which are approved for other uses, have been, and are being, tested clinically for the treatment of cocaine dependence and relapse.

Cocaine users presumed to have preexisting ADHD or mood disorders have been treated with methylphenidate (Ritalin) and lithium (Eskalith), respectively. Those drugs are of little or no benefit in patients without the disorders, and clinicians should adhere strictly to maximal diagnostic criteria before using either of them in the treatment of cocaine dependence. In patients with ADHD, slow-release forms of methylphenidate may be less likely to trigger cocaine craving, but the impact of such pharmacotherapy on cocaine use remains to be demonstrated.

Many pharmacological agents have been explored on the premise that chronic cocaine use alters the function of multiple neurotransmitter systems, especially the dopaminergic and serotonergic transmitters regulating hedonic tone, and that cocaine induces a state of relative dopaminergic deficiency. Although the evidence for such alterations in dopaminergic function has been growing, it has been difficult to demonstrate that agents theoretically capable of modifying dopamine function can alter the course of treatment.

Tricyclic antidepressant drugs yielded some positive results when used early in treatment with minimally drug-dependent patients; however, they are of little or no use inducing abstinence in moderate or severe cases.

Also tried but not confirmed effective in controlled studies are other antidepressants, such as bupropion, MAOIs, SSRIs, antipsychotics, lithium, several different calcium channel inhibitors, and anticonvulsants. One study found that 300 mg a day of phenytoin (Dilantin) reduced cocaine use; this study requires further replication.

Several agents are being developed that have not been tried in human studies. These include agents that would selectively block or stimulate dopamine receptor subtypes (e.g., selective D_1 agonists) and drugs that can selectively block the access of cocaine to the dopamine transporters but still permit the transporters to remove cocaine from the synapse. Another approach is aimed at preventing cocaine from reaching the brain by using antibodies to bind cocaine in the bloodstream (a so-called "cocaine vaccine"). Such cocaine-binding antibodies do reduce the reinforcing effects of cocaine in animal models. Also under study are catalytic antibodies that accelerate the hydrolysis of cocaine, and butyrylcholinesterase (pseudocholinesterase), which appears to hydrolyze cocaine selectively and is normally present in the body.

Vigabatrin is a drug that has been used as a treatment for refractory pediatric epilepsy, which appears to function by significantly elevating brain GABA levels. In animals, vigabatrin was also noted to attenuate cocaine, nicotine, heroin, alcohol, and methamphetamine-induced increases in extracellular nucleus accumbens dopamine as well as drug-seeking behaviors associated with these biochemical changes. Preliminary clinical studies suggest efficacy for the treatment of cocaine and methamphetamine dependence. Large-scale clinical trials for this indication are needed, however.

▲ 16.10 Tobacco-Related Disorders

Tobacco use disorder is among the most prevalent, deadly, and costly of substance dependencies. It is also one of the most ignored, particularly by psychiatrists, because despite recent research that shows commonalities between tobacco dependence and other substance use disorders, tobacco dependence differs from other substance dependencies in unique ways. Tobacco does not cause behavioral problems; therefore, few tobacco-dependent persons seek or are referred for psychiatric treatment. Tobacco is a legal drug and most persons who stop tobacco use have done so without treatment. Thus a common, but erroneous, view is that, unlike alcohol and other illicit drugs, most smokers do not need treatment.

Several recent events may reverse the reluctance of psychiatrists to play a role in treating tobacco dependence: (1) the growing recognition that most psychiatric patients smoke and many die from tobacco dependence; (2) remaining smokers will be more and more likely to have psychiatric problems, which suggests that many need more intensive treatments; and (3) the development of multiple pharmacological agents to aid smokers in quitting.

EPIDEMIOLOGY

The *2004 Monitoring the Future Survey* concluded that, despite the demonstrated health risk associated with cigarette smoking, young Americans continue to smoke. However, 30-day smoking rates among high school students declined from peaks reached in 1996 for eighth-graders (21.0 percent) and tenth-graders (30.4 percent) and in 1997 for seniors (36.5 percent). In 2011, 30-day rates reached the lowest levels ever reported by *Monitoring the Future* surveys for eighth-graders (6.1 percent), tenth-graders (11.8 percent), and twelfth-graders (18.7 percent), with tenth-graders showing the most significant decline. Of high school seniors, 19 percent reported smoking during the month preceding their responses to the survey.

The decrease in smoking rates among young Americans corresponds to several years in which increased proportions of teens said they believe a "great" health risk is associated with cigarette smoking and expressed disapproval of smoking one or more packs of cigarettes a day. Students' personal disapproval of smoking had risen for some years. In 2011, 88 percent of eighth-graders, 85.8 percent of tenth-graders, and 83 percent of twelfth-graders stated that they "disapprove" or "strongly disapprove" of people smoking one or more packs of cigarettes per day. In addition, eighth-graders and tenth-graders reported significant increases in the perceived harmfulness of smoking one or more packs of cigarettes per day.

The World Health Organization (WHO) estimates that there are 1 billion smokers worldwide, and they smoke 6 trillion cigarettes a year. The WHO also estimates that tobacco kills more than 3 million persons each year. Although the number of persons in the United States who smoke is decreasing, the number of persons smoking in developing countries is increasing. The rate of quitting smoking has been highest among well-educated white men and lowest among women, blacks, teenagers, and those with low levels of education.

Tobacco is smoked most commonly in cigarettes, and then, in descending order, cigars, snuff, chewing tobacco, and in pipes. About 3 percent of all persons in the United States currently use snuff or chewing tobacco, and about 6 percent of young adults aged 18 to 25 use those forms of tobacco.

Currently, about 17 of every 100 US adults aged 18 years or older (16.8 percent) currently smoke cigarettes. This means an estimated 40 million adults in the United States smoke. The mean age of onset of smoking is 16 years, and few persons start smoking after 20. Dependence features appear to develop quickly. Classroom and other programs to prevent initiation are only mildly effective, but increased taxation does decrease initiation.

More than 75 percent of smokers have tried to quit, and about 40 percent try to quit each year. On a given attempt, only 30 percent remain abstinent for even 2 days, and only 5 to 10 percent stop permanently. Most smokers make 5 to 10 attempts, however, so eventually 50 percent of "ever smokers" quit. In the past, 90 percent of successful attempts to quit involved no treatment. With the advent of over-the-counter (OTC) and nonnicotine medications in 1998, about one-third of all attempts involved the use of medication.

In terms of the diagnosis of tobacco use disorder per se, about 20 percent of the population develops tobacco dependence at some point, making it one of the most prevalent psychiatric disorders. Approximately 85 percent of current daily smokers are tobacco dependent. Tobacco withdrawal occurs in about 50 percent of smokers who try to quit.

According to the Centers of Disease Control and Prevention (CDC), regional differences exist in smoking throughout the United States. The 13 states with the highest prevalence of current smoking are Kentucky, West Virginia, Oklahoma, Mississippi, Indiana, Missouri, Alabama, Louisiana, Nevada, Tennessee, Alaska, North Carolina, and Ohio. Those states with lowest prevalence are Utah, California, Washington, Massachusetts, Rhode Island, District of Columbia, Hawaii, Maryland, Connecticut, New Hampshire, New Jersey, and Arizona. Utah had the lowest prevalence for men (10.6 percent) and for women (7.9 percent).

Education

Level of education attainment correlated with tobacco use. Of adults who had not completed high school, 37 percent smoked cigarettes, whereas only 17 percent of college graduates smoked.

Psychiatric Patients

Psychiatrists must be particularly concerned and knowledgeable about tobacco dependence because of the high proportion of psychiatric patients who smoke. Approximately 50 percent of all psychiatric outpatients, 70 percent of outpatients with bipolar I disorder, almost 90 percent of outpatients with schizophrenia, and 70 percent of patients with substance use disorder smoke. Moreover, data indicate that patients with depressive disorders or anxiety disorders are less successful in their attempts to quit smoking than other persons; thus, a holistic health approach for these patients probably includes helping them address their smoking habits in addition to the primary mental disorder. The high percentage of patients with schizophrenia who smoke has been attributed to tobacco's ability to reduce their extraordinary sensitivity to outside sensory stimuli and to increase their concentration. In that sense, such patients are self-monitoring to relieve distress.

Death

Death is the primary adverse effect of cigarette smoking. Tobacco use is associated with approximately 400,000 premature deaths each year in the United States—25 percent of all deaths. The causes of death include chronic bronchitis and emphysema (51,000 deaths), bronchogenic cancer (106,000 deaths), 35 percent of fatal myocardial infarctions (115,000 deaths), cerebrovascular disease, cardiovascular disease, and almost all cases of chronic obstructive pulmonary disease and lung cancer. The increased use of chewing tobacco and snuff (smokeless tobacco) has been associated with the development of oropharyngeal cancer, and the resurgence of cigar smoking is likely to lead to an increase in the occurrence of this type of cancer.

Researchers have found that 30 percent of cancer deaths in the United States are caused by tobacco smoke, the single most lethal carcinogen in the United States. Smoking (mainly cigarette smoking) causes cancer of the lung, upper respiratory tract, esophagus, bladder, and pancreas and probably of the stomach, liver, and kidney. Smokers are eight times more likely than nonsmokers to develop lung cancer, and lung cancer has surpassed breast cancer as the leading cause of cancer-related deaths in women. Even secondhand smoke (discussed below) causes a few thousand cancer deaths each year in the United States, about the same number as are caused by radon exposure. Despite these staggering statistics, smokers can dramatically lower their chances of developing smoke-related cancers simply by quitting.

NEUROPHARMACOLOGY

The psychoactive component of tobacco is nicotine, which affects the CNS by acting as an agonist at the nicotinic subtype of acetylcholine receptors. About 25 percent of the nicotine inhaled during smoking reaches the bloodstream, through which nicotine reaches the brain within 15 seconds. The half-life of nicotine is about 2 hours. Nicotine is believed to produce its positive reinforcing and addictive properties by activating the dopaminergic pathway projecting from the ventral tegmental area to the cerebral cortex and the limbic system. In addition to activating this dopamine reward system, nicotine causes an increase in the concentrations of circulating norepinephrine and epinephrine and an increase in the release of vasopressin, β-endorphin, adrenocorticotropic hormone (ACTH), and cortisol. These hormones are thought to contribute to the basic stimulatory effects of nicotine on the CNS.

DIAGNOSIS

Tobacco Use Disorder

The fifth edition of the *Diagnostic and Statistical Manual of Mental Disorder* (DSM-5) includes a diagnosis for tobacco use disorder characterized by craving, persistent and recurrent use, tolerance, and withdrawal if tobacco is stopped. Dependence on tobacco develops quickly, probably because nicotine activates the ventral tegmental area dopaminergic system, the same system affected by cocaine and amphetamine. The development of dependence is enhanced by strong social factors that encourage smoking in some settings and by the powerful effects of tobacco company advertising. Persons are likely to smoke if their parents or siblings smoke and serve as role models. Several recent studies have also suggested a genetic diathesis toward tobacco dependence. Most persons who smoke want to quit and have tried many times to quit but have been unsuccessful.

Tobacco Withdrawal

The DSM-5 does not have a diagnostic category for tobacco intoxication, but it does have a diagnostic category for nicotine withdrawal. Withdrawal symptoms can develop within 2 hours of smoking the last cigarette; they generally peak in the first 24 to 48 hours and can last for weeks or months. The common symptoms include an intense craving for tobacco, tension, irritability, difficulty concentrating, drowsiness and paradoxical trouble sleeping, decreased heart rate and blood pressure, increased appetite and weight gain, decreased motor performance, and increased muscle tension. A mild syndrome of tobacco withdrawal can appear when a smoker switches from regular to low-nicotine cigarettes.

CLINICAL FEATURES

Behaviorally, the stimulatory effects of nicotine produce improved attention, learning, reaction time, and problem-solving ability. Tobacco users also report that cigarette smoking lifts their mood, decreases tension, and lessens depressive feelings. Results of studies of the effects of nicotine on cerebral blood flow (CBF) suggest that short-term nicotine exposure increases CBF without changing cerebral oxygen metabolism, but long-term nicotine exposure decreases CBF. In contrast to its stimulatory CNS effects, nicotine acts as a skeletal muscle relaxant.

Adverse Effects

Nicotine is a highly toxic alkaloid. Doses of 60 mg in an adult are fatal secondary to respiratory paralysis; doses of 0.5 mg are delivered by smoking an average cigarette. In low doses, the signs and symptoms of nicotine toxicity include nausea, vomiting, salivation, pallor (caused by peripheral vasoconstriction), weakness, abdominal pain (caused by increased peristalsis), diarrhea, dizziness, headache, increased blood pressure, tachycardia, tremor, and cold sweats. Toxicity is also associated with an inability to concentrate, confusion, and sensory disturbances. Nicotine is further associated with a decrease in the user's amount of rapid eye movement (REM) sleep. Tobacco use during pregnancy has been associated with an increased incidence of low–birth-weight babies and an increased incidence of newborns with persistent pulmonary hypertension.

Health Benefits of Smoking Cessation

Smoking cessation has major and immediate health benefits for persons of all ages and provides benefits for persons with and without smoking-related diseases. Former smokers live longer than those who continue to smoke. Smoking cessation decreases the risk for lung cancer and other cancers, myocardial infarction, cerebrovascular diseases, and chronic lung diseases. Women who stop smoking before pregnancy or during the first 3 to 4 months of pregnancy reduce their risk for having low-birth-weight infants to that of women who never smoked. The health benefits of smoking cessation substantially exceed any risks from the average 5-lb (2.3-kg) weight gain or any adverse psychological effects after quitting.

TREATMENT

Strategies to prevent tobacco use in children and adolescents are listed in Table 16.10–1. For those who already smoke, psychiatrists should advise them to quit smoking. For patients who are ready to stop smoking, it is best to set a "quit date." Most clinicians and smokers prefer abrupt cessation, but because no good data indicate that abrupt cessation is better than gradual cessation, patient preference for gradual cessation should be

Table 16.10–1
Primary Care Interventions to Prevent Tobacco Use in Children and Adolescents Clinical Summary of U.S. Preventive Services Task Force Recommendation

Population	School-aged children and adolescents
Recommendation	Provide interventions to prevent initiation of tobacco use
Risk assessment	The strongest factors associated with smoking initiation in children and adolescents are parental smoking and parental nicotine dependence. Other factors include low levels of parental monitoring, easy access to cigarettes, perception that peers smoke, and exposure to tobacco promotions
Behavioral counseling interventions	Behavioral counseling interventions, such as face-to-face or phone interaction with a health care provider, print materials, and computer applications, can reduce the risk for smoking initiation in school-aged children and adolescents. The type and intensity of effective behavioral interventions substantially varies
Balance of benefits and harms	There is a moderate net benefit to providing primary care interventions to prevent tobacco use in school-aged children and adolescents
Other relevant USPSTF recommendations	The USPSTF has made recommendations on counseling and interventions to prevent tobacco use and tobacco-caused disease in adults and pregnant women. These recommendations are available at www.uspreventiveservicestaskforce.org

For a summary of the evidence systematically reviewed in making this recommendation, the full recommendation statement, and supporting documents, please go to www.uspreventiveservicestaskforce.org.
From Primary Care Interventions to Prevent Tobacco Use in Children and Adolescents, Topic Page, 2013. U.S. Preventive Services Task Force. http://www.uspreventiveservicestaskforce.org/uspstf/uspstbac.htm

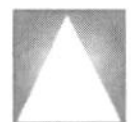

Table 16.10–2
Typical Quit Rates of Common Therapies

Therapy	Rate (%)
Self-quit	5
Self-help books	10
Physician advice	10
Over-the-counter patch or gum	15
Medication plus advice	20
Behavior therapy alone	20
Medication plus group therapy	30

respected. Brief advice should focus on the need for medication or group therapy, weight gain concerns, high-risk situations, making cigarettes unavailable, and so forth. Because relapse is often rapid, the first follow-up phone call or visit should be 2 to 3 days after the quit date. These strategies have been shown to double self-initiated quit rates (Table 16.10–2).

Ms. H was a 45-year-old patient with schizophrenia who smoked 35 cigarettes per day. She began her cigarette use at approximately 20 years of age during the prodromal stages of her first psychotic break. During the first 20 years of treatment, no psychiatrist or physician advised her to stop smoking.

When the patient was 43 years of age, her primary physician recommended smoking cessation. Ms. H attempted to stop on her own but lasted only 48 hours, partly because her housemates and friends smoked. During a routine medication check, her psychiatrist recommended that she stop smoking, and Ms. H described her prior attempts. The psychiatrist and Ms. H discussed ways to avoid smokers and had the patient announce her intent to quit and request that her friends try not to smoke around her and to offer encouragement for her attempt to quit. The psychiatrist also noted that Ms. H became irritable, slightly depressed, and restless, and that she had insomnia during prior cessation attempts, and thus recommended medications. Ms. H chose to use a nicotine patch plus nicotine gum as needed.

The psychiatrist had Ms. H call 2 days after her attempt to quit smoking. At this point, Ms. H stated that the patch and gum were helping. One week later, the patient returned after having relapsed back to smoking. The psychiatrist praised Ms. H for not smoking for 4 days. He suggested that Ms. H contact him again if she wished to try to stop again. Seven months later, during another medication check, the psychiatrist again asked Ms. H to consider cessation, but she was reluctant.

Two months later, Ms. H called and said she wished to try again. This time, the psychiatrist and Ms. H listed several activities that she could do to avoid being around friends who smoked, phoned Ms. H's boyfriend to ask him to assist her in stopping, asked the nurses on the inpatient ward to call Ms. H to encourage her, plus enrolled Ms. H in a support group for the next 4 weeks. This time the psychiatrist prescribed the non-nicotine medication varenicline (Chantix). Ms. H was followed with 15-minute visits for each of the first 3 weeks. She had two "slips" but did not go back to smoking and remained an ex-smoker. *(Adapted from John R. Hughes, M.D.)*

Psychosocial Therapies

Behavior therapy is the most widely accepted and well-proved psychological therapy for smoking. Skills training and relapse prevention identify high-risk situations and plan and practice behavioral or cognitive coping skills for those situations in which smoking occurs. Stimulus control involves eliminating cues for smoking in the environment. Aversive therapy has smokers smoke repeatedly and rapidly to the point of nausea, which associates smoking with unpleasant, rather than pleasant, sensations. Aversive therapy appears to be effective but requires a good therapeutic alliance and patient compliance.

Hypnosis

Some patients benefit from a series of hypnotic sessions. Suggestions about the benefits of not smoking are offered and assimilated into the patient's cognitive framework as a result. Posthypnotic suggestions that cause cigarettes to taste bad or to produce nausea when smoked are also used.

Psychopharmacological Therapies

Nicotine Replacement Therapies. All nicotine replacement therapies double cessation rates, presumably because they reduce nicotine withdrawal. These therapies can also be used to reduce withdrawal in patients on smoke-free wards. Replacement therapies use a short period of maintenance of 6 to 12 weeks, often followed by a gradual reduction period of another 6 to 12 weeks.

Nicotine polacrilex gum (Nicorette) is an OTC product that releases nicotine via chewing and buccal absorption. A 2-mg variety for those who smoke fewer than 25 cigarettes a day and a 4-mg variety for those who smoke more than 25 cigarettes a day are available. Smokers are to use one to two pieces of gum per hour up to a maximum of 24 pieces per day after abrupt cessation. Venous blood concentrations from the gum are one-third to one-half the between-cigarette levels. Acidic beverages (coffee, tea, soda, and juice) should not be used before, during, or after gum use because they decrease absorption. Compliance with the gum has often been a problem. Adverse effects are minor and include bad taste and sore jaws. About 20 percent of those who quit use the gum for long periods, but 2 percent use gum for longer than a year; long-term use does not appear to be harmful. The major advantage of nicotine gum is its ability to provide relief in high-risk situations.

Nicotine lozenges (Commit) deliver nicotine and are also available in 2- and 4-mg forms; they are useful especially for patients who smoke a cigarette immediately on awakening. Generally, 9 to 20 lozenges a day are used during the first 6 weeks, with decrease in dosage thereafter. Lozenges offer the highest level of nicotine of all nicotine replacement products. Users must suck the lozenge until dissolved and not swallow it. Side effects include insomnia, nausea, heartburn, headache, and hiccups.

Nicotine patches, also sold OTC, are available in a 16-hour, no-taper preparation (Nicotrol) and a 24- or 16-hour tapering preparation (Nicoderm CQ). Patches are administered each morning and produce blood concentrations about half those of smoking. Compliance is high, and the only major adverse effects are rashes and, with 24-hour wear, insomnia. Using gum and patches in high-risk situations increases quit rates by another 5 to 10 percent. No studies have been done to determine the relative efficacies of 24- or 16-hour patches or of taper and no-taper patches. After 6 to 12 weeks, the patch is discontinued because it is not for long-term use.

Nicotine nasal spray (Nicotrol), available only by prescription, produces nicotine concentrations in the blood that are more similar to those from smoking a cigarette, and it appears to be especially helpful for heavily dependent smokers. The spray, however, causes rhinitis, watering eyes, and coughing in more than 70 percent of patients. Although initial data suggested abuse liability, further trials have not found this.

The nicotine inhaler, a prescription product, was designed to deliver nicotine to the lungs, but the nicotine is actually absorbed in the upper throat. It delivers 4 mg per cartridge and resultant nicotine levels are low. The major asset of the inhaler is that it provides a behavioral substitute for smoking. The inhaler doubles quit rates. These devices require frequent puffing—about 20 minutes to extract 4 mg of nicotine—and have minor adverse effects.

Non-nicotine Medications. Non-nicotine therapy may help smokers who object philosophically to the notion of replacement therapy and smokers who fail replacement therapy. Bupropion (Zyban) (marketed as Wellbutrin for depression) is an antidepressant medication that has both dopaminergic and adrenergic actions. Bupropion is started at 150 mg per day for 3 days and increased to 150 mg twice a day for 6 to 12 weeks. Daily dosages of 300 mg doubles the quit rates in smokers with and without a history of depression. In one study, combined bupropion and nicotine patch had higher quit rates than either alone. Adverse effects include insomnia and nausea, but these are rarely significant. Seizures have not occurred in smoking trials. Of interest, nortriptyline (Pamelor) appears to be effective for smoking cessation and is recommended as a second-line drug.

Clonidine (Catapres) decreases sympathetic activity from the locus ceruleus and, thus, is thought to abate withdrawal symptoms. Whether given as a patch or orally, 0.2 to 0.4 mg a day of clonidine appears to double quit rates; however, the scientific database for the efficacy of clonidine is neither as extensive nor as reliable as that for nicotine replacement; also, clonidine can cause drowsiness and hypotension. Some patients benefit from benzodiazepine therapy (10 to 30 mg per day) for the first 2 to 3 weeks of abstinence.

A nicotine vaccine that produces nicotine-specific antibodies in the brain is under investigation at the NIDA.

Combined Psychosocial and Pharmacological Therapy

Several studies have shown that combining nicotine replacement and behavior therapy increases quit rates over either therapy alone.

Smoke-Free Environment

Secondhand smoke can contribute to lung cancer death and coronary heart disease in adult nonsmokers. Each year, an estimated 3,000 lung cancer deaths and 62,000 deaths from coronary artery disease in adult nonsmokers are attributed to secondhand smoke. Among children, secondhand smoke is implicated in sudden infant death syndrome, low birth weight, chronic middle ear infections, and respiratory illnesses (e.g., asthma, bronchitis, and pneumonia). Two national health objectives for 2010 are to reduce cigarette smoking among adults to 12 percent and the proportion of nonsmokers exposed to environment tobacco smoke to 45 percent.

Involuntary exposure to secondhand smoke remains a common public health hazard that is preventable by appropriate regulatory policies. Bans on smoking in public places reduce exposure to secondhand smoke and the number of cigarettes smoked by smokers. Support is nearly universal for bans in schools and daycare centers and strong support for bans in indoor work areas and restaurants. Clean indoor air policies are one way to change social norms about smoking and reduce tobacco consumption. Bans on outdoor smoking in areas, such as public parks, are increasing and in 2006 one municipality in California banned smoking entirely within city limits except in one's own home or car and windows had to remain closed. Currently over 600 municipalities have smoke-free park laws, including New York City, which banned smoking in all its public parks, including famed Central Park, in 2011.

▲ 16.11 Anabolic–Androgenic Steroid Abuse

The anabolic–androgenic steroids (AAS) are a family of hormones that includes testosterone, the natural male hormone, which together with numerous synthetic analogs of testosterone have been developed over the last 70 years (Table 16.11–1). These drugs exhibit various degrees of anabolic (muscle building) and androgenic (masculinizing) effects; none of these drugs display purely anabolic effects in the absence of androgenic effects. It is

Table 16.11–1
Examples of Commonly Used Anabolic Steroids

Compounds usually administered orally
- Fluoxymesterone (Halotestin, Android-F, Ultandren)
- Methandienone (formerly called methandrostenolone; Dianabol)
- Methyltestosterone (Android, Testred, Virilon)
- Mibolerone (Cheque Drops[a])
- Oxandrolone (Anavar)
- Oxymetholone (Anadrol, Hemogenin)
- Mesterolone (Mestoranum, Proviron)
- Stanozolol (Winstrol)

Compounds usually administered intramuscularly
- Nandrolone decanoate (Deca-Durabolin)
- Nandrolone phenpropionate (Durabolin)
- Methenolone enanthate (Primobolan Depot)
- Boldenone undecylenate (Equipoise[a])
- Stanozolol (Winstrol-V[a])
- Testosterone esters blends (Sustanon, Sten)
- Testosterone cypionate
- Testosterone enanthate (Delatestryl)
- Testosterone propionate (Testoviron, Androlan)
- Testosterone undecanoate (Andriol, Restandol)
- Trenbolone acetate (Finajet, Finaplix[a])
- Trenbolone hexahydrobencylcarbonate (Parabolan)

Note: Many of the brand names listed above are foreign, but are included because of the widespread illicit use of foreign steroid preparations in the United States.
[a]Veterinary compound.

important not to confuse the AAS (testosterone-like hormones) with corticosteroids (cortisol-like hormones such as hydrocortisone and prednisone). Corticosteroids are hormones secreted by the adrenal gland, rather than by the testes. Corticosteroids have no muscle-building properties and, hence, little abuse potential; they are widely prescribed to treat numerous inflammatory conditions such as poison ivy or asthma. AAS, by contrast, have only limited legitimate medical applications, such as in the treatment of hypogonadal men, the wasting syndrome associated with HIV infection, and a few specific diseases such as hereditary angioedema and Fanconi's anemia. AAS, however, are widely used illicitly, especially by boys and young men seeking to gain increased muscle mass and strength, either for athletic purposes or simply to improve personal appearance.

AAS does not have its own diagnostic category in the fifth edition of the American Psychiatric Association's *Diagnostic and Statistical Manual of Mental Disorders* (DSM-5); rather it is coded as one of the other or unknown substance-related disorders.

EPIDEMIOLOGY

Use of AAS is widespread among men in the United States, but are much less frequently used by women. Approximately 890,000 American men and approximately 190,000 American women reported having used AAS at some time during their lives. Approximately 286,000 men and 26,000 women are estimated to use steroids each year. Among this number, nearly one-third, or 98,000, were between 12 and 17 years of age. Various studies of high school students in the United States have produced even higher estimates of the prevalence of anabolic steroid use among adolescents. Across studies of high school students, it is estimated that 3 to 12 percent of males and 0.5 to 2.0 percent of females have used AAS during their lifetimes.

The current high rates of steroid use among younger individuals appear to represent an important shift in the epidemiology of steroid use. In the 1970s, use of these drugs was largely confined to competition bodybuilders, other elite weight-training athletes, and elite athletes in other sports. Since then, however, it appears that an increasing number of young men, and occasionally even young women, may be using these drugs purely to enhance personal appearance rather than for any athletic purpose.

PHARMACOLOGY

All steroid drugs—including AAS, estrogens, and corticosteroids—are synthesized in vivo from cholesterol and resemble cholesterol in their chemical structure. Testosterone has a four-ring chemical structure containing 19 carbon atoms.

Normal testosterone plasma concentrations for men range from 300 to 1,000 ng/dL. Generally, 200 mg of testosterone cypionate taken every 2 weeks restores physiological testosterone concentrations in a hypogonadal male. A eugonadal male who initiates physiological dosages of testosterone has no net gain in testosterone concentrations because exogenously administered AAS shut down endogenous testosterone production via feedback inhibition of the hypothalamic-pituitary-gonadal axis. Consequently, illicit users take higher than therapeutic dosages to achieve supraphysiological effects. The dose–response curve for anabolic effects may be logarithmic, which could explain why illicit users generally take 10 to 100 times the therapeutic dosages. Doses in this range are most easily achieved by taking combinations of oral and injected AAS, which illicit AAS users often do. Transdermal testosterone, available by prescription for testosterone replacement therapy, may also be used.

Therapeutic Indications

The AAS are indicated primarily for testosterone deficiency (male hypogonadism), hereditary angioedema (a congenital skin disorder), and some uncommon forms of anemia caused by bone marrow or renal failure. In women, AAS are given, although not as first-choice agents, for metastatic breast cancer, osteoporosis, endometriosis, and adjunctive treatment of menopausal symptoms. In men, they have been used experimentally as a male contraceptive and for treating major depressive disorder and sexual disorders in eugonadal men. Recently, they have been used to treat wasting syndromes associated with AIDS. Controlled studies have also suggested that testosterone has antidepressant effects in some men infected with HIV with major depressive disorder, and is also a supplementary (augmentation) treatment in some depressed men with low endogenous testosterone levels who are refractory to conventional antidepressants.

Adverse Reactions

The most common adverse medical effects of AAS involve the cardiovascular, hepatic, reproductive, and dermatological systems.

The AAS produce an adverse cholesterol profile by increasing levels of low-density lipoprotein cholesterol and decreasing levels of high-density lipoprotein cholesterol. High-dose use of AAS can also activate hemostasis and increase blood pressure. Isolated case reports of myocardial infarction, cardiomyopathy, left ventricular hypertrophy, and stroke among users of AAS, including fatalities, have appeared,

Among the AAS-induced endocrine effects in men are testicular atrophy and sterility, both usually reversible after discontinuing AAS, and gynecomastia, which may persist until surgical removal. In women, shrinkage of breast tissue, irregular menses (diminution or cessation), and masculinization (clitoral hypertrophy, hirsutism, and deepened voice) can occur. Masculinizing effects in women may be irreversible. Androgens taken during pregnancy could cause masculinization of a female fetus. Dermatological effects include acne and male pattern baldness. Abuse of AAS by children has led to concerns that AAS-induced premature closure of bony epiphyses could cause shortened stature. Other uncommon adverse effects include edema of the extremities caused by water retention, exacerbation of tic disorders, sleep apnea, and polycythemia.

ETIOLOGY

The major reason for taking illicit AAS is to enhance either athletic performance or physical appearance. Taking AAS is reinforced because they can produce the athletic and physical effects that users desire, especially when combined with proper diet and training. Further reinforcement derives from winning competitions and from social admiration for physical appearance.

AAS users also perceive that they can train more intensively for longer durations with less fatigue and with decreased recovery times between workouts.

Although the anabolic or muscle-building properties of AAS are clearly important to those seeking to enhance athletic performance and physical appearance, psychoactive effects may also be important in the persistent and dependent use of AAS. Anecdotally, some AAS users report feelings of power, aggressiveness, and euphoria, which become associated with, and can reinforce, AAS taking.

In general, males are more likely to take AAS than females, and athletes are more likely to take AAS than nonathletes. Some male and female weightlifters may have muscle dysmorphia, a form of body dysmorphic disorder in which the individual feels that he or she is not sufficiently muscular and lean.

DIAGNOSIS AND CLINICAL FEATURES

Steroids may initially induce euphoria and hyperactivity. After relatively short periods, however, their use can become associated with increased anger, arousal, irritability, hostility, anxiety, somatization, and depression (especially during times when steroids are not used). Several studies have demonstrated that 2 to 15 percent of anabolic steroid abusers experience hypomanic or manic episodes, and a smaller percentage may have clearly psychotic symptoms. Also disturbing is a correlation between steroid abuse and violence ("roid rage" in the parlance of users). Steroid abusers with no record of antisocial behavior or violence have committed murders and other violent crimes.

Steroids are addictive substances. When abusers stop taking steroids, they can become depressed, anxious, and concerned about the physical state of their bodies. Some similarities have been noted between athletes' views of their muscles and the views of patients with anorexia nervosa about their bodies; to an observer, both groups seem to distort realistic assessment of the body.

Iatrogenic addiction is a consideration in view of the increasing number of geriatric patients who are receiving testosterone from their physicians in an attempt to increase libido and reverse some aspects of aging.

Mr. A is a 26-year-old single man. He is 69 inches tall and presently weighs 204 pounds, with a body fat of 11 percent. He reports that he began lifting weights at age 17, at which time he weighed 155 pounds. About 2 years after beginning his weight lifting, he began taking AAS, which he obtained through a friend at his gymnasium. His first "cycle" (course) of AAS, lasting for 9 weeks, involved methandienone (Methanabol), 30 mg a day, orally, and testosterone cypionate, 600 mg a week, intramuscularly. During these 9 weeks he gained 20 pounds of muscle mass. He was so pleased with these results that he took five further cycles of AAS over the course of the next 6 years. During his most ambitious cycle, approximately 1 year ago, he used testosterone cypionate, 600 mg per week; nandrolone decanoate, 400 mg a week; stanozolol (Winstrol), 12 mg a day; and oxandrolone (Anavar), 10 mg a day.

During each of the cycles Mr. A has noted euphoria, irritability, and grandiose feelings. These symptoms were most prominent during his most recent cycle, when he felt "invincible." During this cycle he also noted a decreased need for sleep, racing thoughts, and a tendency to spend excessive amounts of money. For example, he impulsively purchased a $2,700 stereo system when he realistically could not afford to spend more than $500. He also became uncharacteristically irritable with his girlfriend, and on one occasion put his fist through the side window of her car during an argument, an act inconsistent with his normally mild-mannered personality. After this cycle of AAS ended, he became mildly depressed for about 2 months.

Mr. A has used a number of drugs to lose weight in preparation for bodybuilding contests. These include ephedrine, amphetamine, triiodothyronine, and thyroxin. Recently, he has also begun to use the opioid agonist–antagonist nalbuphine intravenously (IV) to treat muscle aches from weightlifting. He also used oral opioids, such as controlled-release oxycodone (OxyContin), at least once a week. He uses oral opioids sometimes to treat muscle aches, but often simply to get high. He reports that use of nalbuphine and other opioids is widespread among other AAS users of his acquaintance.

Mr. A exhibits characteristic features of muscle dysmorphia. He checks his appearance dozens of times a day in mirrors, or when he sees his reflection in a store window or even in the back of a spoon. He becomes anxious if he misses even one day of working out at the gym, and acknowledges that his preoccupation with weightlifting has cost him both social and occupational opportunities. Although he has a 48-inch chest and 19-inch biceps, he has frequently declined invitations to go to the beach or a swimming pool for fear that he would look too small when seen in a bathing suit. He is anxious because he has lost some weight since the end of his previous cycle of AAS and is eager to resume another cycle of AAS in the near future. *(Adapted from Harrison G. Pope, Jr., M.D. and Kirk J. Brower, M.D.)*

TREATMENT

Abstinence is the treatment goal of choice for patients manifesting AAS abuse or dependence. To the extent that users of AAS abuse other addictive substances (including alcohol), traditional treatment approaches for substance-related disorders may be used. Nevertheless, AAS users may differ from other addicted patients in several ways that have implications for treatment. First, the euphorigenic and reinforcing effects of AAS may only become apparent after weeks or months of use in conjunction with intensive exercising. When compared with immediately and passively reinforcing drugs, such as cocaine, heroin, and alcohol, AAS use may entail more delayed gratification. Second, AAS users may manifest greater commitment to culturally endorsed values of physical fitness, success, victory, and goal directness than users of other illicit drugs. Finally, AAS users are often preoccupied with their physical attributes and may rely excessively on these attributes for self-esteem. Treatment therefore depends on a therapeutic alliance that is based on a thorough and nonjudgmental understanding of the patient's values and motivations for using AAS.

AAS Withdrawal

Supportive therapy and monitoring are essential for treating AAS withdrawal because suicidal depressions can occur. Hospitalization may be required when suicidal ideation is severe. Patients should be educated about the possible course of withdrawal and reassured that symptoms are time-limited and manageable. Antidepressant agents are best reserved for patients whose depressive symptomatology persists for several weeks after AAS discontinuation and who meet criteria for major depressive disorder. SSRIs are the preferred agents because of their favorable adverse effect profile and their effectiveness in the only reported case series of treated AAS users with major depressive disorder. Physical withdrawal symptoms are not life-threatening and do not ordinarily require pharmacotherapy. Nonsteroidal anti-inflammatory drugs (NSAIDs) may be useful to treat musculoskeletal pain and headaches.

ANABOLIC STEROID–INDUCED MOOD DISORDERS

Irritability, aggressiveness, hypomania, and frank mania associated with anabolic steroid use probably represent one of the most important public health issues associated with these drugs. Although athletes using these drugs have long recognized that syndromes of anger and irritability could be associated with AAS use, these syndromes were little recognized in the scientific literature until the late 1980s and 1990s. Since then, a series of observational field studies of athletes has suggested that some AAS users develop prominent hypomanic or even manic symptoms during AAS use.

A possible serious consequence of AAS-induced mood disorders may be violent or even homicidal behavior. Several published reports have anecdotally described individuals with no apparent history of psychiatric disorder, no criminal record, and no history of violence, who committed violent crimes, including murder, while under the influence of AAS. In a number of cases, AAS use has been cited in criminal trials as a possible mitigating factor in the defense of such individuals. Although a causal link is difficult to establish in these cases, evidence of AAS use has frequently been presented in forensic settings as a possible mitigating factor in criminal behavior.

Depressive syndromes induced by AAS have occurred and suicide is a risk. A brief and self-limited syndrome of depression occurs on AAS withdrawal, probably as a result of the depression of the hypothalamic-pituitary-gonadal axis after exogenous AAS administration.

ANABOLIC STEROID–INDUCED PSYCHOTIC DISORDER

Psychotic symptoms are rare in association with anabolic steroid use, but they have been described in a few cases, primarily in individuals who were using the equivalent of more than 1,000 mg of testosterone a week. Usually, these symptoms have consisted of grandiose or paranoid delusions, generally occurring in the context of a manic episode, although occasionally occurring in the absence of a frank manic syndrome. In most reported cases, psychotic symptoms have disappeared promptly (within a few weeks) after the discontinuation of the offending agent, although temporary treatment with antipsychotic agents was sometimes required.

OTHER ANABOLIC STEROID–RELATED DISORDERS

Symptoms of anxiety disorders, such as panic disorder and social phobia, can occur during AAS use. AAS use may serve as a "gateway to the use of opioid agonist or antagonists, such as nalbuphine, or to use of frank opioid agonists, such as heroin." A study of men admitted for substance-dependence treatment in Massachusetts produced similar findings.

DEHYDROEPIANDROSTERONE AND ANDROSTENEDIONE

Dehydroepiandrosterone (DHEA), a precursor hormone for both estrogens and androgens, is available over the counter. Recent years have seen an interest in DHEA for improving cognition, depression, sex drive, and general well-being in elderly adults. Some reports suggest that DHEA in dosages of 50 to 100 mg per day increases the sense of physical and social well-being in women aged 40 to 70 years. Reports also exist of androgenic effects, including irreversible hirsutism, hair loss, voice deepening, and other undesirable sequelae. In addition, DHEA has at least a theoretical potential of enhancing tumor growth in persons with latent, hormone-sensitive malignancies, such as prostate, cervical, and breast cancer. Despite its significant popularity, few controlled data exist on the safety or efficacy of DHEA.

▲ 16.12 Cannabis-Related Disorders

Cannabis is the most widely used illegal drug in the world, with an estimate 19 million users in 2012. Cannabis has become a common part of youth culture in most developed societies, with first use now occurring in the mid- to late teenage years. Cannabis is the fourth most commonly used psychoactive drug among adults in the United States, after caffeine, alcohol, and nicotine.

CANNABIS PREPARATIONS

Cannabis preparations are obtained from the plant *Cannabis sativa,* which has been used in China, India, and the Middle East for approximately 8,000 years, primarily for its fibers and secondarily for its medicinal properties. The plant occurs in male and female forms. The female plant contains the highest concentrations of more than 60 cannabinoids that are unique to the plant. Delta-9-tetrahydrocannabinol (Δ9-THC) is the cannabinoid that is primarily responsible for the psychoactive effects of cannabis. The most potent forms of cannabis come from the flowering tops of the plants or from the dried, black-brown, resinous exudate from the leaves, which are referred to as hashish or hash. The cannabis plant is usually cut, dried, chopped, and rolled into cigarettes (commonly called "joints"), which are then smoked. The common names for cannabis are marijuana, grass, pot, weed, tea, and Mary Jane. Other names, which describe cannabis types of various strengths, are hemp, charas, bhang, ganja, dagga, and sinsemilla. The potency of marijuana preparations has increased in recent years because of improved agricultural techniques used in cultivation so that plants may contain up to 15 or 20 percent THC.

EPIDEMIOLOGY

Prevalence and Recent Trends

Based on the 2012 NSDUH, an estimated 19 million persons aged 12 years and older (7 percent) had used marijuana in the past month. Of this age group, 2.4 million initiated use within the last year, 57 percent of which initiated use before age 18 years. Since then, use has increased markedly, especially among young adults 18 to 25.

The *Monitoring the Future* survey of adolescents in school indicates recent increases in lifetime, annual, current (within the past 30 days), and daily use of marijuana by eighth and tenth graders, continuing a trend that began in the early 1990s. In 1996, about 23 percent of eighth graders and about 40 percent of tenth graders reported having used marijuana and, in 1998 and 1999, more than a quarter of marijuana initiates were aged 14 years or younger. The average age was 17. Approximately 1 percent of eighth graders, 4 percent of tenth graders, and 7 percent of twelfth graders reported daily use of marijuana.

Demographic Correlates

The rate of past year and current marijuana use by males was almost twice the rate for females overall among those aged 26 and older. This gap between the sexes narrows with younger users; at ages 12 to 17, there are no significant differences.

Race and ethnicity were also related to marijuana use, but the relationships varied by age group. Among those aged 12 to 17, whites had higher rates of lifetime and past-year marijuana use than blacks. Among those 17 to 34 years of age, whites reported higher levels of lifetime use than blacks and Hispanics. But among those 35 and older, whites and blacks reported the same levels of use. The lifetime rates for black adults were significantly higher than those for Hispanics.

NEUROPHARMACOLOGY

As stated above, the principal component of cannabis is Δ9-THC; however, the cannabis plant contains more than 400 chemicals, of which about 60 are chemically related to Δ9-THC. In humans, Δ9-THC is rapidly converted into 11-hydroxy-Δ9-THC, the metabolite that is active in the CNS.

A specific receptor for the cannabinols has been identified, cloned, and characterized. The cannabinoid receptor, a member of the G-protein-linked family of receptors, is linked to the inhibitory G protein (Gi), which is linked to adenylyl cyclase in an inhibitory fashion. The cannabinoid receptor is found in highest concentrations in the basal ganglia, the hippocampus, and the cerebellum, with lower concentrations in the cerebral cortex. This receptor is not found in the brainstem, a fact consistent with cannabis's minimal effects on respiratory and cardiac functions. Studies in animals have shown that the cannabinoids affect the monoamine and GABA neurons.

According to most studies, animals do not self-administer cannabinoids as they do most other substances of abuse. Moreover, some debate questions whether the cannabinoids stimulate the so-called reward centers of the brain, such as the dopaminergic neurons of the ventral tegmental area. Tolerance to cannabis does develop, however, and psychological dependence has been found, although the evidence for physiological dependence is not strong. Withdrawal symptoms in humans are limited to modest increases in irritability, restlessness, insomnia, and anorexia and mild nausea; all these symptoms appear only when a person abruptly stops taking high doses of cannabis.

When cannabis is smoked, the euphoric effects appear within minutes, peak in about 30 minutes, and last 2 to 4 hours. Some motor and cognitive effects last 5 to 12 hours. Cannabis can also be taken orally when it is prepared in food, such as brownies and cakes. About two to three times as much cannabis must be taken orally to be as potent as cannabis taken by inhaling its smoke. Many variables affect the psychoactive properties of cannabis, including the potency of the cannabis used, the route of administration, the smoking technique, the effects of pyrolysis on the cannabinoid content, the dose, the setting, and the user's past experience, expectations, and unique biological vulnerability to the effects of cannabinoids.

DIAGNOSIS AND CLINICAL FEATURES

The most common physical effects of cannabis are dilation of the conjunctival blood vessels (red eye) and mild tachycardia. At high doses, orthostatic hypotension may appear. Increased appetite—often referred to as "the munchies"—and dry mouth are common effects of cannabis intoxication. That no clearly documented case of death caused by cannabis intoxication alone reflects the substance's lack of effect on the respiratory rate. The most serious potential adverse effects of cannabis use are those caused by inhaling the same carcinogenic hydrocarbons present in conventional tobacco, and some data indicate that heavy cannabis users are at risk for chronic respiratory disease and lung cancer. The practice of smoking cannabis-containing cigarettes to their very ends, so-called "roaches," further increases the intake of tar (particulate matter). Many reports indicate that long-term cannabis use is associated with cerebral atrophy, seizure susceptibility, chromosomal damage, birth defects, impaired immune reactivity, alterations in testosterone concentrations, and dysregulation of menstrual cycles; these reports, however, have not been conclusively replicated, and the association between these findings and cannabis use is uncertain.

Cannabis Use Disorder

The fifth edition of the *Diagnostic and Statistical Manual of Mental Disorders* (DSM-5) includes the diagnosis of cannabis use disorder. People who use cannabis daily over weeks to months are most likely to become dependent. The risk of developing dependence is around one in ten for anyone who uses cannabis. The earlier the age of first use, the more often cannabis has been used, and the longer it has been used, the higher the risk of dependence.

Cannabis Intoxication. Cannabis intoxication commonly heightens users' sensitivities to external stimuli, reveals new details, makes colors seem brighter and richer, and subjectively slows the appreciation of time. In high doses, users may experience depersonalization and derealization. Motor skills are impaired by cannabis use, and the impairment in motor skills remains after the subjective, euphoriant effects have resolved. For 8 to 12 hours after using cannabis, users' impaired motor skills interfere with the operation of motor vehicles and other heavy machinery. Moreover, these effects are additive to those of alcohol, which is commonly used in combination with cannabis.

Mr. M was an unemployed 20-year-old man who lived with his parents. He was brought to a hospital by some friends in a state of anxiety and agitation. He had been out for the evening with some friends at a restaurant, and after a couple of beers, he decided to have some cannabis. He had smoked cannabis on previous occasions; however, this time he ate a lump of cannabis despite warnings from his friends. After about half an hour, Mr. M appeared tense and anxious and complained that everything was changing. He could see the faces of his friends increasing to about three times their natural size. The room became distorted, and its proportions and colors kept altering. He felt that the other guests in the restaurant were talking about him and his friends in a menacing way, so he suddenly rushed outside because he felt that he was in danger. He became increasingly agitated and started running down the middle of the street, dodging in and out among the traffic. Eventually, his friends were able to catch him. They were unable to quiet his anxiety, however, and had a hard time persuading him to go with them to the hospital.

On examination Mr. M appeared tense and apprehensive, looking around the room as if he felt uneasy with the surroundings, but he denied perceptual symptoms and did not really believe that he was the subject of persecution. He was fully aware of his surroundings, but his attention was fleeting, and he did not always answer questions. There was no marked impairment of memory, and he was fully oriented.

Physical examination revealed conjunctival injection and an increased pulse rate of 120 beats per minute, but otherwise no abnormalities were found. Neurological examination also revealed no abnormalities. In the course of a few hours, he quieted down. When he felt recovered, he left the hospital with his friends.

Cannabis Intoxication Delirium

The delirium associated with cannabis intoxication is characterized by marked impairment on cognition and performance tasks. Even modest doses of cannabis impair memory, reaction time, perception, motor coordination, and attention. High doses that also impair users' levels of consciousness have marked effects on cognitive measures.

Cannabis Withdrawal

Studies have shown that cessation of use in daily cannabis users results in withdrawal symptoms within 1 to 2 weeks of cessation. Withdrawal symptoms include irritability, cannabis cravings, nervousness, anxiety, insomnia, disturbed or vivid dreaming, decreased appetite, weight loss, depressed mood, restlessness, headache, chills, stomach pain, sweating, and tremors.

Cannabis-Induced Psychotic Disorder

Cannabis-induced psychotic disorder is diagnosed in the presence of a cannabis-induced psychosis. Cannabis-induced psychotic disorder is rare; transient paranoid ideation is more common.

Florid psychosis is somewhat common in countries in which some persons have long-term access to cannabis of particularly high potency. The psychotic episodes are sometimes referred to as "hemp insanity." Cannabis use rarely causes a "bad-trip" experience, which is often associated with hallucinogen intoxication. When cannabis-induced psychotic disorder does occur, it may be correlated with a preexisting personality disorder in the affected person.

Cannabis-Induced Anxiety Disorder

Cannabis-induced anxiety disorder is a common diagnosis for acute cannabis intoxication, which in many persons induces short-lived anxiety states often provoked by paranoid thoughts. In such circumstances, panic attacks may be induced, based on ill-defined and disorganized fears. The appearance of anxiety symptoms is correlated with the dose and is the most frequent adverse reaction to the moderate use of smoked cannabis. Inexperienced users are much more likely to experience anxiety symptoms than are experienced users.

A 35-year-old white married male who was naïve to cannabis use was given two "joints" by a friend. He smoked the first of the two in the same manner that he normally smoked a cigarette (in about 3 to 5 minutes). Noting no major effects, he proceeded immediately to smoke the second in the same amount of time. Within 30 minutes, he began to experience rapid heartbeat, dry mouth, mounting anxiety and the delusional belief that his throat was closing up and that he was going to die. That belief induced further panic and the patient was brought to the emergency room in the midst of the experience. Reassurance that he would not die had no effect. He was sedated with diazepam and some of his anxiety diminished. He eventually went to sleep and on awakening in about 5 hours he was asymptomatic with full recall of previous events.

Unspecified Cannabis-Related Disorders

DSM-5 includes the category unspecified cannabis-related disorders for cannabis disorders that cannot be classified as cannabis use disorder, cannabis intoxication, cannabis intoxication delirium, cannabis withdrawal, cannabis-induced psychotic disorder, or cannabis-induced anxiety disorder. Cannabis intoxication can be associated with depressive symptoms, although such symptoms may suggest long-term cannabis use. Hypomania, however, is a common symptom in cannabis intoxication.

When either sleep disorder or sexual dysfunction symptoms are related to cannabis use, they almost always resolve within days or a week after cessation of cannabis use.

Flashbacks. There are case reports of persons who have experienced—at times significantly—sensations related to cannabis intoxication after the short-term effects of the substance have disappeared. Continued debate concerns whether flashbacks are related to cannabis use alone or to the concomitant use of hallucinogens or of cannabis tainted with PCP.

Cognitive Impairment. Clinical and experimental evidence indicates that the long-term use of cannabis may produce subtle forms of cognitive impairment in the higher cognitive functions of memory, attention, and organization and in the integration of complex information. This evidence suggests that the longer the period of heavy cannabis use, the more pronounced the cognitive impairment. Nonetheless, because the impairments in performance are subtle, it remains to be determined how significant they are for everyday functioning. It also remains to be investigated whether these impairments can be reversed after an extended period of abstinence from cannabis.

Amotivational Syndrome. A controversial cannabis-related syndrome is *amotivational syndrome.* Whether the syndrome is related to cannabis use or reflects characterological traits in a subgroup of persons regardless of cannabis use is under debate. Traditionally, the amotivational syndrome has been associated with long-term heavy use and has been characterized by a person's unwillingness to persist in a task—be it at school, at work, or in any setting that requires prolonged attention or tenacity. Persons are described as becoming apathetic and anergic, usually gaining weight, and appearing slothful.

TREATMENT AND REHABILITATION

Treatment of cannabis use rests on the same principles as treatment of other substances of abuse—abstinence and support. Abstinence can be achieved through direct interventions, such as hospitalization, or through careful monitoring on an outpatient basis by the use of urine drug screens, which can detect cannabis for up to 4 weeks after use. Support can be achieved through the use of individual, family, and group psychotherapies. Education should be a cornerstone for both abstinence and support programs. A patient who does not understand the intellectual reasons for addressing a substance-abuse problem has little motivation to stop. For some patients, an antianxiety drug may be useful for short-term relief of withdrawal symptoms. For other patients, cannabis use may be related to an underlying depressive disorder that may respond to specific antidepressant treatment.

Medical Use of Marijuana

Marijuana has been used as a medicinal herb for centuries, and cannabis was listed in the US Pharmacopeia until the end of the 19th century as a remedy for anxiety, depression, and gastrointestinal disorders, among others. Currently, cannabis is a controlled substance with a high potential for abuse and no medical use recognized by the DEA; however, it is used to treat various disorders, such as the nausea secondary to chemotherapy, multiple sclerosis (MS) chronic pain, AIDS, epilepsy, and glaucoma. In 1996, California residents approved the California Compensation Use Act that allowed state residents to grow and use marijuana for these disorders: in 2001, however, the U.S. Supreme Court ruled 8 to 0 that the manufacture and distribution of marijuana are illegal under any circumstances. In addition, the Court held that patients using marijuana for medical purposes can be prosecuted; however, as of 2013, 20 states—Alaska, Arizona, California, Colorado, Connecticut, Delaware, Hawaii, Illinois, Maine, Massachusetts, Michigan, Montana, Nevada, New Hampshire, New Jersey, New Mexico, Oregon, Rhode Island, Vermont, and Washington—and the District of Columbia have passed laws exempting patients who use cannabis under a physician's supervision from state criminal penalties.

In addition to the Supreme Court ruling, periodically the federal government attempts to prosecute doctors who prescribe the drug for medical use with the threat of loss of licensure or jail sentences. In a strongly worded editorial, the *New England Journal of Medicine* urged that "Federal authorities should rescind their prohibition of the medical use of marijuana for seriously ill patients and allow physicians to decide which patients to treat." The editorial concluded by commenting on the role of the physician: "Some physicians will have the courage to challenge the continued proscription of marijuana for the sick. Eventually, their actions will force the courts to adjudicate between the rights of those at death's door and the absolute power of bureaucrats whose decisions are based more on reflexive ideology and political correctness than on compassion."

Dronabinol, a synthetic form of THC, has been approved by the FDA; some researchers believe, however, that when taken orally, it is not as effective as smoking the entire plant product. In 2006, regulatory officials authorized the first U.S. clinical trial investigating the efficacy of Sativex, an oral spray consisting of natural cannabis extracts, for the treatment of cancer pain. Sativex is currently available by prescription in Canada and on a limited basis in Spain and Great Britain for patients with neuropathic pain, multiple sclerosis, and other conditions. Sativex can be prescribed in the United States only with a special exemption granted by the FDA for use in certain patients. In 2013, a product called Epidiolex which contains cannabidiol was granted orphan drug status for the treatment of certain rare, intractable types of epilepsy in children.

New York State Medical Marijuana Program. In 2016, New York State licensed physicians who completed special training to become prescribers of marijuana to patients with severe, debilitating or life-threatening conditions: cancer, HIV infection or AIDS, amyotrophic lateral sclerosis (ALS), spinal cord injury with spasticity, epilepsy, inflammatory bowel disease, neuropathy, and Huntington's disease. No psychiatric disorders are currently on the list of conditions; however, there are reports of marijuana being of use in alleviating anxiety and depression in certain patients with those disorders. It has been approved in some states for use in post traumatic stress disorder (PTSD). The program will be closely monitored and should provide a wealth of data about its effectiveness.

▲ 16.13 Other Substance Use and Addictive Disorders

This section considers a diverse set of drugs not covered in the previous sections that are not easily categorized and grouped with other substances. The fifth edition of the *Diagnostic and Statistical Manual of Mental Disorders* (DSM-5) includes a diagnostic category for these substances called unknown or unspecified substance-related disorders. Some of these are discussed in the following.

γ-HYDROXYBUTYRATE

γ-Hydroxybutyrate (GHB) is a naturally occurring neurotransmitter in the brain that is related to sleep regulation. GHB increases dopamine levels in the brain. In general, GHB is a central nervous system (CNS) depressant with effects through the endogenous opioid system. It is used to induce anesthesia and long-term sedation, but its unpredictable duration of action limits its use. GHB has been evaluated recently for the treatment of alcohol and opioid withdrawal and narcolepsy.

Until 1990, GHB was sold in U.S. health food stores, and bodybuilders used it as a steroid alternative. Reports indicate, however, that GHB is abused for its intoxicating effects and consciousness-altering properties. It is variously referred to as "GBH" and "liquid ecstasy," and it is sold illicitly in various forms (e.g., powder and liquid). Similar chemicals, which the body converts to GBH, include γ-butyrolactone (GBL) and 1,4-butanediol. Adverse effects include nausea, vomiting, respiratory problems, seizures, coma, and death. In some reports, GHB abuse has been linked to a syndrome similar to Wernicke–Korsakoff syndrome.

NITRITE INHALANTS

The nitrite inhalants include amyl, butyl, and isobutyl nitrites, all of which are called "poppers" in popular jargon. The intoxication syndromes seen with nitrites can differ markedly from the syndromes seen with the standard inhalant substances, such as lighter fluid and airplane glue. Nitrite inhalants are used by persons seeking the associated mild euphoria, altered sense of time, feeling of fullness in the head, and, possibly, increased sexual feelings. The nitrite compounds are used by some gay men and users of other drugs to heighten sexual stimulation during orgasm and, in some cases, to relax the anal sphincter for penile penetration. Under such circumstances, a person may use the substance for a few or a dozen times within several hours.

Adverse reactions include a toxic syndrome characterized by nausea, vomiting, headache, hypotension, drowsiness, and irritation of the respiratory tract. Some evidence indicates that nitrite inhalants can adversely affect immune function. Because sildenafil (Viagra) and its congeners are lethal when combined with nitrite compounds, persons at risk should be cautioned never to use the two together.

NITROUS OXIDE

Nitrous oxide, commonly known as "laughing gas," is a widely available anesthetic agent that is subject to abuse because of its ability to produce feelings of lightheadedness and of floating, sometimes experienced as pleasurable or specifically as sexual. With long-term abuse patterns, nitrous oxide use has been associated with delirium and paranoia. Female dental assistants exposed to high levels of nitrous oxide have reportedly experienced reduced fertility.

A 35-year-old male dentist with no history of other substance problems complained of problems with nitrous oxide abuse for 10 years. This had begun as experimentation with what he had considered a harmless substance. His rate of use increased over several years, however, eventually becoming almost daily for months at a time. He felt a craving before sessions of use. Then, using the gas while alone in his office, he immediately felt numbness, a change in his temperature and heart rate, and alleviation of depressed feelings. "Things would go through my mind. Time was erased." He sometimes fell asleep. Sessions might last a few minutes or up to 8 hours. They ended when the craving and euphoria ended. He had often tried to stop or cut down, sometimes consulting a professional about the problem.

OTHER SUBSTANCES

Nutmeg

Nutmeg can be ingested in a number of preparations. When nutmeg is taken in sufficiently high doses, it can induce depersonalization, derealization, and a feeling of heaviness in the limbs. In sufficiently high doses, morning glory seeds can produce a syndrome resembling that seen with lysergic acid diethylamide (LSD), characterized by altered sensory perceptions and mild visual hallucinations.

Catnip

Catnip can produce cannabis-like intoxication in low doses and LSD-like intoxication in high doses.

Betel Nuts

Betel nuts, when chewed, can produce a mild euphoria and a feeling of floating in space.

Kava

Kava, derived from a pepper plant native to the South Pacific, produces sedation and incoordination and is associated with hepatitis, lung abnormalities, and weight loss.

Over-the-Counter Drugs

Some persons abuse over-the-counter and prescription medications, such as cortisol, antiparkinsonian agents, and antihistamines.

Ephedra

Ephedra, a natural substance found in herbal tea, acts like epinephrine and, when abused, produces cardiac arrhythmia and fatalities.

Chocolate

A controversial possible substance of abuse is chocolate derived from the cacao bean. Anandamide, an ingredient in chocolate, stimulates the same receptors as marijuana. Other compounds in chocolate include tryptophan, the precursor of serotonin, and phenylalanine, an amphetamine-like substance, both of which improve mood. So-called chocoholics may be self-medicating because of a depressive diathesis.

POLYSUBSTANCE-RELATED DISORDER

Substance users often abuse more than one substance. A diagnosis of polysubstance dependence is appropriate if, for a period of at least 12 months, a person has repeatedly used substances from at least three categories (not including nicotine and caffeine), even if the diagnostic criteria for a substance-related disorder are not met for any single substance, as long as, during this period, the criteria for substance dependence have been met for the substances considered as a group.

TREATMENT AND REHABILITATION

Treatment approaches for the substances covered in this section vary according to substances, patterns of abuse, availability of psychosocial support systems, and patients' individual features. Two major treatment goals for substance abuse have been determined: the first is abstinence from the substance and the second is the physical, psychiatric, and psychosocial well-being of the patient. Significant damage has often been done to a patient's support systems during prolonged periods of substance abuse. For a patient to stop a pattern of substance abuse successfully, adequate psychosocial supports must be in place to foster the difficult change in behavior.

In some rare cases, it may be necessary to initiate treatment on an inpatient unit. Although an outpatient setting is more desirable than an inpatient setting, the temptations available to an outpatient for repeated use may present too high a hurdle for the initiation of treatment. Inpatient treatment is also indicated in the case of severe medical or psychiatric symptoms, a history of failed outpatient treatments, a lack of psychosocial supports, or a particularly severe or long-term history of substance abuse. After an initial period of detoxification, patients need a sustained period of rehabilitation. Throughout treatment, individual, family, and group therapies can be effective. Education about substance abuse and support for patients' efforts are essential factors in treatment.

17

Neurocognitive Disorders

▲ 17.1 Introduction and Overview

Advances in molecular biology diagnostic techniques and medication management have significantly improved the ability to recognize and treat cognitive disorders. Cognition includes memory, language, orientation, judgment, conducting interpersonal relationships, performing actions (praxis), and problem solving. Cognitive disorders reflect disruption in one or more of these domains and are frequently complicated by behavioral symptoms. Cognitive disorders exemplify the complex interface among neurology, medicine, and psychiatry in that medical or neurological conditions often lead to cognitive disorders that, in turn, are associated with behavioral symptoms. It can be argued that of all psychiatric conditions, cognitive disorders best demonstrate how biological insults result in behavioral symptomatology. The clinician must carefully assess the history and context of the presentation of these disorders before arriving at a diagnosis and treatment plan.

This century-old distinction between organic and functional disorders is outdated and has been deleted from the nomenclature. Every psychiatric disorder has an organic (i.e., biological or chemical) component. Because of this reassessment, the concept of functional disorders has been determined to be misleading, and the term *functional* and its historical opposite, *organic,* are no longer used in the current *Diagnostic and Statistical Manual of Mental Disorders* (DSM) nomenclature. A further indication that the dichotomy is no longer valid is the revival of the term *neuropsychiatry,* which emphasizes the somatic substructure on which mental operations and emotions are based; it is concerned with the psychopathological accompaniments of brain dysfunction as observed in seizure disorders, for example. Neuropsychiatry focuses on the psychiatric aspects of neurological disorders and the role of brain dysfunction in psychiatric disorders.

Cognitive disorders tend to defy Occam's razor—the law of parsimony—challenging clinicians and nosologists with multiplicity, comorbidity, and unclear boundaries. These concerns are most true in elderly adults, the demographic group most at risk for cognitive disorders. Dementias of late life are particularly problematic in this regard. Existing, although often unrecognized, dementia is a major risk factor for superimposed delirium. Moreover, certain dementias, such as dementia with Lewy bodies or late stages of Alzheimer's disease, may have chronic clinical presentations virtually indistinguishable from delirium except for temporal onset and the lack of an identifiable acute source. Similarly, the course of nearly all subjects developing a progressive dementia is complicated by the onset of one or more distinct behavioral syndromes, including anxiety, depression, sleep problems, psychosis, and aggression. These symptoms can be as distressing and disabling as the primary cognitive disorder. Some of these behavioral syndromes, such as psychosis, may themselves result from independent underlying biologies and may be additive with the primary neurodegenerative process.

The boundaries between types of dementia and between dementia and normal aging can be similarly diffuse. Neuropathologic studies of both clinical and population samples have revealed a surprising truth. The most common neuropathologic presentation associated with dementia reveal mixtures of Alzheimer's disease, vascular, and Lewy body pathologies. Pure syndromes are relatively less common, although often the dementia is ascribed to one of the coexisting pathologies. Strategies regarding how to understand or reconcile multiple pathologies in the clinic are needed, although they lag behind.

DEFINITION

Delirium

Delirium is marked by short-term confusion and changes in cognition. There are four subcategories based on several causes: (1) general medical condition (e.g., infection), (2) substance induced (e.g., cocaine, opioids, phencyclidine [PCP]), (3) multiple causes (e.g., head trauma and kidney disease), and (4) other or multiple etiologies (e.g., sleep deprivation, mediation). Delirium is discussed in Section 17.2.

Dementia (Major Neurocognitive Disorder)

Dementia, also referred to as major neurocognitive disorder in DSM-5, is marked by severe impairment in memory, judgment, orientation, and cognition. The subcategories are (1) dementia of the Alzheimer's type, which usually occurs in persons older than 65 years of age and is manifested by progressive intellectual disorientation and dementia, delusions, or depression; (2) vascular dementia, caused by vessel thrombosis or hemorrhage; (3) human immunodeficiency virus (HIV) disease; (4) head trauma; (5) Pick's disease or frontotemporal lobar degeneration; (6) Prion disease such as Creutzfeldt–Jakob disease, which is caused by a slow-growing transmittable virus; (7) substance induced, caused by toxin or medication (e.g., gasoline fumes, atropine); (8) multiple etiologies; and (9) not specified (if cause is unknown).

In DSM-5, a less severe form of dementia called mild neurocognitive disorder is listed. Dementia is discussed in Section 17.3.

Amnestic Disorder or Major Neurocognitive Disorder Caused by Other Medical Conditions

Amnestic disorders (a DSM-IV term) are classified in DSM-5 as *major neurocognitive disorders caused by other medical conditions.* They are marked primarily by memory impairment—hence the term amnestic—in addition to other cognitive symptoms. They may be caused by (1) medical conditions (hypoxia), (2) toxins or medications (e.g., marijuana, diazepam), and (3) unknown causes. These disorders are discussed in Section 17.4.

CLINICAL EVALUATION

During the history taking, the clinician seeks to elicit the development of the illness. Subtle cognitive disorders, fluctuating symptoms, and progressing disease processes may be tracked effectively. The clinician should obtain a detailed rendition of changes in the patient's daily routine involving such factors as self-care, job responsibilities, and work habits; meal preparation; shopping and personal support; interactions with friends; hobbies and sports; reading interests; religious, social, and recreational activities; and ability to maintain personal finances. Understanding the past life of each patient provides an invaluable source of baseline data regarding changes in function, such as attention and concentration, intellectual abilities, personality, motor skills, and mood and perception. The examiner seeks to find the particular pursuits that the patient considers most important, or central, to his or her lifestyle and attempts to discern how those pursuits have been affected by the emerging clinical condition. Such a method provides the opportunity to appraise both the impact of the illness and the patient-specific baseline for monitoring the effects of future therapies.

Mental Status Examination

After taking a thorough history, the clinician's primary tool is the assessment of the patient's mental status. As with the physical examination, the mental status examination is a means of surveying functions and abilities to allow a definition of personal strengths and weakness. It is a repeatable, structured assessment of symptoms and signs that promotes effective communication among clinicians. It also establishes the basis for future comparison, essential for documenting therapeutic effectiveness, and it allows comparisons between different patients, with a generalization of findings from one patient to another. Table 17.1–1 lists the components of a comprehensive neuropsychiatric mental status examination.

Cognition

When testing cognitive functions, the clinician should evaluate memory; visuospatial and constructional abilities; and reading, writing, and mathematical abilities. Assessment of abstraction ability is also valuable, although a patient's performance on

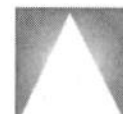

Table 17.1–1
Neuropsychiatric Mental Status Examination

A. General Description
   1. General appearance, dress, sensory aids (glasses, hearing aid)
   2. Level of consciousness and arousal
   3. Attention to environment
   4. Posture (standing and seated)
   5. Gait
   6. Movements of limbs, trunk, and face (spontaneous, resting, and after instruction)
   7. General demeanor (including evidence of responses to internal stimuli)
   8. Response to examiner (eye contact, cooperation, ability to focus on interview process)
   9. Native or primary language
B. Language and Speech
   1. Comprehension (words, sentences, simple and complex commands, and concepts)
   2. Output (spontaneity, rate, fluency, melody or prosody, volume, coherence, vocabulary, paraphasic errors, complexity of usage)
   3. Repetition
   4. Other aspects
      a. Object naming
      b. Color naming
      c. Body part identification
      d. Ideomotor praxis to command
C. Thought
   1. Form (coherence and connectedness)
   2. Content
      a. Ideational (preoccupations, overvalued ideas, delusions)
      b. Perceptual (hallucinations)
D. Mood and Affect
   1. Internal mood state (spontaneous and elicited; sense of humor)
   2. Future outlook
   3. Suicidal ideas and plans
   4. Demonstrated emotional status (congruence with mood)
E. Insight and Judgment
   1. Insight
      a. Self-appraisal and self-esteem
      b. Understanding of current circumstances
      c. Ability to describe personal psychological and physical status
   2. Judgment
      a. Appraisal of major social relationships
      b. Understanding of personal roles and responsibilities
F. Cognition
   1. Memory
      a. Spontaneous (as evidenced during interview)
      b. Tested (incidental, immediate repetition, delayed recall, cued recall, recognition; verbal, nonverbal; explicit, implicit)
   2. Visuospatial skills
   3. Constructional ability
   4. Mathematics
   5. Reading
   6. Writing
   7. Fine sensory function (stereognosis, graphesthesia, two-point discrimination)
   8. Finger gnosis
   9. Right-left orientation
   10. "Executive functions"
   11. Abstraction

Courtesy of Eric D. Caine, M.D. and Jeffrey M. Lyness, M.D.

tasks such as proverb interpretation may be a useful bedside projective test in some patients, the specific interpretation may result from a variety of factors, such as poor education, low intelligence, and failure to understand the concept of proverbs, as well as from a broad array of primary and secondary psychopathological disturbances.

PATHOLOGY AND LABORATORY EXAMINATION

As with all medical tests, psychiatric evaluations such as the mental status examination must be interpreted in the overall context of thorough clinical and laboratory assessment. Psychiatric and neuropsychiatric patients require careful physical examination, especially when issues exist that involve etiologically related or comorbid medical conditions. When consulting internists and other medical specialists, the clinician must ask specific questions to focus on the differential diagnostic process and use the consultation most effectively. In particular, most systemic medical or primary cerebral diseases that lead to psychopathological disturbances also manifest with a variety of peripheral or central abnormalities.

A screening laboratory evaluation is sought initially and may be followed by a variety of ancillary tests to increase the diagnostic specificity. Table 17.1–2 lists such procedures, some of which are described below.

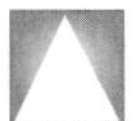

Table 17.1–2
Screening Laboratory Tests

General Tests
Complete blood cell count
Erythrocyte sedimentation rate
Electrolytes
Glucose
Blood urea nitrogen and serum creatinine
Liver function tests
Serum calcium and phosphorus
Thyroid function tests
Serum protein
Levels of all drugs
Urinalysis
Pregnancy test for women of childbearing age
Electrocardiography
Ancillary Laboratory Tests
Blood
Blood cultures
Rapid plasma reagin test
Human immunodeficiency virus (HIV) testing (enzyme-linked immunosorbent assay [ELISA] and Western blot)
Serum heavy metals
Serum copper
Ceruloplasmin
Serum B_{12}, red blood cell (RBC) folate levels
Urine
Culture
Toxicology
Heavy metal screen
Electrography
Electroencephalography
Evoked potentials
Polysomnography
Nocturnal penile tumescence
Cerebrospinal fluid
Glucose, protein
Cell count
Cultures (bacterial, viral, fungal)
Cryptococcal antigen
Venereal Disease Research Laboratory test
Radiography
Computed tomography
Magnetic resonance imaging
Positron emission tomography
Single photon emission computed tomography

Courtesy of Eric D. Caine, M.D. and Jeffrey M. Lyness, M.D.

ELECTROENCEPHALOGRAPHY

Electroencephalography (EEG) is an easily accessible, noninvasive test of brain dysfunction that has high sensitivity for many disorders but relatively low specificity. Beyond its recognized uses in epilepsy, EEG's greatest utility is in detecting altered electrical rhythms associated with mild delirium, space-occupying lesions, and continuing complex partial seizures (in which the patient remains conscious, although behaviorally impaired). EEG is also sensitive to metabolic and toxic states, often showing a diffuse slowing of brain activity.

COMPUTED TOMOGRAPHY AND MAGNETIC RESONANCE IMAGING

Computed tomography (CT) and magnetic resonance imaging (MRI) have proved to be powerful neuropsychiatric research tools. Recent developments in MRI allow the direct measurement of structures such as the thalamus, basal ganglia, hippocampus, and amygdala, as well as temporal and apical areas of the brain and the structures of the posterior fossa. MRI has largely replaced CT as the most utilitarian and cost-effective method of imaging in neuropsychiatry. Patients with acute cerebral hemorrhages or hematomas must continue to be assessed using CT, but these patients present infrequently in psychiatric settings. MRI better discriminates the interface between gray and white matter and is useful in detecting a variety of white matter lesions in the periventricular and subcortical regions. The pathophysiological significance of such findings remains to be defined. White matter abnormalities are detected in younger patients with multiple sclerosis or human immunodeficiency virus (HIV) infection and in older patients with hypertension, vascular dementia, or dementia of the Alzheimer's type. The prevalence of these abnormalities is also increased in healthy, aging individuals who have no defined disease process. As with CT, the greatest utility of MRI in the evaluation of patients with dementia arises from what it may exclude (tumors, vascular disease) rather than what it can demonstrate specifically.

BRAIN BIOPSY

Brain needle biopsy is used to diagnose a variety of disorders: Alzheimer's disease, autoimmune encephalopathies, and tumors. It is conducted stereotactically and indicated when no other investigative techniques such as MRI or lumbar puncture have been sufficient to make a diagnosis. The procedure is not without risk in that seizures may occur if scar tissue forms at the biopsy site.

NEUROPSYCHOLOGICAL TESTING

Neuropsychological testing provides a standardized, quantitative, reproducible evaluation of a patient's cognitive abilities. Such procedures may be useful for initial evaluation and periodic assessment. Tests are available that assess abilities across the broad array of cognitive domains, and many offer comparative normative groups or adjusted scores based on normative samples. The clinician seeking neuropsychological consultation should understand enough about the strengths and weaknesses of selected procedures to benefit fully from the results obtained.

▲ 17.2 Delirium

Delirium is characterized by an acute decline in both the level of consciousness and cognition with particular impairment in attention. A life threatening, yet potentially reversible disorder of the central nervous system (CNS), delirium often involves perceptual disturbances, abnormal psychomotor activity, and sleep cycle impairment. Delirium is often underrecognized by health care workers. Part of the problem is that the syndrome has a variety of other names (Table 17.2–1).

The hallmark symptom of delirium is an impairment of consciousness, usually occurring in association with global impairments of cognitive functions. Abnormalities of mood, perception, and behavior are common psychiatric symptoms. Tremor, asterixis, nystagmus, incoordination, and urinary incontinence are common neurological symptoms. Classically, delirium has a sudden onset (hours or days), a brief and fluctuating course, and rapid improvement when the causative factor is identified and eliminated, but each of these characteristic features can vary in individual patients. Physicians must recognize delirium to identify and treat the underlying cause and to avert the development of delirium-related complications such as accidental injury because of the patient's clouded consciousness.

EPIDEMIOLOGY

Delirium is a common disorder, with most incidence and prevalence rates reported in elderly adults. In community studies, 1 percent of elderly persons aged 55 years or older have delirium (13 percent in the age group 85 years and older in the community). Among elderly emergency department patients, 5 to 10 percent have been reported to have delirium. At the time of admission to medical wards, between 15 and 21 percent of older patients meet criteria for delirium-prevalent cases. Of patients free of delirium at time of hospital admission, 5 to 30 percent reported subsequent incidences of delirium during hospitalization. Delirium has been reported in 10 to 15 percent of general surgical patients, 30 percent of open heart surgery patients, and more than 50 percent of patients treated for hip fractures. Delirium occurs in 70 to 87 percent of those in intensive care units and in up to 83 percent of all patients at the end of life care. Sixty percent of patients in nursing homes or postacute care settings have delirium. An estimated 21 percent of patients with severe burns and 30 to 40 percent of patients with acquired immune deficiency syndrome (AIDS) have episodes of delirium while they are hospitalized. Delirium develops in 80 percent of terminally ill patients. The causes of postoperative delirium include the stress of surgery, postoperative pain, insomnia, pain medication, electrolyte imbalances, infection, fever, and blood loss. The incidence and prevalence rates for delirium across settings are shown in Table 17.2–2.

Table 17.2–1
Delirium by Other Names

Intensive care unit psychosis
Acute confusional state
Acute brain failure
Encephalitis
Encephalopathy
Toxic metabolic state
Central nervous system toxicity
Paraneoplastic limbic encephalitis
Sundowning
Cerebral insufficiency
Organic brain syndrome

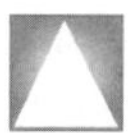

Table 17.2–2
Delirium Incidence and Prevalence in Multiple Settings

Population	Prevalence Range (%)	Incidence Range (%)
General medical inpatients	10–30	3–16
Medical and surgical inpatients	5–15	10–55
General surgical inpatients	N/A	9–15 postoperatively
Critical care unit patients	16	16–83
Cardiac surgery inpatients	16–34	7–34
Orthopedic surgery patients	33	18–50
Emergency department	7–10	N/A
Terminally ill cancer patients	23–28	83
Institutionalized elderly	44	33

N/A, not available.

Risk for delirium could be conceptualized into two categories, predisposing and precipitating factors (Tables 17.2–3 and 17.2–4). Current approaches to delirium focus primarily on the precipitation factors and do little to address the predisposing factors. Managing predisposing factors for delirium becomes essential in decreasing future episodes of delirium and the morbidity and mortality associated with it.

Advanced age is a major risk factor for the development of delirium. Approximately 30 to 40 percent of hospitalized patients older than age 65 years have an episode of delirium, and another 10 to 15 percent of elderly persons exhibit delirium on admission to the hospital. Of nursing home residents older than age 75 years, 60 percent have repeated episodes of delirium. Male gender is also an independent risk factor for delirium.

Delirium is a poor prognostic sign. Rates of institutionalization are increased threefold for patients 65 years and older who exhibit delirium while in the hospital. The 3-month mortality rate of patients who have an episode of delirium is estimated to be 23 to 33 percent. The 1-year mortality rate for patients who have an episode of delirium may be as high as 50 percent. Elderly patients who experience delirium while hospitalized have a 21 to 75 percent mortality rate during that hospitalization.

Table 17.2–3
Predisposing Factors for Delirium

Demographic characteristics
Age 65 years and older
Male sex
Cognitive status
Dementia
Cognitive impairment
History of delirium
Depression
Functional status
Functional dependence
Immobility
History of falls
Low level of activity
Sensory impairment
Hearing
Visual
Decreased oral intake
Dehydration
Malnutrition
Drugs
Treatment with psychoactive drugs
Treatment with drugs with anticholinergic properties
Alcohol abuse
Coexisting medical conditions
Severe medical diseases
Chronic renal or hepatic disease
Stroke
Neurological disease
Metabolic derangements
Infection with human immunodeficiency virus
Fractures or trauma
Terminal diseases

Adapted from Inouye SK. Delirium in older persons. *N Engl J Med.* 2006; 354(11):1157.

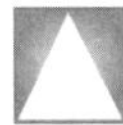

Table 17.2–4
Precipitating Factors for Delirium

Drugs
Sedative–hypnotics
Narcotics
Anticholinergic drugs
Treatment with multiple drugs
Alcohol or drug withdrawal
Primary neurologic diseases
Stroke, nondominant hemispheric
Intracranial bleeding
Meningitis or encephalitis
Intercurrent illnesses
Infections
Iatrogenic complications
Severe acute illness
Hypoxia
Shock
Anemia
Fever or hypothermia
Dehydration
Poor nutritional status
Low serum albumin levels
Metabolic derangements
Surgery
Orthopedic surgery
Cardiac surgery
Prolonged cardiopulmonary bypass
Noncardiac surgery
Environmental
Admission to intensive care unit
Use of physical restraints
Use of bladder catheter
Use of multiple procedures
Pain
Emotional stress
Prolonged sleep depravation

Adapted from Inouye SK. Delirium in older persons. *N Engl J Med.* 2006; 354(11):1157.

After discharge, up to 15 percent of these persons die within a 1-month period, and 25 percent die within 6 months.

ETIOLOGY

The major causes of delirium are CNS disease (e.g., epilepsy), systemic disease (e.g., cardiac failure), and either intoxication or withdrawal from pharmacological or toxic agents (Table 17.2–5). When evaluating patients with delirium, clinicians should assume that any drug that a patient has taken may be etiologically relevant to the delirium.

DIAGNOSIS AND CLINICAL FEATURES

The syndrome of delirium is almost always caused by one or more systemic or cerebral derangements that affect brain function.

A 70-year-old woman, Mrs. K, was brought to the emergency department by the police. The police had responded to complaints from neighbors that Mrs. K was wandering the neighborhood and was not taking care of herself. When the police found Mrs. K in her apartment, she was dirty, foul smelling, and wearing nothing but a bra. Her apartment was also filthy with garbage and rotting food everywhere.

When interviewed, Mrs. K would not look at the interviewer and was confused and unresponsive to most of the questions asked. She knew her name and address but not the date. She was unable to describe the events that led to her admission.

The next day, the supervising psychiatrist attempted to interview Mrs. K. Her facial expression was still unresponsive, and she still did not know the month or the name of the hospital she was in. She explained that the neighbors called the police because she was "sick" and that she did indeed feel sick and weak, with pains in her shoulder. She also reported not eating for 3 days. She denied ever being in a psychiatric hospital or hearing voices but acknowledged seeing a psychiatrist at one point because she had trouble sleeping. She said the doctor had prescribed medication, but she could not remember the name.

The core features of delirium include altered consciousness, such as decreased level of consciousness; altered attention, which can include diminished ability to focus, sustain, or shift attention; impairment in other realms of cognitive function, which can manifest as disorientation (especially to time and space) and decreased memory; relatively rapid onset (usually hours to days); brief duration (usually days to weeks); and often marked, unpredictable fluctuations in severity and other clinical manifestations during the course of the day, sometimes worse at

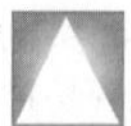

Table 17.2–5
Common Causes of Delirium

Central nervous system disorder	Seizure Migraine Head trauma, brain tumor, subarachnoid hemorrhage, subdural, epidural hematoma, abscess, intracerebral hemorrhage, cerebellar hemorrhage, nonhemorrhagic stroke, transient ischemia
Metabolic disorder	Electrolyte abnormalities Diabetes, hypoglycemia, hyperglycemia, or insulin resistance
Systemic illness	Infection (e.g., sepsis, malaria, erysipelas, viral, plague, Lyme disease, syphilis, or abscess) Trauma Change in fluid status (dehydration or volume overload) Nutritional deficiency Burns Uncontrolled pain Heat stroke High altitude (usually >5,000 m)
Medications	Pain medications (e.g., postoperative meperidine [Demerol] or morphine [Duramorph]) Antibiotics, antivirals, and antifungals Steroids Anesthesia Cardiac medications Antihypertensives Antineoplastic agents Anticholinergic agents Neuroleptic malignant syndrome
Serotonin syndrome	
Over-the-counter preparations	Herbals, teas, and nutritional supplements
Botanicals	Jimsonweed, oleander, foxglove, hemlock, dieffenbachia, and *Amanita phalloides*
Cardiac	Cardiac failure, arrhythmia, myocardial infarction, cardiac assist device, cardiac surgery
Pulmonary	Chronic obstructive pulmonary disease, hypoxia, SIADH, acid–base disturbance
Endocrine	Adrenal crisis or adrenal failure, thyroid abnormality, parathyroid abnormality
Hematological	Anemia, leukemia, blood dyscrasia, stem cell transplant
Renal	Renal failure, uremia, SIADH
Hepatic	Hepatitis, cirrhosis, hepatic failure
Neoplasm	Neoplasm (primary brain, metastases, paraneoplastic syndrome)
Drugs of abuse	Intoxication and withdrawal
Toxins	Intoxication and withdrawal Heavy metals and aluminum

SIADH, syndrome of inappropriate secretion of antidiuretic hormone.

night (sundowning), which may range from periods of lucidity to severe cognitive impairment and disorganization.

Associated clinical features are often present and may be prominent. They can include disorganization of thought processes (ranging from mild tangentiality to frank incoherence), perceptual disturbances such as illusions and hallucinations, psychomotor hyperactivity and hypoactivity, disruption of the sleep–wake cycle (often manifested as fragmented sleep at night, with or without daytime drowsiness), mood alterations (from subtle irritability to obvious dysphoria, anxiety, or even euphoria), and other manifestations of altered neurological function (e.g., autonomic hyperactivity or instability, myoclonic jerking, and dysarthria). The EEG usually shows diffuse slowing of background activity, although patients with delirium caused by alcohol or sedative–hypnotic withdrawal have low-voltage fast activity.

The major neurotransmitter hypothesized to be involved in delirium is acetylcholine, and the major neuroanatomical area is the reticular formation. The reticular formation of the brainstem is the principal area regulating attention and arousal; the major pathway implicated in delirium is the dorsal tegmental pathway, which projects from the mesencephalic reticular formation to the tectum and thalamus. Several studies have reported that a variety of delirium-inducing factors result in decreased acetylcholine activity in the brain. One of the most common causes of delirium is toxicity from too many prescribed medications with anticholinergic activity. Researchers have suggested other pathophysiological mechanisms for delirium. In particular, the delirium associated with alcohol withdrawal has been associated with hyperactivity of the locus ceruleus and its noradrenergic neurons. Other neurotransmitters that have been implicated are serotonin and glutamate.

PHYSICAL AND LABORATORY EXAMINATIONS

Delirium is usually diagnosed at the bedside and is characterized by the sudden onset of symptoms. A bedside mental status examination—such as the mini-mental state examination, the mental status examination, or neurological signs—can be used to document the cognitive impairment and to provide a baseline from which to measure the patient's clinical course. The physical examination often reveals clues to the cause of the delirium (Table 17.2–6). The presence of a known physical illness or a history of head trauma or alcohol or other substance dependence increases the likelihood of the diagnosis.

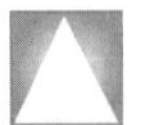

Table 17.2–6
Physical Examination of the Delirious Patient

Parameter	Finding	Clinical Implication
1. Pulse	Bradycardia	Hypothyroidism Stokes–Adams syndrome Increased intracranial pressure
	Tachycardia	Hyperthyroidism Infection Heart failure
2. Temperature	Fever	Sepsis Thyroid storm Vasculitis
3. Blood pressure	Hypotension	Shock Hypothyroidism Addison's disease
	Hypertension	Encephalopathy Intracranial mass
4. Respiration	Tachypnea	Diabetes Pneumonia Cardiac failure Fever Acidosis (metabolic)
	Shallow	Alcohol or other substance intoxication
5. Carotid vessels	Bruits or decreased pulse	Transient cerebral ischemia
6. Scalp and face	Evidence of trauma	
7. Neck	Evidence of nuchal rigidity	Meningitis Subarachnoid hemorrhage
8. Eyes	Papilledema	Tumor Hypertensive encephalopathy
	Pupillary dilatation	Anxiety Autonomic overactivity (e.g., delirium tremens)
9. Mouth	Tongue or cheek lacerations	Evidence of generalized tonic–clonic seizures
10. Thyroid	Enlarged	Hyperthyroidism
11. Heart	Arrhythmia	Inadequate cardiac output, possibility of emboli
	Cardiomegaly	Heart failure Hypertensive disease
12. Lungs	Congestion	Primary pulmonary failure Pulmonary edema Pneumonia
13. Breath	Alcohol	
	Ketones	Diabetes
14. Liver	Enlargement	Cirrhosis Liver failure
15. Nervous system		
a. Reflexes—muscle stretch	Asymmetry with Babinski's signs	Mass lesion Cerebrovascular disease Preexisting dementia
	Snout	Frontal mass Bilateral posterior cerebral artery occlusion
b. Abducent nerve (sixth cranial nerve)	Weakness in lateral gaze	Increased intracranial pressure
c. Limb strength	Asymmetrical	Mass lesion Cerebrovascular disease
d. Autonomic	Hyperactivity	Anxiety Delirium

From Strub RL, Black FW. *Neurobehavioral Disorders: A Clinical Approach*. Philadelphia, PA: FA Davis; 1981:121.

The laboratory workup of a patient with delirium should include standard tests and additional studies indicated by the clinical situation (Table 17.2–7). In delirium, the EEG characteristically shows a generalized slowing of activity and may be useful in differentiating delirium from depression or psychosis. The EEG of a delirious patient sometimes shows focal areas of hyperactivity. In rare cases, it may be difficult to differentiate delirium related to epilepsy from delirium related to other causes.

DIFFERENTIAL DIAGNOSIS

Delirium versus Dementia

A number of clinical features help distinguish delirium from dementia (Table 17.2–8). The major differential points between dementia and delirium are the time to development of the condition and the fluctuation in level of attention in delirium compared with relatively consistent attention in dementia. The time to development of symptoms is usually short in delirium,

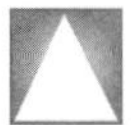

Table 17.2–7
Laboratory Workup of the Patient with Delirium

Standard studies
Blood chemistries (including electrolytes, renal and hepatic indexes, and glucose)
Complete blood count with white cell differential
Thyroid function tests
Serologic tests for syphilis
Human immunodeficiency virus (HIV) antibody test
Urinalysis
Electrocardiogram
Electroencephalogram
Chest radiograph
Blood and urine drug screens
Additional tests when indicated
Blood, urine, and cerebrospinal fluid cultures
B_{12}, folic acid concentrations
Computed tomography or magnetic resonance imaging brain scan
Lumbar puncture and CSF examination

and except for vascular dementia caused by stroke, it is usually gradual and insidious in dementia. Although both conditions include cognitive impairment, the changes in dementia are more stable over time and, for example, usually do not fluctuate over the course of a day. A patient with dementia is usually alert; a patient with delirium has episodes of decreased consciousness. Occasionally, delirium occurs in a patient with dementia, a condition known as *beclouded dementia.* A dual diagnosis of delirium can be made when there is a definite history of preexisting dementia.

Delirium versus Schizophrenia or Depression

Delirium must also be differentiated from schizophrenia and depressive disorder. Some patients with psychotic disorders, usually schizophrenia or manic episodes, can have periods of extremely disorganized behavior difficult to distinguish from delirium. In general, however, the hallucinations and delusions of patients with schizophrenia are more constant and better organized than those of patients with delirium. Patients with schizophrenia usually experience no change in their level of consciousness or in their orientation. Patients with hypoactive symptoms of delirium may appear somewhat similar to severely depressed patients, but they can be distinguished on the basis of an EEG. Other psychiatric diagnoses to consider in the differential diagnosis of delirium are brief psychotic disorder, schizophreniform disorder, and dissociative disorders. Patients with factitious disorders may attempt to simulate the symptoms of delirium but usually reveal the factitious nature of their symptoms by inconsistencies on their mental status examinations, and an EEG can easily separate the two diagnoses.

Table 17.2–8
Frequency of Clinical Features of Delirium Contrasted with Dementia

Feature	Dementia	Delirium
Onset	Slow	Rapid
Duration	Months to years	Hours to weeks
Attention	Preserved	Fluctuates
Memory	Impaired remote memory	Impaired recent and immediate memory
Speech	Word-finding difficulty	Incoherent (slow or rapid)
Sleep–wake cycle	Fragmented sleep	Frequent disruption (e.g., day–night reversal)
Thoughts	Impoverished	Disorganized
Awareness	Unchanged	Reduced
Alertness	Usually normal	Hypervigilant or reduced vigilance

Adapted from Lipowski ZJ. *Delirium: Acute Confusional States.* Oxford: Oxford University Press; 1990.

COURSE AND PROGNOSIS

Although the onset of delirium is usually sudden, prodromal symptoms (e.g., restlessness and fearfulness) can occur in the days preceding the onset of florid symptoms. The symptoms of delirium usually persist as long as the causally relevant factors are present, although delirium generally lasts less than 1 week. After identification and removal of the causative factors, the symptoms of delirium usually recede over a 3- to 7-day period, although some symptoms may take up to 2 weeks to resolve completely. The older the patient and the longer the patient has been delirious, the longer the delirium takes to resolve. Recall of what transpired during a delirium, once it is over, is characteristically spotty; a patient may refer to the episode as a bad dream or a nightmare only vaguely remembered. As stated in the discussion on epidemiology, the occurrence of delirium is associated with a high mortality rate in the ensuing year, primarily because of the serious nature of the associated medical conditions that lead to delirium.

Whether delirium progresses to dementia has not been demonstrated in carefully controlled studies, although many clinicians believe that they have seen such a progression. A clinical observation that has been validated by some studies, however, is that periods of delirium are sometimes followed by depression or posttraumatic stress disorder.

TREATMENT

In treating delirium, the primary goal is to treat the underlying cause. When the underlying condition is anticholinergic toxicity, the use of physostigmine salicylate (Antilirium), 1 to 2 mg intravenously or intramuscularly, with repeated doses in 15 to 30 minutes may be indicated. The other important goal of treatment is to provide physical, sensory, and environmental support. Physical support is necessary so that delirious patients do not get into situations in which they may have accidents. Patients with delirium should be neither sensory deprived nor overly stimulated by the environment. They are usually helped by having a friend or relative in the room or by the presence of a regular sitter. Familiar pictures and decorations; the presence of a clock or a calendar; and regular orientations to person, place, and time help make patients with delirium comfortable. Delirium can sometimes occur in older patients wearing eye patches after cataract surgery ("black-patch delirium"). Such patients can be helped by placing pinholes in the patches to let in some stimuli or by occasionally removing one patch at a time during recovery.

Table 17.2–9
Pharmacological Treatment

Pharmacological Agent	Dosage	Side Effects	Comments
Typical Antipsychotics			
Haloperidol (Haldol)	0.5–1 mg p.o. twice a day (may be given every 4–6 hr as needed, too)	Extrapyramidal side (EPS) effects Prolonged QTc	Most commonly used Can be given intramuscularly
Atypical Antipsychotics		All can prolong QTc duration	
Risperidone (Risperdal)	0.5–1 mg a day	EPS concerns	Limited data in delirium
Olanzapine (Zyprexa)	5–10 mg a day	Metabolic syndrome	Higher mortality in dementia patients
Quetiapine (Seroquel)	25–150 mg a day	More sedating	
Benzodiazepine			
Lorazepam (Ativan)	0.5–3 mg a day and as needed every 4 hr	Respiratory depression, paradoxical agitation	Best use in delirium secondary to alcohol or benzodiazepine withdrawal Can worsen delirium

Pharmacotherapy

The two major symptoms of delirium that may require pharmacological treatment are psychosis and insomnia. A commonly used drug for psychosis is haloperidol (Haldol), a butyrophenone antipsychotic drug. Depending on a patient's age, weight, and physical condition, the initial dose may range from 2 to 6 mg intramuscularly, repeated in an hour if the patient remains agitated. As soon as the patient is calm, oral medication in liquid concentrate or tablet form should begin. Two daily oral doses should suffice, with two-thirds of the dose being given at bedtime. To achieve the same therapeutic effect, the oral dose should be approximately 1.5 times the parenteral dose. The effective total daily dose of haloperidol may range from 5 to 40 mg for most patients with delirium. Haloperidol has been associated with prolongation of QT interval. Clinicians should evaluate baseline and periodic electrocardiograms as well as monitor cardiac status of the patient. Droperidol (Inapsine) is a butyrophenone available as an alternative intravenous (IV) formulation, although careful monitoring of the electrocardiogram may be prudent with this treatment. The U.S. Food and Drug Administration (FDA) has issued a black box warning because cases of QT prolongation and torsades de pointes have been reported in patients receiving droperidol. Because of its potential for serious proarrhythmic effects and death, it should be used only in patients who do not respond well to other treatments. Phenothiazines should be avoided in delirious patients because these drugs are associated with significant anticholinergic activity.

Use of second-generation antipsychotics, such as risperidone (Risperdal), clozapine, olanzapine (Zyprexa), quetiapine (Seroquel), ziprasidone (Geodon), and aripiprazole (Abilify), may be considered for delirium management, but clinical trial experience with these agents for delirium is limited. Ziprasidone appears to have an activating effect and may not be appropriate in delirium management. Olanzapine is available for intramuscular (IM) use and as a rapidly disintegrating oral preparation. These routes of administration may be preferable for some patients with delirium who are poorly compliant with medications or who are too sedated to safely swallow medications.

Insomnia is best treated with benzodiazepines with short or intermediate half-lives (e.g., lorazepam [Ativan] 1 to 2 mg at bedtime). Benzodiazepines with long half-lives and barbiturates should be avoided unless they are being used as part of the treatment for the underlying disorder (e.g., alcohol withdrawal). Clinicians should be aware that there is no conclusive evidence to support the use of benzodiazepines in non–alcohol-related delirium. There have been case reports of improvement in or remission of delirious states caused by intractable medical illnesses with electroconvulsive therapy (ECT); however, routine consideration of ECT for delirium is not advised. If delirium is caused by severe pain or dyspnea, a physician should not hesitate to prescribe opioids for both their analgesic and sedative effects (Table 17.2–9).

Current trials are ongoing to see if dexmedetomidine (Precedex) is a more effective medication than haloperidol in the treatment of agitation and delirium in patients receiving mechanical ventilation in an intensive care unit.

Treatment in Special Populations

Parkinson's Disease. In Parkinson's disease, the antiparkinsonian agents are frequently implicated in causing delirium. If a coexistent dementia is present, delirium is twice as likely to develop in patients with Parkinson's disease with dementia receiving antiparkinsonian agents than in those without dementia. Decreasing the dosage of the antiparkinsonian agent has to be weighed against a worsening of motor symptoms. If the antiparkinsonian agents cannot be further reduced, or if the delirium persists after attenuation of the antiparkinsonian agents, clozapine is recommended. If a patient is not able to tolerate clozapine or the required blood monitoring, alternative antipsychotic agents should be considered. Quetiapine has not been as rigorously studied as clozapine and may have parkinsonian side effects, but it is used in clinical practice to treat psychosis in Parkinson's disease.

Terminally Ill Patients. When delirium occurs in the context of a terminal illness, issues about advanced directives and the existence of a health care proxy become more significant. This scenario emphasizes the importance of early development of advance directives for health care decision making while a person has the capacity to communicate the wishes regarding the extent of aggressive diagnostic tests at life's end. The focus may change from an aggressive search for the etiology of the delirium to one of palliation, comfort, and assistance with dying.

▲ 17.3 Dementia (Major Neurocognitive Disorder)

Dementia refers to a disease process marked by progressive cognitive impairment in clear consciousness. Dementia does not refer to low intellectual functioning or intellectual disability because these are developmental and static conditions, and the cognitive deficits in dementia represent a decline from a previous level of functioning. Dementia involves multiple cognitive domains and cognitive deficits cause significant impairment in social and occupational functioning. There are several types of dementias based on etiology: Alzheimer's disease, dementia of Lewy bodies, vascular dementia, frontotemporal dementia, traumatic brain injury (TBI), HIV, prion disease, Parkinson's disease, and Huntington's disease. Dementia can also be caused by other medical and neurological conditions or can be caused by various substances. (See Section 17.4.)

The critical clinical points of dementia are the identification of the syndrome and the clinical workup of its cause. The disorder can be progressive or static; permanent or reversible. An underlying cause is always assumed, although, in rare cases, it is impossible to determine a specific cause. The potential reversibility of dementia is related to the underlying pathological condition and to the availability and application of effective treatment. Approximately 15 percent of people with dementia have reversible illnesses if treatment is initiated before irreversible damage takes place.

EPIDEMIOLOGY

With the aging population, the prevalence of dementia is rising. The prevalence of moderate to severe dementia in different population groups is approximately 5 percent in the general population older than 65 years of age, 20 to 40 percent in the general population older than 85 years of age, 15 to 20 percent in outpatient general medical practices, and 50 percent in chronic care facilities.

Of all patients with dementia, 50 to 60 percent have the most common type of dementia, dementia of the Alzheimer's type (Alzheimer's disease). Dementia of the Alzheimer's type increases in prevalence with increasing age. For persons age 65 years, men have a prevalence rate of 0.6 percent and women of 0.8 percent. At age 90, rates are 21 percent. For all of these figures, 40 to 60 percent of cases are moderate to severe. The rates of prevalence (men to women) are 11 and 14 percent at age 85, 21 and 25 percent at age 90 years and 36 and 41 percent at age 95 years. Patients with dementia of the Alzheimer's type occupy more than 50 percent of nursing home beds. More than 2 million persons with dementia are cared for in these homes. By 2050, current predictions suggest that there will be 14 million Americans with Alzheimer's disease and therefore more than 18 million people with dementia.

The second most common type of dementia is vascular dementia, which is causally related to cerebrovascular diseases. Hypertension predisposes a person to the disease. Vascular dementias account for 15 to 30 percent of all dementia cases. Vascular dementia is most common in persons between the ages of 60 and 70 and is more common in men than in women. Approximately 10 to 15 percent of patients have coexisting vascular dementia and dementia of the Alzheimer's type.

Other common causes of dementia, each representing 1 to 5 percent of all cases, include head trauma; alcohol-related dementias; and various movement disorder-related dementias, such as Huntington's disease and Parkinson's disease. Because dementia is a fairly general syndrome, it has many causes, and clinicians must embark on a careful clinical workup of a patient with dementia to establish its cause.

ETIOLOGY

The most common causes of dementia in individuals older than 65 years of age are (1) Alzheimer's disease, (2) vascular dementia, and (3) mixed vascular and Alzheimer's dementia. Other illnesses that account for approximately 10 percent include Lewy body dementia; Pick's disease; frontotemporal dementias; normal-pressure hydrocephalus (NPH); alcoholic dementia; infectious dementia, such as HIV or syphilis; and Parkinson's disease. Many types of dementias evaluated in clinical settings can be attributable to reversible causes, such as metabolic abnormalities (e.g., hypothyroidism), nutritional deficiencies (e.g., vitamin B_{12} or folate deficiencies), or dementia syndrome caused by depression. See Table 17.3–1 for a review of possible etiologies of dementia.

Dementia of the Alzheimer's Type

In 1907, Alois Alzheimer first described the condition that later assumed his name. He described a 51-year-old woman with a 4½-year course of progressive dementia. The final diagnosis of Alzheimer's disease requires a neuropathological examination of the brain; nevertheless, dementia of the Alzheimer's type is commonly diagnosed in the clinical setting after other causes of dementia have been excluded from diagnostic consideration.

Genetic Factors. Although the cause of dementia of the Alzheimer's type remains unknown, progress has been made in understanding the molecular basis of the amyloid deposits that are a hallmark of the disorder's neuropathology. Some studies have indicated that as many as 40 percent of patients have a family history of dementia of the Alzheimer's type; thus, genetic factors are presumed to play a part in the development of the disorder, at least in some cases. Additional support for a genetic influence is the concordance rate for monozygotic twins, which is higher than the rate for dizygotic twins (43 percent vs. 8 percent, respectively). In several well-documented cases, the disorder has been transmitted in families through an autosomal dominant gene, although such transmission is rare. Alzheimer's type dementia has shown linkage to chromosomes 1, 14, and 21.

AMYLOID PRECURSOR PROTEIN. The gene for amyloid precursor protein is on the long arm of chromosome 21. The process of differential splicing yields four forms of amyloid precursor protein. The β/A4 protein, the major constituent of senile plaques, is a 42-amino acid peptide that is a breakdown product of amyloid precursor protein. In Down syndrome (trisomy 21) are found three copies of the amyloid precursor protein gene, and in a disease in which a mutation is found at codon 717 in the amyloid precursor protein gene, a pathological process results

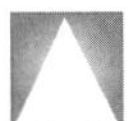

Table 17.3–1
Possible Etiologies of Dementia

Degenerative dementias
Alzheimer's disease
Frontotemporal dementias (e.g., Pick's disease)
Parkinson's disease
Lewy body dementia
Idiopathic cerebral ferrocalcinosis (Fahr's disease)
Progressive supranuclear palsy
Miscellaneous
Huntington's disease
Wilson's disease
Metachromatic leukodystrophy
Neuroacanthocytosis
Psychiatric
Pseudodementia of depression
Cognitive decline in late-life schizophrenia
Physiologic
Normal-pressure hydrocephalus
Metabolic
Vitamin deficiencies (e.g., vitamin B_{12}, folate)
Endocrinopathies (e.g., hypothyroidism)
Chronic metabolic disturbances (e.g., uremia)
Tumor
Primary or metastatic (e.g., meningioma or metastatic breast or lung cancer)
Traumatic
Dementia pugilistica, posttraumatic dementia
Subdural hematoma
Infection
Prion diseases (e.g., Creutzfeldt–Jakob disease, bovine spongiform encephalitis, Gerstmann–Sträussler syndrome)
Acquired immune deficiency syndrome (AIDS)
Syphilis
Cardiac, vascular, and anoxia
Infarction (single or multiple or strategic lacunar)
Binswanger's disease (subcortical arteriosclerotic encephalopathy)
Hemodynamic insufficiency (e.g., hypoperfusion or hypoxia)
Demyelinating diseases
Multiple sclerosis
Drugs and toxins
Alcohol
Heavy metals
Irradiation
Pseudodementia because of medications (e.g., anticholinergics)
Carbon monoxide

in the excessive deposition of β/A4 protein. Whether the processing of abnormal amyloid precursor protein is of primary causative significance in Alzheimer's disease is unknown, but many research groups are studying both the normal metabolic processing of amyloid precursor protein and its processing in patients with dementia of the Alzheimer's type in an attempt to answer this question.

MULTIPLE E4 GENES. One study implicated gene E4 in the origin of Alzheimer's disease. People with one copy of the gene have Alzheimer's disease three times more frequently than do those with no E4 gene, and people with two E4 genes have the disease eight times more frequently than do those with no E4 gene. Diagnostic testing for this gene is not currently recommended because it is found in persons without dementia and not found in all cases of dementia.

Neuropathology. The classic gross neuroanatomical observation of a brain from a patient with Alzheimer's disease is diffuse atrophy with flattened cortical sulci and enlarged cerebral ventricles. The classic and pathognomonic microscopic findings are senile plaques, neurofibrillary tangles, neuronal loss (particularly in the cortex and the hippocampus), synaptic loss (perhaps as much as 50 percent in the cortex), and granulovascular degeneration of the neurons. Neurofibrillary tangles are composed of cytoskeletal elements, primarily phosphorylated tau protein, although other cytoskeletal proteins are also present. Neurofibrillary tangles are not unique to Alzheimer's disease; they also occur in Down syndrome, dementia pugilistica (punch-drunk syndrome), Parkinson-dementia complex of Guam, Hallervorden–Spatz disease, and the brains of normal people as they age. Neurofibrillary tangles are commonly found in the cortex, the hippocampus, the substantia nigra, and the locus ceruleus.

Senile plaques, also referred to as *amyloid plaques,* more strongly indicate Alzheimer's disease, although they are also seen in Down syndrome and, to some extent, in normal aging. Senile plaques are composed of a particular protein, β/A4, and astrocytes, dystrophic neuronal processes, and microglia. The number and the density of senile plaques present in postmortem brains have been correlated with the severity of the disease that affected the persons.

Neurotransmitters. The neurotransmitters that are most often implicated in the pathophysiological condition of Alzheimer's disease are acetylcholine and norepinephrine, both of which are hypothesized to be hypoactive in Alzheimer's disease. Several studies have reported data consistent with the hypothesis that specific degeneration of cholinergic neurons is present in the nucleus basalis of Meynert in persons with Alzheimer's disease. Other data supporting a cholinergic deficit in Alzheimer's disease demonstrate decreased acetylcholine and choline acetyltransferase concentrations in the brain. Choline acetyltransferase is the key enzyme for the synthesis of acetylcholine, and a reduction in choline acetyltransferase concentration suggests a decrease in the number of cholinergic neurons present. Additional support for the cholinergic deficit hypothesis comes from the observation that cholinergic antagonists, such as scopolamine and atropine, impair cognitive abilities, whereas cholinergic agonists, such as physostigmine and arecoline, enhance cognitive abilities. Decreased norepinephrine activity in Alzheimer's disease is suggested by the decrease in norepinephrine-containing neurons in the locus ceruleus found in some pathological examinations of brains from persons with Alzheimer's disease. Two other neurotransmitters implicated in the pathophysiological condition of Alzheimer's disease are the neuroactive peptides somatostatin and corticotropin; decreased concentrations of both have been reported in persons with Alzheimer's disease.

Other Causes. Another theory to explain the development of Alzheimer's disease is that an abnormality in the regulation of membrane phospholipid metabolism results in membranes that are less fluid—that is, more rigid—than normal. Several investigators are using molecular resonance spectroscopic imaging to assess this hypothesis directly in patients with dementia of the Alzheimer's type. Aluminum toxicity has also been hypothesized to be a causative factor because high levels of aluminum have been found in the brains of some patients with Alzheimer's disease, but this is no longer considered a significant etiological factor. Excessive stimulation by the transmitter glutamate that may damage neurons is another theory of causation.

Familial Multiple System Tauopathy with Presenile Dementia. A recently discovered type of dementia, familial multiple system tauopathy, shares some brain abnormalities found in people with Alzheimer's disease. The gene that causes the disorder is thought to be carried on chromosome 17. The symptoms of the disorder include short-term memory problems and difficulty maintaining balance and walking. The onset of disease occurs in the 40s and 50s, and persons with the disease live an average of 11 years after the onset of symptoms.

As in patients with Alzheimer's disease, tau protein builds up in neurons and glial cells of persons with familial multiple system tauopathy. Eventually, the protein buildup kills brain cells. The disorder is not associated with the senile plaques seen with Alzheimer's disease.

Mr. J, a 70-year-old retired businessman, was brought to psychiatric services on referral by the family physician. His wife claimed that Mr. J had become so forgetful that she was afraid to leave him alone, even at home. Mr. J retired at age 62 years after experiencing a decline in work performance during the previous 5 years. He also slowly gave up hobbies he once enjoyed (photography, reading, golf) and became increasingly quiet. However, his growing forgetfulness went basically unnoticed at home. Then one day while walking in an area he knew well, he could not find his way home. From then on his memory failure began to increase. He would forget appointments, misplace things, and lose his way around the neighborhood he resided in for 40 years. He failed to recognize people, even those he knew for many years. His wife had to start bathing and dressing him because he forgot how to do so himself.

On examination, Mr. J was disoriented in time and place. He was only able to recall his name and place of birth. Mr. J seemed lost during the interview, only responding to questions with an occasional shrug of his shoulders. When asked to name objects or to recall words or numbers, Mr. J appeared tense and distressed. Mr. J had difficulty following instructions and was unable to dress or undress himself. His general medical condition was good. Laboratory examinations showed abnormalities on Mr. J's EEG and CT scans.

Vascular Dementia

The primary cause of vascular dementia, formerly referred to as *multi-infarct dementia,* is presumed to be multiple areas of cerebral vascular disease, resulting in a symptom pattern of dementia. Vascular dementia most commonly is seen in men, especially those with preexisting hypertension or other cardiovascular risk factors. The disorder affects primarily small- and medium-sized cerebral vessels, which undergo infarction and produce multiple parenchymal lesions spread over wide areas of the brain. The causes of the infarctions can include occlusion of the vessels by arteriosclerotic plaques or thromboemboli from distant origins (e.g., heart valves). An examination of a patient may reveal carotid bruits, funduscopic abnormalities, or enlarged cardiac chambers.

Binswanger's Disease

Binswanger's disease, also known as *subcortical arteriosclerotic encephalopathy,* is characterized by the presence of many small infarctions of the white matter that spare the cortical regions. Although Binswanger's disease was previously considered a rare condition, the advent of sophisticated and powerful imaging techniques, such as MRI, has revealed that the condition is more common than previously thought.

Frontotemporal Dementia (Pick's Disease)

In contrast to the parietal–temporal distribution of pathological findings in Alzheimer's disease, Pick's disease is characterized by a preponderance of atrophy in the frontotemporal regions. These regions also have neuronal loss, gliosis, and neuronal Pick's bodies, which are masses of cytoskeletal elements. Pick's bodies are seen in some postmortem specimens but are not necessary for the diagnosis. The cause of Pick's disease is unknown, but the disease constitutes approximately 5 percent of all irreversible dementias. It is most common in men, especially those who have a first-degree relative with the condition. Pick's disease is difficult to distinguish from dementia of the Alzheimer's type, although the early stages of Pick's disease are more often characterized by personality and behavioral changes, with relative preservation of other cognitive functions, and it typically begins before 75 years of age. Familial cases may have an earlier onset, and some studies have shown that approximately half of the cases of Pick's disease are familial. Features of Klüver–Bucy syndrome (e.g., hypersexuality, placidity, and hyperorality) are much more common in Pick's disease than in Alzheimer's disease.

Lewy Body Disease

Lewy body disease is a dementia clinically similar to Alzheimer's disease and often characterized by hallucinations, parkinsonian features, and extrapyramidal signs (Table 17.3–2).

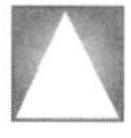

Table 17.3–2
Clinical Criteria for Dementia with Lewy Bodies (DLB)

The patient must have sufficient cognitive decline to interfere with social or occupational functioning. Of note early in the illness, memory symptoms may not be as prominent as attention, frontosubcortical skills, and visuospatial ability. Probable DLB requires two or more core symptoms, whereas possible DLB only requires one core symptom.

Core features
Fluctuating levels of attention and alertness
Recurrent visual hallucinations
Parkinsonian features (cogwheeling, bradykinesia, and resting tremor)

Supporting features
Repeated falls
Syncope
Sensitivity to neuroleptics
Systematized delusions
Hallucinations in other modalities (e.g., auditory, tactile)

Adapted from McKeith LG, Galasko D, Kosaka K. Consensus guidelines for the clinical and pathologic diagnosis of dementia with Lewy bodies (DLB): Report of the consortium on DLB international workshop. *Neurology.* 1996;47:1113–1124.

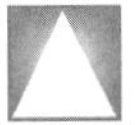

Table 17.3–3
Distinguishing Features of Subcortical and Cortical Dementias

Characteristic	Subcortical Dementia	Cortical Dementia	Recommended Tests
Language	No aphasia (anomia, if severe)	Aphasia early	FAS test Boston Naming Test WAIS-R vocabulary test
Memory	Impaired recall (retrieval) > recognition (encoding)	Recall and recognition impaired	Wechsler memory scale; Symbol Digit Paired Associate Learning (Brandt)
Attention and immediate recall	Impaired	Impaired	WAIS-R digit span
Visuospatial skills	Impaired	Impaired	Picture arrangement, object assembly and block design; WAIS subtests
Calculation	Preserved until late	Involved early	Mini-mental state
Frontal system abilities (executive function)	Disproportionately affected	Degree of impairment consistent with other involvement	Wisconsin Card Sorting Test; Odd Man Out test; Picture Absurdities
Speed of cognitive processing	Slowed early	Normal until late in disease	Trail making A and B: Paced Auditory Serial Addition Test (PASAT)
Personality	Apathetic, inert	Unconcerned	MMPI
Mood	Depressed	Euthymic	Beck and Hamilton depression scales
Speech	Dysarthric	Articulate until late	Verbal fluency (Rosen, 1980)
Posture	Bowed or extended	Upright	
Coordination	Impaired	Normal until late	
Motor speed and control	Slowed	Normal	Finger-tap; grooved pegboard
Adventitious movements	Chorea, tremor tics, dystonia	Absent (Alzheimer's dementia—some myoclonus)	
Abstraction	Impaired	Impaired	Category test (Halstead Battery)

From Pajeau AK, Román GC. HIV encephalopathy and dementia. In: J Biller, RG Kathol, eds. *The Psychiatric Clinics of North America: The Interface of Psychiatry and Neurology.* Vol 15. Philadelphia, PA: WB Saunders; 1992:457.

Lewy inclusion bodies are found in the cerebral cortex. The exact incidence is unknown. These patients often have Capgras syndrome (reduplicative paramnesia) as part of the clinical picture.

Huntington's Disease

Huntington's disease is classically associated with the development of dementia. The dementia seen in this disease is the subcortical type of dementia, characterized by more motor abnormalities and fewer language abnormalities than in the cortical type of dementia (Table 17.3–3). The dementia of Huntington's disease exhibits psychomotor slowing and difficulty with complex tasks, but memory, language, and insight remain relatively intact in the early and middle stages of the illness. As the disease progresses, however, the dementia becomes complete; the features distinguishing it from dementia of the Alzheimer's type are the high incidence of depression and psychosis in addition to the classic choreathetoid movement disorder.

Parkinson's Disease

As with Huntington's disease, parkinsonism is a disease of the basal ganglia, commonly associated with dementia and depression. An estimated 20 to 30 percent of patients with Parkinson's disease have dementia, and an additional 30 to 40 percent have measurable impairment in cognitive abilities. The slow movements of persons with Parkinson's disease are paralleled in the slow thinking of some affected patients, a feature that clinicians may refer to as *bradyphrenia.*

Mr. M, 77 years of age, came for a neurological examination because he noticed his memory was slipping and he was having difficulty concentrating, which interfered with his work. He complained of slowness and losing his train of thought. His wife stated that he was becoming withdrawn and was more reluctant to participate in activities he usually enjoyed. He denied symptoms of depression other than feeling mildly depressed about his disabilities. Two years prior, Mr. M developed an intermittent resting tremor in his right hand and a shuffling gait. Although a psychiatrist considered a diagnosis of Parkinson's disease, it was not confirmed by a neurologist and therefore was never treated.

During an initial neurological examination, Mr. M's spontaneous speech was hesitant and unclear (dysarthric). Cranial nerve examination was normal. Motor tone was increased slightly in the neck and all limbs. He performed alternating movements in his hands slowly. He had a slight intermittent tremor of his right arm at rest. Reflexes were symmetrical. A neuropsychological examination was performed 3 weeks later. It was found that Mr. M showed impairment of memory, naming, and constructional abilities.

HIV-Related Dementia

Encephalopathy in HIV infection is associated with dementia and is termed *acquired immune deficiency syndrome* (AIDS) *dementia complex,* or *HIV dementia.* Patients infected with HIV experience dementia at an annual rate of approximately 14 percent. An estimated 75 percent of patients with AIDS have involvement of the CNS at the time of autopsy. The development of dementia in people infected with HIV is often paralleled

Table 17.3–4
Criteria for Clinical Diagnosis of HIV Type 1-Associated Dementia Complex

Laboratory evidence for systemic human immunodeficiency virus (HIV) type 1 infection with confirmation by Western blot, polymerase chain reaction, or culture.

Acquired abnormality in at least *two* cognitive abilities for a period of at least 1 month: attention and concentration, speed of processing information, abstraction and reasoning, visuospatial skills, memory and learning, and speech and language. The decline should be verified by reliable history and mental status examination. History should be obtained from an informant, and examination should be supplemented by neuropsychological testing.

Cognitive dysfunction causes impairment in social or occupational functioning. Impairment should not be attributable solely to severe systemic illness.

At least *one* of the following:

Acquired abnormality in motor function verified by clinical examination (e.g., slowed rapid movements, abnormal gait, incoordination, hyperreflexia, hypertonia, or weakness), neuropsychological tests (e.g., fine motor speed, manual dexterity, or perceptual motor skills), or both.

Decline in motivation or emotional control or a change in social behavior. This may be characterized by a change in personality with apathy, inertia, irritability, emotional lability, or a new onset of impaired judgment or disinhibition.

This does not exclusively occur in the context of a delirium.

Evidence of another etiology, including active central nervous system opportunistic infection, malignancy, psychiatric disorders (e.g., major depression), or substance abuse, if present, is *not* the cause of the previously mentioned symptoms and signs.

Adapted from Working Group of the American Academy of Neurology AIDS Task Force. Nomenclature and research case definitions for neurologic manifestations of human immunodeficiency virus–type 1 (HIV-1) infection. *Neurology.* 1991;41:778–785.

by the appearance of parenchymal abnormalities in MRI scans. Other infectious dementias are caused by *Cryptococcus* or *Treponema pallidum.*

The diagnosis of AIDS dementia complex is made by confirmation of HIV infection and exclusion of alternative pathology to explain cognitive impairment. The American Academy of Neurology AIDS Task Force developed research criteria for the clinical diagnosis of CNS disorders in adults and adolescents (Table 17.3–4). The AIDS Task Force criteria for AIDS dementia complex require laboratory evidence for systemic HIV, at least two cognitive deficits, and the presence of motor abnormalities or personality changes. Personality changes may be manifested by apathy, emotional lability, or behavioral disinhibition. The AIDS Task Force criteria also require the absence of clouding of consciousness or evidence of another etiology that could produce the cognitive impairment. Cognitive, motor, and behavioral changes are assessed using physical, neurological, and psychiatric examinations, in addition to neuropsychological testing.

Head Trauma-Related Dementia

Dementia can be a sequela of head trauma. The so-called punch-drunk syndrome (dementia pugilistica) occurs in boxers after repeated head trauma over many years. It is characterized by emotional lability, dysarthria, and impulsivity. It has also been observed in professional football players who developed dementia after repeated concussions over many years.

Mrs. S, 75 years of age, was brought to the emergency department after being found wandering her neighborhood in a confused and disoriented state. She was in good health until a few months prior when her husband was hospitalized for 10 days for minor surgery. About a month after her husband returned home, he and their two adult children, who do not reside with them, reported a noticeable change in Mrs. S's mental status. Mrs. S became hyperactive and appeared to have excessive energy, was agitated and irritable, and had difficulty sleeping at night.

At examination, Mrs. S was disoriented to time and place, agitated, and confused. Her husband revealed upon interview that Mrs. S has for many years suffered from dizziness and lightheadedness upon standing and occasionally suffered from falls, none of which caused any major damage. Not long before her confused symptoms began, Mrs. S had apparently suffered a fall one night, and her husband found her the next morning lying next to the bed in a confused state. Because of her history of falls, neither Mr. S nor Mrs. S thought much of the incident. A CT scan revealed the presence of a subdural hematoma, which was then evacuated. Afterward, Mrs. S's confusion and disorientation cleared and she returned to her normal state of functioning.

DIAGNOSIS AND CLINICAL FEATURES

The DSM-5 diagnostic criteria are based on deficits of cognitive functions such as learning and memory, orientation, attention and language among others. The full panoply of signs and symptoms is described below. DSM-5 makes a distinction between major and minor cognitive disorder based upon levels of functioning, but the underlying etiology is similar.

The diagnosis of dementia is based on the clinical examination, including a mental status examination, and on information from the patient's family, friends, and employers. Complaints of a personality change in a patient older than age 40 years suggest that a diagnosis of dementia should be carefully considered.

Clinicians should note patients' complaints about intellectual impairment and forgetfulness as well as evidence of patients' evasion, denial, or rationalization aimed at concealing cognitive deficits. Excessive orderliness, social withdrawal, or a tendency to relate events in minute detail can be characteristic, and sudden outbursts of anger or sarcasm can occur. Patients' appearance and behavior should be observed. Lability of emotions; sloppy grooming; uninhibited remarks; silly jokes; or a dull, apathetic, or vacuous facial expression and manner suggest the presence of dementia, especially when coupled with memory impairment.

Memory impairment is typically an early and prominent feature in dementia, especially in dementias involving the cortex, such as dementia of the Alzheimer's type. Early in the course of dementia, memory impairment is mild and usually most marked for recent events; people forget telephone numbers, conversations, and events of the day. As the course of dementia progresses, memory impairment becomes severe, and only the earliest learned information (e.g., a person's place of birth) is retained.

Inasmuch as memory is important for orientation to person, place, and time, orientation can be progressively affected during the course of a dementing illness. For example, patients with dementia may forget how to get back to their rooms after going to the bathroom. No matter how severe the disorientation seems, however, patients show no impairment in their level of consciousness.

Dementing processes that affect the cortex, primarily dementia of the Alzheimer's type and vascular dementia, can affect patients' language abilities.

Psychiatric and Neurological Changes

Personality. Changes in the personality of a person with dementia are especially disturbing for their families. Preexisting personality traits may be accentuated during the development of a dementia. Patients with dementia may also become introverted and seem to be less concerned than they previously were about the effects of their behavior on others. Persons with dementia who have paranoid delusions are generally hostile to family members and caretakers. Patients with frontal and temporal involvement are likely to have marked personality changes and may be irritable and explosive.

Hallucinations and Delusions. An estimated 20 to 30 percent of patients with dementia (primarily patients with dementia of the Alzheimer's type) have hallucinations, and 30 to 40 percent have delusions, primarily of a paranoid or persecutory and unsystematized nature, although complex, sustained, and well-systematized delusions are also reported by these patients. Physical aggression and other forms of violence are common in demented patients who also have psychotic symptoms.

Mood. In addition to psychosis and personality changes, depression and anxiety are major symptoms in an estimated 40 to 50 percent of patients with dementia, although the full syndrome of depressive disorder may be present in only 10 to 20 percent. Patients with dementia also may exhibit pathological laughter or crying—that is, extremes of emotions—with no apparent provocation.

Cognitive Change. In addition to the aphasias in patients with dementia, apraxias and agnosias are common. Other neurological signs that can be associated with dementia are seizures, seen in approximately 10 percent of patients with dementia of the Alzheimer's type and in 20 percent of patients with vascular dementia, and atypical neurological presentations, such as nondominant parietal lobe syndromes. Primitive reflexes, such as the grasp, snout, suck, tonic-foot, and palmomental reflexes, may be present on neurological examination, and myoclonic jerks are present in 5 to 10 percent of patients.

Patients with vascular dementia may have additional neurological symptoms, such as headaches, dizziness, faintness, weakness, focal neurological signs, and sleep disturbances, possibly attributable to the location of the cerebrovascular disease. Pseudobulbar palsy, dysarthria, and dysphagia are also more common in vascular dementia than in other dementing conditions.

Catastrophic Reaction. Patients with dementia also exhibit a reduced ability to apply what Kurt Goldstein called the "abstract attitude." Patients have difficulty generalizing from a single instance, forming concepts, and grasping similarities and differences among concepts. Furthermore, the ability to solve problems, to reason logically, and to make sound judgments is compromised. Goldstein also described a catastrophic reaction marked by agitation secondary to the subjective awareness of intellectual deficits under stressful circumstances. Persons usually attempt to compensate for defects by using strategies to avoid demonstrating failures in intellectual performance; they may change the subject, make jokes, or otherwise divert the interviewer. Lack of judgment and poor impulse control appear commonly, particularly in dementias that primarily affect the frontal lobes. Examples of these impairments include coarse language, inappropriate jokes, neglect of personal appearance and hygiene, and a general disregard for the conventional rules of social conduct.

Sundowner Syndrome. Sundowner syndrome is characterized by drowsiness, confusion, ataxia, and accidental falls. It occurs in older people who are overly sedated and in patients with dementia who react adversely to even a small dose of a psychoactive drug. The syndrome also occurs in demented patients when external stimuli, such as light and interpersonal orienting cues, are diminished.

Vascular Dementia

The general symptoms of vascular dementia are the same as those for dementia of the Alzheimer's type, but the diagnosis of vascular dementia requires either clinical or laboratory evidence in support of a vascular cause of the dementia. Vascular dementia is more likely to show a decremental, stepwise deterioration than is Alzheimer's disease.

Substance-Induced Persisting Dementia

To facilitate the clinician's thinking about differential diagnosis, substance-induced persisting dementia is listed in two places, with the dementias and with the substance-related disorders. The specific substances that cross references are alcohol, inhalants, sedatives, hypnotics, or anxiolytics, and other or unknown substances.

Alcohol-Induced Persisting Dementia. To make the diagnosis of alcohol-induced persisting dementia, the criteria for dementia must be met. Because amnesia can also occur in the context of Korsakoff's psychosis, it is important to distinguish between memory impairment accompanied by other cognitive deficits (i.e., dementia) and amnesia caused by thiamine deficiency. To complicate matters, however, evidence also suggests that other cognitive functions, such as attention and concentration, may also be impaired in Wernicke–Korsakoff syndrome. In addition, alcohol abuse is frequently associated with mood changes, so poor concentration and other cognitive symptoms often observed in the context of a major depression must also be ruled out. Prevalence rates differ considerably according to the population studied and the diagnostic criteria used, although alcohol-related dementia has been estimated to account for approximately 4 percent of dementias.

PATHOLOGY, PHYSICAL FINDINGS, AND LABORATORY EXAMINATION

A comprehensive laboratory workup must be performed when evaluating a patient with dementia. The purposes of the workup are to detect reversible causes of dementia and to provide the patient and family with a definitive diagnosis. The range of possible causes of dementia mandates selective use of laboratory tests. The evaluation should follow informed clinical suspicion based on the history and physical and mental status examination results. The continued improvements in brain imaging techniques, particularly MRI, have made differentiation between dementia of the Alzheimer's type and vascular dementia, in some cases, somewhat more straightforward than in the past. An active area of research is the use of single-photon emission computed tomography (SPECT) to detect patterns of brain metabolism in various types of dementias; the use of SPECT images may soon help in the clinical differential diagnosis of dementing illnesses.

A general physical examination is a routine component of the workup for dementia. It may reveal evidence of systemic disease causing brain dysfunction, such as an enlarged liver and hepatic encephalopathy, or it may demonstrate systemic disease related to particular CNS processes. The detection of Kaposi's sarcoma, for example, should alert the clinician to the probable presence of AIDS and the associated possibility of AIDS dementia complex. Focal neurological findings, such as asymmetrical hyperreflexia or weakness, are seen more often in vascular than in degenerative disease. Frontal lobe signs and primitive reflexes occur in many disorders and often point to greater progression.

DIFFERENTIAL DIAGNOSIS

Dementia of the Alzheimer's Type versus Vascular Dementia

Classically, vascular dementia has been distinguished from dementia of the Alzheimer's type by the decremental deterioration that can accompany cerebrovascular disease over time. Although the discrete, stepwise deterioration may not be apparent in all cases, focal neurological symptoms are more common in vascular dementia than in dementia of the Alzheimer's type, as are the standard risk factors for cerebrovascular disease.

Vascular Dementia versus Transient Ischemic Attacks

Transient ischemic attacks (TIAs) are brief episodes of focal neurological dysfunction lasting less than 24 hours (usually 5 to 15 minutes). Although a variety of mechanisms may be responsible, the episodes are frequently the result of microembolization from a proximal intracranial arterial lesion that produces transient brain ischemia, and the episodes usually resolve without significant pathological alteration of the parenchymal tissue. Approximately one-third of persons with untreated TIAs experience a brain infarction later; therefore, recognition of TIAs is an important clinical strategy to prevent brain infarction.

Clinicians should distinguish episodes involving the vertebrobasilar system from those involving the carotid arterial system. In general, symptoms of vertebrobasilar disease reflect a transient functional disturbance in either the brainstem or the occipital lobe; carotid distribution symptoms reflect unilateral retinal or hemispheric abnormality. Anticoagulant therapy, antiplatelet agglutinating drugs such as aspirin, and extracranial and intracranial reconstructive vascular surgery are effective in reducing the risk of infarction in patients with TIAs.

Delirium

In general, delirium is distinguished by rapid onset, brief duration, cognitive impairment fluctuation during the course of the day; nocturnal exacerbation of symptoms; marked disturbance of the sleep–wake cycle; and prominent disturbances in attention and perception.

Depression

Some patients with depression have symptoms of cognitive impairment difficult to distinguish from symptoms of dementia. The clinical picture is sometimes referred to as *pseudodementia,* although the term *depression-related cognitive dysfunction* is preferable and more descriptive. Patients with depression-related cognitive dysfunction generally have prominent depressive symptoms, more insight into their symptoms than do demented patients, and often a history of depressive episodes.

Factitious Disorder

Persons who attempt to simulate memory loss, as in factitious disorder, do so in an erratic and inconsistent manner. In true dementia, memory for time and place is lost before memory for person, and recent memory is lost before remote memory.

Schizophrenia

Although schizophrenia can be associated with some acquired intellectual impairment, its symptoms are much less severe than are the related symptoms of psychosis and thought disorder seen in dementia.

Normal Aging

Aging is not necessarily associated with any significant cognitive decline, but minor memory problems can occur as a normal part of aging. These normal occurrences are sometimes referred to as *benign senescent forgetfulness, age-associated memory impairment,* or *normal benign age-related senescence.* They are distinguished from dementia by their minor severity and because they do not interfere significantly with a person's social or occupational behavior. See Section 17.6 for a discussion of mild cognitive impairment.

Other Disorders

Intellectual disability, which does not include memory impairment, occurs in childhood. Amnestic disorder is characterized by circumscribed loss of memory and no deterioration. Major depression in which memory is impaired responds to antidepressant medication. Malingering and pituitary disorder must be ruled out, but they are unlikely.

COURSE AND PROGNOSIS

The classic course of dementia is an onset in the patient's 50s or 60s, with gradual deterioration over 5 to 10 years, leading eventually to death. The age of onset and the rapidity of deterioration vary among different types of dementia and within individual diagnostic categories. The average survival expectation for patients with dementia of the Alzheimer's type is approximately 8 years, with a range of 1 to 20 years. Data suggest that in persons with an early onset of dementia or with a family history of dementia, the disease is likely to have a rapid course. In a recent study of 821 persons with Alzheimer's disease, the median survival time was 3.5 years. After dementia is diagnosed, patients must have a complete medical and neurological workup because 10 to 15 percent of all patients with dementia have a potentially reversible condition if treatment is initiated before permanent brain damage occurs.

The most common course of dementia begins with a number of subtle signs that may, at first, be ignored by both the patient and the people closest to the patient. A gradual onset of symptoms is most commonly associated with dementia of the Alzheimer's type, vascular dementia, endocrinopathies, brain tumors, and metabolic disorders. Conversely, the onset of dementia resulting from head trauma, cardiac arrest with cerebral hypoxia, or encephalitis can be sudden. Although the symptoms of the early phase of dementia are subtle, they become conspicuous as the dementia progresses, and family members may then bring a patient to a physician's attention. People with dementia may be sensitive to the use of benzodiazepines or alcohol, which can precipitate agitated, aggressive, or psychotic behavior. In the terminal stages of dementia, patients become empty shells of their former selves—profoundly disoriented, incoherent, amnestic, and incontinent of urine and feces.

With psychosocial and pharmacological treatment and possibly because of the self-healing properties of the brain, the symptoms of dementia may progress slowly for a time or may even recede somewhat. Symptom regression is certainly a possibility in reversible dementias (dementias caused by hypothyroidism, NPH, and brain tumors) after treatment is initiated. The course of the dementia varies from a steady progression (commonly seen with dementia of the Alzheimer's type) to an incrementally worsening dementia (commonly seen with vascular dementia) to a stable dementia (as may be seen in dementia related to head trauma).

Psychosocial Determinants

The severity and course of dementia can be affected by psychosocial factors. The greater a person's premorbid intelligence and education, the better the ability to compensate for intellectual deficits. People who have a rapid onset of dementia use fewer defenses than do those who experience an insidious onset. Anxiety and depression can intensify and aggravate the symptoms. Pseudodementia occurs in depressed people who complain of impaired memory but, in fact, have a depressive disorder. When the depression is treated, the cognitive defects disappear.

TREATMENT

The first step in the treatment of dementia is verification of the diagnosis. Accurate diagnosis is imperative because the progression may be halted or even reversed if appropriate therapy is provided. Preventive measures are important, particularly in vascular dementia. Such measures might include changes in diet, exercise, and control of diabetes and hypertension. Pharmacological agents might include antihypertensive, anticoagulant, or antiplatelet agents. Blood pressure control should aim for the higher end of the normal range because that has been demonstrated to improve cognitive function in patients with vascular dementia. Blood pressure below the normal range has been demonstrated to further impair cognitive function in patients with dementia. The choice of antihypertensive agent can be significant in that β-adrenergic receptor antagonists have been associated with exaggeration of cognitive impairment. Angiotensin-converting enzyme (ACE) inhibitors and diuretics have not been linked to exaggeration of cognitive impairment and are thought to lower blood pressure without affecting cerebral blood flow, which is presumed to be correlated with cognitive function. Surgical removal of carotid plaques may prevent subsequent vascular events in carefully selected patients. The general treatment approach to patients with dementia is to provide supportive medical care; emotional support for the patients and their families; and pharmacological treatment for specific symptoms, including disruptive behavior.

Psychosocial Therapies

The deterioration of mental faculties has significant psychological meaning for patients with dementia. The experience of a sense of continuity over time depends on memory. Recent memory is lost before remote memory in most cases of dementia, and many patients are highly distressed by clearly recalling how they used to function while observing their obvious deterioration. At the most fundamental level, the self is a product of brain functioning. Patients' identities begin to fade as the illness progresses, and they can recall less and less of their past. Emotional reactions ranging from depression to severe anxiety to catastrophic terror can stem from the realization that the sense of self is disappearing.

Patients often benefit from a supportive and educational psychotherapy in which the nature and course of their illness are clearly explained. They may also benefit from assistance in grieving and accepting the extent of their disability and from attention to self-esteem issues. Any areas of intact functioning should be maximized by helping patients identify activities in which successful functioning is possible. A psychodynamic assessment of defective ego functions and cognitive limitations can also be useful. Clinicians can help patients find ways to deal with the defective ego functions, such as keeping calendars for orientation problems, making schedules to help structure activities, and taking notes for memory problems.

Psychodynamic interventions with family members of patients with dementia may be of great assistance. Those who take care of a patient struggle with feelings of guilt, grief, anger, and exhaustion as they watch a family member gradually deteriorate. A common problem that develops among caregivers involves their self-sacrifice in caring for a patient. The gradually developing resentment from this self-sacrifice is often suppressed because of the guilt feelings it produces. Clinicians can help caregivers understand the complex mixture of feelings associated with seeing a loved one decline and can provide understanding as well as permission to express these feelings. Clinicians must also be aware of the caregivers' tendencies to blame themselves or others for patients' illnesses and must appreciate the role that patients with dementia play in the lives of family members.

Pharmacotherapy

Clinicians may prescribe benzodiazepines for insomnia and anxiety, antidepressants for depression, and antipsychotic drugs for delusions and hallucinations, but they should be aware of possible idiosyncratic drug effects in older people (e.g., paradoxical excitement, confusion, and increased sedation). In general, drugs with high anticholinergic activity should be avoided.

Donepezil (Aricept), rivastigmine (Exelon), galantamine (Reminyl), and tacrine (Cognex) are cholinesterase inhibitors used to treat mild to moderate cognitive impairment in Alzheimer's disease. They reduce the inactivation of the neurotransmitter acetylcholine and thus potentiate the cholinergic neurotransmitter, which in turn produces a modest improvement in memory and goal-directed thought. These drugs are most useful for persons with mild to moderate memory loss who have sufficient preservation of their basal forebrain cholinergic neurons to benefit from augmentation of cholinergic neurotransmission.

Donepezil is well tolerated and widely used. Tacrine is rarely used because of its potential for hepatotoxicity. Fewer clinical data are available for rivastigmine and galantamine, which appear more likely to cause gastrointestinal (GI) and neuropsychiatric adverse effects than does donepezil. None of these medications prevents the progressive neuronal degeneration of the disorder. Prescribing information for anticholinesterase inhibitors can be found in Section 36.14.

Memantine (Namenda) protects neurons from excessive amounts of glutamate, which may be neurotoxic. The drug is sometimes combined with donepezil. It has been known to improve dementia.

Other Treatment Approaches. Other drugs being tested for cognitive-enhancing activity include general cerebral metabolic enhancers, calcium channel inhibitors, and serotonergic agents. Some studies have shown that selegiline (Eldepryl), a selective type B monoamine oxidase (MAO_B) inhibitor, may slow the advance of this disease. Ondansetron (Zofran), a 5-HT_3 receptor antagonist, is under investigation.

Estrogen replacement therapy may reduce the risk of cognitive decline in postmenopausal women; however, more studies are needed to confirm this effect. Complementary and alternative medicine studies of ginkgo biloba and other phytomedicinals are required to see if they have a positive effect on cognition. Reports have appeared of patients using nonsteroidal anti-inflammatory agents having a lower risk of developing Alzheimer's disease. Vitamin E has not been shown to be of value in preventing the disease. Exercise is purported to delay the onset of cognitive deterioration in general.

▲ 17.4 Major or Minor Neurocognitive Disorder due to Another Medical Condition (Amnestic Disorders)

The amnestic disorders—the DSM-IV term for these conditions—are coded in the DSM-5 as "major or minor neurocognitive disorders due to another medical condition." All of these disorders cause impairment in memory as the major sign and symptom, although other signs of cognitive decline may coexist. The authors of *Synopsis* believe amnestic disorder to be a clinically useful descriptive category of illness and both terms are used interchangeably in this section, but they are coded in DSM-5 as a *neurocognitive disorder due to another medical condition* with the specific medical condition noted.

These disorders are a broad category that results from a variety of diseases and conditions that have amnesia as the major complaint. The syndrome is defined primarily by impairment in the ability to create new memories. Three different etiologies exist: caused by a general medical condition (e.g., head trauma), caused by substances (e.g., carbon monoxide poisoning or chronic alcohol consumption), and a category not otherwise specified for cases in which the etiology is unclear.

EPIDEMIOLOGY

No adequate studies have reported on the incidence or prevalence of amnestic disorders. Amnesia is most commonly found in alcohol use disorders and in head injury. In general practice and hospital settings, the frequency of amnesia related to chronic alcohol abuse has decreased, and the frequency of amnesia related to head trauma has increased.

ETIOLOGY

The major neuroanatomical structures involved in memory and in the development of an amnestic disorder are particular diencephalic structures such as the dorsomedial and midline nuclei of the thalamus and midtemporal lobe structures such as the hippocampus, the mamillary bodies, and the amygdala. Although amnesia is usually the result of bilateral damage to these structures, some cases of unilateral damage result in an amnestic disorder, and evidence indicates that the left hemisphere may be more critical than the right hemisphere in the development of memory disorders. Many studies of memory and amnesia in animals have suggested that other brain areas may also be involved in the symptoms accompanying amnesia. Frontal lobe involvement can result in such symptoms as confabulation and apathy, which can be seen in patients with amnestic disorders.

Amnestic disorders have many potential causes (Table 17.4–1). Thiamine deficiency, hypoglycemia, hypoxia (including carbon monoxide poisoning), and herpes simplex encephalitis all have a predilection to damage the temporal lobes, particularly the hippocampi, and thus can be associated with the development of amnestic disorders. Similarly, when tumors, cerebrovascular diseases, surgical procedures, or multiple sclerosis plaques involve the diencephalic or temporal regions of the brain, the

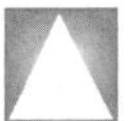

Table 17.4–1
Major Causes of Amnestic Disorders

Thiamine deficiency (Korsakoff's syndrome)
Hypoglycemia
Primary brain conditions
Seizures
Head trauma (closed and penetrating)
Cerebral tumors (especially thalamic and temporal lobe)
Cerebrovascular diseases (especially thalamic and temporal lobe)
Surgical procedures on the brain
Encephalitis due to herpes simplex
Hypoxia (including nonfatal hanging attempts and carbon monoxide poisoning)
Transient global amnesia
Electroconvulsive therapy
Multiple sclerosis
Substance-related causes
Alcohol use disorders
Neurotoxins
Benzodiazepines (and other sedative–hypnotics)
Many over-the-counter preparations

symptoms of an amnestic disorder may develop. General insults to the brain, such as seizures, ECT, and head trauma, can also result in memory impairment. Transient global amnesia is presumed to be a cerebrovascular disorder involving transient impairment in blood flow through the vertebrobasilar arteries.

Many drugs have been associated with the development of amnesia, and clinicians should review all drugs taken, including nonprescription drugs, in the diagnostic workup of a patient with amnesia. The benzodiazepines are the most commonly used prescription drugs associated with amnesia. All benzodiazepines can be associated with amnesia, especially if combined with alcohol. When triazolam (Halcion) is used in doses of 0.25 mg or less, which are generally equivalent to standard doses of other benzodiazepines, amnesia is no more often associated with triazolam than with other benzodiazepines. With alcohol and higher doses, anterograde amnesia has been reported.

DIAGNOSIS

The recognition of amnestic disorder occurs when impairment in the ability to learn new information or to recall previously learned information results in significant impairment in social or occupational functioning. It is caused by a general medical condition (including physical trauma). Amnestic disorder may be transient, lasting for hours or days or chronic lasting weeks or months. A diagnosis of substance-induced persisting amnestic disorder is made when evidence suggests that the symptoms are causatively related to the use of a substance. The DSM-5 refers clinicians to specific diagnoses within substance-related disorders: alcohol-induced disorder; sedative-, hypnotic-, or anxiolytic-induced disorder; and other (or unknown) substance-induced disorder.

CLINICAL FEATURES AND SUBTYPES

The central symptom of amnestic disorders is the development of a memory disorder characterized by an impairment in the ability to learn new information (anterograde amnesia) and an inability to recall previously remembered knowledge (retrograde amnesia). The symptom must result in significant problems for patients in their social or occupational functioning. The time in which a patient is amnestic can begin directly at the point of trauma or include a period before the trauma. Memory for the time during the physical insult (e.g., during a cerebrovascular event) may also be lost.

Short-term and recent memories are usually impaired. Patients cannot remember what they had for breakfast or lunch, the name of the hospital, or their doctors. In some patients, the amnesia is so profound that the patient cannot orient himself or herself to city and time, although orientation to person is seldom lost in amnestic disorders. Memory for overlearned information or events from the remote past, such as childhood experiences, is good, but memory for events from the less remote past (over the past decade) is impaired. Immediate memory (tested, e.g., by asking a patient to repeat six numbers) remains intact. With improvement, patients may experience a gradual shrinking of the time for which memory has been lost, although some patients experience a gradual improvement in memory for the entire period.

The onset of symptoms can be sudden, as in trauma, cerebrovascular events, and neurotoxic chemical assaults, or gradual, as in nutritional deficiency and cerebral tumors. The amnesia can be of short duration.

A variety of other symptoms can be associated with amnestic disorders. For patients with other cognitive impairments, a diagnosis of dementia or delirium is more appropriate than a diagnosis of an amnestic disorder. Both subtle and gross changes in personality can accompany the symptoms of memory impairment in amnestic disorders. Patients may be apathetic, lack initiative, have unprovoked episodes of agitation, or appear to be overly friendly or agreeable. Patients with amnestic disorders can also appear bewildered and confused and may attempt to cover their confusion with confabulatory answers to questions. Characteristically, patients with amnestic disorders do not have good insight into their neuropsychiatric conditions.

A 73-year-old survivor of the Holocaust was admitted to the psychiatric unit from a local nursing home. She was born in Germany to a middle-class family. Her education was truncated because of internment in a concentration camp. She immigrated to Israel after liberation from the concentration camp and later to the United States, where she married and raised a family. Premorbidly, she was described as a quiet, intelligent, and loving woman who spoke several languages. At 55 years of age, she had a significant carbon monoxide exposure when a gas line leaked while she and her husband slept. Her husband died of carbon monoxide poisoning, but the patient survived after a period of coma. After being stabilized, she displayed significant cognitive and behavioral problems. She had difficulty with learning new information and making appropriate plans. She retained the ability to perform activities of daily living but could not be relied on to pay bills, buy food, cook, or clean, despite appearing to have retained the intellectual ability to do these tasks. She was admitted to a nursing home after several difficult years at home and in the homes of relatives. In the nursing home, she was able to learn her way about the facility. She displayed little interest in scheduled group activities, hobbies, reading, or television. She had frequent behavioral problems. She repeatedly pressed staff to get her sweets and snacks and cursed them vociferously with racial epithets and disparaging comments on their weight and dress. On one occasion, she scratched the cars of several staff with a key. Neuropsychological testing demonstrated severe deficits in delayed recall; intact performance on language and general knowledge measures; and moderate deficits on domains of executive function, such as concept formation and cognitive flexibility. She was noted to respond immediately to firmly set limits and rewards, but deficits in memory prevented long-term incorporation of these boundaries. Management involved development of a behavioral plan that could be implemented at the nursing home and empirical trials of medications aimed at amelioration of irritability.

Cerebrovascular Diseases

Cerebrovascular diseases affecting the hippocampus involve the posterior cerebral and basilar arteries and their branches. Infarctions are rarely limited to the hippocampus; they often involve the occipital or parietal lobes. Thus, common accompanying symptoms of cerebrovascular diseases in this region are focal neurological signs involving vision or sensory modalities. Cerebrovascular diseases affecting the bilateral medial thalamus, particularly the anterior portions, are often associated with symptoms of amnestic disorders. A few case studies report amnestic disorders from rupture of an aneurysm of the anterior communicating artery, resulting in infarction of the basal forebrain region.

Multiple Sclerosis

The pathophysiological process of multiple sclerosis involves the seemingly random formation of plaques within the brain parenchyma. When the plaques occur in the temporal lobe and the diencephalic regions, symptoms of memory impairment can occur. In fact, the most common cognitive complaints in patients with multiple sclerosis involve impaired memory, which occurs in 40 to 60 percent of patients. Characteristically, digit span memory is normal, but immediate recall and delayed recall of information are impaired. The memory impairment can affect both verbal and nonverbal material.

Korsakoff's Syndrome

Korsakoff's syndrome is an amnestic syndrome caused by thiamine deficiency, most commonly associated with the poor nutritional habits of people with chronic alcohol abuse. Other causes of poor nutrition (e.g., starvation), gastric carcinoma, hemodialysis, hyperemesis gravidarum, prolonged IV hyperalimentation, and gastric plication can also result in thiamine deficiency. Korsakoff's syndrome is often associated with Wernicke's encephalopathy, which is the associated syndrome of confusion, ataxia, and ophthalmoplegia. In patients with these thiamine deficiency–related symptoms, the neuropathological findings include hyperplasia of the small blood vessels with occasional hemorrhages, hypertrophy of astrocytes, and subtle changes in neuronal axons. Although the delirium clears up within a month or so, the amnestic syndrome either accompanies or follows untreated Wernicke's encephalopathy in approximately 85 percent of all cases.

Patients with Korsakoff's syndrome typically demonstrate a change in personality as well, such that they display a lack of initiative, diminished spontaneity, and a lack of interest or concern. These changes appear frontal lobe–like, similar to the personality change ascribed to patients with frontal lobe lesions or degeneration. Indeed, such patients often demonstrate *executive function* deficits on neuropsychological tasks involving attention, planning, set shifting, and inferential reasoning consistent with frontal pattern injuries. For this reason, Korsakoff's syndrome is not a pure memory disorder, although it certainly is a good paradigm of the more common clinical presentations for the amnestic syndrome.

The onset of Korsakoff's syndrome can be gradual. Recent memory tends to be affected more than remote memory, but this feature is variable. Confabulation, apathy, and passivity are often prominent symptoms in the syndrome. With treatment, patients may remain amnestic for up to 3 months and then gradually improve over the ensuing year. Administration of thiamine may prevent the development of additional amnestic symptoms, but the treatment seldom reverses severe amnestic symptoms when they are present. Approximately one-third to one-fourth of all patients recover completely, and approximately one-fourth of all patients have no improvement of their symptoms.

Alcoholic Blackouts

Some persons with severe alcohol abuse may exhibit the syndrome commonly referred to as an alcoholic blackout. Characteristically, these persons awake in the morning with a conscious awareness of being unable to remember a period the night before during which they were intoxicated. Sometimes specific behaviors (hiding money in a secret place and provoking fights) are associated with the blackouts.

Electroconvulsive Therapy

Electroconvulsive therapy treatments are usually associated with retrograde amnesia for a period of several minutes before the treatment and anterograde amnesia after the treatment. The anterograde amnesia usually resolves within 5 hours. Mild memory deficits may remain for 1 to 2 months after a course of ECT treatments, but the symptoms are completely resolved 6 to 9 months after treatment.

Head Injury

Head injuries (both closed and penetrating) can result in a wide range of neuropsychiatric symptoms, including dementia, depression, personality changes, and amnestic disorders. Amnestic disorders caused by head injuries are commonly associated with a period of retrograde amnesia leading up to the traumatic incident and amnesia for the traumatic incident itself. The severity of the brain injury correlates somewhat with the duration and severity of the amnestic syndrome, but the best correlate of eventual improvement is the degree of clinical improvement in the amnesia during the first week after the patient regains consciousness.

Transient Global Amnesia

Transient global amnesia is characterized by the abrupt loss of the ability to recall recent events or to remember new information.

The syndrome is often characterized by mild confusion and a lack of insight into the problem; a clear sensorium; and, occasionally, the inability to perform some well-learned complex tasks. Episodes last from 6 to 24 hours. Studies suggest that transient global amnesia occurs in 5 to 10 cases per 100,000 persons per year, although, for patients older than age 50 years, the rate may be as high as 30 cases per 100,000 persons per year. The pathophysiology is unknown, but it likely involves ischemia of the temporal lobe and the diencephalic brain regions. Several studies of patients with SPECT have shown decreased blood flow in the temporal and parietotemporal regions, particularly in the left hemisphere. Patients with transient global amnesia almost universally experience complete improvement, although one study found that approximately 20 percent of patients may have recurrence of the episode, and another study found that approximately 7 percent of patients may have epilepsy. Patients with transient global amnesia have been differentiated from patients with transient ischemic attacks in that fewer patients have diabetes, hypercholesterolemia, and hypertriglyceridemia, but more have hypertension and migrainous episodes.

PATHOLOGY AND LABORATORY EXAMINATION

Laboratory findings diagnostic of amnestic disorder may be obtained using quantitative neuropsychological testing. Standardized tests also are available to assess recall of well-known historical events or public figures to characterize an individual's inability to remember previously learned information. Performance on such tests varies among individuals with amnestic disorder. Subtle deficits in other cognitive functions may be noted in individuals with amnestic disorder. Memory deficits, however, constitute the predominant feature of the mental status examination and account largely for any functional deficits. No specific or diagnostic features are detectable on imaging studies such as MRI or CT. Damage of midtemporal lobe structures is common, however, and may be reflected in enlargement of third ventricle or temporal horns or in structural atrophy detected by MRI.

DIFFERENTIAL DIAGNOSIS

Table 17.4–1 lists the major causes of amnestic disorders. To make the diagnosis, clinicians must obtain a patient's history, conduct a complete physical examination, and order all appropriate laboratory tests. Other diagnoses, however, can be confused with the amnestic disorders.

Dementia and Delirium

Amnestic disorders can be distinguished from delirium because they occur in the absence of a disturbance of consciousness and are striking for the relative preservation of other cognitive domains.

Table 17.4–2 outlines the key distinctions between Alzheimer's dementia and amnestic disorders. Both disorders can have an insidious onset with slow progression, as in a Korsakoff's psychosis in a chronic drinker. Amnestic disorders, however, can also develop precipitously, as in Wernicke's encephalopathy, transient global amnesia, or anoxic insults. Although Alzheimer's dementia progresses relentlessly, amnestic disorders tend to remain static or even improve after the offending cause has been removed. In terms of the actual memory deficits, the amnestic disorder and Alzheimer's disease still differ. Alzheimer's disease has an impact on retrieval in addition to encoding and consolidation. The deficits in Alzheimer's disease extend beyond memory to general knowledge (semantic memory), language, praxis, and general function. These are spared in amnestic disorders. The dementias associated with Parkinson's disease, AIDS, and other subcortical disorders demonstrate disproportionate impairment of retrieval, but relatively intact encoding and consolidation and thus can be distinguished from amnestic disorders. The subcortical pattern dementias are also likely to display motor symptoms, such as bradykinesia, chorea, or tremor, that are not components of the amnestic disorders.

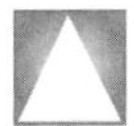

Table 17.4–2
Comparison of Syndrome Characteristics in Alzheimer's Disease and Amnestic Disorder

Characteristic	Alzheimer's Dementia	Amnestic Disorder
Onset	Insidious	Can be abrupt
Course	Progressive deterioration	Static or improvement
Anterograde memory	Impaired	Impaired
Retrograde memory	Impaired	Temporal gradient
Episodic memory	Impaired	Impaired
Semantic memory	Impaired	Intact
Language	Impaired	Intact
Praxis or function	Impaired	Intact

Normal Aging

Some minor impairment in memory may accompany normal aging, but the requirement that the memory impairment cause significant impairment in social or occupational functioning should exclude normal aging from the diagnosis.

Dissociative Disorders

The dissociative disorders can sometimes be difficult to differentiate from the amnestic disorders. Patients with dissociative disorders, however, are more likely to have lost their orientation to self and may have more selective memory deficits than do patients with amnestic disorders. For example, patients with dissociative disorders may not know their names or home addresses, but they are still able to learn new information and remember selected past memories. Dissociative disorders are also often associated with emotionally stressful life events involving money, the legal system, or troubled relationships.

Factitious Disorders

Patients with factitious disorders who are mimicking an amnestic disorder often have inconsistent results on memory tests and have no evidence of an identifiable cause. These findings, coupled with evidence of primary or secondary gain for a patient, should suggest a factitious disorder.

COURSE AND PROGNOSIS

The course of an amnestic disorder depends on its etiology and treatment, particularly acute treatment. Generally, the amnestic disorder has a static course. Little improvement is seen over time, but also no progression of the disorder occurs. The exceptions are the acute amnesias, such as transient global amnesia, which resolves entirely over hours to days, and the amnestic disorder associated with head trauma, which improves steadily in the months subsequent to the trauma. Amnesia secondary to processes that destroy brain tissue, such as stroke, tumor, and infection, are irreversible, although, again, static, after the acute infection or ischemia has been staunched.

TREATMENT

The primary approach to treating amnestic disorders is to treat the underlying cause. Although a patient is amnestic, supportive prompts about the date, the time, and the patient's location can be helpful and can reduce the patient's anxiety. After resolution of the amnestic episode, psychotherapy of some type (cognitive, psychodynamic, or supportive) may help patients incorporate the amnestic experience into their lives.

Psychotherapy

Psychodynamic interventions may be of considerable value for patients who have amnestic disorders that result from insults to the brain. Understanding the course of recovery in such patients helps clinicians to be sensitive to the narcissistic injury inherent in damage to the CNS.

The first phase of recovery, in which patients are incapable of processing what happened because the ego defenses are overwhelmed, requires clinicians to serve as a supportive auxiliary ego who explains to a patient what is happening and provides missing ego functions. In the second phase of recovery, as the realization of the injury sets in, patients may become angry and feel victimized by the malevolent hand of fate. They may view others, including the clinician, as bad or destructive, and clinicians must contain these projections without becoming punitive or retaliatory. Clinicians can build a therapeutic alliance with patients by explaining slowly and clearly what happened and by offering an explanation for a patient's internal experience. The third phase of recovery is integrative. As a patient accepts what has happened, a clinician can help the patient form a new identity by connecting current experiences of the self with past experiences. Grieving over the lost faculties may be an important feature of the third phase.

Most patients who are amnestic because of brain injury engage in denial. Clinicians must respect and empathize with the patient's need to deny the reality of what has happened. Insensitive and blunt confrontations destroy any developing therapeutic alliance and can cause patients to feel attacked. In a sensitive approach, clinicians help patients accept their cognitive limitations by exposing them to these deficits bit by bit over time. When patients fully accept what has happened, they may need assistance in forgiving themselves and any others involved, so that they can get on with their lives. Clinicians must also be wary of being seduced into thinking that all of the patient's symptoms are directly related to the brain insult. An evaluation of preexisting personality disorders, such as borderline, antisocial, and narcissistic personality disorders, must be part of the overall assessment; many patients with personality disorders place themselves in situations that predispose them to injuries. These personality features may become a crucial part of the psychodynamic psychotherapy.

Recently, centers for cognitive rehabilitation have been established whose rehabilitation-oriented therapeutic milieu is intended to promote recovery from brain injury, especially that from traumatic causes. Despite the high cost of extended care at these sites, which provide both long-term institutional and daytime services, no data have been developed to define therapeutic effectiveness for the heterogeneous groups of patients who participate in such tasks as memory retaining.

▲ 17.5 Neurocognitive and Other Disorders due to a General Medical Condition

Increasingly, scientific views of mental illness recognize that, whether caused by an identifiable anomaly (e.g., brain tumor), a neurotransmitter disturbance of unclear origin (e.g., schizophrenia), or a consequence of deranged upbringing or environment (e.g., personality disorder), all mental disorders ultimately share one common underlying theme: aberration in brain function. Treatments for those conditions, whether psychological or biological, attempt to restore normal brain chemistry.

The differential diagnosis for a mental syndrome in a patient should always include consideration of (1) any general medical condition that a patient may have and (2) any prescription, nonprescription, or illegal substances that a patient may be taking. Although some specific medical conditions have classically been associated with mental syndromes, a much larger number of general medical conditions have been associated with mental syndromes in case reports and small studies.

The mental disorders caused by a general medical condition span the entire spectrum of diagnostic categories. Thus, one can have a cognitive disorder, mood disorder, sleep disorder, anxiety disorder, and psychotic disorder to mention but a few that are caused or aggravated by a medical condition. In this section, neurocognitive disorders due to a general medical condition are described, including epilepsy, autoimmune disorders and AIDS, of which psychiatrists should be aware.

SPECIFIC DISORDERS

Epilepsy

Epilepsy is the most common chronic neurological disease in the general population and affects approximately 1 percent of the population in the United States. For psychiatrists, the major concerns about epilepsy are consideration of an epileptic diagnosis in psychiatric patients, the psychosocial ramifications of a diagnosis of epilepsy for a patient, and the psychological and cognitive effects of commonly used anticonvulsant drugs. With regard to the first of these concerns, 30 to 50 percent of all persons with epilepsy have psychiatric difficulties sometime during the course of their illness. The most common behavioral symptom of epilepsy is a change in personality. Psychosis and violence occur much less commonly than was previously believed.

Definitions. A seizure is a transient paroxysmal pathophysiological disturbance of cerebral function caused by a spontaneous, excessive discharge of neurons. Patients are said to have epilepsy if they have a chronic condition characterized by recurrent seizure. The ictus, or ictal event, is the seizure itself. The nonictal periods are categorized as preictal, postictal, and interictal. The symptoms during the ictal event are determined primarily by the site of origin in the brain for the seizure and by the pattern of the spread of seizure activity through the brain. Interictal symptoms are influenced by the ictal event and other neuropsychiatric and psychosocial factors, such as coexisting psychiatric or neurological disorders, the presence of psychosocial stressors, and premorbid personality traits.

Classification. The two major categories of seizures are partial and generalized. Partial seizures involve epileptiform activity in localized brain regions. Generalized seizures involve the entire brain. A classification system for seizures is outlined in Table 17.5–1.

GENERALIZED SEIZURES. Generalized tonic–clonic seizures exhibit the classic symptoms of loss of consciousness, generalized tonic–clonic movements of the limbs, tongue biting, and incontinence. Although the diagnosis of the ictal events of the seizure is relatively straightforward, the postictal state, characterized by a slow, gradual recovery of consciousness and cognition, occasionally presents a diagnostic dilemma for a psychiatrist in an emergency department. The recovery period from a generalized tonic–clonic seizure ranges from a few minutes to many hours, and the clinical picture is that of a gradually clearing delirium. The most common psychiatric problems associated with generalized seizures involve helping patients adjust to a chronic neurological disorder and assessing the cognitive or behavioral effects of anticonvulsant drugs.

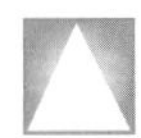

Table 17.5–1
International Classification of Epileptic Seizures

I. Partial seizures (seizures beginning locally)
  A. Partial seizures with elementary symptoms (generally without impairment of consciousness)
    1. With motor symptoms
    2. With sensory symptoms
    3. With autonomic symptoms
    4. Compound forms
  B. Partial seizures with complex symptoms (generally with impairment of consciousness; temporal lobe or psychomotor seizures)
    1. With impairment of consciousness only
    2. With cognitive symptoms
    3. With affective symptoms
    4. With psychosensory symptoms
    5. With psychosensory symptoms (automatisms)
    6. Compound forms
  C. Partial seizures secondarily generalized
II. Generalized seizures (bilaterally symmetrical and without local onset)
  A. Absences (petit mal)
  B. Myoclonus
  C. Infantile spasms
  D. Clonic seizures
  E. Tonic seizures
  F. Tonic–clonic seizures (grand mal)
  G. Atonic seizures
  H. Akinetic seizures
III. Unilateral seizures
IV. Unclassified seizures (because of incomplete data)

Adapted from Gastaut H. Clinical and electroencephalographical classification of epileptic seizures. *Epilepsia.* 1970;11:102.

ABSENCE SEIZURE (PETIT MAL). A difficult type of generalized seizure for a psychiatrist to diagnose is an absence, or petit mal, seizure. The epileptic nature of the episodes may go unrecognized because the characteristic motor or sensory manifestations of epilepsy may be absent or so slight that they do not arouse suspicion. Petit mal epilepsy usually begins in childhood between the ages of 5 and 7 years and ceases by puberty. Brief disruptions of consciousness, during which the patient suddenly loses contact with the environment, are characteristic of petit mal epilepsy, but the patient has no true loss of consciousness and no convulsive movements during the episodes. The EEG produces a characteristic pattern of three-per-second spike-and-wave activity. In rare instances, petit mal epilepsy begins in adulthood. Adult-onset petit mal epilepsy can be characterized by sudden, recurrent psychotic episodes or deliriums that appear and disappear abruptly. The symptoms may be accompanied by a history of falling or fainting spells.

PARTIAL SEIZURES. Partial seizures are classified as either simple (without alterations in consciousness) or complex (with an alteration in consciousness). Somewhat more than half of all patients with partial seizures have complex partial seizures. Other terms used for complex partial seizures are temporal lobe epilepsy, psychomotor seizures, and limbic epilepsy; these terms, however, are not accurate descriptions of the clinical situation. Complex partial epilepsy, the most common form of epilepsy in adults, affects approximately 3 of 1,000 persons. About 30 percent of patients with complex partial seizures have major mental illness such as depression.

Symptoms

PREICTAL SYMPTOMS. Preictal events (auras) in complex partial epilepsy include autonomic sensations (e.g., fullness in the stomach, blushing, and changes in respiration); cognitive sensations (e.g., *déjà vu, jamais vu,* forced thinking, dreamy states); affective states (e.g., fear, panic, depression, elation); and, classically, automatisms (e.g., lip smacking, rubbing, chewing).

ICTAL SYMPTOMS. Brief, disorganized, and uninhibited behavior characterizes the ictal event. Although some defense attorneys may claim otherwise, rarely does a person exhibit organized, directed violent behavior during an epileptic episode. The cognitive symptoms include amnesia for the time during the seizure and a period of resolving delirium after the seizure. A seizure focus can be found on an EEG in 25 to 50 percent of all patients with complex partial epilepsy. The use of sphenoidal or anterior temporal electrodes and sleep-deprived EEGs may increase the likelihood of finding an EEG abnormality. Multiple normal EEGs are often obtained for a patient with complex partial epilepsy; therefore, normal EEGs cannot be used to exclude a diagnosis of complex partial epilepsy. The use of long-term EEG recordings (usually 24 to 72 hours) can help clinicians detect a seizure focus in some patients. Most studies show that the use of nasopharyngeal leads does not add much to the sensitivity of an EEG, but they do add to the discomfort of the procedure for the patient.

INTERICTAL SYMPTOMS

Personality Disturbances. The most frequent psychiatric abnormalities reported in patients with epilepsy are personality disorders, and they are especially likely to occur in patients with epilepsy of temporal lobe origin. The most common features are religiosity, a heightened experience of emotions—a quality usually called *viscosity of personality*—and changes in sexual behavior. The syndrome in its complete form is relatively rare even in those with complex partial seizures of temporal lobe origin. Many patients are not affected by personality disturbances; others have a variety of disturbances that differ strikingly from the classic syndrome.

A striking religiosity may be manifested not only by increased participation in overtly religious activities but also by unusual concern for moral and ethical issues, preoccupation with right and wrong, and heightened interest in global and philosophical concerns. The hyperreligious features can sometimes seem like the prodromal symptoms of schizophrenia and can result in a diagnostic problem in an adolescent or a young adult.

The symptom of viscosity of personality is usually most noticeable in a patient's conversation, which is likely to be slow, serious, ponderous, pedantic, overly replete with nonessential details, and often circumstantial. The listener may grow bored but be unable to find a courteous and successful way to disengage from the conversation. The speech tendencies, often mirrored in the patient's writing, result in a symptom known as *hypergraphia,* which some clinicians consider virtually pathognomonic for complex partial epilepsy.

Changes in sexual behavior may be manifested by hypersexuality; deviations in sexual interest, such as fetishism and transvestism; and, most commonly, hyposexuality. The hyposexuality is characterized both by a lack of interest in sexual matters and by reduced sexual arousal. Some patients with the onset of complex partial epilepsy before puberty may fail to reach a normal level of sexual interest after puberty, although this characteristic may not disturb the patient. For patients with the onset of complex partial epilepsy after puberty, the change in sexual interest may be bothersome and worrisome.

Psychotic Symptoms. Interictal psychotic states are more common than ictal psychoses. Schizophrenia-like interictal episodes can occur in patients with epilepsy, particularly those with temporal lobe origins. An estimated 10 percent of all patients with complex partial epilepsy have psychotic symptoms. Risk factors for the symptoms include female gender, left-handedness, the onset of seizures during puberty, and a left-sided lesion.

The onset of psychotic symptoms in epilepsy is variable. Classically, psychotic symptoms appear in patients who have had epilepsy for a long time, and the onset of psychotic symptoms is preceded by the development of personality changes related to the epileptic brain activity. The most characteristic symptoms of the psychoses are hallucinations and paranoid delusions. Patients usually remain warm and appropriate in affect, in contrast to the abnormalities of affect commonly seen in patients with schizophrenia. The thought disorder symptoms in patients with psychotic epilepsy are most commonly those involving conceptualization and circumstantiality rather than the classic schizophrenic symptoms of blocking and looseness.

Violence. Episodic violence has been a problem in some patients with epilepsy, especially epilepsy of temporal and frontal lobe origin. Whether the violence is a manifestation of the seizure itself or is of interictal psychopathological origin is uncertain. Most evidence points to the extreme rarity of violence as an ictal phenomenon. Only in rare cases should violence in the patient with epilepsy be attributed to the seizure itself.

Mood Disorder Symptoms. Mood disorder symptoms, such as depression and mania, are seen less often in epilepsy than are schizophrenia-like symptoms. The mood disorder symptoms that do occur tend to be episodic and appear most often when the epileptic foci affect the temporal lobe of the nondominant cerebral hemisphere. The importance of mood disorder symptoms may be attested to by the increased incidence of attempted suicide in people with epilepsy.

Diagnosis. A correct diagnosis of epilepsy can be particularly difficult when the ictal and interictal symptoms of epilepsy are severe manifestations of psychiatric symptoms in the absence of significant changes in consciousness and cognitive abilities. Psychiatrists, therefore, must maintain a high level of suspicion during the evaluation of a new patient and must consider the possibility of an epileptic disorder even in the absence of the classic signs and symptoms. Another differential diagnosis to consider is pseudoseizure, in which a patient has some conscious control over mimicking the symptoms of a seizure (Table 17.5–2).

For patients who have previously received a diagnosis of epilepsy, the appearance of new psychiatric symptoms should be considered as possibly representing an evolution in their epileptic symptoms. The appearance of psychotic symptoms, mood disorder symptoms, personality changes, or symptoms of anxiety (e.g., panic attacks) should cause a clinician to evaluate the control of the patient's epilepsy and to assess the patient for the presence of an independent mental disorder. In such circumstances, the clinician should evaluate the patient's compliance with the anticonvulsant drug regimen and should consider whether the psychiatric symptoms could be adverse effects from

Table 17.5–2
Differentiating Features of Pseudoseizures and Epileptic Seizures

Feature	Epileptic Seizures	Pseudoseizure
Clinical features		
Nocturnal seizure	Common	Uncommon
Stereotyped aura	Usually	None
Cyanotic skin changes during seizures	Common	None
Self-injury	Common	Rare
Incontinence	Common	Rare
Postictal confusion	Present	None
Body movements	Tonic or clonic or both	Nonstereotyped and asynchronous
Affected by suggestion	No	Yes
EEG features		
Spike and waveforms	Present	Absent
Postictal slowing	Present	Absent
Interictal abnormalities	Variable	Variable

EEG, electroencephalogram.
From Stevenson JM, King JH. Neuropsychiatric aspects of epilepsy and epileptic seizures. In: Hales RE, Yodofsky SC, eds. *American Psychiatric Press Textbook of Neuropsychiatry.* Washington, DC: American Psychiatric Press; 1987:220.

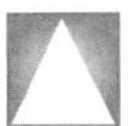

Table 17.5–3
Commonly Used Anticonvulsant Drugs

Drug	Use	Maintenance Dosage (mg/day)
Carbamazepine (Tegretol, Carbatrol)	Generalized tonic–clonic, partial	600–1,200
Clonazepam (Klonopin)	Absence, atypical myoclonic	2–12
Ethosuximide (Zarontin)	Absence	1,000–2,000
Gabapentin (Neurontin)	Complex partial seizures (augmentation)	900–3,600
Lamotrigine (Lamictal)	Complex partial seizures, generalized (augmentation)	300–500
Oxcarbazepine (Trileptal)	Partial	600–2,400
Phenobarbital	Generalized tonic–clonic	100–200
Phenytoin (Dilantin)	Generalized tonic–clonic, partial, status epilepticus	300–500
Primidone (Mysoline)	Partial	750–1,000
Tiagabine (Gabitril)	Generalized	32–56
Topiramate (Topamax)	Complex partial seizures (augmentation)	200–400
Valproate	Absence, myoclonic generalized tonic–clonic akinetic, partial seizures	750–1,000
Zonisamide (Zonegran)	Generalized	400–600

the antiepileptic drugs themselves. When psychiatric symptoms appear in a patient who has had epilepsy diagnosed or considered as a diagnosis in the past, the clinician should obtain results of one or more EEG examinations.

In patients who have not previously received a diagnosis of epilepsy, four characteristics should cause a clinician to be suspicious of the possibility: the abrupt onset of psychosis in a person previously regarded as psychologically healthy, the abrupt onset of delirium without a recognized cause, a history of similar episodes with abrupt onset and spontaneous recovery, and a history of previous unexplained falling or fainting spells.

Treatment. First-line drugs for generalized tonic–clonic seizures are valproate and phenytoin (Dilantin). First-line drugs for partial seizures include carbamazepine, oxcarbazepine (Trileptal), and phenytoin. Ethosuximide (Zarontin) and valproate are first-line drugs for absence (petit mal) seizures. The drugs used for various types of seizures are listed in Table 17.5–3. Carbamazepine and valproic acid may be helpful in controlling the symptoms of irritability and outbursts of aggression, as are the typical antipsychotic drugs. Psychotherapy, family counseling, and group therapy may be useful in addressing the psychosocial issues associated with epilepsy. In addition, clinicians should be aware that many antiepileptic drugs cause mild to moderate cognitive impairment, and an adjustment of the dosage or a change in medications should be considered if symptoms of cognitive impairment are a problem in a patient.

Brain Tumors

Brain tumors and cerebrovascular diseases can cause virtually any psychiatric symptom or syndrome, but cerebrovascular diseases, by the nature of their onset and symptom pattern, are rarely misdiagnosed as mental disorders. In general, tumors are associated with fewer psychopathological signs and symptoms than are cerebrovascular diseases affecting a similar volume of brain tissue. The two key approaches to the diagnosis of either condition are a comprehensive clinical history and a complete neurological examination. Performance of the appropriate brain imaging technique is usually the final diagnostic procedure; the imaging should confirm the clinical diagnosis.

Clinical Features, Course, and Prognosis. Mental symptoms are experienced at some time during the course of illness in approximately 50 percent of patients with brain tumors. In approximately 80 percent of these patients with mental symptoms, the tumors are located in frontal or limbic brain regions rather than in parietal or temporal regions. Whereas meningiomas are likely to cause focal symptoms by compressing a limited region of the cortex, gliomas are likely to cause diffuse symptoms. Delirium is most often a component of rapidly growing, large, or metastatic tumors. If a patient's history and a physical examination reveal bowel or bladder incontinence, a frontal lobe tumor should be suspected; if the history and examination reveal abnormalities in memory and speech, a temporal lobe tumor should be suspected. But there are no pathognomonic signs or symptoms that can localize a brain tumor with any degree of precision.

COGNITION. Impaired intellectual functioning often accompanies the presence of a brain tumor, regardless of its type or location.

LANGUAGE SKILLS. Disorders of language function may be severe, particularly if tumor growth is rapid. In fact, defects of language function often obscure all other mental symptoms.

MEMORY. Loss of memory is a frequent symptom of brain tumors. Patients with brain tumors exhibit Korsakoff's syndrome and retain no memory of events that occurred since the illness began. Events of the immediate past, even painful ones, are lost. Patients, however, retain old memories and are unaware of their loss of recent memory.

PERCEPTION. Prominent perceptual defects are often associated with behavioral disorders, especially because patients must integrate tactile, auditory, and visual perceptions to function normally.

AWARENESS. Alterations of consciousness are common late symptoms of increased intracranial pressure caused by a brain tumor. Tumors arising in the upper part of the brainstem can produce a unique symptom called *akinetic mutism,* or *vigilant coma.* The patient is immobile and mute yet alert.

Colloid Cysts. Although they are not brain tumors, colloid cysts located in the third ventricle can exert physical pressure on structures within the diencephalon and produce such mental symptoms as depression, emotional lability, psychotic symptoms, and personality changes. The classic associated neurological symptoms are position-dependent intermittent headaches.

Head Trauma

Head trauma can result in an array of mental symptoms and lead to a diagnosis of dementia due to head trauma or to mental disorder not otherwise specified due to a general medical condition (e.g., postconcussional disorder). The postconcussive syndrome remains controversial because it focuses on the wide range of psychiatric symptoms, some serious, that can follow what seems to be minor head trauma.

Pathophysiology. Head trauma is a common clinical situation; an estimated 2 million incidents involve head trauma each year. Head trauma most commonly occurs in people 15 to 25 years of age and has a male-to-female predominance of approximately 3 to 1. Gross estimates based on the severity of the head trauma suggest that virtually all patients with serious head trauma, more than half of patients with moderate head trauma and about 10 percent of patients with mild head trauma have ongoing neuropsychiatric sequelae resulting from the head trauma. Head trauma can be divided grossly into penetrating head trauma (e.g., trauma produced by a bullet) and blunt trauma, in which there is no physical penetration of the skull. Blunt trauma is far more common than penetrating head trauma. Motor vehicle accidents account for more than half of all the incidents of blunt CNS trauma; falls, violence, and sports-related head trauma account for most of the remaining cases Whereas brain injury from penetrating wounds is usually localized to the areas directly affected by the missile, brain injury from blunt trauma involves several mechanisms. During the actual head trauma, the head usually moves back and forth violently, so that the brain hits repeatedly against the skull as it and the skull are mismatched in their rapid deceleration and acceleration. This crashing results in focal contusions, and the stretching of the brain parenchyma produces diffuse axonal injury. Later developing processes such as edema and hemorrhaging which can result in further damage to the brain.

Symptoms. The two major clusters of symptoms related to head trauma are those of cognitive impairment and of behavioral sequelae. After a period of posttraumatic amnesia, there is usually a 6- to 12-month period of recovery, after which the remaining symptoms are likely to be permanent. The most common cognitive problems are decreased speed in information processing, decreased attention, increased distractibility, deficits in problem-solving and in the ability to sustain effort, and problems with memory and learning new information. A variety of language disabilities can also occur.

Behaviorally, the major symptoms involve depression, increased impulsivity, increased aggression, and changes in personality. These symptoms can be further exacerbated by the use of alcohol, which is often involved in the head trauma event itself. A debate has ensued about how preexisting character and personality traits affect the development of behavioral symptoms after head trauma. The critical studies needed to answer the question definitively have not yet been done, but the weight of opinion is leaning toward a biologically and neuroanatomically based association between the head trauma and the behavioral sequelae.

Treatment. The treatment of the cognitive and behavioral disorders in patients with head trauma is basically similar to the treatment approaches used in other patients with these symptoms. One difference is that patients with head trauma may be particularly susceptible to the side effects associated with psychotropic drugs; therefore, treatment with these agents should be initiated in lower dosages than usual, and they should be titrated upward more slowly than usual. Standard antidepressants can be used to treat depression, and either anticonvulsants or antipsychotics can be used to treat aggression and impulsivity. Other approaches to the symptoms include lithium, calcium channel blockers, and β-adrenergic receptor antagonists.

Clinicians must support patients through individual or group psychotherapy and should support the major caretakers through couples and family therapy. Patients with minor and moderate head trauma often rejoin their families and restart their jobs; therefore, all involved parties need help to adjust to any changes in the patient's personality and mental abilities.

Demyelinating Disorders

Multiple sclerosis (MS) is the major demyelinating disorder. Other demyelinating disorders include amyotrophic lateral sclerosis (ALS), metachromatic leukodystrophy, adrenoleukodystrophy, gangliosidoses, subacute sclerosing panencephalitis, and Kufs' disease. All of these disorders can be associated with neurological, cognitive, and behavioral symptoms.

Multiple Sclerosis

MS is characterized by multiple episodes of symptoms, pathophysiologically related to multifocal lesions in the white matter of the CNS. The cause remains unknown, but studies have focused on slow viral infections and disturbances in the immune system. The estimated prevalence of MS in the Western Hemisphere is 50 per 100,000 people. The disease is much more frequent in cold and temperate climates than in the tropics and subtropics and more common in women than in men; it is predominantly a disease of young adults. In most patients, the onset occurs between the ages of 20 and 40 years.

The neuropsychiatric symptoms of MS can be divided into cognitive and behavioral types. Research reports have found that 30 to 50 percent of patients with MS have mild cognitive impairment and that 20 to 30 percent of them have serious cognitive impairments. Although evidence indicates that patients with MS experience a decline in their general intelligence, memory is the most commonly affected cognitive function. The severity of the memory impairment does not seem to be correlated with the severity of the neurological symptoms or the duration of the illness.

The behavioral symptoms associated with MS are varied and can include euphoria, depression, and personality changes. Psychosis is a rare complication. Approximately 25 percent of persons with MS exhibit a euphoric mood that is not hypomanic but somewhat more cheerful than their situation warrants and not necessarily in character with their disposition before the onset of MS. Only 10 percent of patients with MS have a sustained and elevated mood, although it is still not truly hypomanic. Depression, however, is common; it affects 25 to 50 percent of patients with MS and results in a higher rate of suicide than is seen in the general population. Risk factors for suicide in patients with MS are male sex, onset of MS before age 30 years, and a relatively recent diagnosis of the disorder. Personality changes are also common in patients with MS; they affect 20 to 40 percent of patients and are often characterized by increased irritability or apathy.

Amyotrophic Lateral Sclerosis

ALS is a progressive, noninherited disease of asymmetrical muscle atrophy. It begins in adult life and progresses over months or years to involve all the striated muscles except the cardiac and ocular muscles. In addition to muscle atrophy, patients have signs of pyramidal tract involvement. The illness is rare and occurs in approximately 1.6 persons per 100,000 annually. A few patients have concomitant dementia. The disease progresses rapidly, and death generally occurs within 4 years of onset.

Infectious Diseases

Herpes Simplex Encephalitis. Herpes simplex encephalitis, the most common type of focal encephalitis, most commonly affects the frontal and temporal lobes. The symptoms often include anosmia, olfactory and gustatory hallucinations, and personality changes and can also involve bizarre or psychotic behaviors. Complex partial epilepsy may also develop in patients with herpes simplex encephalitis. Although the mortality rate for the infection has decreased, many patients exhibit personality changes, symptoms of memory loss, and psychotic symptoms.

Rabies Encephalitis. The incubation period for rabies ranges from 10 days to 1 year, after which symptoms of restlessness, overactivity, and agitation can develop. Hydrophobia, present in up to 50 percent of patients, is characterized by an intense fear of drinking water. The fear develops from the severe laryngeal and diaphragmatic spasms that the patients experience when they drink water. When rabies encephalitis develops, the disease is fatal within days or weeks.

Neurosyphilis. Neurosyphilis (also known as general paresis) appears 10 to 15 years after the primary *Treponema* infection. Since the advent of penicillin, neurosyphilis has become a rare disorder, although AIDS is associated with reintroducing neurosyphilis into medical practice in some urban settings. Neurosyphilis generally affects the frontal lobes and results in personality changes, development of poor judgment, irritability, and decreased care for self. Delusions of grandeur develop in 10 to 20 percent of affected patients. The disease progresses with the development of dementia and tremor until patients are paretic. The neurological symptoms include Argyll Robertson pupils, which are small, irregular, and unequal and have light-near reflex dissociation, tremor, dysarthria, and hyperreflexia. Cerebrospinal fluid (CSF) examination shows lymphocytosis, increased protein, and a positive result on a venereal disease research laboratory (VDRL) test.

Chronic Meningitis. Chronic meningitis is now seen more often than in the recent past because of the immunocompromised condition of people with AIDS. The usual causative agents are *Mycobacterium tuberculosis, Cryptococcus* spp., and *Coccidioides* spp. The usual symptoms are headache, memory impairment, confusion, and fever.

Subacute Sclerosing Panencephalitis. Subacute sclerosing panencephalitis is a disease of childhood and early adolescence, with a 3-to-1 male-to-female ratio. The onset usually follows either an infection with measles or a vaccination for measles. The initial symptoms may be behavioral change, temper tantrums, sleepiness, and hallucinations, but the classic symptoms of myoclonus, ataxia, seizures, and intellectual deterioration eventually develop. The disease progresses relentlessly to coma and death in 1 to 2 years.

Lyme Disease. Lyme disease is caused by infection with the spirochete *Borrelia burgdorferi* transmitted through the bite of the deer tick (*Ixodes scapularis*), which feeds on infected deer and mice. About 16,000 cases are reported annually in the United States.

A characteristic bull's-eye rash is found at the site of the tick bite followed shortly thereafter by flulike symptoms. Impaired cognitive functioning and mood changes are associated with the illness and may be the presenting complaint. These include memory lapses, difficulty concentrating, irritability, and depression.

No clear-cut diagnostic test is available. About 50 percent of patients become seropositive to *B. burgdorferi.* Prophylaxis vaccine is not always effective and is controversial. Treatment consists of a 14- to 21-day course of doxycycline (Vibramycin), which results in a 90 percent cure rate. Specific psychotropic drugs can be targeted to treat the psychiatric sign or symptom (e.g., diazepam [Valium] for anxiety). Left untreated, about 60 percent of persons develop a chronic condition. Such patients may be given an erroneous diagnosis of a primary depression rather than one secondary to the medical condition. Support groups for patients with chronic Lyme disease are important. Group members provide each other with emotional support that helps improve their quality of life.

Prion Disease

Prion disease is a group of related disorders caused by a transmissible infectious protein known as a *prion.* Included in this group are Creutzfeldt–Jakob disease (CJD), Gerstmann–Straussler–Scheinker disorder (GSS), fatal familial insomnia (FFI), and kuru. A variant of CJD (vCJD), also called "mad cow disease," appeared in 1995 in the United Kingdom and is attributed to the transmission of bovine spongiform encephalopathy (BSE) from cattle to humans. Collectively, these disorders are also known as *subacute spongiform encephalopathy* because of shared neuropathological changes that consist of (1) spongiform vacuolization, (2) neuronal loss, and (3) astrocyte proliferation in the cerebral cortex. Amyloid plaques may or may not be present.

ETIOLOGY. Prions are transmissible agents but differ from viruses in that they lack nucleic acid. Prions are mutated proteins generated from the human prion protein gene (PrP), which is located on the short arm of chromosome 20. No direct link exists between prion disease and Alzheimer's disease, which has been traced to chromosome 21.

The PrP mutates into a disease-related isoform PrP-Super-C (PrP^{Sc}), which can replicate and is infectious. The neuropathological changes that occur in prion disease are presumed to be caused by direct neurotoxic effects of PrP^{Sc}.

The specific prion disease that develops depends on the mutation of PrP that occurs. Mutations at PrP 178N/129V cause CJD, mutations at 178N/129M cause FFI, and mutations at 102L/129M cause GSS and kuru. Other mutations of PrP have been described, and research continues in this important area of genomic identification. Some mutations are both fully penetrant and autosomal dominant and account for inherited forms of prion disease. For example, both GSS and FFI are inherited disorders, and about 10 percent of cases of CJD are also inherited. Prenatal testing for the abnormal PrP gene is available; whether or not such testing should be routinely done is open to question at this time.

CREUTZFELDT–JAKOB DISEASE. First described in 1920, CJD is an invariably fatal, rapidly progressive disorder that occurs mainly in middle-aged or older adults. It manifests initially with fatigue, flulike symptoms, and cognitive impairment. As the disease progresses, focal neurological findings such as aphasia and apraxia occur. Psychiatric manifestations are protean and include emotional lability, anxiety, euphoria, depression, delusions, hallucinations, or marked personality changes. The disease progresses over months, leading to dementia, akinetic mutism, coma, and death.

The rates of CJD range from one to two cases per 1 million persons a year worldwide. The infectious agent self-replicates and can be transmitted to humans by inoculation with infected tissue and sometimes by ingestion of contaminated food. Iatrogenic transmission has been reported via transplantation of contaminated cornea or dura mater or to children via contaminated supplies of human growth hormone derived from infected persons. Neurosurgical transmission has also been reported. Household contacts are not at greater risk for developing the disease than the general population unless there is direct inoculation.

Diagnosis requires pathological examination of the cortex, which reveals the classic triad of spongiform vacuolation, loss of neurons, and astrocyte cell proliferation. The cortex and basal ganglia are most affected. An immunoassay test for CJD in the CSF shows promise in supporting the diagnosis; however, this needs to be tested more extensively. Although not specific for CJD, EEG abnormalities are present in nearly all patients, consisting of a slow and irregular background rhythm with periodic complex discharges. CT and MRI studies may reveal cortical atrophy later in the course of disease. SPECT and positron emission tomography (PET) reveal heterogeneously decreased uptake throughout the cortex.

No known treatment exists for CJD. Death usually occurs within 6 months after diagnosis.

VARIANT CJD. In 1995, a variant of CJD (vCJD) appeared in the United Kingdom. The patients affected all died; they were young (younger than age 40 years), and none had risk factors of CJD. At autopsy, prion disease was found. The disease was attributed to the transmission in the United Kingdom of BSE between cattle and from cattle to humans in the 1980s. BSE appears to have originated from sheep scrapie–contaminated feed given to cattle. Scrapie is a spongiform encephalopathy found in sheep and goats that has not been shown to cause human disease; however, it is transmissible to other animal species.

The mean age of onset is 29 years, and about 150 people worldwide had been infected as of 2006. Clinicians must be alert to the diagnosis in young people with behavioral and psychiatric abnormalities in association with cerebellar signs such as ataxia or myoclonus. The psychiatric presentation of vCJD is not specific. Most patients have reported depression, withdrawal, anxiety, and sleep disturbance. Paranoid delusions have occurred. Neuropathological changes are similar to those in vCJD, with the addition of amyloid plaques.

Epidemiological data are still being gathered. The incubation period for vCJD and the amount of infected meat product required to cause infection are unknown. One patient was reported to have been a vegetarian for 5 years before his disease was diagnosed. vCJD can be diagnosed antemortem by examining the tonsils with Western blot immunostains to detect PrP^{Sc} in lymphoid tissue. Diagnosis relies on the development of progressive neurodegenerative features in persons who have ingested contaminated meat or brains. No cure exists, and death usually occurs within 2 to 3 years after diagnosis. Prevention is dependent on careful monitoring of cattle for disease and feeding them grain instead of meat byproducts.

KURU. Kuru is an epidemic prion disease found in New Guinea that is caused by cannibalistic funeral rituals in which the brains of the deceased are eaten. Women are more affected by the disorder than men, presumably because they participate in the ceremony to a greater extent. Death usually occurs within 2 years after symptoms develop. Neuropsychiatric signs and symptoms consist of ataxia, chorea, strabismus, delirium, and dementia. Pathological changes are similar to those with other prion disease: neuronal loss, spongiform lesions, and astrocytic proliferation. The cerebellum is most affected. Iatrogenic transmission of kuru has occurred when cadaveric material such as dura mater and corneas were transplanted into normal recipients. Since the cessation of cannibalism in New Guinea, the incidence of the disease has decreased drastically.

GERSTMANN–STRAUSSLER–SCHEINKER DISEASE. First described in 1928, GSS is a neurodegenerative syndrome characterized by ataxia, chorea, and cognitive decline leading to dementia. It is caused by a mutation in the PrP gene that is fully penetrant and autosomal dominant; thus, the disease is inherited, and affected families have been identified over several generations. Genetic testing can confirm the presence of the abnormal genes before onset. Pathological changes characteristic of prion disease are present: spongiform lesions, neuronal loss, and astrocyte proliferation. Amyloid plaques have been found in the cerebellum. Onset of the disease occurs between 30 and 40 years of age. The disease is fatal within 5 years of onset.

FATAL FAMILIAL INSOMNIA. FFI is an inherited prion disease that primarily affects the thalamus. A syndrome of insomnia and autonomic nervous system dysfunction consisting of fever, sweating, labile blood pressure, and tachycardia occurs that is debilitating. Onset is in middle adulthood, and death usually occurs in 1 year. No treatment currently exists.

FUTURE DIRECTIONS. Determining how prions mutate to produce disease phenotypes and determining how they are transmitted between different mammalian species are major areas of research. Public health measures to prevent transmission of animal disease to humans are ongoing and must be relentless, especially because these disorders are invariably fatal within a few years of onset. Developing genetic interventions that prevent or repair damage to the normal prion gene offers the best hope of cure. Psychiatrists are faced with having to manage cases of persons who actually have the disease and those with hypochondriacal fears of having contracted the disease. In some patients, such fears can reach delusional proportions. Treatment is symptomatic and involves anxiolytics, antidepressants, and psychostimulants, depending on symptoms. Supportive psychotherapy may be of use in early stages to help patients and family cope with the illness.

Preventing unintentional human-to-human or animal-to-human transmission of prions remains the best way to limit the scope of these diseases. Sporadic cases of CJD will still appear, however, because of the rare spontaneous mutation of the normal prion protein into the abnormal form. At present, little exists to offer patients with prion disease other than supportive treatment and emotional support.

Immune Disorders

The major immune disorders in contemporary society is HIV and AIDS, but other immune disorders such as lupus erythematosus and autoimmune disorders that affect brain neurotransmitters (discussed below) can also present diagnostic and treatment challenges to mental health clinicians.

HIV Infection and AIDS

HIV is a retrovirus related to the human T cell leukemia viruses (HTLV) and to retroviruses that infect animals, including

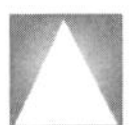

Table 17.5–4
AIDS Safe-Sex Guidelines

Remember: Any activity that allows for the exchange of body fluids of one person through the mouth, anus, vagina, bloodstream, cuts, or sores of another person is considered unsafe at this time.

Safe-sex practices
Massage, hugging, body-to-body rubbing
Dry social kissing
Masturbation
Acting out sexual fantasies (that do not include any unsafe-sex practices)
Using vibrators or other instruments (provided they are not shared)

Low-risk sex practices
These activities are not considered completely safe:
French (wet) kissing (without mouth sores)
Mutual masturbation
Vaginal and anal intercourse while using a condom
Oral sex, male (fellatio), while using a condom
Oral sex, female (cunnilingus), while using a barrier
External contact with semen or urine, provided there are no breaks in the skin

Unsafe-sex practices
Vaginal or anal intercourse without a condom
Semen, urine, or feces in the mouth or the vagina
Unprotected oral sex (fellatio or cunnilingus)
Blood contact of any kind
Sharing sex instruments or needles

AIDS, acquired immunodeficiency syndrome.
From Moffatt B, Spiegel J, Parrish S, Helquist M. *AIDS: A Self-Care Manual.* Santa Monica, CA: IBS Press; 1987:125.

nonhuman primates. At least two types of HIV have been identified, HIV-1 and HIV-2. HIV-1 is the causative agent for most HIV-related diseases; HIV-2, however seems to be causing an increasing number of infections in Africa. Other types of HIV may exist, which are now classified as HIV-O. HIV is present in blood; semen; cervical and vaginal secretions; and, to a lesser extent, in saliva, tears, breast milk, and the CSF of those who are infected. HIV is most often transmitted through sexual intercourse or the transfer of contaminated blood from one person to another. Health providers should be aware of the guidelines for safe sexual practices and should advise their patients to practice safe sex (Table 17.5–4). The Centers for Disease Control and Prevention guidelines for the prevention of HIV from infected to uninfected persons is listed in Table 17.5–5.

After infection with HIV, AIDS is estimated to develop in 8 to 11 years, although this time is gradually increasing because of early treatment. When a person is infected with HIV, the virus primarily targets T4 (helper) lymphocytes, so-called CD4+ lymphocytes, to which the virus binds because of a glycoprotein (gp120) on the viral surface has a high affinity for the CD4 receptor on T4 lymphocytes. After binding, the virus can inject its ribonucleic acid (RNA) into the infected lymphocyte, where the RNA is transcribed into deoxyribonucleic acid (DNA) by the action of reverse transcriptase. The resultant DNA can then be incorporated into the host cell's genome and translated and eventually transcribed when the lymphocyte is stimulated to divide. After viral proteins have been produced by lymphocytes, the various components of the virus assemble, and new mature viruses bud off from the host cell.

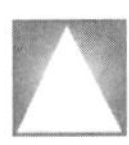

Table 17.5–5
Centers for Disease Control and Prevention Guidelines for the Prevention of HIV Transmission from Infected to Uninfected Persons

Infected persons should be counseled to prevent the further transmission of HIV by:

1. Informing prospective sex partners of their infection with HIV so they can take appropriate precautions. Abstention from sexual activity with another person is one option that would eliminate any risk of sexually transmitted HIV infection.
2. Protecting a partner during any sexual activity by taking appropriate precautions to prevent that person's coming into contact with the infected person's blood, semen, urine, feces, saliva, cervical secretions, or vaginal secretions. Although the efficacy of using condoms to prevent infections with HIV is still under study, the consistent use of condoms should reduce the transmission of HIV by preventing exposure to semen and infected lymphocytes.
3. Informing previous sex partners and any persons with whom needles were shared of their potential exposure to HIV and encouraging them to seek counseling and testing.
4. For IV drug abusers, enrolling or continuing in programs to eliminate the abuse of IV substances. Needles, other apparatus, and drugs must never be shared.
5. Never sharing toothbrushes, razors, or other items that could become contaminated with blood.
6. Refraining from donating blood, plasma, body organs, other tissue, or semen.
7. Avoiding pregnancy until more is known about the risks of transmitting HIV from the mother to the fetus or newborn.
8. Cleaning and disinfecting surfaces on which blood or other body fluids have spilled in accordance with previous recommendations.
9. Informing physicians, dentists, and other appropriate health professionals of antibody status when seeking medical care, so that the patient can be appropriately evaluated.

HIV, human immunodeficiency virus; IV, intravenous.
From Centers for Disease Control (CDC). Additional recommendations to reduce sexual and drug abuse-related transmission of human T-lymphotropic virus type III/lymphadenopathy-associated virus. *MMWR Morb Mortal Wkly Rep.* 1986;35:152.

Diagnosis

SERUM TESTING. Techniques are now widely available to detect the presence of anti-HIV antibodies in human. The conventional test uses blood (time to result, 3 to 10 days) and the rapid test uses an oral swab (time to result, 20 minutes). Both tests are 99.9 percent sensitive and specific. Health care workers and their patients must understand that the presence of HIV antibodies indicate infection, not immunity to infection. Those who test positive have been exposed to the virus, have the virus within their bodies, have the potential to transmit the virus to another person, and will almost certainly eventually develop AIDS. Those who test negative have either not been exposed to the HIV virus and are not infected or were exposed to the HIV virus but have not yet developed the antibodies, which is a possibility if the exposure occurred less than 1 year before testing. Seroconversion most commonly occurs 6 to 12 weeks after infection, although in rare cases seroconversion can take 6 to 12 months.

COUNSELING. Although specific groups of persons are at high risk for contracting HIV and should be tested, any person who wants to be tested should probably be tested. The reason for requesting a test should be ascertained to detect unspoken concerns and motivations that may merit psychotherapeutic intervention.

Past practices that may have put the testee at risk for HIV infection and safe sexual practices should be discussed. During posttest counseling, counselors should explain that a negative test finding implies that safe sexual behavior and the avoidance of shared hypodermic needles are recommended for the person to remain free of HIV infection. Those with positive results must receive counseling about safe practices and potential treatment options. They may need additional psychotherapeutic interventions if anxiety or depressive disorders develop after they discover that they are infected. A person may react to a positive HIV test finding with a syndrome similar to posttraumatic stress disorder. Adjustment disorder with anxiety or depressed mood may develop in as many as 25 percent of those informed of a positive HIV test result.

CONFIDENTIALITY. No one should be given an HIV test without previous knowledge and consent, although various jurisdictions and organizations, such as the military, now require HIV testing for all inhabitants or members. The results of an HIV test can be shared with other members of a medical team, although the information should be provided to no one else except for special circumstances. The patient should be advised against disclosing the result of HIV testing too readily to employers, friends, and family members; the information could result in discrimination in employment, housing, and insurance.

The major exception to restriction of disclosure is the need to notify potential and past sexual or IV substance use partners. If a treating physician knows that a patient who is HIV infected is putting another person at risk of becoming infected, the physician may try either to hospitalize the infected person involuntarily (to prevent danger to others) or to notify the potential victim. Clinicians should be aware of the laws about such issues, which vary among the states. These guidelines also apply to inpatient psychiatric wards when a patient with HIV infection is believed to be sexually active with other patients.

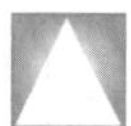

Table 17.5–6
Conditions Associated with Human Immunodeficiency Virus (HIV) Infection

Bacterial infections, multiple or recurrent[a]
Candidiasis of bronchi, trachea, or lungs
Candidiasis, esophageal
Cervical cancer, invasive[b]
Coccidioidomycosis, disseminated or extrapulmonary
Cryptococcosis, extrapulmonary
Cryptosporidiosis, chronic intestinal (>1 month's duration)
Cytomegalovirus disease (other than liver, spleen, or nodes)
Cytomegalovirus retinitis (with loss of vision)
Encephalopathy, HIV-related
Herpes simplex, chronic ulcers (>1 month's duration); or bronchitis, pulmonitis, or esophagitis
Histoplasmosis, disseminated or extrapulmonary
Isosporiasis, chronic intestinal (>1 month's duration)
Kaposi's sarcoma
Lymphoid interstitial pneumonia or pulmonary lymphoid hyperplasia[a]
Lymphoma, Burkitt's (or equivalent term)
Lymphoma, immunoblastic (or equivalent term)
Lymphoma, primary, of brain
Mycobacterium avium complex or *Mycobacterium kansasii,* disseminated or extrapulmonary
Mycobacterium tuberculosis, any site (pulmonary[b] or extrapulmonary)
Mycobacterium, other species or unidentified species, disseminated or extrapulmonary
Pneumocystis carinii pneumonia
Pneumonia, recurrent[b]
Progressive multifocal leukoencephalopathy
Salmonella septicemia, recurrent
Toxoplasmosis of brain
Wasting syndrome due to HIV

[a]Children younger than 13 years old.
[b]Added in the 1993 expansion of the AIDS surveillance case definition for adolescents and adults.
Adapted from 1993 revised classification system for HIV infection and expanded surveillance, case definition for AIDS among adolescents and adults. *MMWR Recomm Rep.* 1992:41.

Clinical Features

NONNEUROLOGICAL FACTORS. About 30 percent of persons infected with HIV experience a flulike syndrome 3 to 6 weeks after becoming infected; most never notice any symptoms immediately or shortly after their infection. The flulike syndrome includes fever, myalgia, headaches, fatigue, GI symptoms, and sometimes a rash. The syndrome may be accompanied by splenomegaly and lymphadenopathy.

The most common infection in persons affected with HIV who have AIDS is *Pneumocystis carinii* pneumonia, which is characterized by a chronic, nonproductive cough, and dyspnea, sometimes sufficiently severe to result in hypoxemia and its resultant cognitive effects. For psychiatrists, the importance of these nonneurological, nonpsychiatric complications lies in their biological effects on patients' brain function (e.g., hypoxia in *P. carinii* pneumonia) and their psychological effects on patients' moods and anxiety states.

NEUROLOGICAL FACTORS. An extensive array of disease processes can affect the brain of a patient infected with HIV (Table 17.5–6). The most important diseases for mental health workers to be aware of are *HIV mild neurocognitive disorder* and *HIV-associated dementia.*

PSYCHIATRIC SYNDROMES. HIV-associated dementia presents with the typical triad of symptoms seen in other subcortical dementias—memory and psychomotor speed impairments, depressive symptoms, and movement disorders. Patients may initially notice slight problems with reading, comprehension, memory, and mathematical skills, but these symptoms are subtle and may be overlooked or discounted as fatigue and illness. The Modified HIV Dementia Scale is a useful bedside screen and can be administered serially to document disease progression. The development of dementia in HIV-infected patients is generally a poor prognostic sign, and 50 to 75 percent of patients with dementia die within 6 months.

HIV-associated neurocognitive disorder (also known as HIV encephalopathy) is characterized by impaired cognitive functioning and reduced mental activity that interferes with work, domestic, and social functioning. No laboratory findings are specific to the disorder, and it occurs independently of depression and anxiety. Progression to HIV-associated dementia usually occurs but may be prevented by early treatment.

Delirium can result from the same causes that lead to dementia in patients with HIV. Clinicians have classified delirious states characterized by both increased and decreased activity. Delirium in patients infected with HIV is probably underdiagnosed, but it should always precipitate a medical workup of a patient infected with HIV to determine whether a new CNS-related process has begun.

Patients with HIV infection may have any of the anxiety disorders, but generalized anxiety disorder, posttraumatic stress disorder, and obsessive-compulsive disorder (OCD) are particularly common.

Adjustment disorder with anxiety or depressed mood has been reported in 5 to 20 percent of HIV-infected patients. The incidence of adjustment disorder in HIV-infected patients is higher than usual in some special populations, such as military recruits and prison inmates.

Depression is a significant problem in HIV and AIDS. Approximately 4 to 40 percent of HIV-infected patients meet the criteria for depressive disorders. Major depression is a risk factor for HIV infection by virtue of its impact on behavior, intensification of substance abuse, exacerbation of self-destructive behaviors, and promotion for poor partner choice in relationships. The pre-HIV infection prevalence of depressive disorders may be higher than usual in some groups who are at risk for contracting HIV. Depression has been shown to hinder effective treatment in infected persons. Patients with major depression are at increased risk for disease progression and death. HIV increases the risk of developing major depression through a variety of mechanisms, including direct injury to subcortical areas of the brain, chronic stress, worsening social isolation, and intense demoralization. Depression is higher in women than in men.

Mania can occur at any stage of HIV infection for individuals with preexisting bipolar disorder. AIDS mania is a type of mania that most commonly occurs in late-stage HIV infections and is associated with cognitive impairment. AIDS mania has a somewhat different clinical profile than bipolar mania. Patients tend to have cognitive slowing or dementia, and irritability is more characteristic than euphoria. AIDS mania is usually quite severe in its presentation and malignant in its course. It seems to be more chronic than episodic, has infrequent spontaneous remissions, and usually relapses with cessation of treatment. One clinically significant presentation is the delusional belief that one has discovered the cure for HIV or has been cured, which may result in high-risk behaviors and the spread of the HIV infection.

Substance abuse is a primary vector for the spread of HIV. This impact is directed not only at those who use IV drugs and their sexual partners but also at those who are disinhibited or cognitively impaired by intoxication and are driven by addiction to impulsive behaviors and unsafe sexual practices. Ongoing substance abuse has grave medical implications for HIV-infected patients. The accumulation of medical sequelae from chronic substance abuse can accelerate the process of immunocompromise and amplify the progressive burdens of the HIV infection itself. In addition to the direct physical effects cause by drugs, active substance use is highly associated with both nonadherence and reduced access to antiretroviral medication.

Suicidal ideation and suicide attempts may increase in patients with HIV infection and AIDS. The risk factors for suicide among persons infected with HIV are having friends who died from AIDS, recent notification of HIV seropositivity, relapses, difficult social issues relating to homosexuality, inadequate social and financial support, and the presence of dementia or delirium.

Psychotic symptoms are usually later-stage complications of HIV infection. They require immediate medical and neurological evaluation and often require management with antipsychotic medications.

The worried well are persons in high-risk groups who, although they tested negative and are disease free, are anxious about contracting the virus. Some are reassured by repeated negative test results, but others cannot be reassured. Their worried well-status can progress quickly to generalized anxiety disorder, panic attacks, illness anxiety disorder and OCD.

Treatment. Prevention is the primary approach to HIV infection. Primary prevention involves protecting persons from getting the disease; secondary prevention involves modification of the disease's course. All persons with any risk of HIV infection should be informed about safe-sex practices and about the necessity to avoid sharing contaminated hypodermic needles. The assessment of patients infected with HIV should include a complete sexual and substance-abuse history, a psychiatric history, and an evaluation of the support systems available to them.

PHARMACOTHERAPY. A growing list of agents that act at different points in viral replication has raised the hope that HIV might be permanently suppressed or actually eradicated from the body. These agents are divided into five major drug classes. Reverse transcriptase inhibitors (RTIs) interfere with the critical step during the HIV life cycle known as reverse transcription. There are two types of RTIs: nucleoside/nucleotide RTIs (NRTIs), which are faulty DNA building blocks, and non-nucleoside RTIs (NNRTIs), which bind to RT, interfering with its ability to convert the HIV RNA into HIV DNA. Protease inhibitors interfere with the protease enzyme that HIV uses to produce infectious viral particles. Fusion or entry inhibitors interfere with the virus' ability to fuse with the cellular membrane, thereby blocking entry into the host cell. Integrase inhibitors block integrase, the enzyme HIV uses to integrate genetic material of the virus into its target host cell. Multidrug combination products combine drugs from more than one class into a single product. The most common of this class of drugs is the highly active antiretroviral therapy (HAART). Table 17.5–7 lists the available agents in each of these categories.

The antiretroviral agents have many adverse effects. Of importance to psychiatrists is that protease inhibitors can increase levels of certain psychotropic drugs such as bupropion (Wellbutrin), meperidine (Demerol), various benzodiazepines, and selective serotonin reuptake inhibitors (SSRIs). Caution must be taken in prescribing psychotropic drugs to persons taking protease inhibitors.

PSYCHOTHERAPY. Major psychodynamic themes for patients infected with HIV involved self-blame, self-esteem, and issues regarding death. The entire range of psychotherapeutic approaches may be appropriate for patients with HIV-related disorders. Both individual and group therapy can be effective. Individual therapy may be either short term or long term and may be supportive, cognitive, behavioral, or psychodynamic. Group therapy techniques can range from psychodynamic to completely supportive in nature. Direct counseling regarding

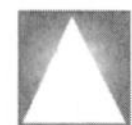

Table 17.5–7
Antiretroviral Agents

Generic Names	Trade Name	Usual Abbreviation
Reverse Transcriptase Inhibitors		
Nucleoside/nucleotide reverse transcriptase inhibitors		
Lamivudine and zidovudine	Combivir	
Emtricitabine	Emtriva	FTC
Lamivudine	Epivir	3TC
Abacavir and lamivudine	Epzicom	
Zidovudine, azidothymidine	Retrovir	ZDV or AZT
Abacavir, zidovudine, and lamivudine	Trizivir	
Tenofovir disoproxil fumarate and emtricitabine	Truvada	
Didanosine, dideoxyinosine	Videx	ddl
Enteric-coated didanosine	Videx EC	ddl EC
Tenofovir disoproxil fumarate	Viread	TDF
Stavudine	Zerit	d4t
Abacavir sulfate	Ziagen	ABC
Nonnucleoside Reverse Transcriptase Inhibitors		
Rilpivirine	Edurant	
Etravirine	Intelence	
Delavirdine	Rescriptor	DLV
Efavirenz	Sustiva	EFV
Nevirapine	Viramune	NVP
Protease Inhibitors		
Amprenavir	Agenerase	APV
Tipranavir	Aptivus	TPV
Indinavir	Crixivan	IDV
Saquinavir mesylate	Invirase	SQV
Lopinavir and ritonavir	Kaletra	LPV/RTV
Fosamprenavir calcium	Lexiva	FOS-APV
Ritonavir	Norvir	RTV
Darunavir	Prezista	
Atazanavir sulfate	Reyataz	ATV
Nelfinavir mesylate	Viracept	NFV
Fusion/Entry Inhibitors		
Enfuvirtide	Fuzeon	T-20
Maraviroc	Selzentry	
Multi-class Combination Products		
Efavirenz, emtricitabine, and tenofovir disoproxil fumarate	Atripla	
Emtricitabine, rilpivirine, and tenofovir disoproxil fumarate	Complera	

substance use and its potential adverse effects on health of the patient who is HIV infected is indicated. Specific treatments for particular substance-related disorders should be initiated if necessary for the total well-being of the patient.

Systemic Lupus Erythematosus. Systemic lupus erythematosus (SLE) is an autoimmune disease that involves inflammation of multiple organ systems. The officially accepted diagnosis of SLE requires a patient to have 4 of 11 criteria that have been defined by the American Rheumatism Association. Between 5 and 50 percent of patients with SLE have mental symptoms at the initial presentation, and approximately 50 percent eventually show neuropsychiatric manifestations. The major symptoms are depression, insomnia, emotional lability, nervousness, and confusion. Treatment with steroids commonly induces further psychiatric complications, including mania and psychosis.

Autoimmune Disorders Affecting Brain Neurotransmitters

A group of autoimmune receptor-seeking disorders have been identified that cause an encephalitis that mimics schizophrenia. Among those is anti-NMDA(N-methyl D-aspartate)-receptor encephalitis that causes dissociative symptoms, amnesia and vivid hallucinations. The disorder occurs mostly in women and was described in a memoir entitled *Brain on Fire.* There is no treatment although intravenous immunogloblins have proved useful. Recovery does occur but some patients might require prolonged intensive care. There is increasing interest in the role of the immune system not only in schizophrenia-like illnesses but also in mood and bipolar disorders.

Endocrine Disorders

Thyroid Disorders. Hyperthyroidism is characterized by confusion; anxiety; and an agitated, depressive syndrome. Patients may also complain of being easily fatigued and of feeling generally weak. Insomnia, weight loss despite increased appetite, tremulousness, palpitations, and increased perspiration are also common symptoms. Serious psychiatric symptoms include impairments in memory, orientation, and judgment; manic excitement; delusions; and hallucinations.

In 1949, Irvin Asher named hypothyroidism "myxedema madness." In its most severe form, hypothyroidism is characterized by paranoia, depression, hypomania, and hallucinations. Slowed thinking and delirium can also be symptoms. The physical symptoms include weight gain, a deep voice, thin and dry hair, loss of the lateral eyebrow, facial puffiness, cold intolerance, and impaired hearing. Approximately 10 percent of all patients have residual neuropsychiatric symptoms after hormone replacement therapy.

Parathyroid Disorders. Dysfunction of the parathyroid gland results in the abnormal regulation of calcium metabolism. Excessive secretion of parathyroid hormone causes hypercalcemia, which can result in delirium, personality changes, and apathy in 50 to 60 percent of patients and cognitive impairments in approximately 25 percent of patients. Neuromuscular excitability, which depends on proper calcium ion concentration, is reduced, and muscle weakness may appear.

Hypocalcemia can occur with hypoparathyroid disorders and can result in neuropsychiatric symptoms of delirium and personality changes. If the calcium level decreases gradually, clinicians may see the psychiatric symptoms without the characteristic tetany of hypocalcemia. Other symptoms of hypocalcemia are cataract formation, seizures, extrapyramidal symptoms, and increased intracranial pressure.

Adrenal Disorders. Adrenal disorders disturb the normal secretion of hormones from the adrenal cortex and produce significant neurological and psychological changes. Patients with chronic adrenocortical insufficiency (Addison's disease), which is most frequently the result of adrenocortical atrophy or granulomatous invasion caused by tuberculous or fungal infection, exhibit mild mental symptoms, such as apathy, easy fatigability, irritability, and depression. Occasionally, confusion or psychotic reactions develop. Cortisone or one of its synthetic derivatives is effective in correcting such abnormalities.

Excessive quantities of cortisol produced endogenously by an adrenocortical tumor or hyperplasia (Cushing's syndrome) lead to a secondary mood disorder, a syndrome of agitated depression, and often suicide. Decreased concentration and memory deficits may also be present. Psychotic reactions, with schizophrenia-like symptoms, are seen in a few patients. The administration of high doses of exogenous corticosteroids typically leads to a secondary mood disorder similar to mania. Severe depression can follow the termination of steroid therapy.

Pituitary Disorders. Patients with total pituitary failure can exhibit psychiatric symptoms, particularly postpartum women who have hemorrhaged into the pituitary, a condition known as *Sheehan's syndrome.* Patients have a combination of symptoms, especially of thyroid and adrenal disorders, and can show virtually any psychiatric symptom.

Metabolic Disorders

A common cause of organic brain dysfunction, metabolic encephalopathy can produce alterations in mental processes, behavior, and neurological functions. The diagnosis should be considered whenever recent and rapid changes in behavior, thinking, and consciousness have occurred. The earliest signals are likely to be impairment of memory, particularly recent memory, and impairment of orientation. Some patients become agitated, anxious, and hyperactive; others become quiet, withdrawn, and inactive. As metabolic encephalopathies progress, confusion or delirium gives way to decreased responsiveness; stupor; and, eventually, death.

Hepatic Encephalopathy. Severe hepatic failure can result in hepatic encephalopathy, characterized by asterixis, hyperventilation, EEG abnormalities, and alterations in consciousness. The alterations in consciousness can range from apathy to drowsiness to coma. Associated psychiatric symptoms are changes in memory, general intellectual skills, and personality.

Uremic Encephalopathy. Renal failure is associated with alterations in memory, orientation, and consciousness. Restlessness, crawling sensations on the limbs, muscle twitching, and persistent hiccups are associated symptoms. In young people with brief episodes of uremia, the neuropsychiatric symptoms tend to be reversible; in elderly people with long episodes of uremia, the neuropsychiatric symptoms can be irreversible.

Hypoglycemic Encephalopathy. Hypoglycemic encephalopathy can be caused either by excessive endogenous production of insulin or by excessive exogenous insulin administration. The premonitory symptoms, which do not occur in every patient, include nausea, sweating, tachycardia, and feelings of hunger, apprehension, and restlessness. As the disorder progresses, disorientation, confusion, and hallucinations, as well as other neurological and medical symptoms, can develop. Stupor and coma can occur, and a residual and persistent dementia can sometimes be a serious neuropsychiatric sequela of the disorder.

Diabetic Ketoacidosis. Diabetic ketoacidosis begins with feelings of weakness, easy fatigability, and listlessness and increasing polyuria and polydipsia. Headache and sometimes nausea and vomiting appear. Patients with diabetes mellitus have an increased likelihood of chronic dementia with general arteriosclerosis.

Acute Intermittent Porphyria. The porphyrias are disorders of heme biosynthesis that result in excessive accumulation of porphyrins. The triad of symptoms is acute, colicky abdominal pain; motor polyneuropathy; and psychosis. Acute intermittent porphyria is an autosomal dominant disorder that affects more women than men and has its onset between ages 20 and 50 years. The psychiatric symptoms include anxiety, insomnia, lability of mood, depression, and psychosis. Some studies have found that between 0.2 and 0.5 percent of chronic psychiatric patients may have undiagnosed porphyrias. Barbiturates precipitate or aggravate the attacks of acute porphyria, and the use of barbiturates for any reason is absolutely contraindicated in a person with acute intermittent porphyria and in anyone who has a relative with the disease.

Nutritional Disorders

Niacin Deficiency

Dietary insufficiency of niacin (nicotinic acid) and its precursor tryptophan is associated with pellagra, a globally occurring nutritional deficiency disease seen in association with alcohol abuse, vegetarian diets, and extreme poverty and starvation. The neuropsychiatric symptoms of pellagra include apathy, irritability, insomnia, depression, and delirium; the medical symptoms include dermatitis, peripheral neuropathies, and diarrhea. The course of pellagra has traditionally been described as "five Ds": dermatitis, diarrhea, delirium, dementia, and death. The response to treatment with nicotinic acid is rapid, but dementia from prolonged illness may improve only slowly and incompletely.

Thiamine Deficiency

Thiamine (vitamin B_1) deficiency leads to beriberi, characterized chiefly by cardiovascular and neurological changes, and to Wernicke–Korsakoff syndrome, which is most often associated with chronic alcohol abuse. Beriberi occurs primarily in Asia and in areas of famine and poverty. The psychiatric symptoms include apathy, depression, irritability, nervousness, and poor concentration; severe memory disorders can develop with prolonged deficiencies.

Cobalamin Deficiency

Deficiencies in cobalamin (vitamin B_{12}) arise because of the failure of the gastric mucosal cells to secrete a specific substance, intrinsic factor, required for the normal absorption of vitamin B_{12} in the ileum. The deficiency state is characterized by the development of a chronic macrocytic megaloblastic anemia (pernicious anemia) and by neurological manifestations resulting from degenerative changes in the peripheral nerves, the spinal cord, and the brain. Neurological changes are seen in approximately 80 percent of all patients. These changes are commonly associated with megaloblastic anemia, but they occasionally precede the onset of hematological abnormalities.

Mental changes, such as apathy, depression, irritability, and moodiness, are common. In a few patients, encephalopathy and its associated delirium, delusions, hallucinations, dementia, and sometimes paranoid features are prominent and are sometimes called *megaloblastic madness.* The neurological manifestations of vitamin B_{12} deficiency can be rapidly and completely arrested by early and continued administration of parenteral vitamin therapy.

Toxins

Environmental toxins are becoming an increasingly serious threat to physical and mental health in contemporary society.

Mercury

Mercury poisoning can be caused by either inorganic or organic mercury. Inorganic mercury poisoning results in the "mad hatter" syndrome (previously seen in workers in the hat industry who softened felt by putting it in their mouths), with depression, irritability, and psychosis. Associated neurological symptoms are headache, tremor, and weakness. Organic mercury poisoning can be caused by contaminated fish or grain and can result in depression, irritability, and cognitive impairment. Associated symptoms are sensory neuropathies, cerebellar ataxia, dysarthria, paresthesias, and visual field defects. Mercury poisoning in pregnant women causes abnormal fetal development. No specific therapy is available, although chelation therapy with dimercaprol has been used in acute poisoning.

Lead

Lead poisoning occurs when the amount of lead ingested exceeds the body's ability to eliminate it. It takes several months for toxic symptoms to appear.

The signs and symptoms of lead poisoning depend on the level of lead in the blood. When lead reaches levels above 200 mg/L, symptoms of severe lead encephalopathy occur, with dizziness, clumsiness, ataxia, irritability, restlessness, headache, and insomnia. Later, an excited delirium occurs, with associated vomiting and visual disturbances, and progresses to convulsions, lethargy, and coma.

Treatment of lead encephalopathy should be instituted as rapidly as possible, even without laboratory confirmation, because of the high mortality rate. The treatment of choice to facilitate lead excretion is intravenous administration of calcium disodium edetate (calcium disodium versenate) daily for 5 days.

Manganese

Early manganese poisoning (sometimes called *manganese madness*) causes symptoms of headache, irritability, joint pains, and somnolence. An eventual picture appears of emotional lability, pathological laughter, nightmares, hallucinations, and compulsive and impulsive acts associated with periods of confusion and aggressiveness. Lesions involving the basal ganglia and pyramidal system result in gait impairment, rigidity, monotonous or whispering speech, tremors of the extremities and tongue, masked facies (manganese mask), micrographia, dystonia, dysarthria, and loss of equilibrium. The psychological effects tend to clear 3 or 4 months after the patient's removal from the site of exposure, but neurological symptoms tend to remain stationary or to progress. No specific treatment exists for manganese poisoning, other than removal from the source of poisoning. The disorder is found in persons working in refining ore, brick workers, and those making steel casings.

Arsenic

Chronic arsenic poisoning most commonly results from prolonged exposure to herbicides containing arsenic or from drinking water contaminated with arsenic. Arsenic is also used in the manufacture of silicon-based computer chips. Early signs of toxicity are skin pigmentation, GI complaints, renal and hepatic dysfunction, hair loss, and a characteristic garlic odor to the breath. Encephalopathy eventually occurs, with generalized sensory and motor loss. Chelation therapy with dimercaprol has been used successfully to treat arsenic poisoning.

▲ 17.6 Mild Cognitive Impairment

The past decade has seen the emergence of a new concept, *mild cognitive impairment* (MCI), which is defined as the presence of mild cognitive decline not warranting the diagnosis of dementia but with preserved basic activities of daily living.

In the DSM-5, MCI is classified as *mild neurocognitive disorder due to multiple etiologies or unspecified neurocognitive disorder.* It will most likely receive more attention in future revisions of the DSM.

DEFINITION

Although the term *mild cognitive impairment* has been in use for more than 25 years, it was suggested as a diagnostic category designed to fill the gap between cognitive changes associated with aging and cognitive impairment suggestive of dementia. The criteria proposed by the Mayo Clinic Alzheimer's Disease Research Center (MCADRC) are (1) memory complaint, preferably qualified by an informant; (2) objective memory impairment for age and education; (3) preserved general cognitive function; (4) intact activities of daily living; and (5) not demented (Table 17.6–1). However, at this time there are no international diagnostic criteria for MCI.

Historical Perspective

The imprecise border between normal aging-related cognitive decline and dementia-related cognitive impairment has been described for several decades. Thus, in 1962, Kral introduced the terms *benign senescent forgetfulness* (forgetfulness for less important facts and awareness of problems) and *malignant senescent forgetfulness* (memory problems for recent events and lack of awareness). In 1986, the National Institutes of Mental Health (NIMH) recommended the term *age associated memory impairment* for age-related normal memory changes. In 1994, the International Psychogeriatrics Association presented the concept of *age-associated cognitive decline,* which described cognitive deficits including but not limited to memory impairment in the absence of dementia or other affecting cognitive conditions. *Cognitive impairment no dementia* was introduced in 1997 by the Canadian Study of Health and Aging to describe the presence of nondemented cognitive impairment regardless of the underlying process (neurological, psychiatric, medical). Several other classifications, including age-consistent memory impairment and late-life forgetfulness, are defined on the bases of performance on various cognitive tests.

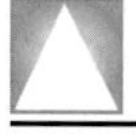

Table 17.6–1
Mild Cognitive Impairment Original Criteria

1. Memory complaint, preferably qualified by an informant
2. Memory impairment for age and education
3. Preserved general cognitive function
4. Intact activities of daily living
5. Not demented

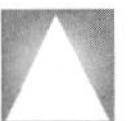

Table 17.6–2
Terms Related to Mild Cognitive Impairment

Term	Author(s)	Year	Inclusion Criteria	Observations
Malignant senescent forgetfulness (MSF)	VA Kral	1962	Memory difficulties for recent events Lack of awareness regarding the memory deficit	Two-year follow-up showed a faster evolution of patients with MSF toward dementia
Age associated memory impairment (AAMI)	NIMH (Crook, Bartus, and Ferris)	1986	Age-related memory disturbances leading to (1) subjective concern; (2) functional problem No underlying neurological illness	Memory tests were validated on young populations, leading to high rates of AAMI in elderly adults
Age-associated cognitive decline (AACD)	International Psychogeriatric Association and World Health Organization (Levy)	1994	Cognitive deficits not meeting the criteria for dementia	Does not include prognosis regarding evolution to dementia Includes several kinds of cognitive decline (not exclusive memory decline)
Cognitively impaired no dementia (CIND)	Canadian Study of Health and Aging	1997	Age 65 years and older	Includes static encephalopathies

The exact place of MCI in the psychiatric nosology will be challenging. Based on the current definition of MCI, functional impairment is an exclusion criterion for MCI, but the same "functional impairment" is one of the standard criteria for defining psychiatric disorders. Further developments in finding biological markers for MCI will probably contribute to a more solid conceptualization and, hopefully, treatment of patients with prodromal dementia (Table 17.6–2).

EPIDEMIOLOGY AND ETIOLOGY OF MCI

The recognition that Alzheimer's disease pathology may exist in the brain long before the presence of clinical symptoms led to the focus on preclinical stages, with the purpose of characterizing initial impairments that are associated with an increased risk of progression to Alzheimer's disease.

The clinical expression of MCI can be viewed as a result of the interaction among several risk factors and several protective factors. The most significant risk factors are related to the different types of neurodegeneration witnessed in dementias. These are clinically expressed in different subtypes of MCI, especially those associated with amnesia. Other risk factors include the APOE4 allele status and cerebrovascular events in the form of either cerebrovascular accident or lacunar disease. The role of chronic exposure to high levels of cortisol, as seen in late-life depression, is also hypothesized to increase the risk for cognitive impairment through hippocampal volume reduction. The notion of "brain reserve" suggests that effects of brain size and neuron density may be protective against dementia despite the presence of neurodegeneration (a larger number of neurons and a bigger brain volume would protect against clinical manifestations of Alzheimer's disease despite the presence of neurodegeneration).

CLINICAL PRESENTATION

The clinical picture of MCI is a function of the criteria used to define it. Memory impairment is necessary but has been difficult to quantify. One measure has been objective loss of memory or other cognitive domain that is more than 1.5 standard deviations below the mean for individuals of similar age and education. Some have suggested subjective complaints of memory loss be used as a marker, but this runs the risk of many false-positive diagnoses.

Assessment

Neuropsychological Assessment. Most experts agree that earlier deficits are noted in episodic (vs. semantic) memory. There is no consensus among experts with regard to which memory tests and which cutoffs to use. There is a lack of norms, test scores do not have normal distributions, and test performance is influenced by multiple demographic characteristics. Several experts have proposed that a scale such as the delayed recall task from the Consortium to Establish a Registry for Alzheimer's Disease might be useful in detecting Alzheimer's disease in the earliest stages. Brief mental status instruments (e.g., the mini–mental state examination) are relatively insensitive for the detection of memory problems in MCI.

Biomarkers. Several markers of progression from MCI to Alzheimer's disease have been studied in the past decade. Among these, apolipoprotein E4 (ApoE4) allele carrier status has been one of the most prominent variables. For the amnestic MCI, ApoE4 has been shown to be a risk factor for a more rapid progression to Alzheimer's disease. Several CSF markers have also been identified as possible predictors of disease progression: Pathological low concentrations of $A\beta_{42}$ (the 42 amino acid form of β-amyloid) as well as pathological high concentrations of total tau (t-tau) and phospho tau (p-tau) may differentiate early Alzheimer's disease from normal aging. Locating alterations in the expression of proteins involved in the pathogenetic pathways of Alzheimer's disease (proteomic approach) is another approach used to help early detection of Alzheimer's disease. Several proteins (cystatin C, β-2 microglobulin, and BEGF polypeptides) have been detected through new techniques, and currently there are a number of proteins from both CSF and blood that are implicated in Alzheimer's disease pathology.

Genetics. Because MCI is regarded as the prodromal stage for several disorders (Alzheimer's disease, frontotemporal or vascular dementia), different genes are probably related to MCI. Four genes have been described in relationship with Alzheimer's disease: the amyloid precursor protein (*APP*) gene, presenilin-1 (*PSEN1*), presenilin-2 (*PSEN2*), and the apolipoprotein E (*APOE*) gene. Because the first three genes are involved in rare autosomal dominant forms of Alzheimer's disease, screening for each of these mutations will have very limited value for the diagnosis of MCI in the general population. The *APOE* gene, a common genetic risk factor for early as well as for late-onset Alzheimer's disease, has been studied more thoroughly in relationship to MCI, but the results have been inconsistent. Because the etiology of MCI is heterogenous, it is likely that a very large number of different genes underlie the pathology of MCI. Most of these genes are yet to be discovered.

Neuroimaging. Advances in neuroimaging studies aim to develop measures allowing the differentiation between MCI and healthy aging as well as within MCI among subjects who will convert to Alzheimer's disease or will remain stable over time.

Structural studies of volumetric MCI showed early changes in the medial temporal structures, including neuronal atrophy, decreased synaptic density, and overall neuronal loss. Atrophy of the hippocampal volume and entorhinal cortex has been described in MCI. Atrophy of the hippocampal formation was also reported to predict the rate of progression from MCI to Alzheimer's disease. Three-dimensional modeling techniques have localized shape alteration and specific regions of atrophy within the hippocampus. Other methods such as tensor-based morphometry allow tracking brain changes in detail, quantifying tissue growth or atrophy throughout the brain, and indicating the local rate at which tissue is being lost. Other innovations in neuroimaging include MR relaxometry, imaging of iron deposition, diffusion tensor imaging, and high-field MRI scanning.

Perhaps the most promising development has been the advent of PET tracer compounds that visualize amyloid plaques and neurofibrillary tangles. These new compounds—Pittsburgh Compound B (carbon-11-PIB) and fluorine-18-FDDNP—track pathology changes in the preclinical stages of Alzheimer's disease. These specific tracers allow investigators to visualize the pathological process and are also used to monitor progression from MCI to Alzheimer's disease. However, the burden of β-amyloid plaques does not always correlate with the clinical stages because some MCI subjects can present with minimal burden similar to healthy control participants, but others have amyloid burden comparable to Alzheimer's disease participants. A single biomarker will probably be insufficient to identify incipient Alzheimer's disease. Thus, the combination of several markers further increases the accuracy of the prediction and will probably become the norm as described by recent studies (combination of decreased parietal rCBF and CSF biomarkers as Aβ42, t-tau, and p-tau).

Diagnostic Differential: The Cognitive Continuum

The cognitive continuum describes the subtle pathway from age-related cognitive decline to MCI to dementia. Per this model, there is an overlap at both ends of MCI, which indicates that it can be quite challenging to identify the transition points. In practice, differentiating MCI from age-related cognitive decline resides mainly on neuropsychological testing, showing a cognitive decline more severe for age and less education. The main differentiation between MCI and Alzheimer's disease resides in the lack of functional impairment in MCI.

COURSE AND PROGNOSIS

The typical rate at which MCI patients progress to Alzheimer's disease is 10 to 15 percent per year and is associated with progressive loss of function. However, several studies have indicated that the diagnosis is not stable in both directions; patients can either convert to Alzheimer's disease or revert back to normal. This variability in course is related to the heterogeneous source of the subjects (clinical vs. community) as well as to the heterogeneous definition criteria used by different studies. Amnestic MCI has been associated with increased morbidity compared with reference subjects.

TREATMENT

There are no FDA-approved treatments for MCI at this time. MCI treatment involves adequate screening and diagnosis. Ideally, MCI treatment would also include improvement of memory loss together with prevention of further cognitive decline to dementia. Cognitive training programs have been reported as mildly beneficial for compensating memory difficulties in MCI. Controlling for vascular risk factors (high blood pressure, hypercholesterolemia, and diabetes mellitus) may be a beneficial preventive method for those MCI cases underlying vascular pathology. Currently, sensitive tools (imaging techniques or biomarkers) are not available for MCI screening in the general population.

In primary care setting, clinicians should maintain a high suspicion for subjective cognitive complaints and should corroborate these complaints with collateral information whenever possible. Also, identifying reversible causes of cognitive impairment (hypothyroidism, vitamin B_{12} deficiency, medication-induced cognitive impairment, depression) can further benefit some of the prodromal dementia MCI cases.

Currently, there is no evidence for long-term efficacy of pharmacotherapies in reversing MCI. Several epidemiological studies indicated a reduced risk of dementia in persons taking antihypertensive medications, cholesterol-lowering drugs, antioxidants, and anti-inflammatory and estrogen therapy, but no randomized controlled trials verify these data. With regard to cognitive enhancers, as of 2007, there have been seven trials designed for amnestic MCI, with ambiguous results (Table 17.6–3). Most of these studies were confronted with several problems, including (1) obtaining homogeneous samples and identifying potential beneficiaries of treatment; (2) treating a wider population, which led to large percentages of negative responses and problematic side effects; and (3) translation of the

Table 17.6–3
Treatment Trials for Mild Cognitive Impairment

Study	Patients (n)	Duration	Primary Outcome	Results	OBS	Sponsor
Donepezil + vitamin E (Thall et al., 1999)	769	3 years	Conversion to AD	Partially positive (reduced risk of developing AD in the active arm group for the first 12 months)	Amnestic MCI status and the presence of APOE4 allele–predictive of rate of progression to AD	ADCS
Donepezil (Salloway et al., 2004)	269	24 weeks	ADAS-Cog total score; NYUPTIR	Negative	Positive results in secondary outcome measures (ADAS-Cog13)	Pfizer (The Donepezil "401" Study Group)
Rivastigmine (Feldman et al., 2007)	1,018	48 months	Conversion to AD	Negative		Novartis
Galantamine (Johnson and Johnson, 2004)	2,048	2 years	Progression of CDR score (from 0.5 to 1)	Negative	Attention assessed by DSST favored galantamine in both studies	Johnson & Johnson
Rofecoxib (Thall et al., 2005)	1,457	3–4 years	Conversion to AD	Negative	Primary outcome favored placebo while secondary outcomes (ADS-cog, CDR) did not differentiate between rofecoxib and placebo	Merck
Piracetam	675	12 months	Composite score extracted from eight tests	Negative		UCB Pharma

AD, Alzheimer's disease; ADCS, Alzheimer Disease Cooperative Study; CDR, Clinical Dementia Rating; DSST, Digit Symbol Substitution test; MCI, mild cognitive impairment; MCI, mild cognitive impairment; NYU PTIR, New York University Paragraph Test Immediate Recall.

MCI construct into multiple cultures and languages and using Alzheimer's disease diagnosis as the primary outcome, given the variability of this diagnosis in different countries.

Advances in MCI detection will be paramount for early detection and treatment of patients with Alzheimer's disease; experts agree that disease-modifying treatments for Alzheimer's disease will focus on cognitively intact individuals at increased risk. The field of identifying sensitive and specific biomarkers (biological and neuroimaging markers) will probably witness exponential development in the coming years.

18 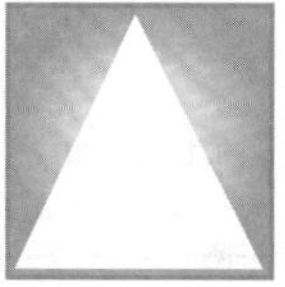

Personality Disorders

INTRODUCTION

The understanding of personality and its disorders distinguishes psychiatry fundamentally from all other branches of medicine. A person is a self-aware human being, as C. Robert Cloninger said, not "a machine-like object that lacks self-awareness." Personality refers to all of the characteristics that adapt in unique ways to ever-changing internal and external environments.

Personality disorders are common and chronic. They occur in 10 to 20 percent of the general population, and their duration is expressed in decades. Approximately 50 percent of all psychiatric patients have a personality disorder, which is frequently comorbid with other clinical syndromes. Personality disorder is also a predisposing factor for other psychiatric disorders (e.g., substance use, suicide, affective disorders, impulse-control disorders, eating disorders, and anxiety disorders) in which it interferes with treatment outcomes of many clinical syndromes and increases personal incapacitation, morbidity, and mortality of these patients.

Persons with personality disorders are far more likely to refuse psychiatric help and to deny their problems than persons with anxiety disorders, depressive disorders, or obsessive-compulsive disorder. In general, personality disorder symptoms are ego syntonic (i.e., acceptable to the ego, as opposed to ego dystonic) and alloplastic (i.e., adapt by trying to alter the external environment rather than themselves). Persons with personality disorders do not feel anxiety about their maladaptive behavior. Because they do not routinely acknowledge pain from what others perceive as their symptoms, they often seem disinterested in treatment and impervious to recovery.

CLASSIFICATION

The fifth edition of the *Diagnostic and Statistical Manual of Mental Disorders* (DSM-5) defines a general personality disorder as an enduring pattern of behavior and inner experiences that deviates significantly from the individual's cultural standards; is rigidly pervasive; has an onset in adolescence or early adulthood; is stable through time; leads to unhappiness and impairment; and manifests in at least two of the following four areas: cognition, affectivity, interpersonal function, or impulse control. When personality traits are rigid and maladaptive and produce functional impairment or subjective distress, a personality disorder may be diagnosed.

Personality disorder subtypes classified in DSM-5 are *schizotypal, schizoid,* and *paranoid* (Cluster A); *narcissistic, borderline, antisocial,* and *histrionic* (Cluster B); and *obsessive-compulsive, dependent,* and *avoidant* (Cluster C). The three clusters are based on descriptive similarities. Cluster A includes three personality disorders with odd, aloof features (paranoid, schizoid, and schizotypal). Cluster B includes four personality disorders with dramatic, impulsive, and erratic features (borderline, antisocial, narcissistic, and histrionic). Cluster C includes three personality disorders sharing anxious and fearful features (avoidant, dependent, and obsessive-compulsive). Individuals frequently exhibit traits that are not limited to a single personality disorder. When a patient meets the criteria for more than one personality disorder, clinicians should diagnose each.

ETIOLOGY

Genetic Factors

The best evidence that genetic factors contribute to personality disorders comes from investigations of more than 15,000 pairs of twins in the United States. The concordance for personality disorders among monozygotic twins was several times that among dizygotic twins. Moreover, according to one study, monozygotic twins reared apart are about as similar as monozygotic twins reared together. Similarities include multiple measures of personality and temperament, occupational and leisure-time interests, and social attitudes.

Cluster A personality disorders are more common in the biological relatives of patients with schizophrenia than in control groups. More relatives with schizotypal personality disorder occur in the family histories of persons with schizophrenia than in control groups. Less correlation exists between paranoid or schizoid personality disorder and schizophrenia.

Cluster B personality disorders apparently have a genetic base. Antisocial personality disorder is associated with alcohol use disorders. Depression is common in the family backgrounds of patients with borderline personality disorder. These patients have more relatives with mood disorders than do control groups, and persons with borderline personality disorder often have a mood disorder as well. A strong association is found between histrionic personality disorder and somatization disorder (Briquet's syndrome); patients with each disorder show an overlap of symptoms.

Cluster C personality disorders may also have a genetic base. Patients with avoidant personality disorder often have high anxiety levels. Obsessive-compulsive traits are more common in monozygotic twins than in dizygotic twins, and patients with obsessive-compulsive personality disorder show some signs associated with depression—for example, shortened rapid eye movement (REM) latency period, and abnormal dexamethasone-suppression test (DST) results.

Biological Factors

Hormones. Persons who exhibit impulsive traits also often show high levels of testosterone, 17-estradiol, and estrone. In nonhuman primates, androgens increase the likelihood of aggression and sexual behavior, but the role of testosterone in human aggression is unclear. DST results are abnormal in some patients with borderline personality disorder who also have depressive symptoms.

Platelet Monoamine Oxidase. Low platelet monoamine oxidase (MAO) levels have been associated with activity and sociability in monkeys. College students with low platelet MAO levels report spending more time in social activities than students with high platelet MAO levels. Low platelet MAO levels have also been noted in some patients with schizotypal disorders.

Smooth Pursuit Eye Movements. Smooth pursuit eye movements are saccadic (i.e., jumpy) in persons who are introverted, who have low self-esteem and tend to withdraw, and who have schizotypal personality disorder. These findings have no clinical application, but they do indicate the role of inheritance.

Neurotransmitters. Endorphins have effects similar to those of exogenous morphine, such as analgesia and the suppression of arousal. High endogenous endorphin levels may be associated with persons who are phlegmatic. Studies of personality traits and the dopaminergic and serotonergic systems indicate an arousal-activating function for these neurotransmitters. Levels of 5-hydroxyindoleacetic acid (5-HIAA), a metabolite of serotonin, are low in persons who attempt suicide and in patients who are impulsive and aggressive.

Raising serotonin levels with serotonergic agents such as fluoxetine (Prozac) can produce dramatic changes in some character traits of personality. In many persons, serotonin reduces depression, impulsiveness, and rumination and can produce a sense of general well-being. Increased dopamine concentrations in the central nervous system produced by certain psychostimulants (e.g., amphetamines) can induce euphoria. The effects of neurotransmitters on personality traits have generated much interest and controversy about whether personality traits are inborn or acquired.

Electrophysiology. Changes in electrical conductance on the electroencephalogram (EEG) occur in some patients with personality disorders, most commonly antisocial and borderline types; these changes appear as slow-wave activity on EEGs.

Psychoanalytic Factors

Sigmund Freud suggested that personality traits are related to a fixation at one psychosexual stage of development. For example, those with an oral character are passive and dependent because they are fixated at the oral stage, when the dependence on others for food is prominent. Those with an anal character are stubborn, parsimonious, and highly conscientious because of struggles over toilet training during the anal period.

Wilhelm Reich subsequently coined the term *character armor* to describe persons' characteristic defensive styles for protecting themselves from internal impulses and from interpersonal anxiety in significant relationships. Reich's theory has had a broad influence on contemporary concepts of personality and personality disorders. For example, each human being's unique stamp of personality is considered largely determined by his or her characteristic defense mechanisms. Each personality disorder has a cluster of defenses that help psychodynamic clinicians recognize the type of character pathology present. Persons with paranoid personality disorder, for instance, use projection, whereas schizoid personality disorder is associated with withdrawal.

When defenses work effectively, persons with personality disorders master feelings of anxiety, depression, anger, shame, guilt, and other affects. Their behavior is ego syntonic; that is, it creates no distress for them even though it may adversely affect others. They may also be reluctant to engage in a treatment process; because their defenses are important in controlling unpleasant affects, they are not interested in surrendering them.

In addition to characteristic defenses in personality disorders, another central feature is internal object relations. During development, particular patterns of the self in relation to others are internalized. Through introjection, children internalize a parent or another significant person as an internal presence that continues to feel like an object rather than a self. Through identification, children internalize parents and others in such a way that the traits of the external object are incorporated into the self and the child "owns" the traits. These internal self-representations and object representations are crucial in developing the personality and, through externalization and projective identification, are played out in interpersonal scenarios in which others are coerced into playing a role in the person's internal life. Hence, persons with personality disorders are also identified by particular patterns of interpersonal relatedness that stem from these internal object relations patterns.

Defense Mechanisms. To help those with personality disorders, psychiatrists must appreciate patients' underlying defenses, the unconscious mental processes that the ego uses to resolve conflicts among the four lodestars of the inner life: instinct (wish or need), reality, important persons, and conscience. When defenses are most effective, especially in those with personality disorders, they can abolish anxiety and depression at the conscious level. Thus, abandoning a defense increases conscious awareness of anxiety and depression—a major reason that those with personality disorders are reluctant to alter their behavior.

Although patients with personality disorders may be characterized by their most dominant or rigid mechanism, each patient uses several defenses. Therefore, the management of defense mechanisms used by patients with personality disorders is discussed here as a general topic and not as an aspect of the specific disorders. Many formulations presented here in the language of psychoanalytic psychiatry can be translated into principles consistent with cognitive and behavioral approaches.

FANTASY. Many persons who are often labeled schizoid—those who are eccentric, lonely, or frightened—seek solace and satisfaction within themselves by creating imaginary lives, especially imaginary friends. In their extensive dependence on fantasy, these persons often seem to be strikingly aloof. Therapists must understand that the unsociableness of these patients rests on a fear of intimacy. Rather than criticizing them or feeling rebuffed by their rejection, therapists should maintain a quiet, reassuring, and considerate interest without insisting on reciprocal responses. Recognition of patients' fear of closeness and respect for their eccentric ways are both therapeutic and useful.

DISSOCIATION. Dissociation or denial is a Pollyanna-like replacement of unpleasant affects with pleasant ones. Persons who frequently dissociate are often seen as dramatizing and emotionally shallow; they may be labeled histrionic personalities. They behave like anxious adolescents who, to erase anxiety, carelessly expose themselves to exciting dangers. Accepting such patients as exuberant and seductive is to overlook their anxiety, but confronting them with their vulnerabilities and defects makes them still more defensive. Because these patients seek appreciation of their courage and attractiveness, therapists should not behave with inordinate reserve. While remaining calm and firm, clinicians should realize that these patients are often inadvertent liars, but they benefit from ventilating their own anxieties and may in the process "remember" what they "forgot." Often therapists deal best with dissociation and denial by using displacement. Thus, clinicians may talk with patients about an issue of denial in an unthreatening circumstance. Empathizing with the denied affect without directly confronting patients with the facts may allow them to raise the original topic themselves.

ISOLATION. Isolation is characteristic of controlled, orderly persons who are often labeled obsessive-compulsive personalities. Unlike those with histrionic personality, persons with obsessive-compulsive personality remember the truth in fine detail but without affect. In a crisis, patients may show intensified self-restraint, overly formal social behavior, and obstinacy. Patients' quests for control may annoy clinicians or make them anxious. Often, such patients respond well to precise, systematic, and rational explanations and value efficiency, cleanliness, and punctuality as much as they do clinicians' effective responsiveness. Whenever possible, therapists should allow such patients to control their own care and should not engage in a battle of wills.

PROJECTION. In projection, patients attribute their own unacknowledged feelings to others. Patients' excessive faultfinding and sensitivity to criticism may appear to therapists as prejudiced, hypervigilant injustice collecting but should not be met by defensiveness and argument. Instead, clinicians should frankly acknowledge even minor mistakes on their part and should discuss the possibility of future difficulties. Strict honesty; concern for patients' rights; and maintaining the same formal, concerned distance as used with patients who use fantasy defenses are all helpful. Confrontation guarantees a lasting enemy and early termination of the interview. Therapists need not agree with patients' injustice collecting, but they should ask whether both can agree to disagree.

The technique of counter projection is especially helpful. Clinicians acknowledge and give paranoid patients full credit for their feelings and perceptions; they neither dispute patients' complaints nor reinforce them but agree that the world described by patients is conceivable. Interviewers can then talk about real motives and feelings, misattributed to someone else, and begin to cement an alliance with patients.

SPLITTING. In splitting, persons toward whom patients' feelings are, or have been, ambivalent are divided into good and bad. For example, in an inpatient setting, a patient may idealize some staff members and uniformly disparage others. This defense behavior can be highly disruptive on a hospital ward and can ultimately provoke the staff to turn against the patient. When staff members anticipate the process, discuss it at staff meetings, and gently confront the patient with the fact that no one is all good or all bad, the phenomenon of splitting can be dealt with effectively.

PASSIVE AGGRESSION. Persons with passive-aggressive defense turn their anger against themselves. In psychoanalytic terms, this phenomenon is called *masochism* and includes failure, procrastination, silly or provocative behavior, self-demeaning clowning, and frankly self-destructive acts. The hostility in such behavior is never entirely concealed. Indeed, in a mechanism such as wrist cutting, others feel as much anger as if they themselves had been assaulted and view the patient as a sadist, not a masochist. Therapists can best deal with passive aggression by helping patients to ventilate their anger.

ACTING OUT. In acting out, patients directly express unconscious wishes or conflicts through action to avoid being conscious of either the accompanying idea or the affect. Tantrums, apparently motiveless assaults, child abuse, and pleasureless promiscuity are common examples. Because the behavior occurs outside reflective awareness, acting out often appears to observers to be unaccompanied by guilt, but when acting out is impossible, the conflict behind the defense may be accessible. The clinician faced with acting out, either aggressive or sexual, in an interview situation must recognize that the patient has lost control, that anything the interviewer says will probably be misheard, and that getting the patient's attention is of paramount importance. Depending on the circumstances, a clinician's response may be, "How can I help you if you keep screaming?" Or, if the patient's loss of control seems to be escalating, say, "If you continue screaming, I'll leave." An interviewer who feels genuinely frightened of the patient can simply leave and, if necessary, ask for help from ward attendants or the police.

PROJECTIVE IDENTIFICATION. The defense mechanism of projective identification appears mainly in borderline personality disorder and consists of three steps. First, an aspect of the self is projected onto someone else. The projector then tries to coerce the other person into identifying with what has been projected. Finally, the recipient of the projection and the projector feel a sense of oneness or union.

PARANOID PERSONALITY DISORDER

Persons with paranoid personality disorder are characterized by long-standing suspiciousness and mistrust of persons in general. They refuse responsibility for their own feelings and assign responsibility to others. They are often hostile, irritable, and angry. Bigots, injustice collectors, pathologically jealous spouses, and litigious cranks often have paranoid personality disorder.

Epidemiology

Data suggest that the prevalence of paranoid personality disorder is 2 to 4 percent of the general population. Those with the disorder rarely seek treatment themselves; when referred to treatment by a spouse or an employer, they can often pull themselves together and appear undistressed. Relatives of patients with schizophrenia show a higher incidence of paranoid personality disorder than control participants. Some evidence suggest a more specific familial relationship with delusional disorder, persecutory type. The disorder is more commonly diagnosed in men than in women in clinical samples. The prevalence among persons who are homosexual is no higher than usual, as was once thought, but it is believed to be higher among minority groups, immigrants, and persons who are deaf than it is in the general population.

Diagnosis

On psychiatric examination, patients with paranoid personality disorder may be formal in manner and act baffled about having to seek psychiatric help. Muscular tension, an inability to relax, and a need to scan the environment for clues may be evident, and the patient's manner is often humorless and serious. Although some premises of their arguments may be false, their speech is goal directed and logical. Their thought content shows evidence of projection, prejudice, and occasional ideas of reference.

Clinical Features

The hallmarks of paranoid personality disorder are excessive suspiciousness and distrust of others expressed as a pervasive tendency to interpret actions of others as deliberately demeaning, malevolent, threatening, exploiting, or deceiving. This tendency begins by early adulthood and appears in a variety of contexts. Almost invariably, those with the disorder expect to be exploited or harmed by others in some way. They frequently dispute, without any justification, friends' or associates' loyalty or trustworthiness. Such persons are often pathologically jealous and, for no reason, question the fidelity of their spouses or sexual partners. Persons with this disorder externalize their own emotions and use the defense of projection; they attribute to others the impulses and thoughts that they cannot accept in themselves. Ideas of reference and logically defended illusions are common.

Persons with paranoid personality disorder are affectively restricted and appear to be unemotional. They pride themselves on being rational and objective, but such is not the case. They lack warmth and are impressed with, and pay close attention to, power and rank. They express disdain for those they see as weak, sickly, impaired, or in some way defective. In social situations, persons with paranoid personality disorder may appear business-like and efficient, but they often generate fear or conflict in others.

Differential Diagnosis

Paranoid personality disorder can usually be differentiated from delusional disorder by the absence of fixed delusions. Unlike persons with paranoid schizophrenia, those with personality disorders have no hallucinations or formal thought disorder. Paranoid personality disorder can be distinguished from borderline personality disorder because patients who are paranoid are rarely capable of overly involved in tumultuous relationships with others. Patients with paranoia lack the long history of antisocial behavior of persons with antisocial character. Persons with schizoid personality disorder are withdrawn and aloof and do not have paranoid ideation.

Course and Prognosis

No adequate, systematic long-term studies of paranoid personality disorder have been conducted. In some, paranoid personality disorder is lifelong; in others, it is a harbinger of schizophrenia. In still others, paranoid traits give way to reaction formation, appropriate concern with morality, and altruistic concerns as they mature or as stress diminishes. In general, however, those with paranoid personality disorder have lifelong problems working and living with others. Occupational and marital problems are common.

Treatment

Psychotherapy. Psychotherapy is the treatment of choice for those with paranoid personality disorder. Therapists should be straightforward in all their dealings with these patients. If a therapist is accused of inconsistency or a fault, such as lateness for an appointment, honesty and an apology are preferable to a defensive explanation. Therapists must remember that trust and toleration of intimacy are troubled areas for patients with this disorder. Individual psychotherapy thus requires a professional and not overly warm style from therapists. Clinicians' overzealous use of interpretation—especially interpretation about deep feelings of dependence, sexual concerns, and wishes for intimacy—increases patients' mistrust significantly. Patients who are paranoid usually do not do well in group psychotherapy, although it can be useful for improving social skills and diminishing suspiciousness through role playing. Many cannot tolerate the intrusiveness of behavior therapy, also used for social skills training.

At times, patients with paranoid personality disorder behave so threateningly that therapists must control or set limits on their actions. Delusional accusations must be dealt with realistically but gently and without humiliating patients. Patients who are paranoid are profoundly frightened when they feel that those trying to help them are weak and helpless; therefore, therapists should never offer to take control unless they are willing and able to do so.

Pharmacotherapy. Pharmacotherapy is useful in dealing with agitation and anxiety. In most cases, an antianxiety agent such as diazepam (Valium) suffices. It may be necessary, however, to use an antipsychotic such as haloperidol (Haldol) in small dosages and for brief periods to manage severe agitation or quasi-delusional thinking. The antipsychotic drug pimozide (Orap) has successfully reduced paranoid ideation in some patients.

SCHIZOID PERSONALITY DISORDER

Schizoid personality disorder is characterized by a lifelong pattern of social withdrawal. Persons with schizoid personality disorder are often seen by others as eccentric, isolated, or lonely. Their discomfort with human interaction; their introversion; and their bland, constricted affect are noteworthy.

Epidemiology

The prevalence of schizoid personality disorder is not clearly established, but the disorder may affect 5 percent of the general population. The sex ratio of the disorder is unknown; some studies report a 2-to-1 male-to-female ratio. Persons with the disorder tend to gravitate toward solitary jobs that involve little or no contact with others. Many prefer night work to day work so that they need not deal with many persons.

Diagnosis

On an initial psychiatric examination, patients with schizoid personality disorder may appear ill at ease. They rarely tolerate eye contact, and interviewers may surmise that such patients are eager for the interview to end. Their affect may be constricted, aloof, or inappropriately serious, but underneath the aloofness, sensitive clinicians can recognize fear. These patients find it difficult to be lighthearted: Their efforts at humor may seem adolescent and off the mark. Their speech is goal directed, but they are likely to give short answers to questions and to avoid spontaneous conversation. They may occasionally use unusual figures of speech, such as an odd metaphor, and may be fascinated with inanimate objects or metaphysical constructs. Their mental content may reveal an unwarranted sense of intimacy with persons they do not know well or whom they have not seen for a long time. Their sensorium is intact, their memory functions well, and their proverb interpretations are abstract.

Clinical Features

Persons with schizoid personality disorder seem to be cold and aloof; they display a remote reserve and show no involvement with everyday events and the concerns of others. They appear quiet, distant, seclusive, and unsociable. They may pursue their own lives with remarkably little need or longing for emotional ties, and they are the last to be aware of changes in popular fashion.

The life histories of such persons reflect solitary interests and success at noncompetitive, lonely jobs that others find difficult to tolerate. Their sexual lives may exist exclusively in fantasy, and they may postpone mature sexuality indefinitely. Men may not marry because they are unable to achieve intimacy; women may passively agree to marry an aggressive man who wants the marriage. Persons with schizoid personality disorder usually reveal a lifelong inability to express anger directly. They can invest enormous affective energy in nonhuman interests, such as mathematics and astronomy, and they may be very attached to animals. Dietary and health fads, philosophical movements, and social improvement schemes, especially those that require no personal involvement, often engross them.

Although persons with schizoid personality disorder appear self-absorbed and lost in daydreams, they have a normal capacity to recognize reality. Because aggressive acts are rarely included in their repertoire of usual responses, most threats, real or imagined, are dealt with fantasized omnipotence or resignation. They are often seen as aloof, yet such persons can sometimes conceive, develop, and give to the world genuinely original, creative ideas.

Differential Diagnosis

Schizoid personality disorder is distinguished from schizophrenia, delusional disorder, and affective disorder with psychotic features based on periods with positive psychotic symptoms, such as delusions and hallucinations in the latter. Although patients with paranoid personality disorder share many traits with those with schizoid personality disorder, the former exhibit more social engagement, a history of aggressive verbal behavior, and a greater tendency to project their feelings onto others. If just as emotionally constricted, patients with obsessive-compulsive and avoidant personality disorders experience loneliness as dysphoric, possess a richer history of past object relations, and do not engage as much in autistic reverie. Theoretically, the chief distinction between a patient with schizotypal personality disorder and one with schizoid personality disorder is that the patient who is schizotypal is more similar to a patient with schizophrenia in oddities of perception, thought, behavior, and communication. Patients with avoidant personality disorder are isolated but strongly wish to participate in activities, a characteristic absent in those with schizoid personality disorder. Schizoid personality disorder is distinguished from autistic disorder and Asperger's syndrome by more severely impaired social interactions and stereotypical behaviors and interests than in those two disorders.

Course and Prognosis

The onset of schizoid personality disorder usually occurs in early childhood or adolescence. As with all personality disorders, schizoid personality disorder is long lasting but not necessarily lifelong. The proportion of patients who incur schizophrenia is unknown.

Treatment

Psychotherapy. The treatment of patients with schizoid personality disorder is similar to that of those with paranoid personality disorder. Patients who are schizoid tend toward introspection; however, these tendencies are consistent with psychotherapists' expectations, and such patients may become devoted, if distant, patients. As trust develops, patients who are schizoid may, with great trepidation, reveal a plethora of fantasies, imaginary friends, and fears of unbearable dependence—even of merging with the therapist.

In group therapy settings, patients with schizoid personality disorder may be silent for long periods; nonetheless, they do become involved. The patients should be protected against aggressive attack by group members for their proclivity to be silent. With time, the group members become important to patients who are schizoid and may provide the only social contact in their otherwise isolated existence.

Pharmacotherapy. Pharmacotherapy with small dosages of antipsychotics, antidepressants, and psychostimulants has benefitted some patients. Serotonergic agents may make patients less sensitive to rejection. Benzodiazepines may help diminish interpersonal anxiety.

SCHIZOTYPAL PERSONALITY DISORDER

Persons with schizotypal personality disorder are strikingly odd or strange, even to laypersons. Magical thinking, peculiar notions, ideas of reference, illusions, and derealization are part of a schizotypal person's everyday world.

Epidemiology

Schizotypal personality disorder occurs in about 3 percent of the population. The sex ratio is unknown; however, it is frequently diagnosed in females with fragile X syndrome. DSM-5 suggests the disorder may be slightly more common in males. A greater association of cases exists among the biological relatives of patients with schizophrenia than among control participants and a higher incidence among monozygotic twins than among dizygotic twins (33 percent vs. 4 percent in one study).

Etiology

Adoption, family, and twin studies demonstrate an increased prevalence of schizotypal features in the families of schizophrenic patients, especially when schizotypal features were not associated with comorbid affective symptoms.

Diagnosis

Schizotypal personality disorder is diagnosed on the basis of the patients' peculiarities of thinking, behavior, and appearance. Taking a history may be difficult because of the patients' unusual way of communicating.

Clinical Features

Patients with schizotypal personality disorder exhibit disturbed thinking and communicating. Although frank thought disorder is absent, their speech may be distinctive or peculiar, may have meaning only to them, and often needs interpretation. As with patients with schizophrenia, those with schizotypal personality disorder may not know their own feelings and yet are exquisitely sensitive to, and aware of, the feelings of others, especially negative affects such as anger. These patients may be superstitious or claim powers of clairvoyance and may believe that they have other special powers of thought and insight. Their inner world may be filled with vivid imaginary relationships and child-like fears and fantasies. They may admit to perceptual illusions or macropsia and confess that other persons seem wooden and all the same.

Because persons with schizotypal personality disorder have poor interpersonal relationships and may act inappropriately, they are isolated and have few, if any, friends. Patients may show features of borderline personality disorder, and indeed, both diagnoses can be made. Under stress, patients with schizotypal personality disorder may decompensate and have psychotic symptoms, but these are usually brief. Patients with severe cases of the disorder may exhibit anhedonia and severe depression.

Differential Diagnosis

Theoretically, persons with schizotypal personality disorder can be distinguished from those with schizoid and avoidant personality disorders by the presence of oddities in their behavior, thinking, perception, and communication and perhaps by a clear family history of schizophrenia. Patients with schizotypal personality disorder can be distinguished from those with schizophrenia by their absence of psychosis. If psychotic symptoms do appear, they are brief and fragmentary. Some patients meet the criteria for both schizotypal personality disorder and borderline personality disorder. Patients with paranoid personality disorder are characterized by suspiciousness but lack the odd behavior of patients with schizotypal personality disorder.

Course and Prognosis

According to current clinical thinking, the schizotype is the premorbid personality of the patient with schizophrenia. Some, however, maintain a stable schizotypal personality throughout their lives and marry and work, despite their oddities. A long-term study by Thomas McGlashan reported that 10 percent of those with schizotypal personality disorder eventually committed suicide.

Treatment

Psychotherapy. The principles of treatment of schizotypal personality disorder do not differ from those of schizoid personality disorder, but clinicians must deal sensitively with the former. These patients have peculiar patterns of thinking, and some are involved in cults, strange religious practices, and the occult. Therapists must not ridicule such activities or be judgmental about these beliefs or activities.

Pharmacotherapy. Antipsychotic medication may be useful in dealing with ideas of reference, illusions, and other symptoms of the disorder and can be used in conjunction with psychotherapy. Antidepressants are useful when a depressive component of the personality is present.

ANTISOCIAL PERSONALITY DISORDER

Antisocial personality disorder is an inability to conform to the social norms that ordinarily govern many aspects of a person's adolescent and adult behavior. Although characterized by continual antisocial or criminal acts, the disorder is not synonymous with criminality.

Epidemiology

The 12-month prevalence rates of antisocial personality disorder are between 0.2 and 3 percent according to DSM-5. It is more common in poor urban areas and among mobile residents of these areas. The highest prevalence of antisocial personality disorder is found among the most severe samples of men with alcohol use disorder (over 70 percent) and in prison populations, where the prevalence may be as high as 75 percent. It is much more common in males than in females. Boys with the disorder come from larger families than girls with the disorder. The onset of the disorder is before the age of 15 years. Girls usually have symptoms before puberty and boys even earlier. A familial pattern is present; the disorder is five times more common among first-degree relatives of men with the disorder than among control participants.

Diagnosis

Patients with antisocial personality disorder can fool even the most experienced clinicians. In an interview, patients can appear composed and credible, but beneath the veneer (or, to use Hervey Cleckley's term, *the mask of sanity*) lurks tension, hostility, irritability, and rage. A stress interview, in which patients are vigorously confronted with inconsistencies in their histories, may be necessary to reveal the pathology.

A diagnostic workup should include a thorough neurological examination. Because patients often show abnormal EEG results and soft neurological signs suggesting minimal brain damage in childhood, these findings can be used to confirm the clinical impression.

Clinical Features

Patients with antisocial personality disorder can often seem to be normal and even charming and ingratiating. Their histories, however, reveal many areas of disordered life functioning. Lying, truancy, running away from home, thefts, fights, substance abuse, and illegal activities are typical experiences that patients report as beginning in childhood. These patients often impress opposite-sex clinicians with the colorful, seductive aspects of their personalities, but same-sex clinicians may regard them as manipulative and demanding. Patients with antisocial personality disorder exhibit no anxiety or depression, a lack that may seem grossly incongruous with their situations, although suicide threats and somatic preoccupations may be common. Their own explanations of their antisocial behavior make it seem mindless, but their mental content reveals the complete absence of delusions and other signs of irrational thinking. In fact, they frequently have a heightened sense of reality testing and often impress observers as having good verbal intelligence.

Persons with antisocial personality disorder are highly representative of so-called con men. They are extremely manipulative and can frequently talk to others into participating in schemes for easy ways to make money or to achieve fame or notoriety. These schemes may eventually lead the unwary to financial ruin or social embarrassment or both. Those with this disorder do not tell the truth and cannot be trusted to carry out any task or adhere to any conventional standard of morality. Promiscuity, spousal abuse, child abuse, and drunk driving are common events in their lives. A notable finding is a lack of remorse for these actions; that is, they appear to lack a conscience.

Differential Diagnosis

Antisocial personality disorder can be distinguished from illegal behavior in that antisocial personality disorder involves many areas of a person's life. When illegal behavior is only for gain and is not accompanied by the rigid, maladaptive, and persistent personality traits characteristic of a personality disorder, it is classified as criminal behavior not associated with a personality disorder according to DSM-5.

Dorothy Lewis found that many of these persons have a neurological or mental disorder that has been either overlooked or undiagnosed. More difficult is the differentiation of antisocial personality disorder from substance abuse. When both substance abuse and antisocial behavior begin in childhood and continue into adult life, both disorders should be diagnosed. When, however, the antisocial behavior is clearly secondary to premorbid alcohol abuse or other substance abuse, the diagnosis of antisocial personality disorder is not warranted.

In diagnosing antisocial personality disorder, clinicians must adjust for the distorting effects of socioeconomic status, cultural background, and sex. Furthermore, the diagnosis of antisocial personality disorder is not warranted when intellectual disability, schizophrenia, or mania can explain the symptoms.

Course and Prognosis

When an antisocial personality disorder develops, it runs an unremitting course, with the height of antisocial behavior usually occurring in late adolescence. The prognosis varies. Some reports indicate that symptoms decrease as persons grow older. Many patients have somatization disorder and multiple physical complaints. Depressive disorders, alcohol use disorders, and other substance abuse are common.

Treatment

Psychotherapy. If patients with antisocial personality disorder are immobilized (e.g., placed in hospitals), they often become amenable to psychotherapy. When patients feel that they are among peers, their lack of motivation for change disappears. Perhaps for this reason, self-help groups have been more useful than jails in alleviating the disorder.

Before treatment can begin, firm limits are essential. Therapists must find ways of dealing with patients' self-destructive behavior. And to overcome patients' fear of intimacy, therapists must frustrate patients' desire to run from honest human encounters. In doing so, therapists face the challenge of separating control from punishment and of separating help and confrontation from social isolation and retribution.

Pharmacotherapy. Pharmacotherapy is used to deal with incapacitating symptoms such as anxiety, rage, and depression, but because patients are often substance abusers, drugs must be used judiciously. If a patient shows evidence of attention-deficit/hyperactivity disorder, psychostimulants such as methylphenidate (Ritalin) may be useful. Attempts have been made to alter catecholamine metabolism with drugs and to control impulsive behavior with antiepileptic drugs, for example, carbamazepine (Tegretol) or valproate (Depakote), especially if abnormal waveforms are noted on an EEG. β-Adrenergic receptor antagonists have been used to reduce aggression.

BORDERLINE PERSONALITY DISORDER

Patients with borderline personality disorder stand on the border between neurosis and psychosis, and they are characterized by extraordinarily unstable affect, mood, behavior, object relations, and self-image. The disorder has also been called *ambulatory schizophrenia, as-if personality* (a term coined by Helene Deutsch), *pseudoneurotic schizophrenia* (described by Paul Hoch and Phillip Politan), and *psychotic character disorder* (described by John Frosch). The 10th revision of the *International Classification of Diseases* 10 (ICD-10) uses the term *emotionally unstable personality disorder* instead of borderline personality disorder.

Table 18–1
Signs and Symptoms of Borderline Personality

Fear of being abandoned
Suicidal ideation or attempts
Self-mutilating or cutting behavior
Impulsivity
Unaware of consequences of actions
Low frustration tolerance
Outburst of anger or violence
Unstable or labile mood
Chaotic sexual behavior, pansexuality
Disturbances in body image
Feelings of emptiness, isolation
Intense and unstable relationships
Lack of clear self-identity
Pan-neuroses: anxiety, depression, depersonalization, phobia
Ambivalence in thought, feeling and relationships

Epidemiology

No definitive prevalence studies are available, but borderline personality disorder is thought to be present in about 1 to 2 percent of the population and is twice as common in women as in men. An increased prevalence of major depressive disorder, alcohol use disorders, and substance abuse is found in first-degree relatives of persons with borderline personality disorder.

Diagnosis

According to DSM-5, the diagnosis of borderline personality disorder is characterized primarily by unstable relationships, poor self-esteem, severe impulsivity, and labile mood. In addition, there are myriad signs and symptoms present in patients with this disorder. While not all of them occur in every case, the clinician will find a majority of them present (Table 18–1). Biological studies may aid in the diagnosis; some patients with borderline personality disorder show shortened REM latency and sleep continuity disturbances, abnormal DST results, and abnormal thyrotropin-releasing hormone test results. Those changes, however, are also seen in some patients with depressive disorders. Generally, the diagnosis is made on the basis of the clinical examination.

Clinical Features

Persons with borderline personality disorder almost always appear to be in a state of crisis. Mood swings are common. Patients can be argumentative at one moment, depressed the next, and later complain of having no feelings. Patients can have short-lived psychotic episodes (so-called *micropsychotic episodes*) rather than full-blown psychotic breaks, and the psychotic symptoms of these patients are almost always circumscribed, fleeting, or doubtful. The behavior of patients with borderline personality disorder is highly unpredictable, and their achievements are rarely at the level of their abilities. The painful nature of their lives is reflected in repetitive self-destructive acts. Such patients may slash their wrists and perform other self-mutilations to elicit help from others, to express anger, or to numb themselves to overwhelming affect.

Because they feel both dependent and hostile, persons with this disorder have tumultuous interpersonal relationships. They can be dependent on those with whom they are close and, when frustrated, can express enormous anger toward their intimate friends. Patients with borderline personality disorder cannot tolerate being alone, and they prefer a frantic search for companionship, no matter how unsatisfactory, to their own company. To assuage loneliness, if only for brief periods, they accept a stranger as a friend or behave promiscuously. They often complain about chronic feelings of emptiness and boredom and the lack of a consistent sense of identity (identity diffusion); when pressed, they often complain about how depressed they usually feel, despite the flurry of other affects.

Otto Kernberg described the defense mechanism of projective identification that occurs in patients with borderline personality disorder. In this primitive defense mechanism, intolerable aspects of the self are projected onto another; the other person is induced to play the projected role, and the two persons act in unison. Therapists must be aware of this process so they can act neutrally toward such patients.

Most therapists agree that these patients show ordinary reasoning abilities on structured tests, such as the Wechsler Adult Intelligence Scale, and show deviant processes only on unstructured projective tests, such as the Rorschach test.

Functionally, patients with borderline personality disorder distort their relationships by considering each person to be either all good or all bad. They see persons as either nurturing attachment figures or as hateful, sadistic figures who deprive them of security needs and threaten them with abandonment whenever they feel dependent. As a result of this splitting, the good person is idealized and the bad person devalued. Shifts of allegiance from one person or group to another are frequent. Some clinicians use the concepts of panphobia, pananxiety, panambivalence, and chaotic sexuality to delineate these patients' characteristics.

Differential Diagnosis

The disorder is differentiated from schizophrenia on the basis that the patient with borderline personality lacks prolonged psychotic episodes, thought disorder, and other classic schizophrenic signs. Patients with schizotypal personality disorder show marked peculiarities of thinking, strange ideation, and recurrent ideas of reference. Those with paranoid personality disorder are marked by extreme suspiciousness. Patients with borderline personality disorder generally have chronic feelings of emptiness and short-lived psychotic episodes; they act impulsively and demand extraordinary relationships; they may mutilate themselves and make manipulative suicide attempts.

Course and Prognosis

Borderline personality disorder is fairly stable; patients change little over time. Longitudinal studies show no progression toward schizophrenia, but patients have a high incidence of major depressive disorder episodes. The diagnosis is usually made before the age of 40 years, when patients are attempting to make occupational, marital, and other choices and are unable to deal with the normal stages of the life cycle.

Treatment

Psychotherapy. Psychotherapy for patients with borderline personality disorder is an area of intensive investigation and has been the treatment of choice. For best results, pharmacotherapy has been added to the treatment regimen.

Psychotherapy is difficult for the patient and therapist alike. Patients regress easily, act out their impulses, and show labile or fixed negative or positive transferences, which are difficult to analyze. Projective identification may also cause countertransference problems when therapists are unaware that patients are unconsciously trying to coerce them to act out a particular behavior. The splitting defense mechanism causes patients to alternately love and hate therapists and others in the environment. A reality-oriented approach is more effective than in-depth interpretations of the unconscious.

Therapists have used behavior therapy to control patients' impulses and angry outbursts and to reduce their sensitivity to criticism and rejection. Social skills training, especially with videotape playback, helps enable patients to see how their actions affect others and thereby improve their interpersonal behavior.

Patients with borderline personality disorder often do well in a hospital setting in which they receive intensive psychotherapy on both an individual and a group basis. In a hospital, they can also interact with trained staff members from a variety of disciplines and can be provided with occupational, recreational, and vocational therapy. Such programs are especially helpful when the home environment is detrimental to a patient's rehabilitation because of intrafamilial conflicts or other stresses, such as parental abuse. Within the protected environment of the hospital, patients who are excessively impulsive, self-destructive, or self-mutilating can be given limits, and their actions can be observed. Under ideal circumstances, patients remain in the hospital until they show marked improvement, up to 1 year in some cases. Patients can then be discharged to special support systems, such as day hospitals, night hospitals, and halfway houses.

DIALECTICAL BEHAVIOR THERAPY. A particular form of psychotherapy called dialectical behavior therapy (DBT) has been used for patients with borderline personality disorder, especially those with parasuicidal behavior, such as frequent cutting. For further discussion of DBT, see Section 24.5.

MENTALIZATION-BASED TREATMENT. Another type of psychotherapy for borderline personality disorder is called mentalization-based therapy (MBT). Mentalization is a social construct that allows a person to be attentive to the mental states of oneself and of others; it comes from a person's awareness of mental processes and subjective states that arise in interpersonal interactions. MBT is based on a theory that borderline personality symptoms, such as difficulty regulating emotions and managing impulsivity, are a result of patients' reduced capacities to mentalize. Thus, it is believed that recovery of mentalization helps patients build relationship skills as they learn to better regulate their thoughts and feelings. MBT was found to be effective for borderline personality disorder in several randomized, controlled research trials.

TRANSFERENCE-FOCUSED PSYCHOTHERAPY. Transference-focused psychotherapy (TFP) is a modified form of psychodynamic psychotherapy used for the treatment of borderline personality disorder that is based on Otto Kernberg's object relations theory. The therapist relies on two major processes in working with the patient: The first is clarification, in which the transference is analyzed more directly than in traditional psychotherapy so that the patient becomes quickly aware his or her distortions about the therapist. The second is confrontation, whereby the therapist points out how these transferential distortions interfere with interpersonal relations toward others (objects). The mechanism of splitting used by borderline patients is characterized by their having a good object and a bad object and is used as a defense against anxiety. If therapy is successful, then the need for splitting diminishes, object relations are improved, and a more normal level of functioning is achieved. Studies comparing TFP, DBT, psychodynamic psychotherapy, and supportive psychotherapy show that all are useful and all show varying degrees of success. As yet, no consensus has been reached as to which, if any, of these is superior to the others.

Pharmacotherapy. Pharmacotherapy is useful to deal with specific personality features that interfere with patients' overall functioning. Antipsychotics have been used to control anger, hostility, and brief psychotic episodes. Antidepressants improve the depressed mood common in patients with borderline personality disorder. The MAO inhibitors (MAOIs) have successfully modulated impulsive behavior in some patients. Benzodiazepines, particularly alprazolam (Xanax), help anxiety and depression, but some patients show a disinhibition with this class of drugs. Anticonvulsants, such as carbamazepine, may improve global functioning for some patients. Serotonergic agents such as selective serotonin reuptake inhibitors (SSRIs) have been helpful in some cases.

HISTRIONIC PERSONALITY DISORDER

Persons with histrionic personality disorder are excitable and emotional and behave in a colorful, dramatic, extroverted fashion. Accompanying their flamboyant aspects, however, is often an inability to maintain deep, long-lasting attachments.

Epidemiology

Limited data from general population studies suggest a prevalence of histrionic personality disorder of about 1 to 3 percent. Rates of about 10 to 15 percent have been reported in inpatient and outpatient mental health settings when structured assessment is used. The disorder is diagnosed more frequently in women than in men. Some studies have found an association with somatization disorder and alcohol use disorders.

Diagnosis

In interviews, patients with histrionic personality disorder are generally cooperative and eager to give a detailed history. Gestures and dramatic punctuation in their conversations are common; they may make frequent slips of the tongue, and their language is colorful. Affective display is common, but when pressed to acknowledge certain feelings (e.g., anger, sadness, and sexual wishes), they may respond with surprise, indignation, or denial. The results of the cognitive examination are usually normal, although a lack of perseverance may be shown on arithmetic or concentration tasks, and the patients' forgetfulness of affect-laden material may be astonishing.

Clinical Features

Persons with histrionic personality disorder show a high degree of attention-seeking behavior. They tend to exaggerate their thoughts and feelings and make everything sound more important than it really is. They display temper tantrums, tears, and accusations when they are not the center of attention or are not receiving praise or approval.

Seductive behavior is common in both sexes. Sexual fantasies about persons with whom patients are involved are common, but patients are inconsistent about verbalizing these fantasies and may be coy or flirtatious rather than sexually aggressive. In fact, histrionic patients may have a psychosexual dysfunction; women may be anorgasmic, and men may be impotent. Their need for reassurance is endless. They may act on their sexual impulses to reassure themselves that they are attractive to the other sex. Their relationships tend to be superficial, however, and they can be vain, self-absorbed, and fickle. Their strong dependence needs make them overly trusting and gullible.

The major defenses of patients with histrionic personality disorder are repression and dissociation. Accordingly, such patients are unaware of their true feelings and cannot explain their motivations. Under stress, reality testing easily becomes impaired.

Differential Diagnosis

Distinguishing between histrionic personality disorder and borderline personality disorder is difficult, but in borderline personality disorder, suicide attempts, identity diffusion, and brief psychotic episodes are more likely. Although both conditions may be diagnosed in the same patient, clinicians should separate the two. Somatization disorder (Briquet's syndrome) may occur in conjunction with histrionic personality disorder. Patients with brief psychotic disorder and dissociative disorders may warrant a coexisting diagnosis of histrionic personality disorder.

Course and Prognosis

With age, persons with histrionic personality disorder show fewer symptoms, but because they lack the energy of earlier years, the difference in number of symptoms may be more apparent than real. Persons with this disorder are sensation seekers, and they may get into trouble with the law, abuse substances, and act promiscuously.

Treatment

Psychotherapy. Patients with histrionic personality disorder are often unaware of their own real feelings; clarification of their inner feelings is an important therapeutic process. Psychoanalytically oriented psychotherapy, whether group or individual, is probably the treatment of choice for histrionic personality disorder.

Pharmacotherapy. Pharmacotherapy can be adjunctive when symptoms are targeted (e.g., the use of antidepressants for depression and somatic complaints, antianxiety agents for anxiety, and antipsychotics for derealization and illusions).

NARCISSISTIC PERSONALITY DISORDER

Persons with narcissistic personality disorder are characterized by a heightened sense of self-importance, lack of empathy, and grandiose feelings of uniqueness. Underneath, however, their self-esteem is fragile and vulnerable to even minor criticism.

Epidemiology

According to DSM-5, estimates of the prevalence of narcissistic personality disorder range from less than 1 to 6 percent in community samples. Persons with the disorder may impart an unrealistic sense of omnipotence, grandiosity, beauty, and talent to their children; thus, offspring of such parents may have a higher than usual risk for developing the disorder themselves.

Diagnosis and Clinical Features

Persons with narcissistic personality disorder have a grandiose sense of self-importance; they consider themselves special and expect special treatment. Their sense of entitlement is striking. They handle criticism poorly and may become enraged when someone dares to criticize them, or they may appear completely indifferent to criticism. Persons with this disorder want their own way and are frequently ambitious to achieve fame and fortune. Their relationships are tenuous, and they can make others furious by their refusal to obey conventional rules of behavior. Interpersonal exploitiveness is commonplace. They cannot show empathy, and they feign sympathy only to achieve their own selfish ends. Because of their fragile self-esteem, they are susceptible to depression. Interpersonal difficulties, occupational problems, rejection, and loss are among the stresses that narcissists commonly produce by their behavior—stresses they are least able to handle.

Differential Diagnosis

Borderline, histrionic, and antisocial personality disorders often accompany narcissistic personality disorder, so a differential diagnosis is difficult. Patients with narcissistic personality disorder have less anxiety than those with borderline personality disorder; their lives tend to be less chaotic, and they are less likely to attempt suicide. Patients with antisocial personality disorder have a history of impulsive behavior, often associated with alcohol or other substance abuse, which frequently gets them into trouble with the law. Patients with histrionic personality disorder show features of exhibitionism and interpersonal manipulativeness that resemble those of patients with narcissistic personality disorder.

Course and Prognosis

Narcissistic personality disorder is chronic and difficult to treat. Patients with the disorder must constantly deal with blows to their narcissism resulting from their own behavior or from life experience. Aging is handled poorly; patients value beauty, strength, and youthful attributes, to which they cling inappropriately. They may be more vulnerable, therefore, to midlife crises than are other groups.

Treatment

Psychotherapy. Because patients must renounce their narcissism to make progress, the treatment of narcissistic personality disorder is difficult. Psychiatrists such as Kernberg and Heinz Kohut have advocated using psychoanalytic approaches to effect change, but much research is required to validate the diagnosis and to determine the best treatment. Some clinicians advocate group therapy for their patients so they can learn how to share with others and, under ideal circumstances, can develop an empathic response to others.

Pharmacotherapy. Lithium (Eskalith) has been used with patients whose clinical picture includes mood swings. Because patients with narcissistic personality disorder tolerate rejection poorly and are susceptible to depression, antidepressants, especially serotonergic drugs, may also be of use.

AVOIDANT PERSONALITY DISORDER

Persons with avoidant personality disorder show extreme sensitivity to rejection and may lead socially withdrawn lives. Although shy, they are not asocial and show a great desire for companionship, but they need unusually strong guarantees of uncritical acceptance. Such persons are commonly described as having an inferiority complex.

Epidemiology

The prevalence of the disorder is suggested to be about 2 to 3 percent of the general population according to DSM-5. No information is available on sex ratio or familial pattern. Infants classified as having a timid temperament may be more susceptible to the disorder than those who score high on activity-approach scales.

Diagnosis and Clinical Features

In clinical interviews, patients' most striking aspect is anxiety about talking with an interviewer. Their nervous and tense manner appears to wax and wane with their perception of whether an interviewer likes them. They seem vulnerable to the interviewer's comments and suggestions and may regard a clarification or interpretation as criticism.

Hypersensitivity to rejection by others is the central clinical feature of avoidant personality disorder, and patients' main personality trait is timidity. These persons desire the warmth and security of human companionship but justify their avoidance of relationships by their alleged fear of rejection. When talking with someone, they express uncertainty, show a lack of self-confidence, and may speak in a self-effacing manner. Because they are hypervigilant about rejection, they are afraid to speak up in public or to make requests of others. They are apt to misinterpret other persons' comments as derogatory or ridiculing. The refusal of any request leads them to withdraw from others and to feel hurt.

In the vocational sphere, patients with avoidant personality disorder often take jobs on the sidelines. They rarely attain much personal advancement or exercise much authority but seem shy and eager to please. These persons are generally unwilling to enter relationships unless they are given an unusually strong guarantee of uncritical acceptance. Consequently, they often have no close friends or confidants.

Differential Diagnosis

Patients with avoidant personality disorder desire social interaction, unlike patients with schizoid personality disorder, who want to be alone. Patients with avoidant personality disorder are not as demanding, irritable, or unpredictable as those with borderline and histrionic personality disorders. Avoidant personality disorder and dependent personality disorder are similar. Patients with dependent personality disorder are presumed to have a greater fear of being abandoned or unloved than those with avoidant personality disorder, but the clinical picture may be indistinguishable.

Course and Prognosis

Many persons with avoidant personality disorder are able to function in a protected environment. Some marry, have children, and live their lives surrounded only by family members. If their support system fails, however, they are subject to depression, anxiety, and anger. Phobic avoidance is common, and patients with the disorder may give histories of social phobia or incur social phobia in the course of their illness.

Treatment

Psychotherapy. Psychotherapeutic treatment depends on solidifying an alliance with patients. As trust develops, a therapist must convey an accepting attitude toward the patient's fears, especially the fear of rejection. The therapist eventually encourages a patient to move out into the world to take what are perceived as great risks of humiliation, rejection, and failure. But therapists should be cautious when giving assignments to exercise new social skills outside therapy; failure can reinforce a patient's already poor self-esteem. Group therapy may help patients understand how their sensitivity to rejection affects them and others. Assertiveness training is a form of behavior therapy that may teach patients to express their needs openly and to enlarge their self-esteem.

Pharmacotherapy. Pharmacotherapy has been used to manage anxiety and depression when they are associated with the disorder. Some patients are helped by β-adrenergic receptor antagonists, such as atenolol (Tenormin), to manage autonomic nervous system hyperactivity, which tends to be high in patients with avoidant personality disorder, especially when they approach feared situations. Serotonergic agents may help rejection sensitivity. Theoretically, dopaminergic drugs might engender novelty-seeking behavior in these patients; however, the patient must be psychologically prepared for any new experience that might result.

DEPENDENT PERSONALITY DISORDER

Persons with dependent personality disorder subordinate their own needs to those of others, get others to assume responsibility for major areas of their lives, lack self-confidence, and may experience intense discomfort when alone for more than a brief period. The disorder has been called *passive-dependent personality*. Freud described an oral-dependent personality dimension characterized by dependence, pessimism, fear of sexuality, self-doubt, passivity, suggestibility, and lack of perseverance; his description is similar to the DSM-5 categorization of dependent personality disorder.

Epidemiology

Dependent personality disorder is more common in women than in men. DSM-5 reports an estimated prevalence of 0.6 percent. One study diagnosed 2.5 percent of all personality disorders as falling into this category. It is more common in young children than in older ones. Persons with chronic physical illness in childhood may be most susceptible to the disorder.

Diagnosis and Clinical Features

Dependent personality disorder is characterized by a pervasive pattern of dependent and submissive behavior. Persons with the disorder cannot make decisions without an excessive amount of advice and reassurance from others. They avoid positions of responsibility and become anxious if asked to assume a leadership role. They prefer to be submissive. When on their own, they find it difficult to persevere at tasks but may find it easy to perform these tasks for someone else. In interviews, patients appear compliant. They try to cooperate, welcome specific questions, and look for guidance.

Because persons with the disorder do not like to be alone, they seek out others on whom they can depend; their relationships, thus, are distorted by their need to be attached to another person. In folie à deux (shared psychotic disorder), one member of the pair usually has dependent personality disorder; the submissive partner takes on the delusional system of the more aggressive, assertive partner on whom he or she depends.

Pessimism, self-doubt, passivity, and fears of expressing sexual and aggressive feelings all typify the behavior of persons with dependent personality disorder. An abusive, unfaithful, or alcoholic spouse may be tolerated for long periods to avoid disturbing the sense of attachment.

Differential Diagnosis

The traits of dependence are found in many psychiatric disorders, so the differential diagnosis is difficult. Dependence is a prominent factor in patients with histrionic and borderline personality disorders, but those with dependent personality disorder usually have a long-term relationship with one person rather than a series of persons on whom they are dependent, and they do not tend to be overtly manipulative. Patients with schizoid and schizotypal personality disorders may be indistinguishable from those with avoidant personality disorder. Dependent behavior can also occur in patients with agoraphobia, but these patients tend to have a high level of overt anxiety or even panic.

Course and Prognosis

Little is known about the course of dependent personality disorder. Occupational functioning tends to be impaired because persons with the disorder cannot act independently and without close supervision. Social relationships are limited to those on whom they can depend, and many suffer physical or mental abuse because they cannot assert themselves. They risk major depressive disorder if they lose the person on whom they depend, but with treatment, the prognosis is favorable.

Treatment

Psychotherapy. The treatment of dependent personality disorder is often successful. Insight-oriented therapies enable patients to understand the antecedents of their behavior, and with the support of a therapist, patients can become more independent, assertive, and self-reliant. Behavioral therapy, assertiveness training, family therapy, and group therapy have all been used, with successful outcomes in many cases.

A pitfall may arise in treatment when a therapist encourages a patient to change the dynamics of a pathological relationship (e.g., supports a physically abused wife in seeking help from the police). At this point, patients may become anxious and unable to cooperate in therapy; they may feel torn between complying with the therapist and losing a pathological external relationship. Therapists must show great respect for these patients' feelings of attachment, no matter how pathological these feelings may seem.

Pharmacotherapy. Pharmacotherapy has been used to deal with specific symptoms, such as anxiety and depression, which are common associated features of dependent personality disorder. Patients who experience panic attacks or who have high levels of separation anxiety may be helped by imipramine (Tofranil). Benzodiazepines and serotonergic agents have also been useful. If a patient's depression or withdrawal symptoms respond to psychostimulants, they may be used.

OBSESSIVE-COMPULSIVE PERSONALITY DISORDER

Obsessive-compulsive personality disorder is characterized by emotional constriction, orderliness, perseverance, stubbornness, and indecisiveness. The essential feature of the disorder is a pervasive pattern of perfectionism and inflexibility.

Epidemiology

DSM-5 reports an estimated prevalence ranging from 2 to 8 percent. It is more common in men than in women and is diagnosed most often in oldest siblings. The disorder also occurs more frequently in first-degree biological relatives of persons with the disorder than in the general population. Patients often have backgrounds characterized by harsh discipline. Freud hypothesized that the disorder is associated with difficulties in the anal stage of psychosexual development, generally around the age of 2 years, but various studies have failed to validate this theory.

Diagnosis and Clinical Features

In interviews, patients with obsessive-compulsive personality disorder may have a stiff, formal, and rigid demeanor. Their affect is not blunted or flat but can be described as constricted.

They lack spontaneity, and their mood is usually serious. Such patients may be anxious about not being in control of the interview. Their answers to questions are unusually detailed. The defense mechanisms they use are rationalization, isolation, intellectualization, reaction formation, and undoing.

Persons with obsessive-compulsive personality disorder are preoccupied with rules, regulations, orderliness, neatness, details, and the achievement of perfection. These traits account for the general constriction of the entire personality. They insist that rules be followed rigidly and cannot tolerate what they consider infractions. Accordingly, they lack flexibility and are intolerant. They are capable of prolonged work, provided it is routinized and does not require changes to which they cannot adapt.

Persons with obsessive-compulsive personality disorder have limited interpersonal skills. They are formal and serious and often lack a sense of humor. They alienate persons, are unable to compromise, and insist that others submit to their needs. They are eager to please those whom they see as more powerful than they are, however, and they carry out these persons' wishes in an authoritarian manner. Because they fear making mistakes, they are indecisive and ruminate about making decisions. Although a stable marriage and occupational adequacy are common, persons with obsessive-compulsive personality disorder have few friends. Anything that threatens to upset their perceived stability or the routine of their lives can precipitate much anxiety otherwise bound up in the rituals that they impose on their lives and try to impose on others.

Differential Diagnosis

When recurrent obsessions or compulsions are present, obsessive-compulsive disorder should be noted. Perhaps the most difficult distinction is between outpatients with some obsessive-compulsive traits and those with obsessive-compulsive personality disorder. The diagnosis of personality disorder is reserved for those with significant impairments in their occupational or social effectiveness. In some cases, delusional disorder coexists with personality disorders and should be noted.

Course and Prognosis

The course of obsessive-compulsive personality disorder is variable and unpredictable. From time to time, persons may develop obsessions or compulsions in the course of their disorder. Some adolescents with obsessive-compulsive personality disorder evolve into warm, open, and loving adults; in others, the disorder can be either the harbinger of schizophrenia or—decades later and exacerbated by the aging process—major depressive disorder.

Persons with obsessive-compulsive personality disorder may flourish in positions demanding methodical, deductive, or detailed work, but they are vulnerable to unexpected changes, and their personal lives may remain barren. Depressive disorders, especially those of late onset, are common.

Treatment

Psychotherapy. Unlike patients with the other personality disorders, those with obsessive-compulsive personality disorder are often aware of their suffering, and they seek treatment on their own. Overtrained and oversocialized, these patients value free association and no-directive therapy highly. Treatment, however, is often long and complex, and countertransference problems are common.

Group therapy and behavior therapy occasionally offer certain advantages. In both contexts, it is easy to interrupt the patients in the midst of their maladaptive interactions or explanations. Preventing the completion of their habitual behavior raises patients' anxiety and leaves them susceptible to learning new coping strategies. Patients can also receive direct rewards for change in group therapy, something less often possible in individual psychotherapies.

Pharmacotherapy. Clonazepam (Klonopin), a benzodiazepine with anticonvulsant use, has reduced symptoms in patients with severe obsessive-compulsive disorder. Whether it is of use in the personality disorder is unknown. Clomipramine (Anafranil) and such serotonergic agents as fluoxetine, usually at dosages of 60 to 80 mg a day, may be useful if obsessive-compulsive signs and symptoms break through. Nefazodone (Serzone) may benefit some patients.

OTHER SPECIFIED PERSONALITY DISORDER

In DSM-5, the category other specified personality disorder is reserved for disorders that do not fit into any of the personality disorder categories described above. Passive-aggressive personality and depressive personality are examples. A narrow spectrum of behavior or a particular trait—such as oppositionalism, sadism, or masochism—can also be classified in this category. A patient with features of more than one personality disorder but without the complete criteria of any one disorder can be assigned this classification.

Passive-Aggressive Personality

Passive-Aggressive Personality was once considered a psychiatric diagnosis but is no longer classified as such. It is included here because persons with this personality type are not uncommon. Persons with passive-aggressive personality are characterized by covert obstructionism, procrastination, stubbornness, and inefficiency. Such behavior is a manifestation of passively expressed underlying aggression.

Epidemiology. No data are available about epidemiology. Sex ratio, familial patterns, and prevalence have not been adequately studied.

Clinical Features. Patients with passive-aggressive personality characteristically procrastinate, resist demands for adequate performance, find excuses for delays, and find fault with those on whom they depend, yet they refuse to extricate themselves from the dependent relationships. They usually lack assertiveness and are not direct about their own needs and wishes. They fail to ask needed questions about what is expected of them and may become anxious when forced to succeed or when their usual defense of turning anger against themselves is removed.

In interpersonal relationships, these persons attempt to manipulate themselves into a position of dependence, but others often experience this passive, self-detrimental behavior as punitive and manipulative. Persons with this personality type expect others to do their errands and to carry out their routine responsibilities. Friends and clinicians may become enmeshed in trying to assuage the patients' many claims of unjust treatment. The close relationships of persons with passive-aggressive personality, however, are rarely tranquil or happy. Because they are bound to their resentment more closely than to their satisfaction, they may never even formulate goals for finding enjoyment in life. Persons with passive-aggressive personality lack self-confidence and are typically pessimistic about the future.

Differential Diagnosis. Passive-aggressive personality must be differentiated from histrionic and borderline personality disorders. Passive-aggressive patients, however, are less flamboyant, dramatic, affective, and openly aggressive than those with histrionic and borderline personality disorders.

Course and Prognosis. In a follow-up study averaging 11 years of 100 inpatients diagnosed with passive-aggressive disorder, Ivor Small found that the primary diagnosis in 54 was passive-aggressive personality disorder; 18 were also alcohol abusers, and 30 could be clinically labeled as depressed. Of the 73 former patients located, 58 (79 percent) had persistent psychiatric difficulties, and 9 (12 percent) were considered symptom free. Most seemed irritable, anxious, and depressed; somatic complaints were numerous. Only 32 (44 percent) were employed full time as workers or homemakers. Although neglect of responsibility and suicide attempts were common, only one patient had committed suicide in the interim. Twenty-eight (38 percent) had been readmitted to a hospital, but only three had been diagnosed as having schizophrenia.

Treatment. Even though no longer considered a disorder, persons with a passive-aggressive personality will often seek out treatment because of poor social or occupational functioning that may result from these traits. Psychotherapy for these patients has many pitfalls. Fulfilling their demands often supports their pathology, but refusing their demands rejects them. Therapy sessions, thus, can become a battleground on which a patient expresses feelings of resentment against a therapist on whom the patient wishes to become dependent. If interpersonal problems become severe, depression may result and suicidal ideation may occur. With these patients, clinicians must treat suicide gestures as any covert expression of anger and not as object loss in major depressive disorder. Therapists must point out the probable consequences of passive-aggressive behaviors as they occur. Such confrontations may be more helpful than a correct interpretation in changing patients' behavior.

Antidepressants should be prescribed only when clinical indications of depression and the possibility of suicide exist. Otherwise, medication is not indicated.

Depressive Personality

Persons with depressive personality are characterized by lifelong traits that fall along the depressive spectrum. They are pessimistic, anhedonic, duty bound, self-doubting, and chronically unhappy. Melancholic personality was described by early 20th century European psychiatrists such as Ernst Kretschmer.

Epidemiology. No epidemiological data are currently available; however, depressive personality type seems to be common, to occur equally in men and women, and to occur in families in which depressive disorders are found.

Etiology. The cause of depressive personality is unknown, but the same factors involved in dysthymic disorder and major depressive disorder may be at work. Psychological theories involve early loss, poor parenting, punitive superegos, and extreme feelings of guilt. Biological theories involve the hypothalamic-pituitary-adrenal-thyroid axis, including the noradrenergic and serotonergic amine systems. Genetic predisposition, as indicated by Stella Chess studies of temperament, may also play a role.

Clinical Features. Patients with depressive personality feel little of the normal joy of living and are inclined to be lonely and solemn, gloomy, submissive, pessimistic, and self-deprecatory. They are prone to express regrets and feelings of inadequacy and hopelessness. They are often meticulous, perfectionistic, overconscientious, and preoccupied with work; feel responsibility keenly; and are easily discouraged under new conditions. They are fearful of disapproval; tend to suffer in silence; and perhaps to cry easily, although usually not in the presence of others. A tendency to hesitation, indecision, and caution betrays an inherent feeling of insecurity.

More recently, Hagop Akiskal described seven groups of depressive traits: (1) quiet, introverted, passive, and nonassertive; (2) gloomy, pessimistic, serious, and incapable of fun; (3) self-critical, self-reproachful, and self-derogatory; (4) skeptical, critical of others, and hard to please; (5) conscientious, responsible, and self-disciplined; (6) brooding and given to worry; and (7) preoccupied with negative events, feelings of inadequacy, and personal shortcomings.

Patients with depressive personality complain of chronic feelings of unhappiness. They admit to low self-esteem and difficulty finding anything in their lives about which they are joyful, hopeful, or optimistic. They are self-critical and derogatory and are likely to denigrate their work, themselves, and their relationships with others. Their physiognomy often reflects their mood—poor posture, depressed facies, hoarse voice, and psychomotor retardation.

Differential Diagnosis. Dysthymic disorder is a mood disorder characterized by greater fluctuations in mood than occur in depressive personality. Dysthymic disorder is episodic, can occur at any time, and usually has a precipitating stressor. The depressive personality can be conceptualized as part of a spectrum of affective conditions in which dysthymic disorder and major depressive disorder are more severe variants. Patients with avoidant personality disorder are introverted and dependent, but they tend to be more anxious than depressed compared with persons with depressive personality.

Course and Prognosis. Persons with depressive personality may be at great risk for dysthymic disorder and major depressive disorder. In a study by Donald Klein and Gregory Mills, subjects with depressive personality exhibited significantly higher rates of current mood disorder, lifetime mood disorder, major depression, and dysthymia than subjects without depressive personality.

Treatment. Psychotherapy is the treatment of choice for depressive personality. Patients respond to insight-oriented psychotherapy, and because their reality testing is good, they can gain insight into the psychodynamics of their illness and appreciate its effects on their interpersonal relationships. Treatment is likely to be long term. Cognitive therapy helps patients understand the cognitive manifestations of their low self-esteem and pessimism. Group psychotherapy and interpersonal therapy are also useful. Some persons respond to self-help measures.

Psychopharmacological approaches include the use of antidepressant medications, especially such serotonergic agents as sertraline (Zoloft), 50 mg a day. Some patients respond to small dosages of psychostimulants, such as amphetamine, 5 to 15 mg a day. In all cases, psychopharmacological agents should be combined with psychotherapy to achieve maximum effects.

Sadomasochistic Personality

Some personality types are characterized by elements of sadism or masochism or a combination of both. Sadomasochistic personality is listed here because it is of major clinical and historical interest in psychiatry. It is not an official diagnostic category in DSM-5, but it can be diagnosed as personality disorder not otherwise classified.

Sadism is the desire to cause others pain by being either sexually abusive or generally physically or psychologically abusive. It is named for the Marquis de Sade, a late 18th century writer of erotica, describing persons who experienced sexual pleasure while inflicting pain on others. Freud believed that sadists ward off castration anxiety and are able to achieve sexual pleasure only when they can do to others what they fear will be done to them.

Masochism, named for Leopold von Sacher-Masoch, a 19th century German novelist, is the achievement of sexual gratification by inflicting pain on the self. So-called moral masochists generally seek humiliation and failure rather than physical pain. Freud believed that masochists' ability to achieve orgasm is disturbed by anxiety and guilt feelings about sex, which are alleviated by suffering and punishment.

Clinical observations indicate that elements of both sadistic and masochistic behavior are usually present in the same person. Treatment with insight-oriented psychotherapy, including psychoanalysis, has been effective in some cases. As a result of therapy, patients become aware of the need for self-punishment secondary to excessive unconscious guilt and come to recognize their repressed aggressive impulses, which originate in early childhood.

Sadistic Personality

Sadistic personality is not included in DSM-5, but it still appears in the literature and may be of descriptive use. Beginning in early adulthood, persons with sadistic personality show a pervasive pattern of cruel, demeaning, and aggressive behavior that is directed toward others. Physical cruelty or violence is used to inflict pain on others, not to achieve another goal, such as mugging a person to steal. Persons with sadistic personality like to humiliate or demean persons in front of others and have usually treated or disciplined persons uncommonly harshly, especially children. In general, persons with sadistic personality are fascinated by violence, weapons, injury, or torture. To be included in this category, such persons cannot be motivated solely by the desire to derive sexual arousal from their behavior; if they are so motivated, the paraphilia of sexual sadism should be diagnosed.

PERSONALITY CHANGE DUE TO A GENERAL MEDICAL CONDITION

Personality change due to a general medical condition is a significant occurrence. ICD-10 includes the category personality and behavioral disorders due to brain disease, damage, and dysfunction, which includes organic personality disorder, postencephalitic syndrome, and postconcussional syndrome. Personality change due to a general medical condition is characterized by a marked change in personality style and traits from a previous level of functioning. Patients must show evidence of a causative organic factor antedating the onset of the personality change.

Etiology

Structural damage to the brain is usually the cause of the personality change, and head trauma is probably the most common cause. Cerebral neoplasms and vascular accidents, particularly of the temporal and frontal lobes, are also common causes. The conditions most often associated with personality change are listed in Table 18–2.

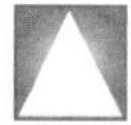

Table 18–2
Medical Conditions Associated with Personality Change

Head trauma
Cerebrovascular diseases
Cerebral tumors
Epilepsy (particularly, complex partial epilepsy)
Huntington's disease
Multiple sclerosis
Endocrine disorders
Heavy metal poisoning (manganese, mercury)
Neurosyphilis
Acquired immune deficiency syndrome (AIDS)

Diagnosis and Clinical Features

A change in personality from previous patterns of behavior or an exacerbation of previous personality characteristics is notable. Impaired control of the expression of emotions and impulses is a cardinal feature. Emotions are characteristically labile and shallow, although euphoria or apathy may be prominent. The euphoria may mimic hypomania, but true elation is absent, and patients may admit to not really feeling happy. There is a hollow and silly ring to their excitement and facile jocularity, particularly when the frontal lobes are involved. Also associated with damage to the frontal lobes, the so-called frontal lobe syndrome, consists of prominent indifference and apathy, characterized by a lack of concern for events in the immediate environment. Temper outbursts, which can occur with little or no provocation, especially after alcohol ingestion, can result in violent behavior. The expression of impulses may be manifested by inappropriate jokes; a coarse manner; improper sexual advances; and antisocial conduct resulting in conflicts with the law, such as assaults on others, sexual misdemeanors, and shoplifting. Foresight and the ability to anticipate the social or legal consequences of actions are typically diminished. Persons with temporal lobe epilepsy characteristically show humorlessness, hypergraphia, hyperreligiosity, and marked aggressiveness during seizures.

Persons with personality change due to a general medical condition have a clear sensorium. Mild disorders of cognitive function often coexist but do not amount to intellectual deterioration. Patients may be inattentive, which may account for disorders of recent memory. With some prodding, however, patients are likely to recall what they claim to have forgotten. The diagnosis should be suspected in patients who show marked changes in behavior or personality involving emotional lability and impaired impulse control, who have no history of mental disorder, and whose personality changes occur abruptly or over a relatively brief time.

Anabolic Steroids. An increasing number of high school and college athletes and bodybuilders are using anabolic steroids as a shortcut to maximize physical development. Anabolic steroids include oxymetholone (Anadrol), somatropin (Humatrope), stanozolol (Winstrol), and testosterone.

It is unclear whether a personality change caused by steroid abuse is better diagnosed as personality change due to a general medical condition or as one of the other (or unknown) substance use disorders. It is mentioned here because anabolic steroids can cause persistent alterations of personality and behavior. Anabolic steroid abuse is discussed in Section 12.13.

Differential Diagnosis

Dementia involves global deterioration in intellectual and behavioral capacities, of which personality change is just one category. A personality change may herald a cognitive disorder that eventually will evolve into dementia. In these cases, as deterioration begins to encompass significant memory and cognitive deficits, the diagnosis of the disorder changes from personality change caused by a general medical condition to dementia. In differentiating the specific syndrome from other disorders in which personality change may occur—such as schizophrenia, delusional disorder, mood disorders, and impulse control disorders—physicians must consider the most important factor, the presence in personality change disorder of a specific organic causative factor.

Course and Prognosis

Both the course and the prognosis of personality change due to a general medical condition depend on its cause. If the disorder results from structural damage to the brain, the disorder tends to persist. The disorder may follow a period of coma and delirium in cases of head trauma or vascular accident and may be permanent. The personality change can evolve into dementia in cases of brain tumor, multiple sclerosis, and Huntington's disease. Personality changes produced by chronic intoxication, medical illness, or drug therapy (such as levodopa [Larodopa] for parkinsonism) may be reversed if the underlying cause is treated. Some patients require custodial care or at least close supervision to meet their basic needs, avoid repeated conflicts with the law, and protect themselves and their families from the hostility of others and from destitution resulting from impulsive and ill-considered actions.

Treatment

Management of personality change disorder involves treatment of the underlying organic condition when possible. Psychopharmacological treatment of specific symptoms may be indicated in some cases, such as imipramine or fluoxetine for depression.

Patients with severe cognitive impairment or weakened behavioral controls may need counseling to help avoid difficulties at work or to prevent social embarrassment. As a rule, patients' families need emotional support and concrete advice on how to help minimize patients' undesirable conduct. Alcohol should be avoided, and social engagements should be curtailed when patients tend to act in a grossly offensive manner.

PSYCHOBIOLOGICAL MODEL OF TREATMENT

The psychobiological model of treatment combines psychotherapy and pharmacotherapy and is based on the established structural, clinical, and postulated neurochemical characteristics of temperament and character. Pharmacotherapy and psychotherapy can be systematically matched to the personality structure and stage of character development of each patient—clearly a unique advantage over other available approaches.

The newest development is treating personality disorders pharmacologically. Target symptoms are identified, and particular drugs with known effects on personality traits (e.g., harm avoidance) are used. Table 18–3 summarizes drug choices for various target symptoms of personality disorders.

In his book, *Listening to Prozac,* Peter Kramer described dramatic personality changes when serotonin levels are raised by fluoxetine administration, such as decreased sensitivity to rejection, increased assertiveness, improved self-esteem, and the ability to tolerate stress. These changes in personality traits occur in patients with a wide range of psychiatric conditions as well as in persons without diagnosable mental disorders. Using medications to treat specific traits in a person who is otherwise normal (i.e., does not meet the criteria for a full-blown personality disorder) is controversial. It has been called "cosmetic psychopharmacology" by its critics.

Temperament

Temperament refers to the body's biases in the modulation of conditioned behavioral responses to prescriptive physical stimuli. Behavioral conditioning (i.e., procedural learning) involves presemantic sensations that elicit basic emotions, such as fear or anger, independent of conscious recognition, descriptive observation, reflection, or reasoning. Pioneering work by A. Thomas and S. Chess conceptualized temperament as the stylistic component ("how") of behavior, as differentiated from the motivation ("why") and the content ("what") of behavior. Modern concepts of temperament, however, emphasize its emotional, motivational, and adaptive aspects. Specifically, four major temperament traits have been identified and subjected to extensive neurobiological, psychosocial, and clinical investigation: harm avoidance, novelty seeking, reward dependence, and persistence. It is remarkable that this four-factor model of temperament can, in retrospect, be seen as a modern interpretation of the ancient four temperaments: Individuals differ in the degree to which they are melancholic (harm avoidance), choleric (novelty seeking), sanguine (reward dependence), and phlegmatic (persistence). However, the four temperaments are now understood to be genetically independent dimensions that occur in all possible combinations within the same individual rather than as mutually exclusive categories.

Biological Character Traits. Four character traits have been described, each with certain neurochemical and neurophysiological substrates. They share a common source of covariation that is strong and invariant regardless of changes in the environment and past experience. Table 18–4 summarizes contrasting sets of behaviors that distinguish extreme scorers on the four dimensions of temperament. Note that each extreme of these dimensions has specific adaptive advantages and disadvantages, so that neither high nor low scores inherently mean better adaptation. Each of the four temperament dimensions has unique genetic determinants according to family and twin studies, as well as studies of genetic associations with specific DNA markers. Some workers postulate specific genes for some traits, such as a novelty-seeking gene.

HARM AVOIDANCE. Harm avoidance involves a heritable bias in the inhibition of behavior in response to signals of punishment and nonreward. High harm avoidance is observed as fear of uncertainty, social inhibition, shyness with strangers, rapid

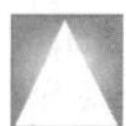

Table 18–3
Pharmacotherapy of Target Symptom Domains of Personality Disorders

Target Symptom	Drug of Choice	Contraindication[a]
I. Behavior dyscontrol		
Aggression or impulsivity		
Affective aggression (hot temper with normal EEG)	Lithium[a]	Benzodiazepines
	Serotonergic drugs[a]	Stimulants
	Anticonvulsants[a]	
	Low-dosage antipsychotics	
Predatory aggression (hostility or cruelty)	Antipsychotics[a]	Benzodiazepines
	Lithium	Stimulants
	β-Adrenergic receptor antagonists	
Organic-like aggression	Imipramine[a]	
	Cholinergic agonists (donepezil)	
Ictal aggression (abnormal EEG)	Carbamazepine[a]	Antipsychotics
	Diphenylhydantoin[a]	Stimulants
	Benzodiazepines	
II. Mood dysregulation		
Emotional lability	Lithium[a]	Tricyclic drugs
	Antipsychotics	
Depression		
Atypical depression, dysphoria	MAOIs[a]	
	Serotonergic drugs[a]	
	Antipsychotics	
Emotional detachment	Serotonin-dopamine antagonists[a]	Tricyclic drugs
	Atypical antipsychotics	
III. Anxiety		
Chronic cognitive	Serotonergic drugs[a]	Stimulants
	MAOIs[a]	
	Benzodiazepines	
Chronic somatic	MAOIs[a]	
	β-Adrenergic receptor antagonists	
Severe anxiety	Low-dose antipsychotics	
	MAOIs	
IV. Psychotic symptoms		
Acute and psychosis	Antipsychotics[a]	Stimulants
Chronic and low-level psychotic-like symptoms	Low-dose antipsychotics[a]	

[a]Drug of choice or major contraindication.
EEG, electroencephalogram; MAOI, monamine oxidase inhibitor.

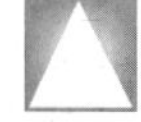

Table 18–4
Descriptors of Individuals Who Score High or Low on the Four Temperament Dimensions

	Descriptors of Extreme Variants	
Temperament dimension	High	Low
Harm avoidance	Pessimistic	Optimistic
	Fearful	Daring
	Shy	Outgoing
	Fatigable	Energetic
Novelty seeking	Exploratory	Reserved
	Impulsive	Deliberate
	Extravagant	Thrifty
	Irritable	Stoical
Reward dependence	Sentimental	Detached
	Open	Aloof
	Warm	Cold
	Affectionate	Independent
Persistence	Industrious	Lazy
	Determined	Spoiled
	Enthusiastic	Underachiever
	Perfectionist	Pragmatist

fatigability, and pessimistic worry in anticipation of problems even in situations that do not worry other persons. Persons low in harm avoidance are carefree, courageous, energetic, outgoing, and optimistic even in situations that worry most persons.

The psychobiology of harm avoidance is complex. Benzodiazepines disinhibit avoidance by γ-aminobutyric acid (GABA)-ergic inhibition of serotonergic neurons originating in the dorsal raphe nuclei.

Positron emission tomography (PET) at the National Institute of Mental Health (NIMH) with [^{18}F]-deoxyglucose (FDG) in 31 healthy adult volunteers during a simple, continuous performance task showed that harm avoidance was associated with increased activity in the anterior paralimbic circuit, specifically the right amygdala and insula, the right orbitofrontal cortex, and the left medial prefrontal cortex.

High GABA concentrations in plasma have also been correlated with low harm avoidance. Plasma GABA concentration has also been correlated with other measures of anxiety susceptibility, and it correlates highly with GABA concentration in the brain. Finally, a gene on chromosome 17q12 that regulates the expression of the serotonin transporter accounts for 4 to 9 percent of the total variance in harm avoidance. These findings support a role for both GABA and serotonergic projections from the dorsal raphe underlying individual differences in behavioral inhibition as measured by harm avoidance. Persons given serotonin drugs show decreased harm avoidance behavior.

NOVELTY SEEKING. Novelty seeking reflects a heritable bias in the initiation or activation of appetitive approach in response to novelty, approach to signals of reward, active avoidance of conditioned signals of punishment, and escape from unconditioned punishment (all of which are hypothesized to covary as part of one heritable system of learning). Novelty seeking is observed as exploratory activity in response to novelty, impulsiveness, extravagance in approach to cues of reward, and active avoidance of frustration. Individuals high in novelty seeking are quick tempered, curious, easily bored, impulsive, extravagant, and disorderly. Persons low in novelty seeking are slow tempered, uninquiring, stoical, reflective, frugal, reserved, tolerant of monotony, and orderly.

Dopaminergic projections have a crucial role in novelty seeking. Novelty seeking involves increased reuptake of dopamine at presynaptic terminals, thereby requiring frequent stimulation to maintain optimal levels of postsynaptic dopaminergic stimulation. Novelty seeking leads to various pleasure-seeking behaviors, including cigarette smoking, which may explain the frequent observation of low platelet MAO type B (MAO_B) activity because cigarette smoking inhibits MAO_B activity in platelets and brain.

Studies of genes involved in dopamine neurotransmission, such as the dopamine transporter gene (*DAT1*) and the type 4 dopamine receptor gene (*DRD4*), have provided evidence of association with novelty seeking or risk-taking behavior.

REWARD DEPENDENCE. Reward dependence reflects maintenance of behavior in response to cues of social reward. Individuals high in reward dependence are tender hearted, sensitive, socially dependent, and sociable. Individuals low in reward dependence are practical, tough minded, cold, socially insensitive, irresolute, and indifferent if alone.

Noradrenergic projections from the locus ceruleus and serotonergic projections from the median raphe are thought to influence such reward conditioning. High reward dependence is associated with increased activity in the thalamus. The 3-methoxy-4-hydroxyphenylglycol (MHPG) concentration is low in persons with high reward dependence.

PERSISTENCE. Persistence reflects maintenance of behavior despite frustration, fatigue, and intermittent reinforcement. Highly persistent persons are hard-working, perseverant, and ambitious overachievers who tend to intensify their effort in response to anticipated rewards and view frustration and fatigue as personal challenges. Individuals low in persistence are indolent, inactive, unstable, and erratic; they tend to give up easily when faced with frustration, rarely strive for higher accomplishments, and manifest little perseverance even in response to intermittent reward.

Recent work in rodents related the integrity of the partial reinforcement extinction effect to hippocampal connections and glutamate metabolism. Persistence may be enhanced by psychostimulants.

Psychobiology of Temperament. Temperament traits of harm avoidance, novelty seeking, reward dependence, and persistence are defined as heritable differences underlying automatic responses to danger, novelty, social approval, and intermittent reward, respectively. The component traits ("facets") for each of the four temperament dimensions have distinct learning characteristics and correlate more strongly with one another than with other components of temperament. The most comprehensive neurobiological model of learning in animals that has been systematically related to the structure of human temperament is summarized in Table 18–5. This model distinguishes four dissociable brain systems for behavioral inhibition (harm avoidance), behavioral activation (novelty seeking), social attachment (reward dependence), and partial reinforcement (persistence).

Individual differences in temperament and basic emotions modify the processing of sensory information and shape early

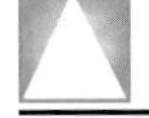

Table 18–5
Four Dissociable Brain Systems Influencing Stimulus–Response Patterns Underlying Temperament

Brain System (Related Personality Dimension)	Principal Neuromodulators	Relevant Stimuli	Behavioral Response
Behavioral inhibition (harm avoidance)	GABA Serotonin (dorsal raphe)	Aversive conditioning (pairing CS and UCS) Conditioned signals for punishment and frustrative nonreward	Formation of aversive CS Passive avoidance Extinction
Behavioral activation (novelty seeking)	Dopamine	Novelty CS of reward CS or UCS of relief of monotony or punishment	Exploratory pursuit Appetitive approach Active Avoidance Escape
Social attachment (reward dependence)	Norepinephrine		
Serotonin (median raphe)	Reward conditioning (pairing CS and UCS)	Formation of appetitive CS	
Partial reinforcement (persistence)	Glutamate Serotonin (dorsal raphe)	Intermittent (partial) reinforcement	Resistance to extinction

CS, conditioned stimulus; GABA, γ-aminobutyric acid; UCS, unconditioned stimulus.
Adapted from Cloninger CR. A systematic method for clinical description and classification of personality variables. *Arch Gen Psychiatry.* 1987;44:573.

learning characteristics, especially associative conditioning of unconscious behavior responses. Temperament is conceptualized in terms of heritable biases in emotionality and learning that underlie the acquisition of emotion-based, automatic behavioral traits and habits observable early in life and relatively stable over an individual's lifespan.

Each of the four major dimensions is a normally distributed quantitative trait, moderately heritable, observable early in childhood, relatively stable in time, and moderately predictive of adolescent and adult behavior. The four dimensions have been shown to be genetically homogeneous and independently inherited from one another in large, independent twin studies in the United States, Australia, and Japan. Temperamental differences, which are not very stable initially, tend to stabilize during the second and third years of life. Accordingly, ratings of these four temperament traits at age 10 to 11 years were moderately predictive of personality traits at ages 15, 18, and 27 years in a large sample of Swedish children.

The four dimensions have been repeatedly shown to be universal across different cultures, ethnic groups, and political systems on every inhabited continent. In summary, these aspects of personality are called temperament because they are heritable, manifest early in life, are developmentally stable, and are consistent in different cultures. Temperament traits are similar to crystallized intelligence in that they do not show the rapid changes with increasing age or across birth cohorts that are observed for fluid intelligence and character traits.

19

Emergency Psychiatric Medicine

▲ 19.1 Suicide

Suicide is derived from the Latin word for "self-murder." It is a fatal act that represents the person's wish to die. There is a range, however, between thinking about suicide and acting it out. Some plan for days, weeks, or even years before acting, while others take their lives seemingly on impulse without premeditation. Lost in the definition are intentional misclassifications of the cause of death, accidents of undetermined cause, and so-called chronic suicide (e.g., deaths through alcohol and substance abuse and consciously poor adherence to medical regimens for addiction, obesity, and hypertension). For other terms in the literature on suicide, see Table 19.1–1.

In psychiatry, suicide is the primary emergency, with homicide and failure to diagnose an underlying potentially fatal illness representing other, less common psychiatric emergencies. Suicide is to the psychiatrist as cancer is to the internist—the psychiatrist may provide optimal care, yet the patient may die by suicide nonetheless. Thus, suicide is impossible to predict, but numerous clues can be seen. There are also some generally accepted standards of care that facilitate risk reduction, as well as lessen the likelihood of successful litigation, should a patient death occur and a lawsuit be filed. Suicide also needs to be considered in terms of the devastating legacy that it leaves for those who have survived a loved one's suicide, the impact it has on the treating physician, and the ramification for the clinicians who cared for the decedents. Perhaps the most important concept regarding suicide is that it is almost always the result of mental illness, usually depression, and is amenable to psychological and pharmacological treatment.

Table 19.1–1
Terms Comprising Suicidal Ideation and Behavior

Aborted suicide attempt: Potentially self-injurious behavior with explicit or implicit evidence that the person intended to die but stopped the attempt before physical damage occurred.
Deliberate self-harm: Willful self-inflicting of painful, destructive, or injurious acts without intent to die.
Lethality of suicidal behavior: Objective danger to life associated with a suicide method or action. Note that lethality is distinct from and may not always coincide with an individual's expectation of what is medically dangerous.
Suicidal ideation: Thought of serving as the agent of one's own death; seriousness may vary depending on the specificity of suicidal plans and the degree of suicidal intent.
Suicidal intent: Subjective expectation and desire for a self-destructive act to end in death.
Suicide attempt: Self-injurious behavior with a nonfatal outcome accompanied by explicit or implicit evidence that the person intended to die.
Suicide: Self-inflicted death with explicit or implicit evidence that the person intended to die.

EPIDEMIOLOGY

There are about 40,000 deaths per year in the United States attributed to suicide. This is in contrast to approximately 20,000 deaths annually from homicide. It is estimated that there is a 25 to 1 ratio between suicide attempts and completed suicides. Although significant shifts were seen in the suicide death rates for certain subpopulations during the past century (e.g., increase adolescent and decreased elderly rates), the rate remains fairly constant, averaging about 12–13 per 100,000 through the 20th century and into the first decade of the 21st century. Suicide is currently ranked the tenth overall cause of death in the United States, after heart disease, cancer, chronic lower respiratory diseases, cerebrovascular diseases, accidents, Alzheimer's disease, diabetes, influenza and pneumonia, and kidney disease.

Suicide rates in the United States are the midpoint of the rates for industrialized countries. Internationally, suicide rates range from highs of more than 25 per 100,000 persons in Lithuania, South Korea, Sri Lanka, Russia, Belarus, and Guyana to fewer than 10 per 100,000 in Portugal, the Netherlands, Australia, Spain, South Africa, Italy, Egypt, and others.

A state-by-state analysis of suicides in the past decade revealed that New Jersey had the nation's lowest suicide rate for both sexes and Montana had the nation's highest rate. Montana and Wyoming had the highest rates for men, and Alaska and Idaho had the highest rates for women. The prime suicide site in the world is the Golden Gate Bridge in San Francisco, with 1,600 suicides committed there since the bridge opened in 1937.

Risk Factors

Gender Differences. Men commit suicide more than four times as often as women, regardless of age or race, in the United States—despite the fact that women attempt suicide or have suicidal thoughts three times as often as men. Although this disparity remains unclear, it may be related to the methods used. Men are more likely than women to commit suicide using firearms, hanging, or jumping from high places. Women, on the other hand, more commonly take an overdose of psychoactive substances or poison. The use of firearms among women, however, is increasing. In states with gun control laws, the use of firearms has decreased as a method of suicide. Globally, the most common method of suicide is hanging.

Age. For all groups, suicide is rare before puberty. Suicide rates increase with age and underscore the significance of the midlife crisis. Among men, suicides peak after age 45; among women, the greatest number of completed suicides occurs after age 55. Rates of 29 per 100,000 population occur in men age 65 or older. Older persons attempt suicide less often than younger persons, but are more often successful. Although they represent only 13 percent of the total population, older persons account for 16 percent of suicides.

The suicide rate, however, is rising among young persons. Suicide is the third leading cause of death in those aged 15 to 24 years, after accidents and homicides. Attempted suicides in this age group number between 1 million and 2 million annually. Most suicides now are among those aged 35 to 64.

Race. Suicide rates among white men and women are approximately two to three times as high as for African American men and women across the life cycle. Among young persons who live in inner cities and certain Native American and Alaskan Native groups, suicide rates have greatly exceeded the national rate. Suicide rates among immigrants are higher than those in the native-born population.

Religion. Historically, Protestants and Jews in the United States have had higher suicide rates than Catholics. Muslims have much lower rates. The degree of orthodoxy and integration may be a more accurate measure of risk in this category than simple institutional religious affiliation.

Marital Status. Marriage lessens the risk of suicide significantly, especially if there are children in the home. Single, never-married persons register an overall rate nearly double that of married persons. Divorce increases suicide risk, with divorced men three times more likely to kill themselves as divorced women. Widows and widowers also have high rates. Suicide occurs more frequently than usual in persons who are socially isolated and have a family history of suicide (attempted or real). Persons who commit so-called anniversary suicides take their lives on the day a member of their family did. Homosexual men and women appear to have higher rates of suicide than heterosexuals.

Occupation. The higher the person's social status, the greater the risk of suicide, but a drop in social status also increases the risk. Work, in general, protects against suicide. Among occupational rankings, professionals, particularly physicians, have traditionally been considered to be at greatest risk. Other high-risk occupations include law enforcement, dentists, artists, mechanics, lawyers, and insurance agents. Suicide is higher among the unemployed than among employed persons. The suicide rates increase during economic recessions and depressions and decrease during times of high employment and during wars.

PHYSICIAN SUICIDES. The weight of current evidence supports the conclusion that both male and female physicians in the United States have elevated rates of suicide. It is estimated that approximately 400 physicians commit suicide each year in the United States. United Kingdom and Scandinavian data show that the suicide rate for male physicians is two to three times that found in the general male population of the same age. Female physicians have a higher risk of suicide than other women. In the United States, the annual suicide rate for female physicians is about 41 per 100,000, compared with 12 per 100,000 among all white women over 25 years of age. Studies show that physicians who commit suicide have a mental disorder, most often depressive disorder, substance dependence, or both. Both male and female physicians commit suicide significantly more often by substance overdoses and less often by firearms than persons in the general population; drug availability and knowledge about toxicity are important factors in physician suicides. Among physicians, psychiatrists are considered to be at greatest risk, followed by ophthalmologists and anesthesiologists, but all specialties are vulnerable.

Climate. No significant seasonal correlation with suicide has been found. Suicides increase slightly in spring and fall but, contrary to popular belief, not during December and holiday periods.

Physical Health. The relation of physical health and illness to suicide is significant. Previous medical care appears to be a positively correlated risk indicator of suicide: About one-third of all persons who commit suicide have had medical attention within 6 months of death, and a physical illness is estimated to be an important contributing factor in about half of all suicides.

Factors associated with illness that contribute to both suicides and suicide attempts are loss of mobility, especially when physical activity is important to occupation or recreation; disfigurement, particularly among women; and chronic, intractable pain. Patients on hemodialysis are at high risk. In addition to the direct effects of illness, the secondary effects—for example, disruption of relationships and loss of occupational status—are prognostic factors.

Certain drugs can produce depression, which may lead to suicide in some cases. Among these drugs are reserpine (Serpasil), corticosteroids, antihypertensives, and some anticancer agents. Alcohol-related illnesses, such as cirrhosis, are associated with higher suicide rates.

Mental Illness. Almost 95 percent of all persons who commit or attempt suicide have a diagnosed mental disorder. Depressive disorders account for 80 percent of this figure, schizophrenia accounts for 10 percent, and dementia or delirium for 5 percent. Among all persons with mental disorders, 25 percent are also alcohol dependent and have dual diagnoses. Persons with delusional depression are at the highest risk of suicide. A history of impulsive behavior or violent acts increases the risk of suicide as does previous psychiatric hospitalization for any reason. Among adults who commit suicide, significant differences between young and old exist for both psychiatric diagnoses and antecedent stressors. Diagnoses of substance abuse and antisocial personality disorder occurred most often among suicides in persons less than 30 years of age and diagnoses of mood disorders and cognitive disorders most often among suicides in those aged 30 and above. Stressors associated with suicide in those under 30 were separation, rejection, unemployment, and legal troubles; illness stressors most often occurred among suicide victims over age 30.

Psychiatric Patients. Psychiatric patients' risk for suicide is 3 to 12 times that of nonpatients. The degree of risk varies, depending on age, sex, diagnosis, and inpatient or outpatient status. Male and female psychiatric patients who have at some time been inpatients have five and ten times higher suicide risks, respectively, than their counterparts in the general population. For male and female outpatients who have never been admitted to a hospital for psychiatric treatment, the suicide risks are three and four times greater, respectively, than those of their counterparts in the general population. The higher suicide risk for psychiatric patients who have been inpatients reflects that patients with severe mental disorders tend to be hospitalized—for example, patients with depressive disorder who require electroconvulsive therapy (ECT). The psychiatric diagnosis with greatest risk of suicide in both sexes is a mood disorder.

Those in the general population who commit suicide tend to be middle aged or older, but studies increasingly report that psychiatric patients who commit suicide tend to be relatively young. In one study, the mean age of male suicides was 29.5 years and that of women 38.4 years. The relative youthfulness in these suicide cases was partly attributed to two early-onset, chronic mental disorders—schizophrenia and recurrent major depressive disorder—which account for just over half of these suicides, and so reflects an age and diagnostic pattern found in most studies of psychiatric patient suicides.

A small, but significant, percentage of psychiatric patients who commit suicide do so while they are inpatients. Most of these do not kill themselves in the psychiatric ward itself, but on the hospital grounds, while on a pass or weekend leave, or when absent without leave. For both sexes, the suicide risk is highest in the first week of the psychiatric admission; after 3 to 5 weeks, inpatients have the same risk as the general population. Times of staff rotation, particularly of the psychiatric residents, are periods associated with inpatient suicides. Epidemics of inpatient suicides tend to be associated with periods of ideological change on the ward, staff disorganization, and staff demoralization.

The period after discharge from the hospital is also a time of increased suicide risk. A follow-up study of 5,000 patients discharged from an Iowa psychiatric hospital showed that in the first 3 months after discharge, the rate of suicide for female patients was 275 times that of all Iowa women; the rate of suicide for male patients was 70 times that of all Iowa men. Studies show that one-third or more of depressed patients who commit suicide do so within 6 months of leaving a hospital; presumably they have relapsed.

The main risk groups are patients with depressive disorders, schizophrenia, and substance abuse and patients who make repeated visits to the emergency room. Patients, especially those with panic disorder, who frequent emergency services, also have an increased suicide risk. Thus, mental health professionals working in emergency services must be well trained in assessing suicidal risk and making appropriate dispositions. They must also be aware of the need to contact patients at risk who fail to keep follow-up appointments.

DEPRESSIVE DISORDERS. Mood disorders are the ones most closely linked to suicide. Approximately 60 to 70 percent of suicide victims suffered a significant depression at the time of their deaths. The lifetime risk of death by suicide among individuals with bipolar disorder is approximately 15 to 20 percent, and suicide is more likely during depressed states rather than manic states.

More patients with depressive disorders commit suicide early in the illness rather than later; more depressed men than women commit suicide; and the chance of depressed persons' killing themselves increases if they are single, separated, divorced, widowed, or recently bereaved. Patients with depressive disorder in the community who commit suicide tend to be middle aged or older.

Social isolation enhances suicidal tendencies among depressed patients. This finding is in accord with the data from epidemiological studies showing that persons who commit suicide may be poorly integrated into society. Suicide among depressed patients is likely at the onset or the end of a depressive episode. As with other psychiatric patients, the months after discharge from a hospital are a time of high risk.

Regarding outpatient treatment, most depressed suicidal patients had a history of therapy; however, less than half were receiving psychiatric treatment at the time of suicide. Of those who were in treatment, studies have shown that some treatment was less than adequate. For example, most patients who received antidepressants were prescribed subtherapeutic doses of the medication. In other cases, however, treatment was considered optimal and other explanations must be sought (see below under discussion of unevitable).

SCHIZOPHRENIA. The suicide risk is high among patients with schizophrenia: Up to 10 percent die by committing suicide. In the United States, an estimated 4,000 patients with schizophrenia commit suicide each year. The onset of schizophrenia is typically in adolescence or early adulthood, and most of these patients who commit suicide do so during the first few years of their illness; therefore, those patients with schizophrenia who commit suicide are young.

Thus, the risk factors for suicide among patients with schizophrenia are young age, male gender, single marital status, a previous suicide attempt, a vulnerability to depressive symptoms, and a recent discharge from a hospital. Having three or four hospitalizations during their 20s probably undermines the social, occupational, and sexual adjustment of possibly suicidal patients with schizophrenia. Consequently, potential suicide victims are likely to be male, unmarried, unemployed, socially isolated, and living alone—perhaps in a single room. After discharge from their last hospitalization, they may experience a new adversity or return to ongoing difficulties. As a result, they become dejected, experience feelings of helplessness and hopelessness, reach a depressed state, and have, and eventually act on, suicidal ideas. Only a small percentage committed suicide because of hallucinated instructions or a need to escape persecutory delusions. Up to 50 percent of suicides among patients with schizophrenia occur during the first few weeks and months after discharge from a hospital; only a minority commit suicide while inpatients.

ALCOHOL DEPENDENCE. Up to 15 percent of all alcohol-dependent persons commit suicide. The suicide rate for those who are alcoholic is estimated to be about 270 per 100,000 annually; in the United States, between 7,000 and 13,000 alcohol-dependent persons commit suicide each year.

About 80 percent of all alcohol-dependent suicide victims are male, a percentage that largely reflects the sex ratio for alcohol dependence. Alcohol-dependent suicide victims tend to be white, middle aged, unmarried, friendless, socially isolated, and currently drinking. Up to 40 percent have made a previous suicide attempt. Up to 40 percent of all suicides by persons who are alcohol dependent occur within a year of the patient's last hospitalization; older alcohol-dependent patients are at particular risk during the post discharge period.

Studies show that many alcohol-dependent patients who eventually commit suicide are rated depressed during hospitalization and up to two-thirds are assessed as having mood disorder symptoms during the period in which they commit suicide. As many as 50 percent of all alcohol-dependent suicide victims have experienced the loss of a close, affectionate relationship during the previous year. Such interpersonal losses and other types of undesirable life events are probably brought about by the alcohol dependence and contribute to the development of the mood disorder symptoms, which are often present in the weeks and months before the suicide.

The largest group of male alcohol-dependent patients is composed of those with an associated antisocial personality disorder. Studies show that such patients are particularly likely to attempt suicide; to abuse other substances; to exhibit impulsive, aggressive, and criminal behaviors; and to be found among alcohol-dependent suicide victims.

OTHER SUBSTANCE DEPENDENCE. Studies in various countries have found an increased suicide risk among those who abuse substances. The suicide rate for persons who are heroin dependent is about 20 times the rate for the general population. Adolescent girls who use intravenous substances also have a high suicide rate. The availability of a lethal amount of substances, intravenous use, associated antisocial personality disorder, a chaotic lifestyle, and impulsivity are some of the factors that predispose substance-dependent persons to suicidal behavior, particularly when they are dysphoric, depressed, or intoxicated.

PERSONALITY DISORDERS. A high proportion of those who commit suicide have various associated personality difficulties or disorders. Having a personality disorder may be a determinant of suicidal behavior in several ways: by predisposing to major mental disorders such as depressive disorders or alcohol dependence; by leading to difficulties in relationships and social adjustment; by precipitating undesirable life events; by impairing the ability to cope with a mental or physical disorder; and by drawing persons into conflicts with those around them, including family members, physicians, and hospital staff members.

An estimated 5 percent of patients with antisocial personality disorder commit suicide. Suicide is three times more common among prisoners than among the general population. More than one-third of prisoner suicides have had past psychiatric treatment, and half have made a previous suicide threat or attempt, often in the previous 6 months.

ANXIETY DISORDER. Uncompleted suicide attempts are made by almost 20 percent of patients with a panic disorder and social phobia. If depression is an associated feature, however, the risk of completed suicide rises.

Previous Suicidal Behavior. A past suicide attempt is perhaps the best indicator that a patient is at increased risk of suicide. Studies show that about 40 percent of depressed patients who commit suicide have made a previous attempt. The risk of a second suicide attempt is highest within 3 months of the first attempt.

Depression is associated with both completed suicide and serious attempts at suicide. The clinical feature most often associated with the seriousness of the intent to die is a diagnosis of a depressive disorder. This is shown by studies that relate the clinical characteristics of suicidal patients with various measures of the medical seriousness of the attempt or of the intent to die. Also, intent-to-die scores correlate significantly with both suicide risk scores and the number and severity of depressive symptoms. Patients having high suicide intent are more often male, older, single or separated, and living alone than those with low intent. In other words, depressed patients who seriously attempt suicide more closely resemble suicide victims than they do suicide attempters.

ETIOLOGY

Sociological Factors: Durkheim's Theory

The first major contribution to the study of the social and cultural influences on suicide was made at the end of the 19th century by the French sociologist Emile Durkheim. In an attempt to explain statistical patterns, Durkheim divided suicides into three social categories: egoistic, altruistic, and anomic. Egoistic suicide applies to those who are not strongly integrated into any social group. The lack of family integration explains why unmarried persons are more vulnerable to suicide than married ones and why couples with children are the best protected group. Rural communities have more social integration than urban areas and, thus, fewer suicides. Protestantism is a less cohesive religion than Roman Catholicism, and so Protestants have a higher suicide rate than Catholics.

Altruistic suicide applies to those susceptible to suicide stemming from their excessive integration into a group, with suicide being the outgrowth of the integration—for example, a Japanese soldier who sacrifices his life in battle. Anomic suicide applies to persons whose integration into society is disturbed so that they cannot follow customary norms of behavior. Anomie explains why a drastic change in economic situation makes persons more vulnerable than they were before their change in fortune. In Durkheim's theory, anomie also refers to social instability and a general breakdown of society's standards and values.

Psychological Factors

Freud's Theory. Sigmund Freud offered the first important psychological insight into suicide. He described only one patient who made a suicide attempt, but he saw many depressed patients. In his paper "Mourning and Melancholia," Freud stated his belief that suicide represents aggression turned inward against an introjected, ambivalently cathected love object. Freud doubted that there would be a suicide without an earlier repressed desire to kill someone else.

Menninger's Theory. Building on Freud's ideas, Karl Menninger, in *Man against Himself,* conceived of suicide as inverted homicide because of a patient's anger toward another person. This retroflexed murder is either turned inward or used as an excuse for punishment. He also described a self-directed death instinct (Freud's concept of Thanatos) plus three components of hostility in suicide: the wish to kill, the wish to be killed, and the wish to die.

Recent Theories. Contemporary suicidologists are not persuaded that a specific psychodynamic or personality structure is associated with suicide. They believe that much can be learned about the psychodynamics of suicidal patients from their fantasies about what would happen and what the consequences would be if they commit suicide. Such fantasies often include wishes for revenge, power, control, or punishment; atonement, sacrifice, or restitution; escape or sleep; rescue, rebirth, reunion with the dead; or a new life. The suicidal patients most likely to act out suicidal fantasies may have lost a love object or received a narcissistic injury, may experience overwhelming affects like rage and guilt, or may identify with a suicide victim. Group dynamics underlie mass suicides such as those at Masada, at Jonestown, and by the Heaven's Gate cult.

Depressed persons may attempt suicide just as they appear to be recovering from their depression. A suicide attempt can cause a long-standing depression to disappear, especially if it fulfills a patient's need for punishment. Of equal relevance, many suicidal patients use a preoccupation with suicide as a way of fighting off intolerable depression and a sense of hopelessness. A study by Aaron Beck showed that hopelessness was one of the most accurate indicators of long-term suicidal risk.

Biological Factors

Diminished central serotonin plays a role in suicidal behavior. A group at the Karolinska Institute in Sweden first noted that low concentrations of the serotonin metabolite 5-hydroxyindoleacetic acid (5-HIAA) in the lumbar cerebrospinal fluid (CSF) were associated with suicidal behavior. This finding has been replicated many times and in different diagnostic groups. Postmortem neurochemical studies have reported modest decreases in serotonin itself or 5-HIAA in either the brainstem or the frontal cortex of suicide victims. Postmortem receptor studies have reported significant changes in presynaptic and postsynaptic serotonin binding sites in suicide victims. Together, these CSF, neurochemical, and receptor studies support the hypothesis that reduced central serotonin is associated with suicide. Recent studies also report some changes in the noradrenergic system of suicide victims.

Low concentrations of 5-HIAA in CSF also predict future suicidal behavior. For example, the Karolinska group examined completed suicide in a sample of 92 depressed patients who had attempted suicide. They found that 8 of the 11 patients who committed suicide within 1 year belonged to the subgroup with below-median concentrations of 5-HIAA in CSF. The suicide risk in that subgroup was 17 percent, compared with 7 percent among those with above-median concentrations of 5-HIAA in CSF. Also, the cumulative number of patient-months survived during the first year after attempted suicide was significantly lower in the subgroup with low 5-HIAA concentrations. The Karolinska group concluded that low 5-HIAA concentrations in CSF predict short-range suicide risk in the high-risk group of depressed patients who have attempted suicide. Low 5-HIAA concentrations in CSF have also been demonstrated in adolescents who kill themselves.

Genetic Factors

Suicidal behavior, as with other psychiatric disorders, tends to run in families. In psychiatric patients, a family history of suicide increases the risk of attempted suicide and that of completed suicide in most diagnostic groups. In medicine, the strongest evidence for involvement of genetic factors comes from twin and adoption studies and from molecular genetics. Such studies in suicide are reviewed below.

Twin Studies. A landmark study in 1991 investigated 176 twin pairs in which one twin had committed suicide. In nine of these twin pairs, both twins had committed suicide. Seven of these nine pairs concordant for suicide were found among the 62 monozygotic pairs, whereas two pairs concordant for suicide were found among the 114 dizygotic twin pairs. This twin group difference for concordance for suicide (11.3 vs. 1.8 percent) is statistically significant ($P < 0.01$).

Another study collected a group of 35 twin pairs in which one twin had committed suicide and the living co-twin was interviewed. Ten of the 26 living monozygotic co-twins had themselves attempted suicide, compared with 0 of the 9 living dizygotic co-twins ($P < 0.04$). Although monozygotic and dizygotic twins may have some differing developmental experiences, these results show that monozygotic twin pairs have significantly higher concordance for both suicide and attempted suicide, which suggests that genetic factors may play a role in suicidal behavior.

Danish-American Adoption Studies. The strongest evidence suggesting the presence of genetic factors in suicide comes from adoption studies carried out in Denmark. A screening of the registers of causes of death revealed that 57 of 5,483 adoptees in Copenhagen eventually committed suicide. They were matched with adopted controls. Searches of the causes of death revealed that 12 of the 269 biological relatives of these 57 adopted suicide victims had themselves committed suicide, compared with only 2 of the 269 biological relatives of the 57 adopted controls. This is a highly significant difference for suicide between the two groups of relatives. None of the adopting relatives of either the suicide or control group had committed suicide.

In a further study of 71 adoptees with mood disorder, adoptee suicide victims with a situational crisis or impulsive suicide attempt or both (particularly) had more biological relatives who had committed suicide than controls had. This led to the suggestion that a genetic factor lowering the threshold for suicidal behavior may lead to an inability to control impulsive behavior. Psychiatric disorders or environmental stress may serve "as potentiating mechanisms which foster or trigger the impulsive behavior, directing it toward a suicidal outcome."

Molecular Genetic Studies. Tryptophan hydroxylase (TPH) is an enzyme involved in the biosynthesis of serotonin. A polymorphism in the human *TPH* gene has been identified, with two alleles—U and L. Because low concentrations of 5-HIAA in CSF are associated with suicidal behavior, it was hypothesized that such individuals may have alterations in genes controlling serotonin synthesis and metabolism. It was found that impulsive alcoholics, who had low CSF 5-HIAA concentrations, had more LL and UL genotypes. Furthermore, a history of suicide attempts was significantly associated with TPH genotype in all the violent alcoholics; 34 of the 36 violent subjects who attempted suicide had either the UL or LL genotype. Thus, it was concluded that the presence of the L allele was associated with an increased risk of suicide attempts.

Also, a history of multiple suicide attempts was found most often in subjects with the LL genotype and to a lesser extent among those with the UL genotype. This led to the suggestion that the L allele was associated with repetitive suicidal behavior. The presence of one TPH*L allele may indicate a reduced capacity to hydroxylate tryptophan to 5-hydroxytryptophan in the synthesis of serotonin, producing low central serotonin turnover and, thus, a low concentration of 5-HIAA in CSF.

Parasuicidal Behavior. *Parasuicide* is a term introduced to describe patients who injure themselves by self-mutilation (e.g., cutting the skin), but who usually do not wish to die. Studies show that about 4 percent of all patients in psychiatric hospitals have cut themselves; the female-to-male ratio is almost 3 to 1. The incidence of self-injury in psychiatric patients is estimated to be more than 50 times that in the general population. Psychiatrists note that so-called cutters have cut themselves over several years. Self-injury is found in about 30 percent of all abusers of oral substances and 10 percent of all intravenous users admitted to substance-treatment units.

These patients are usually in their 20s and may be single or married. Most cut delicately, not coarsely, usually in private with a razor blade, knife, broken glass, or mirror. The wrists, arms, thighs, and legs are most commonly cut; the face, breasts, and abdomen are cut infrequently. Most persons who cut themselves claim to experience no pain and give reasons for this behavior such as anger at themselves or others, relief of tension, and the wish to die. Most are classified as having personality disorders and are significantly more introverted, neurotic, and hostile than controls. Alcohol abuse and other substance abuse are common, and most cutters have attempted suicide. Self-mutilation has been viewed as localized self-destruction, with mishandling of aggressive impulses caused by a person's unconscious wish to punish himself or herself or an introjected object.

PREDICTION

Clinicians must assess an individual patient's risk for suicide on the basis of a clinical examination. The predictive items associated with suicide risk are listed in Table 19.1–2. Suicide is grouped into high-risk–related and low-risk–related factors (Table 19.1–3). High-risk characteristics include more than 45 years of age, male gender, alcohol dependence (the suicide rate is 50 times higher in alcohol-dependent persons than in those who are not alcohol dependent), violent behavior, previous suicidal behavior, and previous psychiatric hospitalization.

It is important that questions about suicidal feelings and behaviors be asked, often directly. Asking depressed patients whether or not they have had thoughts of wanting to kill themselves does not plant the seed of suicide. To the contrary, it may be the first opportunity a patient has had to talk about suicidal ideation that may have been present for some time.

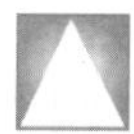

Table 19.1–2
Variables Enhancing Risk of Suicide among Vulnerable Groups

Adolescence and late life
Bisexual or homosexual gender identity
Criminal behavior
Cultural sanctions for suicide
Delusions
Disposition of personal property
Divorced, separated, or single marital status
Early loss or separation from parents
Family history of suicide
Hallucinations
Homicide
Hopelessness
Hypochondriasis
Impulsivity
Increasing agitation
Increasing stress
Insomnia
Lack of future plans
Lack of sleep
Lethality of previous attempt
Living alone
Low self-esteem
Male sex
Physical illness or impairment
Previous attempts that could have resulted in death
Protestant or nonreligious status
Recent childbirth
Recent loss
Repression as a defense
Secondary gain
Severe family pathology
Severe psychiatric illness
Sexual abuse
Signals of intent to die
Suicide epidemics
Unemployment
White race

From Slaby AE. Outpatient management of suicidal patients in the era of managed care. *Prim Psychiatry*. 1995;Apr:43.

The American Psychiatric Association (APA) developed practice guidelines for treating patients with suicidal behaviors.

TREATMENT

Most suicides among psychiatric patients are preventable, because evidence indicates that inadequate assessment or treatment is often associated with suicide. Some patients experience suffering so great and intense, or so chronic and unresponsive to treatment, that their eventual suicides may be perceived as inevitable. Such patients are relatively uncommon, however (see discussion of inevitable suicide below). Other patients have severe personality disorders, are highly impulsive, and commit suicide spontaneously, often when dysphoric, intoxicated, or both.

The evaluation for suicide potential involves a complete psychiatric history; a thorough examination of the patient's mental state; and an inquiry about depressive symptoms, suicidal thoughts, intents, plans, and attempts. A lack of future plans, giving away personal property, making a will, and having recently experienced a loss all imply increased risk of suicide.

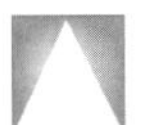

Table 19.1–3
Evaluation of Suicide Risk

Variable	High Risk	Low Risk
Demographic and social profile		
Age	Over 45 years	Below 45 years
Sex	Male	Female
Marital status	Divorced or widowed	Married
Employment	Unemployed	Employed
Interpersonal relationship	Conflictual	Stable
Family background	Chaotic or conflictual	Stable
Health		
Physical	Chronic illness	Good health
	Hypochondriac	Feels healthy
	Excessive substance intake	Low substance use
Mental	Severe depression	Mild depression
	Psychosis	Neurosis
	Severe personality disorder	Normal personality
	Substance abuse	Social drinker
	Hopelessness	Optimism
Suicidal activity		
Suicidal ideation	Frequent, intense, prolonged	Infrequent, low intensity, transient
Suicide attempt	Multiple attempts	First attempt
	Planned	Impulsive
	Rescue unlikely	Rescue inevitable
	Unambiguous wish to die	Primary wish for change
	Communication internalized (self-blame)	Communication externalized (anger)
	Method lethal and available	Method of low lethality or not readily available
Resources		
Personal	Poor achievement	Good achievement
	Poor insight	Insightful
	Affect unavailable or poorly controlled	Affect available and appropriately controlled
Social	Poor rapport	Good rapport
	Socially isolated	Socially integrated
	Unresponsive family	Concerned family

From Adam K. Attempted suicide. *Psychiatr Clin North Am.* 1985;8:183.

The decision to hospitalize a patient depends on diagnosis, depression severity and suicidal ideation, the patient's and the family's coping abilities, the patient's living situation, availability of social support, and the absence or presence of risk factors for suicide.

Inpatient versus Outpatient Treatment

Whether to hospitalize patients with suicidal ideation is the most important clinical decision to be made. Not all such patients require hospitalization; some can be treated on an outpatient basis. But the absence of a strong social support system, a history of impulsive behavior, and a suicidal plan of action are indications for hospitalization. To decide whether outpatient treatment is feasible, clinicians should use a straightforward clinical approach: Ask patients who are considered suicidal to agree to call when they become uncertain about their ability to control their suicidal impulses. Patients who can make such an agreement with a doctor with whom they have a relationship reaffirm the belief that they have sufficient strength to control such impulses and to seek help.

In return for a patient's commitment, clinicians should be available to the patient 24 hours a day. If a patient who is considered seriously suicidal cannot make the commitment, immediate emergency hospitalization is indicated; both the patient and the patient's family should be so advised. If, however, the patient is to be treated on an outpatient basis, the therapist should note the patient's home and work telephone numbers for emergency reference; occasionally, a patient hangs up unexpectedly during a late night call or gives only a name to the answering service. If the patient refuses hospitalization, the family must take the responsibility to be with the patient 24 hours a day.

According to Edwin S. Shneidman, a clinician has several practical preventive measures for dealing with a suicidal person: reducing the psychological pain by modifying the patient's stressful environment, enlisting the aid of the spouse, the employer, or a friend; building realistic support by recognizing that the patient may have a legitimate complaint; and offering alternatives to suicide.

Many psychiatrists believe that any patient who has attempted suicide, despite its lethality, should be hospitalized. Although most of these patients voluntarily enter a hospital, the danger to self is one of the few clear-cut indications currently acceptable in all states for involuntary hospitalization. In a hospital, patients can receive antidepressant or antipsychotic medications as indicated; individual therapy, group therapy, and family therapy are available, and patients receive the hospital's social support and sense of security. Other therapeutic measures depend on patients' underlying diagnoses. For example, if alcohol dependence is an associated problem, treatment must be directed toward alleviating that condition.

Although patients classified as acutely suicidal may have favorable prognoses, chronically suicidal patients are difficult to treat, and they exhaust the caretakers. Constant observation by special nurses, seclusion, and restraints cannot prevent suicide when a patient is resolute. ECT may be necessary for some severely depressed patients, who may require several treatment courses.

Ketamine is being used to treat acutely suicidal patients with some success. Infusions of ketamine are given daily or weekly with reports of a decrease in suicidal ideation. Results are not long-lasting however and the treatment is not FDA approved. Further studies are ongoing.

Useful measures for the treatment of depressed suicidal inpatients include searching patients and their belongings on arrival in the ward for objects that could be used for suicide and repeating the search at times of exacerbation of the suicidal ideation. Ideally, suicidally depressed inpatients should be treated on a locked ward where the windows are shatterproof, and the patient's room should be located near the nursing station to maximize observation by the nursing staff. The treatment team must assess how much to restrict the patient and whether to make regular checks or use continuous direct observation.

Vigorous treatment with antidepressant or antipsychotic medication should be initiated, depending on the underlying disorder. Some medications (e.g., risperidone [Risperdal]) have both antipsychotic and antidepressant effects and are useful when the patient has signs and symptoms of both psychosis and depression.

Supportive psychotherapy by a psychiatrist shows concern and may alleviate some of a patient's intense suffering. Some patients may be able to accept the idea that they are suffering from a recognized illness and that they will probably make a complete recovery. Patients should be dissuaded from making major life decisions while they are suicidally depressed, because such decisions are often morbidly determined and may be irrevocable. The consequences of such bad decisions can cause further anguish and misery when the patient has recovered.

Patients recovering from a suicidal depression are at particular risk. As the depression lifts, patients become energized and, thus, are able to put their suicidal plans into action (paradoxical suicide). A further complication is the activating effect of serotonergic drugs, such as fluoxetine (Prozac), which are effective antidepressants, especially with suicidally depressed patients. Such agents may improve psychomotor withdrawal, thus permitting the patient to act on preexisting suicidal impulses because they have more energy. Sometimes, depressed patients, with or without treatment, suddenly appear to be at peace with themselves because they have reached a secret decision to commit suicide. Clinicians should be especially suspicious of such a dramatic clinical change, which may portend a suicide attempt. Although rare, some patients lie to the psychiatrist about their suicidal intent, thus subverting the most careful clinical assessment.

A patient may commit suicide even when in the hospital. According to one survey, about 1 percent of all suicides were committed by patients who were being treated in general medical-surgical or psychiatric hospitals, but the annual suicide rate in psychiatric hospitals is only 0.003 percent.

Legal and Ethical Factors

Liability issues stemming from suicides in psychiatric hospitals frequently involve questions about a patient's rate of deterioration, the presence during hospitalization of clinical signs indicating risk, and psychiatrists' and staff members' awareness of, and response to, these clinical signs.

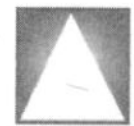

Table 19.1–4
Goals to Reduce Suicide

Promote awareness that suicide is a public health problem that is preventable
Develop broad-based support for suicide prevention
Develop and implement strategies to reduce the stigma associated with being a consumer of mental health, substance abuse, and suicide prevention services
Develop and implement suicide prevention programs
Promote efforts to reduce access to lethal means and methods of self-harm
Implement training for recognition of at-risk behavior and delivery of effective treatment
Develop and promote effective clinical and professional practices
Improve access to, and community linkages with, mental health and substance abuse services
Improve reporting and portrayals of suicidal behavior, mental illness, and substance abuse in the entertainment and news media
Promote and support research on suicide and suicide prevention
Improve and expand surveillance systems

In about half of the cases in which suicides occur while patients are on a psychiatric unit, a lawsuit results. Courts expect suicides to occur; do not require zero suicide rates, but do require periodic patient evaluation for suicidal risk, formulation of a treatment plan with a high level of security, and having staff members follow the treatment plan.

Currently, suicide and attempted suicide are variously viewed as a felony and a misdemeanor, respectively; in some states, the acts are not considered crimes but unlawful under common law and statutes. Aiding and abetting a suicide adds another dimension to the legal morass; some court decisions have held that although neither suicide nor attempted suicide is punishable, anyone who assists in the act may be punished.

National Strategy for Suicide Prevention

In 2001, Surgeon General David Satcher organized the National Strategy for Suicide Prevention, under the auspices of the National Institutes of Health (NIH). The National Strategy for Suicide Prevention has set specific goals and objectives to reduce suicide (Table 19.1–4).

The National Strategy for Suicide Prevention creates a framework for suicide prevention for the nation. It is designed to encourage and empower groups and individuals to work together. The stronger and broader the support and collaboration on suicide prevention, the greater the chance of success for this public health initiative. Suicide and suicidal behaviors can be reduced as the general public gains more understanding about (1) the extent to which suicide is a problem, (2) the ways in which it can be prevented, and (3) the roles individuals and groups can play in prevention efforts.

SUICIDES INVOLVING OTHER DEATHS

Victim-Precipitated Homicide

The phenomenon of using others, usually police, to kill oneself is well known to law enforcement personnel. Described by Marvin Wolfgang, the classic situation is exemplified by a person holding up a gas station or all-night store and brandishing a gun, which he threatens to use on the police when they arrive. They then shoot him, thinking that it is in self-defense. The psychology of such victims is not clear, except that they apparently believe this is the only way they can die.

A 25-year-old white divorced father of twin 3-year-old boys had been threatening to his wife, and, consequently, she had an order of restraint placed on him. Nonetheless, one evening, he went to her home, carrying a realistic-looking toy pistol in his pocket "to give her a scare." She refused to admit him, and, when he began to create a scene, she called the police. When three police officers arrived, he refused to leave, pointed the toy pistol at them and taunted them to shoot him. They drew their revolvers, ordered him to drop his "weapon" (which he did), and restrained him. They took him to a local emergency department, where the nurse's admission note read: "divorced and angry man threatened others with a toy pistol." The on-call psychiatrist saw him briefly; the patient denied suicidal or homicidal intent; and the psychiatrist concluded that it was safe to discharge him (as a "situational problem–marital issues"). The following day, he killed himself by using carbon monoxide. Although this was not a case of "completed" victim-precipitated homicide, hospital staff failed to perceive that this represented "attempted" victim-precipitated homicide and was an act of high risk. Noting that he "threatened others with a toy pistol" trivialized the gravity of pointing what appears to be a genuine gun at armed police and telling them to shoot. In effect, he had given up control over this life-threatening situation to the police, and only their self-restraint protected him from being killed that evening.

Murder-Suicides

Murder-suicides receive a disproportionate amount of attention because they are dramatic and tragic. Unless it is a pact between two truly consenting adults, such events testify to the enormous amount of aggression inherent in many suicides—in addition to the depression. Furthermore, what appears to be a pact is often, in fact, more of a coercion (or flat-out murder) than a true pact among equals. Pacts tend to be made more often by females or elderly couples.

Terrorist Suicides. Terrorist-bomber suicides represent a special category of murder-suicides, one in which there is no question of willingness of the victim's part and in which the victims are unknown to the perpetrators except in some generic, group sense (e.g., Jews, Westerners). Some suicide experts do not classify these as "true" suicides because they differ in so many domains from typical suicides (Table 19.1–5).

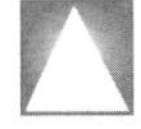

Table 19.1–5
Differences between Terrorist-Bomber Suicides and Typical Suicides

	Terrorist Bombers	Typical Suicides
Goal	To create terror	Death or escape
Expectations	Entry into paradise	Death
Motivation	Vengeance and mass murder	Sadness or escape
Psychological/ Psychiatric disorder	Rarely evident	Present in most cases

Although many terrorists are recruited from poorer and less-educated classes, it is surprising that a very large proportion of terrorist bombers are instead from middle-class, well-educated, and possibly less-fundamentalist populations. Because suicide means to take one's life, it is hard to exclude these terrorist deaths from such a classification.

INEVITABLE SUICIDE: A NEW PARADIGM

Not all suicides are preventable; some may be inevitable. In fact, over one-third of all completed suicides occur in persons who are receiving treatment for a psychiatric disorder, most commonly depression, bipolar disorder, or schizophrenia. It is not unreasonable to assume that some of those patients received the best care available, but their suicides could not be prevented.

Some clinicians believe that viewing certain suicides as being inevitable may lead to therapeutic nihilism, others feel it may cause both clinicians and patients to lose hope. But inevitable suicide can only be determined a posteriori, after all known facts of a particular suicide have been analyzed and synthesized. And if it cannot be predicted there is no reason for therapeutic nihilism or for treatment efforts to be influenced negatively; indeed viewing some suicides as possibly inevitable may encourage clinicians to increase their therapeutic zeal to prevent or postpone the inevitable from happening.

Certain criteria must be met for a particular suicide to be considered inevitable. Most important is a strong genetic history of suicide in one or more family members as well as heavy genetic loading for mental illness. Although a strong genetic diathesis for suicide is associated with completed suicide, it is not, in and of itself, sufficient. Other risk factors must also be present, numerous, and at the extreme end of profound pathology. Among the many risk factors (as described above) are a history of physical, emotional, or sexual abuse, especially during childhood; divorce; unemployment; male gender; recent discharge from a psychiatric hospital; prior suicide attempts; alcoholism or other substance abuse; a history of panic attacks; and the presence of a medical illness. Persistent suicidal thoughts, especially coupled with a plan, are particularly dangerous. As mentioned above, inevitability presumes that these risk factors are numerous, severe, and present in severe degrees.

Finally, to consider suicide inevitable the patient must have received the highest standard of treatment and that treatment must have failed. Inevitability assumes, among many other factors, that everything that could have been done was done—and done correctly—yet the patient died.

The case of Ernest Hemingway may be an example of inevitable suicide. Including Ernest, five people committed suicide in the Hemingway family. His father, brother, sister, and granddaughter all killed themselves. In addition, one of his sons suffered from major depression and underwent several courses of ECT during his lifetime.

Toward the end of his life, Hemingway had several hospitalizations for depression accompanied by suicide attempts. His last hospitalization was in 1961 at the Mayo Clinic, where he had been admitted in a severely depressed state after yet another suicide attempt. He was delusional (thinking that people were following him with deadly intent), had cognitive difficulties that prevented him from writing creatively, was physically ill with cardiovascular disease, and had been drinking heavily. He was hospitalized for 7 weeks, during which time he was treated with antidepressants, ECT, and psychotherapy. On June 26, 1961, he was discharged from the hospital. As Hemingway was leaving the hospital, in a last conversation, he was purported to have said, "You and I both know what I am going to do to myself one day."

On July 2, 1961, at 7:30 in the morning, 6 days after discharge, Hemingway put a shotgun to his head and pulled the trigger.

Hemingway had all of the biopsychosocial determinants of an inevitable suicide. There was heavy genetic loading for suicide, severe psychiatric disorder characterized by persecutory delusions, substance abuse, and other risk factors such as profound suicidal ideation and prior suicide attempts. In addition, Hemingway was the victim of severe childhood trauma, which increased his vulnerability to suicide.

As yet, there are insufficient data to predict the inevitability of a particular suicide. The paradigm of inevitability, however, may serve as a stimulus to increase root cause analysis into this phenomenon. The history of medicine is replete with disorders that inexorably led to death but which are now curable and suicide may one day join those ranks.

SURVIVING SUICIDE

To be a *suicide survivor* refers to those who have lost a loved one to suicide, not to someone who has attempted suicide but lived. The toll on suicide survivors appears greater than that by other deaths, mainly because the opportunities for guilt are so great. Survivors feel that the loved one intentionally and willfully took his or her life and that if only the survivor had done something differently, the decedent would still be here. Because the decedent cannot tell them otherwise, survivors are at the mercy of their often merciless consciences.

What is generally more accurate is that the decedents were not entirely willful but were themselves victims of their own genetic or lifetime experience predispositions to depression and suicide. For children, in particular, the loss of a parent to suicide feels like a shameful abandonment for which the child may blame himself or herself. For parents of children who have killed themselves, their grief is compounded not only by having lost a part of themselves, but also by having failed in what they perceive as their responsibility for the total feelings of their child. To provide mutual support, survivors of suicide groups have appeared throughout the United States, generally led by nonprofessional survivors themselves. Therapists who have lost patients to suicide comprise another survivor group—one too often ignored and unsupported, despite their own considerable suffering and sense of guilt and compounded by the specter of litigation potentially being brought to bear.

▲ 19.2 Psychiatric Emergencies in Adults

A psychiatric emergency is any disturbance in thoughts, feelings, or actions for which immediate therapeutic intervention is necessary. For a variety of reasons—such as the growing incidence of violence, the increased appreciation of the role of medical disease in altered mental status, and the epidemic of alcoholism and other substance use disorders—the number of emergency patients is on the rise. The widening scope of emergency psychiatry goes beyond general psychiatric practice to include such specialized problems as the abuse of substances, children, and spouses; violence in the form of suicide, homicide, and rape; and such social issues as homelessness, aging, competence, and acquired immune deficiency syndrome (AIDS). The emergency psychiatrist must be up to date on medicolegal issues and managed care. This section provides an overview of psychiatric emergencies in general and in adults in particular. Section 19.3 covers psychiatric emergencies in children.

TREATMENT SETTINGS

Most emergency psychiatric evaluations are done by nonpsychiatrists in a general medical emergency room setting, but specialized psychiatric services are increasingly favored. Regardless of the type of setting, an atmosphere of safety and security must prevail. An adequate number of staff members—including psychiatrists, nurses, aides, and social workers—must be present at all times. Additional personnel to help out in times of overcrowding should be available. Specific responsibilities, such as the use of restraints, should be clearly defined and practiced by the entire emergency team. Clear communication and lines of authority are essential. The organization of the staff into multidisciplinary teams is desirable.

Children and young adolescents are best served in a pediatric setting (see Section 19.3). Unless there is a risk of behavioral problems or of their leaving the hospital against advice, they need not be sent to the adult psychiatric emergency service.

Immediate access to the medical emergency room and to appropriate diagnostic services is necessary because one-third of medical conditions present with psychiatric manifestations. The full spectrum of psychopharmacological options should be available to the psychiatrist.

Violence in the emergency service cannot be condoned or tolerated. The code of conduct expected of staff members and patients must be posted and understood from the time of the patient's arrival in the emergency room. Security is best managed as a clinical issue by the clinical staff, not by law enforcement personnel. Whenever possible, agitated and threatening patients should be sequestered from the nonagitated. Seclusion and restraint rooms should be located close to the nursing station for close observation.

The entire staff must understand that patients in physical and emotional distress are fragile and that various expectations and fantasies, often unrealistic, influence their responses to treatment. For example, a man with impaired reality testing who is brought in by the police against his will may not understand that the clinician is interested in helping him. Other patients, influenced by previous unsatisfactory treatment experiences, may be hostile. A high percentage of patients believe that psychiatrists can read minds or are only interested in admitting patients to lock them away. Such people see little point in openly discussing their problems. Many people have an inaccurate understanding of their rights as patients. All clinical interventions must take those expectations and attitudes into account to minimize the possibility of misunderstanding and consequent problems.

EPIDEMIOLOGY

Psychiatric emergency rooms are used equally by men and women and more by single than by married persons. About 20 percent of these patients are suicidal, and about 10 percent are violent. The most common diagnoses are mood disorders (including depressive disorders and manic episodes), schizophrenia, and alcohol dependence. About 40 percent of all patients seen in psychiatric emergency rooms require hospitalization. Most visits occur during the night hours, but usage difference is not based on the day of the week or the month of the year. Contrary to popular belief, studies have not found that use of psychiatric emergency rooms increases during the full moon or the Christmas season.

EVALUATION

The primary goal of an emergency psychiatric evaluation is the timely assessment of the patient in crisis. To that end, the physician must make an initial diagnosis, identify the precipitating factors and immediate needs, and begin treatment or refer the patient to the most appropriate treatment setting. In view of the unpredictable nature of emergency room work, with many patients presenting both physical and emotional complaints, and in view of the limited space and the competition for ancillary services, a pragmatic approach to the patient is required. Sometimes, moving the patient out of the emergency room into the most appropriate diagnostic or treatment setting is best for the patient. Medical emergencies are generally better managed elsewhere in the system. Keeping the number of emergency patients in one place to a minimum reduces the chance of agitation and violence.

The standard psychiatric interview—consisting of a history, a mental status examination, and, when appropriate and depending on the rules of the emergency room, a full physical examination and ancillary tests—is the cornerstone of the emergency room evaluation. The emergency room psychiatrist, however, must be ready to introduce modifications as needed. For example, the emergency psychiatrist may have to structure the interview with a rambling manic patient, medicate or restrain an agitated patient, or forgo the usual rules of confidentiality to assess an adolescent's risk of suicide. In general, any strategy introduced in the emergency room to accomplish the goal of assessing the patient is considered consistent with good clinical practice as long as the rationale for the strategy is documented in the medical record.

What constitutes a psychiatric emergency is highly subjective. The emergency room has increasingly come to serve as an admitting area, a holding room, a detoxification center, and a private medical office. Such medical conditions as head traumas, acute intoxications, withdrawal states, and AIDS encephalopathies may present with acute psychiatric manifestations. The emergency psychiatrists must rapidly assess and distinguish the truly emergency psychiatric patients from those who are less acutely ill and from nonpsychiatric emergencies. A triage system using psychiatrists, nurses, and psychiatric social workers is an efficient and effective way to identify emergency, urgent, and nonurgent patients, who can then be prioritized for care.

In one model, every patient who comes to the emergency room is assessed by a triage nurse on arrival to ascertain the patient's chief complaint, clinical condition, and vital signs. The psychiatrist then briefly meets the patient and other significant people involved in the case—family members, emergency medical service technicians, and police—to assign the patient to one of the three categories—emergency, urgent, and nonurgent—or to refer the patient to an appropriate treatment setting, such as the medical emergency room. Having a senior clinician perform that task ensures rapid identification of the most urgent and troublesome cases, an appropriate allocation of resources, and an answer to the most common question heard in the emergency room: "When am I going to see a doctor?"

The psychiatrist then assigns clinical responsibility for each patient to the appropriate personnel. As the evaluation often stretches over more than one shift, a careful procedure to transfer responsibility and to pass along information from tour to tour must be built into the system by using visual, oral, and written communications. A request for old records should be made automatically for every patient who is assigned to the emergency room. Each emergency should be judged on its own merits, but information from previous records and from workers in the field and family members can be of crucial importance in assessing patients, especially patients who are psychotic, frightened, or otherwise unable or unwilling to cooperate in giving a good history.

A multilingual staff and a hospital language bank that lists bilingual staff members and other translation services should be readily available to the psychiatrist. The use of the patient's friends or family members as translators is not desirable because of the possibility of unconscious or deliberate denial or distortion of the clinical picture stemming from their involvement with the patient.

An initial assessment of the patient's total biopsychosocial needs is optimal, but the patient's emergency status, other patients waiting to be seen, and the constraints of the emergency room setting often make such a full assessment a moot point. At a minimum, the emergency evaluation should address the following five questions before any disposition is decided on: (1) Is it safe for the patient to be in the emergency room? (2) Is the problem organic, functional, or a combination? (3) Is the patient psychotic? (4) Is the patient suicidal or homicidal? (5) To what degree is the patient capable of self-care? Table 19.2–1 provides a general strategy for evaluating patients.

Patient Safety

Physicians should consider the question of the patient's safety before evaluating every patient. The answer must address the issues of the emergency room's physical layout, staffing patterns and communication, and patient population. Psychiatrists must then take stock of themselves: Are they in the proper frame of mind to conduct an evaluation? Do any issues in the case spark countertransference reactions? The self-assessment should go on throughout the evaluation. The physical and emotional safety of the patient takes priority over all other considerations. If verbal interventions fail or are contraindicated, the use of medication or restraints must be considered and, if necessary, ordered. Careful attention to the possible outbreak of agitation or disruptive behavior beyond acceptable limits is often the best insurance against untoward occurrences.

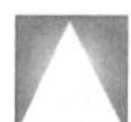

Table 19.2–1
General Strategy in Evaluating the Patient

I. Self-protection
A. Know as much as possible about the patients before meeting them.
B. Leave physical restraint procedures to those who are trained.
C. Be alert to risks of impending violence.
D. Attend to the safety of the physical surroundings (e.g., door access, room objects).
E. Have others present during the assessment if needed.
F. Have others in the vicinity.
G. Attend to developing an alliance with the patient (e.g., do not confront or threaten patients with paranoid psychoses).

II. Prevent harm
A. Prevent self-injury and suicide. Use whatever methods are necessary to prevent patients from hurting themselves during the evaluation.
B. Prevent violence toward others. During the evaluation, briefly assess the patient for the risk of violence. If the risk is deemed significant, consider the following options:
1. Inform the patient that violence is not acceptable.
2. Approach the patient in a nonthreatening manner.
3. Reassure, calm, or assist the patient's reality testing.
4. Offer medication.
5. Inform the patient that restraint or seclusion will be used if necessary.
6. Have teams ready to restrain the patient.
7. When patients are restrained, always closely observe them, and frequently check their vital signs. Isolate restrained patients from surrounding agitating stimuli. Immediately plan a further approach—medication, reassurance, medical evaluation.

III. Rule out organic mental disorders.

IV. Rule out impending psychosis.

Medical or Psychiatric?

The most important question for the emergency psychiatrist to address is whether the problem is medical, psychiatric, or both. Medical conditions—such as diabetes mellitus, thyroid disease, acute intoxications, withdrawal states, AIDS, and head traumas—can present with prominent mental status changes that mimic common psychiatric illnesses. Such conditions may be life-threatening if not treated promptly. Generally, the treatment of a medical illness is more definitive and the prognosis is better than for a functional psychiatric disorder. The psychiatrist must consider all casual possibilities.

Once patients are labeled psychiatric, their complaints may not be taken seriously by nonmental health professionals, however, and such patients' conditions may deteriorate, especially if they have a major Axis I syndrome. Because of such factors as deinstitutionalization, homelessness, and chronic alcoholism, the mentally ill are at great risk of tuberculosis, vitamin deficiencies, and other easily overlooked, but easily treated, conditions. Symptoms such as paranoia, internal preoccupation, and acute psychosis can make a routine medical diagnosis exceedingly difficult. Each patient must be assessed for the possibility that an organic illness is combined with an underlying psychiatric illness. A young man who comes to the emergency room intoxicated or in alcohol withdrawal two or three times a month may one day come with a subdural hematoma as a result of a fall. Table 19.2–2 lists features that point to a medical cause of a mental disorder.

Table 19.2–2
Features That Point to a Medical Cause of a Mental Disorder

Acute onset (within hours or minutes, with prevailing symptoms)
First episode
Geriatric age
Current medical illness or injury
Significant substance abuse
Nonauditory disturbances of perception
Neurological symptoms—loss of consciousness, seizures, head injury, change in headache pattern, change in vision
Classic mental status signs—diminished alertness, disorientation, memory impairment, impairment in concentration and attention, dyscalculia, concreteness
Other mental status signs—speech, movement, or gait disorders
Constructional apraxia—difficulties in drawing clock, cube, intersecting pentagons, Bender gestalt design

SPECIFIC INTERVIEW SITUATIONS

Psychosis

Whether the patient is psychotic refers not so much to the diagnosis as to the severity of the patient's symptoms and the degree of life disruption. The patient's degree of withdrawal from objective reality, level of affectivity, intellectual functioning, and degree of regression are other important parameters. Impairment in any of those areas may lead to difficulties in conducting an evaluation. Agitated, assaultive behavior or failure to comply with treatment recommendations may also result. A paranoid, hypervigilant patient may misperceive a staff member's offer of help as an attack and may lash out in self-defense. Command auditory hallucinations may cause a patient to deny symptoms and to throw prescriptions in the garbage immediately after leaving the emergency room. The psychiatrist should be alert to the complications that can arise with patients whose reality testing is impaired and the psychiatrist should modify the approach accordingly.

All communication with patients must be straightforward. All clinical interventions should be briefly explained in language the patient can understand. Psychiatrists should not assume that the patient trusts or believes them or even wants their help. Clinicians must be prepared to structure or to terminate an interview to limit the potential for agitation and regression.

Depression and Potentially Suicidal Patients

The clinician should always ask about suicidal ideas as part of every mental status examination, especially if the patient is depressed. The patient may not realize that such symptoms as waking during the night and increased somatic complaints are related to depressive disorders. The patient should be asked directly, "*Are you or have you ever been suicidal?*" "*Do you want to die?*" "*Do you feel so bad that you might hurt yourself?*" Eight of ten persons who eventually kill themselves give warnings of their intent. If the patient admits to a plan of action, that is a particularly dangerous sign. If a patient who has been threatening suicide becomes quiet and less agitated than before, that may be an ominous sign. The clinician

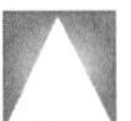

Table 19.2–3
History, Signs, and Symptoms of Suicidal Risk

Previous attempt or fantasized suicide
Anxiety, depression, exhaustion
Availability of means of suicide
Concern for effect of suicide on family members
Verbalized suicidal ideation
Preparation of a will, resignation after agitated depression
Proximal life crisis, such as mourning or impending surgery
Family history of suicide
Pervasive pessimism or hopelessness

should be especially concerned with the factors listed in Table 19.2–3.

A suicide note, a family history of suicide, or previous suicidal behavior on the part of the patient increases the risk of suicide. Evidence of impulsivity or of pervasive pessimism about the future also places the patient at risk. If the physician decides that the patient is in imminent risk for suicidal behavior, the patient must be hospitalized or otherwise protected. A difficult situation arises when the risk does not seem to be immediate but the potential for suicide is present as long as the patient remains depressed. If the psychiatrist decides not to hospitalize the patient immediately, the doctor should insist that the patient promise to call whenever the suicidal pressure mounts.

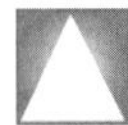

Table 19.2–4
Assessing and Predicting Violent Behavior

1. Signs of impending violence
   a. Very recent acts of violence, including property violence
   b. Verbal or physical threats (menacing)
   c. Carrying weapons or other objects that may be used as weapons (e.g., forks, ashtrays)
   d. Progressive psychomotor agitation
   e. Alcohol or drug intoxication
   f. Paranoid features in a psychotic patient
   g. Command violent auditory hallucinations—some but not all patients are at high risk
   h. Organic mental disorders, global or with frontal lobe findings; less commonly with temporal lobe findings (controversial)
   i. Patients with catatonic excitement
   j. Certain patients with mania
   k. Certain patients with agitated depression
   l. Personality disorder patients prone to rage, violence, or impulse dyscontrol
2. Assess the risk of violence
   a. Consider violent ideation, wish, intention, plan, availability of means, implementation of plan, wish for help.
   b. Consider demographics—sex (male), age (15–24), socioeconomic status (low), social supports (few).
   c. Consider past history: violence, nonviolent antisocial acts, impulse dyscontrol (e.g., gambling, substance abuse, suicide or self-injury, psychosis).
   d. Consider overt stressors (e.g., marital conflict, real or symbolic loss).

Violent Patients

Patients may be violent for many reasons, and the interview with a violent patient must attempt to ascertain the underlying cause of the violent behavior, because cause determines intervention. The differential diagnosis of violent behavior includes psychoactive substance-induced organic mental disorder, antisocial personality disorder, catatonic schizophrenia, medical infections, cerebral neoplasms, decompensating obsessive-compulsive personality disorder, dissociative disorders, impulse control disorders, sexual disorders, alcohol idiosyncratic intoxication, delusional disorder, paranoid personality disorder, schizophrenia, temporal lobe epilepsy, bipolar disorder, and uncontrollable violence secondary to interpersonal stress. The psychiatric interview must include questions that attempt to sort out the differential for violent behavior and questions directed toward the prediction of violence.

The best predictors of violent behavior are (1) excessive alcohol intake; (2) a history of violent acts, with arrests or criminal activity; and (3) a history of childhood abuse. Table 19.2–4 lists some of the most significant factors in assessing and predicting violence.

Rape and Sexual Abuse

Rape is the forceful coercion of an unwilling victim to engage in a sexual act, usually sexual intercourse, although anal intercourse and fellatio can also be acts of rape. As with other acts of violence, rape is a psychiatric emergency that requires immediate, appropriate intervention. Rape victims may suffer sequelae that persist for a lifetime. Rape is a life-threatening experience in which the victim has almost always been threatened with physical harm, often with a weapon. In addition to rape, other forms of sexual abuse include genital manipulation with foreign objects, infliction of pain, and forced sexual activity.

Most rapists are male, and most victims are female. Male rape does occur, however, often in institutions where men are detained (e.g., prisons). Women between the ages of 16 and 24 years are in the highest risk category, but female victims as young as 15 months and as old as 82 years have been raped. More than a third of all rapes are committed by rapists known to the victim, 7 percent by close relatives. A fifth of all rapes involve more than one rapist (gang rape).

Typical reactions in both rape and sexual abuse victims include shame, humiliation, anxiety, confusion, and outrage. Many victims wonder whether they are partly responsible and somehow invited the assault. In fact, victim behavior is less important in precipitating a rape than it is in precipitating a homicide or a robbery. Rape and sexual abuse victims are often confused after the assault. Clinicians should be reassuring, supportive, and nonjudgmental. Inform the patient about the availability of medical and legal services and about rape crisis centers that provide multidisciplinary services.

If possible, a female clinician should evaluate the patient, because the victim may find it easier to talk with a woman than with a man. The evaluation should take place in private. When rape or sexual abuse has not been acknowledged openly, it is usually because many victims hesitate to discuss the assault and thus avoid the topic. If the patient appears to be anxious when questioned about sexual history and avoids the discussion, it is important to validate the patient's avoidance. Recognize that the rape victim has undergone an unanticipated, life-threatening stress.

It is legally and therapeutically important to take a detailed and complete history of the attack.

With the patient's written consent, collect evidence, such as semen and pubic hair, that may be used to identify the rapist. Take photographs of the evidence, if possible. The medical record may be used as evidence in criminal proceedings; therefore, meticulous objective documentation of all aspects of the evaluation is essential.

TREATMENT OF EMERGENCIES

Psychotherapy

In an emergency psychiatric intervention, all attempts are made to help patients' self-esteem. Empathy is critical to healing in a psychiatric emergency. The acquired knowledge of how biogenetic, situational, developmental, and existential forces converge at one point in history to create a psychiatric emergency is tantamount to the maturation of skill in emergency psychiatry. Adjustment disorder in all age groups may result in tantrum-like outbursts of rage. These outbursts are particularly common in marital quarrels, and police are often summoned by neighbors distressed by the sounds of a violent altercation. Such family quarrels should be approached with caution, because they may be complicated by alcohol use and the presence of dangerous weapons. The warring couple frequently turns their combined fury on an unwary outsider. Wounded self-esteem is a major issue, and clinicians must avoid patronizing or contemptuous attitudes and try to communicate an attitude of respect and an authentic peacemaking concern.

In family violence, psychiatrists should note the special vulnerability of selected close relatives. A wife or husband may have a curious masochistic attachment to the spouse and can provoke violence by taunting and otherwise undermining a partner's self-esteem. Such relationships often end in the murder of the provoking partner and sometimes in the suicide of the other partner—the dynamics behind most so-called suicide pacts. As with many suicidal patients, many violent patients require hospitalization and usually accept the offer of inpatient care with a sense of relief.

More than one psychotherapist or type of psychotherapy is frequently used in emergency therapy. For example, a 28-year-old man, depressed and suicidal after a colostomy for intractable colitis, whose wife was threatening to leave him because of his irritability and their constant altercations, may be referred to a psychiatrist for supportive psychotherapy and antidepressant medication, to a marital therapist with his wife to improve their marital functioning, and to a colostomy support group to learn ways of coping with a colostomy. Emergency psychiatric clinicians are pragmatic; they use every necessary mode of therapeutic intervention available to resolve the crisis and facilitate value exploration and growth, with less concern than usual about diluting a therapeutic relationship. Emergency therapy emphasizes how various psychiatric modalities act synergistically to enhance recovery.

No single approach is appropriate for all persons in similar situations. What does a doctor say to a patient and a family experiencing a psychiatric emergency, such as a suicide attempt or a schizophrenic break? For some, a genetic rationale helps; the information that an illness has a strong biological component relieves some persons. For others, however, this approach underlines a lack of control and increases depression and anxiety. All feel helpless because neither the family nor the patient can alter the behavior to minimize the likelihood of recurrence. Some persons may benefit from an explanation of family or individual dynamics. Others only want someone to listen to them; in time, they reach their own understanding.

In an emergency situation as in any other psychiatric situation, when a clinician does not know what to say, the best approach is to listen. Persons in crisis reveal how much they need support, denial, ventilation, and words to conceptualize the meaning of their crisis and to discover paths to resolution.

Pharmacotherapy

The major indications for the use of psychotropic medication in an emergency room include violent or assaultive behavior, massive anxiety or panic, and extrapyramidal reactions, such as dystonia and akathisia as adverse effects of psychiatric drugs. Laryngospasm is a rare form of dystonia, and psychiatrists should be prepared to maintain an open airway with intubation if necessary.

Persons who are paranoid or in a state of catatonic excitement require tranquilization. Episodic outbursts of violence respond to haloperidol (Haldol), β-adrenergic receptor antagonists (β-blockers), carbamazepine (Tegretol), and lithium (Eskalith). If a history suggests a seizure disorder, use clinical studies to confirm the diagnosis and an evaluation to ascertain the cause. If the findings are positive, anticonvulsant therapy is initiated or appropriate surgery is provided (e.g., in the case of a cerebral mass). Conservative measures may suffice for intoxication from drugs of abuse. Sometimes, drugs such as haloperidol (5 to 10 mg every half-hour to an hour) are needed until a patient is stabilized. Benzodiazepines may be used instead of, or in addition to, antipsychotics (to reduce the antipsychotic dosage). When a recreational drug has strong anticholinergic properties, benzodiazepines are more appropriate than antipsychotics. Persons with allergic or aberrant responses to antipsychotics and benzodiazepines are treated with amobarbital (Amytal; 130 mg orally or intramuscularly [IM]), paraldehyde, or diphenhydramine (Benadryl; 50 to 100 mg orally or IM).

Violent, struggling patients are subdued most effectively with an appropriate sedative or antipsychotic. Diazepam (Valium; 5 to 10 mg) or lorazepam (Ativan; 2 to 4 mg) may be given slowly intravenously (IV) over 2 minutes. Clinicians must give IV medication with great care to avoid respiratory arrest. Patients who require IM medication can be sedated with haloperidol (5 to 10 mg IM). If the furor is caused by alcohol or is part of a postseizure psychomotor disturbance, the sleep produced by a relatively small amount of an IV medication may go on for hours. On awakening, patients are often entirely alert and rational and typically have complete amnesia about the violent episode.

If the disturbance is part of an ongoing psychotic process and returns as soon as the IV medication wears off, continuous medication may be given. It is sometimes better to use small IM or oral doses at half-hour to 1-hour intervals (e.g., haloperidol, 2 to 5 mg, or diazepam, 20 mg) until the patient is controlled than to use large dosages initially, which can result in an overmedicated

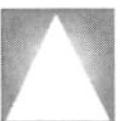

Table 19.2–5
Use of Restraints

Preferably five or a minimum of four persons should be used to restrain the patient. Leather restraints are the safest and surest type of restraint.
Explain to the patient why he or she is going into restraints.
A staff member should always be visible and reassuring the patient who is being restrained. Reassurance helps alleviate the patient's fear of helplessness, impotence, and loss of control.
Patients should be restrained with legs spread-eagled and one arm restrained to one side and the other arm restrained over the patient's head.
Restraints should be placed so that intravenous fluids can be given, if necessary.
The patient's head is raised slightly to decrease the patient's feelings of vulnerability and to reduce the possibility of aspiration.
The restraints should be checked periodically for safety and comfort.
After the patient is in restraints, the clinician begins treatment, using verbal intervention.
Even in restraints, most patients still take antipsychotic medication in concentrated form.
After the patient is under control, one restraint at a time should be removed at 5-minute intervals until the patient has only two restraints on. Both of the remaining restraints should be removed at the same time, because it is inadvisable to keep a patient in only one restraint.
Always thoroughly document the reason for the restraints, the course of treatment, and the patient's response to treatment while in restraints.

Data from Dubin WR, Weiss KJ. Emergency psychiatry. In: Michaels R, Cooper A, Guze SB, et al., eds. *Psychiatry*. Vol 2. Philadelphia: Lippincott; 1991.

patient. As the disturbed behavior is brought under control, successively smaller and less frequent doses should be used. During the preliminary treatment, a patient's blood pressure and other vital signs should be monitored.

Restraints

Restraints are used when patients are so dangerous to themselves or others that they pose a severe threat that cannot be controlled in any other way. Patients may be restrained temporarily to receive medication or for long periods if medication cannot be used. Usually, patients in restraints quiet down after a time. On a psychodynamic level, such patients may even welcome the control of their impulses provided by restraints. Table 19.2–5 provides a summary of the use of restraints.

Disposition

In some cases, the usual option of admitting or discharging the patient is not considered optimal. Suspected toxic psychoses, brief decompensations in a patient with a personality disorder, and adjustment reactions to traumatic events, for example, may be best managed in an extended-observation setting. Allowing the patient additional time in a secure environment can result in sufficient improvement or clarification of the issues to make traditional inpatient treatment unnecessary. It can also spare the patient the trauma and stigma of a psychiatric admission and can free up bed space for needier patients. Crisis intervention for victims of rape and other traumas can also be done in an extended-observation setting.

When the decision is to admit the patient to the hospital, it is preferable to do so on a voluntary basis. Allowing patients that option gives them a sense of control over their lives and of participation in the treatment decisions. Patients who clearly meet involuntary admission criteria on the basis of dangerousness to themselves or to others cannot leave the hospital without further review and can always be converted to involuntary status if warranted.

Because the initial evaluation is often inconclusive, definitive treatment is best deferred until the patient can be further assessed in the inpatient unit or in the outpatient department. When the diagnosis is clear, however, and the patient's response to previous treatment is known, nothing is gained by delay. For example, a patient with chronic schizophrenia that has decompensated after discontinuing the usual regimen of antipsychotic medication is best served by prompt resumption of treatment.

Even if patients feel comfortable coming to the emergency room in times of need, the emergency psychiatrist should always direct or redirect them to the most appropriate treatment setting. Patients in the psychopharmacology clinic who have missed their regular appointments should be given only enough medication to sustain them until they can be seen in the clinic. Feedback to others treating them should be a matter of course.

The emergency room is often the gateway to the department of psychiatry or the general hospital. First impressions carry a great deal of weight. The kind of attention and concern shown to patients on arrival in the emergency room strongly affects how they will respond to staff members and treatment recommendations and even their treatment compliance long after they have left the emergency room.

Documentation

In the interests of good care, respect for patients' rights, cost control, and medicolegal concerns, documentation has become a central focus for the emergency physician. The medical record should convey a concise picture of the patient, highlighting all pertinent positive and negative findings. Gaps in information and their reason should be mentioned. The names and the telephone numbers of interested parties should be noted. A provisional diagnosis or differential diagnosis must be made. An initial treatment plan or recommendations should clearly follow from the findings of the patient's history, mental status examination and other diagnostic tests, and the medical evaluation. The writing must be legible. The emergency physician has unusual latitude under the law to perform an adequate initial assessment; however, all interventions and decisions must be thought out, discussed, and documented in the patient's record.

Specific Psychiatric Emergencies

Table 19.2–6 outlines common psychiatric emergencies in alphabetical order. Readers are referred to the index and to specific chapters of this textbook for a thorough discussion of each disorder.

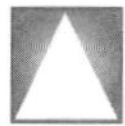

Table 19.2–6
Common Psychiatric Emergencies

Syndrome	Emergency Manifestations	Treatment Issues
Abuse of child or adult	Signs of physical trauma	Management of medical problems; psychiatric evaluation; report to authorities
Acquired immune deficiency syndrome (AIDS)	Changes in behavior secondary to organic causes; changes in behavior secondary to fear and anxiety; suicidal behavior	Management of neurological illness; management of psychological concomitants; reinforcement of social support
Adolescent crises	Suicidal attempts and ideation; substance abuse, truancy, trouble with law, pregnancy, running away; eating disorders; psychosis	Evaluation of suicidal potential, extent of substance abuse, family dynamics; crisis-oriented family and individual therapy; hospitalization if necessary; consultation with appropriate extrafamilial authorities
Agoraphobia	Panic; depression	Alprazolam (Xanax), 0.25 mg to 2 mg; propranolol (Inderal); antidepressant medication
Agranulocytosis (clozapine [Clozaril]-induced)	High fever, pharyngitis, oral and perianal ulcerations	Discontinue medication immediately; administer granulocyte colony-stimulating factor
Akathisia	Agitation, restlessness, muscle discomfort; dysphoria	Reduce antipsychotic dosage; propranolol (30 to 120 mg a day); benzodiazepines; diphenhydramine (Benadryl) orally or IV; benztropine (Cogentin) IM
Alcohol-related emergencies		
Alcohol delirium	Confusion, disorientation, fluctuating consciousness and perception, autonomic hyperactivity; may be fatal	Chlordiazepoxide (Librium); haloperidol (Haldol) for psychotic symptoms may be added if necessary
Alcohol intoxication	Disinhibited behavior, sedation at high doses	With time and protective environment, symptoms abate
Alcohol persisting amnestic disorder	Confusion, loss of memory even for all personal identification data	Hospitalization; hypnosis; amobarbital (Amytal) interview; rule out organic cause
Alcohol persisting dementia	Confusion, agitation, impulsivity	Rule out other causes for dementia; no effective treatment; hospitalization if necessary
Alcohol psychotic disorder with hallucinations	Vivid auditory (at times visual) hallucinations with affect appropriate to content (often fearful); clear sensorium	Haloperidol for psychotic symptoms
Alcohol seizures	Grand mal seizures; rarely status epilepticus	Diazepam (Valium), phenytoin (Dilantin); prevent by using chlordiazepoxide (Librium) during detoxification
Alcohol withdrawal	Irritability, nausea, vomiting, insomnia, malaise, autonomic hyperactivity, shakiness	Fluid and electrolytes maintained; sedation with benzodiazepines; restraints; monitoring of vital signs; 100 mg thiamine IM
Idiosyncratic alcohol intoxication	Marked aggressive or assaultive behavior	Generally no treatment required other than protective environment
Korsakoff's syndrome	Alcohol stigmata, amnesia, confabulation	No effective treatment; institutionalization often needed
Wernicke's encephalopathy	Oculomotor disturbances, cerebellar ataxia; mental confusion	Thiamine, 100 mg IV or IM, with $MgSO_4$ given before glucose loading
Amphetamine (or related substance) intoxication	Delusions, paranoia; violence; depression (from withdrawal); anxiety, delirium	Antipsychotics; restraints; hospitalization if necessary; no need for gradual withdrawal; antidepressants may be necessary
Anorexia nervosa	Loss of 25% of body weight of the norm for age and sex	Hospitalization; electrocardiogram (ECG), fluid and electrolytes; neuroendocrine evaluation
Anticholinergic intoxication	Psychotic symptoms, dry skin and mouth, hyperpyrexia, mydriasis, tachycardia, restlessness, visual hallucinations	Discontinue drug, IV physostigmine (Antilirium), 0.5 to 2 mg, for severe agitation or fever, benzodiazepines; antipsychotics contraindicated
Anticonvulsant intoxication	Psychosis; delirium	Dosage of anticonvulsant is reduced
Benzodiazepine intoxication	Sedation, somnolence, and ataxia	Supportive measures; flumazenil (Romazicon), 7.5 to 45 mg a day, titrated as needed, should be used only by skilled personnel with resuscitative equipment available
Bereavement	Guilt feelings, irritability; insomnia; somatic complaints	Must be differentiated from major depressive disorder; antidepressants not indicated; benzodiazepines for sleep; encouragement of ventilation
Borderline personality disorder	Suicidal ideation and gestures; homicidal ideations and gestures; substance abuse; micropsychotic episodes; burns, cut marks on body	Suicidal and homicidal evaluation (if great, hospitalization); small dosages of antipsychotics; clear follow-up plan
Brief psychotic disorder	Emotional turmoil, extreme lability; acutely impaired reality testing after obvious psychosocial stress	Hospitalization often necessary; low dosage of antipsychotics may be necessary but often resolves spontaneously

Table 19.2–6
Common Psychiatric Emergencies (Continued)

Syndrome	Emergency Manifestations	Treatment Issues
Bromide intoxication	Delirium; mania; depression; psychosis	Serum levels obtained (>50 mg a day); bromide intake discontinued; large quantities of sodium chloride IV or orally; if agitation, paraldehyde or antipsychotic is used
Caffeine intoxication	Severe anxiety, resembling panic disorder; mania; delirium; agitated depression; sleep disturbance	Cessation of caffeine-containing substances; benzodiazepines
Cannabis intoxication	Delusions; panic; dysphoria; cognitive impairment	Benzodiazepines and antipsychotics as needed; evaluation of suicidal or homicidal risk; symptoms usually abate with time and reassurance
Catatonic schizophrenia	Marked psychomotor disturbance (either excitement or stupor); exhaustion; can be fatal	Rapid tranquilization with antipsychotics; monitor vital signs; amobarbital may release patient from catatonic mutism or stupor but can precipitate violent behavior
Cimetidine psychotic disorder	Delirium; delusions	Reduce dosage or discontinue drug
Clonidine withdrawal	Irritability; psychosis; violence; seizures	Symptoms abate with time, but antipsychotics may be necessary; gradual lowering of dosage
Cocaine intoxication and withdrawal	Paranoia and violence; severe anxiety; manic state; delirium: schizophreniform psychosis; tachycardia, hypertension, myocardial infarction, cerebrovascular disease; depression and suicidal ideation	Antipsychotics and benzodiazepines; antidepressants or electroconvulsive therapy (ECT) for withdrawal depression if persistent; hospitalization
Delirium	Fluctuating sensorium; suicidal and homicidal risk; cognitive clouding; visual, tactile, and auditory hallucinations; paranoia	Evaluate all potential contributing factors and treat each accordingly; reassurance, structure, clues to orientation; benzodiazepines and low-dosage, high-potency antipsychotics must be used with extreme care because of their potential to act paradoxically and increase agitation
Delusional disorder	Most often brought into emergency room involuntarily; threats directed toward others	Antipsychotics if patient will comply (IM if necessary); intensive family intervention; hospitalization if necessary
Dementia	Unable to care for self; violent outbursts; psychosis; depression and suicidal ideation; confusion	Small dosages of high-potency antipsychotics; clues to orientation; organic evaluation, including medication use; family intervention
Depressive disorders	Suicidal ideation and attempts; self-neglect; substance abuse	Assessment of danger to self; hospitalization if necessary, nonpsychiatric causes of depression must be evaluated
L-Dopa intoxication	Mania; depression; schizophreniform disorder, may induce rapid cycling in patients with bipolar I disorder	Lower dosage or discontinue drug
Dystonia, acute	Intense involuntary spasm of muscles of neck, tongue, face, jaw, eyes, or trunk	Decrease dosage of antipsychotic; benztropine or diphenhydramine IM
Group hysteria	Groups of people exhibit extremes of grief or other disruptive behavior	Group is dispersed with help of other health care workers; ventilation, crisis-oriented therapy; if necessary, small dosages of benzodiazepines
Hallucinogen-induced psychotic disorder with hallucinations	Symptom picture is result of interaction of type of substance, dose taken, duration of action, user's premorbid personality, setting; panic; agitation; atropine psychosis	Serum and urine screens; rule out underlying medical or mental disorder; benzodiazepines (2 to 20 mg) orally; reassurance and orientation; rapid tranquilization; often responds spontaneously
Homicidal and assaultive behavior	Marked agitation with verbal threats	Seclusion, restraints, medication
Homosexual panic	Not seen with men or women who are comfortable with their sexual orientation; occurs in those who adamantly deny having any homoerotic impulses; impulses are aroused by talk, a physical overture, or play among same-sex friends, such as wrestling, sleeping together, or touching each other in a shower or hot tub; panicked person sees others as sexually interested in him or her and defends against them	Ventilation, environmental structuring, and, in some instances, medication for acute panic (e.g., alprazolam, 0.25 to 2 mg) or antipsychotics may be required; opposite-sex clinician should evaluate the patient whenever possible, and the patient should not be touched save for the routine examination; patients have attacked physicians who were examining an abdomen or performing a rectal examination (e.g., on a man who harbors thinly veiled unintegrated homosexual impulses)

(*continued*)

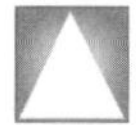

Table 19.2–6
Common Psychiatric Emergencies (Continued)

Syndrome	Emergency Manifestations	Treatment Issues
Hypertensive crisis	Life-threatening hypertensive reaction secondary to ingestion of tyramine-containing foods in combination with monoamine oxidase inhibitors (MAOIs); headache, stiff neck, sweating, nausea, vomiting	α-Adrenergic blockers (e.g., phentolamine [Rogitine]); nifedipine (Procardia) 10 mg orally; chlorpromazine (Thorazine); make sure symptoms are not secondary to hypotension (side effect of MAOIs alone)
Hyperthermia	Extreme excitement or catatonic stupor or both; extremely elevated temperature; violent hyperagitation	Hydrate and cool; may be drug reaction, so discontinue any drug; rule out infection
Hyperventilation	Anxiety, terror, clouded consciousness; giddiness, faintness; blurring vision	Shift alkalosis by having patient breathe into paper bag; patient education; antianxiety agents
Hypothermia	Confusion; lethargy; combativeness; low body temperature and shivering; paradoxical feeling of warmth	IV fluids and rewarming, cardiac status must be carefully monitored; avoidance of alcohol
Incest and sexual abuse of child	Suicidal behavior; adolescent crises; substance abuse	Corroboration of charge, protection of victim; contact social services; medical and psychiatric evaluation; crisis intervention
Insomnia	Depression and irritability; early morning agitation; frightening dreams; fatigue	Hypnotics only in short term (e.g., triazolam [Halcion], 0.25 to 0.5 mg, at bedtime); treat any underlying mental disorder; rules of sleep hygiene
Intermittent explosive disorder	Brief outbursts of violence; periodic episodes of suicide attempts	Benzodiazepines or antipsychotics for short term; long-term evaluation with computed tomography (CT) scan, sleep-deprived electroencephalogram (EEG), glucose tolerance curve
Jaundice	Uncommon complication of low-potency phenothiazine use (e.g., chlorpromazine)	Change drug to low dosage of a low-potency agent in a different class
Leukopenia and agranulocytosis	Side effects within the first 2 months of treatment with antipsychotics	Patient should call immediately for sore throat, fever, etc., and obtain immediate blood count; discontinue drug; hospitalize if necessary
Lithium (Eskalith) toxicity	Vomiting; abdominal pain; profuse diarrhea; severe tremor, ataxia; coma; seizures; confusion; dysarthria; focal neurological signs	Lavage with wide-bore tube; osmotic diuresis; medical consultation; may require intensive care unit treatment
Major depressive episode with psychotic features	Major depressive episode symptoms with delusions; agitation, severe guilt; ideas of reference; suicide and homicide risk	Antipsychotics plus antidepressants; evaluation of suicide and homicide risk; hospitalization and ECT if necessary
Manic episode	Violent, impulsive behavior; indiscriminate sexual or spending behavior; psychosis; substance abuse	Hospitalization; restraints if necessary; rapid tranquilization with antipsychotics; restoration of lithium levels
Marital crises	Precipitant may be discovery of an extramarital affair, onset of serious illness, announcement of intent to divorce, or problems with children or work; one or both members of the couple may be in therapy or may be psychiatrically ill; one spouse may be seeking hospitalization for the other	Each should be questioned alone regarding extramarital affairs, consultations with lawyers regarding divorce, and willingness to work in crisis-oriented or long-term therapy to resolve the problem; sexual, financial, and psychiatric treatment histories from both, psychiatric evaluation at the time of presentation; may be precipitated by onset of untreated mood disorder or affective symptoms caused by medical illness or insidious-onset dementia; referral for management of the illness reduces immediate stress and enhances the healthier spouse's coping capacity; children may give insights available only to someone intimately involved in the social system
Migraine	Throbbing, unilateral headache	Sumatriptan (Imitrex) 6 mg IM
Mitral valve prolapse	Associated with panic disorder; dyspnea and palpitations; fear and anxiety	Echocardiogram; alprazolam or propranolol
Neuroleptic malignant syndrome	Hyperthermia; muscle rigidity; autonomic instability; parkinsonian symptoms; catatonic stupor; neurological signs; 10–30% fatality; elevated creatine phosphokinase (CPK)	Discontinue antipsychotic; IV dantrolene (Dantrium); bromocriptine (Parlodel) orally; hydration and cooling; monitor CPK levels
Nitrous oxide toxicity	Euphoria and light-headedness	Symptoms abate without treatment within hours of use
Nutmeg intoxication	Agitation; hallucinations; severe headaches; numbness in extremities	Symptoms abate within hours of use without treatment
Opioid intoxication and withdrawal	Intoxication can lead to coma and death; withdrawal is not life-threatening	IV naloxone, narcotic antagonist; urine and serum screens; psychiatric and medical illnesses (e.g., AIDS) may complicate picture

Table 19.2–6
Common Psychiatric Emergencies (Continued)

Syndrome	Emergency Manifestations	Treatment Issues
Panic disorder	Panic, terror; acute onset	Must differentiate from other anxiety-producing disorders, both medical and psychiatric; ECG to rule out mitral valve prolapse; propranolol (10 to 30 mg); alprazolam (0.25 to 2.0 mg); long-term management may include an antidepressant
Paranoid schizophrenia	Command hallucinations; threat to others or themselves	Rapid tranquilization; hospitalization; long-acting depot medication; threatened persons must be notified and protected
Parkinsonism	Stiffness, tremor, bradykinesia, flattened affect, shuffling gait, salivation, secondary to antipsychotic medication	Oral antiparkinsonian drug for 4 weeks to 3 months; decrease dosage of the antipsychotic
Perioral (rabbit) tremor	Perioral tumor (rabbit-like facial grimacing) usually appearing after long-term therapy with antipsychotics	Decrease dosage or change to a medication in another class
Phencyclidine (or phencyclidine-like intoxication)	Paranoid psychosis; can lead to death; acute danger to self and others	Serum and urine assay; benzodiazepines may interfere with excretion; antipsychotics may worsen symptoms because of anticholinergic side effects; medical monitoring and hospitalization for severe intoxication
Phenelzine-induced psychotic disorder	Psychosis and mania in predisposed people	Reduce dosage or discontinue drug
Phenylpropanolamine toxicity	Psychosis; paranoia; insomnia; restlessness; nervousness; headache	Symptoms abate with dosage reduction or discontinuation (found in over-the-counter diet aids and oral and nasal decongestants)
Phobias	Panic, anxiety; fear	Treatment same as for panic disorder
Photosensitivity	Easy sunburning secondary to use of antipsychotic medication	Patient should avoid strong sunlight and use high-level sunscreens
Pigmentary retinopathy	Reported with dosages of thioridazine (Mellaril) of 800 mg a day or above	Remain below 800 mg a day of thioridazine
Postpartum psychosis	Childbirth can precipitate schizophrenia, depression, reactive psychoses, mania, and depression; affective symptoms are most common; suicide risk is reduced during pregnancy but increased in the postpartum period	Danger to self and others (including infant) must be evaluated and proper precautions taken; medical illness presenting with behavioral aberrations is included in the differential diagnosis and must be sought and treated; care must be paid to the effects on father, infant, grandparents, and other children
Posttraumatic stress disorder	Panic, terror; suicidal ideation; flashbacks	Reassurance; encouragement of return to responsibilities; avoid hospitalization if possible to prevent chronic invalidism; monitor suicidal ideation
Priapism (trazodone [Desyrel]-induced)	Persistent penile erection accompanied by severe pain	Intracorporeal epinephrine; mechanical or surgical drainage
Propranolol toxicity	Profound depression; confusional states	Reduce dosage or discontinue drug; monitor suicidality
Rape	Not all sexual violations are reported; silent rape reaction is characterized by loss of appetite, sleep disturbance, anxiety, and, sometimes, agoraphobia; long periods of silence, mounting anxiety, stuttering, blocking, and physical symptoms during the interview when the sexual history is taken; fear of violence and death and of contracting a sexually transmitted disease or being pregnant	Rape is a major psychiatric emergency; victim may have enduring patterns of sexual dysfunction; crisis-oriented therapy, social support, ventilation, reinforcement of healthy traits, and encouragement to return to the previous level of functioning as rapidly as possible; legal counsel; thorough medical examination and tests to identify the assailant (e.g., obtaining samples of pubic hairs with a pubic hair comb, vaginal smear to identify blood antigens in semen); if a woman, methoxyprogesterone or diethylstilbestrol orally for 5 days to prevent pregnancy; if menstruation does not commence within 1 week of cessation of the estrogen, all alternatives to pregnancy, including abortion, should be offered; if the victim has contracted a venereal disease, appropriate antibiotics; witnessed written permission is required for the physician to examine, photograph, collect specimens, and release information to the authorities; obtain consent, record the history in the patient's own words, obtain required tests, record the results of the examination, save all clothing, defer diagnosis, and provide protection against disease, psychic trauma, and pregnancy; men's and women's responses to rape affectively are reported similarly, although men are more hesitant to talk about homosexual assault for fear they will be assumed to have consented

(continued)

Table 19.2–6
Common Psychiatric Emergencies (Continued)

Syndrome	Emergency Manifestations	Treatment Issues
Reserpine intoxication	Major depressive episodes; suicidal ideation; nightmares	Evaluation of suicidal ideation; lower dosage or change drug; antidepressants of ECT may be indicated
Schizoaffective disorder	Severe depression; manic symptoms; paranoia	Evaluation of dangerousness to self or others; rapid tranquilization if necessary; treatment of depression (antidepressants alone can enhance schizophrenic symptoms); use of antimanic agents
Schizophrenia	Extreme self-neglect; severe paranoia; suicidal ideation or assaultiveness; extreme psychotic symptoms	Evaluation of suicidal and homicidal potential; identification of any illness other than schizophrenia; rapid tranquilization
Schizophrenia in exacerbation	Withdrawn; agitation; suicidal and homicidal risk	Suicide and homicide evaluation; screen for medical illness; restraints and rapid tranquilization if necessary; hospitalization if necessary; reevaluation of medication regimen
Sedative, hypnotic, or anxiolytic intoxication and withdrawal	Alterations in mood, behavior, thought—delirium; derealization and depersonalization; untreated, can be fatal; seizures	Naloxone (Narcan) to differentiate from opioid intoxication; slow withdrawal with phenobarbital (Luminal) or sodium thiopental or benzodiazepine; hospitalization
Seizure disorder	Confusion; anxiety; derealization and depersonalization; feelings of impending doom; gustatory or olfactory hallucinations; fugue-like state	Immediate EEG; admission and sleep-deprived and 24-hour EEG; rule out pseudoseizures; anticonvulsants
Substance withdrawal	Abdominal pain; insomnia, drowsiness; delirium; seizures; symptoms of tardive dyskinesia may emerge; eruption of manic or schizophrenic symptoms	Symptoms of psychotropic drug withdrawal disappear with time or disappear with reinstitution of the substance; symptoms of antidepressant withdrawal can be successfully treated with anticholinergic agents, such as atropine; gradual withdrawal of psychotropic substances over 2 to 4 weeks generally obviates development of symptoms
Sudden death associated with antipsychotic medication	Seizures; asphyxiation; cardiovascular causes; postural hypotension; laryngeal-pharyngeal dystonia; suppression of gag reflex	Specific medical treatments
Sudden death of psychogenic origin	Myocardial infarction after sudden psychic stress; voodoo and hexes; hopelessness, especially associated with serious physical illness	Specific medical treatments; folk healers
Suicide	Suicidal ideation; hopelessness	Hospitalization, antidepressants, ketamine infusions
Sympathomimetic withdrawal	Paranoia; confusional states; depression	Most symptoms abate without treatment; antipsychotics; antidepressants if necessary
Tardive dyskinesia	Dyskinesia of mouth, tongue, face, neck, and trunk; choreoathetoid movements of extremities; usually but not always appearing after long-term treatment with antipsychotics, especially after a reduction in dosage; incidence highest in the elderly and brain damaged; symptoms are intensified by antiparkinsonian drugs and masked but not cured by increased dosages of antipsychotic	No effective treatment reported; may be prevented by prescribing the least amount of drug possible for as little time as is clinically feasible and using drug-free holidays for patients who need to continue taking the drug; decrease or discontinue drug at first sign of dyskinetic movements
Thyrotoxicosis	Tachycardia; gastrointestinal dysfunction; hyperthermia; panic, anxiety, agitation; mania; dementia; psychosis	Thyroid function test (T_3, T_4, thyroid-stimulating hormone [TSH]); medical consultation
Toluene abuse	Anxiety; confusion; cognitive impairment	Neurological damage is nonprogressive and reversible if toluene use in discontinued early
Vitamin B_{12} deficiency	Confusion; mood and behavior changes; ataxia	Treatment with vitamin B_{12}
Volatile nitrates	Alternations of mood and behavior; light-headedness; pulsating headache	Symptoms abate with cessation of use

▲ 19.3 Psychiatric Emergencies in Children

Few children or adolescents seek psychiatric intervention on their own, even during crisis; thus, most of their emergency evaluations are initiated by parents, relatives, teachers, therapists, physicians, and child protective service workers. Some referrals are for the evaluation of life-threatening situations for the child or for others, such as suicidal behavior, physical abuse, and violent or homicidal behavior. Other urgent but non–life-threatening referrals pertain to children and adolescents with exacerbations of clear-cut serious psychiatric disorders, such as mania, depression, florid psychosis, and school referral. Less diagnostically obvious situations occur when children and adolescents present with a history of a wide range of disruptive, aberrant behaviors, and are accompanied by an overwhelmed, anxious, and distraught adult who perceives the child's actions as an emergency, despite the absence of life-threatening behavior of an obvious psychiatric disorder. In those cases, the spectrum of contributing factors is not immediately clear, and the emergency psychiatrist must assess the entire family or system involved with the child. Familial stressors and parental discord can contribute to the evolution of a crisis for a child. For example, immediate evaluations are sometimes legitimately indicated for a child caught in the crossfire of feuding parents or in a seemingly irreconcilable conflict between a set of parents and a school, therapist, or protective service worker regarding the needs of the child (Table 19.3–1).

An emergency setting is often the site of an initial evaluation of a chronic problem behavior. For example, an identified problem—such as severe tantrums, violence, and destructive behavior in a child—may have been present for months or even years. Yet the initial contact with the mental health system in the emergency room or private office may be the first opportunity for the child or adolescent to disclose underlying stressors, such as physical or sexual abuse.

In view of the integral relation of severe family dysfunction to childhood behavioral disturbance, the emergency psychiatrist must assess familial discord and psychiatric disorder in family members during an urgent evaluation. One way to make the assessment is to interview the child and the individual family members, both alone and together, and to obtain a history from informants outside the family whenever possible. Noncustodial parents, therapists, and teachers may add valuable information regarding the child's daily functioning. Many families, especially those with mental illness and severe dysfunction, may have little or no inclination to seek psychiatric help on a nonurgent basis; therefore, the emergency evaluation becomes the only way to engage them in an extensive psychiatric treatment program.

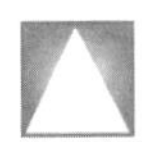

Table 19.3–1
Familial Risk Factors

Physical and sexual abuse
Recent family crisis: loss of a parent, divorce, loss of job, family move
Severe family dysfunction, including parental mental illness

LIFE-THREATENING EMERGENCIES

Suicidal Behavior

Assessment. Suicidal behavior is the most common reason for an emergency evaluation in adolescents. Despite the minimal risk for a complete suicide in a child less than 12 years of age, suicidal ideation or behavior in a child of any age must be carefully evaluated, with particular attention to the psychiatric status of the child and the ability of the family or the guardians to provide the appropriate supervision. The assessment must determine the circumstances of the suicidal ideation or behavior, its lethality, and the persistence of the suicidal intention. An evaluation of the family's sensitivity, supportiveness, and competence must be done to assess their ability to monitor the child's suicidal potential. Ultimately, during the course of an emergency evaluation, the psychiatrist must decide whether the child may return home to a safe environment and receive outpatient follow-up care or whether hospitalization is necessary. A psychiatric history, a mental status examination, and an assessment of family functioning help establish the general level of risk.

Management. When self-injurious behavior has occurred, the adolescent likely requires hospitalization in a pediatric unit for treatment of the injury or for the observation of medical sequelae after a toxic ingestion. If the adolescent is medically clear, the psychiatrist must decide whether the adolescent needs psychiatric admission. If the patient persists in suicidal ideation and shows signs of psychosis, severe depression (including hopelessness), or marked ambivalence about suicide, psychiatric admission is indicated. An adolescent who is taking drugs or alcohol should not be released until an assessment can be done when the patient is in a nonintoxicated state. Patients with high-risk profiles—such as late-adolescent males, especially those with substance abuse and aggressive behavior disorders, and those who have severe depression or who have made prior suicide attempts, particularly with lethal weapons—warrant hospitalization. Young children who have made suicide attempts, even when the attempt had a low lethality, need psychiatric admission if the family is so chaotic, dysfunctional, and incompetent that follow-up treatment is unlikely.

Violent Behavior and Tantrums

Assessment. The first task in an emergency evaluation of a violent child or adolescent is to make sure that both the child and the staff members are physically protected so that nobody gets hurt. If the child appears to be calming down in the emergency area, the clinician may indicate to the child that it would be helpful if the child recounted what happened and may ask whether the child feels in sufficient control to do so. If the child agrees and the clinician judges the child to be in good control, the clinician may approach the child with the appropriate backup close at hand. If not, the clinician may either give the child several minutes to calm down before reassessing the situation or, with an adolescent, suggest that a medication may help the adolescent relax.

If the adolescent is clearly combative, physical restraint may be necessary before anything else is attempted. Some rageful children and adolescents brought to an emergency setting by overwhelmed families are able to regain control of themselves without the use of physical or pharmacological restraint. Children and adolescents are most likely to calm down if approached calmly in a nonthreatening manner and given a chance to tell their side of the story to a nonjudgmental adult. At this time, the psychiatrist should look for any underlying psychiatric disorder that may be mediating the aggression. The psychiatrist should speak to family members and others who have been witnessing the episode to understand the context in which it occurred and the extent to which the child has been out of control.

Management. Prepubertal children, in the absence of major psychiatric illness, rarely require medication to keep them safe, because they are generally small enough to be physically restrained if they begin to hurt themselves or others. It is not immediately necessary to administer medication to a child or an adolescent who was in a rage but is in a calm state when examined. Adolescents and older children who are assaultive, extremely agitated, or overtly self-injurious and who may be difficult to subdue physically may require medication before a dialogue can take place.

Children who have a history of repeated, self-limited, severe tantrums may not require admission to a hospital if they are able to calm down during the course of the evaluation. Yet the pattern, no doubt, will reoccur unless ongoing outpatient treatment for the child and the family is arranged. For adolescents who continue to pose a danger to themselves or others during the evaluation period, admission to a hospital is necessary.

Fire Setting

Assessment. A sense of emergency and panic often surrounds the parents of a child who has set a fire. Parents or teachers often request an emergency evaluation, even for a very young child who has accidentally lit a fire. Many children, during the course of normal development, become interested in fire, but in most cases, a school-aged child who has set a fire has done so accidentally while playing with matches and seeks help to put it out. When a child has a strong interest in playing with matches, the level of supervision by family members must be clarified, so that no further accidental fires occur. The clinician must distinguish between a child who accidentally or even impulsively sets a single fire and a child who engages in repeated fire setting with premeditation and subsequently leaves the fire without making any attempt to extinguish it. In repeated fire setting, the risk is obviously greater than in a single occurrence, and the psychiatrist must determine whether underlying psychopathology exists in the child or in the family members. The psychiatrist should also evaluate family interactions, because any factors that interfere with effective supervision and communication—such as high levels of marital discord and harsh, punitive parenting styles—can impede appropriate intervention.

Fire setting is one of a triad of symptoms—enuresis, cruelty to animals, and fire setting—that were believed, some years ago, to be typical of children with conduct disorders; however, no evidence indicates that the three symptoms are truly linked, although conduct disorder is the most frequent psychiatric disorder that occurs with pathological fire setting.

Management. The critical component of management and treatment for fire setters is to prevent further incidents while treating any underlying psychopathology. In general, fire setting alone is not an indication for hospitalization, unless a continued direct threat exists that the patient will set another fire. The parents of children with a pattern of fire setting must be emphatically counseled that the child must not be left alone at home and should never be left to take care of younger siblings without direct adult supervision. Children who exhibit a pattern of concurrent aggressive behaviors and other forms of destructive behavior are likely to have a poor outcome. Outpatient treatment should be arranged for children who repeatedly set fires. Behavioral techniques that involve both the child and the family are helpful in decreasing the risk for further fire setting, as is positive reinforcement for alternate behaviors.

Child Abuse: Physical and Sexual

Physical and sexual abuse occurs in girls and boys of all ages, in all ethnic groups, and at all socioeconomic levels. The abuses vary widely with respect to severity and duration, but any form of continued abuse constitutes an emergency situation for a child. No single psychiatric syndrome is a *sine qua non* of physical or sexual abuse, but fear, guilt, anxiety, depression, and ambivalence regarding disclosure commonly surround the child who has been abused.

Young children who are being sexually abused may exhibit precocious sexual behavior with peers and present a detailed sexual knowledge that reflects exposure beyond their developmental level. Children who endure sexual or physical abuse often display sadistic and aggressive behaviors themselves. Children who are abused in any manner are likely to have been threatened with severe and frightening consequences by the perpetrator if they reveal the situation to anyone. Frequently, an abused child who is victimized by a family member is placed in the irreconcilable position of having either to endure continued abuse silently or to defy the abuser by disclosing the experiences and be responsible for destroying the family and risk being disbelieved or abandoned by the family.

In cases of suspected abuse, the child and other family members must be interviewed individually to give each member a chance to speak privately. If possible, the clinician should observe the child with each parent individually to get a sense of the spontaneity, warmth, fear, anxiety, or other prominent features of the relationships. One observation is generally not sufficient to make a final judgment about the family relationship, however; abused children almost always have mixed emotions toward abusive parents.

Physical indicators of sexual abuse in children include sexually transmitted diseases (e.g., gonorrhea); pain, irritation, and itching of the genitalia and the urinary tract; and discomfort while sitting and walking. In many instances of suspected sexual abuse, however, physical evidence is not present. Thus, a careful history is essential. The physician should speak directly about the issues without leading the child in any direction, because already frightened children may be easily influenced to endorse what they think the examiner wants to hear. Furthermore, children who have been abused often retract all or part of what has been disclosed during the course of an interview.

The use of anatomically correct dolls in the assessment of sexual abuse can help the child identify body parts and show what has happened, but no conclusive evidence supports sexual play with dolls as a means of validating abuse.

Neglect: Failure to Thrive

Assessment. In child neglect, a child's physical, mental, or emotional condition has been impaired because of the inability of a parent or caretaker to provide adequate food, shelter, education, or supervision. Similar to abuse, any form of continued neglect is an emergency situation for the child. Parents who neglect their children range widely and may include parents who are very young and ignorant about the emotional and concrete needs of a child, parents with depression and significant passivity, substance-abusing parents, and parents with a variety of incapacitating mental illnesses.

In its extreme form, neglect can contribute to failure to thrive—that is, an infant, usually under 1 year of age, becomes malnourished in the absence of an organic cause. Failure to thrive typically occurs under circumstances in which adequate nourishment is available, but a disturbance within the relationship between the caretaker and the child results in a child who does not eat sufficiently to grow and develop. A negative pattern may exist between the mother and the child in which the child refuses feedings and the mother feels rejected and eventually withdraws. She may then avoid offering food as frequently as the infant needs it. Observation of the mother and the child together may reveal a nonspontaneous, tense interaction, with withdrawal on both sides, resulting in a seeming apathy in the mother. Both the mother and the child may seem depressed.

A rare form of failure to thrive in children who are at least several years old and are not necessarily malnourished is the syndrome of psychosocial dwarfism. In that syndrome, marked growth retardation and delayed epiphyseal malnutrition accompany a disturbed relationship between the parent and the child, along with bizarre social and eating behaviors in the child. Those behaviors sometimes include eating from garbage cans, drinking toilet water, binging and vomiting, and diminished outward response to pain. Half of the children with the syndrome have decreased growth hormone. Once the children are removed from the troubled environment and placed in another setting, such as a psychiatric hospital with appropriate supervision and guidance regarding meals, the endocrine abnormalities normalize, and the children begin to grow at a more rapid rate.

Management. In cases of child neglect, as with physical and sexual abuse, the most important decision to be made during the initial evaluation is whether the child is safe in the home environment. Whenever neglect is suspected, it must be reported to the local child protective service agency. In mild cases, the decision to refer the family for outpatient services, as opposed to hospitalizing the child, depends on the clinician's conviction that the family is cooperative and willing to be educated and to enter into treatment and that the child is not in danger. Before a neglected child is released from an emergency setting, a follow-up appointment must be made.

Education for the family must begin during the evaluation; the family must be told, in a nonthreatening manner, that failure to thrive can become life-threatening, that the entire family needs to monitor the child's progress, and that they will receive some help in overcoming the many possible obstacles interfering with the child's emotional and physical well-being.

Anorexia Nervosa

Anorexia nervosa occurs in females about ten times as often as in males. It is characterized by the refusal to maintain body weight, leading to a weight at least 15 percent below the expected weight, by a distorted body image, by a persistent fear of becoming fat, and by the absence of at least three menstrual cycles. The disorder usually begins after puberty, but it has occurred in children of 9 to 10 years of age, in whom expected weight gain does not occur, rather than a loss of 15 percent of body weight. The disorder reaches medical emergency proportions when the weight loss approaches 30 percent of body weight or when metabolic disturbances become severe. Hospitalization then becomes necessary to control the ongoing process of starvation, potential dehydration, and the medical complications of starvation, including electrolyte imbalances, cardiac arrhythmias, and hormonal changes.

Acquired Immune Deficiency Syndrome

Assessment. AIDS, which is caused by the human immunodeficiency virus (HIV), occurs in neonate through perinatal transmission from an infected mother, in children and adolescents secondary to sexual abuse by an infected person, and in adolescents through intravenous drug abuse with an infected person or through intravenous drug abuse with infected needles and through sexual activities with infected partners. Child and adolescent hemophiliac patients may contract AIDS through tainted blood transfusions.

Children and adolescents may present for emergency evaluations at the urging of a family member of a peer; in some cases, they take the initiative themselves when they are faced with anxiety or panic about high-risk behavior. Early screening of high-risk persons may lead to the treatment of asymptomatic infected patients with such drugs as azidothymidine (AZT) and possibly other new medications that may slow the course of the disease. During the assessment of the risks for HIV infection, an educational process can be initiated with both the patient and the rest of the family so that an adolescent who is not infected, but exhibits high-risk behavior, can be counseled about that behavior and about safe-sex practices.

In children, the brain is often a primary site for HIV infection; encephalitis, decreased brain development, and such neuropsychiatric symptoms as impairment in memory, concentration, and attention span may be present before the diagnosis is made. The virus can be present in the cerebrospinal fluid before it shows up in the bloodstream. Changes in cognitive function, frontal lobe disinhibition, social withdrawal, slowed information processing, and apathy constitute some common symptoms of the AIDS dementia complex. Organic mood disorders, organic personality disorder, and frank psychosis can also occur in patients infected with HIV.

URGENT NON–LIFE-THREATENING SITUATIONS

School Refusal

Assessment. Refusal to go to school may occur in a young child who is first entering school or in an older child or adolescent who is making a transition into a new grade or school, or it may emerge in a vulnerable child without an obvious external stressor. In any case, school refusal requires immediate intervention, because the longer the dysfunctional pattern continues, the more difficult it is to interrupt.

School refusal is generally associated with separation anxiety, in which the child's distress is related to the consequences of being separated from the parent, so the child resists going to school. School refusal can also occur in children with school phobia, in which the fear and the distress are targeted on the school itself. In either case, a serious disruption of the child's life occurs. Although mild separation anxiety is universal, particularly among very young children who are first facing school, treatment is required when a child actually cannot attend school. Severe psychopathology, including anxiety and depressive disorders, is often present when school refusal occurs for the first time in an adolescent. Children with separation anxiety disorder typically present extreme worries that catastrophic events will befall their mothers, attachment, or themselves as a result of the separation. Children with separation anxiety disorder may also exhibit many other fears and symptoms of depression, including such somatic complaints such as headaches, stomachaches, and nausea. Severe tantrums and desperate pleas may ensue when preoccupation that a parent will be harmed during the separation is frequently verbalized; in adolescents, the stated reasons for refusing to go to school are often physical complaints.

As part of an urgent assessment, the psychiatrist must ascertain the duration of the patient's absence from school and must assess the parents' ability to participate in a treatment plan that will undoubtedly involve firm parental guidelines to ensure the child's return to school. The parents of a child with separation anxiety disorder often exhibit excessive separation anxiety or other anxiety disorders themselves, thereby compounding the child's problem. When the parents are unable to participate in a treatment program from home, hospitalization should be considered.

Management. When school refusal caused by separation anxiety is identified during an emergency evaluation, the underlying disorder can be explained to the family, and an intervention can be started immediately. In severe cases, however, a multidimensional, long-term family-oriented treatment plan is necessary. Whenever possible, a separation-anxious child should be brought back to school the next school day, despite the distress, and a contact person within the school (counselor, guidance counselor, or teacher) should be involved to help the child stay in school while praising the child for tolerating the school situation.

When school refusal has been going on for months or years or when the family members are unable to cooperate, a treatment program to move the child back to school from the hospital should be considered. When the child's anxiety is not diminished by behavioral methods alone, tricyclic antidepressants, such as imipramine (Tofranil), are helpful. Medication is generally prescribed not at the initial evaluation but after a behavioral intervention has been tried.

Munchausen Syndrome by Proxy

Munchausen syndrome by proxy, essentially, is a form of child abuse in which a parent, usually the mother, or a caretaker repeatedly fabricates or actually inflicts injury or illness in a child for whom medical intervention is then sought, often in an emergency setting. Although it is a rare scenario, mothers who inflict injury often have some prior knowledge of medicine, leading to sophisticated symptoms; the mothers sometimes engage in inappropriate camaraderie with the medical staff regarding the treatment of the child. Careful observation may reveal that the mothers often do not exhibit appropriate signs of distress on hearing the details of the child's medical symptoms. Prototypically, such mothers tend to present themselves as highly accomplished professionals in ways that seem inflated or blatantly untrue.

The illnesses appearing in the child can involve any organ system, but certain symptoms are commonly presented: bleeding from one or may sites, including the gastrointestinal (GI) tract, the genitourinary system, and the respiratory system; seizures; and central nervous system (CNS) depression. At times, the illness is simulated, rather than actually inflicted.

OTHER CHILDHOOD DISTURBANCES

Posttraumatic Stress Disorder

Children who have been subjected to a severe catastrophic or traumatic event may present for a prompt evaluation because they have extreme fears of the specific trauma occurring again or sudden discomfort with familiar places, people, or situations that previously did not evoke anxiety. Within weeks of a traumatic event, a child may re-create the event in play, in stories, and in dreams that directly replay the terrifying situation. A sense of reliving the experience may occur, including hallucinations and flashback (dissociative) experiences, and intrusive memories of the event come and go. Many traumatized children, over time, go on to reproduce parts of the event through their own victimization behaviors toward others, without being aware that those behaviors reflect their own traumatic experiences.

Dissociative Disorders

Dissociative states—including the extreme form, multiple personality disorder—are believed most likely to occur in children who have been subjected to severe and repetitive physical, sexual, or emotional abuse. Children with dissociative symptoms may be referred for evaluation because family members or teachers observe that the children sometimes seem to be spaced out or distracted or act like different persons. Dissociative states are occasionally identified during the evaluation of violent and aggressive behavior, particularly in patients who truly do not remember chunks of their own behavior.

When a child who dissociates is violent or self-destructive or endangers others, hospitalization is necessary. A variety of psychotherapy methods have been used in the complex treatment of children with dissociative disorders, including play techniques and, in some cases, hypnosis.

20

Complementary and Alternative Medicine in Psychiatry

INTRODUCTION

The science and art of "healing" as well as the concept of "illness" have always been significantly influenced by the cultural context in which they developed. What most Western medical practitioners conceive of as "health care" is actually quite in its infancy compared with many practices aimed at curing or ameliorating illness that developed across the world for many centuries past. Major advances in biomedical research and in the scientific method in general over the past century have brought that discovery of revolutionary medical interventions that have saved countless lives, most notably through the treatment of infectious illnesses. Yet, many practitioners and patients alike sense that the biological and reductionist concepts of illness and its treatment that have come to guide much of Western medical care often minimize the role of psychosocial factors in health and wellness. Psychiatry itself, supposed champion among medical fields in addressing psychosocial etiologies of illness, has also become increasingly biological in its focus. Although this approach has undoubtedly benefited persons with mental illness and has increased public awareness that the brain is no less a physical organ than the heart or kidney (susceptible to maladies at times through no fault of the person suffering mental illness), some mental health practitioners worry that the "listening care" in psychiatry will become increasingly marginalized. After all, addressing psychosocial aspects of health is almost always more time-consuming than biological interventions and thus, in a short-sighted vision of health outcomes, often seems inefficient and expensive.

The term *complementary and alternative medicine* (CAM) refers to the various disease-treating or disease-preventing practices whose methods and efficacies differ from traditional or conventional biomedical treatment. Other terms used to describe these therapeutic approaches are *integrative medicine* and *holistic medicine.* This is not a new concept in psychiatry. The idea of emphasizing the whole patient and the need to evaluate psychosocial, environmental, and lifestyle factors in health and disease is subsumed under the heading of psychosomatic or mind–body medicine.

Traditional medicine, as practiced in the United States and elsewhere in the Western world, is based on the scientific method—the use of experiments to validate a hypothesis or determine the probability of a theory being correct. Traditional medicine presumes that the body is a biological and physiological system and that disorders have a cause that can be treated with medications, surgery, and complex technological methods to produce a cure. Traditional medicine is thus also referred to as *biomedicine* or *technomedicine.*

Traditional medicine is also known as *allopathic medicine.* The term *allopathy,* derived from the Greek word *allos* ("other"), refers to the use of outside agents or medications to counteract the signs and symptoms of disease; for example, antipyretics to treat fever. *Allopathy* is the type of medicine taught in medical schools in the United States. Samuel Hahnemann (1755–1843), a German physician, coined the term to distinguish this form of medicine from *homeopathy* (derived from the Greek word *homos* ["same"]), in which specially formulated medicinal remedies, different from allopathic medicine, are used. Allopathy is the most prevalent form of medicine practiced in the Western world. (Homeopathy is discussed more fully later in this chapter.)

NATIONAL CENTER FOR COMPLEMENTARY MEDICINE AND ALTERNATIVE MEDICINE

The widespread adoption of CAM practices led the US government to establish the National Center for Complementary Medicine and Alternative Medicine (NCCAM) within the National Institutes of Health (NIH). NCCAM's mission is to evaluate the usefulness and safety of a broad range of unrelated, nonorthodox healing practices and provide scientific explanations for their possible effectiveness, train CAM researchers, and disseminate information to the public. NCCAM has proposed changing its name to the National Center for Research on Complementary and Integrative Health Care (NCRCI).

An NCCAM study in 2011 revealed that close to 40 percent of Americans used some form of CAM within a 12-month period. When prayer was included, the percentage rose to more than 60 percent. Prayer for one's own health was most prominent, followed by prayer by others for one's own health, natural products, deep-breathing exercises, group prayer, meditation, chiropractic care, yoga, massage, and diet-based therapies. Echinacea, ginseng, Ginkgo biloba, garlic supplements, glucosamine, and St. John's wort were among the most common natural products used. Back, head, and neck pain were the most common conditions treated. The CAM practices were most likely to be embraced by those with more education, women, former smokers, and those who had been recently hospitalized. Most users of CAM practices believed the greatest benefits were achieved in combination with conventional treatment.

NCCAM conducts clinical trials at the NIH and academic research institutions to investigate the benefits of various CAM practices on a spectrum of diseases and disorders, ranging from psychiatric conditions to cancer, osteoporosis, and multiple sclerosis, among others. Some completed studies have validated the following: acupuncture is beneficial to treat functional impairment and osteoarthritic pain of the knee; no prophylactic benefit was found for low-dose *Echinacea angustifolia* in the prevention of cold symptoms; combined glucosamine and chondroitin sulfate supplements do not provide significant relief for osteoarthritic pain in most cases, but does benefit a smaller subset with more severe pain; and St. John's wort (*Hypericum perforatum*) is no more effective for treating major depression of moderate severity than placebo. St. John's wort is being further investigated as a treatment for posttraumatic stress disorder (PTSD), anxiety, and minor depression (see "Herbal Medicine" below).

The NCCAM has compiled a classification of alternative medical practices designed to support research (Table 20–1). Including a practice in the classification does not imply an endorsement of the method. Indeed, many complementary and alternative health practices are based on no known scientific principles and are considered quackery.

Many systems of treatment discussed in this chapter are centuries old, and it would be presumptuous for traditional biomedical practitioners to dismiss them lightly as worthless. Nevertheless, without rigorous scientific evidence to the contrary, physicians must approach many of these treatments with skepticism. The influence of the mind on the body and the effect of psychological factors in health and disease are well known to physicians, especially to psychiatrists. Suggestion is a potent remedy, and the well-established placebo effect, in which an inert substance is effective in curing a disorder, serves to confirm the importance of mind–body interaction in health and disease.

Currently, more than half of the medical schools in the United States offer some form of complementary and alternative medicine education. Several have developed centers for alternative medicine research, with professors of mind–body or integrative medicine drawn largely from the ranks of such traditional specialties as internal medicine and psychiatry. This trend is likely to continue, with the goal of determining which of the many existing alternative medical systems have scientific merit. Only when and if they can withstand rigorous clinical trials can these techniques be integrated into traditional medicine.

Listed below in alphabetical order are some of the most visible complementary and alternative health practices that have been used in the treatment of (broadly defined) psychiatric conditions. The discussion of therapies should not be considered definitive; new therapies continue to emerge. The number of alternative healing practices available in the United States is unknown and probably soars into the hundreds and their practitioners into the tens of thousands, and there are no national standards set to credential such practitioners.

ACUPRESSURE AND ACUPUNCTURE

Acupressure and acupuncture are Chinese healing techniques that are mentioned in ancient medical texts dating back to 5000 BC and continue to be an important medical intervention in the East. A basic tenet of Chinese medicine is the belief that vital energy (*qi* or *chi*) flows along specific pathways (meridians) that have about 350 major points (acupoints) whose manipulation corrects imbalances by stimulating or removing blockages to energy flow. Another fundamental concept is the idea of two opposing energy fields (*yin* and *yang*) that must be in balance for health to be sustained. In acupressure, the acupoints are manipulated by the fingers; in acupuncture, sterilized silver or gold needles (some the diameter of a human hair) are inserted into the skin to varying depths (0.5 mm to 1.5 cm) and

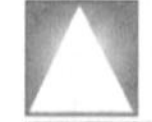

Table 20–1
Complementary and Alternative Medicine Practices

Whole Medical Systems	Biologically Based Practices	Manipulative and Body-Based Practice
Anthroposophically extended medicine	Cell treatment	Acupressure or acupuncture
	Chelation therapy	Alexander technique
Ayurveda	Diet	
Environmental medicine	Atkins diet	Aromatherapy
Homeopathy	Macrobiotic diet	Biofield therapeutics
Kampo medicine	Ornish diet	Chiropractic medicine
Native American medicine	Pritikin diet	Feldenkrais method
Naturopathic medicine	Vegetarian diet	Massage therapy
Tibetan medicine	Zone diet	Osteopathic medicine
Mind–Body Interventions	Dietary supplements	Reflexology
Art therapy	Gerson therapy	Rolfing
Biofeedback	Herbal products	Therapeutic touch
Dance therapy	Echinacea	Trager method
Guided imagery	St. John's wort	**Energy Medicine**
Humor therapy	Ginkgo biloba extract	Blue light treatment and artificial treatment
Meditation	Ginseng root	Electroacupuncture
Mental healing	Garlic supplements	Electromagnetic field therapy
Past life therapy	Peppermint	Electrostimulation and neuromagnetic stimulation
Prayer and counseling Psychotherapy	Metabolic therapy Megavitamin	Magnetoresonance therapy *Qi gong Reiki*
Sound, music therapy	Nutritional supplements	Therapeutic touch Zone therapy
Yoga exercise	Oxidizing agents (ozone, hydrogen peroxide)	
Traditional Chinese medicine		

are rotated or left in place for varying periods to correct any imbalance of *qi*.

In the West, acupressure and acupuncture are explained on the basis of nerve stimulation that releases endogenous neurotransmitters, endorphins, and enkephalins to help cure illness. The benefits of acupuncture have been validated in a variety of conditions, most notably pain management, postoperative nausea and vomiting, osteoarthritis of the knee, fibromyalgia, and headaches. Other conditions treated with these techniques are asthma, dysmenorrhea, cervical pain, insomnia, anxiety, depression, and substance abuse, including smoking cessation (see the description of moxibustion below). Most pain management clinics in the United Kingdom use acupuncture treatment. A variation of acupuncture, which uses mild electric current to augment therapeutic effects (electroacupuncture), is most often used for analgesia or during surgery. Acupuncture applied to the ear (auricolocupuncture) is also common.

ALEXANDER TECHNIQUE

The Alexander technique was developed by F. M. Alexander (1869–1955), who was born in Tasmania and eventually became a well-known stage actor. After developing aphonia, he experimented on himself by changing his body posture and eventually regained his voice. Alexander developed a theory of the proper use of body musculature to help alleviate somatic and mental illnesses. Alexander's approach is an educational process that reduces habitual, unnecessary muscular tension in everyday movements (i.e., unintentionally straining the neck while sitting at a computer) by improving sensory awareness and conscious control of these maladaptive physical habits. Treatment improves cardiovascular, respiratory, and gastrointestinal functioning as well as mood. A small, devoted group of Alexander practitioners is found in the United States and throughout the world. The Alexander technique holds promise as an approach to pain management; it has been shown to be effective in treating chronic back pain in several recent independent studies.

ANTHROPOSOPHICALLY EXTENDED MEDICINE

Anthroposophically extended medicine is a form of healing developed by the Austrian philosopher Rudolf Steiner (1861–1925). The healing process involves the use of conscious understanding, which Steiner called anthroposophy, or the "wisdom of life." Anthroposophy focuses on mental exercises that enable persons to find a balance between mind and body to ensure health maintenance. Steiner founded a school of thought represented in this country by the Rudolf Steiner School, which teaches children these concepts as they apply to civilization, besides a standard educational curriculum.

AROMATHERAPY

Aromatherapy is the therapeutic use of plant oils. Named by the French chemist Maurice René-Maurice Gattefossé in 1928, aromatherapy is one of the fastest growing alternative therapies in the United States and Europe. The essential oils of plants are organic compounds that are benzene derivatives. Aromatic substances were used in ancient civilization as both medicines and perfumes. Today, plant oils are inhaled using atomizers or are absorbed through the skin using massage (aromatherapy massage). Plant oils have many therapeutic effects—analgesic, psychological, antimicrobial—some of which have been demonstrated scientifically. One NCCAM study, for example, found the scent of lavender helped promote sleep. Aromatherapy is used to reduce stress and anxiety and to alleviate gastrointestinal and musculoskeletal disorders. In psychiatry, olfactory stimulation has been used to elicit feeling tones, memories, and emotions during psychotherapy. Aromatherapy can cause skin irritation or allergic reactions in some people. Table 20–2 lists the essential oils and their effects.

Pheromones are chemical substances secreted and smelled by humans, which affect their physiological and behavioral responses, usually related to sex. Women who are exposed to the smell of androstenol, which occurs in male underarm sweat, show increased social exchanges with men, heightened sexual arousal, and improved mood. Androstenol also affects the length and timing of the menstrual cycle as a result of changes in the level and release of gonadotrophic-releasing hormone (GnRH) and luteinizing hormone (LH). Female pheromones, known as copulins, are present in female underarm sweat and in vaginal secretions. Males perceive the odor of copulins as most pleasant during the woman's ovulatory cycle when such odors are most volatile. The synchronization of the menstrual cycle of women living together (a well-documented phenomenon) is also related to the effect of copulins. Olfactory sexual signaling is being investigated extensively, and whether these studies show therapeutic potential remains to be seen.

AYURVEDA

Ayurveda means "knowledge of life." The technique originated in India about 3000 BC and is believed to be one of the oldest and most comprehensive medical systems in the world. Ayurveda is similar to Chinese medicine in its beliefs about energy points on the body and a vital force (*prana*) that must be in balance to maintain health. Ayurveda practitioners diagnose illness by examining the pulse, the urine, and the heat or coldness of the body. Treatment relies on diet, medicines, purification, enemas, and bloodletting. (See also "Tibetan Medicine" below.)

BATES METHOD

The Bates method, designed to treat vision problems, was devised by William H. Bates. It is aimed at naturally strengthening the eye muscles and includes the following basic exercises: splashing closed eyes 20 times with warm water, then 20 times with cold water; alternately focusing on near and distant objects; focusing on an object while gently swaying the body; remembering objects in the mind's eye to facilitate the actual perception of these objects in reality; and closing the eyes, cupping them with the palms of both hands (without touching the eyes), and focusing on pleasant thoughts. Bates practitioners claim that persons who need glasses to correct refraction errors will not need them if these methods are followed rigorously.

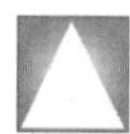

Table 20–2
Common Aromatherapies

Compound	Possible Properties	Purported Psychiatric Use	Other Purported Uses	Aroma
Angelica	Sedative, muscle relaxant, antibiotic, antifungal	Anorexia, anxiety, insomnia	Gastrointestinal (GI) spasm, ulcers, asthma, gout, bronchitis	Woody, pepper, sweet
Basil	Antispasmotic, active on sympathetic nervous system, narcotic, antiviral, insect repellant, aphrodisiac, anti-inflammative, stimulant for the adrenal cortex, GI and urogenital tracts, cerebral or memory stimulator, hepatostimulative	Fatigue, memory problems, depression, anxiety, delirium, alcoholism	Prostatitis, hair loss, asthma, coronary spasm, epilepsy	Warm, spicy, sweet, woody
Bergamot	Antidepressant, sedative, antiseptic, anti-inflammatory	Depression, hyperactivity, anxiety, insomnia	Acne, cold sores, eczema, psoriasis	Citrus, floral
Frankincense or oil of olibanum	Antitumor, antidepressant, expectorant, immunostimulant, anti-inflammatory	Depression	Asthma, bronchitis, pain relief	Woody, fruity
Geranium	Pancreatic stimulant, anti-inflammatory, antibiotic, relaxant, hemostatic	Anxiety, agitation, fatigue	Premenstrual syndrome (PMS), menopause	Floral, dry
Jasmine	Antidepressant, stimulant, analgesic	Depression, stress, fatigue	Menstrual problems, headaches	Floral, musky
Lavender	Sedative, muscular relaxant, anti-inflammatory	Depression, jet lag, insomnia, restlessness	Acne, burns, hiccups, ulcers	Powder, floral
Mandarin	Antispasmodic, sedative, hypnotic	Hyperactivity, anxiety, insomnia	Cardiovascular spasm, pain, dyspnea	Sweet, fruity
Marjoram	Diuretic, analgesic, spasmolytic, parasympathotonic	Anxiety, excessive sexual desire, psychosis, insomnia	Hyperthyroid, cardiovascular disease, vertigo, epilepsy	Nutty, woody, warm
Melissa	Sedative, anti-inflammatory, antispasmodic	Anger, agitation, insomnia	Herpes, hypertension, asthma	Citrus, herb
Myrrh	Anti-inflammatory, analgesic, antifungal	Sexual overexcitation	Dysentery, hemorrhoids	Fruity, clean
Neroli	Antidepressant, stimulant	Depression, fatigue, insomnia, anxiety, postpartum depression	Hemorrhoids, tuberculosis	Floral, powder, spicy
Spikenard	Sedative, antifungal, antiseptic, insect repellent	Insomnia, depression, anxiety	Psoriasis, epilepsy	Earthy, woody
Tuberose	Anxiety, sedative, analgesic	Agitation	Pain	Earthy, tropical

Table by Marissa Kaminsky, M.D.

BIOENERGETICS

Bioenergetics, based on the belief that dammed-up energy produces maladaptive behavioral patterns, evolved from the work of the Austrian psychoanalyst Wilhelm Reich (1897–1957), who studied with Sigmund Freud. Reich believed that energy fields were propelled by sexual impulses called ergs and that satisfactory orgasms indicated healthy bodily functioning. Modern-day practitioners look for areas of muscular tension in the body that are thought to be associated with repressed memories and emotions. Therapists try to bring these repressions to consciousness through a variety of relaxation techniques, including massage.

CHELATION

Chelation therapy is a traditional medical procedure used to treat accidental poisoning with heavy metals, such as lead, arsenic, and mercury. A chelating agent (ethylenediaminetetraacetic acid [EDTA]) is infused into the bloodstream and binds to the metal, which is then excreted from the body. As an alternative medical practice, chelation therapy is used as a form of preventive medicine to remove lead, cadmium, and aluminum from the body. These substances are presumed by some to be associated with premature aging, memory loss, and the symptoms of Alzheimer's disease. Chelation therapy has also been used to treat atherosclerosis and coronary artery disease. One NCCAM study showed that chelation treatments reduced cardiovascular events such as heart attacks and death in patients with diabetes; however, chelation therapy is not yet approved by the U.S. Food and Drug Administration (FDA) as a treatment for this condition.

CHIROPRACTIC

Chiropractic is concerned with the diagnosis and treatment of disorders of the musculoskeletal system, especially those of the spine. It was developed by a Canadian, Daniel David Palmer (1845–1913), who moved to the United States in 1895. Palmer believed that disease could be attributed to spinal misalignment, leading to abnormal nerve transmission.

Chiropractors diagnose illness by clinical examination and x-ray. Treatment involves manual manipulation of bones, joints, and musculature to restore biomechanical function. Chiropractic is the largest independent alternative health profession in the Western world, with more than 50,000 chiropractors in the United States. They are recognized by government and insurance agencies and treat more than 20 million persons in the United States annually.

COLONIC IRRIGATION

Colonic irrigation is a technique known since antiquity that consists of flushing the intestinal colon with large quantities of water, sometimes with minerals or other substances (e.g., coffee) added. It is a method used to eliminate autointoxication, a concept originating from the Pasteur Institute in France in 1908 that holds that retained fecal matter and undigested food ferment in the bowel producing toxins that cause disease. Special colon hydrotherapy machines force fluids via the rectum to clean the colon of this matter, thus eliminating such toxins. Colon cleansing using powerful laxatives and enemas is an alternative way of achieving the same result. Anecdotal reports of improved general health as a result of such practices are common; however, there are risks of electrolyte imbalance and intestinal perforation. The practice is poorly regulated, although some states attempt to monitor therapists and equipment.

COLOR THERAPY

In color therapy, different colors are thought to affect mood, and this has been used to address specific health problems. For example, blue is believed to be sedating, and red, excitatory. A Swiss psychologist, Max Lüscher, devised a color test in which a subject's mood at a particular time is determined by exposing the subject to various colors. Lüscher also experimented with the effect of color on the autonomic nervous system and found that pure red is sympathomimetic and can cause an increase in blood pressure, heart rate, and respiration. Blue is parasympathomimetic and produces the opposite effects.

DANCE THERAPY

Dance therapy was formally recognized in 1942, with the hiring of pioneer dance therapist Marian Chace (1896–1970) at St. Elisabeth's Hospital in Washington, D.C. The terms *dance* and *movement* are used synonymously; however, each actually describes a point of view. *Movement* encompasses the world of physical motion, whereas *dance* is a specific creative act within that world. The American Dance Therapy Association defines dance therapy as "the psychotherapeutic use of movement which furthers the emotional and physical integration of the individual." Dance therapy sessions have four basic goals: the development of body awareness; the expression of feelings; the fostering of interaction and communication; and the integration of the physical, emotional, and social experiences that result in a sense of increased self-confidence and contentment.

DIET AND NUTRITION

Nutritional methods to prevent or cure disease have an important place in modern medicine, and their efficacy has been proved by scientific evidence. The federal government has established recommended daily allowances (RDAs) to meet the nutritional needs of average persons in the United States. Table 20–3 depicts the recommendations for a 40-year-old sedentary man. Whole grain, lean meat, and green vegetable consumption are encouraged, and excess intake of unrefined sugar products is discouraged. Critics have faulted the federal guidelines for being unduly influenced by the meat and dairy industries. Nutritional experts and dieticians have developed alternate recommendations, especially for children, adolescents, diabetics, and pregnant women.

Many alternative diets exist, and specific vitamin and mineral supplementation programs have been developed to deal with specific diseases or bodily processes. Diets low in fat have been recommended for the treatment of cardiovascular disease and diabetes. The Pritikin diet developed by Nathan Pritikin is extremely low in fat (less than 10 percent of daily calories), high in complex carbohydrates, and high in fiber. The Ornish diet, developed by physician Dean Ornish, is vegetarian: No meat, poultry, or fish is allowed, and only 10 percent

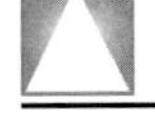

Table 20–3
United States Department of Agriculture Food Guide for a 40-Year-Old Sedentary Male

Grains	Vegetables	Fruits	Milk	Meat and Beans
8 Ounces	**3 Cups**	**2 Cups**	**3 Cups**	**6.5 Ounces**
Make half your grains whole Aim for at least 4 ounces of whole grains a day	Vary your veggies Aim for these amounts each week Dark green veggies = 3 cups Orange veggies = 2 cups Dry beans & peas = 3 cups Starchy veggies = 6 cups Other veggies = 7 cups	Focus on fruits Eat a variety of fruit Go easy on fruit juices	Get your calcium-rich foods Go low-fat or fat-free when you choose milk, yogurt, or cheese	Go lean with protein Choose low-fat or lean meats and poultry Vary your protein routine—choose more fish, beans, peas, nuts, and seeds
Find your balance between food and physical activity. Be physically active for at least 30 minutes most days of the week. Your results are based on a 2,400 calorie pattern.			Know your limits on fats, sugars, and sodium. Your allowance for oils is 7 teaspoons a day. Limit extras—solid fats and sugars—to 360 calories a day.	

Referenced from USDA site: http://www.mypyramid.gov.

of calories are obtained from fat. The low-carbohydrate, high-protein diet developed by Robert Atkins, M.D. (1930–2003) has proved effective in short-term weight loss, most likely because of increased compliance. Concern exists around the risk of ketoacidosis and the lack of long-term studies on health. This diet has also been used to treat refractory childhood epilepsy. All of these diets include an exercise program, a component proved to increase cardiac performance. Studies have shown that weight loss alone can reduce cholesterol, decrease blood pressure, and eliminate the need for drugs in newly diagnosed cases of adult-onset diabetes.

Diets from other cultures may have certain health benefits. In Asia, diets are low in fat, and there is a low incidence of cardiac disease; diets in Mediterranean countries are high in olive oil, garlic, and grains and are associated with a low incidence of colon cancer and cardiac disease. Food allergies have been implicated in many conditions: arthritis, asthma, hyperactivity, and ulcerative colitis, among others.

DIETARY SUPPLEMENTS

In addition to herbs (discussed below), a variety of dietary supplements are used to promote health. Dietary supplements are products that contain vitamins, minerals, or amino acids. In many cases, the supplement is actually an extract, metabolite, or combination of those. They are intended to *supplement* a healthy diet; they do not comprise a diet or meal. Nutritional supplements have long been familiar to Americans in the form of multivitamins, but they are now available in a vast array of other compounds that can be purchased in grocery stores, pharmacies, health food stores, and over the Internet. Annual sales of dietary supplements in the United States exceed $20 billion. Of Americans, 75 percent currently use some form of nutritional supplement on a regular basis. Although medicinal benefits are well documented in some supplements, especially vitamins, others vary greatly in safety and consistency. As a general rule, supplements should not be taken by pregnant or lactating women. In psychiatry, nutritional supplements are being used to treat a wide spectrum of illness including cognitive, mood, psychotic, sleep, and conduct disorders; however, little scientific evidence currently supports their efficacy. Table 20–4 lists some of the more common supplements being used to treat psychiatric illness.

Nutritional status has long been deemed important in mental health, and vitamin deficiencies can produce psychiatric symptoms. Severe niacin deficiency results in pellagra with its characteristic triad of skin lesions, gastrointestinal disorders, and psychiatric symptoms. The psychiatric symptoms include irritability and emotional instability progressing to severe depression and then to disorientation, memory impairment, hallucinations, and paranoia. Folic acid deficiency is associated with depression and dementia, whereas vitamin B_{12} deficiency is associated with cognitive impairment, depression, and other affective symptoms. Severe malnutrition can result in apathy and emotional instability.

In 1968, the eminent chemist and Nobel Prize winner Linus Pauling coined the term *orthomolecular* to refer to the connection between the mind and nutrition. In his book *Orthomolecular Psychiatry,* research articles were compiled supporting the notion that taking many times the recommended minimal daily dose of vitamins is useful in the treatment of schizophrenia and other psychiatric disorders. As mentioned, some severe vitamin deficiencies can result in syndromes with a psychiatric component; however, empirical data and an American Psychiatric Association (APA) task force failed to find evidence supporting the notion that schizophrenia and other disorders respond to vitamin therapies.

Thiamine, Vitamin B_{12}, and Folate

In industrialized societies, severe vitamin deficiencies are rarely encountered except in certain populations. Those who are elderly, alcohol dependent, or chronically ill or who have certain types of gastrointestinal surgeries are at greatest risk. Among the forms of vitamin deficiency most commonly encountered in the emergency room is acute thiamine depletion from alcohol dependence. Whereas the chronic forms of thiamine deficiency that lead to beriberi are rarely seen in the Western world, the fulminant depletion of already low stores of thiamine results in Wernicke's encephalopathy and Korsakoff's syndrome.

Wernicke's encephalopathy classically presents with the triad of ataxia, ophthalmoplegia, and mental confusion, but confusion and a staggering gait are perhaps most common. Although Wernicke's encephalopathy is an acute process, Korsakoff's syndrome may be the permanent residue of this encephalopathy. Patients with Korsakoff's syndrome exhibit a well-circumscribed retrograde and anterograde amnesia that results from destruction of the mammillary bodies, and psychotic symptoms are also reported. Wernicke's encephalopathy is a medical emergency that responds to short-term treatment with 50 mg of thiamine intravenously followed by 250-mg intramuscular injections daily until a normal diet is attained. The treatment of uncomplicated acute thiamine deficiencies usually involves 100 mg given orally one to three times a day.

Vitamin B_{12} deficiency or pernicious anemia is often seen in elderly adults, patients who have had gastric surgery, and malnourished depressed patients. The most typical psychiatric presentations include apathy, malaise, depressed mood, confusion, and memory deficits. Vitamin B_{12} concentrations of 150 mg/mL of serum are sometimes associated with these symptoms. Vitamin B_{12} deficiency is a more common cause of reversible dementia and is typically assessed in dementia evaluations. The treatment of pernicious anemia usually involves daily intramuscular injections of 1,000 mg of vitamin B_{12} for approximately 1 week, followed by maintenance doses of 1,000 mg every 1 to 2 months.

Folate deficiency has been associated with depression, paranoia, psychosis, agitation, and dementia. Folate deficiency can result from anorexia in depressed patients and can also contribute to depression by interfering with the synthesis of norepinephrine and serotonin. Folate deficiency has been associated with anticonvulsant use, particularly phenytoin (Dilantin), primidone (Mysoline), and phenobarbital (Solfoton), and the sex steroids, including oral contraceptives and estrogen replacement. The most common cause of folate deficiency is the malnourishment associated with alcoholism. Many folate deficiencies respond to 1 mg of folate orally per day; however, some more severe forms may require dosages of 5 mg up to three times a day. Folate deficiency in pregnancy is associated with neural tube defects (e.g., spina bifida, anencephaly).

Table 20–4
Some Dietary Supplements Used in Psychiatry

Name	Ingredients/What Is It?	Uses	Adverse Effects	Interactions	Dosage	Comments
Docosahexaenoic acid (DHA)	Omega-3 polyunsaturated fatty acid	ADD, dyslexia, cognitive impairment, dementia	Anticoagulant properties, mild GI distress	Warfarin	Varies with indication	Stop using prior to surgery
Choline	Choline	Fetal brain development, manic conditions, cognitive disorders, tardive dyskinesia, cancers	Restrict in patients with primary genetic trimethylaminuria, sweating, hypotension, depression	Methotrexate, works with B_6, B_{12}, and folic acid in metabolism of homocysteine	300–1,200 mg doses >3 g associated with fishy body odor	Needed for structure and function of all cells
L-α-Glycerylphosphorylcholine (α-GPC)	Derived from soy lecithin	To increase growth hormone secretion, cognitive disorders	None known	None known	500 mg–1 g daily	Remains poorly understood
Phosphatidylcholine	Phospholipid that is part of cell membranes	Manic conditions, Alzheimer's disease and cognitive disorders, tardive dyskinesia	Diarrhea, steatorrhea in those with malabsorption, avoid with antiphospholipid antibody syndrome	None known	3–9 g per day in divided doses	Soybeans, sunflower, rapeseed are major sources
Phosphatidylserine	Phospholipid isolated from soya and egg yolks	Cognitive impairment including Alzheimer's disease, may reverse memory problems	Avoid with antiphospholipid antibody syndrome, GI side effects	None known	For soya-derived variety, 100 mg tid	Type derived from bovine brain carries hypothetical risk of bovine spongiform encephalopathy
Zinc	Metallic element	Immune impairment, wound healing, cognitive disorders, prevention of neural tube defects	GI distress, high doses can cause copper deficiency, immunosuppression	Bisphosphonates, quinolones, tetracycline, penicillamine, copper, cysteine-containing foods, caffeine, iron	Typical dose 15 mg per day, adverse effects >30 mg	Claims that zinc can prevent and treat the common cold are supported in some studies but not in others; more research needed
Acetyl-L-carnitine	Acetyl ester of L-carnitine	Neuroprotection, Alzheimer's disease, Down's syndrome, strokes, antiaging, depression in geriatric patients	Mild GI distress, seizures, increased agitation in some with Alzheimer's disease	Nucleoside analogs, valproic acid and pivalic acid–containing antibiotics	500 mg–2 g daily in divided doses	Found in small amounts in milk and meat
Huperzine A	Plant alkaloid derived from Chinese club moss	Alzheimer's disease, age-related memory loss, inflammatory disorders	Seizures, arrhythmias, asthma, irritable bowel disease	Acetylcholinesterase inhibitors and cholinergic drugs	60–200 µg per day	*Huperzia serrata* has been used in Chinese folk medicine for the treatment of fevers and inflammation
NADH (nicotinamide adenine dinucleotide)	Dinucleotide located in mitochondria and cytosol of cells	Parkinson's disease, Alzheimer's disease, chronic fatigue, CV disease	GI distress	None known	5 mg per day or 5 mg bid	Precursor of NADH is nicotinic acid
S-Adenosyl-L-methionine (SAMe)	Metabolite of essential amino acid L-methionine	Mood elevation, osteoarthritis	Hypomania, hyperactive muscle movement, caution in patients with cancer	None known	200–1,600 mg daily in divided doses	Several trials demonstrate some efficacy in the treatment of depression
5-Hydroxytryptophan (5-HTP)	Immediate precursor of serotonin	Depression, obesity, insomnia, fibromyalgia, headaches	Possible risk of serotonin syndrome in those with carcinoid tumors or taking MAOIs	SSRIs, MAOIs, methyldopa, St. John's wort, phenoxybenzamine, 5-HT antagonists, 5-HT receptor agonists	100 mg–2 g daily, safer with carbidopa	5-HTP along with carbidopa is used in Europe for the treatment of depression

(*continued*)

Table 20–4
Some Dietary Supplements Used in Psychiatry (Continued)

Name	Ingredients/What Is It?	Uses	Adverse Effects	Interactions	Dosage	Comments
Phenylalanine	Essential amino acid	Depression, analgesia, vitiligo	Contraindicated in patients with PKU, may exacerbate tardive dyskinesia or hypertension	MAOIs and neuroleptic drugs	Comes in 2 forms: 500 mg–1.5 g daily for DL-phenylalanine, 375 mg–2.25 g for DL-phenylalanine	Found in vegetables, juices, yogurt, and miso
Myo-inositol	Major nutritionally active form of inositol	Depression, panic attacks, OCD	Caution in patients with bipolar disorder, GI distress	Possible additive effects with SSRIs and 5-HT receptor agonists (sumatriptan)	12 g in divided doses for depression and panic attacks	Studies have *not* shown effectiveness in treating Alzheimer's disease, autism, or schizophrenia
Vinpocetine	Semisynthetic derivative of vincamine (plant derivative)	Cerebral ischemic stroke, dementias	GI distress, dizziness, insomnia, dry mouth, tachycardia, hypotension, flushing	Warfarin	5–10 mg daily with food, no more than 20 mg per day	Used in Europe, Mexico, and Japan as pharmaceutical agent for treatment of cerebrovascular and cognitive disorders
Vitamin E family	Essential fat-soluble vitamin, family made of tocopherols and tocotrienols	Immune-enhancing, antioxidant, some cancers, protection in CV disease, neurologic disorders, diabetes, premenstrual syndrome	May increase bleeding in those with propensity to bleed, possible increased risk of hemorrhagic stroke, thrombophlebitis	Warfarin, antiplatelet drugs, neomycin, may be additive with statins	Depends on form: tocotrienols, 200–300 mg daily with food; tocopherols, 200 mg per day	Stop members of vitamin E family 1 month prior to surgical procedures
Glycine	Amino acid	Schizophrenia, alleviating spasticity and seizures	Avoid in those who are anuric or have hepatic failure	Additive with antispasmodics	1 g per day in divided doses for supplement; 40–90 g per day for schizophrenia	
Melatonin	Hormone of pineal gland	Insomnia, sleep disturbances, jet lag, cancer	May inhibit ovulation in 1 g doses, seizures, grogginess, depression, headache, amnesia	Aspirin, NSAIDs, β-blockers, INH, sedating drugs, corticosteroids, valerian, kava kava, 5-HTP, alcohol	0.3–3 mg hs for short periods of time	Melatonin sets the timing of circadian rhythms and regulates seasonal responses
Fish oil	Lipids found in fish	Bipolar disorder, lowering triglycerides, hypertension, decrease blood clotting	Caution in hemophiliacs, mild GI upset, "fishy"-smelling excretions	Coumadin, aspirin, NSAIDs, garlic, ginkgo	Varies depending on form and indication—usually about 3–5 g daily	Stop prior to any surgical procedure

ADD, attention-deficit disorder; CV, cardiovascular; OCD, obsessive-compulsive disorder; GI, gastrointestinal; MAOIs, monamine oxidase inhibitors; PKU, phenylketonuria; SSRIs, selective serotonin reuptake inhibitors; NSAIDs, nonsteroidal anti-inflammatory drugs; INH, isoniazid; 5-HTP, 5-hydroxytryptophan.
Table by Mercedes Blackstone, M.D.

Mr. S was diagnosed with dysthymic disorder by a psychiatrist in his early 20s and was started on sertraline (Zoloft). After 4 weeks Mr. S's mood improved dramatically, but he experienced night sweats and reduced libido. Over the ensuing years he was tried on paroxetine (Paxil), citalopram (Celexa), and fluoxetine (Prozac). Although his mood improved, his sex drive did not. Mr. S heard about an integrative mental health clinic that offered conventional medications, herbal medications, acupuncture, and *Reiki.* Mr. S was interviewed by a Western physician who had also studied Chinese medicine. The Chinese pulse diagnosis of stagnant liver *qi* was consistent with his Western diagnosis of moderate depressed mood. The doctor ordered a thyroid panel, red blood cell (RBC) folate, and B_{12} levels and suggested an integrative treatment plan including supplementation with folate, B_{12}, omega-3 fatty acids, and S-Adenosyl-L-methionine (SAMe), regular exercise, and acupuncture. The initial treatment plan consisted of daily exercise, SAMe (titrating to 400 mg twice daily), folate 5 mg, B_{12} 800 μg, and omega-3s (eicosapentaenoic acid [EPA] 2 g per day). Three weeks later, Mr. S was frustrated at his lack of progress, remained depressed, and had not started to exercise. His RBC folate level was low, and the other studies were within normal limits. Mr. S had been taking an inexpensive generic brand of SAMe and had stayed at 200 mg per day. He was encouraged to follow the original treatment plan. Two weeks later, Mr. S appeared brighter. He was exercising daily and taking the B vitamins and a quality brand of SAMe at 400 mg twice daily without significant adverse effects. *(Adapted from James H. Lake, M.D.)*

ENVIRONMENTAL MEDICINE

The field of environmental medicine began to emerge in the 1950s when physicians such as Theron Randolf, professor of allergy and immunology at Northwestern University School of Medicine, began to examine some persons' allergic reactions to various foods. Other workers studied the effects on the body of pollutants in water and air, and eventually the field expanded to include the total environment in which humans exist. As a result, environmental medicine now concerns itself with issues such as food additives; electromagnetic fields from electric utility wires; fertilizers and hormones used in food production; microwaves from appliances such as microwave ovens, television sets, and cellular telephones; and nuclear radiation. Practitioners of environmental medicine believe that many persons are extraordinarily sensitive to environmental contaminants that can trigger a disease process. Some issues are highly controversial. For instance, despite claims to the contrary, studies fail to demonstrate a higher incidence of cancer in persons exposed to electromagnetic fields; however, a correlation exists between higher cancer rates and living near oil refineries and chemical plants. Environmental medicine is a form of preventative medicine that focuses on increased individual awareness of environmental hazards and the control or elimination of these hazards. (See also "Naturopathy" below.)

EXERCISE

Exercise improves quality of life through better physical function, reduced morbidities, and improved mental health. The positive effects of exercise on immune system functions are well documented. These benefits extend to the cognitive and emotional realms and, thus, validate the mind–body connection that is central to many CAM physical practices—yoga, *tai chi, qi gong.* Exercise has been shown to ameliorate depression, anxiety, and PTSD; improve cognitive function and self-esteem; and reduce psychotic symptoms in schizophrenic populations. These effects can be accounted for neurochemically, because exercise promotes secretion of neurotransmitters, such serotonin, adrenaline, and endogenous opiates. Studies have also associated weight loss with increased social interaction, distraction from stress, recreational enjoyment, and mastery of challenge.

Exercise offers many benefits to people with serious mental illness because they more likely suffer from serious medical conditions, such as obesity, diabetes, and hypertension; live sedentary lifestyles; and smoke. Studies of adults with schizophrenia have shown a moderate exercise program reduces body mass index, improves aerobic fitness, raises self-esteem, and results in fewer psychiatric symptoms. Exercise may prove useful in remediating the weight gain from antipsychotic medications and improve compliance.

Although presently underused, exercise holds significant potential benefit as a therapeutic intervention in the mental health care setting. A structured aerobic exercise program consisting of 45-minute sessions three times per week showed significant gains in cardiovascular fitness, self-esteem, and quality of life and in altering mood and depression. Unstructured programs benefited those who adhere to the exercise regimen. No drawbacks are found to moderate exercise, and the health gains are significant.

FELDENKRAIS METHOD

The Feldenkrais method was developed by Moshé Feldenkrais (1904–1984), a Russian-born physicist who developed a theory evolved from Freud's work. Feldenkrais thought that the body should be emphasized as much as the mind and that proprioception (somatic sensations from muscles and other organs) can influence behavior. He believed that posture and the positions of the body reflected conflict; therefore, retraining the body was part of his treatment program. Practitioners of the Feldenkrais method are active throughout the world. Those learning the Feldenkrais method are referred to as students rather than patients, to reinforce the view that the work is primarily an educational process. Lessons generally last from 30 to 60 minutes and consist of structured movement that involves thinking, sensing, moving, and imagining. The method has been used in central nervous system disorders, such as multiple sclerosis, cerebral palsy, and stroke. Older persons who use the method claim that they retain or regain their ability to move without strain or discomfort.

HERBAL MEDICINE

Herbal medicine relies on plants to cure illnesses and to maintain health. Probably the oldest known system of medicine, it originated in China about 4000 BC. Ancient texts of Chinese medicine are still in use, and modern Chinese medicine relies on herbs in addition to other methods, such as acupuncture, massage, diet, and exercise, to correct imbalances in the body. A Greco-Roman medical text by Pedanius Dioscorides, *De Materia Medica,* describes the use of more than 500 plants and herbs to cure disease.

The decline of herbal medicine in the late 20th century was related to scientific and technological advances that led to the use of synthetic pharmaceuticals; nevertheless, according to some estimates, at least 25 percent of current medicines are derived from the active ingredients of plants. The examples are many: digitalis from foxglove; ephedrine from ephedra; morphine from the opium poppy; paclitaxel (Taxol) from the yew tree; and quinine from the bark of the cinchona tree.

Herbal medicine is becoming more and more popular. Approximately $4 billion a year is spent in the United States on herbal medicines, which are classified as dietary supplements. Western herbalists use plants to treat various disorders related to the respiratory, gastrointestinal, cardiovascular, and nervous systems; as with most prescription medicines, these plants contain active compounds that produce physiological effects. As a result, they must be used in appropriate doses if toxic results are to be prevented. They are not subject to FDA approval, and no uniform standards exist for quality control or potency in herbal preparations. Indeed, some preparations have no active ingredients or are adulterated. Herbal supplement producers need only prove safety and truth in labeling, not efficacy, to be sold. The herbal industry attempts to regulate itself through organizations such as the Council for Responsible Nutrition and the American Herbal Association, but according to the Federal Trade Commission, fraudulent practices and false advertising still exist. In 2003, the FDA banned ephedra (ma huang)-based diet products because of significant risk to cardiovascular health. There is now a *Physicians Desk Reference* for both herbal products and nutritional supplements.

One herb that has caught the attention of Western psychiatry is St. John's wort (*Hypericum*) for the treatment of major depressive disorders. St. John's wort has been used in folk medicine for hundreds of years and is still commonly used in Europe. In Germany, several million prescriptions for *Hypericum* are obtained annually and covered by insurance for the treatment of depression, anxiety, and sleep problems. Studies have compared St. John's wort with placebo, tricyclic drugs, and selective serotonin reuptake inhibitors (SSRIs) and found that *Hypericum* extracts were more effective than placebo in the treatment of mild to moderate depression. Many of these studies lacked rigor in the diagnosis of depression, sample size, and the assessment of efficacy. NCCAM sponsored studies and other researchers are working to determine the active ingredients, effective dosing, and toxicities associated with this plant and other biologically derived supplements using spectrographic and other scientific analyses.

Mrs. J, a 68-year-old retired schoolteacher in good health, was experiencing anhedonia after the death of her spouse and was started on a low-dose SSRI by her psychiatrist. After several weeks, her symptoms began to improve. One morning, while at the local health food store, she inquired if there were any natural products that improved mood. The store manager informed her that St. John's wort "works just like an SSRI." The patient proceeded to take the recommended daily dose of three capsules that day, each containing 300 mg of 0.3 percent *Hypericin*. Later that evening, she began to feel anxious and could not fall asleep. After several hours of doing needlework to pass the time, she began to sweat profusely. She became concerned for her health when she felt her heart racing. She drove herself to the emergency room of a local hospital. On examination, she was observed to be extremely anxious and hyperactive, tachycardic, and mildly hypertensive. She was given a short-acting, fast-onset benzodiazepine. After 4 hours, the patient reported feeling calm and her vital signs had returned to baseline. The emergency room physician informed Mrs. J that although she had only taken a single daily dose of St. John's wort, she had most likely experienced the side effects of an interaction between the plant extract and the SSRI. Known interactions include a manic reaction and serotonin syndrome. The patient agreed to discontinue the St. John's wort. She was discharged and a follow-up appointment was scheduled with her psychiatrist to discuss treatment options.

Psychoactive Herbs

Many phytomedicinals (from the Greek *phyto,* meaning "plant") have psychoactive properties that are used, or have been used, to treat a variety of psychiatric conditions. Adverse effects are possible, and toxic interactions with other drugs can occur with all phytomedicinals. Clinicians should always attempt to obtain a history of herbal use during the psychiatric evaluation. Adulteration is common, and no consistent standard preparations are available for most herbs. Safety profiles and knowledge of adverse effects of most of these substances are lacking; many, if not all, of these herbs are secreted in breast milk and are contraindicated during lactation and should be avoided during pregnancy.

Many cultures have used hallucinogens, including mescaline, psilocybin, and ergots, for thousands of years to gain spiritual and personal insight. Lysergic acid diethylamide (LSD), synthesized in the 1930s, was marketed to psychiatrists and other practitioners in the late 1940s under the trade name Delysid as a tool for understanding psychosis and for facilitating psychotherapy. Using LSD reportedly helped patients capture repressed memories and deal with anxiety, and it allowed patients to gain insight through an analysis of the primary process induced by the hallucinogen. Oral doses of 150 to 250 mg were administered occasionally by psychiatrists throughout the 1950s and early 1960s to facilitate psychotherapy with some patients. In the 1960s, Timothy Leary advocated the widespread use of hallucinogens, but the drugs were outlawed as class I controlled substances in 1965.

Although no longer used for therapeutic purposes in the United States, LSD has fulfilled part of its early promise as a probe for psychosis. More recent understanding of the pharmacology of LSD and its affinity to serotonin (5-hydroxytryptamine [5-HT]) type 2 (5-HT2) receptors has supported the interest in developing serotonin-dopamine antagonists (atypical antipsychotics) with the 5-HT2-receptor blocking properties. Recently, studies using methylenedioxymethamphetamine (MDMA, "ecstasy") have been approved by the NIH to determine whether psychotherapy is facilitated when the patient is under the influence of the drug, which can affect interpersonal relationships positively by promoting feelings of empathy.

It is important not to be judgmental in dealing with patients who use phytomedicinals. They are used for various reasons: (1) as part of their cultural tradition, (2) because patients mistrust physicians or are dissatisfied with conventional medicine, or (3) because they experience relief of symptoms. If psychotropic agents are prescribed, the clinician must be extraordinarily alert to the possibility of adverse effects as a result of drug–drug interactions, because many phytomedicinals have ingredients that produce physiological changes in the body. More than 200 herbal drugs are in use; only those with psychoactive properties are listed in Table 20–5.

Table 20–5
Phytomedicinals with Psychoactive Effect

Name	Ingredients	Use	Adverse Effects[a]	Interactions	Dosage[a]	Comments
Areca, areca nut, betel nut, *L. Areca catechu*	Arecoline, guvacoline	For alteration of consciousness to reduce pain and elevate mood	Parasympathomimetic overload; increased salivation, tremors, bradycardia, spasms, gastrointestinal disturbances, ulcers of the mouth	Avoid with parasympathomimetic drugs; atropine-like compounds reduce effect	Undetermined; 8–10 g is toxic dose for humans	Used by chewing the nut; used in the past as a chewing balm for gum disease and as a vermifuge; long-term use may result in malignant tumors of the oral cavity
Belladonna, *L. Atropa belladonna,* deadly nightshade	Atropine, scopolamine, flavonoids[b]	Anxiolytic	Tachycardia, arrhythmias, xerostomia, mydriasis, difficulties with micturition and constipation	Synergistic with anticholinergic drugs; avoid with tricyclic antidepressants, amantadine, and quinidine	0.05–0.10 mg a day; maximum single dose is 0.20 mg	Has a strong smell, tastes sharp and bitter, and is poisonous
Bitter orange flower, *Citrus aurantium*	Flavonoids, limonene	Sedative, anxiolytic, hypnotic	Photosensitization	Undetermined	Tincture 2–3 g per day, drug 4–6 g per day, extract 1–2 g per day	Contradictory evidence; some refer to it as a gastric stimulant
Black cohosh, *L. Cimicifuga racemosa*	Triterpenes, isoferulic acid	For premenstrual syndrome, menopausal symptoms, dysmenorrhea	Weight gain, gastrointestinal disturbances	Possible adverse interaction with male or female hormones	1–2 g per day; over 5 g can cause vomiting, headache, dizziness, cardiovascular collapse	Estrogen-like effects questionable because root may act as estrogen-receptor blocker
Black haw, cramp bark, *L. Viburnum prunifolium*	Scopoletin, flavonoids, caffeic acids, triterpenes	Sedative, antispasmodic action on uterus; for dysmenorrhea	Undetermined	Anticoagulant-enhanced effects	1–3 g per day	
California poppy, *L. Eschscholzia californica*	Isoquinoline alkaloids, cyanogenic glycosides	Sedative, hypnotic, anxiolytic; for depression	Lethargy	Combination of California poppy, valerian, St. John's wort, and passion flowers can result in agitation	2 g per day	Clinical or experimental documentation of effects is unavailable
Catnip, *L. Nepeta cataria*	Valeric acid	Sedative, antispasmodic; for migraine	Headache, malaise, nausea, hallucinogenic effects	Undetermined	Undetermined	Delirium produced in children
Chamomile, *L. Matricaria chamomilla*	Flavonoids	Sedative, anxiolytic	Allergic reaction	Undetermined	2–4 g per day	May be GABAergic
Corydalis, *L. Corydalis cava*	Isoquinoline alkaloids	Sedative, antidepressant; for mild depression	Hallucination, lethargy	Undetermined	Undetermined	Clonic spasms and muscular tremor with overdose
Cyclamen, *L. Cyclamen europaeum*	Triterpene	Anxiolytic; for menstrual complaints	Small doses (e.g., 300 mg) can lead to nausea, vomiting, and diarrhea	Undetermined	Undetermined	High doses can lead to respiratory collapse
Echinacea, *L. Echinacea purpurea*	Flavonoids, polysaccharides, caffeic acid derivatives, alkamides	Stimulates immune system; for lethargy, malaise, respiratory and lower urinary tract infections	Allergic reaction, fever, nausea, vomiting	Undetermined	1–3 g per day	Use in HIV and AIDS patients is controversial; potential for immunosuppression with long-term use. NCCAM studied.

(continued)

Table 20–5
Phytomedicinals with Psychoactive Effect (Continued)

Name	Ingredients	Use	Adverse Effects[a]	Interactions	Dosage[a]	Comments
Ephedra, ma-huang *L. Ephedra sinica*	Ephedrine, pseudoephedrine	Stimulant; for lethargy, malaise, diseases of respiratory tract	Sympathomimetic overload; arrhythmias, increased blood pressure, headache, irritability, nausea, vomiting	Synergistic with sympathomimetics, serotonergic agents; avoid with MAOIs	1–2 g per day	Administer for short periods as tachyphylaxis and dependence can occur; risk of myocardial ischemia and stroke. Banned in US diet supplement.
Ginkgo, *L. Ginkgo biloba*	Flavonoids, ginkgolide A, B	Symptomatic relief of delirium, dementia; improves concentration and memory deficits; possible antidote to SSRI-induced sexual dysfunction	Allergic skin reactions, gastrointestinal upset, muscle spasms, headache	Anticoagulant: use with caution because of its inhibitory effect on PAF; increased bleeding possible	120–240 mg per day	Studies indicate improved cognition in Alzheimer's patients after 4–5 weeks of use, possibly because of increased blood flow
Ginseng, *L. Panax ginseng*	Triterpenes, ginsenosides	Stimulant; for fatigue, elevation of mood, immune system	Insomnia, hypertonia, and edema (called ginseng abuse syndrome)	Not to be used with sedatives, hypnotic agents, MAOIs, antidiabetic agents, or steroids; has anticoagulant action (discontinue 7 days before surgery)	1–2 g per day	Several varieties exist: Korean (most highly valued), Chinese, Japanese, American (*Panax quinquefolius*)
Heather, *L. Calluna vulgaris*	Flavonoids, catechin, triterpenes, β-sitosterol	Anxiolytic, hypnotic	Undetermined	Undetermined	Undetermined	Efficacy for claimed uses is not documented
Hops, *L. Humulus lupulus*	Humulone, lupulone, flavonoids	Sedative, anxiolytic, hypnotic; for mood disturbances, restlessness	Contraindicated in patients with estrogen-dependent tumors (breast, uterine, cervical)	Hyperthermia effects with phenothiazine antipsychotics and with CNS depressants	0.5 g per day	May decrease plasma levels of drugs metabolized by CPY450 system
Horehound, *L. Ballota nigra*	Diterpenes, tannins	Sedative	Arrhythmias, diarrhea, hypoglycemia, possible spontaneous abortions	May enhance serotonergic drug effects, may augment hypoglycemic effects of drugs	1–4 g per day	May cause abortion
Jambolan, *L. Syzygium cumini*	Oleic acid, myristic acid, palmitic and linoleic acid, tannins	Anxiolytic, antidepressant	Undetermined	Undetermined	1–2 g per day	In folk medicine, a single dose is 30 seeds (1.9 g) of powder
Kava kava, *L. Piper methysticum*	Kava lactones, kava pyrone	Sedative, hypnotic antispasmodic	Lethargy, impaired cognition, dermatitis with long-term unreported usage	Synergistic with anxiolytics, alcohol; avoid with levodopa and dopaminergic agents	600–800 mg per day	May be GABAergic; contraindicated in patients with endogenous depression; may increase the danger of suicide
Lavender, *L. Lavandula angustifolia*	Hydroxycoumarin, tannins, caffeic acid	Sedative, hypnotic	Headache, nausea, confusion	Synergistic with other sedatives	3–5 g per day	May cause death in overdose
Lemon balm, sweet Mary, *L. Melissa officinalis*	Flavonoids, caffeic acid, triterpenes	Hypnotic, anxiolytic, sedative	Undetermined	Potentiates CNS depressant; adverse reaction with thyroid hormone	8–10 g per day	

Mistletoe, *L. Viscum album*	Flavonoids, triterpenes, lectins, polypeptides	Anxiolytic; for mental and physical exhaustion	Berries said to have emetic and laxative effects	Contraindicated in patients with chronic infections (e.g., tuberculosis)	10 per day	Berries have caused death in children
Mugwort, *L. Artemisia vulgaris*	Lactones, flavonoids	Sedative, antidepressant, anxiolytic	Anaphylaxis, contact dermatitis	Potentiates anticoagulants	5–15 g per day	May stimulate uterine contractions
Nux vomica, *L. strychnos nux vomica,* poison nut	Indole alkaloids: strychnine and brucine, polysaccharides	Antidepressant; for migraine, menopausal symptoms	Convulsions, liver damage, death; severely toxic because of strychnine	Undetermined	0.02–0.05 g per day	Symptoms of poisoning can occur after ingestion of one bean; lethal dose is 1–2 g
Oats, *L. Avena sativa*	Flavonoids, oligo- and polysaccharides	Anxiolytic, hypnotic; for stress, insomnia, opium and tobacco withdrawal	Bowel obstruction or other bowel dysmotility syndromes, flatulence	Undetermined	3 g per day	Oats have sometimes been contaminated with aflatoxin, a fungal toxin linked with some cancers
Passion flower, *L. Passiflora incarnata*	Flavonoids, cyanogenic glycosides	Anxiolytic, sedative, hypnotic	Cognitive impairment	Undetermined	4–8 g per day	Overdose causes depression
St. John's wort, *L. Hypericum perforatum*	Hypericin, flavonoids, xanthones	Antidepressant, sedative, anxiolytic	Headaches, photosensitivity (may be severe), constipation	Report of manic reaction when used with sertraline (Zoloft); do not combine with SSRIs or MAOIs: possible serotonin syndrome; do not use with alcohol, opioids; discontinue 5 days before surgery	100–950 mg per day	Under investigation by the NIH; may act as MAOI or SSRI; 4- to 6-week trial for mild depressive moods if no apparent improvement, another therapy should be tried
Scarlet pimpernel, *L. Anagallis arvensis*	Flavonoids, triterpenes, cucurbitacins, caffeic acids	Antidepressant	Overdose or long-term doses may lead to gastroenteritis and nephritis	Undetermined	1.8 g of powder 4 times a day	Flowers are poisonous
Skullcap, *L. Scutellaria lateriflora*	Flavonoid, monoterpenes	Anxiolytic, sedative, hypnotic	Cognitive impairment, hepatotoxicity	Disulfiram-like reaction may occur if used with alcohol	1–2 g per day	Little information exists to support the use of this herb in humans
Strawberry leaf, *L. Fragaria vesca*	Flavonoids, tannins	Anxiolytic	Contraindicated with strawberry allergy	Undetermined	1 g per day	Little information exists to support the use of this herb in humans
Tarragon, *L. Artemisia dracunculus*	Flavonoids, hydroxycoumarins	Hypnotic, appetite stimulant	Undetermined	Undetermined	Undetermined	Little information exists to support the use of this herb in humans
Valerian, *L. Valeriana officinalis*	Valepotriates, valerenic acid, caffeic acid	Sedative, muscle relaxant, hypnotic	Cognitive and motor impairment, gastrointestinal upset, hepatotoxicity; long-term use: contact allergy, headache, restlessness, insomnia, mydriasis, cardiac dysfunction	Avoid concomitant use with alcohol or CNS depressants	1–2 g per day	May be chemically unstable

[a]No reliable, consistent, or valid data exist on dosages or adverse affects of most phytomedicinals.

[b]Flavonoids are common to many herbs. They are plant by-products that act as antioxidants (i.e., agents that prevent the deterioration of material such as DNA [deoxyribonucleic acid] via oxidation).

AIDS, acquired immunodeficiency syndrome; CNS, central nervous system; GABA, γ-aminobutyric acid; HIV, human immunodeficiency virus; MAOIs, monamine oxidase inhibitors; NIH, National Institutes of Health; PAF, platelet-activating factor; SSRIs, serotonin reuptake inhibitors; NCCAM, National Center for Complementary Medicine and Alternative Medicine.

HOMEOPATHY

Homeopathic healing was developed in the early 1800s by Samuel Hahnemann, a German physician. It is based on the concept that self-healing is a basic characteristic of human life and that special medications can aid this inherent process. The homeopathic pharmacopoeia is unique in several ways. First, it contains more than 2,000 medications, including those from plants, such as aconite, ergot, and hellebore; minerals, such as silver, copper, gold, and iodine; and animals, such as snake and jellyfish venom and tissue extracts. Second, medications are prepared as tinctures (i.e., mixed with 95 percent grain alcohol) or as pills with lactose fillers. Finally, medications are dispersed in infinitesimally dilute solutions, such as 1 to 1,020,000, which prevents the medication from being detected by conventional chemical methods. Homeopaths claim that the therapeutic effect is based on "molecular medicine."

Hahnemann based his drug treatment on the following assumptions: medical substances elicit a standard array of signs and symptoms in healthy people, and the medicine whose effect in normal persons most closely resembles the illness being treated is the one most likely to initiate a curative response. Thus, a medication that produces nausea would be used to treat nausea, except that it would be given in dilute amounts. This law of similars—*Similia similibus curantur* ("Let like be cured by like")—led to coining of the word *homeopathy* ("similar experiences"). In traditional medicine, such highly dilute substances are considered to have no effect, and no pharmacological research studies demonstrate otherwise.

Homeopathic medical schools are no longer found in the United States (the last one was Hahnemann University Medical School, which closed in 1994); nevertheless, the practice of homeopathy is increasing in the United States and around the world. In 2012 over 5 million adults and one million children used homeopathic medicines according to the National Health Interview Survey (NHIS). In Europe, homeopathy is extraordinarily popular. Homeopathic medicines are sold over the counter in the United States. Homeopathic remedies sold in the United States must meet the standards of monographs in the Homeopathic Pharmacopoeia of the United States (HPUS), which was recognized in the Food, Drug and Cosmetic Act with authority equivalent to that of the United States Pharmacopeia (USP).

LIGHT AND MELATONIN THERAPY

Light therapy is based on the concept that humans are subject to circadian rhythms (from the Latin words *circa* ["around"] and *dies* ["day"]) that affect physiological processes in predictable ways. There are 24-hour cycles of rest and activity that include changing levels of corticosteroids, electrolyte excretion, and physiological processes; for instance, blood pressure is higher during the day than at night. By varying light exposure, circadian rhythms can be altered. The concentration of the hormone melatonin, produced by the pineal gland, is highest in the bloodstream at night and is low or absent during the daylight. Melatonin is believed to regulate sleep, and exogenous melatonin (available over the counter) produces drowsiness in normal people. Artificial bright-light therapy (over 2,500 lux) is a proven method used to treat depressive disorder with seasonal pattern, which is seen during the winter months when daylight hours are reduced.

MACROBIOTICS

Macrobiotics (from the Greek words *makros* ["long"] and *bios* ["life"]) is a health practice that focuses on living in harmony with nature, using mainly a balanced diet. Macrobiotics became associated with the biblical patriarchs, the Chinese sages, and the Ethiopians of Africa, who were said to live 120 years or more. In 1797, a German physician and philosopher, Christoph W. Hufeland wrote an influential book on diet and health, *Macrobiotics or the Art of Prolonging Life.*

Macrobiotic foods are classified as *yin* (cold and wet) and *yang* (hot and dry); the goal is to keep *yin* and *yang* in balance. The diet consists of 50 percent grain products, 25 percent cooked or raw vegetables, 10 percent protein, 10 percent vegetable or fish soup, and 5 percent teas and fruits. Prolonged use of the diet can result in vitamin and mineral deficiencies.

MASSAGE

Massage is a treatment that involves manipulation of the soft tissues and the surfaces of the body. It was prescribed for the treatment of diseases more than 5,000 years ago by Chinese physicians, and Hippocrates considered it to be a method of maintaining health.

Massage is believed to affect the body in several ways: it increases blood circulation, improves the flow of lymph through the lymphatic vessels, improves the tone of the musculoskeletal system, and has a tranquilizing effect on the mind. Massage techniques have been described in various ways: stroking, kneading, pinching, rubbing, knuckling, tapping, or applying friction. Massage is most often done with the hands and fingers, but vibrating machines and electrical stimulation are also used. The different types of massage therapies that have evolved over the years are more similar than different. These include Swedish, Oriental, Shiatsu, and Esalen massages. Studies have proved massage useful to reduce anxiety and pain perception. Most persons who experience massage find it physically and mentally restorative. NCCAM studies have shown massage to be of benefit in the treatment of pain, especially pain related to joint disease.

MEDITATION

Meditation is a technique that involves entering a trance state by focusing thought on a word or sound (a mantra), an object (e.g., a burning candle), or a movement (e.g., an oscillating disk). During the trance, the person experiences a state of calm. A meditative trance has physiological effects, all associated with decreased anxiety: heart and respiratory rates slow, blood pressure decreases, and alpha brain waves increase.

Transcendental meditation (TM), developed by the Indian mystic Maharishi Mahesh Yogi, was introduced into the United States in the 1950s. TM uses mantras based on personal characteristics to induce a trance state. In the 1960s, a physician, Herbert Benson, developed the relaxation response, which used mantras and breath control as a treatment for stress and stress-related disorders.

Mindfulness Meditation

Mindfulness meditation is derived from Buddhist practices of meditation and refers to paying attention to the present and being aware of the present using all sensory modalities. As thoughts flow through the mind during meditation, they are viewed nonjudgmentally, accepted for what they are, reflective of our "true nature." It is a process of self-exploration and self-inquiry. NCCAM studies have shown changes in brain, particularly left side anterior activation during meditation also associated with significant improvement in subjective and objective symptoms of anxiety and panic. One study reported improvement in women with irritable bowel syndrome.

Mindfulness Therapy

The concept of mindfulness has been translated into a type of psychotherapy in which therapist's and patient's focus are on the here and now rather than past events. Patients are encouraged to become aware of how they are feeling and what they are thinking in the moment. As they examine their experienced emotion about current events or conflicts, insights leading to change in behavior or attitudes occur.

MOXIBUSTION

Moxibustion is based on theories of Oriental medicine in which energy forces are balanced by applying heat to stimulate specific acupoints. The heat is generated by burning dry mugwort leaves (*Artemisia vulgaris,* known as *moxa*). Heat is applied either directly or indirectly. In the direct method, dried moxa is rolled into small cones and placed on the skin. The tops of the cones are lit, but they are extinguished as soon as heat is felt. In the indirect method, a burning cigar-like moxa is held near the skin at acupoints. More recently glass cups have been used with vacuum pumps. It gained popularity in 2016 when many Olympic athletes were treated with this method.

Moxibustion is used in musculoskeletal disorder, arthritis, asthma, and eczema. As with many other alternative therapies, however, no scientific clinical trials are available to show its effectiveness.

NATUROPATHY

Naturopathy is a health care system intended to ensure a healthy mind and body based on maintaining healthy nutrition, pollution-free air and water supplies, and exercising regularly. The treatment is based on the belief that the body has the power to heal itself; it requires the patient's active participation in the health maintenance program.

Naturopathy developed in Germany in the later 19th century under the guidance of Benedict Lust, who prescribed hydrotherapy (alternating hot and cold water) as a form of natural healing. Lust came to the United States, became an osteopathic physician, and founded the American School of Naturopathy in 1902. Since then, naturopathic medicine has grown into a major form of health care, which uses an eclectic group of methods in addition to hydrotherapy. These methods include eating specialized diets, homeopathy, breathing ionized air, using fomentations (the application of hot and cold compresses), taking colonic irrigations and enemas, drinking pollution-free water, eating foods grown organically, and using massage therapy, herbs, and rest therapy. Naturopathic physicians are licensed in several states (Alaska, Connecticut, New Hampshire, among others), but because no standard regulation of the field exists, persons with minimal or no educational background set up practices.

ORIENTAL MEDICINE

Oriental medicine is a broad term covering the traditional medicines of China, Korea, Japan, Vietnam, Tibet, and other Asian countries. In general, the techniques of Oriental medicine were first developed in China and include acupuncture, moxibustion, herbology, massage, cupping, *gua sha* (scraping away toxins), breath work, *qi gong* (see below), and exercise (*tai chi*). Chinese medicine is a coherent and independent system of thought and practice based on ancient texts. It is the result of a continuous process of critical thinking, extensive clinical observation, and testing, and it represents a thorough exposition of material by respected clinicians and theoreticians. It is rooted in philosophy, logic, sensibility, and habits of civilization foreign to Western civilization and, therefore, is difficult for Western physicians to understand. The basic theory is that a life force, called *chi* energy, flows in us in a harmonious, balanced way. This harmony and balance signify health. When the life force does not flow properly, disharmony and imbalance, or illness, result.

OSTEOPATHIC MEDICINE

The scope of osteopathic medicine is similar to allopathic medicine and is best indicated by the fact that doctors of osteopathy (DO) are licensed to practice in every state and are accepted into medical, surgical, and psychiatric residency programs and the military on the same basis as medical doctors (MD); they are qualified to practice in every branch of clinical medicine and take the same licensure examinations as MDs. Their medical education is identical to that of MDs, except that they have additional training in disorders of the musculoskeletal system, in which DOs consider themselves more knowledgeable than MDs.

As of 2012 there were 29 osteopathic medical schools in the United States. Approximately 82,000 osteopaths treat about 30 million patients each year. Osteopathy was developed by Andrew Taylor Still, M.D. (1828–1917), who founded the American School of Osteopathy in Kirksville, Missouri (now Kirksville College of Osteopathic Medicine), in 1892. Disease is viewed in the same way as in allopathic medicine; however, special emphasis is placed on proper musculoskeletal alignment as a prerequisite for health maintenance. Osteopaths may rely on the manipulation of body parts, particularly the craniosacral spinal axis, as part of a treatment plan. Osteopathic manipulation therapy is perceived as an adjunct, not a substitute, to traditional medical, surgical, and pharmacological intervention.

OZONE THERAPY

Ozone, which acts as an antioxidant and disinfectant, is used conventionally for water purification, odor control, and air purification. Ozone therapy is based on the assumption that most illness is caused by viral and bacterial infection; ozone is used to treat medical conditions that range from influenza to cancer and acquired immunodeficiency syndrome (AIDS). The first ozone generators were developed by Werner von Siemens in Germany in 1857, and ozone was used therapeutically to purify blood shortly thereafter in Germany and other European countries.

Ozone therapy introduces ozone into the body in various ways. These include drinking ozonated water; ozone limb bagging, in which ozone is pumped into an airtight bag that covers an arm or leg; breathing ozone bubbled through olive oil or topically applying ozonated olive oil; insufflations, in which a catheter is inserted into the rectum or vagina with ozone administered at a slow flow rate; and autohemotherapy, in which a person's own ozonized blood is reintroduced into the body.

PAST LIFE MEDICINE

In past life medicine, the healing process is aided by contact with spiritual beings that are believed to have the ability to reverse illness and maintain health. The spirits are approached through the use of altered states of consciousness, so-called *channeling,* higher states of awareness, and transmissions from spiritually evolved beings. Past life regression using hypnosis allows a person to experience past life events (via imagery).

A 40-year-old man, in good health, with an obsessive fear of death was referred to an integrative psychiatrist to deal with his preoccupations about dying. The patient was placed in a trance state under hypnosis and asked to imagine and describe a past life. He described himself as an itinerant silk merchant living in 16th-century France. He was married, had eight children, and was content with his life. He was asked to describe his death and proceeded to do so. He was 90 years old when he died, surrounded by his family who were at his bedside. He knew he was dying and described the process as a "peaceful falling away." Following the session, his fears about dying diminished; when he became anxious about death, he remembered the past life narrative and was able to relax.

PRAYER

The pervasive interest in faith healing, the curative anecdotes of television evangelists, and the millions of hopeful individuals visiting religious shrines in search of relief give witness to the continuing interest in, and prevalence of, prayer and spirituality in the process of healing. Some religious groups specifically recommend against standard psychiatric therapies and offer their own approach as the only valid alternative for mental and spiritual health. Others view prayer as a form of distant healing defined by the psychic Elizabeth Targ as any purely mental effort undertaken by one person with the intention of improving the physical or emotional well-being of another.

Some advocate the use of shared prayer, silent prayer, and distant or "intercessory" prayer (praying on behalf of someone else for a specific purpose) to benefit patients. Studies to date are inconclusive, however, on the impact of prayer on medical outcomes. Surveys indicate that 92 percent of a sample of inner-city homeless women reported one or more spiritual or religious practices. Some 48 percent reported that prayer was significantly related to less use of alcohol or street drugs or both and fewer perceived worries and depression. Recent epidemiological research indicates that religious beliefs and practices are negatively correlated with substance abuse and positively correlated with health status. Also 12-step programs have a long history of successfully incorporating prayer and spirituality in the treatment of addictive behavior. Personal belief in religion and active attendance at worship has been correlated with a moderately decreased incidence of depression and hypertension.

QI GONG

Chinese *qi gong* has been practiced for more than 2,000 years. Translated directly, *qi gong* means the skill or work (*gong*) of cultivating energy (*qi*). It is a Chinese exercise system that attracts and directs the vital life energy (see "Oriental Medicine" above), enabling practitioners to build up their health, prevent illness, and increase vitality. "Still" *qi gong* is practiced as a motionless meditation with the emphasis on breath and intentional thoughts. "Moving" *qi gong* involves external movements under the conscious direction of the mind. Electroencephalogram studies have detected measurable differences in the brain patterns of practitioners. Purported benefits include increased autoimmune cell production, reduced hypertension, and decreased incidence of falls in the elderly.

REFLEXOLOGY

Reflexology is the gentle massaging of the feet, hands, and ears to stimulate the body's natural healing power. It is used to alleviate tension by clearing crystalline deposits under the skin that may interfere with the natural flow of the body's energy. Reflexologists believe that all body parts can be mapped out on the soles or sides of the feet; for instance, the tip of the second toe represents the eye. Applying pressure to a particular area of the foot can relieve disorders related to the represented body parts. NCCAM studies have shown some benefit from reflexology in patients with irritable bowel syndrome.

REIKI

Reiki is a Japanese word with the general meaning of "healing." (*Rei* means "universal" or "spiritual," and *ki* is "life force energy.") It was developed by Mikao Usui in 1922. The two degrees of *Reiki* healing are as follows. First-degree *Reiki* practitioners use light, nonmanipulative touch to the head and torso to precipitate a flow of healing energy, called *Reiki,* drawn and into the patient according to the recipient's needs. Second-degree healing enables practitioners to access this energy for distant healing when touch is impossible. *Reiki* treatment typically creates an almost immediate feeling of relaxation, which may reduce the biochemical effects of prolonged stress. First-degree *Reiki* is easily learned and is a method that patients use to decrease stress, anxiety, insomnia, and pain. *Reiki* is also used in hospices for pain management, to support a peaceful death, and to provide emotional support for family members. It is also beneficial in cardiovascular disease as a means to lower blood pressure and reduce cardiac arrhythmias. The mechanism of action is unknown, however, the autonomic nervous system is involved, especially parasympathetic impulses.

ROLFING

Rolfing is a type of massage that was developed by an American biochemist, Ida Rolf (1896–1979), to relieve tension in muscle, connective tissue, and fascia, which she believed caused musculoskeletal diseases, such as arthritis and fibromyalgia. Therapy consists of deep, sometimes painful, massage to produce flexible planes between muscle groups throughout the body. Rolf discovered that she could achieve remarkable changes in posture and structure by manipulating the body's myofascial system; as various parts of the body are massaged, past memories and emotional states are often released. In this sense, Rolfing is a psychophysiological experience. No NCCAM studies on Rolfing have been performed.

SHAMANISM

A shaman is an individual who is believed to have the power to heal the sick and communicate with the spirit world. Individuals having this designation can be found in many parts of the world, including American aboriginal groups (Native Americans and Alaskan natives). Qualifications of a medicine man (or woman) are determined by a series of initiatory trials and teaching and "certification" by qualified, recognized elders. Shamanistic practices often include cleansing ceremonies, such as fasting or sweating, and so-called vision quests, which are accompanied by hallucinations. The ceremony is sometimes facilitated by rhythmic sounds, dancing, physical pain or privation, and the use of "spiritual herbs." Through this process, the shaman escorts the soul of the dying to the afterlife. Shamanistic practices are also used to provide solutions to insolvable personal or social problems.

SNOEZELEN

This is a term for a system of multisensory stimulation (e.g., lighting effects, tactile surfaces, meditative music, and smell of essential oils) generally conducted in special rooms for 30 to 60 minutes per session. Snoezelen originated in the Netherlands in the field of learning disability and autism with children but has been adapted for use in dementia. Snoezelen may also improve behavioral disturbances such as apathy, mood, and restless or repetitive behaviors. One study showed Snoezelen to be comparable to "reminiscence therapy" (e.g., using newspapers of nostalgic items to allow a person to talk about old memories) for acute agitation in dementia. Lack of widespread availability and potentially high costs for maintaining the therapy may limit its applicability.

SOUND AND MUSIC THERAPY

Sound therapy is an ancient technique in which sounds (e.g., chants, bell rings, or drum beats) are used to create vibrations in the body and believed to have healing powers. Practitioners claim that a sense of relaxation can also be achieved. Sound therapy is used in Ayurveda to promote health, with claims of reducing tumor growth by using certain sounds known as *Sama Veda.* Music therapy uses the sound of musical instruments, such as the flute, to achieve similar results. In the Bible, David attempted to treat King Saul's depression by playing the harp. The effect of music and sound on psychophysiological processes is under investigation at various academic centers.

TAI CHI

Tai chi, or *tai chi chuan,* is one of the most popular Asian movement arts used in the West. This ancient Chinese technique is designed to increase the life force in the body through a series of slow circular movements. It is a moving form of meditation and is based, as are other Chinese methods, on the search for perfect balance between *yin* and *yang* energies.

The practitioner performs sequences of movements that last from 5 to 30 minutes. A session may last a couple of hours and is typically performed in early morning. The practitioner is expected to focus on breathing and its precise synchronization with the movements. *Tai chi chuan* is believed to help mainly stress-related problems and conditions and so is primarily used to treat anxiety, depression, muscular tension, high blood pressure, and other cardiovascular conditions. NCCAM studies have shown improvement in exercise tolerance in patients with cardiovascular disease who practice *tai chi.*

THERAPEUTIC TOUCH

Therapeutic touch is the technique of healing with hands. It was developed by a nurse, Dolores Krieger, in the 1970s. Energy is believed to be transferred by laying the hands over specific parts of the body to aid in the process of healing. Therapeutic touch has gained popularity in the nursing profession, as well as among some physicians. NCCAM studies have shown therapeutic touch to be of value in patients with chronic neck pain.

TIBETAN MEDICINE

The Tibetan health system dates to about the 7th century AD. The Tibetan king Songsten Gampo is credited with its creation from the synthesis of various, more ancient sources. It has elements of Arabic, Indian, and Chinese health systems. In Tibet, its practice is closely related to religion and magic. Disease is believed to be the result of imbalance between the three components or humors of the living organism: wind (breathing and movement in general), bile (related to digestion and temperament), and phlegm (related to sleep, joint mobility, and skin elasticity). Imbalance can be caused by ignorance of health principles, environmental assaults, or improper diet. Treatment consists of restoring the balance between the different humors through the use of herbal medicine and accessory therapies, such as massage, moxibustion, acupuncture, appropriate diet, religious rituals, and purification techniques.

TRAGER METHOD

The Trager method, developed by Milton Trager, a Chicago physician, is a technique of movement reduction to aid individuals suffering from polio and other neuromuscular disorders. The client, typically in 60- to 90-minute sessions, is instructed to relax all conscious muscles and to allow the unconscious to choose natural, less restrictive body movements, as guided by the practitioner. This method is particularly suitable to individuals with back pain and severely restricted movement.

YOGA

Yoga ("yoking" or "union" in Sanskrit) is a comprehensive philosophical system with the goal of preparing an individual to unite with the supreme being. The technique of early yoga seeks to bring into balance all the disparate aspects of body, mind, and personality. Early evidence of yoga practice dates back to 5,000 years ago in India, and it has been practiced as a religion and health system ever since. The West grew familiar with yoga through the practice of Hatha Yoga and an emphasis on the physical collection of *asanas* (postures). The other aspects of the system, *pranayama* (breathing exercises) and *dhyana* (meditation), and other forms of yoga are gaining adoption.

Recent studies in people with chronic low-back pain suggest that yoga poses may help reduce pain and improve function. Other health benefits such as reducing heart rate and blood pressure and reducing anxiety and depression have been reported.

According to the 2007 National Health Interview Survey (NHIS), yoga is the sixth most commonly used complementary health practice among adults. More than 13 million adults practice yoga. There are many training programs for yoga teachers throughout the country. These programs range from a few days to more than 2 years. Standards for teacher training vary and certification differs depending on the style of yoga.

INTEGRATIVE PSYCHIATRY

A new type of psychiatry, called *integrative psychiatry,* selectively incorporates elements of complementary and alternative medicine into practice methods. It emphasizes treatment rather than diagnosis and views the patient holistically, taking into account not only mind–body issues and interactions but spiritual values as well. Integrative psychiatry is also concerned with prevention of illness, emphasized by having the patient pay attention to lifestyle factors such as diet and exercise. Stress reduction involves use of yoga, meditation, or other relaxation exercises. Attention is paid to stress factors related to work and interpersonal relationships.

History

At one time, hypnosis and biofeedback were considered alternative therapies out of the mainstream of traditional psychiatric practice. These modalities are now incorporated into standard psychiatric practice. Hypnosis, for example, is used by psychiatrists for a variety of disorders, and dynamically oriented psychiatrists use hypnotherapy in their work to enable a patient to recover feelings and memories that are repressed and not otherwise available for analysis. In the middle of the 20th century, workers such as Paul Schilder, in his book *The Image and Appearance of the Human Body,* described how one's physiology and physiognomy could be influenced by psychological experiences during various developmental stages. More recently, mainstream psychiatrists, such as Brian Weiss, have described their use of past life regression as a therapeutic method and a means of accessing unconscious material.

Methods

Any of the complementary methods described in this section can be integrated into standard psychotherapeutic practice, although some lend themselves better than others. For example, during a *Reiki* treatment, a patient tends to be in a relaxed state and may have feeling tones, images, or thoughts that would not ordinarily be discussed. In an integrative therapy session, those mental and physical phenomena would be verbalized and subject to analysis and interpretation. Similarly, a patient having past life regression may have an elaborate narrative about his or her past life that would be carefully examined by the integrative psychiatrist for its relevance to current life experiences. Most integrative psychiatrists view past-life narratives as dynamic representations of the patient's unconscious wishes and fears; some view them as representations of actual past lives. In either case, the material is used to help patients gain greater insight and understanding of themselves in their current life.

Complementary and alternative techniques that involve body manipulation (e.g., craniosacral manipulation, massage, or the Alexander technique) lend themselves to integrative psychiatric therapy. As mentioned, the image persons have of their body and the way in which the body is held (e.g., stooped posture) are heavily influenced both by genetics and by life experiences. Depressive facies, Veraguth's folds, and other physiologic correlates of mood have long been recognized in the psychiatric literature. The integrative psychiatrist uses this and other bodily markers as a way to gain access to previously unrecognized neurotic conflict. Patients with somatic symptom disorders or dysmorphophobia are often helped by such approaches, as are patients with eating disorders who have major body image distortions.

Any technique that involves manipulation of a body part can potentially elicit an image, thought, or feeling related to the experience. A patient experiencing a back rub may have myriad associations to the experience that are examined in the session. Some patients cannot tolerate being touched, a trait that is almost always related to some past traumatic experience. Body manipulation can be geared to correcting abnormalities. In the Alexander technique, careful attention is paid to posture and body alignment. As the corrective procedures unfold, patients may gain understanding and insight into what caused the defective or inefficient postural attitude in the first place.

Finally, spiritual beliefs derived from Judeo-Christian, Native American, and Eastern religious thought can be integrated into traditional psychotherapy. Workers such as Alan Watts incorporated Zen Buddhism into Western psychotherapy more than 50 years ago. Psychiatrists are working with Native American healers to help patients diminish anxiety, especially regarding death and dying.

Other Issues

Ideally, the psychiatrist practicing integrative therapy should be schooled in one or more of the complementary methods he or she plans to employ. In some cases, a complementary practitioner may work in conjunction with the psychiatrist, especially if the psychiatrist is not schooled in a particular method. At times, patients may be expert in a field (e.g., yoga) and seek out the integrative psychiatrist to enlarge on their experience. Integrative psychiatrists may use psychoactive herbs and homeopathic medicinals alone or in conjunction with traditional psychopharmacologic agents, mindful of the possibility of adverse drug–drug interactions.

Ethical Issues

The same standards that apply to traditional psychiatric practice and psychotherapy apply to integrative psychiatry. Because some of the techniques involve a laying on of hands or place the patient in a more dependent and vulnerable state than traditional psychotherapy techniques, boundary issues must be carefully evaluated. Currently, no standards of practice exist for this method other than those to which physicians have always been held, including doing no harm. As in complementary and alternative medicine generally, careful outcome studies are needed if this new amalgam is to prove its worth.

21

Other Conditions That May Be a Focus of Clinical Attention

INTRODUCTION

In the fifth edition of *Diagnostic and Statistical Manual of Mental Disorders* (DSM-5), in a section called Other Conditions That May Be a Focus of Clinical Attention, there is a list of conditions that are not mental disorders but that have led to contact with the mental health care system. In some instances, one of these conditions will be noted during the course of a psychiatric evaluation (e.g., divorce), although no mental disorder has been found. In other instances, the diagnostic evaluation reveals no mental disorder, but a need is seen to note the primary reason for contact with the mental health care system (e.g., homelessness).

In some cases, a mental disorder may eventually be found, but the focus of attention or treatment is on a condition that is not caused by a mental disorder. For example, a patient with an anxiety disorder may receive treatment for a marital problem that is unrelated to the anxiety disorder itself.

Table 21–1 lists the many conditions that may be a focus of clinical attention or that may influence the diagnosis, treatment, or course of a mental disorder that is contained in DSM-5. The list of conditions that make up this category cover the entire life cycle from infancy through childhood, adolescence, adulthood, and old age. The list of conditions covers almost every conceivable life circumstance from divorce to problems related to being in military service. In one sense, they represent the vicissitudes of life or, as Shakespeare has Hamlet state, "the slings and arrows of outrageous fortune." Each of these conditions or circumstances is capable of having a profound input on a particular mental illness or on the human experience in general.

The conditions discussed in this chapter include the following: (1) malingering, (2) bereavement, (3) occupational problems, (4) adult antisocial behavior, (5) religious or spiritual problem, (6) acculturation problem, (7) phase of life problem, (8) noncompliance with treatment for a mental disorder, and (9) relational problems. Problems related to the maltreatment and abuse of children is covered in Section 27.19 c, and problems related to the physical and sexual abuse of adults is covered in Chapter 22.

MALINGERING

Malingering is the deliberate falsification of physical or psychological symptoms in an attempt to achieve a secondary gain such as avoiding military duty, avoiding work, obtaining financial compensation, evading criminal prosecution, or obtaining drugs. Under some circumstances, malingering may represent adaptive behavior—for example, as mentioned below, feigning illness while a captive of the enemy during wartime.

Malingering should be strongly suspected if any combination of the following is noted: (1) medicolegal context of presentation (e.g., the person is referred by an attorney to the clinician for examination or is incarcerated), (2) evident discrepancy between the individual's claimed stress or disability and the objective findings, (3) lack of cooperation during the diagnostic evaluation and in complying with the prescribed treatment regimen, and (4) the presence of antisocial personality disorder.

Epidemiology

A 1 percent prevalence of malingering has been estimated among mental health patients in civilian clinical practice, with the estimate rising to 5 percent in the military. In a litigious context, during interviews of criminal defendants, the estimated prevalence of malingering is much higher—between 10 and 20 percent. Approximately 50 percent of children presenting with conduct disorders are described as having serious lying-related issues.

Although no familial or genetic patterns have been reported and no clear sex bias or age at onset has been delineated, malingering does appear to be highly prevalent in certain military, prison, and litigious populations and, in Western society, in men from youth through middle age. Associated disorders include conduct disorder and anxiety disorders in children and antisocial, borderline, and narcissistic personality disorders in adults.

Etiology

Although no biological factors have been found to be causally related to malingering, its frequent association with antisocial personality disorder raises the possibility that hypoarousability may be an underlying metabolic factor. Still, no predisposing genetic, neurophysiological, neurochemical, or neuroendocrinological forces are presently known.

Diagnosis and Clinical Features

Avoidance of Criminal Responsibility, Trial, and Punishment. Criminals may pretend to be incompetent to avoid standing trial; they may feign insanity at the time of

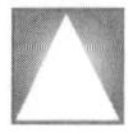

Table 21–1
Conditions That May Be a Focus of Clinical Attention

- I. Relational Problems
  - 1. Problems Related to Family Upbringing
    - i. Parent–Child Problem
    - ii. Sibling Problem
    - iii. Upbringing Away from Parents
    - iv. Parental Relationship Distress
  - 2. Other Problems Related to Primary Support System
    - i. Relationship Distress with Spouse or Partner
    - ii. Separation or Divorce
    - iii. Emotional Distress within Family
    - iv. Uncomplicated Bereavement
- II. Abuse and Neglect
  - 1. Problems of Child Maltreatment and Neglect
    - i. Child Physical Abuse
    - ii. Child Sexual Abuse
    - iii. Child Neglect
    - iv. Child Psychological Abuse
  - 2. Problems of Adult Maltreatment and Neglect
    - i. Physical Violence of Spouse or Partner
    - ii. Sexual Violence of Spouse or Partner
    - iii. Spouse or Partner Neglect
    - iv. Psychological Spouse or Partner Abuse
    - v. Adult Abuse by Nonspouse or Nonpartner (e.g., Physical, Sexual, Psychological)
- III. Educational and Occupational Problems
  - 1. Educational Problems
  - 2. Occupational Problems
    - i. Related to Current Military Deployment Status
    - ii. Other (e.g., job change, loss of job, stress)
- IV. Housing and Economic Problems
  - 1. Housing Problems
    - i. Homelessness
    - ii. Inadequate Housing (e.g., lack of heat or electricity, insect or rodent infestation)
    - iii. Neighbor, Lodger, or Landlord Discord
    - iv. Residential Institution (does not include psychological reaction to change in living situation; see Adjustment Disorder)
  - 2. Economic Problems
    - i. Lack of Adequate Food or Safe Drinking Water
    - ii. Extreme Poverty
    - iii. Low Income
- V. Other Problems Related to the Social Environment
  - 1. Phase of Life Problem
  - 2. Acculturation Difficulty
  - 3. Social Exclusion or Rejection
  - 4. Discrimination or Persecution
- VI. Problems Related to Crime or Interaction with the Legal System (e.g., Victim of Crime, Imprisonment, Release from Prison)
- VII. Other Health Service Encounters for Counseling and Medical Advice (e.g., Sexual Counseling)
- VIII. Problems Related to Other Psychological, Personal, and Environmental Circumstances
  - 1. Religious or Spiritual Problem
  - 2. Victim of Terrorism or Torture
  - 3. Exposure to Disaster or War
- IX. Other Circumstances of Personal History
  - 1. Adult Antisocial Behavior
  - 2. Child or Adolescent Antisocial Behavior
  - 3. Problems Related to Access to Medical and Other Health Care
  - 4. Nonadherence to Medical Treatment (e.g., Overweight or Obesity, Malingering, Wandering Associated with a Mental Disorder)
  - 5. Borderline Intellectual Functioning

Adapted from *Diagnostic and Statistical Manual of Mental Disorders*, 5th edition, American Psychiatric Association, 2013.

perpetration of the crime, malinger symptoms to receive a less harsh penalty, or attempt to act too incapacitated (incompetent) to be executed.

Avoidance of Military Service or of Particularly Hazardous Duties. Persons may malinger to avoid conscription into the armed forces and, after being conscripted, they may feign illness to escape from particularly onerous or hazardous duties.

Financial Gain. Modern malingerers may seek financial gain in the form of undeserved disability insurance, veterans' benefits, workers' compensation, or tort damages for purported psychological injury.

Avoidance of Work, Social Responsibility, and Social Consequences. Individuals may malinger to escape from unpleasant vocational or social circumstances or to avoid the social and litigation-related consequences of vocational or social improprieties.

An owner of a previously successful photographic equipment supplier declared bankruptcy in a way that the government maintained was illegal. Subsequently, the government indicted the defendant on various counts of fraud. The defendant's counsel maintained that the defendant was too depressed to cooperate with him and that, because of that depression, he experienced memory loss that made it impossible to understand what had occurred and therefore impossible to provide a meaningful defense. The government's forensic psychiatrist evaluated the defendant to ascertain the nature of his depression and to determine whether it was causing cognitive problems.

When asked early in his evaluation when his birthday was, he responded, "Oh, what does it matter? It was in the 40s or 50s." Similarly, when queried about where he was born, he said, "Some place in Hungary." Even when pressed for more specifics, he refused to elaborate. Yet, at many points later in his evaluation, he responded with complete, often detailed, information about transactions not related to those for which he had been indicted. It was the impression of the evaluator that the defendant was malingering in a gross and inconsistent fashion, incompatible with the kinds of decreases in cognitive skills that occasionally attend major depression. *(Adapted from case of Mark J. Mills, J.D., M.D. and Mark S. Lipian, M.D., Ph.D.)*

Facilitation of Transfer from Prison to Hospital. Prisoners may malinger (fake bad) with the goal of obtaining a transfer to a psychiatric hospital from which they may hope to escape or in which they expect to do "easier time." The prison context may also give rise to dissimulation (faking good), however; the prospect of an indeterminate number of days on a mental health ward may prompt an inmate with true psychiatric symptoms to make every effort to conceal them.

Admission to a Hospital. In this era of deinstitutionalization and homelessness, individuals may malinger in an effort to gain admission to a psychiatric hospital. Such institutions may be seen as providing free room and board, a safe haven from the police, or refuge from rival gang members or disgruntled drug cronies who have made street life even more unbearable and hazardous than it usually is.

A robust, neatly attired man presented to the psychiatric emergency department in the early-morning hours. He stated that "the voices" were worse and that he wished to be readmitted to the hospital. When the psychiatrist challenged him, observing that he had just been discharged that afternoon, that he routinely left the hospital in the morning and demanded rehospitalization at night, and that, despite multiple hospitalizations, his reported history of hallucinations had been increasingly doubted, the man became belligerent. When the psychiatrist still refused to admit him, the patient grabbed the psychiatrist's clothes, threatening him but inflicting no harm. The psychiatrist asked the hospital police to escort him off the grounds. The patient was told he could seek readmission to his regular ward during the day. Subsequent contact with the patient's ward revealed that their diagnoses were substance abuse and homelessness; his apparent schizophrenia appeared never to have been an actual issue in his treatment. *(Courtesy of Mark J. Mills, J.D., M.D. and Mark S. Lipian, M.D., Ph.D.)*

Drug Seeking. Malingerers may feign illness in an effort to obtain favored medications, either for personal use or, in a prison setting, as currency to barter for cigarettes, protection, or other inmate-provided favors.

The plaintiff, a woman in her late 20s, was injured while dancing at a club. Although her claim initially appeared bona fide, subsequent investigation cast doubt on the mechanism of injury that she claimed—namely, that a misplaced electrical cord under a carpet caused her to slip. This was true, she claimed, even though she had to been dancing in a particularly jerky manner that could have easily caused problems without tripping.

Subsequently, she sought medical and surgical treatment for torn cartilage in her injured knee. Even though the initial surgery went well, she kept reinjuring the knee with various "slips." As a result, she requested narcotic analgesics. A careful medical record review revealed that she was obtaining such medications from multiple practitioners and that she had apparently forged at least one prescription.

In reviewing the case before binding arbitration, it was the opinion of the orthopedic and psychiatric consultants that, although the initial injury and reported pain were real, the plaintiff consciously elaborated her injuries to obtain the desired narcotic analgesics. *(Courtesy of Mark J. Mills, J.D., M.D. and Mark S. Lipian, M.D., Ph.D.)*

Child Custody. Minimizing difficulties or faking good for the sake of obtaining child custody can occur when one party accurately accuses the other of being an unfit parent because of psychological conditions. The accused party may feel compelled to minimize symptoms or to portray him- or herself in a positive light to reduce chances of being deemed unfit and losing custody.

Differential Diagnosis

Malingering must be differentiated from the actual physical or psychiatric illness suspected of being feigned. Furthermore, the possibility of partial malingering, which is an exaggeration of existing symptoms, must be entertained. Also, the possibility exists of unintentional, dynamically driven misattribution of genuine symptoms (e.g., of depression) to an incorrect environmental cause (e.g., to sexual harassment rather than to narcissistic injury).

Table 21–2
Factors Aiding in the Differentiation between Malingering and Conversion Disorder

1. Malingerers are more likely to be suspicious, uncooperative, aloof, and unfriendly; patients with conversion disorder are likely to be friendly, cooperative, appealing, dependent, and clinging.
2. Malingerers may try to avoid diagnostic evaluations and refuse recommended treatment; patients with conversion disorder likely welcome evaluation and treatment, "searching for an answer."
3. Malingerers likely refuse employment opportunities designed to circumvent their disability; patients with conversion disorder likely accept such opportunities.
4. Malingerers are more likely to provide extremely detailed and exacting descriptions of events precipitating their "illness"; patients with conversion disorder are more likely to report historical gaps, inaccuracies, and vagaries.

It should also be remembered that a real psychiatric disorder and malingering are not mutually exclusive.

Factitious disorder is distinguished from malingering by motivation (sick role vs. tangible pain), whereas the somatoform disorders involve no conscious volition. In conversion disorder, as in malingering, objective signs cannot account for subjective experience, and differentiation between the two disorders can be difficult. Table 21–2 lists some variables that may aid in distinguishing between these two conditions.

Course and Prognosis

Malingering persists as long as the malingerer believes it will likely produce the desired rewards. In the absence of concurrent diagnoses, after the rewards have been attained, the feigned symptoms disappear. In some structured settings, such as the military or prison units, ignoring the malingered behavior may result in its disappearance, particularly if an expectation of continued productive performance, despite complaints, is made clear. In children, malingering is most likely associated with a predisposing anxiety or conduct disorder; proper attention to this developing problem may alleviate the child's propensity to malinger.

Treatment

The appropriate stance for the psychiatrist is clinical neutrality. If malingering is suspected, a careful differential investigation should ensue. If, at the conclusion of the diagnostic evaluation, malingering seems most likely, the patient should be tactfully but firmly confronted with the apparent outcome. The reasons underlying the ruse need to be elicited, however, and alternative pathways to the desired outcome explored. Coexisting psychiatric disorders should be thoroughly assessed. Only if the patient is utterly unwilling to interact with the physician under any terms other than manipulation should the therapeutic (or evaluative) interaction be abandoned.

BEREAVEMENT

Normal bereavement begins immediately after or within a few months of the loss of a loved one. Typical signs and symptoms include feelings of sadness, preoccupation with thoughts about the deceased, tearfulness, irritability, insomnia, and difficulties concentrating and carrying out daily activities. On the basis of the cultural group, bereavement is limited to a varying time, usually 6 months, but it can be longer. Normal bereavement, however, can lead to a full depressive disorder that requires treatment. Some grieving individuals present with symptoms characteristic of a major depressive episode such as depressed mood, insomnia, anorexia, and weight loss. The duration of grief and bereavement vary considerably among different cultural groups and with the same cultural group. The diagnosis of depressive disorder is generally not given unless the symptoms are still present 2 months after the loss. However, the presence of certain symptoms that are not characteristic of a "normal" grief reaction may be helpful in differentiating bereavement from depression. These include (1) guilt about things other than actions taken or not taken by the survivor at the time of the death, (2) thoughts of death other than the survivor feeling that he or she would be better off dead or should have died with the deceased person, (3) morbid preoccupation with worthlessness, (4) marked psychomotor retardation, (5) prolonged and marked functional impairment, and (6) hallucinatory experiences other than thinking that he or she hears the voice of or transiently sees the image of the deceased person.

OCCUPATIONAL PROBLEMS

Occupational problems often arise during stressful changes in work, namely, at initial entry into the workforce or when making job changes within the same organization to a higher position because of good performance or to a parallel position because of corporate need. Distress occurs particularly if these changes are not sought and no preparatory training has taken place, as well as during layoffs and at retirement, especially if retirement is mandatory and the person is unprepared for this event. Work distress can result if initially agreed-to conditions change to work overload or lack of challenge and opportunity to experience work satisfaction, if an individual feels unable to fulfill conflicting expectations or feels that work conditions prevent accomplishing assignments because of lack of legitimate power, or if an individual believes he or she works in a hierarchy with harsh and unreasonable superiors.

Work Choices and Changes

Young adults without role models or guidance from families, mentors, or others in their communities too often underestimate their lifetime potential abilities to learn a trade or earn a college or postgraduate degree. In addition, women and members of minority groups often feel less prepared to accept work challenges, fear rejection, and do not apply for jobs for which they are qualified. On the other hand, men, in fields in which they are underrepresented, often and confidently move up the career ladder faster (glass elevator). As part of initial interviews for evaluation of occupational problems, patients should be encouraged to consider their heretofore unrecognized, unadmitted talents; long-held, yet unexpressed, dreams and goals regarding work; actual successes in work and school; and motivation to risk learning what they would find satisfying.

Minorities and those in low-paying and low-skilled jobs too often have less job security. Business and institutional reorganization and consequent downsizing, factory closings, and moves affect many, often leaving these workers feeling hopeless and helpless about future employment, on welfare, angry, and depressed.

With ongoing and often sudden downsizing of corporations and businesses, men and women continue to struggle with unexpected job loss and premature retirement even when finances are not an issue. In addition, men, in particular, define themselves by their work roles, and thus experience more occupational distress from these changes. Women may adjust faster to retirement, but they often have less financial security than men do (white women earn approximately 80 cents on the dollar, and African American and Hispanic women earn even less for comparable work); women have generally been in lower status work positions, find themselves widowed more often than men, and are more likely to be caring for children, grandchildren, and elderly relatives. Women represent more of the single working parent group and the working poor.

Stress and the Workplace

More than 30 percent of workers report that they are under stress at work. Workplace distress is implicated in at least 15 percent of occupational disability claims. Expected distress follows recognized and uncontrollable work changes—downsizing; mergers and acquisitions; work overload; and chronic physical strains, including work noise, temperature, bodily injuries, and strain from performing computer work. According to one study, the top ten most stressful jobs in 1998 were (1) president of the United States, (2) firefighter, (3) senior corporate executive, (4) race car driver, (5) taxi driver, (6) surgeon, (7) astronaut, (8) police officer, (9) football player, and (10) air traffic controller. People who work under deadlines, such as bus drivers, are subject to hypertension.

Work frustration can also arise from an individual worker's unrecognized (and therefore unresolved) psychodynamic issues, such as working appropriately with superiors and not relating to one's supervisor as a parent figure. Other developmental issues include unresolved problems with competition, assertiveness, envy, fear of success, and inability to communicate verbally in a constructive manner.

After the September 11, 2001, World Trade Center tragedy, a 32-year-old, married male firefighter, who had been away on vacation that day with his wife and children, began to exhibit changed behaviors at home and at work. At home, he appeared not to listen to his two children and, instead, focused his attention on television sporting events. At work, he also appeared to be more focused on cooking the same dinners for his peers and watching television than on interacting verbally with his remaining peers and the new chief. In the course of several months, a chaplain visited the station several times and talked to the firefighters about survivor guilt and the 9/11 tragedy, and the firefighter began to return somewhat to his former healthier behaviors. *(Courtesy of Leah J. Dickstein, M.D.)*

Often, work conflicts reflect similar conflicts in the worker's personal life, and referral for treatment, unless there is insight, is in order. Some studies have found that massage therapy, meditation, and yoga at intervals during the work day relieve stress when used on a regular basis. Approaches using cognitive therapy have also helped people reduce work pressure.

Suicide Risk

Some occupations—health professionals, financial service workers, and police, the first and latter groups because of easier access to lethal drugs and weapons—both attract persons with a high suicide risk and involve increased chronic distress that may lead to higher suicide rates.

Career and Job Problems of Women

Most women work outside the home out of necessity to support themselves or their dependents (whether children or adults) or as part of a working couple. With the divorce rate remaining at the 50 percent level, many women find themselves economically poorer after a divorce than when married, although divorced men usually find their economic status improved. Despite more than four decades of increasing knowledge about and concern for women's status in the workplace, unique gender issues, bias, and lack of accommodation to their unique needs at certain life stages (i.e., pregnancy and postpartum, major responsibility for young healthy and ill children) continue. Yet, women were the largest group establishing new small businesses in the 1990s. Many have left large corporations where they were not valued for their efforts because of their gender. Women experience problems when they are the sole woman in a man's field. Despite increasing recognition of the need for men in relationships with women to assume home and family responsibilities, fewer than 25 percent of men do so equitably.

Women of childbearing and child-rearing ages continue to find themselves in conflict with job expectations, opportunities, and personal responsibilities. High-quality, on-site, dependent-care facilities with extended hours are rare and often out of range financially. Major unresolved work issues that are unique to women at certain life stages include flextime and paid and unpaid dependent leave options. Beyond dependent care issues, women in the workforce continue to experience distress after chronic and repeated sexual harassment, despite its illegality and media attention. Increasingly, more women have travel responsibilities, work long hours, work shifts beyond daylight hours, and experience personal workplace violence.

Among dual-career families and partners, the woman is more likely to move when the man chooses to move for a work opportunity than vice versa. Consequently, a woman's career is interrupted more often. Less reluctance is seen, however, to have the two members of a relationship work for the same organization than previously, albeit usually in different departments. Work distress may also stem from continuous miscommunication, especially that based on gender.

Working Teenagers

With unemployment increasing, many teenagers work part time while attending high school. Consequently, stress can arise because of less parent–teenager interaction and constructive parental control issues about teens' use of earnings, time spent away from home, and consequent behaviors both in and outside the home. When both parents or a single parent, as well as the teenager, work outside the home, often on different schedules, parent–teen verbal communication must be proactive, clear, and ongoing.

Working within the Home

Although most women with children of all ages must work outside the home, at times they may be home full time or part time or may work at home. When their husbands or partners work full time outside the home, problems may develop from each one's perceived expectations of the other. Women who care for children and their home exclusively may be seen by their partners as not only economically dependent and inferior but also not as competent and not understanding of the man's stressors and needs. Ongoing respectful listening and verbal communication must be encouraged.

People in organizations are increasingly taking work home as their work expectations increase. This work-at-home experience can and does interfere with personal lives and satisfaction, which can then have further repercussions at work.

Chronic Illness

As general and other medical and psychiatric treatments for chronic diseases improve, employers have been increasingly concerned about accommodating patients with acquired immunodeficiency syndrome (AIDS), diabetes mellitus, and other disorders. The issue of mandatory testing for AIDS and substance abuse (alcohol and other illegal substances) continues to be of concern. Employee assistance programs offering education about general and mental health topics have proved timely and cost effective.

Domestic Violence

Although occurring in the home, signs and symptoms that interfere with work often trigger identification of those who experience domestic violence. Trained professionals must question all employees experiencing work distress about domestic violence and, when indicated, refer individuals for assistance, which includes safety in the workplace.

Job Loss

Regardless of the reason for job loss, most people experience distress, at least temporarily, including symptoms of normal grief, loss of self-esteem, anger, and reactive depressive and anxiety symptoms, as well as somatic symptoms and possibly the onset of or increase in substance abuse or domestic violence. Timely education, support programs, and vocational guidance should be instituted and access to treatment made available if indicated.

Vocational Rehabilitation

Rehabilitation is often necessary for those traumatized by stresses in the workplace, those who had to take a leave of absence because of medical or psychiatric reasons, and those who have been fired. Individual or group counseling enables persons to improve personal relationships, raise self-esteem, or learn new work skills. Patients with schizophrenia may benefit from sheltered workshops in which they perform work that is geared to their level of function. Some patients with schizophrenia or autism do well in tasks that are repetitive or require obsessive concern with details.

ADULT ANTISOCIAL BEHAVIOR

Characterized by activities that are illegal, immoral, or both, antisocial behavior usually begins in childhood and often persists throughout life. The term *antisocial behavior* somewhat confusingly applies both to persons' actions that are not due to a mental disorder and to actions by those who never received a neuropsychiatric workup to determine the presence or absence of a mental disorder. As Dorothy Lewis noted, the term can apply to behavior by normal persons who "struggle to make a dishonest living."

Epidemiology

Depending on the criteria and the sampling, estimates of the prevalence of adult antisocial behavior range from 5 to 15 percent of the population. Within prison populations, investigators report prevalence figures between 20 and 80 percent. Men account for more adult antisocial behavior than do women.

Etiology

Antisocial behaviors in adulthood are characteristic of a variety of persons, ranging from those with no demonstrable psychopathology to those who are severely impaired and have psychotic disorders, cognitive disorders, and retardation, among other conditions. A comprehensive neuropsychiatric assessment of antisocial adults is indicated and may reveal potentially treatable psychiatric and neurological impairments that can easily be overlooked. Only in the absence of mental disorders can patients be categorized as displaying adult antisocial behavior. Adult antisocial behavior may be influenced by genetic and social factors.

Genetic Factors. Data supporting the genetic transmission of antisocial behavior are based on studies that found a 60 percent concordance rate in monozygotic twins and about a 30 percent concordance rate in dizygotic twins. Adoption studies show a high rate of antisocial behavior in the biological relatives of adoptees identified with antisocial behavior and a high incidence of antisocial behavior in the adopted-away offspring of those with antisocial behavior. The prenatal and perinatal periods of those who subsequently display antisocial behavior often are associated with low birth weight, mental retardation, and prenatal exposure to alcohol and other drugs of abuse.

Social Factors. Studies have shown that in neighborhoods in which families with low socioeconomic status (SES) predominate, the sons of unskilled workers are more likely to commit more offenses and more serious criminal offenses than do the sons of middle-class and skilled workers, at least during adolescence and early adulthood. These data are not as clear for women, but the findings are generally similar in studies from many countries. Areas of family training differ by SES group. Middle-SES parents use love-oriented techniques in discipline. They withdraw affection rather than impose physical punishment as is done in low-SES groups. Negative parental attitudes toward aggressive behavior, attempts to curb aggressive behavior, and the ability to communicate parental values are more characteristic of middle- and high-SES groups than of low ones. Adult antisocial behavior is associated with the use and abuse of alcohol and other substances and with the easy availability of handguns.

Diagnosis and Clinical Features. The diagnosis of adult antisocial behavior is one of exclusion. Substance dependence in such behavior often makes it difficult to separate the antisocial behavior related primarily to substance dependence from disordered behaviors that occurred either before substance use or during episodes unrelated to substance dependence.

During the manic phases of bipolar I disorder, certain aspects of behavior, such as wanderlust, sexual promiscuity, and financial difficulties, can be similar to adult antisocial behavior. Patients with schizophrenia may have episodes of adult antisocial behavior, but the symptom picture is usually clear, especially regarding thought disorder, delusions, and hallucinations on the mental status examination.

Neurological conditions can be associated with adult antisocial behavior, and electroencephalograms (EEGs), computed tomography (CT) scans, magnetic resonance imaging (MRI), and complete neurological examinations are indicated. Temporal lobe epilepsy should be considered in the differential diagnosis. When a clear-cut diagnosis of temporal lobe epilepsy or encephalitis can be made, the disorder may be considered to contribute to the adult antisocial behavior. Abnormal EEG findings are prevalent among violent offenders: An estimated 50 percent of aggressive criminals have abnormal EEG findings.

Persons with adult antisocial behavior have difficulties in work, marriage, and money matters and conflicts with various authorities. The symptoms of adult antisocial behavior are summarized in Table 21–3. (Antisocial personality disorder is discussed in Chapter 18.)

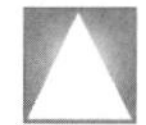

Table 21–3
Symptoms of Adult Antisocial Behavior

Life Area	Antisocial Patients with Significant Problems in Area (%)
Work problems	85
Marital problems	81
Financial dependence	79
Arrests	75
Alcohol abuse	72
School problems	71
Impulsiveness	67
Sexual behavior	64
Wild adolescence	62
Vagrancy	60
Belligerence	58
Social isolation	56
Military record (of those serving)	53
Lack of guilt	40
Somatic complaints	31
Use of aliases	29
Pathological lying	16
Drug abuse	15
Suicide attempts	11

Data from Robins L. *Deviant Children Grown Up: A Sociological and Psychiatric Study of Sociopathic Personality*. Baltimore: Williams & Wilkins; 1966.

Treatment

In general, therapists are pessimistic about treating adult antisocial behavior. They have little hope of changing a pattern that has been present almost continuously throughout a person's life. Psychotherapy has not been effective, and no major breakthroughs with biological treatments, including medications, have occurred.

Therapists show more enthusiasm for the use of therapeutic communities and other forms of group treatment, although the data provide little basis for optimism. Many adult criminals who are incarcerated in institutional settings have shown some response to group therapy approaches. The history of violence, criminality, and antisocial behavior has shown that such behaviors seem to decrease after age 40 years. Recidivism in criminals, which can reach 90 percent in some studies, also decreases in middle age.

Prevention. Because antisocial behavior often begins during childhood, the major focus must be on delinquency prevention. Any measure that improves the physical and mental health of socioeconomically disadvantaged children and their families is likely to reduce delinquency and violent crime. Often, recurrently violent persons have sustained many insults to the central nervous system (CNS) prenatally and throughout childhood and adolescence. Consequently, programs must be developed to educate parents about the dangers to their children of CNS injury from maltreatment, including the effects of psychoactive substances on the brains of growing fetuses. Public education about the releasing effect of alcohol on violent behaviors (as well as its contribution to vehicular homicide) may also reduce crime.

In a Surgeon General's Report on Violence and Public Health, the Committee on the Prevention of Assault and Homicide emphasized the importance of discouraging corporal punishment in the home, forbidding it in the schools, and even abolishing capital punishment by the state, saying that all are models and sanctions for violence. Since that time, capital punishment has been instituted in states that did not have it, such as New York. No evidence indicates that capital punishment reduces crime in states that have it. Opponents of capital punishment see it as "vengeance," not punishment.

Although persons disagree about the contribution of violence in the media to violent crime, the propaganda potential of the media is universally recognized. The extent to which the media, such as television, can be used to transmit positive social values has not yet been realized. The guidelines issued by the television industry to indicate the amount of sex and violence in programs is an attempt to deal with the issue; however, program content that espouses traditional societal values would be beneficial.

The most successful preventive measures within the field of medicine have come from community-wide public health programs (e.g., campaigns against smoking) and from programs that detect individual vulnerabilities (e.g., individual monitoring of blood pressure). Studies of adult antisocial behavior reveal the contribution of broad cultural factors and constellations of individual biopsychosocial vulnerabilities. Prevention programs must recognize and address both kinds of factors.

RELIGIOUS OR SPIRITUAL PROBLEM

A religious or spiritual problem can bring the person to the psychiatrist under one of several circumstances. For example, a person may begin to question his or her faith and choose not to discuss the problem with a spiritual advisor. Or a person may wish to convert to a new faith in order to marry or to create harmony in a marriage in which husband and wife are of different faiths.

Psychiatrists must enable and assist patients to distinguish religious thought or experience from psychopathology and, if this is a problem, encourage patients to work through the issues independently or with assistance. Religious imagery may be recognized in mental illness when persons state they believe they have been commanded by God to take a dangerous or grandiose action.

Religious experience may factor into a person's life in unexpected ways as in the following case. A midcareer male surgeon who was very successful but long overcommitted to his private practice and his academic responsibilities revealed to his often-neglected wife that, at age 9 years, he was approached by his religious leader to get close physically and ultimately engaged in sexual acts over several years. Believing it was his fault, he never told anyone and decided never to have children. After telling his wife about the experience, they engaged in family therapy to work through the stresses the confession produced in their marriage.

Cults

Recently, cults have appeared to be less popular and less attractive to naïve late adolescents and young adults seeking assistance in discovering who they are as they struggle to develop more mature relationships with their parents. Cults are led by charismatic leaders, often out of control themselves, with inappropriate and often unethical values but purporting to offer acceptance and guidance to troubled followers. Cult members are strongly controlled and forced to dissolve allegiance to family and others to serve the cult leader's directives and personal needs. These young members often come from educated families who then seek professional help in persuading their children to leave the cult and enter deprogramming therapy to restore personal psychological stability to the former cult members. Deprogramming and adjustment back into family, society, and an independent life are time intensive and long term with resultant posttraumatic stress disorder (PTSD), which must be recognized and treated.

ACCULTURATION PROBLEM

Acculturation is the process whereby a person from one culture undergoes a change in manner, customs, and dress among others to adapt to a different culture. It leads to assimilation in which the person has identified with the new culture, usually without conflict or ambivalence. In some cases, however, major cultural change can evoke severe distress, termed *culture shock*. This condition arises when individuals suddenly find themselves in a new culture in which they feel completely alien. They may also feel conflict over which lifestyles to maintain, change, or adopt. Children and young adult immigrants often adapt more easily than do middle-aged and elderly immigrants. Younger immigrants often learn the new language more easily and continue to mature in the new culture, but those who are more senior, having had more stability and unchanging routines in their former culture, struggle more to adapt. Culture shock from immigration clearly differs from the restless and continuous moving of psychiatric patients secondary to their illness.

Culture shock can occur within a person's own country with geographic, school, and work changes, such as joining the military, experiencing school abusing, moving across country, or moving to a vastly different neighborhood or from a rural area to a metropolis. Reactive symptoms, which are understandable, include anxiety, depression, isolation, fear, and a sense of loss of identity as the person adjusts. If the person is part of a family or group making this transition and the move is positive and planned, stress can be lower. Furthermore, if selected cultural mores can be safely maintained as persons integrate into the new culture, stress is also minimized.

Constant geographic moves because of chosen work opportunities or necessity involve a large proportion of workers in the United States. Joining activities in the new community and actively trying to meet neighbors and coworkers can lessen the culture shock.

An 18-year-old, first-year female college student offered an academic scholarship by a small Southern college with a major in her field of interest realized on her return home to the Midwest for winter break that she felt like a misfit among her dorm peers. They were friendly yet generally kept their distance from her after class. At home, she discussed her experiences with high school friends, who replied that they had heard about such cultural dissonance from peers at their Midwestern colleges. The student returned to college feeling that it was not her fault or imagination and slowly began to reach out more assertively to her peers so they could get to know her beyond stereotypical beliefs and so she could do the same.

Brainwashing

First practiced by the Chinese Communists on American prisoners during the Korean War, *brainwashing* is the deliberate creation of culture shock. Individuals are isolated, intimidated, and made to feel different and out of place to break their spirits and destroy their coping skills. When a person appears mentally weak and helpless, the aggressors impose new ideas on them that they would never have accepted in their normal state. As with those involved in cults, on release and return to their homes, brainwashed individuals with PTSD require deprogramming treatment, including reeducation and ongoing supportive psychotherapy, both on an individual and group basis. Treatment is usually long term to rebuild healthy self-esteem and coping skills. (See also Section 23.4.)

Prisoners of War and Torture Victims

Prisoners who survive war or torture experiences do so because of personal inner strengths developed in their earlier lives, beginning within their emotionally strong and caring families; if they come from troubled families, they are more likely to commit suicide during imprisonment and torture. Prisoners must constantly cope with ongoing anxiety, fear, isolation from known lives, and complete loss of all control over their lives. Those who appear to cope best believe they must survive for a reason (e.g., to tell others what they experienced or to find and return to loved ones). Prisoners who cope best describe living simultaneously on two levels—coping in the here and now to survive the situation while maintaining constant mental connections to their past values and experiences and those important to them.

Beyond the surviving prisoner's personal difficulties, including PTSD disorder, if and when his or her survival behavior continues, his or her family may be affected by the surviving prisoner's inordinate fear of police and strangers, overprotection and overburdening of children to replace those significant others lost, lack of sharing of the past, continued isolation from current communities, or inappropriate expressed anger. Thus, another generation (i.e., children of survivors) can be affected in their personal development and psychological functioning and may require psychiatric evaluation and treatment. (See also Chapter 8 for further discussion of these topics.)

A 75-year-old, Catholic, female survivor of the Pawiak prison in Warsaw, Poland, and then of a concentration camp after her capture as a member of the underground in World War II stated that she had wanted to become a painter. In camp, she carved the Madonna and Child on her toothbrush and sent it home to her mother. She made other clandestine carvings for several women in her barracks to send home to their families, which pleased everyone. After the war, she became a well-known sculptress with exhibits throughout Europe. Many of her art pieces taught people about suffering and respect for others who are of different religions and cultures.

PHASE OF LIFE PROBLEM

Phase of life problems may occur at any point along the life cycle: the first day of school as a child, the divorce of a parent during adolescence, starting college as a young adult, marriage, having children, illness, caring for aged parents, and many others. Although, on some level, adults recognize that life events will intrude on expected plans in the course of a lifetime, unexpected, multiple, major negative occurrences, especially if they are chronic, overwhelm a person's ability to recover and function constructively. Common phase of life problems include relationship changes, such as a changed significant personal relationship or its loss, job crises, and parenthood.

Because of sex role socialization and consequent cultural expectations, whereas men appear externally better able to handle these phases of life problems, women, people with lower SES, and minority group members appear more vulnerable to negative experiences, perhaps because they feel less empowered psychologically. Major life changes precipitate distress in the form of anxiety and depressive symptoms, an inability to express reactive emotions directly, and often difficulties in coping with ongoing or changed life responsibilities.

Individuals with positive attitudes, strong family and personal relationships, and mature defense mechanisms and coping styles, including basic trust in self and others, good verbal communication skills, a capacity for creative and positive thinking, and the ability to be flexible, reliable, and energetic, appear to be best able to cope with phase of life problems. Furthermore, a capacity for sublimation; adequate financial and work status; solid values; and healthy, feasible goals can enable people to face, accept, and deal realistically with expected and unexpected life problems and changes.

NONCOMPLIANCE WITH TREATMENT

Compliance is the degree to which a patient carries out the recommendations of the treating physician. It is fostered when the doctor–patient relationship is a positive one, but even in those circumstances, the patient may be reluctant to comply with a physician's advice. In psychiatry, a major concern is medication noncompliance, which may result from discomforting side effects, expense, personal value judgments, and denial of illness, among many others. This category should be used only when the problem is sufficiently severe to warrant independent clinical attention.

RELATIONAL PROBLEMS

An adult's psychological health and sense of well-being depend to a significant degree on the quality of his or her important relationships—that is, on patterns of interaction with a partner and children, parents and siblings, and friends and colleagues. Problems in the interaction between any of these significant others can lead to clinical symptoms and impaired functioning among one or more members of the relational unit. Relational problems may be a focus of clinical attention (1) when a relational unit is distressed and dysfunctional or threatened with dissolution and (2) when the relational problems precede, accompany, or follow other psychiatric or medical disorders. Indeed, other medical or psychiatric symptoms can be influenced by the relational context of the patient. Conversely, the functioning of a relational unit is affected by a member's general and other medical or psychiatric illness. Relational disorders require a different clinical approach than other disorders. Instead of focusing primarily on the link between symptoms, signs, and the workings of the individual mind, the clinician must also focus on interactions between the individuals involved and how these interactions are related to the general and other medical or psychiatric symptoms in a meaningful way.

Definition

Relational problems are patterns of interaction between members of a relational unit that are associated with significantly impaired functioning in one or more individual members. Thus one may have parent–child problems, sibling-related problems, or other dyad or triad impairments. At times the entire unit such as the family itself, may be dysfunctional.

Epidemiology

No reliable figures are available on the prevalence of relational problems. They can be assumed to be ubiquitous; however, most relational problems resolve without professional intervention. The nature, frequency, and effects of the problem on those involved are elements that must be considered before a diagnosis of relational problem is made. For example, divorce, which occurs in just under 50 percent of marriages, is a problem between partners that is resolved through the legal remedy of divorce and need not be diagnosed as a relational problem. If the persons cannot resolve their disputation and continue to live together in a sadomasochistic or pathologically depressed relationship with unhappiness and abuse, then they should be so labeled. Relationship problems between involved persons that cannot be resolved by friends, family, or clergy require professional intervention by psychiatrists, clinical psychologists, social workers, and other mental health professionals.

Relational Problem Related to a Mental Disorder or General Medical Condition

When a family member is ill either from a psychiatric or medical illness, there are reverberations throughout the family unit. Studies indicate that whereas satisfying relationships may have a health-protective influence, relationship distress tends to be associated with an increased incidence of illness. The influence of relational systems on health has been explained through psychophysiological mechanisms that link the intense emotions generated in human attachment systems to vascular reactivity and immune processes. Thus, stress-related psychological or physical symptoms can be an expression of family dysfunction.

Adults must often assume responsibility for caring for aging parents while they are still caring for their own children, and this dual obligation can create stress. When adults take care of their parents, both parties must adapt to a reversal of their former roles, and the caretakers not only face the potential loss of their parents but also must cope with evidence of their own mortality.

Some caretakers abuse their aging parents, a problem that is now receiving attention. Abuse is most likely to occur when the caretaking offspring have substance abuse problems, are under economic stress, and have no relief from their caretaking duties or when the parent is bedridden or has a chronic illness requiring constant nursing attention. More women are abused than men, and most abuse occurs in persons older than age 75 years.

The development of a chronic illness in a family member stresses the family system and requires adaptation by both the sick person and the other family members. The person who has become sick must frequently face a loss of autonomy, an increased sense of vulnerability, and sometimes a taxing medical regimen. The other family members must experience the loss of the person as he or she was before the illness, and they usually have substantial caretaking responsibility—for example, in debilitating neurological diseases, including dementia of the Alzheimer's type, and in diseases such as AIDS and cancer. In these cases, the whole family must deal with the stress of prospective death as well as the current illness. Some families use the anger engendered by such situations to create support organizations, increase public awareness of the disease, and rally around the sick member. But chronic illness frequently produces depression in family members and can cause them to withdraw from or attack one another. The burden of caring for ill family members falls disproportionately on the women in a family—mothers, daughters, and daughters-in-law.

Chronic emotional illness also requires major adaptations by families. For instance, family members may react with chaos or fear to the psychotic productions of a family member with schizophrenia. The regression, exaggerated emotions, frequent hospitalizations, and economic and social dependence of a person with schizophrenia can stress the family system. Family members may react with hostile feelings (referred to as expressed emotion) that are associated with a poor prognosis for the person who is sick. Similarly, a family member with bipolar I disorder can disrupt a family, particularly during manic episodes.

Family devastation can occur when illness (1) suddenly strikes a previously healthy person, (2) occurs earlier than expected in the life cycle (some impairment of physical capacities is expected in old age, although many older persons are healthy), (3) affects the economic stability of the family, and (4) when little can be done to improve or ease the condition of the sick family member.

Parent–Child Relational Problem

Parents differ widely in sensing the needs of their infants. Some quickly note their child's moods and needs; others are slow to respond. Parental responsiveness interacts with the children's temperament to affect the quality of the attachment between child and parent. The diagnosis of parent–child relational problem applies when the focus of clinical attention is a pattern of interaction between parent and child that is associated with clinically significant impairment in individual or family functioning or with clinically significant symptoms. Examples include impaired communication, overprotection, and inadequate discipline.

Research on parenting skills has isolated two major dimensions: (1) a permissive–restrictive dimension and (2) a warm and accepting versus a cold and hostile dimension. A typology that separates parents on these dimensions distinguishes among *authoritarian* (restrictive and cold), *permissive* (minimally restrictive and accepting), and *authoritative* (restrictive as needed but also warm and accepting) parenting styles. Children of authoritarian parents tend to be withdrawn or conflicted; those of permissive parents are likely to be more aggressive, impulsive, and low achievers; and children of authoritative parents seem to function at the highest level, socially and cognitively. Yet, switching from an authoritarian to a permissive mode may create a negative reinforcement pattern.

Difficulties in many situations stress the usual parent–child interaction. Substantial evidence indicates that marital discord leads to problems in children, from depression and withdrawal to conduct disorder and poor performance at school. This negative effect may be partly mediated through *triangulation* of the parent–child relationships, which is a process in which conflicted parents attempt to win the sympathy and support of their child, who is recruited by one parent as an ally in the struggle with the partner. Divorces and remarriages stress the parent–child relationship and may create painful loyalty conflicts. Stepparents often find it difficult to assume a parental role and may resent the special relationship that exists between their new marital partner and the children from that partner's previous marriages. The resentment of a stepparent by a stepchild and the favoring of a natural child are usual reactions in a new family's initial phases of adjustment. When a second child is born, both familial stress and happiness may result, although happiness is the dominant emotion in most families. The birth of a child can also be troublesome when parents had adopted a child in the belief that they were infertile. Single-parent families usually consist of a mother and children, and their relationship is often affected by financial and emotional problems.

Other situations that can produce a parent–child problem are the development of fatal, disabling, or chronic illness, such as leukemia, epilepsy, sickle-cell anemia, or spinal cord injury, in either the parent or child. The birth of a child with congenital defects, such as cerebral palsy, blindness, or deafness, may also produce parent–child problems. These situations, which are not rare, challenge the emotional resources of those involved. Parents and the child must face present and potential loss and must adjust their day-to-day lives physically, economically, and emotionally. These situations can strain the healthiest families and produce parent–child problems not only with the sick person but also with the unaffected family members. In a family with a severely sick child, parents may resent, prefer, or neglect the other children because the ill child requires so much time and attention.

Parents with children who have emotional disorders face particular problems, depending on the child's illness. In families with a child with schizophrenia, family treatment is beneficial and improves the social adjustment of the patient. Similarly, family therapy is useful when a child has a mood disorder. In families with a substance-abusing child or adolescent, family involvement is crucial to help control the drug-seeking behavior and to allow family members to verbalize the feelings of frustration and anger that are invariably present.

Normal developmental crises can also be related to parent–child problems. For instance, adolescence is a time of frequent conflict as the adolescent resists rules and demands increasing autonomy and at the same time elicits protective control by displaying immature and dangerous behavior.

The parents of sons ages 18, 15, and 11 years presented with distress about the behavior of their middle child. The family had been cohesive with satisfactory relationships among all members until 6 months before this consultation. At that time, the 15-year-old son began seeing a girl from a comparatively unsupervised household. Frequent arguments had developed between parents and son regarding going out on school nights, curfews, and neglect of schoolwork. The son's combativeness and lowered academic achievement upset his parents a great deal. They had not experienced similar conflicts with their oldest child. The adolescent, however, maintained a good relationship with his siblings and friends, did not have behavior problems at school, continued to participate on the school basketball team, and was not a substance user.

Day Care Centers

Quality of care during the first 3 years of life is crucial to neuropsychological development. The National Institute of Child Health and Human Development does not consider day care harmful to children, especially when the caregivers and day care teachers provide consistent, empathetic, nurturing care. Not all day care centers can meet that level of care, however, especially those located in poor urban areas. Children receiving less than optimal caring exhibit decreased intellectual and verbal skills that indicate delayed neurocognitive development. They may also become irritable, anxious, or depressed, which interferes with the parent–child bonding experience, and they are less assertive and less effectively toilet trained by the age of 5 years.

Currently, more than 55 percent of women are in the workforce, many of whom have no choice but to place their children in day care centers. Close to 50 percent of entering medical students are women; few medical centers, however, make adequate provisions for on-site day care centers for their students or staff. Similarly, corporations need to provide on-site, high-quality care for the children of their employees. Not only will that approach benefit the children, but also corporate economic benefits will accrue as a result of reduced absenteeism, increased productivity, and happier working mothers. Such programs have the added benefit of decreasing stresses on marriages.

Partner Relational Problem

Partner relational problem are characterized by negative communication (e.g., criticisms), distorted communication (e.g., unrealistic expectations), or noncommunication (e.g., withdrawal) associated with clinically significant impairment in individual or family functioning or symptoms in one or both partners.

When persons have partner relational problems, psychiatrists must assess whether a patient's distress arises from the relationship or from a mental disorder. Mental disorders are more common in single persons—those who never married or who are widowed, separated, or divorced—than among married persons. Clinicians should evaluate developmental, sexual, and occupational and relationship histories, for purposes of diagnosis. (Couples therapy is discussed in Section 24.4.)

Marriage demands a sustained level of adaptation from both partners. In a troubled marriage, a therapist can encourage the partners to explore areas such as the extent of communication between the partners, their ways of solving disputes, their attitudes toward child bearing and child rearing, their relationships with their in-laws, their attitudes toward social life, their handling of finances, and their sexual interaction. The birth of a child, an abortion or miscarriage, economic stresses, moves to new areas, episodes of illness, major career changes, and any situations that involve a significant change in marital roles can precipitate stressful periods in a relationship. Illness in a child exerts the greatest strain on a marriage, and marriages in which a child has died through illness or accident more often than not end in divorce. Complaints of lifelong anorgasmia or impotence by marital partners usually indicate intrapsychic problems, although sexual dissatisfaction is involved in many cases of marital maladjustment.

Adjustment to marital roles can be a problem when partners are from different backgrounds and have grown up with different value systems. For example, members of low SES groups perceive a wife as making most of the decisions in the family, and they accept physical punishment as a way to discipline children. Middle-class persons perceive family decision-making processes as shared, with the husband often being the final arbiter, and they prefer to discipline children verbally. Problems involving conflicts in values, adjustment to new roles, and poor communication are handled most effectively when therapist and partners examine the couple's relationship, as in marital therapy.

Epidemiological surveys show that unhappy marriages are a risk factor for major depressive disorder. Marital discord also affects physical health. For example, in a study of women age 30 to 65 years with coronary artery disease, marital stress worsened the prognosis 2.9 times for recurrent coronary events. Marital conflict was also associated with a 46 percent higher relative death risk among female patients having hemodialysis and with elevations in serum epinephrine, norepinephrine, and corticotrophin levels in both men and women. In one study, high levels of hostile marital behavior were associated with slower healing of wounds, lower production of proinflammatory cytokines, and higher cytokine production in peripheral blood. Overall, women show greater psychological and physiological responsiveness to conflict than men.

Physician Marriages. Physicians have a higher risk of divorce than other occupational groups. The incidence of divorce among physicians is about 25 to 30 percent. Specialty choice influenced divorce. The highest rate of divorce occurred in psychiatrists (50 percent) followed by surgeons (33 percent) and internists, pediatricians, and pathologists (31 percent). The average age at first marriage was 26 years among all groups.

It is not clear why physicians are at high risk for divorce. Factors implicated include the stresses of dealing with dying patients, making life-and-death decisions, working long hours, and the constant risk of malpractice litigation. Such stressors may predispose physicians to a variety of emotional ills, with the most common being depression and substance abuse, including alcoholism. Such persons generally cannot deal with the complex interactions required to maintain successful long-term relationships of any kind, and marriage requires the most interpersonal skills of all.

Sibling Relational Problem

Sibling relationships tend to be characterized by competition, comparison, and cooperation. Intense sibling rivalry can occur with the birth of a child and can persist as the children grow up, compete for parental approval, and measure their accomplishments against one another. Alliances between siblings are equally common. Siblings may learn to protect one another against parental control or aggression. In households with three children, one pair tends to become closely involved with one another, leaving the extra child in the position of outsider.

Relational problems can arise when siblings are not treated equally; for instance, when one child is being idealized while another is cast in the role of the family scapegoat. Differences in gender roles and expectations expressed by the parents can underlie sibling rivalry. Parent–child relationships also are dependent on personality interactions. A child's resentment directed at a parental figure or a child's own disavowed dark emotions can be projected onto a sibling and can fuel an intense hate relationship.

A child's general, other medical or psychiatric condition always stresses the sibling relationships. Parental concern and attention to the sick child can elicit envy in the siblings. In addition, chronic disability can leave the sick child feeling devalued and rejected by siblings, and the latter may develop a sense of superiority and may feel embarrassed about having a disabled sister or brother. Twin relationships have become an area of increasing study. Preliminary data show that twins are more likely to be cooperative than competitive. Whether or not identical twins should be dressed differently during their toddler years in an effort to ensure a separate identity is open to question as is the issue of whether or not they should be in separate classrooms when they begin school.

Other Relational Problems

People, across the life cycle, may become involved in relational problems with leaders and others in their communities at large. In such relationships, conflicts are common and can bring about stress-related symptoms. Many relational problems of children occur in the school setting and involve peers. Impaired peer relationships can be the chief complaint in attention-deficit or conduct disorders, as well as in depressive and other psychiatric disorders of childhood, adolescence, and adulthood.

Racial, ethnic, and religious prejudices and ignorance cause problems in interpersonal relationships. In the workplace and in communities at large, sexual harassment is often a combination of inappropriate sexual interactions; inappropriate displays of abuse of power and dominance; and expressions of negative gender stereotypes, primarily toward women and gay men, although it is also geared toward children and adolescents of both sexes.

22

Physical and Sexual Abuse of Adults

INTRODUCTION

Violence is an important public health concern in the United States. The majority of Americans fall victim to a violent crime during their lifetime. Besides mortality, violence creates a heavy toll in medical costs, disability, and psychiatric sequelae.

Assault can be viewed in the context of two variables. The first involves who is being assaulted, and the second is where the assault occurs. With these parameters assault can be classified into several categories, the most common being violent crimes (aggravated and simple assault, robbery), rape, domestic violence, workplace violence, and torture. The prevalence of the different types of assaults is most often reported by two different data collection systems: (1) the Federal Bureau of Investigation's Uniform Crime Report (UCR), which collects reported crime information from local law enforcement agencies and (2) the Bureau of Justice Statistics' National Crime Victimization Survey (NCVS), which generates estimates of the likelihood of victimization from different types of assaults.

VIOLENT CRIME

Violent crime is defined as murder and nonnegligent manslaughter, forcible rape, robbery, and aggravated assault. These categories exclude simple assault, which is defined as an assault not involving a weapon and in which the victim was not seriously harmed. Simple assault has also been defined as stalking, intimidating, coercing, or hazing.

Prevalence

In 2013, the UCR reported over 1.6 million violent crimes occurred within the United States. Aggravated assault accounted for approximately 750,000 of this total, and robberies accounted for approximately 350,000. Ten-year trends show a decrease of 16 percent in violent crime since 2002. Aggravated assault was the most reported violent crime (62 percent), followed by robbery (29 percent), forcible rape (7 percent), and murder (1 percent). Also in 2011, firearms were found to be used in 21 percent of aggravated assaults and 41 percent of robberies.

Risk Factors

Gender and age play large roles in the rate of risk for assaults of all types. Males between the ages of 15 and 34 years are more likely to be assaulted than females and are 11 times more likely to be assaulted by strangers than by someone they know. Research suggests that race is an important factor as well, with African Americans being at greater risk of violence and having a death rate that is four or five times higher than age-matched whites during aggravated assaults. The NCVS found that males and females in households earning less than $15,000 in annual income were twice as likely to be robbed and 1.5 times as likely to suffer a physical assault. Homelessness has also been shown to be a factor in increased physical assaults. Finally, substance abuse has been shown in multiple studies to increase the risk of victimization.

RAPE

Rape is the forceful coercion of an unwilling victim to engage in a sexual act, usually sexual intercourse, although anal intercourse and fellatio can also be acts of rape. The legal definition of rape varies from state to state. Some states strictly define rape, whereas other states describe any sex crime as varying degrees of sexual misconduct or sexual assault. Rape can occur between married partners and between persons of the same sex. Forced acts of fellatio and anal penetration, although they frequently accompany rape, are legally considered sodomy.

In some states the definition of rape has been changed to substitute the word *person* for *female.* In most states, male rape is legally defined as sodomy. Like other violent crimes, sexual assault is declining; however, every 2 minutes someone in the United States is sexually assaulted. Although much of the population believes in the stereotype of the culprit being a stranger, research has shown that only about 26 percent of all rapes are committed by a stranger.

Prevalence

Unfortunately, accurate statistics are difficult to obtain because of underreporting and unacknowledgment. The Rape, Abuse, and Incest National Network (RAINN) estimates that over half of rapes go unreported. Although in the United States, rapes have fallen in number since 1993, as of 2013 there is an average of 207,754 rapes and sexual assaults per year. RAINN estimates that 1 in 6 US women and 1 in 33 US men are victims of sexual assault.

In addition to being underreported, there are many rapes that go unacknowledged by the victim, who often refer to the assault in more benign terms such as a misunderstanding, despite the fact that it meets the legal definition of rape. Research has reported that this percentage is substantial; more than 50 percent of sexual assaults may go unacknowledged and, thus, unreported. Research has further revealed that victims who fail to acknowledge having been raped usually believe that rape

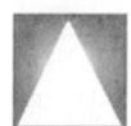

Table 22–1
Violence Against Women Act (VAWA)

VAWA has **improved the criminal justice response** to violence against women by:

- ▲ Holding rapists accountable for their crimes by strengthening federal penalties for repeat sex offenders and creating a federal "rape shield law," which is intended to prevent offenders from using victims' past sexual conduct against them during a rape trial;
- ▲ Mandating that victims, no matter their income levels, are not forced to bear the expense of their own rape exams or for service of a protection order;
- ▲ Keeping victims safe by requiring that a victim's protection order will be recognized and enforced in all state, tribal, and territorial jurisdictions within the United States;
- ▲ Increasing rates of prosecution, conviction, and sentencing of offenders by helping communities develop dedicated law enforcement and prosecution units and domestic violence dockets;
- ▲ Ensuring that police respond to crisis calls and judges understand the realities of domestic and sexual violence by training law enforcement officer, prosecutors, victim advocates and judges; VAWA funds train over 500,000 law enforcement officers, prosecutors, judges, and other personnel every year;
- ▲ Providing additional tools for protecting women in Indian country by creating a new federal habitual offender crime and authorizing warrantless arrest authority for federal law enforcement officers who determine there is probably cause when responding to domestic violence cases.

VAWA has ensured that victims and their families have access to the services they need to achieve safety and rebuild their lives by:

- ▲ Responding to urgent calls for help by establishing the National Domestic Violence Hotline, which has answered over 3 million calls and receives over 22,000 calls every month; 92% of callers report that it is their first call for help;
- ▲ Improving safety and reducing recidivism by developing coordinated community responses that bring together diverse stakeholders to work together to prevent and respond to violence against women;
- ▲ Focusing attention on the needs of underserved communities, including creating legal relief for battered immigrants so that abusers cannot use the victim's immigration status to prevent victims from calling the police or seeking safety, and supporting tribal governments in building their capacity to protect American Indian and Alaska Native women.

VAWA has **created positive change.** Since VAWA was passed:

- ▲ Fewer people are experiencing domestic violence.
  - ▲ Between 1993 and 2010, the rate of intimate partner violence declined 67%;
  - ▲ Between 1993 and 2007, the rate of intimate partner homicides of females decreased 35% and the rate of intimate partner homicides of males decreased 46%.
- ▲ More victims are reporting domestic and sexual violence to police, and reports to police are resulting in more arrests.
- ▲ States have reformed their laws to take violence against women more seriously:
  - ▲ All states have reformed laws that previously treated date or spousal rape as a lesser crime than stranger rape;
  - ▲ All states have passed laws making stalking a crime;
  - ▲ All states have authorized warrantless arrests in misdemeanor domestic violence cases where the responding officer determines that probable cause exists;
  - ▲ All states provide for criminal sanctions for the violation of a civil protection order;
  - ▲ Many states have passed laws prohibiting polygraphing of rape victims;
  - ▲ Over 35 states, the District of Columbia, and the US Virgin Islands have adopted laws addressing domestic and sexual violence and stalking in the workplace. These laws vary widely and may offer a victim time off from work to address the violence in their lives, protect victims from employment discrimination related to the violence, and provide unemployment insurance to survivors who must leave their jobs because of the abuse.

From U.S. Government Fact Sheet, Washington, D.C.

involves two strangers and greater force, as opposed to the views of those who acknowledge their having been sexually assaulted.

Statistics show that most men who commit rapes are between 25 and 44 years of age; 51 percent are white and tend to rape white victims, 47 percent are black and tend to rape black victims, and the remaining 2 percent come from all other races. Alcohol is involved in 34 percent of all forcible rapes. Homosexual rape is much more frequent among men than among women and occurs frequently in closed institutions such as prisons and maximum security hospitals.

Risk Factors

Although women are usually the victim of rape and sexual assault, greater than 10 percent of victims are estimated to be men. Furthermore, most experts believe that men underreport more than women. Nevertheless, young women have four times the risk of any group of becoming a victim of sexual assault. Persons who are raped can be of any age. Cases have been reported in which the victims were as young as 15 months and as old as 82 years. However, 80 percent of all rape victims are under the age of 30 years and the Bureau of Justice statistics indicate that women age 16 to 24 years are at the greatest risk for rape in the United States. Having been a victim of childhood abuse or previous assault increases the likelihood of further assault of all types. Most rapes are premeditated; about half are committed by strangers and half by men known, to varying degrees, by the victims.

The Violence Against Women Act has had an important role to play in reducing rape and other types of violence (Table 22–1).

Perpetrators

In general, rape is considered a crime of power and aggression, not one of sexuality. Male rapists can be categorized into separate groups: sexual sadists, who are aroused by the pain of their victims; exploitive predators, who use their victims as objects for their gratification in an impulsive way; inadequate men, who believe that no woman would voluntarily sleep with them and who are obsessed with fantasies about sex; and men for whom rape is a displaced expression of anger and rage. Seven percent of all rapes are perpetrated by close relatives of the victim; 10 percent of rapes involve more than one attacker.

Rape often accompanies another crime. Rapists always threaten victims, with fists, a knife, or a gun, and frequently harm them in nonsexual ways as well. Victims can be beaten, wounded, and killed.

In cases of male or homosexual rape, the dynamics are identical to those of heterosexual rape. The crime enables the rapist to discharge aggression and to aggrandize himself. The victim is usually smaller than the rapist, is always perceived as passive and unmanly (weaker), and is used as an object. A rapist selecting male victims may be heterosexual, bisexual, or homosexual. The most common act is anal penetration of the victim; the second most common is fellatio.

SEXUAL COERCION

Sexual coercion is a term used for incidents in which a person dominates another by force or compels the other person to perform a sexual act.

STALKING

Stalking is defined as a pattern of harassing or menacing behavior coupled with a threat to do harm. The first antistalking law was passed in 1990 in California. Now most states prohibit stalking, although some will not intervene unless an act of violence has occurred. In states with stalking laws, the person can be arrested on the basis of a pattern of harassment and can be charged with either a misdemeanor or felony. Some stalkers continue the activity for years; others, for only a few months. The court may mandate that stalkers undergo counseling sessions. The best means of deterrent is to report all stalkers to law enforcement agencies. Most stalkers are men, but women who stalk are just as likely as men to attack their victims violently.

SEXUAL HARASSMENT

Sexual harassment refers to sexual advances, requests for sexual favors, or verbal or physical conduct of a sexual nature—all of which are unwelcomed by the victim. In more than 95 percent of cases the perpetrator is a man and the victim is a woman. If a man is being harassed, it is almost always by another man. A woman sexually harassing a man is an extremely rare event. The victim of harassment reacts to the experience in various ways. Some blame themselves and become depressed; others become anxious and angry. In general, harassment most commonly occurs in the workplace, and many organizations have developed procedures to deal with the problem. All too often, however, the victim is unwilling to step forward and lodge a complaint because of fear of retribution, of being humiliated, of being accused of lying, or ultimately of being fired from the job.

The types of behaviors that make up sexual harassment are broad. They include abusive language, requests for sexual favors, sexual jokes, staring, ogling, and giving massages, among others.

To reduce harassment, organizations may distribute educational material. Employees are obligated to investigate every complaint, which most often are addressed to the Equal Employment Opportunity Commission. Appropriate organizational responses range from a written warning to firing the offender.

DOMESTIC VIOLENCE

Domestic violence (also known as *spouse abuse*) is defined as physical assault within the home in which one spouse is repeatedly assaulted by the other. It has been estimated that domestic violence occurs in one of every four families in the United States. Often domestic violence is broken down into two categories: "high-severity abuse," which includes being threatened or hurt with a weapon, burned, choked, hit, or kicked, resulting in broken bones and head or internal injuries; and "low-severity abuse," which includes being slapped, hit, or kicked without injury, but also could include bruising, minor cuts, and sprains.

Unfortunately, domestic violence does not end when a woman becomes pregnant. In fact, the surgeon general's office has identified pregnancy as a high-risk period for battering; 15 to 25 percent of pregnant women are physically abused while pregnant, and the abuse often results in birth defects. In addition, pregnant and recently pregnant women are more likely to die from homicide than any other cause.

Some husband-beating wives have also been reported. Husbands complain of fear of ridicule if they expose the problem; they fear charges of counterassault and often feel unable to leave the situation because of financial difficulties. Husband abuse also been reported when a frail, elderly man is married to a much younger woman.

Prevalence

Estimates of the prevalence of domestic violence in the United States vary widely, and many studies include psychological or emotional abuse. Worldwide estimates state that one in every three women has experienced some form of physical or sexual abuse from a domestic partner. One study based on several internal medicine practices found that approximately 6 percent of women had experienced domestic violence in the year prior to presentation. It was found that of the women currently experiencing abuse, 49 percent experience high-severity abuse and 51 percent experience low-severity abuse.

Risk Factors

Domestic violence occurs in families of every racial and religious background and in all socioeconomic strata. Any person in an intimate relationship can be at risk. It is most frequently found in families with problems of substance abuse, particularly alcohol and crack abuse. Another risk factor is a history of childhood abuse. About 50 percent of battered wives grew up in violent homes and their most common trait is dependence. Abusive men are also likely to have come from violent homes where they witnessed wife beating or were abused themselves as children.

Women face risks when they leave an abusive husband; they have a 75 percent greater chance of being killed by their batterers than women who stay. New York State prepared a physician reference card to alert and guide doctors about domestic violence (Table 22–2).

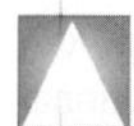

Table 22–2
Physician Reference Card

RECOGNIZING AND TREATING VICTIMS OF DOMESTIC VIOLENCE BASED ON THE AMERICAN MEDICAL ASSOCIATION'S DIAGNOSTIC AND TREATMENT GUIDELINES ON DOMESTIC VIOLENCE

If you treat women, whether in private practice or a hospital setting, you are almost certainly treating some patients who are victims of domestic violence.

The following decision tree is designed to help you assess a patient's risk of domestic violence and offer appropriate help to those in need of it.

Identifying Victims of Domestic Violence

Although many women who are victims of abuse will not volunteer any information, they will discuss it if asked simple, direct questions in a nonjudgmental way and in a confidential setting. *The patient should be interviewed alone, without her partner present.*

You may want to offer a statement such as: "Because violence is so common in many women's lives, I've begun to ask about it routinely." Then you can ask a direct question, such as: "At any time, has your partner hit, kicked, or otherwise hurt or frightened you?"

If Patient Answers Yes, the Following Steps Are Suggested:

1. Encourage her to talk about it:
   "Would you like to talk about what has happened to you?"
   "How do you feel about it?"
   "What would you like to do about this?"
2. Listen nonjudgmentally:
   This serves both to begin the healing process for the woman and to give you an idea of what kind of referrals she needs.
3. Validate:
   Victims of domestic violence are frequently not believed, and the fear they report is minimized. The physician can express support through simple statements such as:
   - ▲ "You are not alone."
   - ▲ "You don't deserve to be treated this way."
   - ▲ "You are not to blame."
   - ▲ "You are not crazy."
   - ▲ "What happened to you is a crime."
   - ▲ "Help is available for you."
4. *Document:*
   - ▲ The patient's complaints and symptoms as well as the results of the observation and assessment. (Complaints should be described in the patient's own words whenever possible.)
   - ▲ The patient's complete medical and trauma history and relevant social history.
   - ▲ A detailed description of the injuries, including type, number, size, location, resolution, possible causes, and explanations given.
   - ▲ An opinion on whether the injuries were inconsistent with the patient's explanation.
   - ▲ Results of all pertinent laboratory and other diagnostic procedures.
   - ▲ Color photographs and imaging studies, if applicable.
   - ▲ If the police are called, the name of the investigating officer and any action taken (the police should be called only if the patient requests this or exhibits a reportable injury).
   - ▲ Child abuse and neglect are reportable offenses. If you suspect that children in the patient's home are also being abused, you are mandated to report the situation to the Department of Social Services.
5. *Assess the danger to your patient:*
   - ▲ Assess your patient's safety *before she leaves the medical setting.* The most important determinants of risk are the woman's level of fear and her appraisal of her immediate and future safety. Discussing the following indicators with the patient can help you determine if she is in escalating danger:
   - ▲ an increase in the frequency or severity of the assaults
   - ▲ increasing or new threats of homicide or suicide by the partner
   - ▲ threats to her children
   - ▲ the presence or availability of a firearm
6. *Provide appropriate treatment referral and support:*
   - ▲ Treat the patient's injuries as indicated. In prescribing medication, keep in mind that medications which hinder the patient's ability to protect herself or to flee from a violent partner may endanger her life.
   - ▲ If your patient is in imminent danger, determine if she has friends or family with whom she can stay. If this is not an option, ask if she wants immediate access to a shelter for battered women. If none is available, can she be admitted to the hospital?
   - ▲ If she doesn't need immediate access to a shelter, offer written information about shelters and other community resources. Remember that it may be dangerous for the woman to have these in her possession. Don't insist that she take them if she is reluctant to do so. Give your patient the telephone number of the local domestic violence hotline or the toll-free Domestic Violence hotline. It may be safest for your patient if you write the number on a prescription blank or an appointment card. You may wish to give her the opportunity to call from a private phone in your office.

If the Patient Answers No, or Will Not Discuss the Topic:

1. Be aware of clinical findings that may indicate abuse:
   - ▲ injury to the head, neck, torso, breasts, abdomen, or genitals
   - ▲ bilateral or multiple injuries
   - ▲ delay between onset of injury and seeking treatment
   - ▲ explanation by the patient which is inconsistent with the type of injury
   - ▲ any injury during pregnancy, especially to the abdomen or breasts
   - ▲ prior history of trauma
   - ▲ chronic pain symptoms for which no etiology is apparent
   - ▲ psychological distress, such as depression, suicidal ideation, anxiety, and/or sleep disorders
   - ▲ a partner who seems overly protective or who will not leave the woman's side

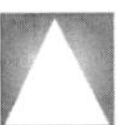

Table 22–2
Physician Reference Card (Continued)

2. *If any of the above clinical signs is present, it is appropriate to ask more specific questions. Be sure that the patient's partner is not present.* Some examples of questions that may elicit more information about the patient's situation are:
   ▲ "It looks as though someone may have hurt you. Could you tell me how it happened?"
   ▲ "Sometimes when people come for health care with physical symptoms like yours, we find that there may be trouble at home. We are concerned that someone is hurting or abusing you. Is this happening?"
   ▲ "Sometimes when people feel the way you do, it's because they may have been hurt or abused at home. Is this happening to you?"

   If patient answers YES:
   See the suggestions for assessment and treatment that begin on the other side of this card.

   If patient answers NO:
   If the patient denies abuse, but you strongly suspect that it is taking place, you can let her know that your office can provide referrals to local programs, should she choose to pursue such options in the future.

   ▲ You may want to write the Domestic Violence hotline number on a prescription blank or on an appointment card.
   Don't judge the success of the intervention by the patient's action. A woman is most at risk of serious injury or even homicide when she attempts to leave an abusive partner, and it may take her a long time before she can finally do so. It is frustrating for the physician when a patient stays in an abusive situation. Be reassured that if you have acknowledged and validated her situation and offered appropriate referrals, you have done what you can to help her.

Adapted from the New York State Office for Prevention of Domestic Violence, Medical Society of the State of New York, New York State Department of Health, with permission.

Perpetrators

The perpetrators of domestic violence come from all races and socioeconomic levels. However, having been a victim of abuse or witnessing abuse in the home increases the risk of someone becoming an abuser. Alcohol abuse is usually involved in most offenses. The act of abuse itself is reinforcing; once a man has beaten his wife, he is likely to do so again. Many abusers are noted to be charming in public but cruel to their intimates.

Abusive husbands tend to be immature, dependent, and nonassertive and to suffer from strong feelings of inadequacy. The husband's aggression is bullying behavior designed to humiliate their wives and to buildup their own low self-esteem. Impatient, impulsive, abusive husbands physically displace aggression provoked by others onto their wives. The abuse most likely occurs when a man feels threatened or frustrated at home, at work, or with his peers. The dynamics include identification with an aggressor (father, boss), testing behavior ("Will she stay with me, no matter how I treat her?"), distorted desires to express manhood, and dehumanization of women. As with rape, aggression is deemed permissible when a woman is perceived as property.

When an abused wife tries to leave her husband, he often becomes doubly intimidating and threatens to "get" her. If the woman has small children to care for, her problem is compounded. The abusive husband wages a conscious campaign to isolate his wife and make her feel worthless.

Some men feel remorse and guilt after an episode of violent behavior and so become particularly loving. If this behavior gives the wife hope, she remains until the next inevitable cycle of violence.

WORKPLACE VIOLENCE

Acts of violence at work are defined as simple assault, aggravated assault, robbery, rape/sexual abuse, and homicide.

Prevalence

Workplace violence accounts for approximately 15 percent of all violent crimes in the United States. According to the NCVS, in 2009 there were approximately 572,000 acts of violence committed against persons at work. During the same time, over 500 work-related homicides occurred. Approximately 78 percent of workplace assaults did not involve weapons, and 80 percent of workplace homicides involved firearms. With some variation, violent crime in the workplace has decline approximately 35 percent since 2002.

Risk Factors

Gender and race are important risk factors in workplace violence. The workplace violence rate for women has decreased approximately 43 percent since 2002, while the rate for men has decreased approximately 30 percent. Approximately two-thirds of all workplace assaults (excluding rape/sexual assault) are committed against men. Workplace crime rates are higher among whites than other races.

An important component of workplace violence is the relationship between the risk of violence and the type of occupation. The NCVS found that police officers are at the highest risk for victimization (78 per 1,000) and constituted 9 percent of all workplace assaults. Other high-risk occupations include security guard (65 per 1,000), correction officer (33 per 1,000), bartender (80 per 1,000), technical/industrial schoolteacher (55 per 1,000), mental health custodial worker (38 per 1,000), gas station attendant (30 per 1,000), and mental health professionals (17 per 1,000).

Perpetrators

There are several distinct characteristics among offenders, of which gender is the most pronounced. As reported by victims, four-fifths of all violent workplace crime is committed by men, and this is regardless of the victim's gender. The race of the offenders is most often white, followed by black, and most of the attacks are interracial. Unlike domestic violence, workplace violence is more often perpetrated by strangers or casual acquaintances than by known intimates. Mental health and teaching are the only fields in which attacks occur more often at the hands of a known perpetrator than by a stranger.

SEQUELAE OF VIOLENCE AND ASSAULT

Survivors of violence have varied reactions, but they are similar to those exposed to other types of trauma. Furthermore, the severity of the sequelae varies with the individual. However, multiple studies have shown that many of the people who experience violence have decreased physical and mental health, resulting in higher utilization of health care services.

The most common reported sequelae after sexual assault in women are posttraumatic stress disorder (PTSD), mood disorders, substance abuse, eating disorders, and sexual disorders. One of the most protective factors in ameliorating the development of PTSD is social support. Furthermore, the lack of social support and the perception of being treated differently can be quite detrimental to the survivor, causing an increase in PTSD symptoms.

Domestic violence has been associated with depression, anxiety, low self-esteem, substance abuse, sexual dysfunction, functional gastrointestinal disorder, headaches, chronic pain, and multiple somatic symptoms. Physical symptoms associated with current abuse include loss of appetite; frequent or serious bruises; nightmares; vaginal discharge; eating binges or self-induced vomiting; diarrhea; broken bones; sprains or serious cuts; pain in the pelvic or genital area; fainting; abdominal pain; breast pain; frequent or severe headaches; difficulty passing urine; chest pain; problems with sleeping; shortness of breath; and constipation. Many studies have shown that survivors of domestic violence attempt suicide more frequently than those who have not experienced violence.

Substance abuse seems to be a significant factor for both the survivor and the batterer. It is both a risk factor for abuse and a consequence of it.

The relationship between childhood abuse and adult abuse is complex. Childhood abuse is a risk factor for abuse as an adult, and childhood abuse increases both physical and mental health sequelae of adult abuse. Survivors of sexual assault or domestic violence who are older and without a history of childhood abuse have fewer symptoms

TREATMENT ISSUES

Initial Evaluation

Many victims of assault initially present to a medical doctor for treatment of their injuries. In emergency departments, patients may often be treated for their injuries without the assault being recognized or addressed. Consequently, it is important to consider any concerning injuries as being a potential stigmata of assault. The patient may initially be avoidant when asked about the cause of injuries that appear related to assault. This may be further complicated by the need to complete specific tasks (i.e., rape kit, photo documentation, reporting of legal concerns) that require the patient to describe and relive the recent assault. It is paramount to build rapport with the patient while continuing to complete a thorough evaluation. To facilitate this process, it is important to reduce the victim's stress and anxiety regarding discussion of the event. The initial evaluation process should be explained to the patient before beginning. Allowing the patient some say in dictating the pace and content of the interview is preferable to having a patient feel a lack of control over the process. The crime may represent a time when the patient lacked control, and similar feelings in the initial interview can lead to a triggering of traumatic or anxious responses. Finally, the physician should remain attuned to nonverbal patient responses that signify discomfort and conduct the interview accordingly. Furthermore, when a patient discloses domestic violence, this should be documented in his or her chart for future follow-up and possible future legal documentation.

Safety

After an assault, it is imperative that a safety assessment be performed on the victim. The patient needs to be evaluated for suicidal and homicidal ideation as it pertains to the recent assault. The patient's safety from further assault also needs to be addressed, especially in a setting in which the perpetrator was a loved one or known acquaintance. Finally, the patient needs to be screened for severe psychological symptoms that would cause difficulty in self-care. These would include acute mood deterioration or affective instability, self-destructive behaviors, dissociative symptoms, or psychosis. If the evaluation shows that any of these areas are inadequate to ensure patient safety, then a plan needs to be developed. This plan should provide for the patient's physical safety and give the patient a place to sleep, recuperate, and eat.

Hospitalization

In the event that the patient's safety cannot be guaranteed, hospitalization of the assault victim may be necessary. Common indications for hospitalization include (1) severe medical injuries, (2) suicidality or homicidality, (3) dissociative or psychotic symptoms, (4) mood instability or affective dysregulation, (5) self-destructive behaviors, and (6) a continued serious threat to the patient's life or well-being. If the victim is admitted to the hospital, then an individualized multidisciplinary treatment plan should be developed. Safety, milieu therapy, mood stabilization, and medication evaluation are the primary treatment modalities provided in the hospital and reflect the short-stay nature of most psychiatric facilities. Because the assault victim will likely need longer treatment than what can be provided in the hospital, it is important that there is a coordinated inpatient-to-outpatient transition in which psychiatric, medical, and social work issues all being addressed prior to discharge.

Legal Issues

A physician evaluating an assault victim needs to adhere to mandatory reporting requirements for the state in which he or she is practicing. Mandatory reporting of child abuse, abuse of developmentally disabled children, and abuse of the elderly exist in all 50 states. In cases of assault secondary to domestic violence, states do not usually require mandatory reporting. However, many states do require physicians to report serious injuries due to acts of criminal violence. Thus, in the setting of injury secondary to domestic violence, this can sometimes be considered a de facto mandatory reporting situation.

Psychotherapy Treatment

After the patient's safety has been ensured and the initial evaluation is complete, there are a variety of psychological interventions that can be initiated. Cognitive–behavioral approaches are the most researched techniques demonstrating efficacy. Exposure therapy is a variant of cognitive–behavioral therapy (CBT) that has been shown to help victims emotionally process the assault by decreasing their fear to memories or cues of the event. There is evidence in the literature that brief early CBT may accelerate recovery in victims manifesting acute PTSD. Eye movement desensitization and reprocessing (EMDR) is another alternative treatment for the processing of distressing memories. These individual psychotherapies may be augmented with group psychotherapy, art therapy, dance and movement therapy, music therapy, and body-oriented approaches if they prove beneficial to the patient.

Psychopharmacological Treatment

Although medication is not recommended in the acute treatment of all assault victims, it may be beneficial in certain circumstances. The clinician may decide to medicate a patient with incapacitating anxiety, extreme aggression toward themselves or others, or dissociation or psychoses immediately after the assault. The patient's safety and the safety of those around the patient will help to decide the need for pharmacologic intervention. Most medication treatment will be initiated much later after the assault as the patient develops symptoms of PTSD, depression, anxiety, obsessive-compulsive disorder, or psychosis. Although medication may be useful in symptom management, they should not be viewed as a replacement for psychotherapy aimed at trauma symptom resolution.

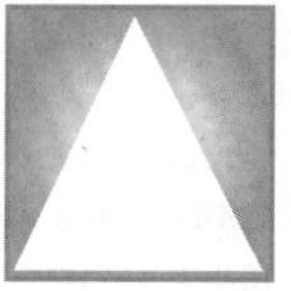

23

Psychiatry and Reproductive Medicine

INTRODUCTION

Reproductive events and processes have both physiological and psychological concomitants. Likewise, psychological states affect reproductive physiology and modulate reproductive events. This chapter examines these bidirectional relationships with the goal of introducing fundamental concepts related to the classic reproductive events, such as menarche, pregnancy, delivery, postpartum, and menopause. The fields of psychiatry and reproductive medicine continue to define the multiple mechanisms by which psyche and soma interact to determine a woman's gynecological and psychological health. For instance, premenstrual dysphoric disorder—the impairing symptoms and severe mood, cognitive, and behavioral changes that occur in association with the menstrual cycle—exemplifies a disorder in which biological changes occurring in the soma trigger changes in psychological state. In contrast, functional forms of hypothalamic anovulation represent psychosomatic illness that originates in the brain but alters somatic functioning.

REPRODUCTIVE PHYSIOLOGY

The physiological processes associated with menarche, menstrual cycling, pregnancy, postpartum, and menopause occur within the context of a woman's physiological and interpersonal life, interfacing with psychosocial functioning throughout adolescence, young adulthood, midlife, and late life. The fields of psychiatry and reproductive medicine are just beginning to elaborate the multiple mechanisms by which psyche and soma interact to determine a woman's gynecological and psychological function. This chapter illustrates how reproductive processes interact with psychosocial events and aims ultimately to improve the approach to both gynecologic and psychiatric treatments.

Menstrual Cycles

Menstrual cyclicity results directly from ovarian cyclicity. Each ovarian cycle starts with the development of a group or cohort of follicles, one of which becomes dominant. The follicles are composed of an oocyte surrounded by granulosa cells, which, in turn, are surrounded by theca cells.

As shown at the top of Figure 23–1, follicular development is initiated by the hypothalamic release of gonadotropin-releasing hormones (GnRH) at a pulse frequency of approximately one pulse every 90 minutes. GnRH stimulates the release of the pituitary gonadotropins, luteinizing hormone (LH), and follicle-stimulating hormone (FSH). In turn, LH stimulates ovarian theca cells to synthesize and secrete androgens; FSH induces granulosa cell development, including the enzyme aromatase, which converts the thecally produced androgens to estrogens. In the presence of a constant GnRH pulse frequency of one pulse each 90 minutes, the secretion of LH and FSH in the follicular phase will be regulated primarily by estradiol feedback at the level of the pituitary. Rising estradiol concentrations suppress FSH, thereby limiting the number of follicles that become mature oocytes capable of ovulating.

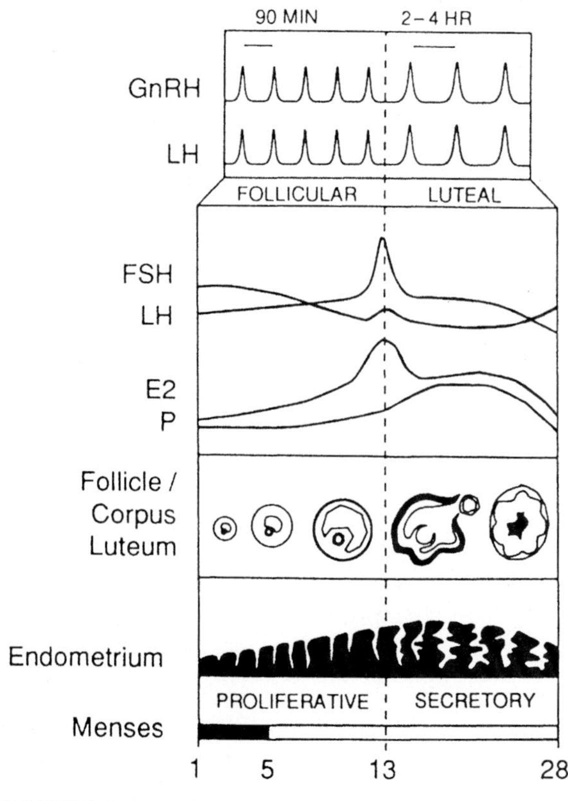

FIGURE 23–1

Schematization of the human menstrual cycle. Es, estradiol; FSH, follicle-stimulating hormone; GnRH, gonadotropin-releasing hormone; LH, luteinizing hormone; P, progesterone.

As illustrated in the middle panel of Figure 23–1, when estradiol concentrations rise exponentially to exceed a critical threshold and remain elevated for at least 36 hours, which is the pattern one fully mature follicle produces, an LH surge is triggered and ovulation (release of the ovum from the follicle sac) ensues approximately 36 hours later. Thereafter, granulosa cells transform into progesterone-secreting luteal cells, and the ovulated follicle is then referred to as the *corpus luteum,* which secretes progesterone.

Figure 23–1 displays the levels of LH, FSH, estradiol, and progesterone throughout the menstrual cycle and corresponding follicular events. The target tissues for ovarian steroids include the endometrium, whose developmental sequence is illustrated along the bottom panel, and the hypothalamic GnRH pulse generator, whose frequency, as indicated in the top right panel, is slowed dramatically by the combination of estrogen and progesterone secreted during the postovulatory or luteal phase of the menstrual cycle. This inhibition of GnRH is followed by decreased secretion of LH and FSH so that new follicular development is prevented until the corpus luteum regresses. As progesterone concentrations decline, GnRH pulsatility increases, and gonadotropin, especially FSH, secretion rises. The phases of the menstrual cycle can be termed *follicular* and *luteal* in reference to ovarian events or *proliferative* and *secretory* in reference to endometrial events.

PREGNANCY

Biology of Pregnancy

The first presumptive sign of pregnancy is the absence of menses for 1 week. Other presumptive signs are breast engorgement and tenderness, changes in breast size and shape, nausea with or without vomiting (morning sickness), frequent urination, and fatigue. A diagnosis can be made 10 to 15 days after fertilization by testing for human chorionic gonadotropin (hCG), which is produced by the placenta. The definitive diagnosis requires a doubling of hCG levels and the presence of fetal heart sounds. Transvaginal ultrasound scanning can reveal a pregnant uterus as early as 4 weeks after fertilization, by visualization of a gestational sac.

Stages of Pregnancy

Pregnancy is commonly divided into three trimesters, starting from the first day of the last menstrual cycle and ending with the delivery of a baby. During the first trimester, the woman must adapt to changes in her body, such as fatigue, nausea and vomiting, breast tenderness, and mood lability. The second trimester is often the most rewarding for women. A return of energy and the end of nausea and vomiting allow women to feel better and experience the excitement of starting to look pregnant. The third trimester is associated with physical discomfort for many women. All systems—cardiovascular, renal, pulmonary, gastrointestinal, and endocrine—have undergone profound changes that can produce a heart murmur, weight gain, exertional dyspnea, and heartburn. Some women require reassurance that those changes are not evidence of disease and that they will return to normal shortly after delivery—generally in 4 to 6 weeks.

Psychology of Pregnancy

Pregnant women undergo marked psychological changes. Their attitudes toward pregnancy reflect deeply felt beliefs about all aspects of reproduction, including whether the pregnancy was planned and whether the baby is wanted. The relationship with the infant's father, the age of the mother, and her sense of identity also affect a woman's reaction to prospective motherhood. Prospective fathers also face psychological challenges.

Psychologically healthy women often find pregnancy a means of self-realization. Many women report that being pregnant is a creative act gratifying a fundamental need. Other women use pregnancy to diminish self-doubts about femininity or to reassure themselves that they can function as women in the most basic sense. Still others view pregnancy negatively; they may fear childbirth or feel inadequate about mothering.

During early stages of their own development, women must undergo the experience of separating from their mothers and of establishing an independent identity; this experience later affects their own success at mothering. If a woman's mother was a poor role model, a woman's sense of maternal competence may be impaired, and she may lack confidence before and after her baby's birth. Women's unconscious fears and fantasies during early pregnancy often center on the idea of fusion with their own mothers.

Psychological attachment to the fetus begins in utero and, by the beginning of the second trimester, most women have a mental picture of the infant. Even before being born, the fetus is viewed as a separate being, endowed with a prenatal personality. Many mothers talk to their unborn children. Recent evidence suggests that emotional talk with the fetus is related not only to early mother–infant bonding but also to the mother's efforts to have a healthy pregnancy, for example, by giving up cigarettes and caffeine. According to psychoanalytic theorists, the child-to-be is a blank screen on which a mother projects her hopes and fears. In rare instances, these projections account for postpartum pathological states, such as a mother's desire to harm her infant, whom she views as a hated part of herself. Normally, however, giving birth to a child fulfills a woman's need to create and nurture life.

Fathers are also profoundly affected by pregnancy. Impending parenthood demands a synthesis of such developmental issues as gender role and identity, separation or individuation from a man's own father, sexuality, and, as Erik Erikson proposed, generativity. Pregnancy fantasies in men and wishes to give birth in boys reflect early identification with their mothers as well as the wish to be as powerful and creative as they perceive mothers to be. For some men, getting a woman pregnant is proof of their potency, a dynamic that plays a large part in adolescent fatherhood.

Marriage and Pregnancy

The prospective mother–wife and father–husband must redefine his or her roles as a couple and as an individual. They face readjustments in their relationships with friends and relatives and must deal with new responsibilities as caretakers of the newborn and each other. Both parents may experience anxiety about their adequacy as parents; one or both partners may be consciously or unconsciously ambivalent about the addition of the child to the family and about the effects on the dyadic (two-person) relationship. A husband may feel guilty about his wife's discomfort during pregnancy and parturition, and some men experience jealousy or envy of the experience of pregnancy. Accustomed to gratifying each other's dependency needs, the couple must attend to the unremitting needs of a new infant and a developing child. Although most couples respond positively to these demands, some do not. Under ideal conditions, the decision to become a parent and have a child should be agreed on by both partners, but sometimes parenthood is rationalized as a way to achieve intimacy in a conflicted marriage or to avoid having to deal with other life circumstance problems.

Attitudes Toward the Pregnant Woman

In general, others' attitudes toward a pregnant woman reflect a variety of factors: intelligence, temperament, cultural practices, and myths of the society and the subculture into which the person was born. Married men's responses to pregnancy are generally positive. For some men, however, reactions vary from a misplaced sense of pride that they are able to impregnate the woman to fear of increased responsibility and subsequent termination of the relationship. A woman's risk of abuse by her husband or boyfriend increases during pregnancy, particularly during the first trimester. One study found that 6 percent of pregnant women are abused. Domestic abuse adds significantly to the cost of health care during pregnancy, and abused women are more likely than nonabused controls to have histories of miscarriage, abortion, and neonatal death. The reasons for abuse vary. Some men fear being neglected and not having excessive dependency needs gratified; others may see the fetus as a rival. In most cases, however, one finds a history of abuse before the woman became pregnant.

Same-Sex Partnering, Marriage, and Pregnancy

Some lesbian couples decide that one partner should become pregnant through artificial insemination. Societal attitudes may put stress on this arrangement, but if the two women have a secure relationship, they tend to bond strongly together as a family unit. Men in committed gay relationships are fathering children through artificial insemination with surrogate mothers. Recent studies show that children raised in same sex couple households are not measurably different from children raised by heterosexual parents with respect to personality development, psychological development, and gender identity. These children are also not more likely to be gay or lesbian themselves.

Some single, never-married women who do not wish to marry but do want to become pregnant may do so through artificial or natural insemination. Such women constitute a group who believe that motherhood is the fulfillment of female identity, without which they view their lives to be incomplete. Most of these women have considered the consequence of single parenthood and feel able to rise to the challenges.

Sexual Behavior

The effects of pregnancy on sexual behavior vary. Some women experience an increased sex drive as pelvic vasocongestion produces a more sexually responsive state. Others are more responsive than before the pregnancy, because they no longer fear becoming pregnant. Some have diminished desire or lose interest in sexual activity altogether. Libido may be decreased because of higher estrogen levels or feelings of unattractiveness. Avoidance of sex may also result from physical discomfort or an association of motherhood with asexuality. Men with a Madonna complex view pregnant women as sacred and not to be defiled by the sexual act. Either a man or a woman may erroneously consider intercourse potentially harmful to the developing fetus and, thus, something to be avoided. Men who have extramarital affairs during their wives' pregnancies usually do so during the last trimester.

Coitus. Most obstetricians place no prohibitions on coitus during pregnancy. Some suggest that sexual intercourse cease 4 to 5 weeks antepartum. If bleeding occurs early in pregnancy, an obstetrician may prohibit coitus temporarily as a therapeutic measure. Bleeding in the first 20 days of pregnancy occurs in 20 to 25 percent of women and approximately half of that group experience spontaneous abortion. Maternal death resulting from forcibly blowing air into the vagina during cunnilingus has been reported; the deaths presumably result from air emboli in the placental–maternal circulation.

Parturition

Fears regarding pain and bodily harm during delivery are universal and, to some extent, warranted. Preparation for childbirth affords a sense of familiarity and can ease anxieties, which facilitates delivery. Continuous emotional support during labor reduces the rate of cesarean section and forceps deliveries, the need for anesthesia, the use of oxytocin (Pitocin), and the duration of labor. A technically difficult or even painful delivery, however, does not appear to influence the decision to bear additional children.

Men's responses to pregnancy and labor have not been well studied, but the recent trend toward inclusion of fathers in the birth process eases their anxieties and elicits a fuller sense of participation. Fathers do not parent the same way as mothers, and new mothers sometimes need to be encouraged to respect these differences and view them positively.

Lamaze Method. Also known as natural childbirth, the Lamaze method originated with the French obstetrician Fernand Lamaze. In this method, women are fully conscious during labor and delivery, and no analgesic or anesthetic is used. The expectant mother and father attend special classes, during which they are taught relaxation and breathing exercises designed to facilitate the birth process. Women who have such training often report minimal pain during labor and delivery. Participating in the birth process may help a fearful or ambivalent father bond with his newborn infant.

Prenatal Screening

Prenatal screening for potential or actual fetal malformation is conducted in most pregnant women. Sonograms are noninvasive and can detect structural fetal abnormalities. Maternal α-fetoprotein (AFP) is measured between 15 and 20 weeks, screening for neural tube defects and Down syndrome. The sensitivity of Down syndrome testing is increased when a triple screen is done (AFP, hCG, and estriol). Amniocentesis is indicated for women over 35 years, those with a sibling or parent with a known chromosome anomaly, and those with abnormal AFP or any other risk for severe genetic disorder. Amniocentesis is usually done between 16 and 18 weeks and carries a risk that 1 in 300 women will miscarry after the procedure. In the first trimester, chorionic villus sampling (CVS) can be done, which reveals the same information concerning chromosomal status, enzyme levels, and DNA (deoxyribonucleic acid) patterns. With CVS, there is a risk that 1 in 100 women will have a spontaneous abortion after the procedure.

Screening in the first trimester allows women to choose early termination, which may be physically and emotionally easier on the woman. Profound ethical questions are involved in whether or not to abort a fetus with a known defect. Some women choose not to terminate and report a strong loving bond that lasts throughout the life of the child, who usually predeceases the parent.

Lactation

Lactation occurs because of a complex psychoneuroendocrine cascade that is triggered by the abrupt decline in estrogen and progesterone concentrations at parturition. In general, babies should be fed as needed, rather than by schedule. Breast-feeding has many benefits. The composition of breast milk supports timely neuronal development, confers passive immunity, and reduces food allergies in the child. In subsistence-level cultures in which children are allowed to nurse as long as they want (a practice supported by La Leche League, a breast-feeding advocacy group), most babies will wean themselves between ages 3 and 5 if not encouraged by the mother to do so earlier. Women who decide to breast-feed need good teaching and social support, which if lacking may lead to frustration and feelings of inadequacy. Women must not feel pressured or coerced into breast-feeding if they are opposed or ambivalent. In the long term, no discernible difference exists between bottle-fed and breast-fed children as adults.

An incidental finding about lactation is that some women experience sexual sensations during lactation, which in rare cases can lead to orgasm. In the early 1990s a woman who called a help line about such feelings was put in jail and had her infant taken from her on allegations of sexual abuse. Common sense ultimately prevailed, however, and mother and infant were reunited.

Perinatal Death

Perinatal death, defined as death sometime between the 20th week of gestation and the first month of life, includes spontaneous abortion (miscarriage), fetal demise, stillbirth, and neonatal death. In previous years, the intense bond between the expectant or new parent and the fetus or neonate was underestimated, but perinatal loss is now recognized as a significant trauma for both parents. Parents who experience such a loss go through a period of mourning much as that experienced when any loved one is lost.

Intrauterine fetal death, which can occur at any time during the pregnancy, is an emotionally traumatic experience. In the early months of pregnancy, a woman is usually unaware of fetal death and learns of it only from her doctor. Later in pregnancy, after fetal movements and heart tones have been experienced, a woman may be able to detect fetal demise. When given the diagnosis of fetal death, most women want the dead fetus removed; depending on the trimester, labor may be induced, or the woman may have to wait for spontaneous expulsion of the uterine contents. Many couples consider sexual relations during the period of waiting not only undesirable but psychologically unacceptable as well.

A sense of loss also accompanies the birth of a stillborn child and induced abortion of an abnormal fetus detected by antenatal diagnosis. As mentioned, attachment to an unborn child begins before birth, and grief and mourning occur after a loss at any time. The grief experienced after a third-trimester loss, however, is generally greater than that experienced after a first-trimester loss. Some parents do not wish to view a stillborn child, and their wishes should be respected. Others wish to hold the stillborn, and this act can assist the mourning process. A subsequent pregnancy may diminish overt feelings of grief, but it does not eliminate the need to mourn. So-called replacement children are at risk for overprotection and future emotional problems.

CONCEPTION

Infertility

Infertility is the inability of a couple to conceive after 1 year of coitus without the use of a contraceptive. In the United States, about 15 percent of married couples are unable to have children. In the past, women were blamed when couples did not have children, and feelings of guilt, depression, and inadequacy frequently accompanied the perception of being barren. Today, it is known that causes of infertility are attributed to disorders in men in 40 percent of cases, disorders in women in 40 percent, and disorders of both in 20 percent. Separate histories obtained for each partner (Table 23–1) and tests in an infertility workup (Table 23–2) usually reveal the specific cause; however, 10 to 20 percent of couples have no identifiable cause.

The inability to have a child can produce severe psychological stress on one or both partners in a marriage. Self-blame increases the likelihood of psychological problems. Women—but not men—are at increased risk for psychological distress if they are older and do not already have biological children. If one or both partners are unwilling to take advantage of assisted reproductive techniques, the marriage may falter. A psychiatric evaluation of the couple may be advisable. Marital disharmony or emotional conflicts about intimacy, sexual relations, or parenting roles can directly affect endocrine function and such physiological processes as erection, ejaculation, and ovulation. No evidence exists, however, for any simple, causal relation between stress and infertility.

When pre-existing conflict gives rise to problems of identity, self-esteem, and guilt, the disturbance may be severe and may manifest through regression; extreme dependence on a physician, mate, or parent; diffuse anger; impulsive behavior; or depression. The problem is further complicated when hormone therapy is used to treat the infertility, because the therapy may temporarily increase depression in some patients. Mood and cognition can be altered by pharmacological agents used to treat disorders of ovulation or to hyperstimulate the ovaries.

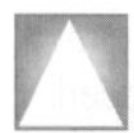

Table 23–1
Focused History for Infertility Workup

Medical History	Female Partner	Male Partner
Medical history and review of systems	Current medical problems and medication, allergies, hirsutism, thyroid dysfunction, weight gain, diabetes mellitus	Current medical problems and medication, allergies, erectile function, exposure to high temperatures
Surgical history	Fallopian tube surgery, ectopic pregnancy, appendectomy, pelvic surgery	Hernia repair, testicular or varicocele surgery
Sexual history	Frequency of intercourse, timing of intercourse with ovulation kit, dyspareunia	History of contraception use, excessive use of lubricants
Infertility history	Prior fertility, history of infertility treatments, duration of infertility	Prior fertility or infertility
Social history	Use of tobacco, caffeine, tetrahydrocannabinol (THC), recreational drugs, exposure to chemotherapy or radiation, psychosocial stressors	Use of tobacco, caffeine, THC, recreational drugs, exposure to chemotherapy or radiation
Developmental history	Menarche, breast development, dysmenorrhea, history of sexually transmitted diseases, use of prior contraception, diethylstilbestrol (DES) exposure, history of abnormal Papanicolaou smear and subsequent treatment	Degree of virilization, testicular infections, genital trauma, undescended testes, pubertal development, history of sexually transmitted diseases

Adapted from Frey KA, Patel KS. Initial evaluation and management of infertility. *Mayo Clin Proc*. 2004;79(11):1439–1443, with permission.

Persons who have difficulty conceiving may experience shock, disbelief, and a general sense of helplessness, and they develop an understandable preoccupation with the problem. Involvement in the infertility workup and the development of expertise about infertility can be a constructive defense against feelings of inadequacy and the humiliating, sometimes painful aspects of the workup itself. Worries about attractiveness and sexual desirability are common. Partners may feel ugly or impotent, and episodes of sexual dysfunction and loss of desire are reported. These problems are aggravated when a couple is scheduling sexual relations according to temperature charts or ovulatory cycles. Treatments for infertility (Table 23–3) are expensive and consume much time and energy. Both men and women can be overwhelmed by complexity, cost, invasiveness, and uncertainty associated with medical intervention.

Single persons who are aware of their own infertility may shy away from relationships for fear of being rejected once their "defect" is known. Persons who are infertile may have particular difficulty in their adult relationships with their own parents. The identification and equality that come from sharing the experience of parenthood must be replaced by internal reserves and other generative aspects of their lives.

Professional intervention may be necessary to help infertile couples ventilate their feelings and go through the process of mourning for their lost biological functions and the children they cannot have. Couples who remain infertile must cope with an actual loss. Couples who decide not to pursue parenthood may develop a renewed sense of love, dedication, and identity as a pair. Others may need help in exploring the options of husband or donor insemination, laboratory implantation, and adoption.

Family Planning and Contraception

Family planning is the process of choosing when, and if, to bear children. One form of family planning is contraception, the prevention of fecundation, or fertilization of the ovum. The choice

Table 23–2
Tests in the Infertility Workup

Possible Cause	Test	Comments
Anovulation	Basal body temperature chart	Patient must do each morning
	Endometrial biopsy	Office procedure in the late luteal phase
	Serum progesterone	Single or multiple blood tests
	Urinary ovulation detection kit	Home use at midcycle to time intercourse
	Ultrasound	Visualizes ovarian follicles and their rupture
Anatomic disorder	Hysterosalpingography	X-ray done in the proliferative phase, in which a radio-opaque dye is introduced through the cervix into the uterus to define intrauterine contours and tubal patency
	Sonohysterography	Transvaginal ultrasound examination with instillation of saline into the uterine cavity to define contours
	Diagnostic laparoscopy	Views external surfaces of internal structures
	Hysteroscopy	Visualizes endometrial cavity directly
Abnormal spermatogenesis	Semen analysis	Normal value >20 million/mL, 2 mL volume, 60% motility
	Postcoital test	Midcycle timing to look at sperm–cervical mucus interaction
Immunological disorder	Antisperm antibodies	Male semen test
Azoospermia	Testicular biopsy	Determines eligibility for intracytoplasmic sperm injection
	Semen analysis for fructose	Determines if the vas deferens are patent

Adapted from Beckmann CRB, Ling FW, Barzansky BM, et al. *Obstetrics and Gynecology for Medical Students*. Baltimore, MD: Williams Wilkins; 1992.

Table 23–3
Assisted Reproduction Techniques

Method	Comments
Ovulation induction or augmentation (multiple agents, particularly recombinant or highly purified gonadotropins)	Stimulates multifollicular development and ovulation; may produce multiple births; used in anovulation, luteal phase deficiency, unexplained infertility, and assisted reproduction
Induction of spermatogenesis	Used in men with idiopathic hypothalamic hypogonadism of functional or organic nature
Artificial insemination	Donor sperm is injected into the uterine cavity or the fallopian tubes; the sperm of the male partner may be used if healthy
Gamete intrafallopian transfer	Transfer of collected oocytes and sperm into the fallopian tubes; zygote may also be transferred; used for infertility from endometriosis and unexplained infertility
In vitro fertilization and embryo transfer	Transfer of developing embryos into the uterus after extracorporeal incubation of collected sperm with oocytes retrieved by laparoscopic surgery or by ultrasound-guided transvaginal aspiration; used with occlusion of the fallopian tubes or significant sperm dysfunction; permits preimplantation genetic diagnosis
Intracytoplasmic sperm injection	Injection in vitro of sperm head or sperm DNA (deoxyribonucleic acid) to cause fertilization and production of embryos for transfer to receptive endometrium; may be used even if sperm are barely viable; genetic causes of male infertility may be transmitted to offspring
Gamete donors	Donation of sperm or oocytes to another couple; can include oocytes only, oocyte cytoplasm only to restore reproductive competence to aged oocyte, donor sperm alone, or any combination; cytoplasmic transfer considered unethical and is illegal in some states
Surrogate mother	Surrogate mother receives donated embryo and carries the baby to term; a highly controversial technique with unclear legal ramifications

Data are taken in part from Susman V. *Pregnancy in Behavioral Sciences for Medical Students*. Baltimore, MD: Williams & Wilkins; 1993. Table by S. L. Berga, M.D., B. L. Parry, M.D., and E. L. Moses-Kolko, M.D.

of a contraceptive method (Table 23–4) is a complex decision involving both women and their partners. Factors influencing the decision include a woman's age and medical condition, her access to medical care, the couple's religious beliefs, and the need for coital spontaneity. The woman and her partner can weigh the risks and benefits of the various forms of contraception and make their decision on the basis of their current lifestyle and other factors. The success of contraceptive technology has enabled career-minded couples to delay child-bearing into their 30s and 40s. Such a delay, however, may increase infertility problems. Consequently, many women with careers feel their biological clocks ticking and plan to have children while in their early 30s to avoid the risk of not being able to have them at all.

Sterilization

Sterilization is a procedure that prevents a man or a woman from producing offspring. In a woman, the procedure is usually salpingectomy, ligation of the fallopian tubes, a procedure with low morbidity and low mortality. A man is usually sterilized by vasectomy, excision of part of the vas deferens, which is a simpler procedure than salpingectomy and can be performed in a physician's office. Voluntary sterilization, especially vasectomy, has become the most popular form of birth control in couples married for more than 10 years.

A small proportion of patients who elect sterilization may suffer from neurotic poststerilization syndrome, which can manifest through hypochondriasis, pain, loss of libido, sexual unresponsiveness, depression, and concerns about masculinity or femininity. One study of a group of women who regretted sterilization reported they had chosen the procedure while in poor relationships, frequently with abusive partners. Regret is most prevalent when a woman forms a new relationship and wishes to have a child with a new partner. Psychiatric consultation may be necessary to separate persons seeking sterilization for irrational or psychotic reasons from those who have made the decision after some time and thought.

The operative procedures for sterilization, namely vasectomy and tubal ligation, have assumed less importance than in the past because of the advent of contraceptives and the relative ease of obtaining abortions. Nonetheless, sterilization procedures are still chosen by men and women who, for a variety of reasons, want to permanently end their ability to produce children.

Abortion

Induced abortion is the planned termination of a pregnancy. About 1.3 million abortions are performed in the United States each year—246 abortions for every 1,000 live births. The various types of abortion are listed in Table 23–5. Over the past decade, the number of abortions has declined by about 15 percent. Family planning experts believe that more sex education and greater availability of contraceptive devices keep the number of abortions down. In Western countries, most women who obtain abortions are young, unmarried, and primiparous; in emerging countries, abortion is most common among married women with two or more children.

Of abortions, 60 percent are performed before 8 weeks of gestation, 88 percent are performed before 13 weeks, and 4.1 percent between 16 and 20 weeks, with 1.4 percent occurring after 21 weeks. Table 23–6 summarizes the most common abortion techniques, and Table 23–7 compares medical and surgical abortion techniques.

Abortion has become a political and philosophical issue in the United States. The country is sharply divided between pro-choice and pro-life factions. In recent years, antiabortion demonstrators have picketed abortion clinics and have provoked

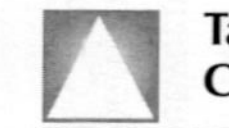

Table 23–4
Current Methods of Contraception

Type	Efficacy[a]	Advantages	Disadvantages	Potential Complications[b]
Spermicidal agents	Moderate	Readily available and easy to use	Messy; loss of spontaneity; requires forethought	Allergic reactions
Diaphragm, cervical cap	Moderate	Inexpensive; does not interfere with menstrual cycle	User familiarity required; prescription and fitting required; may interfere with spontaneity; requires forethought	Recurrent urinary tract infections with diaphragm; allergic reactions to latex or spermicide
Male condom	Moderate	Readily available and easy to use; protects against sexually transmitted infections	May interfere with spontaneity; requires forethought	Allergic reactions to latex or spermicide
Female condom	Moderate	Inconvenient to use; protects against sexually transmitted infections	May interfere with spontaneity; requires forethought	Allergic reactions to latex or spermicide
Hormonal (suppresses ovulation and/or impairs endometrial development)				
Oral contraceptives, contraceptive patches, and intravaginal rings	High	Protect against uterine and ovarian cancer, some sexually transmitted infections	Pharmacological side effects; require daily or weekly use, regardless of frequency of sex; must be prescribed and monitored by health care professional	Depression; breast tenderness; nausea; headaches; may be contraindicated in some medical conditions; can be taken continuously to achieve greater ovarian suppression and amenorrhea and to treat medical conditions
Postcoital steroids	High	Can be used after intercourse; inexpensive	Must be initiated within 72 hours; requires some medical supervision	Side effects, particularly nausea and headache; not universally available
Contraceptive implants (rods)	High	Implantable device that provides contraception for up to 1 year; once in place, no forethought required	Irregular bleeding and spotting due to endometrial effects and suppression of ovarian function; must be surgically placed and removed	Bone loss, depression; other medical sequelae of associated hormonal alterations unclear
Injectable steroids	High	Injectable progestin or combination of estrogen and progestin that prevents ovulation and suppresses ovarian activity; given intramuscularly at an interval that depends on the product	Slow return of ovarian activity after last dose; not removable	Bone loss and depression greater with progestin-only injections due to induction of greater hypoestrogenism; other consequences of hypoestrogenism unclear
Antiprogestins (RU-486)	High	Easy to use; does not disrupt menstrual cycle when administered in luteal phase; can be used postcoitally	Currently not available in the United States; must have predictable cycles	Impairs implantation rather than preventing conception
Sterilization				
Male sterilization (vasectomy)	High	Failure very rare; 20-minute office procedure	Morbidity in 1–2% of patients includes infections, clots	Can be reversed in only 80% of cases; rare neurotic impotence reaction; used by 10.4% of men
Female sterilization	High	Almost 100% protection; no impairment of sexual function or pleasure	More complex procedure than vasectomy; reversal is complicated and difficult	Surgical morbidity; used by 13.6% of women
Other				
Intrauterine device	High	Once in place, no forethought required; impairs endometrial receptivity	May cause nonbacterial endometritis or heavy menses; requires professional insertion	Likelihood of pelvic infection may be increased and tubal damage with infertility may result; uterine perforation or spontaneous expulsion
Rhythm	Low	No cost	Imposed coital timing	None
Natural family planning	Moderate	Readily available	User must monitor cervical mucus and body temperature closely; imposed coital timing	None
Withdrawal, coitus interruptus	Low	Readily available	Difficult to implement	None

[a]Estimates of efficacy are those associated with use rather than theoretically derived. High, <5% chance of contraceptive failure during the first year of use; moderate, <20% chance; low, >20% chance.
[b]Other than failure (pregnancy).
Table by S. L. Berga, M.D., B. L. Parry, M.D., and E. L. Moses-Kolko, M.D.

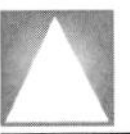

Table 23–5
Types of Abortion

Spontaneous	Spontaneous expulsion of the products of conception before viability (500 g or approximately 24 weeks from last menses)
Recurrent	Three or more spontaneous abortions
Missed	Abnormal development of an intrauterine pregnancy; usually caused by the presence of a blighted ovum and lack of fetal development
Threatened	Uterine bleeding or cramping and positive pregnancy test; must be distinguished from an ectopic (usually tubal) pregnancy
Incomplete	Spontaneous passage of a portion of the products of conception and the retention of placental fragments that result in ongoing bleeding
Elective	Induced by medical or surgical techniques before fetal viability; techniques include dilation, evacuation, and curettage; suction curettage; injection into the amniotic sac of saline or prostaglandins; hysterotomy; prostaglandins with antiprogestins (RU-486) or methotrexate; medical indications include the detection of fetal abnormalities by ultrasound or amniocentesis

Table by S. L. Berga, M.D., B. L. Parry, M.D., and E. L. Moses-Kolko, M.D.

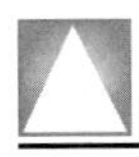

Table 23–6
Abortion Techniques

Type	Benefits	Risks
Cervical dilation and evacuation of uterine contents by curettage or vacuum aspiration	Most commonly performed procedure for termination of pregnancy; can be done before 24 weeks' gestation	Uterine perforation, adhesions, hemorrhage, infection, incomplete removal of fetus and placenta (all rare)
Menstrual aspiration (mini-abortion)	Can be done within 1–3 weeks of missed period	Implanted zygote not removed, uterine perforation (rare), failure to recognize ectopic pregnancy
Medical induction (cervical dilation with laminaria followed by intravaginal prostaglandin or intravenous oxytocin)	Can be used for second-trimester abortion	Water intoxication, uterine rupture, infection
Intra-amniotic hyperosmotic solutions (salting out)	Can be used for second-trimester abortions	Hyperosmolar crisis, heart failure, peritonitis, hemorrhage, water intoxication, myometrial necrosis
Prostaglandin (oral, intravaginal, cervical, or intra-amniotic)	Noninvasive procedure; can be used in conjunction with antiprogestins (RU-486) or methotrexate	Expulsion of live fetus, missed ectopic, hemorrhage, incomplete abortion
Antiprogestins (RU-486) with or without concomitant prostaglandin use	Nonsurgical; first trimester only	Incomplete abortion, hemorrhage
Methotrexate with or without prostaglandin use	Nonsurgical; first trimester only	Leukopenia, hemorrhage, incomplete results

Table by S. L. Berga, M.D., B. L. Parry, M.D., and E. L. Moses-Kolko, M.D.

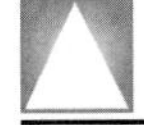

Table 23–7
Comparison of Medical and Surgical Pregnancy Termination

Termination	Medical	Surgical
Timing	Up to 9 weeks' gestation	As soon as intrauterine pregnancy confirmed, as early as 5 weeks
Anesthesia	None	Required
Side effects	Pain, bleeding expected	Usually minimal side effects
Efficacy	92–98% effective	98–99% effective
Privacy	Termination likely to occur at home	Procedure in surgical suite or office

Adapted from Brigham and Women's Hospital. *Contraception and Family Planning: A Guide to Counseling and Management*. Boston, MA: Brigham and Women's Hospital; 2005:15.

angry confrontations with patients. The atmosphere of moral condemnation and intimidation may make the decision to terminate a pregnancy difficult.

Psychological Reactions to Abortion. Recent studies demonstrate that most women who have an abortion for an unwanted pregnancy (i.e., induced abortion) were satisfied with their decision, with few, if any, negative psychological sequelae. Women who had miscarriages, however (i.e., spontaneous abortion), reported a high rate of dysphoric reactions. The difference can be explained, in part, by the fact that most women who induced abortion did so because they did not want the child. Women who spontaneously miscarried presumably wanted their babies. In the long term, however, about 10 percent of women who had induced abortion regretted having had the procedure.

Second-trimester abortions are more psychologically traumatic than first-trimester abortions. The most common reason for late abortions is the discovery (via amniocentesis or ultrasound) of an abnormal karyotype or fetal anomaly. Thus, late abortions usually involve the loss of a wanted child with whom the mother has already formed a bond.

Before the legalization of abortion in the United States in 1973, many women sought illegal abortions, often performed by untrained practitioners under nonsterile conditions. Considerable morbidity and mortality were associated with these abortions, and women who were denied abortion sometimes chose suicide over continuation of an unwanted pregnancy. In general, however, the risk of suicide is low in pregnant women, even in those who do not want a child but who carry the baby to term. When a woman is forced to carry a fetus to term, even though the risk of suicide is low, the risk increases for infanticide, abandonment, and neglect of the unwanted newborn.

Abortion can also be a significant experience for men. If a man has a close relationship with the woman, he may wish to play an active role in the abortion by accompanying her to the hospital or abortion clinic and providing emotional support. Fathers may experience considerable grief over the termination of a wanted pregnancy.

Reproductive Senescence

Both men and women age and experience an age-related decline in reproductive capacity, but only women experience complete gonadal cessation. Loss of reproductive capacity may present a psychological challenge to those who are not reconciled to the loss of fertility. Even with gonadal failure, however, the availability of donor oocytes and sperm means that pregnancy can be initiated in a menopausal woman with an intact uterus who elects to pursue that option. Studies have shown that older men may develop a genetic sperm mutation, giving rise to a higher incidence of autistic or schizophrenic offspring.

Menopause

Menopause, the cessation of ovulation, generally occurs between 47 and 53 years of age. The hypoestrogenism that follows can lead to hot flashes, sleep disturbances, vaginal atrophy and dryness, and cognitive and affective disturbances. Women are at increased risk for osteoporosis, dementia, and cardiovascular disease. Depression at menopause has been attributed to the "empty nest syndrome." Many women, however, report an enhanced sense of well-being and enjoy opportunities to pursue goals postponed because of child rearing.

PSYCHIATRIC ASPECTS OF PREGNANCY

Postpartum Depression

Many women experience some affective symptoms during the postpartum period, 4 to 6 weeks following delivery. Most of these women report symptoms consistent with "baby blues," a transient mood disturbance characterized by mood lability, sadness, dysphoria, subjective confusion, and tearfulness. These feelings, which may last several days, have been ascribed to rapid changes in women's hormonal levels, the stress of childbirth, and the awareness of the increased responsibility that motherhood brings. No professional treatment is required other than education and support for the new mother. If the symptoms persist longer than 2 weeks, evaluation is indicated for postpartum depression.

Postpartum depression (coded as a subtype of major depressive disorder in the fifth edition of *Diagnostic and Statistical Manual of Mental Disorders* [DSM-5]) is characterized by a depressed mood, excessive anxiety, insomnia, and change in weight. The onset is generally within 12 weeks after delivery. No conclusive evidence indicates that "baby blues" will lead to a subsequent episode of depression. Several studies do indicate that an episode of postpartum depression increases the risk of lifetime episodes of major depression. Treatment of postpartum depression is not well studied because of the risk of transmitting antidepressants to newborns during lactation. Table 23–8 differentiates postpartum "baby blues" from postpartum depression.

A syndrome described in fathers is characterized by mood changes during their wives' pregnancies or after the babies are born. These fathers are affected by several factors: added responsibility, diminished sexual outlet, decreased attention from his wife, and the belief that the child is a binding force in an unsatisfactory marriage.

Postpartum Psychosis

Postpartum psychosis (sometimes called *puerperal psychosis*) is an example of a psychotic disorder that occurs in women who have recently delivered a baby. The syndrome is often characterized by the mother's depression, delusions, and thoughts of harming either herself or her infant. Such ideation of suicide or infanticide must be carefully monitored; although rare, some mothers have acted on these ideas. Most available data suggest a close relation between postpartum psychosis and mood disorders, particularly bipolar disorder and major depressive disorder. It is coded as a subtype of bipolar disorder in DSM-5.

The incidence of postpartum psychosis is about 1 to 2 per 1,000 childbirths. About 50 to 60 percent of affected women have just had their first child, and about 50 percent of cases involve deliveries associated with nonpsychiatric perinatal complications. About 50 percent of the affected women have a family history of mood disorders. The most robust data indicate that an episode of postpartum psychosis is essentially an episode of a mood disorder, usually a bipolar disorder but possibly a depressive disorder. Relatives of those with postpartum

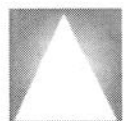

Table 23–8
Comparison of "Baby Blues" and Postpartum Depression

Characteristic	"Baby Blues"	Postpartum Depression
Incidence	30–75% of women who give birth	10–15% of women who give birth
Time of onset	3–5 days after delivery	Within 3–6 months after delivery
Duration	Days to weeks	Months to years, if untreated
Associated stressors	No	Yes, especially lack of support
Sociocultural influence	No; present in all cultures and socioeconomic classes	Strong association
History of mood disorder	No association	Strong association
Family history of mood disorder	No association	Some association
Tearfulness	Yes	Yes
Mood lability	Yes	Often present, but sometimes mood is uniformly depressed
Anhedonia	No	Often
Sleep disturbance	Sometimes	Nearly always
Suicidal thoughts	No	Sometimes
Thoughts of harming the baby	Rarely	Often
Feelings of guilt, inadequacy	Absent or mild	Often present and excessive

From Miller LJ. How "baby blues" and postpartum depression differ. *Women's Psychiatric Health*. 1995:13, with permission. Copyright 1995, The KSF Group.

psychosis have an incidence of mood disorders that is similar to the incidence in relatives of persons with mood disorders. As many as two-thirds of the patients have a second episode of an underlying affective disorder during the year after a baby's birth. The delivery process may best be seen as a nonspecific stress that causes the development of an episode of a major mood disorder, perhaps through a major hormonal mechanism.

The symptoms of postpartum psychosis can often begin within days of the delivery, although the mean time to onset is within 2 to 3 weeks and almost always within 8 weeks of delivery. Characteristically, patients begin to complain of fatigue, insomnia, and restlessness, and they may have episodes of tearfulness and emotional lability. Later, suspiciousness, confusion, incoherence, irrational statements, and obsessive concerns about the baby's health and welfare may be present. Delusional material may involve the idea that the baby is dead or defective. Patients may deny the birth and express thoughts of being unmarried, virginal, persecuted, influenced, or perverse. Hallucinations with similar content may involve voices telling the patient to kill the baby or herself. Complaints regarding the inability to move, stand, or walk are also common.

The onset of florid psychotic symptoms is usually preceded by prodromal signs such as insomnia, restlessness, agitation, lability of mood, and mild cognitive deficits. Once the psychosis occurs, the patient may be a danger to herself or to her newborn, depending on the content of her delusional system and her degree of agitation. In one study, 5 percent of patients committed suicide and 4 percent committed infanticide. A favorable outcome is associated with a good premorbid adjustment and a supportive family network. Subsequent pregnancies are associated with an increased risk of another episode, sometimes as high as 50 percent.

As with any psychotic disorder, clinicians should consider the possibility of either a psychotic disorder caused by a general medical condition or a substance-induced psychotic disorder. Potential general medical conditions include hypothyroidism and Cushing's syndrome. Substance-induced psychotic disorder can be associated with the use of pain medications such as pentazocine (Talwin) or of antihypertensive drugs during pregnancy. Other potential medical causes include infections, toxemia, and neoplasms.

Postpartum psychosis is a psychiatric emergency. Antipsychotic medications and lithium (Eskalith), often in combination with an antidepressant, are the treatments of choice. No pharmacological agents should be prescribed to a woman who is breast-feeding. Suicidal patients may require transfer to a psychiatric unit to help prevent a suicide attempt.

The mother is usually helped by contact with her baby if she so desires, but the visits must be closely supervised, especially if the mother is preoccupied with harming the infant. Psychotherapy is indicated after the period of acute psychosis, and therapy is usually directed at helping the patient accept and be at ease with the mothering role. Changes in environmental factors may also be indicated, such as increased support from the husband and others in the environment. Most studies report high rates of recovery from the acute illness.

Mrs. Z is a 30-year-old high school teacher living in Lagos, Nigeria. She is married and has five children. The birth of her last child was complicated by hemorrhage and sepsis, and she was still hospitalized on the gynecology service for 13 days after delivery when her gynecologist requested a psychiatric consultation. Mrs. Z was agitated and seemed to be in a daze. She said to the psychiatrist: "I am a sinner. I have to die. My time is past. I cannot be a good Christian again. I need to be reborn. Jesus Christ should help me. He is not helping me." A diagnosis of postpartum psychosis was made. An antipsychotic drug, chlorpromazine (Thorazine), was prescribed, and Mrs. Z was soon well enough to go home. Three weeks later, she was readmitted, this time to the psychiatric ward, claiming she "had had a vision of the spirits" and was "wrestling with the spirits." Her relatives reported that at home she had been fasting and "keeping a vigil" through the nights and was not sleeping. She had complained to the neighbors that there was a witch in her house. The witch turned out to be her mother. Mrs. Z's husband, who was studying engineering in Europe, hurriedly returned and took over the running of the household, sending his mother-in-law

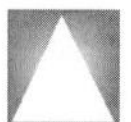

Table 23–9
Food and Drug Administration Rating of Drug Safety in Pregnancy

Category	Definition	Drug Examples
A	No fetal risks in controlled human studies	Iron
B	No fetal risk in animal studies, but no controlled human studies or fetal risk in animals, but no risk in well-controlled human studies	Acetaminophen
C	Adverse fetal effects in animals and no human data available	Aspirin, haloperidol, chlorpromazine
D	Human fetal risk seen (may be used in life-threatening situation)	Lithium, tetracycline, ethanol
X	Proved fetal risk in humans (no indication for use, even in life-threatening situations)	Valproic acid, thalidomide

away and supervising Mrs. Z's treatment himself. She improved rapidly on an antidepressant medication and was discharged in 2 weeks. Her improvement, however, was short-lived. She threw away her medications and began to attend mass whenever one was given, pursuing the priests to ask questions about scriptures. Within 1 week, she was readmitted. On the ward, she accused the psychiatrist of shining powerful torchlights on her and taking pictures of her, opening her chest, using her as a guinea pig, poisoning her food, and planning to bury her alive. She claimed to receive messages from Mars and Jupiter and announced that there was a riot in town. She clutched her Bible to her breast and accused all the doctors of being "idol worshippers," calling down the wrath of her god on all of them. After considerable resistance, Mrs. Z was finally convinced to accept electroconvulsive treatment, and she became symptom free after six treatments. At this point, she attributed her illness to a difficult childbirth, the absence of her husband, and her unreasonable mother. She saw no further role for doctors, called for her priest, and began to speak of her illness as a religious experience that was similar to the experience of religious leaders throughout history. However, her symptoms did not return, and she was discharged after 6 weeks of hospitalization. *(Courtesy of Bushra Naz, M.D., Laura J. Fochtmann, M.D., and Evelyn J. Bromet, Ph.D.)*

Psychotropic Medications in Pregnancy

No definitive answers exist to the questions of which psychotropic medications are safest during pregnancy and lactation. In patients with worsening psychiatric illness during pregnancy, outpatient psychotherapy, hospitalization, and milieu therapy should be attempted before routine use of psychotropic medication. The risks and benefits of treatment with psychotropics versus maternal psychiatric illness must be carefully evaluated on an individual basis. If the patient, her psychiatrist, and her obstetrician decide to continue psychiatric medications throughout pregnancy, the dosage should be calibrated to the physiological changes each trimester. Although no antidepressant medications have been associated with intrauterine death or major birth defects, both selective serotonin reuptake inhibitors (SSRIs) and tricyclic antidepressants (TCAs) are associated with a transient perinatal syndrome. Studies demonstrate that fluoxetine (Prozac) has been found in amniotic fluid. Mood stabilizers are associated with more consequential teratogenic risks, namely cardiac anomalies and neural tube defects, but women with bipolar disorder are at a significant risk of relapse without medication maintenance. Lithium has been associated with an increased risk of Ebstein's anomaly, a congenital downward displacement of the tricuspid valve into the right ventricle.

The U.S. Food and Drug Administration (FDA) rates drugs in five categories of safety for use in pregnancy, with categories of risk coded A, B, C, D, and X (Table 27–9). In general, all medications that are not absolutely essential should be avoided during pregnancy.

Teratogens

Teratogens are drugs or other agents that cause abnormal fetal development. Infections such as varicella, toxoplasmosis, and herpes simplex, among others, can interfere with normal development. Pregnant women who smoke are subject to premature births, and congenital defects are more common in smokers than in nonsmokers. Alcohol abuse is associated with fetal alcohol syndrome (see Section 16.2). Other drugs of abuse, such as cocaine and heroin, produce drug-dependent newborns. In general, pregnant women should not use prescription and over-the-counter drugs and phytomedicinals. Drugs given in the third trimester are rarely teratogenic. Retinoids (used to treat acne) taken early in pregnancy have been associated with fetal abnormalities.

Premenstrual Dysphoric Disorder

Premenstrual dysphoric disorder (PMDD) is a somatopsychic illness triggered by changing levels of sex steroids that accompany an ovulatory menstrual cycle. It occurs about 1 week before the onset of menses and is characterized by irritability, emotional lability, headache, anxiety, and depression. Somatic symptoms include edema, weight gain, breast pain, syncope, and paresthesias. Approximately 5 percent of women have the disorder. Treatment is symptomatic and includes analgesics for pain and sedatives for anxiety and insomnia. Some patients respond to short courses of SSRIs. Fluid retention is relieved with diuretics.

The generally recognized syndrome involves mood symptoms (e.g., lability, irritability), behavior symptoms (e.g., changes in eating patterns, insomnia), and physical symptoms (e.g., breast tenderness, edema, and headaches). This pattern of symptoms occurs at a specific time during the menstrual cycle, and the symptoms resolve for some period of time between menstrual cycles. The hormonal changes that occur during the

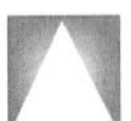

Table 23–10
Diagnostic Criteria for Premenstrual Syndrome

Psychological Symptoms	Somatic Symptoms
Depression	Breast tenderness
Irritability	Abdominal bloating
Anxiety	Headache
Confusion	Swelling of extremities
Social withdrawal	

Adapted from American College of Obstetricians and Gynecologists [ACOG]. Practice Bulletin #15, April 2000.

menstrual cycle are probably involved in producing the symptoms, although the exact etiology is unknown.

Because of the absence of generally agreed-upon diagnostic criteria, the epidemiology of premenstrual dysphoria is not known with certainty. Up to 80 percent of all women experience some alteration in mood, sleep, or somatic symptoms during the premenstrual period, and about 40 percent of these women have at least mild to moderate premenstrual symptoms prompting them to seek medical advice. Only 3 to 7 percent of women have symptoms that meet the full diagnostic criteria for PMDD.

Given that most women who experience changes in affect or somatic symptoms during the premenstrual period are not severely functionally impaired, it is important to distinguish these women from those who are diagnosed with PMDD. Premenstrual syndrome (PMS) is distinguished from PMDD by the severity and number of symptoms, as well as the degree to which function is impaired. Table 23–10 lists the diagnostic criteria for PMS in which the patient reports at least one of the affective or somatic symptoms during the 5 days before menses in each of the three prior menstrual cycles.

The course and the prognosis of PMDD have not been studied sufficiently to reach any reasonable conclusions. Anecdotally, the symptoms tend to be chronic unless effective treatment is initiated. Treatment of PMDD includes support for the patient about the presence and recognition of the symptoms. SSRIs (e.g., fluoxetine) and alprazolam (Xanax) have been reported to be effective, although no treatment has been conclusively demonstrated to be effective in multiple, well-controlled trials. If symptoms are present throughout the menstrual cycle, with no intercycle symptom relief, clinicians should consider one of the nonmenstrual cycle–related mood disorders and anxiety disorders. The presence of especially severe symptoms, even if cyclical, should prompt clinicians to consider other mood disorders and anxiety disorders. A thorough medical workup is necessary to rule out medical or surgical conditions to account for symptoms (e.g., endometriosis).

OTHER ISSUES

Sexually Transmitted Diseases

A sexually transmitted disease (STD) is a contagious disease acquired as a result of a physical sexual interaction. From the 1950s through 1970s, the infections were considered treatable and not life-threatening. That was before acquired immune deficiency syndrome (AIDS) was recognized, which is caused by infection with human immunodeficiency virus (HIV) and is currently incurable, life-threatening, and transmissible from mother to fetus.

A sequela of STDs, such as gonorrhea and chlamydia, is pelvic inflammatory disease (PID). Untreated, PID can develop into bilateral tubo-ovarian abscesses and necessitate hysterectomy and bilateral salpingo-oophorectomy. Early antibiotic treatment is advocated to prevent development of the abscesses and to reduce the likelihood of infertility, chronic pelvic pain, and ectopic pregnancy from tubal damage. These infections also can lead to obstruction of the vas deferens and chronic prostatitis and subsequent male infertility.

Another STD that can have serious consequences is venereal warts, or human papillomavirus (HPV). Genital infections with certain subtypes of HPV can lead to premalignant changes of the penis, vulva, vagina, and cervix and are thought to cause cervical cancer. Venereal warts can be removed chemically or surgically but are difficult to eradicate completely. Women who contract HPV are encouraged to have regular gynecological examinations and Papanicolaou smears to detect premalignant lesions. An HPV vaccine exists, which is recommended for all girls 11 to 12 years of age to decrease the incidence of certain strains of HPV virus. This vaccine would then decrease the incidence of genital warts and cervical cancer.

Sexual monogamy and abstinence, which will prevent most STDs, are advocated as public health measures. Libidinal impulses, however, can be difficult to control and restrict. Therefore, measures such as condom use are strongly recommended as an alternative public health measure. Adolescents, in particular, need to know the potential consequences of sexual activity with regard to STDs and pregnancy. Admonishing teens to remain chaste is unlikely to be completely effective and may be counterproductive. The risks of sexual intercourse may be forgotten or seem minimal in comparison to the need for affection or escape. Persons with low self-esteem or under stress may view sex as a means of bolstering their self-image or escaping their stresses. The reinforcing properties of sex ensure that the problem of STDs will endure. Studies in Europe, especially Holland, have shown that easy availability of condoms (e.g., in schools) reduces both STDs and unwanted pregnancies.

Pelvic Pain

Pelvic pain can have many causes, including endometriosis, pelvic adhesions, ovarian or adnexal masses, hernias, and bowel or rectal disease. Pelvic pain can also be secondary to psychogenic causes such as guilt, fertility, or fears of infertility, and the emotional disturbances associated with ongoing or past incest or sexual abuse. Pelvic pain should not be attributed to psychogenic causes unless a thorough evaluation has excluded organic causes. In most instances, the evaluation should include a diagnostic laparoscopy. Likewise, dyspareunia or pain with intercourse should not be assumed to have a psychogenic origin unless all anatomical causes have been excluded.

Pseudocyesis

Pseudocyesis (false pregnancy) is the development of the classic symptoms of pregnancy—amenorrhea, nausea, breast enlargement and pigmentation, abdominal distention, and labor pains—in a nonpregnant woman. Pseudocyesis demonstrates the ability of the psyche to dominate the soma, probably via central input at the level of the hypothalamus. Predisposing psychological processes are thought to include a pathological wish for, and fear of, pregnancy; ambivalence or conflict regarding gender, sexuality, or childbearing; and a grief reaction to loss following a miscarriage, tubal ligation, or hysterectomy. The patient may have a true somatic delusion that is not subject to reality testing, but often a negative pregnancy test result or pelvic ultrasound scan leads to resolution. Psychotherapy is recommended during or after a presentation of pseudocyesis to evaluate and treat the underlying psychological dysfunction. A related event, couvade, occurs in some cultures in which the father of the child undergoes simulated labor, as though he were giving birth. In those societies couvade is a normal phenomenon.

Miss S, aged 16, thought she had become pregnant after her first coital experience, which occurred without contraception. Shortly after she read about the signs and symptoms of pregnancy, her menses stopped. She related that she felt tingling in her breasts, which she believed were enlarged. She also reported nausea and vomiting in the morning, which was observed by her mother. On examination, the uterus was enlarged, breasts were developed with dark areola and contained milk, and a pigmented line was observed from the umbilicus to the pubis. The abdomen was not enlarged, but she believed she felt fetal movement. A pregnancy test had negative results and the patient was so informed; however, she could not be dissuaded of her belief that she was pregnant. She entered psychotherapy, and within 2 months her menses returned and she accepted the fact that she was not pregnant.

Hyperemesis Gravidarum

Hyperemesis gravidarum is differentiated from morning sickness in that vomiting is chronic, persistent, and frequent, leading to ketosis, acidosis, weight loss, and dehydration. The prognosis is excellent for both mother and fetus with prompt treatment. Most women can be treated as outpatients, with changing to smaller meals, discontinuing iron supplements, and avoiding certain foods. In severe cases, hospitalization may be necessary. Although the cause is unknown, a psychological component may exist. Women with histories of anorexia nervosa or bulimia nervosa may be at risk.

Pica

Pica is the repeated ingestion of nonnutritive substances, such as dirt, clay, starch, sand, and feces. This eating disorder is most often seen in young children, but is common in pregnant women in some subcultures, most notably among African-American women in the rural South, who may eat clay or starch (e.g., Argo). The cause of pica is unknown, but it may be related to nutritional deficiencies in the mother.

24 Psychotherapies

24.1 Psychoanalysis and Psychoanalytic Psychotherapy

As broadly practiced today, psychoanalytic treatment encompasses a wide range of uncovering strategies used in varied degrees and blends. Despite the inevitable blurring of boundaries in actual application, the original modality of classic psychoanalysis and major modes of psychoanalytic psychotherapy (expressive and supportive) are delineated separately here (Table 24.1–1). Analytical practice in all its complexity resides on a continuum. Individual technique is always a matter of emphasis, as the therapist titrates the treatment according to the needs and capacities of the patient at every moment.

Psychoanalysis is virtually synonymous with the renowned name of its founding father, Sigmund Freud. It is also referred to as "classic" or "orthodox" psychoanalysis to distinguish it from more recent variations known as *psychoanalytic psychotherapy* (discussed below).

Psychoanalysis is based on the theory of sexual repression and traces the unfulfilled infantile libidinal wishes in the individual's unconscious memories. It remains unsurpassed as a method to discover the meaning and motivation of behavior, especially the unconscious elements that inform thoughts and feelings.

PSYCHOANALYSIS

Psychoanalytic Process

The psychoanalytic process involves bringing to the surface repressed memories and feelings by means of a scrupulous unraveling of hidden meanings of verbalized material and of the unwitting ways in which the patient wards off underlying conflicts through defensive forgetting and repetition of the past.

The overall process of analysis is one in which unconscious neurotic conflicts are recovered from memory and verbally expressed, reexperienced in the transference, reconstructed by the analyst, and, ultimately, resolved through understanding. Freud referred to these processes as *recollection, repetition,* and *working through,* which make up the totality of remembering, reliving, and gaining insight. *Recollection* entails the extension of memory back to early childhood events, a time in the distant past when the core of neurosis was formed. The actual reconstruction of these events comes through reminiscence, associations, and autobiographical linking of developmental events. *Repetition* involves more than mere mental recall; it is an emotional replay of former interactions with significant individuals in the patient's life. The replay occurs within the special context of the analyst as projected parent, a fantasized object from the patient's past with whom the latter unwittingly reproduces forgotten, unresolved feelings and experiences from childhood. Finally, *working through* is both an affective and cognitive integration of previously repressed memories that have been brought into consciousness and through which the patient is gradually set free (cured of neurosis). The analytical course can be subdivided into three major stages (Table 24.1–2).

Indications and Contraindications

In general, all of the so-called *psychoneuroses* are suitable for psychoanalysis. These include anxiety disorders, obsessional thinking, compulsive behavior, conversion disorder, sexual dysfunction, depressive states, and many other nonpsychotic conditions, such as personality disorders. Significant suffering must be present so that patients are motivated to make the sacrifices of time and financial resources required for psychoanalysis. Patients who enter analysis must have a genuine wish to understand themselves, not a desperate hunger for symptomatic relief. They must be able to withstand frustration, anxiety, and other strong affects that emerge in analysis without fleeing or acting out their feelings in a self-destructive manner. They must also have a reasonable, mature superego that allows them to be honest with the analyst. Intelligence must be at least average, and above all, they must be psychologically minded in the sense that they can think abstractly and symbolically about the unconscious meanings of their behavior.

Many contraindications for psychoanalysis are the flip side of the indications. The absence of suffering, poor impulse control, inability to tolerate frustration and anxiety, and low motivation to understand are all contraindications. The presence of extreme dishonesty or antisocial personality disorder contraindicates analytic treatment. Concrete thinking or the absence of psychological mindedness is another contraindication. Some patients who might ordinarily be psychologically minded are not suitable for analysis because they are in the midst of a major upheaval or life crisis, such as a job loss or a divorce. Serious physical illness can also interfere with a person's ability to invest in a long-term treatment process. Patients of low intelligence generally do not understand the procedure or cooperate in the process. An age older than 40 years was once considered a contraindication, but today analysts recognize that patients are malleable and analyzable in their 60s or 70s. One final contraindication is a close relationship with the analyst. Analysts should avoid analyzing friends, relatives, or persons with whom they have other involvements.

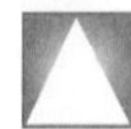

Table 24.1–1
Scope of Psychoanalytic Practice: A Clinical Continuum[a]

		Psychoanalytic Psychotherapy	
Feature	**Psychoanalysis**	**Expressive Mode**	**Supportive Mode**
Frequency	Regular four to five times per week; "50-minute hour"	Regular one to three times per week; half to full hour	Flexible one time per week or less; or as needed half to full hour
Duration	Long-term; usually 3 to 5+ years	Short or long term; several sessions to months or years	Short or intermittent long term; single session to lifetime
Setting	Patient primarily on couch with analyst out of view	Patient and therapist face to face; occasional use of couch	Patient and therapist face to face; couch contraindicated
Modus operandi	Systematic analysis of all positive and negative transference and resistance; primary focus on analyst and intrasession events; transference neurosis facilitated; regression encouraged	Partial analysis of dynamics and defenses; focus on current interpersonal events and transference to others outside of sessions; analysis of negative transference; positive transference left unexplored unless impedes progress; limited regression encouraged	Formation of therapeutic alliance and real object relationship; analysis of transference contraindicated with rare exceptions; focus on conscious external events; regression discouraged
Analyst/Therapist role	Absolute neutrality; frustration of patient; reflector/mirror role	Modified neutrality; implicit gratification of patient and greater activity	Neutrality suspended; limited explicit gratification, direction, and disclosure
Mutative change agents	Insight predominates within relatively deprived environment	Insight within more empathic environment; identification with benevolent object	Auxiliary or surrogate ego as temporary substitute; holding environment; insight to degree possible
Patient population	Neuroses; mild character psychopathology	Neuroses; mild to moderate character psychopathology, especially narcissistic and borderline disorders	Severe character disorders, latent or manifest psychoses, acute crises, physical illness
Patient requisites	High motivation, psychological mindedness; good previous object relationships; ability to maintain transference neurosis; good frustration tolerance	Moderate to high motivation and psychological mindedness; ability to form therapeutic alliance; some frustration tolerance	Some degree of motivation and ability to form therapeutic alliance
Basic goals	Structural reorganization of personality; resolution of unconscious conflicts; insight into intrapsychic events; symptom relief an indirect result	Partial reorganization of personality and defenses; resolution of preconscious and conscious derivatives of conflicts; insight into current interpersonal events; improved object relations; symptom relief	Reintegration of self and ability to cope; stabilization or restoration of pre-existing equilibrium; strengthening of defenses; better adjustment or acceptance of pathology; symptom relief and environmental restructuring as primary goals
Major techniques	Free association method predominates; full dynamic interpretation (including confrontation, clarification, and working through), with emphasis on genetic reconstruction	Limited free association; confrontation, clarification, and partial interpretation predominate, with emphasis on here-and-now interpretation and limited genetic interpretation	Free association method contraindicated; suggestion (advise) predominates; abreaction useful; confrontation, clarification, and interpretation in the here-and-now secondary; genetic interpretation contraindicated
Adjunct treatment	Primarily avoided; if applied, all negative and positive meanings and implications are thoroughly analyzed	May be necessary (e.g., psychotropic drugs as temporary measure); if applied, its negative implications explored and diffused	Often necessary (e.g., psychotropic drugs, family rehabilitative therapy, or hospitalization); if applied, its positive implications are emphasized

[a]This division is not categorical; all practice resides on a clinical continuum.

Patient Requisites

The most important patient requisites for psychoanalysis are listed in Table 24.1–3.

Ms. M, a 29-year-old unmarried woman who worked in a low-level capacity for a magazine, presented for consultation with the chief complaints of considerable sadness and distress over her parent's reaction when they found that she had had a homosexual relationship. She also realized that she had been working far below her potential. She had never sought any treatment before. She was clearly intelligent, sensitive, self-reflective, and insightful. When the possibility of psychoanalysis was presented to her, she worried that meant she was "sicker." Ms. M, however, began reading Freud, realized that analysis was actually recommended for those who are higher functioning, and became intrigued by the idea. She agreed to come 4 days a week for 50-minute sessions.

She was the oldest of three children and the only girl. Ms. M's father, a successful professional, was described as very demanding and intrusive, someone who never thought anything was good

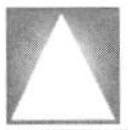

Table 24.1–2
Stages of Psychoanalysis

Stage one: Patient becomes familiar with the methods, routines, and requirements of analysis, and a realistic therapeutic alliance is formed between patient and analyst. Basic rules are established; the patient describes his or her problems; there is some review of history, and the patient gains initial relief through catharsis and a sense of security before delving more deeply into the source of the illness. The patient is primarily motivated by the wish to get well.

Stage two: Transference neurosis emerges that substitutes for the actual neurosis of the patient and in which the wish for health comes into direct conflict with the simultaneous wish to receive emotional gratification from the analyst. There is a gradual surfacing of unconscious conflicts; an increased irrational attachment to the analyst, with regressive and dependent concomitants of that bond; a developmental return to earlier forms of relating (sometimes compared with that of mother and infant); and a repetition of childhood patterns and recall of traumatic memories through transfer to the analyst of unresolved libidinal wishes.

Stage three: The termination phase is marked by the dissolution of the analytical bond as the patient prepares for leave-taking. The irrational attachment to the analyst in the transference neurosis has subsided because it has been worked through, and more rational aspects of the psyche preside, providing greater mastery and more mature adaptation to the patient's problems. Termination is not a hard-and-fast event, and the patient invariably has to continue to work through any problems outside of the therapy situation without the analyst or may need intermittent assistance after analysis has technically terminated.

Courtesy of T. Byram Karasu, M.D.

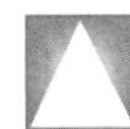

Table 24.1–3
Patient Prerequisites for Psychoanalysis

1. *High motivation.* The patient needs a strong motivation to persevere, in light of the rigors of intense and lengthy treatment. The desire for health and self-understanding must surpass the neurotic need for unhappiness. The patient must be willing to face issues of time and money and to endure the pain and frustration associated with sacrificing rapid relief in favor of future cure and with foregoing the secondary gains of illness.
2. *Ability to form a relationship.* The capacity to form and maintain, as well as to detach from, a trusting object relationship is essential. The patient also has to withstand a frustrating and regressive transference without decompensating or becoming excessively attached. Patients with a history of impaired or transient interpersonal relations who cannot establish a viable connection to another human make poor candidates for psychoanalysis.
3. *Psychological mindedness and capacity for insight.* As an introspective process, psychoanalysis requires curiosity about oneself and the capacity for self-scrutiny. Those who are unable to articulate and comprehend their inner thoughts and feelings cannot negotiate with the fundamental analytical coin words and their meanings. The inability to examine one's own motivations and behaviors precludes benefits from the analytical method.
4. *Ego strength.* Ego strength is the integrative capacity to oscillate appropriately between two antithetical types of ego functioning. On the one hand, the patient must be able to reflect temporarily, to relinquish reality for fantasy, and to be dependent and passive. On the other hand, the patient has to be able to accept analytical rules, to integrate interpretations, to defer important decisions, to shift perspectives to become an observer of his or her intrapsychic processes, and to function in a sustained interpersonal relationship as a responsible adult.

Courtesy of T. Byram Karasu, M.D.

enough. He had always expected his children to do the "extra credit" assignments as part of their regular work. Ms. M, however, was very proud of her father's accomplishments. She spoke of her mother in conflicting terms as well: She was a homemaker, weak, and sometimes acquiescent to the powerful father but also a woman in her own right who was involved in community volunteer work and could be a powerful public speaker.

Just prior to beginning her analysis, Ms. M had had her wallet stolen. In her first analytic session, she spoke of losing all of her identification cards, and to her it seemed as if she were starting analysis "with a completely new identity." Initially, she was somewhat hesitant to use the couch because she wanted to see her analyst's reactions, but she quickly appreciated that she could associate more easily without seeing the analyst.

As her analysis proceeded, through dreams and free associations, Ms. M became quite focused on the analyst. She became extremely curious about the analyst's life. What emerged from her associations to seeing the analyst's appointment book on the desk was that she felt "slotted in." Whenever Ms. M saw other patients, she felt the office was "like an assembly line." Further associations led to her feeling slotted in by her parents as they ran from one activity to another. Her resistance manifested itself in Ms. M's often coming as much or more than 15 minutes late to her sessions. Her associations led to her admitting that she did not want her analyst to think that she was "too eager." Ms. M was able to see that she needed to devalue her analyst and her importance to Ms. M as a defense against an overwhelming positive and even erotic transference toward her.

For example, Ms. M wanted to improve her appearance so that the therapist, who she called a "role model," would find her more attractive. Her negative transference, however, was never far from the surface, and she denigrated the analyst by wondering if the analyst were a "clotheshorse" who was financing her wardrobe with the patient's payments.

Her conflicts about her sexual orientation were a central preoccupation in the course of her analysis, particularly because her father was so homophobic. Early on, Ms. M felt awkward and uncomfortable when she went to a lesbian bar, and when asked if she qualified for the "lesbian discount," she said she did not. At one point, she began seeing several men, including a male psychologist. The analyst made the transference interpretation, which Ms. M accepted, that a date with this man seemed as if it were a date with the analyst and sleeping with him would be equivalent to sleeping with the analyst. Ms. M was also able to see that her transient choice of dating a male therapist was a defensive compromise. Although her homosexual object choice was multidetermined, Ms. M came to appreciate, through her work in analysis, that at least a part of her conflicts about homosexuality stemmed from her relationship toward her father. It was a means of securing his attention as well as infuriating him.

Over the course of 4 years, Ms. M began to do considerably better at work and was promoted to a job commensurate with her potential. She was also able to deal better with both her parents, and particularly her father, regarding her sexual orientation. She became much more comfortable with her "new identity" and became involved in a relationship with a professional woman. At the end of therapy, Ms. M and this woman were committed to each other and were thinking of adopting a child. *(Courtesy of T. Byram Karasu, M.D., and S. R. Karasu, M.D.)*

Goals

Stated in developmental terms, psychoanalysis aims at the gradual removal of amnesias rooted in early childhood based on the assumption that when all gaps in memory have been filled, the morbid condition will cease because the patient no longer needs to repeat or remain fixated to the past. The patient should be better able to relinquish former regressive patterns and to develop new, more adaptive ones, particularly as he or she learns the reasons for his or her behavior. A related goal of psychoanalysis is for the patient to achieve some measure of self-understanding or insight.

Psychoanalytic goals are often considered formidable (e.g., a total personality change), involving the radical reorganization of old developmental patterns based on earlier affects and the entrenched defenses built up against them. Goals may also be elusive, framed as they are in theoretical intrapsychic terms (e.g., greater ego strength) or conceptually ambiguous ones (resolution of the transference neurosis). Criteria for successful psychoanalysis may be largely intangible and subjective and they are best regarded as conceptual endpoints of treatment that must be translated into more realistic and practical terms.

In practice, the goals of psychoanalysis for any patient naturally vary, as do the many manifestations of neuroses. The form that the neurosis takes—unsatisfactory sexual or object relationships, inability to enjoy life, underachievement, and fear of work or academic success, or excessive anxiety, guilt, or depressive ideation—determines the focus of attention and the general direction of treatment, as well as the specific goals. Such goals may change at any time during the course of analysis, especially as many years of treatment may be involved.

Major Approach and Techniques

Structurally, *psychoanalysis* usually refers to individual (dyadic) treatment that is frequent (four or five times per week) and long term (several years). All three features take their precedent from Freud himself.

The dyadic arrangement is a direct function of the Freudian theory of neurosis as an intrapsychic phenomenon, which takes place within the person as instinctual impulses continually seek discharge. Because dynamic conflicts must be internally resolved if structural personality reorganization is to take place, the individual's memory and perceptions of the repressed past are pivotal.

Freud initially saw patients 6 days a week for 1 hour each day, a routine now reduced to four or five sessions per week of the classic 50-minute hour, which leaves time for the analyst to take notes and organize relevant thoughts before the next patient. Long intervals between sessions are avoided so that the momentum gained in uncovering conflictual material is not lost and confronted defenses do not have time to restrengthen.

Freud's belief that successful psychoanalysis always takes a long time because profound changes in the mind occur slowly still holds. The process can be likened to the fluid sense of time that is characteristic of our unconscious processes. Moreover, because psychoanalysis involves a detailed recapitulation of present and past events, any compromise in time presents the risk of losing pace with the patient's mental life.

Psychoanalytic Setting. As with other forms of psychotherapy, psychoanalysis takes place in a professional setting, apart from the realities of everyday life, in which the patient is offered a temporary sanctuary in which to ease psychic pain and reveal intimate thoughts to an accepting expert. The psychoanalytic environment is designed to promote relaxation and regression. The setting is usually spartan and sensorially neutral, and external stimuli are minimized.

USE OF THE COUCH. The couch has several clinical advantages that are both real and symbolic: (1) the reclining position is relaxing because it is associated with sleep and so eases the patient's conscious control of thoughts; (2) it minimizes the intrusive influence of the analyst, thus curbing unnecessary cues; (3) it permits the analyst to make observations of the patient without interruption; and (4) it holds symbolic value for both parties, a tangible reminder of the Freudian legacy that gives credibility to the analyst's professional identity, allegiance, and expertise. The reclining position of the patient with analyst nearby can also generate threat and discomfort, however, as it recalls anxieties derived from the earlier parent–child configuration that it physically resembles. It may also have personal meanings—for some, a portent of dangerous impulses or of submission to an authority figure; for others, a relief from confrontation by the analyst (e.g., fear of use of the couch and overeagerness to lie down may reflect resistance and, thus, need to be analyzed). Although the use of the couch is requisite to analytical technique, it is not applied automatically; it is introduced gradually and can be suspended whenever additional regression is unnecessary or countertherapeutic.

FUNDAMENTAL RULE. The fundamental rule of free association requires patients to tell the analyst everything that comes into their heads—however disagreeable, unimportant, or nonsensical—and to let themselves go as they would in a conversation that leads from "cabbages to kings." It differs decidedly from ordinary conversation—instead of connecting personal remarks with a rational thread, the patient is asked to reveal those very thoughts and events that are objectionable precisely because of being averse to doing so.

This directive represents an ideal because free association does not arise freely but is guided and inhibited by a variety of conscious and unconscious forces. The analyst must not only encourage free association through the physical setting and a nonjudgmental attitude toward the patient's verbalizations, but also examine those very instances when the flow of associations is diminished or comes to a halt—they are as important analytically as the content of the associations. The analyst should also be alert to how individual patients use or misuse the fundamental rule.

Aside from its primary purpose of eliciting recall of deeply hidden early memories, the fundamental rule reflects the analytical priority placed on verbalization, which translates the patient's thoughts into words so they are not channeled physically or behaviorally. As a direct concomitant of the fundamental rule, which prohibits action in favor of verbal expression, patients are expected to postpone making major alterations in their lives, such as marrying or changing careers, until they discuss and analyze them within the context of treatment.

PRINCIPLE OF EVENLY SUSPENDED ATTENTION. As a reciprocal corollary to the rule that patients communicate everything that occurs to them without criticism or selection, the principle of evenly suspended attention requires the analyst to suspend judgment and to give impartial attention to every detail equally. The method consists simply of making no effort to concentrate on anything specific, while maintaining a neutral, quiet attentiveness to all that is said.

ANALYST AS MIRROR. A second principle is the recommendation that the analyst be impenetrable to the patient and, as a mirror, reflects only what is shown. Analysts are advised to be neutral blank screens and not to bring their own personalities into treatment. This means that they are not to bring their own values or attitudes into the discussion or to share personal reactions or mutual conflicts with their patients, although they may sometimes be tempted to do so. The bringing in of reality and external influences can interrupt or bias the patient's unconscious projections. Neutrality also allows the analyst to accept without censure all forbidden or objectionable responses.

RULE OF ABSTINENCE. The fundamental rule of abstinence does not mean corporal or sexual abstinence, but refers to the frustration of emotional needs and wishes that the patient may have toward the analyst or part of the transference. It allows the patient's longings to persist and serve as driving forces for analytical work and motivation to change. Freud advised that the analyst carry through the analytical treatment in a state of renunciation. The analyst must deny the patient who is longing for love the satisfaction he or she craves.

Limitations. At present, the predominant treatment constraints are often economic, relating to the high cost in time and money, both for patients and in the training of future practitioners. In addition, because clinical requirements emphasize such requisites as psychological mindedness, verbal and cognitive ability, and stable life situation, psychoanalysis may be unduly restricted to a diagnostically, socioeconomically, or intellectually advantaged patient population. Other intrinsic issues pertain to the use and misuse of its stringent rules, whereby overemphasis on technique may interfere with an authentic human encounter between analyst and patient, and to the major long-term risk of interminability, in which protracted treatment may become a substitute for life. Reification of the classic analytical tradition may interfere with a more open and flexible application of its tenets to meet changing needs. It may also obstruct a comprehensive view of patient care that includes a greater appreciation of other treatment modalities in conjunction with, or as an alternative to, psychoanalysis.

Ms. A, a 25-year-old articulate and introspective medical student, began analysis complaining of mild, chronic anxiety, dysphoria, and a sense of inadequacy, despite above-average intelligence and performance. She also expressed difficulty in long-term relationships with her male peers.

Ms. A began the initial phase of analysis with enthusiastic self-disclosure, frequent reports of dreams and fantasies, and overidealization of the analyst; she tried to please him by being a compliant, good patient, just as she had been a good daughter to her father (a professor of medicine) by going to medical school.

Over the next several months, Ms. A gradually developed a strong attachment to the analyst and settled into a phase of excessive preoccupation with him. Simultaneously, however, she began dating an older psychiatrist and proceeded to complain about the analyst's coldness and unresponsiveness, even considering dropping out of analysis because he did not meet her demands.

In the course of analysis, through dreams and associations, Ms. A recalled early memories of her ongoing competition with her mother for her father's attention and realized that, failing to obtain his exclusive love, she had tried to become like him. She was also able to see how her increasing interest in becoming a psychiatrist (rather than following her original plan to be a pediatrician), as well as her recent choice of a man to date, were recapitulations of the past vis-à-vis the analyst. As this repeated pattern was recognized, the patient began to relinquish her intense erotic and dependent tie to the analyst, viewing him more realistically and beginning to appreciate the ways in which his quiet presence reminded her of her mother. She also became less disturbed by the similarities she shared with her mother and was able to disengage from her father more comfortably. By the fifth year of analysis, she was happily married to a classmate, was pregnant, and was a pediatric chief resident. Her anxiety was now attenuated and situation specific (i.e., she was concerned about motherhood and the termination of analysis). *(Courtesy of T. Byram Karasu, M.D.)*

PSYCHOANALYTIC PSYCHOTHERAPY

Psychoanalytic psychotherapy, which is based on fundamental dynamic formulations and techniques that derive from psychoanalysis, is designed to broaden its scope. Psychoanalytic psychotherapy, in its narrowest sense, is the use of insight-oriented methods only. As generically applied today to an ever-larger clinical spectrum, it incorporates a blend of uncovering and suppressive measures.

The strategies of psychoanalytic psychotherapy currently range from expressive (insight-oriented, uncovering, evocative, or interpretive) techniques to supportive (relationship-oriented, suggestive, suppressive, or repressive) techniques. Although those two types of methods are sometimes regarded as antithetical, their precise definitions and the distinctions between them are by no means absolute.

The duration of psychoanalytic psychotherapy is generally shorter and more variable than in psychoanalysis. Treatment may be brief, even with an initially agreed-upon or fixed time limit, or may extend to a less definite number of months or years. Brief treatment is chiefly used for selected problems or highly focused conflict, whereas longer treatment may be applied for more chronic conditions or for intermittent episodes that require ongoing attention to deal with pervasive conflict or recurrent decompensation. Unlike psychoanalysis, psychoanalytic psychotherapy rarely uses the couch; instead, patient and therapist sit face to face. This posture helps to prevent regression because it encourages the patient to look on the therapist as a real person from whom to receive direct cues, even though transference and fantasy will continue. The couch is considered unnecessary because the free-association method is rarely used, except when the therapist wishes to gain access to fantasy material or dreams to enlighten a particular issue.

Expressive Psychotherapy

Indications and Contraindications. Diagnostically, psychoanalytic psychotherapy in its expressive mode is suited to a range of psychopathology with mild to moderate ego weakening, including neurotic conflicts, symptom complexes, reactive conditions, and the whole realm of nonpsychotic character disorders, including those disorders of the self that are among the more transient and less profound on the severity-of-illness spectrum, such as narcissistic behavior disorders and narcissistic personality disorders. It is also one of the treatments recommended for patients with borderline personality disorders, although special variations may be required to deal with the associated turbulent personality characteristics, primitive defense mechanisms, tendencies toward regressive episodes, and irrational attachments to the analyst.

Ms. B, an intelligent and verbal 34-year-old divorced woman, presented with complaints of being unappreciated at work. Always angry and irritable, she considered quitting her job and even leaving the city. Her social life was also being negatively affected; her boyfriend had threatened to leave her because of her extremely hostile, clinging behavior (the same reason her ex-husband had given when he left her 9 years earlier after only 16 months of marriage).

Her past included promiscuity and experimentation with various drugs, and, currently, she indulged in heavy drinking on weekends and occasionally smoked marijuana. She had held many jobs and had lived in various cities. The eldest of three children of a middle-class family, she came from an unhappy and unstable home: her brother had been in and out of psychiatric hospitals; her sister had left home at the age of 16 after becoming pregnant and being forced to marry; and her overly controlling parents had subjected their children to psychological (and occasionally physical) abuse, alternating between heated arguments and passionate reconciliations.

Initially, Ms. B attempted to contain her rage in treatment, but it frequently surfaced and alternated with child-like helplessness; she interrogated the psychiatrist regarding his credentials, ridiculed psychodynamic concepts, constantly challenged statements, and would demand practical advice but then denigrate or fail to follow the guidance given. The psychiatrist remained unprovoked by her aggression and explored with her the need to engage him negatively. Her response was to question and test his continued concern.

When her boyfriend left her, she attempted suicide (she cut her wrists superficially), was briefly hospitalized, and, on discharge, was placed on selective serotonin reuptake inhibitors (SSRIs) for 6 months for her minor, but protracted, depression. The psychiatrist maintained their regular frequency of sessions despite her greater demands. Although she was puzzled by the steadiness of his interest, she gradually felt safe enough to express her vulnerabilities. As they explored her lack of full commitment to work, friends, and therapy, she began to understand the meaning of her anger in terms of the early abusive relationship with her parents and her tendency to bring it into contemporary relationships. With the psychiatrist's encouragement, she also began to seek work and make small strides in relationship-oriented efforts. By the end of her second year of treatment, she had decided to remain in the city, to stay at her place of employment, and to continue therapy. She needed to experience and practice her somewhat fragile new self, which included greater intimacy in relationships, additional mastery of work skills, and a more cohesive sense of self. *(Courtesy of T. Byram Karasu, M.D.)*

The persons best suited for the expressive psychotherapy approach have fairly well integrated egos and the capacity to both sustain and detach from a bond of dependency and trust. They are, to some degree, psychologically minded and self-motivated, and they are generally able, at least temporarily, to tolerate doses of frustration without decompensating. They must also have the ability to manage the rearousal of painful feelings outside the therapy hour without additional contact. Patients must have some capacity for introspection and impulse control, and they should be able to recognize the cognitive distinction between fantasy and reality.

Goals. The overall goals of expressive psychotherapy are to increase the patient's self-awareness and to improve object relations through exploration of current interpersonal events and perceptions. In contrast to psychoanalysis, major structural changes in ego function and defenses are modified in light of patient limitations. The aim is to achieve a more limited and, thus, select and focused understanding of one's problems. Rather than uncovering deeply hidden and past motives and tracing them back to their origins in infancy, the major thrust is to deal with preconscious or conscious derivatives of conflicts as they became manifest in present interactions. Although insight is sought, it is less extensive; instead of delving to a genetic level, greater emphasis is on clarifying recent dynamic patterns and maladaptive behaviors in the present.

Major Approach and Techniques. The major modus operandi involves establishment of a therapeutic alliance and early recognition and interpretation of negative transference. Only limited or controlled regression is encouraged, and positive transference manifestations are generally left unexplored, unless they are impeding therapeutic progress; even here, the emphasis is on shedding light on current dynamic patterns and defenses.

Limitations. A general limitation of expressive psychotherapy, as of psychoanalysis, is the problem of emotional integration of cognitive awareness. The major danger for patients who are at the more disorganized end of the diagnostic spectrum, however, may have less to do with the overintellectualization that is sometimes seen in neurotic patients than with the threat of decompensation from, or acting out of, deep or frequent interpretations that the patient is unable to integrate properly.

Some therapists fail to accept the limitations of a modified insight-oriented approach and so apply it inappropriately to modulate the techniques and goals of psychoanalysis. Overemphasis on dreams and fantasies, zealous efforts to use the couch, indiscriminate deep interpretations, and continual focus on the analysis of transference may have less to do with the patient's needs than with those of a therapist who is unwilling or unable to be flexible.

Ms. S was an attractive 30-year-old unmarried woman working as a secretary when she presented for consultation. Her chief complaints at the time were feeling "only anger and tension" and an inability to apply herself to studying voice, "which is one of the most important things to me."

In obtaining a history, the therapist noted that Ms. S had never completed anything: She had dropped out of college; never pursued a music degree; and switched from job to job, and even city to city. What initially seemed like a woman with diverse interests (e.g., jobs as a research assistant, freelance copyeditor, part-time radio announcer; manager of data entry for a software company; and, most recently, secretary) really reflected a woman with a chaotic lifestyle and serious difficulties committing to anyone or anything. Although obviously intelligent, Ms. S presented with unrealistic expectations regarding her consultation. For example, after the first consultative session, Ms. S said she felt good afterward but felt there were "no revelations yet." Because of Ms. S's inability to commit and her somewhat disorganized life, the therapist recommended a course of psychotherapy, beginning twice a week, rather than something more intense like psychoanalysis. The therapist also realized over the course of the consultation that Ms. S would have difficulty with free association without getting disorganized. The therapist also thought that Ms. S might regress unproductively on the couch without visual contact with the therapist.

Ms. S was the second oldest of four children—two brothers and a younger sister, with whom she was most competitive and who clearly seemed the mother's favorite. She described her mother as a successful professor who was demanding and critical, as if she had a "raised eyebrow" in disapproval. For example, much to her mother's chagrin, Ms. S had once wanted a sandwich "with everything on it." Ms. S was also disappointed when she was given one piece of luggage rather than a complete set for a Christmas gift. She was able to accept the therapist's interpretation that she felt "part of a set" by being one of four siblings. Ms. S initially idealized her father, who was active in the family church, but eventually saw him as disappointing and rejecting.

Ms. S's ideal therapist would be "flexible," by which she meant a therapist who might do hypnosis one session, psychotherapy the next, and, maybe, analysis another session. In fact, within the first week of beginning therapy, Ms. S had simultaneously consulted a hypnotherapist, which she mentioned in passing only weeks later, for her neck pain and tension. Although she did not pursue hypnosis, she did maintain a chiropractor for most of her therapy, also something she mentioned many months after beginning therapy. She did speak of wanting to be "on best behavior" and "follow the rules." Her tremendous sense of entitlement, however, was evident: She had an expectation of getting "cut-rate prices" on everything from haircuts and car repairs to doctors' visits. Her initial fee was a much-reduced one, which she paid late and begrudgingly.

Although she was seen only twice a week, Ms. S developed intense feelings for her therapist. Mostly she experienced rage when she saw evidence of the therapist's other patients, such as footprints on the waiting room floor after a snowstorm or a coat hanger turned around. She expressed the wish to keep some of her things, like bobby pins and hairspray, in the therapist's bathroom. She vacillated between feelings she wanted to move in and feelings that the therapist did not exist. For example, before she took a plane flight, she wondered who would tell her therapist if something happened to her. She had never given the therapist's name to anyone, nor did she have her name in her weekly appointment book. The therapist interpreted that she had a simultaneous wish to devalue her and not to share her with anyone else. Associations to a dream with an image of a string of baroque pearls led to thoughts that these pearls—irregular and imperfect—defective and even lopsided, represented how she viewed herself.

Over the course of the next few years, Ms. S was able to commit to coming regularly to therapy, although the course was somewhat tumultuous, with many threats of quitting and much withholding of information. At one point, she even tried to provoke the therapist by seeking a consultation with another therapist in order to "tattle" on her, just as she had tattled on her siblings. Her therapist remained unprovoked and continued to provide a safe environment for Ms. S to explore her ambivalence to the therapist and the therapeutic situation. The therapist was also able to contain Ms. S's tendency to regress, particularly with separations, by providing her with the therapist's telephone number.

She had actually entered therapy with an unconscious wish to become a world-famous singer who would win her mother's approval and praise. Her narcissism and sense of entitlement made it difficult for her to give up on that fantasy despite repeated evidence that she did not have sufficient talent. She was finally able to settle on a compromise: She began to work diligently and closely as a research assistant to her mother, who was writing a book, and as Ms. S became more focused and organized over time, she even thought she might write a book about the church. (*Courtesy of T. Byram Karasu, M.D., and S. R. Karasu, M.D.*)

Supportive Psychotherapy

Supportive psychotherapy aims at the creation of a therapeutic relationship as a temporary buttress or bridge for the deficient patient. It has roots in virtually every therapy that recognizes the ameliorative effects of emotional support and a stable, caring atmosphere in the management of patients. As a nonspecific attitude toward mental illness, it predates scientific psychiatry, with foundations in 18th-century moral treatment, whereby for the first time patients were treated with understanding and kindness in a humane, interpersonal environment free from mechanical restraints.

Supportive psychotherapy has been the chief form used in the general practice of medicine and rehabilitation, frequently to augment extratherapeutic measures, such as prescriptions of medication to suppress symptoms, rest to remove the patient from excessive stimulation, or hospitalization to provide a structured therapeutic environment, protection, and control of the patient. It can be applied as primary or ancillary treatment. The global perspective of supportive psychotherapy (often part of a combined treatment approach) places major etiological emphasis on external rather than intrapsychic events, particularly on stressful environmental and interpersonal influences on a severely damaged self.

Indications and Contraindications. Supportive psychotherapy is generally indicated for those patients for whom classic psychoanalysis or insight-oriented psychoanalytic psychotherapy is typically contraindicated—those who have poor ego strength and whose potential for decompensation is high. Amenable patients fall into the following major areas: (1) individuals in acute crisis or a temporary state of disorganization and inability to cope (including those who might otherwise be well functioning) whose intolerable life circumstances have produced extreme anxiety or sudden turmoil (e.g., individuals going through grief reactions, illness, divorce, job loss, or who were victims of crime, abuse, natural disaster, or accident); (2) patients with chronic severe pathology with fragile or deficient ego functioning (e.g., those with latent psychosis, impulse disorder, or severe character disturbance); (3) patients whose cognitive deficits and physical symptoms make them particularly vulnerable and, thus, unsuitable for an insight-oriented approach (e.g., certain psychosomatic or medically ill persons); and (4) individuals who are psychologically unmotivated, although not necessarily characterologically resistant to a depth approach (e.g., patients who come to treatment in response to family or agency pressure and are interested only in immediate relief or those who need assistance in very specific problem areas of social adjustment as a possible prelude to more exploratory work).

Mr. C, a 50-year-old married man with two sons, the owner of a small construction company, was referred by his internist after recovery from bypass surgery because of frequent, unfounded physical complaints. He was taking minor tranquilizers in increasing doses, not complying with his daily regimen, avoiding sexual contact with his wife, and had dropped out of group therapy for postsurgical patients after one session.

He came to his first appointment 20 minutes late, after having "forgotten" two previous appointments. He was extremely anxious, often lost in his train of thought, and was semidelusional about his wife and sons, suggesting that they might want to have him locked up. He briefly told his life history, which included his coming from a strict and hard-working but caring middle-class family and the death of his mother when he was only 11 years old. He had joined his father's business (taking over after his father's death 2 years earlier), with both of his sons as associates. Describing himself as successful in work and marriage, he claimed that "the only test I ever failed was the stress test."

Mr. C explained his lack of compliance with diet restrictions as a lack of will and his constant contact with the internist as his having real physical problems not yet diagnosed; he rejected the idea of addiction to tranquilizers, insisting that he could quit any time. He had no fantasy life, remembered no dreams, made it clear that he had entered treatment on his internist's instruction only, and started each session by stating that he had nothing to talk about.

After suggesting that Mr. C was coming to sessions just to pass the "sanity test" and that there was no reason to have him locked up, the psychiatrist encouraged the patient to join him in figuring out the real reasons for his anxiety. Initial sessions were devoted to discussing the patient's medical condition and providing factual information about heart and bypass surgery. The therapist likened the patient's condition to that of an older house getting new plumbing, trying to allay his unrealistic fears of impending death. As Mr. C's anxiety declined, he became less defensive and more psychologically accessible. As the therapist began to explore his difficulty in accepting help, Mr. C was able to talk about his inability to admit problems (i.e., weaknesses). The therapist's explicit recognition of the patient's strength in admitting his weaknesses encouraged the patient to reveal more about himself—how he had welcomed his father's death and his belief that perhaps his illness was punishment. The psychiatrist also encouraged him to speak about his unrealistic guilt and, at the same time, helped him recognize his suspicion of his sons as the reflection of his own wishes concerning his father and his lack of commitment to his medical regimen as a wish to die so as to expiate guilt. After steady urging by the therapist, Mr. C returned to work. He agreed to meet monthly with the psychiatrist and to taper off his use of tranquilizers. He even agreed that he might see the psychiatrist for "deep analysis" in the future because his wife now jokingly complained of his obsessive dieting, his uncompromising exercise regimens, and his regularly scheduled sexual activities. *(Courtesy of T. Byram Karasu, M.D.)*

Because support forms a tacit part of every therapeutic modality, it is rarely contraindicated as such. The typical attitude regards better-functioning patients as unsuitable not because they will be harmed by a supportive approach, but because they will not be sufficiently benefited by it. In aiming to maximize the patient's potential for further growth and change, supportive therapy tends to be regarded as relatively restricted and superficial and, thus, is not recommended as the treatment of choice if the patient is available for, and capable of, a more in-depth approach.

Goals. The general aim of supportive treatment is the amelioration or relief of symptoms through behavioral or environmental restructuring within the existing psychic framework. This often means helping the patient to adapt better to problems and to live more comfortably with his or her psychopathology. To restore the disorganized, fragile, or decompensated patient to a state of relative equilibrium, the major goal is to suppress or control symptomatology and to stabilize the patient in a protective and reassuring benign atmosphere that militates against overwhelming external and internal pressures. The ultimate goal is to maximize the integrative or adaptive capacities so that the patient increases the ability to cope, while decreasing vulnerability by reinforcing assets and strengthening defenses.

Major Approach and Techniques. Supportive therapy uses several methods, either singly or in combination, including warm, friendly, strong leadership; partial gratification of dependency needs; support in the ultimate development of legitimate independence; help in developing pleasurable activities (e.g., hobbies); adequate rest and diversion; removal of excessive strain, when possible; hospitalization, when indicated; medication to alleviate symptoms; and guidance and advice in dealing with current issues. This therapy uses techniques to help patients feel secure, accepted, protected, encouraged, safe, and not anxious.

Limitations. To the extent that much supportive therapy is spent on practical, everyday realities and on dealing with the external environment of the patient, it may be viewed as more mundane and superficial than depth approaches. Because those patients are seen intermittently and less frequently, the interpersonal commitment may not be as compelling on the part of either the patient or the therapist. Greater severity of illness (and possible psychoses) also makes such treatment potentially more erratic, demanding, and frustrating. The need for the therapist to deal with other family members, caretakers, or agencies (auxiliary treatment, hospitalization) can become an additional complication, because the therapist comes to serve as an ombudsman to negotiate with the outside world of the patient and with other professional peers. Finally, the supportive therapist must be able to accept personal limitations and the patient's limited psychological resources and to tolerate the often unrewarded efforts until small gains are made.

Mr. W was a 42-year-old widowed businessman who was referred by his internist because of the sudden death of his wife, who had had an intracranial hemorrhage, about 2 months earlier. Mr. W had two children, a boy and a girl, ages 10 and 8 years, respectively.

Mr. W had never been to a psychiatrist before, and when he arrived he admitted he was not certain what a psychiatrist could do for him. He just had to get over his wife's death. He was not sure how talking about anything could really help. He had been married for 15 years. He admitted to having difficulty sleeping, particularly awakening in the middle of the night with considerable anxiety about the future. One of his relatives had given him some of her own Klonopin for his anxiety, which helped tremendously, but he feared getting dependent on it. He was also drinking more than he thought he should. He was most concerned about raising his children alone and felt somewhat overwhelmed by the responsibility. He was beginning to appreciate just how wonderful a mother his wife had been and now saw how critical he had been of her for spending so much time with the children. "It really does take a lot of effort," he said.

Mr. W did admit to feelings of guilt. For one thing, he admitted to some sense that he could now start over. He had been somewhat restless in the marriage recently before his wife's death and had actually been unfaithful for a brief period early in the marriage. He also felt some guilt that had he been awake the night of his wife's hemorrhage, maybe he could have saved his wife. In reality, there was nothing he could have done.

Mr. W agreed to come for a few sessions to talk about his wife. At this point, only 2 months after her death, he seemed to have an uncomplicated mourning reaction. Although he talked easily in session, he was clearly worried that he might like "being here too much." The therapist chose not to interpret his dependency conflicts. Mr. W seemed to have good coping skills and used humor as a high-functioning defense. For example, in giving a eulogy for his wife (who had been a very popular member of their congregation), he looked around at the enormous crowd of people at the church service and said he had never seen so many people attending church before, adding, "Sorry, Reverend."

After about four sessions, Mr. W said he that felt better and no longer saw the need for further sessions. He was sleeping better and had stopped drinking excessively. The therapist suggested that he might want to continue to talk more about his guilt and his life as he went forward without his wife. The therapist was also reassuring that there seemed to be nothing else Mr. W could have done to save his wife. He also encouraged the patient to begin dating when he felt ready, something that Mr. W's in-laws were clearly not encouraging. For now, however, Mr. W was not interested in any further therapy. He was appreciative of the therapist and felt that talking about his wife's death had been helpful. The therapist accepted his wish to discontinue their sessions but encouraged Mr. W to keep in touch to let him know how he was doing. *(Courtesy of T. Byram Karasu, M.D., and S. R. Karasu, M.D.)*

Corrective Emotional Experience. The relationship between therapist and patient gives a therapist an opportunity to display behavior different from the destructive or unproductive behavior of a patient's parent. At times, such experiences seem to neutralize or reverse some effects of the parents' mistakes. If the patient had overly authoritarian parents, the therapist's friendly, flexible, nonjudgmental, nonauthoritarian—but at times firm and limit setting—attitude gives the patient an opportunity to adjust to, be led by, and identify with a new parent figure. Franz Alexander described this process as a corrective emotional experience. It draws on elements of both psychoanalysis and psychoanalytic psychotherapy.

Relationship Therapy

Relationship therapy was developed by Robert Steward, M.D. and Maurice Levine, M.D. at the Chicago Institute of Psychoanalysis in the 1960s. The treatment stands somewhat between supportive psychotherapy and the techniques of psychoanalysis and other types of insight-oriented psychotherapy. The therapy requires that doctor and patient develop and maintain a relationship—a state of being connected—for a prolonged period of time. During that time there is interplay of feeling and communication that provide an experience in which new insights are acquired that allow the patient to deal with vicissitudes of life in an effective and meaningful way. Relationship therapy contains strong elements of support and may be considered a protracted form of supportive psychotherapy, but with deeper dimensions. Its methods and goals are somewhat more complicated than those involved, for example, in supporting a fairly well-adjusted person through some current crisis.

In relationship therapy, the therapist avoids being judgmental and is accepting of patient's behavior while, at the same time, examining that behavior as appropriate or inappropriate. A fairly consistent attitude toward the patient is maintained which has been described as "good and deeply helpful." Often the transference takes the form of the patient viewing the therapist as a benevolent family member, be it father, mother, or older brother or sister. In that sense, relationship therapy provides the therapist with frequent opportunities to behave in a fashion different from the destructive or unproductive behavior of significant figures in the past. If the patient had overly authoritarian parents, for example, the therapist's friendly, flexible, nonjudgmental attitude provides opportunities to experience and identify with a new type of parent figure. Similarly, patients who had parents who were overly indulgent or seductive can begin to see that limit-setting is not punitive and intimacy and seductiveness are vastly different psychological processes.

Relationship therapy relies heavily on the corrective emotional experience which holds that the doctor's attitudes and responses to the patient's idea and impulses are different from those important figures in the patient's past life. Ideally, the therapist's responses are more suitable, more mature, more realistic and potentially more productive. At times the therapist, using knowledge of the patient's past life is explicit in comparing those differences as in the following example.

A 50-year-old man recalled his father whipping him severely whenever he misbehaved as a child. When the therapist described this behavior as abusive rather than corrective, the patient was taken aback, felt that he deserved to be whipped as a form of punishment (even for minor infractions) and began to defend his father's behavior as representing how one should raise a child. The therapist explained how this abusive experience contributed to the patient's personality which was marked by his being deferential and intimidated by persons in authority and which interfered with his asserting himself appropriately with anyone older such as his boss or other authority figures. In time, the patient began to test reality more appropriately.

As mentioned above, relationship therapy is characterized by a warm and friendly interaction between doctor and patient; but it is not one that fosters dependency. To the contrary, the therapist attempts to provide a setting in which the patient can develop autonomy as expressed in free interchange between the two, interchange that is not censored by intimidation or fear. That free exchange also allows for greater self-disclosure by the therapist as compared to other forms of talk therapy, certainly compared to psychoanalysis in which the analyst is often perceived as a "blank screen." Self-disclosure allows for identification to unfold as an important therapeutic process. The therapist is a role model for the patient; however, it is not deliberate role playing. Relationship therapy requires that the doctor be scrupulously honest. The therapist may or may not choose to reveal personal information but there is no room for dissembling to facilitate—erroneously—the role of modeling process. The therapist must not deliberately or artificially alter his or her usual behavior toward the patient to provide the patient with a corrective emotional experience.

Relationship therapy is suitable for a variety of psychiatric disorders in which anxiety or depression accompanies the disorder. It is not a substitute for pharmacotherapy; rather it is an adjunctive process. It is especially useful for transitional period in the life span—adolescence to adulthood, early adulthood to late adulthood, late adulthood to old age, and so on. Transitional periods often take years to master during which time relationship therapy can offer comfort and guidance dealing with the vagaries of emotion that accompany such passages. Its use as corrective emotional experience has already been mentioned.

▲ 24.2 Brief Psychodynamic Psychotherapy

The growth of psychotherapy in general and of dynamic psychotherapies derived from the psychoanalytic framework in particular represents a landmark achievement in the history of psychiatry. Brief psychodynamic psychotherapy has gained widespread popularity, partly because of the great pressure on health care professionals to contain treatment costs. It is also easier to evaluate treatment efficacy by comparing groups of persons who have had short-term therapy for mental illness with control groups than it is to measure the results of long-term psychotherapy. Thus, short-term therapies have been the subject of much research, especially on outcome measures, which have found them to be effective. Other short-term methods include interpersonal therapy (discussed in Section 24.10) and cognitive–behavioral therapy (CBT) (discussed in Section 24.7).

Brief psychodynamic psychotherapy is a time-limited treatment (10 to 12 sessions) that is based on psychoanalysis and psychodynamic theory. It is used to help persons with depression, anxiety, and posttraumatic stress disorder, among others. There are several methods, each having its own treatment technique and specific criteria for selecting patients; however, they are more similar than different.

In 1946, Franz Alexander and Thomas French identified the basic characteristics of brief psychodynamic psychotherapy. They described a therapeutic experience designed to put patients at ease, to manipulate the transference, and to use trial interpretations flexibly. Alexander and French conceived psychotherapy as a corrective emotional experience capable of repairing traumatic events of the past and convincing patients that new ways of thinking, feeling, and behaving are possible. At about the same time, Eric Lindemann established a consultation service at Massachusetts General Hospital in Boston for persons experiencing a crisis. He developed new treatment methods to deal with these situations and eventually applied these techniques to persons who were not in crisis, but who were experiencing various kinds of emotional distress. Since then, the field has been influenced by many workers such as David Malan in England, Peter Sifneos in the United States, and Habib Davanloo in Canada.

TYPES

Brief Focal Psychotherapy (Tavistock—Malan)

Brief focal psychotherapy was originally developed in the 1950s by the Balint team at the Tavistock Clinic in London. Malan, a member of the team, reported the results of the therapy. Malan's selection criteria for treatment included eliminating absolute contraindications, rejecting patients for whom certain dangers seemed inevitable, clearly assessing patients' psychopathology, and determining patients' capacities to consider problems in emotional terms, face disturbing material, respond to interpretations, and endure the stress of the treatment. Malan found that high motivation invariably correlated with a successful outcome. Contraindications to treatment were serious suicide attempts, substance dependence, chronic alcohol abuse, incapacitating chronic obsessional symptoms, incapacitating chronic phobic symptoms, and gross destructive or self-destructive acting out.

Requirements and Techniques. In Malan's routine, therapists should identify the transference early and interpret it and the negative transference. They should then link the transferences to patients' relationships with their parents. Both patients and therapists should be willing to become deeply involved and to bear the ensuing tension. Therapists should formulate a circumscribed focus and set a termination date in advance, and patients should work through grief and anger about termination. An experienced therapist should allow about 20 sessions as an average length for the therapy; a trainee should allow about 30 sessions. Malan himself did not exceed 40 interviews with his patients.

Time-Limited Psychotherapy (Boston University—Mann)

A psychotherapeutic model of exactly 12 interviews focusing on a specified central issue was developed at Boston University by James Mann and his colleagues in the early 1970s. In contrast with Malan's emphasis on clear-cut selection and rejection criteria, Mann has not been as explicit about the appropriate candidates for time-limited psychotherapy. Mann considered the major emphases of his theory to be determining a patient's central conflict reasonably correctly and exploring young persons' maturational crises with many psychological and somatic complaints. Mann's exceptions, similar to his rejection criteria, include persons with major depressive disorder that interferes with the treatment agreement, those with acute psychotic states, and desperate patients who need, but cannot tolerate, object relations.

Requirements and Techniques. Mann's technical requirements included strict limitation to 12 sessions, positive transference predominating early, specification and strict adherence to a central issue involving transference, positive identification, making separation a maturational event for patients, absolute prospect of termination to avoid development of dependence, clarification of present and past experiences and resistances, active therapists who support and encourage patients, and education of patients through direct information, reeducation, and manipulation. The conflicts likely to be encountered included independence versus dependence, activity versus passivity, unresolved or delayed grief, and adequate versus inadequate self-esteem.

Short-Term Dynamic Psychotherapy (McGill University—Davanloo)

As conducted by Davanloo at McGill University, short-term dynamic psychotherapy encompasses nearly all varieties of brief psychotherapy and crisis intervention. Patients treated in Davanloo's series are classified as those whose psychological conflicts are predominantly oedipal, those whose conflicts are not oedipal, and those whose conflicts have more than one focus. Davanloo also devised a specific psychotherapeutic technique for patients with severe, long-standing neurotic problems, specifically those with incapacitating obsessive–compulsive disorders and phobias.

Davanloo's selection criteria emphasize evaluating those ego functions of primary importance to psychotherapeutic work: the establishment of a psychotherapeutic focus; the psychodynamic formulation of the patient's psychological problems; the ability to interact emotionally with evaluators; a history of give-and-take relationships with a significant person in the patient's life; the patient's ability to experience and tolerate anxiety, guilt, and depression; and the patient's motivations for change, psychological mindedness, and an ability to respond to interpretation and to link evaluators with persons in the present and past. Both Malan and Davanloo emphasized a patient's responses to interpretation as an important selection and prognostic criterion.

Requirements and Techniques. The highlights of Davanloo's psychotherapeutic approach are flexibility (therapists should adapt the technique to the patient's needs), control, the patient's regressive tendencies, active intervention to avoid having the patient develop overdependence on a therapist, and the patient's intellectual insight and emotional experiences in the transference. These emotional experiences become corrective as a result of the interpretation.

Ana, a divorced 60-year-old woman, sought psychiatric help following a severe depressive episode lasting several months. This episode, which was one of many in her life, was especially severe in terms of loss of energy, interest, and motivation, as well as in terms of the intensity of her sadness and her wish to die. Only her profound religious convictions protected her from acting on these wishes. Ana had lost a lot of weight, had trouble sleeping, experienced many nightmares, and had difficulty with concentration. She was plagued by pervasive feelings of hatred for her mother, who was very old, ill, and dependent on Ana, who was unable to forgive her for abandoning her in an orphanage when she was 5 or 6 years of age.

After an extensive assessment, the dynamic formulation of Ana's problem was represented as follows:

1. *Life problems:* Recurrent depressive episodes plagued by feelings of guilt and self-reproach; problems with men involving choosing partners who are commonly cold, distant, or otherwise unavailable; involuntary and painful emotional distance from her children, friends, and other close relationships; and unproductive and unrewarding work life, despite considerable intellectual gifts.
2. *Dynamics:* Ambivalent relationship with her mother, whom she blames for most of the tragedies of her life; guilt and need for punishment in relation to her unrelenting hatred for her mother; and pathological grief reaction for the loss of an idealized and more optimal relationship with her mother, the one she remembers she had prior to her orphanage placement. From this focus there flows a melancholic conviction of the inevitable failure of human relationships.
3. *Pathogenic foci:* Grief and inability to mourn the loss of her mother after she was placed in the orphanage, with attendant rage and guilt; pathological grief for the loss of her father, who, because of severe alcoholism, abandoned the family first, a move that caused the mother to place her children in an orphanage in order to be able to work and ultimately recover their care. Unconsciously, she blamed her mother for the family catastrophe, thus "protecting" an idealized view of her father, to whom she was profoundly attached.

For Ana, the initial phase of treatment focused on the clarification and the experience of her destructive impulses toward her mother, which, as they were worked through, made possible the appearance of a modicum of empathy with her mother's painful life situation around the time she placed Ana and her sisters in the orphanage. Next, the therapy focused on Ana's father. Deep feelings of idealization, disappointment, anger, and grief were experienced with increasing clarity and intensity, frequently via displaced feelings in the transference and after overcoming considerable resistance. The last phase of treatment permitted the development of realistic feelings of empathy and appreciation for her mother, now without anger or emotional distancing, and the reawakening within Ana of feelings of joy and hope, as well as professional ambition. *(Courtesy of M. Trujillo, M.D.)*

Short-Term Anxiety-Provoking Psychotherapy (Harvard University—Sifneos)

Sifneos developed short-term anxiety-provoking psychotherapy at the Massachusetts General Hospital in Boston during the 1950s. He used the following criteria for selection: a circumscribed chief complaint (implying a patient's ability to select one of a variety of problems to be given top priority and the patient's desire to resolve the problem in treatment), one meaningful or give-and-take relationship during early childhood, the ability to interact flexibly with an evaluator and to express feelings appropriately, above-average psychological sophistication (implying not only above-average intelligence but also an ability to respond to interpretations), a specific psychodynamic formulation (usually a set of psychological conflicts underlying a patient's difficulties and centering on an oedipal focus), a contract between therapist and patient to work on the specified focus and the formulation of minimal expectations of outcome, and good to excellent motivation for change, not just for symptom relief.

Chris, a 31-year-old single man, sought help for a moderate depressive episode precipitated by the loss of his relationship with his girlfriend, Joanna. She had broken off the relationship after approximately 1 year, tired of Chris's erratic work ethic and emotional instability and discouraged by his fear of commitment to the future of their relationship. This cycle of infatuation, increasing fear of commitment, and relationship loss had become a pattern in Chris's interpersonal life. His work life was plagued with similar problems. Jobs were frequently lost because of serious conflict and threatening confrontations with his superiors. As conflicts arose at both work and home, Chris typically suffered increasing anxiety and episodic panic attacks. After the loss of each relationship, Chris usually confronted moderate depressive feelings, at times accompanied by suicidal ideation.

After an assessment, the dynamic hologram for Chris was represented as follows:

1. *Life problems:* Recurrent episodes of anxiety and depression; work problems; unstable interpersonal relationships; conflict with authority figures; antagonism toward, and emotional distance from, his father, brother, and male friends; and fears of heterosexual intimacy and of commitment.
2. *Dynamic forces:* Ongoing hostility and envy toward males, authority figures, and successful people, and compulsive and possessive seeking of female love objects with a serious inability to consider, fulfill, or tolerate their independent needs.
3. *Genetic pathogenic foci:* Unconscious loss of maternal objects precipitated by birth of a brother when Chris was age 2 years; uncontrolled grief for that loss with a compulsive drive to experience child-like possession of love objects; and compulsive hostility toward others perceived as rivals.

The therapist's active inquiry yielded additional confirmation of the persistence of repressed sexual feelings toward his mother and the presence of hostile feelings toward all rivals for his mother's affection. A memory suffused with very visceral feelings emerged in this phase as a result of the therapist's active inquiry. In this memory, Chris saw himself in his mother's arms in a dark room. He remembered vividly the intense pleasure of the contact with the warm skin of his mother, the texture of her clothes, and the smell of her perfume. While narrating this memory to the therapist, Chris was so absorbed in the experience that he blushed intensely. He also described the painful termination of this moment of pleasure by his father's sudden and disruptive opening of the door and the flood of light that disturbed his pleasurable absorption. This sequence gave way to the experience of grief at the loss of the intense and exclusive bond with his mother after his brother's birth and to a reexperiencing of a sense of anger, impotence, and loneliness. These feelings were all too familiar in his present life when his romantic attachments would be threatened or lost. The affective link between this childhood experience and his intimacy problems in the present became very obvious to Chris, and the acceptance of this link enhanced his capacity to work through this essential component of his pathology. A parallel conflict appeared in the transference as the patient resented the "intrusion" of the inquiring therapist into the zealously guarded privacy of this primal fantasy of material possession. *(Courtesy of M. Trujillo, M.D.)*

Requirements and Techniques. Treatment can be divided into four major phases: patient–therapist encounter, early therapy, height of treatment, and evidence of change and termination. Therapists use the following techniques during the four phases.

PATIENT–THERAPIST ENCOUNTER. A therapist establishes a working alliance by using the patient's quick rapport with, and positive feelings for, the therapist that appear in this phase. Judicious use of open-ended and forced-choice questions enables the therapist to outline and concentrate on a therapeutic focus. The therapist specifies the minimal expectations of outcome to be achieved by the therapy.

EARLY THERAPY. In transference, feelings for the therapist are clarified as soon as they appear, a technique that leads to the establishment of a true therapeutic alliance.

HEIGHT OF THE TREATMENT. Height of treatment emphasizes active concentration on the oedipal conflicts that have been chosen as the therapeutic focus; repeated use of anxiety-provoking questions and confrontations; avoidance of pregenital characterological issues, which the patient uses defensively to avoid dealing with the therapist's anxiety-provoking techniques; avoidance at all costs of a transference neurosis; repetitive demonstration of the patient's neurotic ways or maladaptive patterns of behavior; concentration on the anxiety-laden material, even before the defense mechanisms have been clarified; repeated demonstrations of parent–transference links by the use of properly timed interpretations based on material given by the patient; establishment of a corrective emotional experience; encouragement and support of the patient, who becomes anxious while struggling to understand the conflicts; new learning and problem-solving patterns; and repeated presentations and recapitulations of the patient's psychodynamics until the defense mechanisms used in dealing with oedipal conflicts are understood.

EVIDENCE OF CHANGE AND TERMINATION OF PSYCHOTHERAPY. The final phase of therapy emphasizes the tangible demonstration of change in the patient's behavior outside therapy, evidence that adaptive patterns of behavior are being used, and initiation of talk about terminating the treatment.

OVERVIEW AND RESULTS

The shared techniques of all the brief psychotherapies described above outdistance their differences. They share the therapeutic alliance or dynamic interaction between therapist and patient, the use of transference, the active interpretation of a therapeutic focus or central issue, the repetitive links between parental and transference issues, and the early termination of therapy.

The outcomes of these brief treatments have been investigated extensively. Contrary to prevailing ideas that the therapeutic factors in psychotherapy are nonspecific, controlled studies and other assessment methods (e.g., interviews with unbiased evaluators, patients' self-evaluations) point to the importance of the specific techniques used. The capacity for genuine recovery in certain patients is far greater than was thought. A certain type of patient receiving brief psychotherapy can benefit greatly from a practical working-through of his or her nuclear conflict in the transference. Such patients can be recognized in advance through a process of dynamic interaction, because they are responsive, motivated, and able to face disturbing feelings and because a circumscribed focus can be formulated for them. The more radical the technique in terms of transference, depth of interpretation, and the link to childhood, the more radical the therapeutic effects will be. For some disturbed patients, a carefully chosen partial focus can be therapeutically effective.

▲ 24.3 Group Psychotherapy, Combined Individual and Group Psychotherapy, and Psychodrama

Group psychotherapy is a modality that employs a professionally trained leader who selects, composes, organizes, and leads a collection of members to work together toward the maximal attainment of the goals for each individual in the group and for the group itself. Certain properties present in groups, such as mutual support, can be harnessed in the service of providing relief from psychological suffering and supply peer support to counter isolation experienced by many who seek psychiatric help. Similarly, homogeneously composed small groups are ideal settings for the dissemination of accurate information about a condition shared by group members. Medical illness, substance abuse, and chronic and persistent severe psychiatric conditions, including schizophrenia and major affective disorders, are cases in point.

A widely accepted psychiatric treatment modality, group psychotherapy uses therapeutic forces within the group, constructive interactions among members, and interventions of a trained leader to change the maladaptive behaviors, thoughts, and feelings of emotionally distressed individuals. In an era of increasingly stringent financial constraints, decreasing emphasis on individual psychotherapies, and expanding use of psychopharmacological approaches, more patients have been treated with group psychotherapy than with any other form of verbal therapy. Group therapy is applicable to inpatient and outpatient settings, institutional work, partial hospitalization units, halfway houses, community settings, and private practice. Group psychotherapy is also widely used by those who are not mental health professionals in the adjuvant treatment of physical disorders. The principles of group psychotherapy have also been applied with success in the fields of business and education in the form of training, sensitivity, and role-playing.

Group psychotherapy is a treatment in which carefully selected persons who are emotionally ill meet in a group guided by a trained therapist and help one another effect personality change. By using a variety of technical maneuvers and theoretical constructs, the leader directs group members' interactions to bring about changes.

CLASSIFICATION

Group therapy at present has many approaches. Some clinicians work within a psychoanalytic frame of reference. Others use therapy techniques, such as transactional group therapy, which was devised by Eric Berne and emphasizes the here-and-now interactions among group members; behavioral group therapy, which relies on conditioning techniques based on learning theory; Gestalt group therapy, which was created from the theories of Frederick Perls, enables patients to abreact and express themselves fully; and client-centered group psychotherapy, which was developed by Carl Rogers and is based on the nonjudgmental expression of feelings among group members. Table 24.3–1 outlines the major group psychotherapy approaches.

PATIENT SELECTION

To determine a patient's suitability for group psychotherapy, a therapist needs a great deal of information, which is gathered in a screening interview. The psychiatrist should take a psychiatric history and perform a mental status examination to obtain certain dynamic, behavioral, and diagnostic information. Table 24.3–2 outlines the general criteria for the selection of patients for group therapy.

Authority Anxiety

Those patients whose primary problem is their relationship to authority and who are extremely anxious in the presence of authority figures may do well in group therapy because they are more comfortable in a group and more likely to do better in a group than in a dyadic (one-to-one) setting. Patients with a great deal of authority anxiety may be blocked, anxious, resistant, and unwilling to verbalize thoughts and feelings in an individual setting, generally for fear of the therapist's censure or disapproval. Thus, they may welcome the suggestion of group psychotherapy to avoid the scrutiny of the dyadic situation. Conversely, if a patient reacts negatively to the suggestion of group psychotherapy or openly resists the idea, the therapist should consider the possibility that the patient has high peer anxiety.

Peer Anxiety

Patients with conditions such as borderline and schizoid personality disorders who have destructive relationships with their peer groups or who have been extremely isolated from peer group contact generally react negatively or anxiously when placed in a group setting. When such patients can work through their anxiety, however, group therapy can be beneficial.

Robert entered therapy seeking to understand why he was unable to maintain close or lasting relationships. A handsome and successful businessman, he had made a painful and courageous transition away from self-centered, dysfunctional parents early in his life. Although he made good initial impressions in his jobs, he was always puzzled and disappointed when his superiors gradually lost interest in him and his colleagues avoided him. In one-on-one therapy, he was charming and entertaining, but was easily injured by perceived narcissistic slights and would become angry and attacking. Group psychotherapy was suggested when his transference feelings remained intense and therapy was at a seeming impasse. Initially, Robert charmed the group and strove to be the center of attention. Visibly annoyed whenever he felt the group leader was paying more attention to other members, Robert was especially critical and hostile toward older people in the group and displayed little empathy for others. After repeated and forceful confrontations from the group about his antagonistic behavior, he gradually realized that he was repeating childhood patterns in his family of desperately seeking the attention of unloving parents and then entering violent rages when they lost interest. *(Courtesy of Normund Wong, M.D.)*

Table 24.3–1
Comparison of Types of Group Psychotherapy

Parameters	Supportive Group Therapy	Analytically Oriented Group Therapy	Psychoanalysis of Groups	Transactional Group Therapy	Behavioral Group Therapy
Frequency	Once a week	One to three times a week	One to five times a week	One to three times a week	One to three times a week
Duration	Up to 6 months	1–3+ years	1–3+ years	1–3 years	Up to 6 months
Primary indications	Psychotic and anxiety disorders	Anxiety disorders, borderline states, personality disorders	Anxiety disorders, personality disorders	Anxiety and psychotic disorders	Phobias, passivity, sexual problems
Individual screening interview	Usually	Always	Always	Usually	Usually
Communication content	Primarily environmental factors	Present and past life situations, intragroup and extragroup relationships	Primarily past life experiences, intragroup relationships	Primarily intragroup relationships; rarely, history; here and now stressed	Specific symptoms without focus on causality
Transference	Positive transference encouraged to promote improved functioning	Positive and negative transference evoked and analyzed	Transference neurosis evoked and analyzed	Positive relationships fostered, negative feelings analyzed	Positive relationships fostered, no examination of transference
Dreams	Not analyzed	Analyzed frequently	Always analyzed and encouraged	Analyzed rarely	Not used
Dependence	Intragroup dependence encouraged; members rely on leader to great extent	Intragroup dependence encouraged; dependence on leader variable	Intragroup dependence not encouraged; dependence on leader variable	Intragroup dependence encouraged; dependence on leader not encouraged	Intragroup dependence not encouraged; reliance on leader is high
Therapist activity	Strengthen existing defenses, active, give advice	Challenge defenses, active, give advice or personal response	Challenge defense, passive, give no advice or personal response	Challenge defenses, active, give personal response, rather than advice	Create new defenses, active and directive
Interpretation	No interpretation of unconscious conflict	Interpretation of unconscious conflict	Interpretation of unconscious conflict extensive	Interpretation of current behavioral patterns in the here and now	Not used
Major group processes	Universalization, reality testing	Cohesion, transference, reality testing	Transference, ventilation, catharsis, reality testing	Abreaction, reality testing	Cohesion, reinforcement, conditioning
Socialization outside of group	Encouraged	Generally discouraged	Discouraged	Variable	Discouraged
Goals	Improved adaptation to environment	Moderate reconstruction of personality dynamics	Extensive reconstruction of personality dynamics	Alteration of behavior through mechanism of conscious control	Relief of specific psychiatric symptoms

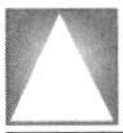

Table 24.3–2
Therapist's Role in Group Therapy

1. Size of group
2. Frequency of sessions
3. Patient composition
4. Confidentiality
5. Goals
6. Preparation of patients
7. Determine group processes

Diagnosis

The diagnosis of patients' disorders is important in determining the best therapeutic approach and in evaluating patients' motivations for treatment, capacities for change, and personality structure strengths and weaknesses. Few contraindications exist to group therapy. Antisocial patients generally do poorly in a heterogeneous group setting because they cannot adhere to group standards; but if the group is composed of other antisocial patients, they may respond better to peers than to perceived authority figures. Depressed patients profit from group therapy after they have established a trusting relationship with the therapist. Patients who are actively suicidal or severely depressed should not be treated solely in a group setting. Patients who are manic are disruptive but, once under pharmacological control, do well in the group setting. Patients who are delusional and who may incorporate the group into their delusional system should be excluded, as should patients who pose a physical threat to other members because of uncontrollable aggressive outbursts.

PREPARATION

Patients prepared by a therapist for a group experience tend to continue in treatment longer and report less initial anxiety than those who are not prepared. The preparation consists of having a therapist explain the procedure in as much detail as possible and answer the patient's questions before the first session.

STRUCTURAL ORGANIZATION

Table 24.3–2 summarizes some of the critical tasks that a group therapist must face when organizing a group.

Size

Group therapy has been successful with as few as 3 members and as many as 15, but most therapists consider 8 to 10 members the optimal size. Interaction may be insufficient with fewer members unless they are especially verbal, and with more than 10 members, the interaction may be too great for the members or the therapist to follow.

Frequency and Length of Sessions

Most group psychotherapists conduct group sessions once a week. Maintaining continuity in sessions is important. When there are alternate sessions, the group meets twice a week, once with and once without the therapist. Group sessions generally last anywhere from 1 to 2 hours, but the time limit should be constant.

Marathon groups were most popular in the 1970s but are much less common today. In time-extended therapy (marathon group therapy), the group meets continuously for 12 to 72 hours. Enforced interactional proximity and, during the longest time-extended sessions, sleep deprivation break down certain ego defenses, release affective processes, and theoretically promote open communication. Time-extended sessions, however, can be dangerous for patients with weak ego structures, such as persons with schizophrenia or borderline personality disorder.

Homogeneous versus Heterogeneous Groups

Most therapists believe that groups should be as heterogeneous as possible to ensure maximal interaction. Members with different diagnostic categories and varied behavioral patterns; from all races, social levels, and educational backgrounds; and of varying ages and both sexes should be brought together. Patients between the ages of 20 and 65 years can be included effectively in the same group. Age differences help in developing parent–child and brother–sister models, and patients have the opportunity to relive and rectify interpersonal difficulties that may have appeared insurmountable.

Both children and adolescents are best treated in groups comprising mostly persons in their own age groups. Some adolescent patients are capable of assimilating the material of an adult group, regardless of content, but they should not be deprived of a constructive peer experience that they might otherwise not have.

Open versus Closed Groups

Closed groups have a set number and composition of patients. If members leave, no new members are accepted. In open groups, membership is more fluid, and new members are taken on whenever old members leave.

MECHANISMS

Group Formation

Each patient approaches group therapy differently and, in this sense, groups are microcosms. Patients use typical adaptive abilities, defense mechanisms, and ways of relating, and when these tactics are ultimately reflected back to them by the group, they learn to be introspective about their personality functioning. A process inherent in group formation requires that patients suspend their previous ways of coping. In entering the group, they allow their executive ego functions—reality testing, adaptation to and mastery of the environment, and perception—to be assumed, to some degree, by the collective assessment provided by the total membership, including the leader.

Therapeutic Factors

Table 24.3–3 outlines 20 significant therapeutic factors that account for change in group psychotherapy.

ROLE OF THE THERAPIST

Although opinions differ about how active or passive a group therapist should be, the consensus is that the therapist's role is

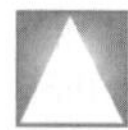

Table 24.3–3
Twenty Therapeutic Factors in Group Psychotherapy

Factor	Definition
Abreaction	A process by which repressed material, particularly a painful experience or conflict, is brought back to consciousness. In the process, the person not only recalls but relives the material, which is accompanied by the appropriate emotional response; insight usually results from the experience.
Acceptance	The feeling of being accepted by other members of the group; differences of opinion are tolerated, and there is an absence of censure.
Altruism	The act of one member helping another; putting another person's need before one's own and learning that there is value in giving to others. The term was originated by Auguste Comte (1798–1857), and Sigmund Freud believed it was a major factor in establishing group cohesion and community feeling.
Catharsis	The expression of ideas, thoughts, and suppressed material that is accompanied by an emotional response that produces a state of relief in the patient.
Cohesion	The sense that the group is working together toward a common goal; also referred to as a sense of "we-ness"; believed to be the most important factor related to positive therapeutic effects.
Consensual validation	Confirmation of reality by comparing one's own conceptualizations with those of other group members; interpersonal distortions are thereby corrected. The term was introduced by Harry Stack Sullivan; Trigant Burrow had used the phrase "consensual observation" to refer to the same phenomenon.
Contagion	The process in which the expression of emotion by one member stimulates the awareness of a similar emotion in another member.
Corrective familial experience	The group recreates the family of origin for some members who can work through original conflicts psychologically through group interaction (e.g., sibling rivalry, anger toward parents).
Empathy	The capacity of a group member to put himself or herself into the psychological frame of reference of another group member and thereby understand his or her thinking, feeling, or behavior.
Identification	An unconscious defense mechanism in which the person incorporates the characteristics and the qualities of another person or object into his or her ego system.
Imitation	The conscious emulation or modeling of one's behavior after that of another (also called *role modeling*); also known as spectator therapy, as one patient learns from another.
Insight	Conscious awareness and understanding of one's own psychodynamics and symptoms of maladaptive behavior. Most therapists distinguish two types: (1) intellectual insight—knowledge and awareness without any changes in maladaptive behavior; (2) emotional insight—awareness and understanding leading to positive changes in personality and behavior.
Inspiration	The process of imparting a sense of optimism to group members; the ability to recognize that one has the capacity to overcome problem; also known as instillation of hope.
Interaction	The free and open exchange of ideas and feelings among group members; effective interaction is emotionally charged.
Interpretation	The process during which the group leader formulates the meaning or significance of a patient's resistance, defenses, and symbols; the result is that the patient has a cognitive framework within which to understand his or her behavior.
Learning	Patients acquire knowledge about new areas, such as social skills and sexual behavior; they receive advice, obtain guidance, and attempt to influence and are influenced by other group members.
Reality testing	Ability of the person to evaluate objectively the world outside the self; includes the capacity to perceive oneself and other group members accurately. *See also* Consensual validation.
Transference	Projection of feelings, thoughts, and wishes onto the therapist, who has come to represent an object from the patient's past. Such reactions, while perhaps appropriate for the condition prevailing in the patient's earlier life, are inappropriate and anachronistic when applied to the therapist in the present. Patients in the group may also direct such feelings toward one another, a process called *multiple transferences*.
Universalization	The awareness of the patient that he or she is not alone in having problems; others share similar complaints or difficulties in learning; the patient is not unique.
Ventilation	The expression of suppressed feelings, ideas, or events to other group members; the sharing of personal secrets that ameliorate a sense of sin or guilt (also referred to as *self-disclosure*).

primarily facilitative. Ideally, the group members themselves are the primary source of cure and change. The climate produced by the therapist's personality is a potent agent of change. The therapist is more than an expert applying techniques; he or she exerts a personal influence that taps such variables as empathy, warmth, and respect.

INPATIENT GROUP PSYCHOTHERAPY

Group therapy is an important part of hospitalized patients' therapeutic experiences. Groups can be organized in many ways on a ward. In a community meeting, an entire inpatient unit meets with all the staff members (e.g., psychiatrists, psychologists, and nurses). In team meetings, 15 to 20 patients and staff members meet; a regular or small group comprising 8 to 10 patients may meet with 1 or 2 therapists, as in traditional group therapy. Although the goals of each group vary, they all have common purposes: to increase patients' awareness of themselves through their interactions with the other group members, who provide feedback about their behavior; to provide patients with improved interpersonal and social skills; to help the members adapt to an inpatient setting; and to improve communication between patients and staff. In addition, one type of group meeting is attended only by inpatient hospital staff and is meant to improve communication among the staff members and to provide mutual support and encouragement in their day-to-day work with patients. Community meetings and team meetings are more helpful for dealing with patient treatment problems than they are for providing insight-oriented therapy, which is the province of the small-group therapy meeting.

Group Composition

Two key factors of inpatient groups common to all short-term therapies are the heterogeneity of the members and the rapid turnover of patients. Outside the hospital, therapists have large caseloads from which to select patients for group therapy. On the ward, therapists have a limited number of patients to choose from and are further restricted to those patients who are both willing to participate and suitable for a small-group experience. In certain settings, group participation may be mandatory (e.g., in substance abuse and alcohol dependence units), but mandatory attendance does not usually apply in a general psychiatry unit. In fact, most group experiences are more productive when the patients themselves choose to enter them.

More sessions are preferable to fewer. During patients' hospital stays, groups may meet daily to allow interactional continuity and the carryover of themes from one session to the next. A new member of a group can be brought up to date quickly, either by the therapist in an orientation meeting or by one of the members. A newly admitted patient has often learned many details about the small-group program from another patient before actually attending the first session. The less frequently the group sessions are held, the greater the need for a therapist to structure the group and be active in it.

Inpatient versus Outpatient Groups

Although the therapeutic factors that account for change in small inpatient groups are similar to those in the outpatient settings, there are qualitative differences. For example, the relatively high turnover of patients in inpatient groups complicates the process of cohesion. But the fact that all the group members are together in the hospital aids cohesion, as do the therapists' efforts to foster the process. Sharing of information, universalization, and catharsis are the main therapeutic factors at work in inpatient groups. Although insight more likely occurs in outpatient groups because of their long-term nature, some patients can obtain a new understanding of their psychological makeup within the confines of a single group session. A unique quality of inpatient groups is the patients' extragroup contacts, which are extensive because they live together on the same ward. Verbalizing their thoughts and feelings about such contacts in the therapy sessions encourages interpersonal learning. In addition, conflicts between patients or between patients and staff members can be anticipated and resolved.

Twelve former psychiatric inpatients who attended the monthly medication clinic would meet for 1 hour before their individual appointments with the psychiatrist to review their current social situation and medications. All had been treated by the same ward doctor and had known one another while on the inpatient service. The psychiatrist who performed the medication reviews also served as the group leader. Periodically, he was assisted by a staff member who was also familiar with the patients. Coffee was available, and the patients often brought pastries from home. The patients socialized with one another during the hour and frequently exchanged helpful ideas and tips about job opportunities. Those without cars shared rides with other members. The group was open ended and well attended. Most of the patients were single and had a long history of psychotic illness. For most, this meeting was their only opportunity to socialize and be among peers. Frequently, on learning that a member had been rehospitalized, many in the group would visit their colleague on the ward. *(Courtesy of Normund Wong, M.D.)*

SELF-HELP GROUPS

Self-help groups comprise persons who are trying to cope with a specific problem or life crisis and are usually organized with a particular task in mind. Such groups do not attempt to explore individual psychodynamics in great depth or to change personality functioning significantly, but self-help groups have improved the emotional health and well-being of many persons.

A distinguishing characteristic of the self-help groups is their homogeneity. The members have the same disorders and share their experiences—good and bad, successful and unsuccessful—with one another. By so doing, they educate one another, provide mutual support, and alleviate the sense of alienation usually felt by persons drawn to this kind of group.

Self-help groups emphasize cohesion, which is exceptionally strong in these groups. Because the group members have similar problems and symptoms, they develop a strong emotional bond. Each group may have its unique characteristics, to which the members can attribute magical qualities of healing. Examples of self-help groups are Alcoholics Anonymous (AA), Gamblers Anonymous (GA), and Overeaters Anonymous (OA).

The self-help group movement is presently in ascendancy. These groups meet their members' needs by providing acceptance, mutual support, and help in overcoming maladaptive patterns of behavior or states of feeling that traditional mental health and medical professionals have not generally dealt with successfully. Self-help groups and therapy groups have begun to converge. Self-help groups have enabled their members to give up patterns of unwanted behavior; therapy groups have helped their members understand why and how they got to be the way they were or are.

COMBINED INDIVIDUAL AND GROUP PSYCHOTHERAPY

In combined individual and group psychotherapy, patients see a therapist individually and also take part in group sessions. The therapist for the group and individual sessions is usually the same person. Groups can vary in size from 3 to 15 members, but the most helpful size is 8 to 10. Patients must attend all group sessions. Attendance at individual sessions is also important, and failure to attend either group or individual sessions should be examined as part of the therapeutic process.

Combined therapy is a particular treatment modality, not a system by which individual therapy is augmented by an occasional group session or a group therapy in which a participant meets alone with a therapist from time to time. Rather, it is an ongoing plan in which meaningful integration of the group experience with the individual sessions yields reciprocal feedback to help form an integrated therapeutic experience. Although the one-to-one doctor–patient relationship makes a deep examination of the transference reaction possible for some patients, it may not provide other patients with the corrective emotional experiences necessary for therapeutic change. The group gives patients a variety of persons with whom they can have transferential reactions. In the microcosm of the group, patients can relive and work through familial and other important influences.

Techniques

Differing techniques based on varying theoretical frameworks have been used in the combined therapy format. Some clinicians increase the frequency of individual sessions to encourage the emergence of the transference neurosis. In the behavioral model, individual sessions are scheduled regularly, but they tend to be less frequent than in other approaches. Whether patients use a couch or a chair during individual sessions depends on a therapist's orientation. Techniques such as alternate meetings or "after-sessions" without the therapist present may be used. A combined therapy approach called *structured interactional group psychotherapy* has a different group member as the focus of each weekly group session who is discussed in depth by the other members.

Results

Most workers in the field believe that combined therapy has the advantages of both dyadic and group settings, without sacrificing the qualities of either. Generally, the dropout rate in combined therapy is lower than that in group therapy alone. In many cases, combined therapy appears to bring problems to the surface and to resolve them more quickly than might be possible with either method alone.

PSYCHODRAMA

Psychodrama is a method of group psychotherapy originated by the Viennese-born psychiatrist Jacob Moreno in which personality makeup, interpersonal relationships, conflicts, and emotional problems are explored by means of special dramatic methods. Therapeutic dramatization of emotional problems includes the protagonist or patient, the person who acts out problems with the help of auxiliary egos, persons who enact varying aspects of the patient, and the director, psychodramatist, or therapist, the person who guides those in the drama toward the acquisition of insight.

Roles

Director. The director is the leader or therapist and so must be an active participant. He or she has a catalytic function by encouraging the members of the group to be spontaneous. The director must also be available to meet the group's needs without superimposing his or her values. Of all the group psychotherapies, psychodrama requires the most participation from the therapist.

Protagonist. The protagonist is the patient in conflict. The patient chooses the situation to portray in the dramatic scene, or the therapist chooses it if the patient so desires.

Auxiliary Ego. An auxiliary ego is another group member who represents something or someone in the protagonist's experience. The auxiliary egos help account for the great range of therapeutic effects available in psychodrama.

Group. The members of the psychodrama and the audience make up the group. Some are participants, and others are observers, but all benefit from the experience to the extent that they can identify with the ongoing events. The concept of spontaneity in psychodrama refers to the ability of each member of the group, especially the protagonist, to experience the thoughts and feelings of the moment and to communicate emotion as authentically as possible.

Techniques

The psychodrama can focus on any special area of functioning (a dream, a family, or a community situation), a symbolic role, an unconscious attitude, or an imagined future situation. Such symptoms as delusions and hallucinations can also be acted out in the group. Techniques to advance the therapeutic process and to increase productivity and creativity include the soliloquy (a recital of overt and hidden thoughts and feelings), role reversal (the exchange of the patient's role for the role of a significant person), the double (an auxiliary ego acting as the patient), the multiple double (several egos acting as the patient did on varying occasions), and the mirror technique (an ego imitating the patient and speaking for him or her). Other techniques include the use of hypnosis and psychoactive drugs to modify the acting behavior in various ways.

ETHICAL AND LEGAL ISSUES

Confidentiality

Except where disclosure is required by law, the group therapist legally and ethically gives information about the group members to others only after obtaining appropriate patient consent. The therapist is obligated to take appropriate steps to be responsible to society, as well as to patients, when patients pose a danger to themselves or to others. The guidelines for ethics of the American Group Psychotherapy Association state that therapists must obtain specific permission to confer with the referring therapist or with the individual therapist when the patient is in conjoint therapy.

Although the group members, as well as the therapist, should protect the identity of the members and maintain confidentiality, the group members are not legally bound to do so. During the preparation of patients for group psychotherapy, therapists should routinely instruct the prospective members to keep all material discussed in the group confidential. Theoretically, in a legal case, one member of a group can be asked to testify against another, but such a situation has not yet occurred.

A therapist must exercise clinical judgment and caution in placing a patient in a group if he or she thinks that the burdens of maintaining secrets will be too great for some potential members or if a prospective group patient harbors a secret of such magnitude or notoriety that membership in a group would not be wise.

Violence and Aggression

Although reports of violence and aggression are rare, the potential exists that a group member may physically attack another patient or a therapist. The attack may occur within the group or outside the group. The likelihood of such an event can be diminished through the careful selection of group members. Patients with a demonstrated history of assaultive behavior and psychotic patients who pose a potential for violence should not be placed in a group. In institutional settings, in which group therapy is commonly practiced, sufficient safeguards must be in place to discourage any physical danger to others—for example, guards or attendants can act as observers.

Sexual Behavior

For therapists, sexual intercourse with a patient or a former patient is unethical; in many states, such behavior is considered a criminal act. The issue is complicated in group psychotherapy, however, because members may engage in sexual activities with one another. The issues of pregnancy, rape, and the transmission of acquired immunodeficiency syndrome (AIDS) by group members are open questions. If a patient is injured as a result of sexual activity by group members, the therapist could be held accountable for not preventing such behavior. The therapist should advise prospective group members that each patient is responsible for reporting any sexual contact between members. The therapist cannot anticipate every group sexual encounter or prevent sexual relationships from developing, but he or she is obligated to provide patients with guidelines of acceptable behavior. The therapist should identify sexual, vulnerable, or exploitive patients in the selection and preparation of patients for the group. Sociopathic patients who sexually exploit others should be informed that such behavior is explicitly not acceptable in the group and that such behavior should be verbalized rather than acted out. The group must be conducted in such a way that the therapist does not encourage or tacitly allow sexual activity. Patients with AIDS are encouraged to reveal that they harbor the virus. To protect members if sexual relationships occur, some therapists do not accept patients with AIDS into a group unless they agree to reveal their condition. In those situations, the therapist discusses the issue of AIDS with the patient and the group into which the patient is to be placed.

▲ 24.4 Family Therapy and Couples Therapy

FAMILY THERAPY

The family is the foundation on which most societies are built. The study of families in different cultures has been a subject of fascination and scientific interest from viewpoints as diverse as sociology, group dynamics, anthropology, ethnicity, race, evolutionary biology, and, of course, the mental health field. The confluence of information gleaned from family studies has set the backdrop against which the contemporary practice of family therapy has evolved.

Family therapy can be defined as any psychotherapeutic endeavor that explicitly focuses on altering the interactions between or among family members and seeks to improve the functioning of the family as a unit, or its subsystems, and the functioning of individual members of the family. Both family therapy and couple therapy aim at some change in relational functioning. In most cases, they also aim at some other change, typically in the functioning of specific individuals in the family. Family therapy meant to heal a rift between parents and their adult children is an example of the use of family therapy centered on relationship goals. Family therapy aimed at increasing the family's coping with schizophrenia and at reducing the family's expressed emotion is an example of family therapy aimed at individual goals (in this case, the functioning of the person with schizophrenia), as well as family goals. In the early years of family therapy, change in the family system was seen as being sufficient to produce individual change. More recent treatments aimed at change in individuals, as well as in the family system, tend to supplement the interventions that focus on interpersonal relationships with specific strategies that focus on individual behavior.

Indications

The presence of a relational difficulty is a clear indication for family and couple therapies. Couples and family therapies are the only treatments that have been shown to be efficacious for such problems as marital maladjustment, and other methods, such as individual therapy, have been shown to often have deleterious effects in these situations. Couples and family therapies have also been demonstrated to have a clear and important role in the treatment of numerous specific psychiatric disorders, often as a component within a multimethod treatment.

Of course, as with any therapy, the indications for family and couple therapies are broad and vary from case to case. Family therapy is a therapeutic collage of ideas regarding the underpinnings of family and individual stability and change, psychopathology, and problems in living, as well as relational ethics. Family therapy might better be called *systemically sensitive therapy* and, in this sense, reflects a basic worldview as much as a clinical treatment methodology. For therapists thus inclined, then, all clinical problems involve salient interactional components; thus, some kind of family (or other functionally significant other's) involvement in therapy is always called for, even in treatment that emphasizes individual problems.

An impressive array now exists of common clinical disorders and problems, including child, adolescent, and adult disorders, for which research has demonstrated family or couple treatment methods to be effective. In a few instances, couple and family interventions are probably even the treatment of choice, and for several disorders, the research argues for family intervention to be an essential part of treatment.

Techniques

Initial Consultation. Family therapy is familiar enough to the general public for families with a high level of conflict to request it specifically. When the initial complaint is about an individual family member, however, pretreatment work may

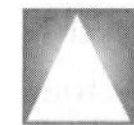

Table 24.4–1
Rationale for Family-Life Chronology

The family therapist enters a session knowing little or nothing about the family.
The therapist may know who the identified patient is and what symptoms the patient manifests, but that is usually all. So the therapist must get clues about the meaning of the symptom.
The therapist may know that pain exists in the marital relationship, but needs to get clues about how the pain shows itself.
The therapist needs to know how the mates have tried to cope with their problems.
The therapist may know that the mates both operate from models (from what they saw going on between their own parents), but needs to find out how those models have influenced each mate's expectations about how to be a mate and how to be a parent.
The family therapist enters a session knowing that the family, in fact, has had a history, but that is usually all.
Every family, as a group, has gone through or jointly experienced many events. Certain events (e.g., deaths, childbirth, sickness, geographical moves, and job changes) occur in almost all families.
Certain events primarily affect the mates and only indirectly the children. (Maybe the children were not born yet or were too young to fully comprehend the nature of an event as it affected their parents. They may have only sensed periods of parental remoteness, distraction, anxiety, or annoyance.)
The therapist can profit from answers to just about every question asked.
Family members enter therapy with a great deal of fear.
Therapist structuring helps decrease the threats. It says, "I am in charge of what will happen here. I will see to it that nothing catastrophic happens here."
All members are covertly feeling to blame that nothing seems to have turned out right (even though they may overtly blame the identified patient or the other mate).
Parents, especially, need to feel that they did the best they could as parents. They need to tell the therapist, "This is why I did what I did. This is what happened to me."
A family-life chronology that deals with such facts as names, dates, labeled relationships, and moves, seems to appeal to the family. It asks questions that members can answer, questions that are relatively nonthreatening. It deals with life as the family understands it.
Family members enter therapy with a great deal of despair.
Therapist structuring helps stimulate hope.
As far as family members are concerned, past events are part of them. They now can tell the therapist, "I existed." And they can also say, "I am not just a big blob of pathology. I succeeded in overcoming many handicaps."
If the family knew what questions needed asking, they would not need to be in therapy. So the therapist does not say, "Tell me what you want to tell me." Family members will simply tell the therapist what they have been telling themselves for years. The therapist's questions say, "I know what to ask. I take responsibility for understanding you. We are going to go somewhere."
The family therapist also knows that, to some degree, the family has focused on the identified patient to relieve marital pain. The therapist also knows that, to some degree, the family will resist any effort to change that focus. A family-life chronology is an effective, nonthreatening way to change from an emphasis on the "sick" or "bad" family member to an emphasis on the marital relationship.
The family-life chronology serves other useful therapy purposes, such as providing the framework within which a reeducation process can take place. The therapist serves as a model in checking out information or correcting communication techniques and placing questions and eliciting answers to begin the process. In addition, when taking the chronology, the therapist can introduce in a relatively nonfrightening way some of the crucial concepts to induce change.

Adapted from Satir V. *Conjoint Family Therapy*. Palo Alto, CA: Science and Behavior; 1967:57, with permission.

be needed. Underlying resistance to a family approach typically includes fears by parents that they will be blamed for their child's difficulties, that the entire family will be pronounced sick, that a spouse will object, and that open discussion of one child's misbehavior will have a negative influence on siblings. Refusal by an adolescent or young adult patient to participate in family therapy is frequently a disguised collusion with the fears of one or both parents.

Interview Technique. The special quality of a family interview springs from two important facts. A family comes to treatment with its history and dynamics firmly in place. To a family therapist, the established nature of the group, more than the symptoms, constitutes the clinical problem. Family members usually live together and, at some level, depend on one another for their physical and emotional well-being. Whatever transpires in the therapy session is known to all. Central principles of technique also derive from these facts. For example, the therapist must carefully channel the catharsis of anger by one family member toward another. The person who is the object of the anger will react to the attack, and the anger may escalate into violence and fracture relationships, with one or more member withdrawing from therapy. For another example, free association is inappropriate in family therapy because it can encourage one person to dominate a session. Thus, therapists must always control and direct the family interview.

Table 24.4–1 summarizes the principles in which the history of the family is examined in an effort to understand how that history informs the current familial interactions.

Frequency and Length of Treatment. Unless an emergency arises, sessions are usually held no more than once a week. Each session, however, may require as much as 2 hours. Long sessions can include an intermission to give the therapist time to organize the material and plan a response. A flexible schedule is necessary when geography or personal circumstances make it physically difficult for the family to get together. The length of treatment depends both on the nature of the problem and on the therapeutic model. Therapists who use problem-solving models exclusively may accomplish their goals in a few sessions, whereas therapists using growth-oriented models may work with a family for years and may schedule sessions at long intervals. Table 24.4–2 summarizes one model for treatment termination.

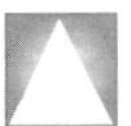

Table 24.4–2
Criteria for Treatment Termination

Treatment is completed:
When family members can complete transactions, check, ask
When they can interpret hostility
When they can see how others see them
When they can see how they see themselves
When one member can tell others how they manifest themselves
When one member can tell others what is hoped, feared, and expected from them
When they can disagree
When they can make choices
When they can learn through practice
When they can free themselves from the harmful effects of past models
When they can give clear messages—that is, be congruent in their behavior—with a minimum of difference between feelings and communication and with a minimum of hidden messages.

Adapted from Satir V. *Conjoint Family Therapy*. Palo Alto, CA: Science and Behavior; 1967:133, with permission.

Models of Intervention

Many models of family therapy exist, none of which is superior to the others. The particular model used depends on the training received, the context in which therapy occurs, and the personality of the therapist.

Psychodynamic-Experiential Models. Psychodynamic-experiential models emphasize individual maturation in the context of the family system and are free from unconscious patterns of anxiety and projection rooted in the past. Therapists seek to establish an intimate bond with each family member, and sessions alternate between the therapist's exchanges with the members and the members' exchanges with one another. Clarity of communication and honestly admitted feelings are given high priority. Toward this end, family members may be encouraged to change their seats, to touch each other, and to make direct eye contact. Their use of metaphor, body language, and parapraxes helps reveal the unconscious pattern of family relationships. The therapist may also use family sculpting, in which family members physically arrange one another in tableaus depicting their personal view of relationships, past or present. The therapist both interprets the living sculpture and modifies it in a way to suggest new relationships. In addition, the therapist's subjective responses to the family are given great importance. At appropriate moments, the therapist expresses these responses to the family to form yet another feedback loop of self-observation and change.

Bowen Model. Murray Bowen called his model *family systems,* but in the family therapy field it rightfully carries the name of its originator. The hallmark of the Bowen model is persons' differentiation from their family of origin, their ability to be their true selves in the face of familial or other pressures that threaten the loss of love or social position. Problem families are assessed on two levels: the degree of their enmeshment versus the degree of their ability to differentiate and the analysis of emotional triangles in the problem for which they seek help.

An emotional triangle is defined as a three-party system (and many of these can exist within a family) arranged so that the closeness of two members expressed as either love or repetitive conflict tends to exclude a third. When the excluded third person attempts to join with one of the other two or when one of the involved parties shifts in the direction of the excluded one, emotional cross-currents are activated. The therapist's role is, first, to stabilize or shift the "hot" triangle—the one producing the presenting symptoms—and, second, to work with the most psychologically available family members, individually if necessary, to achieve sufficient personal differentiation so that the hot triangle does not recur. To preserve his or her neutrality in the family's triangles, the therapist minimizes emotional contact with family members.

Bowen also originated the *genogram,* a theoretical tool that is a historical survey of the family, going back several generations.

Structural Model. In a structural model, families are viewed as single, interrelated systems assessed in terms of significant alliances and splits among family members, hierarchy of power (parents in charge of children), clarity and firmness of boundaries between the generations, and family tolerance for one another. The structural model uses concurrent individual and family therapy.

General Systems Model. Based on general systems theory, a general systems model holds that families are systems and that every action in a family produces a reaction in one or more of its members. Families have external boundaries and internal rules. Every member is presumed to play a role (e.g., spokesperson, persecutor, victim, rescuer, symptom bearer, or nurturer), which is relatively stable, but which member fills each role may change. Some families try to scapegoat one member by blaming him or her for the family's problems (the identified patient). If the identified patient improves, another family member may become the scapegoat. The general systems model overlaps with some of the other models presented, particularly the Bowen and structural models.

Modifications of Techniques

Family Group Therapy. Family group therapy combines several families into a single group. Families share mutual problems and compare their interactions with those of the other families in the group. Treatment of schizophrenia has been effective in multiple family groups. Parents of disturbed children may also meet together to share their situations.

Social Network Therapy. In social network therapy, the social community or network of a disturbed patient meets in group sessions with the patient. The network includes those with whom the patient comes into contact in daily life, not only the immediate family but also relatives, friends, tradespersons, teachers, and coworkers.

Paradoxical Therapy. With the paradoxical therapy approach, which evolved from the work of Gregory Bateson, a therapist suggests that the patient intentionally engage in the unwanted behavior (called the paradoxical injunction) and, for example, avoid a phobic object or perform a compulsive ritual. Although paradoxical therapy and the use of paradoxical injunctions seem to be counterintuitive, the therapy can create new insights for some patients. It is used in individual therapy as well as in family therapy.

Reframing. Reframing, also known as *positive connotation,* is a relabeling of all negatively expressed feelings or behavior as positive. When the therapist attempts to get family members to view behavior from a new frame of reference, "This child is impossible" becomes "This child is desperately trying to distract and protect you from what he or she perceives as an unhappy marriage." Reframing is an important process that allows family members to view themselves in new ways that can produce change.

Goals

Family therapy has several goals: to resolve or reduce pathogenic conflict and anxiety within the matrix of interpersonal relationships; to enhance the perception and fulfillment by family members of one another's emotional needs; to promote appropriate role relationships between the sexes and generations; to strengthen the capacity of individual members and the family as a whole to cope with destructive forces inside and outside the surrounding environment; and to influence family identity and values so that members are oriented toward health and growth. The therapy ultimately aims to integrate families into the large systems of society, extended family, and community groups and social systems, such as schools, medical facilities, and social, recreational, and welfare agencies.

COUPLES (MARITAL) THERAPY

Couples or marital therapy is a form of psychotherapy designed to psychologically modify the interaction of two persons who are in conflict with each other over one parameter or a variety of parameters—social, emotional, sexual, or economic. In couples therapy, a trained person establishes a therapeutic contract with a patient-couple and, through definite types of communication, attempts to alleviate the disturbance, to reverse or change maladaptive patterns of behavior, and to encourage personality growth and development.

Marriage counseling may be considered more limited in scope than marriage therapy; Only a particular familial conflict is discussed, and the counseling is primarily task oriented, geared to solving a specific problem, such as child rearing. Marriage therapy, by contrast, emphasizes restructuring a couple's interaction and sometimes explores the psychodynamics of each partner. Both therapy and counseling stress helping marital partners cope effectively with their problems. Most important is the definition of appropriate and realistic goals, which may involve extensive reconstruction of the union or problem-solving approaches or a combination of both.

Types of Therapies

Individual Therapy. In individual therapy, the partners may consult different therapists, who do not necessarily communicate with each other and indeed may not even know each other. The goal of treatment is to strengthen each partner's adaptive capacities. At times, only one of the partners is in treatment; and, in such cases, it is often helpful for the person who is not in treatment to visit the therapist. The visiting partner may give the therapist data about the patient that may otherwise be overlooked; overt or covert anxiety in the visiting partner as a result of change in the patient can be identified and dealt with; irrational beliefs about treatment events can be corrected; and conscious or unconscious attempts by the partner to sabotage the patient's treatment can be examined.

Individual Couples Therapy. In individual couples therapy, each partner is in therapy, which is either concurrent, with the same therapist, or collaborative, with each partner seeing a different therapist.

Conjoint Therapy. In conjoint therapy, the most common treatment method in couples therapy, either one or two therapists treat the partners in joint sessions. Cotherapy with therapists of both sexes prevents a particular patient from feeling ganged up on when confronted by two members of the opposite sex.

Four-Way Session. In a four-way session, each partner is seen by a different therapist, with regular joint sessions in which all four persons participate. A variation of the four-way session is the roundtable interview, developed by William Masters and Virginia Johnson for the rapid treatment of sexually dysfunctional couples. Two patients and two opposite-sex therapists meet regularly.

Group Psychotherapy. Group therapy for couples allows a variety of group dynamics to affect the participants. Groups usually consist of three to four couples and one or two therapists. The couples identify with one another and recognize that others have similar problems; each gains support and empathy from fellow group members of the same or opposite sex. They explore sexual attitudes and have an opportunity to gain new information from their peer groups, and each receives specific feedback about his or her behavior, either negative or positive, which may have more meaning and be better assimilated coming from a neutral, nonspouse member, for example, than from the spouse or the therapist.

During the middle phase of a couples group comprising four couples, the theme of whether to have children arose. One couple had just come from a visit to the gynecologist, who informed them that they were running out of time because of the wife's age. The woman in the couple did not want to have children, but her husband did. His complaint about the marriage was that his wife never was demonstrative in showing her loving feelings for him. He felt her to be detached, distant, and sexually inhibited.

The prevailing sentiment among the other couples who had children was that children only added additional stress to an already stressed relationship. One other couple, however, voiced their different view by describing how their children had enriched their lives.

As the talk about going forward and getting pregnant progressed, the group leader noted the nonverbal communication between the ambivalent couple. Whenever the tone of the group leaned toward having children, the wife would reach out and grasp the hand of her husband in a tender way. This invariably had the effect of stopping him from pursuing the topic for fear of the withdrawal of the affection he hungered for. All this occurred without words. Once identified, this repetitive nonverbal pattern was available for examination in the group, and the supportive elements provided by other members and the leader encouraged a frank, direct, and open conversation between the partners, who eventually chose to go forward and attempt to have a child. *(Courtesy of H. I. Spitz, M.D., and S. Spitz, ACSW.)*

Combined Therapy. Combined therapy refers to all or any of the preceding techniques used concurrently or in combination. Thus, a particular patient-couple may begin treatment with one or both partners in individual psychotherapy, continue in conjoint therapy with the partner, and terminate therapy after a course of treatment in a married couples' group. The rationale for combined therapy is that no single approach to marital problems has been shown to be superior to another. A familiarity with a variety of approaches thus allows therapists a flexibility that provides maximal benefit for couples in distress.

Indications

Whatever the specific therapeutic technique, initiation of couples therapy is indicated when individual therapy has failed to resolve the relationship difficulties, when the onset of distress in one or both partners is clearly a relational problem, and when couples therapy is requested by a couple in conflict. Problems in communication between partners are a prime indication for couples therapy. In such instances, one spouse may be intimidated by the other, may become anxious when attempting to tell the other about thoughts or feelings, or may project unconscious expectations onto the other. The therapy is geared toward enabling each partner to see the other realistically.

Conflicts in one or several areas, such as the partners' sexual life, are also indications for treatment. Similarly, difficulty in establishing satisfactory social, economic, parental, or emotional roles implies that a couple needs help. Clinicians should evaluate all aspects of the marital relationship before attempting to treat only one problem, which could be a symptom of a pervasive marital disorder.

Contraindications

Contraindications for couples therapy include patients with severe forms of psychosis, particularly patients with paranoid elements and those in whom the marriage's homeostatic mechanism is a protection against psychosis, marriages in which one or both partners really want to divorce, and marriages in which one spouse refuses to participate because of anxiety or fear.

Goals

Nathan Ackerman defined the aims of couples therapy as follows: The goals of therapy for partner relational problems are to alleviate emotional distress and disability and to promote the levels of well-being of both partners together and of each as an individual. Ideally, therapists move toward these goals by strengthening the shared resources for problem solving, by encouraging the substitution of adequate controls and defenses for pathogenic ones, by enhancing both the immunity against the disintegrative effects of emotional upset and the complementarity of the relationship, and by promoting the growth of the relationship and of each partner.

Part of a therapist's task is to persuade each partner in the relationship to take responsibility in understanding the psychodynamic makeup of personality. Each person's accountability for the effects of behavior on his or her own life, the life of the partner, and the lives of others in the environment is emphasized, and the result is often a deep understanding of the problems that created the marital discord.

Couples therapy does not ensure the maintenance of any marriage or relationship. Indeed, in certain instances, it may show the partners that they are in a nonviable union that should be dissolved. In these cases, couples may continue to meet with therapists to work through the difficulties of separating and obtaining a divorce, a process that has been called *divorce therapy.*

▲ 24.5 Dialectical Behavior Therapy

Dialectical behavior therapy (DBT) is the psychosocial treatment that has received the most empirical support for patients with borderline personality disorder (BPD). Put simply, the overarching goal of DBT is to help create a life worth living for patients who often suffer tremendously from chronic and pervasive problems across many areas of their lives. DBT is a type of psychotherapy that was originally developed for chronically self-injurious patients with BPD and parasuicidal behavior. In recent years, its use has extended to other forms of mental illness. The method is eclectic, drawing on concepts derived from supportive, cognitive, and behavioral therapies. Some elements can be traced to Franz Alexander's view of therapy as a corrective emotional experience and other elements from certain Eastern philosophical schools (e.g., Zen).

Patients are seen weekly, with the goal of improving interpersonal skills and decreasing self-destructive behavior using techniques involving advice, metaphor, storytelling, and confrontation, among others. Patients with BPD especially are helped to deal with the ambivalent feelings that are characteristic of the disorder. Marsha Linehan, Ph.D., developed the treatment method, based on her theory that such patients cannot identify emotional experiences and cannot tolerate frustration or rejection. As with other behavioral approaches, DBT assumes all behavior (including thoughts and feelings) is learned and that patients with BPD behave in ways that reinforce or even reward their behavior, regardless of how maladaptive it is.

FUNCTIONS OF DBT

As described by its originator, there are five essential "functions" in treatment: (1) to enhance and expand the patient's repertoire of skillful behavioral patterns; (2) to improve patient motivation to change by reducing reinforcement of maladaptive behavior, including dysfunctional cognition and emotion; (3) to ensure that new behavioral patterns generalize from the therapeutic to the natural environment; (4) to structure the environment so that effective behaviors, rather than dysfunctional behaviors, are reinforced; and (5) to enhance the motivation and capabilities of the therapist so that effective treatment is rendered.

The four modes of treatment in DBT are as follows: (1) group skills training, (2) individual therapy, (3) phone consultation, and (4) consultation team. These are described below. Other ancillary treatments used are pharmacotherapy and hospitalization, when needed.

Group Skills Training

In group format, patients learn specific behavioral, emotional, cognitive, and interpersonal skills. Unlike traditional group therapy, observations about others in the group are discouraged. Rather, a didactic approach, using specific exercises taken from a skills training manual, is used, many exercises of which are geared toward control of emotional dysregulation and impulsive behavior.

Individual Therapy

Sessions in DBT are held weekly, generally for 50 to 60 minutes, in which skills learned during group training are reviewed and life events from the previous week are examined. Particular attention is paid to episodes of pathological behavioral patterns that could have been corrected if learned skills had been put into effect. Patients are encouraged to record their thoughts, feelings, and behaviors on diary cards, which are analyzed in the session.

Telephone Consultation

Therapists are available for phone consultation 24 hours a day. Patients are encouraged to call when they feel themselves heading toward some crisis that might lead to injurious behavior to themselves or others. Calls are intended to be brief and usually last about 10 minutes.

Consultation Team

Therapists meet in weekly meetings to review their work with their patients. By doing so, they provide support for one another and maintain motivation in their work. The meetings enable them to compare techniques used and to validate those that are most effective (Table 24.5–1).

Table 24.5–1
Consultation Team Agreements in Dialectical Behavior Therapy

Meet weekly for 1–2 hours
Discuss cases according to the treatment hierarchy (i.e., self-injurious/life-threatening behavior, behaviors that interfere with treatment or quality of life)
Accept a dialectical philosophy
Consult with the patient on how to interact with other therapists, but do not tell other therapists how to interact with the patient
Consistency of therapists with one another (even across the same patient) is not expected
All therapists observe their own limits without fear of judgmental reactions from other consultation group members
Search for nonpejorative empathic interpretation of the patient's behavior
All therapists are fallible

RESULTS

Several studies evaluating the effect of DBT for patients with BPD found that such therapy was positive. Patients had a low dropout rate from treatment; the incidence of parasuicidal behaviors declined; self-report of angry affect decreased; and social adjustment and work performance improved. The method is now being applied to other disorders, including substance abuse, eating disorders, schizophrenia, and posttraumatic stress disorder.

▲ 24.6 Biofeedback

Biofeedback involves the recording and display of small changes in the physiological levels of the feedback parameter. The display can be visual, such as a big meter or a bar of lights, or auditory. Patients are instructed to change the levels of the parameter, using the feedback from the display as a guide. Biofeedback is based on the idea that the autonomic nervous system can come under voluntary control through operant conditioning. Biofeedback can be used by itself or in combination with relaxation. For example, patients with urinary incontinence use biofeedback alone to regain control over the pelvic musculature. Biofeedback is also used in the rehabilitation of neurological disorders. The benefits of biofeedback may be augmented by the relaxation that patients are trained to facilitate.

THEORY

Neal Miller demonstrated the medical potential of biofeedback by showing that the normally involuntary autonomic nervous system can be operantly conditioned by use of appropriate feedback. By means of instruments, patients acquire information about the status of involuntary biological functions, such as skin temperature and electrical conductivity, muscle tension, blood pressure, heart rate, and brain wave activity. Patients then learn to regulate one or more of these biological states that affect symptoms. For example, a person can learn to raise the temperature of his or her hands to reduce the frequency of migraines, palpitations, or angina pectoris. Presumably, patients lower the sympathetic activation and voluntarily self-regulate arterial smooth muscle vasoconstrictive tendencies.

METHODS

Instrumentation

The feedback instrument used depends on the patient and the specific problem. The most effective instruments are the electromyogram (EMG), which measures the electrical potentials of muscle fibers; the electroencephalogram (EEG), which measures alpha waves that occur in relaxed states; the galvanic skin response (GSR) gauge, which shows decreased skin conductivity during a relaxed state; and the thermistor, which measures skin temperature (which drops during tension because of peripheral vasoconstriction). Patients are attached to one of the instruments that measures a physiological function and translates the measurement into an audible or visual signal that patients use to gauge their responses. For example, in the treatment of bruxism, an EMG is attached to the masseter muscle. The EMG emits a high tone when the muscle is contracted and a low tone when at rest. Patients can learn to alter the tone to indicate relaxation. Patients receive feedback about the masseter muscle, the tone reinforces the learning, and the condition ameliorates—all of these events interacting synergistically.

Many less-specific clinical applications (e.g., treating insomnia, dysmenorrhea, and speech problems; improving athletic performance; treating volitional disorders; achieving altered states of consciousness; managing stress; and supplementing psychotherapy for treating anxiety associated with somatic symptom and related disorders) use a model in which frontalis muscle EMG biofeedback is combined with thermal biofeedback and verbal instructions in progressive relaxation. Table 24.6–1 outlines some important clinical applications of biofeedback and shows that a wide variety of biofeedback modalities have been used to treat numerous conditions.

Relaxation Therapy

Muscle relaxation is used as a component of treatment programs (e.g., systematic desensitization) or as treatment in its own right (relaxation therapy). Relaxation is characterized by (1) immobility of the body, (2) control over the focus of attention, (3) low muscle tone, and (4) cultivation of a specific frame of mind, described as contemplative, nonjudgmental, detached, or mindful.

Progressive relaxation was developed by Edmund Jacobson in 1929. Jacobson observed that when an individual lies "relaxed," in the ordinary sense, the following clinical signs reveal the presence of residual tension: respiration is slightly irregular in time or force; the pulse rate, although often normal, is in some instances moderately increased as compared with later tests; voluntary or local reflex activities are revealed in such slight marks as wrinkling of the forehead, frowning, movements of the eyeballs frequent or rapid winking, restless shifting of the head, a limb, or even a finger; and finally, the mind continues to be active, and once started, worry or oppressive emotion will persist. It is amazing that a faint degree of tension can be responsible for all of this.

Learning relaxation, therefore, involves cultivating a muscle sense. To develop the muscle sense further, patients are taught to isolate and contract specific muscles or muscle groups, one at a time. For example, patients flex the forearm while the therapist holds it back to observe tenseness in the biceps muscle.

Table 24.6–1
Biofeedback Applications

Condition	Effects
Asthma	Both frontal electromyogram (EMG) and airway resistance biofeedback have been reported as producing relaxation from the panic associated with asthma, as well as improving air flow rate.
Cardiac arrhythmias	Specific biofeedback of the electrocardiogram has permitted patients to lower the frequency of premature ventricular contractions.
Fecal incontinence and enuresis	The timing sequence of internal and external anal sphincters has been measured, using triple-lumen rectal catheters providing feedback to incontinent patients to allow them to reestablish normal bowel habits in a relatively small number of biofeedback sessions. An actual precursor of biofeedback dating to 1938 was a buzzer sounding for sleeping enuretic children at the first sign of moisture (the pad and bell).
Grand mal epilepsy	A number of electroencephalogram (EEG) biofeedback procedures have been used experimentally to suppress seizure activity prophylactically in patients not responsive to anticonvulsant medication. The procedures permit patients to enhance the sensorimotor brain wave rhythm or to normalize brain activity as computed in real-time power spectrum displays.
Hyperactivity	EEG biofeedback procedures have been used with children with attention-deficit/hyperactivity disorder to train them to reduce their motor restlessness.
Idiopathic hypertension and orthostatic hypotension	A variety of specific (direct) and nonspecific biofeedback procedures—including blood pressure feedback, galvanic skin response, and foot–hand thermal feedback combined with relaxation procedures—have been used to teach patients to increase or decrease their blood pressure. Some follow-up data indicate that the changes may persist for years and often permit the reduction or elimination of antihypertensive medications.
Migraine	The most common biofeedback strategy with classic or common vascular headaches has been thermal biofeedback from a digit accompanied by autogenic self-suggestive phrases encouraging hand warming and head cooling. The mechanism is thought to help prevent excessive cerebral artery vasoconstriction, often accompanied by an ischemic prodromal symptom, such as scintillating scotomata, followed by rebound engorgement of arteries and stretching of vessel wall pain receptors.
Myofacial and temporomandibular joint (TMJ) pain	High levels of EMG activity over the powerful muscles associated with bilateral TMJs have been decreased, using biofeedback in patients who are jaw clenchers or have bruxism.
Neuromuscular rehabilitation	Mechanical devices or an EMG measurement of muscle activity displayed to a patient increases the effectiveness of traditional therapies, as documented by relatively long clinical histories in peripheral nerve–muscle damage, spasmodic torticollis, selected cases of tardive dyskinesia, cerebral palsy, and upper motor neuron hemiplegias.
Raynaud's syndrome	Cold hands and cold feet are frequent concomitants of anxiety and also occur in Raynaud's syndrome, caused by vasospasm of arterial smooth muscle. A number of studies report that thermal feedback from the hand, an inexpensive and benign procedure compared with surgical sympathectomy, is effective in about 70% of cases of Raynaud's syndrome.
Tension headaches	Muscle contraction headaches are most frequently treated with two large active electrodes spaced on the forehead to provide visual or auditory information about the levels of muscle tension. The frontal electrode placement is sensitive to EMG activity regarding the frontalis and occipital muscles, which the patient learns to relax.

(Jacobson used the word "tenseness" rather than "tension" to emphasize the patient's role in tensing the muscles.) Once this sensation is reported, Jacobson would say, "This is your doing! What we wish is the reverse of this—simply not doing." Patients are repeatedly reminded that relaxation involves no effort. In fact "making an effort is being tense and therefore is not to relax." As the session progresses, patients are instructed to let go further and further, even past the point when the body part seems perfectly relaxed.

Patients would work in this fashion with different muscle groups, often over more than 50 sessions. For example, an entire session might be devoted to relaxing the biceps muscle. Another feature of Jacobson's method was that instructions were given tersely so they would not interfere with a patient's focus on muscle sensations; suggestions commonly used today (e.g., "*Your arm is becoming limp*") were avoided. Patients were also frequently left alone, while the therapist attended to other patients.

In psychiatry, relaxation therapy is mainly used as a component of multifaceted broad-spectrum programs. Its use in desensitization was mentioned previously. Relaxing breathing exercises are often helpful for patients with panic disorder, especially when considered to be related to hyperventilation. In the treatment of patients with anxiety disorders, relaxation can serve as an occasion-setting stimulus (i.e., as a context of safety in which other specific intervention can be confidently tried).

Later Adaptation of Progressive Muscular Relaxation

Joseph Wolpe chose progressive relaxation as a response incompatible with anxiety when designing his systematic desensitization treatment (discussed below). For this purpose, Jacobson's original method was too lengthy to be practical. Wolpe abbreviated the program to 20 minutes during the first six sessions (devoting the remainder of these sessions to other things, such as behavioral analysis). In a later modification of progressive relaxation, patients completed work with all the principal muscle groups in one session. The specific muscle groups and instructions for this type of progressive relaxation are listed in Table 24.6–2. Once patients have mastered this procedure (typically after three sessions), these groups are combined into larger groups. Finally, patients practice relaxation by recall (i.e., without tensing the muscles).

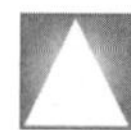

Table 24.6–2
Outline of Initial Progressive Relaxation Session, All Muscle Groups

Muscle Group	Instruction
Dominant hand and forearm	Make a tight fist, now
Dominant biceps, triceps	Make your upper arm tense by counter-posing muscles
Nondominant arm, forearm	Make a tight fist, now
Nondominant biceps	Make your upper arm tense by counter-posing muscles
Forehead	Lift eyebrows
Orbital and nose muscles	Squint and wrinkle your nose
Lower cheeks and jaws	Bite your teeth together and pull the corners of your mouth back
Neck and throat	Pull your chin toward your chest, but prevent it from happening by counter-posing muscles in front and back
Chest, shoulders, upper back	Take a deep breath, hold it, and pull the shoulder blades upward (if sitting) or backward (if supine)
Abdominal or stomach region	Make your stomach hard, as if you were going to hit yourself
Dominant thigh	Counter-pose extensors and flexors
Dominant lower leg	Dorsiflex foot
Dominant foot	Curl toes upward (not down to avoid cramps)
Nondominant thigh	Counter-pose extensors and flexors
Nondominant calf	Dorsiflex foot
Nondominant foot	Curl toes upward (not down, to avoid cramps)

Adapted from Bernstein DA, Borkovec TD. *Progressive Relaxation Training: A Manual for the Helping Professions*. Champaign, IL: Research Press; 1973.

Autogenic Training

Autogenic training is a method of self-suggestion that originated in Germany. It involves the patients directing their attention to specific bodily areas and hearing themselves think certain phrases reflecting a relaxed state. In the original German version, patients progressed through six themes over many sessions. The six areas are listed in Table 24.6–3 along with representative autogenic phrases. Autogenic relaxation is an American modification of autogenic training, in which all six areas are covered in one session.

Applied Tension

Applied tension is a technique that is the opposite of relaxation; applied tension can be used to counteract the fainting response. The treatment extends over four sessions. In the first session, patients learn to tense the muscles of the arms, legs, and torso for 10 to 15 seconds (as if they were bodybuilders). The tension is maintained long enough for a sensation of warmth to develop in the face. The patients then release the tension, but do not progress to a state of relaxation. The maneuver is repeated five times at half-minute intervals. This method can be augmented with feedback of the patient's blood pressure during the muscle contraction; increased blood pressure suggests that appropriate muscle tension was achieved. The patients continue to practice the technique five times a day. An adverse effect of treatment that sometimes develops is headache. In this case, the intensity of the muscle contraction and the frequency of treatment are reduced.

Patients with blood and injury phobia show a unique, biphasic response when exposed to a phobic stimulus. The first

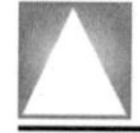

Table 24.6–3
Sample Autogenic Phrases

Theme	Examples of Self-Statements
Heaviness	"My left arm is heavy."
Warmth	"My left arm is warm."
Cardiac regulation	"My heartbeat is calm and regular."
Breathing adjustment	"It breathes me."
Solar plexus	"My solar plexus is warm."
Forehead	"My forehead is cool."

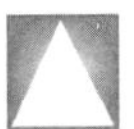

Table 24.6–4
Steps in Applied Relaxation

Technique	Instructions
Progressive relaxation	Session 1: hands, arms, face, neck, and shoulders Session 2: back, chest, stomach, breathing, hips, legs, and feet
Release-only relaxation	As with progressive relaxation, except that the tension phase is omitted; when release-only relaxation is mastered, the patient can relax within 5–7 minutes.
Cue-controlled relaxation	A stimulus—the word *relax*—is presented just before exhalation; patients focus on their breathing while already in a relaxed state; the therapist says the word *inhale* just before each inhalation and the word *relax* just before each exhalation; after approximately five cycles, the patient mentally says these words (optionally dropping the *inhale*).
Differential relaxation	Patients can remain relaxed and move at the same time by differentially keeping muscles unrelated to the movement in a relaxed state; after achieving a relaxed state, patients lift an arm or a leg or look around in the room, while keeping movements and tension in other body parts at a minimum; patients also perform differential relaxation in other settings, including sitting in different chairs, sitting at a desk while writing, talking on the phone, and walking.
Rapid relaxation	Patients relax by taking one to three breaths with slow exhalations, thinking the word *relax* before each exhalation and scanning their bodies for areas of tension; with this practice, relaxation is shortened to 20–30 seconds; patients are instructed to relax in this manner 15–20 times per day at certain predetermined events in their natural environment (e.g., when they look at a watch or make a telephone call. As a reminder, colored dots might be taped on the watch or phone. After some time, the dots are changed to a different color to keep their reminding power fresh).
Application training	Patients relax just before entering the target situation; they stay in the situation for 10–15 minutes, using their relaxation skills as a coping technique; patients may initially be accompanied by the therapist; alternatively, if the patient's problem is panic attacks or generalized anxiety, imagery or physical exercise is used to induce fearful sensations, which then are used for application training.

phase is associated with increased heart rate and blood pressure. In the second phase, however, blood pressure suddenly falls and the patient faints. To treat the problem, patients are shown a series of slides that are provocative (e.g., mutilated bodies). They are coached in identifying early warning signs of fainting, such as queasiness, cold sweats, or dizziness, and in applying the learned muscle tension response quickly, contingent on these warning signs. Patients can also perform applied tension while donating blood or watching a surgical operation. The technique of isometric tension raises blood pressure, which prevents fainting.

Applied Relaxation

Applied relaxation involves eliciting a relaxation response in the stressful situation itself. The previous discussion showed that this is not advisable right away because of the possible ironic effects of relaxation. Therefore, patients should first practice relaxation in nonstressful circumstances. The method developed by Lars-Göran Öst and coworkers in Sweden has been proven efficacious for panic disorder and generalized anxiety disorder. Establishing the relaxation response in the patient's natural environment consists of seven phases of one to two sessions each: progressive relaxation, release-only relaxation, cue-controlled relaxation, differential relaxation, rapid relaxation, application training, and maintenance. Details are provided in Table 24.6–4.

RESULTS

Biofeedback, progressive relaxation, and applied tension have been shown to be effective treatment methods for a broad range of disorders. They form one basis of behavioral medicine in which the patient changes (or learns how to change) behavior that contributes to illness. They form a basis on which many complementary and alternative medical procedures are effective (e.g., yoga and Reiki) in which relaxation is an important component. Relaxation also informs more mainstream treatments, such as hypnosis.

▲ 24.7 Cognitive Therapy

A central feature of the cognitive theory of emotional disorders is its emphasis on the psychological significance of people's beliefs about themselves, their personal world (including the people in their lives), and their future—the "cognitive triad." When people experience excessive, maladaptive emotional distress, it is linked to their problematic, stereotypic, biased interpretations pertinent to this cognitive triad of the self, the world, and the future. For example, clinically depressed patients may be prone to believe that they are incapable and helpless and to view others as being judgmental and critical and the future as being bleak and unrewarding. Similarly, patients with anxiety disorders may be apt to see themselves as highly vulnerable, others as more capable, and the future as likely to be characterized by personal disasters.

Although the patient's viewpoints are flawed and dysfunctional, they nonetheless tend to be perpetuated by cognitive processes that maintain them. Cognitive therapy is a short-term, structured therapy that uses active collaboration between patient and therapist to achieve its therapeutic goals, which are oriented toward current problems and their resolution. Cognitive therapy is used with depression, panic disorder, obsessive–compulsive disorder, personality disorders, and somatoform disorders. Therapy is usually conducted on an individual basis, although group methods are sometimes helpful. A therapist may also prescribe drugs in conjunction with therapy.

The treatment of depression can serve as a paradigm of the cognitive approach. Cognitive therapy assumes that perception and experiencing, in general, are active processes that involve both inspective and introspective data. The patient's cognitions represent a synthesis of internal and external stimuli. The way persons appraise a situation is generally evident in their cognitions (thoughts and visual images). Those cognitions constitute their stream of consciousness or phenomenal field, which reflects their configuration of themselves, their world, their past, and their future.

Alterations in the content of their underlying cognitive structures affect their affective state and behavioral pattern. Through psychological therapy, patients can become aware of their cognitive distortions. Correction of faulty dysfunctional constructs can lead to clinical improvement.

COGNITIVE THEORY OF DEPRESSION

According to the cognitive theory of depression, cognitive dysfunctions are the core of depression, and affective and physical changes, and other associated features of depression are consequences of cognitive dysfunctions. For example, apathy and low energy result from a person's expectation of failure in all areas. Similarly, paralysis of will stems from a person's pessimism and feelings of hopelessness. From a cognitive perspective, depression can be explained by the cognitive triad, which explains that negative thoughts are about the self, the world, and the future.

The goal of therapy is to alleviate depression and to prevent its recurrence by helping patients to identify and test negative cognitions, to develop alternative and more flexible schemas, and to rehearse both new cognitive and behavioral responses. Changing the way a person thinks can alleviate the psychiatric disorder.

STRATEGIES AND TECHNIQUES

Therapy is relatively short and lasts about 25 weeks. If a patient does not improve in this time, the diagnosis should be reevaluated. Maintenance therapy can be carried out over the years. As with other psychotherapies, therapists' attributes are important to successful therapy. Therapists must exude warmth, understand the life experience of each patient, and be genuine and honest with themselves and with their patients. They must be able to relate skillfully and interactively with their patients. Cognitive therapists set the agenda at the beginning of each session, assign homework to be performed between sessions, and teach new skills. Therapist and patient collaborate actively (Table 24.7–1). The three components of cognitive therapy are didactic aspects, cognitive techniques, and behavioral techniques.

Didactic Aspects

The therapy's didactic aspects include explaining to patients the cognitive triad, schemas, and faulty logic. Therapists must tell patients that they will formulate hypotheses together and test them over the course of the treatment. Cognitive therapy requires a full explanation of the relation between depression and thinking, affect, and behavior, as well as the rationale for all aspects of treatment. This explanation contrasts with psychoanalytically oriented therapies, which require little explanation.

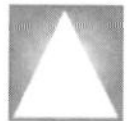

Table 24.7–1
Cognitive Psychotherapy

Goal	Identify and alter cognitive distortions that maintain symptoms
Selection criteria	Primarily used in dysthymic disorder Nonendogenous depressive disorders Symptoms not sustained by pathological family
Duration	Time-limited, usually 15–25 weeks, once-weekly meetings
Techniques	Collaborative empiricism Structured and directive Assigned readings Homework and behavioral techniques Identification of irrational beliefs and automatic thoughts Identification of attitudes and assumptions underlying negatively biased thoughts

Reprinted from Ursano RJ, Silberman EK. Individual psychotherapies. In: Talbott JA, Hales RE, Yudofsky SC, eds. *The American Psychiatric Press Textbook of Psychiatry*. Washington, DC: American Psychiatric Press; 1988:872.

Cognitive Techniques

The therapy's cognitive approach includes four processes: eliciting automatic thoughts, testing automatic thoughts, identifying maladaptive underlying assumptions, and testing the validity of maladaptive assumptions.

Eliciting Automatic Thoughts. Automatic thoughts, also called *cognitive distortions,* are cognitions that intervene between external events and a person's emotional reaction to the event. For example, the belief that "people will laugh at me when they see how badly I bowl" is an automatic thought that occurs to someone who has been asked to go bowling and responds negatively. Another example is the thought "She doesn't like me" when someone passes in the hall without saying "Hello." Every psychopathological disorder has its own specific cognitive profile of distorted thought, which, if known, provides a framework for specific cognitive interventions (Table 24.7–2).

Testing Automatic Thoughts. Acting as a teacher, a therapist helps a patient test the validity of automatic thoughts. The goal is to encourage the patient to reject inaccurate or exaggerated automatic thoughts after careful examination. Patients often blame themselves when things that are outside their control go awry. The therapist reviews the entire situation with the patient and helps reassign the blame or cause of the unpleasant events. Generating alternative explanations for events is another way of undermining inaccurate and distorted automatic thoughts.

Identifying Maladaptive Assumptions. As the patient and therapist continue to identify automatic thoughts, patterns usually become apparent. The patterns represent rules or maladaptive general assumptions that guide a patient's life. Samples of such rules are "In order to be happy, I must be perfect" and "If anyone doesn't like me, I'm not lovable." Such rules inevitably lead to disappointments and failure and, ultimately, to depression.

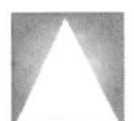

Table 24.7–2
Cognitive Profile of Psychiatric Disorders

Disorder	Core Belief
Depressive disorder	Negative view of self, experience, and future
Hypomanic episode	Inflated view of self, experience, and future
Anxiety disorders	Fear of physical or psychological danger
Panic disorder	Catastrophic misinterpretation of bodily and mental experiences
Phobias	Danger in specific, avoidable situations
Paranoid personality disorder	Negative bias, interference, and so forth by others
Conversion disorder	Concept of motor or sensory abnormality
Obsessive–compulsive disorder	Repeated warning or doubting about safety and repetitive acts to ward off threat
Suicidal behavior	Hopelessness and deficit in problem solving
Anorexia nervosa	Fear of being fat or unshapely
Hypochondriasis	Attribution of serious medical disorder

Courtesy of Aaron Beck, M.D., and A. John Rush, M.D.

Testing the Validity of Maladaptive Assumptions. Testing the accuracy of maladaptive assumptions is similar to testing the validity of automatic thoughts. In a particularly effective test, therapists ask patients to defend the validity of their assumptions. For example, patients may state that they should always work up to their potential, and a therapist may ask "*Why is that so important to you?*"

A woman presented for therapy with anger control problems. She had sent a slew of hostile voice mail and e-mail messages to a colleague, had alienated her neighbors with her complaints about noise, and had been asked to leave her bowling league after two physical altercations with members of other teams. A careful review of the patient's thoughts and beliefs surrounding these situations revealed a common denominator of a sense of *mistrust* and *entitlement.* In each situation, she believed that the persons who were the objects of her anger had gone out of their way to mistreat her. Furthermore, she had an exaggerated sense of self-importance represented by beliefs such as, "Nobody has the right to treat me that way," "I shouldn't have to deal with these people and their stupidity," and "I have to show them they can't ever push me around." To this patient, her anger was justified, as she was trying to defend herself from the misbehavior of others. However, to the outside observer, the patient was a "loose cannon" who took offense at the drop of a hat and whose behavior was outrageous and indefensible. In therapy, the patient at first was not open to viewing her anger problem in the manner just described. However, as she learned to recognize the activation of her schemas of *mistrust* and *entitlement,* she became more willing to consider ways in which she could modify her viewpoints and behaviors. This positive change was facilitated by the therapist's empathic responses to the patient's more credible stories of mistreatment she had received from her family, whose abusive behavior gave her the message that she should never trust anyone and that she should never put up with being mistreated again. *(Courtesy of C.F. Newman, Ph.D., and A.T. Beck, M.D.)*

Behavioral Techniques

Behavioral and cognitive techniques go hand in hand; behavioral techniques test and change maladaptive and inaccurate cognitions. The overall purposes of such techniques are to help patients understand the inaccuracy of their cognitive assumptions and learn new strategies and ways of dealing with issues.

Among the behavioral techniques in cognitive therapy are scheduling activities, mastery and pleasure, graded task assignments, cognitive rehearsal, self-reliance training, role playing, and diversion techniques. One of the first things done in therapy is to schedule activities on an hourly basis. Patients keep records of the activities and review them with the therapist. In addition to scheduling activities, patients are asked to rate the amount of mastery and pleasure their activities bring them. Patients are often surprised to learn that they have much more mastery of activities and enjoy them more than they had thought.

To simplify the situation and allow mini accomplishments, therapists often break tasks into subtasks, as in graded task assignments, to show patients that they can succeed. In cognitive rehearsal, patients imagine and rehearse the various steps in meeting and mastering a challenge.

Patients (especially inpatients) are encouraged to become self-reliant by doing such simple things as making their own beds, doing their own shopping, and preparing their own meals. This process is called self-reliance training. Role playing is a particularly powerful and useful technique to elicit automatic thoughts and to learn new behaviors. Diversion techniques are useful in helping patients get through difficult times and include physical activity, social contact, work, play, and visual imagery.

Imagery or thought stoppage can treat impulsive or obsessive behavior. For instance, patients imagine a stop sign with a police officer nearby or another image that evokes inhibition at the same time that they recognize an impulse or obsession that is alien to the ego. Similarly, obesity can be treated by having patients visualize themselves as thin, athletic, trim, and well muscled, and then training them to evoke this image whenever they have an urge to eat. Hypnosis or autogenic training can enhance such imagery. In a technique called guided imagery, therapists encourage patients to have fantasies that can be interpreted as wish fulfillments or attempts to master disturbing affects or impulses.

EFFICACY

Cognitive therapy can be used alone in the treatment of mild to moderate depressive disorders or in conjunction with antidepressant medication for major depressive disorder. Studies have clearly shown that cognitive therapy is effective and in some cases is superior or equal to medication alone. It is one of the most useful psychotherapeutic interventions currently available for depressive disorders, and it shows promise in the treatment of other disorders.

Cognitive therapy has also been studied as a way of increasing compliance with lithium (Eskalith) prescription by patients with bipolar I disorder and as an adjunct in treating withdrawal from heroin. Table 24.7–3 outlines Beck's criteria for determining when cognitive therapy is indicated.

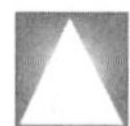

Table 24.7–3
Indications for Cognitive Therapy

Criteria that justify the administration of cognitive therapy alone:
Failure to respond to adequate trials of two antidepressants
Partial response to adequate dosages of antidepressants
Failure to respond or only a partial response to other psychotherapies
Diagnosis of dysthymic disorder
Variable mood reactive to environmental events
Variable mood that correlates with negative cognitions
Mild somatoform disorders (sleep, appetite, weight, libidinal)
Adequate reality testing (i.e., no hallucinations or delusions), span of concentration, and memory function
Inability to tolerate medication effects or evidence that excessive risk is associated with pharmacotherapy
Features that suggest cognitive therapy alone is not indicated:
Evidence of coexisting schizophrenia, dementia, substance-related disorders, mental retardation
Patient has medical illness or is taking medication that is likely to cause depression
Obvious memory impairment or poor reality testing (hallucinations, delusions)
History of manic episode (bipolar I disorder)
History of family member who responded to antidepressant
History of family member with bipolar I disorder
Absence of precipitating or exacerbating environmental stresses
Little evidence of cognitive distortions
Presence of severe somatoform disorders (e.g., pain disorder)
Indications for combined therapies (medication plus cognitive therapy):
Partial or no response to trial of cognitive therapy alone
Partial but incomplete response to adequate pharmacotherapy alone
Poor compliance with medication regimen
Historical evidence of chronic maladaptive functioning with depressive syndrome on intermittent basis
Presence of severe somatoform disorders and marked cognitive distortions (e.g., hopelessness)
Impaired memory and concentration and marked psychomotor difficulty
Major depressive disorder with suicidal danger
History of first-degree relative who responded to antidepressants
History of manic episode in relative or patient

Adapted from Beck AT, Rush AJ, Shaw BF, Emery G. *Cognitive Therapy of Depression*. New York: Guilford; 1979:42.

▲ 24.8 Behavior Therapy

The term *behavior* in *behavior therapy* refers to a person's observable actions and responses. Behavior therapy involves changing the behavior of patients to reduce dysfunction and to improve quality of life. Behavior therapy includes a methodology, referred to as *behavior analysis,* for the strategic selection of behaviors to change, and a technology to bring about behavior change, such as modifying antecedents or consequences or giving instructions. Behavior therapy has not only influenced mental health care, but, under the rubric of behavioral medicine, it has also made inroads into other medical specialties.

Behavior therapy represents clinical applications of the principles developed in learning theory. Behavioral psychology, or behaviorism, arose in the early 20th century in reaction to the method of introspection that dominated psychology at the time. John B. Watson, the father of behaviorism, had initially studied animal psychology. This background made it a small conceptual leap to argue that psychology should concern itself only with publicly observable phenomena (i.e., overt behavior). According to behavioristic thinking, because mental content is not publicly observable, it cannot be subjected to rigorous scientific inquiry. Consequently, behaviorists developed a focus on overt behaviors and their environmental influences.

Today, different behavioral schools continue to share a focus on verifiable behavior. Behavioral views differ from cognitive views in holding that physical, rather than mental, events control behavior. According to behaviorism, mental phenomena or speculations about them are of little or no scientific interest.

HISTORY

As early as the 1920s, scattered reports about the application of learning principles to the treatment of behavioral disorders began to appear, but they had little effect on the mainstream of psychiatry and clinical psychology. Not until the 1960s did behavior therapy emerge as a systematic and comprehensive approach to psychiatric (behavioral) disorders; at that time, it arose independently on three continents. Joseph Wolpe and his colleagues in Johannesburg, South Africa, used Pavlovian techniques to produce and eliminate experimental neuroses in cats. From this research, Wolpe developed systematic desensitization, the prototype of many current behavioral procedures for the treatment of maladaptive anxiety produced by identifiable stimuli in the environment. At about the same time, a group at the Institute of Psychiatry of the University of London, particularly Hans Jurgen Eysenck and M. B. Shapiro, stressed the importance of an empirical, experimental approach to understanding and treating individual patients, using controlled, single-case experimental paradigms and modern learning theory. The third origin of behavior therapy was work inspired by the research of Harvard psychologist B. F. Skinner. Skinner's students began to apply his operant-conditioning technology, developed in animal-conditioning laboratories, to human beings in clinical settings.

SYSTEMATIC DESENSITIZATION

Developed by Wolpe, systematic desensitization is based on the behavioral principle of counterconditioning, whereby a person overcomes maladaptive anxiety elicited by a situation or an object by approaching the feared situation gradually, in a psychophysiological state that inhibits anxiety. In systematic desensitization, patients attain a state of complete relaxation and are then exposed to the stimulus that elicits the anxiety response. The negative reaction of anxiety is inhibited by the relaxed state, a process called *reciprocal inhibition.* Rather than using actual situations or objects that elicit fear, patients and therapists prepare a graded list or hierarchy of anxiety-provoking scenes associated with a patient's fears. The learned relaxation state and the anxiety-provoking scenes are systematically paired in treatment. Thus, systematic desensitization consists of three steps: relaxation training, hierarchy construction, and desensitization of the stimulus.

Relaxation Training

Relaxation produces physiological effects opposite to those of anxiety: slow heart rate, increased peripheral blood flow, and neuromuscular stability. A variety of relaxation methods have been developed. Some, such as yoga and Zen, have been known for centuries. Most methods use so-called progressive relaxation, developed by the psychiatrist Edmund Jacobson. Patients relax major muscle groups in a fixed order, beginning with the small muscle groups of the feet and working cephalad or vice versa. Some clinicians use hypnosis to facilitate relaxation or use tape-recorded exercise to allow patients to practice relaxation on their own. Mental imagery is a relaxation method in which patients are instructed to imagine themselves in a place associated with pleasant, relaxed memories. Such images allow patients to enter a relaxed state or experience (as Herbert Benson termed it) the *relaxation response.*

The physiological changes that take place during relaxation are the opposite of those induced by the adrenergic stress responses that are part of many emotions. Muscle tension, respiration rate, heart rate, blood pressure, and skin conductance decrease. Finger temperature and blood flow to the finger usually increase. Relaxation increases respiratory heart rate variability, an index of parasympathetic tone.

Hierarchy Construction

When constructing a hierarchy, clinicians determine all the conditions that elicit anxiety, and then patients create a hierarchy list of 10 to 12 scenes in order of increasing anxiety. For example, an acrophobic hierarchy may begin with a patient's imagining standing near a window on the second floor and end with being on the roof of a 20-story building, leaning on a guard rail and looking straight down.

Desensitization of the Stimulus

In the final step, called *desensitization,* patients proceed systematically through the list from the least to the most anxiety-provoking scene while in a deeply relaxed state. The rate at which patients progress through the list is determined by their responses to the stimuli. When patients can vividly imagine the most anxiety-provoking scene of the hierarchy with equanimity, they experience little anxiety in the corresponding real-life situation.

Adjunctive Use of Drugs. Clinicians have used various drugs to hasten relaxation, but drugs should be used cautiously and only by clinicians trained and experienced in potential adverse effects. Either the ultrarapidly acting barbiturate sodium methohexital (Brevital) or diazepam (Valium) is given intravenously in subanesthetic doses. If the procedural details are followed carefully, almost all patients find the procedure pleasant, with few unpleasant side effects. The advantages of pharmacological desensitization are that preliminary training in relaxation can be shortened, almost all patients can relax adequately, and the treatment itself seems to proceed more rapidly than without the drugs. Best practices require that these procedures be conducted with an anesthetist in attendance.

Indications. Systematic desensitization works best in cases of a clearly identifiable anxiety-provoking stimulus. Phobias, obsessions, compulsions, and certain sexual disorders have been treated successfully with this technique.

THERAPEUTIC-GRADED EXPOSURE

Therapeutic-graded exposure is similar to systematic desensitization, except that relaxation training is not involved and treatment is usually carried out in a real-life context. This means that the individual must be brought in contact with (i.e., be exposed to) the warning stimulus to learn firsthand that no dangerous consequences will ensue. Exposure is graded according to a hierarchy. Patients afraid of cats, for example, might progress from looking at a picture of a cat to holding one.

FLOODING

Flooding (sometimes called *implosion*) is similar to graded exposure in that it involves exposing the patient to the feared object in vivo; however, there is no hierarchy. Flooding is based on the premise that escaping from an anxiety-provoking experience reinforces the anxiety through conditioning. Thus, clinicians can extinguish the anxiety and prevent the conditioned avoidance behavior by not allowing patients to escape the situation. Clinicians encourage patients to confront feared situations directly, without a gradual buildup, as in systematic desensitization or graded exposure. No relaxation exercises are used, as in systematic desensitization. Patients experience fear, which gradually subsides after a time. The success of the procedure depends on having patients remain in the fear-generating situation until they are calm and feel a sense of mastery. Prematurely withdrawing from the situation or prematurely terminating the fantasized scene is equivalent to an escape, which then reinforces both the conditioned anxiety and the avoidance behavior and produces the opposite of the desired effect. In a variant, called *imaginal flooding,* the feared object or situation is confronted only in the imagination, not in real life. Many patients refuse flooding because of the psychological discomfort involved. It is also contraindicated when intense anxiety would be hazardous to a patient (e.g., those with heart disease or fragile psychological adaptation). The technique works best with specific phobias. An example of in vivo flooding is presented in the case study.

The patient was a 33-year-old woman with social fears of eating in public. In particular, she was afraid of being observed by others when chewing and swallowing, particularly at dinner parties. A contrived situation was arranged in which the patient came to the session with a prepared meal and drink. She entered a conference room in which five persons in professional attire were already seated along a table. The patient was instructed to eat her meal in front of these individuals. Between bites, she was instructed to look at them often, and they had been instructed to avoid staring contests. She was not to distract herself from her anxiety symptoms. She was to eat her meal slowly, paying attention to the behavior of the observers and to her anxiety symptoms (e.g., dry mouth or difficulty swallowing). No conversation between the patient and observers was permitted. The observers would look at her and observe her chewing and swallowing behaviors, at times writing comments in a notebook. Occasionally, observers would communicate by whispering to each other, exchanging written notes, or giving knowing glances and smiles.

The only other communication occurred between the patient and therapist, and this was limited to the patient providing her subjective units of distress rating. The session lasted 90 minutes. **Note:** This situation may seem quite traumatizing. Because the exposure session is long and continues until ratings decline, the patient becomes desensitized. *(Courtesy of Rolf G. Jacob, M.D., and William H. Pelham, M.D.)*

PARTICIPANT MODELING

In participant modeling, patients learn a new behavior by imitation, primarily by observation, without having to perform the behavior until they feel ready. Just as irrational fears can be acquired by learning, they can be unlearned by observing a fearless model confront the feared object. The technique has been useful with phobic children who are placed with other children of their own age and sex who approach the feared object or situation. With adults, a therapist may describe the feared activity in a calm manner that a patient can identify. Or, the therapist may act out the process of mastering the feared activity with a patient. Sometimes a hierarchy of activities is established, with the least anxiety-provoking activity being dealt with first. The participant-modeling technique has been used successfully with agoraphobia by having a therapist accompany a patient into the feared situation. In a variant of the procedure, called *behavior rehearsal,* real-life problems are acted out under a therapist's observation or direction.

The following is a self-report by a patient with a contamination phobia, who is afraid to touch objects for fear of being infected or contaminated. She describes her reactions.

[The therapist] started touching everything very slowly. I was told to follow behind and touch everything she touched. It was like we were spreading the contamination. She touched doorknobs, light switches, walls, pictures, and woodwork. She opened drawers in each bedroom and touched the contents. She opened closets and touched clothes hanging on the rods. She touched the towels and sheets in the linen closet. She went through the children's rooms, touching dolls, stuffed animals, models, Star Wars figures, Transformers, and books.

[The therapist] kept talking to me quietly and calmly all the time we went along. I had been anxious when we started, but as we continued, my anxiety level decreased. At one point, when I had begun to think the worst was over, she pointed to the attic door and said we were going inside. I said, "No, that's where the mice were." She told me I didn't want to have a place in my home that was off limits. I agreed but became very anxious. It was very hard for me to go inside. I began touching the boxes too, but I was very upset. Then, she put her hands down on the floor and wanted me to do the same. I said, "I can't. I just can't." [The therapist] said, "Yes you can."

[The therapist] spent several hours with me that day. Before she left, she made a list of things for me to do by myself. Twice a day I was to go through the house touching everything the way she had done with me. I was to invite a friend of mine who had a pet to come and visit and also friends of my children who had pets. *(Courtesy of Rolf G. Jacobs, M.D., and William H. Pelham, M.D.)*

EXPOSURE TO STIMULI PRESENTED IN VIRTUAL REALITY

Advances in computer technology have made it possible to present environmental cues in virtual reality for exposure treatment. Beneficial effects have been reported with virtual reality exposure of patients with height phobia, fear of flying, spider phobia, and claustrophobia. Much experimental work is being done in the field. One model uses an avatar of the patient walking through a crowded supermarket filled with other avatars (including one of the therapists) as a way of conquering agoraphobia.

ASSERTIVENESS TRAINING

Assertiveness is defined as assertive behavior that enables a person to act in his or her own best interest, to stand up for herself or himself without undue anxiety, to express honest feelings comfortably, and to exercise personal rights without denying the rights of others.

Two types of situations frequently call for assertive behaviors: (1) setting limits on pushy friends or relatives and (2) commercial situations, such as countering a sales pitch or being persistent when returning defective merchandise. Early assertiveness training programs tended to define specific behaviors as assertive or nonassertive. For example, individuals were encouraged to assert themselves if somebody got in front of them in a supermarket checkout line. Increasing attention is now given to context, that is, what would be assertive behavior in this situation depends on circumstances.

SOCIAL SKILLS TRAINING

The negative symptoms in patients with schizophrenia constitute behavioral deficits that go beyond difficulties with assertiveness. These patients have inadequate expressive behaviors and inappropriate stimulus control of their social behaviors (i.e., they do not pick up social cues). Similarly, patients with depression often experience a lack of social reinforcement because of a lack of social skills, and social skills training has been found

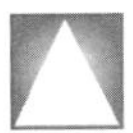

Table 24.8–1
Daily Monitoring of Rituals

Each day, record the amount of time spent doing rituals in the morning, afternoon, and evening							
	Tuesday	**Wednesday**	**Thursday**	**Friday**	**Saturday**	**Sunday**	**Monday**
Morning	2 hours	1.5 hours					
Afternoon	3 hours	2 hours					
Evening	1.5 hours	3 hours					

Once a day, record the following details about an episode of rituals:						
Day	**Time**	**Situation**	**Feelings**	**Thoughts (Obsessions)**	**Type of Ritual**	**Feelings after Rituals**
Saturday	8 AM	Finished breakfast	Afraid Scared Worried	Shouldn't have thrown away my napkin Might have left something under my plate What if I lost something important?	Checking through trash Looking under plate Staring to see if I lost something	Better For now, I think I have not lost anything
Sunday	2 PM	At the store; signed a check	Worried Anxious	Did I sign my name correctly? Did I write the correct amount? What if I give them the check and it is wrong?	Staring at the check Tracing the lines I wrote Standing there	Anxious because I couldn't finish checking

Courtesy of M. A. Stanley, Ph.D., and D. C. Beidel, Ph.D.

to be efficacious for depression. Patients with social phobia similarly often have not acquired adolescents' social skills. In fact, their social defensive behaviors (e.g., avoiding eye contact, making brief statements, and minimizing self-disclosure) increase the probability of the rejection that they fear.

Social skills training programs for patients with schizophrenia cover skills in the following areas: conversation, conflict management, assertiveness, community living, friendship and dating, work and vocation, and medication management. Each of these skills has several components. For example, assertiveness skills include making requests, refusing requests, making complaints, responding to complaints, expressing unpleasant feelings, asking for information, making apologies, expressing fear, and refusing alcohol and street drugs. Each component involves specific steps. For example, conflict management includes skills in negotiating, compromising, tactful disagreeing, responding to untrue accusations, and leaving overly stressful situations. A situation in which conflict management skills might be used is when the patient and a friend decide to go to a movie and their choice of movie differs.

Negotiating and compromising, for example, involves the following steps:

1. Explain one's viewpoint briefly.
2. Listen to the other person's viewpoint.
3. Repeat the other person's viewpoint.
4. Suggest a compromise.

At his initial appointment, Phillip described very serious symptoms of obsessive-compulsive disorder (OCD). He was 23 years old and living at home because he was no longer able to work or go to school. His days were consumed with behaviors related to checking, repeating, and hoarding. Phillip was unable to throw away anything—he saved junk mail, used tissues and napkins, old papers and magazines, and any kind of receipt for fear that he might lose something important. Phillip spent many hours checking his trash, his car, and his home to be sure that he had not thrown away anything important. He also checked everything he wrote (e.g., checks, school exams and papers, letters and e-mails) to be sure that he had not made a mistake, and he read and reread books, magazines, and articles to be sure he understood the written material adequately. Phillip worried constantly that he had done something wrong and would disappoint his parents. He was also depressed because he was unable to function well in life, and he had tremendous social anxiety that had plagued him for many years, making it difficult to make and keep friends.

By the end of Phillip's second session, his therapist was beginning to get a good idea of the general nature and severity of his symptoms and some of the maintaining factors. However, to plan the treatment in more detail and to get a better idea of how the symptoms occurred during his daily life, she asked Phillip to keep daily records over the next week using a form that she had prepared for him. The form had a place for recording the amount of time he spent doing rituals each morning, afternoon, and evening, as well as another place to record more details about at least one episode of rituals each day (e.g., what was happening before, during, and after the rituals; see Table 24.8–1).

Phillip's therapist determined that his difficulties with obsessions, rituals, depression, and social fears reflected a core fear of negative evaluation. Phillip was overly concerned with making mistakes, being imperfect, and disappointing others. Even as a child, Phillip was concerned about not doing well enough, and he had difficulty making friends for fear that others would not like him. His parents, who were highly anxious, provided much adulation when Phillip did things well (e.g., learned to ride a bike, got good grades in school), and they spent much time instructing him about how to improve his performance when an activity or grade was not perfect. As Phillip took on more responsibility at school and with part-time work, he became more concerned about doing things right. He learned that going back and checking his work relieved his anxiety. He also learned that saving his papers for future checking reassured him that he would be able to fix any unrecognized mistakes at a later time. His parents helped him to reduce his anxiety when he was uncertain about his work by reassuring him that he was doing okay. As Phillip progressed from elementary school to junior high school to high school, his workload and anxiety gradually increased, but he was able to manage things with some moderate checking and saving. When he began attending college, however, the workload increased extensively, and he found himself doing even more checking and hoarding to reduce his fears about making mistakes. Phillip began to feel that these behaviors were getting out of control, but he could not stop them. He had to check and recheck to be sure that he was not making mistakes. The cycle of anxiety-ritual-reduced anxiety was so powerfully reinforcing that he could not stop. He needed help to break this cycle and to address his persistent fear of negative evaluation.

Phillip's therapist decided to begin treatment with a course of exposure and response prevention (ERP) to get his obsessions and rituals under control and begin to address his core fear of making mistakes and being evaluated negatively. Given that Phillip's depression had grown from the disability associated with his OCD, the therapist expected that a successful course of ERP might also help to reduce his depressive symptoms. ERP for Phillip began with a home visit, where the therapist helped him to complete common daily activities with adherence to his RP plan, which included the following:

- ▲ No more checking: After eating, leave the table immediately without inspecting your plate and the surrounding areas (including under the table and chair) for lost items. Leave the restroom immediately after using it, without checking the toilet, trash, and sink for lost items. When leaving the car, no more checking of seats, floors, and windows. Write everything (papers, checks, etc.) only once; no checking to be sure that letters and words are correct.
- ▲ No more repeating. No more rereading books. No staring repeatedly at items to ensure that nothing is lost.
- ▲ No more saving. Throw tissues away immediately after using. Discard trash and junk mail immediately. Do not look into the trash can for lost items.

Phillip's parents also were asked to stop reassuring him and to discontinue doing rituals for him. This was a very difficult session for Phillip and his family, but they understood the logic of ERP, and they were willing to try anything.

For the next 3 weeks, Phillip and his therapist met three times a week to conduct in vivo exposure sessions that helped him to face his core fears. For many of these sessions, Phillip was asked to bring hoarded items from home and to discard all unnecessary items during the therapy session. At first, this created tremendous anxiety, but over time, Phillip was able to throw things away with less fear of losing something important. He also developed the ability to conduct self-directed exposure at home. Other exposure sessions involved writing letters and mailing them without checking, reading passages from magazines and books only once, and sorting through junk mail to make quick decisions about what to save or discard. As Phillip was able to take on more responsibility for home-based exposure, session frequency decreased to two times per week, and then to once per week. After 3 months of treatment, Phillip's scores on the YBOCS (Yale–Brown Obsessive-Compulsive Scale) and BDI (Beck Depression Inventory) had decreased to 20 and 19, respectively, demonstrating significant improvement in obsessive-compulsive symptoms and depression. His SPAI (Social Phobia and Anxiety Inventory) score, however, remained relatively unchanged, suggesting that he was still experiencing significant social anxiety.

Next, while Phillip worked on maintaining the gains he had made following ERP, he and his therapist conducted some role plays to evaluate his social skills. It was apparent that Phillip had extreme difficulty with initiating and maintaining conversations. His eye contact also was quite poor in social interactions. Thus, the therapist devised a plan for teaching and practicing new skills, which also involved additional exposure to Phillip's core fears as he was asked to resume contact with old friends and identify activities where he could meet new people. He practiced new behaviors first in session with his therapist and then developed a hierarchy of feared social situations in which he could practice his new behaviors. These practice exercises also involved a form of exposure as Phillip was asked to make social contact, which produced fears of negative evaluation. After another 3 months of treatment focused on social skills training (and associated exposure), Phillip's scores on the YBOCS and BDI had decreased further (YBOCS = 15; BDI = 13), and his SPAI score had decreased to 100. Phillip had gone back to school to take one class, he was spending small amounts of time with old friends, and he was volunteering a few hours each week at his church. *(Courtesy of M. A. Stanley, Ph.D., and D. C. Beidel, Ph.D.)*

AVERSION THERAPY

When a noxious stimulus (punishment) is presented immediately after a specific behavioral response, theoretically, the response is eventually inhibited and extinguished. Many types of noxious stimuli are used: electric shocks, substances that induce vomiting, corporal punishment, and social disapproval. The negative stimulus is paired with the behavior, which is thereby suppressed. The unwanted behavior may disappear after a series of such sequences. Aversion therapy has been used for alcohol abuse, paraphilias, and other behaviors with impulsive or compulsive qualities, but this therapy is controversial for many reasons. For example, punishment does not always lead to the expected decreased response and can sometimes be positively reinforcing.

EYE MOVEMENT DESENSITIZATION AND REPROCESSING

Saccadic eye movements are rapid oscillations of the eyes that occur when a person tracks an object that is moved back and forth across the line of vision. A few studies have demonstrated that inducing saccades while a person is imagining or thinking about an anxiety-producing event can yield a positive thought or image that results in decreased anxiety. Eye movement desensitization and reprocessing has been used in posttraumatic stress disorders and phobias.

POSITIVE REINFORCEMENT

When a behavioral response is followed by a generally rewarding event, such as food, avoidance of pain, or praise, it tends to be strengthened and to occur more frequently than before the reward. This principle has been applied in a variety of situations. On inpatient hospital wards, patients with mental disorders receive a reward for performing a desired behavior, such as tokens that they can use to purchase luxury items or certain privileges. The process, known as *token economy,* has successfully altered behavior. Table 24.8–2 gives a summary of some clinical applications of behavior therapy.

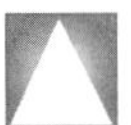

Table 24.8–2
Some Common Clinical Applications of Behavior Therapy

Disorder	Comments
Agoraphobia	Graded exposure and flooding can reduce the fear of being in crowded places. About 60% of patients so treated improve. In some cases, the spouse can serve as the model while accompanying the patient into the fear situation; however, the patient cannot get a secondary gain by keeping the spouse nearby and displaying symptoms.
Alcohol dependence	Aversion therapy in which the alcohol-dependent patient is made to vomit (by adding an emetic to the alcohol) every time a drink is ingested is effective in treating alcohol dependence. Disulfiram (Antabuse) can be given to alcohol-dependent patients when they are alcohol free. Such patients are warned of the severe physiological consequences of drinking (e.g., nausea, vomiting, hypotension, collapse) with disulfiram in the system.
Anorexia nervosa	Observe eating behavior; contingency management; record weight
Bulimia nervosa	Record bulimic episodes; log moods
Hyperventilation	Hyperventilation test; controlled breathing; direct observation
Other phobias	Systematic desensitization has been effective in treating phobias, such as fears of heights, animals, and flying. Social skills training has also been used for shyness and fear of other people.
Paraphilias	Electric shocks or other noxious stimuli can be applied at the time of a paraphilic impulse, and eventually the impulse subsides. Shocks can be administered by either the therapist or the patient. The results are satisfactory but must be reinforced at regular intervals.
Schizophrenia	The token economy procedure, in which tokens are awarded for desirable behavior and can be used to buy ward privileges, has been useful in treating inpatients with schizophrenia. Social skills training teaches patients with schizophrenia how to interact with others in a socially acceptable way so that negative feedback is eliminated. In addition, the aggressive behavior of some patients with schizophrenia can be diminished through those methods.
Sexual dysfunctions	Sex therapy, developed by William Masters and Virginia Johnson, is a behavior therapy technique used for various sexual dysfunctions, especially male erectile disorder, orgasm disorders, and premature ejaculation. It uses relaxation, desensitization, and graded exposure as the primary techniques.
Shy bladder	Inability to void in a public bathroom; relaxation exercises
Type A behavior	Physiological assessment, muscle relaxation, and biofeedback (on electromyogram [EMG])

Charles was a 70-year-old retired business executive. Throughout his life, his work consumed him. Although he married and had a family, his job was his primary focus. He went to the office early and came home late. He enjoyed what he did—it was stimulating and made him feel important and useful. But as he got older, his performance was not what it used to be, and he decided it was time to retire. However, his mood was pretty low when he no longer had a job. He did not have the energy to get more involved in his church or to develop other hobbies, so he sat around all day, without any social contacts. His wife and best friend encouraged him to go talk to someone. The therapist suggested that they try behavioral activation. Charles was somewhat skeptical, as it seemed too simple, but he needed to do something. The therapist spent some time with Charles talking about the kinds of activities that used to make him feel good and some of the things he used to enjoy. They then put together a list of things he might be able do—even if he did not feel much like it—just to see what would happen. The list included looking for volunteer work where he could use his job skills, spending more time with his wife in some of the activities they once had enjoyed (e.g., watching movies, taking walks), and rejuvenating an old hobby from his college days—fishing. Charles initially agreed to do some easy activities—go to one movie a week, take one walk a week, and contact his church activity leader about possible volunteer activities. He was surprised to find that even these "baby steps" helped him feel better. He had the chance to talk with other people and began to see that even in retirement, he could find useful and fun things to do. *(Courtesy of M. A. Stanley, Ph.D., and D. C. Beidel, Ph.D.)*

RESULTS

Behavior therapy has been used successfully for a variety of disorders (Table 24.8–2) and can be easily taught (Table 24.8–3). It requires less time than other therapies and is less expensive to

Table 24.8–3
Social Skills Competence Checklist of Therapist–Trainer Behaviors

1. Actively helps the patient set and elicit specific interpersonal goals.
2. Promotes favorable expectations, a therapeutic orientation, and motivation before role playing begins.
3. Assists the patient in building possible scenes in terms of "What emotion or communication?" "Who is the interpersonal target?" "Where and when?"
4. Structures the role playing by setting the scene and assigning roles to the patient and surrogates.
5. Engages the patient in behavioral rehearsal—getting the patient to role-play with others.
6. Uses self or other group members in modeling appropriate alternatives for the patient.
7. Prompts and cues the patient during the role playing.
8. Uses an active style of training through coaching, shadowing, being physically out of a seat, and closely monitoring and supporting the patient.
9. Gives the patient positive feedback for specific verbal and nonverbal behavioral skills.
10. Identifies the patient's specific verbal and nonverbal behavioral deficits or excesses and suggests constructive alternatives.
11. Ignores or suppresses inappropriate and interfering behavior.
12. Shapes behavioral improvements in small, attainable increments.
13. Solicits from the patient or suggests an alternative behavior for a problem situation that can be used and practiced during the behavioral rehearsal or role playing.
14. Evaluates deficits in social perception and problem solving and remedies them.
15. Gives specific attainable and functional homework assignments.

Courtesy of Robert Paul Liberman, M.D., and Jeffrey Bedell, Ph.D.

administer. Although useful for circumscribed behavioral symptoms, the method cannot be used to treat global areas of dysfunction (e.g., neurotic conflicts, personality disorders). Controversy continues between behaviorists and psychoanalysts, which is epitomized by Eysenck's statement: "Learning theory regards neurotic symptoms as simply learned habits; there is no neurosis underlying the symptoms, but merely the symptom itself. Get rid of the symptom and you have eliminated the neurosis." Analytically oriented theorists have criticized behavior therapy by noting that simple symptom removal can lead to symptom substitution. When symptoms are not viewed as consequences of inner conflicts and the core cause of the symptoms is not addressed or altered, the result is the production of new symptoms. Whether this occurs remains open to question, however.

BEHAVIORAL MEDICINE

Behavioral medicine uses the concepts and methods described above to treat a variety of physical diseases. Emphasis is placed on the role of stress and its influence on the body, particularly on the endocrine system. Attempts to relieve stress are made with the expectation that either the disease state will lessen or the patient's ability to tolerate the disease state will strengthen.

One study measured the effects of a behavioral medicine program on symptoms of AIDS. The treatment group received training in biofeedback, guided imagery, and hypnosis. Results included significant decreases in fever, fatigue, pain, headache, nausea, and insomnia and increased vigor and hardiness.

Another study of immunological and psychological outcomes of a stress reduction program was conducted with patients with malignant melanoma. Results included significant increases in large granular lymphocytes (defined as CD57 with Leu-7) and natural killer (NK) cells (defined as CD16 with Leu-II and CD56 with NKHI), along with indications of increased NK cytotoxic activity. Also noted were significantly lower levels of psychological distress and higher levels of positive coping methods in comparison with patients who were not part of the group.

Many other applications of behavior therapy are used in medical care. In general, most patients feel they benefit from such interventions, especially in their ability to cope with chronic illness.

▲ 24.9 Hypnosis

The concept of hypnosis conjures up myriad perceptions among clinicians and the lay public. Even the term *hypnosis* can be misleading, coming as it does from the Greek root *hypnos* (meaning "sleep"). In reality, hypnosis is not sleep. It is more likely a complex process that requires alert, focused, and receptive attention. Hypnosis is a powerful means of directing innate capabilities of imagination, imagery, and attention. Many also believe the myth that the clinician projects the hypnotic trance onto the patient or has the power to influence the patient. In reality it is the patient who has the hypnotic gift, and the clinician's role is to assess the patient's capacity to capitalize on this asset and to help the patient discover and use it effectively. Patient motivation, personality style, and biological predisposition may contribute to the manifestation of this talent.

During the hypnotic trance, focal attention and imagination are enhanced and simultaneously peripheral awareness is decreased. This trance may be induced by a hypnotist through formalized induction procedures, but it can also occur spontaneously. The capacity to be hypnotized and, relatedly, the occurrence of spontaneous trance states is a trait that varies among individuals but is relatively stable throughout a person's life cycle.

HISTORY

Descriptions of trance states, ecstatic states, and spontaneous dissociative states abound in the Eastern and Western religious, literary, and philosophical traditions. Anton Franz Anton Mesmer (1734–1815) first formally described hypnosis as a therapeutic modality in the 18th century and believed it to be the result of a magnetic energy or an invisible fluid that the therapist channels into the patient to correct imbalances, restoring health. James Braid (1795–1860), an English physician and surgeon, used eye fixation and closure to induce trance states. Later, Jean Martin Charcot (1825–1893) theorized the hypnotic state to be a neurophysiologic phenomenon that was a sign of mental illness. Contemporaneously, Hippolyte Bernheim (1840–1919) believed it to be a function of the normal brain.

Early in his career, Sigmund Freud (1856–1939) used hypnosis as part of his psychoanalysis and noticed that patients in a trance could relive traumatic events, a process called *abreaction.* Later, Freud switched from hypnosis to free association because he wanted to minimize the transference that sometimes accompanies the trance state. Importantly, the switch did not eliminate the occurrence of spontaneous trance during the analysis.

World War I produced many shell-shocked soldiers and Ernst Simmel (1882–1947), a German psychoanalyst, developed a technique for accessing repressed material that he named *hypnoanalysis.* During World War II, hypnosis played a prominent role in the treatment of pain, combat fatigue, and neurosis. Formal recognition of hypnosis as a therapeutic modality did not occur, however, until the 1950s. The British Medical Society recommended its teaching in medical schools in 1955 and the American Medical Association and American Psychiatric Association officially stated its safety and efficacy in 1958.

DEFINITION

Hypnosis is currently understood as a normal activity of a normal mind through which attention is more focused, critical judgment is partially suspended, and peripheral awareness is diminished. The trance state, being a function of the subject's mind, cannot be forcibly projected by an outside person. The hypnotist, however, may aid in the achievement of the state and use its uncritical, intense focus to facilitate the acceptance of new thoughts and feelings, thereby accelerating therapeutic change. For the subject, hypnosis is typified by a feeling of involuntariness and movements seem automatic.

TRAIT OF HYPNOTIZABILITY

A person's degree of hypnotizability is a trait that is relatively stable throughout the life cycle and is measurable. The process of hypnosis takes the hypnotizability trait and transforms it into

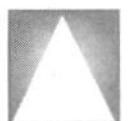

Table 24.9–1
Indicators of Trance Development

Autonomous ideation
Balanced tonicity (catalepsy)
Changed voice quality
Comfort, relaxation
Economy of movement
Eye changes/closure
Facial features ironed out
Feeling distant
Feeling good after trance
Lack of body movement
Lack of startle response
Literalism
Objective and impersonal ideation
Pupillary changes
Response attentiveness
Retardation of reflexes:
  Swallowing
  Blinking
Sensory, muscular, and body changes
Slowing pulse
Slowing and loss of blink reflex
Slowing respiration
Spontaneous hypnotic phenomena:
  Amnesia
  Anesthesia
  Catalepsy
  Regression
Time distortion
Time lag in motor and conceptual behavior

From Erickson M, Rossi EL, Rossi SI. *Hypnotic Realities: The Induction of Clinical Hypnosis and Forms of Indirect Suggestion*. New York: Irvington; 1976:98.

the hypnotized state. Experiencing the hypnotic concentration state requires a convergence of three essential components: absorption, dissociation, and suggestibility.

Absorption is an ability to reduce peripheral awareness that results in a greater focal attention. It can be metaphorically described as a psychological zoom lens that increases attention to the given thought or emotion to the increasing exclusion of all context, even including orientation to time and space.

Dissociation is the separating out from consciousness elements of the patient's identity, perception, memory, or motor response as the hypnotic experience deepens. The result is that components of self-awareness, time, perception, and physical activity can occur without being known to the patient's consciousness and so may seem involuntary.

Suggestibility is the tendency of the hypnotized patient to accept signals and information with a relative suspension of normal critical judgment; it is controversial whether critical judgment can be completely suspended. This trait will vary from an almost compulsive response to input in the highly hypnotizable to a sense of automaticity in the less hypnotizable individual. Table 24.9–1 lists the indicators of trance development.

QUANTIFICATION OF HYPNOTIZABILITY

Quantifying a patient's degree of hypnotizability is useful in a clinical setting because it predicts the effectiveness of hypnosis as a therapeutic modality. Quantification also provides useful information about the way patients relate to themselves and the social environment. Highly hypnotizable patients have an increased incidence of spontaneous trance-like states and so may be unduly influenced by ideas and emotions that are not being appropriately self-critiqued.

NEUROPHYSIOLOGICAL CORRELATES OF HYPNOSIS

Neurological testing of individuals in the hypnotized state and those with a high degree of hypnotizability has led to some interesting findings, but no set of changes has been shown to be sensitive or specific for the trance state or hypnotizability trait.

EEG studies have shown that hypnotized persons exhibit electrical patterns that are similar to those of fully awake and attentive persons and not like those found during sleep. Increased alpha activity and theta power in the left frontal region have been reported in highly hypnotizable patients as compared with those who are less hypnotizable; these differences exist in the trance and nontrance states.

Positron emission tomography (PET) studies that compare regional blood flow in the brain in both hypnotized and nonhypnotized subjects lend further evidence to the hypothesis that hypnosis exerts some of its effects at lower-level modalities of the brain. Hypnotic suggestions to add color to a visual image result in increased blood flow to the lingual and fusiform gyri, the color vision processing centers of the brain; suggestions to remove color have the opposite effect. Similarly, the intensity and noxiousness of pain are believed to be processed by different regions of the brain, because different areas of reduced blood flow result when each is minimized through hypnosis.

The role of the anterior brain regions, such as the frontal lobes, in hypnosis has been shown physiologically by the positive correlation between homovanillic acid concentrations in the cerebrospinal fluid and degree of hypnotizability. The frontal cortex and basal ganglia have a large number of neurons that use dopamine, of which the metabolite is homovanillic acid. This may explain why pharmacological enhancement of hypnotizability, although difficult, is primarily accomplished with dopaminergic agents, such as amphetamine. The increased activation of the basal ganglia may relate to the increased automaticity of hypnotic motor behavior.

CLINICAL ASSESSMENT OF HYPNOTIC CAPACITY

Two major procedures exist to clinically evaluate hypnotic capacity: the Stanford Hypnotic Susceptibility Scale and the Hypnotic Induction Profile (HIP) (Table 24.9–2). The Stanford Hypnotic Susceptibility Scale is a long laboratory-based test that has been modified for clinical evaluation and requires approximately 20 minutes to perform. It primarily measures behavioral compliance and suggestibility. The HIP is a shorter test that uses the eye-roll sign as a biological indicator and measures cognitive flow, which differentiates those with no hypnotic capacity because of mental pathology from those mentally normal patients with any inherent hypnotic capacity.

Table 24.9–2
Hypnotic Induction Profile–Derived Method of Self-Hypnosis

One, look up toward your eyebrows, all the way up; two, close your eyelids slowly and take a deep breath; count to three, exhale, let your eyes relax, and let your body float.

As you feel yourself floating, you permit one hand or the other to feel like a buoyant balloon and allow it to float upward. As it does, your elbow bends, and your forearm floats into an upright position. When your hand reaches this upright position, it becomes a signal for you to enter a state of meditation and to increase your receptivity to new thoughts and feelings.

In this state of meditation, you concentrate on this feeling of imaginary floating and, at the same time, concentrate on the following critical points (e.g., the three critical points to stop smoking in the following discussion).

Reflect on the implications of these critical points, and then bring yourself out of this state of concentration called self-hypnosis by counting backward in this manner: Three, get ready; two, with your eyelids closed, roll up your eyes (do it now); and, one, let your eyelids open slowly. Then, when your eyes are back in focus, slowly make a fist with the hand that is up; and, as you open your fist slowly, your usual sensation and control returns. Let your hand float down. That is the end of the exercise, but you can retain a general overall feeling of floating.

By doing this exercise 10 different times each day, you can float into this state of buoyant repose. Give yourself this island of time, 20 seconds, 10 times a day, in which to use this extra receptivity to reimprint these critical points. Reflect on them, then float back to your usual state of awareness, and then continue with what you ordinarily do.

Courtesy of Herbert Spiegel, M.D., Marcia Greenleaf, Ph.D., and David Spiegel, M.D.

INDUCTION

Many different induction protocols follow the same basic principles and pattern, but may be better suited to the patients with different levels of hypnotizability.

Doctor: Take a long, deep breath—inhale and exhale; now close your eyes and relax. Pay particular attention to the muscles in and about your eyes—relax them to the point that they just won't work. Are you trying to do that? Good. If you really have them relaxed, right at this very moment, no matter how hard you try, they just won't open. Test them. The harder you try, the faster they stick together, just as if they were glued together. That's fine!

Now you can open your eyes; that's good. When I tell you to and not before, open and close your eyes once more, and, when you close them this time, you will be ten times as relaxed as you are right now. Go ahead, open and close, and feel that surge of relaxation go through your whole body, from the top of your head to the tip of your toes. Very good!

Now once again, open and close your eyes, and this time, when you close them, you will double the relaxation that you now have. Fine.

If you have followed my suggestions, right at this very moment, when I lift your hand and let it drop into your lap, it will drop like a wet cloth, heavy and limp. That's very, very good.

You now have good physical relaxation, but medical relaxation consists of two phases: physical, which you now have, and mental, which I will now show you how to achieve.

When I ask you to and not before, I want you to start counting backward from 100. I know you can count; that is not what we're after. I just want you to relax mentally. As you say each number, pause momentarily until you feel a wave of relaxation cover your whole body, from the top of your head to the tip of your toes. When you feel this wave of relaxation, then say the next number, and each time you say a number, you will double the relaxation you had before you said the number. If you do this properly, an interesting thing will happen—as you say the numbers and relax, the succeeding numbers will start to disappear and vanish from your mind. Command your mind to dispel these numbers. Now, aloud and slowly, start counting backward from 100.

Patient: One hundred.

Doctor: Very good.

Patient: Ninety-nine.

Doctor: Make them start to disappear now.

Patient: Ninety-eight.

Doctor: Now they're fading away, and after the next number they'll all be gone. Make them disappear. Let the numbers go.

Patient: Ninety-seven.

Doctor: And now they're all gone. Are they gone? Fine. If there are any numbers still lurking in your mind, when I lift your hand and drop it, they will all disappear. *(Courtesy of William Holt, M.D.)*

INDICATIONS

A patient's degree of hypnotizability and the technique of hypnosis are clinically useful in diagnosis and in treatment, respectively.

The existence of spontaneous, trance-like states in everyday life and the potential of individuals to uncritically accept emotions and information in these states make a person's degree of hypnotizability a factor in the way the world is viewed and processed. A relation is seen between various conditions and hypnotizability. For example, patients with paranoid personality disorder are low and patients who are histrionic are higher on the hypnotizability spectrum. Patients with dissociative identity disorder are highly hypnotizable. Patients with eating disorders are difficult to hypnotize.

A 32-year-old man presented to the emergency department with a severe headache. He was a chronic migraine sufferer and had been unable to control the pain on this occasion with his propranolol (Inderal). The emergency department recognized that he had high hypnotic capacity. The imagery of an icepack being placed on his forehead was suggested. Initially some real ice was placed on his forehead to help. The patient was able to control his pain completely with this imagery. He did not require narcotics, as he had on previous visits. On follow-up several weeks later the patient reported being able to use this strategy to control, as well as prevent, migraine attacks, and he no longer had to rely on frequent emergency department visits for pain relief. *(Courtesy of A. D. Axelrad, M.D., D. Brown, Ph.D., and H. J. Wain, Ph.D.)*

A 22-year-old male patient was brought to the emergency room with bilateral blindness. Following an evaluation by ophthalmology, it was determined that the blindness was psychogenic. After initial evaluation by psychiatry, a therapeutic alliance was developed, and hypnosis was used to take the patient to a safe place and then back to the time immediately prior to the blindness. After two sessions the patient was able to describe seeing his wife in an adulterous relationship. At that moment the patient vocalized a desire to harm his wife and her suitor. Immediately after this vocalization, he became amnesic for the event and blind. On describing this under hypnosis, he was given a suggestion that when he became alert "He would only remember what he felt comfortable remembering." Subsequent to the patient becoming alert, he had no idea what had occurred, and each day after the hypnotic intervention was initiated the patient's anger was reframed. When the patient felt comfortable he then confronted his wife. The patient became aware that the amnesia was being used to prevent him from acting out. Use of a psychodynamic, cognitive reframing approach with a hypnotic milieu helped this patient to gain control and understanding of his symptoms. The patient and his wife were then referred for marital counseling. *(Courtesy of A. D. Axelrad, M.D., D. Brown, Ph.D., and H. J. Wain, Ph.D.)*

Therapeutically, hypnosis's effectiveness in facilitating acceptance of new thoughts and feelings makes it useful in treating habitual problems and also with symptom management. Smoking, overeating, phobias, anxiety, conversion symptoms, and chronic pain are all indications for hypnosis. They can often be treated in a single session, in which a patient is taught to perform self-hypnosis. Hypnosis can also aid in psychotherapy, notably for posttraumatic stress disorder, and it has been used for memory retrieval.

A 29-year-old woman was referred for evaluation and treatment of ongoing facial pain that was not responding to traditional methods of intervention. Neurological evaluation showed no objective physical correlations. Her high midrange performance on the HIP added support to the potential of a psychological mechanism for the pain. Initially the pain was controlled by a hypnotic intervention, but it returned 24 hours later. Her self-hypnotic technique ceased to be effective. A decision was made to explore more completely the meaning of the pain. Age regression under hypnosis was used, and the patient was regressed to a time prior to the pain. She related that her brother had been injured by a car while he was running in the street. The patient was babysitting at the time, and her father was so angered that he hit her. Recently her friend's dog ran away, and she felt responsible. As she began to recognize her need to punish herself because of her guilt over what had occurred, she was able to understand her feelings and reframe her thoughts in a more productive manner. An "affect bridge" was also used, and the patient was asked to go back to a previous time when she felt guilty and was punished. She then was able to describe her feelings of being hit by her alcoholic, abusive father. She continued to gain insight and mastery over the past and was able to ablate her pain. *(Courtesy of A. D. Axelrad, M.D., D. Brown, Ph.D., and H. J. Wain, Ph.D.)*

A 42-year-old married mother of three children had been kidnapped and locked in a large packing trunk. After she had freed herself and broken out, her abductors had stabbed her multiple times, tied her up, put her back in the trunk, and thrown her down a cliff. She had eventually managed to break out and crawl to safety. Eventually she had been picked up by a passerby. She reported that others had seen her lying on the road and appeared frightened to approach her. Eventually 911 had been called and she had been transported to a hospital. Following medical stabilization she had been discharged and found herself developing nightmares, reexperiencing avoidance, and having hyperarousal symptoms. She was referred by her internist for treatment and was initially started on 25 mg of sertraline (Zoloft), which was increased to 50 mg 4 days later. She was evaluated on the HIP and determined to be a mid- to high-range hypnotic subject. She was taught to go to a safe place and to use a split-screen technique. She was also given permission to describe her nightmares, reexperiences, and overwhelming anxieties and fears that she faced while being captive, as well as her feelings of abandonment while lying on the road. She was reinforced for her ingenuity in breaking out of the trunk. Her feeling of blame for her capture was reframed while she was under hypnosis. She was taught to calm herself and to reframe her negative feelings about her helplessness. Hypnotic age regression was used to help her master her experiences and facilitate their becoming like a bad movie. Initially her startle response was used as a signal for her to go to her comfort zone. Age progression was used to help her to rehearse the future. The treatment used the milieu of hypnosis along with exposure, cognitive reframing, psychodynamic approaches, and pharmacology. *(Courtesy of A. D. Axelrad, M.D., D. Brown, Ph.D., and H. J. Wain, Ph.D.)*

CONTRAINDICATIONS

No intrinsic dangers to the hypnotic process exist. Because of the increased dependence that the hypnotized patient has toward the therapist, a strong transference may occur, however, in which the patient exhibits feelings for the therapist that are inappropriate in regard to their relationship. Strong attachments may occur, and it is important that these are respected and properly interpreted. Negative emotions may also be brought out in the patient, especially those who are emotionally fragile or who have poor reality testing. To minimize the likelihood of this negative transference, caution should be taken when choosing patients who have problems with basic trust, such as those who are paranoid or who require high levels of control. The hypnotized patient also has a reduced ability to critically evaluate hypnotic suggestions and, thus, the hypnotist must have a strong ethical value system. Controversy exists about whether patients can perform acts during a trance state that they would otherwise find repugnant or that run contrary to their moral system.

▲ 24.10 Interpersonal Therapy

Interpersonal psychotherapy (ITP), a time-limited treatment for major depressive disorder, was developed in the 1970s, defined in a manual, and tested in randomized clinical trials by Gerald L. Klerman and Myrna Weissman. ITP was initially formulated as an attempt to represent the current practice of psychotherapy for depression. It assumes that the development and maintenance of some psychiatric illnesses occur in a social and interpersonal context and that the onset, response to treatment, and outcomes are influenced by the interpersonal relations between the patient and significant others. The overall goal of ITP is to reduce or eliminate psychiatric symptoms by improving the quality of the patient's current interpersonal relations and social functioning.

The typical course of ITP lasts 12 to 20 sessions over a 4- to 5-month period. ITP moves through three defined phases:

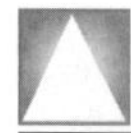

Table 24.10–1
Phases of Interpersonal Psychotherapy

Initial phase: sessions 1–5
Give the syndrome a name; provide information about prevalence and characteristics of the disorder
Describe the rationale and nature of interpersonal psychotherapy
Conduct the interpersonal inventory to identify the current interpersonal problem area(s) associated with the onset or maintenance of the psychiatric symptoms
Review significant relationships, past and present
Identify interpersonal precipitants of episodes of psychiatric symptoms
Select and reach consensus about the interpersonal psychotherapy problem area(s) and treatment plan with patient
Intermediate phase: sessions 6–15
Implement strategies specific to the identified problem area(s)
Encourage and review work on goals specific to the problem area
Illuminate connections between symptoms and interpersonal events during the week
Work with the patient to identify and manage negative or painful affects associated with his or her interpersonal problem area
Relate issues about psychiatric symptoms to the interpersonal problem area
Termination phase: sessions 16–20
Discuss termination explicitly
Educate patient about the end of treatment as a potential time of grieving; encourage patient to identify associated emotions
Review progress to foster feelings of accomplishment and competence
Outline goals for remaining work; identify areas and warning signs of anticipated future difficulty
Formulate specific plans for continued work after termination of treatment

(1) The initial phase is dedicated to identifying the problem area that will be the target for treatment; (2) the intermediate phase is devoted to working on the target problem area(s); and (3) the termination phase is focused on consolidating gains made during treatment and preparing the patients for future work on their own (Table 24.10–1).

TECHNIQUES

Individual Interpersonal Psychotherapy

Initial Phase. Sessions 1 through 5 typically constitute the initial phase of ITP. After assessing the patient's current psychiatric symptoms and obtaining a history of these symptoms, the therapist gives the patient a formal diagnosis. Therapist and patient then discuss the diagnosis, as well as what might be expected from the treatment. Assignment of the sick role during this phase serves the dual function of granting the patient both the permission to recover and the responsibility to recover. The therapist explains the rationale of ITP, underscoring that therapy will focus on identifying and altering dysfunctional interpersonal patterns related to psychiatric symptomatology. To determine the precise focus of treatment, the therapist conducts an interpersonal inventory with the patient and develops an interpersonal formulation based on this. In the interpersonal formulation, the therapist links the patient's psychiatric symptomatology to one of the four interpersonal problem areas—grief, interpersonal deficits, interpersonal role disputes, or role transitions. The patient's concurrence with the therapist's identification of the problem area and agreement to work on this area are essential before beginning the intermediate treatment phase.

Intermediate Phase. The intermediate phase—typically, sessions 6 to 15—constitutes the "work" of the therapy. An essential task throughout the intermediate phase is to strengthen the connections the patient makes between the changes he or she is making in his or her interpersonal life and the changes in his or her psychiatric symptoms. During the intermediate phase, the therapist implements the treatment strategies specific to the identified problem area as specified in Table 24.10–2.

Termination Phase. In the termination phase (usually, sessions 16 through 20), the therapist discusses termination explicitly with the patient and assists him or her in understanding that the end of treatment is a potential time of grief. During this phase, patients are encouraged to describe specific

Table 24.10–2
Treatment of Interpersonal Problem Areas

Problem Area	Description	Goals	Strategies
Grief and loss	Depression after the death of a loved one	Help patient through the mourning process Reestablish interest in new relationships	Explore relationship of patient with the deceased; explore negative and positive feelings associated with the loss
Role transitions	Life-phase transitions such as adolescence, childbirth, aging; or social/economic changes such as getting married, change in career, diagnosis of a medical illness	Deal with the loss of the old role Affirm positive and negative aspects of new roles. Develop self-esteem and mastery	Examine all aspects of old and new roles; examine feelings about what is lost; explore social support system and develop new skills
Interpersonal role disputes	Conflict between the patient and someone else	Identify and modify expectations and faulty communication	Examine how role expectations relate to conflict; examine ways to bring about change in the relationship
Interpersonal deficits	A history of inadequate or unsustaining interpersonal relationships	Enhance quality of existing relationships; encourage the formation of new relationships	Discuss negative and positive feelings regarding the therapist; examine parallel interpersonal relations in patient's life

Based on Treasure J, Schmidt U, van Furth E. *Handbook of Eating Disorders*. 2nd ed. Hoboken, NJ: John Wiley & Sons; 2003:258.

changes in their psychiatric symptoms, especially as they relate to improvements in the identified problem area(s). The therapist also assists the patient in evaluating and consolidating gains, detailing plans for maintaining improvements in the identified interpersonal problem area(s), and outlining remaining work for the patient to continue on his or her own. Patients are also encouraged to identify early warning signs of symptom recurrence and to identify plans of action.

Ms. G is a 51-year-old woman who presented for treatment of binge eating disorder. She is college educated, has her own business, and is a divorced mother of one adult son in his early 20s. Before treatment, she had a body mass index (BMI) of 42 and had been binge eating approximately 10 to 15 days per month for the past 8 years. Along with her current diagnosis of binge eating disorder, Ms. G struggled with recurrent major depression.

During the initial phase, Ms. G and her therapist began to review her history and the interpersonal events that were associated with her binge eating. Ms. G shared that she began overeating and gaining weight at age 14. When she was 18 years of age, she moved to a foreign country with her parents. Soon after the move, Ms. G's father left her and her mother to return to the United States. Ms. G was enraged at her father for leaving them and still gets very tearful and angry when discussing the separation. She and her mother decided to stay abroad because she had started university and her mother was working. Both had developed strong social ties and felt comfortable in their new home. During this time, Ms. G continued to gain weight and started dieting. Shortly after graduating from university, Ms. G met and married a foreign national and, at the age of 28, delivered their only son. Two years later, she and her husband went through a very bitter divorce. Although Ms. G described this as a terrible time in her life, she maintained close ties with her friends and her mother. During this time, she began to diet and reached her lowest adult weight. At the age of 35, when her mother died of a heart condition, Ms. G had her first episode of major depression, which was treated and resolved with antidepressants and a brief course of psychotherapy. Although she had previous cycles of weight loss and weight regain, she did not evidence any sign of eating disturbance at this point. She continued to maintain close social ties and enjoyed her close relationship with her son. When Ms. G was in her early 40s, an economic downturn in her adopted country forced her to return to the United States. Having lost all of her savings, she struggled financially while she looked for work. During this time, she started binge eating and gaining weight. Within 1 year of this move, Ms. G's son decided to return to live with his father (who was very wealthy). Ms. G felt angry and betrayed. Yet, when her son would visit, she would assume a subservient role with him, because she was afraid of losing his affection. He, in turn, became quite demanding and critical of her. Before seeking treatment, her heightened feelings of isolation and loneliness were leading to increased binge eating, depression, and weight gain.

By session 3 of the initial phase, Ms. G's therapist began to consider which problem area would be the focus of the remainder of treatment. Ms. G had a history of important relationship losses and subsequent grief—the loss of her father, her husband, her mother, and, most recently, her son. However, none of these losses was associated with the development of binge eating problems (although her dieting was clearly linked to her feelings of anger after the divorce from her husband and her depression was intimately linked with her mother's death). Ms. G's anger at her son for returning to live with the enemy was clearly a role dispute, yet her binge eating had begun 2 years before his departure (although it clearly worsened after he left). Because neither of these problem areas was directly linked to the onset of the eating disorder, Ms. G's therapist decided that the focus of treatment would be to assist her in managing her role transition. Her move back to the United States, with the subsequent loss of her support and friendship networks, was clearly associated with the onset and continued maintenance of her binge eating. During session 4 of the initial phase, Ms. G's therapist shared her formulation of the problem area with her: "From what you have described, your binge eating really began after you returned to the United States. After that transition, you were more isolated and alone than you have ever been. It seems that binge eating was a way for you to manage that transition and the subsequent feelings of isolation and loneliness. Your transition has also had a negative impact on your relationship with your son. Even though you are a very social person and enjoy the company of others, you have yet to develop the kind of support that you had before you moved. Although you have struggled with some very significant issues over the course of your life—your father leaving, the pain of the divorce, and the death of your mother—your friends and support systems sustained you. If we work together to help you find and develop more intimate and supportive relationships here, I believe you will be much less likely to turn to food and binge eating as a source of support or comfort."

Ms. G agreed with the formulation and worked with her therapist to establish some treatment goals to help her resolve the problem area. First, she was encouraged to become more aware of her feelings (especially isolation and loneliness) when she was binge eating and of how binge eating seemed to be the way she managed those feelings. A second goal was for her to take steps to increase her social contacts and develop more friendships. The third goal, which was identified as a secondary problem area, centered on helping Ms. G resolve the role dispute with her son. Specifically, the therapist developed a goal with her to help her establish a clearer parental role with her son.

During the intermediate phase, the therapist helped Ms. G grieve the loss of her previous role and the extensive support that she once had. Ms. G and her therapist worked to identify several sources of support and friendships of which she had not been aware. Soon after, Ms. G reported significant progress in initiating and establishing relationships with others. This change appeared to help give her confidence in her new roles. In fact, she had begun to receive a few social invitations. She was more attuned to the ways that she would rely on food, especially when she felt lonely or felt that she was not receiving enough time from others. The connection between the lack of supportive contacts and binge eating was becoming very clear to her in these intermediate sessions. During this phase, the therapist also assisted her in setting appropriate limits in her relationship with her adult son and in recognizing his adult-like responses in return. By the termination phase, Ms. G reported that she no longer felt so lonely and isolated and that her binge eating had all but disappeared. She remarked how the quality of her relationship with her son had changed dramatically. He was more supportive and respectful, visited more frequently, and stayed with her for longer periods of time. In the final sessions, she talked about her need to let go of the past and move on with her life as it is now, assuming her new roles more fully. She worked closely with her therapist to develop a plan to maintain the gains that she had made in treatment and used the final session to review the important work that she had accomplished. *(Courtesy of D. E. Wilfley, Ph.D. and R. W. Guynn, M.D.)*

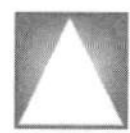

Table 24.10–3
Stages of Group Development in Interpersonal Psychotherapy (ITP)

ITP Phases	Group Stages	Group Process	Group Technique
Initial: sessions 1–5; identify interpersonal problem areas	Engagement: sessions 1–2	Members deal with anxiety and sharing of problems; need for leadership emerges	Therapist should encourage self-disclosure and sharing of experience
	Differentiation: sessions 3–5	As interpersonal differences emerge in the group, members work to manage negative feelings	Members share their feelings in the context of interpersonal activities outside the group
Middle: sessions 6–15; work on goals	Work: sessions 6–15	Members strive toward common goals and work out differences	Connections among members increase as they share common experiences. Therapist encourages the practice of newly acquired interpersonal skills
Final: sessions 16–20; consolidate treatment	Termination: sessions 16–20	Members deal with loss and separation as group disbands	Set goals after leaving group; deal with feelings of loss and grieving

Based on Wilfley DE, MacKenzie KR, Welch RR, et al. *Interpersonal Psychotherapy for Group*. New York: Basic Books; 2000:20.

Interpersonal Psychotherapy Delivered in a Group Format

A recent approach in the ongoing development of ITP has been its use in a group format. ITP delivered in a group format has many potential benefits in comparison with individual treatment. For example, a group format in which membership is based on diagnostic similarity (e.g., depression, social phobia, eating disorders) can help alleviate patients' concerns that they are the only one with a particular psychiatric disorder, while offering a social environment for patients who have become isolated, withdrawn, or disconnected from others. Given the number and different types of interpersonal interactions in a group setting, the interpersonal skills that are developed may be more readily transferable to the patient's outside social life than are the relationship patterns that are addressed in a one-on-one setting. Moreover, a group modality has therapeutic features not present in individual psychotherapy (e.g., interpersonal learning). The group format also facilitates the identification of problems common to many patients and provides a cost-effective alternative to individual treatment. Table 24.10–3 links the phases of ITP to the stages of group development.

Timeline and Structure of Treatment. The typical course of group ITP lasts 20 sessions over a 5-month period. It is recommended that group size range from six to nine members, with one or two group leaders, depending on resources and training needs. The three individual meetings (pregroup, midgroup, and postgroup), sequenced to correspond with critical time points in the three phases of ITP, in combination with other techniques, were designed to maintain the exclusive and strategic focus on individual patients' interpersonal problem areas—the hallmark of ITP.

Pregroup Meeting. The pretreatment meeting is crucial for facilitating a patient's individualized work in the first phase of group ITP. The focus of the 2-hour pretreatment meeting is to identify interpersonal problem areas, establish an explicit treatment contract to work on problem areas, and prepare patients for group treatment. After identifying a patient's interpersonal problem(s) (i.e., interpersonal deficits, role disputes, role transitions, or grief), the therapist works collaboratively with the patient to formulate concrete prescriptions for change, in addition to the specific steps the patient will take to improve social relationships and patterns of relating. These goals of treatment are expressed in language that is as specific and personally meaningful to the patient as possible. Before the start of the group, each group member is given a written summary of his or her goals and told that these goals will guide his or her work in the group.

Another important element of the pregroup meeting involves adequately preparing patients for group treatment. That is, patients are encouraged to think of the group as an "interpersonal laboratory" in which they can experiment with new approaches to handle challenging interpersonal situations. In this regard, patients are informed about the important interpersonal skills that are learned while participating in a group (e.g., interpersonal confrontation, honest communication, expression of feelings) and are encouraged to learn from others as they see changes occur. The therapist stresses to patients the importance of keeping their work in the group focused on changing their current interpersonal situations or intensifying important existing relationships and not using the group as a substitute social network.

Initial Phase. The first five sessions of the group treatment comprise the initial phase in group ITP. During this phase, the therapist works to cultivate positive group norms and group cohesion, while emphasizing the commonality of symptoms among members and how they will be addressed in the group context. During this phase, group members are encouraged to review their goals with the group and begin to make some initial changes in their respective interpersonal problem areas. As members begin to experiment with the changes outlined in their goals, the therapist works collaboratively with each group member to refine and make any alterations in the target areas before the beginning of the intermediate phase.

Intermediate Phase. During the intermediate "work" phase of group ITP (sessions 6 through 15), the therapist works to facilitate connections among members as they share the work on their goals with one another. In contrast to other interactive group approaches, the group interpersonal psychotherapist is much less likely to focus on intragroup processes and relationships unless they are specific to the work on a member's interpersonal problem area (e.g., interpersonal deficits). The therapist, however, consistently and continuously encourages group members to practice newly acquired interpersonal skills both inside and, most importantly, outside the group. As is the case with individual ITP, an essential task throughout the intermediate phase is to strengthen the connections the group members make between difficulties in their interpersonal lives and their psychiatric problems.

Midtreatment Meeting. The midtreatment meeting is held midway (usually between sessions 10 and 11) through the intermediate phase. This meeting provides an opportunity to conduct a detailed review of each group member's progress on his or her individual problems and to refine interpersonal goals. The therapist(s) recontracts with group members during this meeting as a means of outlining and emphasizing the work that remains, both inside and outside of the group, before the conclusion of treatment.

Termination Phase. In the termination phase (sessions 16 through 20), the therapist discusses termination explicitly with the group members and begins to help them recognize that the end of treatment is a time of possible grief and loss. The therapist helps members recognize their own progress and the progress made by other group members. During this phase, group members are encouraged to describe the specific changes in their psychiatric symptoms, especially as they relate to improvements in the identified problem area(s) and relationships. Although it is common for group members to want to keep meeting on their own or to have frequent reunions, group members are encouraged to use this phase of the group to formally say goodbye to one another and to the therapist(s). The therapist(s) also uses this time to encourage members to detail their plans for maintaining improvements in their identified interpersonal problem area(s) and to outline their remaining work.

Posttreatment Meeting. The posttreatment meeting is scheduled within 1 week after the final group session. The therapist(s) uses this final individual meeting to develop an individualized plan for each group member's continued work on his or her interpersonal goals. The therapist(s) reviews the group experience and the changes the patient has made in his or her interpersonal problem area and significant relationships.

▲ 24.11 Narrative Psychotherapy

More than anything else psychiatrists do, they listen to stories. These stories so saturate the clinical encounter that it would be impossible to imagine a clinical encounter without them. In the very first meeting between psychiatrist and patient, the psychiatrist begins with an open-ended invitation to a story: "*What brings you here?*" or "*What seems to be the problem?*" Patients respond to these questions by telling psychiatrists about their lives, their troubles, when the troubles began, what seems to have caused them, how they create difficulty, and what kinds of problem solving they have tried. Such stories may be rudimentary, they may be only partially worked out, and they may even be baffled and confused. The patient may even be perplexed enough to answer "I don't know why I came" or "I'm not really sure what's wrong, my family sent me." Nonetheless, the patient's response to the psychiatrist's initial questions always involves a story.

Narrative psychotherapy emerges out of this increased interest in clinical stories. The two main tributaries that lead to narrative psychotherapy come from the two different sides of psychiatry: narrative medicine and narrative psychotherapy. Narrative psychiatrists are psychiatrists who combine the wisdom of these two domains. Following the lead of narrative medicine, narrative psychiatrists recognize that psychiatric patients, like medical patients, come to clinics with intense stories to tell. Contemporary narrative medicine has developed from 30 years of work in bioethics and medical humanities devoted to humanizing the clinical encounter through a better understanding of patient stories. The term *narrative medicine* comes from Rita Charon, an internist and literary scholar, who used it to describe an approach to medicine that uses narrative approaches to augment scientific understandings of illness. Narrative medicine brings together insights from human-centered medical models, such as George Engel's biopsychosocial model and Eric Cassel's person-centered model, with research and insights from phenomenology, the humanities, and interpretive social sciences.

Narrative medicine uses these resources to better understand the illness experience, "to recognize, absorb, interpret, and be moved by the stories of illness." As Charon argued, when clinicians possess narrative competency, they can enter the clinical setting with a nuanced capacity for "attentive listening..., adopting alien perspectives, following the narrative thread of the story of another, being curious about other people's motives and experiences, and tolerating the uncertainty of stories." She further argued that doctors "*need* rigorous and disciplined training" in narrative reading and writing not just for their own sake (helping them to deal with the strains and traumas of clinical work), but also "*for the sake of their practice.*" Without such narrative competency, clinicians lack the ability to fully understand their client's experience of illness. For Charon and others in narrative medicine, narrative study is not a mere adornment to a doctor's medical training, it is a crucial and basic science that must be mastered for medical practice.

A major task of narrative medicine, and therefore narrative psychotherapy, is to be a good listener and to connect empathically with the patient's story. A narrative psychiatrist, like a narrative physician, seeks to understand the patient first and foremost. This understanding brings patient and clinician together into a shared experience of the patient's world. This narrative understanding is much more than a causal explanation of problem A or problem B that the patient might have. It does not simply abstract from the person's situation a categorical label that groups problems under a well-known abstract grid. Instead, narrative understanding tunes in to the uniqueness of the individual and the unrepeatability of the person's experience and difficulties. Narrative understanding, in short, is a deep appreciation of the person as a whole—what it feels like for this person, in this particular context, going through these particular problems.

In addition to following the lead of narrative medicine colleagues, narrative psychiatrists also follow the lead of contemporary colleagues in narrative psychotherapy. The history of narrative psychotherapy goes back to Sigmund Freud's early work at the inception of psychoanalysis. At that time, Freud lamented about how his case histories sounded more like narrative fictions than hard science.

Contemporary narrative psychotherapy's motivation for returning to the role of narrative comes partly from the broader turn to narrative in humanities, psychology, and social science and partly from the history of psychotherapy since Freud. The past century of psychotherapy has been a century of strife, with one faction after another splitting off from psychoanalysis. Leading alternatives to psychoanalysis included behavioral, humanistic, family, cognitive, feminist, and interpersonal, just to name a few. All of these splits are characterized by further splits within splits, which have fragmented the field of psychotherapy to the point that there are now more than 400 active approaches to psychotherapy. Narrative approaches emerge at this particular moment as part of an important trend away from further fragmentation and toward psychotherapy reintegration. Narrative approaches are invaluable for psychotherapy integration because they provide a metatheoretical orientation from which to understand and practice psychotherapy.

METAPHOR

Metaphor performs this function by allowing us to understand and experience one thing in terms of something else. The metaphor selects, accentuates, and backgrounds aspects of two systems of ideas so that they come to be seen as similar: "Men are seen to be more like wolves after the wolf metaphor is used, and wolves seem to be more human."

Understanding metaphor in this way connects to broader work in continental linguistic philosophy, and that work, as a whole, shifts standard ideas about truth and objectivity. It allows us to sidestep the usual binary traps between relativism (anything goes) and realism (there is only one correct or true way to describe the world). When the role of language is understood as a mediator between our concepts and the world, it no longer makes sense to think in these highly modernist either/or terms. Rather than using the rigid binary distinction between true and false, it becomes possible to think instead in a postmodern language of semiotic realism and pluridimensional consequences.

PLOT

Plot works like metaphor in that it also orders experiences and provides form for narratives. Plot, or the process of emplotment, adds to metaphor two key dimensions: (1) it brings together what would otherwise be separate and heterogeneous elements, and (2) it organizes understanding and experience or time, or what could be called temporal perception.

The critical function of plot for narrative is that plot creates a narrative synthesis between multiple individual events and brings them together into a single story. It allows an intelligible connection to be made between them. Remarkably, plot can create a synthesis between events and elements that are surprisingly incongruous or heterogeneous—events that do not seem to fit together.

Plot also configures these multiple elements into a temporal order. This temporal order is of two sorts. First, each plot comprises a discrete series of incidents, of theoretically infinite *nows*. Second, each plot takes these infinite nows, proceeding one after another in succession, and organizes them into a humanly manageable experience.

CHARACTER

In narrative theory, the concept of character connects directly to contemporary controversy surrounding the related and, some may argue, more basic concept of identity. The controversy around identity may be understood as a tension between essentialist and nonessentialist approaches. Essentialist notions of identity tell us that each person has a fixed personality, perhaps biologically stamped, that authentically belongs to that person and that is at the core of that person's being. This "true self" or "core self" may be distorted or covered over, but it is nonetheless there for the discovery if individuals apply themselves patiently and persistently to the task. Nonessentialist critiques, however, have deconstructed this ideal of identity and its notion of an integral, originary, and unified self. One of the most productive ways to navigate the tension between essentialist and nonessentialist understandings of identity is to draw a comparison between identity (in life) and character (in fiction). Rather than adopting a linear logic that understands identity as a more fundamental concept to character, this approach uses a circular logic to argue that people understand themselves in the same way they understand characters.

Narrative approaches to identity allow people to navigate the tension between essentialist and nonessentialist identities because narrative identity allows for a kind of continuity over time, a relative stability of self, without implying a substantialist or essentialist core to this stability. People's interpretations of themselves use the cultural stories with which they are surrounded to tell a story of self that escapes the two poles of random change and absolute identity. In this way, a narrative identity is also a cultural identification. A person's identification may seem original, but he or she narrates stories with the resources of history, language, and culture.

NARRATIVE THERAPY

Fortunately, one of the most helpful aspects of narrative theory for psychiatry is that it provides an overarching, or metatheoretical, rationale for understanding how these many psychotherapies work. From a narrative perspective, all therapies involve a process of storytelling and story retelling. No matter which style of psychotherapy one uses, the process of therapy involves an initial presentation of problems that the client is unable to resolve. The client and therapist work together to bring additional perspectives to these problems, allowing the client to understand them in a new way. These additional perspectives vary greatly depending on which style of psychotherapy is used. It matters, in other words, whether the therapy is psychodynamic, cognitive, humanistic, feminist, spiritual, or expressive. From the vantage point of narrative theory, however, what these different approaches all have in common is that they rework, or "reauthor," the patient's initial story into a new story. This new story allows new degrees of flexibility for understanding the past and provides new strategies for moving into the future.

FUTURE DIRECTIONS

Recent work in narrative medicine, narrative psychotherapy, and narrative theory has opened the door for the development of narrative psychiatry. This development provides a critical corrective to contemporary psychiatric practice that helps to bring psychiatry back from its current obsessions with science and scientific method. This corrective is not a return to psychoanalysis nor does it demolish the progress of scientific psychiatry. When psychiatrists take a narrative turn, they do not throw out their other skills and knowledge. The shift to narrative is, as much as anything else, an attitude shift and an opening out to additional sources of information. It starts by bringing to the foreground that the clinical encounter is a human encounter, and it follows by opening out to colleagues in the humanities, interpretive social sciences, and the arts to help to better understand this human encounter.

Most of all, narrative psychotherapy joins with other contemporary efforts in psychiatry—such as the recovery movement—to make clinical encounters much more client focused and collaborative. Narrative psychotherapy, at its core, recognizes that there are many ways to tell the story of one's life. The choice among these different options is a key way in which people create their identity. These choices should not be reduced to expert choices or scientific choices because they are always also personal and ethical choices. In the end, they are choices about what kind of life one wants to live.

Furthermore, clinicians must come to understand the value of biography, autobiography, and literature for developing a repertoire of narrative frames and options. In the end, narrative competency in psychiatry means a tremendous familiarity with the many possible stories of psychic pain and psychic difference. The more stories clinicians know, the more likely they are to help their clients find a narrative frame that works for them.

For patients and potential service users, a narrative understanding means that there is a range of possible therapists and healing solutions that might be helpful. An approach that is right for one person may not be right for another. There must be a fit between the person and the approach, and people should feel empowered to take seriously their intuitions and feelings. If the person getting help does not feel this fit, he or she is likely right. There may well be another approach that would work better with the person's proclivities. Like everything else, however, judgment is critical. Therapeutic experiences of all kinds can be frustrating, slow, and uncertain. How, for example, does one know when an approach misses his or her needs and when it is something that will take time, patience, and perseverance to be helpful? From a narrative perspective, there can be no gold standard or simple answers. Only judgment, wisdom, and trial and error can decide.

▲ 24.12 Psychiatric Rehabilitation

Psychiatric rehabilitation denotes a wide range of interventions designed to help people with disabilities caused by mental illness improve their functioning and quality of life, by enabling them to acquire the skills and supports needed to be successful in usual adult roles and in the environments of their choice. Normative adult roles include living independently, attending school, working in competitive jobs, relating to family, having friends, and having intimate relationships. Psychiatric rehabilitation emphasizes independence rather than reliance on professionals, community integration rather than isolation in segregated settings for persons with disabilities, and patient preferences rather than professional goals.

VOCATIONAL REHABILITATION

Impairment of vocational role performance is a common complication related to schizophrenia. Studies across the United States show that less than 15 percent of patients with severe mental illnesses, such as schizophrenia, are employed. Nevertheless, studies also show that competitive employment is a primary goal for 50 to 75 percent of patients with schizophrenia. Because of patient interests and historical factors, vocational rehabilitation has always been a centerpiece of psychiatric rehabilitation.

Antonio is a 45-year-old man who has been a client of a mental health agency for more than 10 years. He attended the rehabilitative day treatment program until it was converted to a supported employment program. His case manager encouraged him to think about the possibility of working part time. Antonio told his case manager that he could not work because of his schizophrenia and because he was helping to raise his two kids and needed to be home at 3 p.m., when they returned from school every day. The case manager explained to Antonio that getting a job does not necessarily mean working 40 hours a week and that lots of people in the agency's supported employment program were working in part-time jobs, even jobs that only require a few hours a week.

Antonio agreed to meet one of the employment specialists to discuss the possibility of work. Over the next couple of weeks, the employment specialist met with Antonio several times, read his clinical record, and talked with his case manager and psychiatrist. The employment specialist learned that Antonio loved to drive his car. He also learned that Antonio had attendance problems in past jobs because he felt unappreciated. The employment specialist found Antonio to be a sociable and likable person.

Antonio told the employment specialist that he was willing to do any job. He did not have one specific job in mind. After discussing options with Antonio and with the team, the employment specialist suggested a job at Meals on Wheels as a driver for the lunch delivery. Antonio was hired and loved it right from the start. Absenteeism was never a problem, because he liked driving around and knew that people were counting on him for their meals. The hours were perfect (10 a.m. to 2 p.m.), so he could be at home when his kids returned from school. He became good friends with the other workers. He told his case manager that it was wonderful to be bringing home a paycheck again. And best of all, he said, was that his kids saw him going to work just like their friends' dads. *(Courtesy of Robert E. Drake, M.D., Ph.D. and Alan S. Bellack, Ph.D.)*

SOCIAL SKILLS REHABILITATION

Social dysfunction is a defining characteristic of schizophrenia. People with the illness have difficulty fulfilling social roles, such as worker, spouse, and friend, and have difficulty meeting their needs when social interaction is required (e.g., negotiating with merchants, requesting assistance to solve problems).

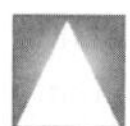

Table 24.12–1
Components of Social Skill

Expressive behaviors
Speech content
Paralinguistic features
Voice volume
Speech rate
Pitch
Intonation
Nonverbal behaviors
Eye contact (gaze)
Posture
Facial expression
Proxemics
Kinesics
Receptive skills (social perception)
Attention to and interpretation of relevant cues
Emotion recognition
Processing skills
Analysis of the situation demands
Incorporation of relevant contextual information
Social problem solving
Interactive behaviors
Response timing
Use of social reinforcers
Turn taking
Situational factors
Social "intelligence" (knowledge of social mores and the demands of the specific situation)

Social dysfunction is semi-independent of symptomatology and plays an important role in the course and outcome of the illness. As shown in Table 24.12–1, social competence is based on three component skills: (1) social perception or receiving skills; (2) social cognition or processing skills; and (3) behavioral response or expressive skills. Social perception is the ability to read or decode social inputs accurately. This includes accurate detection of affect cues, such as facial expressions and nuances of voice, gesture, and body posture, as well as verbal content and contextual information. Social cognition involves effective analysis of the social stimulus, integration of current information with historical information, and planning an effective response. This domain is also referred to as *social problem solving.*

Methods

The primary modality of social skills training is role play of simulated conversations. The trainer first provides instructions on how to perform the skill and then models the behavior to demonstrate how it is performed. After identifying a relevant social situation in which the skill might be used, the patient engages in role play with the trainer. The trainer next provides feedback and positive reinforcement, which are followed by suggestions for how the response can be improved. The sequence of role play followed by feedback and reinforcement is repeated until the patient can perform the response adequately. Training is typically conducted in small groups (six to eight patients), in which case, patients each practice role playing for three to four trials and provide feedback and reinforcement to one another. Teaching is tailored to the individual—for example, a highly impaired group member might simply practice saying "no" to a simple request, whereas a less cognitively impaired peer might learn to negotiate and compromise.

Richard was a single white man first diagnosed with schizophrenia at age 22, when he was a freshman at college. He was hospitalized briefly but was unable to return to school and moved back home with his parents. He attended a day treatment program intermittently over the next 6 years, before he was referred for help with getting a job and dating.

Richard had missed out on a critical period of adult development and had never learned dating skills or the social skills needed to get or maintain a job. He was appropriately groomed and did not present himself as a patient, but he seemed quite uncomfortable in social interactions. He scarcely made eye contact, staring at the floor when he spoke, and did not initiate conversation, responding to questions with brief answers.

Richard was invited to participate in a social skills training group for 3 months with six other patients. The focus of the group was employment skills. Patients were taught critical social skills for getting and maintaining a job, such as how to participate in job interviews; how to approach a supervisor to understand how to do a job or for help with work-related problems; how and when to make requests or explain problems, such as getting to work late because of traffic or needing to leave early to go to a doctor's appointment; and socializing with coworkers. Simultaneously, Richard was enrolled in a supported employment program and worked with a case manager to find a job as a computer support person. He found a 24-hour-per-week job at a small company and continued to attend the skills group, using the sessions to work on interpersonal issues at work, including engaging in casual conversation with coworkers and dealing with unreasonable requests from people.

When the vocational skills group ended, Richard was scheduled for a dating group with seven other male and female patients who had similar interests. This group focused on finding someone to date, dating etiquette, asking someone out (or being asked out), appropriate conversation for dates, sexual interactions, and safe sex practices. In addition to role play and discussion, the group shared ideas on how to meet people and what to do on dates.

Richard responded well to treatment. He had maintained the computer job at follow-up, 6 months after he concluded the dating skills group. His case manger also reported that he had a girlfriend, a woman whom he had met at his church group. He had also expressed an interest in enrolling in college classes at night. He was still living at home with his parents, but, for the first time, was seriously considering what he would need to do to move out. *(Courtesy of Robert E. Drake, M.D., Ph.D. and Alan S. Bellack, Ph.D.)*

Goals

In a treatment setting, there are four major goals of social skills training: (1) improved social skills in specific situations, (2) moderate generalization of acquired skills to similar situations, (3) acquisition or relearning of social and conversational skills, and (4) decreased social anxiety. Learning, however, is tedious or almost nonexistent when patients are floridly ill with positive symptoms and high levels of distractibility.

Some findings limit the applicability of social skills training. It is more difficult to teach complex conversational skills than to teach briefer, more discrete verbal and nonverbal responses in social situations. Because complex behaviors are more critical for generating social support in the community, methods have been developed to improve the learning and durability of conversational skills. These training methods, focusing on training in social skills and information-processing skills, are discussed below.

Training in Social Perception Skills

Recently, efforts have been made to develop strategies for training patients in affect and social cue recognition. Patients with chronic psychotic disorders, such as schizophrenia, often have difficulty perceiving and interpreting the subtle affective and cognitive cues that are critical elements of communication. Social perception abilities are considered the first step in effective interpersonal problem solving; difficulties in this area are likely to lead to a cascade of deficits in social behavior. Training skills in social perception address these deficits and help provide a foundation for developing more specific social and coping skills.

Despite attending several social gatherings, Matt felt apart from the rest of the group. He reported that these events seemed like "a jumble of sights and sounds." His therapist, recognizing Matt's difficulty with social perception, gave him a series of questions designed to help him organize and give meaning to the social stimuli he encountered. For example, when Matt was confused about a conversation someone was having with him, he would ask himself, "What is this person's short-term goal? At what level of disclosure should I be? Should I be talking now or listening?" Identifying the rules and goals of a particular social interaction provided a template for Matt to recognize, and react to, a greater variety of social cues, thus enhancing his behavioral repertoire. *(Courtesy of Robert Paul Liberman, M.D., Alex Kopelowicz, M.D., and Thomas E. Smith, M.D.)*

Information-Processing Model of Training

Methods of training that follow a cognitive perspective teach patients to use a set of generative rules that can be adapted for use in various situations. For example, a six-step problem-solving strategy was developed as an outline for helping patients overcome interpersonal dilemmas: (1) adopt a problem-solving attitude, (2) identify the problem, (3) brainstorm alternative solutions, (4) evaluate solutions and pick one to implement, (5) plan the implementation and carry it out, and (6) evaluate the efficacy of the effort and, if ineffective, choose another alternative. Although the step-wise, structured, linear process of problem solving occurs intuitively, without conscious awareness in normal persons, it can be a useful interpersonal crutch to help cognitively impaired mental patients cope with the information needed to fill their social and personal needs.

MILIEU THERAPY

The locus of milieu is a living, learning, or working environment. The defining characteristics of treatment are the use of a team to provide treatment and the time the patient spends in the environment. Recent adaptations of milieu therapy include 24-hour-a-day programs situated in community locales frequented by patients, which provide in vivo support, case management, and training in living skills.

Most milieu therapy programs emphasize group and social interaction; rules and expectations are mediated by peer pressure for normalization of adaptation. When patients are viewed as responsible human beings, the patient role becomes blurred. Milieu therapy stresses a patient's rights to goals and to have freedom of movement and informal relationship with staff; it also emphasizes interdisciplinary participation and goal-oriented, clear communication.

Token Economy

The use of tokens, points, or credits as secondary or generalized reinforcers can be seen as normalizing a mental hospital or day hospital environment with a program mimicking society's use of money to meet instrumental needs. Token economies establish the rules and culture of a hospital inpatient unit or partial hospitalization program, offering coherence and consistency to the interdisciplinary team as it struggles to promote therapeutic progress in difficult patients. These programs are challenging to establish, however, and their widespread dissemination has suffered because of the organizational prerequisites and the additional resources and rewards needed to create a truly positively reinforcing environment. Table 24.12–2 lists behaviors that can be reinforced by tokens.

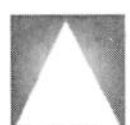

Table 24.12–2
Contingencies of Reinforcement in the Token Economy Used at the Camarillo–UCLA Clinical Research Unit[a]

Token earnings	
Morning rising from bed and getting dressed on time	3
Satisfactory completion of morning activities of daily living	3
Satisfactory participation in a social skills training group or recreational therapy activity	10
Satisfactory participation in individual behavioral therapy session	10
Satisfactory participation in leisure time activities (per activity)	5
Meets criteria for dress and grooming checks during day (per check)	3
Showers satisfactorily	3
Completes assigned jobs or tasks on unit (per job or task)	4
Participates in off-unit vocational rehabilitation or adult education activity (per half-day)	10
Token fines	
Smoking rule violation	5
Lying on floor	5
Stealing	10
Forgery of token credit card	10
Assault or property destruction	20
Late return from grounds privileges	20
Reinforcers available for tokens	
Cigarettes	4
Drinks (coffee, tea, sodas, hot chocolate)	10
Snacks (potato chips, pretzels, ice cream, candy)	10
Grounds privileges (per half hour)	4
Music time (per half hour)	4
Private room time (per half hour)	4
Nintendo, Walkman stereo, private TV (per half hour)	4

[a]This token economy uses a card that can be punched with holes to document token earnings and purchases. The token economy has three levels, which differ in the immediacy and type of reinforcement and privileges. At the highest level of performance, the patient carries a "credit card" and has full access to all unit privileges and rewards without having to pay with tokens.
Courtesy of Robert Paul Liberman, M.D.

COGNITIVE REHABILITATION

Increased recognition of the prevalence and importance of neurocognitive deficits over the past decade has stimulated increasing interest in remediation strategies. Much of the work in this area has focused on psychopharmacological approaches, especially on the new-generation antipsychotics. New-generation medications appear to have a positive effect on neurocognitive test performance, but the effect size for any of the medications is small to medium, and little evidence indicates that these medications have a clinically meaningful impact on neurocognitive functioning in the community. As a result, a parallel interest has arisen in the potential for *rehabilitation* or *cognitive remediation.* This body of work is distinguished from CBT and cognitive therapy, which focus on reducing psychotic symptoms.

A study at the National Institutes of Health (NIH) found that patients with schizophrenia were unable to benefit from explicit instructions and practice on the Wisconsin Card Sorting Test (WCST), a widely used test of executive functioning. The study was linked to data demonstrating that patients had diminished prefrontal blood flow in dorsolateral prefrontal cortex while responding to the WCST, implying that schizophrenia was marked by an unmodifiable abnormality of the dorsolateral prefrontal cortex. The NIH work stimulated a series of mostly successful laboratory demonstrations that WCST performance deficits, albeit widespread, are neither endemic to the illness nor immutable. For example, one study demonstrated that WCST performance could be enhanced by financial reinforcement and specific instructions. Other laboratories have since produced comparable and enduring effects using similar training strategies and extended practice alone.

ETHICAL ISSUES

The ethics of conducting rehabilitation strategies are generally the same as for conducting other psychotherapies. Two issues come up regularly, however: avoiding infantilization and maintaining confidentiality. The first concerns the risk of viewing the patient as unable to make adult choices such as whether to participate in rehabilitation, where to live, whether or not to work, and whether or not to use drugs and alcohol. Although it may be more of a value than an ethical standard, psychiatric rehabilitation is based on the assumption that the practitioner and the patient are in a partnership to facilitate recovery and improve quality of life. The basic model involves collaboration and shared decision making and does not portray the practitioner as an authority or parental figure. When patients make what appear to be bad choices, the practitioner must consider the patient's right to choose and whether the choice is dangerous versus simply not the choice the practitioner would make. If the choice, in fact, is potentially harmful, a collaborative process of considering alternatives is more likely to produce good choices than an authoritative, admonitory approach.

Failure to consider the patient as a partner also leads to violations of confidentiality. Practitioners sometimes assume that they are the primary arbiters of what information to share with parents, other clinicians, and other agencies. In fact, in most circumstances that do not involve the safety of patients or others, the patient should be the arbiter of what information is shared with whom. For example, in supported employment, the patients always determine whether to disclose information about their illnesses to employers.

▲ 24.13 Combined Psychotherapy and Pharmacotherapy

The use of psychotropic drugs in combination with psychotherapy has become widespread. In fact, it has become the standard of care for many patients seen by psychiatrists. In this therapeutic approach, psychotherapy is augmented by the use of pharmacological agents. It should not be a system in which the therapist meets with the patient on an occasional or irregular basis to monitor the effects of medication or to make notations on a rating scale to assess progress or side effects; rather, it should be a system in which both therapies are integrated and synergistic. In many cases, it has been demonstrated that the results of combined therapy are superior to either type of therapy used alone. The term *pharmacotherapy-oriented psychotherapy* is used by some practitioners to refer to the combined approach. The methods of psychotherapy used can vary immensely, and all can be combined with pharmacotherapy when indicated.

INDICATIONS FOR COMBINED THERAPY

A major indication for using medication when conducting psychotherapy, particularly for those patients with major mental disorders, such as schizophrenia or bipolar disorder, is that psychotropics reduce anxiety and hostility. This improves the patient's capacity to communicate and to participate in the psychotherapeutic process. Another indication for combined therapy is to relieve distress when the signs and the symptoms of the patient's disorder are so prominent that they require more rapid amelioration than psychotherapy alone may be able to offer. In addition, each technique may facilitate the other; psychotherapy may enable the patient to accept a much-needed pharmacological agent, and the psychoactive drug may enable the patient to overcome resistance to entering or continuing psychotherapy (Table 24.13–1).

The reduction of symptoms, especially anxiety, does not decrease the patient's motivation for psychoanalysis or other insight-oriented psychotherapy. In practice, drug-induced symptom reduction improves communication and motivation. All therapies have a cognitive base, and anxiety generally interferes with the patient's ability to gain cognitive understanding of the illness. Drugs that decrease anxiety facilitate cognitive understanding. They can improve attention, concentration, memory, and learning in patients who suffer from anxiety disorders.

NUMBER OF TREATING CLINICIANS

Any number of clinicians can be involved in treatment of a psychiatric disorder. In *one-person therapy,* the psychia-

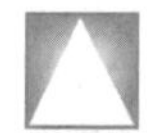

Table 24.13–1
Benefits of Combined Therapy

Improved medication compliance
Better monitoring of clinical status
Decreased number and length of hospitalizations
Decreased risk of relapse
Improved social and occupational functioning

trist provides individual psychotherapy and medication treatment. Multiperson therapy is a form of treatment in which one therapist (who may be a psychiatrist, psychologist, or a social worker) conducts psychotherapy, while the other therapist (always a psychiatrist) prescribes medications. Other therapists may oversee marriage or family therapy or group therapy. The terms *cotherapy* or *triangular therapy* are sometimes used to describe permutations of multiperson therapy.

COMMUNICATION AMONG THERAPISTS

Whenever more than one clinician is involved in treatment, there should be regular exchanges of information. Some patients split the transference between the two; one therapist may be seen as giving and nurturing, and the other may be seen as withholding and aloof. Similarly, countertransference issues, such as one therapist identifying with the patient's idealized or devalued image of the other therapist, can interfere with therapy. Those issues must be worked out, and the cotherapists must be compatible and respectful of each other's orientation, so that the therapy program can succeed.

A therapist may have some concerns about the quality of the psychopharmacology or that the existing regimen needs to be reconsidered. For example, a patient may not be doing well on medication, experiencing significant side effects, or showing lack of sufficient improvement. Some patients may also be taking many different medications. When and if it is deemed in the patient's interest to question the medication regimen or the prescriber's skill, these misgivings should not be shared with the patient without first conferring with the prescribing physician.

If the therapist or pharmacologist, after a good-faith effort to understand the methods and course of treatment, still has misgivings about treatment, he or she should inform his or her counterpart that a second opinion would be useful. This should then be suggested to the patient without necessarily raising undue alarm. Communication between treating clinicians should take place as frequently as needed. No standard exists for how frequent that should be.

ORIENTATIONS OF TREATING CLINICIANS

The orientation of the treating psychiatrist or other clinician can influence the therapeutic process during combination treatment. Clinicians invariably bring a theoretical bias to the treatment setting. Some, for example, are oriented, by preference and training, to practice a specific form of psychotherapy such as psychoanalysis, CBT, or group therapy. To these clinicians, psychotherapy is seen as the primary treatment modality, with pharmacological agents being used as an adjunct. Conversely, to a psychopharmacologically oriented psychiatrist, psychotherapy is seen as augmenting the use of medication. Although disagreement may arise on which approach represents the most active ingredient in clinical response, the optimal use of both modalities should complement each other.

In addition to having extensive training in one or more psychoanalytic or psychotherapeutic techniques, the psychiatrist who practices pharmacotherapy-oriented psychotherapy must have a comprehensive knowledge of psychopharmacology. That knowledge must include a thorough understanding of the indications for the use of each drug, the contraindications, the pharmacokinetics and pharmacodynamics, the drug–drug interactions (with all pharmacological agents, not only the psychoactive agents), and the adverse effects of medications. The psychiatrist must be able both to identify adverse effects and to treat them.

Table 24.13–2
Clinical Situations in Which It Is Advantageous for One Psychiatrist to Provide Medication and Psychotherapy

Patients with schizophrenia and other psychotic disorders who are not compliant with prescribed medication
Patients with bipolar I disorder who deny illness and do not cooperate with the treatment plan
Patients with serious or unstable medical conditions
Patients with severe borderline personality disorders
Impulsive and severely suicidal patients who are likely to require hospitalization
Patients with eating disorders who present complicated management problems
Patients who present a clinical picture in which the need for medication is unclear, thus requiring ongoing assessment

Nonpsychiatric physicians often use psychoactive agents inaccurately (too small or too large a dose for too short or too long a course), because they lack the requisite psychopharmacological knowledge, training, and experience. Psychotherapists who work with primary care physicians instead of psychiatrists should understand the limitations in depth of knowledge that these practitioners have and should seek a consultation with a psychiatrist if a patient is not responding to, or tolerating, medication. In some situations, it is preferable for psychotherapy and pharmacotherapy to be carried out by the same clinician; however, this is often not possible for a variety of reasons, including therapist availability, time limitations, and economic restraints, among others (Table 24.13–2).

Therapist Attitudes

Psychiatrists trained primarily as psychotherapists may prescribe medication more reluctantly than those who are more oriented toward biological psychiatry. Conversely, those who view medication as the preferred intervention for most psychiatric disorders may be reluctant to refer patients for psychotherapy. Therapists who are pessimistic about the value of psychotherapy or who misjudge the patient's motivation may prescribe medications because of their own beliefs; others may withhold medication if they overvalue psychotherapy or undervalue pharmacological treatments. When a patient is in psychotherapy with someone other than the clinician prescribing medication, it is important to recognize treatment bias and to avoid contentious turf battles that put the patient in the middle of such conflict.

Linkage Phenomenon

At some point, patients may view the improvement being made in therapy as the result of a conscious or unconscious linkage between the psychopharmacological agent and the therapist. In fact, after being weaned from medication, patients often carry a pill with them for reassurance. In that sense, the pill acts as a transitional object between the patient and the therapist. Some patients with anxiety disorders, for example, may carry a single benzodiazepine tablet, which they take when they think they are about to have an anxiety attack. Then, the patient may report that the attack was aborted—before the medication could even have been absorbed into the bloodstream. In other cases, the pill is never taken, because the patient knows that the pill is available and gains reassurance from that fact. The linkage phenomenon is usually not seen unless the patient is in a positive transference to the therapist. Indeed, the therapist may use this phenomenon to his or her advantage by suggesting that the patient carry medication to use as needed. Eventually, the behavior has to be analyzed, and it is often found that the patient has attributed magical properties to the therapist that are then transferred to the medication. Some clinicians believe the effect to be the result of conditioning. After repeated trials, the sight of the medicine can decrease anxiety. The positive transference may also cause *transference cure* or *flight into health,* in which the patient feels better in an unconscious attempt to meet the presumed expectations of the prescribing physician. Therapists should consider this phenomenon, if the patient reports rapid improvement well before a particular medication may reach its therapeutic level.

Rachel, a 25-year-old white woman, presented with depressive symptoms and abdominal pain. After an extensive psychiatric and medical evaluation, she was diagnosed with major depression of moderate severity and irritable bowel disorder. She began a course of CBT targeting her negative attributional style and low self-esteem, and she was taught relaxation and distraction techniques for her pain. After a 12-week trial, she experienced only partial remission of her symptoms and was offered an antidepressant, citalopram (Celexa) at 20 mg per day. Her depressive symptoms remitted within 1 month, and she was able to function better at work, but socially remained hesitant to engage with her peers. Her abdominal pain persisted and she began to exhibit a pattern of disordered eating, severely restricting her intake to 500 calories per day due to the "pain." She experienced a 15-pound weight loss over the next several months. An intensive behavioral plan to target eating was begun, as well as continued probing of her negative cognitions relating to eating, pain, and newly emerging concerns that she would regain the weight too quickly and would become "fat." She did not meet weight loss criteria for anorexia nervosa, although her cognitive distortions about her body image were extreme. These new concerns resulted in a relapse of her depressive symptoms, including suicidal ideation, and her citalopram was increased to 40 mg per day. She reported severe akathisia on this dose and refused to take any more medication, including an antidepressant of another class. Rachel did agree to intensify her therapy to twice weekly, and this allowed her to explore some of her conflicts, feelings, and thoughts that fostered her treatment-refractory illness. A combination of psychotherapy and hypnosis was used for this work. Over the next 6 months, Rachel revealed that she had been sexually abused as a child and this made her feel that she did not "deserve" to live or to eat, and that the pain served to "punish" her for being bad. She also admitted that she resisted the medication "psychologically" because she felt that she did not deserve to get well. Her newly found insight, as well as the coping skills she developed in therapy, resulted in a reduction of her depressive symptoms, marked improvement in her eating habits with normalization of her weight, and decreased abdominal pain. She maintained these gains over the next year, including normalization of her daily functioning, a promotion at work, and the ability to tolerate the intimacy of a boyfriend. *(Courtesy of E. M. Szigethy, M.D., Ph.D. and E. S. Friedman, M.D.)*

COMPLIANCE AND PATIENT EDUCATION

Compliance

Compliance is the degree to which a patient carries out the recommendations of the treating physician. Compliance is fostered when the doctor–patient relationship is a positive one, and the patient's refusal to take medication may provide insight into a negative transferential situation. In some cases, the patient acts out hostilities by noncompliance, rather than by becoming aware of, and ventilating such negative feelings toward the doctor. Medication noncompliance may provide the psychiatrist with the first clue that a negative transference is present in an otherwise compliant patient who had appeared to be agreeable and cooperative.

Education

Patients should know the target signs and symptoms that the drug is supposed to reduce, the length of time they will be taking the drug, the expected and unexpected adverse effects, and the treatment plan to be followed if the current drug is unsuccessful. Although some psychiatric disorders interfere with patients' abilities to comprehend that information, the psychiatrist should relay as much of the information as possible. The clear presentation of such material is often less frightening than are patients' fantasies about drug treatment. The psychiatrist should tell patients when they may expect to begin to receive benefits from the drug. That information is most critical when the patient has a mood disorder and may not observe any therapeutic effects for 3 to 4 weeks.

Some patients' ambivalent attitudes toward drugs often reflect the confusion about drug treatment that exists in the field of psychiatry. Patients often believe that taking a psychotherapeutic drug means they are not in control of their lives or they may become addicted to the drug and have to take it forever. Psychiatrists should explain the difference between drugs of abuse that affect the normal brain and psychiatric drugs that are used to treat emotional disorders. They should also point out to patients that antipsychotics, antidepressants, and antimanic drugs are not addictive in the way in which, for example, heroin is addictive. The psychiatrist's clear and honest explanation of how long the patient should take the drug helps the patient adjust to the idea of chronic maintenance medication, if that is the treatment plan. In some cases, the psychiatrist may appropriately give the patient increasing responsibility for adjusting the medications as the treatment progresses. Doing so often helps the patient feel less controlled by the drug and supports a collaborative role with the therapist.

ATTRIBUTION THEORY

Attribution theory is concerned with how persons perceive the causes of behavior. According to attribution theory, persons are likely to attribute changes in their own behavior to external events, but are likely to attribute another's behavior to internal dispositions, such as that person's personality traits. Research on drug effects by attribution theorists has shown that, when patients take medication and their behaviors change, they attribute it to the drug and not to any changes that occur within themselves. Accordingly, it may be unwise to describe a drug as extremely strong or effective, because if it does have the desired effect, the patient may believe that is the only reason he or she got better; if the drug does not work, the patient may assume his or her condition is incurable. Therapists do best by presenting the use of drugs and psychotherapy as complementary or adjunctive, as neither standing alone and both being needed for improvements or cure to occur.

MENTAL DISORDERS

Depressive Disorders

Some patients and clinicians fear that medication covers over the depression and that psychotherapy is impeded. Instead, medication should be viewed as a facilitator in overcoming the anergia that can inhibit the communication process between doctor and patient. The psychiatrist should explain to the patient that depression interferes with interpersonal activity in a variety of ways. For instance, depression produces withdrawal and irritability, which alienate significant others who may otherwise gratify the strong dependency needs that make up much of depressive psychodynamics.

If medication is stopped, the psychiatrist should be alert for signs and symptoms of a recurrent major depressive episode. Medication may have to be reinstituted. Before doing so, however, carefully review any stress, especially rejections, that could have precipitated recurrent major depressive disorder. A new episode of depression may occur because the patient is in a stage of negative transference, and the psychiatrist must try to elicit negative feelings. In many cases, the ventilation of angry feelings toward the therapist without an angry response can serve as a corrective emotional experience, and a major depressive episode necessitating medication can thereby be forestalled. Depressed patients are generally maintained on their medication for 6 months or longer after clinical improvement. The cessation of pharmacotherapy before that time is likely to result in a relapse.

Combined treatment has been shown to be superior to either therapy used alone in the treatment of major depression. It is associated with improved social and occupational functioning and improved quality of life compared with either therapy alone.

Bipolar I Disorder

Patients taking lithium (Eskalith) or other treatments for bipolar I disorder are usually medicated for an indefinite period of time to prevent episodes of mania or depression. Most psychotherapists insist that patients with bipolar I disorder be medicated before starting any insight-oriented therapy. Without such premedication, most patients with bipolar I disorder are unable to make the necessary therapeutic alliance. When those patients are depressed, their abulia seriously disrupts their flow of thoughts, and the sessions are nonproductive. When they are manic, their flow of associations can be rapid, and their speech can be so pressured that the therapist could be flooded with material and may be unable to make appropriate interpretations or to assimilate the material into the patient's disrupted cognitive framework.

The practice guideline of the American Psychiatric Association (APA) for bipolar disorder recommends combined therapy as the best approach. It increases compliance, decreases relapse, and reduces the need for hospitalization.

Substance Abuse

Patients who abuse alcohol or drugs present the most difficult challenge in combined therapy. They are often impulsive, and although they may promise not to abuse a substance, they may do so repeatedly. In addition, they frequently withhold information from the psychiatrist about episodes of abuse. For that reason, some psychiatrists do not prescribe any medication to such patients, especially not those substances with a high abuse potential, such as benzodiazepines, barbiturates, and amphetamines. Drugs with no abuse potential, such as amitriptyline (Elavil) and fluoxetine (Prozac), have an important role in treating the anxiety or depression that almost always accompanies substance-related disorders. The psychiatrist conducting psychotherapy with such patients should have no reservations about sending the patient to a laboratory for random urine toxicological tests.

Anxiety Disorders

Anxiety disorders encompass OCD, posttraumatic stress disorder (PTSD), generalized anxiety disorder, phobic disorders, and panic disorder with or without agoraphobia. Many drugs are effective in managing distressing signs and symptoms. As the symptoms are controlled by medication, patients are reassured and develop confidence that they will not be incapacitated by the disorder. That effect is particularly strong in panic disorder, which is often associated with anticipatory anxiety about the attack. Depression can also complicate the symptom picture in patients with anxiety disorders and has to be addressed pharmacologically and psychotherapeutically. Studies have shown that patients with anxiety disorders who receive ongoing psychotherapy are less likely to experience relapse compared with patients who receive medication alone.

Schizophrenia and Other Psychotic Disorders

Included in the group of schizophrenia and other disorders are schizophrenia, delusional disorder, schizoaffective disorder, schizophreniform disorder, and brief psychotic disorder. Drug treatment for those disorders is always indicated, and hospitalization is often necessary for diagnostic purposes to stabilize medication, to prevent danger to self or others, and to establish a psychosocial treatment program that may include individual psychotherapy. In attempting individual psychotherapy, the therapist must establish a treatment relationship and a therapeutic alliance with the patient. The patient with schizophrenia defends against closeness and trust and often becomes suspicious, anxious, hostile, or regressed in therapy. Before the advent of psychotropics, many psychiatrists were fearful for their own safety when working with such patients. Indeed, many assaults have occurred.

Individual psychotherapy for schizophrenia is labor intensive, expensive, and not often attempted. The recognition that combined psychotherapy and pharmacotherapy have a greater chance of success than either type of therapy alone may reverse that situation. The psychiatrist who conducts such combined therapy must be especially empathic and must be able to tolerate the bizarre manifestations of the illness. The patient with schizophrenia is exquisitely sensitive to rejection, and individual psychotherapy should never be started unless the therapist is willing to make a total commitment to the process.

OTHER ISSUES

Evidence suggests that therapy can induce physical changes in the nervous system. Eric Kandel has provided elegant proof, winning the Nobel Prize for demonstrating that environmental stimuli produce lasting changes in the synaptic architecture of living organisms. Imaging studies have begun to show that patients who show clinical improvement from psychotherapy show changes in brain metabolism that are similar to that seen in patients successfully treated with medications.

Still, some patients do well on only one form of treatment. Even with identical diagnoses, not all patients respond to the same treatment regimens. Success may be as dependent on the knowledge and quality of the clinician as on the potential benefit of a particular drug.

A real dilemma when combining treatment is the additional direct costs of two treatments. Although successful treatment results in reduced costs to society, the cost of treatment is usually narrowly defined by the patient as out-of-pocket expenses and by insurance and managed care companies as payments to the physician or hospital. Restrictions placed on the frequency and cost of visits to mental health professionals by managed care organizations, however, encourage the use of medication rather than psychotherapy.

▲ 24.14 Genetic Counseling

Medical geneticists and specially trained and qualified genetic counselors have traditionally provided genetic counseling to patients in need of such help. Many psychiatrists, however, are also well placed to provide genetic education and counseling, because they often have knowledge of their clients' needs and family histories and have ongoing therapeutic relationships. The ideal approach for providing psychiatric genetic counseling is through a multidisciplinary team approach, with collaboration between genetics and mental health professionals. Genetic professionals often seek collaboration with a psychiatrist for those with difficult psychiatric medical or family histories. Genetic professionals also seek collaboration or referral for persons with a psychiatric disorder; those who are having difficulty adapting to a genetic-related diagnosis; those dealing with the death of a family member; or those who are experiencing persistent difficulty with decision making regarding prenatal diagnosis or genetic testing. In turn, genetic professionals can be available for professional consultation regarding risk assessment, the collection and construction of complicated family medical histories, and the availability and limitations of genetic or genomic testing.

DEFINITIONS

Genetic counseling is the process of helping people to understand and adapt to the medical, psychological, and familial implications of genetic contributions to disease. According to the National Society of Genetic Counseling, it integrates three factors: (1) interpretation of family and medical histories to assess the chance of disease occurrence or recurrence; (2) education about inheritance, testing, management, prevention, resources, and research; and (3) counseling to promote informed choices and adaptation to the risk or condition. The process aims to minimize distress and facilitate adaptation, to increase one's feeling of personal control, and to facilitate informed decision making and life planning.

Genetic counseling is not limited to considerations of the genetic contributions of disease. Genetic counseling also considers *environmental* components of the presenting disease along with *genetic* ones. Table 24.14–1 lists common terminology used in the field of genetic counseling.

GENETICS AND MENTAL HEALTH

Disorders can recur in families for many reasons, including the functioning of genes (single genes vs. polygenic) (Table 24.14–2), shared environmental exposures, a combination of genetic and environmental factors (multifactorial), and cultural transmission. *Single gene disorders* are caused by defects in one particular gene, and they often have simple and predictable inheritance patterns. By contrast, most psychiatric disorders are *multifactorial* in etiology, influenced by multiple genes as well as environmental factors, making them more difficult to predict.

Two phenomena that further complicate genetic counseling include penetrance and expressivity. *Penetrance* refers to the portion of individuals with a specific genotype who also manifest that genotype at the phenotype level. If all individuals who carry the dominant gene show any phenotype of the gene, the gene is said to be *completely penetrant.* Currently, only rare examples exist of known genes for mental disorders that demonstrate complete penetrance of symptoms in the presence of a single gene. One such example is early-onset familial Alzheimer's disease resulting from mutations in the amyloid precursor protein (APP) located on the long arm of chromosome 21. In contrast, *expressivity* refers to the extent to which a genotype is expressed. In the case of variable expressivity, the trait can vary in expression from mild to severe, but is never completely unexpressed in individuals who have the gene. The genes that result in most mental disorders are believed to regulate a wide spectrum of traits demonstrating variability of expression (spectrum disorders).

COMPONENTS OF THE GENETIC COUNSELING PROCESS

Requests for genetic counseling are often initiated by the client's or relatives' questions about the disorder that is present in the family. In the case of mental illness, the questions are often posed to the treating psychiatrist. The client's questions are most effectively addressed through an interactive process that provides the client, as well as the professional, with information pertinent to the next step in the communication process. The basic components of genetic counseling are outlined in Table 24.14–3.

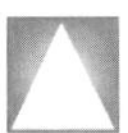

Table 24.14–1
Genetic Terminology

Absolute risk	One's risk of developing a disease over a specified time period (e.g., the empirical risk for autism in a sibling of an individual with idiopathic autism is about 6–8%; related term: relative risk)
Allele	One of the variant forms of a gene at a particular locus or location on a chromosome
Assortative mating	Nonrandom mating in which individuals preferentially mate with others with similar traits
Consultand	Person seeking genetic counseling
Complex (or multifactorial)	Traits, diseases, or disorders resulting from the interactions of genetic and environmental factors
Familial	Disorder recurring in a family that may result from a combination of shared genotype and environment
First-degree relatives	Biological relatives sharing 50% of their genetic makeup (e.g., parents, siblings, children)
Gene of major effect	As found in true dominant and recessive genetic disorders, a gene that is able independently to cause a phenotype, with little influence from the environment or other genetic contributions
Genome	All of the DNA (deoxyribonucleic acid) within a cell or organism; nuclear and mitochondrial
Genotype	Genetic makeup; most often referring to the allelic contribution at a particular locus
Heritability	Proportion of phenotypic variance attributable to genetic variance
Morbid or lifetime risk	The probability that subjects under study will develop an illness if they live long enough; takes into consideration that a susceptible subject may not have onset at the time of examination or may die of another cause before onset
Phenotype	Clinical presentation of the disorder
Polygenic	Traits resulting from the interaction of multiple genes
Presymptomatic	Unaffected individual known to carry a mutation that is very likely to result in the expression of the disorder
Proband	The affected person bringing the family to medical attention
Recurrence risk	Probability that a disorder will recur in other family members
Relative risk	One's risk of developing a disease when compared with a referent group (e.g., if the probability of developing idiopathic autism among siblings of an affected person is 6–8% compared with the risk in the general population of 0.1%, then the relative risk of autism in siblings of an affected individual is about 70; related term: absolute risk)
Second-degree relative	Biological relatives sharing 25% of their genetic makeup (e.g., grandparents, grandchildren, nephews, nieces)
Susceptibility	Increased risk, owing to the presence of deleterious allele, of developing a disease or disorder compared with the general population
Spectrum disorders	Disease or disorders in which the phenotypic expression is characterized by a broad range of variance (e.g., autism spectrum disorders)

Contracting

Contracting is a vital portion of the psychiatric genetic counseling session. Often, the goals of the session will vary based on the consultant's histories and reason(s) for concern. The provider should work with the consultant at the beginning of the session to define mutual goals.

Documentation of Diagnosis, Collection, and Review of Family Medical History

A family medical history (FMH) is collected, and at least a three-generation pedigree is constructed. The collection of

Table 24.14–2
Examples of Psychiatric Disorders Recognized as Having a Genetic Component to Their Etiology

Psychotic disorders: Schizophrenia, schizoaffective disorder
Mood disorders: Bipolar disorder, recurrent unipolar depression
Personality disorders: Antisocial personality disorder, schizotypal disorder
Anxiety disorders: Generalized anxiety disorder, obsessive-compulsive disorder, panic disorder, phobia
Substance-related disorders: Substance dependence and abuse
Eating disorders: Anorexia nervosa, bulimia
Childhood disorders: Attention-deficit/hyperactivity disorder, autism, chronic tic disorders, including Tourette's disorder
Memory disorders: Alzheimer's disease

Table 24.14–3
Steps and Process of Genetic Counseling

Solicit and clarify the client's presenting questions and goals for genetic counseling
Collect and review medical and family medical history
Identify support systems
Verify diagnoses in proband and other affected family members when possible
Address issues and concerns identified through the genetic counseling process
Assess the client's emotional and intellectual capacity before proceeding to determine the approach to the provision of education and counseling
Provide information at cognitively appropriate levels
Note that the processing of emotional reactions is intertwined with the provision of information
Assess the personal meaning of the information and the client's willingness to negotiate various risks and burdens
When applicable, assist the client in arriving at a decision by discussing available options; discuss benefits and limitations of each alternative
Assist the client with adapting to the risk status in the family
Assist in formulating a plan that the client is able to carry out
Provide follow-up counseling and support. Continue to assess the client's and family's understanding of the information and the effect of the information, risks, or decisions

Table 24.14–4
Topics Included in the Family Medical History

A. Any psychiatric diagnosis, whether childhood, adult, postpartum, or geriatric
   1. Age of symptom onset and at diagnosis
   2. Subjective assessment of illness severity and treatment response
   3. Potentially important environmental exposures (e.g., birth trauma, cannabis use, head injury)
B. Symptomatic, undiagnosed individuals
   1. Suggest a psychiatric evaluation
C. Undiagnosed individuals treated with psychiatric medications
D. Developmental history (e.g., has the individual achieved normal milestones for age, such as independent living and employment for adults?)
E. Social history
F. Substance abuse
G. Suicide
H. Birth defects, mental retardation or learning disabilities, and unusual medical conditions
I. The age and sex of at-risk family members (which may play a role in risk assessment)

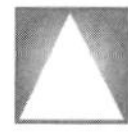

Table 24.14–5
Issues That Can Hinder an Accurate Psychiatric Family History

▲ Stigma and shame may limit what a consultand is willing to share.
▲ Stigma and shame may limit what family history has been shared with the consultand by other family members.
▲ Many affected individuals have not been diagnosed.
▲ Diagnoses change over time for reasons including patients' evolving illness course, changes in diagnostic criteria, and interprofessional variation in diagnosis.
▲ Highly symptomatic individuals may not be able to provide a comprehensive and accurate family history.

FMH begins with the individual seeking information. The *consultand* (or client) is the individual seeking information. *Proband* is the term used to identify the affected person within the family who first brought the family to medical attention. The FMH should be comprehensive, and include the following information: ages (or dates of birth) of each family member, the age at which the diagnosis was made for individuals with the disorder, pregnancy losses (including the gestational length along with the recognized cause, if known), the recognized cause and age of any deceased family members, and ethnic backgrounds (Table 24.14–4).

Confirmation or clarification of the diagnosis is essential to the provision of valid information within the session. This usually requires obtaining medical records to clarify or to confirm the suspected diagnosis in the relatives. Depending on the situation, genetic testing may be available for at-risk members in families with single-gene disorders; but because DNA (deoxyribonucleic acid) testing for most mental disorders is not yet an option, risk assessment is based solely on analysis of the pedigree.

The collection and review of the FMH with the patient might elicit or recall intense feelings of sadness, guilt, anxiety, or anger. Furthermore, the graphic presentation of the family history may bring to light a more concrete realization of an individual's risks; therefore, attention to the patient's affect is important throughout the process. Specific issues that may hinder an accurate psychiatric family history and may increase consultants affect related to family history are listed in Table 24.14–5.

Communication of Risk and Decision Making

Individuals vary in their level of understanding risks. The provision of risk information is best approached in a balanced and accurate manner that is tailored to the patient as much as possible. There is the temptation to use nonnumeric phrases of probability (e.g., often, rarely, most likely); however, the meaning of these nonnumeric phrases is highly subjective and their use in the genetic counseling session introduces the potential for bias.

Ideally, risks should be presented in several different ways, taking clues from interactions with the client that inform the approach. Some examples of approaches to assist the client's understanding of risks include stating numeric risks as percentages (25 percent) and as fractional risks (one-in-four chance). It is important to frame risks from the perspective of a negative and a positive outcome; for example, there is a 1 percent chance that the test will result in a complication and a 99 percent chance that there will be no complication.

Owing to the high rate of co-occurring disorders and the wide phenotypic range of psychiatric disorders, patients should be informed of potential risks for disorders other than those that brought them to genetic counseling. An example of this is the risk to first-degree relatives of an individual diagnosed with bipolar disorder. In this situation, the risk for bipolar disorder is increased for first-degree relatives, as are the risks for unipolar disorder, schizoaffective disorder, and cyclothymia.

It should be made clear that the risks are determined from populations and not derived from individuals, and therefore are estimates at best. Table 24.14–6 provides a compilation of recurrence risks from various referenced sources in the literature.

PSYCHOSOCIAL COUNSELING AND SUPPORT

Setting the stage for the inclusion of psychological and emotional issues can occur early in the process by verbalizing the intent to provide factual information, as well as fostering a discussion of the client's reaction to the information. Insight into the client's perspective and experiences with the disorder, values, beliefs, and family dynamics can begin to be obtained through asking what brings the client to the genetic counseling session. Eliciting this personal information provides a relational context from which the provider can assess concerns and emotional issues. Collection of the FMH can also provide a backdrop of the client's and family's experiences with the disorder. The exchange of information that occurs during the collection of the FMH can identify underlying risk and perceptions, family beliefs or myths regarding the disorder, and existing support system within the family.

Table 24.14–6
Empirical Risks for Selected Mental Disorders

			Unipolar Major Depressive Disorder						Alcohol Dependence				
	Schizophrenia	Bipolar Disorder	Men	Women	Schizoaffective Disorder	Obsessive-Compulsive Disorder	Panic Disorder	Generalized Anxiety Disorder	Men	Women	Phobia	Anorexia Nervosa	ADHD
Affected relative													
General population	1%[a]	0.8–1.6%[b,c,d,e]	1–15%[b,c]	2–23%[b,c]	0.5–<1%[b,c,d]	1.5–3%[a,f]	1.5–3.5%[a,g]	3.5%[a]	14%[a]	3%[a]	4–11%[a]	0.1%[a]	3–5%[h]
First degree (pooled)	9%[a]	5–20%[b,c,e]	9%[a]	18%[a]	1–10%[b,c,d]	17–25%[a,f]	15–25%[a,g]	20%[a]	27%[a]	5%[a]	12–31%[a]	5–10%[a]	15–60%[i]
Siblings	9–16%[d,j,k,l]	5–20%[b,c,e,m,j]	5–30%[b,c,m,j]	5–30%[b,c,m,j]	—	25–35%[n]	—	—	—	—	—	—	17–25%[o]
Parent	5–13%[o,j,k,l,p]	15%[c,d,e,m,q]	7–19%[m,j]	7–19%[m,j]	—	25–35%[n]	—	—	—	—	—	—	—
Both parents	45%[m,j]	50–75% for affective disorder[b,d,m,j]	—	—	—	—	—	—	—	—	—	—	—
Second degree (pooled)	2–6%[m,j]	5%[m]	—	—	—	—	—	—	—	—	—	—	3–9%[i]
Uncle/aunt	1–4%[j,k]	—	—	—	—	—	—	—	—	—	—	—	—
Nephew/niece	2–4%[j,k,p]	—	—	—	—	—	—	—	—	—	—	—	—
Grandparent	2–8%[j,k]	—	—	—	—	—	—	—	—	—	—	—	—
Half-sibling	4%[j,k]	—	—	—	—	—	—	—	—	—	—	—	—
Third degree	—	—	—	—	—	—	—	—	—	—	—	—	—
First cousin	2–6%[j,k]	—	—	—	—	—	—	—	—	—	—	—	—
Risks for additional mental disorders	Spectrum disorders (schizoaffective disorder, schizotypal personality disorder, paranoid personality disorder); unipolar and major depression	Unipolar disorder, substance dependence, schizoaffective disorder, cyclothymia, anxiety disorder, FDR; RR any affective disorder: ~20–30%	Anxiety disorders, alcohol dependence, dysthymia, ADHD		Schizophrenia, other psychotic disorders, bipolar disorder, unipolar depression, FDR; RR mood or psychotic disorder <30%	Tourette's disorder chronic tics, unipolar depression	—	Unipolar major depression	—		—	—	Unipolar depression, bipolar disorder, oppositional disorder, conduct disorder, anxiety disorders

(continued)

Table 24.14–6
Empirical Risks for Selected Mental Disorders (Continued)

			Unipolar Major Depressive Disorder						Alcohol Dependence				
	Schizophrenia	Bipolar Disorder	Men	Women	Schizoaffective Disorder	Obsessive-Compulsive Disorder	Panic Disorder	Generalized Anxiety Disorder	Men	Women	Phobia	Anorexia Nervosa	ADHD
Notes:	Early onset and severe phenotype may increase RR	Early onset may increase RR; female relatives at greatest risk for any affective disorder	Early onset and recurrent episodes may increase RR in first-degree relatives; male-to-female ratio is 1:2–3		—	Early onset may increase RR	Early onset may increase RR	—	Males may have greater sensitivity to genetic risk factors		—	—	RR higher for male relatives than female relatives; continuation of symptoms into adulthood may indicate increased RR

ADHD, attention-deficit/hyperactivity disorder; FDR, first-degree relative; RR, recurrence risk.

[a]Moldin SO. Psychiatric genetic counseling. In: Guze SB, ed. *Washington University Adult Psychiatry.* Mosby-Year Book; 1997.
[b]Duffy A, Grof P. The implications of genetic studies of major mood disorders for clinical practice. *J Clin Psychiatry.* 2000;61: 630–637.
[c]Gershon ES. A family study of schizoaffective, bipolar I, bipolar II, unipolar and normal control probands. *Arch Gen Psychiatry.* 1982;39:1157–1167.
[d]Gershon ES. A controlled family study of chronic psychosis. *Arch Gen Psychiatry.* 1988;45:328–336.
[e]Potash JB. Searching high and low: A review of the genetics of bipolar disorder. *Bipolar Disord.* 2000;2:8–26.
[f]Swedo SE, Rapoport IL, Leonard H. Obsessive-compulsive disorder children and adolescence. *Arch Gen Psychiatry.* 1989;46: 335–341.
[g]Crowe RR, Noyes R, Pauls DL. A family study of panic disorder. *Arch Gen Psychiatry.* 1983;40:1065.
[h]Barkley RA. Attention deficit hyperactivity disorder. *Sci Am.* 1998;9:66.
[i]National Society of Genetic Counselors Psychiatric Special Interest Group. At a glance empiric risk data. Available at: www.nsgc.org/members_only/sig/sig_psyc_empiric.cfm.
[j]Nurnberger J Jr, Berrettini W. *Psychiatric Genetics.* 1st ed. London: Chapman Hall; 1998:164.
[k]Hodgkinson KA. Genetic counseling for schizophrenia in the era of molecular genetics. *Can J Psychiatry.* 2001;46:123–130.
[l]Kendler KS, McGuire M. An epidemiologic, clinical and family study of simple schizophrenia in County Roscommon, Ireland. *Am J Psychiatry.* 1994;151:27–34.
[m]Harper PS. *Practical Genetic Counseling.* 4th ed. Oxford: Butterworth-Heinemann; 1994:348.
[n]Rasmussen SA, Tsuang MT. The epidemiology of obsessive-compulsive disorder. *J Clin Psychiatry.* 1984;45:450–457.
[o]Biederman, Faraone SV, Keenan K, et al. Further evidence for family-genetic risk factors in attention deficit hyperactivity disorder. Patterns of comorbidity in probands and relatives psychiatrically and pediatrically referred samples. *J Arch Gen Psychiatry.* 1992;49:728–738.
[p]Gottesman II, Shields J. *Schizophrenia: The Epigenetic Puzzle.* New York, NY: Cambridge University Press; 1982.
[q]Goodwin FK, Jamison KR. *Manic Depressive Illness.* New York, NY: Oxford University Press; 1990:938.
Asarnow RF. Schizophrenia and schizophrenia spectrum personality disorders in the first-degree relatives of children with schizophrenia: The UCLA family study. *Arch Gen Psychiatry.* 2001;58:581–588.
Kendler KS, Gardner CO. The risk for psychiatric disorders in relatives of schizophrenic and control probands: A comparison of three independent studies. *Psychol Med.* 1997;27:411–419.
Kendler KS, Walsh D. Schizophreniform disorder, delusional disorder and psychotic disorder not otherwise specified: Clinical features, outcome and familial psychopathology. *Acta Psychiatry Scand.* 1995;91:370–378.
McGuffin P. The heritability of bipolar affective disorder and the genetic relationship to unipolar depression. *Arch Gen Psychiatry.* 2003;60:497–502.
National Institutes of Mental Health. *Genetics and Mental Disorders.* 1999. Available at: www.nimh.nih.gov/research/genetics.htm.

A couple in their mid-30s with a 10-year history of infertility had been trying to adopt a child for a number of years. Recently, the adoption agency they were working with told them of a baby who was being placed for adoption because the biological mother was affected with bipolar disorder and did not feel that she could provide adequate care for the baby. The FMH collected on the newborn baby did not identify others in his family with mental disorders. The recurrence risk for bipolar disorder to the newborn was, therefore, estimated to be between 5 and 20 percent, with additional risks for other mental disorders. The couple individually reacted quite disparately to the estimated risks. In attempting to help them clarify the factors contributing to their feelings regarding the risks, the husband shared his experience with a childhood neighbor who had "some kind of mental illness" and detailed the "torment and agony" that the child brought to the family. Retorting, the woman shared the fact that her coworker also had bipolar disorder and did "just fine" at work with the help of medication. She therefore did not feel that the risks for mental disorders were of concern. The psychiatrist facilitated the couple's discussion of the spectrum and meaning of mental illness, along with recurrence risks in the context of a genetic education and counseling session. Although the couple did not come to agreement at that meeting over the potential for adopting the child, they did feel that the information and sharing of experiences and perspectives about mental disorders were beneficial. They agreed to return in 1 week after further considering the issues in an effort to reach a decision regarding the adoption. *(Courtesy of Holly L. Peay, M.S. and Donald W. Hadley, M.S.)*

CHALLENGES POSED BY PRESYMPTOMATIC AND SUSCEPTIBILITY GENETIC TESTING

Psychiatrists will be on the front line for receiving requests for genetic counseling and testing, because of their established relationship between patients and families with mental disorders. The identification of these risks will most likely occur before the discovery or availability of preventative options. The option of knowing risks without preventative options raises concerns regarding the impact of such knowledge on the individual's mood, anxiety, distress, self-image, reproductive decisions, career decisions, family relationships, insurability, employment, and potentially other areas.

A model for the provision of presymptomatic genetic testing is provided through the protocol developed for Huntington's disease (see the Hereditary Disease Foundation website at www.hdfoundation.org). This model recommends conducting education, counseling, and evaluative sessions over an extended period of time (3 to 4 months), during which time information is provided, questions are addressed, and counseling is initiated, thus maximizing informed decision making. The process is most appropriately undertaken in the absence of other stressful events (e.g., death of a family member, diagnosis of the disease in another family member, job loss, and divorce).

Studies suggest that most individuals receiving information of their increased risk for the disease in their family experience significantly more anxiety, depression, and psychological distress and have poorer perception of their health over the short term (within 1 month after receiving test results) compared with their baseline levels, but no difference over the long term (as long as 1 year after the receipt of results) compared with pretest levels. Consideration should also be given to the impact of such information on the spouse, because initial studies have suggested that the spouse may experience higher levels of depression related to the presymptomatic diagnosis than the client. Furthermore, partners of gene-positive individuals may experience increased levels of intrusive thoughts, avoidance, and hopelessness over the short and long term compared with baseline levels.

ETHICAL, LEGAL, AND SOCIAL CONSIDERATIONS

Certain individuals and families may experience significant levels of stigma associated with the identification of a genetic disorder, a situation already familiar to individuals and families with mental illness. The added knowledge of a hereditary component may heighten stigmatization. Conversely, having an identified biological basis may supplant current public perceptions that mental illness is somehow a personal or family failure in moral, spiritual, or attitudinal perspectives.

Questions frequently arise about the privacy of an individual's genetic information, the ability of employers or insurers to access such information, and the potential of using the information against them by denying insurance, raising rates to unreasonable levels, or denying jobs and a host of other possible concerns. Currently, no overarching federal laws comprehensively protect citizens of the United States from the potential of these abuses, although significant efforts are continuing in this regard. The status of existing and proposed state and federal laws can be reviewed through the website of the National Human Genome Research Institute (www.genome.gov).

▲ 24.15 Mentalization-Based Therapy and Mindfulness

Mentalization is a relatively new term that has been defined as the process of thinking and feeling about oneself and others. *Mindfulness* is somewhat similar except that it applies only to oneself. In both modalities the person attempts to stay aware of thoughts, feelings, affects, moods, and somatic sensations; but in mentalization, that exercise extends to another person as well. It is an interpersonal transaction. The origins of mentalization-based therapy (MBT) have been attributed to two psychologists, Jon Allen and Peter Fonagy, and one psychiatrist, Anthony Batemen, who described the process in their book *Mentalizing in Clinical Practice*.

From a theoretical perspective, MBT is eclectic in that it combines theories from a number of analytic and nonanalytic schools of thought: Sigmund Freud and psychoanalysis; John Bowlby and attachment theory; Aaron Beck and cognitive therapy; Carl Rogers and client-centered therapy; and Gerald Klerman and interpersonal therapy. The amalgam of these techniques developed into the unique method of treatment known as mentalization.

Mindfulness has its origins in Buddhist philosophy and the term was used in the 19th century to refer to a meditative technique in which the person stayed in the moment focusing on innermost feelings and states of mind. Mindfulness and mentalization rely on the same process; the person focuses on being in the "here and now." Some have described the differences between MBT and mindfulness by stating that in MBT one is "mindful of mindfulness."

The novel focus of a mindfulness approach is on present-moment, nonjudgmental awareness of consciousness, that is, noticing one's thoughts and feelings in the moment and accepting them without judging or trying to change them. In many ways, mindfulness is a variation of self-monitoring in which patients attend to and increase awareness of thoughts, feelings, and behaviors. However, increased awareness of these phenomena from a mindfulness perspective does not involve analyzing them to determine how best to modify them. Instead, patients might be asked to imagine their thoughts and feelings as if they were written on cards carried by marchers in a parade or as if they were pieces of luggage on a conveyor belt. They are asked to observe internal phenomena without reaction.

THERAPEUTIC APPROACHES

Freud believed that all action was preceded by thought (conscious or unconscious), and in mentalization the therapist helps the patient "capture" the thought so that actions are understood more fully. Bowlby saw attachment of the infant to the mother or to the primary caregiver as the basis for a sense of security later in life. In mentalization, the therapist relies on a secure attachment with the patient to enable him or her to explore the inner world of emotions and the outer world of action, both of which elicit anxiety. Beck proposed that cognitive distortions of the self (e.g., "She doesn't like me") could be reversed by positive cognitions (e.g., "I don't know if she likes me; many people do"). The mentalization therapist corrects distortions through interpretation and helps the patient test the validity of negative thoughts. The patient is encouraged to use the mechanism of empathy to step into the shoes of the other and to experience what that person may be thinking or feeling. It is the antithesis of self-centeredness. Klerman emphasized transferential distortions—a Freudian concept—that interfere with interpersonal relationships. The mentalization therapist attempts to strengthen the patient's capacity to see the other as he or she really is by not "mind reading" or fantasizing about what the other person thinks. Rogers emphasized the autonomy of the patient vis-à-vis the therapist who was not to be seen as all knowing and omnipotent. The mentalization therapist relies on a certain degree of self-disclosure to reinforce that concept. In that sense, the therapist serves as a role model for coping with the anxieties of daily living and the vicissitudes of life. The task of the therapist is neither to judge nor advise. He or she takes a "mentalizing stance," which is neutral and allows the patient to resolve conflict using innate resources that were previously unrecognized. MBT also allows the patient to mentalize the future by anticipating events and his or her reactions to them. In MBT emotion is experienced in a controlled and modulated manner, which can be a valuable therapeutic experience for persons whose affect is restricted because of fear. Fonagy has described what he calls the *mentalizing stance* as "an attitude of openness, inquisitiveness and curiosity about what's going on in the others' mind and in your own." In that sense, the use and development of empathy is a core component of the process.

Mindfulness is the practice of paying attention in a particular way—on purpose, in the present moment, and without judgment. Mindfulness skills include the ability to observe, describe, and participate fully in one's actions in a nonjudgmental, mindful, and effective manner. Some of the work in mindfulness-based approaches centers on decreasing what is known as *experiential avoidance* or the unwillingness to experience negative feelings, thoughts, and sensations. Persons who are skilled and well practiced in mindfulness are more adept at taking their automatic thoughts "with a grain of salt." Upset by a series of interpersonal disappointments, a person may think "I am never going to let myself care about people ever again." However, as he or she takes stock of this thought, the individual quickly concludes that this self-statement is neither realistic nor constructive. Instead, the person recognizes that the emotional pain of the moment is tied up in biased thinking, and that the solution to recovering from negative life events requires learning from the difficult situations and moving on.

Mindfulness approaches are aimed at improving patients' abilities to regulate their emotions and tolerating distress may then be considered, in effect, exposure exercises. Although techniques that increase patients' nonjudgmental awareness of internal sensations may be considered at odds with attempts to change thoughts in a way that is typical within cognitive therapy, the techniques may be considered comparable to exposure-based procedures that help patients to reduce anxiety and distress associated with certain types of thoughts and images through repeated exposure to those thoughts and images. The overlap between cognitive–behavioral treatments and mindfulness based approaches continues to be hotly debated.

INDICATIONS

Mentalization has been applied to a number of clinical disorders, one of which is autism. In autism, both child and adult are impaired socially because they are less sensitive to emotional cues given by others. They have difficulty empathizing, which makes their social interactions awkward and stilted. Mentalization focuses on teaching empathy and improving social engagement with others.

Patients with antisocial personality disorder may also benefit from MBT. Such patients are manipulative, give no thought to the results of their actions, lack the capacity for loyalty, and are unable or unwilling to empathize with others. MBT focuses on the core issues of their psychopathology. If a secure attachment can be made between patient and therapist, the basic trust that is lacking in the antisocial person may be developed for the first time. MBT has also been of use in patients with borderline personality disorder.

Mindfulness-based treatments have been demonstrated to be effective for a wide range of psychological problems, including borderline personality disorder, anxiety, chronic pain, depression, and stress. The approaches also have been used to reduce dysfunction in patients with medical conditions (e.g., cancer, multiple sclerosis) and to increase general well-being. Patients also learn to develop a greater tolerance for feelings of anxiety or depression and recognize that those states are often transitory, which may enable them to deal with conflict with greater confidence.

25

Psychopharmacological Treatment

GENERAL PRINCIPLES OF PSYCHOPHARMACOLOGY

Greater understanding about the role of neurotransmitters and neural pathways in the brain as the basis of mental and cognitive dysfunction has dramatically expanded the parameters of psychiatric treatments. The discovery of new receptor subtypes and their mechanism, brain imaging and modulation of gene expression have led to greater understanding of psychiatric disorders and consequently the development of receptor-specific targeted psychotropic drugs that are more efficacious, less toxic, and better tolerated. In fact the term neuropsychopharmacology may be a more accurate and appropriate term to use considering the role of neurotransmitters, ligands, neuropeptides, and specific drugs being developed to target and manipulate these systems.

With the ever-increasing sophistication and array of treatment options, clinicians, however, must remain aware of potential adverse effects, drug–drug (and drug–food or drug–supplement) interactions, and how to manage the emergence of unwanted or unintended consequences. Newer drugs could ultimately lead to side effects that are not recognized initially. Keeping up with the latest research findings is increasingly important as these findings proliferate. A thorough understanding of the management of medication-induced side effects (either through treating the effect with another agent or substituting another primary agent) is necessary.

Classification

Medications used to treat psychiatric disorders are referred to as *psychotropic drugs*. These drugs are commonly described by their major clinical application, for example, *antidepressants, antipsychotics, mood stabilizers, anxiolytics, hypnotics, cognitive enhancers,* and *stimulants*. A problem with this approach is that, in many instances, drugs have multiple indications. For example, drugs such as the selective serotonin reuptake inhibitors (SSRIs) are both antidepressants and anxiolytics, and the serotonin-dopamine antagonists (SDAs) are antipsychotics, mood stabilizers, and antidepressants. Psychotropic drugs have also been organized according to structure (e.g., tricyclic), mechanism (e.g., monoamine oxidase inhibitor [MAOI]), history (e.g., first generation, traditional), uniqueness (e.g., atypical), or indication (e.g., antidepressant). A further problem is that many drugs used to treat medical and neurological conditions are routinely used to treat psychiatric disorders.

The first pharmaceutical agents used to treat schizophrenia were termed *tranquilizers*. When newer drugs emerged as therapies for anxiety, a distinction was drawn between *major* and *minor tranquilizers*. At first, antidepressants were tricyclic antidepressants (TCAs) or MAOIs. In the 1970s and 1980s, as newer antidepressant drugs emerged, they were labeled as *second-* or *third-generation antidepressants*. More recently, older agents used as treatments for psychosis became known as *typical, conventional,* or *traditional neuroleptics*. Newer ones became *atypical neuroleptics*. In addition, the same class of drugs has interchangeable names (major tranquilizer, neuroleptic, and antipsychotic) adding to the confusion.

During the last decade, the definition of psychotropic drugs has evolved and instead of describing them by their clinical indication, the better approach has been to classify them based on mechanism of action. This approach is more practical and easier for clinicians when prescribing for on- and off-label use. In order to eliminate much of this confusion, drugs in this section are presented according to shared mechanism of action or by similarity of structure to provide consistency, ease of reference, and comprehensiveness.

Pharmacological Actions

Both genetic and environmental factors influence individual response to, and tolerability of, psychotropic agents. Thus, a drug that may not prove effective in many patients with a disorder can dramatically improve symptoms in others. In these cases, identification of characteristics that might predict potential candidates for that drug becomes important, but often remains elusive.

Drugs, even within the same class, are distinguished from one another by often subtle differences in molecular structure, types of interactions with neurotransmitter systems, differences in pharmacokinetics, the presence or absence of active metabolites, and protein binding. These differences, combined with the biochemistry of the patient, account for the profile of efficacy, tolerability, and safety and the risk-to-benefit ratio for the individual. These multiple variables, some poorly understood, make it difficult to predict a drug's effect with certainty. Nevertheless, knowledge of the nature of each property increases the likelihood of successful treatment. The clinical effects of drugs are best understood in terms of pharmacokinetics, which describes *what the body does to a drug,* and pharmacodynamics, which describes *what the drug does to the body.*

Pharmacokinetics and pharmacodynamics need to be seen in the context of the underlying variability among patients with respect to how drug effects are expressed clinically. Patients differ in their therapeutic response to a drug and the experience of side effects. It is increasingly clear that these differences have a strong genetic basis. Pharmacogenetics research is attempting to identify the role of genetics in drug response.

Pharmacogenomic Testing

Genetics play an important and pivotal role in understanding illnesses as well as response to medications. Pharmacogenomics is defined as an individual's genetic variability to drug response and is an emerging and evolving field in psychiatry. The field of genetics in behavioral health so far has mostly been limited to epidemiology within the context of understanding heredity risk factors and chromosomal aberrations with no specific markers elicited to date. Its utility in clinical practice is limited by the fact that data is not universally substantiated by research nor validated or accepted by insurance companies, or third party payers. In psychiatry, pharmacogenomic testing has some utility for psychotropic drugs though clinicians (psychiatrists) have not yet incorporated this into daily practice for numerous reasons including cost barriers; and furthermore, it has not been recommended by the FDA or endorsed by any expert panels.

The principles of pharmacogenomic testing are similar to basic psychopharmacology as they are categorized into pharmacodynamic and pharmacokinetic genes. The former set of genes illustrate the effect of the drug on the body and help in identifying drug candidate selection while the latter indicates the effect of the body on the drug through metabolism and determines drug dosage. A few examples of pharmacodynamics gene testing include serotonin transporter (SLC6A4), which predicts response and adverse effects of SSRI and SNRI antidepressants. Another serotonin receptor 2C (5-HT_{2C}) mutation may predict weight gain with atypical antipsychotics. The list is evolving, but to mention a few, others include the dopaminergic (COMT), opioid (OPRM1) and glutamate (GRIK1) system.

The pharmacokinetic genes CYP450 (CYP1A2, CYP2B6, CYP2C9, CYP2C19, CYP2D6, CYP3A4/5) are particularly important and clinically relevant as they predict rate of metabolism of medications and predict dose adjustment.

Despite the limitations and current utility, pharmacogenomics will continue to evolve, the data will accumulate and mature, and eventually this new emerging field will integrate into practice. For now, psychiatrists should familiarize themselves with genetic terminology, genes and alleles affecting various psychotropic medications as well as understanding metabolizing factors that may impact the use of psychotropic medicines and inform the patients about potential issues and individualizing treatment choices.

In summary, this testing can offer a more personalized treatment without trial and error approach and help both the clinician and the patient address patient symptoms more objectively with the appropriate therapy and identify the risk of side effects.

Drug Selection

Although all U.S. Food and Drug Administration (FDA)-approved psychotropics are similar in overall effectiveness for their indicated disorder, they differ considerably in their pharmacology and in their efficacy and adverse effects on individual patients. The ability of a drug to prove effective, thus, is only partially predictable and is dependent on poorly understood patient variables. Nevertheless, it is possible that some drugs have a niche in which they can be uniquely helpful for a subgroup of patients, without demonstrating any overall superiority in efficacy. No drug is universally effective, and no evidence indicates the unambiguous superiority of any single agent as a treatment for any major psychiatric disorders. The only exception, clozapine (Clozaril), has been approved by the FDA as a treatment for cases of treatment-refractory schizophrenia.

Decisions about drug selection and use are made on a case-by-case basis, relying on the individual judgment by the physician. Other factors in drug selection are the characteristics of the drug and the nature of the patient's illness. Each of these components affects the probability of a successful outcome.

Drug Factors

Pharmacodynamics. The time course and intensity of a drug's effects are referred to as its *pharmacodynamics.* Major pharmacodynamic considerations include receptor mechanisms, the dose–response curve, the therapeutic index, and the development of tolerance, dependence, and withdrawal phenomena. Drug mechanism of action is subsumed under pharmacodynamics. The clinical response to a drug, including adverse reactions, results from an interaction between that drug and a patient's susceptibility to those actions. Pharmacogenetic studies are beginning to identify genetic polymorphisms linked to individual differences in treatment response and sensitivity to side effects.

Mechanisms. The mechanisms through which most psychotropic drugs produce their therapeutic effects remain poorly understood. Standard explanations focus on ways that drugs alter synaptic concentrations of dopamine, serotonin, norepinephrine, histamine, γ-aminobutyric acid (GABA), or acetylcholine. These changes are said to result from receptor antagonists or agonists, interference with neurotransmitter reuptake, enhancement of neurotransmitter release, or inhibition of enzymes. Specific drugs are associated with permutations or combinations of these actions. For example, a drug can be an agonist for a receptor, thus stimulating the specific biological activity of the receptor, or an antagonist, thus inhibiting the biological activity. Some drugs are partial agonists, because they are not capable of fully activating a specific receptor. Some psychotropic drugs also produce clinical effects through mechanisms other than receptor interactions. For example, lithium (Eskalith) can act by directly inhibiting the enzyme inositol-1-phosphatase. Some effects are closely linked to a specific synaptic effect. For example, most medications that treat psychosis share the ability to block the dopamine type 2 (D_2) receptor. Similarly, benzodiazepine agonists bind a receptor complex that contains benzodiazepine and GABA receptors.

Further illustrating the fact that the mechanisms of action of psychotropic drugs remain only partially understood is based on the observations that medications that do not directly target monoamine neurotransmitters can be remarkably effective in treating some psychiatric disorders. For example, ketamine (Ketalar), an anesthetic agent that targets glutamate, can rapidly and dramatically alleviate symptoms of depression when given as a slow infusion. Another example involves the antibiotic minocycline (Solodyn), which has been shown to have

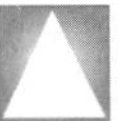

Table 25–1
Glossary of Receptor Drug Interactions

Receptor Interaction	Definition	Examples and Comments
Agonist (full agonist)	A drug or medication that binds to a specific receptor producing an effect identical to that usually produced by the neurotransmitter affecting that receptor. Drugs are often designed as receptor agonists to treat a variety of diseases and disorders in which the original neurotransmitter is missing or diminished.	Full agonists include opioids such as morphine, methadone, oxycodone, hydrocodone, heroin, codeine, meperidine, propoxyphene, and fentanyl. Benzodiazepines act as agonists at the GABA receptor complex.
Antagonist	A compound that binds to a receptor that blocks or reduces the action of another substance (agonist) at the receptor site involved. Antagonists that compete with an agonist for a receptor are *competitive antagonists*. Those that antagonize by other means are *noncompetitive antagonists*.	Flumazenil is a competitive benzodiazepine receptor antagonist. It competitively inhibits the activity at the benzodiazepine recognition site on the GABA/benzodiazepine receptor complex. It is the purest antagonist synthesized. Drugs used in the treatment of schizophrenia block dopamine type 2 receptors. Examples of opioid antagonists include naltrexone and naloxone.
Partial agonist (mixed agonist)	A compound that (even when fully occupying a receptor) possesses affinity for a receptor, but elicits a partial pharmacological response at the receptor involved. Partial agonists are often structural analogs of agonist molecules. If neurotransmitter concentrations are low, partial agonists may behave as an agonist. This is why these medications are sometimes called mixed agonists.	Buprenorphine is a partial agonist that produces typical opioid agonist effects and side effects, such as euphoria and respiratory depression, but its maximal effects are less than those of full agonists like heroin and methadone. When used at low doses buprenorphine produces sufficient agonist effect to enable opioid-addicted individuals to discontinue the drugs with fewer withdrawal symptoms.
Inverse agonist	An inverse agonist is an agent that binds to the same receptor as an agonist for that receptor but produces the opposite pharmacological effect.	Several inverse agonists are currently in clinical development. One particular example is R015–4513, which is the inverse agonist of the benzodiazepine class of drugs. R015–4513 and the benzodiazepines both utilize the same GABA-binding site on neurons, yet R015–4513 has the opposite effect, producing severe anxiety rather than the sedative and anxiolytic effects associated with benzodiazepines. Cannabinoid inverse agonists have been found to reduce appetite, the opposite of the craving effect associated with cannabis.

GABA, γ-aminobutyric acid.
Table by Norman Sussman, M.D.

antidepressant effects. Along with other findings, this suggests that the immune system and inflammatory responses may underlie some mood disorders.

Accounts of so-called mechanisms of action should nevertheless be kept in perspective. Explanations of how psychotropic drugs actually work that focus on synaptic elements represent an oversimplification of a complex series of events. If merely raising or lowering levels of neurotransmitter activity is associated with the clinical effects of a drug, then all drugs that cause these changes should produce equivalent benefits. This is not the case. Multiple obscure actions, several steps removed from events at neuronal receptor sites, are probably responsible for the therapeutic effects of psychotropic drugs. These *downstream* elements are postulated to represent the actual reasons that these drugs produce clinical improvement. A glossary of terms related to receptor drug interactions is given in Table 25–1.

Side Effects. Side effects are an unavoidable risk of medication treatment. Although it is impossible to have an encyclopedic knowledge of all possible adverse drug effects, prescribing clinicians should be familiar with the more common adverse effects, as well as those with serious medical consequences. No single text or document, including the product information, contains a complete list of possible treatment-emergent events.

Side effect considerations include the probability of its occurrence, its impact on a patient's quality of life, its time course, and its cause. Just as no one drug is certain to produce clinical improvement in all patients, no side effect, no matter how common, occurs in every patient. When concurrent medical disorders or a history of a similar adverse reaction puts a patient at increased risk for a side effect, it is logical to consider prescribing a compound not typically associated with that adverse reaction.

Side effects can result from the same pharmacological action that is responsible for a drug's therapeutic activity or from an unrelated property. In examples of the latter, some of the most common adverse effects of the TCAs are caused by blockade of muscarinic acetylcholine receptors or histamine 2 receptors. If a patient is sensitive to these effects, alternative agents without these properties should be prescribed. When side effects are manifestations of the drug's presumed mechanism of action, side effects may be unavoidable. Thus, blockade of serotonin reuptake by SSRIs can cause nausea and sexual dysfunction. The D_2 blockade of drugs used to treat psychosis can cause extrapyramidal side effects (EPS). Agonist action of benzodiazepine receptors can cause ataxia and daytime sleepiness. In these cases, additional medications are frequently used to make the primary agent better tolerated.

Time Course. Adverse effects differ in terms of their onset and duration. Some side effects appear at the outset of treatment and then rapidly diminish. Nausea occurring with SSRIs or venlafaxine (Effexor) and sedation occurring with mirtazapine (Remeron) are good examples of early, time-limited side effects. Early-onset, but persistent, side effects include dry mouth that is associated with noradrenergic reuptake inhibition or antimuscarinic activity. Some side effects appear later in treatment (*late-appearing side effects*) and, sometimes, may be just the opposite of adverse events early in treatment. For example, patients may typically lose weight during early treatment with SSRIs, only to find, over time, a reversal occurs, so that they gain weight. Similarly, early activation or agitation may be followed by constant fatigue or apathy. Because most data about new drugs come from short-term studies, generally 8 weeks in duration, early-onset side effects are overrepresented in product information and descriptions of newly marketed information. It is essential that clinicians follow the letters to the editor sections of journals and other sources of information to update their understanding of the true side effect profile of a drug.

Adverse effects differ in their impact on compliance and potential to cause harm. Depending on a patient's threshold of tolerance for a side effect and the impact on quality of life, side effects can lead to drug discontinuation. Examples of serious side effects include agranulocytosis (clozapine), Stevens–Johnson syndrome (lamotrigine [Lamictal]), hepatic failure (nefazodone [Serzone]), stroke (phenelzine [Nardil]), and heart block (thioridazine [Mellaril]). Overall, the risk of life-threatening side effects with psychotropics is low. Drugs that carry such a risk should be monitored more closely, and the prescribing physician should take into account whether the potential clinical benefits justify the additional risk. Any drug with a serious risk, as reflected in a black box warning, is generally used less extensively than would otherwise be the case.

In the case of haloperidol (Haldol) and other dopamine receptor antagonists (DRAs), long-term complications, such as tardive dyskinesia, have been well documented. Emerging evidence also suggests that the use of dopamine antagonists is associated with a small increase in the risk of breast cancer and that this is related to larger cumulative doses. In cases in which serious risk is associated with a drug, closer medical monitoring of medication treatment is warranted. Because the most widely used psychotropics, such as the SSRIs and SDAs, have only been in use since the 1980s or 1990s, there is less certainty about long-term effects, but no evidence indicates that side effects are not merely extensions of those already evident during initial therapy. It should also be kept in mind that most drugs used in the treatment of chronic medical disorders have not been in use sufficiently long to provide assurances about unintended long-term adverse effects.

Suicidal Ideation and Antidepressant Treatment. The issue of antidepressant-associated suicide has become front-page news, the result of an analysis suggesting a link between medication use and suicidal ideation among children, adolescents, and adults up to age 24 in short-term (4 to 16 weeks), placebo-controlled trials of nine newer antidepressant drugs. The data from trials involving more than 4,400 patients suggested that the average risk of suicidal thinking or behavior (suicidality) during the first few months of treatment in those receiving antidepressants was 4 percent, twice the placebo risk of 2 percent. No suicides occurred in these trials. The analysis also showed no increase in suicide risk among the 25 to 65 age group. Antidepressants reduced suicidality among those over age 65.

Following public hearings on the subject, in October 2004, the FDA requested the addition of black box warnings—the most serious warning placed on the labeling of a prescription medication—to all antidepressant drugs, old and new. This action raised alarm among parents and physicians and prompted an explosion of advertisements by malpractice attorneys. Most important, antidepressant prescriptions written for adolescents declined, whereas those for adults flattened, after years of growth.

A large study of real world patients published in the January 2006 issue of the *American Journal of Psychiatry* raised serious doubt about true antidepressants and suicidality and about the wisdom of the FDA's decision to change the labeling. The study examined suicides and hospitalizations for suicide attempts in the medical records of 65,103 members of a nonprofit insurer in the Pacific Northwest that covers about 500,000 people who received antidepressants from 1992 to 2003. It found that (1) newer antidepressants were associated with a more rapid and greater reduction in risk than older types of antidepressants and (2) patients were significantly more likely to attempt or commit suicide in the month before they began drug therapy than in the 6 months after starting it.

This is not the first time credible evidence has contradicted a significant link between antidepressant use and increased risk of suicide. At the hearings that led to the black box warning, John Mann of Columbia University presented population data showing that since 1987, the year before fluoxetine (Prozac) became the first marketed SSRI, suicide rates in the United States began dropping, and that areas in the United States with the highest SSRI prescription rates had the biggest decline in suicides. For every 10 percent increase in prescription rates, the US suicide rate declined 3 percent.

Another study, a review of 588 case files of patients aged 10 to 19, found that a 1 percent increase in antidepressant use was associated with a decrease of 0.23 suicides per 100,000 adolescents per year.

A more important question, given how slight the risk may be, if indeed it exists, is whether as a result of the FDA's ill-considered actions, some depressed patients are not getting potentially life-saving treatment. Epidemiological findings from several countries, including the United States, have shown that decreased prescribing of antidepressants for depressed children and adolescents resulted in an increase in suicide rates in those populations.

Side Effects Associated with Newer Medications. All medications are associated with side effects. The clinician should be aware of these, be able to recognize them, and take appropriate measures to treat them.

SOMNOLENCE. Sedation is often an intended effect of many psychotropic drugs, especially when used to treat insomnia, anxiety, or agitation. Daytime sleepiness, or somnolence, is also an unwanted adverse event, however. It is important for the clinician to alert patients to the possibility of sedation and to document that the person was advised to exercise caution when operating any type of vehicle or mechanical equipment. Some somnolence results from a carryover of nighttime use of drugs as hypnotics. Even with drugs, such as the SSRIs, which are activating to many patients, somnolence can be problematic. In some instances, it results from impairment of sleep quality. Chronic use of SSRIs can cause some patients to experience a subjective sense of fatigue, exhaustion, or yawning, even with adequate amounts of sleep. Management of unwanted somnolence includes adjustment of dose or timing of administration, switching to alternative medications, addition of small doses of stimulants, or the addition of modafinil (Provigil).

GASTROINTESTINAL DISTURBANCES. The major gastrointestinal (GI) side effects of the older antidepressant and antipsychotic drugs consisted primarily of constipation and dry mouth, a consequence of their antimuscarinic activity. Most of the newer drugs have little antimuscarinic activity, but do have effects on the serotonin system. Most of the body's serotonin is in the GI tract, and serotonergic drugs often cause varying degrees of stomach pain, nausea, flatulence, and diarrhea. In most cases, these side effects are transient, but some persons never accommodate and must switch to another class of drugs. Initial use of lower doses or use of delayed-release preparations are the most effective strategies for minimizing GI side effects.

MOVEMENT DISORDERS. The introduction of SDAs has greatly reduced the incidence of medication-induced movement disorders, but varying degrees of dose-related parkinsonism, akathisia, and dystonia still occur. Risperidone (Risperdal) most closely resembles the older agents in terms of these side effects. Olanzapine (Zyprexa) also causes more extrapyramidal effects than clinical trials suggested. Aripiprazole (Abilify) causes severe akathisia. There have been rare reports of SSRI-induced movement disorders, ranging from akathisia to tardive dyskinesia.

SEXUAL DYSFUNCTION. The use of psychiatric drugs can be associated with sexual dysfunction—decreased libido, impaired ejaculation and erection, and inhibition of female orgasm. In clinical trials with the SSRIs, the extent of sexual side effects was grossly underestimated, because data were based on spontaneous reports by patients. The rate of sexual dysfunction in the original fluoxetine product information, for example, was less than 5 percent. In subsequent studies in which information about sexual side effects was elicited by specific questions, the rate of SSRI-associated sexual dysfunction was found to be between 35 and 75 percent. In clinical practice, patients are not likely to report sexual dysfunction spontaneously to the physician, so it is important to ask about this side effect. Also, some sexual dysfunctions may be related to the primary psychiatric disorder. Nevertheless, if sexual dysfunction emerges after pharmacotherapy has begun and the primary response to treatment has been positive, it may be worthwhile to attempt to treat the symptoms. Long lists of possible antidotes to these side effects have evolved, but few interventions are consistently effective, and few have more than anecdotal evidence to support their use. The clinician and patient should consider the possibility of sexual side effects with a patient when selecting a drug and switching treatment to another drug that is less or not at all associated with sexual dysfunction if this adverse effect is not acceptable to the patient.

WEIGHT GAIN. Weight gain accompanies the use of many psychotropic drugs as a result of retained fluid, increased caloric intake, decreased exercise, or altered metabolism. Weight gain can also occur as a symptom of disorder, as in bulimia or atypical depression, or as a sign of recovery from an episode of illness. Treatment-emergent increase in body weight is a common reason for noncompliance with a drug regimen. No specific mechanisms have been identified as causing weight gain, and it appears that the histamine and serotonin systems mediate changes in weight associated with many drugs used to treat depression and psychosis. Metformin (Glucophage) has been reported to facilitate weight loss among patients whose weight gain is attributed to use of serotonin-dopamine reuptake inhibitors and valproic acid (Depakene). Valproate (Depacon), as well as olanzapine, has been linked to the development of insulin resistance, which could induce appetite increase, with subsequent weight increase. Weight gain is a noteworthy side effect of clozapine (Clozaril) and olanzapine. Genetic factors that regulate body weight, as well as the related problem of diabetes mellitus, seem to involve the 5-HT_{2C} receptor. There is a genetic polymorphism of the promoter region of this receptor, with significantly less weight gain in patients with the variant allele than in those without this allele. Drugs with a strong 5-HT_{2C} affinity would be expected to have a greater impact on body weight of patients with a polymorphism of the 5-HT_{2C} receptor promoter region.

WEIGHT LOSS. Initial weight loss is associated with SSRI treatment but is usually transient, with most weight being regained within the first few months. Bupropion (Wellbutrin) has been shown to cause modest weight loss that is sustained. When combined with diet and lifestyle changes, bupropion can facilitate more significant weight loss. Topiramate (Topamax) and zonisamide (Zonegran), marketed as treatments for epilepsy, sometimes produce substantial, sustained loss of weight.

GLUCOSE CHANGES. Increased risk of glucose abnormalities, including diabetes mellitus, is associated with weight increase during psychotropic drug therapy. Clozapine and olanzapine are associated with a greater risk than other SDAs of abnormalities in fasting glucose levels, as well as hyperosmolar diabetes and ketoacidosis. This dysregulation of glucose homeostasis appears to be drug induced and increases glucagon.

HYPONATREMIA. Hyponatremia is associated with oxcarbazepine (Trileptal) and SSRI treatment, especially in elderly patients. Confusion, agitation, and lethargy are common symptoms.

COGNITIVE IMPAIRMENT. Cognitive impairment means a disturbance in the capacity to think. Some agents, such as the benzodiazepine agonists, are recognized as causes of cognitive impairment. Other widely used psychotropics, such as the SSRIs, lamotrigine (Lamictal), gabapentin (Neurontin), lithium, TCAs, and bupropion, however, are also associated with varying degrees of memory impairment and word-finding difficulties. In contrast to the benzodiazepine-induced anterograde amnesia, these agents cause a more subtle type of absent-mindedness. Drugs with anticholinergic properties are likely to worsen memory performance.

SWEATING. Severe perspiration unrelated to ambient temperature is associated with TCAs, SSRIs, and venlafaxine. This side effect is often socially disabling. Attempts can be made to treat this side effect with alpha agents, such as terazosin (Hytrin) and oxybutynin (Ditropan).

CARDIOVASCULAR DISTURBANCES. Newer agents are less likely to have direct cardiac effects. Many older agents, such as TCAs and phenothiazines, affected blood pressure (BP) and cardiac conduction. Thioridazine (Mellaril), which has been in use for decades, has been shown to prolong the QTc interval in a dose-related manner and may increase the risk of sudden death by delaying ventricular repolarization and causing torsades de pointes. Similar issues of slight QTc effects noted with ziprasidone (Geodon) delayed the marketing of that drug. Though newer drugs are now routinely scrutinized for evidence of cardiac effects, clinicians should be aware that first-generation antipsychotics as well as coadministration with some antibiotics can prolong the QTc and increase the risk for torsade de pointes. Clozapine can cause myocarditis and cardiomyopathy in rare cases of which the clinician should be aware.

RASH. Any medication is a potential source of a drug rash. Some psychotropics, such as carbamazepine (Equetro, Tegretol) and lamotrigine, have been linked to an increased risk of serious exfoliative dermatitis. Commonly referred to as Stevens–Johnson syndrome, this condition is a systemic, immune-mediated reaction that can prove fatal or result in permanent scarring or blindness. All patients should be informed about the potential seriousness of lesions that are widespread, that occur above the neck, that involve the mucous membranes, and that may be associated with fever and lymphadenopathy. If such symptoms manifest, a patient should be instructed at the time that the medication is prescribed to go immediately to an emergency department.

Idiosyncratic and Paradoxical Drug Responses.

Idiosyncratic reactions occur in a very small percentage of patients taking a drug. The reactions are not related to the known pharmacologic properties, and most likely represent a genetically based abnormal sensitivity to a drug. A paradoxical response represents the manifestation of a clinical effect the opposite of what is expected. In March 2007, the FDA reported dissociative-like states associated with certain sedative hypnotics. These included behaviors such as sleepwalking, binge eating, aggressive outbursts, and night driving of which the patient was unaware. Table 25–2 lists the drugs required to have warning labels for that effect.

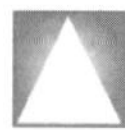

Table 25–2
Sedative Hypnotics Cited by the U.S. Food and Drug Administration

Drug	Manufacturer
Zolpidem (Ambien/Ambien CR)	Sanofi Aventis
Butabarbital (Butisol Sodium)	MedPointe Pharmaceuticals
Pentobarbital and carbromal (Carbrital)	Parke-Davis
Flurazepam (Dalmane)	Valeant Pharmaceuticals
Quazepam (Doral)	Questcor Pharmaceuticals
Triazolam (Halcion)	Pfizer
Eszopiclone (Lunesta)	Sepracor
Ethchlorvynol (Placidyl)	Abbott
Estazolam (Prosom)	Abbott
Temazepam (Restoril)	Tyco Healthcare
Ramelteon (Rozerem)	Takeda
Secobarbital (Seconal)	Lilly
Zaleplon (Sonata)	King Pharmaceuticals

Therapeutic Index.

Therapeutic index is a relative measure of the toxicity or safety of a drug and is defined as the ratio of the median toxic dose to the median effective dose. The median toxic dose is the dose at which 50 percent of patients experience a specific toxic effect, and the median effective dose is the dose at which 50 percent of patients have a specified therapeutic effect. When the therapeutic index is high, as it is for haloperidol, it is reflected by the wide range of dosages in which that drug is prescribed. Conversely, the therapeutic index for lithium is quite low, thus requiring careful monitoring of serum lithium levels in patients for whom the drug is prescribed.

Overdose.

Safety in overdose is always a consideration in drug selection. Almost all of the newer agents, however, have a wide margin of safety when taken in overdose. By contrast, a 1-month supply of TCAs could be fatal. The depressed patients they were used to treat are the group most at risk to attempt suicide. Because even the safest drugs can sometimes produce severe medical complications, especially when combined with other agents, clinicians must recognize that the prescribed medication can be used in an attempt to commit suicide. Although it is prudent to write nonrefillable prescriptions for small quantities, this practice passes along increased copay costs to the patient. In fact, many pharmacy benefit management programs encourage the prescribing of a 3-month supply of medication.

In cases in which suicide is a major concern, an attempt should be made to verify that medication is not being hoarded for a later overdose attempt. Random pill counts or asking a family member to dispense daily doses may be helpful. Some patients attempt suicide just as they are beginning to recover. Large quantities of medications with a low therapeutic index should be prescribed judiciously. Another reason to limit the number of pills prescribed is the possibility of accidental ingestion of medications by children in the household. Psychotherapeutic medications should be kept in a safe place.

Physicians who work in emergency rooms should know which drugs can be hemodialyzed. The issues involved are complex and are not based on any single chemical property of the drug. For example, it is generally presumed that drugs with low protein binding are good candidates for dialysis. Venlafaxine, however, is only 27 percent protein bound and is too large as a molecule dialyzed. Hemodialysis is effective for treating overdose of valproic acid.

Pharmacokinetics.

Pharmacokinetic drug interactions are the effects of drugs on the plasma concentrations of each other, and *pharmacodynamic drug interactions* are the effects of drugs on the biological activities of each other. Pharmacokinetic concepts are used to describe and predict the time course of drug concentrations in different parts of the body, such as plasma, adipose tissue, and the central nervous system (CNS). From a clinical perspective, pharmacokinetic methods help explain or predict the onset and duration of drug activity and interactions between drugs that alter their metabolism or excretion.

Pharmacogenetic research focuses on finding variant alleles that alter drug pharmacokinetics and pharmacodynamics. Researchers are attempting to identify genetic differences in how enzymes metabolize psychotropics, as well as CNS proteins directly involved in drug action. Likely, identification of patient genotypes will facilitate prediction of clinical response to different types of drugs.

Most clinicians need to consult charts or computer programs to determine when potential interactions may occur and, if so, how clinically relevant they may be. Whenever possible, it is preferable to use a medication that produces minimal risk of drug interactions. Also, it is recommended that prescribers know the interaction profiles of the drugs they most commonly prescribe.

Examples of pharmacokinetic interactions include one drug increasing or decreasing the concentrations of a coadministered compound. These types of interactions can also lead to altered concentrations of metabolites. In some cases, there may also be interference with the conversion of a drug to its active metabolite. Enormous variability exists among patients with respect to pharmacokinetic parameters, such as drug absorption and metabolism. Another type of interaction is represented by interactions involving the kidney. Commonly used medications, such as angiotensin-converting enzyme inhibitors (ACEIs), nonsteroidal anti-inflammatory drugs (NSAIDs), and thiazides, decrease renal clearance of lithium, increasing the likelihood of severe elevations of lithium. Drug interactions can occur pharmacokinetically or pharmacodynamically.

Patient-Related Factors

Response to medication and sensitivity to side effects are influenced by factors related to the patient. This is why there is no one-size-fits-all approach to pharmacological treatment. Patient-related variables include diagnosis, genetic factors, lifestyle, overall medical status, concurrent disorders, and history of drug response. A patient's attitude toward medication in general, aversion to certain types of side effects, and preference for a specific agent also need to be considered.

Diagnosis. Failure to correctly diagnose a disorder diminishes the likelihood of optimal drug selection. Misdiagnosis not only can result in a missed opportunity, but it also can, at times, produce worsening of symptoms. Inadvertently diagnosing a patient in the depressed phase of bipolar disorder as having unipolar depression can induce mania or rapid cycling. Treatment failure or exacerbation of symptoms should prompt a reassessment of the working diagnosis.

Past Treatment Response. A specific drug should be selected according to the patient's history of drug response (compliance, therapeutic response, adverse effects), the patient's family history of drug response, the profile of adverse effects for that drug with regard to the particular patient, and the prescribing clinician's usual practice. If a drug has previously been effective in treating a patient or a family member, the same drug should be used again. For reasons that are not understood, however, some patients fail to respond to a previously effective agent when challenged again. A history of severe adverse effects from a specific drug is a strong indicator that the patient would not be compliant with that particular drug.

It is helpful if patients can recall the details of past psychotropic drug treatment: the drugs prescribed, in what dosages, for how long, and in what combinations. Because of their mental disorders, many patients, however, are poor historians. If possible, patients' medical records should be obtained to confirm their reports. Family members are a good source of collateral information.

Response in Family Members. It is widely held that drug responses cluster in families. Thus, response to a drug in a relative is an indicator of whether a patient might also benefit from that medication. Although no conclusive evidence supports this as a consideration in drug selection, existing studies do confirm that a history of positive response to treatment with a drug should be considered in making treatment decisions.

Concurrent Medical or Psychiatric Disorders. Initial assessment should elicit information about coexisting medical disorders. In some cases, a medical disorder may be responsible for the symptoms. Patients with thyroid disease who are not adequately treated may appear depressed. Sleep apnea produces depression and cognitive impairment. Rare conditions, such as Kleine–Levin syndrome, can mimic bipolar disorder. A drug should be selected that minimally exacerbates any preexisting medical problems that a particular patient may have.

Recreational drug use, excessive consumption of alcohol, and frequent ingestion of caffeine-containing beverages can complicate and even undermine psychotropic drug treatment. These compounds possess significant psychoactive properties and, in some cases, may represent the source of the patient's symptoms. It is reasonable to ask patients to abstain from use of these substances, at least until the benefits of psychotropic drug treatment have been unequivocally established. Gradual reintroduction of moderate amounts of alcohol, tea, and coffee can then take place. Patients can then observe for themselves whether there are any untoward effects on their clinical status.

Informed Consent and Patient Education

Establishing trust and providing motivation to comply with the medication regimen are essential components of successful treatment. Patients should be informed about treatment options and the probable side effects and unique benefits of each treatment. Patient preference should be respected, unless a compelling advantage exists involving efficacy, tolerability, or safety with an alternative agent. If a particular medication is being recommended, the reasons for this recommendation should be explained. Patients are more likely to continue taking their medication if they fully understand the reasons why it is being prescribed.

A strong therapeutic alliance between a clinician and a patient is always helpful. Given the unpredictability of medication response, the frequent occurrence of side effects, and underlying ambivalence about, or fear of taking, medication, a positive, trusting relationship serves to improve patient compliance. Repeated failed trials may be needed before a response is seen. A patient's confidence in the physician's knowledge and judgment enables medication trials and more complex regimens, such as the use of multiple medications.

Discussions about drug selection should be documented in notes, but a signed informed consent is not needed. Surprisingly, patients who are informed of potential adverse effects report a higher incidence of side effects but do not have higher rates of premature discontinuation.

How the patient and family are engaged in the treatment plan can determine the success of treatment. The psychodynamic meaning of pharmacotherapy to the patient and family and environmental influences, psychosocial stressors, and support should be explored. Some patients may view drug treatment as a panacea, and others may view it as the enemy. With the patient's consent, relatives and other clinicians should be instructed about the reasons for the drug treatment, as well as the expected benefits and potential risks.

Dosing, Duration, and Monitoring

Dosing. The clinically effective dose for treatment depends on the characteristics of the drug and patient factors, such as inherited sensitivity and ability to metabolize a drug, concurrent medical disorders, use of concurrent medications, and history of exposure to previous medications.

Plasma concentrations of many psychotropics can vary up to 10-fold. Thus, to some extent, the optimal dose for an individual is ultimately determined by trial and error, guided by the empirical evidence of the usual dose range for that drug. In some cases, it may prove helpful to test patients for genetic polymorphisms involving hepatic enzymes. Patients who are ultrarapid metabolizers of certain drugs may require higher than normal dosing. Slow metabolizers might demonstrate side effects and even toxicity at very low doses.

Some drugs demonstrate a clear relationship between increases in dose and clinical response. This dose–response curve plots the drug concentration against the effects of the drug.

The *potency* of a drug refers to the relative dose required to achieve certain effects, not to its efficacy. Haloperidol, for example, is more potent than chlorpromazine (Thorazine), because approximately 5 mg of haloperidol is required to achieve the same therapeutic effect as 100 mg of chlorpromazine. These drugs, however, are equal in their clinical efficacy—that is, the maximal clinical response achievable by administration of a drug.

Drugs must be used in effective dosages for sufficient periods. Although drug tolerability and safety are always considerations, subtherapeutic doses and incomplete therapeutic trials should be avoided. The use of inadequate doses merely exposes the patient to the risk of side effects, without providing the probability of therapeutic benefit. In view of the wide margin of safety associated with most currently prescribed medications, more risk exists in underdosing than in overshooting the recommended dose range.

Time of dosing is usually based on the plasma half-life of a drug and its side effect profile. Sedating drugs are given all at night or with disproportionate daily doses at night. The opposite is true with activating drugs. The frequency of dosing is less clear-cut. Most dosing regimens of psychotropic drugs, such as once-a-day versus divided doses, are based on measurements of plasma concentrations rather than receptor occupancy in the brain. Evidence suggests a significant dissociation exists between brain and plasma kinetics. Reliance on plasma kinetics as the basis for dosing regimens leads to misunderstanding of necessary schedules.

As a rule, psychotropic drugs should be used continuously. Exceptions are the use of drugs for insomnia, acute agitation, and severe situational anxiety. A common mistake is the use of high-potency benzodiazepines, such as alprazolam (Xanax) and clonazepam (Klonopin), only after an attack has begun. These drugs should be used as part of a regular schedule to prevent attacks.

Some patients who experience sexual dysfunction while being treated with SSRIs take a drug holiday, that is, they skip a daily dose from time to time to facilitate sexual performance.

Intermittent dosing regimens of SSRIs have been found to be effective as a treatment for premenstrual dysphoric disorder (PMDD). The drugs are taken daily during the 2-week luteal phase of the menstrual cycle.

Duration of Treatment. A common question from a patient is "How long do I need to take the medication?" The answer depends on multiple variables, including the nature of the disorder, the duration of symptoms, the family history, and the extent to which the patient tolerates and benefits from the medication. Patients can be given a reasonable explanation of the probabilities but should be told that it is first best to see if the medication works for him or her and whether any side effects are acceptable. Any more definitive discussion of treatment duration can be held once the degree of success is clear. Even patients with a philosophical aversion to the use of psychotropic drugs may elect to stay on medication indefinitely if the magnitude of improvement is great. Most psychiatric disorders have high rates of chronicity and relapse. Because of this, long-term treatment is often needed to prevent recurrence. Nevertheless, the fact remains that psychotropic drugs are not said to cure the disorders they treat but rather to help control the symptoms.

Treatment is conceptually broken down into three phases: the initial therapeutic trial, the continuation, and the maintenance phase. The initial period of treatment should last at least several weeks because of the delay in therapeutic effects that characterizes most classes of psychotropic drugs. The required duration of a *therapeutic trial* of a drug should be discussed at the outset of treatment, so that the patient does not have unrealistic expectations of an immediate improvement in symptoms. Patients are more likely to experience side effects early in the course of pharmacotherapy than any relief from their disorder. In some cases, medication may even exacerbate some symptoms. Patients should be counseled that a poor initial reaction to medication is not an indicator of the ultimate outcome of treatment. For instance, many patients with panic disorder develop jitteriness or an increase in panic attacks after starting on tricyclic or SSRI treatment. Benzodiazepine agonists are an exception to the rule that clinical onset is delayed. In most cases, their hypnotic and antianxiety effects are evident immediately.

Ongoing use of medication, however, does not provide absolute protection against relapse. Continuation therapy provides clinically and statistically significant protective effects against relapse. The optimal duration of continuation or maintenance therapy is variable and dependent on the clinical history of the patient. Early-onset chronic major depression, for example, has a more severe course and greater comorbidity than late-onset chronic major depression. In addition to early onset, a history of multiple past episodes and severity and length of a current episode would make longer, even indefinite, treatment appropriate.

Frequency of Visits. Until an unequivocal response to treatment occurs, patients should be seen as frequently as circumstances warrant. The frequency of follow-up or monitoring visits is determined by clinical judgment. In severely ill patients, this might mean several times a week. Patients on maintenance therapy, even when stable, need monitoring, but no consensus exists on the frequency of follow-up therapy. Three months is a reasonable interval between visits, but 6 months may be adequate after long-standing treatment.

Laboratory Tests and Therapeutic Blood Monitoring

Laboratory testing and therapeutic blood monitoring should be based on clinical circumstances and the drugs being used. For most commonly used psychotropic drugs, routine testing is not required. No currently available laboratory test can confirm the diagnosis of a mental disorder.

Pretreatment tests are routine as part of a workup to establish baseline values and to rule out underlying medical problems that may be causing the psychiatric symptoms or that might complicate treatment with drugs. Results of recently performed tests should be obtained. With agents known to cause cardiac conduction changes, a pretreatment electrocardiogram (ECG) should be obtained before initiating treatment. With lithium and clozapine, the possibility of serious changes in thyroid, renal, hepatic, or hematological functions requires pretreatment and ongoing monitoring with appropriate laboratory tests.

As a result of both anecdotal and research findings of sometimes severe glucose dysregulation during treatment primarily with SDAs, the FDA has suggested that patients being treated with any atypical antipsychotic be monitored for the emergence dyslipidemia and diabetes.

Certain circumstances present in which it is necessary or useful to use plasma concentrations to monitor a patient's condition. These include the monitoring of drugs with narrow therapeutic indexes, such as lithium; drugs with a therapeutic window, the optimal dose range for a therapeutic response; drug combinations that can lead to interactions that raise drug concentrations of medications or their metabolites, which can cause toxicity; unexplained toxicity at normal therapeutic doses; and failure to respond in a patient who may be noncompliant. A clinician should have no reservations about requesting random urine toxicological tests in a patient who abuse substances.

Treatment Outcomes

The goal of psychotropic treatment is to eliminate all manifestations of a disorder, thus enabling the patient to regain the ability to function as well and to enjoy life as fully as before he or she became ill. This degree of improvement to below the syndromal threshold is defined as *remission*.

Response and Remission. Remission is the preferred outcome of treatment, not only because of the immediate impact on functioning and state of mind, but also because emerging evidence suggests that patients in remission are less likely to experience relapse and recurrence of their disorder.

Patients who improve but do not experience a full resolution are considered to be responders. They may exhibit significant improvement but continue to experience symptoms. In depression studies, *response* is usually defined as a 50 percent or greater decrease from baseline on a standard rating scale, such as the Hamilton Depression (HAM-D) Scale or the Montgomery-Asberg Depression Rating Scale (MADRS). *Remission* is defined as an absolute score of 7 or less on the HAM-D or 10 or less on the MADRS. Expectations about the likely degree of improvement should be based on what is known about the responsiveness of specific disorders to medication therapy. Obsessive-compulsive disorder (OCD) and schizophrenia, for example, are more likely to be associated with residual manifestations of illness than major depression or panic disorder. The probability of full remission from OCD with SSRI treatment alone over a 2-year period is less than 12 percent, and the probability of partial remission is approximately 47 percent.

Treatment Failure. The initial treatment plan should anticipate the possibility that the medication may be ineffective. A next-step strategy should be in place at the initiation of treatment. Repeated drug failures should prompt reassessment of the patient. First, was the original diagnosis correct? In answering this question, the clinician should include the possibility of an undiagnosed medical condition or recreational drug use as the cause of the psychiatric symptoms.

Second, are the observed symptoms related to the original disorder, or are they actually adverse effects of the drug treatment? Some antipsychotic drugs, for example, can produce akinesia, which resembles psychotic withdrawal, or akathisia and neuroleptic malignant syndrome, which resemble increased psychotic agitation. Long-term use of SSRIs can produce emotional blunting, which can mimic depression.

Intolerance of side effects may be the most common reason for treatment failure. Third, was the drug administered at an appropriate dosage for a sufficient length of time? Because absorption and metabolism of drugs can vary greatly in patients, the clinician may need to measure plasma levels of a drug to ensure a sufficient dose of the drug.

Fourth, did a pharmacokinetic or pharmacodynamic interaction with another drug that the patient was taking reduce the efficacy of the newly prescribed drug?

Fifth, did the patient take the drug as directed? Drug noncompliance is a common clinical problem that arises as a result of complicated drug regimens (more than one drug in more than one daily dosage), adverse effects (especially if unnoticed by the clinician), and poor patient education about the drug treatment plan. Patients may discontinue medication when they recover, thinking that they are cured and no longer benefiting from the medication.

Treatment Resistance. Some patients fail to respond to repeated trials of medication. No single factor can explain the ineffectiveness of the various interventions in these cases. Strategies in these cases include the use of drug combinations, high-dose therapy, and use of unconventional drugs. Limited evidence is available on the comparative success rates associated with any given strategy.

Tolerance. The development of tolerance is marked by a need, over time, to use increased doses of a drug for it to maintain a clinical effect. This decreased responsiveness to a drug occurs after repeated doses. Tolerance also describes decreased sensitivity to adverse effects of the drug, such as nausea. This phenomenon is used as the basis for starting some drugs at subtherapeutic doses, with the plan to adjust the schedule once the patient can tolerate higher doses. Clinical tolerance appears to represent changes in the CNS, such as altered receptor configuration or density. Drugs with similar pharmacological actions often exhibit cross-tolerance.

Sensitization. Clinically manifested as the reverse of tolerance, sensitization is said to occur when sensitivity to a drug effect increases over time. In these cases, the same dose typically produces more pronounced effects as treatment progresses.

Withdrawal. The development of physiological adaptation to a drug, with a subsequent risk of withdrawal symptoms, has been reported for many classes of psychotropic drugs. Technically, withdrawal should be considered a side effect. The probability and severity of these reactions are remote with most drugs and more common with others. As a general rule, the more abruptly a drug is stopped and the shorter its elimination half-life, the more likely it is that clinically significant withdrawal symptoms will occur. When using some short-acting drugs, withdrawal reactions can result from missed doses and during daily intervals between doses. Gradual tapering of medications after prolonged use is recommended whenever possible. Although this reduces the risk of withdrawal reactions, it does not ensure they will not occur. The so-called sedative hypnotics and opiates are the agents most often associated with mentally and physically distressing discontinuation reactions. In some cases, such as barbiturate use, withdrawal can be fatal.

Marked differences are found among agents, even within a given class, with respect to the probability and severity of discontinuation effects. For example, among the benzodiazepines, alprazolam and triazolam (Halcion) commonly produce more immediate and intense withdrawal symptoms than other compounds. Among the SSRIs, there is a well-described withdrawal syndrome that appears to be more frequent and severe with paroxetine (Paxil). It can, however, occur with any SSRI. Even fluoxetine can be associated with discontinuation symptoms, but the symptoms may be delayed and attenuated because of the long elimination half-life of its active metabolite. These manifestations are subtle and are delayed for weeks after the last dose. Venlafaxine also produces a severe SSRI-like withdrawal syndrome.

In addition to half-life, many variables can influence the likelihood and degree of discontinuation symptoms. Changes in the rate of drug metabolism, as an example, can play a role. Paroxetine is primarily metabolized by the cytochrome P450 (CYP) 2D6 isoenzyme, however, it is also a potent inhibitor of CYP 2D6. This results in *autoinhibition,* a dose-dependent inhibition of its own metabolism, with a subsequent increase in plasma concentrations of paroxetine. If the dose of paroxetine is decreased or the drug is stopped, the decline in its plasma concentrations can be steep, causing withdrawal to occur. Withdrawal can occur in rare cases in which the dose of a drug is not decreased, but a second agent, which had been inhibiting its metabolism, was stopped. For example, alprazolam is metabolized via the CYP 3A3/4 enzyme system. Nefazodone inhibits that enzyme. If a patient taking both agents for several weeks discontinues the nefazodone, it could result in a rapid increase in the rate of alprazolam metabolism and a consequent drop in plasma concentrations.

The development of sustained-release versions of drugs, such as alprazolam, paroxetine, and venlafaxine, has not reduced the severity of their withdrawal reactions. The prolonged half-life of those agents results from delayed absorption rather than prolongation of the elimination phase. The frequency of drug dosing is reduced but not the rate of falloff in plasma concentrations.

Poor bioavailability with a generic agent may account for unexpected loss of clinical effect in emergence of withdrawal symptoms. The occurrence of these events soon after refilling a prescription should prompt examination of the new medication. It should be confirmed whether the dispensed medication and dose are both correct. It is difficult to ascertain whether generic medications are truly equivalent, so the possibility exists that differences in potency may underlie adverse changes in clinical status.

Withdrawal symptoms invariably occur hours or days after dose reduction or discontinuation. Symptoms resolve within a few weeks, so the persistence of symptoms argues against withdrawal. Although depletion studies have been shown to provoke rapid return of symptoms, in clinical practice, psychotic and mood symptoms do not usually reappear abruptly after long-term treatment.

Combination of Drugs

According to the American Psychiatric Association Practice Guidelines for the Treatment of Psychiatric Disorders, "the use of multiple agents should be avoided if possible" in the treatment of psychiatric disorders. Although *monotherapy* represents the ideal, *polypharmacy,* the simultaneous use of psychotropic medications, has been commonplace since chlorpromazine was combined with reserpine (Diupres) in the early 1950s. The practice of combining drugs and the merits of various *augmentation* or *combination* strategies are routinely discussed in the literature and at scientific meetings. The mean number of simultaneously prescribed medications has increased in recent decades. Among psychiatric inpatients, the mean number of psychotropics prescribed is approximately three. Fixed combinations—drugs that contain more than one active ingredient—have been successfully marketed in the past, and research on new combinations is ongoing. A fluoxetine-olanzapine fixed combination has been approved as a treatment for bipolar disorder. The use of such drugs may increase the patients' compliance by simplifying the drug regimen. A problem with combination drugs, however, is that the clinician has less flexibility in adjusting the dosage of one of the components; that is, the use of combination drugs can cause two drugs to be administered when only one drug continues to be necessary for therapeutic efficacy (Table 25–3).

Sometimes distinctions are made between augmentation and combination therapy. When two psychotropics with the same approved indications are used concurrently, this is termed

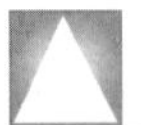

Table 25–3
Combination Drugs Used in Psychiatry

Ingredients	Preparation	Amount of Each	Recommended Dosage	Indications
Perphenazine and amitriptyline	—	Tablet: 2:25, 4:25, 4:50, 2:10, 4:10	Initial therapy: tablet of 2:25 or 4:25 qid Maintenance therapy: tablet 2:25 or 4:25 bid or qid	Depression and associated anxiety
Dextroamphetamine and amphetamine	Adderall	Tablet: 5, 7.5, 10.0, 12.5, 15.0, 20.0, 30.0 mg	3–5 yrs: 2.5 mg/day; 6 yrs and older: 5 mg/day	Attention-deficit/hyperactivity disorder
	Adderall XR	Capsule: 5, 10, 15, 20, 25, 30 mg	—	—
Chlordiazepoxide and clidinium bromide	—	Capsule: 5:25	One or two capsules tid or qid before meals and at bedtime	Peptic ulcer, gastritis, duodenitis, irritable bowel syndrome, spastic colitis, and mild ulcerative colitis
Chlordiazepoxide and amitriptyline	—	Tablet: 5.0:12.5, 10:25	Tablet of 5:12.5 tid or qid; tablet of 10:25 tid or qid, initially, then may increase to six tablets daily as required	Depression and associated anxiety
Olanzapine and fluoxetine	Symbyax	Capsule: 6:25, 6:50, 12:25, 12:50	Once daily in the evening in a dose range of olanzapine 6–12 mg and fluoxetine 25–50 mg	Depressive episodes associated with bipolar I disorder

qid, four times daily; bid, twice daily; tid, three times daily.

combination therapy. Adding a drug with another indication is termed *augmentation.* Augmentation often entails use of a drug that is not primarily considered a psychotropic. For example, in treating depression, it is not common to add thyroid hormone to an approved antidepressant.

Almost all patients with bipolar disorder are taking more than one psychotropic agent. Combination treatment with drugs that treat depression and DRA or SDA has long been held as preferable in patients with psychotic depression. Similarly, SSRIs typically produce partial improvement in patients with OCD, so the addition of an SDA may be helpful.

Medications also can be combined to counteract side effects, to treat specific symptoms, and as a temporary measure to transition from one drug to another. It is common practice to add a new medication without the discontinuation of a prior drug, particularly when the first drug has provided partial benefit. This can be done as part of a plan to transition from an agent that is not producing a satisfactory response or as an attempt to maintain the patient on combined therapy.

Advantages of combining drugs include building on existing response, which may be less demoralizing, and the possibility that combinations produce new mechanisms that no single agent can provide. One limitation is that noncompliance and adverse effects increase, and the clinician may not be able to determine whether it was the second drug alone or the combination of drugs that resulted in a therapeutic success or a particular adverse effect. Combining drugs can create a broad-spectrum effect and also changes the ratio of metabolites.

Combined Psychotherapy and Pharmacotherapy

Many psychiatrists believe that patients are best treated with a combination of medication and psychotherapy. Studies have demonstrated that the results of combined therapy are superior to those of either type of therapy alone. When pharmacotherapy and psychotherapy are used together, the approach should be coordinated, integrated, and synergistic. If the psychotherapy and the pharmacotherapy are directed by two separate clinicians, the clinicians must communicate with each other clearly and often.

Special Populations

Although every patient brings a unique combination of demographic and clinical variables to the clinical setting, certain patient populations require special consideration. When treating the young, the elderly, those with medical disorders, and women who want to conceive, are pregnant, or are nursing, awareness of risks associated with medication assumes increased importance. Data derived from clinical trials are of limited value in guiding many decisions, because populations in these studies consisted of healthy young adults and, until recently, excluded many women of child-bearing age. Studies of children and adolescents have become more common, so understanding of treatment effects in this population has grown.

Children. Understanding of the safety and efficacy of most psychotropic drugs when used to treat children is based more on clinical experience than on evidence from large clinical trial data. Other than attention-deficit/hyperactivity disorder (ADHD) and OCD, commonly used psychotropic drugs have no labeling for pediatric use, so results from adult studies are extrapolated to children. This is not necessarily appropriate because of developmental differences in pharmacokinetics and pharmacodynamics. Dosing is another special consideration in drug use with children. Although the small volume of distribution suggests the use of lower doses than those used in adults, a child's higher rate of metabolism suggests that a higher ratio of milligrams of drug to kilograms of body weight should be used.

In practice, it is best to begin with a small dose and to increase it until clinical effects are observed. The clinician should not hesitate, however, to use adult dosages in children if these dosages are effective and the adverse effects are acceptable.

The paucity of research data is a legacy of many years in which manufacturers avoided conducting trials in children because of liability concerns, small market share, and, hence, limited profit potential represented by this population. To correct this problem, the FDA Modernization Act (FDAMA) of 1997 provided for special encouragement and incentives to study drugs for pediatric use.

Pregnant and Nursing Women. No definitive assurances exist that any drug is completely without risk during pregnancy and lactation. No psychotropic medication is absolutely contraindicated during pregnancy, although drugs with known risks of birth defects, premature birth, or neonatal complications should be avoided if acceptable alternatives are available.

Women who are pregnant or lactating are excluded from clinical trials, and it is only recently that women of child-bearing age have been able to participate in these studies. As a result, there are large gaps in knowledge of the effects of psychotropic agents on the developing fetus and on the neonate. Most of what is known is the result of anecdotal reports or data from registries. The basic rule is to avoid administering any drug to a woman who is pregnant (particularly during the first trimester) or who is breastfeeding a child, unless the mother's psychiatric disorder is severe and it is determined that the therapeutic value of the drug outweighs the theoretical adverse effects on the fetus or newborn. A woman may elect to continue on medication, because she does not want to chance a possible recurrence of painful or disabling symptoms.

Among the newer antidepressants, paroxetine is the only one to carry a warning from the FDA, the result of an increased risk of cardiac malformation. The agents with the most well-documented risk of specific birth defects are lithium, carbamazepine, and valproate. Lithium administration during pregnancy is associated with Ebstein's anomaly, a serious abnormality in cardiac development, although recent evidence suggests that the risk is not as great as previously believed. Carbamazepine and valproic acid are associated with neural tube defects, which can be prevented by use of folate during pregnancy. Lamotrigine may cause oral clefts when used during the first trimester. Some experts advise that all women of child-bearing age who are treated with psychotropics take supplemental folate.

The administration of psychotherapeutic drugs at or near delivery can cause the baby to be overly sedated at delivery, thus requiring a respirator, or to be physically dependent on the drug, requiring detoxification and the treatment of a withdrawal syndrome. Reports exist of a neonatal withdrawal syndrome associated with third trimester use of SSRIs in pregnant women. They have also been implicated in producing pulmonary hypertension in newborns.

Virtually all psychiatric drugs are secreted in the milk of a nursing mother; therefore, mothers on those agents should be advised not to breastfeed their infants.

Elderly Patients. The two major concerns when treating geriatric patients with psychotherapeutic drugs are that elderly persons may be more susceptible to adverse effects (particularly cardiac effects) and may metabolize and excrete drugs more slowly, thus requiring lower dosages of medication. In practice, clinicians should begin treating geriatric patients with a small dose, usually approximately half of the usual starting dose. The dose should be raised in small increments, more slowly than for middle-aged adults, until a clinical benefit is achieved or unacceptable adverse effects appear. Although many geriatric patients require a small dose of medication, many others require a full therapeutic dose.

Elderly patients account for approximately one-third of all prescription drug use and a substantial percentage of over-the-counter preparations as well. Even more significant is the incidence of polypharmacy. Recent surveys have found that elderly patients in the community are taking between three and five medications, and that hospitalized elderly patients are treated with an average of ten drugs. Nearly half of all patients in long-term care facilities are prescribed one or more psychotropic agents. In view of these statistics, clinicians need to consider potential types and likelihood of drug interactions when selecting medications.

Psychotropic drugs have been shown to be causally related to falls in the elderly. Discontinuation of psychotropic drugs results in an estimated 40 percent risk reduction for falls. This association between psychotropics and falls and hip fractures may weaken as newer agents become widely used. As a rule, new-generation compounds produce less unwanted sedation, dizziness, parkinsonism, and postural hypotension.

Age-related changes in renal clearance and hepatic metabolism make it more important to be conservative with the starting doses of medication as well as the rate of dose titration. Within any class of psychotropic agents, those with potentially serious consequences, such as hypotension, cardiac conduction abnormalities, anticholinergic activity, and respiratory depression, are not suitable choices. Drugs that cause cognitive impairment, such as benzodiazepines and anticholinergics, can mimic or exacerbate symptoms of dementia. Similarly, DRAs can worsen or induce Parkinson's disease, another age-related disorder. Some side effects, such as SSRI-associated syndrome of inappropriate secretion of antidiuretic hormone (SIADH) and oxcarbazepine-associated hyponatremia, occur more commonly in older patients.

A common ethical dilemma with the medically ill elderly or those with dementia is the question of their capacity to give informed consent before treatment with psychotropic drugs or electroconvulsive therapy (ECT).

Medically Ill Patients. There are special considerations, diagnostic and therapeutic, when administering psychiatric drugs to medically ill patients. The medical disorder should be ruled out as a cause of the psychiatric symptoms. For example, patients with neurological or endocrine disorders or those infected with human immunodeficiency virus (HIV) may experience disturbances of mood and cognition. Common medications, such as corticosteroids and L-dopa, are associated with induction of mania.

A patient with diabetes mellitus is better treated with an agent without the risk of weight gain or glucose dysregulation. Depending on the diagnosis, drugs that might treat the primary psychiatric disorder and also cause weight loss, drugs such as bupropion, topiramate, and zonisamide, should be prescribed for these patients. Patients with obstructive pulmonary disease should not be given sedating drugs, which raise the arousal threshold and suppress respiration. Patients with medical disorders are also taking other medications, which can result in pharmacodynamic and pharmacokinetic interactions. Combined treatment with an inducer of multiple CYP enzymes and a drug that is a substrate for those enzymes could result in subtherapeutic levels, leading to inadequate symptom control. Use of the tuberculosis treatment rifampicin (Rifadin) with carbamazepine is an example of this. Use of drugs that inhibit CYP 2D6, agents such as paroxetine and fluoxetine, can prevent the conversion of hydrocodone (Robidone) and other opiates into an active analgesic form. NSAIDs are also a rare cause of perceptual disturbances and psychotic symptoms.

Other issues include a potentially increased sensitivity to adverse effects, including increased or decreased metabolism and excretion of the drug, and interactions with other medications. Drug interactions are an obvious concern when drugs with a narrow therapeutic range are being used. Any change in the rate of metabolism or interference with the formation and elimination of metabolites can profoundly influence the activity of that drug. Similarly, interactions that interfere with drug metabolism can produce an increase in side effects and toxicity.

As with children and geriatric patients, the most reasonable clinical practice is to begin with a small dosage, to increase it slowly, and to watch for clinical benefit and adverse effects. Determining the plasma drug concentrations may be helpful for such patients, but therapeutic blood concentrations for most psychotropic drugs are neither necessary nor routinely available.

Substance Abuse. Many patients who seek or need treatment for a psychiatric disorder engage in chronic use of illicit substances or drink excessive amounts of alcohol. Marijuana is the most commonly used illicit (in most states) drug in the United States.

Discontinuation of chronic drug or alcohol use can result not only in craving, but also in clinically significant psychiatric and physiological withdrawal symptoms. For many patients, successful treatment of their underlying psychiatric disorder may not be possible in the presence of ongoing marijuana, cocaine, and alcohol use. If several trials of medications fail, hospitalization for detoxification may be necessary. Little research and no consensus exist about how to use psychotropic agents in patients who are regular users of cocaine, marijuana, or other recreational drugs.

Regulatory Issues

The FDA has the authority to approve a drug for clinical use and to ensure that product labeling is truthful and contains all information pertinent to the safe and effective use of that drug.

Product information that is FDA approved for marketed drugs appears as a package insert that lists potential side effects, drug interactions, the need for special monitoring, and restrictions for use. In some cases, these adverse reactions and potential safety hazards warrant a special warning label called a black box label. The FDA typically negotiates final labeling language with the company; however, in cases where a company refuses to satisfy the FDA, the agency may initiate proceedings to remove the drug from clinical use. In recent years, warning labels have been applied to entire classes of psychotropic drugs, including the SDAs and antidepressants such as the SSRIs.

The product information may also contain a "Contraindications" heading. This section describes instances in which the drug should not be used because the risk of using it clearly outweighs the benefit. If no contraindications are known, this section of the labeling will state "None known."

A precautions section may contain precautions for most individuals taking the drug, as well as for specific groups, such as pregnant women, nursing mothers, or children. In this section, one will find recommendations for patients to ensure safe and effective use of the drug. For example, there may be precautions about driving when taking the medication or using substances such as other drugs, food, or alcohol that may have harmful effects if taken while using the medication. The Precautions section also provides information about laboratory tests needed to track responses or to identify adverse reactions to the drug or about known interactions with other drugs, foods, or ingredients.

Every product label has an Adverse Reaction section that lists the frequency of undesirable effects that may be associated with use of a drug. Causes of adverse reactions can include medication errors, such as overdosage, or interactions between different drugs or between drugs and certain foods.

Nonapproved Dosages and Uses

It is now common practice to treat psychiatric disorders with drugs that are approved for nonpsychiatric conditions. Some examples include propranolol (Inderal) for social anxiety and treatment of lithium-induced tremor; verapamil (Calan, Isoptin) for mania and treatment of MAOI-induced hypertensive crisis; levothyroxine (Levoxyl) for antidepressant augmentation; clonidine (Catapres) and guanfacine (Tenex) for ADHD and posttraumatic stress disorder (PTSD); dextroamphetamine (Dexedrine) for antidepressant augmentation; and riluzole (Rilutek) for self-injurious behavior. Off-label use of a drug is not a violation of law or a departure from good medical practice. The FDA does not limit the manner in which a physician may use an approved drug. Medications can be prescribed for any reason shown to be medically indicated for the welfare of the patient. Once a drug is approved for commercial use, a physician can, as part of the practice of medicine, lawfully prescribe a different dosage for a patient or may otherwise vary the conditions of use from what is approved in the package labeling without notifying the FDA or obtaining its approval.

Failure to follow the information on the drug label does not in itself impose liability and should not preclude a physician from using good clinical judgment in the service of the patient. Physicians are permitted to use a drug for indications not included on the drug's official labeling without violating the FDA rules. This fact, however, does not absolve the physician of responsibility for an untoward result from treatment. Patients can still sue for possible medical malpractice with the reasoning that the failure to follow the FDA-approved label can be interpreted as deviating from the prevailing standard of care.

When using a drug for an unapproved indication or in a dose outside the usual range, good clinical practice is to explain to the patient and to document in the chart why a drug is being used instead of an approved agent. In cases of doubt about a plan to use a drug off label, a consultation with a colleague should be obtained.

In some cases, a drug has obtained a limited approval for an indication. Divalproex (Depakote), quetiapine (Seroquel), and risperidone, for example, are approved by the FDA for the acute, but not long-term, treatment of mania. Nevertheless, these drugs are routinely used for long-term prevention of recurrences of mania and bipolar disorder. In the case of lamotrigine, it was accepted as a first-choice agent for the treatment of bipolar disorder long before the FDA granted approval for that indication.

Placebos

Pharmacologically inactive substances have long been known to sometimes produce significant clinical benefits. A patient who believes that a compound is helpful may often derive considerable benefit from taking that substance, whether it is known to be pharmacologically active or not. For many psychiatric disorders, including mild to moderate depression and some anxiety disorders, well over 30 percent of patients can exhibit significant improvement or remission of symptoms on a placebo. For other conditions, such as schizophrenia, manic episodes, and psychotic depression, the placebo response rate is very low. Whereas suggestion is undoubtedly important in the efficacy of placebos (and active drugs), placebos can produce biological effects. For example, placebo-induced analgesia may sometimes be blocked by naloxone (Narcan), which suggests that endorphins may mediate the analgesia derived from taking a placebo. It is conceivable that placebos may also stimulate endogenous anxiolytic and antidepressant factors, resulting in clinical improvement in patients with depression and anxiety disorders.

Just as placebos can produce benefit, they can also have adverse effects. In many studies, some adverse effects are likely to be more common with placebos than with the active drug. Some patients will not tolerate placebos despite the fact that they are supposedly inert, and they exhibit adverse effects (called the *nocebo phenomenon*). It is easy to discount such patients as overly suggestible; however, if beneficial endogenous factors can be stimulated by placebos, perhaps toxic endogenous factors can also be produced.

Prudence is needed in contemplating the use of a placebo in clinical practice. Treating a patient with a placebo without consent can seriously undermine a patient's confidence in the physician if, and when, it is discovered.

MEDICATION-INDUCED MOVEMENT DISORDERS

Medication-induced movement disorders are commonly associated with the use of psychotropic drugs. Although most frequently associated with drugs that block dopamine type 2 (D_2) receptors, abnormal motor activity may occur with other types of medications as well. Sometimes it can be difficult to determine if abnormal motor movements are an adverse event or a symptom of an underlying disorder. For example, anxiety can resemble akathisia, and alcohol or benzodiazepine withdrawal can cause tremor. The American Psychiatric Association has decided to retain the term *neuroleptic* when discussing side effects associated with drugs used to treat psychosis—the DRAs and second-generation antipsychotics (SGAs). The rationale for continued use of the term is that it was originally used to describe the tendency of these drugs to cause abnormal movements.

The most common neuroleptic-related movement disorders are parkinsonism, acute dystonia, and acute akathisia. Neuroleptic malignant syndrome is a life-threatening and often misdiagnosed condition. Neuroleptic-induced tardive dyskinesia is a late-appearing adverse effect of neuroleptic drugs and can be irreversible; recent data, however, indicate that the syndrome, although still serious and potentially disabling, is less pernicious than was previously thought in patients taking DRAs. The newer antipsychotics, the SDAs, block binding to dopamine receptors to a much lesser degree and thereby are presumed to be less likely to produce such movement disorders. Nevertheless, this risk remains and vigilance is still required when these drugs are prescribed.

Table 25–4 lists the selected medications associated with movement disorders and their impact on relevant neuroreceptors.

Neuroleptic-Induced Parkinsonism and Other Medication-Induced Parkinsonism

Diagnosis, Signs, and Symptoms. Symptoms of neuroleptic-induced parkinsonism and other medication-induced parkinsonism include muscle stiffness (lead pipe rigidity), cogwheel rigidity, shuffling gait, stooped posture, and drooling. The pill-rolling tremor of idiopathic parkinsonism is rare, but a regular, coarse tremor similar to essential tremor may be present. The so-called *rabbit syndrome,* a tremor affecting the lips and perioral muscles, is another parkinsonian effect seen with antipsychotics, although perioral tremor is more likely than other tremors to occur late in the course of treatment.

Epidemiology. Parkinsonian adverse effects typically occur within 5 to 90 days of the initiation of treatment. Patients who are elderly and female are at the highest risk for neuroleptic-induced parkinsonism, although the disorder can occur at all ages.

Etiology. Neuroleptic-induced parkinsonism is caused by the blockade of D_2 receptors in the caudate at the termination of the nigrostriatal dopamine neurons. All antipsychotics can cause the symptoms, especially high-potency drugs with low levels of anticholinergic activity, most notably haloperidol (Haldol).

Differential Diagnosis. Included in the differential diagnosis are idiopathic parkinsonism, other organic causes of parkinsonism, and depression, which can also be associated with parkinsonian symptoms. Decreased psychomotor activity and blunted facial expression are symptoms of depression and idiopathic parkinsonism.

Treatment. Parkinsonism can be treated with anticholinergic agents, benztropine (Cogentin), amantadine (Symmetrel), or diphenhydramine (Benadryl) (Table 25–5). Anticholinergics should be withdrawn after 4 to 6 weeks to assess whether tolerance to the parkinsonian effects has developed; about half of patients with neuroleptic-induced parkinsonism require continued treatment. Even after the antipsychotics are withdrawn, parkinsonian symptoms can last up to 2 weeks and even up to 3 months in elderly patients. With such patients, the clinician may continue the anticholinergic drug after the antipsychotic has been stopped until the parkinsonian symptoms resolve completely.

Table 25–4
Selected Medications Associated with Movement Disorders: Impact on Relevant Neuroreceptors

Type (Subtype)	Name (Brand)	D_2 Blockade	5-HT_2 Blockade	mACh Blockade
Antipsychotics				
Phenothiazine (aliphatic)	Chlorpromazine (Thorazine)	Low	High	High
Phenothiazine (piperidines)	Thioridazine (Mellaril)	Low	Med	High
	Mesoridazine (Serentil)	Low	Med	High
Phenothiazine (piperazines)	Trifluoperazine (Stelazine)	Med	Med	Med
	Fluphenazine (Prolixin)	High	Low	Low
	Perphenazine (Trilafon)	High	Med	Low
Thioxanthenes	Thiothixene (Navane)	High	Med	Low
	Chlorprothixene (Taractan)	Med	High	Med
Dibenzoxazepines	Loxapine (Loxitane)	Med	High	Low
Butyrophenones	Haloperidol (Haldol)	High	Low	Low
	Droperidol (Inapsine)	High	Med	—
Diphenyl-butylpiperidines	Pimozide (Orap)	High	Med	Low
Dihydroindolones	Molindone (Moban)	Med	Low	Low
Dibenzodiazepines	Clozapine (Clozaril)	Low	High	High
Benzisoxazole	Risperidone (Risperdal)	High	High	Low
Thienobenzodiazepines	Olanzapine (Zyprexa)	Low	High	High
Dibenzothiazepines	Quetiapine (Seroquel)	Low/med	Low/med	Low
Benzisothiazolvils	Ziprasidone (Geodon)	Med	High	Low
Quinolones	Aripiprazole (Abilify)	High (as partial agonist)	High	Low
Nonantipsychotic psychotropics	Lithium (Eskalith)	N/A	N/A	N/A
Anticonvulsants		Low	Low	Low
Antidepressants		Low (except amoxapine)	(Varies)	(Varies)
Nonpsychotropics	Prochlorperazine (Compazine)	High	Med	Low
	Metoclopramide (Reglan)	High	High	—

D_2, dopamine type 2; 5-HT_2, 5-hydroxytryptomine type 2; mACh, muscarinic acetylcholine; N/A, not applicable.
Adapted from Jantcak PG, David JM, Preshorn SH, et al. *Principles and Practice of Psychopharmacotherapy*. 3rd ed. Philadelphia, PA: Lippincott Williams & Wilkins; 2001.

Neuroleptic Malignant Syndrome

Diagnosis, Signs, and Symptoms. *Neuroleptic malignant syndrome* is a life-threatening complication that can occur anytime during the course of antipsychotic treatment. The motor and behavioral symptoms include muscular rigidity and dystonia, akinesia, mutism, obtundation, and agitation. The autonomic symptoms include hyperthermia, diaphoresis, and increased pulse and BP. Laboratory findings include an increased white blood cell (WBC) count and increased levels of creatinine phosphokinase, liver enzymes, plasma myoglobin, and myoglobinuria, occasionally associated with renal failure.

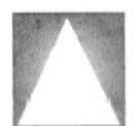

Table 25–5
Drug Treatment of Extrapyramidal Disorders

Generic Name	Trade Name	Usual Daily Dosage	Indications
Anticholinergics			
Benztropine	Cogentin	PO 0.5–2 mg tid; IM or IV 1–2 mg	Acute dystonia, parkinsonism, akinesia, akathisia
Biperiden	Akineton	PO 2–6 mg tid; IM or IV 2 mg	
Procyclidine	Kemadrin	PO 2.5–5 mg bid-qid	
Trihexyphenidyl	Artane, Tremin	PO 2–5 mg tid	
Orphenadrine	Norflex, Disipal	PO 50–100 mg bid-qid; IV 60 mg	Rabbit syndrome
Antihistamine			
Diphenhydramine	Benadryl	PO 25 mg qid; IM or IV 25 mg	Acute dystonia, parkinsonism, akinesia, rabbit syndrome
Amantadine	Symmetrel	PO 100–200 mg bid	Parkinsonism, akinesia, rabbit syndrome
β-Adrenergic antagonist			
Propranolol	Inderal	PO 20–40 mg tid	Akathisia, tremor
α-Adrenergic antagonist			
Clonidine	Catapres	PO 0.1 mg tid	Akathisia
Benzodiazepines			
Clonazepam	Klonopin	PO 1 mg bid	Akathisia, acute dystonia
Lorazepam	Ativan	PO 1 mg tid	
Buspirone	BuSpar	PO 20–40 mg qid	Tardive dyskinesia
Vitamin E	—	PO 1,200–1,600 IU/day	Tardive dyskinesia

PO, orally; IM, intramuscularly; IV, intravenously; qd, per day; bid, twice a day; tid, three times a day; qid; four times a day.

Table 25–6
Treatment of Neuroleptic Malignant Syndrome

Intervention	Dosing	Effectiveness
Amantadine	200–400 mg PO/day in divided doses	Beneficial as monotherapy or in combination; decrease in death rate
Bromocriptine	2.5 mg PO bid or tid, may increase to a total of 45 mg/day	Mortality reduced as a single or combined agent
Levodopa/carbidopa	Levodopa 50–100 mg/day IV as continuous infusion	Case reports of dramatic improvement
Electroconvulsive therapy	Reports of good outcome with both unilateral and bilateral treatments; response may occur in as few as three treatments	Effective when medications have failed; also may treat underlying psychiatric disorder
Dantrolene	1 mg/kg/day for 8 days, then continue as PO for 7 additional days	Benefits may occur in minutes or hours as a single agent or in combination
Benzodiazepines	1–2 mg IM as test dose; if effective, switch to PO; consider use if underlying disorder has catatonic symptoms	Has been reported effective when other agents have failed
Supportive measures	IV hydration, cooling blankets, ice packs, ice water enema, oxygenation, antipyretics	Often effective as initial approach early in the episode

PO, orally; bid, twice a day; tid, three times a day; IV, intravenously; IM, intramuscularly.
Adapted from Davis JM, Caroif SN, Mann SC. Treatment of neuroleptic malignant syndrome. *Psychiatr Ann*. 2000;30:325–331.

Epidemiology. About 0.01 to 0.02 percent of patients treated with antipsychotics develop neuroleptic malignant syndrome. Men are affected more frequently than women, and young patients are affected more commonly than elderly patients. The mortality rate can reach 10 to 20 percent or even higher when depot antipsychotic medications are involved.

Course and Prognosis. The symptoms usually evolve over 24 to 72 hours, and the untreated syndrome lasts 10 to 14 days. The diagnosis is often missed in the early stages, and the withdrawal or agitation may mistakenly be considered to reflect an exacerbation of the psychosis.

Treatment. In addition to supportive medical treatment, the most commonly used medications for the condition are dantrolene (Dantrium) and bromocriptine (Parlodel), although amantadine (Symmetrel) is sometimes used (Table 25–6). Bromocriptine and amantadine pose direct DRA effects and may serve to overcome the antipsychotic-induced dopamine receptor blockade. The lowest effective dosage of the antipsychotic drug should be used to reduce the chance of neuroleptic malignant syndrome. High-potency drugs, such as haloperidol, pose the greatest risk. Antipsychotic drugs with anticholinergic effects seem less likely to cause neuroleptic malignant syndrome. ECT has been used.

Medication-Induced Acute Dystonia

Diagnosis, Signs, and Symptoms. *Dystonias* are brief or prolonged contractions of muscles that result in obviously abnormal movements or postures, including oculogyric crises, tongue protrusion, trismus, torticollis, laryngeal–pharyngeal dystonias, and dystonic postures of the limbs and trunk. Other dystonias include blepharospasm and glossopharyngeal dystonia; the latter results in dysarthria, dysphagia, and even difficulty in breathing, which can cause cyanosis. Children are particularly likely to evidence opisthotonos, scoliosis, lordosis, and writhing movements. Dystonia can be painful and frightening and often results in noncompliance with future drug treatment regimens.

Epidemiology. The development of acute dystonic symptoms is characterized by their early onset during the course of treatment with neuroleptics. There is a higher incidence of acute dystonia in men, in patients younger than age 30 years, and in patients given high dosages of high-potency medications.

Etiology. Although it is most common with intramuscular (IM) doses of high-potency antipsychotics, dystonia can occur with any antipsychotic. The mechanism of action is thought to be dopaminergic hyperactivity in the basal ganglia that occurs when CNS levels of the antipsychotic drug begin to fall between doses.

Differential Diagnosis. The differential diagnosis includes seizures and tardive dyskinesia.

Course and Prognosis. Dystonia can fluctuate spontaneously and respond to reassurance, so the clinician gets the false impression that the movement is hysterical or completely under conscious control.

Treatment. Prophylaxis with anticholinergics or related drugs (outlined in Table 25–5) usually prevents dystonia, although the risks of prophylactic treatment weigh against that benefit. Treatment with IM anticholinergics or intravenous or IM diphenhydramine (Benadryl) (50 mg) almost always relieves the symptoms. Diazepam (Valium) (10 mg intravenously), amobarbital (Amytal), caffeine sodium benzoate, and hypnosis have also been reported to be effective. Although tolerance for the adverse effects usually develops, it is prudent to change the antipsychotic if the patient is particularly concerned that the reaction may recur.

Medication-Induced Acute Akathisia

Diagnosis, Signs, and Symptoms. *Akathisia* is subjective feelings of restlessness, objective signs of restlessness, or both. Examples include a sense of anxiety, inability to relax, jitteriness, pacing, rocking motions while sitting, and rapid alternation of sitting and standing. Akathisia has been associated with the use of a wide range of psychiatric drugs, including antipsychotics, antidepressants, and sympathomimetics. Once akathisia is recognized and diagnosed, the antipsychotic dose should be reduced to the minimal effective level. Akathisia may be associated with a poor treatment outcome.

Epidemiology. Middle-aged women are at increased risk of akathisia, and the time course is similar to that for neuroleptic-induced parkinsonism.

Treatment. Three basic steps in the treatment of akathisia are reducing medication dosage, attempting treatment with appropriate drugs, and considering changing the neuroleptic. The most efficacious drugs are β-adrenergic receptor antagonists, although anticholinergic drugs, benzodiazepines, and cyproheptadine (Periactin) may benefit some patients. In some cases of akathisia, no treatment seems to be effective.

Tardive Dyskinesia

Diagnosis, Signs, and Symptoms. *Tardive dyskinesia* is a delayed effect of antipsychotics; it rarely occurs until after 6 months of treatment. The disorder consists of abnormal, involuntary, irregular choreoathetoid movements of the muscles of the head, limbs, and trunk. The severity of the movements ranges from minimal—often missed by patients and their families—to grossly incapacitating. Perioral movements are the most common and include darting, twisting, and protruding movements of the tongue; chewing and lateral jaw movements; lip puckering; and facial grimacing. Finger movements and hand clenching are also common. Torticollis, retrocollis, trunk twisting, and pelvic thrusting occur in severe cases. In the most serious cases, patients may have breathing and swallowing irregularities that result in aerophagia, belching, and grunting. Respiratory dyskinesia has also been reported. Dyskinesia is exacerbated by stress and disappears during sleep.

Epidemiology. Tardive dyskinesia develops in about 10 to 20 percent of patients who are treated for more than a year. About 20 to 40 percent of patients who require long-term hospitalization have tardive dyskinesia. Women are more likely to be affected than men. Children, patients who are more than 50 years of age, and patients with brain damage or mood disorders are also at high risk.

Course and Prognosis. Between 5 and 40 percent of all cases of tardive dyskinesia eventually remit, and between 50 and 90 percent of all mild cases remit. Tardive dyskinesia is less likely to remit in elderly patients than in young patients, however.

Treatment. The three basic approaches to tardive dyskinesia are prevention, diagnosis, and management. Prevention is best achieved by using antipsychotic medications only when clearly indicated and in the lowest effective doses. The atypical antipsychotics are associated with less tardive dyskinesia than the older antipsychotics. Clozapine (Clozaril) is the only antipsychotic to have minimal risk of tardive dyskinesia and can even help improve preexisting symptoms of tardive dyskinesia. This has been attributed to its low affinity for D_2 receptors and high affinity for 5-hydroxytryptamine (5-HT) receptor antagonism. Patients who are receiving antipsychotics should be examined regularly for the appearance of abnormal movements, preferably with the use of a standardized rating scale (Table 25–7). Patients frequently experience an exacerbation of their symptoms when the DRA is withheld, whereas substitution of an SDA may limit

Table 25–7
Abnormal Involuntary Movement Scale (AIMS) Examination Procedure

Patient Identification	Date

Rated by

Either before or after completing the examination procedure, observe the patient unobtrusively at rest (e.g., in waiting room).
The chair to be used in this examination should be a hard, firm one without arms.
After observing the patient, rate him or her on a scale of 0 (none), 1 (minimal), 2 (mild), 3 (moderate), and 4 (severe), according to the severity of the symptoms.
Ask patient whether there is anything in his or her mouth (e.g., gum, candy) and, if so, to remove it.
Ask patient about the current condition of his or her teeth. Ask patient if he or she wears dentures. Do teeth or dentures bother patient now?
Ask patient whether he or she notices movement in mouth, face, hands, or feet. If yes, ask patient to describe and indicate to what extent movements currently bother patient or interfere with his or her activities.
0 1 2 3 4 Have patient sit in chair with hands on knees, legs slightly apart, and feet flat on floor. (Look at entire body for movement while in this position.)
0 1 2 3 4 Ask patient to sit with hands hanging unsupported—If male, between legs; if female and wearing a dress, hanging over knees. (Observe hands and other body areas.)
0 1 2 3 4 Ask patient to open mouth. (Observe tongue at rest within mouth.) Do this twice.
0 1 2 3 4 Ask patient to protrude tongue. (Observe abnormalities of tongue movement.) Do this twice.
0 1 2 3 4 Ask patient to tap thumb, with each finger, as rapidly as possible for 10–15 seconds; separately with right hand, then with left hand. (Observe facial and leg movements.)
0 1 2 3 4 Flex and extend patient's left and right arms. (One at a time.)
0 1 2 3 4 Ask patient to stand up. (Observe in profile. Observe all body areas again, hips included.)
0 1 2 3 4 [a]Ask patient to extend both arms outstretched in front with palms down. (Observe trunk, legs, and mouth.)
0 1 2 3 4 [a]Have patient walk a few paces, turn, and walk back to chair. (Observe hands and gait.)
Do this twice.

[a]Activated movements.

the abnormal movements without worsening the progression of the dyskinesia.

Once tardive dyskinesia is recognized, the clinician should consider reducing the dose of the antipsychotic or even stopping the medication altogether. Alternatively, the clinician may switch the patient to clozapine or to one of the new SDAs. In patients who cannot continue taking any antipsychotic medication, lithium (Eskalith), carbamazepine (Tegretol), or benzodiazepines may effectively reduce the symptoms of both the movement disorder and the psychosis.

Tardive Dystonia and Tardive Akathisia

On occasion, dystonia and akathisia emerge late in the course of treatment. These symptoms may persist for months or years despite drug discontinuation or dose reduction.

Medication-Induced Postural Tremor

Diagnosis, Signs, and Symptoms. *Tremor* is a rhythmic alteration in movement that is usually faster than one beat per second. Fine tremor (8 to 12 Hz) is most common.

Epidemiology. Typically, tremors decrease during periods of relaxation and sleep and increase with stress or anxiety.

Etiology. Whereas all the above diagnoses specifically include an association with a neuroleptic, a range of psychiatric medications can produce tremor—most notably, lithium, stimulants, antidepressants, caffeine, and valproate (Depakene).

Treatment. The treatment involves four principles:

1. The lowest possible dose of the psychiatric drug should be taken.
2. Patients should minimize caffeine consumption.
3. The psychiatric drug should be taken at bedtime to minimize the amount of daytime tremor.
4. β-adrenergic receptor antagonists (e.g., propranolol [Inderal]) can be given to treat drug-induced tremors.

Other Medication-Induced Movement Disorders

Nocturnal Myoclonus. *Nocturnal myoclonus* consists of highly stereotyped, abrupt contractions of certain leg muscles during sleep. Patients lack any subjective awareness of the leg jerks. The condition may be present in about 40 percent of persons over 65 years of age. The cause is unknown, but it is a rare side effect of SSRIs.

The repetitive leg movements occur every 20 to 60 seconds, with extensions of the large toe and flexion of the ankle, the knee, and the hips. Frequent awakenings, unrefreshing sleep, and daytime sleepiness are major symptoms. No treatment for nocturnal myoclonus is universally effective. Treatments that may be useful include benzodiazepines, levodopa (Larodopa), quinine, and, in rare cases, opioids.

Restless Leg Syndrome. In *restless leg syndrome*, persons feel deep sensations of creeping inside the calves whenever sitting or lying down. The dysesthesias are rarely painful but are agonizingly relentless and cause an almost irresistible urge to move the legs; thus, this syndrome interferes with sleep and with falling asleep. It peaks in middle age and occurs in 5 percent of the population. The cause is unknown, but it is a rare side effect of SSRIs.

Symptoms are relieved by movement and by leg massage. The dopamine receptor agonists ropinirole (Requip) and pramipexole (Mirapex) are effective in treating this syndrome. Other treatments include the benzodiazepines, levodopa, quinine, opioids, propranolol, valproate, and carbamazepine.

Hyperthermic Syndromes

All the medication-induced movement disorders may be associated with hyperthermia. Table 25–8 lists the various conditions associated with hyperthermia.

α_2-ADRENERGIC RECEPTOR AGONISTS, α_1-ADRENERGIC RECEPTOR ANTAGONISTS: CLONIDINE, GUANFACINE, PRAZOSIN, AND YOHIMBINE

Clonidine (Catapres) was developed initially as an antihypertensive medication because of its noradrenergic effects. It is an α_2-adrenergic receptor agonist and reduces plasma norepinephrine. It has been studied in many neurologic and psychiatric conditions, including ADHD, tic disorders, opiates and alcohol withdrawal, and PTSD. Its use has been somewhat limited by sedation and hypotension, which are common, and in children, its use is limited by its cardiac effects. Guanfacine (Tenex), another α_2-adrenergic receptor agonist, has been preferentially used because of its differential affinity for certain α_2-adrenergic receptor subtypes, resulting in less sedation and hypotension. However, there have been fewer clinical studies of guanfacine than of clonidine.

Prazosin (Minipress) is an α_1-postsynaptic antagonist. It reduces BP through vasodilation. Prazosin has shown benefits in treating sleep disorders associated with PTSD.

Clonidine and Guanfacine

Pharmacological Actions. Guanfacine is an agonist on presynaptic α_2-receptors. It inhibits sympathetic outflow and causes vasodilation of blood vessels. It is marketed as a treatment for high BP. It is more selective and less potent than clonidine, the other widely used α_2-agonist. Clonidine and guanfacine are well absorbed from the GI tract and reach peak plasma levels 1 to 3 hours after oral administration. The half-life of clonidine is 6 to 20 hours and that of guanfacine is 10 to 30 hours.

The agonist effects of clonidine and guanfacine on presynaptic α_2-adrenergic receptors in the sympathetic nuclei of the brain result in a decrease in the amount of norepinephrine released from the presynaptic nerve terminals. This serves generally to reset the body's sympathetic tone at a lower level and decrease arousal.

Therapeutic Indications. There is considerably more experience in clinical psychiatry with clonidine than with

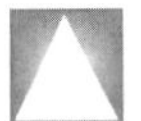

Table 25–8
Drug-Induced Central Hyperthermic Syndromes[a]

Condition (and Mechanism)	Common Drug Causes	Frequent Symptoms	Possible Treatment[b]	Clinical Course
Hyperthermia (↓ heat dissipation) (↑ heat production)	Atropine, lidocaine, meperidine NSAID toxicity, pheochromocytoma, thyrotoxicosis	Hyperthermia, diaphoresis, malaise	Acetaminophen per rectum (325 mg every 4 hrs), diazepam oral or per rectum (5 mg every 8 hrs) for febrile seizures	Benign, febrile seizures in children
Malignant hyperthermia (↑ heat production)	NMJ blockers (succinylcholine), halothane	Hyperthermia muscle rigidity, arrhythmias, ischemia,[c] hypotension, rhabdomyolysis; disseminated intravascular coagulation	Dantrolene sodium (1–2 mg/kg/min IV infusion)[d]	Familial, 10% mortality if untreated
Tricyclic overdose (↑ heat production)	Tricyclic antidepressants, cocaine	Hyperthermia, confusion, visual hallucinations, agitation, hyperreflexia, muscle relaxation, anticholinergic effects (dry skin, pupil dilation), arrhythmias	Sodium bicarbonate (1 mEq/kg IV bolus) if arrhythmia is present, physostigmine (1–3 mg IV) with cardiac monitoring	Fatalities have occurred if untreated
Autonomic hyperreflexia (↑ heat production)	CNS stimulants (amphetamines)	Hyperthermia excitement, hyperreflexia	Trimethaphan (0.3–7 mg/min IV infusion)	Reversible
Lethal catatonia (↓ heat dissipation)	Lead poisoning	Hyperthermia, intense anxiety, destructive behavior, psychosis	Lorazepam (1–2 mg IV every 4 hrs), antipsychotics may be contraindicated	High mortality if untreated
Neuroleptic malignant syndrome (mixed; hypothalamic, ↓ heat dissipation, ↑ heat production)	Antipsychotics (neuroleptics), methyldopa, reserpine	Hyperthermia, muscle rigidity, diaphoresis (60%), leukocytosis, delirium, rhabdomyolysis, elevated CPK, autonomic deregulation, extrapyramidal symptoms	Bromocriptine (2–10 mg every 8 hrs orally or nasogastric tube), lisuride (0.02– 0.1 mg/hr IV infusion), carbidopa-levodopa (Sinemet) (25/100 PO every 8 hrs), dantrolene sodium (0.3–1 mg/kg IV every 6 hrs)	Rapid onset, 20% mortality if untreated

NSAID, nonsteroidal anti-inflammatory drug; NMJ, neuromuscular junction; CNS, central nervous system; CPK, creatine phosphokinase; PO, orally; IV, intravenously.
[a]Boldface indicates features that may be used to distinguish one syndrome from another.
[b]Gastric lavage and supportive measures, including cooling, are required in most cases.
[c]Oxygen consumption increases by 7% for every 1°F increase in body temperature.
[d]Has been associated with idiosyncratic hepatocellular injury, as well as severe hypotension in one case.
From Theoharides TC, Harris RS, Weckstein D. Neuroleptic malignant-like syndrome due to cyclobenzaprine? *J Clin Psychopharmacol* 1995;15:79–81, with permission.

guanfacine. There is recent interest in the use of guanfacine for the same indications that respond to clonidine due to guanfacine's longer half-life and relative lack of sedative effects.

WITHDRAWAL FROM OPIOIDS, ALCOHOL, BENZODIAZEPINES, OR NICOTINE. Clonidine and guanfacine are effective in reducing the autonomic symptoms of rapid opioid withdrawal (e.g., hypertension, tachycardia, dilated pupils, sweating, lacrimation, and rhinorrhea) but not the associated subjective sensations. Clonidine administration (0.1 to 0.2 mg two to four times a day) is initiated before detoxification and is then tapered off over 1 to 2 weeks (Table 25–9).

Clonidine and guanfacine can reduce symptoms of alcohol and benzodiazepine withdrawal, including anxiety, diarrhea, and tachycardia. They can reduce craving, anxiety, and the irritability symptoms of nicotine withdrawal. The transdermal patch formulation of clonidine is associated with better long-term compliance for purposes of detoxification than is the tablet formulation.

TOURETTE'S DISORDER. Clonidine and guanfacine are effective drugs for the treatment of Tourette's disorder. Most clinicians begin treatment for Tourette's disorder with the standard DRAs haloperidol (Haldol) and pimozide (Orap) and the SDAs risperidone (Risperdal) and olanzapine (Zyprexa). However, if concerned about the adverse effects of these drugs, the clinician may begin treatment with clonidine or guanfacine. The starting dose of clonidine for children is 0.05 mg a day; it can be increased to 0.3 mg a day in divided doses. Up to 3 months are needed before the beneficial effects of clonidine can be seen in patients with Tourette's disorder. The response rate has been reported to be up to 70 percent.

OTHER TIC DISORDERS. Clonidine and guanfacine reduce the frequency and severity of tics in persons with tic disorder with or without comorbid ADHD.

HYPERACTIVITY AND AGGRESSION IN CHILDREN. Clonidine and guanfacine can be useful alternatives for the treatment of

Table 25–9
Oral Clonidine Protocols for Opioid Detoxification

Clonidine 0.1–0.2 mg PO four times a day; hold for systolic BP <90 mm Hg or bradycardia; stabilize for 2–3 days, then taper over 5–10 days
OR
Clonidine 0.1–0.2 mg PO q4–6h as needed for withdrawal signs or symptoms; stabilize for 2–3 days, then taper over 5–10 days
OR
Test dose with clonidine 0.1–0.2 mg PO or SL (for patients weighing over 200 lb); check BP after 1 hr. If diastolic BP >70 mm Hg and no symptoms of hypotension, begin treatment as follows:

Weight (lb)	Number of Clonidine Patches
<110	1 patch
110–160	2 patches
160–200	2 patches
>200	2 patches

OR
Test dose of oral clonidine 0.1 mg; check BP after 1 hr (if systolic BP <90 mm Hg, do not give patch)
Place two TTS-2 clonidine patches (or three patches if patient weighs >150 lb) on hairless area of upper body; then
For first 23 hrs after patch application, give oral clonidine 0.2 mg q6h; then
For next 24 hrs, give oral clonidine 0.1 mg q6h
Change patches weekly
After 2 weeks of two patches, switch to one patch (or two patches if patient weighs >150 lb)
After 1 week of one patch, discontinue patches

BP, blood pressure; PO, oral; q, every; SL, sublingual; TTS, through the skin.
From American Society of Addiction Medicine. Detoxification: Principle and protocols. In: *The Principles Update Series: Topics in Addiction Medicine* (Section 11). American Society of Addiction, 1997, with permission.

ADHD. They are used in place of sympathomimetics and antidepressants, which may produce paradoxical worsening of hyperactivity in some children with intellectual disability, aggression, or features on the spectrum of autism. Clonidine and guanfacine can improve mood, reduce activity level, and improve social adaptation. Some impaired children may respond favorably to clonidine, but others may simply become sedated. The starting dose is 0.05 mg a day; it can be raised to 0.3 mg a day in divided doses. The efficacy of clonidine and guanfacine for control of hyperactivity and aggression often diminishes over several months of use.

Clonidine and guanfacine can be combined with methylphenidate (Ritalin) or dextroamphetamine (Dexedrine) to treat hyperactivity and inattentiveness, respectively. A small number of cases have been reported of sudden death of children taking clonidine together with methylphenidate; however, it has not been conclusively demonstrated that these medications contributed to these deaths. The clinician should explain to the family that the efficacy and safety of this combination have not been investigated in controlled trials. Periodic cardiovascular assessments, including vital signs and ECGs, are warranted if this combination is used.

POSTTRAUMATIC STRESS DISORDER. Acute exacerbations of PTSD may be associated with hyperadrenergic symptoms such as hyperarousal, exaggerated startle response, insomnia, vivid nightmares, tachycardia, agitation, hypertension, and perspiration. Preliminary reports suggested that these symptoms may respond to the use of clonidine or, especially for overnight benefit, to the use of guanfacine. More recent studies have failed to demonstrate that guanfacine produces an improvement in PTSD symptoms.

OTHER DISORDERS. Other potential indications for clonidine include other anxiety disorders (panic disorder, phobias, obsessive-compulsive disorder, and generalized anxiety disorder) and mania, in which it may be synergistic with lithium (Eskalith) or carbamazepine (Tegretol). Anecdotal reports have noted the efficacy of clonidine in schizophrenia and tardive dyskinesia. A clonidine patch can reduce the hypersalivation and dysphagia caused by clozapine. Low-dose use has been reported effective in hallucinogen-persisting perceptive disorders.

Precautions and Adverse Reactions. The most common adverse effects associated with clonidine are dry mouth and eyes, fatigue, sedation, dizziness, nausea, hypotension, and constipation, which result in discontinuation of therapy by about 10 percent of all persons taking the drug. Some persons also experience sexual dysfunction. Tolerance may develop to these adverse effects. A similar but milder adverse profile is seen with guanfacine, especially in doses of 3 mg or more per day. Clonidine and guanfacine should not be taken by adults with BP below 90/60 mm Hg or with cardiac arrhythmias, especially bradycardia. Development of bradycardia warrants gradual, tapered discontinuation of the drug. Clonidine in particular is associated with sedation, and tolerance does not usually develop to this adverse effect. Uncommon CNS adverse effects of clonidine include insomnia, anxiety, and depression; rare CNS adverse effects include vivid dreams, nightmares, and hallucinations. Fluid retention associated with clonidine treatment can be treated with diuretics.

The transdermal patch formulation of clonidine may cause local skin irritation, which can be minimized by rotating the sites of application.

Overdose. Persons who take an overdose of clonidine may present with coma and constricted pupils, symptoms similar to those of an opioid overdose. Other symptoms of overdose are decreased BP, pulse, and respiratory rate. Guanfacine overdose produces a milder version of these symptoms. Clonidine and guanfacine should be avoided during pregnancy and by nursing mothers. Elderly persons are more sensitive to the drug than are younger adults. Children are susceptible to the same adverse effects as are adults.

Withdrawal. Abrupt discontinuation of clonidine can cause anxiety, restlessness, perspiration, tremor, abdominal pain, palpitations, headache, and a dramatic increase in BP. These symptoms may appear about 20 hours after the last dose of clonidine, and these may also be seen if one or two doses are skipped. A similar set of symptoms occasionally occurs 2 to 4 days after discontinuation of guanfacine, but the usual course is gradual return to baseline BP over 2 to 4 days. Because of the possibility of discontinuation symptoms, doses of clonidine and guanfacine should be tapered slowly.

Drug Interactions. Clonidine and guanfacine cause sedation, especially early in therapy, and when administered with other centrally active depressants, such as barbiturates, alcohol, and benzodiazepines, the potential for additive sedative effects should be considered. Dose reduction may be required in patients receiving agents that interfere with atrioventricular (AV) node and sinus node conduction such as β-blockers, calcium channel blockers (CCBs), and digitalis. This combination increases the risk of AV block and bradycardia. Clonidine should not be given with TCAs, which can inhibit the hypotensive effects of clonidine.

Laboratory Interferences. No known laboratory interferences are associated with the use of clonidine or guanfacine.

Dosage and Clinical Guidelines. Clonidine is available in 0.1-, 0.2-, and 0.3-mg tablets. The usual starting dosage is 0.1 mg orally twice a day; the dosage can be raised by 0.1 mg a day to an appropriate level (up to 1.2 mg per day). Clonidine must always be tapered when it is discontinued to avoid rebound hypertension, which may occur about 20 hours after the last clonidine dose. A weekly transdermal formulation of clonidine is available at doses of 0.1, 0.2, and 0.3 mg per day. The usual starting dosage is the 0.1-mg-a-day patch, which is changed each week for adults and every 5 days for children; the dose can be increased, as needed, every 1 to 2 weeks. Transition from the oral to the transdermal formulations should be accomplished gradually by overlapping them for 3 to 4 days.

Guanfacine is available in 1- and 2-mg tablets. The usual starting dosage is 1 mg before sleep, and this can be increased to 2 mg before sleep after 3 to 4 weeks, if necessary. Regardless of the indication for which clonidine or guanfacine is being used, the drug should be withheld if a person becomes hypotensive (BP below 90/60 mm Hg).

An extended-release preparation of guanfacine (Intuniv) is also available. Extended-release guanfacine should be dosed once daily. Tablets should not be crushed, chewed, or broken before swallowing because this will increase the rate of guanfacine release. It should not be administered with high fat meals due to increased exposure. The extended-release formulation should not be substituted for immediate-release guanfacine tablets on a milligram-per-milligram basis because of differing pharmacokinetic profiles. If switching from immediate-release guanfacine, discontinue that treatment, and titrate with extended-release guanfacine according to the following recommended schedule:

1. Begin at a dose of 1 mg/day, and adjust in increments of no more than 1 mg/wk, for both monotherapy and adjunctive therapy to a psychostimulant.
2. Maintain the dose within the range of 1 to 4 mg once daily, depending on clinical response and tolerability, for both monotherapy and adjunctive therapy to a psychostimulant. In clinical trials, patients were randomized or dose optimized to doses of 1, 2, 3, or 4 mg and received extended-release guanfacine once daily in the morning in monotherapy trials and once daily in the morning or the evening in the adjunctive therapy trial.
3. In monotherapy trials, clinically relevant improvements were observed beginning at doses in the range 0.05 to 0.08 mg/kg once daily. Efficacy increased with increasing weight-adjusted dose (mg/kg). If well tolerated, doses up to 0.12 mg/kg once daily may provide additional benefit. Doses above 4 mg/day have not been systematically studied in controlled clinical trials.
4. In the adjunctive trial, the majority of subjects reached optimal doses in the 0.05 to 0.12 mg/kg/day range.

In clinical trials, there were dose-related and exposure-related risks for several clinically significant adverse reactions (e.g., hypotension, bradycardia, sedative events). Thus, consideration should be given to dosing an extended-release preparation of guanfacine on a milligram-per-kilogram basis in order to balance the exposure-related potential benefits and risks of treatment.

Yohimbine

Yohimbine (Yocon) is an α_2-adrenergic receptor antagonist that is used as a treatment for both idiopathic and medication-induced erectile disorder. Currently, sildenafil (Viagra) and its congeners and alprostadil (Impulse, Edex) are considered more efficacious for this indication than yohimbine. Yohimbine is derived from an alkaloid found in *Rubaceae* and related trees and in the *Rauwolfia serpentina* plant.

Pharmacological Actions. Yohimbine is erratically absorbed after oral administration, with bioavailability ranging from 7 to 87 percent. There is extensive hepatic first-pass metabolism. Yohimbine affects the sympathomimetic autonomic nervous system by increasing plasma concentrations of norepinephrine. The half-life of yohimbine is 0.5 to 2 hours. Clinically, yohimbine produces increased parasympathetic (cholinergic) tone.

Therapeutic Indications. Yohimbine has been used to treat erectile dysfunction. Penile erection has been linked to cholinergic activity and to α_2-adrenergic blockade, which theoretically results in increased penile inflow of blood, decreased penile outflow of blood, or both. Yohimbine is reported to help counteract the loss of sexual desire and the orgasmic inhibition caused by some serotonergic antidepressants (e.g., SSRIs). It has not been found useful in women for these indications.

Precautions. The side effects of yohimbine include anxiety, elevated BP and heart rate, increased psychomotor activity, irritability, tremor, headache, skin flushing, dizziness, urinary frequency, nausea, vomiting, and sweating. Patients with panic disorder show heightened sensitivity to yohimbine and experience increased anxiety, increased BP, and increased plasma 3-methoxy-4-hydroxyphenylglycol (MHPG).

Yohimbine should be used with caution in female patients and should not be used in patients with renal disease, cardiac disease, glaucoma, or a history of gastric or duodenal ulcer.

Drug Interactions. Yohimbine blocks the effects of clonidine, guanfacine, and other α_2-receptor agonists.

Laboratory Interferences. No known laboratory interferences are associated with yohimbine use.

Table 25–10
α_2-Adrenergic Receptor Agonists Used in Psychiatry[a]

Drug	Preparations	Usual Child Starting Dosage	Usual Child Dosage Range	Usual Adult Starting Dosage	Usual Adult Dosage
Clonidine tablets (Catapres)	0.1, 0.2, 0.3 mg	0.05 mg/day	Up to 0.3 mg/day tablets in divided doses	0.1–0.2 mg, two to four times a day (0.2–0.8 mg/day)	0.3–1.2 mg/day, two to three times a day (1.2 mg/day maximal dosage)
Clonidine transdermal system (Catapres-TTS)	0.1, 0.2, 0.3 mg/day	0.05 mg/day	Up to 0.3 mg/day patch every 5 days (0.5 mg/day every 5 days maximal dosage)	0.1 mg/day every 7 days	0.1 mg/day patch per week 0.6 mg/day every 7 days
Guanfacine (Tenex)	1- and 2-mg tablets	1 mg/day at bedtime	1–2 mg/day at bedtime (3 mg/day maximal dosage)	1 mg/day at bedtime	1–2 mg at bedtime (3 mg/day maximal dosage)

[a]Dosages for medical indications, such as hypertension, vary.

Dosage and Clinical Guidelines. Yohimbine is available in 5.4-mg tablets. The dosage of yohimbine in the treatment of erectile disorder is approximately 16 mg a day given in doses that range from 2.7 to 5.4 mg three times a day. In the event of significant adverse effects, dose should first be reduced and then gradually increased again. Yohimbine should be used judiciously in psychiatric patients because it may have an adverse effect on their mental status. Because yohimbine has no consistent effect on erectile dysfunction, its use remains controversial. Phosphodiesterase-5 (PDE-5) inhibitors are the preferred medication for this disorder.

Prazosin

Prazosin (Minipress) is a quinazoline derivative and one of a new chemical class of antihypertensives. It is an α_1-adrenergic receptor antagonist as opposed to the drugs mentioned above, which are α_2-blockers.

Pharmacological Actions. The exact mechanism of the hypotensive action or prazosin is unknown, particularly as it effects nightmare suppression. Prazosin causes a decrease in total peripheral resistance that is related to its action as an α_1-adrenergic receptor antagonist. BP is lowered in both the supine and standing positions. This effect is most pronounced on the diastolic BP. After oral administration, human plasma concentrations reach a peak at about 3 hours with a plasma half-life of 2 to 3 hours. The drug is highly bound to plasma protein. Tolerance has not been observed to develop with long-term therapy.

Therapeutic Action. Prazosin is used in psychiatry to suppress nightmares, particularly those associated with PTSD.

Precautions and Adverse Reactions. During clinical trials and subsequent marketing experience, the most frequent reactions were dizziness (10.3 percent); headache (7.8 percent); drowsiness (7.6 percent); lack of energy (6.9 percent); weakness (6.5 percent); palpitations (5.3 percent); and nausea (4.9 percent). In most instances, side effects disappeared with continued therapy or have been tolerated with no decrease in dose of drug. Prazosin should not be used in nursing mothers or during pregnancy.

Drug Interactions. No adverse drug interactions have been reported.

Laboratory Interferences. No laboratory interferences have been reported.

Dosage and Clinical Guidelines. The drug is supplied in 1-, 2-, and 5-mg capsules and a nasal spray. The therapeutic dosages most commonly used have ranged from 6 to 15 mg daily given in divided doses. Doses higher than 20 mg do not increase efficacy. When adding a diuretic or other antihypertensive agent, the dose should be reduced to 1 or 2 mg three times a day and retitration then carried out. Concomitant use with a PDE-5 inhibitor can result in additive BP lowering effects and symptomatic hypotension; therefore, PDE-5 inhibitor therapy should be initiated at the lowest dose in patients taking prazosin.

Table 25–10 provides a summary of α_2-adrenergic receptor agonists used in psychiatry.

β-ADRENERGIC RECEPTOR ANTAGONISTS

Because of the innervations of many, if not most, peripheral organs and vasculature by the sympathetic division of the autonomic nervous system, their functions are ultimately controlled, in part, by one of the two major classes of adrenergic receptors: α-receptors and β-receptors. These receptors are further subdivided based on their action and location, and they are located both peripherally and in the CNS. Shortly after being introduced for cardiac indications, propranolol (Inderal) was reported to be useful for agitation, and its use in psychiatry spread rapidly. The five most commonly used β-receptor antagonists in psychiatry are propranolol, nadolol (Corgard), metoprolol (Lopressor, Toprol), pindolol (Visken), and atenolol (Tenormin) (Table 25–11).

Pharmacological Actions

The β-receptor antagonists differ with regard to lipophilicities, metabolic routes, β-receptor selectivity, and half-lives. The absorption of the β-receptor antagonists from the GI tract is variable. The agents that are most soluble in lipids (i.e., are lipophilic) are likely to cross the blood–brain barrier and enter

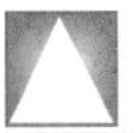

Table 25–11
β-Adrenergic Drugs Used in Psychiatry

Drug	Pregnancy Category	Trade Name	Protein Binding (%)	Lipophilic	ISA	Metabolism	Receptor Selectivity	Half-Life (hrs)	Usual Starting Dosage (mg)	Usual Maximal Dosage (mg)
Atenolol (Tenormin)	D	Tenormin	6–16	No		Renal	$\beta_1 > \beta_2$	6–9	50 OD	50–100 OD
Metoprolol (Lopressor)	C	Lopressor	5–10	Yes		Hepatic	$\beta_1 > \beta_2$	3–4	50 bid	75–150 bid
Nadolol (Corgard)	C	Corgard	30	No		Renal	$\beta_1 = \beta_2$	14–24	40 OD	80–240 OD
Propranolol (Inderal)	C	Inderal	>90	Yes		Hepatic	$\beta_1 = \beta_2$	3–6	10–20 bid/tid	80–140 tid
Pindolol (Visken)	B	Visken	40	Yes	Minimal	Hepatic	$\beta_1 > \beta_2$	3–4	5 tid/qid	60 bid/tid

ISA, intrinsic sympathomimetic activity; OD, once daily; bid, twice a day; tid, three times a day; qid, four times a day.

the brain; those agents that are least lipophilic are less likely to enter the brain. When CNS effects are desired, a lipophilic drug may be preferred; when only peripheral effects are desired, a less lipophilic drug may be indicated.

Whereas propranolol, nadolol, pindolol, and labetalol (Normodyne, Trandate) have essentially equal potency at both the β_1- and β_2-receptors, metoprolol and atenolol have greater affinity for the β_1-receptor than for the β_2-receptor. Relative β_1-selectivity confers few pulmonary and vascular effects of these drugs, although they must be used with caution in persons with asthma because the drugs retain some activity at the β_2-receptors.

Pindolol has sympathomimetic effects in addition to its β-antagonist effects, which has allowed its use for augmentation of antidepressant drugs. Pindolol, propranolol, and nadolol possess some antagonist activity at the serotonin 5-HT_{1A} receptors.

Therapeutic Indications

Anxiety Disorders. Propranolol is useful for the treatment of social phobia, primarily of the performance type (e.g., disabling anxiety before a musical performance). Data are also available for its use in treatment of panic disorder, posttraumatic stress disorder, and generalized anxiety disorder. In social phobia, the common treatment approach is to take 10 to 40 mg of propranolol 20 to 30 minutes before the anxiety-provoking situation. The β-receptor antagonists are less effective for the treatment of panic disorder than are benzodiazepines or SSRIs.

Lithium-Induced Postural Tremor. The β-receptor antagonists are beneficial for lithium-induced postural tremor and other medication-induced postural tremors—for example, those induced by tricycle antidepressants (TCAs) and valproate (Depakene). The initial approach to this movement disorder includes lowering the dose of lithium (Eskalith), eliminating aggravating factors, such as caffeine, and administering lithium at bedtime. If these interventions are inadequate, however, propranolol in the range of 20 to 160 mg a day given two or three times daily is generally effective for the treatment of lithium-induced postural tremor.

Neuroleptic-Induced Acute Akathisia. Many studies have shown that β-receptor antagonists can be effective in the treatment of neuroleptic-induced acute akathisia. They are generally more effective for this indication than are anticholinergics and benzodiazepines. The β-receptor antagonists are not effective in the treatment of such neuroleptic-induced movement disorders as acute dystonia and parkinsonism.

Aggression and Violent Behavior. The β-receptor antagonists may be effective in reducing the number of aggressive and violent outbursts in persons with impulse disorders, schizophrenia, and aggression associated with brain injuries such as trauma, tumors, anoxic injury, encephalitis, alcohol dependence, and degenerative disorders (e.g., Huntington's disease).

Alcohol Withdrawal. Propranolol is reported to be useful as an adjuvant to benzodiazepines but not as a sole agent in the treatment of alcohol withdrawal. The following dose schedule is suggested: no propranolol for a pulse rate below 50 beats per minute; 50-mg propranolol for a pulse rate between 50 and 79 beats per minute; and 100-mg propranolol for a pulse rate of 80 beats per minute or above.

Antidepressant Augmentation. Pindolol has been used to augment and hasten the antidepressant effects of SSRIs, tricyclic drugs, and ECT. Small studies have shown that pindolol administered at the onset of antidepressant therapy may shorten the usual 2- to 4-week latency of antidepressant response by several days. Because the β-receptor antagonists may possibly induce depression in some persons, augmentation strategies with these drugs need to be further clarified in controlled trials.

Other Disorders. A number of case reports and controlled studies have reported data indicating that β-receptor antagonists may be of modest benefit for persons with schizophrenia and manic symptoms. They have also been used in some cases of stuttering (Table 25–12).

Precautions and Adverse Reactions

The β-receptor antagonists are contraindicated for use in people with asthma, insulin-dependent diabetes, congestive heart failure, significant vascular disease, persistent angina, and hyperthyroidism. The contraindication in diabetic persons is because of the drugs' antagonizing the normal physiologic response to

Table 25–12
Psychiatric Uses for β-Adrenergic Receptor Antagonists

Definitely effective
Performance anxiety
Lithium-induced tremor
Neuroleptic-induced akathisia
Probably effective
Adjunctive therapy for alcohol withdrawal and other substance-related disorders
Adjunctive therapy for aggressive or violent behavior
Possibly effective
Antipsychotic augmentation
Antidepressant augmentation

Table 25–13
Adverse Effects and Toxicity of β-Adrenergic Receptor Antagonists

Cardiovascular
Hypotension
Bradycardia
Congestive heart failure (in patients with compromised myocardial function)
Respiratory
Asthma (less risk with β_1-selective drugs)
Metabolic
Worsened hypoglycemia in diabetic patients on insulin or oral agents
Gastrointestinal
Nausea
Diarrhea
Abdominal pain
Sexual function
Impotence
Neuropsychiatric
Lassitude
Fatigue
Dysphoria
Insomnia
Vivid nightmares
Depression (rare)
Psychosis (rare)
Other (rare)
Raynaud's phenomenon
Peyronie's disease
Withdrawal syndrome
Rebound worsening of preexisting angina pectoris when β-adrenergic receptor antagonists are discontinued

hypoglycemia. The β-receptor antagonists can worsen AV conduction defects and lead to complete AV heart block and death. If the clinician decides that the risk-to-benefit ratio warrants a trial of a β-receptor antagonist in a person with one of these coexisting medical conditions, a β_1-selective agent should be the first choice, and the patient should be monitored. All currently available β-receptor antagonists are excreted in breast milk and should be administered with caution to nursing women.

The most common adverse effects of β-receptor antagonists are hypotension and bradycardia. In persons at risk for these adverse effects, a test dosage of 20 mg a day of propranolol can be given to assess the reaction to the drug. Depression has been associated with lipophilic β-receptor antagonists, such as propranolol, but it is probably rare. Nausea, vomiting, diarrhea, and constipation can also be caused by treatment with these agents. The β-receptor antagonists may blunt cognition in some people. Serious CNS adverse effects (e.g., agitation, confusion, and hallucinations) are rare. Table 25–13 lists the possible adverse effects of β-receptor antagonists.

Drug Interactions

Concomitant administration of propranolol results in increases in plasma concentrations of antipsychotics, anticonvulsants, theophylline (Theo-Dur, Slo-bid), and levothyroxine (Synthroid). Other β-receptor antagonists may have similar effects. The β-receptor antagonists that are eliminated by the kidneys may have similar effects on drugs that are also eliminated by the renal route. Barbiturates, phenytoin (Dilantin), and cigarette smoking increase the elimination of β-receptor antagonists that are metabolized by the liver. Several reports have associated hypertensive crises and bradycardia with the coadministration of β-receptor antagonists and MAOIs. Depressed myocardial contractility and AV nodal conduction can occur from concomitant administration of a β-receptor antagonist and calcium channel inhibitors.

Laboratory Interferences

The β-receptor antagonists do not interfere with standard laboratory tests.

Dosage and Clinical Guidelines

Propranolol is available in 10-, 20-, 40-, 60-, 80-, and 90-mg tablets; 4-, 8-, and 80-mg/mL solutions; and 60-, 80-, 120-, and 160-mg sustained-release capsules. Nadolol is available in 20-, 40-, 80-, 120-, and 160-mg tablets. Pindolol is available in 5- and 10-mg tablets. Metoprolol is available in 50- and 100-mg tablets and 50-, 100-, and 200-mg sustained-release tablets. Atenolol is available in 25-, 50-, and 100-mg tablets. Acebutolol is available in 200- and 400-mg capsules.

For the treatment of chronic disorders, propranolol administration is usually initiated at 10 mg by mouth three times a day or 20 mg by mouth twice daily. The dosage can be raised by 20 to 30 mg a day until a therapeutic effect emerges. The dosage should be leveled off at the appropriate range for the disorder under treatment. The treatment of aggressive behavior sometimes requires dosages up to 80 mg a day, and therapeutic effects may not be seen until the person has been receiving the maximal dosage for 4 to 8 weeks. For the treatment of social phobia, primarily the performance type, the patient should take 10 to 40 mg of propranolol 20 to 30 minutes before the performance.

Pulse and BP readings should be taken regularly, and the drug should be withheld if the pulse rate is below 50 beats per minute or the systolic BP is below 90 mm Hg. The drug should be temporarily discontinued if it produces severe dizziness, ataxia, or wheezing. Treatment with β-receptor antagonists should never be discontinued abruptly. Propranolol should be tapered by 60 mg a day until a dosage of 60 mg a day is reached, after which the drug should be tapered by 10 to 20 mg a day every 3 or 4 days.

The clinical guidelines for the other drugs listed in this chapter are similar to propranolol, taking into consideration the different doses used. For example, if propranolol is prescribed initially at the lowest available dose (e.g., 10 mg) then metoprolol should be prescribed at its lowest available dose (e.g., 50 mg).

ANTICHOLINERGIC AGENTS

In the clinical practice of psychiatry, the anticholinergic drugs are primarily used to treat medication-induced movement disorders, particularly neuroleptic-induced Parkinsonism, neuroleptic-induced acute dystonia, and medication-induced postural tremor.

Anticholinergics

Pharmacological Actions. All anticholinergic drugs are well absorbed from the GI tract after oral administration, and all are sufficiently lipophilic to enter the CNS. Trihexyphenidyl (Artane) and benztropine (Cogentin) reach peak plasma concentrations in 2 to 3 hours after oral administration, and their duration of action is 1 to 12 hours. Benztropine is absorbed equally rapidly by IM and intravenous (IV) administration; IM administration is preferred because of its low risk for adverse effects.

All six anticholinergic drugs listed in this section (Table 25–14) block muscarinic acetylcholine receptors, and benztropine has some antihistaminergic effects. None of the available anticholinergic drugs has any effect on the nicotinic acetylcholine receptors. Of these drugs, trihexyphenidyl is the most stimulating agent, perhaps acting through dopaminergic neurons, and benztropine is the least stimulating and thus is least associated with abuse potential.

Therapeutic Indications. The primary indication for the use of anticholinergics in psychiatric practice is for the treatment of *neuroleptic-induced parkinsonism,* characterized by tremor, rigidity, cogwheeling, bradykinesia, sialorrhea, stooped posture, and festination. All of the available anticholinergics are equally effective in the treatment of parkinsonian symptoms. Neuroleptic-induced parkinsonism is most common in elderly persons and is most frequently seen with high-potency DRAs, for example, haloperidol (Haldol). The onset of symptoms usually occurs after 2 or 3 weeks of treatment. The incidence of neuroleptic-induced parkinsonism is lower with the newer antipsychotic drugs of the SDA class.

Another indication for the use of anticholinergics is for the treatment of *neuroleptic-induced acute dystonia,* which is most common in young men. The syndrome often occurs early in the course of treatment; is commonly associated with high-potency DRAs (e.g., haloperidol); and most commonly affects the muscles of the neck, tongue, face, and back. Anticholinergic drugs are effective both in the short-term treatment of dystonias and in prophylaxis against neuroleptic-induced acute dystonias.

Akathisia is characterized by a subjective and objective sense of restlessness, anxiety, and agitation. Although a trial of anticholinergics for the treatment of neuroleptic-induced acute akathisia is reasonable, these drugs are not generally considered as effective as the β-adrenergic receptor antagonists, the benzodiazepines, and clonidine (Catapres).

Application in Depressive Disorders. During the last few years, the role of anticholinergic medications has expanded to include treatment of depressive disorders. Numerous studies since then have shown depressive symptoms associated with increased cholinergic activity while the inverse is true for improvement in major depression. Among the anticholinergic medications, scopolamine in particular has been shown to improve symptoms of moderate to severe depression. Numerous studies suggest that scopolamine as monotherapy as well as when used as an adjunct is a safe and effective strategy in major depressive disorders (MDDs) and seems to be an appropriate treatment option for difficult to treat patients with major and bipolar depression.

Precautions and Adverse Reactions. The adverse effects of the anticholinergic drugs result from blockade of muscarinic acetylcholine receptors. Anticholinergic drugs should be used cautiously, if at all, by persons with prostatic hypertrophy, urinary retention, and narrow-angle glaucoma. The anticholinergics are occasionally used as drugs of abuse because of their mild mood-elevating properties, most notably, trihexyphenidyl. They may also impact cognition particularly in older patients.

The most serious adverse effect associated with anticholinergic toxicity is anticholinergic intoxication, which can be characterized by delirium, coma, seizures, agitation, hallucinations, severe hypotension, supraventricular tachycardia, and peripheral manifestations (flushing, mydriasis, dry skin, hyperthermia, and decreased bowel sounds). Treatment should begin with the immediate discontinuation of all anticholinergic drugs. The syndrome of anticholinergic intoxication can be diagnosed and treated with physostigmine (Antilirium, Eserine), an inhibitor of anticholinesterase, 1 to 2 mg IV (1 mg every 2 minutes) or

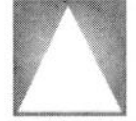

Table 25–14
Anticholinergic Drugs

Generic Name	Brand Name	Tablet Size	Injectable	Usual Daily Oral Dosage	Short-Term Intramuscular or Intravenous Dosage
Benztropine	Cogentin	0.5, 1, 2 mg	1 mg/mL	1–4 mg one to three times	1–2 mg
Biperiden	Akineton	2 mg	5 mg/mL	2 mg one to three times	2 mg
Ethopropazine	Parsidol	10, 50 mg	—	50–100 mg one to three times	—
Orphenadrine	Norflex, Disipal	100 mg	30 mg/mL	50–100 mg three times	60 mg IV given over 5 min
Procyclidine	Kemadrin	5 mg	—	2.5–5 mg three times	—
Trihexyphenidyl	Artane, Trihexane, Trihexy-5	2, 5 mg elixir 2 mg/5 mL	—	2–5 mg two to four times	—

IV, intravenous.

IM every 30 or 60 minutes. Because physostigmine can lead to severe hypotension and bronchial constriction, it should be used only in severe cases and only when emergency cardiac monitoring and life-support services are available.

Drug Interactions. The most common drug–drug interactions with the anticholinergics occur when they are coadministered with psychotropics that also have high anticholinergic activity, such as DRAs, tricyclic and tetracyclic drugs, and MAOIs. Many other prescription drugs and over-the-counter cold preparations also induce significant anticholinergic activity. The coadministration of those drugs can result in a life-threatening anticholinergic intoxication syndrome. In addition, anticholinergic drugs can delay gastric emptying, thereby decreasing the absorption of drugs that are broken down in the stomach and usually absorbed in the duodenum (e.g., levodopa [Larodopa] and DRAs).

Laboratory Interferences. No known laboratory interferences have been associated with anticholinergics.

Dosage and Clinical Guidelines. The six anticholinergic drugs discussed in this chapter are available in a range of preparations (see Table 25–14).

NEUROLEPTIC-INDUCED PARKINSONISM. For the treatment of neuroleptic-induced parkinsonism, the equivalent of 1 to 3 mg of benztropine should be given one to two times daily. The anticholinergic drug should be administered for 4 to 8 weeks, and then it should be discontinued to assess whether the person still requires the drug. Anticholinergic drugs should be tapered over a period of 1 to 2 weeks.

Treatment with anticholinergics as prophylaxis against the development of neuroleptic-induced parkinsonism is usually not indicated, because the onset of its symptoms is usually sufficiently mild and gradual to allow the clinician to initiate treatment only after it is clearly indicated. In young men, prophylaxis may be indicated, however, especially if a high-potency DRA is being used. The clinician should attempt to discontinue the antiparkinsonian agent in 4 to 6 weeks to assess whether its continued use is necessary.

NEUROLEPTIC-INDUCED ACUTE DYSTONIA. For the short-term treatment and prophylaxis of neuroleptic-induced acute dystonia, 1 to 2 mg of benztropine or its equivalent in another drug should be given IM. The dose can be repeated in 20 to 30 minutes, as needed. If the person still does not improve in another 20 to 30 minutes, a benzodiazepine (e.g., 1 mg IM or IV lorazepam [Ativan]) should be given. Laryngeal dystonia is a medical emergency and should be treated with benztropine, up to 4 mg in a 10-minute period, followed by 1 to 2 mg of lorazepam, administered slowly by the IV route.

Prophylaxis against dystonias is indicated in persons who have had one episode or in persons at high risk (young men taking high-potency DRAs). Prophylactic treatment is given for 4 to 8 weeks and then gradually tapered over 1 to 2 weeks to allow assessment of its continued need. The prophylactic use of anticholinergics in persons requiring antipsychotic drugs has largely become a moot issue because of the availability of SDAs, which are relatively free of parkinsonian effects.

AKATHISIA. As mentioned, anticholinergics are not the drugs of choice for this syndrome. The β-adrenergic receptor antagonists and perhaps the benzodiazepines and clonidine are preferable drugs to try initially.

ANTICONVULSANTS

The newer anticonvulsants described in this section were developed for the treatment of epilepsy, but were also found to have beneficial effects in psychiatric disorders. In addition, these agents are used as skeletal muscle relaxants and in neurogenic pain. These drugs have a variety of mechanisms including increasing GABAergic function or decreasing glutamatergic function. This chapter includes six of the newer anticonvulsants: gabapentin (Neurontin), levetiracetam (Keppra), pregabalin (Lyrica), tiagabine (Gabitril), topiramate (Topamax), and zonisamide (Zonegran), as well as one of the first used anticonvulsants, phenytoin (Dilantin). Carbamazepine (Tegretol), valproate (Depakene, Depakote), lamotrigine (Lamictal), and oxcarbazepine (Trileptal) are discussed in separate sections.

In 2008, the FDA issued a warning that these drugs may increase the risk of suicidal ideation or act in some persons compared with placebo; however, the relative risk for suicidality was higher in patients with epilepsy compared with those with psychiatric disorders. However, some published data contradict the warning by the FDA regarding the use of anticonvulsants and the risk of suicidal thoughts. These studies suggest that anticonvulsants may have a protective effect on suicidal thoughts in bipolar disorder. Considering the inherent increased risk of suicide in persons with bipolar disorder, clinicians should be aware of these warnings.

Gabapentin

Gabapentin was first introduced as an antiepileptic drug and was found to have sedative effects that were useful in some psychiatric disorders, especially insomnia. It was also found to be beneficial in reducing neuropathic pain, including postherpetic neuralgia. It is used in anxiety disorders (social phobia and panic disorder), but not as a main intervention in mania or treatment-resistant mood disorders.

Pharmacological Actions. Gabapentin circulates in the blood largely unbound and is not appreciably metabolized in humans. It is eliminated unchanged by renal excretion and can be removed by hemodialysis. Food only moderately affects the rate and extent of absorption. Clearance is decreased in elderly persons, requiring dosage adjustments. Gabapentin appears to increase cerebral GABA and may inhibit glutamate synthesis as well. It increases human whole blood serotonin concentrations and modulates calcium channels to reduce monoamine release. It has antiseizure as well as antispastic activity and antinociceptive effects in pain.

Therapeutic Indications. In neurology, gabapentin is used for the treatment of both general and partial seizures. It is effective in reducing the pain of postherpetic neuralgia and other pain syndromes associated with diabetic neuropathy, neuropathic cancer pain, fibromyalgia, meralgia paresthetica, amputation, and headache. It has been found to be effective in some cases of chronic pruritus.

In psychiatry, gabapentin is used as a hypnotic agent because of its sedating effects. It has anxiolytic properties and benefits patients with social anxiety and panic disorder. It may decrease the craving for alcohol in some patients and improve mood as well; hence, it may have some use in depressed patients. Some bipolar patients have benefited when gabapentin is used adjunctively with mood stabilizers.

Precautions and Adverse Reactions. Adverse effects are mild, with the most common being daytime somnolence, ataxia, and fatigue, which are usually dose related. Overdose (over 45 g) has been associated with diplopia, slurred screech, lethargy, and diarrhea, but all patients recovered. The drug is classified as pregnancy Category C and is excreted in breast milk, so it is best to avoid in pregnant women and nursing mothers.

Drug Interactions. Gabapentin bioavailability may decrease as much as 20 percent when administered with antacids. In general, there are no drug interactions. Chronic use does not interfere with lithium administration.

Laboratory Interferences. Gabapentin does not interfere with any laboratory tests, although spontaneous reports of false-positive or positive drug toxicology screenings for amphetamines, barbiturates, benzodiazepines, and marijuana have been reported.

Dosages and Clinical Guidelines. Gabapentin is well tolerated, and the dosage can be increased to the maintenance range within a few days. A general approach is to start with 300 mg on day 1, increase to 600 mg on day 2, 900 mg on day 3, and subsequently increase up to 1,800 mg per day in divided doses as needed to relieve symptoms. Final total daily doses tend to be between 1,200 and 2,400 mg per day but occasionally results may be achieved with dosages as low as 200 to 300 mg per day, especially in elderly persons. Sedation is usually the limiting factor in determining the dosage. Some patients have taken dosages as high as 4,800 mg per day.

Gabapentin is available as 100-, 300-, and 400-mg capsules and as 600- and 800-mg tablets. A 250-mg/5-mL oral solution is also available. Although abrupt discontinuation of gabapentin does not cause withdrawal effects, use of all anticonvulsant drugs should be gradually tapered.

Topiramate

Topiramate (Topamax) was developed as an anticonvulsant and was found useful in a variety of psychiatric and neurologic conditions, including migraine prevention, treatment of obesity, bulimia, binge eating, and alcohol dependence.

Pharmacological Actions. Topiramate has GABAergic effects and increases cerebral GABA in humans. It has 80 percent oral bioavailability and is not significantly altered by food. It is 15 percent protein bound, and about 70 percent of the drug is eliminated by renal excretion. With renal insufficiency topiramate clearance decreases about 50 percent, so the dosage needs to be decreased. It has a half-life of around 24 hours.

Therapeutic Indications. Topiramate is used mainly as an antiepileptic medication and has been found superior to placebo as monotherapy in patients with seizure disorders. It is also used in the prevention of migraine, smoking cessation, pain syndromes (e.g., low back pain), PTSD, and essential tremor. The drug has been associated with weight loss, and that fact has been used to counteract the weight gain caused by many psychotropic drugs. It has also been used in general obesity and in the treatment of bulimia and binge-eating disorder. Self-mutilating behavior may be decreased in borderline personality disorder. It is of little or no benefit in the treatment of psychotic disorders. In one study, the combination of topiramate with bupropion (Wellbutrin) showed some efficacy in bipolar depression, but double-blind, placebo-controlled trials failed to demonstrate topiramate monotherapy efficacy in acute mania in adults.

Precautions and Adverse Reactions. The most common adverse effects of topiramate include paresthesias, weight loss, somnolence, anorexia, dizziness, and memory problems. Sometimes disturbances in the sense of taste occur. In many cases, the adverse effects are mild to moderate and can be attenuated by decreasing the dose. No deaths have been reported during overdose. The drug affects acid–base balance (low serum bicarbonate), which can be associated with cardiac arrhythmias, and the formation of renal calculi in about 1.5 percent of cases. Patients taking the drug should be encouraged to drink plenty of fluids. It is not known if the drug passes through the placenta or is present in breast milk, and it should be avoided by pregnant women or nursing mothers.

Drug Interactions. Topiramate has few drug interactions with other anticonvulsant drugs. Topiramate may increase phenytoin concentrations up to 25 percent and valproic acid 11 percent; it does not affect the concentration of carbamazepine, phenobarbital (Luminal), or primidone. Topiramate concentrations are decreased by 40 to 48 percent, with concomitant administration of carbamazepine or phenytoin. Topiramate should not be combined with carbonic anhydrase inhibitors, such as acetazolamide (Diamox) or dichlorphenamide (Daranide), because this could increase the risk of nephrolithiasis or heat-related problems (oligohidrosis and hyperthermia).

Laboratory Interferences. Topiramate does not interfere with any laboratory tests.

Dosages and Clinical Guidelines. Topiramate is available as unscored 25-, 100-, and 200-mg tablets. To reduce the risk of adverse cognitive and sedative effects, topiramate dosage is titrated gradually over 8 weeks to a maximum of 200 mg twice a day. Off-label topiramate is typically used adjunctively, starting with 25 mg at bedtime and increasing weekly by 25 mg as necessary and tolerated. Final doses in efforts to promote weight loss are often between 75 and 150 mg per day at bedtime. Doses higher than 400 mg are not associated with increased efficacy. All of the dose can be given at bedtime to take advantage of the sedative effects. Persons with renal insufficiency should reduce doses by half.

Tiagabine

Tiagabine was introduced as a treatment for epilepsy in 1997 and was found to have efficacy in some psychiatric conditions, including acute mania. However, safety concerns (see later) along with a lack of controlled data have limited the use of tiagabine in disorders other than epilepsy.

Pharmacological Actions. Tiagabine is well absorbed with a bioavailability of about 90 percent and is extensively (96 percent) bound to plasma proteins. Tiagabine is a cytochrome P450 (CYP)3A substrate and is extensively transformed into inactive 5-oxo-tiagabine and glucuronide metabolites, with only 2 percent being excreted unchanged in the urine. The remainder is excreted as metabolites in the feces (65 percent) and the urine (25 percent). Tiagabine blocks uptake of the inhibitory amino acid neurotransmitter GABA into neurons and glia, enhancing the inhibitory action of GABA at both $GABA_A$ and $GABA_B$ receptors, putatively yielding anticonvulsant and antinociceptive effects, respectively. It has mild blocking effects on histamine 1 (H_1), serotonin type 1B ($5\text{-}HT_{1B}$), benzodiazepine, and chloride channel receptors.

Therapeutic Indications. Tiagabine is rarely used for psychiatric disorders, and then it is used only for generalized anxiety disorder and insomnia. Its main indication is in generalized epilepsy.

Precautions and Adverse Reactions. Tiagabine may cause withdrawal seizures, cognitive or neuropsychiatric problems (impaired concentration, speech or language problems, somnolence, and fatigue), status epilepticus, and sudden unexpected death in epilepsy (SUDEP). Acute oral overdoses of tiagabine have been associated with seizures, status epilepticus, coma, ataxia, confusion, somnolence, drowsiness, impaired speech, agitation, lethargy, myoclonus, stupor, tremors, disorientation, vomiting, hostility, temporary paralysis, and respiratory depression. Deaths have been reported in polydrug overdoses involving tiagabine. Cases of serious rash may occur, including Stevens–Johnson syndrome.

Tiagabine is classified as pregnancy Category C because fetal loss and teratogenicity have been demonstrated in animals. It is not known if the drug is excreted in breast milk. Pregnant women and nursing mothers should not be given the drug.

Laboratory Tests. Tiagabine does not interfere with any laboratory tests.

Dosage and Administration. Tiagabine should not be rapidly loaded or rapidly initiated because of the risk of serious adverse effects. In adults and adolescents 12 years of age or older with epilepsy who are also taking enzyme inducers, tiagabine should be initiated at 4 mg per day and increased weekly by 4 mg per day during the first month. The dose should then be increased weekly by 4 to 8 mg per day for weeks 5 and 6, yielding 24 to 32 mg per day administered in two to four divided doses by week 6. In adults (but not adolescents), tiagabine doses may be further increased weekly by 4 to 8 mg per day to as high as 56 mg per day. Plasma concentrations in patients with epilepsy commonly range between 20 and 100 ng/mL, but do not appear to be systematically related to antiseizure effects and thus are not routinely monitored.

Levetiracetam

Initially developed as a nootropic (memory enhancing) drug, levetiracetam proved to be a potent anticonvulsant and marketed as a treatment for partial seizures. It has been used to treat acute mania and anxiety and to augment antidepressant drug therapy.

Pharmacological Actions. The CNS effects are not well understood, but it appears to indirectly enhance GABA inhibition. It is rapidly and completely absorbed, and peak concentrations are reached in 1 hour. Food delays the rate of absorption and decreases the amount of absorption. Levetiracetam is not significantly plasma protein bound and is not metabolized through the hepatic CYP system. Its metabolism involves hydrolysis of the acetamide group. Serum concentrations are not correlated with therapeutic effects.

Therapeutic Indications. The major indication is for the treatment of convulsive disorders, including partial-onset seizures, myoclonic seizures, and idiopathic generalized epilepsy. In psychiatry, levetiracetam has been used off label to treat acute mania, as an add-on treatment for major depression, and as an anxiolytic agent.

Precautions and Adverse Reactions. The most common side effects of levetiracetam include drowsiness, dizziness, ataxia, diplopia, memory impairment, apathy, and paresthesias. Some patients develop behavioral disturbances during treatment, and hallucinations may occur. Suicidal patients may become agitated. It should not be used in pregnant or lactating women.

Drug Interactions. There are few if any interactions with other drugs, including other anticonvulsants. There is no interaction with lithium.

Laboratory Interferences. No laboratory interferences have been reported.

Dosages and Clinical Guidelines. The drug is available as 250-, 500-, 750-, and 1,000-mg tablets; 500-mg extended-release tablets; a 100-mg/mL oral solution; and a 100-mg/mL intravenous solution. In epilepsy, the typical adult daily dose is 1,000 mg.

In view of its renal clearance, dosages should be reduced in patients with impaired renal function.

Zonisamide

Used originally as an anticonvulsant for the treatment of seizure disorders, zonisamide was also found to be useful in bipolar disorder, obesity, and binge-eating disorder.

Pharmacological Actions. Zonisamide blocks sodium channels and may weakly potentiate dopamine and serotonin activity. It also inhibits carbonic anhydrase. Some evidence suggests that it may block calcium channels. Zonisamide is metabolized by the hepatic CYP3A system, so enzyme-inducing agents such as carbamazepine, alcohol, and phenobarbital increase the clearance and reduce the availability of the drug. Zonisamide does not affect the metabolism of other drugs. It has a long half-life of 60 hours, so it is easily dosed once daily, preferably at nighttime.

Therapeutic Indications. Its main use is in the treatment of generalized seizure disorders and in refractory partial seizures. In psychiatry, controlled studies found it to be of use in obesity and binge-eating disorder. Uncontrolled trials have found it useful in bipolar disorder, particularly mania; however, further studies are warranted for this indication.

Precautions and Adverse Reactions. Zonisamide is a sulfonamide and thus may cause fatal rash and blood dyscrasias, although these events are rare. About 4 percent of patients develop kidney stones. The most common side effects are drowsiness, cognitive impairment, insomnia, ataxia, nystagmus, paresthesia, speech abnormalities, constipation, diarrhea, nausea, and dry mouth. Weight loss is also a common side effect, which has been exploited as a therapy for patients who have gained weight during treatment with psychotropics or, as mentioned above, have ongoing difficulty controlling their eating. Zonisamide should not be used in pregnant women or breastfeeding mothers.

Drug Interactions. Zonisamide does not inhibit CYP isoenzymes and does not instigate drug interactions. It is important not to combine carbonic anhydrase inhibitors with zonisamide because of an increased risk of nephrolithiasis related to increased blood levels of urea.

Laboratory Interferences. Zonisamide can elevate hepatic alkaline phosphatase and increase blood urea nitrogen and creatinine.

Dosages and Clinical Guidelines. Zonisamide is available in 100- and 200-mg capsules. In epilepsy, the dosage range is 100 to 400 mg per day, with side effects becoming more pronounced at doses above 300 mg. Because of its long half-life, zonisamide can be given once a day.

Pregabalin

Pregabalin is pharmacologically similar to gabapentin. It is believed to work by inhibiting the release of excess excitatory neurotransmitters. It increases neuronal GABA levels, its binding affinity is six times greater than that of gabapentin, and it has a longer half-life.

Pharmacological Actions. Pregabalin exhibits linear pharmacokinetics. It is rapidly absorbed in proportion to its dose. The time to maximal plasma concentration is about 1 hour and that to steady state is within 24 to 48 hours. Pregabalin demonstrates high bioavailability, and it has a mean elimination half-life of about 6.5 hours. Food does not affect absorption. Pregabalin does not bind to plasma proteins and is excreted virtually unchanged (<2 percent metabolism) by the kidneys. It is not subject to hepatic metabolism and does not induce or inhibit liver enzymes such as the CYP system. Dose reduction may be necessary in patients with creatinine clearance (CLcr) less than 60 mL per minute. Daily doses should be further reduced by approximately 50 percent for each additional 50 percent decrease in CLcr. Pregabalin is highly cleared by hemodialysis, so additional doses may be needed for patients on chronic hemodialysis treatment after each hemodialysis treatment.

Therapeutic Indications. Pregabalin is approved for the management of diabetic peripheral neuropathy and postherpetic neuralgia, and for adjunctive treatment of partial-onset seizures. It has been found to be of benefit to some patients with generalized anxiety disorder. In studies, no consistent dose–response relationship was found, although 300 mg of pregabalin per day was more effective than 150 or 450 mg. Some patients with panic disorder or social anxiety disorder may benefit from pregabalin, but little evidence supports its routine use in treating persons with these disorders. It was most recently approved for the treatment of fibromyalgia.

Precautions and Adverse Reactions. The most common adverse events associated with pregabalin use are dizziness, somnolence, blurred vision, peripheral edema, amnesia or loss of memory, and tremors. Pregabalin potentiates sedating effects of alcohol, antihistamines, benzodiazepines, and other CNS depressants. It remains to be seen if pregabalin is associated with benzodiazepine-type withdrawal symptoms. There are scant data about its use in pregnant women or nursing mothers, and it is best avoided in these patients.

Drug Interactions. In view of the absence of hepatic metabolism, pregabalin lacks metabolic drug interactions.

Laboratory Interferences. There are no effects on laboratory tests.

Dosage and Clinical Guidelines. The recommended dose for postherpetic neuralgia is 50 or 100 mg orally three times a day. The recommended dose for diabetic peripheral neuropathy is 100 to 200 mg orally three times a day. Patients with fibromyalgia may require up to 450 to 600 mg per day given in divided doses. Pregabalin is available as 25-, 50-, 75-, 100-, 150-, 200-, 225-, and 300-mg capsules.

Phenytoin

Phenytoin sodium (Dilantin) is an antiepileptic drug and is related to the barbiturates in chemical structure. It is indicated for the control of generalized tonic–clonic (grand mal) and complex partial (psychomotor, temporal lobe) seizures and prevention and treatment of seizures occurring during or after neurosurgery. Studies have shown comparable efficacy of phenytoin to other anticonvulsants in bipolar disorder, but clinicians should take into account the danger of gingival hyperplasia, leukopenia, or anemia and the danger of toxicity caused by nonlinear pharmacokinetics.

Pharmacological Action. Similar to other anticonvulsants, phenytoin causes blockade of voltage-activated sodium channels and hence is efficacious as an antimanic agent. The plasma half-life after oral administration averages 22 hours, with a range of 7 to 42 hours. Steady-state therapeutic levels are achieved at least 7 to 10 days (5 to 7 half-lives) after initiation of therapy, with recommended doses of 300 mg per day. Serum level should be obtained at least 5 to 7 half-lives after treatment initiation. Phenytoin is excreted in the bile, which is then reabsorbed from the intestinal tract and excreted in the urine. Urinary excretion of phenytoin occurs partly with glomerular filtration and by tubular secretion. Small incremental doses of phenytoin may increase the half-life and produce very substantial increases in serum levels. Patients should adhere strictly to the prescribed dosage, and serial monitoring of phenytoin levels is recommended.

Therapeutic Indications. Apart from its indication in generalized tonic–clonic (grand mal) and complex partial (psychomotor, temporal lobe) seizures, phenytoin is also used for the treatment of acute mania in bipolar disorder.

Precautions and Adverse Reactions. The most common adverse reactions reported with phenytoin therapy are usually dose related and include nystagmus, ataxia, slurred speech, decreased coordination, and mental confusion. Other side effects include dizziness, insomnia, transient nervousness, motor twitching, and headaches. There have been rare reports of phenytoin-induced dyskinesias, similar to those induced by phenothiazine and other neuroleptic drugs. More serious side effects include thrombocytopenia, leukopenia, agranulocytosis, and pancytopenia, with or without bone marrow suppression.

A number of reports have suggested the development of lymphadenopathy (local or generalized), including benign lymph node hyperplasia, pseudolymphoma, lymphoma, and Hodgkin's disease. Prenatal exposure to phenytoin may increase the risks for congenital malformations, and a potentially life-threatening bleeding disorder related to decreased levels of vitamin K–dependent clotting factors may occur in newborns exposed to phenytoin in utero. Hyperglycemia has been reported with phenytoin use; in addition, the agent may increase the serum glucose level in patients with diabetes.

Drug Interactions. Acute alcohol intake, amiodarone, chlordiazepoxide, cimetidine, diazepam, disulfiram, estrogens, fluoxetine, H_2-antagonists, isoniazid, methylphenidate, phenothiazines, salicylates, and trazodone may increase phenytoin serum levels. Drugs that may lower phenytoin levels include carbamazepine, chronic alcohol abuse, and reserpine.

Laboratory Interferences. Phenytoin may decrease serum concentrations of thyroxine. It may cause increased serum levels of glucose, alkaline phosphatase, and γ-glutamyl transpeptidase.

Dosage and Clinical Guidelines. Patients may be started on one 100-mg extended oral capsule three times daily, and the dosage then adjusted to suit individual requirements. Patients may then be switched to once-a-day dosing, which is more convenient. In this case, extended-release capsules may be used. Serial monitoring of phenytoin levels is recommended, and the normal range is usually 10 to 20 μg/mL.

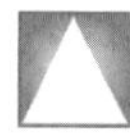

Table 25–15
Histamine Antagonists Commonly Used in Psychiatry

Generic Name	Trade Name	Duration of Action (hrs)
Diphenhydramine	Benadryl	4–6
Hydroxyzine	Atarax, Vistaril	6–24
Promethazine	Phenergan	4–6
Cyproheptadine	Periactin	4–6

ANTIHISTAMINES

Antihistamines are frequently used in the treatment of a variety of psychiatric disorders because of their sedative and anticholinergic activities. Certain antihistamines (antagonists of histamine H_1 receptors) are used to treat neuroleptic-induced parkinsonism and neuroleptic-induced acute dystonia and as hypnotics and anxiolytics. Diphenhydramine (Benadryl) is used to treat neuroleptic-induced parkinsonism and neuroleptic-induced acute dystonia and sometimes as a hypnotic. Hydroxyzine hydrochloride (Atarax) and hydroxyzine pamoate (Vistaril) are used as anxiolytics. Promethazine (Phenergan) is used for its sedative and anxiolytic effects. Cyproheptadine (Periactin) has been used for the treatment of anorexia nervosa and inhibited male and female orgasms caused by serotonergic agents. The antihistamines most commonly used in psychiatry are listed in Table 25–15. Second-generation, "nonsedating" H_1 blockers, such as fexofenadine (Allegra), loratadine (Claritin), and cetirizine (Zyrtec) are less commonly used in psychiatric practice. The newer H_2-receptor antagonists, such as cimetidine, work primarily on gastric mucosa, inhibiting gastric secretion.

Table 25–16 lists antihistaminic drugs not used in psychiatry but that may have psychiatric adverse effects or drug–drug interactions.

Pharmacological Actions

The H_1 antagonists used in psychiatry are well absorbed from the GI tract. The antiparkinsonian effects of IM diphenhydramine have their onset in 15 to 30 minutes, and the sedative effects of diphenhydramine peak in 1 to 3 hours. The sedative effects of hydroxyzine and promethazine begin after 20 to 60 minutes and last for 4 to 6 hours. Because all three drugs are metabolized in the liver, persons with hepatic disease, such as cirrhosis, may

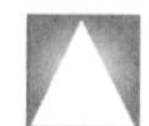

Table 25–16
Other Histamine Antagonists Often Prescribed

Class	Generic Name	Trade Name
Second-generation histamine 1 receptor antagonists	Cetirizine	Zyrtec
	Loratadine	Claritin
	Fexofenadine	Allegra
Histamine 2 receptor antagonists	Nizatidine	Axid
	Famotidine	Pepcid
	Ranitidine	Zantac
	Cimetidine	Tagamet

attain high plasma concentrations with long-term administration. Cyproheptadine is well absorbed after oral administration, and its metabolites are excreted in the urine.

Activation of H_1 receptors stimulates wakefulness; therefore, receptor antagonism causes sedation. All four agents also possess some antimuscarinic cholinergic activity. Cyproheptadine is unique among the drugs because it has both potent antihistamine and serotonin 5-HT_2-receptor antagonist properties.

Therapeutic Indications

Antihistamines are useful as a treatment for neuroleptic-induced parkinsonism, neuroleptic-induced acute dystonia, and neuroleptic-induced akathisia. They are an alternative to anticholinergics and amantadine for these purposes. The antihistamines are relatively safe hypnotics, but they are not superior to the benzodiazepines, which have been much better studied in terms of efficacy and safety. The antihistamines have not been proven effective for long-term anxiolytic therapy; therefore, the benzodiazepines, buspirone (BuSpar), or SSRIs are preferable for such treatment. Cyproheptadine is sometimes used to treat impaired orgasms, especially delayed orgasm resulting from treatment with serotonergic drugs.

Because it promotes weight gain, cyproheptadine may be of some use in the treatment of eating disorders, such as anorexia nervosa. Cyproheptadine can reduce recurrent nightmares with posttraumatic themes. The antiserotonergic activity of cyproheptadine may counteract the serotonin syndrome caused by concomitant use of multiple serotonin-activating drugs, such as SSRIs and MAOIs.

Precautions and Adverse Reactions

Antihistamines are commonly associated with sedation, dizziness, and hypotension, all of which can be severe in elderly persons, who are also likely to experience the anticholinergic effects of those drugs. Paradoxical excitement and agitation is an adverse effect seen in a small number of persons. Poor motor coordination can result in accidents; therefore, persons should be warned about driving and operating dangerous machinery. Other common adverse effects include epigastric distress, nausea, vomiting, diarrhea, and constipation. Because of mild anticholinergic activity, some people experience dry mouth, urinary retention, blurred vision, and constipation. For this reason also, antihistamines should be used only at very low doses, if at all, by persons with narrow-angle glaucoma or obstructive GI, prostate, or bladder conditions. A central anticholinergic syndrome with psychosis may be induced by either cyproheptadine or diphenhydramine. The use of cyproheptadine in some persons has been associated with weight gain, which may contribute to its reported efficacy in some persons with anorexia nervosa.

In addition to the above adverse effects, antihistamines have some potential for abuse. The coadministration of antihistamines and opioids can increase the euphoria experienced by persons with substance dependence. Overdoses of antihistamines can be fatal. Antihistamines are excreted in breast milk, so their use should be avoided by nursing mothers. Because of some potential for teratogenicity, pregnant women should avoid the use of antihistamines.

Drug Interactions

The sedative property of antihistamines can be additive with other CNS depressants, such as alcohol, other sedative–hypnotic drugs, and many psychotropic drugs, including tricyclic drugs and DRAs. Anticholinergic activity can also be additive with that of other anticholinergic drugs and may sometimes result in severe anticholinergic symptoms or intoxication.

Laboratory Interferences

H_1 antagonists may eliminate the wheal and induration that form the basis of allergy skin tests. Promethazine may interfere with pregnancy tests and may increase blood glucose concentrations. Diphenhydramine may yield a false-positive urine test result for phencyclidine (PCP). Hydroxyzine use can falsely elevate the results of certain tests for urinary 17-hydroxycorticosteroids.

Dosage and Clinical Guidelines

The antihistamines are available in a variety of preparations (Table 25–17). IM injections should be deep, because superficial administration can cause local irritation.

Intravenous (IV) administration of 25 to 50 mg of diphenhydramine is an effective treatment for neuroleptic-induced acute dystonia, which may immediately disappear. Treatment with 25 mg three times a day—up to 50 mg four times a day, if necessary—can be used to treat neuroleptic-induced parkinsonism, akinesia, and buccal movements. Diphenhydramine can be used as a hypnotic at a 50-mg dose for mild transient insomnia. Doses of 100 mg have not been shown to be superior to doses of 50 mg, but they produce more anticholinergic effects than doses of 50 mg.

Hydroxyzine is most commonly used as a short-term anxiolytic. Hydroxyzine should not be given IV because it is irritating to the blood vessels. Dosages of 50 to 100 mg given orally four times a day for long-term treatment or 50 to 100 mg IM every 4 to 6 hours for short-term treatment are usually effective.

SSRI-induced anorgasmia may sometimes be reversed with 4 to 16 mg a day of cyproheptadine taken by mouth 1 or 2 hours before anticipated sexual activity. A number of case reports and small studies have also reported that cyproheptadine may be of some use in the treatment of eating disorders, such as anorexia nervosa. Cyproheptadine is available in 4-mg tablets and a 2-mg/5-mL solution. Children and elderly patients are more sensitive to the effects of antihistamines than are young adults.

BARBITURATES AND SIMILARLY ACTING DRUGS

The first barbiturate to be used in medicine was barbital (Veronal), which was introduced in 1903. It was followed by phenobarbital (Luminal), amobarbital (Amytal), pentobarbital (Nembutal), secobarbital (Seconal), and thiopental (Pentothal). Many others have been synthesized, but only a handful has been used clinically (Table 25–18). Many problems are associated with these drugs, including high abuse and addiction potential, a narrow therapeutic range with low therapeutic index, and

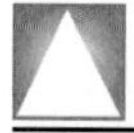

Table 25–17
Dosage and Administration of Common Histamine Antagonists

Medication	Route	Preparation	Common Dosage
Diphenhydramine (Benadryl)	PO	Capsules and tablets: 25 mg, 50 mg	Adults: 25–50 mg three to four times per day
		Liquid: 12.5 mg/5.0 mL	Children: 5 mg/kg three to four times per day, not to exceed 300 mg/day
	Deep IM or IV	Solution: 10 or 50 mg/mL	Same as oral
Hydroxyzine Hydrochloride (Atarax)	PO	Tablets: 10, 25, 50, and 100 mg	Adults: 50–100 mg three to four times daily
		Syrup: 10 mg/5 mL	Children younger than 6 yrs of age: 2 mg/kg/day in divided doses Children older than 6 yrs of age: 12.5–25.0 mg three to four times daily
	IM	Solution: 25 or 50 mg/mL	Same as oral
Pamoate (Vistaril)	PO	Suspension: 25 mg/mL Capsules: 25, 50, and 100 mg	Same as dosages for hydrochloride
Promethazine (Phenergan)	PO	Tablets: 15.2, 25.0, and 50.0 mg	Adults: 50–100 mg three to four times daily for sedation
		Syrup: 3.25 mg/5 mL	Children: 12.5–25.0 mg at night for sedation
	Rectal	Suppositories: 12.5, 25.0, and 50.0 mg	
	IM	Solution: 25 and 50 mg/mL	
Cyproheptadine (Periactin)	PO	Tablets: 4 mg Syrup: 2 mg/5 mL	Adults: 4–20 mg/day Children 2–7 yrs of age: 2 mg two to three times daily (maximum, 12 mg/day) Children 7–14 yrs of age: 4 mg two to three times daily (maximum of 16 mg/day)

IM, intramuscular; IV, intravenous; PO, oral.

unfavorable side effects. The use of barbiturates and similar compounds such as meprobamate (Miltown) has practically been eliminated by the benzodiazepines and hypnotics, such as zolpidem (Ambien), eszopiclone (Lunesta), and zaleplon (Sonata), which have a lower abuse potential and a higher therapeutic index than the barbiturates. Nevertheless, the barbiturates still have an important role in the treatment of certain mental and convulsive disorders.

Pharmacological Actions

The barbiturates are well absorbed after oral administration. The binding of barbiturates to plasma proteins is high, but lipid solubility varies. The individual barbiturates are metabolized by the liver and excreted by the kidneys. The half-lives of specific barbiturates range from 1 to 120 hours. The barbiturates may also induce hepatic enzymes (cytochrome P450, CYP), thereby reducing the levels of

Table 25–18
Barbiturate Dosages (Adult)

Drug	Trade Name	Available Preparations	Hypnotic Dose Range	Anticonvulsant Dose Range
Amobarbital	Amytal	200 mg	50–300 mg	65–500 mg IV
Aprobarbital	Alurate	40-mg/5-mL elixir	40–120 mg	Not established
Butabarbital	Butisol	15-, 30-, and 50-mg tablets 30-mg/5-mL elixir	45–120 mg	Not established
Mephobarbital	Mebaral	32-, 50-, and 100-mg tablets	100–200 mg	200–600 mg
Methohexital	Brevital	500 mg/50 mL	1 mg/kg for electroconvulsive therapy	Not established
Pentobarbital	Nembutal	50- and 100-mg capsules 50-mg/mL injection or elixir 30-, 60-, 120-, and 200-mg suppository	100–200 mg	100 mg IV, each minute up to 500 mg
Phenobarbital	Luminal	Tablets range from 15 to 100 mg 20-mg/5-mL elixir 30–130 mg/mL injection	30–150 mg	100–300 mg IV, up to 600 mg/day
Secobarbital	Seconal	100-mg capsule, 50-mg/mL injection	100 mg	5.5 mg/kg IV

IV, intravenous.

both the barbiturate and any other concurrently administered drugs metabolized by the liver. The mechanism of action of barbiturates involves the GABA receptor–benzodiazepine receptor–chloride ion channel complex.

Therapeutic Indications

Electroconvulsive Therapy. Methohexital (Brevital) is commonly used as an anesthetic agent for ECT. It has lower cardiac risks than other barbiturate anesthetics. Used intravenously (IV), methohexital produces rapid unconsciousness, and because of its rapid redistribution, it has a brief duration of action (5 to 7 minutes). Typical dosing for ECT is 0.7 to 1.2 mg/kg. Methohexital can also be used to abort prolonged seizures in ECT or to limit postictal agitation.

Seizures. Phenobarbital (Solfoton, Luminal), the most commonly used barbiturate for the treatment of seizures, has indications for the treatment of generalized tonic–clonic and simple partial seizures. Parenteral barbiturates are used in the emergency management of seizures independent of cause. Intravenous phenobarbital should be administered slowly at 10 to 20 mg/kg for status epilepticus.

Narcoanalysis. Amobarbital (Amytal) has been used historically as a diagnostic aid in a number of clinical conditions, including conversion reactions, catatonia, hysterical stupor, and unexplained muteness, and to differentiate stupor of depression, schizophrenia, and structural brain lesions.

The *Amytal interview* is performed by placing the patient in a reclining position and administering amobarbital IV at 50 mg a minute. Infusion is continued until lateral nystagmus is sustained or drowsiness is noted, usually at 75 to 150 mg. After this, 25 to 50 mg can be administered every 5 minutes to maintain narcosis. The patient should be allowed to rest for 15 to 30 minutes after the interview before attempting to walk.

Because of the risk of laryngospasm with IV amobarbital, diazepam has become the drug of choice for narcoanalysis.

Sleep. The barbiturates reduce sleep latency and the number of awakenings during sleep, although tolerance to these effects generally develops within 2 weeks. Discontinuation of barbiturates often leads to rebound increases on electroencephalographic (EEG) measures of sleep and a worsening of the insomnia.

Withdrawal from Sedative Hypnotics

Barbiturates are sometimes used to determine the extent of tolerance to barbiturates or other hypnotics to guide detoxification. After intoxication has resolved, a test dose of pentobarbital (200 mg) is given orally. One hour later, the patient is examined. Tolerance and dose requirements are determined by the degree to which the patient is affected. If the patient is not sedated, another 100 mg of pentobarbital can be administered every 2 hours, up to three times (maximum, 500 mg over 6 hours). The amount needed for mild intoxication corresponds to the approximate daily dose of barbiturate used. Phenobarbital (30 mg) may then be substituted for each 100 mg of pentobarbital. This daily dose requirement can be administered in divided doses and gradually tapered by 10 percent a day, with adjustments made according to withdrawal signs.

Precautions and Adverse Reactions

Some adverse effects of barbiturates are similar to those of benzodiazepines, including paradoxical dysphoria, hyperactivity, and cognitive disorganization. Rare adverse effects associated with barbiturate use include the development of Stevens–Johnson syndrome, megaloblastic anemia, and neutropenia.

Prior to the advent of benzodiazepines, the widespread use of barbiturates as hypnotics and anxiolytics made them the most common cause of acute porphyria reactions. Severe attacks of porphyria have decreased largely because barbiturates are now seldom used and are contraindicated in patients with the disease.

A major difference between the barbiturates and the benzodiazepines is the low therapeutic index of the barbiturates. An overdose of barbiturates can easily prove fatal. In addition to narrow therapeutic indexes, the barbiturates are associated with a significant risk of abuse potential and the development of tolerance and dependence. Barbiturate intoxication is manifested by confusion, drowsiness, irritability, hyporeflexia or areflexia, ataxia, and nystagmus. The symptoms of barbiturate withdrawal are similar to, but more marked than, those of benzodiazepine withdrawal.

Ten times the daily dose or 1 g of most barbiturates causes severe toxicity; 2 to 10 g generally proves fatal. Manifestations of barbiturate intoxication may include delirium, confusion, excitement, headache, and CNS and respiratory depression, ranging from somnolence to coma. Other adverse reactions include Cheyne–Stokes respiration, shock, miosis, oliguria, tachycardia, hypotension, hypothermia, irritability, hyporeflexia or areflexia, ataxia, and nystagmus. Treatment of overdose includes induction of emesis or lavage, activated charcoal, and saline cathartics; supportive treatment, including maintaining airway and respiration and treating shock as needed; maintaining vital signs and fluid balance; alkalinizing the urine, which increases excretion; forced diuresis if renal function is normal, or hemodialysis in severe cases.

Because of some evidence of teratogenicity, barbiturates should not be used by pregnant women or women who are breastfeeding. Barbiturates should be used with caution by patients with a history of substance abuse, depression, diabetes, hepatic impairment, renal disease, severe anemia, pain, hyperthyroidism, or hypoadrenalism. Barbiturates are also contraindicated in patients with acute intermittent porphyria, impaired respiratory drive, or limited respiratory reserve.

Drug Interactions

The primary area for concern about drug interactions is the potentially dangerous effects of respiratory depression. Barbiturates should be used with great caution with other prescribed CNS drugs (including antipsychotic and antidepressant drugs) and nonprescribed CNS agents (e.g., alcohol). In addition, caution must be exercised when prescribing barbiturates to patients who are taking other drugs that are metabolized in the liver, especially cardiac drugs and anticonvulsants. Because individual patients have a wide range of sensitivities to barbiturate-induced enzyme induction, it is not possible to predict the degree to which the metabolism of concurrently administered medications may be affected. Drugs that have their metabolism enhanced by barbiturate administration include opioids, antiarrhythmic agents, antibiotics, anticoagulants, anticonvulsants, antidepressants, β-adrenergic receptor antagonists, DRAs, contraceptives, and immunosuppressants.

Laboratory Interferences

No known laboratory interferences are associated with the administration of barbiturates.

Dose and Clinical Guidelines

Barbiturates and other drugs described later begin to act within 1 to 2 hours of administration. The doses of barbiturates vary, and treatment should begin with low doses that are increased to achieve a clinical effect. Children and older people are more sensitive to the effects of the barbiturates than are young adults. The most commonly used barbiturates are available in a variety of dose forms. Barbiturates with half-lives in the 15- to 40-hour range are preferable, because long-acting drugs tend to accumulate in the body. Clinicians should instruct patients clearly about the adverse effects and the potential for dependence associated with barbiturates.

Although determining plasma concentrations of barbiturates is rarely necessary in psychiatry, monitoring of phenobarbital concentrations is standard practice when the drug is used as an anticonvulsant. The therapeutic blood concentrations for phenobarbital in this indication range from 15 to 40 mg/L, although some patients may experience significant adverse effects in that range.

Barbiturates are contained in combination products with which the clinician should be familiar.

Other Similarly Acting Drugs

A number of agents that act similarly to the barbiturates have been used in the treatment of anxiety and insomnia. Three such available drugs are paraldehyde (Paral), meprobamate, and chloral hydrate (Noctec). These drugs are rarely used because of their abuse potential and potential toxic effects.

Paraldehyde. Paraldehyde is a cyclic ether and was first used in 1882 as a hypnotic. It has also been used to treat epilepsy, alcohol withdrawal symptoms, and delirium tremens. Because of its low therapeutic index, it has been supplanted by the benzodiazepines and other anticonvulsants.

PHARMACOLOGICAL ACTIONS. Paraldehyde is rapidly absorbed from the GI tract and from IM injections. It is primarily metabolized to acetaldehyde by the liver, and unmetabolized drug is expired by the lungs. Reported half-lives range from 3.4 to 9.8 hours. The onset of action is 15 to 30 minutes.

THERAPEUTIC INDICATIONS. Paraldehyde is not indicated as an anxiolytic or a hypnotic and has little place in current psychopharmacology.

PRECAUTIONS AND ADVERSE REACTIONS. Paraldehyde frequently causes foul breath because of expired unmetabolized drug. It can inflame pulmonary capillaries and cause coughing. It can also cause local thrombophlebitis with IV use. Patients may experience nausea and vomiting with oral use. Overdose leads to metabolic acidosis and decreased renal output. There is risk of abuse among drug addicts.

DRUG INTERACTIONS. Disulfiram (Antabuse) inhibits acetaldehyde dehydrogenase and reduces metabolism of paraldehyde, leading to possible toxic concentration of paraldehyde. Paraldehyde has addictive sedating effects in combination with other CNS depressants such as alcohol or benzodiazepines.

LABORATORY INTERFERENCES. Paraldehyde can interfere with the metyrapone, phentolamine, and urinary 17-hydroxycorticosteroid tests.

DOSING AND CLINICAL GUIDELINES. Paraldehyde is available in 30-mL vials for oral, IV, or rectal use. For seizures in adults, up to 12 mL (diluted to a 10 percent solution) can be administered by gastric tube every 4 hours. For children, the oral dose is 0.3 mg/kg.

Meprobamate. Meprobamate, a carbamate, was introduced shortly before the benzodiazepines, specifically to treat anxiety. It is also used for muscle relaxant effects.

PHARMACOLOGICAL ACTIONS. Meprobamate is rapidly absorbed from the GI tract and from IM injections. It is metabolized primarily by the liver, and a small portion is excreted unchanged in urine. The plasma half-life is approximately 10 hours.

THERAPEUTIC INDICATIONS. Meprobamate is indicated for short-term treatment of anxiety disorders. It has also been used as a hypnotic and is prescribed as a muscle relaxant.

PRECAUTIONS AND ADVERSE REACTIONS. Meprobamate can cause CNS depression and death in overdose and carries the risk of abuse by patients with drug or alcohol dependence. Abrupt cessation after long-term use can lead to withdrawal syndrome, including seizures and hallucinations. Meprobamate can exacerbate acute intermittent porphyria. Other rare side effects include hypersensitivity reactions, wheezing, hives, paradoxical excitement, and leukopenia. It should not be used in patients with hepatic compromise.

DRUG INTERACTIONS. Meprobamate has additive sedating effects in combination with other CNS depressants, such as alcohol, barbiturates, or benzodiazepines.

LABORATORY INTERFERENCES. Meprobamate can interfere with the metyrapone, phentolamine, and urinary 17-hydroxycorticosteroid tests.

DOSING AND CLINICAL GUIDELINES. Meprobamate is available in 200-, 400-, and 600-mg tablets; 200- and 400-mg extended-release capsules; and various combinations, for example, aspirin, 325 mg and 200 mg of meprobamate (Equagesic) for oral use. For adults, the usual dose is 400 to 800 mg twice daily. Elderly patients and children aged 6 to 12 years require half the adult dose.

Chloral Hydrate. Chloral hydrate is a hypnotic agent rarely used in psychiatry because numerous safer options, such as benzodiazepines, are available.

PHARMACOLOGICAL ACTIONS. Chloral hydrate is well absorbed from the GI tract. The parent compound is metabolized within minutes by the liver to the active metabolite trichloroethanol, which has a half-life of 8 to 11 hours. A dose of chloral hydrate induces sleep in about 30 to 60 minutes and maintains sleep for 4 to 8 hours. It probably potentiates GABAergic neurotransmission, which suppresses neuronal excitability.

THERAPEUTIC INDICATIONS. The major indication for chloral hydrate is to induce sleep. It should be used for no more than 2 or 3 days because longer-term treatment is associated with an increased incidence and severity of adverse effects. Tolerance develops to the hypnotic effects of chloral hydrate after 2 weeks of treatment. The benzodiazepines are superior to chloral hydrate for all psychiatric uses.

PRECAUTIONS AND ADVERSE REACTIONS. Chloral hydrate has adverse effects on the CNS, GI system, and skin. High doses (>4 g) may be associated with stupor, confusion, ataxia, falls, or coma. The GI effects include nonspecific irritation, nausea, vomiting, flatulence, and an unpleasant taste. With long-term use and overdose, gastritis and gastric ulceration can develop. In addition to the development of tolerance, dependence on chloral hydrate can occur, with symptoms similar to those of alcohol dependence. With a lethal dose between 5,000 and 10,000 mg, chloral hydrate is a particularly poor choice for potentially suicidal persons.

DRUG INTERACTIONS. Because of metabolic interference, chloral hydrate should be strictly avoided with alcohol, a notorious concoction known as a *Mickey Finn.* Chloral hydrate may displace warfarin (Coumadin) from plasma proteins and enhance anticoagulant activity; this combination should be avoided.

LABORATORY INTERFERENCES. Chloral hydrate administration can lead to false-positive results for urine glucose determinations that use cupric sulfate (e.g., Clinitest) but not in tests that use glucose oxidase (e.g., Clinistix and Tes-Tape). Chloral hydrate can also interfere with the determination of urinary catecholamines in 17-hydroxycorticosteroids.

DOSING AND CLINICAL GUIDELINES. Chloral hydrate is available in 500-mg capsules; 500-mg/5-mL solution; and 324-, 500-, and 648-mg rectal suppositories. The standard dose of chloral hydrate is 500 to 2,000 mg at bedtime. Because the drug is a GI irritant, it should be administered with excess water, milk, other liquids, or antacids to decrease gastric irritation.

Propofol. Propofol (Diprivan) is a $GABA_A$ agonist that is used as an anesthetic. It induces presynaptic release of GABA and dopamine (the latter possibility through an action on $GABA_B$ receptors) and is a partial agonist at dopamine D_2 and N-methyl-D-aspartate (NMDA) receptors. Because it is very lipid soluble, it crosses the blood–brain barrier readily and induces anesthesia in less than 1 minute. Rapid redistribution from the CNS results in offset of action within 3 to 8 minutes after the infusion is discontinued. It is well tolerated when used for conscious sedation, but it has a potential for acute adverse effects, including respiratory depression, apnea, and bradyarrhythmias, and prolonged infusion can cause acidosis and mitochondrial myopathies. The carrier used for the infusion is a soybean emulsion that can be a culture medium for various organisms. In addition, the carrier can impair macrophage function and cause hematologic and lipid abnormalities and anaphylactic reactions.

Etomidate. Etomidate is a carboxylated imidazole that acts at the β_2 and β_3 subunits of the $GABA_A$ receptor. It has a rapid onset (1 minute) and short duration (less than 5 minutes) of action. The propylene glycol vehicle has been linked to hyperosmolar metabolic acidosis. It has both proconvulsant and anticonvulsant properties, and it inhibits cortisol release, with possible adverse consequences after long-term use.

BENZODIAZEPINES AND DRUGS ACTING ON GABA RECEPTORS

The first benzodiazepine to be introduced was chlordiazepoxide (Librium), in 1959. In 1963, diazepam (Valium) became available. Over the next three decades, superior safety and tolerability helped the benzodiazepines replace the older antianxiety and hypnotic medications, such as the barbiturates and meprobamate (Miltown). Dozens of benzodiazepines and drugs acting on benzodiazepine receptors have been synthesized and marketed worldwide. Many of these agents are not in the United States, and some benzodiazepines have been discontinued because of lack of use. Table 25–19 lists agents currently available in the United States.

The benzodiazepines derive their name from their molecular structure. They share a common effect on receptors that have been termed benzodiazepine receptors, which in turn modulate GABA activity. Nonbenzodiazepine agonists, such as zolpidem (Ambien), zaleplon (Sonata), and eszopiclone (Lunesta)—the so-called "Z drugs"—are discussed in this chapter because their clinical effects result from binding domains located close to benzodiazepine receptors. Flumazenil (Romazicon), a benzodiazepine receptor antagonist used to reverse benzodiazepine-induced sedation and in emergency care of benzodiazepine overdosage, is also covered here.

Because benzodiazepines have a rapid anxiolytic sedative effect, they are most commonly used for acute treatment of insomnia, anxiety, agitation, or anxiety associated with any psychiatric disorder. In addition, the benzodiazepines are used as anesthetics, anticonvulsants, and muscle relaxants and as the preferred treatment for catatonia. Because of the risk of psychological and physical dependence associated with long-term use of benzodiazepines, ongoing assessment should be made as to the continued clinical need for these drugs in treating patients. In most patients, given the nature of their disorders, it is often best if benzodiazepine agents are used in conjunction with psychotherapy and when alternative agents have been tried and proven ineffective or poorly tolerated. In many forms of chronic anxiety disorders, antidepressant drugs such as the SSRI and serotonin–norepinephrine reuptake inhibitors (SNRIs) are now used as primary treatments, with benzodiazepines used as adjuncts. Benzodiazepine abuse is rare, usually found in patients who abuse multiple prescription and recreational drugs.

Pharmacological Actions

All benzodiazepines except clorazepate (Tranxene) are completely absorbed after oral administration and reach peak serum

Table 25–19
Preparations and Doses of Medications Acting on the Benzodiazepine Receptor Available in the United States

Medication	Brand Name	Dose Equivalent	Usual Adult Dose (mg)	How Supplied
Diazepam	Valium	5	2.5–40.0	2-, 5-, and 10-mg tablets 15-mg slow-release tablets
Clonazepam	Klonopin	0.25	0.5–4.0	0.5-, 1.0-, and 2.0-mg tablets
Alprazolam	Xanax	0.5	0.5–6.0	0.25-, 0.5-, 1.0-, and 2.0-mg tablets 1.5-mg sustained-release tablet
Lorazepam	Ativan	1	0.5–6.0	0.5-, 1.0-, and 2.0-mg tablets 4 mg/mL parenteral
Oxazepam	Serax	15	15–120	7.5-, 10.0-, 15.0-, and 30.0-mg capsules 15-mg tablets
Chlordiazepoxide	Librium	25	10–100	5-, 10-, and 25-mg capsules and tablets
Clorazepate	Tranxene	7.5	15–60	3.75-, 7.50-, and 15.00-mg tablets 11.25- and 22.50-mg slow-release tablets
Midazolam	Versed	0.25	1–50	5 mg/mL parenteral 1-, 2-, 5-, and 10-mL vials
Flurazepam	Dalmane	15	15–30	15- and 30-mg capsules
Temazepam	Restoril	15	7.5–30.0	7.5-, 15.0-, and 30.0-mg capsules
Triazolam	Halcion	0.125	0.125–0.250	0.125- and 0.250-mg tablets
Estazolam	ProSom	1	1–2	1- and 2-mg tablets
Quazepam	Doral	5	7.5–15.0	7.5- and 15.0-mg tablets
Zolpidem	Ambien	10	5–10	5- and 10-mg tablets
	Ambien CR	5	6.25–12.5	6.25- and 12.5-mg tablets
Zaleplon	Sonata	10	5–20	5- and 10-mg capsules
Eszopiclone	Lunesta	1	1–3	1-, 2- and 3-mg tablets
Flumazenil	Romazicon	0.05	0.2–0.5 per min	0.1 mg/mL 5- and 10-mL vials

levels within 30 minutes to 2 hours. Metabolism of clorazepate in the stomach converts it to desmethyldiazepam, which is then completely absorbed.

The absorption, the attainment of peak concentrations, and the onset of action are quickest for diazepam (Valium), lorazepam (Ativan), alprazolam (Xanax), triazolam (Halcion), and estazolam (ProSom). The rapid onset of effects is important to persons who take a single dose of a benzodiazepine to calm an episodic burst of anxiety or to fall asleep rapidly. Several benzodiazepines are effective after intravenous (IV) injection, but only lorazepam and midazolam (Versed) have rapid and reliable absorption after IM administration.

Diazepam, chlordiazepoxide, clonazepam (Klonopin), clorazepate, flurazepam (Dalmane), and quazepam (Doral) have plasma half-lives of 30 hours to more than 100 hours and are technically described as long-acting benzodiazepines. The plasma half-lives of these compounds can be as high as 200 hours in persons whose metabolism is genetically slow. Because the attainment of steady-state plasma concentrations of the drugs can take up to 2 weeks, persons may experience symptoms and signs of toxicity after only 7 to 10 days of treatment with a dosage that seemed initially to be in the therapeutic range.

Clinically, half-life alone does not necessarily determine the duration of therapeutic action for most benzodiazepines. The fact that all benzodiazepines are lipid soluble to varying degrees means that benzodiazepines and their active metabolites bind to plasma proteins. The extent of this binding is proportional to their lipid solubility. The amount of protein binding varies from 70 to 99 percent. Distribution, onset, and termination of action after a single dose are thus largely determined by benzodiazepine lipid solubility, not elimination half-life. Preparations with high lipid solubility, such as diazepam and alprazolam, are absorbed rapidly from the GI tract and distribute rapidly to the brain by passive diffusion along a concentration gradient, resulting in a rapid onset of action. However, as the concentration of the medication increases in the brain and decreases in the bloodstream, the concentration gradient reverses itself, and these medications leave the brain rapidly, resulting in fast cessation of drug effect. Drugs with longer elimination half-lives, such as diazepam, may remain in the bloodstream for a substantially longer period of time than their actual pharmacologic action at benzodiazepine receptors because the concentration in the brain decreases rapidly below the level necessary for a noticeable effect. In contrast, lorazepam, which has a shorter elimination half-life than diazepam but is less lipid soluble, has a slower onset of action after a single dose because the drug is absorbed and enters the brain more slowly. However, the duration of action after a single dose is longer because it takes longer for lorazepam to leave the brain and for brain levels to decrease below the concentration that produces an effect. In chronic dosing, some of these differences are not as apparent because brain levels are in equilibrium with higher and more consistent steady-state blood levels, but additional doses still produce a more rapid but briefer action with diazepam than with lorazepam. Benzodiazepines are distributed widely in adipose tissue. As a result, medications may persist in the body after discontinuation longer than would be predicted from their elimination half-lives. In addition, the dynamic half-life (i.e., duration of action on the receptor) may be longer than the elimination half-life.

The advantages of long–half-life drugs over short–half-life drugs include less frequent dosing, less variation in plasma concentration, and less severe withdrawal phenomena. The disadvantages include drug accumulation, increased risk of daytime psychomotor impairment, and increased daytime sedation.

The half-lives of lorazepam, oxazepam (Serax), temazepam (Restoril), and estazolam are between 8 and 30 hours. Alprazolam has a half-life of 10 to 15 hours, and triazolam has the shortest half-life (2 to 3 hours) of all the orally administered benzodiazepines. Rebound insomnia and anterograde amnesia are thought to be more of a problem with the short–half-life drugs than with the long–half-life drugs.

Because administration of medications more frequently than the elimination half-life leads to drug accumulation, medications such as diazepam and flurazepam accumulate with daily dosing, eventually resulting in increased daytime sedation.

Some benzodiazepines (e.g., oxazepam) are conjugated directly by glucuronidation and are excreted. Most benzodiazepines are oxidized first by CYP3A4 and CYP2C19, often to active metabolites. These metabolites may then be hydroxylated to another active metabolite. For example, diazepam is oxidized to desmethyldiazepam, which, in turn, is hydroxylated to produce oxazepam. These products undergo glucuronidation to inactive metabolites. A number of benzodiazepines (e.g., diazepam, chlordiazepoxide) have the same active metabolite (desmethyldiazepam), which have an elimination half-life of more than 120 hours. Flurazepam (Dalmane), a lipid-soluble benzodiazepine used as a hypnotic that has a short elimination half-life, has an active metabolite (desalkylflurazepam) with a half-life greater than 100 hours. This is another reason that the duration of action of a benzodiazepine may not correspond to the half-life of the parent drug.

Zaleplon, zolpidem, and eszopiclone are structurally distinct and vary in their binding to the GABA receptor subunits. Benzodiazepines activate all three specific GABA–benzodiazepine (GABA–BZ)-binding sites of the $GABA_A$-receptor, which opens chloride channels and reduces the rate of neuronal and muscle firing. Zolpidem, zaleplon, and eszopiclone have selectivity for certain subunits of the GABA receptor. This may account for their selective sedative effects and relative lack of muscle relaxant and anticonvulsant effects.

Zolpidem, zaleplon, and eszopiclone are rapidly and well absorbed after oral administration, although absorption can be delayed by as long as 1 hour if they are taken with food. Zolpidem reaches peak plasma concentrations in 1.6 hours and has a half-life of 2.6 hours. Zaleplon reaches peak plasma concentrations in 1 hour and has a half-life of 1 hour. If taken immediately after a high-fat or heavy meal, the peak is delayed by approximately 1 hour, reducing the effects of eszopiclone on sleep onset. The terminal-phase elimination half-life is approximately 6 hours in healthy adults. Eszopiclone is weakly bound to plasma protein (52 to 59 percent).

The rapid metabolism and lack of active metabolites of zolpidem, zaleplon, and eszopiclone avoid the accumulation of plasma concentrations compared with the long-term use of benzodiazepines.

Therapeutic Indications

Insomnia. Because insomnia may be a symptom of a physical or psychiatric disorder, hypnotics should not be used for more than 7 to 10 consecutive days without a thorough investigation of the cause of the insomnia. However, many patients have long-standing sleep difficulties and benefit greatly from long-term use of hypnotic agents. Temazepam, flurazepam, and triazolam are benzodiazepines with a sole indication for insomnia. Zolpidem, zaleplon, and eszopiclone are also indicated only for insomnia. Although these "Z drugs" are not usually associated with rebound insomnia after the discontinuation of their use for short periods, some patients experience increased sleep difficulties the first few nights after discontinuing their use. Use of zolpidem, zaleplon, and eszopiclone for periods longer than 1 month is not associated with the delayed emergence of adverse effects. No development of tolerance to any parameter of sleep measurement was observed over 6 months in clinical trials of eszopiclone.

Flurazepam, temazepam, quazepam, estazolam, and triazolam are the benzodiazepines approved for use as hypnotics. The benzodiazepine hypnotics differ principally in their half-lives; flurazepam has the longest half-life, and triazolam has the shortest. Flurazepam may be associated with minor cognitive impairment on the day after its administration, and triazolam may be associated with mild rebound anxiety and anterograde amnesia. Quazepam may be associated with daytime impairment when used for a long time. Temazepam or estazolam may be a reasonable compromise for most adults. Estazolam produces rapid onset of sleep and a hypnotic effect for 6 to 8 hours.

γ-Hydroxybutyrate (GHB, Xyrem), which is approved for the treatment of narcolepsy and improves slow-wave sleep, is also an agonist at the $GABA_A$ receptor, where it binds to specific GHB receptors. GHB has the capacity both to reduce drug craving and to induce dependence, abuse, and absence seizures as a result of complex actions on tegmental dopaminergic systems.

Anxiety Disorders

GENERALIZED ANXIETY DISORDER. Benzodiazepines are highly effective for the relief of anxiety associated with generalized anxiety disorder (GAD). Most persons should be treated for a predetermined, specific, and relatively brief period. However, because GAD is a chronic disorder with a high rate of recurrence, some persons with GAD may warrant long-term maintenance treatment with benzodiazepines.

PANIC DISORDER. Alprazolam and clonazepam, both high-potency benzodiazepines, are commonly used medications for panic disorder with or without agoraphobia. Although the SSRIs are also indicated for the treatment of panic disorder, the benzodiazepines have the advantage of working quickly and not causing significant sexual dysfunction and weight gain. However, the SSRIs are still often preferred because they target common comorbid conditions, such as depression or OCD. Benzodiazepines and SSRIs can be initiated together to treat acute panic symptoms; use of the benzodiazepine can be tapered after 3 to 4 weeks after the therapeutic benefits of the SSRI have emerged.

SOCIAL PHOBIA. Clonazepam has been shown to be an effective treatment for social phobia. In addition, several other benzodiazepines (e.g., diazepam) have been used as adjunctive medications for the treatment of social phobia.

OTHER ANXIETY DISORDERS. Benzodiazepines are used adjunctively for the treatment of adjustment disorder with anxiety, pathological anxiety associated with life events (e.g., after an accident), OCD, and posttraumatic stress disorder.

ANXIETY ASSOCIATED WITH DEPRESSION. Depressed patients often experience significant anxiety, and antidepressant drugs may cause initial exacerbation of these symptoms. Accordingly, benzodiazepines are indicated for the treatment of anxiety associated with depression.

BIPOLAR I AND II DISORDERS. Clonazepam, lorazepam, and alprazolam are effective in the management of acute manic episodes and as an adjuvant to maintenance therapy in lieu of antipsychotics. As an adjuvant to lithium (Eskalith) or lamotrigine (Lamictal), clonazepam may result in an increased time between cycles and fewer depressive episodes. Benzodiazepines may help patients with bipolar disorder sleep better.

Catatonia. Lorazepam, sometimes in low doses (less than 5 mg per day) and sometimes in very high doses (12 mg per day or more), is regularly used to treat acute catatonia, which is more frequently associated with bipolar disorder than with schizophrenia. Other benzodiazepines have also been said to be helpful. However, there are no valid controlled trials of benzodiazepines in catatonia. Chronic catatonia does not respond as well to benzodiazepines. The definitive treatment for catatonia is ECT.

Akathisia. The first-line drug for akathisia is most commonly a β-adrenergic receptor antagonist. However, benzodiazepines are also effective in treating some patients with akathisia.

Parkinson's Disease. A small number of persons with idiopathic Parkinson's disease respond to long-term use of zolpidem with reduced bradykinesia and rigidity. Zolpidem dosages of 10 mg four times daily may be tolerated without sedation for several years.

Other Psychiatric Indications. Chlordiazepoxide (Librium) and clorazepate (Tranxene) are used to manage the symptoms of alcohol withdrawal. The benzodiazepines (especially IM lorazepam) are used to manage substance-induced and psychotic agitation in the emergency department. Benzodiazepines have been used instead of amobarbital (Amytal) for drug-assisted interviewing.

Flumazenil for Benzodiazepine Overdosage. Flumazenil is used to reverse the adverse psychomotor, amnestic, and sedative effects of benzodiazepine receptor agonists, including benzodiazepines, zolpidem, and zaleplon. Flumazenil is administered IV and has a half-life of 7 to 15 minutes. The most common adverse effects of flumazenil are nausea, vomiting, dizziness, agitation, emotional lability, cutaneous vasodilation, injection-site pain, fatigue, impaired vision, and headache. The most common serious adverse effect associated with the use of flumazenil is the precipitation of seizures, which is especially likely to occur in persons with seizure disorders, those who are physically dependent on benzodiazepines, and those who have ingested large quantities of benzodiazepines. Flumazenil alone may impair memory retrieval.

In mixed-drug overdosage, the toxic effects (e.g., seizures and cardiac arrhythmias) of other drugs (e.g., TCAs) may emerge with the reversal of the benzodiazepine effects of flumazenil. For example, seizures caused by an overdosage of TCAs may have been partially treated in a person who had also taken an overdosage of benzodiazepines. With flumazenil treatment, the tricyclic-induced seizures or cardiac arrhythmias may appear and result in a fatal outcome. Flumazenil does not reverse the effects of ethanol, barbiturates, or opioids.

For the initial management of a known or suspected benzodiazepine overdosage, the recommended initial dosage of flumazenil is 0.2 mg (2 mL) administered IV over 30 seconds. If the desired consciousness is not obtained after 30 seconds, a further dose of 0.3 mg (3 mL) can be administered over 30 seconds. Further doses of 0.5 mg (5 mL) can be administered over 30 seconds at 1-minute intervals up to a cumulative dose of 3.0 mg. The clinician should not rush the administration of flumazenil. A secure airway and IV access should be established before the administration of the drug. Persons should be awakened gradually.

Most persons with a benzodiazepine overdosage respond to a cumulative dose of 1 to 3 mg of flumazenil; doses above 3 mg of flumazenil do not reliably produce additional effects. If a person has not responded 5 minutes after receiving a cumulative dose of 5 mg of flumazenil, the major cause of sedation is probably not benzodiazepine receptor agonists, and additional flumazenil is unlikely to have an effect.

Sedation can return in 1 to 3 percent of persons treated with flumazenil. It can be prevented or treated by giving repeated dosages of flumazenil at 20-minute intervals. For repeat treatment, no more than 1 mg (given as 0.5 mg a minute) should be given at any one time, and no more than 3 mg should be given in any 1 hour.

Precautions and Adverse Reactions

The most common adverse effect of the benzodiazepines is drowsiness, which occurs in about 10 percent of all persons. Because of this adverse effect, persons should be advised to be careful while driving or using dangerous machinery when taking the drugs. Drowsiness can be present during the day after the use of a benzodiazepine for insomnia the previous night, the so-called residual daytime sedation. Some persons also experience ataxia (fewer than 2 percent) and dizziness (less than 1 percent). These symptoms can result in falls and hip fractures, especially in elderly persons. The most serious adverse effects of the benzodiazepines occur when other sedative substances, such as alcohol, are taken concurrently. These combinations can result in marked drowsiness, disinhibition, or even respiratory depression. Infrequently, benzodiazepine receptor agonists cause mild cognitive deficits that may impair job performance. Persons taking benzodiazepine receptor agonists should be advised to exercise additional caution when driving or operating dangerous machinery.

High-potency benzodiazepines, especially triazolam, can cause anterograde amnesia. A paradoxical increase in aggression has been reported in persons with preexisting brain damage. Allergic reactions to the drugs are rare, but a few studies report maculopapular rashes and generalized itching. The symptoms of benzodiazepine intoxication include confusion, slurred speech, ataxia, drowsiness, dyspnea, and hyporeflexia.

Triazolam has received significant attention in the media because of an alleged association with serious aggressive behavioral manifestations. Therefore, the manufacturer recommends that the drug be used for no more than 10 days for the treatment of insomnia and that physicians carefully evaluate the emergence of any abnormal thinking or behavioral changes in persons treated with triazolam, giving appropriate consideration to all potential causes. Triazolam was banned in Great Britain in 1991.

Zolpidem (Ambien) has also been associated with automatic behavior and amnesia.

Persons with hepatic disease and elderly persons are particularly likely to have adverse effects and toxicity from the benzodiazepines, including hepatic coma, especially when the drugs are administered repeatedly or in high dosages. Benzodiazepines can produce clinically significant impairment of respiration in persons with chronic obstructive pulmonary disease and sleep apnea. Alprazolam may exert a direct appetite stimulant effect and may cause weight gain. The benzodiazepines should be used with caution by persons with a history of substance abuse, cognitive disorders, renal disease, hepatic disease, porphyria, CNS depression, or myasthenia gravis.

Some data indicate that benzodiazepines are teratogenic; therefore, their use during pregnancy is not advised. Moreover, the use of benzodiazepines in the third trimester can precipitate a withdrawal syndrome in newborns. The drugs are secreted in the breast milk in sufficient concentrations to affect newborns. Benzodiazepines may cause dyspnea, bradycardia, and drowsiness in nursing babies.

Zolpidem and zaleplon are generally well tolerated. At zolpidem dosages of 10 mg per day and zaleplon dosages above 10 mg per day, a small number of persons will experience dizziness, drowsiness, dyspepsia, or diarrhea. Zolpidem and zaleplon are secreted in breast milk and are therefore contraindicated for use by nursing mothers. The dosage of zolpidem and zaleplon should be reduced in elderly persons and persons with hepatic impairment.

In rare cases, zolpidem may cause hallucinations and behavioral changes. The coadministration of zolpidem and SSRIs may extend the duration of hallucinations in susceptible patients.

Eszopiclone exhibits a dose–response relationship in elderly adults for the side effects of pain, dry mouth, and unpleasant taste.

Tolerance, Dependence, and Withdrawal. When benzodiazepines are used for short periods (1 to 2 weeks) in moderate dosages, they usually cause no significant tolerance, dependence, or withdrawal effects. The short-acting benzodiazepines (e.g., triazolam) may be an exception to this rule because some persons have reported increased anxiety the day after taking a single dose of the drug and then stopping its use. Some persons also report a tolerance for the anxiolytic effects of benzodiazepines and require increased doses to maintain the clinical remission of symptoms.

The appearance of a withdrawal syndrome, also called a discontinuation syndrome, depends on the length of time the person has been taking a benzodiazepine, the dosage the person has been taking, the rate at which the drug is tapered, and the half-life of the compound. Benzodiazepine withdrawal syndrome consists of anxiety, nervousness, diaphoresis, restlessness, irritability, fatigue, lightheadedness, tremor, insomnia, and weakness (Table 25–20). Abrupt discontinuation of benzodiazepines, particularly those with short half-lives, is associated with severe withdrawal symptoms, which may include depression, paranoia, delirium, and seizures. These severe symptoms are more likely to occur if flumazenil is used for rapid reversal of the benzodiazepine receptor agonist effects. Some features of the syndrome may occur in as many as 90 percent of persons treated with the drugs. The development of a severe withdrawal syndrome is seen only in persons who have taken high dosages for long periods. The appearance of the syndrome may be delayed for 1 or 2 weeks in persons who had been taking benzodiazepines with long half-lives. Alprazolam seems to be particularly associated with an immediate and severe withdrawal syndrome and should be tapered gradually.

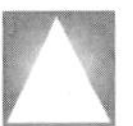

Table 25–20
Signs and Symptoms of Benzodiazepine Withdrawal

Anxiety	Tremor
Irritability	Depersonalization
Insomnia	Hyperesthesia
Hyperacusis	Myoclonus
Nausea	Delirium
Difficulty concentrating	Seizures

When the medication is to be discontinued, the drug must be tapered slowly (25 percent a week); otherwise, recurrence or rebound of symptoms is likely. Monitoring of any withdrawal symptoms (possibly with a standardized rating scale) and psychological support of the person are helpful in the successful accomplishment of benzodiazepine discontinuation. Concurrent use of carbamazepine (Tegretol) during benzodiazepine discontinuation has been reported to permit a more rapid and better tolerated withdrawal than does a gradual taper alone. The dosage range of carbamazepine used to facilitate withdrawal is 400 to 500 mg a day. Some clinicians report particular difficulty in tapering and discontinuing alprazolam, especially in persons who have been receiving high dosages for long periods. There have been reports of successful discontinuation of alprazolam by switching to clonazepam, which is then gradually withdrawn.

Zolpidem and zaleplon can produce a mild withdrawal syndrome lasting 1 day after prolonged use at higher therapeutic dosages. Rarely, a person taking zolpidem has self-titrated up the daily dosage to 30 to 40 mg a day. Abrupt discontinuation of such a high dosage of zolpidem may cause withdrawal symptoms for 4 or more days. Tolerance does not develop to the sedative effects of zolpidem and zaleplon.

Drug Interactions

The most common and potentially serious benzodiazepine receptor agonist interaction is excessive sedation and respiratory depression occurring when benzodiazepines, zolpidem, or zaleplon are administered concomitantly with other CNS depressants, such as alcohol, barbiturates, tricyclic and tetracyclic drugs, DRAs, opioids, and antihistamines. Ataxia and dysarthria may be likely to occur when lithium, antipsychotics, and clonazepam are combined. The combination of benzodiazepines and clozapine (Clozaril) has been reported to cause delirium and should be avoided. Cimetidine (Tagamet), disulfiram (Antabuse), isoniazid, estrogen, and oral contraceptives increase the plasma concentration of diazepam, chlordiazepoxide, clorazepate, and flurazepam. Cimetidine increases the plasma concentrations of zaleplon. However, antacids may reduce the GI absorption of benzodiazepines. The plasma concentrations of triazolam and alprazolam are increased to potentially toxic concentrations by nefazodone (Serzone) and fluvoxamine (Luvox). The manufacturer of nefazodone recommends that the dosage of triazolam be lowered by 75 percent and the dosage of alprazolam be lowered by 50 percent when given concomitantly with nefazodone. Over-the-counter preparations of kava plant, advertised as a "natural tranquilizer," can potentiate the action of benzodiazepine receptor agonists through synergistic overactivation of GABA receptors. Carbamazepine can lower the plasma concentration of alprazolam. Antacids and food may decrease the plasma concentrations of benzodiazepines, and smoking may increase the metabolism of benzodiazepines. Rifampin (Rifadin), phenytoin (Dilantin), carbamazepine, and phenobarbital (Solfoton, Luminal) significantly increase the metabolism of zaleplon. The benzodiazepines may increase the plasma concentrations of phenytoin and digoxin (Lanoxin). The SSRIs may prolong and exacerbate the severity of zolpidem-induced hallucinations. Deaths have been reported when parental lorazepam is given with parental olanzapine.

The CYP3A4 and CYP2E1 enzymes are involved in the metabolism of eszopiclone. Eszopiclone did not show any inhibitory potential on CYP450 1A2, 2A6, 2C9, 2C19, 2D6, 2E1, and 3A4 in cryopreserved human hepatocytes. Coadministration of 3 mg of eszopiclone to subjects receiving 400 mg of ketoconazole, a potent inhibitor of CYP3A4, resulted in a 2.2-fold increase in exposure to eszopiclone.

Laboratory Interferences

No known laboratory interferences are associated with the use of the benzodiazepines, zolpidem, and zaleplon.

Dosage and Clinical Guidelines

The clinical decision to treat an anxious person with a benzodiazepine should be carefully considered. Medical causes of anxiety (e.g., thyroid dysfunction, caffeinism, and prescription medications) should be ruled out. Benzodiazepine use should be started at a low dosage, and the person should be instructed regarding the drug's sedative properties and abuse potential. An estimated length of therapy should be decided at the beginning of therapy, and the need for continued therapy should be reevaluated at least monthly because of the problems associated with long-term use. However, certain persons with anxiety disorders are unresponsive to treatments other than benzodiazepines in long-term use.

Benzodiazepines are available in a wide range of formulations. Clonazepam is available in a wafer formulation that facilitates its use in patients who have trouble swallowing pills. Alprazolam is available in an extended-release form, which reduces the frequency of dosing. Some benzodiazepines are more potent than others in that one compound requires a relatively smaller dosage than another compound to achieve the same effect. For example, clonazepam requires 0.25 mg to achieve the same effect as 5 mg of diazepam; thus, clonazepam is considered a high-potency benzodiazepine. Conversely, oxazepam has an approximate dosage equivalence of 15 mg and is a low-potency drug.

Zaleplon is available in 5- and 10-mg capsules. A single 10-mg dose is the usual adult dose. The dose can be increased to a maximum of 20 mg as tolerated. A single dose of zaleplon can be expected to provide 4 hours of sleep with minimal residual impairment. For persons older than age 65 years or persons with hepatic impairment, an initial dose of 5 mg is advised.

Eszopiclone is available in 1-, 2-, and 3-mg tablets. The starting dose should not exceed 1 mg in patients with severe hepatic impairment or those taking potent CYP3A4 inhibitors. The recommended dosing to improve sleep onset or maintenance is 2 or 3 mg for adult patients (ages 18 to 64 years) and 2 mg for older adult patients (ages 65 years and older). The 1-mg dose is for sleep onset in older adult patients whose primary complaint is difficulty falling asleep.

Table 25–19 lists preparations and doses of medications discussed in this chapter.

BUPROPION

Bupropion (Wellbutrin, Wellbutrin SR, Wellbutrin XL, Zyban) is an antidepressant drug that inhibits the reuptake of norepinephrine and, possibly, dopamine. Most significantly, it does not act on the serotonin system like SSRI antidepressants. This results in a side effect profile characterized by a low risk of sexual dysfunction and sedation and with modest weight loss during acute and long-term treatment. No withdrawal syndrome has been linked to discontinuation of bupropion. Although increasingly used as first-line monotherapy, a significant percentage of bupropion use occurs as add-on therapy to other antidepressants, usually SSRIs. Bupropion has been marketed under the name Zyban for use in smoking cessation regimens, clinicians should make note and remind the patients not to combine these two formulations as this may increase the risk of adverse effects particularly seizures.

Pharmacological Actions

Three formulations of bupropion are available: immediate release (taken three times daily), sustained release (taken twice daily), and extended release (taken once daily). The different versions of the drug contain the same active ingredient but differ in their pharmacokinetics and dosing. There have been reports of inconsistencies in bioequivalence between various branded and generic versions of bupropion. Any changes with this drug in tolerability or clinical efficacy in a patient who had been doing well should prompt an inquiry about whether these changes correspond to a switch to a new formulation.

Immediate-release bupropion is well absorbed from the GI tract. Peak plasma concentrations of bupropion are usually reached within 2 hours of oral administration, and peak levels of the sustained-release version are seen after 3 hours. The mean half-life of the compound is 12 hours, ranging from 8 to 40 hours. Peak levels of extended-release bupropion occur 5 hours after ingestion. This provides a longer time to maximum plasma concentration (t_{max}) but comparable peak and trough plasma concentrations. The 24-hour exposure occurring after administration of the extended-release version of 300 mg once daily is equivalent to that provided by sustained release of 150 mg twice daily. Clinically, this permits the drug to be taken once a day in the morning. Plasma levels are also reduced in the evening, making it less likely for some patients to experience treatment-related insomnia.

The mechanism of action for the antidepressant effects of bupropion is presumed to involve the inhibition of dopamine and norepinephrine reuptake. Bupropion binds to the dopamine transporter in the brain. The effects of bupropion on smoking cessation may be related to its effects on dopamine reward pathways or to inhibition of nicotinic acetylcholine receptors.

Therapeutic Indications

Depression. Although overshadowed by the SSRIs as first-line treatment for major depression, the therapeutic efficacy of bupropion in depression is well established in both outpatient and inpatient settings. Observed rates of response and remission are comparable to those seen with the SSRIs. Bupropion has been found to prevent seasonal major depressive episodes in patients with a history of seasonal pattern or affective disorder.

Smoking Cessation. As the brand name Zyban, bupropion is indicated for use in combination with behavioral modification programs for smoking cessation. It is intended to be used in patients who are highly motivated and who receive some form of structured behavioral support. Bupropion is most effective when combined with nicotine substitutes (Nico-Derm, Nicotrol).

Bipolar Disorders. Bupropion is less likely than TCAs to precipitate mania in persons with bipolar I disorder and less likely than other antidepressants to exacerbate or induce rapid-cycling bipolar II disorder; however, the evidence about use of bupropion in the treatment of patients with bipolar disorder is limited.

Attention-Deficit/Hyperactivity Disorder. Bupropion is used as a second-line agent, after the sympathomimetics, for the treatment of ADHD. It has not been compared with proven ADHD medications such as methylphenidate (Ritalin) or atomoxetine (Strattera) for childhood and adult ADHD. Bupropion is an appropriate choice for persons with comorbid ADHD and depression or persons with comorbid ADHD, conduct disorder, or substance abuse. It may also be considered for use in patients who develop tics when treated with psychostimulants.

Cocaine Detoxification. Bupropion may be associated with a euphoric feeling; thus, it may be contraindicated in persons with histories of substance abuse. However, because of its dopaminergic effects, bupropion has been explored as a treatment to reduce the cravings for cocaine in persons who have withdrawn from the substance. Results have been inconclusive, with some patients showing a reduction in drug craving and others finding their cravings increased.

Hypoactive Sexual Desire Disorder. Bupropion is often added to drugs such as SSRIs to counteract sexual side effects and may be helpful as a treatment for nondepressed individuals with hypoactive sexual desire disorder. Bupropion may improve sexual arousal, orgasm completion, and sexual satisfaction.

Precautions and Adverse Reactions

Headache, insomnia, dry mouth, tremor, and nausea are the most common side effects. Restlessness, agitation, and irritability may also occur. Patients with severe anxiety or panic disorder should not be prescribed bupropion. Most likely because of its potentiating effects on dopaminergic neurotransmission, bupropion can cause psychotic symptoms, including hallucinations, delusions, and catatonia, as well as delirium. Most notable about bupropion is the absence of significant drug-induced orthostatic hypotension, weight gain, daytime drowsiness, and anticholinergic effects. Some persons, however, may experience dry mouth or constipation and weight loss. Hypertension may occur in some patients, but bupropion causes no other significant cardiovascular or clinical laboratory changes. Bupropion exerts indirect sympathomimetic activity, producing positive inotropic effects in human myocardium, an effect that may reflect catecholamine release. Some patients experience cognitive impairment, most notably word-finding difficulties.

Concern about seizure has deterred some physicians from prescribing bupropion. The risk of seizure is dose dependent. Studies show that at dosages of 300 mg a day or less of sustained-release bupropion, the incidence of seizures is 0.05 percent, which is no worse than the incidence of seizures with other antidepressants. The risk of seizures increases to about 0.1 percent with dosages of 400 mg a day.

Changes in EEG waveforms have been reported to be associated with bupropion use. About 20 percent of individuals treated with bupropion exhibit spike waves, sharp waves, and focal slowing. The likelihood of women having sharp waves is higher than for men. The presence of these waveforms in individuals taking a medication known to lower the seizure threshold may be a risk factor for developing seizures. Other risk factors for seizures include a history of seizures, use of alcohol, recent benzodiazepine withdrawal, organic brain disease, head trauma, or pretreatment epileptiform discharges on EEG.

The use of bupropion by pregnant women is not associated with specific risk of increased rate of birth defects. Bupropion is secreted in breast milk, so the use of bupropion in nursing women should be based on the clinical circumstances of the patient and the judgment of the clinician.

Few deaths have been reported after overdoses of bupropion. Poor outcomes are associated with cases of huge doses and mixed-drug overdoses. Seizures occur in about one-third of all overdoses and are dose dependent, with those having seizures ingesting a significantly higher median dose. Fatalities can involve uncontrollable seizures, sinus bradycardia, and cardiac arrest. Symptoms of poisoning most often involve seizures, sinus tachycardia, hypertension, GI symptoms, hallucinations, and agitation. All seizures are typically brief and self-limited. In general, however, bupropion is safer in overdose cases than are other antidepressants except perhaps SSRIs.

Drug Interactions

Given the fact that bupropion is frequently combined with SSRIs or venlafaxine, potential interactions are significant. Bupropion has been found to have an effect on the pharmacokinetics of venlafaxine. One study noted a significant increase in venlafaxine levels and a consequent decrease in its main metabolite O-desmethylvenlafaxine during combined treatment with sustained-release bupropion. Bupropion hydroxylation is weakly inhibited by venlafaxine. No significant changes in plasma levels of the SSRIs paroxetine and fluoxetine have been reported. However, few case reports indicate that the combination of bupropion and fluoxetine (Prozac) may be associated with panic, delirium, or seizures. Bupropion in combination with lithium (Eskalith) may rarely cause CNS toxicity, including seizures.

Because of possibility of inducing a hypertensive crisis, bupropion should not be used concurrently with MAOIs. At least 14 days should pass after the discontinuation of an MAOI before initiating treatment with bupropion. In some cases, the addition of bupropion may permit persons taking antiparkinsonian medications to lower the doses of their dopaminergic drugs. However, delirium, psychotic symptoms, and dyskinetic movements may be associated with the coadministration of bupropion and dopaminergic agents such as levodopa (Larodopa), pergolide (Permax), ropinirole (Requip), pramipexole (Mirapex), amantadine (Symmetrel), and bromocriptine (Parlodel). Sinus bradycardia may occur when bupropion is combined with metoprolol.

Carbamazepine (Tegretol) may decrease plasma concentrations of bupropion, and bupropion may increase plasma concentrations of valproic acid (Depakene).

In vitro biotransformation studies of bupropion have found that formation of a major active metabolite, hydroxybupropion, is mediated by CYP2B6. Bupropion has a significant inhibitory effect on CYP2D6.

Laboratory Interferences

A report has appeared indicating that bupropion may give a false-positive result on urinary amphetamine screens. No other reports have appeared of laboratory interferences clearly associated with bupropion treatment. Clinically nonsignificant changes in the ECG (premature beats and nonspecific ST-T changes) and decreases in the WBC count (by about 10 percent) have been reported in a small number of persons.

Dosage and Clinical Guidelines

Immediate-release bupropion is available in 75-, 100-, and 150-mg tablets. Sustained-release bupropion is available in 100-, 150-, 200-, and 300-mg tablets. Extended-release bupropion comes in 150- and 300-mg strengths.

There have been problems associated with one of the extended-release generic versions called Budeprion XL 300-mg tablets, which was found not to be therapeutically equivalent to Bupropion XL 300 mg and was removed from the market.

Initiation of immediate-release bupropion in the average adult person should be 75 mg orally twice a day. On the fourth day of treatment, the dosage can be increased to 100 mg three times a day. Because 300 mg is the recommended dose, the person should be maintained on this dose for several weeks before increasing it further. The maximum dosage, 450 mg a day, should be given as 150 mg three times a day. Because of the risk of seizures, increases in dose should never exceed 100 mg in a 3-day period; a single dose of immediate-release bupropion should never exceed 150 mg, and the total daily dosage should not exceed 450 mg. The maximum of 400 mg of the sustained-release version should be used as a twice-a-day regimen of either 200 mg twice daily or 300 mg in the morning and 100 mg in the afternoon. A starting dosage of the sustained-release version, 100 mg once a day, can be increased to 100 mg twice a day after 4 days. Then 150 mg twice a day may be used. A single dose of sustained-release bupropion should never exceed 300 mg. The maximum dosage is 200 mg twice a day of the immediate-release or extended-release formulations. An advantage of the extended-release preparation is that after appropriate titration, a total of 450 mg can be given all at once in the morning.

For smoking cessation, the patient should start taking 150 mg a day of sustained-release bupropion 10 to 14 days before quitting smoking. On the fourth day, the dosage should be increased to 150 mg twice daily. Treatment generally lasts 7 to 12 weeks.

BUSPIRONE

Buspirone hydrochloride (BuSpar) is classified as an azapirone and is chemically distinct from other psychotropic agents. It acts on two types of receptors, serotonin (5-HT) and dopamine (D). It has high affinity for the 5-HT_{1A} serotonin receptor, acting as an agonist or partial agonist, and moderate affinity for the D_2 dopamine receptor, acting as both an agonist and an antagonist. The approved indication for this psychotropic drug is for the treatment of GAD. It was initially believed to be a better alternative to the benzodiazepine drug group because buspirone does not possess anticonvulsant and muscle relaxant effects. Reports continue to appear that some patients benefit from the addition of buspirone to their antidepressant regimen. Its use in this role is more common than its use as an anxiolytic. Interestingly, the antidepressant drug vilazodone (Viibryd) inhibits 5-HT reuptake and acts as a 5-HT_{1A} receptor partial agonist.

Pharmacological Actions

Buspirone is well absorbed from the GI tract, but absorption is delayed by food ingestion. Peak plasma levels are achieved 40 to 90 minutes after oral administration. At doses of 10 to 40 mg, single-dose linear pharmacokinetics are observed. Nonlinear pharmacokinetics are observed after multiple doses. Because of its short half-life (2 to 11 hours), buspirone is dosed three times daily. An active metabolite of buspirone, 1-pyrimidinylpiperazine (1-PP), is about 20 percent less potent than buspirone but is up to 30 percent more concentrated in the brain than the parent compound. The elimination half-life of 1-PP is 6 hours.

Buspirone has no effect on the GABA-associated chloride ion channel or the serotonin reuptake transporter, targets of other drugs that are effective in GAD. Buspirone also has activity at 5-HT_2 and dopamine type 2 (D_2) receptors, although the significance of the effects at these receptors is unknown. At D_2 receptors, it has properties of both an agonist and an antagonist.

Therapeutic Indications

Generalized Anxiety Disorder. Buspirone is a narrow-spectrum antianxiety agent with demonstrated efficacy only in the treatment of GAD. In contrast to the SSRIs or venlafaxine, buspirone is not effective in the treatment of panic disorder, OCD, or social phobia. Buspirone, however, has an advantage over these agents in that it does not typically cause sexual dysfunction or weight gain.

Some evidence suggests that compared with benzodiazepines, buspirone is generally more effective for symptoms of anger and hostility, equally effective for psychic symptoms of anxiety, and less effective for somatic symptoms of anxiety. The full benefit of buspirone is evident only at dosages above 30 mg a day. Compared with the benzodiazepines, buspirone has a delayed onset of action and lacks any euphoric effect. Unlike benzodiazepines, buspirone has no immediate effects, and patients should be told that a full clinical response may take 2 to 4 weeks. If an immediate response is needed, patients can be started on a benzodiazepine and then withdrawn from the drug after buspirone's effects begin. Sometimes the sedative effects of benzodiazepines, which are not found with buspirone, are desirable; however, these sedative effects may cause impaired motor performance and cognitive deficits.

Other Disorders. Many other clinical uses of buspirone have been reported, but most have not been confirmed in controlled trials. Evidence of the efficacy of high-dosage buspirone (30 to 90 mg a day) for depressive disorders is mixed. Buspirone appears to have weak antidepressant activity, which has led to its use as an augmenting agent in patients who have failed standard antidepressant therapy. In a large study, buspirone augmentation of SSRIs worked as well as other commonly used strategies. Buspirone is sometimes used to augment SSRIs in the treatment of OCD. There are reports that buspirone may be beneficial against the increased arousal and flashbacks associated with posttraumatic stress disorder.

Because buspirone does not act on the GABA–chloride ion channel complex, the drug is not recommended for the treatment of withdrawal from benzodiazepines, alcohol, or sedative–hypnotic drugs, except as treatment of comorbid anxiety symptoms.

Scattered trials suggest that buspirone reduces aggression and anxiety in persons with organic brain disease or traumatic brain injury. It is also used for SSRI-induced bruxism and sexual dysfunction, nicotine craving, and ADHD.

Precautions and Adverse Reactions

Buspirone does not cause weight gain, sexual dysfunction, discontinuation symptoms, or significant sleep disturbance. It does not produce sedation or cognitive and psychomotor impairment. The most common adverse effects of buspirone are headache, nausea, dizziness, and (rarely) insomnia. No sedation is associated with buspirone. Some persons may report a minor feeling of restlessness, although that symptom may reflect an incompletely treated anxiety disorder. No deaths have been reported from overdoses of buspirone, and the median lethal dose is estimated to be 160 to 550 times the recommended daily dose. Buspirone should be used with caution by persons with hepatic and renal impairment, pregnant women, and nursing mothers. Buspirone can be used safely by the elderly.

Drug Interactions

The coadministration of buspirone and haloperidol (Haldol) results in increased blood concentrations of haloperidol. Buspirone should not be used with MAOIs to avoid hypertensive episodes, and a 2-week washout period should pass between the discontinuation of MAOI use and the initiation of treatment with buspirone. Drugs or foods that inhibit CYP3A4, for example, erythromycin (E-mycin), itraconazole (Sporanox), nefazodone (Serzone), and grapefruit juice, increase buspirone plasma concentrations.

Laboratory Interferences

Single doses of buspirone can cause transient elevations in growth hormone, prolactin, and cortisol concentrations, although the effects are not clinically significant.

Dosage and Clinical Guidelines

Buspirone is available in single-scored 5- and 10-mg tablets and triple-scored 15- and 30-mg tablets; treatment is usually initiated with either 5 mg orally three times daily or 7.5 mg orally twice daily. The dosage can be raised 5 mg every 2 to 4 days to the usual dosage range of 15 to 60 mg a day.

Buspirone should not be used in patients with past hypersensitivity to buspirone, in cases of diabetes-associated metabolic acidosis, or in patients with severely compromised liver or renal function.

Switching from a Benzodiazepine to Buspirone. Buspirone is not cross-tolerant with benzodiazepines, barbiturates, or alcohol. A common clinical problem, therefore, is how to initiate buspirone therapy in a person who is currently taking benzodiazepines. There are two alternatives. First, the clinician can start buspirone treatment gradually while the benzodiazepine is being withdrawn. Second, the clinician can start buspirone treatment and bring the person up to a therapeutic dosage for 2 to 3 weeks while the person is still receiving the regular dosage of the benzodiazepine and then slowly taper the benzodiazepine dosage. Patients who have received benzodiazepines in the past, especially in recent months, may find that buspirone is not as effective as the benzodiazepines in the treatment of their anxiety. This might be explained by the absence of the immediate mildly euphoric and sedative effects of the benzodiazepines. The coadministration of buspirone and benzodiazepines may be effective in the treatment of persons with anxiety disorders who have not responded to treatment with either drug alone.

CALCIUM CHANNEL BLOCKERS

The intracellular calcium ion regulates activity of multiple neurotransmitters such as serotonin and dopamine, and that action may account for its role as a treatment in mood disorders. Calcium channel inhibitors are used in psychiatry as antimanic agents for persons who are refractory to or cannot tolerate treatment with first-line mood-stabilizing agents such as lithium (Eskalith), carbamazepine (Tegretol), and divalproex (Depakote). Calcium channel inhibitors include nifedipine (Procardia, Adalat), nimodipine (Nimotop), isradipine (DynaCirc), amlodipine (Norvasc, Lotrel), nicardipine (Cardene), nisoldipine (Sular), nitrendipine, and verapamil (Calan). They are used for control of mania and ultradian bipolar disorder (mood cycling in less than 24 hours).

The results of a large genetic study have rekindled interest in the potential clinical uses of CCBs. Two genome-wide findings implicated genes encoding L-type voltage-gated calcium channel subunits as susceptibility genes for bipolar disorder, schizophrenia, MDD, ADHD, and autism.

Table 25–21
Half-Lives, Dosages, and Effectiveness of Selected Calcium Channel Inhibitors in Psychiatric Disorders

	Verapamil (Calan, Isoptin)	Nimodipine (Nimotop)	Isradipine (DynaCirc)	Amlodipine (Norvasc)
Half-Life	Short (5–12 hrs)	Short (1–2 hrs)	Short (1–2 hrs)	Long (30–50 hrs)
Starting Dosage	30 mg TID	30 mg TID	2.5 mg BID	5 mg HS
Peak Daily Dosage	480 mg	240–450 mg	20 mg	10–15 mg
Antimanic	++	++	++	[a]
Antidepressant	±	+	+	[a]
Antiultradian[b]	±	++	(++)	[a]

BID, twice a day; HS, half strength; TID, three times a day.
[a]No systematic studies, only case reports.
[b]Rapid-cycling bipolar disorder.
Table adapted from Robert M. Post, M.D.

Pharmacological Actions

The calcium channel inhibitors are nearly completely absorbed after oral use, with significant first-pass hepatic metabolism. Considerable intra- and interindividual variations are seen in the plasma concentrations of the drugs after a single dose. Peak plasma levels of most of these agents are achieved within 30 minutes. Amlodipine does not reach peak plasma levels for about 6 hours. The half-life of verapamil after the first dose is 2 to 8 hours; the half-life increases to 5 to 12 hours after the first few days of therapy. The half-lives of the other CCBs range from 1 to 2 hours for nimodipine and isradipine to 30 to 50 hours for amlodipine (Table 25–21).

The primary mechanism of action of CCBs in bipolar illness is not known. The calcium channel inhibitors discussed in this section inhibit the influx of calcium into neurons through L-type (long-acting) voltage-dependent calcium channels.

Therapeutic Indications

Bipolar Disorder. Nimodipine and verapamil have been demonstrated to be effective as maintenance therapy in persons with bipolar illness. Patients who respond to lithium appear to also respond to treatment with verapamil. Nimodipine may be useful for ultradian cycling and recurrent brief depression. The clinician should begin treatment with a short-acting drug such as nimodipine or isradipine, beginning with a low dosage and increasing the dosage every 4 to 5 days until a clinical response is seen or adverse effects appear. When symptoms are controlled, a longer-acting drug, such as amlodipine, can be substituted as maintenance therapy. Failure to respond to verapamil does not exclude a favorable response to one of the other drugs. Verapamil has been shown to prevent antidepressant-induced mania. The CCBs can be combined with other agents, such as carbamazepine, in patients who are partial responders to monotherapy.

Depression. None of the CCBs is effective as treatment for depression and may in fact prevent response to antidepressants.

Other Psychiatric Indications. Nifedipine is used to treat hypertensive crises associated with the use of MAOIs. Isradipine may reduce the subjective response to methamphetamine. Calcium channel inhibitors may be beneficial in Tourette's disorder, Huntington's disease, panic disorder, intermittent explosive disorder, and tardive dyskinesia.

Other Medical Uses. These drugs have been used to treat medical conditions such as angina, hypertension, migraine headaches, Raynaud's phenomenon, esophageal spasm, premature labor, and headache. Verapamil has antiarrhythmic activity and has been used to treat superventricular arrhythmias.

Precautions and Adverse Reactions

The most common adverse effects associated with calcium channel inhibitors are those attributable to vasodilation: dizziness, headache, tachycardia, nausea, dysesthesias, and peripheral edema. Verapamil and diltiazem (Cardizem) in particular can cause hypotension, bradycardia, and AV heart block, which necessitate close monitoring and sometimes discontinuation of the drugs. In all patients with cardiovascular disease, the drugs should be used with caution. Other common adverse effects include constipation, fatigue, rash, coughing, and wheezing. Adverse effects noted with diltiazem include hyperactivity, akathisia, and parkinsonism; with verapamil, delirium, hyperprolactinemia, and galactorrhea; with nimodipine, subjective sense of chest tightness and skin flushing; and with nifedipine, depression. The drugs have not been evaluated for safety in pregnant women and are best avoided. Because the drugs are secreted in breast milk, nursing mothers should also avoid the drugs.

Drug Interactions

All CCBs have a potential for drug–drug interactions. The types and risks of these interactions vary by compound. Verapamil raises serum levels of carbamazepine, digoxin, and other CYP3A4 substrates. Verapamil and diltiazem but not nifedipine have been reported to precipitate carbamazepine-induced neurotoxicity. Calcium channel inhibitors should not be used by persons taking β-adrenergic receptor antagonists, hypotensives (e.g., diuretics, vasodilators, and ACEIs), or antiarrhythmic drugs (e.g., quinidine and digoxin) without consultation with an internist or cardiologist. Cimetidine (Tagamet) has been reported to increase plasma concentrations of nifedipine and diltiazem. Some patients who are treated with lithium and calcium channel inhibitors concurrently may be at increased risk for the signs and symptoms of neurotoxicity, and deaths have occurred.

Laboratory Interferences

No known laboratory interferences are associated with the use of calcium channel inhibitors.

Dosage and Clinical Guidelines

Verapamil is available in 40-, 80-, and 120-mg tablets; 120-, 180-, and 240-mg sustained-release tablets; and 100-, 120-, 180-, 200-, 240-, 300-, and 360-mg sustained-release capsules. The starting dosage is 40 mg orally three times a day and can be increased in increments every 4 to 5 days up to 80 to 120 mg three times a day. The patient's BP, pulse, and ECG (in patients older than 40 years old or with a history of cardiac illness) should be routinely monitored.

Nifedipine is available in 10- and 20-mg capsules and 30-, 60-, and 90-mg extended-release tablets. Administration should be started at 10 mg orally three or four times a day and can be increased up to a maximum dosage of 120 mg a day.

Nimodipine is available in 30-mg capsules. It has been used at 60 mg every 4 hours for ultra–rapid-cycling bipolar disorder and sometimes briefly at up to 630 mg per day.

Isradipine is available in 2.5- and 5-mg capsules, with a maximum of 20 mg/day. An extended-release formulation of isradipine has been discontinued.

Amlodipine is available in 2.5-, 5-, and 10-mg tablets. Administration should start at 5 mg once at night and can be increased to a maximum dosage of 10 to 15 mg a day.

Diltiazem is available in 30-, 60-, 90-, and 120-mg tablets; 60-, 90-, 120-, 180-, 240-, 300-, and 360-mg extended-release capsules; and 60-, 90-, 120-, 180-, 240-, 300-, and 360-mg extended-release tablets. Administration should start with 30 mg orally four times a day and can be increased up to a maximum of 360 mg a day.

Elderly persons are more sensitive to the calcium channel inhibitors than are younger adults. No specific information is available regarding the use of the agents for children.

CARBAMAZEPINE AND OXCARBAZEPINE

Carbamazepine (Tegretol) possesses some structural similarity to the tricyclic antidepressant imipramine (Tofranil). It was approved for use in the United States for the treatment of trigeminal neuralgia in 1968 and for temporal lobe epilepsy (complex partial seizures) in 1974. Interestingly, carbamazepine was first synthesized as a potential antidepressant, but because of its atypical profile in a number of animal models, it was initially developed for use in pain and seizure disorders. It is now recognized in most guidelines as a second-line mood stabilizer useful in the treatment and prevention of both phases of bipolar affective disorder. A long-acting sustained-release formulation (Equetro) was approved by the FDA for the treatment of acute mania in 2002.

An analog of carbamazepine, oxcarbazepine (Trileptal), was marketed as an antiseizure medication in the United States in 2000, after being used as a treatment for pediatric epilepsy in Europe since 1990. Because of its similarity to carbamazepine, many clinicians began to use it as a treatment for patients with bipolar disorder. Despite some reports that oxcarbazepine has mood-stabilizing properties, this has not been confirmed in large, placebo-controlled trials.

Carbamazepine

Pharmacological Actions. Absorption of carbamazepine is slow and unpredictable. Food enhances absorption. Peak plasma concentrations are reached 2 to 8 hours after a single dose, and steady-state levels are reached after 2 to 4 days on a steady dosage. It is 70 to 80 percent protein bound. The half-life of carbamazepine ranges from 18 to 54 hours, with an average of 26 hours. However, with chronic administration, the half-life of carbamazepine decreases to an average of 12 hours. This results from induction of hepatic CYP450 enzymes by carbamazepine, specifically autoinduction of carbamazepine metabolism. The induction of hepatic enzymes reaches its maximum level after about 3 to 5 weeks of therapy.

The pharmacokinetics of carbamazepine are different for two long-acting preparations of carbamazepine, each of which uses slightly different technology. One formulation, Tegretol XR, requires food to ensure normal GI transit time. The other preparation, Carbatrol, relies on a combination of intermediate, extended-release, and very slow-release beads, making it suitable for bedtime administration.

Carbamazepine is metabolized in the liver, and the 10,11-epoxide metabolite is active as an anticonvulsant. Its activity in the treatment of bipolar disorders is unknown. Long-term use of carbamazepine is associated with an increased ratio of the epoxide to the parent molecule.

The anticonvulsant effects of carbamazepine are thought to be mediated mainly by binding to voltage-dependent sodium channels in the inactive state and prolonging their inactivation. This secondarily reduces voltage-dependent calcium channel activation and, thus, synaptic transmission. Additional effects include reduction of currents through N-methyl-D-aspartate (NMDA) glutamate-receptor channels, competitive antagonism of adenosine α_1-receptors, and potentiation of CNS catecholamine neurotransmission. Whether any or all of these mechanisms also result in mood stabilization is not known.

Therapeutic Indications

BIPOLAR DISORDER

Acute Mania. The acute antimanic effects of carbamazepine are typically evident within the first several days of treatment. About 50 to 70 percent of all persons respond within 2 to 3 weeks of initiation. Studies suggest that carbamazepine may be especially effective in persons who are not responsive to lithium (Eskalith), such as persons with dysphoric mania, rapid cycling, or a negative family history of mood disorders. The antimanic effects of carbamazepine can be, and often are, augmented by concomitant administration of lithium, valproic acid (Depakene), thyroid hormones, DRAs, or SDAs. Some persons may respond to carbamazepine but not lithium or valproic acid and vice versa.

Prophylaxis. Carbamazepine is effective in preventing relapses, particularly among patients with bipolar II disorder and schizoaffective disorder, and dysphoric mania.

Acute Depression. A subgroup of treatment-refractory patients with acute depression responds well to carbamazepine. Patients with more severe episodic and less chronic depression seem to be better responders to carbamazepine. Nevertheless, carbamazepine remains an alternative drug for depressed persons who have not responded to conventional treatments, including ECT.

OTHER DISORDERS. Carbamazepine helps to control symptoms associated with acute alcohol withdrawal, although benzodiazepines are more effective in this population. Carbamazepine has been suggested as a treatment for the paroxysmal recurrent component of PTSD. Uncontrolled studies suggest that carbamazepine is effective in controlling impulsive, aggressive behavior in nonpsychotic persons of all ages, including children and elderly persons. Carbamazepine is also effective in controlling nonacute agitation and aggressive behavior in patients with schizophrenia and schizoaffective disorder. Persons with prominent positive symptoms (e.g., hallucinations) may be likely to respond, as are persons who display impulsive aggressive outbursts.

Precautions and Adverse Reactions.

Carbamazepine is relatively well tolerated. Mild GI (nausea, vomiting, gastric distress, constipation, diarrhea, and anorexia) and CNS (ataxia, drowsiness) side effects are the most common. The severity of these adverse effects is reduced if the dosage of carbamazepine is increased slowly and kept at the minimal effective plasma concentration. In contrast to lithium and valproate (other drugs used to manage bipolar disorder), carbamazepine does not appear to cause weight gain. Because of the phenomenon of autoinduction, with consequent reductions in carbamazepine concentrations, side effect tolerability may improve over time. Most of the adverse effects of carbamazepine are correlated with plasma concentrations above 9 μg/mL. The rarest but most serious adverse effects of carbamazepine are blood dyscrasias, hepatitis, and serious skin reactions (Table 25–22).

BLOOD DYSCRASIAS. The drug's hematologic effects are not dose related. Severe blood dyscrasias (aplastic anemia, agranulocytosis) occur in about 1 in 125,000 persons treated with carbamazepine. There does not appear to be a correlation between the degree of benign WBC suppression (leukopenia), which is seen in 1 to 2 percent of persons, and the emergence of life-threatening blood dyscrasias. Persons should be warned that the emergence of such symptoms as fever, sore throat, rash, petechiae, bruising, and easy bleeding can potentially herald a serious dyscrasia, and they should seek medical evaluation immediately. Routine hematologic monitoring in carbamazepine-treated persons is recommended at 3, 6, 9, and 12 months. If there is no significant evidence of bone marrow suppression by that time, many experts would reduce the interval of monitoring. However, even assiduous monitoring may fail to detect severe blood dyscrasias before they cause symptoms.

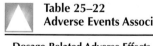

Table 25–22
Adverse Events Associated with Carbamazepine

Dosage-Related Adverse Effects	Idiosyncratic Adverse Effects
Double or blurred vision	Agranulocytosis
Vertigo	Stevens–Johnson syndrome
Gastrointestinal disturbances	Aplastic anemia
Task performance impairment	Hepatic failure
Hematologic effects	Rash
	Pancreatitis

HEPATITIS. Within the first few weeks of therapy, carbamazepine can cause both hepatitis associated with increases in liver enzymes, particularly transaminases, and cholestasis associated with elevated bilirubin and alkaline phosphatase. Mild transaminase elevations warrant observation only, but persistent elevations more than three times the upper limit of normal indicate the need to discontinue the drug. Hepatitis can recur if the drug is reintroduced to the person and can result in death.

DERMATOLOGIC EFFECTS. About 10 to 15 percent of those treated with carbamazepine develop a benign maculopapular rash within the first 3 weeks of treatment. Stopping the medication usually leads to resolution of the rash. Some patients may experience life-threatening dermatologic syndromes, including exfoliative dermatitis, erythema multiforme, Stevens–Johnson syndrome, and toxic epidermal necrolysis. The possible emergence of these serious dermatologic problems causes most clinicians to discontinue carbamazepine use in people who develop any type of rash. The risk of drug rash is about equal between valproic acid and carbamazepine in the first 2 months of use but is subsequently much higher for carbamazepine. If carbamazepine seems to be the only effective drug for a person who has a benign rash with carbamazepine treatment, a retrial of the drug can be undertaken. Many patients can be rechallenged without reemergence of the rash. Pretreatment with prednisone (Deltasone; 40 mg a day) may suppress the rash, although other symptoms of an allergic reaction (e.g., fever and pneumonitis) may develop even with steroid pretreatment.

RENAL EFFECTS. Carbamazepine is occasionally used to treat diabetes insipidus not associated with lithium use. This activity results from direct or indirect effects at the vasopressin receptor. It may also lead to the development of hyponatremia and water intoxication in some patients, particularly elderly persons, or when used in high doses.

OTHER ADVERSE EFFECTS. Carbamazepine decreases cardiac conduction (although less than the tricyclic drugs do) and can thus exacerbate preexisting cardiac disease. Carbamazepine should be used with caution in persons with glaucoma, prostatic hypertrophy, diabetes, or a history of alcohol abuse. Carbamazepine occasionally activates vasopressin receptor function, which results in a condition resembling the syndrome of secretion of inappropriate antidiuretic hormone, characterized by hyponatremia and, rarely, water intoxication. This is the opposite of the renal effects of lithium (i.e., nephrogenic diabetes insipidus). Augmentation of lithium with carbamazepine does not reverse the lithium effect, however. Emergence of confusion, severe weakness, or headache in a person taking carbamazepine should prompt measurement of serum electrolytes.

Carbamazepine use rarely elicits an immune hypersensitivity response consisting of fever, rash, eosinophilia, and possibly fatal myocarditis.

Cleft palate, fingernail hypoplasia, microcephaly, and spina bifida in infants may be associated with the maternal use of carbamazepine during pregnancy. Pregnant women should not use carbamazepine unless absolutely necessary. All women with childbearing potential should take 1 to 4 mg of folic acid daily even if they are not trying to conceive. Carbamazepine is secreted in breast milk.

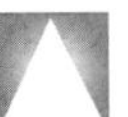

Table 25–23
Carbamazepine: Drug Interactions

Effect of Carbamazepine on Plasma Concentrations of Concomitant Agents	Agents That May Affect Carbamazepine Plasma Concentrations
Carbamazepine may decrease drug plasma concentration of:	*Agents that may increase carbamazepine plasma concentration:*
Acetaminophen	Allopurinol
Alprazolam	Cimetidine
Amitriptyline	Clarithromycin
Bupropion	Danazol
Clomipramine	Diltiazem
Clonazepam	Erythromycin
Clozapine	Fluoxetine
Cyclosporine	Fluvoxamine
Desipramine	Gemfibrozil
Dicumarol	Itraconazole
Doxepin	Ketoconazole
Doxycycline	Isoniazid[a]
Ethosuximide	Itraconazole
Felbamate	Lamotrigine
Fentanyl	Loratadine
Fluphenazine	Macrolides
Haloperidol	Nefazodone
Hormonal contraceptives	Nicotinamide
Imipramine	Propoxyphene
Lamotrigine	Terfenadine
Methadone	Troleandomycin
Methsuximide	Valproate[a]
Methylprednisolone	Verapamil
Nimodipino	Viloxazine
Pancuronium	*Drugs that may decrease carbamazepine plasma concentrations:*
Phensuximide	Carbamazepine (autoinduction)
Phenytoin	Cisplatin
Primidone	Doxorubicin HCl
Theophylline	Felbamate
Valproate	Phenobarbital
Warfarin	Phenytoin
Carbamazepine may increase drug plasma concentrations of:	Primidone
Clomipramine	Rifampin[b]
Phenytoin	Theophylline
Primidone	Valproate

[a]Increased concentrations of the active 10,11-epoxide.
[b]Decreased concentrations of carbamazepine and increased concentrations of the 10,11-epoxide.
Table by Carlos A. Zarate, Jr., M.D., and Mauricio Tohen, M.D.

Drug Interactions. Carbamazepine decreases serum concentrations of numerous drugs as a result of prominent induction of hepatic CYP3A4 (Table 25–23). Monitoring for a decrease in clinical effects is frequently indicated. Carbamazepine can decrease the blood concentrations of oral contraceptives, resulting in breakthrough bleeding and uncertain prophylaxis against pregnancy. Carbamazepine should not be administered with MAOIs, which should be discontinued at least 2 weeks before initiating treatment with carbamazepine. Grapefruit juice inhibits the hepatic metabolism of carbamazepine. When carbamazepine and valproate are used in combination, the dosage of carbamazepine should be decreased because valproate displaces carbamazepine binding on proteins, and the dosage of valproate may need to be increased.

Laboratory Interferences. Circulating levels of thyroxine and triiodothyronine are associated with a decrease in thyroid-stimulating hormone (TSH) and may be associated with treatment. Carbamazepine is also associated with an increase in total serum cholesterol, primarily by increasing high-density lipoproteins. The thyroid and cholesterol effects are not clinically significant. Carbamazepine may interfere with the dexamethasone (Decadron) suppression test and may also cause false-positive pregnancy test results.

Dosing and Administration. The target dose for antimanic activity is 1,200 mg a day, although this varies considerably. Immediate-release carbamazepine needs to be taken three or four times a day, which leads to lapses in compliance. Extended-release formulations are thus preferred because they can be taken once or twice a day. One form of extended-release carbamazepine, Carbatrol, comes as 100-, 200-, and 300-mg capsules. Another form, Equetro, is identical to Carbatrol and is marketed as a treatment for bipolar disorder. Equetro contain tiny beads with three different types of coatings so they dissolve at different times. Capsules should not be crushed or chewed. The contents can be sprinkled over food, however, without affecting the extended-release qualities. This formulation can be taken either with or without meals. The entire daily dose can be given at bedtime. The rate of absorption is faster when it is given with a high-fat meal. Another extended-release form of carbamazepine, Tegretol XR, uses a different drug-delivery system than Carbatrol. It is available in 100-, 200-, and 300-mg tablets.

Preexisting hematologic, hepatic, and cardiac diseases can be relative contraindications for carbamazepine treatment. Persons with hepatic disease require only one-third to one-half the usual dosage; the clinician should be cautious about raising the dosage in such persons and should do so only slowly and gradually. The laboratory examination should include a complete blood count (CBC) with platelet count, liver function tests, serum electrolytes, and an ECG in persons older than 40 years of age or with a preexisting cardiac disease. An electroencephalogram is not necessary before the initiation of treatment, but it may be helpful in some cases for the documentation of objective changes correlated with clinical improvement. Table 25–24 presents a brief user's guide to carbamazepine in bipolar disorder.

Routine Laboratory Monitoring. Serum levels for antimanic efficacy have not been established. The anticonvulsant blood concentration range for carbamazepine is 4 to 12 μg/mL, and this range should be reached before determining that carbamazepine is not effective in the treatment of a mood disorder. A clinically insignificant suppression of the WBC count commonly occurs during carbamazepine treatment. This benign decrease can be reversed by adding lithium, which enhances colony-stimulating factor. Potential serious hematologic effects of carbamazepine, such as pancytopenia, agranulocytosis, and aplastic anemia, occur in about 1 in 125,000 patients. Complete laboratory blood assessments may be performed every 2 weeks for the first 2 months of treatment and quarterly thereafter, but the FDA has revised the package insert for carbamazepine to suggest that blood monitoring be performed at the discretion of the physician. Patients should be informed that fever, sore throat, rash, petechiae, bruising, or unusual bleeding may indicate a hematologic problem and should prompt immediate notification of a

Table 25–24
Carbamazepine in Bipolar Illness: A Brief User's Guide

1. Start with low (200 mg) bedtime dose in depression or euthymia; higher doses (600–800 mg/day in divided doses) in manic inpatients.
2. All bedtime dosing is reasonable with carbamazepine extended-release preparation.
3. Titrate slowly to the individual's response or side effects threshold.
4. Hepatic enzyme CYP450 (3A4) induction and autoinduction occur in 2–3 weeks; slightly higher doses may be needed or tolerated at that time.
5. Warn regarding benign rash, which occurs in 5–10% of those taking the drug; progression to rare, severe rash is unpredictable, so the drug should be discontinued if any rash develops.
6. Benign white blood cell count decreases occur regularly (usually inconsequential).
7. Rarely, agranulocytosis and aplastic anemia may develop (several per million new exposures); warn regarding appearance of fever, sore throat, petechiae, and bleeding gums and to check with physician to obtain an immediate complete blood cell count.
8. Use adequate birth control methods, including higher dosage forms of estrogen (as carbamazepine lowers estrogen levels).
9. Avoid carbamazepine in pregnancy (spina bifida occurs in 0.5%; other severe adverse outcomes occur in about 8%).
10. Some people will respond well to carbamazepine and not other mood stabilizers (lithium) or anticonvulsants (valproic acid).
11. Combination treatment often required to maintain remission and prevent loss of effect via tolerance.
12. Major drug interactions associated with increases in carbamazepine and potential toxicity from 3A4 enzyme inhibition include calcium channel blockers (isradipine and verapamil); erythromycin and related macrolide antibiotics; and valproate.

physician. This approach is probably more effective than is frequent blood monitoring during long-term treatment. It has also been suggested that liver and renal function tests be conducted quarterly, although the benefit of conducting tests this frequently has been questioned. It seems reasonable, however, to assess hematologic status, along with liver and renal functions whenever a routine examination of the person is being conducted. A monitoring protocol is listed in Table 25–25.

Carbamazepine treatment should be discontinued and a consult with a hematologist should be obtained if the following laboratory values are found: total WBC count below 3,000/mm^3, erythrocytes below 4.0×10^6/mm^3, neutrophils below 1,500/mm^3, hematocrit less than 32 percent, hemoglobin less than 11 g/100 mL, platelet count below 100,000/mm^3, reticulocyte count below 0.3 percent, and a serum iron concentration below 150 mg/100 mL.

Oxcarbazepine

Although structurally related to carbamazepine, the usefulness of oxcarbazepine as a treatment for mania has not been established in controlled trials.

Pharmacokinetics. Absorption is rapid and unaffected by food. Peak concentrations occur after about 45 minutes. The elimination half-life of the parent compound is 2 hours, which remains stable over long-term treatment. The monohydroxide has a half-life of 9 hours. Most of the drug's anticonvulsant activity is presumed to result from this monohydroxy derivative.

Side Effects. The most common side effects are sedation and nausea. Less frequent side effects are cognitive impairment, ataxia, diplopia, nystagmus, dizziness, and tremor. In contrast to carbamazepine, oxcarbazepine does not have an increased risk of serious blood dyscrasias, so hematologic monitoring is not necessary. The frequency of benign rash is lower than observed with carbamazepine, and serious rashes are extremely rare. However, about 25 to 30 percent of patients who develop an allergic rash while taking carbamazepine also develop a rash with oxcarbazepine. Oxcarbazepine is more likely to cause hyponatremia than carbamazepine. Approximately 3 to 5 percent of patients taking oxcarbazepine develop this side effect. It is advisable to obtain serum sodium concentrations early in the course of treatment because hyponatremia may be clinically silent. In severe cases, confusion and seizure may occur.

Dosing and Administration. Oxcarbazepine dosing for bipolar disorder has not been established. It is available in 150-, 300-, and 600-mg tablets. The dose range may vary from 150 to 2,400 mg per day given in divided doses twice a day. In clinical trials for mania, the doses typically used were from 900 to 1,200 mg per day with a starting dose of 150 or 300 mg at night.

Drug Interactions. Drugs such as phenobarbital and alcohol, which induce CYP34A, increase the clearance and reduce oxcarbazepine concentrations. Oxcarbazepine induces CYP3A4/5 and inhibits CYP2C19, which may affect the metabolism of drugs that use that pathway. Women taking oral contraceptives should

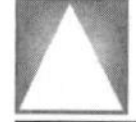

Table 25–25
Laboratory Monitoring of Carbamazepine for Adult Psychiatric Disorders

	Baseline	Weekly to Stability	Monthly for 6 Months	6–12 Months
CBC	+	+	+	+
Bilirubin	+		+	+
Alanine aminotransferase	+		+	+
Aspartate aminotransferase	+		+	+
Alkaline phosphatase	+		+	+
Carbamazepine level	+	+		+

CBC, complete blood count.

be told to consult with their gynecologists because oxcarbazepine may reduce concentrations of their contraceptive and thus decrease its efficacy.

CHOLINESTERASE INHIBITORS AND MEMANTINE

Donepezil (Aricept), rivastigmine (Exelon), and galantamine (Reminyl) are cholinesterase inhibitors used to treat mild to moderate cognitive impairment in dementia of the Alzheimer's type. They reduce the inactivation of the neurotransmitter acetylcholine and, thus, potentiate cholinergic neurotransmission, which in turn produces a modest improvement in memory and goal-directed thought. Memantine (Namenda) is not a cholinesterase inhibitor, producing its effects through blockade of N-methyl-D-aspartate (NMDA) receptors. Unlike the cholinesterase inhibitors, which are indicated for the mild to moderate stages of Alzheimer's disease, memantine is indicated for the moderate to severe stages of the disease. Tacrine (Cognex), the first cholinesterase inhibitor to be introduced, is no longer used because of its multiple daily dosing regimens, its potential for hepatotoxicity, and the consequent need for frequent laboratory monitoring. Routine clinical practice often combines a cholinesterase inhibitor with memantine, and recent studies have shown that this combination may provide beneficial response compared with only cholinesterase inhibitor pharmacotherapy. In December 2014 FDA approved the combination version pill, Memantine hydrochloride extended-release + donepezil hydrochloride (Namzaric). It is specifically indicated for the treatment of moderate to severe dementia of the Alzheimer's type. It is available as a capsule for once daily oral administration and can also be opened to allow the contents to be sprinkled on the food for patient with dysphagia. The most common side effects include diarrhea, dizziness, and headache.

Pharmacological Actions

Donepezil is absorbed completely from the GI tract. Peak plasma concentrations are reached about 3 to 4 hours after oral dosing. The half-life of donepezil is 70 hours in elderly persons, and it is taken only once daily. Steady-state levels are achieved within about 2 weeks. The presence of stable alcoholic cirrhosis reduces clearance of donepezil by 20 percent. Rivastigmine (Exelon) is rapidly and completely absorbed from the GI tract and reaches peak plasma concentrations in 1 hour, but this is delayed by up to 90 minutes if rivastigmine is taken with food. The half-life of rivastigmine is 1 hour, but because it remains bound to cholinesterases, a single dose is therapeutically active for 10 hours, and it is taken twice daily. Galantamine (Reminyl) is an alkaloid similar to codeine and is extracted from daffodils of the plant *Galanthus nivalis.* It is readily absorbed, with maximum concentrations reached after 30 minutes to 2 hours. Food decreases the maximum concentration by 25 percent. The elimination half-life of galantamine is approximately 6 hours.

Tacrine (Cognex) is absorbed rapidly from the GI tract. Peak plasma concentrations are reached about 90 minutes after oral dosing. The half-life of tacrine is about 2 to 4 hours, thereby necessitating four-times-daily dosing.

The primary mechanism of action of cholinesterase inhibitors is reversible, nonacylating inhibition of acetylcholinesterase and butyrylcholinesterase, the enzymes that catabolize acetylcholine in the CNS. The enzyme inhibition increases synaptic concentrations of acetylcholine, especially in the hippocampus and cerebral cortex. Unlike tacrine, which is nonselective for all forms of acetylcholinesterase, donepezil appears to be selectively active within the CNS and has little activity in the periphery. Donepezil's favorable side effect profile appears to correlate with its lack of inhibition of cholinesterases in the GI tract. Rivastigmine appears to have somewhat more peripheral activity than donepezil and is thus more likely to cause GI adverse effects than is donepezil.

Therapeutic Indications

Cholinesterase inhibitors are effective for the treatment of mild to moderate cognitive impairment in dementia of the Alzheimer's type. In long-term use, they slow the progression of memory loss and diminish apathy, depression, hallucinations, anxiety, euphoria, and purposeless motor behaviors. Functional autonomy is less well preserved. Some persons note immediate improvement in memory, mood, psychotic symptoms, and interpersonal skills. Others note little initial benefit but are able to retain their cognitive and adaptive faculties at a relatively stable level for many months. A practical benefit of cholinesterase inhibitor use is a delay or reduction of the need for nursing home placement.

Donepezil and rivastigmine may be beneficial for patients with Parkinson's disease and Lewy body disease and for treatment of cognitive deficits caused by traumatic brain injury. Donepezil is under study for the treatment of mild cognitive impairment that is less severe than that caused by Alzheimer's disease. People with vascular dementia may respond to acetylcholinesterase inhibitors. Occasionally, cholinesterase inhibitors elicit an idiosyncratic catastrophic reaction, with signs of grief and agitation, which is self-limited after the drug is discontinued. Use of cholinesterase inhibitors to improve cognition by nondemented individuals should be discouraged.

Precautions and Adverse Reactions

Donepezil. Donepezil is generally well tolerated at recommended dosages. Fewer than 3 percent of those taking donepezil experience nausea, diarrhea, and vomiting. These mild symptoms are more common with a 10-mg dose than with a 5-mg dose, and when present, they tend to resolve after 3 weeks of continued use. Donepezil may cause weight loss. Donepezil treatment has been infrequently associated with bradyarrhythmias, especially in those with underlying cardiac disease. A small number of persons experience syncope.

Rivastigmine. Rivastigmine is generally well tolerated, but recommended dosages may need to be scaled back in the initial period of treatment to limit GI and CNS adverse effects. These mild symptoms are more common at dosages above 6 mg a day, and when present, they tend to resolve after the dosage is lowered. The most common adverse effects associated with rivastigmine are nausea, vomiting, dizziness, headache, diarrhea, abdominal pain, anorexia, fatigue, and somnolence.

Rivastigmine may cause weight loss, but it does not appear to cause hepatic, renal, hematologic, or electrolyte abnormalities.

Galantamine. The most common side effects of galantamine are dizziness, headache, nausea, vomiting, diarrhea, and anorexia. These side effects tend to be mild and transient.

Tacrine. Tacrine is the least used of the cholinesterase inhibitors but requires more discussion than the others because it is cumbersome to titrate and use, and it poses the risk of potentially significant elevations in hepatic transaminase levels. These increases occur in 25 to 30 percent of persons. Aside from elevated transaminase levels, the most common specific adverse effects associated with tacrine treatment are nausea, vomiting, myalgia, anorexia, and rash, but only nausea, vomiting, and anorexia have been found to have a clear relation to the dosage. Transaminase elevations characteristically develop during the first 6 to 12 weeks of treatment, and cholinergically mediated events are dosage related.

HEPATOTOXICITY. Tacrine is associated with increases in the plasma activities of alanine aminotransferase (ALT) and aspartate aminotransferase (AST). The ALT measurement is the more sensitive indicator of the hepatic effects of tacrine. About 95 percent of patients who develop elevated ALT serum levels do so in the first 18 weeks of treatment. The average length of time for elevated ALT concentrations to return to normal after stopping tacrine treatment is 4 weeks.

For routine monitoring of hepatic enzymes, AST and ALT activities should be measured weekly for the first 18 weeks, every month for the second 4 months, and every 3 months thereafter. Weekly assessments of AST and ALT should be performed for at least 6 weeks after any increase in dosage. Patients with mildly elevated ALT activity should be monitored weekly and not be rechallenged with tacrine until the ALT activity returns to the normal range. For any patient with elevated ALT activity and jaundice, tacrine treatment should be stopped, and the patient should not be given the drug again.

Table 25–26 summarizes the incidence of major adverse side effects associated with each of the cholinesterase inhibitors.

Drug Interactions. All cholinesterase inhibitors should be used cautiously with drugs that also possess cholinomimetic activity, such as succinylcholine (Anectine) and bethanechol (Urecholine). The coadministration of cholinesterase inhibitors and drugs that have cholinergic antagonist activity (e.g., tricyclic drugs) is probably counterproductive. Paroxetine (Paxil) has the most marked anticholinergic effects of any of the newer antidepressant and anxiolytic drugs and should be avoided for that reason, as well as its inhibiting effect on the metabolism of some of the cholinesterase inhibitors.

Donepezil undergoes extensive metabolism via both CYP2D6 and 3A4 isozymes. The metabolism of donepezil may be increased by phenytoin (Dilantin), carbamazepine (Tegretol), dexamethasone (Decadron), rifampin (Rifadin), and phenobarbital (Solfoton). Commonly used agents such as paroxetine, ketoconazole (Nizoral), and erythromycin can significantly increase donepezil concentrations. Donepezil is highly protein bound, but it does not displace other protein-bound drugs, such as furosemide (Lasix), digoxin (Lanoxin), or warfarin (Coumadin). Rivastigmine circulates mostly unbound to serum proteins and has no significant drug interactions.

Similar to donepezil, galantamine is metabolized by both CYP2D6 and 3A4 isozymes and thus may interact with drugs that inhibit these pathways. Paroxetine and ketoconazole should be used with great caution.

Laboratory Interferences. No laboratory interferences have been associated with the use of cholinesterase inhibitors.

Dosage and Clinical Guidelines. Before initiation of cholinesterase inhibitor therapy, potentially treatable causes of dementia should be ruled out and the diagnosis of dementia of the Alzheimer's type established.

Donepezil is available in 5- and 10-mg tablets. Treatment should be initiated at 5 mg each night. If well tolerated and of some discernible benefit after 4 weeks, the dosage should be increased to a maintenance dosage of 10-mg each night. Donepezil absorption is unaffected by meals.

Rivastigmine is available in 1.5-, 3-, 4.5-, and 6-mg capsules. The recommended initial dosage is 1.5 mg twice daily for a minimum of 2 weeks, after which increases of 1.5 mg a day can be made at intervals of at least 2 weeks to a target dosage of 6 mg a day, taken in two equal dosages. If tolerated, the dosage may be further titrated upward to a maximum of 6 mg twice daily. The risk of adverse GI events can be reduced by administration of rivastigmine with food.

Galantamine is available in 4-, 8-, and 16-mg tablets. The suggested dose range is 16 to 32 mg per day given twice a day. The higher dose is actually better tolerated than the lower dose. The initial dosage is 8 mg per day, and after a minimum of 4 weeks, the dose can be raised. All subsequent dosage increases should occur at 4-week intervals and should be based on tolerability.

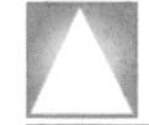

Table 25–26
Incidence of Major Adverse Side Effects with Cholinesterase Inhibitors (%)

Drug	Dose (mg/day)	Nausea	Vomiting	Diarrhea	Dizziness	Muscle Cramps	Insomnia
Donepezil	5	4	3	9	15	9	7
Donepezil	10	17	10	17	13	12	8
Rivastigmine	1–4	14	7	10	15	NR	NR
Rivastigmine	6–12	48	27	17	24	NR	NR
Galantamine	8	5.7	3.6	5	NR	NR	NR
Galantamine	16	13.3	6.1	12.2	NR	NR	NR
Galantamine	24	16.5	9.9	5.5	NR	NR	NR

NR, not reported from clinical trial data; incidence less than 5%.

Tacrine is available in 10-, 20-, 30-, and 40-mg capsules. Before the initiation of tacrine treatment, a complete physical and laboratory examination should be conducted, with special attention to liver function tests and baseline hematologic indexes. Treatment should be initiated at 10 mg four times a day and then raised by increments of 10 mg a dose every 6 weeks up to 160 mg a day; the person's tolerance of each dosage is indicated by the absence of unacceptable side effects and lack of elevation of ALT activity. Tacrine should be given four times daily—ideally 1 hour before meals because the absorption of tacrine is reduced by about 25 percent when it is taken during the first 2 hours after meals. If tacrine is used, the specific guidelines for tacrine-induced ALT listed above should be followed.

Memantine

Pharmacological Actions. Memantine is well absorbed after oral administration, with peak concentrations reached in about 3 to 7 hours. Food has no effect on the absorption of memantine. Memantine has linear pharmacokinetics over the therapeutic dosage range and has a terminal elimination half-life of about 60 to 80 hours. Plasma protein binding is 45 percent.

Memantine undergoes little metabolism, with the majority (57 to 82 percent) of an administered dose excreted unchanged in urine; the remainder is converted primarily to three polar metabolites: the N-gludantan conjugate, 6-hydroxy memantine, and 1-nitroso-deaminated memantine. These metabolites possess minimal NMDA receptor antagonist activity. Memantine is a low- to moderate-affinity NMDA receptor antagonist. It is thought that overexcitation of NMDA receptors by the neurotransmitter glutamate may play a role in Alzheimer's disease because glutamate plays an integral role in the neural pathways associated with learning and memory. Excess glutamate overstimulates NMDA receptors to allow too much calcium into nerve cells, leading to the eventual cell death observed in Alzheimer's disease. Memantine may protect cells against excess glutamate by partially blocking NMDA receptors associated with abnormal transmission of glutamate while allowing for physiologic transmission associated with normal cell functioning.

Therapeutic Indications. Memantine is the only approved therapy in the United States for moderate to severe Alzheimer's disease.

Precautions and Adverse Reactions. Memantine is safe and well tolerated. The most common adverse effects are dizziness, headache, constipation, and confusion. The use of memantine in patients with severe renal impairment is not recommended. In a documented case of an overdose with up to 400 mg of memantine, the patient experienced restlessness, psychosis, visual hallucinations, somnolence, stupor, and loss of consciousness. The patient recovered without permanent sequelae.

Drug Interactions. In vitro studies conducted with marker substrates of CYP450 enzymes (CYP1A2, 2A6, 2C9, 2D6, 2E1, and 3A4) showed minimal inhibition of these enzymes by memantine. No pharmacokinetic interactions with drugs metabolized by these enzymes are expected.

Because memantine is eliminated in part by tubular secretion, coadministration of drugs that use the same renal cationic system, including hydrochlorothiazide triamterene (Dyrenium), cimetidine (Tagamet), ranitidine (Zantac), quinidine, and nicotine, could potentially result in altered plasma levels of both agents. Coadministration of memantine and a combination of hydrochlorothiazide and triamterene did not affect the bioavailability of either memantine or triamterene, and the bioavailability of hydrochlorothiazide decreased by 20 percent.

Urine pH is altered by diet, drugs (e.g., carbonic anhydrase inhibitors, topiramate [Topamax], sodium bicarbonate), and the clinical state of the patient (e.g., renal tubular acidosis or severe infections of the urinary tract). The clearance of memantine is reduced by about 80 percent under alkaline urine conditions at pH 8. Therefore, alterations of urine pH toward the alkaline condition may lead to an accumulation of the drug with a possible increase in adverse effects. Hence, memantine should be used with caution under these conditions.

Laboratory Interferences. No laboratory interferences have been associated with the use of memantine.

Dosage and Clinical Guidelines. Memantine is available in 5- and 10-mg tablets, with a recommended starting dose of 5 mg daily. The recommended target dose is 20 mg per day. The drug is administered twice daily in separate doses with 5-mg increment increases weekly depending on tolerability.

Patients with mild to moderate disease receiving memantine in combination with a cholinesterase inhibitor have not been found to experience significantly greater benefit in cognition or overall function than those who receive a cholinesterase inhibitor alone.

DISULFIRAM AND ACAMPROSATE

Disulfiram (Antabuse) and acamprosate (Campral) are drugs used to treat alcohol dependence. Disulfiram has suffered from a reputation as a dangerous medication only suitable for highly motivated and strictly supervised drinkers because of the severe physical reactions the drug causes after drinking. Experience has shown, however, that at recommended doses it is an acceptable and safe medication for dependent drinkers seeking to sustain abstinence. The properties that constitute disulfiram's main therapeutic effect (i.e., the ability to produce unpleasant symptoms after alcohol intake, also known as disulfiram–alcohol reaction) have created that perception of dangerousness.

In the most severe cases, when disulfiram is combined with alcohol serious clinical conditions can occur. These include respiratory depression, cardiovascular collapse, acute heart failure, convulsions, loss of consciousness, and death in rare cases. These potential complications as well as the development of alternative antialcohol medications have been the limiting factors for the wider use of disulfiram. Unlike disulfiram, acamprosate, the other drug discussed in this section, does not produce aversive side effects. Acamprosate is now prescribed more commonly than disulfiram in outpatient settings, but disulfiram is prescribed more often in inpatient settings because it helps facilitate initial abstinence.

Other drugs that are useful in reducing alcohol consumption include naltrexone (ReVia, Trexan), nalmefene (Revex), topiramate (Topamax), and gabapentin (Neurontin). These agents are discussed in their respective sections.

Disulfiram

Pharmacological Actions. Disulfiram is almost completely absorbed from the GI tract after oral administration. Its half-life is estimated to be 60 to 120 hours. Therefore, 1 or 2 weeks may be needed before disulfiram is totally eliminated from the body after the last dose has been taken.

The metabolism of ethanol proceeds through oxidation via alcohol dehydrogenase to the formation of acetaldehyde, which is further metabolized to acetyl-coenzyme A (acetyl-CoA) by aldehyde dehydrogenase. Disulfiram is an aldehyde dehydrogenase inhibitor that interferes with the metabolism of alcohol by producing a marked increase in blood acetaldehyde concentration. The accumulation of acetaldehyde (to a level up to 10 times higher than occurs in the normal metabolism of alcohol) produces a wide array of unpleasant reactions, called the *disulfiram–alcohol reaction,* characterized by nausea, throbbing headache, vomiting, hypertension, flushing, sweating, thirst, dyspnea, tachycardia, chest pain, vertigo, and blurred vision. The reaction occurs almost immediately after the ingestion of one alcoholic drink and may last from 30 minutes to 2 hours.

Blood Concentrations in Relation to Action. Plasma concentrations of disulfiram vary among individuals because of a number of factors, most notably age and hepatic function. In general, the severity of disulfiram–alcohol reaction has been shown to be proportional to the amount of the ingested disulfiram and alcohol. Nevertheless, disulfiram plasma levels are rarely obtained in clinical practice. The positive correlation between plasma concentrations of alcohol and the intensity of the reaction is described as follows: in sensitive individuals, as little as 5 to 10 mg per 100 mL increase of the plasma alcohol level may produce mild symptoms; fully developed symptoms occur at alcohol levels of 50 mg per 100 mL; and levels as high as 125 to 150 mg per 100 mL result in loss of consciousness and coma.

Therapeutic Indications. The primary indication for disulfiram use is as an aversive conditioning treatment for alcohol dependence. Either the fear of having a disulfiram–alcohol reaction or the memory of having had one is meant to condition the person not to use alcohol. Usually, describing the severity and the unpleasantness of the disulfiram–alcohol reaction graphically enough discourages the person from imbibing alcohol. Disulfiram treatment should be combined with such treatments as psychotherapy, group therapy, and support groups such as Alcoholics Anonymous (AA). Treatment with disulfiram requires careful monitoring because a person can simply decide not to take the medication.

Precautions and Adverse Reactions

WITH ALCOHOL CONSUMPTION. The intensity of the disulfiram–alcohol reaction varies with each person. In extreme cases, it is marked by respiratory depression, cardiovascular collapse, myocardial infarction, convulsions, and death. Therefore, disulfiram is contraindicated for persons with significant pulmonary or cardiovascular disease. In addition, disulfiram should be used with caution, if at all, by persons with nephritis, brain damage, hypothyroidism, diabetes, hepatic disease, seizures, polydrug dependence, or an abnormal electroencephalogram. Most fatal reactions occur in persons who take more than 500 mg a day of disulfiram and who consume more than 3 oz of alcohol. The treatment of a severe disulfiram–alcohol reaction is primarily supportive to prevent shock. The use of oxygen, intravenous vitamin C, ephedrine, and antihistamines has been reported to aid in recovery.

WITHOUT ALCOHOL CONSUMPTION. The adverse effects of disulfiram in the absence of alcohol consumption include fatigue, dermatitis, impotence, optic neuritis, a variety of mental changes, and hepatic damage. A metabolite of disulfiram inhibits dopamine-β-hydroxylase, the enzyme that metabolizes dopamine into norepinephrine and epinephrine, and thus may exacerbate psychosis in persons with psychotic disorders. Catatonic reactions may also occur.

Drug Interactions. Disulfiram increases the blood concentration of diazepam (Valium), paraldehyde, phenytoin (Dilantin), caffeine, tetrahydrocannabinol (the active ingredient in marijuana), barbiturates, anticoagulants, isoniazid (Nydrazid), and tricyclic drugs. Disulfiram should not be administered concomitantly with paraldehyde because paraldehyde is metabolized to acetaldehyde in the liver.

Laboratory Interferences. In rare instances, disulfiram has been reported to interfere with the incorporation of iodine-131 into protein-bound iodine. Disulfiram may reduce urinary concentrations of homovanillic acid, the major metabolite of dopamine, because of its inhibition of dopamine hydroxylase.

Dosage and Clinical Guidelines. Disulfiram is supplied in 250- and 500-mg tablets. The usual initial dosage is 500 mg a day taken by mouth for the first 1 or 2 weeks followed by a maintenance dosage of 250 mg a day. The dosage should not exceed 500 mg a day. The maintenance dosage range is 125 to 500 mg a day.

Persons taking disulfiram must be instructed that the ingestion of even the smallest amount of alcohol will bring on a disulfiram–alcohol reaction, with all of its unpleasant effects. In addition, persons should be warned against ingesting any alcohol-containing preparations, such as cough drops, tonics of any kind, and alcohol-containing foods and sauces. Some reactions have occurred in patients who used alcohol-based lotions, toilet water, colognes, or perfumes and inhaled the fumes; therefore, precautions must be explicit and should include any topically applied preparations containing alcohol, such as perfume.

Disulfiram should not be administered until the person has abstained from alcohol for at least 12 hours. Persons should be warned that the disulfiram–alcohol reaction may occur as long as 1 or 2 weeks after the last dose of disulfiram. Persons taking disulfiram should carry identification cards describing the disulfiram–alcohol reaction and listing the name and telephone number of the physician to be called.

Acamprosate

Pharmacological Actions. Acamprosate's mechanism of action is not fully understood, but it is thought to antagonize neuronal overactivity related to the actions of the excitatory neurotransmitter glutamate. In part, this may result from antagonism of N-methyl-D-aspartate (NMDA) receptors.

Indications. Acamprosate is used for treating alcohol-dependent individuals seeking to continue to remain alcohol free after they have stopped drinking. Its efficacy in promoting abstinence has not been demonstrated in persons who have not undergone detoxification and who have not achieved alcohol abstinence before beginning treatment.

Precautions and Adverse Effects. Side effects are mostly seen early in treatment and are usually mild and transient in nature. The most common side effects are headache, diarrhea, flatulence, abdominal pain, paresthesias, and various skin reactions. No adverse events occur after abrupt withdrawal of acamprosate, even after long-term use. There is no evidence of addiction to the drug. Patients with severe renal impairment (creatinine clearance of less than 30 mL per minute) should not be given acamprosate.

Drug Interactions. The concomitant intake of alcohol and acamprosate does not affect the pharmacokinetics of either alcohol or acamprosate. Administration of disulfiram or diazepam does not affect the pharmacokinetics of acamprosate. Coadministration of naltrexone with acamprosate produces an increase in concentrations of acamprosate. No adjustment of dosage is recommended in such patients. The pharmacokinetics of naltrexone and its major metabolite 6-β-naltrexol were unaffected after coadministration with acamprosate. During clinical trials, patients taking acamprosate concomitantly with antidepressants more commonly reported both weight gain and weight loss compared with patients taking either medication alone.

Laboratory Interferences. Acamprosate has not been shown to interfere with commonly done laboratory tests.

Dosage and Clinical Guidelines. It is important to remember that acamprosate should not be used to treat alcohol withdrawal symptoms. It should only be started after the individual has been successfully weaned off alcohol. Patients should show a commitment to remaining abstinent, and treatment should be part of a comprehensive management program that includes counseling or support group attendance.

Each tablet contains acamprosate calcium 333 mg, which is equivalent to 300 mg of acamprosate. The dose of acamprosate is different for different patients. The recommended dosage is two 333-mg tablets (each dose should total 666 mg) taken three times daily. Although dosing may be done without regard to meals, dosing with meals was used during clinical trials and is suggested as an aid to compliance in patients who regularly eat three meals daily. A lower dose may be effective in some patients. A missed dose should be taken as soon as possible. However, if it is almost time for the next dose, the missed dose should be skipped, and then the regular dosing schedule should be resumed. Doses should not be doubled up. For patients with moderate renal impairment (creatinine clearance of 30- to 50-mL minute), a starting dosage of one 333-mg tablet taken three times daily is recommended. People with severe renal insufficiency should not take acamprosate.

DOPAMINE RECEPTOR AGONISTS AND PRECURSORS

Dopamine agonists activate dopamine receptors in the absence of endogenous dopamine and have been widely used to treat idiopathic Parkinson's disease, hyperprolactinemia, and certain pituitary tumors (prolactinoma). Because dopamine stimulates the heart and increases blood flow to the liver, kidneys, and other organs, low levels of dopamine are associated with low BP and low cardiac input. Dopamine agonist drugs are also administered to treat shock and congestive heart failure.

Their use in psychiatry has been limited to treat such adverse effects of antipsychotic drugs as parkinsonism, extrapyramidal symptoms, akinesia, focal perioral tremors, hyperprolactinemia, galactorrhea, and neuroleptic malignant syndrome. The drugs in this class most commonly prescribed are bromocriptine (Parlodel), levodopa (also called L-Dopa; Larodopa), carbidopa-levodopa (Sinemet), and amantadine (Symmetrel). Amantadine is used primarily for the treatment of medication-induced movement disorders, such as neuroleptic-induced parkinsonism. It is also used as an antiviral agent for the prophylaxis and treatment of influenza A infection and Cotard's syndrome, a rare neuropsychiatric disorder in which a person holds a delusional belief that he or she is dead. There are also a few reports of amantadine's role in augmenting antidepressant medications in patients with treatment-resistant depression.

New dopamine receptor agonists include ropinirole (Requip), pramipexole (Mirapex), apomorphine (Apokyn), and pergolide (Permax). Of these drugs, pramipexole is the most widely prescribed in psychiatry as an augmenter of antidepressants. In 2007, pergolide was removed from the market because of the risk of serious damage to patients' heart valves. In 2012, the FDA notified health care professionals about a possible increased risk of heart failure with pramipexole. This warning was based on studies that suggested a potential risk of heart failure; however, further review is required because of study limitations.

Pharmacological Actions

L-Dopa is rapidly absorbed after oral administration, and peak plasma levels are reached after 30 to 120 minutes. The half-life of L-Dopa is 90 minutes. Absorption of L-Dopa can be significantly reduced by changes in gastric pH and by ingestion with meals. Bromocriptine and ropinirole are rapidly absorbed but undergo first-pass metabolism such that only about 30 to 55 percent of the dose is bioavailable. Peak concentrations are achieved 1.5 to 3 hours after oral administration. The half-life of ropinirole is 6 hours. Pramipexole is rapidly absorbed with little first-pass metabolism and reaches peak concentrations in 2 hours. Its half-life is 8 hours. Oral forms of apomorphine have been studied, but this form is not available in the United States. Subcutaneous apomorphine injection results in rapid and controlled systemic delivery, with linear pharmacokinetics over a dose ranging from 2 to 8 mg.

After L-Dopa enters the dopaminergic neurons of the CNS, it is converted into the neurotransmitter dopamine. Apomorphine, bromocriptine, ropinirole, and pramipexole act directly on dopamine receptors. L-Dopa, pramipexole, and ropinirole bind about 20 times more selectively to dopamine D_3 than D_2 receptors; the corresponding ratio for bromocriptine is less than

2 to 1. Apomorphine binds selectively to D_1 and D_2 receptors, with little affinity for D_3 and D_4 receptors. L-Dopa, pramipexole, and ropinirole have no significant activity at nondopaminergic receptors, but bromocriptine binds to serotonin 5-HT_1 and 5-HT_2 and α_1-, α_2-, and β-adrenergic receptors.

Therapeutic Indications

Medication-Induced Movement Disorders. In present-day clinical psychiatry, dopamine receptor agonists are used for the treatment of medication-induced parkinsonism, extrapyramidal symptoms, akinesia, and focal perioral tremors. Their use has diminished sharply, however, because the incidence of medication-induced movement disorders is much lower with the use of the newer, atypical antipsychotics (SDAs). Dopamine receptor agonists are effective in treating idiopathic restless legs syndrome and may also be helpful when this is a medication side effect. Ropinirole has an indication for restless legs syndrome.

For the treatment of medication-induced movement disorders, most clinicians rely on anticholinergics, amantadine, and antihistamines because they are equally effective and have few adverse effects. Bromocriptine remains in use in the treatment of neuroleptic malignant syndrome; however, the incidence of this disorder is diminishing with the decreased use of DRAs.

Dopamine receptor agonists are also used to counteract the hyperprolactinemic effects of DRAs, which result in the side effects of amenorrhea and galactorrhea.

Mood Disorders. Bromocriptine has long been used to enhance response to antidepressant drugs in refractory patients. Ropinirole has been reported to be useful as augmentation to antidepressant therapy and as a treatment for medication-resistant bipolar II depression. Ropinirole may also be helpful in the treatment of antidepressant-induced sexual dysfunction. Pramipexole is often used in the augmentation of antidepressants in treatment-resistant depression. Some studies have found pramipexole to be superior to sertraline (Zoloft) in the treatment of depression in Parkinson's disease, as well as reducing anhedonia in Parkinson's patients.

Sexual Dysfunction. Dopamine receptor agonists improve erectile dysfunction in some patients. However, they are rarely used because they frequently cause adverse effects at therapeutic dosages. PDE-5 inhibitor agents are better tolerated and more effective.

Precautions and Adverse Reactions

Adverse effects are common with dopamine receptor agonists, thus limiting the usefulness of these drugs. Adverse effects are dosage dependent and include nausea, vomiting, orthostatic hypotension, headache, dizziness, and cardiac arrhythmias. To reduce the risk of orthostatic hypotension, the initial dosage of all dopamine receptor agonists should be quite low, with incremental increases at intervals of at least 1 week. These drugs should be used with caution in persons with hypertension, cardiovascular disease, and hepatic disease. After long-term use, persons, particularly elderly persons, may experience choreiform and dystonic movements and psychiatric disturbances—including hallucinations, delusions, confusion, depression, and mania—and other behavioral changes.

Long-term use of bromocriptine can produce retroperitoneal and pulmonary fibrosis, pleural effusions, and pleural thickening.

In general, ropinirole and pramipexole have a similar but milder adverse effect profile than L-Dopa and bromocriptine. Pramipexole and ropinirole may cause irresistible sleep attacks that occur suddenly without warning and have caused motor vehicle accidents.

The most common adverse effects of apomorphine are yawning, dizziness, nausea, vomiting, drowsiness, bradycardia, syncope, and perspiration. Hallucinations have also been reported. Apomorphine's sedative effects are exacerbated with concurrent use of alcohol or other CNS depressants.

Dopamine receptor agonists are contraindicated during pregnancy, especially for nursing mothers, because they inhibit lactation.

Drug Interactions

DRAs are capable of reversing the effects of dopamine receptor agonists, but this is not usually clinically significant. The concurrent use of tricyclic drugs and dopamine receptor agonists has been reported to cause symptoms of neurotoxicity, such as rigidity, agitation, and tremor. They may also potentiate the hypotensive effects of diuretics and other antihypertensive medications. Dopamine receptor agonists should not be used in conjunction with MAOIs, including selegiline (Eldepryl), and MAOIs should be discontinued at least 2 weeks before the initiation of dopamine receptor agonist therapy.

Benzodiazepines, phenytoin (Dilantin), and pyridoxine may interfere with the therapeutic effects of dopamine receptor agonists. Ergot alkaloids and bromocriptine should not be used concurrently because they may cause hypertension and myocardial infarction. Progestins, estrogens, and oral contraceptives may interfere with the effects of bromocriptine and may raise plasma concentrations of ropinirole. Ciprofloxacin (Cipro) can raise plasma concentrations of ropinirole, and cimetidine (Tagamet) can raise plasma concentrations of pramipexole.

Laboratory Interferences

L-Dopa administration has been associated with false reports of elevated serum and urinary uric acid concentrations, urinary glucose test results, urinary ketone test results, and urinary catecholamine concentrations. No laboratory interferences have been associated with the administration of the other dopamine receptor agonists.

Dosage and Clinical Guidelines

Table 25–27 lists the various dopamine receptor agonists and their formulations. For the treatment of antipsychotic-induced parkinsonism, the clinician should start with a 100-mg dose of levodopa three times a day, which may be increased until the person is functionally improved. The maximum dosage of L-Dopa is 2,000 mg a day, but most persons respond to dosages below 1,000 mg per day. The dosage of the carbidopa component of the L-Dopa-carbidopa formulation should total at least 75 mg a day.

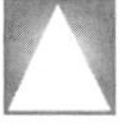

Table 25–27
Available Preparations of Dopamine Receptor Agonists and Carbidopa

Generic Name	Trade Name	Preparations
Amantadine	Symmetrel	100-mg capsule, 50-mg/5-mL syrup (teaspoon)
Bromocriptine	Parlodel	2.5-, 5-mg tablets
Carbidopa	Lodosyn	25 mg[a]
Levodopa (L-Dopa)	Larodopa	100-, 250-, 500-mg tablets
Levodopa-carbidopa (co-careldopa)	Sinemet, Atamet	100/10-mg, 100/25-mg, 250/25-mg tablets; 100/25-, 200/50-mg extended-release tablets
Pramipexole	Mirapex	0.125-, 0.375-, 0.75-, 1.5-, 3-, 4-mg extended-release tablets
Ropinirole	Requip	0.25-, 0.5-, 1-, 2-, 5-mg tablets

[a]Drug only available directly through the manufacturer.

The dosage of bromocriptine for mental disorders is uncertain, although it seems prudent to begin with low dosages (1.25 mg twice daily) and to increase the dosage gradually. Bromocriptine is usually taken with meals to help reduce the likelihood of nausea.

The starting dosage of pramipexole is 0.125 mg three times daily, which is increased to 0.25 mg three times daily in the second week and is increased by 0.25 mg per dose each week until therapeutic benefit or adverse effects emerge. Persons with idiopathic Parkinson's disease usually experience benefit at total daily doses of 1.5 mg, and the maximum daily dose is 4.5 mg.

For ropinirole, the starting dosage is 0.25 mg three times daily and is increased by 0.25 mg per dose each week to a total daily dose of 3 mg, then by 0.5 mg per dose each week to a total daily dose of 9 mg, and then by 1 mg per dose each week to a maximum dosage of 24 mg a day until therapeutic benefit or adverse effects emerge. The average daily dose for persons with idiopathic Parkinson's disease is about 16 mg.

The recommended subcutaneous dose of apomorphine in Parkinson's disease is 0.2 to 0.6 mL subcutaneously during acute hypomobility episodes delivered via metered injector pen. Apomorphine can be administered three times daily, with a maximum dose of 0.6 mL five times daily.

Amantadine

Amantadine is an antiviral drug used for the prophylaxis and treatment of influenza. It was found to have antiparkinsonian properties and is now used to treat that disorder as well as akinesias and other extrapyramidal signs, including focal perioral tremors (rabbit syndrome).

Pharmacological Actions. Amantadine is well absorbed from the GI tract after oral administration, reaches peak plasma concentrations in approximately 2 to 3 hours, has a half-life of about 12 to 18 hours, and attains steady-state concentrations after approximately 4 to 5 days of therapy. Amantadine is excreted unmetabolized in the urine. Amantadine plasma concentrations can be twice as high in elderly persons as in younger adults. Patients with renal failure accumulate amantadine in their bodies.

Amantadine augments dopaminergic neurotransmission in the CNS; however, the precise mechanism for the effect is unknown. The mechanism may involve dopamine release from presynaptic vesicles, blocking reuptake of dopamine into presynaptic nerve terminals, or an agonist effect on postsynaptic dopamine receptors.

Therapeutic Indications. The primary indication for amantadine use in psychiatry is to treat extrapyramidal signs and symptoms, such as parkinsonism, akinesia, and rabbit syndrome (focal perioral tremor of the choreoathetoid type) caused by the administration of DRA or SDA drugs. Amantadine is as effective as the anticholinergics (e.g., benztropine [Cogentin]) for these indications and results in improvement in approximately half of all persons who take it. Amantadine, however, is not generally considered as effective as the anticholinergics for the treatment of acute dystonic reactions and is not effective in treating tardive dyskinesia and akathisia.

Amantadine is a reasonable compromise for persons with extrapyramidal symptoms who would be sensitive to additional anticholinergic effects, particularly those taking a low-potency DRA or the elderly. Elderly persons are susceptible to anticholinergic adverse effects, both in the CNS, such as anticholinergic delirium, and in the peripheral nervous system, such as urinary retention. Amantadine is associated with less memory impairment than are the anticholinergics.

Amantadine has been reported to be of benefit in treating some SSRI–associated side effects, such as lethargy, fatigue, anorgasmia, and ejaculatory inhibition.

Amantadine is used in general medical practice for the treatment of parkinsonism of all causes, including idiopathic parkinsonism.

Precautions and Adverse Effects. The most common CNS effects of amantadine are mild dizziness, insomnia, and impaired concentration (dosage related), which occur in 5 to 10 percent of all persons. Irritability, depression, anxiety, dysarthria, and ataxia occur in 1 to 5 percent of all persons. More severe CNS adverse effects, including seizures and psychotic symptoms, have been reported. Nausea is the most common peripheral adverse effect of amantadine. Headache, loss of appetite, and blotchy spots on the skin have also been reported.

Livedo reticularis of the legs (a purple discoloration of the skin caused by dilation of blood vessels) has been reported in up to 5 percent of persons who take the drug for longer than 1 month. It usually diminishes with elevation of the legs and resolves in almost all cases when drug use is terminated.

Amantadine is relatively contraindicated in persons with renal disease or a seizure disorder. Amantadine should be used with caution in persons with edema or cardiovascular disease. Some evidence indicates that amantadine is teratogenic and therefore should not be taken by pregnant women. Because amantadine is excreted in breast milk, women who are breastfeeding should not take the drug.

Suicide attempts with amantadine overdosages are life-threatening. Symptoms can include toxic psychoses (confusion, hallucinations, aggressiveness) and cardiopulmonary arrest. Emergency treatment beginning with gastric lavage is indicated.

Drug Interactions. Coadministration of amantadine with phenelzine (Nardil) or other MAOIs can result in a significant increase in resting BP. The coadministration of amantadine with CNS stimulants can result in insomnia, irritability, nervousness, and possibly seizures or irregular heartbeat. Amantadine should not be coadministered with anticholinergics because unwanted side effects—such as confusion, hallucinations, nightmares, dry mouth, and blurred vision—may be exacerbated.

Dosage and Clinical Guidelines. Amantadine is available in 100-mg capsules and as a 50-mg per 5-mL syrup. The usual starting dosage of amantadine is 100 mg given orally twice a day, although the dosage can be cautiously increased up to 200 mg given orally twice a day if indicated. Amantadine should be used in persons with renal impairment *only* in consultation with the physician treating the renal condition. If amantadine is successful in the treatment of the drug-induced extrapyramidal symptoms, it should be continued for 4 to 6 weeks and then discontinued to see whether the person has become tolerant to the neurological adverse effects of the antipsychotic medication. Amantadine should be tapered over 1 to 2 weeks after a decision has been made to discontinue the drug. Persons taking amantadine should not drink alcoholic beverages.

DOPAMINE RECEPTOR ANTAGONISTS (FIRST-GENERATION ANTIPSYCHOTICS)

The DRAs represent the first group of effective agents for schizophrenia and other psychotic illnesses. The first of these drugs, the phenothiazine chlorpromazine (Thorazine), was introduced in the early 1950s. Other DRAs include all of the antipsychotics in the following groups: phenothiazines, butyrophenones, thioxanthenes, dibenzoxazepines, dihydroindoles, and diphenylbutylpiperidines. Because these agents are associated with extrapyramidal syndromes (EPSs) at clinically effective dosages, newer antipsychotic drugs—the SDAs—have gradually replaced the older agents in the United States. The SDAs are differentiated from earlier drugs by their lower liability to cause EPS. These newer drugs have other liabilities, most notably a propensity to cause weight gain, lipid elevations, and diabetes. Therefore, a reason to still consider use of the DRAs is their lower risk of causing significant metabolic abnormalities. Intermediate-potency DRAs, such as perphenazine (Trilafon), have been shown to be as effective and well tolerated as the SDAs. Manufacturing of molindone (Moban), the DRA with the lowest risk of weight gain and metabolic side effects, was discontinued in the United States.

Pharmacological Actions

All of the DRAs are well absorbed after oral administration, with liquid preparations being absorbed more efficiently than tablets or capsules. Peak plasma concentrations are usually reached 1 to 4 hours after oral administration and 30 to 60 minutes after parenteral administration. Smoking, coffee, antacids, and food interfere with absorption of these drugs. Steady-state levels are reached in approximately 3 to 5 days. The half-lives of these drugs are approximately 24 hours. All can be given in one daily oral dose, if tolerated, after the patient is in a stable condition. Most DRAs are highly protein bound. Parenteral formulation of the DRAs results in a more rapid and more reliable onset of action. Bioavailability is also up to 10-fold higher with parenteral administration. Most DRAs are metabolized by cytochrome P450 (CYP) CYP2D6 and 3A isozymes. However, there are differences among the specific agents.

Long-acting depot parenteral formulations of haloperidol (Haldol, Decanoate) and fluphenazine are available in the United States. These agents are usually administered once every 1 to 4 weeks, depending on the dose and the patient. It can take up to 6 months of treatment with depot formulations to reach steady-state plasma levels, indicating that oral therapy should be continued during the first month or so of depot antipsychotic treatment.

Antipsychotic activity derives from inhibition of dopaminergic neurotransmission. The DRAs are effective when approximately 72 percent of dopamine D_2 receptors in the brain are occupied. The DRAs also block noradrenergic, cholinergic, and histaminergic receptors, with different drugs having different effects on these receptor systems.

Some generalizations can be made about the DRAs based on their potency. Potency refers to the amount of drug that is required to achieve therapeutic effects. Low-potency drugs such as chlorpromazine and thioridazine (Mellaril), given in doses of several 100 mg per day, typically produce more weight gain and sedation than high-potency agents such as haloperidol and fluphenazine, usually given in doses of less than 10 mg per day. High-potency agents are also more likely to cause EPS. Some factors influencing the pharmacological actions of DRAs are listed in Table 25–28.

Therapeutic Indications

Many types of psychiatric and neurological disorders may benefit from treatment with DRAs. Some of these indications are shown in Table 25–29.

Schizophrenia and Schizoaffective Disorder. The DRAs are effective in both the short-term and long-term

Table 25–28
Factors Influencing the Pharmacokinetics of Antipsychotics

Age	Elderly patients may demonstrate reduced clearance rates.
Medical condition	Decreased hepatic blood flow can reduce clearance.
	Hepatic disease can decrease clearance.
Enzyme inducers	Carbamazepine, phenytoin, ethambutol, barbiturates.
Clearance inhibitors	Include SSRIs, TCAs, cimetidine, β-blockers, isoniazid, methylphenidate, erythromycin, triazolobenzodiazepines, ciprofloxacin, and ketoconazole.
Changes in binding protein	Hypoalbuminemia can occur with malnutrition or hepatic failure.

SSRI, selective serotonin reuptake inhibitor; TCA, tricyclic antidepressant.
Adapted from Ereshefsky L. Pharmacokinetics and drug interactions: Update for new antipsychotics. *J Clin Psychiatry*. 1996;57(Suppl 1)1:12–25.

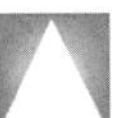

Table 25–29
Indications for Dopamine Receptor Antagonists

Acute psychotic episodes in schizophrenia and schizoaffective disorder
Maintenance treatment in schizophrenia and schizoaffective disorders
Mania
Depression with psychotic symptoms
Delusional disorder
Borderline personality disorder
Substance-induced psychotic disorder
Delirium and dementia
Mental disorders caused by a medical condition
Childhood schizophrenia
Pervasive developmental disorder
Tourette's disorder
Huntington's disease

management of schizophrenia and schizoaffective disorder. They both reduce acute symptoms and prevent future exacerbations. These agents produce their most dramatic effects against the positive symptoms of schizophrenia (e.g., hallucinations, delusions, and agitation). Negative symptoms (e.g., emotional withdrawal and ambivalence) are less likely to improve significantly, and they may appear to worsen, because these drugs produce constriction of facial expression and akinesia, side effects that mimic negative symptoms.

Schizophrenia and schizoaffective disorder are characterized by remission and relapse. DRAs decrease the risk of reemergence of psychosis in patients who have recovered while on medication. After a first episode of psychosis, patients should be maintained on medication for 1 to 2 years; after multiple episodes, for 2 to 5 years.

Mania. DRAs are effective for treating psychotic symptoms of acute mania. Because antimanic agents (e.g., lithium) generally have a slower onset of action than do antipsychotics in the treatment of acute symptoms, it is standard practice to initially combine either a DRA or an SDA with lithium (Eskalith), divalproex (Depakote), lamotrigine (Lamictal), or carbamazepine (Tegretol) and then to gradually withdraw the antipsychotic.

Depression with Psychotic Symptoms. Combination treatment with an antipsychotic and an antidepressant is one of the treatments of choice for MDD with psychotic features; the other is ECT.

Delusional Disorder. Patients with delusional disorder often respond favorably to treatment with these drugs. Some persons with borderline personality disorder who may develop paranoid thinking in the course of their disorder may respond to antipsychotic drugs.

Severe Agitation and Violent Behavior. Severely agitated and violent patients, regardless of diagnosis, may be treated with DRAs. Symptoms such as extreme irritability, lack of impulse control, severe hostility, gross hyperactivity, and agitation respond to short-term treatment with these drugs. Children with mental disabilities, especially those with profound mental retardation and autistic disorder, often have associated episodes of violence, aggression, and agitation that respond to treatment with antipsychotic drugs; however, the repeated administration of antipsychotics to control disruptive behavior in children is controversial.

Tourette's Disorder. DRAs are used to treat Tourette's disorder, a neurobehavioral disorder marked by motor and vocal tics. Haloperidol and pimozide (Orap) are the drugs most frequently used, but other DRAs are also effective. Some clinicians prefer to use clonidine (Catapres) for this disorder because of its lower risk of neurological side effects.

Borderline Personality Disorder. Patients with borderline personality disorder who experience transient psychotic symptoms, such as perceptual disturbances, suspiciousness, ideas of reference, and aggression, may need to be treated with a DRA. This disorder is also associated with mood instability, so patients should be evaluated for possible treatment with mood-stabilizing agents.

Dementia and Delirium. About two-thirds of agitated, elderly patients with various forms of dementia improve when given a DRA. Low doses of high-potency drugs (e.g., 0.5 to 1 mg a day of haloperidol) are recommended. DRAs are also used to treat psychotic symptoms and agitation associated with delirium. The cause of the delirium needs to be determined because toxic deliriums caused by anticholinergic agents can be exacerbated by low-potency DRAs, which often have significant antimuscarinic activity. Orthostasis, parkinsonism, and worsened cognition are the most problematic side effects in this elderly population.

Substance-Induced Psychotic Disorder. Intoxication with cocaine, amphetamines, alcohol, PCP, or other drugs can cause psychotic symptoms. Because these symptoms tend to be time limited, it is preferable to avoid use of a DRA unless the patient is severely agitated and aggressive. Usually, benzodiazepines can be used to calm the patient. Benzodiazepines should be used instead of DRAs in cases of PCP intoxication. When a patient is experiencing hallucinations or delusions as a result of alcohol withdrawal, DRAs may increase the risk of seizure.

Childhood Schizophrenia. Children with schizophrenia benefit from treatment with antipsychotic medication, although considerably less research has been devoted to this population. Studies are currently under way to determine if intervention with medication at the very earliest signs of disturbance in children genetically at risk for schizophrenia can prevent the emergence of more florid symptoms. Careful consideration needs to be given to side effects, especially those involving cognition and alertness.

Other Psychiatric and Nonpsychiatric Indications. The DRAs reduce the chorea in the early stages of Huntington's disease. Patients with this disease may develop hallucinations, delusions, mania, or hypomania. These and other psychiatric symptoms respond to DRAs. High-potency DRAs should be used. However, clinicians should be aware that patients with the rigid form of this disorder may experience acute EPS. The use of DRAs to treat impulse control disorders should be reserved for patients in whom other interventions have failed. Patients with pervasive developmental disorder may exhibit hyperactivity, screaming, and agitation with combativeness. Some of these symptoms respond to high-potency DRAs, but there is little research evidence supporting benefits in these patients.

The rare neurological disorders ballismus and hemiballismus (which affect only one side of the body), characterized by propulsive movements of the limbs away from the body, also respond to treatment with antipsychotic agents. Other miscellaneous indications for the use of DRAs include the treatment of nausea, emesis, intractable hiccups, and pruritus. Endocrine disorders and temporal lobe epilepsy may be associated with psychosis that responds to antipsychotic treatment.

The most common side effects of DRAs are neurological. As a rule, low-potency drugs cause most nonneurological adverse effects, and the high-potency drugs cause most neurological adverse effects.

Precautions and Adverse Reactions

Table 25–30 summarizes the most common adverse events associated with the use of DRAs.

Neuroleptic Malignant Syndrome. A potentially fatal side effect of DRA treatment, neuroleptic malignant syndrome, can occur at any time during the course of DRA treatment. Symptoms include extreme hyperthermia, severe muscular rigidity and dystonia, akinesia, mutism, confusion, agitation, and increased pulse rate and BP. Laboratory findings include increased WBC count, and levels of creatinine phosphokinase, liver enzymes, plasma myoglobin, and myoglobinuria, occasionally associated with renal failure. The symptoms usually evolve over 24 to 72 hours, and the untreated syndrome lasts 10 to 14 days. The diagnosis is often missed in the early stages, and the withdrawal or agitation may mistakenly be considered to reflect increased psychosis. Men are affected more frequently than are women, and young persons are affected more commonly than are elderly persons. The mortality rate can reach 20 to 30 percent, or even higher when depot medications are involved. Rates are also increased when high doses of high-potency agents are used.

If neuroleptic malignant syndrome is suspected, the DRA should be stopped immediately and the following done: medical support to cool the person; monitoring of vital signs, electrolytes, fluid balance, and renal output; and symptomatic treatment of fever. Antiparkinsonian medications may reduce some of the muscle rigidity. Dantrolene (Dantrium), a skeletal muscle relaxant (0.8 to 2.5 mg/kg every 6 hours, up to a total dosage of 10 mg a day) may be useful in the treatment of this disorder. When the person can take oral medications, dantrolene can be given in doses of 100 to 200 mg a day. Bromocriptine (20 to 30 mg a day in four divided doses) or amantadine can be added to the regimen. Treatment should usually be continued for 5 to 10 days. When drug treatment is restarted, the clinician should consider switching to a low-potency drug or an SDA, although these agents—including clozapine—may also cause neuroleptic malignant syndrome.

Seizure Threshold. DRAs may lower the seizure threshold. Chlorpromazine, thioridazine, and other low-potency drugs are thought to be more epileptogenic than are high-potency drugs. The risk of inducing a seizure by drug administration warrants consideration when the person already has a seizure disorder or brain lesion.

Sedation. Blockade of histamine H_1 receptors is the usual cause of sedation associated with DRAs. Chlorpromazine is the most sedating typical antipsychotic. The relative sedative properties of the drugs are summarized in Table 25–30. Giving the entire daily dose at bedtime usually eliminates any problems from sedation, and tolerance for this adverse effect often develops.

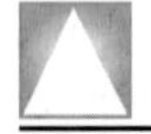

Table 25–30
Dopamine Receptor Antagonists: Potency and Adverse Effects

			Side Effects		
Drug Name	**Chemical Classification**	**Therapeutically Equivalent Oral**	**Sedation**	**Autonomic[a]**	**Extrapyramidal Reactions[b]**
Pimozide[c]	Diphenylbutylpiperidine	1.5	+	+	+++
Fluphenazine	Phenothiazine: piperazine compound	2	+	+	+++
Haloperidol	Butyrophenone	2	+	+	+++
Thiothixene	Thioxanthene	4	+	+	+++
Trifluoperazine	Phenothiazine: piperazine compound	5	++	+	+++
Perphenazine	Phenothiazine: piperazine compound	8	++	+	++/+++
Molindone	Dihydroindolone	10	++	+	+
Loxapine	Dibenzoxazepine	10	++	+/++	++/+++
Prochlorperazine[c]	Phenothiazine: piperazine compound	15	++	+	+++
Acetophenazine	Phenothiazine: piperazine compound	20	++	+	++/+++
Triflupromazine	Phenothiazine: aliphatic compound	25	+++	++/+++	++
Mesoridazine	Phenothiazine: piperidine compound	50	+++	++	+
Chlorpromazine	Phenothiazine: aliphatic compound	100	+++	+++	++
Chlorprothixene	Thioxanthene	100	+++	+++	+/++
Thioridazine	Phenothiazine: piperidine compound	100	+++	+++	+

[a]Anti–α-adrenergic and anticholinergic effects.
[b]Excluding tardive dyskinesia, which appears to be produced to the same degree and frequency by all agents with equieffective antipsychotic dosages.
[c]Pimozide is used principally in the treatment of Tourette's disorder; prochlorperazine is used rarely, if ever, as an antipsychotic agent.
Adapted from American Medical Association. *AMA Drug Evaluations: Annual 1992*. Chicago: American Medical Association, 1992.

Central Anticholinergic Effects. The symptoms of central anticholinergic activity include severe agitation; disorientation to time, person, and place; hallucinations; seizures; high fever; and dilated pupils. Stupor and coma may ensue. The treatment of anticholinergic toxicity consists of discontinuing the causal agent or agents, close medical supervision, and physostigmine (Antilirium, Eserine), 2 mg by slow intravenous (IV) infusion, repeated within 1 hour as necessary. Too much physostigmine is dangerous, and symptoms of physostigmine toxicity include hypersalivation and sweating. Atropine sulfate (0.5 mg) can reverse the effects of physostigmine toxicity.

Cardiac Effects. The DRAs decrease cardiac contractility, disrupt enzyme contractility in cardiac cells, increase circulating levels of catecholamines, and prolong atrial and ventricular conduction time and refractory periods. Low-potency DRAs, particularly the phenothiazines, are usually more cardiotoxic than are high-potency drugs. One exception is haloperidol, which has been linked to abnormal heart rhythm, ventricular arrhythmias, torsades de pointes, and sudden death when injected IV. Pimozide, sulpiride, and droperidol (a butyrophenone) also prolong the QTc interval and have clearly been associated with torsades de pointes and sudden death. In one study, thioridazine was responsible for 28 (61 percent) of the 46 sudden antipsychotic deaths and consequently in July 2000 FDA added a black box warning to its label. In 15 of these cases, it was the only drug ingested. Chlorpromazine also causes prolongation of the QT and PR intervals, blunting of the T waves, and depression of the ST segment. These drugs are thus indicated only when other agents have been ineffective.

Sudden Death. Occasional reports of sudden cardiac death during treatment with DRAs may be the result of cardiac arrhythmias. Other causes may include seizure, asphyxiation, malignant hyperthermia, heat stroke, and neuroleptic malignant syndrome. However, there does not appear to be an overall increase in the incidence of sudden death linked to the use of antipsychotics.

Orthostatic (Postural) Hypotension. Orthostatic (postural) hypotension is most common with low-potency drugs, particularly chlorpromazine, thioridazine, and chlorprothixene. When using IM low-potency DRAs, the clinician should measure the patient's BP (lying and standing) before and after the first dose and during the first few days of treatment.

Orthostatic hypotension is mediated by adrenergic blockade and occurs most frequently during the first few days of treatment. Tolerance often develops for this side effect, which is why initial dosing of these drugs is lower than the usual therapeutic dose. Fainting or falls, although uncommon, may lead to injury. Patients should be warned of this side effect and instructed to rise slowly after sitting and reclining. Patients should avoid all caffeine and alcohol; should drink at least 2 L of fluid a day; and if not under treatment for hypertension, should add liberal amounts of salt to their diet. Support hose may help some persons.

Hypotension can usually be managed by having patients lie down with their feet higher than their heads and pump their legs as if bicycling. Volume expansion or vasopressor agents, such as norepinephrine (Levophed), may be indicated in severe cases. Because hypotension is produced by α-adrenergic blockade, the drugs also block the α-adrenergic stimulating properties of epinephrine, leaving the β-adrenergic stimulating effects untouched. Therefore, the administration of epinephrine results in a paradoxical worsening of hypotension and is contraindicated in cases of antipsychotic-induced hypotension. Pure α-adrenergic pressor agents, such as metaraminol (Aramine) and norepinephrine, are the drugs of choice in the treatment of the disorder.

Hematologic Effects. Temporary leukopenia with a WBC count of about 3,500 is a common but not serious problem. Agranulocytosis, a life-threatening hematologic problem, occurs in about 1 in 10,000 persons treated with DRAs. Thrombocytopenic or nonthrombocytopenic purpura, hemolytic anemias, and pancytopenia may occur rarely in persons treated with DRAs. Although routine CBCs are not indicated, if a person reports a sore throat and fever, a CBC should be done immediately to check for the possibility of a serious blood dyscrasia. If blood index values are low, administration of DRAs should be stopped, and the patient should be transferred to a medical facility. The mortality rate for the complication may be as high as 30 percent.

Peripheral Anticholinergic Effects. Peripheral anticholinergic effects, consisting of dry mouth and nose, blurred vision, constipation, urinary retention, and mydriasis, are common, especially with low-potency DRAs, for example, chlorpromazine, thioridazine, mesoridazine (Serentil). Some persons may also have nausea and vomiting.

Constipation should be treated with the usual laxative preparations, but severe constipation can progress to paralytic ileus. A decrease in the DRA dosage is warranted in such cases. Pilocarpine (Salagen) may be used to treat paralytic ileus, although the relief is only transitory. Bethanechol (Urecholine) (20 to 40 mg a day) may be useful in some persons with urinary retention.

Weight gain is associated with increased mortality and morbidity and with medication noncompliance. Low-potency DRAs may cause significant weight gain but not as much as is seen with the SDAs olanzapine (Zyprexa) and clozapine (Clozaril). Among the DRAs loxapine (Loxitane) appears to be least likely to cause weight gain.

Endocrine Effects. Blockade of the dopamine receptors in the tuberoinfundibular tract results in the increased secretion of prolactin, which can result in breast enlargement, galactorrhea, amenorrhea, and inhibited orgasm in women and impotence in men. The SDAs, with the exception of risperidone (Risperdal), are not particularly associated with an increase in prolactin levels and may be the drugs of choice for persons experiencing disturbing side effects from increased prolactin release.

Sexual Adverse Effects. Both men and women taking DRAs can experience anorgasmia and decreased libido. Up to 50 percent of men who take antipsychotics report ejaculatory and erectile disturbances. Sildenafil (Viagra), vardenafil (Levitra), and tadalafil (Cialis) are often used to treat psychotropic-induced orgasmic dysfunction, but they have not been studied in combination with the DRAs. Clinicians should be aware of the potential for hypotension with these medications particularly in combination with low-potency antipsychotics and those with preexisting cardiac disease as well as those on hypertensive medications. Thioridazine is particularly associated with decreased libido and retrograde ejaculation in men. Priapism and reports of painful orgasms have also been described, both possibly resulting from α_1-adrenergic antagonist activity.

Skin and Eye Effects. Allergic dermatitis and photosensitivity may occur, especially with low-potency agents. Urticarial, maculopapular, petechial, and edematous eruptions may occur early in treatment, generally in the first few weeks, and remit spontaneously. A photosensitivity reaction that resembles a severe sunburn also occurs in some persons taking chlorpromazine. Persons should be warned of this adverse effect, should spend no more than 30 to 60 minutes in the sun, and should use sunscreens. Long-term chlorpromazine use is associated with blue-gray discoloration of skin areas exposed to sunlight. The skin changes often begin with a tan or golden brown color and progress to such colors as slate gray, metallic blue, and purple. These discolorations resolve when the patient is switched to another medication.

Irreversible retinal pigmentation is associated with the use of thioridazine at dosages above 1,000 mg a day. An early symptom of the side effect can sometimes be nocturnal confusion related to difficulty with night vision. The pigmentation can progress even after thioridazine administration is stopped, finally resulting in blindness. It is for this reason that the maximum recommended dosage of thioridazine is 800 mg per day. It also has a black box warning secondary to its effect on QT prolongation.

Patients taking chlorpromazine may develop a relatively benign pigmentation of the eyes, characterized by whitish brown granular deposits concentrated in the anterior lens and posterior cornea and visible only by slit-lens examination. The deposits can progress to opaque white and yellow-brown granules, often stellate. Occasionally, the conjunctiva is discolored by a brown pigment. No retinal damage is seen, and vision is almost never impaired. This condition gradually resolves when chlorpromazine is discontinued.

Jaundice. Elevations of liver enzymes during treatment with a DRA tend to be transient and not clinically significant. When chlorpromazine first came into use, cases of obstructive or cholestatic jaundice were reported, usually in the first month of treatment and heralded by symptoms of upper abdominal pain, nausea, and vomiting. This was followed by fever; rash; eosinophilia; bilirubin in the urine; and increases in levels of serum bilirubin, alkaline phosphatase, and hepatic transaminases. Reported cases are now extremely rare, but if jaundice occurs, the medication should be discontinued.

Overdoses. Overdoses typically consist of exaggerated DRA side effects. Symptoms and signs include CNS depression, EPS, mydriasis, rigidity, restlessness, decreased deep tendon reflexes, tachycardia, and hypotension. The severe symptoms of overdose include delirium, coma, respiratory depression, and seizures. Haloperidol may be among the safest typical antipsychotics in overdose. After an overdose, electroencephalography (EEG) shows diffuse slowing and low voltage. Extreme overdose may lead to delirium and coma, with respiratory depression and hypotension. Life-threatening overdose usually involves ingestion of other CNS depressants, such as alcohol or benzodiazepines.

Activated charcoal, if possible, and gastric lavage should be administered if the overdose is recent. Emetics are not indicated because the antiemetic actions of the DRAs inhibit their efficacy. Seizures can be treated with IV diazepam (Valium) or phenytoin (Dilantin). Hypotension can be treated with either norepinephrine or dopamine but not epinephrine.

Pregnancy and Lactation. There is a low correlation between the use of antipsychotics during pregnancy and congenital malformations. Nevertheless, antipsychotics should be avoided during pregnancy, particularly in the first trimester unless the benefit outweighs the risk. High-potency drugs are preferable to low-potency drugs because the low-potency drugs are associated with hypotension.

DRAs are secreted in the breast milk, although concentrations are low. Women taking these agents should be advised against breastfeeding.

Drug Interactions

Many pharmacokinetic and pharmacodynamic drug interactions are associated with these drugs (Table 25–31). CYP2D6 is the most common hepatic isozyme involved in DRA pharmacokinetic interactions. Other common drug interactions affect the absorption of the DRAs.

Antacids, activated charcoal, cholestyramine (Questran), kaolin, pectin, and cimetidine (Tagamet) taken within 2 hours of antipsychotic administration can reduce the absorption of these drugs. Anticholinergics may decrease the absorption of the DRAs. The additive anticholinergic activity of the DRAs, anticholinergics, and tricyclic drugs may result in anticholinergic toxicity. Digoxin (Lanoxin) and steroids, both of which decrease gastric motility, can increase DRA absorption.

Phenothiazines, especially thioridazine, may decrease the metabolism of and cause toxic concentrations of phenytoin. Barbiturates may increase the metabolism of DRAs.

Tricyclic drugs and SSRIs that inhibit CYP2D6—paroxetine (Paxil), fluoxetine (Prozac), and fluvoxamine (Luvox)—interact with DRAs, resulting in increased plasma concentrations of both drugs. The anticholinergic, sedative, and hypotensive effects of the drugs may also be additive.

Typical antipsychotics may inhibit the hypotensive effects of α-methyldopa (Aldomet). Conversely, typical antipsychotics may have an additive effect on some hypotensive drugs. Antipsychotic drugs have a variable effect on the hypotensive effects of clonidine. Propranolol (Inderal) coadministration increases the blood concentrations of both drugs.

The DRAs potentiate the CNS-depressant effects of the sedatives, antihistamines, opiates, opioids, and alcohol, particularly in persons with impaired respiratory status. When these agents are taken with alcohol, the risk for heat stroke may be increased.

Cigarette smoking may decrease the plasma levels of the typical antipsychotic drugs. Epinephrine has a paradoxical hypotensive effect in persons taking typical antipsychotics. These drugs may decrease the blood concentration of warfarin (Coumadin), resulting in decreased bleeding time. The phenothiazines, thioridazine, and pimozide should not be coadministered with other agents that prolong the QT interval. Thioridazine is contraindicated in

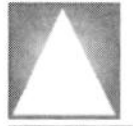

Table 25–31
Antipsychotic Drug Interactions

Interacting Medication	Mechanism	Clinical Effect
Drug interactions assessed to have major severity		
β-Adrenergic receptor antagonists	Synergistic pharmacologic effect; antipsychotic inhibits metabolism of propranolol; antipsychotic increases plasma concentrations	Severe hypotension
Anticholinergics	Pharmacodynamic effects Additive anticholinergic effect	Decreased antipsychotic effect Anticholinergic toxicity
Barbiturates	Phenobarbital induces antipsychotic metabolism	Decreased antipsychotic concentrations
Carbamazepine	Induces antipsychotic metabolism	Up to 50% reduction in antipsychotic concentrations
Charcoal	Reduces GI absorption of antipsychotic and adsorbs drug during enterohepatic circulation	May reduce antipsychotic effect or cause toxicity when used to treat overdose or for GI disturbances
Cigarette smoking	Induction of microsomal enzymes	Reduced plasma concentrations of antipsychotic agents
Epinephrine, norepinephrine	Antipsychotic antagonizes pressor effect	Hypotension
Ethanol	Additive CNS depression	Impaired psychomotor status
Fluvoxamine	Fluvoxamine inhibits metabolism of haloperidol and clozapine	Increased concentrations of haloperidol and clozapine
Guanethidine	Antipsychotic antagonizes guanethidine reuptake	Impaired antihypertensive effect
Lithium	Unknown	Rare reports of neurotoxicity
Meperidine	Additive CNS depression	Hypotension and sedation
Drug interactions assessed to have minor or moderate severity		
Amphetamines, anorexiants	Decreased pharmacologic effect of amphetamine	Diminished weight loss effect; amphetamines may exacerbate psychosis
ACEIs	Additive hypotensive crisis	Hypotension, postural intolerance
Antacids containing aluminum	Insoluble complex formed in GI tract	Possible reduced antipsychotic effect
AD nonspecific	Decreased metabolism of AD through competitive inhibition	Increased AD concentration
Benzodiazepines	Increased pharmacologic effect of the benzodiazepine	Respiratory depression, stupor, hypotension
Bromocriptine	Antipsychotic antagonizes dopamine receptor stimulation	Increased prolactin
Caffeinated beverages	Form precipitate with antipsychotic solutions	Possible diminished antipsychotic effect
Cimetidine	Reduced antipsychotic absorption and clearance	Decreased antipsychotic effect
Clonidine	Antipsychotic potentiates α-adrenergic hypotensive effect	Hypotension or hypertension
Disulfiram	Impairs antipsychotic metabolism	Increased antipsychotic concentrations
Methyldopa	Unknown	BP elevations
Phenytoin	Induction of antipsychotic metabolism; decreased phenytoin metabolism	Decreased antipsychotic concentrations: increased phenytoin levels
SSRIs	Impair antipsychotic metabolism; pharmacodynamic interaction	Sudden onset of extrapyramidal symptoms
Valproic acid	Antipsychotic inhibits valproic acid metabolism	Increased valproic acid half-life and levels

ACEI, angiotensin-converting enzyme inhibitor; AD, antidepressant; BP, blood pressure; CNS, central nervous system; GI, gastrointestinal; SSRI, selective serotonin reuptake inhibitor.
From Ereshosky L, Overman GP, Karp JK. Current psychotropic dosing and monitoring guidelines. *Prim Psychiatry*. 1996;3:21.

patients taking drugs that inhibit the CYP2D6 isoenzyme or in patients with reduced levels of CYP2D6.

Laboratory Interferences

Chlorpromazine and perphenazine (Trilafon) may cause both false-positive and false-negative results in immunological pregnancy tests and falsely elevated bilirubin (with reagent test strips) and urobilinogen (with Ehrlich's reagent test) values. These drugs have also been associated with an abnormal shift in results of the glucose tolerance test, although that shift may reflect the effects of the drugs on the glucose-regulating system. Phenothiazines have been reported to interfere with the measurement of 17-ketosteroids and 17-hydroxycorticosteroids and to produce false-positive results in tests for phenylketonuria.

Dosage and Clinical Guidelines

Contraindications to the use of DRAs include the following: (1) a history of a serious allergic response; (2) the possible ingestion of a substance that will interact with the antipsychotic to induce CNS depression (e.g., alcohol, opioids, barbiturates, and benzodiazepines) or anticholinergic delirium (e.g., scopolamine and possibly PCP); (3) the presence of a severe cardiac abnormality; (4) a high risk for seizures; (5) the presence of narrow-angle glaucoma or prostatic hypertrophy if a drug with high anticholinergic activity is to be used; and (6) the presence or a history of tardive dyskinesia. Antipsychotics should be administered with caution in persons with hepatic disease, because impaired hepatic metabolism may result in high plasma concentrations. The usual assessment should include a CBC with WBC indexes, liver function tests, and electrocardiography (ECG), especially in women older than 40 years of age and men older than 30 years of age. Elderly persons and children are more sensitive to side effects than are young adults, so the dosage of the drug should be adjusted accordingly.

Various patients may respond to widely different dosages of antipsychotics; therefore, there is no set dosage for any given antipsychotic drug. Because of side effects, it is reasonable clinical practice to begin at a low dosage and increase as necessary. It is important to remember that the maximal effects of a particular dosage may not be evident for 4 to 6 weeks. Available preparations and dosages of the DRAs are given in Table 25–32.

Short-Term Treatment. The equivalent of 5 to 20 mg of haloperidol is a reasonable dose for an adult in an acute state. An elderly person may benefit from as little as 1 mg of haloperidol. The administration of more than 25 mg of chlorpromazine in one injection may result in serious hypotension. IM administration results in peak plasma levels in about 30 minutes versus 90 minutes using the oral route. Doses of drugs for IM administration are about half those given by the oral route. In a short-term treatment setting, the person should be observed for 1 hour after the first dose of medication. After that time, most clinicians administer a second dose or a sedative agent (e.g., a benzodiazepine) to achieve effective behavioral control. Possible sedatives include lorazepam (Ativan) (2 mg IM) and amobarbital (50 to 250 mg IM), though its use is highly selective in certain settings.

Rapid Neuroleptization. Rapid neuroleptization (also called psychotolysis) is the practice of administering hourly IM doses of antipsychotic medications until marked sedation is achieved. However, several research studies have shown that merely waiting several more hours after one dose yields the same clinical improvement as is seen with repeated doses. Nevertheless, clinicians must be careful to keep patients from becoming violent while they are psychotic. Clinicians can help prevent violent episodes by using adjuvant sedatives or by temporarily using physical restraints until the persons can control their behavior.

Early Treatment. A full 6 weeks may be necessary to evaluate the extent of the improvement in psychotic symptoms. However, agitation and excitement usually improve quickly with antipsychotic treatment. About 75 percent of persons with a short history of illness show significant improvement in their psychosis. Psychotic symptoms, both positive and negative, usually continue to improve 3 to 12 months after the initiation of treatment.

About 5 mg of haloperidol or 300 mg of chlorpromazine is a usual effective daily dose. In the past, much higher doses were used, but evidence suggests that it resulted in more side effects without additional benefits. A single daily dose is usually given at bedtime to help induce sleep and to reduce the incidence of adverse effects. However, bedtime dosing for elderly persons may increase their risk of falling if they get out of bed during the night. The sedative effects of typical antipsychotics last only a few hours, in contrast to the antipsychotic effects, which last for 1 to 3 days.

Intermittent Medications. It is common clinical practice to order medications to be given intermittently as needed (PRN). Although this practice may be reasonable during the first few days that a person is hospitalized, the amount of time the person takes antipsychotic drugs, rather than an increase in dosage, is what produces therapeutic improvement. Clinicians on inpatient services may feel pressured by staff members to write PRN antipsychotic orders; such orders should include specific symptoms, how often the drugs should be given, and how many doses can be given each day. Clinicians may choose to use small doses for the PRN doses (e.g., 2 mg of haloperidol) or use a benzodiazepine instead (e.g., 2 mg of lorazepam IM). If PRN doses of an antipsychotic are necessary after the first week of treatment, the clinician may want to consider increasing the standing daily dose of the drug.

Maintenance Treatment. The first 3 to 6 months after a psychotic episode are usually considered a period of stabilization. After that time, the dosage of the antipsychotic can be decreased about 20 percent every 6 months until the minimum effective dosage is found. A person is usually maintained on antipsychotic medications for 1 to 2 years after the first psychotic episode. Antipsychotic treatment is often continued for 5 years after a second psychotic episode, and lifetime maintenance is considered after the third psychotic episode, although attempts to reduce the daily dosage can be made every 6 to 12 months.

Antipsychotic drugs are effective in controlling psychotic symptoms, but persons may report that they prefer being off the drugs because they feel better without them. The clinician must discuss maintenance medication with patients and take into account their wishes, the severity of their illnesses, and the quality of their support systems. It is essential for the clinician to know enough about the patient's life to try to predict upcoming stressors that might require increasing the dosage or closely monitoring compliance.

Long-Acting Depot Medications. Long-acting depot preparations may be needed to overcome problems with compliance. IM preparations are typically given once every 1 to 4 weeks.

Two depot preparations, a decanoate and an enanthate, of fluphenazine and a decanoate preparation of haloperidol are available in the United States. The preparations are injected IM into an area of large muscle tissue, from which they are absorbed slowly into the blood. Decanoate preparations can be given less frequently than enanthate preparations because they are absorbed more slowly. Although stabilizing a person on the oral preparation of the specific drugs is not necessary before initiating the depot form, it is good practice to give at least one oral dose of the drug to assess the possibility of an adverse effect, such as severe EPS or an allergic reaction.

It is reasonable to begin with either 12.5 mg (0.5 mL) of fluphenazine preparation or 25 mg (0.5 mL) of haloperidol decanoate. If symptoms emerge in the next 2 to 4 weeks, the person can be treated temporarily with additional oral medications or with additional small depot injections. After 3 to 4 weeks, the depot injection can be increased to a single dose equal to the total of the doses given during the initial period.

A good reason to initiate depot treatment with low doses is that the absorption of the preparations may be faster than usual at the onset of treatment, resulting in frightening episodes of dystonia that eventually discourage compliance with the medication.

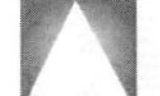

Table 25–32
Dopamine Receptor Antagonists

Name							Adult Dose Range (mg/day)	
Generic or Chemical	Trade	Tablets (mg)	Capsules (mg)	Solution	Parenteral	Rectal Suppositories (mg)	Acute	Maintenance
Chlorpromazine	Thorazine	10, 25, 50, 100, 200	30, 75, 150, 200, 300	10 mg/5 mL, 30 mg/mL, 100 mg/mL	25 mg/mL	25, 100	100–1,600 PO 25–400 IM	50–400 PO
Prochlorperazine	Compazine	5, 10, 25	10, 15, 30	5 mg/5 mL	5 mg/mL	2.5, 5, 25	15–200 PO 40–80 IM	15–60 PO
Perphenazine	Trilafon	2, 4, 8, 16	—	16 mg/5 mL	5 mg/mL	—	12–64 PO 15–30 IM	8–24 PO
Trifluoperazine	Stelazine	1, 2, 5, 10	—	10 mg/mL	2 mg/mL	—	4–40 PO 4–10 IM	5–20 PO
Fluphenazine	Prolixin	1, 2.5, 5, 10	—	2.5 mg/5 mL, 5 mg/mL	2.5 mg/mL (IM only)	—	2.5–40.0 PO 5–20 IM	1.0–15.0 PO 12.5–50.0 IM (decanoate or enanthate, weekly or biweekly)
Fluphenazine decanoate	—	—	—	—	2.5 mg/mL	—	—	—
Fluphenazine enanthate	—	—	—	2.5 mg/mL	—	—	—	—
Thioridazine	Mellaril	10, 15, 25, 50, 100, 150, 200	—	25 mg/5 mL, 100 mg/5 mL, 30 mg/mL, 100 mg/mL	—	—	200–800 PO	100–300 PO
Mesoridazine	Serentil	10, 25, 50, 100	—	25 mg/mL	25 mg/mL	—	100–400 PO 25–200 IM	30–150 PO
Haloperidol	Haldol	0.5, 1, 2, 5, 10, 20	—	2 mg/5 mL	5 mg/mL (IM only)	—	5–20 PO 12.5–25 IM	1–10 PO
Haloperidol decanoate		—	—	—	50 mg/mL, 100 mg/mL (IM only)	—		25–200 IM (decanoate, monthly)
Chlorprothixene	Taractan	10, 25, 50, 100	—	100 mg/5 mL (suspension)	12.5 mg/mL	—	75–600 PO 75–200 IM	50–400
Thiothixene	Navane	—	1, 2, 5, 10, 20	5 mg/mL	5 mg/mL (IM only), 20 mg/mL (IM only)	—	6–100 PO 8–30 IM	6–30
Loxapine	Loxitane	—	5, 10, 25, 50	25 mg/5 mL	50 mg/mL	—	20–250 20–75 IM	20–100
Molindone	Moban	5, 10, 25, 50, 100	—	20 mg/mL	—	—	50–225	5–150
Pimozide	Orap	2	—	—	—	—	0.5–20	0.5–5.0

IM, intramuscular; PO, oral.

Some clinicians keep persons drug free for 3 to 7 days before initiating depot treatment and give small doses of the depot preparations (3.125 mg of fluphenazine or 6.25 mg of haloperidol) every few days to avoid those initial problems.

Plasma Concentrations

Genetic differences among persons and pharmacokinetic interactions with other drugs influence the metabolism of the antipsychotics. If a person has not improved after 4 to 6 weeks of treatment, the plasma concentration of the drug should be determined if feasible. After a patient has been on a particular dosage for at least five times the half-life of the drug and thus approaches steady-state concentrations, blood levels may be helpful. It is standard practice to obtain plasma samples at trough levels—just before the daily dose is given, usually at least 12 hours after the previous dose and most commonly 20 to 24 hours after the previous dose. In fact, most antipsychotics have no well-defined dose–response curve. The best-studied drug is haloperidol, which may have a therapeutic window ranging from 2 to 15 ng/mL. Other therapeutic ranges that have been reasonably well documented are 30 to 100 ng/mL for chlorpromazine and 0.8 to 2.4 ng/mL for perphenazine.

Treatment-Resistant Persons. Unfortunately, 10 to 35 percent of persons with schizophrenia do not obtain significant benefit from the antipsychotic drugs. Treatment resistance is a failure on at least two adequate trials of antipsychotics from two pharmacological classes. It is useful to determine plasma concentrations for such persons because it is possible that they are slow or rapid metabolizers or are not taking their medication. Clozapine has been conclusively shown to be effective when given to patients who have failed multiple trials of DRAs.

Adjunctive Medications. It is common practice to use DRAs in conjunction with other psychotropic agents, either to treat side effects or to further improve symptoms. Most commonly, this involves the use of lithium or other mood-stabilizing agents, SSRIs, or benzodiazepines. It was once held that antidepressant drugs exacerbated psychosis in patients with schizophrenia. In all likelihood, this observation involved patients with bipolar disorder who were misdiagnosed as having schizophrenia. Abundant evidence suggests that antidepressants in fact improve symptoms of depression in patients with schizophrenia. In some cases, amphetamines can be added to DRAs if patients remain withdrawn and apathetic.

Choice of Drug

Given their proven efficacy in managing acute psychotic symptoms and the fact that prophylactic administration of antiparkinsonian medication prevents or minimizes acute motor abnormalities, DRAs are still valuable, especially for short-term therapy. There is a considerable cost advantage to a DRA antiparkinsonian regimen compared with monotherapy with a newer antipsychotic agent. Concern about the development of DRA-induced tardive dyskinesia is the major deterrent to long-term use of these drugs, yet it is not clear that SDAs are completely free of this complication. Thus, DRAs still occupy an important role in psychiatric treatment. DRAs are not predictably interchangeable. For reasons that cannot be explained, some patients do better on one drug than another. Choice of a particular DRA should be based on the known adverse effect profile of the drugs. Other than a significant advantage in terms of medication cost, the choice currently would be an SDA. If a DRA is thought to be preferable, a high-potency antipsychotic is favored, even though it may be associated with more neurological adverse effects, mainly because there is a higher incidence of other adverse effects (e.g., cardiac, hypotensive, epileptogenic, sexual, and allergic) with the low-potency drugs. If sedation is a desired goal, either a low-potency antipsychotic can be given in divided doses or a benzodiazepine can be coadministered.

An unpleasant or dysphoric reaction (a subjective sense of restlessness, oversedation, and acute dystonia) to the first dose of an antipsychotic predicts future poor response and noncompliance. Prophylactic use of antiparkinsonian medications may prevent this reaction. In general, clinicians should be vigilant about serious side effects and adverse events (described above) regardless of which drug is used.

LAMOTRIGINE

Lamotrigine (Lamictal) was developed as a result of screening folate antagonists as anticonvulsants. Lamotrigine proved effective in several animal models of epilepsy, was developed as an antiepileptic drug, and was marketed for the adjunctive treatment of partial seizures in the United States in 1995. Initial, postmarketing, open, clinical experience suggested efficacy in a variety of neurological and psychiatric conditions, coupled with good tolerability (aside from the risk of rash). Later, double-blind, placebo-controlled studies revealed that lamotrigine was useful for some, but not all, of the neurological and psychiatric conditions reported in open studies. Therefore, lamotrigine appeared effective as maintenance treatment for bipolar disorder and was approved for maintenance treatment of bipolar I disorder in 2003. Lamotrigine also appeared to have potential utility in acute bipolar depression, but the magnitude of the effect was too modest to yield consistently superior performance compared with placebo, and hence lamotrigine did not receive approval for the treatment of acute bipolar depression. Similarly, limited data suggested lamotrigine had potential utility in rapid-cycling bipolar disorder. Lamotrigine did not appear to be effective as a main intervention in acute mania. Thus, lamotrigine has emerged as an agent that appears to "stabilize mood from below" in the sense that it may maximally impact the depressive component of bipolar disorders.

Pharmacological Actions

Lamotrigine is completely absorbed, has a bioavailability of 98 percent, and has a steady-state plasma half-life of 25 hours. However, the rate of metabolism of lamotrigine varies over a sixfold range, depending on which other drugs are administered concomitantly. Dosing is escalated slowly to twice-a-day maintenance dosing. Food does not affect its absorption, and it is 55 percent protein bound in the plasma; 94 percent of lamotrigine and its inactive metabolites are excreted in the urine. Among the better-delineated biochemical actions of lamotrigine are blockade of voltage-sensitive sodium channels, which in turn modulates release of glutamate and aspartate, and has a slight effect on calcium channels. Lamotrigine modestly increases plasma serotonin concentrations, possibly through inhibition of serotonin reuptake, and is a weak inhibitor of serotonin 5-HT_3 receptors.

Therapeutic Indications

Bipolar Disorder. Lamotrigine is indicated in the treatment of bipolar disorder and may prolong the time between episodes of depression and mania. It is more effective in lengthening the intervals between depressive episodes than manic episodes. It is also effective as treatment for rapid-cycling bipolar disorder.

Other Indications. There have been reports of therapeutic benefit in the treatment of borderline personality disorder and in the treatment for various pain syndromes.

Precautions and Adverse Reactions

Lamotrigine is remarkably well tolerated. The absence of sedation, weight gain, and other metabolic effects is noteworthy. The most common adverse effects—dizziness, ataxia, somnolence, headache, diplopia, blurred vision, and nausea—are typically mild. Anecdotal reports of cognitive impairment and joint or back pain are common.

The appearance of a rash, which is common and occasionally very severe, is a source of concern. About 8 percent of patients started on lamotrigine develop a benign maculopapular rash during the first 4 months of treatment, and the drug should be discontinued if a rash develops (see Color Plate 29.18–1). Even though these rashes are benign, there is concern that in some cases, they may represent early manifestations of Stevens–Johnson syndrome or toxic epidermal necrolysis. Nevertheless, even if lamotrigine is discontinued immediately upon development of rash or other signs of hypersensitivity reaction, such as fever and lymphadenopathy, this may not prevent subsequent development of a life-threatening rash or permanent disfiguration.

Estimates of the rate of serious rash vary, depending on the source of the data. In some studies, the incidence of serious rashes was 0.08 percent in adult patients receiving lamotrigine as initial monotherapy and 0.13 percent in adult patients receiving lamotrigine as adjunctive therapy. German registry data, based on clinical practice, suggest that the risk of rash may be as low as 1 in 5,000 patients. The appearance of any type of rash necessitates immediate discontinuation of drug administration.

It is known that the likelihood of a rash increases if the recommended starting dose and speed of dose increase exceed what is recommended. Concomitant administration of valproic acid also increases risk and should be avoided if possible. If valproate is used, a more conservative dosing regimen is followed. Children and adolescents younger than age 16 years appear to be more susceptible to rash with lamotrigine. If patients miss more than 4 consecutive days of lamotrigine treatment, they need to restart therapy at the initial starting dose and titrate upward as if they had not already been on the medication.

Laboratory Testing

There is no proven correlation between lamotrigine blood concentrations and either antiseizure effects or efficacy in bipolar disorders. Laboratory tests are not useful in predicting the occurrence of adverse events.

Drug Interactions

Lamotrigine has significant, well-characterized drug interactions involving other anticonvulsants. The most potentially serious lamotrigine drug interaction involves concurrent use of valproic acid, which doubles serum lamotrigine concentrations. Lamotrigine decreases the plasma concentration of valproic acid by 25 percent. Sertraline (Zoloft) also increases plasma lamotrigine concentrations, but to a lesser extent than does valproic acid. Lamotrigine concentrations are decreased by 40 to 50 percent, with concomitant administration of carbamazepine, phenytoin, or phenobarbital. Combinations of lamotrigine and other anticonvulsants have complex effects on the time of peak plasma concentration and the plasma half-life of lamotrigine.

Laboratory Interferences

Lamotrigine and topiramate do not interfere with any laboratory tests.

Dosage and Administration

In the clinical trials leading to the approval of lamotrigine as a treatment for bipolar disorder, no consistent increase in efficacy was associated with doses above 200 mg per day. Most patients should take between 100 and 200 mg a day. In epilepsy, the drug is administered twice daily, but in bipolar disorder, the total dose can be taken once a day, either in the morning or night, depending on whether the patient finds the drug activating or sedating.

Lamotrigine is available as unscored 25-, 100-, 150-, and 200-mg tablets. The major determinant of lamotrigine dosing is minimization of the risk of rash. Lamotrigine should not be taken by anyone younger than 16 years of age. Because valproic acid markedly slows the elimination of lamotrigine, concomitant administration of these two drugs necessitates a much slower titration (Table 25–33). People with renal insufficiency should aim for a lower maintenance dosage. Appearance of any type of rash necessitates immediate discontinuation of lamotrigine administration. Lamotrigine should usually be discontinued gradually over 2 weeks unless a rash emerges, in which case it should be discontinued over 1 to 2 days.

Lamotrigine orally disintegrating tablets (Lamictal ODT) are available for patients who have difficulty swallowing. It is the

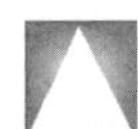

Table 25–33
Lamotrigine Dosing (mg/day)

Treatment	Weeks 1–2	Weeks 3–4	Weeks 4–5
Lamotrigine monotherapy	25	50	100–200 (500 maximum)
Lamotrigine + carbamazepine	50	100	200–500 (700 maximum)
Lamotrigine + valproate	25 every other day	25	50–200 (200 maximum)

only antiepileptic treatment that is available in an orally disintegrating formulation. It is available in 25, 50, 100, and 200 mg strengths and matches the dose of lamotrigine tablets. Chewable dispersible tablets of 2, 5, and 25 mg are also available.

LITHIUM

The effectiveness of lithium for mania and for the prophylactic treatment of manic–depressive disorder was established in the early 1950s as a result of research done by John F.J. Cade, an Australian psychiatrist. Concerns about toxicity-limited initial acceptance of lithium use in the United States, but its use increased gradually in the late 1960s. It was not until 1970 that the FDA approved its labeling for the treatment of mania. The only other approved FDA indication came in 1974, when it was accepted as maintenance therapy in patients with a history of mania. For several decades, lithium was the only drug approved for both acute and maintenance treatment. It is also used as an adjunctive medication in the treatment of MDD.

Lithium (Li), a monovalent ion, is a member of the group IA alkali metals on the periodic table, a group that also includes sodium, potassium, rubidium, cesium, and francium. Lithium exists in nature as both ^{6}Li (7.42 percent) and ^{7}Li (92.58 percent). The latter isotope allows the imaging of lithium by magnetic resonance spectroscopy. Some 300 mg of lithium is contained in 1,597 mg of lithium carbonate (Li_2CO_3). Most lithium used in the United States is obtained from dry lake mining in Chile and Argentina.

Pharmacological Actions

Lithium is rapidly and completely absorbed after oral administration, with peak serum concentrations occurring in 1 to 1.5 hours with standard preparations and in 4 to 4.5 hours with slow-release and controlled-release preparations. Lithium does not bind to plasma proteins, is not metabolized, and is excreted through the kidneys. The plasma half-life is initially 1.3 days, and is 2.4 days after administration for more than 1 year. The blood–brain barrier permits only slow passage of lithium, which is why a single overdose does not necessarily cause toxicity and why long-term lithium intoxication is slow to resolve. The elimination half-life of lithium is 18 to 24 hours in young adults, but is shorter in children and longer in elderly persons. Renal clearance of lithium is decreased with renal insufficiency. Equilibrium is reached after 5 to 7 days of regular intake. Obesity is associated with higher rates of lithium clearance. The excretion of lithium is complex during pregnancy; excretion increases during pregnancy but decreases after delivery. Lithium is excreted in breast milk and in insignificant amounts in the feces and sweat. Thyroid and renal concentrations of lithium are higher than serum levels.

An explanation for the mood-stabilizing effects of lithium remains elusive. Theories include alterations of ion transport and effects on neurotransmitters and neuropeptides, signal transduction pathways, and second messenger systems.

Therapeutic Indications

Bipolar I Disorder

MANIC EPISODES. Lithium controls acute mania and prevents relapse in about 80 percent of persons with bipolar I disorder and in a somewhat smaller percentage of persons with mixed (mania and depression) episodes, rapid-cycling bipolar disorder, or mood changes in encephalopathy. Lithium has a relatively slow onset of action when used and exerts its antimanic effects over 1 to 3 weeks. Thus, a benzodiazepine, DRA, SDA, or valproic acid is usually administered for the first few weeks. Patients with mixed or dysphoric mania, rapid cycling, comorbid substance abuse, or organicity respond less well to lithium than those with classic mania.

BIPOLAR DEPRESSION. Lithium has been shown to be effective in the treatment of depression associated with bipolar I disorder, as well as in the role of add-on therapy for patients with severe MDD. Augmentation of lithium therapy with valproic acid (Depakene) or carbamazepine (Tegretol) is usually well tolerated, with little risk of precipitation of mania.

When a depressive episode occurs in a person taking maintenance lithium, the differential diagnosis should include lithium-induced hypothyroidism, substance abuse, and lack of compliance with the lithium therapy. Possible treatment approaches include increasing the lithium concentration (up to 1 to 1.2 mEq/L); adding supplemental thyroid hormone (e.g., 25 μg a day of liothyronine [Cytomel]), even in the presence of normal findings on thyroid function tests; augmentation with valproate or carbamazepine; the judicious use of antidepressants; or ECT. After the acute depressive episode resolves, other therapies should be tapered in favor of lithium monotherapy, if clinically tolerated.

MAINTENANCE. Maintenance treatment with lithium markedly decreases the frequency, severity, and duration of manic and depressive episodes in persons with bipolar I disorder. Lithium provides relatively more effective prophylaxis for mania than for depression, and supplemental antidepressant strategies may be necessary either intermittently or continuously. Lithium maintenance is almost always indicated after the first episode of bipolar I disorder, depression or mania, and should be considered after the first episode for adolescents or for persons who have a family history of bipolar I disorder. Others who benefit from lithium maintenance are those who have poor support systems, had no precipitating factors for the first episode, have a high suicide risk, had a sudden onset of the first episode, or had a first episode of mania. Clinical studies have shown that lithium reduces the incidence of suicide in bipolar I disorder patients six- or sevenfold. Lithium is also an effective treatment for persons with severe cyclothymic disorder.

Initiating maintenance therapy after the first manic episode is considered a wise approach based on several observations. First, each episode of mania increases the risk of subsequent episodes. Second, among people responsive to lithium, relapses are 28 times more likely after lithium use is discontinued. Third, case reports describe persons who initially responded to lithium, discontinued taking it, and then had a relapse but no longer responded to lithium in subsequent episodes. Continued maintenance treatment with lithium is often associated with increasing efficacy and reduced mortality. Therefore, an episode of depression or mania that occurs after a relatively short time of lithium maintenance does not necessarily represent treatment failure. However, lithium treatment alone may begin to lose its effectiveness after several years of successful use. If this occurs, then supplemental treatment with carbamazepine or valproate may be useful.

Maintenance lithium dosages can often be adjusted to achieve plasma concentration somewhat lower than that needed for the treatment of acute mania. If lithium use is to be discontinued, then the dosage should be slowly tapered. Abrupt discontinuation of lithium therapy is associated with an increased risk of recurrence of manic and depressive episodes.

Major Depressive Disorder. Lithium is effective in the long-term treatment of major depression, but it is not more effective than antidepressant drugs. The most common role for lithium in MDD is as an adjuvant to antidepressant use in persons who have failed to respond to the antidepressants alone. About 50 to 60 percent of antidepressant nonresponders do respond when lithium, 300 mg three times daily, is added to the antidepressant regimen. In some cases, a response may be seen within days, but most often, several weeks are required to see the efficacy of the regimen. Lithium alone may effectively treat depressed persons who have bipolar I disorder but have not yet had their first manic episode. Lithium has been reported to be effective in persons with MDD whose disorder has a particularly marked cyclicity.

Schizoaffective Disorder and Schizophrenia. Persons with prominent mood symptoms—either bipolar type or depressive type—with schizoaffective disorder are more likely to respond to lithium than those with predominant psychotic symptoms. Although SDAs and DRAs are the treatments of choice for persons with schizoaffective disorder, lithium is a useful augmentation agent. This is particularly true for persons whose symptoms are resistant to treatment with SDAs and DRAs. Lithium augmentation of an SDA or DRA treatment may be an effective treatment for persons with schizoaffective disorder even in the absence of a prominent mood disorder component. Some persons with schizophrenia who cannot take antipsychotic drugs may benefit from lithium treatment alone.

Other Indications. Over the years, reports have appeared about the use of lithium to treat a wide range of other psychiatric and nonpsychiatric conditions (Tables 25–34 and 25–35). The effectiveness and safety of lithium for most of these disorders have not been confirmed. Lithium has antiaggressive activity that is separate from its effects on mood. Aggressive outbursts in persons with schizophrenia, violent prison inmates, and children with conduct disorder and aggression, or self-mutilation in persons with mental retardation can sometimes be controlled with lithium.

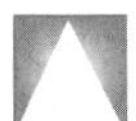

Table 25–34
Psychiatric Uses of Lithium

Historical
Gouty mania
Well established (FDA approved)
Manic episode
Maintenance therapy
Reasonably well established
Bipolar I disorder
Depressive episode
Bipolar II disorder
Rapid-cycling bipolar I disorder
Cyclothymic disorder
Major depressive disorder
Acute depression (as an augmenting agent)
Maintenance therapy
Schizoaffective disorder
Evidence of benefit in particular groups
Schizophrenia
Aggression (episodic), explosive behavior, and self-mutilation
Conduct disorder in children and adolescents
Mental retardation
Cognitive disorders
Prisoners
Anecdotal, controversial, unresolved, or doubtful
Alcohol and other substance-related disorders
Cocaine abuse
Substance-induced mood disorder with manic features
Obsessive-compulsive disorder
Phobias
Posttraumatic stress disorder
ADHD
Eating disorders
Anorexia nervosa
Bulimia nervosa
Impulse-control disorders
Kleine–Levin syndrome
Mental disorders caused by a general medical condition (e.g., mood disorder caused by a general medical condition with manic features)
Periodic catatonia
Periodic hypersomnia
Personality disorders (e.g., antisocial, borderline, emotionally unstable, schizotypal)
Premenstrual dysphoric disorder
Sexual disorders
Transvestism
Exhibitionism
Pathological hypersexuality

FDA, Food and Drug Administration; ADHD, attention-deficit/hyperactivity disorder.

Precautions and Adverse Effects

More than 80 percent of patients taking lithium experience side effects. It is important to minimize the risk of adverse events through monitoring of lithium blood levels and to use appropriate pharmacological interventions to counteract unwanted effects when they occur. The most common adverse effects are summarized in Table 25–36. Patient education can play an important role in reducing the incidence and severity of side effects. Patients taking lithium should be advised that changes in the body's water and salt content can affect the amount of lithium excreted, resulting in either increases or decreases in lithium concentrations. Excessive sodium intake (e.g., a dramatic dietary change) lowers lithium concentrations. Conversely, too little sodium (e.g., fad diets) can lead to potentially toxic concentrations of lithium. Decreases in body fluid (e.g., excessive perspiration) can lead to dehydration and lithium intoxication. Patients should report whenever medications are prescribed by another clinician because many commonly used agents can affect lithium concentrations.

Cardiac Effects. Lithium can cause diffuse slowing, widening of frequency spectrum, and potentiation and disorganization of background rhythm on ECG. Bradycardia and cardiac arrhythmias may occur, especially in people with cardiovascular disease. Lithium infrequently reveals Brugada syndrome, an inherited, life-threatening heart problem that some people

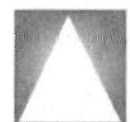

Table 25–35
Nonpsychiatric Uses of Lithium[a]

Historical
Gout and other uric acid diatheses
Lithium bromide as anticonvulsant
Neurological
Epilepsy
Headache (chronic cluster, hypnic, migraine, particularly cyclic)
Ménière's disease (not supported by controlled studies)
Movement disorders
Huntington's disease
L-Dopa–induced hyperkinesias
On–off phenomenon in Parkinson's disease (controlled study found decreased akinesia but development of dyskinesia in a few cases)
Spasmodic torticollis
Tardive dyskinesia (not supported by controlled studies, and pseudoparkinsonism has been reported)
Tourette's disorder
Pain (facial pain syndrome, painful shoulder syndrome, fibromyalgia)
Periodic paralysis (hypokalemic and hypermagnesic but not hyperkalemic)
Hematological
Aplastic anemia
Cancer—chemotherapy induced, radiotherapy induced
Neutropenia (one study found increased risk of sudden death in patients with preexisting cardiovascular disorder)
Drug-induced neutropenia (e.g., from carbamazepine, antipsychotics, immunosuppressives, and zidovudine)
Felty's syndrome
Leukemia
Endocrine
Thyroid cancer as an adjunct to radioactive iodine
Thyrotoxicosis
Syndrome of inappropriate antidiuretic hormone secretion
Cardiovascular
Antiarrhythmic agent (animal data only)
Dermatological
Genital herpes (controlled studies support topical and oral use)
Eczematoid dermatitis
Seborrheic dermatitis (controlled study supports)
Gastrointestinal
Cyclic vomiting
Gastric ulcers
Pancreatic cholera
Ulcerative colitis
Respiratory
Asthma (controlled study did not support)
Cystic fibrosis
Other
Bovine spastic paresis

[a]All the uses listed here are experimental and do not have Food and Drug Administration (FDA)-approved labeling. There are conflicting reports about many of these uses—some have negative findings in controlled studies, and a few involve reports of possible adverse effects.
L-Dopa, levodopa.

may have without knowing it. It can cause a serious abnormal heartbeat and other symptoms (such as severe dizziness, fainting, shortness of breath) that need medical attention right away. Before starting lithium treatment, clinicians should ask about known heart conditions, unexplained fainting, and family history of problems or sudden unexplained death before age 45.

Gastrointestinal Effects. GI symptoms—which include nausea, decreased appetite, vomiting, and diarrhea—can be diminished by dividing the dosage, administering the lithium with food, or switching to another lithium preparation. The lithium preparation least likely to cause diarrhea is lithium citrate. Some lithium preparations contain lactose, which can cause diarrhea in lactose-intolerant persons. Persons taking slow-release formulations of lithium who experience diarrhea caused by unabsorbed medication in the lower part of the GI tract may experience less diarrhea than with standard-release preparations. Diarrhea may also respond to antidiarrheal preparations such as loperamide (Imodium, Kaopectate), bismuth subsalicylate (Pepto-Bismol), or diphenoxylate with atropine (Lomotil).

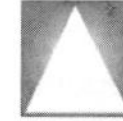

Table 25–36
Adverse Effects of Lithium

Neurological
Benign, nontoxic: dysphoria, lack of spontaneity, slowed reaction time, memory difficulties
Tremor: postural, occasional extrapyramidal
Toxic: coarse tremor, dysarthria, ataxia, neuromuscular irritability, seizures, coma, death
Miscellaneous: peripheral neuropathy, benign intracranial hypertension, myasthenia gravis–like syndrome, altered creativity, lowered seizure threshold
Endocrine
Thyroid: goiter, hypothyroidism, exophthalmos, hyperthyroidism (rare)
Parathyroid: hyperparathyroidism, adenoma
Cardiovascular
Benign T-wave changes, sinus node dysfunction
Renal
Concentrating defect, morphologic changes, polyuria (nephrogenic diabetes insipidus), reduced GFR, nephrotic syndrome, renal tubular acidosis
Dermatological
Acne, hair loss, psoriasis, rash
Gastrointestinal
Appetite loss, nausea, vomiting, diarrhea
Miscellaneous
Altered carbohydrate metabolism, weight gain, fluid retention

GFR, glomerular filtration rate.

Weight Gain. Weight gain results from a poorly understood effect of lithium on carbohydrate metabolism. Weight gain can also result from lithium-induced hypothyroidism, lithium-induced edema, or excessive consumption of soft drinks and juices to quench lithium-induced thirst.

Neurological Effects

TREMOR. A lithium-induced postural tremor may occur that is usually 8 to 12 Hz and is most notable in outstretched hands, especially in the fingers, and during tasks involving fine manipulations. The tremor can be reduced by dividing the daily dosage, using a sustained-release formulation, reducing caffeine intake, reassessing the concomitant use of other medicines, and treating comorbid anxiety. β-Adrenergic receptor antagonists, such as propranolol, 30 to 120 mg a day in divided doses, and primidone (Mysoline), 50 to 250 mg a day, are usually effective in reducing the tremor. In persons with hypokalemia, potassium supplementation may improve the tremor. When a person taking lithium has a severe tremor, the possibility of lithium toxicity should be suspected and evaluated.

COGNITIVE EFFECTS. Lithium use has been associated with dysphoria, lack of spontaneity, slowed reaction times, and impaired memory. The presence of these symptoms should be noted carefully because they are a frequent cause of noncompliance. The differential diagnosis for such symptoms should include depressive disorders, hypothyroidism, hypercalcemia, other illnesses, and other drugs. Some, but not all, persons have reported that fatigue and mild cognitive impairment decrease with time.

OTHER NEUROLOGICAL EFFECTS. Uncommon neurological adverse effects include symptoms of mild parkinsonism, ataxia, and dysarthria, although the last two symptoms may also be attributable to lithium intoxication. Lithium is rarely associated with the development of peripheral neuropathy, benign intracranial hypertension (pseudotumor cerebri), findings resembling myasthenia gravis, and increased risk of seizures.

RENAL EFFECT. The most common adverse renal effect of lithium is polyuria with secondary polydipsia. The symptom is particularly a problem in 25 to 35 percent of persons taking lithium who may have a urine output of more than 3 L a day (reference range: 1 to 2 L a day). The polyuria primarily results from lithium antagonism to the effects of antidiuretic hormone, which thus causes diuresis. When polyuria is a significant problem, the person's renal function should be evaluated and followed up with 24-hour urine collections for creatinine clearance determinations. Treatment consists of fluid replacement, the use of the lowest effective dosage of lithium, and single daily dosing of lithium. Treatment can also involve the use of a thiazide or potassium-sparing diuretic—for example, amiloride (Midamor), spironolactone (Aldactone), triamterene (Dyrenium), or amiloride–hydrochlorothiazide (Moduretic). If treatment with a diuretic is initiated, the lithium dosage should be halved, and the diuretic should not be started for 5 days, because the diuretic is likely to increase lithium retention.

The most serious renal adverse effects, which are rare and associated with continuous lithium administration for 10 years or more, involve appearance of nonspecific interstitial fibrosis, associated with gradual decreases in glomerular filtration rate and increases in serum creatinine concentrations, and rarely with renal failure. Lithium is occasionally associated with nephrotic syndrome and features of distal renal tubular acidosis. Another pathological finding in patients with lithium nephropathy is the presence of microcysts. Magnetic resonance imaging (MRI) can be used to demonstrate renal microcysts secondary to chronic lithium nephropathy and therefore avoid renal biopsy. It is prudent for persons taking lithium to check their serum creatinine concentration, urine chemistries, and 24-hour urine volume at 6-month intervals. If creatinine levels do rise, then more frequent monitoring and MRI might be considered.

Thyroid Effects.

Lithium causes a generally benign and often transient diminution in the concentrations of circulating thyroid hormones. Reports have attributed goiter (5 percent of persons), benign reversible exophthalmos, hyperthyroidism, and hypothyroidism (7 to 10 percent of persons) to lithium treatment. Lithium-induced hypothyroidism is more common in women (14 percent) than in men (4.5 percent). Women are at highest risk during the first 2 years of treatment. Persons taking lithium to treat bipolar disorder are twice as likely to develop hypothyroidism if they develop rapid cycling. About 50 percent of persons receiving long-term lithium treatment have laboratory abnormalities, such as an abnormal thyrotropin-releasing hormone (TRH) response, and about 30 percent have elevated concentrations of TSH. If symptoms of hypothyroidism are present, replacement with levothyroxine (Synthroid) is indicated. Even in the absence of hypothyroid symptoms, some clinicians treat persons with significantly elevated TSH concentrations with levothyroxine. In lithium-treated persons, TSH concentrations should be measured every 6 to 12 months. Lithium-induced hypothyroidism should be considered when evaluating depressive episodes that emerge during lithium therapy.

Cardiac Effects.

The cardiac effects of lithium resemble those of hypokalemia on ECG. They are caused by the displacement of intracellular potassium by the lithium ion. The most common changes on the ECG are T-wave flattening or inversion. The changes are benign and disappear after lithium is excreted from the body.

Lithium depresses the pacemaking activity of the sinus node, sometimes resulting in sinus dysrhythmias, heart block, and episodes of syncope. Lithium treatment, therefore, is contraindicated in persons with sick sinus syndrome. In rare cases, ventricular arrhythmias and congestive heart failure have been associated with lithium therapy. Lithium cardiotoxicity is more prevalent in persons on a low-salt diet, those taking certain diuretics or ACEIs, and those with fluid–electrolyte imbalances or any renal insufficiency.

Dermatological Effects.

Dermatological effects may be dose dependent. They include acneiform, follicular, and maculopapular eruptions; pretibial ulcerations; and worsening of psoriasis. Occasionally, aggravated psoriasis or acneiform eruptions may force the discontinuation of lithium treatment. Alopecia has also been reported. Persons with many of those conditions respond favorably to changing to another lithium preparation and the usual dermatological measures. Lithium concentrations should be monitored if tetracycline is used for the treatment of acne because it can increase the retention of lithium.

Lithium Toxicity and Overdoses.

The early signs and symptoms of lithium toxicity include neurological symptoms, such as coarse tremor, dysarthria, and ataxia; GI symptoms; cardiovascular changes; and renal dysfunction. The later signs and symptoms include impaired consciousness, muscular fasciculations, myoclonus, seizures, and coma. Signs and symptoms of lithium toxicity are outlined in Table 25–37. Risk factors include exceeding the recommended dosage, renal impairment, low-sodium diet, drug interaction, and dehydration. Elderly persons are more vulnerable to the effects of increased serum lithium concentrations. The greater the degree and duration of elevated lithium concentrations, the worse the symptoms of lithium toxicity.

Lithium toxicity is a medical emergency, potentially causing permanent neuronal damage and death. In cases of toxicity (Table 25–38), lithium should be stopped and dehydration treated. Unabsorbed lithium can be removed from the GI tract by ingestion of sodium polystyrene sulfonate (Kayexalate) or polyethylene glycol solution (GoLYTELY), but not activated charcoal. Ingestion of a single large dose may create clumps of medication in the stomach, which can be removed by gastric

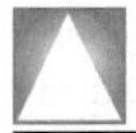

Table 25–37
Signs and Symptoms of Lithium Toxicity

1. Mild to moderate intoxication (lithium level, 1.5–2.0 mEq/L)

GI	Vomiting
	Abdominal pain
	Dryness of mouth
Neurological	Ataxia
	Dizziness
	Slurred speech
	Nystagmus
	Lethargy or excitement
	Muscle weakness

2. Moderate to severe intoxication (lithium level: 2.0–2.5 mEq/L)

GI	Anorexia
	Persistent nausea and vomiting
Neurological	Blurred vision
	Muscle fasciculations
	Clonic limb movements
	Hyperactive deep tendon reflexes
	Choreoathetoid movements
	Convulsions
	Delirium
	Syncope
	Electroencephalographic changes
	Stupor
	Coma
	Circulatory failure (lowered BP, cardiac arrhythmias, and conduction abnormalities)

3. Severe lithium intoxication (lithium level >2.5 mEq/L)
   Generalized convulsions
   Oliguria and renal failure
   Death

lavage with a wide-bore tube. The value of forced diuresis is still debated. In severe cases, hemodialysis rapidly removes excessive amounts of serum lithium. Postdialysis serum lithium concentrations may increase as lithium is redistributed from tissues to blood, so repeat dialysis may be needed. Neurological improvement may lag behind clearance of serum lithium by several days because lithium crosses the blood–brain barrier slowly.

Adolescents. The serum lithium concentrations for adolescents are similar to those for adults. Weight gain and acne associated with lithium use can be particularly troublesome to adolescents.

Elderly Persons. Lithium is a safe and effective drug for elderly persons. However, the treatment of elderly persons taking lithium may be complicated by the presence of other medical illnesses, decreased renal function, special diets that affect lithium clearance, and generally increased sensitivity to lithium. Elderly persons should initially be given low dosages, their dosages should be switched less frequently than those of younger persons, and a longer time must be allowed for renal excretion to equilibrate with absorption before lithium can be assumed to have reached its steady-state concentrations.

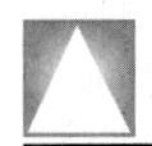

Table 25–38
Management of Lithium Toxicity

1. Contact personal physician or go to a hospital emergency department.
2. Lithium should be discontinued.
3. Vital signs and a neurological examination with complete formal mental status examination.
4. Lithium level, serum electrolytes, renal function tests, and ECG.
5. Emesis, gastric lavage, and absorption with activated charcoal.
6. For any patient with a serum lithium level greater than 4.0 mEq/L, hemodialysis.

ECG, electrocardiography.

Pregnant Women. Lithium should not be administered to pregnant women in the first trimester because of the risk of birth defects. The most common malformations involve the cardiovascular system, most commonly Ebstein's anomaly of the tricuspid valves. The risk of Ebstein's malformation in lithium-exposed fetuses is 1 in 1,000, which is 20 times the risk in the general population. The possibility of fetal cardiac anomalies can be evaluated with fetal echocardiography. The teratogenic risk of lithium (4 to 12 percent) is higher than that for the general population (2 to 3 percent) but appears to be lower than that associated with the use of valproate or carbamazepine. A woman who continues to take lithium during pregnancy should use the lowest effective dosage. The maternal lithium concentration must be monitored closely during pregnancy, and especially after pregnancy, because of the significant decrease in renal lithium excretion as renal function returns to normal in the first few days after delivery. Adequate hydration can reduce the risk of lithium toxicity during labor. Lithium prophylaxis is recommended for all women with bipolar disorder as they enter the postpartum period. Lithium is excreted into breast milk and should be taken by a nursing mother only after careful evaluation of potential risks and benefits. Signs of lithium toxicity in infants include lethargy, cyanosis, abnormal reflexes, and sometimes hepatomegaly.

Miscellaneous Effects. Lithium should be used with caution in diabetic persons, who should monitor their blood glucose concentrations carefully to avoid diabetic ketoacidosis. Benign, reversible leukocytosis is commonly associated with lithium treatment. Dehydrated, debilitated, and medically ill persons are most susceptible to adverse effects and toxicity.

Drug Interactions

Lithium drug interactions are summarized in Table 25–39.

Lithium is commonly used in conjunction with DRAs. This combination is typically effective and safe. However, coadministration of higher dosages of a DRA and lithium may result in a synergistic increase in the symptoms of lithium-induced neurological side effects and neuroleptic extrapyramidal symptoms. In rare instances, encephalopathy has been reported with this combination.

The coadministration of lithium and carbamazepine, lamotrigine, valproate, and clonazepam may increase lithium concentrations and aggravate lithium-induced neurological adverse effects. Treatment with the combination should be initiated at slightly lower dosages than usual, and the dosages should be increased gradually. Changes from one to another treatment for mania should be made carefully, with as little temporal overlap between the drugs as possible.

Most diuretics (e.g., thiazide and potassium sparing) can increase lithium concentrations, when treatment with such a

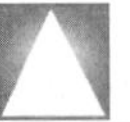

Table 25–39
Drug Interactions with Lithium

Drug Class	Reaction
Antipsychotics	Case reports of encephalopathy, worsening of extrapyramidal adverse effects, and neuroleptic malignant syndrome; inconsistent reports of altered red blood cell and plasma concentrations of lithium, antipsychotic drug, or both
Antidepressants	Occasional reports of a serotonin-like syndrome with potent serotonin reuptake inhibitors
Anticonvulsants	No significant pharmacokinetic interactions with carbamazepine or valproate; reports of neurotoxicity with carbamazepine; combinations helpful for treatment resistance
NSAIDs	May reduce renal lithium clearance and increase serum concentration; toxicity reported (exception is aspirin)
Diuretics	
Thiazides	Well-documented reduced renal lithium clearance and increased serum concentration; toxicity reported
Potassium sparing	Limited data; may increase lithium concentration
Loop	Lithium clearance unchanged (some case reports of increased lithium concentration)
Osmotic (mannitol, urea)	Increase renal lithium clearance and decrease lithium concentration
Xanthine (aminophylline, caffeine, theophylline)	Increase renal lithium clearance and decrease lithium concentration
Carbonic anhydrase inhibitors (acetazolamide)	Increase renal lithium clearance
ACEIs	Reports of reduced lithium clearance, increased concentrations, and toxicity
Calcium channel inhibitors	Case reports of neurotoxicity; no consistent pharmacokinetic interactions
Miscellaneous	
Succinylcholine, pancuronium	Reports of prolonged neuromuscular blockade
Metronidazole	Increased lithium concentration
Methyldopa	Few reports of neurotoxicity
Sodium bicarbonate	Increased renal lithium clearance
Iodides	Additive antithyroid effects
Propranolol	Used for lithium tremor; possible slight increase in lithium concentration

NSAID, nonsteroidal anti-inflammatory drug; ACEI, angiotensin-converting enzyme inhibitor.

diuretic is stopped, the clinician may need to increase the person's daily lithium dosage. Osmotic and loop diuretics, carbonic anhydrase inhibitors, and xanthines (including caffeine) may reduce lithium concentrations to below therapeutic concentrations. Whereas ACEIs may cause an increase in lithium concentrations, the AT_1 angiotensin II receptor inhibitors losartan (Cozaar) and irbesartan (Avapro) do not alter lithium concentrations. A wide range of NSAIDs can decrease lithium clearance, thereby increasing lithium concentrations. These drugs include indomethacin (Indocin), phenylbutazone (Azolid), diclofenac (Voltaren), ketoprofen (Orudis), oxyphenbutazone (Oxalid), ibuprofen (Motrin, Advil), piroxicam (Feldene), and naproxen (Naprosyn). Aspirin and sulindac (Clinoril) do not affect lithium concentrations.

The coadministration of lithium and quetiapine (Seroquel) may cause somnolence but is otherwise well tolerated. The coadministration of lithium and ziprasidone (Geodon) may modestly increase the incidence of tremor. The coadministration of lithium and calcium channel inhibitors should be avoided because of potentially fatal neurotoxicity.

A person taking lithium who is about to undergo ECT should discontinue taking lithium 2 days before beginning ECT to reduce the risk of delirium.

Laboratory Interferences

Lithium does not interfere with any laboratory tests, but lithium-induced alterations include an increased WBC count, decreased serum thyroxine, and increased serum calcium. Blood collected in a lithium–heparin anticoagulant tube will produce falsely elevated lithium concentrations.

Dosage and Clinical Guidelines

Initial Medical Workup. All patients should have a routine laboratory workup and physical examination before being started on lithium. The laboratory tests should include serum creatinine concentration (or a 24-hour urine creatinine if the clinician has any reason to be concerned about renal function), electrolytes, thyroid function (TSH, T_3 [triiodothyronine], and T_4 [thyroxine]), a CBC, ECG, and a pregnancy test in women of childbearing age.

Dosage Recommendations. Lithium formulations include immediate-release 150-, 300-, and 600-mg lithium carbonate capsules (Eskalith and generic), 300-mg lithium carbonate tablets (Lithotabs), 450-mg controlled-release lithium carbonate capsules (Eskalith CR and Lithonate), and 8 mEq/5 mL of lithium citrate syrup.

The starting dosage for most adults is 300 mg of the regular-release formulation three times daily. The starting dosage for elderly persons or persons with renal impairment should be 300 mg once or twice daily. After stabilization, dosages between 900 and 1,200 mg a day usually produce a therapeutic plasma concentration of 0.6 to 1 mEq/L, and a daily dose of 1,200 to 1,800 mg usually produces a therapeutic concentration of 0.8 to 1.2 mEq/L. Maintenance dosing can be given either in two or three divided doses of the regular-release formulation or in a single dosage of the sustained-release formulation equivalent to the combined daily dosage of the regular-release formulation. The use of divided doses reduces gastric upset and avoids single high-peak lithium concentrations. Discontinuation of lithium should be gradual to minimize the risk of early recurrence of mania and to permit recognition of early signs of recurrence.

Laboratory Monitoring. The periodic measurement of serum lithium concentration is an essential aspect of patient care, but it should always be combined with sound clinical judgment. A laboratory report listing the therapeutic range as 0.5 to 1.5 mEq/L may lull a clinician into disregarding early signs of lithium intoxication in patients whose levels are less than 1.5 mEq/L. Clinical toxicity, especially in elderly persons, has been well documented within this so-called therapeutic range.

Regular monitoring of serum lithium concentrations is essential. Lithium levels should be obtained every 2 to 6 months except when there are signs of toxicity, during dosage adjustments, and in persons suspected to be noncompliant with the prescribed dosages. Under these circumstances, levels may be done weekly. Baseline ECG studies are essential, and should be repeated annually.

When obtaining blood for lithium levels, patients should be at steady-state lithium dosing (usually after 5 days of constant dosing), preferably using a twice-daily or thrice-daily dosing regimen, and the blood sample must be drawn 12 hours (±30 minutes) after a given dose. Lithium concentrations 12 hours postdose in persons treated with sustained-release preparations are generally about 30 percent higher than the corresponding concentrations obtained from those taking the regular-release preparations. Because available data are based on a sample population following a multiple-dosage regimen, regular-release formulations given at least twice daily should be used for initial determination of the appropriate dosages. Factors that may cause fluctuations in lithium measurements include dietary sodium intake, mood state, activity level, body position, and use of an improper blood sample tube.

Laboratory values that do not seem to correspond to clinical status may result from the collection of blood in a tube with a lithium–heparin anticoagulant (which can give results falsely elevated by as much as 1 mEq/L) or aging of the lithium ion–selective electrode (which can cause inaccuracies of up to 0.5 mEq/L). After the daily dose has been set, it is reasonable to change to the sustained-release formulation given once daily.

Effective serum concentrations for mania are 1.0 to 1.5 mEq/L, a level associated with 1,800 mg a day. The recommended range for maintenance treatment is 0.4 to 0.8 mEq/L, which is usually achieved with a daily dose of 900 to 1,200 mg. A small number of persons will not achieve therapeutic benefit with a lithium concentration of 1.5 mEq/L, yet will have no signs of toxicity. For such persons, titration of the lithium dosage to achieve a concentration above 1.5 mEq/L may be warranted. Some patients can be maintained at concentrations below 0.4 mEq/L. There may be considerable variation from patient to patient, so it is best to follow the maxim "treat the patient, not the laboratory results." The only way to establish an optimal dose for a patient may be through trial and error.

Package inserts (U.S.) for lithium products list effective serum concentrations for mania between 1.0 and 1.5 mEq/L (usually achieved with 1,800 mg of lithium carbonate daily) and for long-term maintenance between 0.6 and 1.2 mEq/L (usually achieved with 900 to 1,200 mg of lithium carbonate daily). The dose–blood level relationship may vary considerably from patient to patient. The likelihood of achieving a response at levels above 1.5 mEq/L is usually outweighed greatly by the increased risk of toxicity, although rarely a patient may both require and tolerate a higher-than-usual blood concentration.

What constitutes the lower end of the therapeutic range remains a matter of debate. A prospective 3-year study found patients who maintained a concentration between 0.4 and 0.6 mEq/L (mean 0.54) were 2.6 times more likely to relapse than those who maintained between 0.8 and 1.0 mEq/L (mean 0.83). However, the higher blood concentrations produced more adverse effects and were less well tolerated.

If there is no response after 2 weeks at a concentration that is beginning to cause adverse effects, then the person should taper off lithium over 1 to 2 weeks and other mood-stabilizing drugs should be tried.

Patient Education. Lithium has a narrow therapeutic index, and many factors can upset the balance between lithium concentrations that are well tolerated and therapeutic, and those that produce side effects or toxicity. It is thus imperative that persons taking lithium be educated about signs and symptoms of toxicity, factors that affect lithium levels, how and when to obtain laboratory testing, and the importance of regular communication with the prescribing physician. Lithium concentrations can be disrupted by common factors such as excessive sweating from ambient heat or exercise or use of widely prescribed agents such as ACEIs or NSAIDs. Patients may stop taking their lithium because they are feeling well or because they are experiencing side effects. They should be advised against discontinuing or modifying their lithium regimen. Table 25–40 lists some important instructions for patients.

MELATONIN AGONISTS: RAMELTEON AND MELATONIN

There are two melatonin receptor agonists commercially available in the United States: (1) melatonin, a dietary supplement available in various preparations in health food stores, and not under FDA regulations; and (2) ramelteon (Rozerem), an FDA-approved drug for the treatment of insomnia characterized by difficulties with sleep onset. Both exogenous melatonin and ramelteon are thought to exert their effects by interaction with central melatonin receptors.

Ramelteon

Ramelteon (Rozerem) is a melatonin receptor agonist used to treat sleep-onset insomnia. Unlike the benzodiazepines, ramelteon has no appreciable affinity for the GABA receptor complex.

Pharmacological Actions. Ramelteon essentially mimics melatonin's sleep-promoting properties and has high affinity for melatonin MT1 and MT2 receptors in the brain. These receptors are thought to be critical in the regulation of the body's sleep–wake cycle.

Ramelteon is rapidly absorbed and eliminated over a dose range of 4 to 64 mg. Maximum plasma concentration (C_{max}) is reached approximately 45 minutes after administration, and the elimination half-life is 1 to 2.6 hours. The total absorption of ramelteon is at least 84 percent, but extensive first-pass metabolism results in a bioavailability of approximately 2 percent.

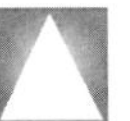

Table 25–40
Instructions to Patients Taking Lithium

Lithium can be remarkably effective in treating your disorder. If not used appropriately and not monitored closely, it can be ineffective and potentially harmful. It is important to keep the following instructions in mind.

Dosing

Take lithium exactly as directed by your doctor—never take more or less than the prescribed dose.

Do not stop taking without speaking to your doctor.

If you miss a dose, take it as soon as possible. If it is within 4 hrs of the next dose, skip the missed dose (about 6 hrs in the case of extended-release or slow-release preparations). Never double up doses.

Blood tests

Comply with the schedule of recommended regular blood tests.

Despite their inconvenience and discomfort, your lithium blood levels, thyroid function, and kidney status need to be monitored as long as you take lithium.

When going to have lithium levels checked, you should have taken your last lithium dose 12 hrs earlier.

Use of other medications

Do not start any prescription or over-the-counter medications without telling your doctor.

Even drugs such as ibuprofen (Advil, Motrin) and naproxen (Aleve) can significantly increase lithium levels.

Diet and fluid intake

Avoid sudden changes in your diet or fluid intake. If you do go on a diet, your doctor may need to increase the frequency of blood tests.

Caffeine and alcohol act as diuretics and can lower your lithium concentrations.

During treatment with lithium, it is recommended that you drink about 2 or 3 quarts of fluid daily and use normal amounts of salt.

Inform your doctor if you start or stop a low-salt diet.

Recognizing potential problems

If you engage in vigorous exercise or have an illness that causes sweating, vomiting, or diarrhea, consult your doctor because these might affect lithium levels.

Nausea, constipation, shakiness, increased thirst, frequency of urination, weight gain, or swelling of the extremities should be reported to your doctor.

Blurred vision, confusion, loss of appetite, diarrhea, vomiting, muscle weakness, lethargy, shakiness, slurred speech, dizziness, loss of balance, inability to urinate, or seizures could indicate severe toxicity and should prompt immediate medical attention.

Ramelteon is metabolized primarily through the cytochrome P450 (CYP)1A2 pathway and eliminated principally in urine. Repeated once-daily dosing does not appear to result in accumulation, likely because of the compound's short half-life.

Therapeutic Indications. Ramelteon was approved by the FDA for the treatment of insomnia characterized by difficulty with sleep onset. Potential off-label use is centered on application in circadian rhythm disorders, predominantly jet lag, delayed sleep phase syndrome, and shift work sleep disorder.

Clinical trials and animal studies have failed to demonstrate evidence of rebound insomnia of withdrawal effects.

Precautions and Adverse Events. Headache is the most common side effect of ramelteon. Other adverse effects may include somnolence, fatigue, dizziness, worsening insomnia, depression, nausea, and diarrhea. The drug should not be used in patients with severe hepatic impairment. It is also not recommended in patients with severe sleep apnea or severe chronic obstructive pulmonary disease. Prolactin levels may be increased in women. The drug should be used with caution, if at all, in nursing mothers and pregnant women.

Ramelteon has been found to sometimes decrease blood cortisol and testosterone and to increase prolactin. Female patients should be monitored for cessation of menses and of galactorrhea, decreased libido, and fertility problems. The safety and effectiveness of ramelteon in children has not been established.

Drug Interactions. CYP1A2 is the major isozyme involved in the hepatic metabolism of ramelteon. Accordingly, fluvoxamine (Luvox) and other CYP1A2 inhibitors may increase side effects of ramelteon.

Ramelteon should be administered with caution in patients taking CYP1A2 inhibitors, strong CYP3A4 inhibitors such as ketoconazole, and strong CYP2C inhibitors such as fluconazole (Diflucan). No clinically meaningful interactions were found when ramelteon was coadministered with omeprazole, theophylline, dextromethorphan, midazolam, digoxin, and warfarin.

Dosing and Clinical Guidelines. The usual dose of ramelteon is 8 mg within 30 minutes of going to bed. It should not be taken with or immediately after high-fat meals.

Melatonin

Melatonin (N-acetyl-5-methoxytryptamine) is a hormone produced mainly at night in the pineal gland. Ingested melatonin can reach and bind to melatonin-binding sites in the brains of mammals, and produce somnolence when used at high doses. Melatonin is available as a dietary supplement and is not a medication. Few well-controlled clinical trials have been conducted to determine its effectiveness in treating such conditions as insomnia, jet lag, and sleep disturbances related to shift work.

Pharmacological Actions. Melatonin's secretion is stimulated by the dark and inhibited by the light. It is naturally synthesized from the amino acid tryptophan, which is converted to serotonin and finally converted to melatonin. The suprachiasmatic nuclei (SCN) of the hypothalamus have melatonin receptors, and melatonin may have a direct action on SCN to influence circadian rhythms, which are relevant for jet lag and sleep disturbances. In addition to the pineal gland, melatonin is also produced in the retina and GI tract.

Melatonin has a very short half-life of 0.5 to 6 minutes. Plasma concentrations are a function of the dose administered and the endogenous rhythm. Approximately 90 percent of melatonin is cleared through first-pass metabolism by way of the CYP1A1 and CYP1A2 pathways. Elimination occurs principally in urine.

Exogenous melatonin interacts with the melatonin receptors that suppress neuronal firing and promote sleep. There does not appear to be a dose–response relationship between exogenous melatonin administrations and sleep effects.

Therapeutic Indications. Melatonin is not regulated by the FDA. Individuals have used exogenous melatonin to address sleep difficulties (insomnia, circadian rhythm disorders), cancer (breast, prostate, colorectal), seizures, depression, anxiety, and seasonal affective disorder. Some studies suggest that exogenous melatonin may have some antioxidant effects and antiaging properties.

Precautions and Adverse Reactions. Adverse events associated with melatonin include fatigue, dizziness, headache, irritability, and somnolence. Disorientation, confusion, sleepwalking, vivid dreams, and nightmares have also been observed, often with effects resolving after melatonin administration was suspended.

Melatonin may reduce fertility in both men and women. In men, exogenous melatonin reduces sperm motility, and long-term administration has been shown to inhibit testicular aromatase levels. In women, exogenous melatonin may inhibit ovarian function and for that reason it has been evaluated as a contraceptive, but with inconclusive results.

Drug Interactions. As a dietary supplement preparation, exogenous melatonin is not regulated by the FDA and has not been subjected to the same type of drug interaction studies that were performed for ramelteon. Caution is suggested in coadministering melatonin with blood thinners (e.g., warfarin [Coumadin], aspirin, and heparin), antiseizure medications, and medications that lower BP.

Laboratory Interference. Melatonin is not known to interfere with any commonly used clinical laboratory tests.

Dosage and Administration. Over-the-counter melatonin is available in the following formulations: 1-, 2.5-, 3-, and 5-mg capsules; 1 mg/4 mL liquid; 0.5- and 3-mg lozenges; 2.5-mg sublingual tablets; and 1-, 2-, and 3-mg timed-release tablets.

Standard recommendations are to take the desired melatonin dose at bedtime, but some evidence from clinical trials suggests that dosing up to 2 hours before habitual bedtime may produce greater improvement in sleep onset.

Agomelatine (Valdoxan)

Agomelatine is structurally related to melatonin and is used in Europe as a treatment for MDD. It acts as an agonist at melatonin (MT1 and MT2) receptors. It also acts as a serotonin antagonist. Analysis of agomelatine clinical trial data raised serious questions about the efficacy and safety of the drug. The drug is not being marketed in the United States.

MIRTAZAPINE

Mirtazapine (Remeron) is unique among drugs used to treat major depression in that it increases both norepinephrine and serotonin through a mechanism other than reuptake blockade (as in the case of tricyclic agents or SSRIs) or monoamine oxidase inhibition (as in the case of phenelzine or tranylcypromine). Mirtazapine is also more likely to reduce rather than cause nausea and diarrhea, the result of its effects on serotonin 5-HT_3 receptors. Characteristic side effects include increased appetite and sedation.

Pharmacological Actions

Mirtazapine is administered orally and is rapidly and completely absorbed. It has a half-life of about 30 hours. Peak concentration is achieved within 2 hours of ingestion, and steady state is reached after 6 days. Plasma clearance may be slowed up to 30 percent in persons with impaired hepatic function, up to 50 percent in those with impaired renal function, up to 40 percent slower in elderly men, and up to 10 percent slower in elderly women.

The mechanism of action of mirtazapine is antagonism of central presynaptic α_2-adrenergic receptors and blockade of postsynaptic serotonin 5-HT_2 and 5-HT_3 receptors. The α_2-adrenergic receptor antagonism causes increased firing of norepinephrine and serotonin neurons. The potent antagonist of serotonin 5-HT_2 and 5-HT_3 receptors serves to decrease anxiety, relieve insomnia, and stimulate appetite. Mirtazapine is a potent antagonist of histamine H_1 receptors and is a moderately potent antagonist at α_1-adrenergic and muscarinic-cholinergic receptors.

Therapeutic Indications

Mirtazapine is effective for the treatment of depression. It is highly sedating, making it a reasonable choice for use in depressed patients with severe or long-standing insomnia. Some patients find the residual daytime sedation associated with initiation of treatment to be quite pronounced. However, the more extreme sedating properties of the drug generally lessen over the first week of treatment. Combined with the tendency to sometimes cause a ravenous appetite, mirtazapine is well suited for depressed patients with melancholic features such as insomnia, weight loss, and agitation. Elderly depressed patients in particular are good candidates for mirtazapine; young adults are more likely to object to this side effect profile.

Mirtazapine's blockade of 5-HT_3 receptors, a mechanism associated with medications used to combat the severe GI side effects of cancer chemotherapy agents, has led to the use of the drug in a similar role. In this population, sedation and stimulation of appetite clearly could be seen as being beneficial instead of unwelcome side effects.

Mirtazapine is often combined with SSRIs or venlafaxine to augment antidepressant response or counteract serotonergic side effects of those drugs, particularly nausea, agitation, and insomnia. Mirtazapine has no significant pharmacokinetic interactions with other antidepressants.

Precautions and Adverse Reactions

Somnolence, the most common adverse effect of mirtazapine, occurs in more than 50 percent of persons (Table 25–41). Persons starting mirtazapine should thus exercise caution when driving or operating dangerous machinery and even when getting out of bed at night. This adverse effect is why mirtazapine is almost always given before sleep. Mirtazapine potentiates the sedative effects of other CNS depressants, so potentially sedating prescription or over-the-counter drugs and alcohol should be avoided during use of mirtazapine. Mirtazapine also causes dizziness in 7 percent of persons. It does not appear to increase the risk for seizures. Mania or

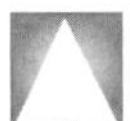

Table 25–41
Adverse Reactions Reported with Mirtazapine

Event	Patients (%)
Somnolence	54
Dry mouth	25
Increased appetite	17
Constipation	13
Weight gain	12
Dizziness	7
Myalgias	5
Disturbing dreams	4

hypomania occurred in clinical trials at a rate similar to that of other antidepressant drugs.

Mirtazapine increases appetite in about one-third of patients. Mirtazapine may also increase serum cholesterol concentration to 20 percent or more above the upper limit of normal in 15 percent of persons and increase triglycerides to 500 mg/dL or more in 6 percent of persons. Elevations of alanine transaminase levels to more than three times the upper limit of normal were seen in 2 percent of mirtazapine-treated persons as opposed to 0.3 percent of placebo control subjects.

In limited premarketing experience, the absolute neutrophil count (ANC) dropped to 500/mm^3 or less within 2 months of the onset of use in 0.3 percent of persons, some of whom developed symptomatic infections. This hematologic condition was reversible in all cases and was more likely to occur when other risk factors for neutropenia were present. Increases in the frequency of neutropenia have not, however, been reported during the extensive postmarketing period. Persons who develop fever, chills, sore throat, mucous membrane ulceration, or other signs of infection should nevertheless be evaluated medically. If a low WBC count is found, mirtazapine should be immediately discontinued, and the infectious disease status should be followed closely.

A small number of persons experience orthostatic hypotension while taking mirtazapine. Although no data exist regarding the effects on fetal development, mirtazapine should be used with caution during pregnancy.

Mirtazapine use by pregnant women has not been studied, but because the drug may be excreted in breast milk, it should not be taken by nursing mothers. Because of the risk of agranulocytosis associated with mirtazapine use, persons should be attuned to signs of infection. Because of the sedating effects of mirtazapine, persons should determine the degree to which they are affected before engaging in driving or other potentially dangerous activities.

Drug Interactions

Mirtazapine can potentiate the sedation of alcohol and benzodiazepines. Mirtazapine should not be used within 14 days of use of an MAOI.

Laboratory Interferences

No laboratory interferences have yet been described for mirtazapine.

Dosage and Administration

Mirtazapine is available in 15-, 30-, and 45-mg scored tablets. Mirtazapine is also available in 15-, 30-, and 45-mg orally disintegrating tablets for persons who have difficulty swallowing pills. If persons fail to respond to the initial dose of 15 mg of mirtazapine before sleep, the dose may be increased in 15-mg increments every 5 days to a maximum of 45 mg before sleep. Lower dosages may be necessary in elderly persons or persons with renal or hepatic insufficiency.

MONOAMINE OXIDASE INHIBITORS

Introduced in the late 1950s, MAOIs were the first class of approved antidepressant drugs. The first of these drugs, isoniazid, was intended to be used as a treatment for tuberculosis, but its antidepressant properties were discovered by chance when some treated patients experienced elevation of mood during treatment. Despite their effectiveness, prescription of MAOIs as first-line agents has always been limited by concern about the development of potentially lethal hypertension and the consequent need for a restrictive diet. Use of MAOIs declined further after the introduction of the SSRIs and other new agents. They are now mainly relegated to use in treatment-resistant cases. Thus, the second-line status of MAOIs has less to do with considerations of efficacy than with concerns for safety. The currently available MAOIs include phenelzine (Nardil), isocarboxazid (Marplan), tranylcypromine (Parnate), rasagiline (Azilect), moclobemide (Manerix), and selegiline (Eldepryl).

Two subsequent advances in the field of antidepressant MAOIs involve the introduction of a selective reversible inhibitor of MAO_A (RIMA), moclobemide (Manerix), in the early 1990s into most countries except the United States, and in 2005, the introduction of a transdermal delivery form of selegiline (Emsam) in the United States that is used for the treatment of parkinsonism and thereafter in 2006 was approved for the treatment of major depressive disorder. Other RIMA agents, including brofaromine (Consonar) and befloxatone, have not been submitted for registration despite favorable outcomes in clinical trials.

Pharmacological Actions

Phenelzine, tranylcypromine, and isocarboxazid are readily absorbed after oral administration and reach peak plasma concentrations within 2 hours. Whereas their plasma half-lives are in the range of 2 to 3 hours, their tissue half-lives are considerably longer. Because they irreversibly inactivate MAOs, the therapeutic effect of a single dose of irreversible MAOIs may persist for as long as 2 weeks. The RIMA moclobemide is rapidly absorbed and has a half-life of 0.5 to 3.5 hours. Because it is a reversible inhibitor, moclobemide has a much briefer clinical effect after a single dose than do irreversible MAOIs.

The MAO enzymes are found on the outer membranes of mitochondria, where they degrade cytoplasmic and extraneuronal monoamine neurotransmitters such as norepinephrine, serotonin, dopamine, epinephrine, and tyramine. MAOIs act in the CNS, the sympathetic nervous system, the liver, and the GI tract. There are two types of MAOs, MAO_A and MAO_B. MAO_A primarily metabolizes norepinephrine, serotonin, and epinephrine; dopamine and tyramine are metabolized by both MAO_A and MAO_B.

The structures of phenelzine and tranylcypromine are similar to those of amphetamine and have similar pharmacologic effects in that they increase the release of dopamine and norepinephrine with attendant stimulant effects on the brain.

Therapeutic Indications

MAOIs are used for the treatment of depression. Some research indicates that phenelzine is more effective than TCAs in depressed patients with mood reactivity, extreme sensitivity to interpersonal loss or rejection, prominent anergia, hyperphagia, and hypersomnia—a constellation of symptoms conceptualized as atypical depression. Evidence also suggests that MAOIs are more effective than TCAs as a treatment for bipolar depression.

Patients with panic disorder and social phobia respond well to MAOIs. MAOIs have also been used to treat bulimia nervosa, PTSD, anginal pain, atypical facial pain, migraine, ADHD, idiopathic orthostatic hypotension, and depression associated with traumatic brain injury.

Precautions and Adverse Reactions

The most frequent adverse effects of MAOIs are orthostatic hypotension, insomnia, weight gain, edema, and sexual dysfunction. Orthostatic hypotension can lead to dizziness and falls. Thus, cautious upward tapering of the dosage should be used to determine the maximum tolerable dosage. Treatment for orthostatic hypotension includes avoidance of caffeine; intake of 2 L of fluid per day; addition of dietary salt or adjustment of antihypertensive drugs (if applicable); support stockings; and in severe cases, treatment with fludrocortisone (Florinef), a mineralocorticoid, 0.1 to 0.2 mg a day. Orthostatic hypotension associated with tranylcypromine use can usually be relieved by dividing the daily dosage.

Insomnia can be treated by dividing the dose, not giving the medication after dinner, and using trazodone (Desyrel) or a benzodiazepine hypnotic if necessary. Weight gain, edema, and sexual dysfunction often do not respond to any treatment and may warrant switching to another agent. When switching from one MAOI to another, the clinician should taper and stop use of the first drug for 10 to 14 days before beginning use of the second drug.

Paresthesias, myoclonus, and muscle pains are occasionally seen in persons treated with MAOIs. Paresthesias may be secondary to MAOI-induced pyridoxine deficiency, which may respond to supplementation with pyridoxine, 50 to 150 mg orally each day. Occasionally, persons complain of feeling drunk or confused, perhaps indicating that the dosage should be reduced and then increased gradually. Reports that the hydrazine MAOIs are associated with hepatotoxic effects are relatively uncommon. MAOIs are less cardiotoxic and less epileptogenic than are the tricyclic and tetracyclic drugs.

The most common adverse effects of the RIMA moclobemide are dizziness, nausea, and insomnia or sleep disturbance. RIMAs cause fewer GI adverse effects than do SSRIs. Moclobemide does not have adverse anticholinergic or cardiovascular effects, and it has not been reported to interfere with sexual function.

MAOIs should be used with caution by persons with renal disease, cardiovascular disease, or hyperthyroidism. MAOIs may alter the dosage of a hypoglycemic agent required by persons with diabetes. MAOIs have been particularly associated with induction of mania in persons in the depressed phase of bipolar I disorder and triggering of a psychotic decompensation in persons with schizophrenia. MAOIs are contraindicated during pregnancy, although data on their teratogenic risk are minimal. MAOIs should not be taken by nursing women because the drugs can pass into the breast milk.

Tyramine-Induced Hypertensive Crisis. The most worrisome side effect of MAOIs is the tyramine-induced hypertensive crisis. The amino acid tyramine is normally transformed via GI metabolism. However, MAOIs inactivate GI metabolism of dietary tyramine, thus allowing intact tyramine to enter the circulation. A hypertensive crisis may subsequently occur as a result of a powerful pressor effect of the amino acid. Tyramine-containing foods should be avoided for 2 weeks after the last dose of an irreversible MAOI to allow resynthesis of adequate concentrations of MAO enzymes.

Accordingly, foods rich in tyramine (Table 25–42) or other sympathomimetic amines, such as ephedrine, pseudoephedrine (Sudafed), or dextromethorphan (Trocal), should be avoided

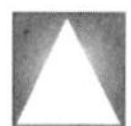

Table 25–42
Tyramine-Rich Foods to Be Avoided in Planning Monoamine Oxidase Inhibitor Diets

High tyramine content[a] (≥2 mg of tyramine a serving)
Cheese: English Stilton, blue cheese, white (3 yr old), extra old, old cheddar, Danish blue, mozzarella, cheese snack spreads
Fish, cured meats, sausage; pâtés and organs, salami, mortadella, air-dried sausage
Alcoholic beverages[b]: Liqueurs and concentrated after-dinner drinks
Marmite (concentrated yeast extract)
Sauerkraut (Krakus)

Moderate tyramine content[a] (0.5–1.99 mg of tyramine a serving)
Cheese: Swiss Gruyere, muenster, feta, parmesan, gorgonzola, blue cheese dressing, Black Diamond
Fish, cured meats, sausage, pâtés and organs: Chicken liver (5 days old): bologna; aged sausage, smoked meat; salmon mousse
Alcoholic beverages: Beer and ale (12 oz per bottle)—Amstel, Export Draft, Blue Light, Guinness Extra Stout, Old Vienna, Canadian, Miller Light, Export, Heineken, Blue Wines (per 4 oz glass)—Rioja (red wine)

Low tyramine content[a] (0.01 to >0.49 mg of tyramine a serving)
Cheese: Brie, Camembert, Cambozola with or without rind
Fish, cured meat, sausage, organs, and pâtés; pickled herring; smoked fish; kielbasa sausage; chicken liver; liverwurst (<2 days old)
Alcoholic beverages: Red wines, sherry, scotch[c]
Others: Banana or avocado (ripe or not), banana peel

[a]Any food left out to age or spoil can spontaneously develop tyramine through fermentation.
[b]Alcohol can produce profound orthostasis interacting with monoamine oxidase inhibitors (MAOIs) but cannot produce direct hypotensive reactions.
[c]White wines, gin, and vodka have no tyramine content.
Table by Jonathan M. Himmelhoch, M.D.

by persons who are taking irreversible MAOIs. Patients should be advised to continue the dietary restrictions for 2 weeks after they stop MAOI treatment to allow the body to resynthesize the enzyme. Bee stings may cause a hypertensive crisis. In addition to severe hypertension, other symptoms may include headache, stiff neck, diaphoresis, nausea, and vomiting. A patient with these symptoms should seek immediate medical treatment.

An MAOI-induced hypertensive crisis should be treated with α-adrenergic antagonists—for example, phentolamine (Regitine) or chlorpromazine (Thorazine). These drugs lower BP within 5 minutes. IV furosemide (Lasix) can be used to reduce fluid load, and a β-adrenergic receptor antagonist can control tachycardia. A sublingual 10-mg dose of nifedipine (Procardia) can be given and repeated after 20 minutes. MAOIs should not be used by persons with thyrotoxicosis or pheochromocytoma.

The risk of tyramine-induced hypertensive crises is relatively low for persons who are taking RIMAs, such as moclobemide and befloxatone. These drugs have relatively little inhibitory activity for MAO_B, and because they are reversible, normal activity of existing MAO_A returns within 16 to 48 hours of the last dose of a RIMA. Therefore, the dietary restrictions are less stringent for RIMAs, applying only to foods containing high concentrations of tyramine, which need be avoided for 3 days after the last dose of a RIMA. A reasonable dietary recommendation for persons taking RIMAs is to avoid eating tyramine-containing foods 1 hour before and 2 hours after taking a RIMA.

Spontaneous, nontyramine-induced hypertensive crisis is a rare occurrence, usually shortly after the first exposure of an MAOI. Persons experiencing such a crisis should avoid MAOIs altogether.

Withdrawal. Abrupt cessation of regular doses of MAOIs may cause a self-limited discontinuation syndrome consisting of arousal, mood disturbances, and somatic symptoms. To avoid these symptoms when discontinuing use to an MAOI, dosages should be gradually tapered over several weeks.

Overdose. There is often an asymptomatic period of 1 to 6 hours after an MAOI overdose before the occurrence of the symptoms of toxicity. MAOI overdose is characterized by agitation that can progress to coma with hyperthermia, hypertension, tachypnea, tachycardia, dilated pupils, and hyperactive deep tendon reflexes. Involuntary movements may be present, particularly in the face and the jaw. Acidification of the urine markedly hastens the excretion of MAOIs, and dialysis can be of some use. Phentolamine or chlorpromazine may be useful if hypertension is a problem. Moclobemide alone in overdosage causes relatively mild and reversible symptoms.

Drug Interactions

The major drug–drug interactions involving MAOIs are listed in Table 25–43. Most antidepressants as well as precursor agents should be avoided. Persons should be instructed to tell any other physicians or dentists who are treating them that they are taking an MAOI. MAOIs may potentiate the action of CNS depressants, including alcohol and barbiturates. MAOIs should not be coadministered with serotonergic drugs, such as SSRIs and clomipramine (Anafranil), because this combination can trigger a serotonin syndrome. Use of lithium or tryptophan with an irreversible MAOI may also induce a serotonin syndrome. Initial symptoms of a serotonin syndrome can include tremor, hypertonicity, myoclonus, and autonomic instability, which can then progress to hallucinosis, hyperthermia, and even death. Fatal reactions have occurred when MAOIs were combined with meperidine (Demerol) or fentanyl (Sublimaze).

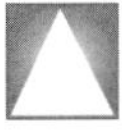

Table 25–43
Drugs to be Avoided During Monoamine Oxidase Inhibitor Treatment (Part of Listing)

Never use
Antiasthmatics
Antihypertensives (methyldopa, guanethidine, reserpine)
Buspirone
Levodopa
Opioids (especially meperidine, dextromethorphan, propoxyphene, tramadol; morphine or codeine may be less dangerous.)
Cold, allergy, or sinus medications containing dextromethorphan or sympathomimetics
SSRIs, clomipramine, venlafaxine, sibutramine
Sympathomimetics (amphetamines, cocaine, methylphenidate, dopamine, epinephrine, norepinephrine, isoproterenol, ephedrine, pseudoephedrine, phenylpropanolamine)
L-Tryptophan
Use carefully
Anticholinergics
Antihistamines
Disulfiram
Bromocriptine
Hydralazine
Sedative hypnotics
Terpin hydrate with codeine
Tricyclics and tetracyclics (avoid clomipramine)

SSRI, selective serotonin reuptake inhibitor.

When switching from an irreversible MAOI to any other type of antidepressant drug, persons should wait at least 14 days after the last dose of the MAOI before beginning use of the next drug to allow replenishment of the body's MAOs. When switching from an antidepressant to an irreversible MAOI, persons should wait 10 to 14 days (or 5 weeks for fluoxetine [Prozac]) before starting use of the MAOI to avoid drug–drug interactions. In contrast, MAO activity recovers completely 24 to 48 hours after the last dose of a RIMA.

The effects of the MAOIs on hepatic enzymes are poorly studied. Tranylcypromine inhibits CYP2C19. Moclobemide inhibits CYP2D6, CYP2C19, and CYP1A2 and is a substrate for 2C19.

Cimetidine (Tagamet) and fluoxetine significantly reduce the elimination of moclobemide. Modest doses of fluoxetine and moclobemide administered concurrently may be well tolerated, with no significant pharmacodynamic or pharmacokinetic interactions.

Laboratory Interferences

MAOIs may lower blood glucose concentrations. MAOIs artificially raise urinary metanephrine concentrations and may cause a false-positive test result for pheochromocytoma or neuroblastoma. MAOIs have been reported to be associated with a minimal false elevation in thyroid function test results.

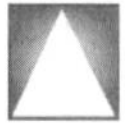

Table 25–44
Typical Dosage Forms and Recommended Dosages for Currently Available Monoamine Oxidase Inhibitors

Drug	Usual Dose (mg/day)	Maximum Dose (mg/day)	Dosage (Oral) Formulation
Isocarboxazid (Marplan)	20–40	60	10-mg tablets
Phenelzine (Nardil)	30–60	90	15-mg tablets
Tranylcypromine (Parnate)	20–60	60	10-mg tablets
Rasagiline	0.5–1.0	1.0	0.5- or 1.0-mg tablets
Selegiline (Eldepryl)	10	30	5-mg tablets
Moclobemide (Manerix)	300–600	600	100- or 150-mg tablets

Dosage and Clinical Guidelines

There is no definitive rationale for choosing one irreversible MAOI over another. Table 25–44 lists MAOI preparations and typical dosages. Phenelzine use should begin with a test dose of 15 mg on the first day. The dosage can be increased to 15 mg three times daily during the first week and increased by 15 mg a day each week thereafter until the dosage of 90 mg a day, in divided doses, is reached by the end of the fourth week. Tranylcypromine and isocarboxazid use should begin with a test dosage of 10 mg and may be increased to 10 mg three times daily by the end of the first week. Many clinicians and researchers have recommended upper limits of 50 mg a day for isocarboxazid and 40 mg a day for tranylcypromine. Administration of tranylcypromine in multiple small daily doses may reduce its hypotensive effects.

Even though coadministration of MAOIs with TCAs, SSRIs, or lithium is generally contraindicated, these combinations have been used successfully and safely to treat patients with refractory depression. However, they should be used with extreme caution.

Hepatic transaminase serum concentrations should be monitored periodically because of the potential for hepatotoxicity, especially with phenelzine and isocarboxazid. Elderly persons may be more sensitive to MAOI adverse effects than are younger adults. MAO activity increases with age, so MAOI dosages for elderly persons are the same as those required for younger adults. The use of MAOIs for children has had minimal study.

Studies have suggested that transdermal selegiline has antidepressant properties. Although selegiline is a type B inhibitor at low doses, it becomes less selective as the dose is increased.

NEFAZODONE, VILAZODONE, AND TRAZODONE

Nefazodone (Serzone) and Trazodone (Desyrel, Oleptro) are mechanistically and structurally related drugs approved as treatments for depression. Nefazodone (Serzone) is an analog of trazodone. When nefazodone was introduced in 1995, there were expectations that it would become widely used because it did not cause the sexual side effects and sleep disruption associated with the selective SSRIs. Although it was devoid of these side effects, it was nevertheless found to produce problematic sedation, nausea, dizziness, and visual disturbances. Consequently, nefazodone was never extensively adopted in clinical practice. This fact, as well as reports of rare cases of sometimes fatal hepatotoxicity, led the original manufacturer to discontinue production of branded nefazodone in 2004. Generic nefazodone remains available in the United States.

Vilazodone (Vibryd)

Vilazodone was approved in 2011 by the FDA for the treatment of major depressive disorder. It has a unique mechanism of action combining selective serotonin reuptake inhibition with partial agonism of the serotonin 5-HT$_{1A}$ receptor and may synergistically increase serotonergic transmission.

Trazodone received FDA approval in 1981 as a treatment for MDD. Its novel triazolopyridine chemical structure distinguished it from the TCAs, and clinical trials suggested improved safety and tolerability compared with TCAs. There were high expectations that it would replace the older drugs as a mainstay of treatment for depression. However, the extreme sedation associated with trazodone, even at subtherapeutic doses, limited the clinical effectiveness of the drug. However, its soporific properties made trazodone a favorite alternative to standard hypnotics as a sleep-inducing agent. Unlike conventional sleeping pills, trazodone is not a controlled substance.

In 2010, the FDA approved an extended-release, once-daily formulation (Oleptro) as a treatment for MDD in adults. In the trial leading to the approval of the extended-release formulation, the most common adverse events were somnolence or sedation, dizziness, constipation, and blurred vision. Surprisingly, only 4 percent of patients in the trazodone group discontinued treatment because of somnolence or sedation.

Nefazodone

Pharmacological Actions. Nefazodone is rapidly and completely absorbed but is then extensively metabolized so that the bioavailability of active compounds is about 20 percent of the oral dose. Its half-life is 2 to 4 hours. Steady-state concentrations of nefazodone and its principal active metabolite, hydroxynefazodone, are achieved within 4 to 5 days. Metabolism of nefazodone in elderly persons, especially women, is about half of that seen in younger persons, so lowered doses are recommended for elderly persons. An important metabolite of nefazodone is meta-chlorophenylpiperazine (mCPP), which has some serotonergic effects and may cause migraine, anxiety, and weight loss.

Although nefazodone is an inhibitor of serotonin uptake and, more weakly, of norepinephrine reuptake, its antagonism of serotonin 5-HT$_A$ receptors is thought to produce its antianxiety and antidepressant effects. Nefazodone is also a mild antagonist of the α_1-adrenergic receptors, which predisposes some persons to orthostatic hypotension but is not sufficiently potent to produce priapism.

Therapeutic Indications. Nefazodone is effective for the treatment of major depression. The usual effective dosage is

300 to 600 mg a day. In direct comparison with SSRIs, nefazodone is less likely to cause inhibition of orgasm or decreased sexual desire. Nefazodone is also effective for the treatment of panic disorder and panic with comorbid depression or depressive symptoms, generalized anxiety disorder, and PMDD and for management of chronic pain. It is not effective for the treatment of OCD. Nefazodone increases rapid eye movement (REM) sleep and increases sleep continuity. Nefazodone is also of use in patients with PTSD and chronic fatigue syndrome. It may also be effective in patients who have been treatment resistant to other antidepressant drugs.

Precautions and Adverse Reactions. The most common reasons for discontinuing nefazodone use are sedation, nausea, dizziness, insomnia, weakness, and agitation. Many patients report no specific side effect but describe a vague sense of feeling medicated. Nefazodone also causes visual trails, in which patients see an afterimage when looking at moving objects or when moving their heads quickly.

A major safety concern with the use of nefazodone is severe elevation of hepatic enzymes, and, in some instances, liver failure. Accordingly, serial hepatic function tests need to be done when patients are treated with nefazodone. Hepatic effects can be seen early in treatment and are more likely to develop when nefazodone is combined with other drugs metabolized in the liver.

Some patients taking nefazodone may experience a decrease in BP that can cause episodes of postural hypotension. Nefazodone should therefore be used with caution by persons with underlying cardiac conditions or history of stroke or heart attack, dehydration, or hypovolemia or by persons being treated with antihypertensive medications. Patients switched from SSRIs to nefazodone may experience an increase in side effects, possibly because nefazodone does not protect against SSRI withdrawal symptoms. One of its metabolites, mCPP, may actually intensify these discontinuation symptoms. Patients have survived nefazodone overdoses in excess of 10 g, but deaths have been reported when it has been combined with alcohol. Nausea, vomiting, and somnolence are the most common signs of toxicity.

The effects of nefazodone in human mothers are not as well understood as those of the SSRIs, mainly because of the paucity of its clinical use. Nefazodone should therefore be used during pregnancy only if the potential benefit to the mother outweighs the potential risks to the fetus. It is not known whether nefazodone is excreted in human breast milk. Therefore, it should be used with caution by lactating mothers. The nefazodone dosage should be lowered in persons with severe hepatic disease, but no adjustment is necessary for persons with renal disease (Table 25–45).

Drug Interactions and Laboratory Interferences. Nefazodone should not be given concomitantly with MAOIs. In addition, nefazodone has particular drug–drug interactions with the triazolobenzodiazepines triazolam (Halcion) and alprazolam (Xanax) because of the inhibition of CYP3A4 by nefazodone. Potentially elevated levels of each of these drugs can develop after administration of nefazodone, but the levels of nefazodone are generally not affected. The dose of triazolam should be lowered by 75 percent, and the dose of alprazolam should be lowered by 50 percent when given concomitantly with nefazodone.

Table 25–45
Adverse Reactions Reported with Nefazodone (300–600 mg a Day)

Reaction	Patients (%)
Headache	36
Dry mouth	25
Somnolence	25
Nausea	22
Dizziness	17
Constipation	14
Insomnia	11
Weakness	11
Lightheadedness	10
Blurred vision	9
Dyspepsia	9
Infection	8
Confusion	7
Scotomata	7

Nefazodone may slow the metabolism of digoxin; therefore, digoxin levels should be monitored carefully in persons taking both medications. Nefazodone also slows the metabolism of haloperidol (Haldol) so that the dosage of haloperidol should be reduced in persons taking both medications. Addition of nefazodone may also exacerbate the adverse effects of lithium carbonate (Eskalith).

There are no known laboratory interferences associated with nefazodone.

Dosage and Clinical Guidelines. Nefazodone is available in 50-, 200-, and 250-mg unscored tablets and 100- and 150-mg scored tablets. The recommended starting dosage of nefazodone is 100 mg twice a day, but 50 mg twice a day may be better tolerated, especially by elderly persons. To limit the development of adverse effects, the dosage should be slowly raised in increments of 100 to 200 mg a day at intervals of no less than 1 week per increase. The optimal dosage is 300 to 600 mg daily in two divided doses. However, some studies report that nefazodone is effective when taken once a day, especially at bedtime. Geriatric persons should receive dosages about two-thirds of the usual nongeriatric dosages, with a maximum of 400 mg a day. Similar to other antidepressants, clinical benefit of nefazodone usually appears after 2 to 4 weeks of treatment. Patients with premenstrual syndrome are treated with a flexible dosage that averages about 250 mg a day.

Vilazodone

Pharmacological Actions. Vilazodone reaches peak plasma concentrations in 4 to 5 hours after administration with a terminal half-life of approximately 25 hours. Food impacts the absorption and the absolute bioavailability of vilazodone with food reaches 72 percent while in a fasting state the AUC and C_{max} can be decreased by approximately 50 percent and 60 percent, respectively. It is important to note that administration without food can result in inadequate drug concentrations and may reduce effectiveness. Clinicians should inform the patients about the importance of taking the medicine with meals. Vilazodone is widely distributed and approximately 96 to 99 percent protein-bound.

Vilazodone inhibits serotonin uptake with minimal or no effect on reuptake of norepinephrine or dopamine. It binds selectively to 5-HT_{1A} receptors and is also a 5-HT_{1A} receptor partial agonist. It has been postulated that 5-HT_{1A} receptor activity may be altered in depression and anxiety and Vilazodone may mitigates depressive symptoms by binding to this receptor.

Therapeutic Indications. Vilazodone is indicated for the treatment of MDD. The usual recommended dose for vilazodone is 40 mg once daily with food. Patients should start with an initial dose of 10 mg once daily for 7 days, followed by 20 mg once daily for an additional 7 days, and then an increase to 40 mg once daily.

Precautions and Adverse Reactions. There are no dose-related adverse effects between 20- and 40-mg dose. The most common adverse effects associated with vilazodone are diarrhea, nausea, and headache. Other less frequent side effects include ventricular extrasystoles, dry eyes, blurred vision, sedation, and night sweats. As with all antidepressants suicidal thoughts should be evaluated, and patients should be monitored for serotonin syndrome, risk for bleeding, seizures, and hyponatremia.

Drug Interactions. There are CYP450 enzyme interactions requiring dosage adjustment. Concomitant administration of CYP3A4 inhibitors may require a maximum dose of 20 mg while CYP3A4 inducers may decrease the C_{max} and AUC by twofold. Viazodone is unlikely to inhibit or induce the metabolism of substrates for CYP1A1, 1A2, 2A6, 2B6, 2C9, 2C19, 2D6, 2E1, 3A4, or 3A5, except for CYP2C8.

Dosage and Clinical Guidelines. Vilazodone is available as 10-, 20-, and 40-mg tablets. The recommended therapeutic dose of vilazodone is 40 mg once daily. Treatment should be titrated, starting with an initial dose of 10 mg once daily for 7 days, followed by 20 mg once daily for an additional 7 days, and then an increase to 40 mg once daily. Vilazodone should be taken with food. If vilazodone is taken without food, inadequate drug concentrations may result and the drug's effectiveness may be diminished. Vilazodone is not approved for use in children. The safety and efficacy of vilazodone in pediatric patients have not been studied. No dose adjustment is recommended on the basis of age. No dose adjustment is recommended in patients with mild or moderate hepatic impairment. Vilazodone has not been studied in patients with severe hepatic impairment. No dose adjustment is recommended in patients with mild, moderate, or severe renal impairment.

Trazodone

Pharmacological Actions. Trazodone is readily absorbed from the GI tract and reaches peak plasma levels in about 1 hour. It has a half-life of 5 to 9 hours. Trazodone is metabolized in the liver, and 75 percent of its metabolites are excreted in the urine.

Trazodone is a weak inhibitor of serotonin reuptake and a potent antagonist of serotonin 5-HT_{2A} and 5-HT_{2C} receptors. The active metabolite of trazodone is mCPP, which is an agonist at 5-HT_{2C} receptors and has a half-life of 14 hours. mCPP has been associated with migraine, anxiety, and weight loss. The adverse effects of trazodone are partially mediated by α_1-adrenergic receptor antagonism.

Therapeutic Indications

DEPRESSIVE DISORDERS. The main indication for the use of trazodone is MDD. There is a clear dose–response relationship, with dosages of 250 to 600 mg a day being necessary for trazodone to have therapeutic benefit. Trazodone increases total sleep time, decreases the number and the duration of nighttime awakenings, and decreases the amount of REM sleep. Unlike tricyclic drugs, trazodone does not decrease stage 4 sleep. Trazodone is thus useful for depressed persons with anxiety and insomnia.

INSOMNIA. Trazodone is a first-line agent for the treatment of insomnia because of its marked sedative qualities and favorable effects on sleep architecture (see above) combined with its lack of anticholinergic effects. Trazodone is effective for insomnia caused by depression or use of drugs. When used as a hypnotic, the usual initial dosage is 25 to 100 mg at bedtime.

ERECTILE DISORDER. Trazodone is associated with an increased risk of priapism. Trazodone can potentiate erections resulting from sexual stimulation. It has thus been used to prolong erectile time and turgidity in some men with erectile disorder. The dosage for this indication is 150 to 200 mg a day. Trazodone-triggered priapism (an erection lasting more than 3 hours with pain) is a medical emergency. The use of trazodone for the treatment of male erectile dysfunction has diminished considerably since the introduction of PDE-5 agents (see Chapter 25).

OTHER INDICATIONS. Trazodone may be useful in low dosages (50 mg a day) for controlling severe agitation in children with developmental disabilities and elderly persons with dementia. At dosages above 250 mg a day, trazodone reduces the tension and apprehension associated with generalized anxiety disorder. It has been used to treat depression in patients with schizophrenia. Trazodone may have a beneficial effect on insomnia and nightmares in persons with PTSD.

Precautions and Adverse Reactions. The most common adverse effects associated with trazodone are sedation, orthostatic hypotension, dizziness, headache, and nausea. Some persons experience dry mouth or gastric irritation. The drug is not associated with anticholinergic adverse effects, such as urinary retention, weight gain, and constipation. A few case reports have noted an association between trazodone and arrhythmias in persons with preexisting premature ventricular contractions or mitral valve prolapse. Neutropenia, usually not of clinical significance, may develop, which should be considered if persons have fever or sore throat.

Trazodone may cause significant orthostatic hypotension 4 to 6 hours after a dose is taken, especially if taken concurrently with antihypertensive agents or if a large dose is taken without food. Administration of trazodone with food slows absorption and reduces the peak plasma concentration, thus reducing the risk of orthostatic hypotension.

Because suicide attempts often involve ingestion of sleeping pills, it is important to be familiar with the symptoms and treatment of trazodone overdose. Patients have survived trazodone overdoses of more than 9 g. Symptoms of overdose include lethargy, vomiting, drowsiness, headache, orthostasis, dizziness, dyspnea, tinnitus, myalgias, tachycardia, incontinence, shivering, and coma. Treatment consists of emesis or lavage and supportive care. Forced diuresis may enhance elimination. Treat hypotension and sedation as appropriate.

Trazodone causes priapism, prolonged erection in the absence of sexual stimuli, in one of every 10,000 men. Trazodone-induced priapism usually appears in the first 4 weeks of treatment but may occur as late as 18 months into treatment. It can appear at any dose. In such cases, trazodone use should be discontinued, and another antidepressant should be used. Painful erections or erections lasting more than 1 hour are warning signs that warrant immediate discontinuation of the drug and medical evaluation. The first step in the emergency management of priapism is intracavernosal injection of an α_1-adrenergic agonist pressor agent, such as metaraminol (Aramine) or epinephrine. In about one-third of reported cases, surgical intervention was required. In some cases, permanent impairment of erectile function or impotence resulted.

The use of trazodone is contraindicated in pregnant and nursing women. Trazodone should be used with caution in persons with hepatic and renal diseases.

Drug Interactions. Trazodone potentiates the CNS depressant effects of other centrally acting drugs and alcohol. Concurrent use of trazodone and antihypertensives may cause hypotension. No cases of hypertensive crisis have been reported when trazodone has been used to treat MAOI-associated insomnia. Trazodone can increase levels of digoxin and phenytoin. Trazodone should be used with caution in combination with warfarin. Drugs that inhibit CYP3A4 can increase levels of trazodone's major metabolite, mCPP, leading to an increase in side effects.

Laboratory Interferences. No known laboratory interferences are associated with the administration of trazodone.

Dosage and Clinical Guidelines. Trazodone is available in 50-, 100-, 150-, and 300-mg tablets. Once-a-day dosing is as effective as divided dosing and reduces daytime sedation. The usual starting dose is 50 mg before sleep. The dosage can be increased in increments of 50 mg every 3 days if sedation or orthostatic hypotension does not become a problem. The therapeutic range for trazodone is 200 to 600 mg a day in divided doses. Some reports indicate that dosages of 400 to 600 mg a day are required for maximal therapeutic effects; other reports indicate that 250 to 400 mg a day is sufficient. The dosage may be titrated up to 300 mg a day; then the person can be evaluated for the need for further dosage increases on the basis of the presence or the absence of signs of clinical improvement.

Once-daily trazodone is available as bisectable tablets of 150 mg or 300 mg. The starting dosage of the extended-release formulation is 150 mg once daily. It may be increased by 75 mg per day every 3 days. The maximum dosage is 375 mg per day. Dosing should be at the same time every day in the late evening, preferably at bedtime, on an empty stomach. Tablets should be swallowed whole or broken in half along the score line.

OPIOID RECEPTOR AGONISTS

Opioid receptor agonists are a structurally diverse group of compounds that are used for pain management. These drugs are also called narcotics. Although highly effective as analgesics, they often cause dependence and are frequently diverted for recreational use. Commonly used opioid agonists for pain relief include morphine, hydromorphone (Dilaudid), codeine, meperidine (Demerol), oxycodone (OxyContin), buprenorphine (Buprenex), hydrocodone (Robidone), tramadol (Ultram), and fentanyl (Durogesic). Heroin is used as a street drug. Methadone is used both for pain management and for the treatment of opiate addiction. This chapter focuses on the μ-opioid receptor agonists that are most likely to be used in the treatment of psychiatric disorders instead of pain management.

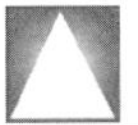

Table 25–46
μ- and κ-Opiate Receptors

Receptor	Agonist Effects	Antagonist Effects
Mu (μ)	Analgesia Euphoria Antidepressant Anxiety	Anxiety Hostility
Kappa (κ)	Analgesia Dysphoria Depression Stress-induced anxiety	Antidepressant

It is now recognized that the pharmacology of the opioid system is complex. There are multiple types of opioid receptors, with μ- and κ-opioid receptors representing functionally opposing endogenous systems (Table 25–46). All of the compounds above, which represent the most extensively used narcotic analgesics, are agonists at μ-opioid receptors. However, analgesic effects also result from antagonist effects on the κ-opioid receptor. Buprenorphine has mixed receptor effects, being primarily a μ-opioid receptor agonist as well as a κ-opioid antagonist.

There is growing interest in the use of some drugs that act on opioid receptors as alternative treatments for a subpopulation of patients with refractory depression, as well as treatment for cutting behavior in patients with borderline personality disorder.

Consideration of such off-label use is tempered by the well-known fact that ongoing, regular use of opioids produces dependence and tolerance and may lead to maladaptive use, functional impairment, and withdrawal symptoms. The prevalence of opioid use, abuse, and dependence, particularly in regard to prescription opioids, has risen in recent years.

Before using opioid receptor agonists with patients who have failed on multiple conventional therapeutic agents, screen carefully for history of drug abuse, document the rationale for off-label use, establish treatment ground rules, obtain written consent, consult with primary care physician, and monitor closely. Avoid replacing "lost" prescriptions and providing early prescription renewals.

Pharmacological Actions

Methadone and buprenorphine are absorbed rapidly from the GI tract. Hepatic first-pass metabolism significantly affects the bioavailability of each of the drugs but in markedly different ways. For methadone, hepatic enzymes reduce the bioavailability of an oral dosage by about half, an effect that is easily managed with dosage adjustments.

For buprenorphine, first-pass intestinal and hepatic metabolism eliminates oral bioavailability almost completely. When used in opioid detoxification, buprenorphine is given sublingually in either a liquid or a tablet formulation.

The peak plasma concentrations of oral methadone are reached within 2 to 6 hours, and the plasma half-life initially is 4 to 6 hours in opioid-naive persons and 24 to 36 hours after steady dosing of any type of opioid. Methadone is highly protein bound and equilibrates widely throughout the body, which ensures little postdosage variation in steady-state plasma concentrations.

Elimination of a sublingual dosage of buprenorphine occurs in two phases: an initial phase with a half-life of 3 to 5 hours and a terminal phase with a half-life of more than 24 hours. Buprenorphine dissociates from its receptor-binding site slowly, which permits an every-other-day dosing schedule.

Methadone acts as pure agonists at μ-opioid receptors and has negligible agonist or antagonist activity at κ- or δ-opioid receptors. Buprenorphine is a partial agonist at μ-receptors, a potent antagonist at κ-receptors, and neither an agonist nor an antagonist at δ-receptors.

Therapeutic Indications

Methadone. Methadone is used for short-term detoxification (7 to 30 days), long-term detoxification (up to 180 days), and maintenance (treatment beyond 180 days) of opioid-dependent individuals. For these purposes, it is only available through designated clinics called methadone maintenance treatment programs (MMTPs) and in hospitals and prisons. Methadone is a schedule II drug, which means that its administration is tightly governed by specific federal laws and regulations.

Enrollment in a methadone program reduces the risk of death by 70 percent; reduces illicit use of opioids and other substances of abuse; reduces criminal activity; reduces the risk of infectious diseases of all types, most importantly HIV and hepatitis B and C infection; and in pregnant women, reduces the risk of fetal and neonatal morbidity and mortality. The use of methadone maintenance frequently requires lifelong treatment.

Some opioid-dependence treatment programs use a stepwise detoxification protocol in which a person addicted to heroin switches first to the strong agonist methadone; then to the weaker agonist buprenorphine; and finally to maintenance on an opioid receptor antagonist, such as naltrexone (ReVia). This approach minimizes the appearance of opioid withdrawal effects, which, if they occur, are mitigated with clonidine (Catapres). However, compliance with opioid receptor antagonist treatment is poor outside of settings using intensive cognitive–behavioral techniques. In contrast, noncompliance with methadone maintenance precipitates opioid withdrawal symptoms, which serve to reinforce the use of methadone and make cognitive–behavioral therapy less than essential. Thus, some well-motivated, socially integrated former heroin addicts are able to use methadone for years without participation in a psychosocial support program.

Data pooled from many reports indicate that methadone is more effective when taken at dosages in excess of 60 mg a day. The analgesic effects of methadone are sometimes used in the management of chronic pain when less addictive agents are ineffective.

PREGNANCY. Methadone maintenance, combined with effective psychosocial services and regular obstetric monitoring, significantly improves obstetric and neonatal outcomes for women addicted to heroin. Enrollment of a heroin-addicted pregnant woman in such a maintenance program reduces the risk of malnutrition, infection, preterm labor, spontaneous abortion, preeclampsia, eclampsia, abruptio placenta, and septic thrombophlebitis.

The dosage of methadone during pregnancy should be the lowest effective dosage, and no withdrawal to abstinence should be attempted during pregnancy. Methadone is metabolized more rapidly in the third trimester, which may necessitate higher dosages. To avoid potentially sedating postdose peak plasma concentrations, the daily dose can be administered in two divided doses during the third trimester. Methadone treatment has no known teratogenic effects.

NEONATAL METHADONE WITHDRAWAL SYMPTOMS. Withdrawal symptoms in newborns frequently include tremor, a high-pitched cry, increased muscle tone and activity, poor sleep and eating, mottling, yawning, perspiration, and skin excoriation. Convulsions that require aggressive anticonvulsant therapy may also occur. Withdrawal symptoms may be delayed in onset and prolonged in neonates because of their immature hepatic metabolism. Women taking methadone are sometimes counseled to initiate breastfeeding as a means of gently weaning their infants from methadone dependence, but they should not breastfeed their babies while still taking methadone.

Buprenorphine. The analgesic effects of buprenorphine are sometimes used in the management of chronic pain when less addictive agents are ineffective. Because buprenorphine is a partial agonist rather than a full agonist at the μ-receptor and is a weak antagonist at the κ-receptor, this agent produces a milder withdrawal syndrome and has a wider margin of safety than the full μ-agonist compounds generally used in treatment. Buprenorphine has a ceiling effect beyond which dose increases prolong the duration of action of the drug without further increasing the agonist effects. Because of this, buprenorphine has a high clinical safety profile, with limited respiratory depression, therefore decreasing the likelihood of lethal overdose. Buprenorphine does have the capacity to cause typical side effects associated with opioids, including sedation, nausea and vomiting, constipation, dizziness, headache, and sweating. A relevant pharmacokinetic consideration when using buprenorphine is the fact that it requires hepatic conversion to become analgesic (*N*-dealkylation catalyzed by CYP3A4). This may explain why some patients do not benefit from buprenorphine. Genetics, grapefruit juice, and many medications (including fluoxetine and fluvoxamine) can reduce a person's ability to metabolize buprenorphine into its bioactive form.

To reduce the likelihood of abusing buprenorphine via the IV route, buprenorphine has been combined with the narcotic antagonist naloxone for sublingual administration. Because naloxone is poorly absorbed by the sublingual route, when the combination drug is taken sublingually, there is no effect of the naloxone on the efficacy of buprenorphine. If an opioid-dependent individual injects the combination medication, the naloxone precipitates a withdrawal reaction, therefore reducing the likelihood of illicit injection use of the sublingual preparation.

Inducting and stabilizing a patient on buprenorphine is analogous to inducting and stabilizing a patient on methadone except that, as a partial agonist, buprenorphine has the potential to cause precipitated withdrawal in patients who have recently taken full agonist opioids. Thus, a patient must abstain from the use of short-acting opioids for 12 to 24 hours before starting buprenorphine and from longer-acting opioids such as methadone for 24 to 48 hours or longer. The physician must assess the patient clinically and determine that the patient is in mild to moderate opioid withdrawal with objectively observable withdrawal signs before initiating buprenorphine.

In most instances, a relatively low dose of buprenorphine (2 to 4 mg) can then be administered with additional doses given in 1 to 2 hours if withdrawal signs persist. The goal for the first 24 hours is to suppress withdrawal signs and symptoms, and the total 24-hour dose to do so can range from 2 to 16 mg on the first day. In subsequent days, the dose can be adjusted upward or downward to resolve withdrawal fully and, as with methadone, to achieve an absence of craving, adequate tolerance to prevent reinforcement from the use of other opioids, and ultimately abstinence from other opioids while minimizing side effects. Dose-ranging studies have demonstrated that dosages of 6 to 16 mg per day are associated with improved treatment outcomes compared with lower doses of buprenorphine (1 to 4 mg). Sometimes patients seem to need dosages higher than 16 mg per day, although there is no evidence for any benefit of dosages beyond 32 mg per day. For the treatment of opioid dependence, a dose of approximately 4 mg of sublingual buprenorphine is the equivalent of a daily dose of 40 mg of oral methadone. It has also been demonstrated that daily, alternate-day, or three-times-per-week administration has equivalent effects in suppressing the symptoms of opioid withdrawal in dependent individuals. The combination tablet is recommended for most clinical purposes, including induction and maintenance. The buprenorphine mono should be used only for pregnant patients or for patients who have a documented anaphylactic reaction to naloxone.

Newer forms of buprenorphine delivery, including a transdermal skin patch, a long-acting depot IM injection that provides therapeutic plasma levels for several weeks, and subcutaneous buprenorphine implants that may provide therapeutic plasma levels for 6 months, are being investigated. The last two delivery systems could obviate the need for taking medications daily while virtually eliminating the risk of medication nonadherence.

Tramadol. There are multiple reports of tramadol's antidepressant effects, both as monotherapy and augmentation agent in treatment-resistant depression. Clinical and experimental data suggest that tramadol has an inherent antidepressant-like activity. Tramadol has a complex pharmacology. It is a weak μ-opioid receptor agonist, a 5-HT releasing agent, a DA-releasing agent, a 5-HT_{2C} receptor antagonist, an norepinephrine reuptake inhibitor, an N-methyl-D-aspartate (NMDA) receptor antagonist, a nicotinic acetylcholine receptor antagonist, a TRPV1 receptor agonist and an M1 and M3 muscarinic acetylcholine receptor antagonist. Consistent with the evidence of its antidepressant effects is the fact that tramadol has a close structural similarity to the antidepressant venlafaxine.

Both venlafaxine and tramadol inhibit norepinephrine/serotonin reuptake and inhibit the reserpine-induced syndrome completely. Both compounds also have an analgesic effect on chronic pain. Venlafaxine may have an opioid component, and naloxone reverses the antipain effect of venlafaxine. Nonopioid activity is demonstrated by the fact that its analgesic effect is not fully antagonized by the μ-opioid receptor antagonist naloxone. Indicative of their structural similarities, venlafaxine may cause false-positive results on liquid chromatography tests to detect urinary tramadol levels.

Another relevant property of tramadol is its relatively long half-life, which reduces the potential for misuse. Its habituating effects are found to be much less than other opiate agonists, but abuse, withdrawal, and dependence are risks. Tramadol requires metabolism to become analgesic: individuals who are CYP2D6 "poor metabolizers" or use drugs that are CYP2D6 inhibitors reduce the efficacy of tramadol (the same is true of codeine).

Precautions and Adverse Reactions

The most common adverse effects of opioid receptor agonists are lightheadedness, dizziness, sedation, nausea, constipation, vomiting, perspiration, weight gain, decreased libido, inhibition of orgasm, and insomnia or sleep irregularities. Opioid receptor agonists are capable of inducing tolerance as well as producing physiologic and psychological dependence. Other CNS adverse effects include depression, sedation, euphoria, dysphoria, agitation, and seizures. Delirium has been reported in rare cases. Occasional non-CNS adverse effects include peripheral edema, urinary retention, rash, arthralgia, dry mouth, anorexia, biliary tract spasm, bradycardia, hypotension, hypoventilation, syncope, antidiuretic hormone–like activity, pruritus, urticaria, and visual disturbances. Menstrual irregularities are common in women, especially in the first 6 months of use. Various abnormal endocrine laboratory indexes of little clinical significance may also be seen.

Most persons develop tolerance to the pharmacologic adverse effects of opioid agonists during long-term maintenance, and relatively few adverse effects are experienced after the induction period.

Overdosage. The acute effects of opioid receptor agonist overdosage include sedation, hypotension, bradycardia, hypothermia, respiratory suppression, miosis, and decreased GI motility. Severe effects include coma, cardiac arrest, shock, and death. The risk of overdosage is greatest in the induction stage of treatment and in persons with slow drug metabolism caused by preexisting hepatic insufficiency. Deaths have been caused during the first week of induction by methadone dosages of only 50 to 60 mg a day.

The risk of overdosage with buprenorphine appears to be lower than with methadone. However, deaths have been caused by use of buprenorphine in combination with benzodiazepines.

Withdrawal Symptoms. Abrupt cessation of methadone use triggers withdrawal symptoms within 3 to 4 days, which usually reach peak intensity on the sixth day. Withdrawal symptoms include weakness, anxiety, anorexia, insomnia, gastric distress, headache, sweating, and hot and cold flashes. The withdrawal symptoms usually resolve after 2 weeks. However, a protracted methadone abstinence syndrome is possible that may include restlessness and insomnia.

The withdrawal symptoms associated with buprenorphine are similar to, but less marked than, those caused by methadone.

In particular, buprenorphine is sometimes used to ease the transition from methadone to opioid receptor antagonists or abstinence because of the relatively mild withdrawal reaction associated with discontinuation of buprenorphine.

Drug–Drug Interactions

Opioid receptor agonists can potentiate the CNS-depressant effects of alcohol, barbiturates, benzodiazepines, other opioids, low-potency DRAs, tricyclic and tetracyclic drugs, and MAOIs. Carbamazepine (Tegretol), phenytoin (Dilantin), barbiturates, rifampin (Rimactane, Rifadin), and heavy long-term consumption of alcohol may induce hepatic enzymes, which may lower the plasma concentration of methadone or buprenorphine and thereby precipitate withdrawal symptoms. In contrast, however, hepatic enzyme induction may increase the plasma concentration of active levomethadyl metabolites and cause toxicity.

Acute opioid withdrawal symptoms may be precipitated in persons on methadone maintenance therapy who take pure opioid receptor antagonists such as naltrexone, nalmefene (Revex), and naloxone (Narcan); partial agonists such as buprenorphine; or mixed agonist–antagonists such as pentazocine (Talwin). These symptoms may be mitigated by use of clonidine, a benzodiazepine, or both.

Competitive inhibition of methadone or buprenorphine metabolism after short-term use of alcohol or administration of cimetidine (Tagamet), erythromycin, ketoconazole (Nizoral), fluoxetine (Prozac), fluvoxamine (Luvox), loratadine (Claritin), quinidine (Quinidex), and alprazolam (Xanax) may lead to higher plasma concentrations or a prolonged duration of action of methadone or buprenorphine. Medications that alkalinize the urine may reduce methadone excretion.

Methadone maintenance may also increase plasma concentrations of desipramine (Norpramin, Pertofrane) and fluvoxamine. Use of methadone may increase zidovudine (Retrovir) concentrations, which increases the possibility of zidovudine toxicity at otherwise standard dosages. Moreover, in vitro human liver microsome studies demonstrate competitive inhibition of methadone demethylation by several protease inhibitors, including ritonavir (Norvir), indinavir (Crixivan), and saquinavir (Invirase). The clinical relevance of this finding is unknown.

Fatal drug–drug interactions with the MAOIs are associated with use of the opioids fentanyl (Sublimaze) and meperidine (Demerol) but not with use of methadone, levomethadyl, or buprenorphine.

Tramadol may interact with drugs that inhibit serotonin reuptake. Such combinations can trigger seizures and serotonin syndrome. These events may also develop during tramadol monotherapy, either at routine or excessive doses. Risk of interactions is increased when tramadol is combined with virtually all classes of antidepressants and with drugs that lower the seizure threshold, especially the antidepressant bupropion.

Laboratory Interferences

Methadone and buprenorphine can be tested for separately in urine toxicology to distinguish them from other opioids. No known laboratory interferences are associated with the use of methadone or buprenorphine.

Dosage and Clinical Guidelines

Methadone. Methadone is supplied in 5-, 10-, and 40-mg dispersible scored tablets; 40-mg scored wafers; 5-mg/5-mL, 10-mg/5-mL, and 10-mg/mL solutions; and a 10-mg/mL parenteral form. In maintenance programs, methadone is usually dissolved in water or juice, and dose administration is directly observed to ensure compliance. For induction of opioid detoxification, an initial methadone dose of 15 to 20 mg will usually suppress craving and withdrawal symptoms. However, some individuals may require up to 40 mg a day in single or divided doses. Higher dosages should be avoided during induction of treatment to reduce the risk of acute toxicity from overdosage.

Over several weeks, the dosage should be raised to at least 70 mg a day. The maximum dosage is usually 120 mg a day, and higher dosages require prior approval from regulatory agencies. Dosages above 60 mg a day are associated with much more complete abstinence from use of illicit opioids than are dosages less than 60 mg a day.

The duration of treatment should not be predetermined but should be based on response to treatment and assessment of psychosocial factors. All studies of methadone maintenance programs endorse long-term treatment (i.e., several years) as more effective than short-term programs (i.e., less than 1 year) for prevention of relapse into opioid abuse. In actual practice, however, a minority of programs are permitted by policy or approved by insurers to provide even 6 months of continuous maintenance treatment. Moreover, some programs actually encourage withdrawal from methadone in less than 6 months after induction. This is quite ill conceived because more than 80 percent of persons who terminate methadone maintenance treatment eventually return to illicit drug use within 2 years. In programs that offer both maintenance and withdrawal treatments, the overwhelming majority of participants enroll in the maintenance treatment.

Buprenorphine. Buprenorphine is supplied as a 0.3-mg/mL solution in 1-mL ampules. Sublingual tablet formulations of buprenorphine containing buprenorphine only or buprenorphine combined with naloxone in a 4:1 ratio are used for opioid maintenance treatment. Buprenorphine is not used for short-term opioid detoxification. Maintenance dosages of 8 to 16 mg thrice weekly have effectively reduced heroin use. Physicians must be trained and certified to carry out this therapy in their private offices. There are a number of approved training programs in the United States.

Tramadol. There are no controlled trials establishing the appropriate dosing schedule for tramadol when used for conditions other than pain. Tramadol is available in many formulations. These range from capsules (regular and extended release) to tablets (regular, extended release, chewable tablets) that can be taken sublingually, suppositories and injectable ampules. It also comes as tablets and capsules containing acetaminophen or aspirin. Doses in case reports of treatment for depression or OCD range from 50 to 200 mg a day and involve short-term use. The long-term use of tramadol in the treatment of psychiatric disorders has not been studied.

OPIOID RECEPTOR ANTAGONISTS: NALTREXONE, NALMEFENE, AND NALOXONE

Naltrexone (Revia, Depade) and naloxone (Narcan) are competitive opioid antagonists. They bind to opioid receptors without causing their activation. Because these drugs induce opioid withdrawal effects in people using full opioid agonists, these drugs are classified as opioid antagonists.

Naltrexone is the most widely used of these drugs. It has a relatively long half-life, is orally effective, is not associated with dysphoria, and is administered once daily. Naloxone, which predated naltrexone to treat narcotic overdose, became less widely used for preventing relapse to opiate use in detoxified opiate addicts. Since its introduction, naltrexone has been tried for the treatment of a wide range of psychiatric disorders, including, among others, eating disorders, autism, self-injurious behavior, cocaine dependence, gambling, and alcoholism. Naltrexone was approved for the treatment of alcohol dependence in 1994. A number of generic formulations are also available. An extended-release, once-a-month injectable suspension (Vivitrol) was also approved in 2006. Nalmefene (Revex) is indicated for the complete or partial reversal of opioid drug effects and in the management of known or suspected opioid overdose. An oral formulation of nalmefene is available in some countries but not in the United States. Nalmefene (Revex) is an opioid receptor antagonist that is sometimes used in the management of alcohol dependence.

Pharmacological Actions

Oral opioid receptor antagonists are rapidly absorbed from the GI tract, but because of first-pass hepatic metabolism, only 60 percent of a dose of naltrexone and 40 to 50 percent of a dose of nalmefene reach the systemic circulation unchanged. Peak concentrations of naltrexone and its active metabolite, 6-β-naltrexol, are achieved within 1 hour of ingestion. The half-life of naltrexone is 1 to 3 hours and the half-life of 6-β-naltrexol is 13 hours. Peak concentrations of nalmefene are achieved in about 1 to 2 hours, and the half-life is 8 to 10 hours. Clinically, a single dose of naltrexone effectively blocks the rewarding effects of opioids for 72 hours. Traces of 6-β-naltrexol may linger for up to 125 hours after a single dose.

Naltrexone and nalmefene are competitive antagonists of opioid receptors. Understanding the pharmacology of opioid receptors can explain the difference in adverse effects caused by naltrexone and nalmefene. Opioid receptors in the body are typed pharmacologically as μ, κ, or δ. Whereas activation of the κ- and δ-receptors is thought to reinforce opioid and alcohol consumption centrally, activation of μ-receptors is more closely associated with central and peripheral antiemetic effects. Because naltrexone is a relatively weak antagonist of κ- and δ-receptors and a potent μ-receptor antagonist, dosages of naltrexone that effectively reduce opioid and alcohol consumption also strongly block μ-receptors and therefore may cause nausea. Nalmefene, in contrast, is an equally potent antagonist of all three opioid receptor types, and dosages of nalmefene that effectively reduce opioid and alcohol consumption have no particularly increased effect on μ-receptors. Thus, nalmefene is associated clinically with few GI adverse effects.

Naloxone has the highest affinity for the μ-receptor but is a competitive antagonist at the μ-, κ-, and δ-receptors.

Whereas the effects of opioid receptor antagonists on opioid use are easily understood in terms of competitive inhibition of opioid receptors, the effects of opioid receptor antagonists on alcohol dependence are less straightforward and probably relate to the fact that the desire for and the effects of alcohol consumption appear to be regulated by several neurotransmitter systems, both opioid and nonopioid.

Therapeutic Indications

The combination of a cognitive–behavioral program plus use of opioid receptor antagonists is more successful than either the cognitive–behavioral program or use of opioid receptor antagonists alone. Naltrexone is used as a screening test to ensure that the patient is opioid-free before the induction of therapy with naltrexone (see "Naloxone Challenge Test" in Table 25–47).

Opioid Dependence. Patients in detoxification programs are usually weaned from potent opioid agonists such as heroin over a period of days to weeks, during which emergent adrenergic withdrawal effects are treated as needed with clonidine

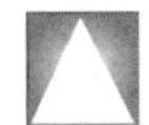

Table 25–47
Naloxone (Narcan) Challenge Test

The naloxone challenge test should not be performed in a patient showing clinical signs or symptoms of opioid withdrawal or in a patient whose urine contains opioids. The naloxone challenge test may be administered by either the intravenous (IV) or the subcutaneous route.

IV challenge: After appropriate screening of the patient, 0.8 mg of naloxone should be drawn into a sterile syringe. If the IV route of administration is selected, 0.2 mg of naloxone should be injected, and while the needle is still in the patient's vein, the patient should be observed for 30 sec for evidence of withdrawal signs or symptoms. If there is no evidence of withdrawal, the remaining 0.6 mg of naloxone should be injected and the patient observed for an additional 20 min for signs and symptoms of withdrawal

Subcutaneous challenge: If the subcutaneous route is selected, 0.8 mg should be administered subcutaneously and the patient observed for signs and symptoms of withdrawal for 20 min.

Conditions and technique for observation of patient: During the appropriate period of observation, the patient's vital signs should be monitored, and the patient should be monitored for signs of withdrawal. It is also important to question the patient carefully. The signs and symptoms of opioid withdrawal include, but are not limited to, the following:

Withdrawal signs: Stuffiness or running nose, tearing, yawning, sweating, tremor, vomiting, or piloerection

Withdrawal symptoms: Feeling of temperature change, joint or bone and muscle pain, abdominal cramps, and formication (feeling of bugs crawling under skin)

Interpretation of the challenge: Warning—the elicitation of the enumerated signs or symptoms indicates a potential risk for the subject, and naltrexone should not be administered. If no signs or symptoms of withdrawal are observed, elicited, or reported, naltrexone may be administered. If there is any doubt in the observer's mind that the patient is not in an opioid-free state or is in continuing withdrawal, naltrexone should be withheld for 24 hrs and the challenge repeated.

(Catapres). A serial protocol is sometimes used in which potent agonists are gradually replaced by weaker agonists followed by mixed agonist–antagonists and then finally by pure antagonists. For example, an abuser of the potent agonist heroin would switch first to the weaker agonist methadone (Dolophine), then to the partial agonist buprenorphine (Buprenex) or levomethadyl acetate (ORLAAM)—commonly called LAAM—and finally, after a 7- to 10-day washout period, to a pure antagonist, such as naltrexone or nalmefene. However, even with gradual detoxification, some persons continue to experience mild adverse effects or opioid withdrawal symptoms for the first several weeks of treatment with naltrexone.

As the opioid receptor agonist potency diminishes, so do the adverse consequences of discontinuing the drug. Thus, because there are no pharmacological barriers to discontinuation of pure opioid receptor antagonists, the social environment and frequent cognitive–behavioral intervention become extremely important factors supporting continued opioid abstinence. Because of poorly tolerated adverse symptoms, most persons not simultaneously enrolled in a cognitive–behavioral program stop taking opioid receptor antagonists within 3 months. Compliance with the administration of an opioid receptor antagonist regimen can also be increased with participation in a well-conceived voucher program.

Issues of medication compliance should be a central focus of treatment. If a person with a history of opioid addiction stops taking a pure opioid receptor antagonist, the person's risk of relapse into opioid abuse is exceedingly high because reintroduction of a potent opioid agonist would yield a very rewarding subjective "high." In contrast, compliant persons do not develop tolerance to the therapeutic benefits of naltrexone even if it is administered continuously for 1 year or longer. Individuals may undergo several relapses and remissions before achieving long-term abstinence.

Persons taking opioid receptor antagonists should also be warned that sufficiently high dosages of opioid agonists can overcome the receptor antagonism of naltrexone or nalmefene, which may lead to hazardous and unpredictable levels of receptor activation (see "Precautions and Adverse Reactions").

Rapid Detoxification. To avoid the 7- to 10-day period of opioid abstinence generally recommended before use of opioid receptor antagonists, rapid detoxification protocols have been developed. Continuous administration of adjunct clonidine—to reduce the adrenergic withdrawal symptoms—and adjunct benzodiazepines, such as oxazepam (Serax)—to reduce muscle spasms and insomnia—can permit use of oral opioid receptor antagonists on the first day of opioid cessation. Detoxification can thus be completed within 48 to 72 hours, at which point opioid receptor antagonist maintenance is initiated. Moderately severe withdrawal symptoms may be experienced on the first day, but they taper off rapidly thereafter.

Because of the potential hypotensive effects of clonidine, the BP of persons undergoing rapid detoxification must be closely monitored for the first 8 hours. Outpatient rapid detoxification settings must therefore be adequately prepared to administer emergency care.

The main advantage of rapid detoxification is that the transition from opioid abuse to maintenance treatment occurs over just 2 or 3 days. The completion of detoxification in as little time as possible minimizes the risk that the person will relapse into opioid abuse during the detoxification protocol.

Alcohol Dependence. Opioid receptor antagonists are also used as adjuncts to cognitive–behavioral programs for the treatment of alcohol dependence. Opioid receptor antagonists reduce alcohol craving and alcohol consumption, and they ameliorate the severity of relapses. The risk of relapse into heavy consumption of alcohol attributable to an effective cognitive–behavioral program alone may be halved with concomitant use of opioid receptor antagonists.

The newer agent nalmefene has a number of potential pharmacological and clinical advantages over its predecessor naltrexone for the treatment of alcohol dependence. Whereas naltrexone may cause reversible transaminase elevations in persons who take dosages of 300 mg a day (which is six times the recommended dosage for treatment of alcohol and opioid dependence [50 mg a day]), nalmefene has not been associated with any hepatotoxicity. Clinically effective dosages of naltrexone are discontinued by 10 to 15 percent of persons because of adverse effects, most commonly nausea. In contrast, discontinuation of nalmefene because of an adverse event is rare at the clinically effective dosage of 20 mg a day and in the range of 10 percent at excessive dosages—that is, 80 mg a day. Because of its pharmacokinetic profile, a given dosage of nalmefene may also produce a more sustained opioid antagonist effect than does naltrexone.

The efficacy of opioid receptor antagonists in reducing alcohol craving may be augmented with an SSRI, although data from large trials are needed to assess this potential synergistic effect more fully.

Precautions and Adverse Reactions

Because opioid receptor antagonists are used to maintain a drug-free state after opioid detoxification, great care must be taken to ensure that an adequate washout period elapses—at least 5 days for a short-acting opioid such as heroin and at least 10 days for longer-acting opioids such as methadone—after the last dose of opioids and before the first dose of an opioid receptor antagonist is taken. The opioid-free state should be determined by self-report and urine toxicology screens. If any question persists of whether opioids are in the body despite a negative urine screen result, then a *naloxone challenge test* should be performed. Naloxone challenge is used because its opioid antagonism lasts less than 1 hour, but those of naltrexone and nalmefene may persist for more than 24 hours. Thus, any withdrawal effects elicited by naloxone will be relatively short lived (see "Dosage and Clinical Guidelines"). Symptoms of acute opioid withdrawal include drug craving, feeling of temperature change, musculoskeletal pain, and GI distress. Signs of opioid withdrawal include confusion, drowsiness, vomiting, and diarrhea. Naltrexone and nalmefene should not be taken if naloxone infusion causes any signs of opioid withdrawal except as part of a supervised rapid detoxification protocol.

A set of adverse effects resembling a vestigial withdrawal syndrome tends to affect up to 10 percent of persons who take opioid receptor antagonists. Up to 15 percent of persons taking naltrexone may experience abdominal pain, cramps, nausea, and vomiting, which may be limited by transiently halving the dosage or altering the time of administration. Adverse CNS effects of naltrexone, experienced by up to 10 percent of persons, include headache, low energy, insomnia, anxiety, and nervousness. Joint and muscle pains may occur in up to 10 percent of persons taking naltrexone, as may rash.

Naltrexone may cause dosage-related hepatic toxicity at dosages well in excess of 50 mg a day; 20 percent of persons taking 300 mg a day of naltrexone may experience serum aminotransferase concentrations 3 to 19 times the upper limit of normal. The hepatocellular injury of naltrexone appears to be a dose-related toxic effect rather than an idiosyncratic reaction. At the lowest dosages of naltrexone required for effective opioid antagonism, hepatocellular injury is not typically observed. However, naltrexone dosages as low as 50 mg a day may be hepatotoxic in persons with underlying liver disease, such as persons with cirrhosis of the liver caused by chronic alcohol abuse. Serum aminotransferase concentrations should be monitored monthly for the first 6 months of naltrexone therapy and thereafter on the basis of clinical suspicion. Hepatic enzyme concentrations usually return to normal after discontinuation of naltrexone therapy.

If analgesia is required while a dose of an opioid receptor antagonist is pharmacologically active, opioid agonists should be avoided in favor of benzodiazepines or other nonopioid analgesics. Persons taking opioid receptor antagonists should be instructed that low dosages of opioids will have no effect but larger dosages could overcome the receptor blockade and suddenly produce symptoms of profound opioid overdosage, with sedation possibly progressing to coma or death. Use of opioid receptor antagonists is contraindicated in persons who are taking opioid agonists, small amounts of which may be present in over-the-counter antiemetic and antitussive preparations; in persons with acute hepatitis or hepatic failure; and in persons who are hypersensitive to the drugs.

Because naltrexone is transported across the placenta, opioid receptor antagonists should only be taken by pregnant women if a compelling need outweighs the potential risks to the fetus. It is not known whether opioid receptor antagonists are distributed into breast milk.

Opioid receptor antagonists are relatively safe drugs, and ingestion of high doses of opioid receptor antagonists should be treated with supportive measures combined with efforts to decrease GI absorption.

Because buprenorphine has a high affinity and slow displacement from the opioid receptors, nalmefene may not completely reverse buprenorphine-induced respiratory depression.

Drug Interactions

Many drug interactions involving opioid receptor antagonists have been discussed earlier, including those with opioid agonists associated with drug abuse as well as those involving antiemetics and antitussives. Because of its extensive hepatic metabolism, naltrexone may affect or be affected by other drugs that influence hepatic enzyme levels. However, the clinical importance of these potential interactions is not known.

One potentially hepatotoxic drug that has been used in some cases with opioid receptor antagonists is disulfiram (Antabuse). Although no adverse effects were observed, frequent laboratory monitoring is indicated when such combination therapy is contemplated. Opioid receptor antagonists have been reported to potentiate the sedation associated with use of thioridazine (Mellaril), an interaction that probably applies equally to all low-potency DRAs.

Intravenous nalmefene has been administered after benzodiazepines, inhalational anesthetics, muscle relaxants, and muscle relaxant antagonists administered in conjunction with general anesthetics without any adverse reactions. Care should be taken when using flumazenil (Romazicon) and nalmefene together because both of these agents have been shown to induce seizures in preclinical studies.

Laboratory Interferences

The potential for a false-positive urine for opiates using less specific urine screens such as enzyme-multiplied immunoassay technique (EMIT) may exist, given that naltrexone and nalmefene are derivatives of oxymorphone. Thin-layer, gas–liquid, and high-pressure liquid chromatographic methods used for the detection of opiates in the urine are not interfered with by naltrexone.

Dosage and Clinical Guidelines

To avoid the possibility of precipitating an acute opioid withdrawal syndrome, several steps should be taken to ensure that the person is opioid free. Within a supervised detoxification setting, at least 5 days should elapse after the last dose of short-acting opioids, such as heroin, hydromorphone (Dilaudid), meperidine (Demerol), or morphine, and at least 10 days should elapse after the last dose of longer-acting opioids, such as methadone, before opioid antagonists are initiated. Briefer periods off opioids have been used in rapid detoxification protocols. To confirm that opioid detoxification is complete, urine toxicological screens should demonstrate no opioid metabolites. However, an individual may have a negative urine opioid screen result, yet still be physically dependent on opioids and thus susceptible to antagonist-induced withdrawal effects. Therefore, after the urine screen result is negative, a naloxone challenge test is recommended unless an adequate period of opioid abstinence can be reliably confirmed by observers (Table 25–47).

The initial dosage of naltrexone for the treatment of opioid or alcohol dependence is 50 mg a day, which should be achieved through gradual introduction, even when the naloxone challenge test result is negative. Various authorities begin with 5, 10, 12.5, or 25 mg and titrate up to the 50-mg dosage over a period ranging from 1 hour to 2 weeks while constantly monitoring for evidence of opioid withdrawal. When a daily dose of 50 mg is well tolerated, it may be averaged over a week by giving 100 mg on alternate days or 150 mg every third day. Such schedules may increase compliance. The corresponding therapeutic dosage of nalmefene is 20 mg a day divided into two equal doses. Gradual titration of nalmefene to this daily dose is probably a wise strategy, although clinical data on dosage strategies for nalmefene are not yet available.

To maximize compliance, it is recommended that family members directly observe ingestion of each dose. Random urine tests for opioid receptor antagonists and their metabolites as well as for ethanol or opioid metabolites should also be taken. Opioid receptor antagonists should be continued until the person is no longer considered psychologically at risk for relapse into opioid or alcohol abuse. This generally requires at least 6 months but may take longer, particularly if there are external stresses.

Nalmefene is available as a sterile solution for intravenous, intramuscular, and subcutaneous administration in two concentrations, containing 100 μg or 1.0 mg of nalmefene free base per milliliter. The 100 μg/mL concentration contains 110.8 μg of nalmefene hydrochloride and the 1.0 mg/mL concentration contains 1.108 mg of nalmefene hydrochloride per milliliter. Both concentrations contain 9.0 mg of sodium chloride per milliliter and the pH is adjusted to 3.9 with hydrochloric acid. Pharmacodynamic studies have shown that nalmefene has a longer duration of action than naloxone at fully reversing opiate activity.

Rapid Detoxification. Rapid detoxification has been standardized using naltrexone, although nalmefene would be expected to be equally effective with fewer adverse effects. In rapid detoxification protocols, the addicted person stops opioid use abruptly and begins the first opioid-free day by taking clonidine, 0.2 mg, orally every 2 hours for nine doses, to a maximum dose of 1.8 mg, during which time the BP is monitored every 30 to 60 minutes for the first 8 hours. Naltrexone, 12.5 mg, is administered 1 to 3 hours after the first dose of clonidine. To reduce muscle cramps and later insomnia, a short-acting benzodiazepine, such as oxazepam, 30 to 60 mg, is administered simultaneously with the first dose of clonidine, and half of the initial dose is readministered every 4 to 6 hours as needed. The maximum daily dosage of oxazepam should not exceed 180 mg. The person undergoing rapid detoxification should be accompanied home by a reliable escort. On the second day, similar doses of clonidine and the benzodiazepine are administered but with a single dose of naltrexone, 25 mg, taken in the morning. Relatively asymptomatic persons may return home after 3 to 4 hours. Administration of the daily maintenance dose of 50 mg of naltrexone is begun on the third day, and the dosages of clonidine and the benzodiazepine are gradually tapered off over 5 to 10 days.

PHOSPHODIESTERASE-5 INHIBITORS

PDE-5 inhibitors, such as sildenafil (Viagra), which was developed in 1998, revolutionized the treatment of the major sexual dysfunction affecting men—erectile disorder. Two congeners have since come on the market—vardenafil (Levitra) and tadalafil (Cialis). All have a similar method of action and have changed people's expectations of sexual functioning. Although indicated only for the treatment of male erectile dysfunction, there is anecdotal evidence of these drugs being effective in women. They are also being misused as recreational drugs to enhance sexual performance. These drugs have been used by more than 20 million men around the world.

The development of sildenafil provided important information about the physiology of erection. Sexual stimulation causes the release of the neurotransmitter nitric oxide (NO), which increases the synthesis of cyclic guanosine monophosphate (cGMP), causing smooth muscle relaxation in the corpus cavernosum that allows blood to flow into the penis and results in turgidity and tumescence. The concentration of cGMP is regulated by the enzyme PDE-5, which, when inhibited, allows cGMP to increase and enhance erectile function. Because sexual stimulation is required to cause the release of NO, PDE-5 inhibitors have no effect in the absence of such stimulation, an important point to understand when providing information to patients about their use. The congeners vardenafil and tadalafil work in the same way, by inhibiting PDE-5, thus allowing an increase in cGMP and enhancing the vasodilatory effects of NO. For this reason, these drugs are sometimes referred to as NO enhancers.

Pharmacological Actions

All three substances are fairly rapidly absorbed from the GI tract, with maximum plasma concentrations reached in 30 to 120 minutes (median, 60 minutes) in the fasting state. Because it is lipophilic, concomitant ingestion of a high-fat meal delays the rate of absorption by up to 60 minutes and reduces the peak concentration by one quarter. These drugs are principally metabolized by the CYP3A4 system, which may lead to clinically significant drug–drug interactions, not all of which have been documented. Excretion of 80 percent of the dose is via feces, and another 13 percent is eliminated in the urine. Elimination is reduced in persons older than age 65 years, which results in plasma concentrations 40 percent higher than in persons age 18 to 45 years. Elimination is also reduced in the presence of severe renal or hepatic insufficiency.

The mean half-lives of sildenafil and vardenafil are 3 to 4 hours, and that of tadalafil is about 18 hours. Tadalafil can be detected in the bloodstream 5 days after ingestion, and because of its long half-life, it has been marketed as effective for up to 36 hours—the so-called weekend pill. The onset of sildenafil occurs about 30 minutes after ingestion on an empty stomach; tadalafil and vardenafil act somewhat more quickly.

Clinicians need to be aware of the important clinical observation that these drugs do not by themselves create an erection. Rather, the mental state of sexual arousal brought on by erotic stimulation must first lead to activity in the penile nerves, which then release NO into the cavernosum, triggering the erectile cascade, the resulting erection being prolonged by the NO enhancers. Thus, full advantage may be taken of a sexually exciting stimulus, but the drug is not a substitute for foreplay and emotional arousal.

Therapeutic Indications

Erectile dysfunctions have traditionally been classified as organic, psychogenic, or mixed. Over the past 20 years, the prevailing view of the cause of erectile dysfunction has shifted away from psychological causes toward organic causes. The latter include diabetes mellitus, hypertension, hypercholesterolemia, cigarette smoking, peripheral vascular disease, pelvic or spinal cord injury, pelvic or abdominal surgery (especially prostate surgery), multiple sclerosis, peripheral neuropathy, and Parkinson's disease. Erectile dysfunction is often induced by alcohol, nicotine, and other substances of abuse and by prescription drugs.

These drugs are effective regardless of the baseline severity of erectile dysfunction, race, or age. Among those responding to sildenafil are men with coronary artery disease, hypertension, other cardiac disease, peripheral vascular disease, diabetes mellitus, depression, coronary artery bypass graft surgery, radical prostatectomy, transurethral resection of the prostate, spina bifida, and spinal cord injury, as well as persons taking antidepressants, antipsychotics, antihypertensives, and diuretics. However, the response rate is variable.

Sildenafil has been reported to reverse SSRI–induced anorgasmia in men. There are anecdotal reports of sildenafil having a therapeutic effect on sexual inhibition in women as well.

Precautions and Adverse Reactions

A major potential adverse effect associated with use of these drugs is myocardial infarction (MI). The FDA distinguished the risk of MI caused directly by these drugs from that caused by underlying conditions such as hypertension, atherosclerotic heart disease, diabetes mellitus, and other atherogenic conditions. The FDA concluded that when used according to the approved labeling, the drugs do not by themselves confer an increased risk of death. However, there is increased oxygen demand and stress placed on the cardiac muscle by sexual intercourse. Thus, coronary perfusion may be severely compromised, and cardiac failure may occur as a result. For that reason, any person with a history of MI, stroke, renal failure, hypertension, or diabetes mellitus and any person older than the age of 70 years should discuss plans to use these drugs with an internist or a cardiologist. The cardiac evaluation should specifically address exercise tolerance and the use of nitrates.

Use of PDE-5 inhibitors is contraindicated in persons who are taking organic nitrates in any form. Also, amyl nitrate (poppers), a popular substance of abuse used by homosexual men to enhance the intensity of orgasm, should not be used with any of the erection-enhancing drugs. The combination of organic nitrates and PDE inhibitors can cause a precipitous lowering of BP and can reduce coronary perfusion to the point of causing MI and death.

Adverse effects are dose dependent, occurring at higher rates with higher dosages. The most common adverse effects are headache, flushing, and stomach pain. Other less common adverse effects include nasal congestion, urinary tract infection, abnormal vision (colored tinge [usually blue], increased sensitivity to light, or blurred vision), diarrhea, dizziness, and rash. No cases of priapism were reported in premarketing trials. Supportive management is indicated in cases of overdosage. Tadalafil has been associated with back and muscle pain in about 10 percent of patients.

Recently, there have been 50 reports and 14 verified cases of a serious condition in men taking sildenafil called nonarteritic anterior ischemic optic neuropathy. This is an eye ailment that causes restriction of blood flow to the optic nerve and can result in permanent vision loss. The first symptoms appear within 24 hours after use of sildenafil and include blurred vision and some degree of vision loss. The incidence of this effect is very rare—1 in 1 million. In the reported cases, many patients had preexisting eye problems that may have increased their risk, and many had a history of heart disease and diabetes, which may indicate vulnerability in these men to endothelial damage.

In addition to vision problems, in 2010, a warning of possible hearing loss was reported based on 29 incidents of the problem since introduction of these drugs. Hearing loss usually occurs within hours or days of using the drug and in some cases is both unilateral and temporary.

No data are available on the effects on human fetal growth and development or testicular morphologic or functional changes. However, because these drugs are not considered an essential treatment, they should not be used during pregnancy.

Treatment of Priapism

Phenylephrine (Neo-Synephrine) is the drug of choice and first-line treatment of priapism because the drug has almost pure α-agonist effects and minimal β activity. In short-term priapism (less than 6 hours), especially for drug-induced priapism, intracavernosal injection of phenylephrine can be used to cause detumescence. A mixture of 1 ampule of phenylephrine (1 mL/1,000 μg) should be diluted with an additional 9 mL of normal saline. Using a 29-gauge needle, 0.3 to 0.5 mL should be injected into the corpora cavernosa, with 10 to 15 minutes between injections. Vital signs should be monitored, and compression should be applied to the area of injection to help prevent hematoma formation.

Phenylephrine can also be used orally, 10 to 20 mg every 4 hours as needed, but it may not be as effective or act as rapidly as the injectable route.

Drug Interactions

The major route of PDE-5 metabolism is through CYP3A4, and the minor route is through CYP2C9. Inducers or inhibitors of these enzymes will therefore affect the plasma concentration and half-life of sildenafil. For example, 800 mg of cimetidine (Tagamet), a nonspecific CYP inhibitor, increases plasma sildenafil concentrations by 56 percent, and erythromycin (E-mycin) increases plasma sildenafil concentrations by 182 percent. Other, stronger inhibitors of CYP3A4 include ketoconazole (Nizoral), itraconazole (Sporanox), and mibefradil (Posicor). In contrast, rifampicin, a CYP3A4 inducer, decreases plasma concentrations of sildenafil.

Laboratory Interferences

No laboratory interferences have been described.

Dosage and Clinical Guidelines

Sildenafil is available as 25-, 50-, and 100-mg tablets. The recommended dose of sildenafil is 50 mg taken by mouth 1 hour before intercourse. However, sildenafil may take effect within 30 minutes. The duration of the effect is usually 4 hours, but in healthy young men, the effect may persist for 8 to 12 hours. Based on effectiveness and adverse effects, the dose should be titrated between 25 and 100 mg. Sildenafil is recommended for use no more than once a day. The dosing guidelines for use by women, an off-label use, are the same as those for men.

Increased plasma concentrations of sildenafil may occur in persons older than 65 years of age and those with cirrhosis or severe renal impairment or using CYP3A4 inhibitors. A starting dose of 25 mg should be used in these circumstances.

An investigational nasal spray formulation of sildenafil has been developed that acts within 5 to 15 minutes of administration. This formulation is highly water soluble, and it is rapidly absorbed directly into the bloodstream. Such a formulation would permit more ease of use.

Vardenafil is supplied in 2.5-, 5-, 10-, and 20-mg tablets. The initial dose is usually 10 mg taken with or without food about 1 hour before sexual activity. The dose can be increased to a maximum of 20 mg or decreased to 5 mg based on efficacy and side effects. The maximum dosing frequency is once per day. As with sildenafil, dosages may have to be adjusted in patients with hepatic impairment or in patients using certain CYP3A4 inhibitors. A 10 mg orally disintegrating form of vardenafil (Staxyn) is available. It is placed on the tongue approximately 60 minutes before sexual activity and should not be used more than once a day.

Tadalafil is available in 2.5-, 5-, or 20-mg tablets for oral administration. The recommended dose of tadalafil is 10 mg before sexual activity, which may be increased to 20 mg or decreased to 5 mg depending on efficacy and side effects. Once-a-day use of the 2.5- or 5-mg pill is acceptable for most patients. Similar cautions apply as mentioned earlier in patients with hepatic impairment and in those taking concomitant potent inhibitors of CYP3A4. As with other PDE-5 inhibitors, concomitant use of nitrates in any form is contraindicated.

SELECTIVE SEROTONIN–NOREPINEPHRINE REUPTAKE INHIBITORS

There are currently four SNRIs approved for use in the United States: venlafaxine (Effexor and Effexor XR), desvenlafaxine succinate (DVS; Pristiq), duloxetine (Cymbalta), and levomilnacipran (Fetzima). A fifth SNRI, milnacipran (Savella), available in other countries as an antidepressant, has FDA approval in the United States as a treatment for fibromyalgia. The term SNRI reflects the belief that the therapeutic effects of these medications are mediated by concomitant blockade of neuronal serotonin (5-HT) and norepinephrine uptake transporters. The SNRIs are also sometimes referred to as dual reuptake inhibitors, a broader functional class of antidepressant medications that includes TCAs such as clomipramine (Anafranil) and, to a lesser extent, imipramine (Tofranil) and amitriptyline (Elavil). What distinguishes the SNRIs from TCAs is their relative lack of affinity for other receptors, especially muscarinic, histaminergic, and the families of α- and β-adrenergic receptors. This distinction is an important one because the SNRIs have a more favorable tolerability profile than the older dual reuptake inhibitors.

Venlafaxine and Desvenlafaxine

Therapeutic Indications. Venlafaxine is approved for the treatment of four disorders: MDD, generalized anxiety disorder, social anxiety disorder, and panic disorder. MDD is currently the only FDA-approved indication for DVS.

DEPRESSION. The FDA does not recognize any class of antidepressant as being more effective than any other. This does not mean that differences do not exist, but no study to date has sufficiently demonstrated such superiority. It has been argued that direct modulation of serotonin and norepinephrine may convey greater antidepressant effects than are exerted by medications that selectively enhance only noradrenergic or serotoninergic neurotransmission. This greater therapeutic benefit could result from an acceleration of postsynaptic adaptation to increased neuronal signaling; simultaneous activation of two pathways for intracellular signal transduction; additive effects on the activity of relevant genes such as brain-derived neurotrophic factor; or, quite simply, broader coverage of depressive symptoms. Clinical evidence supporting this hypothesis first emerged in a pair of studies conducted by the Danish University Antidepressant Group, which found an advantage for the dual reuptake inhibitor clomipramine compared with the SSRIs citalopram (Celexa) and paroxetine (Paxil). Another report, which compared the results of a group of patients prospectively treated with the combination of the TCAs desipramine (Norpramin) and fluoxetine (Prozac) with a historical comparison group treated with desipramine alone, provided additional support. A meta-analysis of 25 inpatient studies comparing the efficacy of TCAs and SSRIs yielded the strongest evidence. Specifically, although the TCAs were found to have a modest overall advantage, superiority versus SSRIs was almost entirely explained by the studies that used the TCAs that are considered to be dual reuptake inhibitors—clomipramine, amitriptyline, and imipramine. Meta-analyses of head-to-head studies suggest that venlafaxine has the potential to induce higher rates of remission in depressed patients than do the SSRIs. This difference of the venlafaxine advantage is about 6 percent. DVS has not been extensively compared with other classes of antidepressants with respect to efficacy.

GENERALIZED ANXIETY DISORDER. The extended-release formulation of venlafaxine is approved for the treatment of generalized anxiety disorder. In clinical trials lasting 6 months, dosages of 75 to 225 mg a day were effective in treating insomnia, poor concentration, restlessness, irritability, and excessive muscle tension related to generalized anxiety disorder.

SOCIAL ANXIETY DISORDER. The extended-release formulation of venlafaxine is approved for the treatment of social anxiety disorder. Its efficacy was established in 12-week studies.

OTHER INDICATIONS. Case reports and uncontrolled studies have indicated that venlafaxine may be beneficial in the treatment of obsessive-compulsive disorder, panic disorder, agoraphobia, social phobia, attention-deficit/hyperactivity disorder, and patients with a dual diagnosis of depression and cocaine dependence. It has also been used in chronic pain syndromes with good effect.

Precautions and Adverse Reactions. Venlafaxine has a safety and tolerability profile similar to that of the more widely prescribed SSRI class. Nausea is the most frequently reported treatment-emergent adverse effect associated with venlafaxine and DVS therapy. Initiating therapy at lower dosages may also attenuate nausea. When extremely problematic, treatment-induced nausea can be controlled by prescribing a selective 5-HT_3 antagonist or mirtazapine (Remeron).

Venlafaxine and DVS therapy is associated with sexual side effects, predominantly decreased libido and a delay to orgasm or ejaculation. The incidence of these side effects may exceed 30 to 40 percent when there is direct, detailed assessment of sexual function.

Other common side effects include headache, insomnia, somnolence, dry mouth, dizziness, constipation, asthenia, sweating, and nervousness. Although several side effects are suggestive of anticholinergic effects, these drugs have no affinity for muscarinic or nicotinic receptors. Thus, noradrenergic agonism is likely to be the culprit.

Higher-dose venlafaxine therapy is associated with an increased risk of sustained elevations of BP. Experience with the instant-release (IR) formulation in studies of depressed patients indicated that sustained hypertension was dose related, increasing from 3 to 7 percent at doses of 100 to 300 mg per day and to 13 percent at doses greater than 300 mg per day. In this dataset, venlafaxine therapy did not adversely affect BP control of patients taking antihypertensives and actually lowered mean values of patients with elevated BP readings before therapy. In controlled studies of the extended-release formulation, venlafaxine therapy resulted in only approximately 1 percent greater risk of high BP when compared with placebo. Arbitrarily capping the upper dose of venlafaxine used in these studies thus greatly attenuated concerns about elevated BP. When higher doses of the extended-release formulation are used, however, monitoring of BP is recommended.

Venlafaxine and DVS are commonly associated with a discontinuation syndrome. This syndrome is characterized by the appearance of a constellation of adverse effects during a rapid taper or abrupt cessation, including dizziness, dry mouth, insomnia, nausea, nervousness, sweating, anorexia, diarrhea, somnolence, and sensory disturbances. It is recommended that, whenever possible, a slow taper schedule should be used when longer-term treatment must be stopped. On occasion, substituting a few doses of the sustained-release formulation of fluoxetine may help to bridge this transition.

There were no overdose fatalities in premarketing trials of venlafaxine, although electrocardiographic changes (e.g., prolongation of QT interval, bundle branch block, QRS interval prolongation), tachycardia, bradycardia, hypotension, hypertension, coma, serotonin syndrome, and seizures were reported. Fatal overdoses have been documented subsequently, typically involving venlafaxine ingestion in combination with other drugs, alcohol, or both.

Information concerning use of venlafaxine and DVS by pregnant and nursing women is not available at this time. Venlafaxine and DVS are excreted in breast milk. Clinicians should carefully weigh the risks and benefits of venlafaxine use by pregnant and nursing women.

Drug Interactions. Venlafaxine is metabolized in the liver primarily by the CYP2D6 isoenzyme. Because the parent drug and principal metabolite are essentially equipotent, medications that inhibit this isoenzyme usually do not adversely affect therapy. Venlafaxine is itself a relatively weak inhibitor of CYP2D6, although it can increase levels of substrates, such as desipramine or risperidone (Risperdal). In vitro and in vivo studies have shown venlafaxine to cause little or no inhibition of CYP1A2, CYP2C9, CYP2C19, and CYP3A4.

Venlafaxine is contraindicated in patients taking MAOIs because of the risk of a pharmacodynamic interaction (i.e., serotonin syndrome). An MAOI should not be started for at least 7 days after stopping venlafaxine. Few data are available regarding the combination of venlafaxine with atypical neuroleptics, benzodiazepines, lithium (Eskalith), and anticonvulsants; therefore, clinical judgment should be exercised when combining medications.

Laboratory Interferences. Data are not currently available on laboratory interferences with venlafaxine.

Dosage and Administration. Venlafaxine is available in 25-, 37.5-, 50-, 75-, and 100-mg tablets and 37.5-, 75-, and 150-mg extended-release capsules. The tablets and the extended-release capsules are equally potent, and persons stabilized with one can switch to an equivalent dosage of the other. Because the immediate-release tablets are rarely used due to their tendency to cause nausea and the need for multiple daily doses, the dosage recommendations that follow refer to use of the extended-release capsules.

In depressed persons, venlafaxine demonstrates a dose–response curve. The initial therapeutic dosage is 75 mg a day given once a day. However, most persons are started at a dosage of 37.5 mg for 4 to 7 days to minimize adverse effects, particularly nausea. A convenient starter kit for the drug contains a 1-week supply of both the 37.5- and 75-mg strengths. If a rapid titration is preferred, the dosage can be raised to 150 mg per day after day 4. As a rule, the dosage can be raised in increments of 75 mg a day every 4 or more days. Although the recommended upper dosage of the extended-release preparation (venlafaxine XR) is 225 mg per day, it is approved by the FDA for use at dosages up to 375 mg a day. The dosage of venlafaxine should be halved in persons with significantly diminished hepatic or renal function. If discontinued, venlafaxine use should be gradually tapered over 2 to 4 weeks to avoid withdrawal symptoms.

There are minor differences in the doses used for major depression, generalized anxiety disorder, and social anxiety disorder. In the treatment of these disorders, for example, a dose–response effect has not been found. In addition, lower mean dosages are typically used, with most patients taking 75 to 150 mg per day.

DVS is available as 50- and 100-mg extended-release tablets. The therapeutic dose for most patients is 50 mg a day. Although some patients may need higher doses, in clinical trials, no greater therapeutic benefit was noted when the dose was increased. At higher doses, adverse event and discontinuation rates were increased.

Duloxetine

Pharmacological Actions. Duloxetine is formulated as a delayed-release capsule to reduce the risk of severe nausea associated with the drug. It is well absorbed, but there is a 2-hour delay before absorption begins. Peak plasma concentrations occur 6 hours after ingestion. Food delays the time to achieve maximum concentrations from 6 to 10 hours and reduces the extent of absorption by about 10 percent. Duloxetine has an elimination half-life of about 12 hours (range, 8 to 17 hours). Steady-state plasma concentrations occur after 3 days. Elimination is mainly through the isozymes CYP2D6 and CYP1A2. Duloxetine undergoes extensive hepatic metabolism to numerous metabolites. About 70 percent of the drug appears in the urine as metabolites and about 20 percent is excreted in the feces. Duloxetine is 90 percent protein bound.

Therapeutic Indications

DEPRESSION. In contrast to venlafaxine, a small number of studies have compared duloxetine with the SSRIs. Although these studies are suggestive of some advantage in efficacy, their findings are limited by the use of fixed, low starting doses of paroxetine and fluoxetine, but dosages of duloxetine in some studies were as high as 120 mg per day. Any inferences on whether duloxetine is superior to the SSRIs in any aspect of treatment for depression thus await more evidence from properly designed trials.

NEUROPATHIC PAIN ASSOCIATED WITH DIABETES AND STRESS URINARY INCONTINENCE. Duloxetine is the first drug to be approved by the FDA as a treatment for neuropathic pain associated with diabetes. The drug has been studied for its effects on physical symptoms, including pain, in depressed patients, but these effects have not been compared with those seen with other widely used agents such as venlafaxine and the TCAs. Duloxetine is currently approved in EU as a treatment for stress urinary incontinence, the inability to voluntarily control bladder voiding, which is the most frequent type of incontinence in women. The action of duloxetine in the treatment of stress urinary incontinence is associated with its effects in the sacral spinal cord, which in turn increase the activity of the striated urethral sphincter. Duloxetine is marketed under the name Yentreve for this indication. It is not yet approved by the FDA for stress urinary incontinence.

Precautions and Adverse Reactions. The most common adverse reactions are nausea, dry mouth, dizziness, constipation, fatigue, decreased appetite, anorexia, somnolence, and increased sweating. Nausea was the most common side effect that led to treatment discontinuation in clinical trials. The true incidence of sexual dysfunction is unknown; the long-term effects on body weight are also unknown. In clinical trials, treatment with duloxetine was associated with mean increases in BP averaging 2 mm Hg systolic and 0.5 mm Hg diastolic versus placebo. No studies have compared the BP effects of venlafaxine and duloxetine at equivalent therapeutic doses.

Close monitoring is suggested when using duloxetine in patients who have or are at risk for diabetes. Duloxetine has been shown to increase blood sugar and hemoglobin A1c levels during long-term treatment.

Patients with substantial alcohol use should not be treated with duloxetine because of possible hepatic effects. It also should not be prescribed for patients with hepatic insufficiency and end-stage renal disease or for patients with uncontrolled narrow-angle glaucoma.

Abrupt discontinuation of duloxetine should be avoided because it may produce a discontinuation syndrome similar to that of venlafaxine. A gradual dose reduction is recommended.

Clinicians should avoid the use of duloxetine by pregnant and nursing women unless the potential benefits justify the potential risks.

Drug Interactions. Duloxetine is a moderate inhibitor of CYP450 enzymes.

Laboratory Interferences. Data are not currently available on laboratory interferences with duloxetine.

Dosage and Administration. Duloxetine is available in 20-, 30-, and 60-mg tablets. The recommended therapeutic, and maximum, dosage is 60 mg per day. The 20- and 30-mg doses are useful for either initial therapy or for twice-daily use as strategies to reduce side effects. In clinical trials, dosages of up to 120 mg per day were studied, but no consistent advantage in efficacy was noted at doses higher than 60 mg per day. Duloxetine thus does not appear to demonstrate a dosage–response curve. However, there were difficulties in tolerability with single doses above 60 mg. Accordingly, when dosages of 80 and 120 mg per day were used, they were administered as 40 or 60 mg twice daily. Because of limited clinical experience with duloxetine, it remains to be seen to what extent dosages above 60 mg per day will be necessary and whether this will actually require divided doses to make the drug tolerable.

Milnacipran and Levomilnacipran

Milnacipran is only FDA approved for the treatment of fibromyalgia. Although some countries have approved milnacipran for general use as an antidepressant, efficacy is not as well established. Compared with venlafaxine, milnacipran is approximately five times more potent for inhibition of norepinephrine uptake than for 5-HT reuptake inhibition. Milnacipran has a half-life of approximately 8 hours and shows linear pharmacokinetics between doses of 50 and 250 mg per day. Metabolized in the liver, milnacipran has no active metabolites. Milnacipran is primarily excreted by the kidneys.

Milnacipran is available as 12.5-, 25-, 50-, and 100-mg tablets. The standard recommended milnacipran dose is as follows: day 1, 12.5 mg once daily; days 2 and 3, 12.5 mg twice daily; days 4 to 7, 25 mg twice daily; and day 7 and beyond, 50 mg twice daily.

Levomilnacipran was approved in 2013 by the FDA as a treatment for MDD in adults. Levomilnacipran is an active enantiomer of the racemic drug milnacipran. In vitro studies have shown that it has greater potency for norepinephrine reuptake inhibition than for serotonin reuptake inhibition and does not directly affect the uptake of dopamine or other neurotransmitters. It is taken once daily as a sustained-release formulation. In clinical trials, doses of 40-, 80-, or 120-mg improved symptoms compared with placebo.

The most common adverse reactions in the placebo-controlled trials were nausea, constipation, hyperhidrosis, increased heart rate, erectile dysfunction, tachycardia, vomiting, and palpitations. Rates of adverse events were generally consistent across the 40- to 120-mg dose range. The only dose-related adverse events were urinary hesitation and erectile dysfunction.

SELECTIVE SEROTONIN REUPTAKE INHIBITORS

Fluoxetine (Prozac), the first SSRI marketed in the United States, rapidly captured the favor of both clinicians and the general public as reports emerged of dramatic patient responses to treatment of depression. Patients no longer experienced such side effects as dry mouth, constipation, sedation, orthostatic hypotension, and tachycardia, common side effects associated with the earlier antidepressant drugs—the TCAs and MAOIs. It was also significantly safer when taken in overdose than any previously available antidepressant. A significant effect of

Table 25–48
Currently Approved Indications of the Selective Serotonin Reuptake Inhibitors in the United States for Adult and Pediatric Populations

	Citalopram (Celexa)	Escitalopram (Lexapro)	Fluoxetine (Prozac)	Fluvoxamine (Luvox)	Paroxetine (Paxil)	Sertraline (Zoloft)	Vilazodone (Viibryd)
Major depressive disorder	Adult	Adult	Adult[a] and pediatric	—	Adult[b]	Adult	Adult
Generalized anxiety disorder	—	Adult	—	—	Adult	—	—
OCD	—	—	Adult and pediatric	Adult and pediatric	Adult	Adult and pediatric	—
Panic disorder	—	—	Adult	—	Adult[b]	Adult	—
PTSD	—	—	—	—	Adult	Adult	—
Social anxiety disorder	—	—	Adult	—	Adult[b]	Adult	—
Bulimia nervosa	—	—	Adult	—	—	—	—
Premenstrual dysphoric disorder	—	—	Adult[c]	—	Adult[d]	Adult	—

[a]Weekly fluoxetine is approved for continuation and maintenance therapy in adults.
[b]Paroxetine-and-paroxetine–controlled release.
[c]Marketed as Sarafem.
[d]Paroxetine-controlled release is approved for premenstrual dysphoric disorder.
OCD, obsessive-compulsive disorder; PTSD, posttraumatic stress disorder.

fluoxetine's popularity was that it helped ameliorate the long-standing stigma of depression and its treatment.

Fluoxetine was followed by other SSRIs. These include sertraline (Zoloft), paroxetine (Paxil), fluvoxamine (Luvox), citalopram (Celexa), escitalopram (Lexapro), and vilazodone (Viibryd). These drugs are all equally effective in treating depression but some are approved by the FDA for multiple indications, such as major depression, OCD, PTSD, PMDD, panic disorder, and social phobia (social anxiety disorder) (Table 25–48). Note that fluvoxamine is not FDA approved as an antidepressant, a fact that is due to a marketing decision. It is considered an antidepressant in other countries.

Although all SSRIs are equally effective, there are meaningful differences in pharmacodynamics, pharmacokinetics, and side effects, differences that might affect clinical responses among individual patients. This would explain why some patients have better clinical responses to a particular SSRI than another. The SSRIs have proven more problematic in terms of some side effects than the original clinical trials suggested. Quality-of-life–associated adverse effects such as nausea, sexual dysfunction, and weight gain sometimes mitigate the therapeutic benefits of the SSRIs. There can also be distressing withdrawal symptoms when SSRIs are stopped abruptly. This is especially true with paroxetine, but also occurs when other SSRIs with short half-lives are stopped.

Pharmacological Actions

Pharmacokinetics. A significant difference among the SSRIs is their broad range of serum half-lives. Fluoxetine has the longest half-life: 4 to 6 days; its active metabolite has a half-life of 7 to 9 days. The half-life of sertraline is 26 hours, and its less active metabolite has a half-life of 3 to 5 days. The half-lives of the other three, which do not have metabolites with significant pharmacological activity, are 35 hours for citalopram, 27 to 32 hours for escitalopram, 21 hours for paroxetine, and 15 hours for fluvoxamine. As a rule, the SSRIs are well absorbed after oral administration and have their peak effects in the range of 3 to 8 hours. Absorption of sertraline may be slightly enhanced by food.

There are also differences in plasma protein–binding percentages among the SSRIs, with sertraline, fluoxetine, and paroxetine being the most highly bound and escitalopram being the least bound.

All SSRIs are metabolized in the liver by the CYP450 enzymes. Because the SSRIs have such a wide therapeutic index, it is rare that other drugs produce problematic increases in SSRI concentrations. The most important drug–drug interactions involving the SSRIs occur as a result of the SSRIs inhibiting the metabolism of the coadministered medication. Each of the SSRIs possesses a potential for slowing or blocking the metabolism of many drugs (Table 25–49). Fluvoxamine is the most problematic of the drugs in this respect. It has a marked effect on several of the CYP enzymes. Examples of clinically significant interactions include fluvoxamine and theophylline (Slo-Bid, Theo-Dur) through CYP1A2 interaction; fluvoxamine and clozapine (Clozaril) through CYP1A2 inhibition; and fluvoxamine with alprazolam (Xanax) or clonazepam (Klonopin) through CYP3A4 inhibition. Fluoxetine and paroxetine also possess significant effects on the CYP2D6 isozyme, which may interfere with the efficacy of opiate analogs, such as codeine and hydrocodone, by blocking the conversion of these agents to their active form. Thus, coadministration of fluoxetine and paroxetine with an opiate interferes with its analgesic effects. Sertraline, citalopram, and escitalopram are least likely to complicate treatment because of interactions.

The pharmacokinetics of vilazodone (5 to 80 mg) are dose proportional. Steady-state plasma levels are achieved in about 3 days. Elimination of vilazodone is primarily by hepatic metabolism with a terminal half-life of approximately 25 hours.

Pharmacodynamics. The SSRIs are believed to exert their therapeutic effects through serotonin reuptake inhibition. They derive their name because they have little effect on reuptake of norepinephrine or dopamine. Often, adequate clinical activity and saturation of the 5-HT transporters are achieved at starting

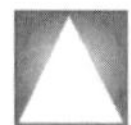

Table 25–49
CYP450 Inhibitory Potential of Commonly Prescribed Antidepressants

Relative Rank	CYP1A2	CYP2C	CYP2D6	CYP3A
Higher	Fluvoxamine (Luvox)	Fluoxetine Fluvoxamine	Bupropion Fluoxetine Paroxetine	Fluvoxamine Nefazodone Tricyclics
Moderate	Tertiary amine tricyclics Fluoxetine (Prozac)	Sertraline	Secondary amine tricyclics Citalopram (Celexa) Escitalopram (Lexapro) Sertraline	Fluoxetine Sertraline
Low or minimal	Bupropion (Wellbutrin) Mirtazapine (Remeron) Nefazodone (Serzone) Paroxetine (Paxil) Sertraline (Zoloft) Venlafaxine	Paroxetine Venlafaxine (Effexor)	Fluvoxamine Mirtazapine Nefazodone Venlafaxine	Citalopram Escitalopram Mirtazapine Paroxetine Venlafaxine

CYP, cytochrome P450.

dosages. As a rule, higher dosages do not increase antidepressant efficacy but may increase the risk of adverse effects.

Citalopram and escitalopram are the most selective inhibitors of serotonin reuptake, with very little inhibition of norepinephrine or dopamine reuptake and very low affinities for histamine H_1, GABA, or benzodiazepine receptors. The other SSRIs have a similar profile except that fluoxetine weakly inhibits norepinephrine reuptake and binds to 5-HT_{2C} receptors, sertraline weakly inhibits norepinephrine and dopamine reuptake, and paroxetine has significant anticholinergic activity at higher dosages and binds to nitric oxide synthase. The SSRI vilazodone has 5-HT_{1A} receptor agonist properties. The clinical implications of the 5-HT_{1A} receptor agonist effects are not yet evident.

A pharmacodynamic interaction appears to underlie the antidepressant effects of combined fluoxetine–olanzapine. When taken together, these drugs increase brain concentrations of norepinephrine. Concomitant use of SSRIs and drugs in the triptan class (sumatriptan [Imitrex], naratriptan [Amerge], rizatriptan [Maxalt], and zolmitriptan [Zomig]) may result in a serious pharmacodynamic interaction—the development of a serotonin syndrome (see "Precautions and Adverse Reactions"). However, many people use triptans while taking low doses of an SSRI for headache prophylaxis without adverse reaction. A similar reaction may occur when SSRIs are combined with tramadol (Ultram).

Therapeutic Indications

Depression. In the United States, all SSRIs other than fluvoxamine have been approved by the FDA for the treatment of depression. Several studies have found that antidepressants with serotonin-norepinephrine activity—drugs such as the MAOIs, TCAs, venlafaxine (Effexor), and mirtazapine (Remeron)—may produce higher rates of remission than SSRIs in head-to-head studies. The continued role of SSRIs as first-line treatment thus reflects their simplicity of use, safety, and broad spectrum of action.

Direct comparisons of individual SSRIs have not revealed any to be consistently superior to another. There nevertheless can be considerable diversity in response to the various SSRIs among individuals. For example, more than 50 percent of people who respond poorly to one SSRI will respond favorably to another. Thus, before shifting to non-SSRI antidepressants, it is most reasonable to try other agents in the SSRI class for persons who did not respond to the first SSRI.

Some clinicians have attempted to select a particular SSRI for a specific person on the basis of the drug's unique adverse effect profile. For example, thinking that fluoxetine is an activating and stimulating SSRI, they may assume it is a better choice for an abulic person than paroxetine, which is presumed to be a sedating SSRI. These differences, however, usually vary from person to person. Analyses of clinical trial data show that the SSRIs are more effective in patients with more severe symptoms of major depression than those with milder symptoms.

SUICIDE. The FDA has issued a black box warning for antidepressants and suicidal thoughts and behavior in children and young adults. This warning is based on a decade-old analysis of clinical trial data. More recent, comprehensive reanalysis of data has shown that suicidal thoughts and behavior decreased over time for adult and geriatric patients treated with antidepressants as compared with placebo. No differences were found for youths. In adults, reduction in suicide ideation and attempts occurred through a reduction in depressive symptoms. In all age groups, severity of depression improved with medication and was significantly related to suicide ideation or behavior. It appears that SSRIs, as well as SNRIs, have a protective effect against suicide that is mediated by decreases in depressive symptoms with treatment. For youths, no significant effects of treatment on suicidal thoughts and behavior were found, although depression responded to treatment. No evidence of increased suicide risk was observed in youths receiving active medication. It is important to keep in mind that SSRIs, like all antidepressants, prevent potential suicides as a result of their primary action, the shortening and prevention of depressive episodes. In clinical practice, a few patients become especially anxious and agitated when started on an SSRI. The appearance of these symptoms could conceivably provoke or aggravate suicidal ideation. Thus, all depressed patients should be closely monitored during the period of maximum risk, the first few days and weeks they are taking SSRIs.

DEPRESSION DURING PREGNANCY AND POSTPARTUM. Rates of relapse of major depression during pregnancy among women who discontinue, attempt to discontinue, or modify their antidepressant regimens are extremely high. Rates range from 68 to 100 percent of patients. Thus, many women need to continue taking their medication during pregnancy and postpartum. The impact of maternal depression on infant development is unknown. There is no increased risk for major congenital malformations after exposure to SSRIs during pregnancy. The exception to this is paroxetine, which has been shown in various studies to cause cardiac malformations, as well as increased overall risk of congenital malformations but the risk of relapse into depression when a newly pregnant mother is taken off SSRIs is several-fold higher than the risk to the fetus of exposure to SSRIs.

There is some evidence suggesting increased rates of special care nursery admissions after delivery for children of mothers taking SSRIs. There is also a potential for a discontinuation syndrome with paroxetine. However, there is an absence of clinically significant neonatal complications associated with SSRI use.

Studies that have followed children into their early school years have failed to find any perinatal complications, congenital fetal anomalies, decreases in global intelligence quotient (IQ), language delays, or specific behavioral problems attributable to the use of fluoxetine during pregnancy.

Postpartum depression (with or without psychotic features) affects a small percentage of mothers. Some clinicians start administering SSRIs if the postpartum blues extend beyond a few weeks or if a woman becomes depressed during pregnancy. The head start afforded by starting SSRI administration during pregnancy if a woman is at risk for postpartum depression also protects the newborn, toward whom the woman may have harmful thoughts after parturition.

Babies whose mothers are taking an SSRI in the later part of pregnancy may be at a slight risk of developing pulmonary hypertension. Data about the risk of this side effect are inconclusive, but it is estimated to involve 1 to 2 babies for 1,000 births. Paroxetine should be avoided during pregnancy.

The FDA has classified paroxetine as a *pregnancy Category D* medication. In 2005, the FDA issued an alert that paroxetine increases the risk of birth defects, particularly heart defects, when women take it during the first 3 months of pregnancy. Paroxetine should usually not be taken during pregnancy, but for some women who have already been taking paroxetine, the benefits of continuing paroxetine may be greater than the potential risk to the baby. Women taking paroxetine who are pregnant, think they may be pregnant, or plan to become pregnant should talk to their physicians about the potential risks of taking paroxetine during pregnancy.

The FDA alert was based on the findings of studies that showed that women who took paroxetine during the first 3 months of pregnancy were about one and a half to two times as likely to have a baby with a heart defect as women who received other antidepressants or women in the general population. Most of the heart defects in these studies were not life-threatening and happened mainly in the inside walls of the heart muscle where repairs can be made if needed (atrial and ventricular septal defects). Sometimes these septal defects resolve without treatment. In one of the studies, the risk of heart defects in babies whose mothers had taken paroxetine early in pregnancy was 2 percent, compared with a 1 percent risk in the whole population. In the other study, the risk of heart defects in babies whose mothers had taken paroxetine in the first 3 months of pregnancy was 1.5 percent, compared with 1 percent in babies whose mothers had taken other antidepressants in the first 3 months of pregnancy. This study also showed that women who took paroxetine in the first 3 months of pregnancy were about twice as likely to have a baby with any birth defect as women who took other antidepressants.

Very small amounts of SSRIs are found in breast milk and no harmful effects have been found in breastfed babies. Concentrations of sertraline and escitalopram are especially low in breast milk. However, in some cases, reported concentrations may be higher than average. No decision regarding the use of an SSRI is risk free. It is thus important to document that communication of potential risks to the patient has taken place.

A recent Canadian study of 145,000 infants found a link between antidepressant (SSRIs) use during pregnancy and an increased risk of autism but only an association and did not show a cause and effect. The use of SSRIs during the second and third trimester increased this risk but the study found the overall risk to be about 0.5 percent. This study does not prove that antidepressants cause autism and clinicians should continue to discuss the risk of maternal depression and high rates of postnatal complications compared to the risks of antidepressants.

DEPRESSION IN ELDERLY AND MEDICALLY ILL PERSONS. The SSRIs are safe and well tolerated when used to treat elderly and medically ill persons. As a class, they have little or no cardiotoxic, anticholinergic, antihistaminergic, or α-adrenergic adverse effects. Paroxetine does have some anticholinergic activity, which may lead to constipation and worsening of cognition. The SSRIs can produce subtle cognitive deficits, prolonged bleeding time, and hyponatremia, all of which may impact the health of this population. The SSRIs are effective in poststroke depression and dramatically reduce the symptom of crying.

DEPRESSION IN CHILDREN. The use of SSRI antidepressants in children and adolescents has been controversial. Few studies have shown clear-cut benefits from the use of these drugs, and studies show that there may be an increase in suicidal or aggressive impulses. However, some children and adolescents do exhibit dramatic responses to these drugs in terms of depression and anxiety. Fluoxetine has most consistently demonstrated effectiveness in reducing symptoms of depressive disorder in both children and adolescents. This may be a function of the quality of the clinical trials involved. Sertraline has been shown to be effective in treating social anxiety disorder in this population, especially when combined with cognitive–behavioral therapy. Given the potential negative effect of untreated depression and anxiety in a young population and the uncertainty about many aspects of how children and adolescents might react to medication, any use of SSRIs should be undertaken only within the context of comprehensive management of the patient.

Anxiety Disorders

OBSESSIVE-COMPULSIVE DISORDER. Fluvoxamine, paroxetine, sertraline, and fluoxetine are indicated for the treatment of OCD in persons older than the age of 18 years. Fluvoxamine and sertraline have also been approved for treatment of children with OCD (ages 6 to 17 years). About 50 percent of persons with OCD begin to show symptoms in childhood or adolescence, and more than half of these respond favorably to medication. Beneficial responses can be dramatic. Long-term data support the model of OCD as a genetically determined, lifelong condition that is best treated continuously with drugs and cognitive–behavioral therapy from the onset of symptoms in childhood throughout the lifespan.

SSRI dosages for OCD may need to be higher than those required to treat depression. Although some response can be seen in the first few weeks of treatment, it may take several months for the maximum effects to become evident. Patients who fail to obtain adequate relief of their OCD symptoms with an SSRI often benefit from the addition of a small dose of risperidone (Risperdal). Apart from the EPS of risperidone, patients should be monitored for increases in prolactin levels when this combination is used. Clinically, hyperprolactinemia may manifest as gynecomastia and galactorrhea (in both men and women) and loss of menses.

A number of disorders are now considered to be within the OCD spectrum. This includes a number of conditions and symptoms characterized by nonsuicidal self-mutilation, such as trichotillomania, eyebrow picking, nose picking, nail biting, compulsive picking of skin blemishes, and cutting. Patients with these behaviors benefit from treatment with SSRIs. Other spectrum disorders include compulsive gambling, compulsive shopping, hypochondriasis, and body dysmorphic disorder.

PANIC DISORDER. Paroxetine and sertraline are indicated for the treatment of panic disorder, with or without agoraphobia. These agents work less rapidly than do the benzodiazepines alprazolam and clonazepam but are far superior to the benzodiazepines for the treatment of panic disorder with comorbid depression. Citalopram, fluvoxamine, and fluoxetine also may reduce spontaneous or induced panic attacks. Because fluoxetine can initially heighten anxiety symptoms, persons with panic disorder must begin taking small dosages (5 mg a day) and increase the dosage slowly. Low doses of benzodiazepines may be given to manage this side effect.

SOCIAL ANXIETY DISORDER. SSRIs are effective agents in the treatment of social phobia. They reduce both symptoms and disability. The response rate is comparable to that seen with the MAOI phenelzine (Nardil), the previous standard treatment. The SSRIs are safer to use than MAOIs or benzodiazepines.

POSTTRAUMATIC STRESS DISORDER. Pharmacotherapy for PTSD must target specific symptoms in three clusters: reexperiencing, avoidance, and hyperarousal. For long-term treatment, SSRIs appear to have a broader spectrum of therapeutic effects on specific PTSD symptom clusters than do TCAs and MAOIs. Benzodiazepine augmentation is useful in the acute symptomatic state. The SSRIs are associated with marked improvement of both intrusive and avoidant symptoms.

GENERALIZED ANXIETY DISORDER. The SSRIs may be useful for the treatment of specific phobias, generalized anxiety disorder, and separation anxiety disorder. A thorough, individualized evaluation is the first approach, with particular attention to identifying conditions amenable to drug therapy. In addition, cognitive–behavioral or other psychotherapies can be added for greater efficacy.

Bulimia Nervosa and Other Eating Disorders. Fluoxetine is indicated for the treatment of bulimia, which is best done in the context of psychotherapy. Dosages of 60 mg a day are significantly more effective than 20 mg a day. In several well-controlled studies, fluoxetine in dosages of 60 mg a day was superior to placebo in reducing binge eating and induced vomiting. Some experts recommend an initial course of cognitive–behavioral therapy alone. If there is no response in 3 to 6 weeks, then fluoxetine administration is added. The appropriate duration of treatment with fluoxetine and psychotherapy has not been determined.

Fluvoxamine was not effective at a statistically significant level in one double-blind, placebo-controlled trial for inpatients with bulimia.

ANOREXIA NERVOSA. Fluoxetine has been used in inpatient treatment of anorexia nervosa to attempt to control comorbid mood disturbances and obsessive-compulsive symptoms. However, at least two careful studies, one of 7-month and one of 24-month duration, failed to find that fluoxetine affected the overall outcome and the maintenance of weight. Effective treatments for anorexia include cognitive–behavioral, interpersonal, psychodynamic, and family therapies in addition to a trial with SSRIs.

OBESITY. Fluoxetine, in combination with a behavioral program, has been shown to be only modestly beneficial for weight loss. A significant percentage of all persons who take SSRIs, including fluoxetine, lose weight initially but later may gain weight. However, all SSRIs may cause initial weight gain.

PREMENSTRUAL DYSPHORIC DISORDER. PMDD is characterized by debilitating mood and behavioral changes in the week preceding menstruation that interfere with normal functioning. Sertraline, paroxetine, fluoxetine, and fluvoxamine have been reported to reduce the symptoms of PMDD. Controlled trials of fluoxetine and sertraline administered either throughout the cycle or only during the luteal phase (the 2-week period between ovulation and menstruation) showed both schedules to be equally effective.

An additional observation of unclear significance was that fluoxetine was associated with changing the duration of the menstrual period by more than 4 days, either lengthening or shortening it. The effects of SSRIs on menstrual cycle length are mostly unknown and may warrant careful monitoring in women of reproductive age.

Off-Label Uses

PREMATURE EJACULATION. The antiorgasmic effects of SSRIs make them useful as a treatment for men with premature ejaculation. The SSRIs permit intercourse for a significantly longer period and are reported to improve sexual satisfaction in couples in which the man has premature ejaculation. Fluoxetine and sertraline have been shown to be effective for this purpose.

PARAPHILIAS. The SSRIs may reduce obsessive-compulsive behavior in people with paraphilias. The SSRIs diminish the average time per day spent in unconventional sexual fantasies, urges, and activities. Evidence suggests a greater response for sexual obsessions than for paraphilic behavior.

AUTISM. Obsessive-compulsive behavior, poor social relatedness, and aggression are prominent autistic features that may respond to serotonergic agents such as SSRIs and clomipramine (Anafranil). Sertraline and fluvoxamine have been shown in controlled and open-label trials to mitigate aggressiveness, self-injurious behavior, repetitive behaviors, some degree of language delay, and (rarely) lack of social relatedness in adults with autistic spectrum disorders. Fluoxetine has been reported to be effective for features of autism in children, adolescents, and adults.

Precautions and Adverse Reactions

SSRI side effects need to be considered in terms of their onset, duration, and severity. For example, nausea and jitteriness are early, generally mild, and time-limited side effects. Although SSRIs share common side effect profiles, individual drugs in this class may cause a higher rate or carry a more severe risk of certain side effects depending on the patient.

Sexual Dysfunction. All SSRIs cause sexual dysfunction, and it is the most common adverse effect of SSRIs associated with long-term treatment. It has an estimated incidence of between 50 and 80 percent. The most common complaints are anorgasmia, inhibited orgasm, and decreased libido. Some studies suggest that sexual dysfunction is dose related, but this has not been clearly established. Unlike most of the other adverse effects of SSRIs, sexual inhibition rarely resolves in the first few weeks of use but usually continues as long as the drug is taken. In some cases, there may be improvement over time.

Strategies to counteract SSRI-induced sexual dysfunction are numerous, and none has been proven to be very effective. Some reports suggest decreasing the dosage or adding bupropion (Wellbutrin) or amphetamine. Reports have described successful treatment of SSRI-induced sexual dysfunction with agents such as sildenafil (Viagra), which are used to treat erectile dysfunction. Ultimately, patients may need to be switched to antidepressants that do not interfere with sexual functioning, drugs such as mirtazapine or bupropion.

Gastrointestinal Adverse Effects. GI side effects are very common and are mediated largely through effects on the serotonin 5-HT_3 receptor. The most frequent GI complaints are nausea, diarrhea, anorexia, vomiting, flatulence, and dyspepsia. Sertraline and fluvoxamine produce the most intense GI symptoms. Delayed-release paroxetine, compared with the immediate-release preparation of paroxetine, has less intense GI side effects during the first week of treatment. However, paroxetine, because of its anticholinergic activity, frequently causes constipation. Nausea and loose stools are usually dose related and transient, usually resolving within a few weeks. Sometimes flatulence and diarrhea persist, especially during sertraline treatment. Initial anorexia may also occur and is most common with fluoxetine. SSRI-induced appetite and weight loss begin as soon as the drug is taken and peak at 20 weeks, after which weight often returns to baseline. Up to one-third of persons taking SSRIs will gain weight, sometimes more than 20 lb. This effect is mediated through a metabolic mechanism, increase in appetite, or both. It happens gradually and is usually resistant to diet and exercise regimens. Paroxetine is associated with more frequent, rapid, and pronounced weight gain than the other SSRIs, especially among young women.

Cardiovascular Effects. All SSRIs can lengthen the QT interval in otherwise healthy people and cause drug-induced long QT syndrome, especially when taken in overdose. The risk of QTc prolongation increases when an antidepressant and an antipsychotic are used in combination, an increasingly common practice. Citalopram stands out as the SSRI with the most pronounced effect QT intervals. A QT study to assess the effects of 20-mg and 60-mg doses of citalopram on the QT interval in adults, compared with placebo, found a maximum mean prolongation in the individually corrected QT intervals were 8.5 milliseconds for 20-mg citalopram and 18.5 milliseconds for 60 mg. For 40 mg, prolongation of the corrected QT interval was estimated to be 12.6 milliseconds. Based on these findings, the FDA has issued the following recommendation regarding citalopram use:

- ▲ Twenty milligrams a day is the maximum recommended dose for patients with hepatic impairment, who are older than 60 years of age, who are CYP2C19 poor metabolizers, or who are taking concomitant cimetidine (Tagamet).
- ▲ No longer prescribe at doses greater than 40 mg a day.
- ▲ Do not use in patients with congenital long QT syndrome.
- ▲ Correct hypokalemia and hypomagnesemia before administering citalopram.
- ▲ Monitor electrolytes as clinically indicated.
- ▲ Consider more frequent ECGs in patients with congestive heart failure, bradyarrhythmias, or patients on concomitant medications that prolong the QT interval.

The fact that citalopram carries greater risk of causing fatal rhythm abnormalities was confirmed in a review of 469 SSRI poisoning admissions. Accordingly, patients should be advised to contact their prescriber immediately if they experience signs and symptoms of an abnormal heart rate or rhythm while taking citalopram.

The effect of vilazodone (20, 40, 60, and 80 mg) on the QTc interval was evaluated and a small effect was observed. The upper bound of the 90 percent confidence interval for the largest placebo-adjusted, baseline-corrected QTc interval was below 10 milliseconds, based on the individual correction method (QTcI). This is below the threshold for clinical concern. However, it is unknown whether 80 mg is adequate to represent a high clinical exposure condition.

Physicians should consider whether the benefits of androgen deprivation therapy outweigh the potential risks in SSRI-treated patients with prostate cancer as reductions in androgen levels can cause QTc interval prolongation.

Dextromethorphan/Quinidine (Nuedexta) is available as a treatment for pseudobulbar affect, which is defined by involuntary, sudden, and frequent episodes of laughing or crying that are generally out of proportion or inappropriate to the situation. Quinidine that can prolong the QT interval is a potent inhibitor of CYP2D6. It should not be used with other medications that prolong the QT interval and are metabolized by CYP2D6. This drug should be used with caution with any medications that can prolong the QT interval and inhibit CYP3A4, particularly in patients with cardiac disease.

Antepartum use of SSRIs is sometimes associated with QTc interval prolongation in exposed neonates. In a review of 52 newborns exposed to SSRIs in the immediate antepartum period and 52 matched control subjects, the mean QTc was significantly longer in the group of newborns exposed to antidepressants as compared with control subjects. Five (10 percent) newborns exposed to SSRIs had a markedly prolonged QTc interval (greater than 460 milliseconds) compared with none of the unexposed newborns. The longest QTc interval observed among exposed newborns was 543 milliseconds. All of the drug-associated repolarization abnormalities normalized in subsequent electrocardiographic tracings.

Headaches. The incidence of headache in SSRI trials was 18 to 20 percent, only 1 percentage point higher than the placebo rate. Fluoxetine is the most likely to cause headache. On the other hand, all SSRIs are effective prophylaxis against both migraine and tension-type headaches in many persons.

Central Nervous System Adverse Effects

ANXIETY. Fluoxetine may cause anxiety, particularly in the first few weeks of treatment. However, these initial effects usually give way to an overall reduction in anxiety after a few weeks. Increased anxiety is caused considerably less frequently by paroxetine and escitalopram, which may be better choices if sedation is desired, as in mixed anxiety and depressive disorders.

INSOMNIA AND SEDATION. The major effect SSRIs exert in the area of insomnia and sedation is improved sleep resulting from treatment of depression and anxiety. However, as many as 25 percent of persons taking SSRIs note trouble sleeping, excessive somnolence, or overwhelming fatigue. Fluoxetine is the most likely to cause insomnia, for which reason it is often taken in the morning. Sertraline and fluvoxamine are about equally likely to cause insomnia as somnolence, and citalopram and especially paroxetine often cause somnolence. Escitalopram is more likely to interfere with sleep than its isomer, citalopram. Some persons benefit from taking their SSRI dose before going to bed, but others prefer to take it the morning. SSRI-induced insomnia can be treated with benzodiazepines, trazodone (Desyrel) (clinicians must explain the risk of priapism), or other sedating medicines. Significant SSRI-induced somnolence often requires switching to use of another SSRI or bupropion.

OTHER SLEEP EFFECTS. Many persons taking SSRIs report recalling extremely vivid dreams or nightmares. They describe sleep as "busy." Other sleep effects of the SSRIs include bruxism, restless legs, nocturnal myoclonus, and sweating.

EMOTIONAL BLUNTING. Emotional blunting is a largely overlooked but frequent side effect associated with chronic SSRI use. Patients report an inability to cry in response to emotional situations, a feeling of apathy or indifference, or a restriction in the intensity of emotional experiences. This side effect often leads to treatment discontinuation, even when the drugs provide relief from depression or anxiety.

YAWNING. Close clinical observation of patients taking SSRIs reveals an increase in yawning. This side effect is not a reflection of fatigue or poor nocturnal sleep but is the result of SSRI effects on the hypothalamus.

SEIZURES. Seizures have been reported in 0.1 to 0.2 percent of all patients treated with SSRIs, an incidence comparable to that reported with other antidepressants and not significantly different from that with placebo. Seizures are more frequent at the highest doses of SSRIs (e.g., fluoxetine 100 mg a day or higher).

EXTRAPYRAMIDAL SYMPTOMS. The SSRIs may rarely cause akathisia, dystonia, tremor, cogwheel rigidity, torticollis, opisthotonos, gait disorders, and bradykinesia. Rare cases of tardive dyskinesia have been reported. Some people with well-controlled Parkinson's disease may experience acute worsening of their motor symptoms when they take SSRIs.

Anticholinergic Effects. Paroxetine has mild anticholinergic activity that causes dry mouth, constipation, and sedation in a dose-dependent fashion. Nevertheless, most persons taking paroxetine do not experience cholinergic adverse effects. Other SSRIs are associated with dry mouth, but this effect is not mediated by muscarinic activity.

Hematologic Adverse Effects. The SSRIs can cause functional impairment of platelet aggregation but not a reduction in platelet number. Easy bruising and excessive or prolonged bleeding manifest this pharmacological effect. When patients exhibit these signs, a test for bleeding time should be performed. Special monitoring is suggested when patients use SSRIs in conjunction with anticoagulants or aspirin. Concurrent use of SSRIs and NSAIDs is associated with a significantly increased risk of gastric bleeding. In cases where this combination is necessary, use of proton pump inhibitors should be considered.

Electrolyte and Glucose Disturbances. The SSRIs may acutely decrease glucose concentrations; therefore, diabetic patients should be carefully monitored. Long-term use may be associated with increased glucose levels, although it remains to be proven whether this is the result of a pharmacological effect. It is possible that antidepressant users have other characteristics that raise their odds of developing diabetes or are more likely to be diagnosed with diabetes or other medical conditions as a result of being in treatment for depression.

Cases of SSRI-associated hyponatremia and the syndrome of inappropriate antidiuretic hormone have been seen in some patients, especially those who are older or treated with diuretics.

Endocrine and Allergic Reactions. The SSRIs can increase prolactin levels and cause mammoplasia and galactorrhea in both men and women. Breast changes are reversible upon discontinuation of the drug, but this may take several months to occur.

Various types of rashes appear in about 4 percent of all patients; in a small subset of these patients, the allergic reaction may generalize and involve the pulmonary system, resulting rarely in fibrotic damage and dyspnea. SSRI treatment may have to be discontinued in patients with drug-related rashes.

Serotonin Syndrome. Concurrent administration of an SSRI with an MAOI, L-tryptophan, or lithium (Eskalith) can raise plasma serotonin concentrations to toxic levels, producing a constellation of symptoms called *serotonin syndrome.* This serious and possibly fatal syndrome of serotonin overstimulation comprises, in order of appearance as the condition worsens, (1) diarrhea; (2) restlessness; (3) extreme agitation, hyperreflexia, and autonomic instability with possible rapid fluctuations in vital signs; (4) myoclonus, seizures, hyperthermia, uncontrollable shivering, and rigidity; and (5) delirium, coma, status epilepticus, cardiovascular collapse, and death.

Treatment of serotonin syndrome consists of removing the offending agents and promptly instituting comprehensive supportive care with nitroglycerine, cyproheptadine (Periactin), methysergide (Sansert), cooling blankets, chlorpromazine (Thorazine), dantrolene (Dantrium), benzodiazepines, anticonvulsants, mechanical ventilation, and paralyzing agents.

Sweating. Some patients experience sweating while being treated with SSRIs. The sweating is unrelated to ambient temperature. Nocturnal sweating may drench bed sheets and require a change of night clothes. Terazosin (Hytrin), 1 or 2 mg per day, is often dramatically effective in counteracting sweating.

Overdose. The adverse reactions associated with overdose of vilazodone at doses of 200 to 280 mg as observed in clinical trials included serotonin syndrome, lethargy, restlessness, hallucinations, and disorientation.

Selective Serotonin Reuptake Inhibitor Withdrawal. The abrupt discontinuance of SSRI use, especially one with a shorter half-life such as paroxetine or fluvoxamine, has been associated with a withdrawal syndrome that may include dizziness, weakness, nausea, headache, rebound depression, anxiety, insomnia, poor concentration, upper respiratory symptoms, paresthesias, and migraine-like symptoms. It usually does not appear until after at least 6 weeks of treatment and usually resolves spontaneously in 3 weeks. Persons who experienced transient adverse effects in the first weeks of taking an SSRI are more likely to experience discontinuation symptoms.

Fluoxetine is the SSRI least likely to be associated with this syndrome because the half-life of its metabolite is more than 1 week, and it effectively tapers itself. Fluoxetine has therefore been used in some cases to treat the discontinuation syndrome caused by termination of other SSRIs. Nevertheless, a delayed and attenuated withdrawal syndrome occurs with fluoxetine as well.

Drug Interactions

The SSRIs do not interfere with most other drugs. A serotonin syndrome (Table 25–50) can develop with concurrent administration of MAOIs, L-tryptophan, lithium, or other antidepressants that inhibit reuptake of serotonin. Fluoxetine, sertraline, and paroxetine can raise plasma concentrations of TCAs, which can cause clinical toxicity. A number of potential pharmacokinetic interactions have been described based on in vitro analyses of the CYP enzymes, but clinically relevant interactions are rare. SSRIs that inhibit CYP2D6 may interfere with the analgesic effects of hydrocodone and oxycodone. These drugs can also reduce the effectiveness of tamoxifen (Nolvadex, Soltamox). Combined use of SSRIs and NSAIDs increases the risk of gastric bleeding.

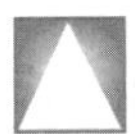

Table 25–50
Serotonin Syndrome Symptoms

Diarrhea	Myoclonus
Diaphoresis	Hyperactive reflexes
Tremor	Disorientation
Ataxia	Lability of mood

The SSRIs, particularly fluvoxamine, should not be used with clozapine because it raises clozapine concentrations, increasing the risk of seizure. The SSRIs may increase the duration and severity of zolpidem (Ambien)-induced side effects, including hallucinations.

Fluoxetine. Fluoxetine can be administered with tricyclic drugs, but the clinician should use low dosages of the tricyclic drug. Because it is metabolized by the hepatic enzyme CYP2D6, fluoxetine may interfere with the metabolism of other drugs in the 7 percent of the population who have an inefficient isoform of this enzyme, the so-called poor metabolizers. Fluoxetine may slow down the metabolism of carbamazepine (Tegretol), antineoplastic agents, diazepam (Valium), and phenytoin (Dilantin). Drug interactions have been described for fluoxetine that may affect the plasma levels of benzodiazepines, antipsychotics, and lithium. Fluoxetine and other SSRIs may interact with warfarin (Coumadin), increasing the risk of bleeding and bruising.

Sertraline. Sertraline may displace warfarin from plasma proteins and may increase the prothrombin time. The drug interaction data on sertraline support a generally similar profile to that of fluoxetine, although sertraline does not interact as strongly with the CYP2D6 enzyme.

Paroxetine. Paroxetine has a higher risk for drug interactions than does either fluoxetine or sertraline because it is a more potent inhibitor of the CYP2D6 enzyme. Cimetidine can increase the concentration of sertraline and paroxetine, and phenobarbital (Luminal) and phenytoin can decrease the concentration of paroxetine. Because of the potential for interference with the CYP2D6 enzyme, the coadministration of paroxetine with other antidepressants, phenothiazines, and antiarrhythmic drugs should be undertaken with caution. Paroxetine may increase the anticoagulant effect of warfarin. Coadministration of paroxetine and tramadol may precipitate serotonin syndrome in elderly persons.

Fluvoxamine. Among the SSRIs, fluvoxamine appears to present the most risk for drug–drug interactions. Fluvoxamine is metabolized by the enzyme CYP3A4, which may be inhibited by ketoconazole (Nizoral). Fluvoxamine may increase the half-life of alprazolam, triazolam (Halcion), and diazepam, and it should not be coadministered with these agents. Fluvoxamine may increase theophylline levels threefold and warfarin levels twofold, with important clinical consequences; thus, the serum levels of the latter drugs should be closely monitored and the doses adjusted accordingly. Fluvoxamine raises concentrations and may increase the activity of clozapine, carbamazepine, methadone (Dolophine, Methadose), propranolol (Inderal), and diltiazem (Cardizem). Fluvoxamine has no significant interactions with lorazepam (Ativan) or digoxin (Lanoxin).

Citalopram. Citalopram is not a potent inhibitor of any CYP enzymes. Concurrent administration of cimetidine increases concentrations of citalopram by about 40 percent. Citalopram does not significantly affect the metabolism of, nor is its metabolism significantly affected by, digoxin, lithium, warfarin, carbamazepine, or imipramine (Tofranil). Citalopram increases the plasma concentrations of metoprolol (Lopressor) twofold, but this usually has no effect on BP or heart rate. Data on coadministration of citalopram and potent inhibitors of CYP3A4 or CYP2D6 are not available.

Escitalopram. Escitalopram is a moderate inhibitor of CYP2D6 and has been shown to significantly raise desipramine (Norpramin) and metoprolol concentrations.

Vilazodone. Vilazodone dose should be reduced to 20 mg when coadministered with CYP3A4 strong inhibitors. Concomitant use with inducers of CYP3A4 can result in inadequate drug concentrations and may diminish effectiveness. The effect of CYP3A4 inducers on systemic exposure of vilazodone has not been evaluated.

Laboratory Interferences

The SSRIs do not interfere with any laboratory tests.

Dosage and Clinical Guidelines

Fluoxetine. Fluoxetine is available in 10- and 20-mg capsules, in a scored 10-mg tablet, as a 90-mg enteric-coated capsule for once-weekly administration, and as an oral concentrate (20 mg/5 mL). Fluoxetine is also marketed as Sarafem for PMDD. For depression, the initial dosage is usually 10 or 20 mg orally each day, usually given in the morning, because insomnia is a potential adverse effect of the drug. Fluoxetine should be taken with food to minimize the possible nausea. The long half-lives of the drug and its metabolite contribute to a 4-week period to reach steady-state concentrations. Twenty milligrams is often as effective as higher doses for treating depression. The maximum dosage recommended by the manufacturer is 80 mg a day. To minimize the early side effects of anxiety and restlessness, some clinicians initiate fluoxetine use at 5 to 10 mg a day either with the scored 10-mg tablet or by using the liquid preparation. Alternatively, because of the long half-life of fluoxetine, its use can be initiated with an every-other-day administration schedule. The dosage of fluoxetine (and other SSRIs) that is effective in other indications may differ from the dosage generally used for depression.

Sertraline. Sertraline is available in scored 25-, 50-, and 100-mg tablets. For the initial treatment of depression, sertraline use should be initiated with a dosage of 50 mg once daily. To limit the GI effects, some clinicians begin at 25 mg a day and increase to 50 mg a day after 3 weeks. Patients who do not respond after 1 to 3 weeks may benefit from dosage increases of 50 mg every week up to a maximum of 200 mg given once daily. Sertraline can be administered in the morning or the evening. Administration after eating may reduce the GI adverse effects. Sertraline oral concentrate (1 mL = 20 mg) has 12 percent alcohol content and must be diluted before use. When used to treat panic disorder, sertraline should be initiated at 25 mg to reduce the risk of provoking a panic attack.

Paroxetine. Immediate-release paroxetine is available in scored 20-mg tablets; in unscored 10-, 30-, and 40-mg tablets; and as an orange-flavored 10-mg/5-mL oral suspension. Paroxetine use for the treatment of depression is usually initiated at a dosage of 10 or 20 mg a day. An increase in the dosage should be considered when an adequate response is not seen in 1 to 3 weeks. At that point, the clinician can initiate upward dose titration in 10-mg increments at weekly intervals to a maximum of 50 mg a day. Persons who experience GI upset may benefit by taking the drug with food. Paroxetine can be taken initially as a single daily dose in the evening; higher dosages may be divided into two doses per day.

A delayed-release formulation of paroxetine, paroxetine CR, is available in 12.5-, 25-, and 37.5-mg tablets. The starting dosages of paroxetine CR are 25 mg per day for depression and 12.5 mg per day for panic disorder.

Paroxetine is the SSRI most likely to produce a discontinuation syndrome because plasma concentrations decrease rapidly in the absence of continuous dosing. To limit the development of symptoms of abrupt discontinuation, paroxetine use should be tapered gradually, with dosage reductions every 2 to 3 weeks.

Fluvoxamine. Fluvoxamine is the only SSRI not approved by the FDA as an antidepressant. It is indicated for social anxiety disorder and OCD. It is available in unscored 25-mg tablets and scored 50- and 100-mg tablets. The effective daily dosage range is 50 to 300 mg a day. A usual starting dosage is 50 mg once a day at bedtime for the first week, after which the dosage can be adjusted according to the adverse effects and clinical response. Dosages above 100 mg a day may be divided into twice-daily dosing. A temporary dosage reduction or slower upward titration may be necessary if nausea develops over the first 2 weeks of therapy. Although fluvoxamine can also be administered as a single evening dose to minimize its adverse effects, its short half-life may lead to interdose withdrawal. An extended-release formulation is available in 100- and 150-mg dose strengths. All fluvoxamine formulations should be swallowed with food without chewing the tablet. Abrupt discontinuation of fluvoxamine may cause a discontinuation syndrome owing to its short half-life.

Citalopram. Citalopram is available in 20- and 40-mg scored tablets and as a liquid (10 mg/5 mL). The usual starting dosage is 20 mg a day for the first week, after which it usually is increased to 40 mg a day. For elderly persons or persons with hepatic impairment, 20 mg a day is recommended, with an increase to 40 mg a day only if there is no response at 20 mg a day. Tablets should be taken once daily in either the morning or the evening with or without food.

Escitalopram. Escitalopram is available as 10- and 20-mg scored tablets, as well as an oral solution at a concentration of 5 mg/5 mL. The recommended dosage of escitalopram is 10 mg per day. In clinical trials, no additional benefit was noted when 20 mg per day was used.

Vilazodone. Vilazodone is available as 10-, 20-, and 40-mg tablets. The recommended therapeutic dose of vilazodone is 40 mg once daily. Treatment should be titrated, starting with an initial dose of 10 mg once daily for 7 days, followed by 20 mg once daily for an additional 7 days, and then an increase to 40 mg once daily. Vilazodone should be taken with food. If vilazodone is taken without food, inadequate drug concentrations may result and the drug's effectiveness may be diminished. Vilazodone is not approved for use in children. The safety and efficacy of vilazodone in pediatric patients have not been studied. No dose adjustment is recommended on the basis of age. No dose adjustment is recommended in patients with mild or moderate hepatic impairment. Vilazodone has not been studied in patients with severe hepatic impairment. No dose adjustment is recommended in patients with mild, moderate, or severe renal impairment.

Pregnancy and Breastfeeding. With the exception of paroxetine, the SSRIs are safe to take during pregnancy when deemed necessary for treatment of the mother. There are no controlled human data regarding vilazodone use during pregnancy nor are there human data regarding drug concentrations in breast milk. Transient QTc prolongation has been noted in newborns whose mother was being treated with an SSRI during pregnancy.

Loss of Efficacy. Some patients report a diminished response or total loss of response to SSRIs with recurrence of depressive symptoms while remaining on a full dose of medication. The exact mechanism of this so-called poop-out is unknown, but the phenomenon is very real. Potential remedies for the attenuation of response to SSRIs include increasing or decreasing the dosage, tapering drug use, and then rechallenging with the same medication, switching to another SSRI or non-SSRI antidepressant, and augmenting with bupropion or another augmentation agent.

Vortioxetine (Brintellix). Vortioxetine works mainly as an inhibitor of serotonin (5-HT) reuptake, but it has a more complex pharmacologic profile than other SSRIs. It also acts as an agonist at 5-HT_{1A} receptors, a partial agonist at 5-HT_{1B} receptors and an antagonist at 5-HT_3, 5-HT_{1D} and 5-HT_7 receptors. The contribution of each of these activities to the drug's antidepressant effect has not been established, but it is the only compound with this combination of pharmacodynamic actions.

Side effects seen during the trials include, but are not limited to, nausea, constipation and vomiting.

The recommended starting dose is 10 mg administered orally once daily without regard to meals. The dose should then be increased to 20 mg/day, as tolerated. A dose of 5 mg/day should be considered for patients who do not tolerate higher doses.

The maximum recommended dose of Vortioxetine is 10 mg/day in known CYP2D6 poor metabolizers. Reduction of the dose of Vortioxetine by one-half is suggested when patients are receiving a CYP2D6 strong inhibitor (e.g., bupropion, fluoxetine, paroxetine, or quinidine) concomitantly. The dose should be increased to the original dose of vortioxetine in patients who stop taking CYP inducers, (e.g., rifampin, carbamazepine, or phenytoin) increasing its dose should be considered. This is especially important when a strong CYP inducer is coadministered for greater than 14 days. The maximum recommended dose should not exceed three times the original dose. The dose of vortioxetine should be reduced to the original level within 14 days, when the inducer is discontinued.

Although vortioxetine can be abruptly discontinued, in placebo-controlled trials patients experienced transient adverse reactions such as headache and muscle tension following abrupt discontinuation of vortioxetine 15 or 20 mg/day. To avoid these adverse reactions, it is recommended that the dose be decreased to 10 mg/day for one week before full discontinuation of vortioxetine 15 or 20 mg/day.

Vortioxetine is available in 5-mg, 10-mg, 15-mg, and 20-mg tablets.

Ketamine

Despite the development of newer antidepressants with a broad neuroreceptor profile, the delay in response has been a challenge for both the clinicians and the patients. Ketamine has been in use for many years since 1970 and is used as an anesthetic agent for diagnostic and surgical procedures. It is also used as an induction agent prior to the administration of general anesthetic agents. It also became a drug of abuse and was popular as a psychedelic club drug. It was not until 2006 when a study by Zarate CA Jr at the National Institute of Mental Health (NIMH) concluded that Ketamine produced a robust and rapid antidepressant effect after a single intravenous infusion with an onset within 2 hours postinfusion and remained significant for a week.

Ketamine hydrochloride is a nonbarbiturate anesthetic chemically designated dl 2-(0-chlorophenyl)-2-(methylamino) cyclohexanone hydrochloride. It is important to note that Ketamine hydrochloride injection should be used by or under the direction and supervision of physicians who are experienced in administering general anesthetics and in maintenance of an airway and in the control of respiration. Of note Ketamine has a wide margin of safety; there have been several cases of overdoses with ketamine hydrochloride (up to 10 times the required dose) that have required prolonged observation but had complete recovery.

Since the landmark study thousands of depressed patients have received off-label Ketamine infusions with mixed results even though the FDA has not approved it. Though it has been found to be safe and effective the benefits are transitory for 1 to 2 weeks and require ongoing regular infusions with varying schedules based on the necessity and acuity of the symptoms. This ongoing infusion therapy is not practical and alternate modes of administration including intranasal and PO formulations are being explored. The oral bioavailability of Ketamine is only 8 to 17 percent secondary to first-pass metabolism and slightly higher with sublingual formulation. Intranasal Ketamine has been used for pain and in migraine headache but its use in depression is in development. Studies looking at intranasal delivery of Ketamine have found rapid response but required administration every 2 to 3 days and may require ongoing intravenous administration as well.

As of now this treatment modality is being practiced by a few psychiatrists as an off-label use for patients who have failed to show response to conventional antidepressant therapy or ECT.

Psilocybin

Psilocybin the active ingredient in mushrooms is being investigated in the treatment of anxiety and depression particularly in the end of life situations like patient with terminal cancer. Numerous studies across the country are looking at this mysterious and magical product that has been used since ancient times in various cultures. A single dose of Psilocybin has been shown to reduce anxiety and depression by altering perception and producing mystical-type experiences with effects lasting up to 6 months. At this time Psilocybin remains confined as a potential treatment for anxiety and depression in controlled research setting under the guidance of well-trained personnel.

SEROTONIN–DOPAMINE ANTAGONISTS AND SIMILARLY ACTING DRUGS (SECOND-GENERATION OR ATYPICAL ANTIPSYCHOTICS)

The SDAs, also known as second-generation or atypical antipsychotic drugs, are a group of pharmacologically diverse drugs that have largely supplanted the older DRAs. The term *atypical* is used because these drugs differ in their side effect profiles, most notably a lower risk of EPS, and have spectra of action that are broader than those of the DRAs. In contrast to the earlier antipsychotic drugs, the SDAs have significant effects on both the dopamine and serotonin systems. Their pharmacology is complex, with individual drugs in this group having multiple neurotransmitter effects. All SDAs are indicated for the treatment of schizophrenia. Most of these SGA drugs have also received approval as monotherapy or adjunctive therapy in the treatment of bipolar disorder. Some have also been approved as adjuncts for treatment of major depression.

As of 2016, 12 SGA drugs were approved by the FDA. These include the following: risperidone (Risperdal), risperidone IM long acting (Consta), olanzapine (Zyprexa), olanzapine for extended-release injectable suspension (Zyprexa, Relprevv), olanzapine sublingual (Zyprexa Zydis), quetiapine (Seroquel), quetiapine XR (Seroquel XR), ziprasidone (Geodon), aripiprazole (Abilify), aripiprazole IM long acting (Abilify Maintena), paliperidone (Invega), paliperidone palmitate (Invega, Invega Sustenna), asenapine (Saphris), lurasidone (Latuda), iloperidone (Fanapt), cariprazine (Vraylar), brexpiprazole (Rexulti), clozapine (Clozaril), and clozapine sublingual (FazaClo).

It is arguable whether the SDAs represent an improvement in overall tolerability than the DRAs. Although there is improvement with respect to a lowered, but not absent, risk of EPS, most of the drugs in this group often produce substantial weight gain, which in turn increases the potential for the development of diabetes mellitus. Olanzapine and clozapine appear to account for most cases of weight gain and drug-induced diabetes mellitus. The other agents pose a smaller risk of these side effects; nevertheless, the FDA has requested that all SDAs carry a warning label that patients taking the drugs be monitored closely, and has recommended the following factors be considered for all patients prescribed SGAs.

1. Personal and family history of obesity, diabetes, dyslipidemia, hypertension, and cardiovascular disease
2. Weight and height (so that body mass index [BMI] can be calculated)
3. Waist circumference (at the level of the umbilicus)
4. BP
5. Fasting plasma glucose level
6. Fasting lipid profile

Patients with preexisting diabetes should have regular monitoring, including hemoglobin A1c (HgA1c) and in some cases insulin levels. Among these drugs, clozapine sits apart. It is not considered a first-line agent because of side effects (hematological) and need for weekly blood tests. Although highly effective in treating both mania and depression, clozapine does not have an FDA indication for these conditions.

Mechanisms of Action

The presumed antipsychotic effects of the SDAs are blockade of D_2 dopamine receptors. Where the SDAs differ from older antipsychotic drugs is their higher ratio interactions with serotonin receptor subtypes, most notably the 5-HT_{2A} subtype, as well as with other neurotransmitter systems. It is hypothesized that these properties account for the distinct tolerability profiles associated with each of the SDAs. All SDAs have different chemical structures, receptor affinities, and side effect profiles. No SDA is identical in its combination of receptor affinities, and the relative contribution of each receptor interaction to the clinical effects is unknown.

Therapeutic Indications

Although initially approved for the treatment of schizophrenia and acute mania, some of these drugs have also been approved for schizoaffective disorder, depressive episodes in bipolar I and as adjunctive therapy in treatment-resistant depression and as adjunctive therapy in MDD. They are also useful in PTSD and anxiety disorders, and although clinicians tend to use them in behavioral disturbances associated with dementia, all SDAs carry an FDA boxed warning regarding adverse effects when used in elderly persons with dementia-related psychoses, because elderly patients with dementia-related psychoses are at an increased risk (1.6 to 1.7 times) of death compared with placebo. All of these agents are considered first-line drugs for schizophrenia as well as acute mania and bipolar disorder except clozapine, which may cause adverse hematological effects that require regular blood sampling based on most recent Risk Evaluation and Mitigation Strategies (REMS) guidelines.

Schizophrenia and Schizoaffective Disorder

The SDAs are effective for treating acute and chronic psychoses such as schizophrenia and schizoaffective disorder, in both adults and adolescents. SDAs are as good as or better than typical antipsychotics (DRAs) for the treatment of positive symptoms in schizophrenia and superior to DRAs for the treatment of negative symptoms. Compared with persons treated with DRAs, persons treated with SDAs have fewer relapses and require less frequent hospitalization, fewer emergency department visits, less phone contact with mental health professionals, and less treatment in day programs.

Because clozapine has potentially life-threatening adverse effects, it is appropriate only for patients with schizophrenia who are resistant to all other antipsychotics, though it is usually prescribed after failure of two antipsychotics that may belong to either first or SGA class. Other indications for clozapine include treatment of persons with severe tardive dyskinesia—which can be reversed with high dosages in some cases—and those with a low threshold for EPS. Persons who tolerate clozapine have done well on long-term therapy. The effectiveness of clozapine may be increased by augmentation with lamotrigine, aripiprazole and risperidone, which raises clozapine concentrations and sometimes results in dramatic clinical improvement.

Mood Disorders. All of the SDAs (except clozapine) are FDA approved for the treatment of acute mania. Some of these agents, including aripiprazole, olanzapine, quetiapine, and quetiapine XR, are also approved for the maintenance treatment in bipolar disorder as monotherapy or adjunctive therapy. The SDAs improve depressive symptoms in schizophrenia, and both clinical experience and clinical trials show that all of the SDAs augment antidepressants in the acute management of major depression. At this time, olanzapine in combination with fluoxetine has been approved for treatment-resistant depression, and aripiprazole and quetiapine XR are indicated for adjunctive therapy to antidepressants in MDDs. Lurasidone, Quetiapine, and quetiapine XR are also approved in bipolar depression. A fixed combination of olanzapine and fluoxetine (Symbyax) is approved as a treatment for acute bipolar depression.

Other Indications. About 10 percent of patients with schizophrenia exhibit outwardly aggressive or violent behavior, and the SDAs are effective for treatment of such aggression. Other off-label indications include acquired immunodeficiency syndrome (AIDS) dementia, autistic spectrum disorders, Tourette's disorder, Huntington's disease, and Lesch–Nyhan syndrome. Risperidone and olanzapine have been used to control aggression and self-injury in children. These drugs have also been coadministered with sympathomimetics, such as methylphenidate (Ritalin) or dextroamphetamine (Dexedrine), to children with ADHD who are comorbid for either oppositional–defiant disorder or conduct disorder. SDAs—especially olanzapine, quetiapine, and clozapine—are useful in persons who have severe tardive dyskinesia. The SDAs are also effective for treating psychotic depression and for psychosis secondary to head trauma, dementia, or treatment drugs.

Treatment with SDAs especially clozapine decreases the risk of suicide and water intoxication (psychogenic polydipsia) in patients with schizophrenia. Patients with treatment-resistant OCD have responded to the SDAs; however, a few persons treated with the SDAs have been noted to develop treatment-emergent symptoms of OCD. Some patients with borderline personality disorder may improve with the SDAs.

Some data suggest that treatment with conventional DRAs has protective effects against the progression of schizophrenia when used during the first episode of psychosis. Ongoing studies are looking at whether the use of SDAs in at-risk patients with early evidence of disease prevents deterioration, thus improving long-term outcome.

Adverse Effects

The SDAs share a similar spectrum of adverse reactions, but differ considerably in terms of frequency or severity of their occurrence. Specific side effects that are more common with an individual SDA are emphasized in the discussion of each drug in subsequent text.

Risperidone (Risperdal)

Indications. Risperidone is indicated for the acute and maintenance treatment of schizophrenia in adults and for the treatment of schizophrenia in adolescents age 13 to 17 years. Risperidone is also indicated for the short-term treatment of acute manic or mixed episodes associated with bipolar I disorder in adults and in children and adolescents age 10 to 17 years. The combination of risperidone with lithium or valproate is indicated for the short-term treatment of acute manic or mixed episodes associated with bipolar I disorder.

Risperidone is also indicated for the treatment of irritability associated with autistic spectrum disorder in children and adolescents age 5 to 16 years, including symptoms of aggression toward others, deliberate self-injuriousness, temper tantrums, and quickly changing moods.

Pharmacology. Risperidone is a benzisoxazole. It undergoes extensive first-pass hepatic metabolism to 9-hydroxy risperidone, a metabolite with equivalent antipsychotic activity. Peak plasma levels of the parent compound occur within 1 hour for the parent compound and 3 hours for the metabolite. Risperidone has a bioactivity of 70 percent. The combined half-life of risperidone and 9-hydroxy risperidone averages 20 hours, so it is effective in once-daily dosing. Risperidone is an antagonist of the serotonin 5-HT_{2A}, dopamine D_2, α_1-adrenergic and α_2-adrenergic, and histamine H_1 receptors. It has a low affinity for α-adrenergic and muscarinic cholinergic receptors. Although it is as potent an antagonist of D_2 receptors, as is haloperidol (Haldol), risperidone is much less likely than haloperidol to cause EPS in humans when the dose of risperidone is below 6 mg per day.

Dosages. The recommended dose range and frequency of risperidone dosing has changed since the drug first came into clinical use. Risperidone is available in 0.25-, 0.5-, 1-, 2-, 3-, and 4-mg tablets and a 1-mg/mL oral solution. The initial dosage is usually 1 to 2 mg at night, which can then be increased to 4 mg per day. Positron emission tomography (PET) studies have shown that dosages of 1 to 4 mg per day provide the required D_2 blockade for a therapeutic effect. At first it was believed that because of its short elimination half-life, risperidone should be given twice a day, but studies have shown equal efficacy with once-a-day dosing. Dosages above 6 mg a day are associated with a higher incidence of adverse effects, particularly EPS. There is no correlation between plasma concentrations and therapeutic effect. Dosing guidelines for adolescents and children are different from those for adults, requiring lower starting dosages; higher dosages are associated with more adverse effects.

Side Effects. The EPS of risperidone are largely dosage dependent, and there has been a trend to using lower doses than initially recommended. Weight gain, anxiety, nausea and vomiting, rhinitis, erectile dysfunction, orgasmic dysfunction, and increased pigmentation are associated with risperidone use. The most common drug-related reasons for discontinuation of risperidone use are EPS, dizziness, hyperkinesias, somnolence, and nausea. Marked elevation of prolactin may occur. Weight gain occurs more commonly with risperidone use in children than in adults.

Risperidone is also available as an orally disintegrating tablet (Risperdal M-Tab), which is available in 0.5, 1, and 2 mg strengths, and in a depot formulation (Risperdal Consta), which is given as an IM injection formulation every 2 weeks. The dose may be 25, 50, or 75 mg. Oral risperidone should be coadministered with Risperdal Consta for the first 3 weeks before being discontinued.

Drug Interactions. Inhibition of CYP2D6 by drugs such as paroxetine and fluoxetine can block the formation of risperidone's active metabolite. Risperidone is a weak inhibitor of CYP2D6 and has little effect on other drugs. Combined use of risperidone and SSRIs may result in significant elevation of prolactin, with associated galactorrhea and breast enlargement.

Paliperidone (Invega)

Indications. Paliperidone is indicated for the acute and maintenance treatment of schizophrenia. Paliperidone is also indicated for the acute treatment of schizoaffective disorder as monotherapy, or as an adjunct to mood stabilizers or antidepressants.

Pharmacology. Paliperidone is a benzisoxazole derivative and is the major active metabolite of risperidone. Peak plasma concentrations (C_{max}) are achieved approximately 24 hours after dosing, and steady-state concentrations of paliperidone are attained within 4 or 5 days. The hepatic isoenzymes CYP2D6 and CYP3A4 play a limited role in the metabolism and elimination of paliperidone, so no dose adjustment is required in patients with mild or moderate hepatic impairment.

Dosage. Paliperidone is available in 3-, 6-, and 9-mg tablets. The recommended dosage is 6 mg once daily administered in the morning. It can be taken with or without food. It is also available as extended-release tablets, which are also available in 3-, 6-, and 9-mg tablets administered once daily. It is recommended that no more than 12 mg should be administered per day. A long-acting formulation of paliperidone (Invega Sustenna) is given by injection once a month. Invega Sustenna is available as a white to off-white sterile aqueous extended-release suspension for IM injection in dose strengths of 39-, 78-, 117-, 156-, and 234-mg paliperidone palmitate. The drug product hydrolyzes to the active moiety, paliperidone, resulting in dose strengths of 25, 50, 75, 100, and 150 mg of paliperidone, respectively.

Invega Sustenna is provided in a prefilled syringe with a plunger stopper and tip cap. The kit also contains two safety needles (a 1½-in 22-gauge safety needle and a 1-in 23-gauge safety needle). It has a half-life of 25 to 49 days. Monthly injections of 117 mg are recommended, although higher or lower dosages can be used depending on the clinical situation. The first two injections should be in the deltoid muscle because plasma concentrations are 28 percent higher with deltoid versus gluteal administration. Subsequent injections can alternate between gluteal and deltoid sites.

Side Effects. The dose of paliperidone should be reduced in patients with renal impairment. It may cause more sensitivity to temperature extremes such as very hot or cold conditions. Paliperidone may cause an increase in QT (QTc) interval and should be avoided in combination with other drugs that cause prolongation of QT interval. It may cause orthostatic hypotension, tachycardia, somnolence, akathisia, dystonia, EPS, and parkinsonism.

Olanzapine (Zyprexa)

Indications. Olanzapine is indicated for the treatment of schizophrenia. Oral olanzapine is indicated for use as monotherapy for the acute treatment of manic or mixed episodes associated with bipolar I disorder and maintenance treatment of bipolar I disorder. Oral olanzapine is also indicated for the treatment of manic or mixed episodes associated with bipolar I disorder as an adjunct to lithium or valproate, and olanzapine can also be used in combination with fluoxetine (Symbyax) for the treatment of depressive episodes associated with bipolar I disorder.

Oral olanzapine and fluoxetine in combination (Symbyax) is indicated for the treatment of treatment-resistant depression. Olanzapine monotherapy is not indicated for the treatment of treatment-resistant depression.

Pharmacology. Approximately 85 percent of olanzapine is absorbed from the GI tract, and about 40 percent of the dosage is inactivated by first-pass hepatic metabolism. Peak concentrations are reached in 5 hours, and the half-life averages 31 hours (range 21 to 54 hours). It is given in once-daily dosing. In addition to 5-HT_{2A} and D_2 antagonism, olanzapine is an antagonist of the D_1, D_4, α_1, 5-HT_{1A}, muscarinic M_1 to M_5, and H_1 receptors.

Dosages. Olanzapine is available in 2.5-, 5-, 7.5-, 10-, 15-, and 20-mg oral and Zydis form (orally disintegrating) tablets. The initial dosage for the treatment of psychosis is usually 5 or 10 mg, and for the treatment of acute mania is usually 10 or 15 mg given once daily. It is also available as 5-, 10-, 15-, and 20-mg orally disintegrating tablets that might be useful for patients who have difficulty swallowing pills or who "cheek" their medication.

A starting daily dose of 5 to 10 mg is recommended. After 1 week, the dosage can be raised to 10 mg a day. Given the long half-life, 1 week must be allowed to achieve each new steady-state blood level. Dosages in clinical use ranges vary, with 5 to 20 mg a day being most commonly used, but 30 to 40 mg a day being needed in treatment-resistant patients. A word of caution, however, is that the higher dosages are associated with increased EPS and other adverse effects, and dosages above 20 mg a day were not studied in the pivotal trials that led to the approval of olanzapine. The parenteral form of olanzapine is indicated for the treatment of acute agitation associated with schizophrenia and bipolar disorder, and the IM dosage is 10 mg. Coadministration with benzodiazepines is not approved.

Other Formulations. Olanzapine is available as an extended-release injectable suspension (Relprevv), which is a long-acting atypical IM injection indicated for the treatment of schizophrenia. It is injected deeply in the gluteal region and should not be administered intravenously or subcutaneously, nor is it approved for deltoid administration. Before administering the injection, the administrator should aspirate the syringe for several seconds to ensure that no blood is visible. It carries a boxed warning for postinjection delirium sedation syndrome (PDSS). Patients are at risk for severe sedation (including coma) and must be observed for 3 hours after each injection in a registered facility. In controlled studies, all patients with PDSS recovered, and there were no deaths reported. It is postulated that PDSS is secondary to increased levels of olanzapine secondary to accidental rupture of a blood vessel, causing extreme sedation or delirium. Patients should be managed as clinically appropriate and, if necessary, monitored in a facility capable of resuscitation. The injection can be given every 2 or 4 weeks depending on the dosing guidelines.

Drug Interactions. Fluvoxamine (Luvox) and cimetidine (Tagamet) increase, whereas carbamazepine and phenytoin decrease serum concentrations of olanzapine. Ethanol increases olanzapine absorption by more than 25 percent, leading to increased sedation. Olanzapine has little effect on the metabolism of other drugs.

Side Effects. Other than clozapine, olanzapine consistently causes a greater amount and more frequent weight gain than other atypicals. This effect is not dose related and continues over time. Clinical trial data suggest it peaks after 9 months, after which it may continue to increase more slowly. Somnolence, dry mouth, dizziness, constipation, dyspepsia, increased appetite, akathisia, and tremor are associated with olanzapine use. A small number of patients (2 percent) may need to discontinue use of the drug because of transaminase elevation. There is a dose-related risk of EPS. The manufacturer recommends "periodic" assessment of blood sugar and transaminases during treatment with olanzapine. There is an FDA-mandated warning about an increased risk of stroke among patients with dementia treated with SDAs, but this risk is small and is outweighed by improved behavioral control that treatment may produce.

Quetiapine (Seroquel)

Indications. Quetiapine is indicated for the treatment of schizophrenia, as well as the acute treatment of manic episodes associated with bipolar I disorder, both as monotherapy and as an adjunct to lithium or divalproex. It is also indicated as monotherapy for the acute treatment of depressive episodes associated with bipolar disorder and maintenance treatment of bipolar I disorder as an adjunct to lithium or divalproex.

Pharmacology. Quetiapine is a dibenzothiazepine structurally related to clozapine, but it differs markedly from that agent in biochemical effects. It is rapidly absorbed from the GI tract, with peak plasma concentrations reached in 1 to 2 hours. The steady-state half-life is about 7 hours, and optimal dosing is two or three times per day. Quetiapine, in addition to being an antagonist of D_2 and 5-HT_2, also blocks 5-HT_6, D_1 and H_1, and α_1 and α_2 receptors. It does not block muscarinic or benzodiazepine receptors. The receptor antagonism for quetiapine is generally lower than that for other antipsychotic drugs, and it is not associated with EPS.

Dosages. Quetiapine is available in 25-, 50-, 100-, 200-, 300-, and 400-mg tablets. Quetiapine dosing should begin at 25 mg twice daily, with doses then increased by 25 to 50 mg per dose every 2 to 3 days, up to a target of 300 to 400 mg a day. Studies have shown efficacy in the range of 300 to 800 mg a day. In reality, more aggressive dosing is both tolerated and more effective. It has become evident that the target dose can be achieved more rapidly, and that some patients benefit from dosages of as much as 1,200 to 1,600 mg a day. When used at higher doses, serial ECG studies are required. Despite its short elimination half-life, quetiapine can be given to many patients once a day. This is consistent with the observation that quetiapine receptor occupancy remains even when concentrations in the blood have markedly declined. Quetiapine in doses of 25 to 300 mg at night has been used for insomnia.

Other Formulations. Quetiapine XR has a comparable bioavailability to an equivalent dose of quetiapine administered two or three times daily. Quetiapine XR is given once daily, preferably in the evening 3 to 4 hours before bedtime without food or a light meal to prevent an increase in C_{max}. The usual starting dose is 300 mg in acute mania, and it may be increased to 400 to 800 mg. In bipolar depression the dosing is gradual with starting dose of 50 mg on day 1 and increasing by day 4 to 300 mg. It has all of the above indications and in addition is indicated for use as adjunctive therapy to antidepressants for the treatment of MDD.

Drug Interactions. The potential interactions between quetiapine and other drugs have been well studied. Phenytoin increases quetiapine clearance fivefold; no major pharmacokinetic interactions have been noted. Avoid use of quetiapine with drugs that increase the QT interval and in patients with risk factors for prolonged QT interval. The FDA has added a new warning about quetiapine cautioning prescribers about potential prolongation of the QT interval when above-recommended amounts of quetiapine are combined with specific drugs. The use of quetiapine should be avoided in combination with other drugs that are known to prolong QTc including class 1A antiarrhythmics (e.g., quinidine, procainamide) or class III antiarrhythmics (e.g., amiodarone, sotalol), antipsychotic medications (e.g., ziprasidone, chlorpromazine, thioridazine), antibiotics (e.g., gatifloxacin, moxifloxacin), or any other class of medications known to prolong the QTc interval (e.g., pentamidine, levomethadyl acetate, methadone). Quetiapine should also be avoided in circumstances that may increase the risk of occurrence of torsade de pointes and/or sudden death including (1) a history of cardiac arrhythmias such as bradycardia; (2) hypokalemia or hypomagnesemia; (3) concomitant use of other drugs that prolong the QTc interval; and (4) presence of congenital prolongation of the QT interval. Postmarketing cases also show increases in QT interval in patients who overdose on quetiapine.

Side Effects. Somnolence, postural hypotension, and dizziness are the most common adverse effects of quetiapine. These are usually transient and are best managed with initial gradual upward titration of the dosage. Quetiapine is the SDA least likely to cause EPS, regardless of dose. This makes it particularly useful in treating patients with Parkinson's disease who develop dopamine agonist–induced psychosis. Prolactin elevation is rare and both transient and mild when it occurs. Quetiapine is associated with modest transient weight gain in some persons, but some patients occasionally gain a considerable amount of weight. The relationship between quetiapine and the development of diabetes is not as clearly established as are the cases involving the use of olanzapine. Small increases in heart rate, constipation, and a transient increase in liver transaminases may also occur. Initial concerns about cataract formation, based on animal studies, have not been borne out since the drug has been in clinical use. Nevertheless, it might be prudent to test for lens abnormalities early in treatment and periodically thereafter.

Ziprasidone (Geodon)

Indications. Ziprasidone is indicated for the treatment of schizophrenia. Ziprasidone is also indicated as monotherapy for the acute treatment of manic or mixed episodes associated with bipolar I disorder and as an adjunct to lithium or valproate for the maintenance treatment of bipolar I disorder.

Pharmacology. Ziprasidone is a benzisothiazole piperazine. Peak plasma concentrations of ziprasidone are reached in 2 to 6 hours. Steady-state levels ranging from 5 to 10 hours are reached between the first and the third days of treatment. The mean terminal half-life at steady state ranges from 5 to 10 hours, which accounts for the recommendation that twice-daily dosing is necessary. Bioavailability doubles when ziprasidone is taken with food, and therefore it should be taken with food.

Peak serum concentrations of IM ziprasidone occur after approximately 1 hour, with a half-life of 2 to 5 hours.

Ziprasidone, similar to the other SDAs, blocks 5-HT_{2A} and D_2 receptors. It is also an antagonist of 5-HT_{1D}, 5-HT_{2C}, D_3, D_4, α_1, and H_1 receptors. It has very low affinity for D_1, M_1, and α_2 receptors. In addition, ziprasidone has agonist activity at the serotonin 5-HT_{1A} receptors and is an SSRI and a norepinephrine reuptake inhibitor. This is consistent with clinical reports that ziprasidone has antidepressant-like effects in nonschizophrenic patients.

Dosages. Ziprasidone is available in 20-, 40-, 60-, and 80-mg capsules. Ziprasidone for IM use comes as a single-use 20 mg/mL vial. Oral ziprasidone dosing should be initiated at 40 mg a day divided into two daily doses. Studies have shown efficacy in the range of 80 to 160 mg a day, divided twice daily. In clinical practice, doses as high as 240 mg a day are being used. The recommended IM dosage for 10 mg is 10 to 20 mg every 2 hours and 20 mg IM every 4 hours for the 20-mg dose. The maximum total daily dose of IM ziprasidone is 40 mg.

Other than interactions with other drugs that prolong the QTc complex, ziprasidone appears to have low potential for clinically significant drug interactions.

Side Effects. Somnolence, headache, dizziness, nausea, and lightheadedness are the most common adverse effects in patients taking ziprasidone. It has almost no significant effects outside the CNS, is associated with almost no weight gain, and does not cause sustained prolactin elevation. Concerns about prolongation of the QTc complex have deterred some clinicians from using ziprasidone as a first choice. The QTc interval has been shown to increase in patients treated with 40 and 120 mg per day. Ziprasidone is contraindicated in combination with other drugs known to prolong the QTc interval. These include, but are not limited to, dofetilide, sotalol, quinidine, other class IA and III antiarrhythmics, mesoridazine, thioridazine, chlorpromazine, droperidol, pimozide, sparfloxacin, gatifloxacin, moxifloxacin, halofantrine, mefloquine, pentamidine, arsenic trioxide, levomethadyl acetate, dolasetron mesylate, probucol, and tacrolimus. Ziprasidone should be avoided in patients with congenital long QT syndrome and in patients with a history of cardiac arrhythmias.

Aripiprazole (Abilify)

Aripiprazole is a potent 5-HT_{2A} antagonist and is indicated for the treatment of both schizophrenia and acute mania. It is also approved for augmentation of antidepressant agents in MDD. Aripiprazole is a D_2 antagonist, but can also act as a partial D_2 agonist. Partial D_2 agonists compete at D_2 receptors for endogenous dopamine, thereby producing a functional reduction of dopamine activity.

Indications. Aripiprazole is indicated for the treatment of schizophrenia. Short-term, 4- to 6-week studies comparing aripiprazole with haloperidol and risperidone in patients with schizophrenia and schizoaffective disorder have shown comparable efficacy. Dosages of 15, 20, and 30 mg a day were found to be effective. Long-term studies suggest that aripiprazole is effective as a maintenance treatment at a daily dose of 15 to 30 mg.

Aripiprazole is also indicated for the acute and maintenance treatment of manic and mixed episodes associated with bipolar I disorder. It is also used as an adjunctive therapy to either lithium or valproate for the acute treatment of manic and mixed episodes associated with bipolar I disorder.

Aripiprazole is indicated for use as an adjunctive therapy to antidepressants for the treatment of MDD. Aripiprazole is also indicated for the treatment of irritability associated with autistic disorder.

Pharmacology. Aripiprazole is well absorbed, reaching peak plasma concentrations after 3 to 5 hours. Absorption is not affected by food. The mean elimination half-life of aripiprazole is about 75 hours. It has a weakly active metabolite with a half-life of 96 hours. These relatively long half-lives make aripiprazole suitable for once-daily dosing. Clearance is reduced in elderly persons. Aripiprazole exhibits linear pharmacokinetics and is primarily metabolized by CYP3A4 and CYP2D6 enzymes. It is 99 percent protein bound. Aripiprazole is excreted in breast milk in lactating rats.

Mechanistically, aripiprazole acts as a modulator, rather than a blocker, and acts on both postsynaptic D_2 receptors and presynaptic autoreceptors. In theory, this mechanism addresses excessive limbic dopamine (hyperdopaminergic) activity, and decreased dopamine (hypodopaminergic) activity in frontal and prefrontal areas—abnormalities that are thought to be present in schizophrenia. The absence of complete D_2 blockade in the striatal areas would be expected to minimize EPS. Aripiprazole is an α_1-adrenergic receptor antagonist, which may cause some patients to experience orthostatic hypotension. Similar to the so-called atypical antipsychotic agents, aripiprazole is a 5-HT_{2A} antagonist.

Other Uses. A study of aggressive children and adolescents with oppositional defiant disorder or conduct disorder found that there was a positive response in about 60 percent of the subjects. In this study, vomiting and somnolence led to a reduction in initial aripiprazole dosage.

Drug Interactions. Whereas carbamazepine and valproate reduce serum concentrations, ketoconazole, fluoxetine, paroxetine, and quinidine increase aripiprazole serum concentrations. Lithium and valproic acid, two drugs likely to be combined with aripiprazole when treating bipolar disorder, do not affect the steady-state concentrations of aripiprazole. Combined use with antihypertensives may cause hypotension. Drugs that inhibit CYP2D6 activity reduce aripiprazole elimination.

Dosage and Clinical Guidelines. Aripiprazole is available as 5-, 10-, 15-, 20-, and 30-mg tablets. The effective dosage range is 10 to 30 mg per day. Although the starting dosage is 10 to 15 mg per day, problems with nausea, insomnia, and akathisia have led to use of lower than recommended starting dosages of aripiprazole. Many clinicians find that an initial dose of 5 mg increases tolerability.

Aripiprazole (Maintena) is a long-acting aripiprazole formulation injected at 4-week intervals. The recommended starting and maintenance dose of Aripiprazole (Maintena) is 400 mg monthly and should not be given earlier than 26 days after the previous injection. It is important to inform the patient that they must continue to take the oral aripiprazole (10 to 20 mg) for 14 days to achieve therapeutic levels of the injection. Clinicians should be aware of the requirement for dosage adjustments that are recommended in patients who are CYP2D6 poor metabolizers and in patients taking concomitant CYP3A4 inhibitors or CYP2D6 inhibitors for greater than 14 days. Patients requiring lower doses should receive in the range of 160 to 200 mg monthly.

Side Effects. The most commonly reported side effects of aripiprazole are headache, somnolence, agitation, dyspepsia, anxiety, and nausea. Although it is not a frequent cause of EPS, aripiprazole does cause akathisia-like activation. Described as restlessness or agitation, it can be highly distressing and often leads to discontinuation of medication. Insomnia is another common complaint. Data so far do not indicate that weight gain or diabetes mellitus have an increased incidence with aripiprazole (Abilify). Prolactin elevation does not typically occur. Aripiprazole does not cause significant QTc interval changes. There have been reports of seizures.

Asenapine (Saphris)

Indications. Asenapine is approved for the acute treatment of adults with schizophrenia and acute treatment of manic or mixed episodes associated with bipolar I disorder with or without psychotic features in adults.

Pharmacology. Asenapine has an affinity for several receptors, including serotonin (5-HT_{2A} and 5-HT_{2C}), noradrenergic (α_2 and α_1), dopaminergic (D_3 and D_4 receptors is higher than its affinity for D_2 receptors), and histamine (H_1). It has negligible affinity for muscarinic-1 cholinergic receptors and hence less incidence of dry mouth, blurred vision, constipation, and urinary retention. The bioavailability is 35 percent via sublingual (preferred) route and it achieves peak plasma concentration in 1 hour. Asenapine is metabolized through glucuronidation and oxidative metabolism by CYP1A2, so coadministration with fluvoxamine and other CYP1A2 inhibitors should be done cautiously.

Dosage. Asenapine is available as 5- and 10-mg sublingual tablets, and should be placed under the tongue. This is because the bioavailability of asenapine is less than 2 percent when swallowed, but is 35 percent when absorbed sublingually. The agent dissolves in saliva within seconds and is absorbed through the oral mucosa. Sublingual administration avoids first-pass hepatic metabolism. Patients should be advised to avoid drinking or eating for 10 minutes after taking asenapine because this may lower the blood levels. The recommended starting and target dose for schizophrenia is 5 mg twice a day. In bipolar disorder, the patient may be started on 10 mg twice a day, and if necessary, the dosage may be lowered to 5 mg twice a day depending on the tolerability issues. In acute schizophrenia treatment there is no evidence of added benefit with a 10 mg twice-daily dose, but there is a clear increase in certain adverse reactions. In both bipolar I disorder and schizophrenia, the maximum dose should not exceed 10 mg two times a day. The safety of doses above 10 mg twice a day has not been evaluated in clinical studies.

Side Effects. The most common side effects observed in schizophrenic and bipolar disorders are somnolence, dizziness, EPS other than akathisia, and increased weight. In clinical trials, the mean weight gain after 52 weeks is 0.9 kg, and there were no clinically relevant differences in lipid profile and blood glucose after 52 weeks. In clinical trials, asenapine was found to increase the QTc interval in a range of 2 to 5 milliseconds compared to placebo. No patients treated with asenapine experienced QTc increases 60 milliseconds or greater from baseline measurements, nor did any experience a QTc of 500 milliseconds or more. Nevertheless, asenapine should be avoided in combination with other drugs known to prolong QTc interval, in patients with congenital prolongation of QT interval or a history of cardiac arrhythmias, and in circumstances that may increase the occurrence of torsades de pointes. Asenapine can elevate prolactin levels, and the elevation can persist during chronic administration. Galactorrhea, amenorrhea, gynecomastia, and impotence may occur.

Clozapine (Clozaril)

Indications. In addition to being the most effective drug treatment for patients who have failed to respond to standard therapies, clozapine has been shown to benefit patients with severe tardive dyskinesia. Clozapine suppresses these dyskinesias, but the abnormal movements return when clozapine is discontinued. This is true even though clozapine, on rare occasions, may cause tardive dyskinesia. Other clinical situations in which clozapine may be used include the treatment of psychotic patients who are intolerant of EPS caused by other agents, treatment-resistant mania, severe psychotic depression, idiopathic Parkinson's disease, Huntington's disease, and suicidal patients with schizophrenia or schizoaffective disorder. Other treatment-resistant disorders that have demonstrated response to clozapine include pervasive developmental disorder, autism of childhood, and OCD (either alone or in combination with an SSRI). Used by itself, clozapine may very rarely induce obsessive-compulsive symptoms.

Pharmacology. Clozapine is a dibenzothiazepine. It is rapidly absorbed, with peak plasma levels reached in about 2 hours. Steady state is achieved in less than 1 week if twice daily dosing is used. The elimination half-life is about 12 hours. Clozapine has two major metabolites, one of which, N-dimethyl clozapine, may have some pharmacological activities. Clozapine is an antagonist of 5-HT_{2A}, D_1, D_3, D_4, and α (especially α_1) receptors. It has relatively low potency as a D_2 receptor antagonist. Data from PET scanning show that whereas 10 mg of haloperidol produces 80 percent occupancy of striatal D_2 receptors, clinically effective dosages of clozapine occupy only 40 to 50 percent of striatal D_2 receptors. This difference in D_2 receptor occupancy is probably why clozapine does not cause EPS. It has also been postulated that clozapine and other SDAs bind more loosely to the D_2 receptor, and because of this "fast dissociation," more normal dopamine neurotransmission is possible.

Dosages. Clozapine is available in 25- and 100-mg tablets. The initial dosage is usually 25 mg one or two times daily, although a conservative initial dosage is 12.5 mg twice daily. The dosage can then be increased gradually (25 mg a day every 2 or 3 days) to 300 mg a day in divided doses, usually two or three times a day. Dosages up to 900 mg a day can be used. Testing for blood concentrations of clozapine may be helpful in patients who fail to respond. Studies have found that plasma concentrations greater than 350 μg/mL are associated with a better likelihood of response.

Drug Interactions. Clozapine should not be used with any other drug that is associated with the development of agranulocytosis or bone marrow suppression. Such drugs include carbamazepine, phenytoin, propylthiouracil, sulfonamides, and captopril (Capoten). Lithium combined with clozapine may increase the risk of seizures, confusion, and movement disorders. Lithium should not be used in combination with clozapine by persons who have experienced an episode of neuroleptic malignant syndrome. Clomipramine (Anafranil) can increase the risk of seizure by lowering the seizure threshold and by increasing clozapine plasma concentrations. Risperidone, fluoxetine, paroxetine, and fluvoxamine increase serum concentrations of clozapine. Addition of paroxetine may precipitate clozapine-associated neutropenia.

Side Effects. The most common drug-related adverse effects are sedation, dizziness, syncope, tachycardia, hypotension, ECG changes, nausea, and vomiting. Other common adverse effects include fatigue, weight gain, various GI symptoms (most commonly constipation), anticholinergic effects, and subjective muscle weakness. Sialorrhea, or hypersalivation, is a side effect that begins early in treatment and is most evident at night. Patients report that their pillows are drenched with saliva. This side effect is most likely the result of impairment of swallowing. Although there are reports that clonidine or amitriptyline may help reduce hypersalivation, the most practical solution is to put a towel over the pillow.

The risk of seizures is about 4 percent in patients taking dosages greater than 600 mg a day. Leukopenia, granulocytopenia, agranulocytosis, and fever occur in about 1 percent of patients. During the first year of treatment, there is a 0.73 percent risk of clozapine-induced agranulocytosis. The risk during the second year is 0.07 percent. For neutropenia, the risk is 2.32 percent and 0.69 percent, respectively, during the first and second years of treatment. The only contraindications to the use of clozapine are a WBC count below 3,500 cells per mm^3; a previous bone marrow disorder; a history of agranulocytosis during clozapine treatment; or the use of another drug that is known to suppress the bone marrow, such as carbamazepine (Tegretol).

Clozapine Risk Evaluation and Mitigation Strategy (REMS). In 2015 FDA announced new requirements for the monitoring, prescribing, and dispensing of clozapine. This requirement led to the new clozapine REMS program with revised prescribing information and will replace the six existing clozapine registries. This will also centralize all the information and have patients, clinicians, and pharmacies enroll in one place.

The REMS program establishes that patients will be monitored for neutropenia using the ANC and WBC will no longer be acceptable. Furthermore the ANC threshold has been lowered so more patients will be able to continue taking the drug.

Patient's treatment will be interrupted if the ANC drops below 1,000 cells/μL with special consideration to patients with African American origin who are more susceptible to develop benign ethnic neutropenia (BEN). These patients treatment will be stopped if the ANC drops below 500 cells/ul. These changes allow clinicians to prescribe clozapine to patients who were previously ineligible to receive the medicine as well as continue treatment for a greater number of patients.

During the first 6 months of treatment, weekly ANC counts are indicated to monitor the patient for the development of agranulocytosis. If the ANC count remains normal, the frequency of testing can be decreased to every 2 weeks. Although monitoring is expensive, early indication of agranulocytosis can prevent a fatal outcome. Clozapine should be discontinued if the ANC count is below 1,000 cells per mm^3 or in case of BEN falls below 500 cells/ul. In addition, a hematological consultation should be obtained, and obtaining bone marrow sample should be considered. FDA further stated, "Patients with agranulocytosis could be rechallenged if the prescriber determines the risk of psychiatric illness is greater than the risk of neutropenia." To avoid situations in which a physician or a patient fails to comply with the required blood tests, clozapine cannot be dispensed without proof of monitoring.

Patients exhibiting symptoms of chest pain, shortness of breath, fever, or tachypnea should be immediately evaluated for myocarditis or cardiomyopathy, an infrequent but serious adverse effect ending in death. Serial CPK-MB (creatine phosphokinase with myocardial band fractions), troponin levels, and EKG studies are recommended, with immediate discontinuation of clozapine.

Iloperidone (Fanapt)

Indications. Iloperidone (Fanapt) is indicated for the acute treatment of schizophrenia in adults. The safety and efficacy of iloperidone in children and adolescents has not been established.

Pharmacology. Iloperidone is not a derivative of another antipsychotic agent. It has complex multiple antagonist effects on several neurotransmitter systems. Iloperidone has a strong affinity for dopamine D_3 receptors, followed by decreasing affinities of α_{2c}-noradrenergic, 5-HT_{1a}, D_{2a}, and 5-HT_6 receptors. Iloperidone has a low affinity for histaminergic receptors. As with other antipsychotics, the clinical significance of this receptor binding affinity is unknown.

Iloperidone has a peak concentration of 2 to 4 hours and a half-life that is dependent on hepatic isoenzyme metabolism. It is metabolized primarily through CYP2D6 and CYP3A4, and the dosage should be reduced by half when administered concomitantly with strong inhibitors of these two isoenzymes. The half-life is 18 to 26 hours in CYP2D6 extensive metabolizers and is 31 to 37 hours in CYP2D6 poor metabolizers. Of note, approximately 7 to 10 percent of whites and 3 to 8 percent of African Americans lack the capacity to metabolize CYP2D6 substrates; hence, dosing should be determined with this caveat in mind. Iloperidone should be used with caution in persons with severe hepatic impairment.

Side Effects. Iloperidone prolongs the QT interval and may be associated with arrhythmia and sudden death. Iloperidone prolongs the QTc interval by 9 milliseconds at dosages of 12 mg twice daily. Concurrent use with other agents that prolong the QTc interval may result in additive effects on the QTc interval. The concurrent use of iloperidone with agents that prolong the QTc interval may result in potentially life-threatening cardiac arrhythmias, including torsades de pointes. Concurrent administration of other drugs that are known to prolong the QTc interval should be avoided. Cardiovascular disease, hypokalemia, hypomagnesemia, bradycardia, congenital prolongation of the QT interval, and concurrent use of inhibitors of CYP3A4 or CYP2D6, which metabolize iloperidone, may increase the risk of QT prolongation.

The most common adverse effects reported are dizziness, dry mouth, fatigue, sedation, tachycardia, and orthostatic hypotension (depending on dosing and titration). Despite being a strong D_2 antagonist, the rates of EPS and akathisia are similar to those of placebo. The mean weight gain in short- and long-term trials is 2.1 kg. Due to its relatively limited use, there is no accurate understanding of iloperidone's effects on weight and lipids. Some patients exhibit elevated prolactin levels. Three cases of priapism have been reported in the premarketing phase.

Dosing. Iloperidone must be titrated slowly to avoid orthostatic hypotension. It is available in a titration pack, and the effective dose (12 mg) should be reached in approximately 4 days based on a twice-a-day dosing schedule. It is usually started on day 1 at 1 mg twice a day and increased daily on a twice-a-day schedule to reach 12 mg by day 4. The maximum recommended dose is 12 mg twice a day (24 mg a day), and it can be administered without regard to food.

Lurasidone HCl (Latuda)

Indications. Lurasidone hydrochloride is an oral, once-daily atypical antipsychotic indicated for the treatment of patients with schizophrenia and depressive episodes associated with bipolar I disorder.

Side Effects. The most commonly observed adverse reactions associated with the use of lurasidone are similar to those seen with other new-generation antipsychotics. These include, but are not limited to somnolence, akathisia, nausea, parkinsonism, and agitation. Based on clinical trial data, lurasidone appears to cause less weight gain and metabolic changes than the two other most recently approved SDAs, asenapine and iloperidone. More extensive clinical experience with the drug is required to determine whether this is in fact the case.

Drug Interactions. When coadministration of lurasidone with a moderate CYP3A4 inhibitor such as diltiazem is considered, the dose should not exceed 40 mg per day. Lurasidone should not be used in combination with a strong CYP3A4 inhibitor (e.g., ketoconazole). Lurasidone also should not be used in combination with a strong CYP3A4 inducer (e.g., rifampin), or grapefruit juice.

Dosages. Lurasidone is available as 20-, 40-, 80-, and 120-mg tablets. For treatment of schizophrenia the initial dose titration is not required. The recommended starting dose is 40 mg once daily, and the medication should be taken with food (at least 350 calories). It has been shown to be effective in a dose range of 40 to 120 mg per day. Although there is no proven added benefit with the 120 mg per day dose, there may be a dose-related increase in adverse reactions. Still, some patients may benefit from the maximum recommended dose of 160 mg per day. Dose adjustment is recommended in patients with renal impairment. The dose in moderate to severe renal impairment should not exceed 80 mg per day. The dose in severe hepatic impairment patients should not exceed 40 mg per day. In bipolar depression the recommended starting dose is 20 mg once daily as monotherapy or as an adjunctive to lithium or valproate. The maximum recommended dose is 120 mg though no additional benefit has been seen with doses higher than 60 mg.

Brexpiprazole (Rexulti)

Brexpiprazole is a new second-generation ("atypical") antipsychotic approved by the FDA in July 2015 for the treatment of schizophrenia and as an add-on treatment to an antidepressant medication to treat adults with MDD.

Pharmacology. It is a partial agonist at 5-HT_{1a}, D_2, and D_3 receptors and an antagonist at 5-HT_{2A}, 5-HT_{2B}, 5-HT_7, α1A, α1B, α1D, and α2C receptors. Though similar in profile to aripiprazole there are a few differences in pharmacological activity between brexpiprazole and aripiprazole. It has lower intrinsic activity for partial agonism at D_2 receptors and less likely to cause akathisia, restlessness, insomnia and nausea. At the same time considering the fact that it has intrinsic activity at the D_2 receptor it is more likely to cause extra pyramidal symptoms (EPS) and prolactin elevation.

Brexpiprazole reaches peaches peak plasma concentration in 4 hours and steady-state concentration in 1 to 12 days. It is highly protein bound >99 percent with a half-life of 91 hours and is metabolized primarily by CYP2D6 and CYP3A4.

Indications. Brexpiprazole is approved for the treatment of schizophrenia and adjunctive treatment of MDD.

Side effects. The most common side effects include akathisia (dose related), increased serum triglycerides, weight gain, headache, drowsiness, and EPS.

Drug Interactions. Concomitant use of medications that are moderate to strong inhibitors of CYP2D6 and CYP3A4 require that dosage of brexpiprazole be reduced by 25 to 50 percent. Clinicians should consult drug interaction checker for an exhaustive list to prevent toxicity and adverse reactions.

Dosage

SCHIZOPHRENIA. Initial starting dose of 1 mg daily from day1 to 4 and dose can be adjusted gradually based on response and tolerability to 2 mg daily for 3 days followed by 4 mg on day 8 with a maximum dose of 4 mg.

MAJOR DEPRESSIVE DISORDER. Initial starting dose is lower, 0.5 mg or 1 mg once daily and then adjust at weekly intervals based on response and tolerability to 1 mg once daily, followed by 2 mg once daily with a maximum daily dose of 3 mg.

Cariprazine (Vraylar)

Cariprazine is the newest atypical antipsychotic approved by the FDA in September 2015 for the treatment of schizophrenia and bipolar I disorder.

Pharmacology. Cariprazine is a partial agonist with high binding affinity at the dopamine D_3 and D_2 receptors and serotonin 5-HT_{1A} receptors. It acts as an antagonist at 5-HT_{2B} and 5-HT_{2A} receptors and also binds to the histamine H_1 receptors. It shows lower binding affinity to the serotonin 5-HT_{2C} and α1A-adrenergic receptors and has no appreciable affinity for cholinergic muscarinic receptors. Though the exact mechanism of action in schizophrenia and bipolar I disorder is unknown, cariprazine mediates its effect through a combination of partial agonist activity at central dopamine D_2 and serotonin 5-HT_{1A} receptors and antagonist activity at serotonin 5-HT_{2A} receptors. The two major metabolites of cariprazine include desmethyl cariprazine (DCAR) and didesmethyl cariprazine (DDCAR). The half-life of cariprazine is 2 to 4 days and increases to 103 weeks for its metabolite. Cariprazine is highly protein bound and is extensively metabolized by CYP3A4 and, to a lesser extent, by CYP2D6. It does not induce any P450 enzymes and has minimal inhibitory activity.

Indications. Cariprazine is an atypical antipsychotic approved by the FDA in September 2015 for the treatment of schizophrenia and acute manic or mixed episodes associated with bipolar I disorder.

Its safety and effectiveness in pediatric patients has not been established.

Side Effects. The most commonly observed adverse reactions associated with the use of cariprazine include extrapyramidal symptoms, akathisia, dyspepsia, vomiting, somnolence, insomnia, agitation, anxiety, and restlessness. Like other SDA's metabolic monitoring is required and long-term open label studies show 4 percent of patients with normal HgA1c developed elevated HgA1c above 6.5 and 8 percent of patients had a 7 percent weight increase or greater.

Drug Interactions. Clinicians should be aware of CYP3A4 enzyme inhibition and make dosage adjustments especially when coadministered strong 3A4 inhibitor.

DOSAGE. Cariprazine is available as a 1.5-, 3-, 4.5-, and 6-mg capsule and is given once daily orally with or without food. The usual starting dosage in schizophrenia and bipolar I disorder is 1.5 mg and can be increased to 3 mg on day 2. Further dose adjustments should be made based on response and tolerability in 1.5 or 3 mg increments up to a maximum dose of 6 mg. In patients with concomitant 3A4 inhibitor, dose should be reduced by half to one-third of the prescribed dosage.

Clinical Guidelines for SDAs

All SDAs are appropriate for the management of an initial psychotic episode, but clozapine is reserved for persons who are refractory to all other antipsychotic drugs. If a person does not respond to the first SDA, other SDAs should be tried. The choice of drug should be based on the patient's clinical status and history of response to medication. Recent studies have challenged the notion that SDAs require 4 to 6 weeks to reach full effectiveness, and it may take up to 8 weeks for the full clinical effects of an SDA to become apparent. The newer meta-analyses suggest that the apparent benefits may be seen as early as 2 to 3 weeks, and early response or failure is an indicator of subsequent response or failure. Nevertheless, it is acceptable practice to augment an SDA with a high-potency DRA or benzodiazepine in the first few weeks of use. Lorazepam (Ativan) 1 to 2 mg orally or IM can be used as needed for acute agitation. Once effective, dosages can be lowered as tolerated. Clinical improvement may take 6 months of treatment with SDAs in some particularly treatment-refractory persons.

Use of all SDAs must be initiated at low dosages and gradually tapered upward to therapeutic dosages. The gradual increase in dosage is necessitated by the potential development of adverse effects. If a person stops taking an SDA for more than 36 hours, drug use should be resumed at the initial titration schedule. After the decision to terminate olanzapine or clozapine use, dosages should be tapered whenever possible to avoid cholinergic rebound symptoms such as diaphoresis, flushing, diarrhea, and hyperactivity.

After a clinician has determined that a trial of an SDA is warranted for a particular person, the risks and benefits of SDA treatment must be explained to the person and the family. In the case of clozapine, an informed consent procedure should be documented in the person's chart. The patient's history should include information about blood disorders, epilepsy, cardiovascular disease, hepatic and renal diseases, and drug abuse. The presence of a hepatic or renal disease necessitates using low starting dosages of the drug. The physical examination should include supine and standing BP measurements to screen for orthostatic hypotension. The laboratory examination should include an ECG and several CBCs with WBC counts, which can then be averaged; and liver and renal function tests. Periodic monitoring of blood glucose, lipids, and body weight is recommended.

Although the transition from a DRA to an SDA may be made abruptly, it is wiser to taper off the DRA slowly while titrating up the SDA. Clozapine and olanzapine both have anticholinergic effects, and the transition from one to the other can usually be accomplished with little risk of cholinergic rebound. The transition from risperidone to olanzapine is best accomplished by tapering the risperidone off over 3 weeks while simultaneously beginning olanzapine at 10 mg a day. Risperidone, quetiapine, and ziprasidone lack anticholinergic effects, and the abrupt transition from a DRA, olanzapine, or clozapine to one of these agents may cause cholinergic rebound, which consists of excessive salivation, nausea, vomiting, and diarrhea. The risk of cholinergic rebound can be mitigated by initially augmenting risperidone, quetiapine, or ziprasidone with an anticholinergic drug, which is then tapered off slowly. Any initiation and termination of SDA use should be accomplished gradually.

It is wise to overlap administration of the new drug with the old drug. Of interest, some people have a more robust clinical response while taking the two agents during the transition and then regressing on monotherapy with the newer drug. Little is known about the effectiveness and safety of a strategy of combining one SDA with another SDA or with a DRA.

Persons receiving regular injections of depot formulations of a DRA who are to switch to SDA use are given the first dose of the SDA on the day the next injection is due.

Persons who developed agranulocytosis while taking clozapine can safely switch to olanzapine use, although initiation of olanzapine use in the midst of clozapine-induced agranulocytosis can prolong the time of recovery from the usual 3 to 4 days up to 11 to 12 days. It is prudent to wait for resolution of agranulocytosis before initiating olanzapine use. Emergence or recurrence of agranulocytosis has not been reported with olanzapine, even in persons who developed it while taking clozapine.

SDA use by pregnant women has not been studied, but consideration should be given to the potential of risperidone to raise prolactin concentrations, sometimes up to three to four times the upper limit of the normal range. Because the drugs can be excreted in breast milk, they should not be taken by nursing mothers. The dosages for selected SDAs are given in Table 25–51.

STIMULANT DRUGS AND ATOMOXETINE

Stimulant drugs increase motivation, mood, energy, focus, attention and wakefulness. They are also called sympathomimetics, because they mimic the physiological effects of the neurotransmitter epinephrine. Several chemical classes are included in this group.

Currently these drugs are most commonly used to treat symptoms of poor concentration and hyperactivity in children and adults with ADHD. Paradoxically, many patients with ADHD find that these drugs can have a calming effect. Sympathomimetics are also approved for use in increasing alertness in narcolepsy.

Amphetamines were the first stimulants to be synthesized. They were created in the late 19th century and were used by Bavarian soldiers in the mid-1880s to maintain wakefulness, alertness, energy, and confidence in combat. They have been used in a similar fashion in most wars since then. They were not widely used clinically until the 1930s, when they were marketed as Benzedrine inhalers for relief of nasal congestion. When their psychostimulant effects were noted, these drugs were used to treat sleepiness associated with narcolepsy. They have been classified as controlled drugs because of their rapid onset, immediate behavioral effects, and propensity to develop tolerance, which leads to the risk of abuse and dependence in vulnerable individuals. Their manufacture, distribution, and use are regulated by state and federal agencies. In 2005, pemoline was withdrawn from the market because of significant risks of treatment-emergent hepatotoxicity.

Sympathomimetics have been widely used in persons with ADHD and narcolepsy because no equally effective agents have been available. They have also been found effective in treating certain cognitive disorders that result in secondary depression or profound apathy (e.g., AIDS, multiple sclerosis, poststroke depression and dementia, closed head injury) as well as in the augmentation of antidepressant medications in specific treatment-resistant depressions.

Atomoxetine is included in this section because it is used to treat ADHD, even though it is not a psychostimulant.

Pharmacological Actions

All of these drugs are well absorbed from the GI tract. Amphetamine (Adderall) and dextroamphetamine (Dexedrine, Dextrostat) reach peak plasma concentrations in 2 to 3 hours and have a half-life of about 6 hours, thereby necessitating once- or twice-daily dosing. Methylphenidate is available in immediate-release (Ritalin), sustained-release (Ritalin SR), and extended-release (Concerta, Quillivant XR) formulations. Immediate-release methylphenidate reaches peak plasma concentrations in 1 to 2 hours and has a short half-life of 2 to 3 hours, thereby necessitating multiple-daily dosing. The sustained-release formulation reaches peak plasma concentrations in 4 to 5 hours and doubles the effective half-life of methylphenidate. The extended-release formulation reaches peak plasma concentrations in 6 to 8 hours and is designed to be effective for 12 hours in once-daily dosing. Dexmethylphenidate (Focalin) reaches peak plasma concentration in about 3 hours and is prescribed twice daily.

Lisdexamfetamine dimesylate, also known as L-lysine-D-amphetamine (Vyvanse), is an amphetamine prodrug. In this formulation, dextroamphetamine is coupled with the amino acid L-lysine. Lisdexamfetamine becomes active upon cleavage of the lysine portion of the molecule by enzymes in the red blood cells. This results in the gradual release of dextroamphetamine into the bloodstream. Apart from having an extended duration of action, this type of formulation reduces its abuse potential. It is the only prodrug of its kind. Lisdexamfetamine is indicated for the treatment of ADHD in children 6 to 12 years and in adults as an integral part of a total treatment program that may include other measures (i.e., psychological, educational, social). The safety and efficacy of lisdexamfetamine dimesylate in patients 3 to 5 years old has not been established. In contrast to Adderall, which contains approximately 75 percent dextroamphetamine and 25 percent levoamphetamine, lisdexamfetamine is a single, dextro-enantiomer amphetamine molecule. In most cases this makes the drug better tolerated, but there are some patients who experience greater benefit from the mixed isomer preparation.

Methylphenidate, dextroamphetamine, and amphetamine are indirectly acting sympathomimetics, with the primary effect causing the release of catecholamines from presynaptic neurons. Their clinical effectiveness is associated with increased release of both dopamine and norepinephrine. Dextroamphetamine and methylphenidate are also weak inhibitors of catecholamine reuptake and inhibitors of monoamine oxidase.

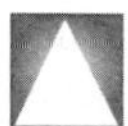

Table 25–51
Comparison of Usual Dosing[a] for Some Available Second-Generation Antipsychotics in Schizophrenia

Antipsychotic	Typical Starting Dosage	Maintenance Therapy Dose Range	Titration	Maximum Recommended Dosage
Aripiprazole (Abilify)	10–15-mg tablets once a day	10–30 mg/day	Dosage increases should not be made before 2 wks	30 mg/day
Asenapine (Saphris)	5 mg twice a day	10 mg twice a day	Titration not necessary	20 mg/day
Clozapine (Clozaril)	12.5-mg tablets once or twice a day	150–300 mg/day in divided doses or 200 mg as a single dose in the evening	The dosage should be increased to 25–50 mg on the second day. Further increases may be made in daily increments of 25–50 mg to a target dosage of 300–450 mg/day. Subsequent dosage increases should be made no more than once or twice weekly in increments of no more than 100 mg.	900 mg/day
Iloperidone (Fanapt)	1 mg twice a day	12–24 mg a day in divided dose	Start at 1 mg twice a day than move to 2, 4, 6, 8 and 12 mg twice a day. Do this over the course of 7 days	24 mg/day
Lurasidone (Latuda)	40 mg/day	40–80 mg/day	Titration not necessary	120 mg/day
Olanzapine (Zyprexa)	5–10-mg/day tablets or orally disintegrating tablets	10–20 mg/day	Dosage increments of 5 mg once a day are recommended when required at intervals of not less than 1 wk.	20 mg/day
Paliperidone (Invega)	3–9-mg extended-release tablets once a day	3–6 mg/day	Plasma concentration rises to a peak approximately 24 hrs after dosing	12 mg/day
Quetiapine (Seroquel)	25-mg tablets twice a day	Lowest dose needed to maintain remission	Increase in increments of 25–50 mg two or three times a day on the second and the third day, as tolerated, to a target dosage of 500 mg daily by the fourth day (given in two or three doses/day). Further dosage adjustments, if required, should be of 25–50 mg twice a day and occur at intervals of not fewer than 2 days.	800 mg/day
Risperidone (Risperdal)	1-mg tablet and oral solution once a day	2–6 mg once a day	Starting dose: 25 mg every 2 wks	50 mg for 2 wks
Risperidone IM long-acting (Consta)	25–50 mg IM injection every 2 wks	Start with oral risperidone for 3 wks	Increase to 2 mg once a day on the second day and 4 mg once a day on the third day. In some patients, a slower titration may be appropriate. When dosage adjustments are necessary, further dosage increments of 1–2 mg/day at intervals of not less than 1 wk are recommended.	1–6 mg/day
Ziprasidone (Geodon)	20-mg capsules twice a day with food	20–80 mg twice a day	Dosage adjustments based on individual clinical status may be made at intervals of not fewer than 2 days.	80 mg twice a day
Ziprasidone (IM)	For acute agitation: 10–20 mg, as required, up to a maximum of 40 mg/day	Not applicable	For acute agitation: Doses of 10 mg may be administered every 2 hours, and doses of 20 mg may be administered every 4 hours up to a maximum of 40 mg/day.	For acute agitation: 40 mg/day, for not more than 3 consecutive days

Note: Information taken from U.S. Prescribing Information for individual agents.
[a]Dosage adjustments may be required in special populations.
IM, intramuscular.

For modafinil, the specific mechanism of action is unknown. Narcolepsy–cataplexy results from deficiency of hypocretin, a hypothalamic neuropeptide. Hypocretin-producing neurons are activated after modafinil administration. Modafinil does not appear to work through a dopaminergic mechanism. It does have α_1-adrenergic agonist properties, which may account for its alerting effects, because the wakefulness induced by modafinil can be attenuated by prazosin, an α_1-adrenergic antagonist. Some evidence suggests that modafinil has some norepinephrine reuptake blocking effects. Armodafinil (Nuvigil) is the R-enantiomer of modafinil. Both drugs have similar clinical effects and side effects.

Therapeutic Indications

Attention-Deficit/Hyperactivity Disorder. Sympathomimetics are the first-line drugs for treatment of ADHD in children and are effective about 75 percent of the time. Methylphenidate and dextroamphetamine are equally effective and work within 15 to 30 minutes. Pemoline (Cylert) requires 3 to

4 weeks to reach its full efficacy; however, because of toxicity, it is rarely used. Sympathomimetic drugs decrease hyperactivity, increase attentiveness, and reduce impulsivity. They may also reduce comorbid oppositional behaviors associated with ADHD. Many persons take these drugs throughout their schooling and beyond. In responsive persons, use of a sympathomimetic may be a critical determinant of scholastic success.

Sympathomimetics improve the core ADHD symptoms of hyperactivity, impulsivity, and inattentiveness and permit improved social interactions with teachers, family, other adults, and peers. The success of long-term treatment of ADHD with sympathomimetics, which are efficacious for most of the various constellations of ADHD symptoms present from childhood to adulthood, supports a model in which ADHD results from a genetically determined neurochemical imbalance that requires lifelong pharmacologic management.

Methylphenidate is the most commonly used initial agent, at a dosage of 5 to 10 mg every 3 to 4 hours. Dosages may be increased to a maximum of 20 mg four times daily or 1 mg/kg a day. Use of the 20-mg sustained-release formulation to achieve 6 hours of benefit and eliminate the need for dosing at school is supported by many experts, although other authorities believe it is less effective than the immediate-release formulation. Dextroamphetamine is about twice as potent as methylphenidate on a per milligram basis and provides 6 to 8 hours of benefit. Some 70 percent of nonresponders to one sympathomimetic may benefit from another. All of the sympathomimetic drugs should be tried before switching to drugs of a different class. The previous dictum that sympathomimetics worsen tics and therefore should be avoided by persons with comorbid ADHD and tic disorders has been questioned. Small dosages of sympathomimetics do not appear to cause an increase in the frequency and severity of tics. Alternatives to sympathomimetics for ADHD include bupropion (Wellbutrin), venlafaxine (Effexor), guanfacine (Tenex), clonidine (Catapres), and tricyclic drugs. Further studies are needed to determine whether modafinil improves the symptoms of ADHD.

Short-term use of the sympathomimetics induces a euphoric feeling; however, tolerance develops for both the euphoric feeling and the sympathomimetic activity.

Narcolepsy and Hypersomnolence. Narcolepsy consists of sudden sleep attacks (*narcolepsy*), sudden loss of postural tone (*cataplexy*), loss of voluntary motor control going into (hypnagogic) or coming out of (hypnopompic) sleep (*sleep paralysis*), and hypnagogic or hypnopompic *hallucinations*. Sympathomimetics reduce narcoleptic sleep attacks and improve wakefulness in other types of hypersomnolent states. Modafinil is approved as an antisomnolence agent for the treatment of narcolepsy, for people who cannot adjust to night shift work, and for those who do not sleep well because of obstructive sleep apnea.

Other sympathomimetics are also used to maintain wakefulness and accuracy of motor performance in persons subject to sleep deprivation, such as pilots and military personnel. Persons with narcolepsy, unlike persons with ADHD, may develop tolerance for the therapeutic effects of the sympathomimetics.

In direct comparison with amphetamine-like drugs, modafinil is equally effective at maintaining wakefulness, with a lower risk of excessive activation.

Depressive Disorders. Sympathomimetics may be used for treatment-resistant depressive disorders, usually as augmentation of standard antidepressant drug therapy. Possible indications for use of sympathomimetics as monotherapy include depression in elderly persons, who are at increased risk for adverse effects from standard antidepressant drugs; depression in medically ill persons, especially persons with AIDS; obtundation caused by chronic use of opioids; and clinical situations in which a rapid response is important but for which ECT is contraindicated. Depressed patients with abulia and anergia may also benefit.

Dextroamphetamine may be useful in differentiating pseudodementia of depression from dementia. A depressed person generally responds to a 5-mg dose with increased alertness and improved cognition. Sympathomimetics are thought to provide only short-term benefit (2 to 4 weeks) for depression, because most persons rapidly develop tolerance for the antidepressant effects of the drugs. However, some clinicians report that long-term treatment with sympathomimetics can benefit some persons.

Encephalopathy Caused by Brain Injury. Sympathomimetics increase alertness, cognition, motivation, and motor performance in persons with neurological deficits caused by strokes, trauma, tumors, or chronic infections. Treatment with sympathomimetics may permit earlier and more robust participation in rehabilitative programs. Poststroke lethargy and apathy may respond to long-term use of sympathomimetics.

Obesity. Sympathomimetics are used in the treatment of obesity because of their anorexia-inducing effects. Because tolerance develops for the anorectic effects and because of the drugs' high abuse potential, their use for this indication is limited. Of the sympathomimetic drugs, phentermine (Adipex-P, Fastin) is the most widely used for appetite suppression. Phentermine was the second half of "fen-phen," an off-label combination of fenfluramine and phentermine, widely used to promote weight loss until fenfluramine and dexfenfluramine were withdrawn from commercial availability because of an association with cardiac valvular insufficiency, primary pulmonary hypertension, and irreversible loss of cerebral serotonergic nerve fibers. The toxicity of fenfluramine is attributed to the fact that it stimulates release of massive amounts of serotonin from nerve endings, a mechanism of action not shared by phentermine. Use of phentermine alone has not been reported to cause the same adverse effects as those caused by fenfluramine or dexfenfluramine.

Careful limitation of caloric intake and judicious exercise are at the core of any successful weight loss program. Sympathomimetic drugs facilitate loss of, at most, an additional fraction of a pound per week. Sympathomimetic drugs are effective appetite suppressants only for the first few weeks of use; then the anorexigenic effects tend to decrease.

Fatigue. Between 70 and 90 percent of individuals with multiple sclerosis experience fatigue. Modafinil, armodafinil, amphetamines, methylphenidate, and the dopamine receptor agonist amantadine (Symmetrel) are sometimes effective in combating this symptom. Other causes of fatigue such as chronic fatigue syndrome respond to stimulants in many cases.

Precautions and Adverse Reactions

The most common adverse effects associated with amphetamine-like drugs are stomach pain, anxiety, irritability, insomnia, tachycardia, cardiac arrhythmias, and dysphoria. Sympathomimetics cause a decreased appetite, although tolerance usually develops for this effect. The treatment of common adverse effects in children with ADHD is usually straightforward (Table 25–52). The drugs can also cause increases in heart rate and BP and may cause palpitations. Less common adverse effects include the possible induction of movement disorders, such as tics, Tourette's disorder–like symptoms, and dyskinesias, all of which are often self-limited over 7 to 10 days. If a person taking a sympathomimetic develops one of these movement disorders, a correlation between the dose of the medication and the severity of the disorder must be firmly established before adjustments are made in the medication dosage. In severe cases, augmentation with risperidone (Risperdal), clonidine (Catapres), or guanfacine (Tenex) is necessary. Methylphenidate may worsen tics in one-third of persons; these persons fall into two groups: those whose methylphenidate-induced tics resolve immediately upon metabolism of the dosage and a smaller group in whom methylphenidate appears to trigger tics that persist for several months but eventually resolve spontaneously.

Table 25–52
Management of Common Stimulant-Induced Adverse Effects in Attention-Deficit/Hyperactivity Disorder

Adverse Effect	Management
Anorexia, nausea, weight loss	▲ Administer stimulant with meals. ▲ Use caloric-enhanced supplements. Discourage forcing meals.
Insomnia, nightmares	▲ Administer stimulants earlier in day. ▲ Change to short-acting preparations. ▲ Discontinue afternoon or evening dosing. ▲ Consider adjunctive treatment (e.g., antihistamines, clonidine, antidepressants).
Dizziness	▲ Monitor BP. ▲ Encourage fluid intake. ▲ Change to long-acting form.
Rebound phenomena	▲ Overlap stimulant dosing. ▲ Change to long-acting preparation or combine long- and short-acting preparations. ▲ Consider adjunctive or alternative treatment (e.g., clonidine, antidepressants).
Irritability	▲ Assess timing of phenomena (during peak or withdrawal phase). ▲ Evaluate comorbid symptoms. ▲ Reduce dose. ▲ Consider adjunctive or alternative treatment (e.g., lithium, antidepressants, anticonvulsants).
Dysphoria, moodiness, agitation	▲ Consider comorbid diagnosis (e.g., mood disorder). ▲ Reduce dosage or change to long-acting preparation. ▲ Consider adjunctive or alternative treatment (e.g., lithium, anticonvulsants, antidepressants).

BP, blood pressure.
From Wilens TE, Blederman J. The stimulants. In: Shaffer D, ed. *The Psychiatric Clinics of North America: Pediatric Psychopharmacology*. Philadelphia, PA: Saunders; 1992, with permission.

Longitudinal studies do not indicate that sympathomimetics cause growth suppression. Sympathomimetics may exacerbate glaucoma, hypertension, cardiovascular disorders, hyperthyroidism, anxiety disorders, psychotic disorders, and seizure disorders.

High dosages of sympathomimetics can cause dry mouth, pupillary dilation, bruxism, formication, excessive ebullience, restlessness, emotional lability, and occasionally seizures. Long-term use of high dosages can cause a delusional disorder that resembles paranoid schizophrenia. Seizures can be treated with benzodiazepines, cardiac effects with β-adrenergic receptor antagonists, fever with cooling blankets, and delirium with DRAs. Overdosages of sympathomimetics result in hypertension, tachycardia, hyperthermia, toxic psychosis, delirium, hyperpyrexia, convulsions, coma, chest pain, arrhythmia, heart block, hypertension or hypotension, shock, and nausea. Toxic effects of amphetamines can be seen at 30 mg, but idiosyncratic toxicity can occur at doses as low as 2 mg. Conversely, survival has been reported up to 500 mg.

The most limiting adverse effect of sympathomimetics is their association with psychological and physical dependence. At the doses used for treatment of ADHD, development of psychological dependence virtually never occurs. A larger concern is the presence of adolescent or adult cohabitants who might confiscate the supply of sympathomimetics for abuse or sale.

The use of sympathomimetics should be avoided during pregnancy, especially during the first trimester. Dextroamphetamine and methylphenidate pass into the breast milk, and it is not known whether modafinil or armodafinil do.

Drug Interactions

The coadministration of sympathomimetics and tricyclic or tetracyclic antidepressants, warfarin (Coumadin), primidone (Mysoline), phenobarbital (Luminal), phenytoin (Dilantin), or phenylbutazone (Butazolidin) decreases the metabolism of these compounds, resulting in increased plasma levels. Sympathomimetics decrease the therapeutic efficacy of many antihypertensive drugs, especially guanethidine (Esimil, Ismelin). The sympathomimetics should be used with extreme caution with MAOIs.

Laboratory Interferences

Dextroamphetamine may elevate plasma corticosteroid levels and interfere with some assay methods for urinary corticosteroids.

Dosage and Administration

Many psychiatrists believe that amphetamine use has been overly regulated by governmental authorities. Amphetamines are listed as schedule II drugs by the Drug Enforcement Agency. Some states keep a registry of patients who receive amphetamines. Such mandates worry both patients and physicians about breaches in confidentiality, and physicians are concerned that their prescribing practices may be misinterpreted by official agencies. Consequently, some physicians may withhold

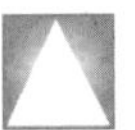

Table 25–53
Sympathomimetics Commonly Used in Psychiatry

Generic Name	Trade Name	Preparations	Initial Daily Dose	Usual Daily Dose for ADHD[a]	Usual Daily Dose for Disorders Associated with Excessive Daytime Somnolence	Maximum Daily Dose
Amphetamine–dextroamphetamine	Adderall	5-, 10-, 20-, and 30-mg tablets	5–10 mg	20–30 mg	5–60 mg	Children: 40 mg Adults: 60 mg
Armodafinil*	Nuvigil	50-, 150-, and 250-mg tablets	50–150 mg	150–250 mg	250 mg	
Atomoxetine	Strattera	10-, 18-, 25-, 40, and 60-mg tablets	20 mg	40–80 mg	Not used	Children: 80 mg Adults: 100 mg
Dexmethylphenidate	Focalin	2.5-, 5-, and 10-mg capsules	5 mg	5–20 mg	Not used	20 mg
Dextroamphetamine	Dexedrine, Dextrostat	5-, 10-, and 15-mg ER capsules; 5- and 10-mg tablets	5–10 mg	20–30 mg	5–60 mg	Children: 40 mg Adults: 60 mg
Lisdexamfetamine	Vyvanse	20-, 30-, 40-, 50-, 60-, and 70-mg capsules	20–30 mg			70 mg
Methamphetamine	Desoxyn	5-mg tablets; 5-, 10-, and 15-mg ER tablets	5–10 mg	20–25 mg	Not generally used	45 mg
Methylphenidate	Ritalin, Methidate, Methylin, Attenade	5-, 10-, and 20-mg tablets; 10- and 20-mg SR tablets	5–10 mg	5–60 mg	20–30 mg	Children: 80 mg Adults: 90 mg
	Concerta	18- and 36-mg ER tablets	18 mg	18–54 mg	Not yet established	54 mg
Methylphenidate hydrochloride	Quillivant XR		20 mg			60 mg
Modafinil*	Provigil	100- and 200-mg tablets	100 mg	Not used	400 mg	400 mg

*Obstructive sleepapnea, narcolepsy, and shift work disorder.
[a]All medications that have dosage for children should be for 6 years or older except "Amphetamine" and "dextramphetamine".
ER, extended release; SR, sustained release.

prescription of sympathomimetics, even from persons who may benefit from the medications.

The dosage ranges and the available preparations for sympathomimetics are presented in Table 25–53. Vyvanse dosing is a special case, because many patients are switched to this formulation after being treated with other stimulants. A conversion table is shown in Table 25–54. It is available in 20-, 30-, 40-, 50-, 60-, and 70-mg capsules. Dosage should be individualized according to the therapeutic needs and response of the patient. Lisdexamfetamine (Vyvanse) should be administered at the lowest effective dosage. In patients who are either starting treatment for the first time or switching from another medication, 30 mg once daily in the morning is the recommended dose. Dosages may go up or down in 10- or 20-mg increments in intervals of approximately 1 week. Afternoon doses should be avoided because of the potential for insomnia. The drug may be taken with or without food.

Dextroamphetamine, methylphenidate, amphetamine, benzphetamine, and methamphetamine are schedule II drugs and in the past, required triplicate prescriptions in some states but since transitioning to electronic medical records this has been replaced by digital signature while prescribing via electronic prescription method. Phendimetrazine (Adipost, Bontril) and phenmetrazine (Prelude) are schedule III drugs, and modafinil, armodafinil, phentermine, diethylpropion (Tenuate), and mazindol (Mazanor, Sanorex) are schedule IV drugs.

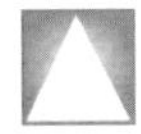

Table 25–54
Lisdexamfetamine (Vyvanse) Dosage Equivalency Conversions

Vyvanse and Adderall XR		
Vyvanse	**Adderall XR**	
20 mg	5 mg	
30 mg	10 mg	
40 mg	15 mg	
50 mg	20 mg	
60 mg	25 mg	
70 mg	30 mg	
Vyvanse, Adderall IR, and Dexedrine		
Vyvanse	**Adderall IR**	**Dexedrine**
70 mg	30 mg	22.5 mg
50 mg	20 mg	15 mg
30 mg	10 mg	7.5 mg

XR, extended release; IR, immediate release.

Pretreatment evaluation should include an evaluation of the patient's cardiac function, with particular attention to the presence of hypertension or tachyarrhythmias. The clinician should also examine the patient for the presence of movement disorders, such as tics and dyskinesia, because these conditions can be exacerbated by the administration of sympathomimetics. If tics are present, many experts will not prescribe sympathomimetics but will instead choose clonidine or antidepressants. However, recent data indicate that sympathomimetics may cause only a mild increase in motor tics and may actually suppress vocal tics. Liver function and renal function should be assessed, and dosages of sympathomimetics should be reduced for persons with impaired metabolism.

Persons with ADHD can take immediate-release methylphenidate at 8 AM, 12 noon, and 4 PM. Dextroamphetamine, Adderall, sustained-release methylphenidate, or 18 mg of extended-release methylphenidate may be taken once at 8 AM. The starting dose of methylphenidate ranges from 2.5 mg of regular to 20 mg of the sustained-release formulation. If this is inadequate, it may be increased to a maximum dose of 80 mg in children and 90 mg daily in adults. The dosage of dextroamphetamine is 2.5 to 40 mg a day up to 0.5 mg/kg a day.

Quillivant XR (methylphenidate hydrochloride) is a once-daily, extended-release liquid formulation of methylphenidate HCl. Quillivant XR is supplied as a liquid solution designed for oral administration and is taken once a day. The recommended dose for patients 6 years and older is 20 mg orally once daily in the morning with or without food. The dose may be titrated weekly in increments of 10 to 20 mg. Daily doses above 60 mg have not been studied and are not recommended. Before administering the dose, vigorously shake the bottle of Quillivant XR for at least 10 seconds, to ensure that the proper dose is administered. The clinical effects of the drug are evident from 45 minutes to 12 hours after dosing.

The starting dosage of modafinil is 200 mg in the morning in medically healthy individuals and 100 mg in the morning in persons with hepatic impairment. Some persons take a second 100- or 200-mg dose in the afternoon. The maximum recommended daily dosage is 400 mg, although dosages of 600 to 1,200 mg a day have been used safely. Adverse effects become prominent at dosages greater than 400 mg a day. Compared with amphetamine-like drugs, modafinil promotes wakefulness but produces less attentiveness and less irritability. Some persons with excessive daytime sleepiness extend the activity of the morning modafinil dose with an afternoon dose of methylphenidate. Armodafinil is virtually identical to modafinil, but is dosed differently, the dosing range being 50 to 250 mg daily.

Atomoxetine (Strattera)

Atomoxetine is the first nonstimulant drug to be approved by the FDA as a treatment of ADHD in children, adolescents, and adults. It is included in this chapter because it shares this indication with the stimulants described earlier.

Pharmacological Actions. Atomoxetine is believed to produce a therapeutic effect through selective inhibition of the presynaptic norepinephrine transporter. It is well absorbed after oral administration and is minimally affected by food. High-fat meals may decrease the rate but not the extent of absorption. Maximum plasma concentrations are reached after approximately 1 to 2 hours. At therapeutic concentrations, 98 percent of atomoxetine in plasma is bound to protein, mainly albumin. Atomoxetine has a half-life of approximately 5 hours and is metabolized principally by the cytochrome P450 (CYP)2D6 pathway. Poor metabolizers of this compound reach a fivefold higher area under the curve and fivefold higher peak plasma concentration than normal or extensive metabolizers. This is important to consider in patients receiving medications that inhibit the CYP2D6 enzyme. For example, the antidepressant-like pharmacology of atomoxetine has led to its use as an add-on to SSRIs or other antidepressants. Drugs such as fluoxetine (Prozac), paroxetine (Paxil), and bupropion (Wellbutrin) are CYP2D6 inhibitors and may raise atomoxetine levels.

Therapeutic Indications. Atomoxetine is used for the treatment of ADHD. It should be considered for use in patients who find stimulants too activating or who experience other intolerable side effects. Because atomoxetine has no abuse potential, it is a reasonable choice in the treatment of patients with both ADHD and substance abuse, patients who complain of ADHD symptoms but are suspected of seeking stimulant drugs, and patients who are in recovery.

Atomoxetine may enhance cognition when used to treat patients with schizophrenia. It may also be used as an alternative or add-on to antidepressants in patients who fail to respond to standard therapies.

Precautions and Adverse Reactions. Common side effects of atomoxetine include abdominal discomfort, decreased appetite with resulting weight loss, sexual dysfunction, dizziness, vertigo, irritability, and mood swings. Minor increases in BP and heart rate have also been observed. There have been cases of severe liver injury in a small number of patients taking atomoxetine. The drug should be discontinued in patients with jaundice (yellowing of the skin or whites of the eyes, itching) or laboratory evidence of liver injury. Atomoxetine should not be taken at the same time as, or within 2 weeks of taking, an MAOI or by patients with narrow-angle glaucoma.

The effects of overdose greater than twice the maximum recommended daily dose in humans are unknown. No specific information is available on the treatment of overdose with atomoxetine.

Dosage and Clinical Guidelines. Atomoxetine is available as 10-, 18-, 25-, 40-, and 60-mg capsules. In children and adolescents who weigh up to 70 kg, atomoxetine should be initiated at a total daily dose of approximately 0.5 mg/kg and increased after a minimum of 3 days to a target total daily dose of approximately 1.2 mg/kg, administered either as a single daily dose in the morning or as evenly divided doses in the morning and late afternoon or early evening. The total daily dose in smaller children and adolescents should not exceed 1.4 mg/kg or 100 mg, whichever is less. Dosing of children and adolescents who weigh more than 70 kg and adults should start at a total daily dose of 40 mg and then be increased after a minimum of 3 days to a target total daily dose of approximately 80 mg. The doses can be administered either as a single daily dose in the morning or as evenly divided doses in the morning and late afternoon or early evening. After 2 to 4 additional weeks, the dose may be increased to a maximum of 100 mg in patients who have not achieved an optimal response. The maximum recommended total daily dose in children and adolescents over 70 kg and adults is 100 mg.

THYROID HORMONES

Thyroid hormones—levothyroxine (Synthroid, Levothroid, Levoxine) and liothyronine (Cytomel)—are used in psychiatry either alone or as augmentation to treat persons with depression or rapid-cycling bipolar I disorder. They can convert an antidepressant-nonresponsive person into an antidepressant-responsive person. Thyroid hormones are also used as replacement therapy for persons treated with lithium (Eskalith) who have developed a hypothyroid state. Successful use of thyroid hormone as an intervention for treatment-resistant patients was first reported in the early 1970s. Study results since then have been mixed; however, most show that patients taking triiodothyronine (T_3) are twice as likely to respond to antidepressant treatment versus placebo. These studies have found that augmentation with T_3 is effective with TCAs and SSRIs. Nevertheless, many endocrinologists object to the use of thyroid hormones as antidepressant augmentation agents, citing such risks as osteoporosis and cardiac arrhythmias.

Pharmacological Actions

Thyroid hormones are administered orally, and their absorption from the GI tract is variable. Absorption is increased if the drug is administered on an empty stomach. Thyroxine (T_4) crosses the blood–brain barrier and diffuses into neurons, where it is converted into T_3, which is the physiologically active form. The half-life of T_4 is 6 to 7 days, and that of T_3 is 1 to 2 days.

The mechanism of action for thyroid hormone effects on antidepressant efficacy is unknown. Thyroid hormone binds to intracellular receptors that regulate the transcription of a wide range of genes, including several receptors for neurotransmitters.

Therapeutic Indications

The major indication for thyroid hormones in psychiatry is as an adjuvant to antidepressants. There is no clear correlation between the laboratory measures of thyroid function and the response to thyroid hormone supplementation of antidepressants. If a patient has not responded to a 6-week course of antidepressants at appropriate dosages, adjuvant therapy with either lithium or a thyroid hormone is an alternative. Most clinicians use adjuvant lithium before trying a thyroid hormone. Several controlled trials have indicated that liothyronine use converts about 50 percent of antidepressant nonresponders to responders.

The dosage of liothyronine is 25 or 50 μg a day added to the patient's antidepressant regimen. Liothyronine has been used primarily as an adjuvant for tricyclic drugs; however, evidence suggests that liothyronine augments the effects of all of the antidepressant drugs.

Thyroid hormones have not been shown to cause particular problems in pediatric or geriatric patients; however, the hormones should be used with caution in elderly persons, who may have occult heart disease.

Precautions and Adverse Reactions

At the dosages usually used for augmentation—25 to 50 μg a day—adverse effects occur infrequently. The most common adverse effects associated with thyroid hormones are transient headache, weight loss, palpitations, nervousness, diarrhea, abdominal cramps, sweating, tachycardia, increased BP, tremors, and insomnia. Osteoporosis may also occur with long-term treatment, but this has not been found in studies involving liothyronine augmentation. Overdoses of thyroid hormones can lead to cardiac failure and death.

Thyroid hormones should not be taken by persons with cardiac disease, angina, or hypertension. The hormones are contraindicated in thyrotoxicosis and uncorrected adrenal insufficiency and in persons with acute myocardial infarctions. Thyroid hormones can be administered safely to pregnant women, provided that laboratory thyroid indexes are monitored. Thyroid hormones are minimally excreted in breast milk and have not been shown to cause problems in nursing babies.

Drug Interactions

Thyroid hormones can potentiate the effects of warfarin (Coumadin) and other anticoagulants by increasing the catabolism of clotting factors. They may increase the insulin requirement for diabetic persons and the digitalis requirement for persons with cardiac disease. Thyroid hormones should not be coadministered with sympathomimetics, ketamine (Ketalar), or maprotiline (Ludiomil) because of the risk of cardiac decompensation. Administration of SSRIs, tricyclic and tetracyclic drugs, lithium, or carbamazepine (Tegretol) can mildly lower serum T_4 and raise serum thyrotropin concentrations in euthyroid persons or persons taking thyroid replacements. This interaction warrants close serum monitoring and may require an increase in the dosage or initiation of thyroid hormone supplementation.

Laboratory Interferences

Levothyroxine has not been reported to interfere with any laboratory test other than thyroid function indexes. Liothyronine, however, suppresses the release of endogenous T_4, thereby lowering the result of any thyroid function test that depends on the measure of T_4.

Thyroid Function Tests

Several thyroid function tests are available, including tests for T_4 by competitive protein binding (T_4 [D]) and by radioimmunoassay (T_4 RIA) involving a specific antigen–antibody reaction. More than 90 percent of T_4 is bound to serum protein and is responsible for TSH secretion and cellular metabolism. Other thyroid measures include the free T_4 index (FT_4I), T_3 uptake, and total serum T_3 measured by radioimmunoassay (T_3 RIA). Those tests are used to rule out hypothyroidism, which can be associated with symptoms of depression. In some studies, up to 10 percent of patients complaining of depression and associated fatigue had incipient hypothyroid disease. Lithium can cause hypothyroidism and, more rarely, hyperthyroidism. Neonatal hypothyroidism results in intellectual disability and is preventable if the diagnosis is made at birth.

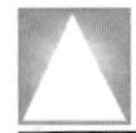

Table 25–55
Tricyclic and Tetracyclic Drug Preparations

Drug	Tablets (mg)	Capsules (mg)	Parenteral (mg/mL)	Solution
Imipramine (Tofranil)	10, 25, and 50	75, 100, 125, and 150	12.5	—
Desipramine (Norpramin, Pertofrane)	10, 25, 50, 75, 100, and 150	—	—	—
Trimipramine (Surmontil)	—	25, 50, and 100	—	—
Amitriptyline (Elavil)	10, 25, 50, 75, 100, and 150	—	10	—
Nortriptyline (Aventyl, Pamelor)	—	10, 25, 50, and 75	—	10 mg/5 mL
Protriptyline (Vivactil)	5 and 10	—	—	—
Amoxapine (Asendin)	25, 50, 100, and 150	—	—	—
Doxepin (Sinequan)	—	10, 25, 50, 75, 100, and 150	—	10 mg/mL
Maprotiline (Ludiomil)	25, 50, and 75	—	—	—
Clomipramine (Anafranil)	—	25, 50, and 75	—	—

Thyrotropin-releasing Hormone Stimulation Test. The TRH stimulation test is indicated for patients who have marginally abnormal thyroid test results with suspected subclinical hypothyroidism, which may account for clinical depression. It is also used in patients with possible lithium-induced hypothyroidism. The procedure entails an intravenous injection of 500 mg of protirelin (TRH), which produces a sharp increase in serum TSH levels that are measured at 15, 30, 60, and 90 minutes. An increase in serum TSH of 5 to 25 mIU/mL above the baseline is normal. An increase of less than 7 mIU/mL is considered a blunted response, which may correlate with a diagnosis of depression. Eight percent of all patients with depression have some thyroid illness.

Dosage and Clinical Guidelines

Liothyronine is available in 5-, 25-, and 50-μg tablets. Levothyroxine is available in 12.5-, 25-, 50-, 75-, 88-, 100-, 112-, 125-, 150-, 175-, 200-, and 300-μg tablets; it is also available in a 200 and 500 μg parenteral form. The dosage of liothyronine is 25 or 50 μg a day added to the person's antidepressant regimen. Liothyronine has been used as an adjuvant for all of the available antidepressant drugs. An adequate trial of liothyronine supplementation should last 2 to 3 weeks. If liothyronine supplementation is successful, it should be continued for 2 months and then tapered off at a rate of 12.5 μg a day every 3 to 7 days.

TRICYCLICS AND TETRACYCLICS

The observation in 1957 that imipramine (Tofranil) had antidepressant effects led to the development of a new class of antidepressant compounds, the tricyclics (TCAs). In turn, the finding that imipramine blocked reuptake of norepinephrine led to research into the role of catecholamines in depression. After the introduction of imipramine, several other antidepressant compounds were developed that shared a basic tricyclic structure and had relatively similar effects. Later, other heterocyclic compounds were also marketed that were somewhat similar in structure and that had relatively comparable secondary properties. At one time, amitriptyline (Elavil, Endep) and imipramine were the two most commonly prescribed antidepressants in the United States, but because of their anticholinergic and antihistaminic side effects, their use declined, and nortriptyline (Aventyl, Pamelor) and desipramine (Norpramin, Pertofrane) became more popular. Nortriptyline has the least effect on orthostatic hypotension, and desipramine is the least anticholinergic. Although introduced as antidepressants, the therapeutic indications for these agents have grown to include panic disorder, GAD, PTSD, OCD, and pain syndromes. The introduction of newer antidepressant agents with more selective actions on neurotransmitters or with unique mechanisms of action has sharply reduced the prescribing of TCAs and tetracyclics. The improved safety profiles of the newer drugs, especially when taken in overdose, also contributed to the decline in use of the older drugs. Nevertheless, the TCAs and tetracyclics remain unsurpassed in terms of their antidepressant efficacy. Table 25–55 lists TCA and tetracyclic drugs and their available preparations.

Pharmacological Actions

The absorption of most TCAs is complete after oral administration, and there is significant metabolism from the first-pass effect. Peak plasma concentrations occur within 2 to 8 hours, and the half-lives of the TCAs vary from 10 to 70 hours; nortriptyline, maprotiline (Ludiomil), and particularly protriptyline (Vivactil) can have longer half-lives. The long half-lives allow all the compounds to be given once daily; 5 to 7 days is needed to reach steady-state plasma concentrations. Imipramine pamoate (Tofranil) is a depot form of the drug for IM administration; indications for the use of this preparation are limited.

The TCAs undergo hepatic metabolism by the CYP450 enzyme system. Clinically relevant drug interactions may result from competition for enzyme CYP2D6 among TCAs and quinidine, cimetidine (Tagamet), fluoxetine (Prozac), sertraline (Zoloft), paroxetine (Paxil), phenothiazines, carbamazepine (Tegretol), and the type IC antiarrhythmics propafenone (Rythmol) and flecainide (Tambocor). Concomitant administration of TCAs and these inhibitors may slow down the metabolism and raise the plasma concentrations of TCAs. Additionally, genetic variations in the activity of CYP2D6 may account for up to a 40-fold difference in plasma TCA concentrations in different persons. The dosage of the TCA may need to be adjusted to correct changes in the rate of hepatic TCA metabolism.

The TCAs block the transporter site for norepinephrine and serotonin, thus increasing synaptic concentrations of these neurotransmitters. Each drug differs in its affinity for each of these transporters, with clomipramine (Anafranil) being the most serotonin selective and desipramine the most norepinephrine selective of the TCAs. Secondary effects of the TCAs include antagonism at the muscarinic acetylcholine, histamine H_1, and α_1- and α_2-adrenergic receptors. The potency of these effects on other receptors largely determines the side effect profile of each drug. Amoxapine, nortriptyline, desipramine, and maprotiline have the least anticholinergic activity; doxepin has the most antihistaminergic activity. Although they are more likely to cause constipation, sedation, dry mouth, or lightheadedness than the SSRIs, the TCAs are less prone to cause sexual dysfunction, significant long-term weight gain, and sleep disturbances than the SSRIs. The half-lives and plasma clearance for most TCAs are very similar.

Therapeutic Indications

Each of the following indications is also an indication for the SSRIs, which have widely replaced the TCAs in clinical practice. However, the TCAs represent a reasonable alternative for persons who cannot tolerate the adverse effects of the SSRIs.

Major Depressive Disorder. The treatment of a major depressive episode and the prophylactic treatment of MDD are the principal indications for using TCAs. Although the TCAs are effective in the treatment of depression in persons with bipolar I disorder, they are more likely to induce mania, hypomania, or cycling than the newer antidepressants, most notably the SSRIs and bupropion. It is thus not advised that TCAs be routinely used to treat depression associated with bipolar I or bipolar II disorder.

Melancholic features, prior major depressive episodes, and a family history of depressive disorders increase the likelihood of a therapeutic response. All of the available TCAs are equally effective in the treatment of depressive disorders. In the case of an individual person, however, one tricyclic or tetracyclic may be effective, and another one may be ineffective. The treatment of a major depressive episode with psychotic features almost always requires the coadministration of an antipsychotic drug and an antidepressant.

Although it is used worldwide as an antidepressant, clomipramine is only approved in the United States for the treatment of OCD.

Panic Disorder with Agoraphobia. Imipramine is the TCA most studied for panic disorder with agoraphobia, but other TCAs are also effective when taken at the usual antidepressant dosages. Because of the potential initial anxiogenic effects of the TCAs, starting dosages should be small, and the dosage should be titrated upward slowly. Small doses of benzodiazepines may be used initially to deal with this side effect.

Generalized Anxiety Disorder. The use of doxepin for the treatment of anxiety disorders is approved by the FDA. Some research data show that imipramine may also be useful. Although rarely used anymore, a chlordiazepoxide–amitriptyline combination (Limbitrol) is available for mixed anxiety and depressive disorders.

Obsessive-Compulsive Disorder. Patients with OCD appear to respond specifically to clomipramine, as well as the SSRIs. Some improvement is usually seen in 2 to 4 weeks, but a further reduction in symptoms may continue for the first 4 to 5 months of treatment. None of the other TCAs appears to be nearly as effective as clomipramine for treatment of this disorder. Clomipramine may also be a drug of choice for depressed persons with marked obsessive features.

Pain. The TCAs are widely used to treat chronic neuropathic pain and in prophylaxis of migraine headache. Amitriptyline is the TCA most often used in this role. During treatment of pain, doses are generally lower than those used in depression; for example, 75 mg of amitriptyline may be effective. These effects also appear more rapidly.

Other Disorders. Childhood enuresis is often treated with imipramine. Peptic ulcer disease can be treated with doxepin, which has marked antihistaminergic effects. Other indications for the TCAs are narcolepsy, nightmare disorder, and PTSD. The drugs are sometimes used for treatment of children and adolescents with ADHD, sleepwalking disorder, separation anxiety disorder, and sleep terror disorder. Clomipramine has also been used to treat premature ejaculation, movement disorders, and compulsive behavior in children with autistic disorders; however, because the TCAs have caused sudden death in several children and adolescents, they should not be used in children.

Precautions and Adverse Reactions

The TCAs are associated with a wide range of problematic side effects and can be lethal when taken in overdose.

Psychiatric Effects. The TCAs can induce a switch to mania or hypomania in susceptible individuals. The TCAs may also exacerbate psychotic disorders in susceptible persons. At high plasma concentrations (levels above 300 ng/mL), the anticholinergic effects of the TCAs can cause confusion or delirium. Patients with dementia are particularly vulnerable to this development.

Anticholinergic Effects. Anticholinergic effects often limit the tolerable dosage to relatively low ranges. Some persons may develop a tolerance for the anticholinergic effects with continued treatment. Anticholinergic effects include dry mouth, constipation, blurred vision, delirium, and urinary retention. Sugarless gum, candy, or fluoride lozenges can alleviate dry mouth. Bethanechol (Urecholine), 25 to 50 mg three or four times a day, may reduce urinary hesitancy and may be helpful in erectile dysfunction when the drug is taken 30 minutes before sexual intercourse. Narrow-angle glaucoma can also be aggravated by anticholinergic drugs, and the precipitation of glaucoma requires emergency treatment with a miotic agent. The TCAs should be avoided in persons with narrow-angle glaucoma, and an SSRI should be substituted. Severe anticholinergic effects can lead to a CNS anticholinergic syndrome with confusion and delirium, especially if the TCAs are administered with DRAs or anticholinergic drugs. IM or IV physostigmine (Antilirium, Eserine) is used to diagnose and treat anticholinergic delirium.

Cardiac Effects. When administered in their usual therapeutic dosages, the TCAs may cause tachycardia, flattened T waves, prolonged QT intervals, and depressed ST segments in the electrocardiographic (EKG) recording. Imipramine has a quinidine-like effect at therapeutic plasma concentrations and may reduce the number of premature ventricular contractions. Because the drugs prolong conduction time, their use in persons with preexisting conduction defects is contraindicated. In persons with a history of any type of heart disease, the TCAs should be used only after SSRIs or other newer antidepressants have been found ineffective, and if used, they should be introduced at low dosages, with gradual increases in dosage and monitoring of cardiac functions. All of the TCAs can cause tachycardia, which may persist for months and is one of the most common reasons for drug discontinuation, especially in younger persons. At high plasma concentrations, as seen in overdoses, the drugs become arrhythmogenic.

Other Autonomic Effects. Orthostatic hypotension is the most common cardiovascular autonomic adverse effect and the most common reason TCAs are discontinued. It can result in falls and injuries in affected persons. Nortriptyline may be the drug least likely to cause this problem. Orthostatic hypotension is treated with avoidance of caffeine, intake of at least 2 L of fluid per day and addition of salt to the diet unless the person is being treated for hypertension. In persons taking antihypertensive agents, reduction of the dosage may reduce the risk of orthostatic hypotension. Other possible autonomic effects are profuse sweating, palpitations, and increased BP. Although some persons respond to fludrocortisone (Florinef), 0.02 to 0.05 mg twice a day, substitution of an SSRI is preferable to addition of a potentially toxic mineralocorticoid such as fludrocortisone. The TCAs' use should be discontinued several days before elective surgery because of the occurrence of hypertensive episodes during surgery in persons receiving TCAs.

Sedation. Sedation is a common effect of the TCAs and may be welcomed if sleeplessness has been a problem. The sedative effect of the TCAs is a result of anticholinergic and antihistaminergic activities. Amitriptyline, trimipramine, and doxepin are the most sedating agents; imipramine, amoxapine, nortriptyline, and maprotiline are less sedating; and desipramine and protriptyline are the least sedating agents.

Neurologic Effects. A fine, rapid tremor may occur. Myoclonic twitches and tremors of the tongue and the upper extremities are common. Rare effects include speech blockage, paresthesia, peroneal palsies, and ataxia.

Amoxapine is unique in causing parkinsonian symptoms, akathisia, and even dyskinesia because of the dopaminergic blocking activity of one of its metabolites. Amoxapine may also cause neuroleptic malignant syndrome in rare cases. Maprotiline may cause seizures when the dosage is increased too quickly or is kept at high levels for too long. Clomipramine and amoxapine may lower the seizure threshold more than other drugs in the class. As a class, however, the TCAs have a relatively low risk for inducing seizures except in persons who are at risk for seizures (e.g., persons with epilepsy and those with brain lesions). Although the TCAs can still be used by such persons, the initial dosages should be lower than usual, and subsequent dosage increases should be gradual.

Allergic and Hematologic Effects. Exanthematous rashes are seen in 4 to 5 percent of all persons treated with maprotiline. Jaundice is rare. Agranulocytosis, leukocytosis, leukopenia, and eosinophilia are rare complications of TCA treatment. However, a person who has a sore throat or a fever during the first few months of TCA treatment should have a CBC done immediately.

Hepatic Effects. Mild and self-limited increases in serum transaminase concentrations may occur and should be monitored. The TCAs can also produce a fulminant acute hepatitis in 0.1 to 1 percent of persons. This can be life threatening, and the antidepressant should be discontinued.

Other Adverse Effects. Modest weight gain is common. Amoxapine exerts a DRA effect and may cause hyperprolactinemia, impotence, galactorrhea, anorgasmia, and ejaculatory disturbances. Other TCAs have also been associated with gynecomastia and amenorrhea. The syndrome of inappropriate secretion of antidiuretic hormone has also been reported with TCAs. Other effects include nausea, vomiting, and hepatitis.

TERATOGENICITY AND PREGNANCY-RELATED RISKS. A definitive link between the tricyclic compounds and tetracyclic compounds and teratogenic effects has not been established, but isolated reports of morphogenesis have been reported. TCAs cross the placenta, and neonatal drug withdrawal can occur. This syndrome includes tachypnea, cyanosis, irritability, and poor sucking reflex. If possible, tricyclic and tetracyclic medications should be discontinued 1 week before delivery. Recently, norepinephrine and serotonin transporters have been identified in the placenta and appear to play an important role in the clearance of these amines in the fetus. The understanding of the effects of reuptake inhibitors on these transporters during pregnancy is limited, but one study compared intelligence and language development in 80 children exposed to TCAs during pregnancy with 84 children exposed to other nonteratogenic agents and found no deleterious effects of the TCAs. The TCAs are excreted in breast milk at concentrations similar to plasma. The actual quantity delivered, however, is small, so drug levels in the infant are usually undetectable or very low. Because the risk of relapse is a serious concern in patients with recurrent depression, and these risks may be increased during pregnancy or the postpartum period, the risks and benefits of continuing or withdrawing treatment need to be discussed with the patient and weighed carefully.

PRECAUTIONS. The TCAs may cause a withdrawal syndrome in newborns consisting of tachypnea, cyanosis, irritability, and poor sucking reflex. The drugs do pass into breast milk but at concentrations that are usually undetectable in the infant's plasma. The drugs should be used with caution in persons with hepatic and renal diseases. The TCAs should not be administered during a course of ECT, primarily because of the risk of serious adverse cardiac effects.

Drug Interactions

Monoamine Oxidase Inhibitors. The TCAs should not be taken within 14 days of administration of an MAOI.

Antihypertensives. The TCAs block the therapeutic effects of antihypertensive medication. The antihypertensive effects of the β-adrenergic receptor antagonists (e.g., propranolol [Inderal] and clonidine [Catapres]) may be blocked by the TCAs. The coadministration of a TCA and α-methyldopa (Aldomet) may cause behavioral agitation.

Antiarrhythmic Drugs. The antiarrhythmic properties of TCAs can be additive to those of quinidine, an effect that is further exacerbated by the inhibition of TCA metabolism by quinidine.

Dopamine Receptor Antagonists. Concurrent administration of TCAs and DRAs increases the plasma concentrations of both drugs. Desipramine plasma concentrations may increase twofold during concurrent administration with perphenazine (Trilafon). The DRAs also add to the anticholinergic and sedative effects of the TCAs. Concomitant use of SDAs also increases those effects.

Central Nervous System Depressants. Opioids, alcohol, anxiolytics, hypnotics, and over-the-counter cold medications have additive effects by causing CNS depression when coadministered with TCAs. Persons should be advised to avoid driving or using dangerous equipment if sedated by TCAs.

Sympathomimetics. Tricyclic drug use with sympathomimetic drugs may cause serious cardiovascular effects.

Oral Contraceptives. Birth control pills may decrease TCA plasma concentrations through the induction of hepatic enzymes.

Other Drug Interactions. Nicotine may reduce TCA concentrations. Plasma concentrations may also be lowered by ascorbic acid, ammonium chloride, barbiturates, cigarette smoking, carbamazepine, chloral hydrate, lithium (Eskalith), and primidone (Mysoline). TCA plasma concentrations may be increased by concurrent use of acetazolamide (Diamox), sodium bicarbonate, acetylsalicylic acid, cimetidine, thiazide diuretics, fluoxetine, paroxetine, and fluvoxamine (Luvox). Plasma concentrations of the TCAs may rise three- to fourfold when administered concurrently with fluoxetine, fluvoxamine, and paroxetine.

Laboratory Interferences

The tricyclic compounds are present at low concentrations and are not likely to interfere with other laboratory assays. It is possible that they may interfere with the determination of conventional neuroleptic blood concentrations because of their structural similarity and the low concentrations of some neuroleptics.

Dosage and Clinical Guidelines

Persons who intend to take TCAs should undergo routine physical and laboratory examinations, including a WBC count with differential, and serum electrolytes with liver function tests. An EKG should be obtained for all persons, especially women older than 40 years of age and men older than 30 years of age. The TCAs are contraindicated in persons with a QT_c greater than

Table 25–56
General Information for the Tricyclic and Tetracyclic Antidepressants

Generic Name	Trade Name	Usual Adult Dosage Range (mg/day)	Therapeutic Plasma Concentrations (mg/mL)
Imipramine	Tofranil	150–300	150–300[a]
Desipramine	Norpramin, Pertofrane	150–300	150–300[a]
Trimipramine	Surmontil	150–300	?
Amitriptyline	Elavil, Endep	150–300	100–250[b]
Nortriptyline	Pamelor, Aventyl	50–150	50–150[a] (maximum)
Protriptyline	Vivactil	15–60	75–250
Amoxapine	Asendin	150–400	[c]
Doxepin	Adapin, Sinequan	150–300	100–250[a]
Maprotiline	Ludiomil	150–230	150–300[a]
Clomipramine	Anafranil	130–250	[c]

[a]Exact range may vary among laboratories.
[b]Includes parent compound and desmethyl metabolite.
[c]Therapeutic plasma levels unknown.

450 milliseconds. The initial dose should be small and should be raised gradually. Because of the availability of highly effective alternatives to TCAs, a newer agent should be used if there is any medical condition that may interact adversely with the TCAs.

Elderly persons and children are more sensitive to TCA adverse effects than are young adults. In children, the EKG should be regularly monitored during use of a TCA.

The available preparations of TCAs are presented in Table 25–55. The dosages and therapeutic blood levels for the TCAs vary among the drugs (Table 25–56). With the exception of protriptyline, all of the TCAs should be started at 25 mg a day and increased as tolerated. Divided doses at first reduce the severity of the adverse effects, although most of the dosage should be given at night to help induce sleep if a sedating drug such as amitriptyline is used. Eventually, the entire daily dose can be given at bedtime. A common clinical mistake is to stop increasing the dosage when the person is tolerating the drug but taking less than the maximum therapeutic dose and does not show clinical improvement. The clinician should routinely assess the person's pulse and orthostatic changes in BP while the dosage is being increased.

Nortriptyline use should be started at 25 mg a day. Most patients need only 75 mg a day to achieve a blood level of 100 mg/nL. However, the dosage may be raised to 150 mg a day if needed. Amoxapine use should be started at 150 mg a day and raised to 400 mg a day. Protriptyline use should be started at 15 mg a day and raised to 60 mg a day. Maprotiline has been associated with an increased incidence of seizures if the dosage is raised too quickly or is maintained at too high a level. Maprotiline use should be started at 25 mg a day and increased over 4 weeks to 225 mg a day. It should be kept at that level for only 6 weeks and then be reduced to 175 to 200 mg a day.

Persons with chronic pain may be particularly sensitive to adverse effects when TCA are started. Therefore, treatment should begin with low dosages that are raised in small increments. However, persons with chronic pain may experience relief on long-term low-dosage therapy, such as amitriptyline or nortriptyline at 10 to 75 mg a day.

The TCAs should be avoided in children except as a last resort. Dosing guidelines in children for imipramine include initiation at 1.5 mg/kg a day. The dosage can be titrated to no more than 5 mg/kg a day. In enuresis, the dosage is usually 50 to 100 mg a day taken at bedtime. Clomipramine use can be initiated at 50 mg a day and increased to no more than 250 mg a day.

When TCA treatment is discontinued, the dosage should first be decreased to three-fourths the maximal dosage for a month. At that time, if no symptoms are present, drug use can be tapered by 25 mg (5 mg for protriptyline) every 4 to 7 days. Slow tapering avoids a cholinergic rebound syndrome consisting of nausea, upset stomach, sweating, headache, neck pain, and vomiting. This syndrome can be treated by reinstituting a small dosage of the drug and tapering more slowly than before. Several case reports note the appearance of rebound mania or hypomania after the abrupt discontinuation of TCA use.

Plasma Concentrations and Therapeutic Drug Monitoring. Clinical determinations of plasma concentrations should be conducted after 5 to 7 days on the same dosage of medication and 8 to 12 hours after the last dose. Because of variations in absorption and metabolism, there may be a 30- to 50-fold difference in the plasma concentrations in persons given the same dosage of a TCA. Nortriptyline is unique in its association with a therapeutic window—that is, plasma concentrations below 50 ng/mL or above 150 ng/mL may reduce its efficacy.

Plasma concentrations may be useful in confirming compliance, assessing reasons for drug failures, and documenting effective plasma concentrations for future treatment. Clinicians should always treat the person and not the plasma concentration. Some persons have adequate clinical responses with seemingly subtherapeutic plasma concentrations, and other persons only respond at supratherapeutic plasma concentrations without experiencing adverse effects. The latter situation, however, should alert the clinician to monitor the person's condition with, for example, serial EKG recordings.

Overdose Attempts. Overdose attempts with TCAs are serious and can often be fatal. Prescriptions for these drugs should be nonrefillable and for no longer than 1 week at a time for patients at risk for suicide. Amoxapine may be more likely than the other TCAs to result in death when taken in overdose. The newer antidepressants are safer in overdose.

Symptoms of overdose include agitation, delirium, convulsions, hyperactive deep tendon reflexes, bowel and bladder paralysis, dysregulation of BP and temperature, and mydriasis. The patient then progresses to coma and perhaps respiratory depression. Cardiac arrhythmias may not respond to treatment. Because of the long half-lives of TCAs, the patients are at risk of cardiac arrhythmias for 3 to 4 days after the overdose, so they should be monitored in an intensive care medical setting.

VALPROATE

Valproate (Depakene, Depakote), or valproic acid, is approved for the treatment of manic episodes associated with bipolar I disorder and is one of the most widely prescribed mood stabilizers in psychiatry. It has a rapid onset of action and is well tolerated, and numerous studies suggest that it reduces the frequency and intensity of recurrent manic episodes over extended periods of time.

Chemistry

Valproate is a simple-chain branch carboxylic acid. It is called valproic acid because it is rapidly converted to the acid form in the stomach. Multiple formulations of valproic acid are marketed. These include valproic acid (Depakene); divalproex sodium (Depakote), an enteric-coated delayed-release 1:1 mixture of valproic acid and sodium valproate available in tablet and sprinkle formulation (can be opened and spread on food); and sodium valproate injection (Depacon). An extended-release preparation is also available. Each of these is therapeutically equivalent because at physiologic pH, valproic acid dissociates into valproate ion.

Pharmacological Actions

Regardless of how it is formulated, valproate is rapidly and completely absorbed 1 to 2 hours after oral administration, with peak concentrations occurring 4 to 5 hours after oral administration. The plasma half-life of valproate is 10 to 16 hours. Valproate is highly protein bound. Protein binding becomes saturated at higher dosages, and concentrations of therapeutically effective free valproate increase at serum concentrations above 50 to 100 μg/mL. The unbound portion of valproate is considered to be pharmacologically active and can cross the blood–brain barrier. The extended-release preparation produces lower peak concentrations and higher minimum concentrations and can be given once a day. Valproate is metabolized primarily by hepatic glucuronidation and mitochondrial β oxidation.

The biochemical basis of valproate's therapeutic effects remains poorly understood. Postulated mechanisms include enhancement of GABA activity, modulation of voltage-sensitive sodium channels, and action on extrahypothalamic neuropeptides.

Therapeutic Indications

Valproate is currently approved as monotherapy or adjunctive therapy of complex partial seizures, monotherapy and adjunctive therapy of simple and complex absence seizures, and adjunctive therapy for patients with multiple seizures that include absence seizures. Divalproex has additional indications for prophylaxis of migraine.

Bipolar I Disorder

ACUTE MANIA. About two-thirds of persons with acute mania respond to valproate. The majority of patients with mania usually respond within 1 to 4 days after achieving valproate serum concentrations above 50 μg/mL. Antimanic response is generally associated with levels greater than 50 μg/mL, in a range of 50 to 150 μg/mL. Using gradual dosing strategies, this serum concentration may be achieved within 1 week of initiation of dosing, but rapid oral loading strategies achieve therapeutic serum concentrations in 1 day and can control manic symptoms within 5 days. The short-term antimanic effects of valproate can be augmented with addition of lithium, carbamazepine

(Tegretol), SDAs, or DRAs. Numerous studies have suggested that the irritable manic subtype respond significantly better to divalproex than lithium or placebo. Because of its more favorable profile of cognitive, dermatologic, thyroid, and renal adverse effects, valproate is preferred to lithium for treatment of acute mania in children and elderly persons.

ACUTE BIPOLAR DEPRESSION. Valproate possesses some activity as a short-term treatment of depressive episodes in bipolar I disorder, but this effect is far less pronounced than for treatment of manic episodes. Among depressive symptoms, valproate is more effective for treatment of agitation than dysphoria. In clinical practice, valproate is most often used as add-on therapy to an antidepressant to prevent the development of mania or rapid cycling.

PROPHYLAXIS. Studies suggest that valproate is effective in the prophylactic treatment of bipolar I disorder, resulting in fewer, less severe, and shorter manic episodes. In direct comparison, valproate is at least as effective as lithium and is better tolerated than lithium. It may be particularly effective in persons with rapid-cycling and ultrarapid-cycling bipolar disorders, dysphoric or mixed mania, and mania caused by a general medical condition as well as in persons who have comorbid substance abuse or panic attacks and in persons who have not had complete favorable responses to lithium treatment.

Schizophrenia and Schizoaffective Disorder. Valproate may accelerate response to antipsychotic therapy in patients with schizophrenia or schizoaffective disorder. Valproate alone is generally less effective in schizoaffective disorder than in bipolar I disorder. Valproate alone is ineffective for treatment of psychotic symptoms and is typically used in combination with other drugs in patients with these symptoms.

Other Mental Disorders. Valproate has been studied for possible efficacy in a broad range of psychiatric disorders. These include alcohol withdrawal and relapse prevention, panic disorder, PTSD, impulse control disorder, borderline personality disorder, and behavioral agitation and dementia. Evidence supporting use in these cases is weak, and any observed therapeutic effects may be related to treatment of comorbid bipolar disorder.

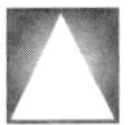

Table 25–57
Black Box Warnings and Other Warnings for Valproate

More Serious Side Effect	Management Considerations
Hepatotoxicity	Rare, idiosyncratic event Estimated risk, 1:118,000 (adults) Greatest risk profile (polypharmacy, younger than 2 yrs of age, mental retardation): 1:800
Pancreatitis	Rare, similar pattern to hepatotoxicity Incidence in clinical trial data is 2 in 2,416 (0.0008%) Postmarketing surveillance shows no increased incidence Relapse with rechallenge Asymptomatic amylase not predictive
Hyperammonemia	Rare; more common in combination with carbamazepine (Tegretol) Associated with coarse tremor and may respond to L-carnitine administration
Associated with urea cycle disorders	Discontinue valproate and protein intake Assess underlying urea cycle disorder Divalproex is contraindicated in patients with urea cycle disorders
Teratogenicity	Neural tube defect: 1–4% with valproate Preconceptual education and folate–vitamin B complex supplementation for all young women of childbearing potential
Somnolence in elderly persons	Slower titration than conventional doses Regular monitoring of fluid and nutritional intake
Thrombocytopenia	Decrease dose if clinically symptomatic (i.e., bruising, bleeding gums) Thrombocytopenia more likely with valproate levels ≥110 μg/mL (women) and ≥135 μg/mL (men)

Precautions and Adverse Reactions

Although valproate treatment is generally well tolerated and safe, it carries quite a few black box warnings and other warnings (Table 25–57). The two most serious adverse effects of valproate treatment affect the pancreas and liver. Risk factors for potentially fatal hepatotoxicity include young age (younger than 3 years); concurrent use of phenobarbital; and the presence of neurologic disorders, especially inborn errors of metabolism. The rate of fatal hepatotoxicity in persons who have been treated with only valproate is 0.85 per 100,000 persons; no persons older than the age of 10 years have been reported to have died from hepatotoxicity. Therefore, the risk of this adverse reaction in adult psychiatric patients is low. Nevertheless, if symptoms of lethargy, malaise, anorexia, nausea and vomiting, edema, and abdominal pain occur in a person treated with valproate, the clinician must consider the possibility of severe hepatotoxicity. A modest increase in liver function test results does not correlate with the development of serious hepatotoxicity. Rare cases of pancreatitis have been reported; they occur most often in the first 6 months of treatment, and the condition occasionally results in death. Pancreatic function can be assessed and followed with serum amylase concentrations. Other potentially serious consequences of treatment include hyperammonemia-induced encephalopathy and thrombocytopenia. Thrombocytopenia and platelet dysfunction occur most commonly at high dosages and result in the prolongation of bleeding times.

There are multiple concerns regarding the use of valproate during pregnancy. Women who require valproate therapy should therefore inform their physicians if they intend to become pregnant. First trimester use of valproate has been associated with a 3 to 5 percent risk of neural tube defects, as well as an increased risk of other malformations affecting the heart and other organ systems. Multiple reports have also indicated that in utero exposure to valproate may negatively affect cognitive development in children of mothers who take valproate during pregnancy. They have lower IQ scores at age 6 years compared with those exposed to other antiepileptic drugs. Fetal valproate exposure has dose-dependent associations with reduced cognitive abilities across a range of domains at 6 years of age. Valproate exposure may also increase the risk of autistic spectrum disorder.

The risk of valproate-induced neural tube defects can be reduced with daily folic acid supplements (1 to 4 mg a day). All women with childbearing potential who take the drug should be given folic acid supplements. Infants breastfed by mothers taking valproate develop serum valproate concentrations 1 to 10 percent of maternal serum concentrations, but no data suggest that this poses a risk to the infant. Valproate is not contraindicated in nursing mothers. Clinicians should not administer the drug to persons with hepatic diseases. Valproate may be especially problematic for adolescent and young women. Cases of polycystic ovarian disease have been reported in women using valproate. Even when the full syndromal criteria for this syndrome are not met, many of these women develop menstrual irregularities, hair loss, and hirsutism. These effects are thought to result from a metabolic syndrome that is driven by insulin resistance and hyperinsulinemia.

The common adverse effects associated with valproate (Table 25–58) are those affecting the GI system, such as nausea, vomiting, dyspepsia, and diarrhea. The GI effects are generally most common in the first month of treatment, particularly if the dosage is increased rapidly. Unbuffered valproic acid (Depakene) is more likely to cause GI symptoms than the enteric-coated "sprinkle" or the delayed-release divalproex sodium formulations. Other common adverse effects involve the nervous system, such as sedation, ataxia, dysarthria, and tremor. Valproate-induced tremor may respond well to treatment with β-adrenergic receptor antagonists or gabapentin. Treatment of the other neurologic adverse effects usually requires lowering the valproate dosage.

Weight gain is a common adverse effect, especially in long-term treatment, and can best be treated by strict limitation of caloric intake. Hair loss may occur in 5 to 10 percent of all persons treated, and rare cases of complete loss of body hair have been reported. Some clinicians have recommended treatment of valproate-associated hair loss with vitamin supplements that contain zinc and selenium. About 5 to 40 percent of persons experience a persistent but clinically insignificant elevation in liver transaminases up to three times the upper limit of normal, which is usually asymptomatic and resolves after discontinuation of the drug. High dosages of valproate (above 1,000 mg a day) may rarely produce mild to moderate hyponatremia, most likely because of some degree of the syndrome of secretion of inappropriate antidiuretic hormone, which is reversible upon lowering of the dosage. Overdoses of valproate can lead to coma and death.

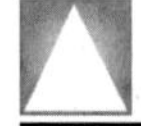

Table 25–58
Adverse Effects of Valproate

Common
GI irritation
Nausea
Sedation
Tremor
Weight gain
Hair loss
Uncommon
Vomiting
Diarrhea
Ataxia
Dysarthria
Persistent elevation of hepatic transaminases
Rare
Fatal hepatotoxicity (primarily in pediatric patients)
Reversible thrombocytopenia
Platelet dysfunction
Coagulation disturbances
Edema
Hemorrhagic pancreatitis
Agranulocytosis
Encephalopathy and coma
Respiratory muscle weakness and respiratory failure

GI, gastrointestinal.

Drug Interactions

Valproate is commonly prescribed as part of a regimen involving other psychotropic agents. The only consistent drug interaction with lithium, if both drugs are maintained in their respective therapeutic ranges, is the exacerbation of drug-induced tremors, which can usually be treated with β-receptor antagonists. The combination of valproate and DRAs may result in increased sedation, as can be seen when valproate is added to any CNS depressant (e.g., alcohol), and an increased severity of extrapyramidal symptoms, which usually responds to treatment with antiparkinsonian drugs. Valproate can usually be safely combined with carbamazepine or SDAs. Perhaps the most worrisome interaction of valproate and a psychotropic drug involves lamotrigine. Since the approval of lamotrigine for the treatment of bipolar disorder, the likelihood that patients will be treated with both agents has increased. Valproate more than doubles lamotrigine concentrations, increasing the risk of a serious rash (Stevens–Johnson syndrome, and toxic epidermal necrolysis).

The plasma concentrations of carbamazepine, diazepam (Valium), amitriptyline (Elavil), nortriptyline (Pamelor), and phenobarbital (Luminal) may also be increased when these drugs are coadministered with valproate, and the plasma concentrations of phenytoin (Dilantin) and desipramine (Norpramin) may be decreased when they are combined with valproate. The plasma concentrations of valproate may be decreased when the drug is coadministered with carbamazepine and may be increased when coadministered with guanfacine (Tenex), amitriptyline, or fluoxetine (Prozac). Valproate can be displaced from plasma proteins by carbamazepine, diazepam, and aspirin. Persons who are treated with anticoagulants (e.g., aspirin and warfarin [Coumadin]) should also be monitored when valproate use is initiated to assess the development of any undesired augmentation of the anticoagulation effects. Interactions of valproate with other drugs are listed in Table 25–59.

Laboratory Interferences

Valproate may cause laboratory increase of serum-free fatty acids. Valproate metabolites may produce a false-positive test result for urinary ketones as well as falsely abnormal thyroid function test results.

Dosage and Clinical Guidelines

When starting valproate therapy, a baseline hepatic panel, CBC and platelet counts, and pregnancy testing should be

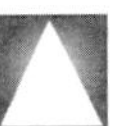

Table 25–59
Interactions of Valproate with Other Drugs

Drug	Interactions Reported with Valproate
Lithium	Increased tremor
Antipsychotics	Increased sedation; increased extrapyramidal effects; delirium and stupor (single report)
Clozapine	Increased sedation; confusional syndrome (single report)
Carbamazepine	Acute psychosis (single report); ataxia, nausea, lethargy (single report); may decrease valproate serum concentrations
Antidepressants	Amitriptyline and fluoxetine may increase valproate serum concentrations
Diazepam	Serum concentration increased by valproate
Clonazepam	Absence status (rare; reported only in patients with preexisting epilepsy)
Phenytoin	Serum concentration decreased by valproate
Phenobarbital	Serum concentration increased by valproate; increased sedation
Other CNS depressants	Increased sedation
Anticoagulants	Possible potentiation of effect

CNS, central nervous system.

ordered. Additional testing should include amylase and coagulation studies if baseline pancreatic disease or coagulopathy is suspected. In addition to baseline laboratory tests, hepatic transaminase concentrations should be obtained 1 month after initiation of therapy and every 6 to 24 months thereafter. However, because even frequent monitoring may not predict serious organ toxicity, it is more prudent to reinforce the need for prompt evaluation of any illnesses when reviewing the instructions with patients. Asymptomatic elevation of transaminase concentrations up to three times the upper limit of normal are common and do not require any change in dosage. Table 25–60 lists the recommended laboratory tests for valproate treatment.

Table 25–60
Recommended Laboratory Tests During Valproate Therapy

Before treatment
Standard chemistry screen with special attention to liver function tests
CBC, including WBC and platelet count

During treatment
Liver function tests at 1 mo; then every 6–24 mo if no abnormalities are found.
Complete blood work with platelet count at 1 mo; then every 6–24 mo if findings are normal.

If liver function test results become abnormal
Mild transaminase elevation (less than three times normal): monitoring every 1–2 wks; if stable and patient is responding to valproate, results are monitored monthly to every 3 mo.
Pronounced transaminase elevation (more than three times normal): dosage reduction or discontinuation of valproate; increase dose or rechallenge if transaminases normalize and if the patient is a valproate responder.

CBC, complete blood count; WBC, white blood cell.

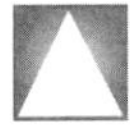

Table 25–61
Valproate Preparations Available in the United States

Generic Name	Trade Name, Form (Doses)	Time to Peak
Valproate sodium injection	Depacon, injection (100 mg valproic acid/mL)	1 hr
Valproic acid	Depakene, syrup (250 mg/5 mL)	1–2 hrs
	Depakene, capsules (250 mg)	1–2 hrs
Divalproex sodium	Depakote, delayed-released tablets (125, 250, 500 mg)	3–8 hrs
Divalproex sodium-coated particles in capsules	Depakote, sprinkle capsules (125 mg)	Compared with divalproex tablets, divalproex sprinkle has earlier onset and slower absorption, with slightly lower peak plasma concentration.

Valproate is available in a number of formulations (Table 25–61). For the treatment of acute mania, an oral loading strategy of initiation with 20 to 30 mg/kg a day can be used to accelerate control of symptoms. This is usually well tolerated but can cause excessive sedation and tremor in elderly persons. Agitated behavior can be rapidly stabilized with IV infusion of valproate. If acute mania is absent, it is best to initiate drug treatment gradually to minimize the common adverse effects of nausea, vomiting, and sedation. The dose on the first day should be 250 mg administered with a meal. The dosage can be raised up to 250 mg orally three times daily over the course of 3 to 6 days. The plasma concentrations can be assessed in the morning before the first daily dose is administered. Therapeutic plasma concentrations for the control of seizures range between 50 and 150 μg/mL, but concentrations up to 200 μg/mL are usually well tolerated. It is reasonable to use the same range for the treatment of mental disorders; most of the controlled studies have used 50 to 125 μg/mL. Most persons attain therapeutic plasma concentrations on a dosage between 1,200 and 1,500 mg a day in divided doses. After a person's symptoms are well controlled, the full daily dose can be taken all at once before sleep.

NUTRITIONAL SUPPLEMENTS AND MEDICAL FOODS

Thousands of herbal and dietary supplements are being marketed today. Some are purported to have psychoactive properties. A number have even shown promise in the treatment of certain psychiatric symptoms. Although certain compounds may be beneficial, in many cases the quantity and quality of data have been insufficient to make definitive conclusions. Nevertheless, some patients prefer to use these substances in place of, or in conjunction with, standard pharmaceutical treatments. If electing to use herbal drugs or nutritional supplements, bear in mind that their use may come at the expense of proven interventions and that adverse effects are possible. Though more research is needed, information published to date is still of clinical interest in diagnosing and treating patients who may be taking dietary supplements.

Additionally, herbal and nonherbal supplements may augment or antagonize the actions of prescription and nonprescription drugs. Thus, it is important for clinicians to remain informed on the latest research involving these substances. Because of the paucity of clinical trials, the clinician must be extraordinarily alert to the possibility of adverse effects as a result of drug–drug interactions, especially if psychotropic agents are prescribed, because many phytomedicinals have ingredients that produce physiological changes in the body.

Nutritional Supplements

In the United States, the term *nutritional supplement* is used interchangeably with the term *dietary supplement.* The Dietary Supplement Health and Education Act (DHSEA) of 1994 defined nutritional supplements as items taken by mouth that contain a "dietary ingredient" meant to supplement the diet. These ingredients may include vitamins, minerals, herbs, botanicals, amino acids, and substances such as enzymes, tissues, glandulars, and metabolites. By law such products must be labeled as supplements and may not be marketed as conventional food.

The DSHEA places dietary supplements in a special category, and therefore the regulations governing them are more lax than those for prescription and over-the-counter drugs. Unlike pharmaceutical drugs, nutritional supplements do not need the approval of the FDA, and the FDA does not evaluate their effectiveness. Because dietary supplements are not regulated by the FDA, the contents and quality on store shelves vary dramatically. Contamination, mislabeling, and misidentification of herbs and supplements are important problems. Table 25–62 provides a list of dietary supplements used in psychiatry.

Medical Foods

In recent years the FDA has introduced a new category of nutritional supplement called *medical foods.* According to the FDA, medical food, as defined in the Orphan Drug Act, is "a food which is formulated to be consumed or administered enterally under the supervision of a physician and which is intended for the specific dietary management of a disease or condition for which distinctive nutritional requirements, based on recognized scientific principles, are established by medical evaluation."

A clear distinction can be made between the regulatory classifications of medical foods and dietary supplements. Medical foods must be shown, by medical evaluation, to meet the distinctive nutritional needs of a specific population of patients with a specific disease being targeted. Dietary supplements, on the other hand, are intended for normal, healthy adults and may not require proof of efficacy of the finished product. Medical foods are distinguished from the broader category of foods for special dietary use and from foods that make health claims by the requirement that medical foods are to be used under medical supervision.

Medical foods do not have to undergo premarket approval by the FDA. But medical food firms must comply with other requirements, such as good manufacturing practices and registration of food facilities. Medical foods do have some additional regulations that dietary supplements do not because medical foods are intended to treat illnesses. For example, a compliance program requires annual inspections of all medical food manufacturers.

In summary, to be considered a medical food a product must, at a minimum, meet the following criteria: (1) The product must be a food for oral or tube feeding; (2) the product must be labeled for the dietary management of a specific medical disorder, disease, or condition for which there is distinctive nutritional requirements; and (3) the product must be intended to be used under medical supervision. The most common medical foods with psychoactive claims are listed in Table 25–63.

Phytomedicinals

The term *phytomedicinals* (from the Greek *phyto,* meaning "plant") refers to herb and plant preparations that are used or have been used for centuries for the treatment of a variety of medical conditions. Phytomedicinals are categorized as dietary supplements, not drug products, and are therefore exempt from the regulations that govern prescription and over-the-counter medications. Manufacturers of phytomedicinals are not required to provide the FDA with safety information before marketing a product or give the FDA postmarketing safety reports. Thousands of herbal drugs are being marketed today; the most common with psychoactive properties are listed in Table 25–64. Ingredients, to the extent they have been identified, are listed, as indications, adverse events, dosages, and comments, particularly on interactions with commonly prescribed drugs used in psychiatry. For example, St. John's wort (*wort* is an old English word meaning "root or herb"), which is used to treat depression, decreases the effectiveness of certain psychotropic drugs such as amitriptyline (Elavil), alprazolam (Xanax), paroxetine (Paxil), and sertraline (Zoloft), among others. Kava kava, which is used to treat anxiety states, has been associated with liver toxicity.

Adverse Effects. Adverse effects are possible, and toxic interactions with other drugs may occur with all phytomedicinals, dietary supplements, and medicinal foods. Adulteration is possible, especially with phytomedicinals. There are few or no consistent standard preparations available for most herbs. Medical foods are not tested by the FDA; however, strict voluntary compliance is required. Safety profiles and knowledge of adverse effects of most of these substances have not been studied rigorously. Because of the paucity of clinical trials, all of these agents should be avoided during pregnancy; some herbs may act as abortifacients, for example. Because most of these substances or their metabolites are secreted in breast milk, they are contraindicated during lactation.

Clinicians should always attempt to obtain a history of herbal use or the use of medical foods or nutritional supplements during the psychiatric evaluation.

It is important to be nonjudgmental in dealing with patients who use these substances. Many do so for various reasons: (1) as part of their cultural tradition, (2) because they mistrust physicians or are dissatisfied with conventional medicine, or (3) because they experience relief of symptoms with the particular substance. Because patients will be more cooperative with traditional psychiatric treatments if they are allowed to continue using their preparations, psychiatrists should try to keep an open mind and not attribute all effects to suggestion. If psychotropic

Table 25–62
Dietary Supplements Used in Psychiatry

Name	Ingredients/What Is It?	Uses	Adverse Effects	Interactions	Dosage	Comments
Docosahexaenoic acid (DHA)	Omega-3 polyunsaturated fatty acid	ADD, dyslexia, cognitive impairment, dementia	Anticoagulant properties, mild GI distress	Warfarin	Varies with indication	Stop using prior to surgery
Choline	Choline	Fetal brain development, manic conditions, cognitive disorders, tardive dyskinesia, cancers	Restrict in patients with primary genetic trimethylaminuria, sweating, hypotension, depression	Methotrexate, works with B_6, B_{12}, and folic acid in metabolism of homocysteine	300–1,200-mg doses >3 g associated with fishy body odor	Needed for structure and function of all cells
L-α-Glyceryl-phosphorylcholine (α-GPC)	Derived from soy lecithin	To increase growth hormone secretion, cognitive disorders	None known	None known	500 mg–1 g daily	Remains poorly understood
Phosphatidylcholine	Phospholipid that is part of cell membranes	Manic conditions, Alzheimer's disease, and cognitive disorders, tardive dyskinesia	Diarrhea, steatorrhea in those with malabsorption, avoid with antiphospholipid antibody syndrome	None known	3–9 g/day in divided doses	Soybeans, sunflower, and rapeseed are major sources.
Phosphatidylserine	Phospholipid isolated from soya and egg yolks	Cognitive impairment including Alzheimer's disease, may reverse memory problems	Avoid with antiphospholipid antibody syndrome, GI side effects	None known	For soya-derived variety, 100 mg tid	Type derived from bovine brain carries hypothetical risk of bovine spongiform encephalopathy
Zinc	Metallic element	Immune impairment, wound healing, cognitive disorders, prevention of neural tube defects	GI distress, high doses can cause copper deficiency, immunosuppression	Bisphosphonates, quinolones, tetracycline, penicillamine, copper, cysteine-containing foods, caffeine, iron	Typical dose 15 mg/day, adverse effects >30 mg	Claims that zinc can prevent and treat the common cold are supported in some studies but not in others; more research needed
Acetyl-L-carnitine	Acetyl ester of L-carnitine	Neuroprotection, Alzheimer's disease, Down syndrome, strokes, antiaging, depression in geriatric patients	Mild GI distress, seizures, increased agitation in some with Alzheimer's disease	Nucleoside analogs, valproic acid, and pivalic acid–containing antibiotics	500 mg–2 g daily in divided doses	Found in small amounts in milk and meat
Huperzine A	Plant alkaloid derived from Chinese club moss	Alzheimer's disease, age-related memory loss, inflammatory disorders	Seizures, arrhythmias, asthma, irritable bowel disease	Acetylcholinesterase inhibitors and cholinergic drugs	60 μg–200 μg/day	*Huperzia serrata* has been used in Chinese folk medicine for the treatment of fevers and inflammation.
NADH (nicotinamide adenine dinucleotide)	Dinucleotide located in mitochondria and cytosol of cells	Parkinson's disease, Alzheimer's disease, chronic fatigue, CV disease	GI distress	None known	5 mg/day or 5 mg bid	Precursor of NADH is nicotinic acid
S-Adenosyl-L-methionine (SAMe)	Metabolite of essential amino acid L-methionine	Mood elevation, osteoarthritis	Hypomania, hyperactive muscle movement, caution in patients with cancer	None known	200–1,600 mg daily in divided doses	Several trials demonstrate some efficacy in the treatment of depression

(*continued*)

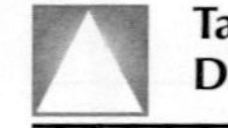

Table 25–62
Dietary Supplements Used in Psychiatry (Continued)

Name	Ingredients/What Is It?	Uses	Adverse Effects	Interactions	Dosage	Comments
5-Hydroxytryptophan (5-HTP)	Immediate precursor of serotonin	Depression, obesity, insomnia, fibromyalgia, headaches	Possible risk of serotonin syndrome in those with carcinoid tumors or taking MAOIs	SSRIs, MAOIs, methyldopa, St. John's wort, phenoxybenzamine, 5-HT antagonists, 5-HT receptor agonists	100 mg–2 g daily, safer with carbidopa	5-HTP along with carbidopa is used in Europe for the treatment of depression.
Phenylalanine	Essential amino acid	Depression, analgesia, vitiligo	Contraindicated in patients with PKU, may exacerbate tardive dyskinesia or hypertension	MAOIs and neuroleptic drugs	Comes in 2 forms: 500 mg–1.5 g daily for DL-phenylalanine, 375 mg–2.25 g for DL-phenylalanine	Found in vegetables, juices, yogurt, and miso
Myoinositol	Major nutritionally active form of inositol	Depression, panic attacks, OCD	Caution in patients with bipolar disorder, GI distress	Possible additive effects with SSRIs and 5-HT receptor agonists (sumatriptan)	12 g in divided doses for depression and panic attacks	Studies have *not* shown effectiveness in treating Alzheimer's disease, autism, or schizophrenia
Vinpocetine	Semisynthetic derivative of vincamine (plant derivative)	Cerebral ischemic stroke, dementias	GI distress, dizziness, insomnia, dry mouth, tachycardia, hypotension, flushing	Warfarin	5–10 mg daily with food, no more than 20 mg/day	Used in Europe, Mexico, and Japan as pharmaceutical agent for treatment of cerebrovascular and cognitive disorders
Vitamin E family	Essential fat-soluble vitamin, family made of tocopherols and tocotrienols	Immune-enhancing, antioxidant, some cancers, protection in CV disease, neurologic disorders, diabetes, premenstrual syndrome	May increase bleeding in those with propensity to bleed, possible increased risk of hemorrhagic stroke, thrombophlebitis	Warfarin, antiplatelet drugs, neomycin, may be additive with statins	Depends on form: tocotrienols, 200–300 mg daily with food; tocopherols, 200 mg/day	Stop members of vitamin E family 1 mo prior to surgical procedures
Glycine	Amino acid	Schizophrenia, alleviating spasticity, and seizures	Avoid in those who are anuric or have hepatic failure	Additive with antispasmodics	1 g/day in divided doses for supplement; 40–90 g/day for schizophrenia	
Melatonin	Hormone of pineal gland	Insomnia, sleep disturbances, jet lag, cancer	May inhibit ovulation in 1 g doses, seizures, grogginess, depression, headache, amnesia	Aspirin, NSAIDs, β-blockers, INH, sedating drugs, corticosteroids, valerian, kava kava, 5-HTP, alcohol	0.3–3 mg HS for short periods of time	Melatonin sets the timing of circadian rhythms and regulates seasonal responses.
Fish oil	Lipids found in fish	Bipolar disorder, lowering triglycerides, hypertension, decrease blood clotting	Caution in hemophiliacs, mild GI upset, "fishy"-smelling excretions	Coumadin, aspirin, NSAIDs, garlic, ginkgo	Varies depending on form and indication—usually about 3–5 g daily	Stop prior to any surgical procedure

ADD, attention-deficit disorder; CV, cardiovascular; OCD, obsessive-compulsive disorder; GI, gastrointestinal; hs, at night; MAOIs, monamine oxidase inhibitors; PKU, phenylketonuria; SSRIs, serotonin reuptake inhibitors; NSAIDs, nonsteroidal anti-inflammatory drugs; INH, isoniazid; 5-HTP, 5-hydroxytryptophan; tid, three times a day; bid, twice a day.
Table by Mercedes Blackstone, M.D.

Table 25–63
Some Common Medical Foods

Medical Food	Indication	Mechanism of Action
Caprylic-triglyceride (Axona)	Alzheimer's disease	Increases plasma concentration of ketones as an alternative energy source in the brain; metabolized in the liver.
L-methylfolate (Deplin)	Depression	Regulates synthesis of serotonin, norepinephrine, and dopamine; adjunctive to selective serotonin reuptake inhibitors (SSRIs); 15 mg/day.
S-adenosyl-L-methionine (SAMe)	Depression	Naturally occurring molecule involved in synthesis of hormones and neurotransmitters including serotonin and norepinephrine.
L-Tryptophane	Sleep disturbance Depression	Essential amino acid; precursor of serotonin; reduces sleep latency; usual dose 4–5 g/day.
Omega-3 fatty acid	Depression Cognition	Eicosapentaenoic (EPA) and docosahexaenoic (DHA) acids; direct effect on lipid metabolism; used for augmentation of antidepressant drugs
Theramine (Sentra)	Sleep disturbances Cognitive enhancer	Cholinergic modulator; increases acetylcholine and glutamate
N-Acetylcysteine	Depression Obsessive-compulsive disorder	Amino acid that attenuates glutamatergic neurotransmission; used to augment SSRIs.
L-Tyrosine	Depression	Amino acid precursor to biogenic amines epinephrine and norepinephrine
Glycine	Depression	Amino acid that activates N-methyl-D-aspartate (NMDA) receptors; may facilitate excitatory transmission in the brain.
Citicoline	Alzheimer's disease Ischemic brain injury	Choline donor involved in synthesis of brain phospholipids and acetylcholine; 300–1,000 mg/day; may improve memory.
Acetyl L-carnitine (Alcar)	Alzheimer's disease Memory loss	Antioxidant that may prevent oxidative damage in the brain.

agents are prescribed, the clinician must be extraordinarily alert to the possibility of adverse effects as a result of drug–drug interactions because many of these compounds have ingredients that produce actual physiological changes in the body.

WEIGHT LOSS DRUGS

Weight management is an important element of psychotropic drug treatment because obesity is common among persons with mental disorders. Thus, medical conditions such as hypertension, diabetes mellitus, and hyperlipidemia need to be taken into account when selecting medications. With few exceptions, most psychotropic drugs used to manage mood disorders, anxiety disorders, and psychosis are associated with significant risk of weight gain as a side effect. Many patients may refuse or discontinue treatment if weight gain occurs, even if the drug is effective in treating their symptoms. For this and other reasons, it is important for clinicians to be well informed about treatment strategies for mitigating drug-induced weight gain and obesity in general.

The standard recommendation for weight loss regimens consists of attempting to manage body weight through consistent dietary modifications and regular physical activity. This may be difficult for patients struggling with psychiatric symptoms because their ability to be disciplined in this effort can be compromised by their mental disorder. Also, the physiologic effects of some psychotropic drugs on regulation of satiety and on body metabolism are difficult, if not impossible, to overcome through diet and exercise alone. For these reasons, it may be necessary to use prescription medications to facilitate weight loss.

In this section, drugs used to manage obesity are categorized in two ways: (1) drugs approved by the FDA as diet pills; and (2) drugs with primary indications other than weight loss but produce weight loss as a side effect.

Drugs with U.S. Food and Drug Administration Approval for Weight Loss

All of the drugs approved by the FDA as weight loss agents are specifically indicated as an adjunct to a reduced calorie diet and increased physical activity for chronic weight management in adult patients with an initial BMI of 30 kg/m^2 or greater (obese) or 27 kg/m^2 or greater (overweight) in the presence of at least one weight-related comorbidity such as hypertension, type 2 diabetes mellitus, or dyslipidemia.

Phentermine. Phentermine hydrochloride (Adipex-P) is a sympathomimetic amine with pharmacological activity similar to the amphetamines. It is indicated as a short-term adjunct in a regimen of weight reduction, but in fact, many patients use the drug for extended periods. As with all sympathomimetics, contraindications include advanced arteriosclerosis, cardiovascular disease, moderate to severe hypertension, hyperthyroidism, known hypersensitivity or idiosyncrasy to the sympathomimetic amines, agitated states, and glaucoma.

The drug should be prescribed with caution to patients with a history of drug abuse. Hypertensive crises may result if phentermine is used during or within 14 days following the administration of MAOIs. Insulin requirements in diabetes mellitus may be altered in association with the use of phentermine hydrochloride and the concomitant dietary regimen. Phentermine hydrochloride may decrease the hypotensive effect of guanethidine. Phentermine is pregnancy Category X and thus contraindicated during pregnancy. Studies have not been performed with phentermine hydrochloride to determine the potential for carcinogenesis, mutagenesis, or impairment of fertility.

Phentermine should be taken on an empty stomach, once daily, prior to breakfast. Tablets may be broken or cut in half but

Table 25–64
Phytomedicinals with Psychoactive Effects

Name	Ingredients	Use	Adverse Effects[a]	Interactions	Dosage[a]	Comments
Arctic weed, golden root	MAOI and β endorphin	Anxiolytic, mood enhancer, antidepressant	No side effect yet documented in trials		100 mg bid to 200 mg tid	Use caution with drugs that mimic MAOIs
Areca, areca nut, betel nut, *L. Areca catechu*	Arecoline, guvacoline	For alteration of consciousness to reduce pain and elevate mood	Parasympathomimetic overload: increased salivation, tremors, bradycardia, spasms, GI disturbances, ulcers of the mouth	Avoid with parasympathomimetic drugs; atropine-like compounds reduce effect	Undetermined; 8–10 g is toxic dose for humans.	Used by chewing the nut; used in the past as a chewing balm for gum disease and as a vermifuge; long-term use may result in malignant tumors of the oral cavity.
Ashwaganda	Also called Indian Winter Cherry or Indian Ginseng, native to India. Flavonoids.	Antioxidant, may decrease anxiety levels. Improved libido in men and women May lower levels of the stress hormone cortisol.	Drowsiness and sleepiness	None	Dosage is 1 tablet twice daily before meals with a gradual increase to 4 tablets per day.	None
Belladonna, *L. Atropa belladonna,* deadly nightshade	Atropine, scopolamine, flavonoids[b]	Anxiolytic	Tachycardia, arrhythmias, xerostomia, mydriasis, difficulties with micturition and constipation	Synergistic with anticholinergic drugs; avoid with TCAs, amantadine, and quinidine	0.05–0.10 mg a day; maximum single dose is 0.20 mg	Has a strong smell, tastes sharp and bitter, and is poisonous
Biota, *Platycladus orientalis*	Plant derivative	Used as a sedative. Other uses are to treat heart palpitations, panic, night sweats, and constipation. May be useful in ADHD.	No known adverse effects.	None	No clear established doses exist.	None
Bitter orange flower, *citrus aurantium*	Flavonoids, limonene	Sedative, anxiolytic, hypnotic	Photosensitization	Undetermined	Tincture, 2–3 g/day; drug, 4–6 g/day; extract, 1–2 g/day	Contradictory evidence; some refer to it as a gastric stimulant
Black cohosh, *L. Cimicifuga racemosa*	Triterpenes, isoferulic acid	For PMS, menopausal symptoms, dysmenorrhea	Weight gain, GI disturbances	Possible adverse interaction with male or female hormones	1–2 g/day; over 5 g can cause vomiting, headache, dizziness, cardiovascular collapse.	Estrogen-like effects questionable because root may act as an estrogen-receptor blocker.
Black haw, cramp bark, *L. Viburnum prunifolium*	Scopoletin, flavonoids, caffeic acids, triterpenes	Sedative, antispasmodic action on uterus; for dysmenorrhea	Undetermined	Anticoagulant-enhanced effects	1–3 g/day	Insufficient data

California poppy, *L. Eschscholtzia californica*	Isoquinoline alkaloids, cyanogenic glycosides	Sedative, hypnotic, anxiolytic; for depression	Lethargy	Combination of California poppy, valerian, St. John's wort, and passion flowers can result in agitation.	2 g/day	Clinical or experimental documentation of effects is unavailable.
Casein	Casein peptides	Used as antistress agent. May improve sleep.	Usually consumed through milk products. May interact with antihypertensive medicine and lower blood pressure. May cause drowsiness and should be avoided when taking alcohol or benzodiazepines.	None	One to two tablets once or twice daily	
Catnip, *L. Nepeta cataria*	Valeric acid	Sedative, antispasmodic; for migraine	Headache, malaise, nausea, hallucinogenic effects	Undetermined	Undetermined	Delirium produced in children
Chamomile, *L. Matricaria chamomilla*	Flavonoids	Sedative, anxiolytic	Allergic reaction	Undetermined	2–4 g/day	May be GABAergic
Coastal water hyssop		Anxiolytic, sedative, epilepsy, asthma	Mild GI discomfort	May stimulate	300–450 mg qid	Insufficient data
Cordyceps sinensis	A genus of fungi that includes about 400 described species, found primarily in the high altitudes of the Tibetan plateau in China. Antioxidant.	Has been used for weakness, fatigue, to improve sexual drive in the elderly.	GI discomfort, dry mouth, and nausea	None	Dosage in ranges of 3–6 g daily	None
Corydalis, *L. Corydalis cava*	Isoquinoline alkaloids	Sedative, antidepressant; for mild depression	Hallucination, lethargy	Undetermined	Undetermined	Clonic spasms and muscular tremor with overdose
Cyclamen, *L. Cyclamen europaeum*	Triterpene	Anxiolytic; for menstrual complaints	Small doses (e.g., 300 mg) can lead to nausea, vomiting, and diarrhea.	Undetermined	Undetermined	High doses can lead to respiratory collapse.
Echinacea, *L. Echinacea purpurea*	Flavonoids, polysaccharides, caffeic acid derivatives, alkamides	Stimulates immune system; for lethargy, malaise, respiratory infections, and lower UTIs	Allergic reaction, fever, nausea, vomiting	Undetermined	1–3 g/day	Use in HIV and AIDS patients is controversial; may not be effective in coryza.
Ephedra, ma-huang *L. Ephedra sinica*	Ephedrine, pseudoephedrine	Stimulant; for lethargy, malaise, diseases of respiratory tract	Sympathomimetic overload: arrhythmias, increased BP, headache, irritability, nausea, vomiting	Synergistic with sympathomimetics, serotonergic agents; avoid with MAOIs	1–2 g/day	Tachyphylaxis and dependence can occur (taken off market).

(continued)

Table 25–64
Phytomedicinals with Psychoactive Effects (Continued)

Name	Ingredients	Use	Adverse Effects[a]	Interactions	Dosage[a]	Comments
Ginkgo, *L. Ginkgo biloba*	Flavonoids, ginkgolide A, B	Symptomatic relief of delirium, dementia; improves concentration and memory deficits; possible antidote to SSRI-induced sexual dysfunction	Allergic skin reactions, GI upset, muscle spasms, headache	Anticoagulant: use with caution because of its inhibitory effect on PAF; increased bleeding possible	120–240 mg/day	Studies indicate improved cognition in persons with Alzheimer's disease after 4–5 wks of use, possibly because of increased blood flow.
Ginseng, *L. Panax ginseng*	Triterpenes, ginsenosides	Stimulant; for fatigue, elevation of mood, immune system	Insomnia, hypertonia, and edema (called ginseng abuse syndrome)	Not to be used with sedatives, hypnotic agents, MAOIs, antidiabetic agents, or steroids	1–2 g/day	Several varieties exist; Korean (most highly valued), Chinese, Japanese, American (*Panox quinquefolius*)
Heather, *L. Calluna vulgaris*	Flavonoids, triterpenes	Anxiolytic, hypnotic	Undetermined	Undetermined	Undetermined	Efficacy for claimed uses is not documented
Holy Basil formula, *Ocimum tenuiflorum*	*Ocimum tenuiflorum*, an aromatic plant native to the tropics, part of the *Lamiaceae* family. Flavonoids.	Used to combat stress, also used for common colds, headaches, stomach disorders, inflammation, heart disease.	No data exists regarding the long-term effects. May prolong clotting time, increase the risk of bleeding during surgery, and lower blood sugar.	None	Dosage depends on the formulation type, recommended dose is 2 softgel capsules taken with 8-oz water daily.	None
Hops, *L. Humulus lupulus*	Humulone, lupulone, flavonoids	Sedative, anxiolytic, hypnotic; for mood disturbances, restlessness	Contraindicated in patients with estrogen-dependent tumors (breast, uterine, cervical)	Hyperthermia effects with phenothiazine antipsychotics and with CNS depressants	0.5 g/day	May decrease plasma levels of drugs metabolized by CYP450 system
Horehound, *L. Ballota nigra*	Diterpenes, tannins	Sedative	Arrhythmias, diarrhea, hypoglycemia, possible spontaneous abortions	May enhance serotonergic drug effects, may augment hypoglycemic effects of drugs	1–4 g/day	May cause abortion
Jambolan, *L. Syzygium cumini*	Oleic acid, myristic acid, palmitic and linoleic acids, tannins	Anxiolytic, antidepressant	Undetermined	Undetermined	1–2 g/day	In folk medicine, a single dose is 30 seeds (1.9 g) of powder
Kanna, *Sceletium tortuosum*	Alkaloid, mesembrine	Anxiolytic, mood enhancer, empathogen, COPD treatment	Sedation, vivid dreams, headache	Potentiates cannabis, PDE inhibitor	50–100 mg	Insufficient data
Kava kava, *L. Piperis methysticum*	Kava lactones, kava pyrone	Sedative, hypnotic antispasmodic	Lethargy, impaired cognition, dermatitis with long-term usage, liver toxicity	Synergistic with anxiolytics, alcohol; avoid with levodopa and dopaminergic agents	600–800 mg/day	May be GABAergic; contraindicated in patients with endogenous depression; may increase the danger of suicide

Kratom, *Mitragyna speciosa*	Alkaloid	Stimulant and depressant	Priapism, testicular enlargement, withdrawal, depression, fatigue, insomnia	Structurally similar to yohimbine	Undetermined	Chewed, extracted into water, tar formulations
Lavender, *L. Lavandula angustifolia*	Hydroxycoumarin, tannins, caffeic acid	Sedative, hypnotic	Headache, nausea, confusion	Synergistic with other sedatives	3–5 g/day	May cause death in overdose
Lemon balm, sweet Mary, *L. Melissa officinalis*	Flavonoids, caffeic acid, triterpenes	Hypnotic, anxiolytic, sedative	Undetermined	Potentiates CNS depressant; adverse reaction with thyroid hormone	8–10 g/day	Insufficient data
L-Methylfolate	Folate is a B vitamin found in some foods, needed to form healthy cells, especially red blood cells. L-methylfolate and levomefolate are names for the active form of folic acid.	Adjunctive L is used for major depression, not an antidepressant when used alone. Folate and L-methylfolate are also used to treat folic acid deficiency in pregnancy, to prevent spinal cord birth defects.	GI side effects reported.	None	15 mg once a day by mouth with or without food	Considered a "medical food" by the FDA and only available by prescription. Safe to take during pregnancy when used as directed.
Mistletoe, *L. Viscum album*	Flavonoids, triterpenes, lectins, polypeptides	Anxiolytic; for mental and physical exhaustion	Berries said to have emetic and laxative effects	Contraindicated in patients with chronic infections (e.g., tuberculosis)	10 per day	Berries have caused death in children.
Mugwort, *L. Artemisia vulgaris*	Sesquiterpene lactones, flavonoids	Sedative, antidepressant, anxiolytic	Anaphylaxis, contact dermatitis, may cause hallucinations.	Potentiates anticoagulants	5–15 g/day	May stimulate uterine contractions, can induce abortion
N-Acetylcysteine (NAC)	Amino acid	Used as an antidote for acetaminophen overdose, augmentation of SSRIs in the treatment of trichoti lomania.	Rash, cramps, and angioedema may occur.	Activated charcoal, ampicillin, carbamazepine, cloxacillin, oxacillin, nitroglycerin, and penicillin G.	1,200–2,400 mg/day	Acts as an antioxidant and a glutamate modulating agent. When used as an antidote for acetaminophen overdose, the doses 20–40 times higher than those used in OCD trials. It has not been shown to be effective in treating schizophrenia.
Nux vomica, *L. Strychnos nux vomica,* poison nut	Indole alkaloids: strychnine and brucine, polysaccharides	Antidepressant; for migraine, menopausal symptoms	Convulsions, liver damage, death; severely toxic because of strychnine	Undetermined	0.02–0.05 g/day	Symptoms of poisoning can occur after ingestion of one bean; lethal dose is 1–2 g.
Oats, *L. Avena sativa*	Flavonoids, oligo and polysaccharides	Anxiolytic, hypnotic; for stress, insomnia, opium, and tobacco withdrawal	Bowel obstruction or other bowel dysmotility syndromes, flatulence	Undetermined	3 g/day	Oats have sometimes been contaminated with aflatoxin, a fungal toxin linked with some cancers.

(continued)

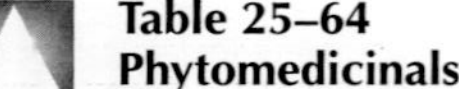

Table 25–64
Phytomedicinals with Psychoactive Effects (Continued)

Name	Ingredients	Use	Adverse Effects[a]	Interactions	Dosage[a]	Comments
Omega-3 fatty acid	Comes in three forms, eicosapentaenoic acid (EPA), docosahexaenoic acid (DHA), and alpha-linolenic acid (LNA)	Used as a supplement in the treatment of heart disease, high cholesterol, high blood pressure. May also be helpful in treatment of depression, bipolar disorder, schizophrenia, and ADHD. May reduce the risk of ulcers when used in conjunction with NSAID pain relievers.	Can cause gas, bloating, belching, and diarrhea.	May increase effectiveness of blood thinners, may increase fasting blood sugar levels when used with diabetes medications such as insulin and metformin.	Doses vary from 1 to 4 g/day.	Can be contaminated with mercury and PCBs.
Passion flower, *L. Passiflora incarnata*	Flavonoids, cyanogenic glycosides	Anxiolytic, sedative, hypnotic	Cognitive impairment	Undetermined	4–8 g/day	Overdose causes depression
Phosphatidylserine and Phosphatidylcholine	Phospholipids	Used for Alzheimer's disease, age-related decline in mental function, improving thinking skills in young people, ADHD, depression, preventing exercise-induced stress, and improving athletic performance.	Insomnia and stomach upset.	None	100 mg three times daily	None
Polygala	Polygala is a genus of about 500 species of flowering plants belonging to the family *Polygalaceae*, commonly known as milkwort or snakeroot.	Used for insomnia, forgetfulness, mental confusion, palpitation, seizures, anxiety, and listlessness.	Contraindicated in patients who have ulcers or gastritis, should not be used long term.	None	Dosage of polygala is 1.5–3 g of dried root, 1.5–3 g of a fluid extract, or 2.5–7.5 g of a tincture. A polygala tea can also be made, with a maximum of three cups per day.	None
Rehmannia	Iridoid glycosides	Stimulates the release of cortisol. Used in lupus, rheumatoid arthritis (RA), fibromyalgia, and multiple sclerosis. May improve asthma and urticaria. Used to treat menopause, hair loss, and impotence.	Loose bowel movements, bloating, nausea, and abdominal cramps.	None	Exact dosage unknown	None
Rhodiola rosea	Potentiator, monoterpene alcohols, flavonoids					

S-Adenosyl-L-methionine (SAMe)	S-adenosyl-L-methionine	Used for arthritis and fibromyalgia, may be effective as an augmentation strategy for SSRI in depression.	GI symptoms, anxiety, nightmares, insomnia, and worsening of Parkinson's symptoms.	Use with SSRIs or SNRIs may result in serotonin syndrome. Interacts with levodopa, meperidine, pentazocine, and tramadol.	400–1,600 mg/day	A naturally occurring molecule made from the amino acid methionine and ATP, serves as a methyl donor in human cellular metabolism.
Scarlet Pimpernel, *L. Anagallis arvensis*	Flavonoids, triterpenes, cucurbitacins, caffeic acids	Antidepressant	Overdose or long-term doses may lead to gastroenteritis and nephritis	Undetermined	1.8 g of powder four times a day	Flowers are poisonous.
Skullcap, *L. Scutellaria lateriflora*	Flavonoid, monoterpenes	Anxiolytic, sedative, hypnotic	Cognitive impairment, hepatotoxicity	Disulfiram-like reaction may occur if used with alcohol	1–2 g/day	Little information exists to support the use of this herb in humans.
St. John's wort, *L. Hypericum perforatum*	Hypericin, flavonoids, xanthones	Antidepressant, sedative, anxiolytic	Headaches, photosensitivity (may be severe), constipation	Report of manic reaction when used with sertraline (Zoloft); do not combine with SSRIs or MAOIs: possible serotonin syndrome; do not use with alcohol, opioids	100–950 mg/day	Under investigation by the NIH; may act as MAOI or SSRI; 4- to 6-wk trial for mild depressive moods; if no apparent improvement, another therapy should be tried.
Strawberry leaf, *L. Fragaria vesca*	Flavonoids, tannins	Anxiolytic	Contraindicated with strawberry allergy	Undetermined	1 g/day	Little information exists to support the use of this herb in humans.
Tarragon, *L. Artemisia dracunculus*	Flavonoids, hydroxycoumarins	Hypnotic, appetite stimulant	Undetermined	Undetermined	Undetermined	Little information exists to support the use of this herb in humans.
Valerian, *L. Valeriana officinalis*	Valepotriates, valerenic acid, caffeic acid	Sedative, muscle relaxant, hypnotic	Cognitive and motor impairment, GI upset, hepatotoxicity; long-term use: contact allergy, headache, restlessness, insomnia, mydriasis, cardiac dysfunction	Avoid concomitant use with alcohol or CNS depressants	1–2 g/day	May be chemically unstable
Wild lettuce, *Lactuca, Virosa*	Flavonoids, coumarins, lactones	Sedative, anesthetic, galactagogue	Tachycardia, tachypnea, visual disturbance, diaphoresis		Undetermined	Bitter taste, added to salad or drinks, active compound closely resembles opium
Winter cherry, *withania, somnifera*	Alkaloids, steroidal lactones	Sedative, treatment for arthritis, possible anticarcinogenic	Thyrotoxicosis, unfavorable effects on heart and adrenal gland		Undetermined	Smoke inhaled

ADHD, attention-deficit/hyperactivity disorder; AIDS, acquired immunodeficiency syndrome; ATP, adenosine triphosphate; bid, twice a day; BP, blood pressure; CNS, central nervous system; COPD, chronic obstructive pulmonary disease; FDA, U.S. Food and Drug Administration; GABA, γ-aminobutyric acid; GI, gastrointestinal; MAOI, monoamine oxidase inhibitor; NIH, National Institutes of Health; PAF, platelet-activating factor; PCB, polychlorinated biphenyl; PDE, phosphodiesterase; PMS, premenstrual syndrome; NSAID, nonsteroidal anti-inflammatory drug; OCD, obsessive-compulsive disorder; qid, four times a day; SNRI, serotonin and norepinephrine reuptake inhibitor; SSRI, selective serotonin reuptake inhibitor; TCA tricyclic antidepressant; tid, three times a day; UTI, urinary tract infection.

[a]There are no reliable, consistent, or valid data exist on dosages or adverse effects of most phytomedicinals.

[b]Flavonoids are common to many herbs. They are plant byproducts that act as antioxidants (i.e., agents that prevent the deterioration of material such as deoxyribonucleic acid [DNA] via oxidation).

should not be crushed. To avoid disrupting normal sleep patterns, it should be dosed early in the day. If taking more than one dose a day, the last dose should be taken approximately 4 to 6 hours prior to going to bed. The recommended dose of phentermine may be different for different patients. Adults under age 60 taking phentermine using 15- to 37.5-mg capsules should take them once per day before breakfast or 1 to 2 hours after breakfast. Instead of taking it once a day, some patients may take 15 to 37.5 mg in divided doses a half hour before meals. An oral resin formulation is available in 15- and 30-mg capsules, which should be taken once per day before breakfast.

Phentermine/Topiramate Extended Release (Qsymia). This drug is a combination of phentermine and topiramate (Topamax). The phentermine/topiramate combination was approved by the FDA in 2012 as an extended-release formulation. Both active agents in this formulation are associated with weight loss through separate mechanisms.

Adverse events associated with the use of this drug may include, but are not limited to, paresthesia, dizziness, dysgeusia, insomnia, constipation, dry mouth, kidney stones, metabolic acidosis, and secondary angle closure glaucoma. Use of this drug is associated with a fivefold increased risk of infants with cleft palate and is classified as pregnancy Category X. As a result, it can only be prescribed by clinicians who have been certified in the use of this drug.

It is available as a tablet and should be administered once daily in the morning with or without food. Avoid dosing with the drug in the evening due to the possibility of insomnia. The recommended dose is as follows: Start treatment with 3.75 mg/23 mg (phentermine/topiramate extended release) daily for 14 days; after 14 days increase the recommended dose to 7.5 mg/46 mg once daily. Evaluate weight loss after 12 weeks of treatment. If at least 3 percent of baseline body weight has not been lost on 7.5 mg/46 mg, discontinue the drug or escalate the dose. To escalate the dose, increase to 11.25 mg/69 mg daily for 14 days; followed by dosing 15 mg/92 mg daily. Evaluate weight loss following dose escalation to 15 mg/92 mg after an additional 12 weeks of treatment. If at least 5 percent of baseline body weight has not been lost on 15 mg/92 mg, discontinue the medication gradually.

Phendimetrazine (Bontril PDM Adipost, Phendiet, Statobex). Phendimetrazine is a sympathomimetic amine that is closely related to the amphetamines. It is classified by the Drug Enforcement Agency (DEA) as a Schedule III controlled substance.

Overall prescribing of this agent is limited. The most commonly used formulation is the 105-mg extended-release capsule, which approximates the action of three 35-mg immediate-release doses taken at 4-hour intervals. The average half-life of elimination when studied under controlled conditions is about 3.7 hours for both the extended-release and immediate-release forms. The absorption half-life of the drug from the immediate-release 35-mg phendimetrazine tablets is appreciably more rapid than the absorption rate of the drug from the extended-release formulation. The major route of elimination is via the kidneys, where most of the drug and metabolites are excreted.

Phendimetrazine contraindications are similar to those of phentermine. They include history of cardiovascular disease (e.g., coronary artery disease, stroke, arrhythmias, congestive heart failure, uncontrolled hypertension, pulmonary hypertension); use during or within 14 days following the administration of MAOIs; hyperthyroidism; glaucoma; agitated states; history of drug abuse; pregnancy; nursing; use in combination with other anorectic agents or CNS stimulants; and known hypersensitivity or idiosyncratic reactions to sympathomimetics. Given the lack of systematic research, phendimetrazine should not be used in combination with over-the-counter preparations and herbal products that claim to promote weight loss.

Phendimetrazine tartrate is considered pregnancy Category X and is contraindicated during pregnancy because weight loss offers no potential benefit to a pregnant woman and may result in fetal harm. Studies with phendimetrazine tartrate sustained release have not been performed to evaluate carcinogenic potential, mutagenic potential, or effects on fertility.

Interactions may occur with MAOIs, alcohol, insulin, and oral hypoglycemic agents. Phendimetrazine may decrease the hypotensive effect of adrenergic neuron blocking drugs. The effectiveness and the safety of phendimetrazine in pediatric patients have not been established. It is not recommended in patients less than 17 years of age.

Adverse reactions reported with phendimetrazine include sweating, flushing, tremor, insomnia, agitation, dizziness, headache, psychosis, and blurred vision. Elevated BP, palpitations, and tachycardia are common. GI side effects include dry mouth, nausea, stomach pain, diarrhea, and constipation. Genitourinary side effects include frequency, dysuria, and changes in libido.

Phendimetrazine tartrate is related chemically and pharmacologically to the amphetamines. Amphetamines and related stimulant drugs have been extensively abused, and the possibility of abuse of phendimetrazine should be kept in mind when evaluating the desirability of including a drug as part of a weight reduction program.

Acute overdose with phendimetrazine may manifest itself by restlessness, confusion, belligerence, hallucinations, and panic states. Fatigue and depression usually follow the central stimulation. Cardiovascular effects include tachycardia, arrhythmias, hypertension or hypotension, and circulatory collapse. GI symptoms include nausea, vomiting, diarrhea, and abdominal cramps. Poisoning may result in convulsions, coma, and death. The management of acute overdose is largely symptomatic. It includes lavage and sedation with a barbiturate. If hypertension is marked, the use of a nitrate or rapid-acting α-receptor–blocking agent should be considered.

Diethylpropion (Tenuate). Diethylpropion preceded its analog, the antidepressant drug bupropion (Wellbutrin). Diethylpropion comes in two formulations: a 25-mg tablet and a 75-mg extended-release tablet (Tenuate Dospan). It is usually taken three times a day, 1 hour before meals (regular tablets), or once a day in midmorning (extended-release tablets). The extended-release tablets should be swallowed whole, never crushed, chewed, or cut. The maximum daily dose is 75 mg.

Side effects include dry mouth, unpleasant taste, restlessness, anxiety, dizziness, depression, tremors, upset stomach, vomiting, and increased urination. Side effects that warrant medical attention include tachycardia, palpitations, blurred vision, skin rash, itching, difficulty breathing, chest pain, fainting, swelling of the ankles or feet, fever, sore throat, chills, and painful urination.

Diethylpropion is classified pregnancy Category B and has a low abuse potential. It is listed as a Schedule IV drug by the DEA.

Orlistat (Xenical, Alli). Orlistat interferes with the absorption of dietary fats, causing reduced caloric intake. It works by inhibiting gastric and pancreatic lipases, the enzymes that break down triglycerides in the intestine. When lipase activity is blocked, triglycerides from the diet are not hydrolyzed into absorbable free fatty acids and are excreted undigested instead. Only trace amounts of orlistat are absorbed systemically; it is almost entirely eliminated through the feces.

The effectiveness of orlistat in promoting weight loss is definite, though modest. When used as part of weight loss program, between 30 and 50 percent of patients can expect a 5 percent or greater decrease in body mass. About 20 percent achieve at least a 10 percent decrease in body mass. After orlistat is stopped, up to a third of people gain the weight they lose.

Among the benefits of orlistat treatment are a decrease in BP and a reduced risk of developing type 2 diabetes.

The most common subjective side effects of orlistat are GI related, and include steatorrhea, flatulence, fecal incontinence, and frequent or urgent bowel movements. To minimize these effects, foods with high fat content should be avoided; a low-fat, reduced calorie diet is advisable. Ironically, orlistat can be used with high-fat content diets to treat constipation that results from treatment with some psychotropic drugs, such as the TCAs. Side effects are most severe when beginning therapy and may decrease in frequency with time. Hepatic and renal injuries are potentially serious side effects of orlistat use. In 2010, new safety information about rare cases of severe liver injury was added to the product label of orlistat. The rate of acute kidney injury is more common among orlistat users than nonusers. It should be used with caution in patients with impaired liver function and renal function, as well as those with an obstructed bile duct and pancreatic disease. Orlistat is contraindicated in malabsorption syndromes, hypersensitivity to orlistat, reduced gallbladder function, and in pregnancy and breastfeeding. Orlistat is rated pregnancy Category X.

Absorption of fat-soluble vitamins and other fat-soluble nutrients is inhibited by the use of orlistat. Multivitamin supplements that contain vitamins A, D, E, K, as well as β-carotene should be taken once a day, preferably at bedtime.

Orlistat can reduce plasma levels of the immunosuppressant cyclosporine (Sandimmune), so the two drugs should therefore not be administered concomitantly. Orlistat can also impair absorption of the antiarrhythmic amiodarone (Nexterone).

At the standard prescription dose of 120 mg three times daily before meals, orlistat prevents approximately 30 percent of dietary fat from being absorbed. Higher doses have not been shown to produce more pronounced effects.

An over-the-counter formulation of orlistat (Alli) is available as 60-mg capsules—half the dosage of prescription orlistat.

Lorcaserin (Belviq). Locaserin is among the newest weight loss drugs approved by the FDA. The exact mechanism of action of lorcaserin is not known, but it most likely decreases food consumption and promotes satiety through selective activation of 5-HT_{2C} receptors on neurons in the hypothalamus.

The effect of multiple oral doses of lorcaserin 15 and 40 mg once daily on QTc interval has been evaluated in healthy subjects. The largest placebo adjusted, baseline-corrected QTc based on QTcI was below 10 milliseconds, the threshold for regulatory concern.

Lorcaserin is absorbed from the GI tract, with peak plasma concentration occurring 1.5 to 2 hours after oral dosing. The absolute bioavailability of lorcaserin has not been determined. Lorcaserin has a plasma half-life of approximately 11 hours; steady state is reached within 3 days after twice daily dosing, and accumulation is estimated to be approximately 70 percent. Lorcaserin can be administered with or without food. Lorcaserin hydrochloride is moderately bound (approximately 70 percent) to human plasma proteins.

It is extensively metabolized in the liver by multiple enzymatic pathways, and the metabolites are excreted in the urine. Lorcaserin and its metabolites are not cleared by hemodialysis. It is not recommended for patients with severe renal impairment (creatinine clearance less than 30 mL per minute) or patients with end-stage renal disease.

The half-life of lorcaserin is prolonged by 59 percent to 19 hours in patients with moderate hepatic impairment. Lorcaserin exposure (area under the curve) is approximately 22 and 30 percent higher in patients with mild and moderate hepatic impairment, respectively. Dose adjustment is not required for patients with mild to moderate hepatic impairment.

The recommended dosage is 10 mg twice a day, clinicians should evaluate weight loss at 12 weeks and if the weight loss is less than 5 percent of body weight the drug should be discontinued.

No dosage adjustment based on gender is necessary because it did not meaningfully affect the pharmacokinetics of lorcaserin. No dosage adjustment is required based on age alone.

Lorcaserin significantly inhibits CYP2D6-mediated metabolism.

Drugs without U.S. Food and Drug Administration Approval for Weight Loss

Topiramate. Topiramate and zonisamide (Zonegran) are discussed more fully on pages 545–547, but are mentioned here because both agents can have a substantial effect on weight loss.

Topiramate is approved as an antiepileptic drug and for prevention in adults of migraine headaches. The degree of weight loss associated with topiramate may be comparable to the weight loss that other FDA-approved antiobesity drugs induce. Small studies and extensive anecdotal reports indicate that topiramate can help to offset weight gain associated with SSRIs and SGA drugs. Its impact on body weight may be due to its effects on both appetite suppression and satiety enhancement. These may be the result of a combination of pharmacological effects including augmenting GABA activity, modulation of voltage-gated ion channels, inhibition of excitatory glutamate receptors, or inhibition of carbonic anhydrase.

The duration and dosage of treatment affect the weight loss benefits of topiramate. Weight loss is higher when the drug is prescribed at doses of 100 to 200 mg per day for more than a month compared with less than a month. In a large study it was shown that compared to those who took placebo, topiramate-treated patients were seven times more likely to lose more than 10 percent of their body weight. In clinical practice, many patients experience weight loss at a starting dose of 25 mg per day.

The most common side effects of topiramate are paresthesias, typically around the mouth, impaired taste (taste perversion), and psychomotor disturbances, including slowed cognition and reduced physical movements. Concentration and memory impairment, often characterized by word finding and name recall problems, is often reported. Some patients may experience emotional lability and mood changes. Medical side effects include increased risk of kidney stones and acute-angle closure glaucoma. Patients should report any change in visual acuity. Those with a history of kidney stones should be instructed to drink adequate amounts of fluid.

Topiramate is available as 25-, 50- 100-, and 200-mg tablets and as 15-, 25-, and 50-mg capsules.

Zonisamide. Zonisamide is a sulfonamide-related drug, similar in many ways to topiramate. Its exact mechanism of action is not known. Like topiramate, it can cause cognitive problems, but the incidence is lower than that with topiramate.

Zonisamide has been assigned to pregnancy Category C. Animal studies have revealed evidence of teratogenicity. Fetal abnormalities or embryo-fetal deaths have been reported in animal tests at zonisamide dosage and maternal plasma levels similar to, or lower than, human therapeutic levels. Therefore, use of this drug in human pregnancy may expose the fetus to significant risk.

The most common side effects include drowsiness, loss of appetite, dizziness, headache, nausea, and agitation or irritability. Zonisamide has also been associated with hypohidrosis. There is a 2 to 4 percent risk of kidney stones. Other drugs known to provoke stones, such as topiramate or acetazolamide (Diamox), should not be combined with zonisamide. Serious, but rare, adverse drug reactions include Stevens–Johnson syndrome, toxic epidermal necrolysis, and metabolic acidosis.

Typical dosing for weight loss has not been established. Generally, zonisamide is started at 100 mg at night for 2 weeks, and increased by 100 mg daily every 2 weeks to a target dose of 200 to 600 mg per day in one or two daily doses.

Metformin (Glucophage). Metformin is a medication for type 2 diabetes mellitus. Its actions include reduction of hepatic glucose production, reduced intestinal glucose absorption, increased insulin sensitivity, and improved peripheral glucose uptake and regulation. It does not increase insulin secretion.

When used as an adjunct to SGAs, it has consistently been shown to reduce body weight and waist circumference. Metformin probably has the best evidence of therapeutic benefit for the treatment of antipsychotic drug–induced metabolic syndrome. In several studies, metformin has been shown to attenuate or reverse some of the weight gain induced by antipsychotics. The degree of effect on body weight compares favorably with the effect of other treatment options that are approved for weight reduction. The weight loss effect of adjunctive metformin appears to be stronger in drug-naive patients treated with SGA medications. This effect is most evident for those being treated with clozapine (Clozaril) and olanzapine (Zyprexa). Based on the existing evidence, if weight gain occurs after SGA initiation, despite lifestyle intervention, metformin should be considered.

Common side effects include nausea, vomiting, abdominal pain, and loss of appetite. GI side effects can be mitigated by dividing the dose, taking the drug after meals, or using delayed-release formulations.

One serious treatment risk is that of lactic acidosis. This side effect is more common in those with reduced renal function. Although very rare (approximately 9 in 100,000 persons per year), it has a 50 percent mortality rate. Alcohol use along with metformin can increase the risk of acidosis. Renal function monitoring and alcohol avoidance are important.

The weight loss effects of metformin are also evident in chronically ill patients with schizophrenia. Long-term use of metformin appears to be safe and effective.

There is no clearly established dose range for metformin when used as an adjunct for weight loss. In most reports, the usual dose ranged from 500 to 2,000 mg per day. The maximum dose used in treating diabetes is 850 mg three times daily. Patients usually start with a low dose to see how the drug affects them.

Metformin is available in 500-, 850-, and 1,000-mg tablets, all now generic. Metformin SR (slow release) or XR (extended release) is available in 500- and 750-mg strengths. These formulations are intended to reduce GI side effects and to increase patient compliance by reducing pill burden.

Amphetamine. Amphetamine is a psychostimulant approved for the treatment of ADHD and narcolepsy. It has the effect of reducing appetite and has been used off label for that purpose for many years. Some of the drugs discussed above have amphetamine-like properties, which account for their effectiveness.

26 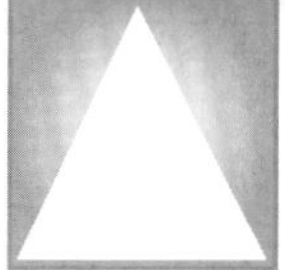

Brain Stimulation Methods

▲ 26.1 Electroconvulsive Therapy

Convulsive therapies for major psychiatric illnesses predate the modern therapeutic era, with the use of camphor reported as early as the 16th century and the existence of several accounts of camphor convulsive therapies from the late 1700s to the mid-1800s.

Unaware of the history of camphor convulsive therapy, the Hungarian neuropsychiatrist Ladislas von Meduna made the observation that the brains of epileptics had greater than normal numbers of glial cells, whereas those of schizophrenics had fewer, and he hypothesized that there might be a biological antagonism between convulsions and schizophrenia. Following animal experimentation, camphor was (again) selected as the appropriate agent to use for the therapeutic induction of seizures. In 1934, the first catatonic psychotic patient was successfully treated using intramuscular injections of camphor in oil to produce therapeutic seizures. Lucio Bini and Ugo Cerletti were interested in the use of electricity to induce seizures, and, after a series of animal experiments and observation of the use of electricity commercially, they were able to safely apply current across the heads of animals for this purpose. In 1938, the first electroconvulsive treatment (ECT) course was administered to a delusional and incoherent patient, who improved with 1 treatment and remitted after 11 treatments. Electrical induction of convulsive therapy could be made more reliable and shorter acting than chemically induced convulsive therapies, and, by the early 1940s, it had replaced them. In 1940, the first use of ECT occurred in the United States.

In an effort to reduce the retrograde memory problems that persisted for some patients after the initial recovery period post-ECT, explorations of nondominant electrode placement and alternative, more efficient waveforms were undertaken in subsequent decades. The practice of ECT also benefited from the introduction of controlled trials methodology, which demonstrated its safety and efficacy, and from refinements made in diagnostic systems and the process of informed consent. In the 1980s and 1990s efforts to ensure uniformly high standards of practice were under way with the publication of recommendations for treatment delivery, education, and training by professional organizations in the United States, England, Scandinavia, and Canada, among others.

With the widespread use of pharmacological agents as first-line treatments for major psychiatric disorders, ECT is now more commonly used for patients with resistance to those treatments, except in the case of life-threatening illness due to inanition, severe suicidal symptoms, or catatonia. Although the failure of subconvulsive stimulation to induce the remission of psychiatric illness and the effectiveness of chemical convulsive therapy suggested that the seizure was necessary and sufficient for therapeutic benefit with ECT, it is now known that there is a dose–response relationship with right unilateral ECT and that bilateral ECT is likely to be ineffective with ultrabrief pulse widths. Work continues to explore the underlying mechanisms and biological characteristics of effective ECT treatments, with interest in having the treatment focus on appropriate neural networks with a more efficient stimulus as a method of reducing cognitive side effects. With the growing understanding that depression is a chronic disease for many patients, more emphasis has been placed on continuation and maintenance treatments following an acute course of ECT. Utilization of ECT has diminished since the middle of the 20th century; but because ECT remains the most effective treatment for major depression and a rapidly effective treatment for life-threatening psychiatric conditions, ECT, unlike its contemporaneous somatic therapies, such as insulin coma, remains in the active treatment portfolio of modern therapeutics. Its use has shifted from public to private institutions, and it is estimated that approximately 100,000 patients have received ECT annually over the past few decades in the United States (Table 26.1–1).

The Nobel laureate Paul Greengard has suggested that the term *electrocortical therapy* might be used to replace the current term electroconvulsive therapy. Greengard has acknowledged that if the mechanism of action of ECT, as yet unknown, turns out to be subcortical, then the term might have limited use. Until that time, however, the authors of this text think Greengard's suggestion deserves consideration. It would help diminish the fear associated with the word convulsion and help destigmatize a very effective treatment method.

ELECTROPHYSIOLOGY IN ELECTROCONVULSIVE THERAPY

Neurons maintain a resting potential across the plasma membrane and may propagate an action potential, which is a transient reversal of the membrane potential. Normal brain activity is desynchronized; that is, neurons fire action potentials asynchronously. A convulsion, or seizure, occurs when a large percentage of neurons fire in unison. Such rhythmical changes in the extracellular potential entrain neighboring neurons, propagate the seizure activity across the cortex and into deeper structures, and eventually engulf the entire brain in high-voltage

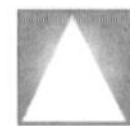

Table 26.1–1
Milestones in the History of Convulsive Therapy

1500s	Paracelsus induces seizures by administering camphor (by mouth) to treat psychiatric illness.
1785	First published report of the use of seizure induction to treat mania, again using camphor.
1934	Ladislaus Meduna begins the modern era of convulsive therapy using intramuscular injection of camphor for catatonic schizophrenia. Camphor is soon replaced with pentylenetetrazol.
1938	Lucio Cerletti and Ugo Bini conduct the first electrical induction of a series of seizures in a catatonic patient and produce a successful treatment response.
1940	ECT is introduced to the United States.
	Curare developed for use as a muscle relaxant at ECT.
1951	Introduction of succinylcholine.
1958	First controlled study of unilateral ECT.
1960	Attenuation of seizure expression with an anticonvulsant agent (lidocaine [Dalcaine]) reduces the efficacy of ECT. Subconvulsive treatment produces only weak clinical responses; the hypothesis that seizure activity is necessary and sufficient for efficacy is upheld.
1960s	Randomized clinical trials of the efficacy of ECT vs. medications in the treatment of depression yield response rates that are significantly higher with ECT.
	Comparisons of neuroleptics and ECT show that neuroleptic medication is superior for acute treatment, although ECT may be more effective in the long term.
1970	The most common electrode positioning for right unilateral ECT developed.
1976	A constant current, brief pulse ECT device, the prototype for modern devices, is developed.
1978	The American Psychiatric Association publishes the first Task Force Report on ECT with the aim of establishing standards for consent and the technical and clinical aspects of the conduct of ECT.
Late 1970s–early 1980s	Randomized, controlled trials demonstrate that ECT is more effective than sham treatment for major depression.
1985	The National Institutes of Health and National Institute of Mental Health Consensus Conference on ECT endorse a role for the use of ECT and advocate research and national standards of practice.
1987	The belief that the seizure in itself is sufficient for clinical response is challenged by H. A. Sackheim and collaborators, who report that the combination of dosage just above seizure threshold and right unilateral electrode placement, while producing a seizure of sufficient duration, is ineffective.
1988	Randomized, controlled clinical trials of ECT vs. lithium (Eskalith) demonstrate them to be equally effective in mania.
2000	In controlled trials, the dose–response relationship for right unilateral ECT is validated; high-dose right unilateral and bilateral ECT show equal response rates in major depression, but right unilateral electrode placement is associated with fewer adverse cognitive effects.
	Convulsive treatment is induced with magnetic stimulation by S. H. Lisanby and colleagues.
2001	The largest modern controlled trial of relapse prevention post-ECT with continuation pharmacotherapy demonstrates a significantly better outcome for combined treatment with a tricyclic antidepressant (nortriptyline) plus lithium compared with nortriptyline alone or placebo during the first 6 months post-ECT.

ECT, electroconvulsive therapy.

synchronous neuronal firing. Cellular mechanisms work to contain the seizure activity and to maintain cellular homeostasis, and the seizure eventually ends. In epilepsy, any of possibly several hundred genetic defects can alter the balance in favor of unrestrained activity. In ECT, seizures are triggered in normal neurons by application through the scalp of pulses of current, under conditions that are carefully controlled to create a seizure of a particular duration over the entire brain.

The qualities of the electricity used in ECT can be described by Ohm's law: $E = IR$, or $I = E/R$, in which E is voltage, I is current, and R is resistance. The intensity or dose of electricity in ECT is measured in terms of charge (milliampere-seconds or millicoulombs) or energy (watt-seconds or joules). Resistance is synonymous with impedance. In ECT, since both electrodes are in contact with the body, the bodily tissues are major determinants of resistance. The skull has a high impedance; the brain has a low impedance. Because scalp tissues are much better conductors of electricity than bone, only about 20 percent of the applied charge actually enters the skull to excite neurons. The ECT machines that are now widely used can be adjusted to administer the electricity under conditions of constant current, voltage, or energy.

MECHANISM OF ACTION

The induction of a bilateral generalized seizure is necessary for both the beneficial and the adverse effects of ECT. Although a seizure superficially seems as though it is an all-or-none event, some data indicate that not all generalized seizures involve all the neurons in deep brain structures (e.g., the basal ganglia and the thalamus); recruitment of these deep neurons may be necessary for full therapeutic benefit. After the generalized seizure, the electroencephalogram (EEG) shows about 60 to 90 seconds of postictal suppression. This period is followed by the appearance of high-voltage delta and theta waves and a return of the EEG to preseizure appearance in about 30 minutes. During the course of a series of ECT treatments, the interictal EEG is generally slower and of greater amplitude than usual, but the EEG returns to pretreatment appearance 1 month to 1 year after the end of the course of treatment.

One research approach to the mechanism of action for ECT has been to study the neurophysiological effects of treatment. Positron emission tomography (PET) studies of both cerebral blood flow and glucose use have shown that, during seizures, cerebral blood flow, use of glucose and oxygen, and permeability of the blood–brain barrier increase. After the seizure, blood flow and glucose metabolism are decreased, perhaps most markedly in the frontal lobes. Some research indicates that the degree of decrease in cerebral metabolism is correlated with therapeutic response.

Seizure foci in idiopathic epilepsy are hypometabolic during interictal periods; ECT itself acts as an anticonvulsant because its administration is associated with an increase in the seizure threshold as treatment progresses. Recent data suggest that for 1 to 2 months following a session of ECT, EEGs record a large increase in slow-wave activity located over the prefrontal cortex in patients who responded well to the ECT. High-intensity, bilateral stimulation produced the best response; low-intensity, unilateral stimulation, the weakest. These data are of unclear significance, however, because the specific EEG correlate disappeared 2 months after ECT, whereas the clinical benefit persisted.

ECT affects the cellular mechanisms of memory and mood regulation and raises the seizure threshold. The latter effect may be blocked by the opiate antagonist naloxone (Narcan).

Neurochemical research into the mechanisms of action of ECT has focused on changes in neurotransmitter receptors and, recently, changes in second-messenger systems. Virtually every neurotransmitter system is affected by ECT, but a series of ECT sessions results in downregulation of postsynaptic β-adrenergic receptors, the same receptor change observed with virtually all antidepressant treatments. The effects of ECT on serotonergic neurons remain controversial. Various research studies have reported an increase in postsynaptic serotonin receptors, no change in serotonin receptors, and a change in the presynaptic regulation of serotonin release. ECT has also been reported to effect changes in the muscarinic, cholinergic, and dopaminergic neuronal systems. In second-messenger systems, ECT has been reported to affect the coupling of G proteins to receptors, the activity of adenylyl cyclase and phospholipase C, and the regulation of calcium entry into neurons.

Recently, there has been increased interest in structural changes in the brain associated with psychiatric syndromes and response to treatment. This has been particularly so for microscopic changes associated with electroconvulsive stimulation, as well as antidepressant and other medications. In animals, mostly rodents, synaptic plasticity in hippocampus, including mossy fiber sprouting, alterations in cytoskeletal structure, increased connectivity in perforant pathways, promotion of neurogenesis, and suppression of apoptosis have been observed. Many of these structural events are also observed, although to a lesser extent, with antidepressant medications such as fluoxetine (Prozac). These reports have also galvanized controversy over various aspects of the technical validity of the observations. It is unknown whether such changes occur clinically and, if they do, what significance to efficacy and cognitive side effects might be discovered.

Table 26.1–2
Indications for the Use of Electroconvulsive Therapy

Diagnoses for which ECT may be indicated

Major diagnostic indications

Major depression, both unipolar and bipolar
Psychotic depression in particular
Mania, including mixed episodes
Schizophrenia with acute exacerbation
Catatonic subtype
Schizoaffective disorder

Other diagnostic indications

Parkinson's disease
Neuroleptic malignant disorder
Clinical indications

Primary use

Rapid definitive response required on medical or psychiatric grounds
Risks of alternative treatments outweigh benefits
Past history of poor response to psychotropics or good response to ECT
Patient preference

Secondary use

Failure to respond to pharmacotherapy in the current episode
Intolerance of pharmacotherapy in the current episode
Rapid definitive response necessitated by deterioration of the patient's condition

ECT, electroconvulsive therapy.

INDICATIONS

Major Depressive Disorder

The most common indication for ECT is major depressive disorder, for which ECT is the fastest and most effective available therapy. ECT should be considered for use in patients who have failed medication trials, have not tolerated medications, have severe or psychotic symptoms, are acutely suicidal or homicidal, or have marked symptoms of agitation or stupor. Controlled studies have shown that up to 70 percent of patients who fail to respond to antidepressant medications may respond positively to ECT. Table 26.1–2 presents the indications for the use of ECT.

ECT is effective for depression in both major depressive disorder and bipolar I disorder. Delusional or psychotic depression has long been considered particularly responsive to ECT; but recent studies have indicated that major depressive episodes with psychotic features are no more responsive to ECT than nonpsychotic depressive disorders. Nevertheless, because major depressive episodes with psychotic features respond poorly to antidepressant pharmacotherapy alone, ECT should be considered much more often as the first-line treatment for patients with the disorder. Major depressive disorder with melancholic features (e.g., markedly severe symptoms, psychomotor retardation, early morning awakening, diurnal variation, decreased appetite and weight, and agitation) is considered likely to respond to ECT. ECT is particularly indicated for persons who are severely depressed, who have psychotic symptoms, who show suicidal intent, or who refuse to eat. Depressed patients less likely to respond to ECT include those with somatization disorder. Elderly patients tend to respond to ECT more slowly than do young patients. ECT is a treatment for major depressive episode and does not provide prophylaxis unless it is administered on a long-term maintenance basis.

Manic Episodes

ECT is at least equal to lithium (Eskalith) in the treatment of acute manic episodes. The pharmacological treatment of manic episodes, however, is so effective in the short term and for prophylaxis that the use of ECT to treat manic episodes is generally limited to situations with specific contraindications to all available pharmacological approaches. The relative rapidity of the ECT response indicates its usefulness for patients whose manic behavior has produced dangerous levels of exhaustion. ECT should not be used for a patient who is receiving lithium, because lithium can lower the seizure threshold and cause a prolonged seizure.

Schizophrenia

Although an effective treatment for the symptoms of acute schizophrenia, ECT is not for those of chronic schizophrenia. Patients with schizophrenia who have marked positive symptoms, catatonia, or affective symptoms are considered most likely to respond to ECT. In such patients, the efficacy of ECT is about equal to that of antipsychotics, but improvement may occur faster.

Other Indications

Small studies have found ECT effective in the treatment of catatonia, a symptom associated with mood disorders, schizophrenia, and medical and neurological disorders. ECT is also reportedly useful to treat episodic psychoses, atypical psychoses, obsessive-compulsive disorder, and delirium and such medical conditions as neuroleptic malignant syndrome, hypopituitarism, intractable seizure disorders, and the on–off phenomenon of Parkinson's disease. ECT may also be the treatment of choice for depressed suicidal pregnant women who require treatment and cannot take medication; for geriatric and medically ill patients who cannot take antidepressant drugs safely; and perhaps even for severely depressed and suicidal children and adolescents who may be less likely to respond to antidepressant drugs than are adults. ECT is not effective in somatization disorder (unless accompanied by depression), personality disorders, and anxiety disorders.

CLINICAL GUIDELINES

Patients and their families are often apprehensive about ECT; therefore, clinicians must explain both beneficial and adverse effects and alternative treatment approaches. The informed-consent process should be documented in the patients' medical records and should include a discussion of the disorder, its natural course, and the option of receiving no treatment. Printed literature and videotapes about ECT may be useful in attempting to obtain a truly informed consent. The use of involuntary ECT is rare today and should be reserved for patients who urgently need treatment and who have a legally appointed guardian who has agreed to its use. Clinicians must know local, state, and federal laws about the use of ECT.

Pretreatment Evaluation

Pretreatment evaluation should include standard physical, neurological, and preanesthesia examinations and a complete medical history. Laboratory evaluations should include blood and urine chemistries, a chest x-ray, and an electrocardiogram (ECG). A dental examination to assess the state of patients' dentition is advisable for elderly patients and patients who have had inadequate dental care. An x-ray of the spine is needed if other evidence of a spinal disorder is seen. Computed tomography (CT) or magnetic resonance imaging (MRI) should be performed if a clinician suspects the presence of a seizure disorder or a space-occupying lesion. Practitioners of ECT no longer consider even a space-occupying lesion to be an absolute contraindication to ECT, but with such patients the procedure should be performed only by experts.

Concomitant Medications

Patients' ongoing medications should be assessed for possible interactions with the induction of a seizure, for effects (both positive and negative) on the seizure threshold, and for drug interactions with the medications used during ECT. The use of tricyclic and tetracyclic drugs, monoamine oxidase inhibitors, and antipsychotics is generally considered acceptable. Benzodiazepines used for anxiety should be withdrawn because of their anticonvulsant activity; lithium should be withdrawn because it can result in increased postictal delirium and can prolong seizure activity; clozapine (Clozaril) and bupropion (Wellbutrin) should be withdrawn because they are associated with the development of late-appearing seizures. Lidocaine (Xylocaine) should not be administered during ECT because it markedly increases the seizure threshold; theophylline (Theo-Dur) is contraindicated because it increases the duration of seizures. Reserpine (Serpasil) is also contraindicated because it is associated with further compromise of the respiratory and cardiovascular systems during ECT.

Premedications, Anesthetics, and Muscle Relaxants

Patients should not be given anything orally for 6 hours before treatment. Just before the procedure, the patient's mouth should be checked for dentures and other foreign objects, and an intravenous (IV) line should be established. A bite block is inserted in the mouth just before the treatment is administered to protect the patient's teeth and tongue during the seizure. Except for the brief interval of electrical stimulation, 100 percent oxygen is administered at a rate of 5 L a minute during the procedure until spontaneous respiration returns. Emergency equipment for establishing an airway should be immediately available in case it is needed.

Muscarinic Anticholinergic Drugs. Muscarinic anticholinergic drugs are administered before ECT to minimize oral and respiratory secretions and to block bradycardias and asystoles, unless the resting heart rate is above 90 beats a minute. Some ECT centers have stopped the routine use of anticholinergics as premedications, although their use is still indicated for patients taking β-adrenergic receptor antagonists and those with ventricular ectopic beats. The most commonly used drug is atropine, which can be administered 0.3 to 0.6 mg intramuscularly (IM) or subcutaneously (SC) 30 to 60 minutes before the anesthetic or 0.4 to 1.0 mg IV 2 or 3 minutes before the anesthetic. An option is to use glycopyrrolate (Robinul) (0.2 to 0.4 mg IM, IV, or SC), which is less likely to cross the blood–brain barrier and less likely to cause cognitive dysfunction and nausea, although it is thought to have less cardiovascular protective activity than does atropine.

Anesthesia. Administration of ECT requires general anesthesia and oxygenation. The depth of anesthesia should be as light as possible, not only to minimize adverse effects but also to avoid elevating the seizure threshold associated with many anesthetics. Methohexital (Brevital) (0.75 to 1.0 mg/kg IV bolus) is the most commonly used anesthetic because of its shorter duration of action and lower association with postictal arrhythmias than thiopental (Pentothal) (usual dose 2 to 3 mg/kg IV), although this difference in cardiac effects is not universally accepted. Four other anesthetic alternatives are etomidate (Amidate), ketamine (Ketalar), alfentanil (Alfenta), and propofol (Diprivan). Etomidate (0.15 to 0.3 mg/kg IV) is sometimes used because it does not increase the seizure threshold; this effect is particularly useful for elderly patients because the seizure threshold increases with age. Ketamine (6 to 10 mg/kg IM) is sometimes used because it does not increase the seizure threshold, although its use is limited by the frequent association of psychotic symptoms with emergence from anesthesia with this drug. Alfentanil (2 to 9 mg/kg IV) is sometimes coadministered with barbiturates to allow the use of low doses of the barbiturate anesthetics and, thus, reduce the seizure threshold less than usual, although its use can be associated with an increased incidence of nausea. Propofol (0.5 to 3.5 mg/kg IV) is less useful because of its strong anticonvulsant properties.

Muscle Relaxants. After the onset of the anesthetic effect, usually within a minute, a muscle relaxant is administered to minimize the risk of bone fractures and other injuries resulting from motor activity during the seizure. The goal is to produce profound relaxation of the muscles, not necessarily to paralyze them, unless the patient has a history of osteoporosis or spinal injury or has a pacemaker and, therefore, is at risk for injury related to motor activity during the seizure. Succinylcholine (Anectine), an ultrafast-acting depolarizing blocking agent, has gained virtually universal acceptance for the purpose. Succinylcholine is usually administered in a dose of 0.5 to 1 mg/kg as an IV bolus or drip. Because succinylcholine is a depolarizing agent, its action is marked by the presence of muscle fasciculations, which move in a rostrocaudal progression. The disappearance of these movements in the feet or the absence of muscle contractions after peripheral nerve stimulation indicates maximal muscle relaxation. In some patients, tubocurarine (3 mg IV) is administered to prevent myoclonus and increases in potassium and muscle enzymes; these reactions can be a problem in patients with musculoskeletal or cardiac disease. To monitor the duration of the convulsion, a blood pressure cuff may be inflated at the ankle to a pressure in excess of the systolic pressure before infusion of the muscle relaxant to allow observation of relatively innocuous seizure activity in the foot muscles.

If a patient has a known history of pseudocholinesterase deficiency, atracurium (Tracrium) (0.5 to 1 mg/kg IV) or curare can be used instead of succinylcholine. In such a patient, the metabolism of succinylcholine is disrupted, and prolonged apnea may necessitate emergency airway management. In general, however, because of the short half-life of succinylcholine, the duration of apnea after its administration is generally shorter than the delay in regaining consciousness caused by the anesthetic and the postictal state.

Electrode Placement. Historically, most practitioners have used bifrontotemporal electrode placement because of its reliability in producing efficacy and its ease of use. This electrode placement is also associated with more short-term and long-term adverse cognitive effects and is more likely to produce delirium, which may require interrupting a course of ECT and perhaps even terminating it before optimal therapeutic effects have been obtained. Hence, when bifrontotemporal ECT is used, attention should be paid to restricting the dose to a moderately suprathreshold level to attenuate adverse cognitive effects as much as possible. It should be emphasized that the combination of ultrabrief pulse and bifrontotemporal electrode placement has not been demonstrated to be effective. Treatment with bilateral electrode placements, particularly a bifrontal configuration, is more likely to manifest EEG seizure without motor seizure, and EEG monitoring can be particularly useful in detecting its occurrence.

Newer electrode placements include bifrontal configuration and asymmetrical placements. There are limitations to these strategies, imposed by the fact that the high impedance of the skull and scalp causes spreading of the electrical stimulus and restricts possibilities for localization of the stimulus. Bifrontal electrode placement, with positioning far enough laterally to minimize interference with impedance relations, has been investigated, and there have been several demonstrations that bifrontal electrode placements are equally effective to bifrontotemporal and adequately dosed right unilateral electrode configurations. Evidence of advantages in sparing of cognitive effects is quite preliminary, and adequately powered investigations with more extensive and sensitive cognitive batteries are needed. Seizure threshold is likely to be relatively higher with bifrontal ECT.

The relatively better cognitive side effect profile of right unilateral ECT should encourage wider use now that the efficacy of this electrode placement can be ensured with adequate dosing strategies. In contrast to bilateral ECT, a dose closer to 500 percent above the seizure threshold is more likely to ensure efficacy. ECT devices in the United States are restricted to an output in the range of 504 to 576 mCi. Approximately 90 percent of patients have seizure thresholds that can accommodate optimal dosing with brief-pulse right unilateral ECT, and the combination of right unilateral electrode placement with ultrabrief pulse width extends the range of US devices so that most patients can be treated within these constraints. Individuals with an exceptionally high seizure threshold may require bilateral electrode placements to remain within the device restrictions. Maximizing interelectrode distance by using the d'Elia placement may also be optimal. Many other right unilateral placements have been described, but there is little work to support their use.

There has been some concern that left-handed patients may require different electrode placement than right-handed patients, especially if unilateral placement is desired. Even when handedness is lateralized to the left, the anatomic localization of language function in 70 percent of left-handed individuals is the same as in those who are right-handed. Furthermore, there is evidence for independent lateralization of affect, with the right hemisphere involved in sustaining depressed mood regardless of handedness. Because of limited indications that affective function and efficacy of ECT are associated with handedness, handedness is not generally used to guide the choice of electrode placement.

Electrical Stimulus

The electrical stimulus must be sufficiently strong to reach the seizure threshold (the level of intensity needed to produce a seizure). The electrical stimulus is given in cycles, and each cycle contains a positive and a negative wave. Old machines use a sine wave; however, this type of machine is now considered obsolete because of the inefficiency of that wave shape. When a sine wave is delivered, the electrical stimulus in the sine wave before the seizure threshold is reached and after the seizure is activated is unnecessary and excessive. Modern ECT machines use a brief pulse waveform that administers the electrical stimulus usually in 1 to 2 milliseconds at a rate of 30 to 100 pulses a second. Machines that use an ultrabrief pulse (0.5 milliseconds) are not as effective as brief pulse machines.

Establishing a patient's seizure threshold is not straightforward. A 40 times variability in seizure thresholds occurs among patients. In addition, during the course of ECT treatment, a patient's seizure threshold may increase 25 to 200 percent. The seizure threshold is also higher in men than in women and higher in older than in younger adults. A common technique is to initiate treatment at an electrical stimulus that is thought to be below the seizure threshold for a particular patient and then to increase this intensity by 100 percent for unilateral placement and by 50 percent for bilateral placement until the seizure threshold is reached. A debate in the literature concerns whether a minimally suprathreshold dose, a moderately suprathreshold dose (one and a half times the threshold), or a high suprathreshold dose (three times the threshold) is preferable. The debate about stimulus intensity resembles the debate about electrode placement. Essentially, the data support the conclusion that doses of three times the threshold are the most rapidly effective and that minimal suprathreshold doses are associated with the fewest and least severe cognitive adverse effects.

Induced Seizures

A brief muscular contraction, usually strongest in a patient's jaw and facial muscles, is seen concurrently with the flow of stimulus current, regardless of whether a seizure occurs. The first behavioral sign of the seizure is often a plantar extension, which lasts 10 to 20 seconds and marks the tonic phase. This phase is followed by rhythmic (i.e., clonic) contractions that decrease in frequency and finally disappear. The tonic phase is marked by high-frequency, sharp EEG activity on which a higher-frequency muscle artifact may be superimposed. During the clonic phase, bursts of polyspike activity occur simultaneously with the muscular contractions but usually persist for at least a few seconds after the clonic movements stop.

Monitoring Seizures. A physician must have an objective measure that a bilateral generalized seizure has occurred after the stimulation. The physician should be able to observe either some evidence of tonic–clonic movements or electrophysiological evidence of seizure activity from the EEG or electromyogram (EMG). Seizures with unilateral ECT are asymmetrical, with higher ictal EEG amplitudes over the stimulated hemisphere than over the nonstimulated hemisphere. Occasionally, unilateral seizures are induced; for this reason, at least a single pair of EEG electrodes should be placed over the contralateral hemisphere when using unilateral ECT. For a seizure to be effective in the course of ECT, it should last at least 25 seconds.

Failure to Induce Seizures. If a particular stimulus fails to cause a seizure of sufficient duration, up to four attempts at seizure induction can be tried during a course of treatment. The onset of seizure activity is sometimes delayed as long as 20 to 40 seconds after the stimulus administration. If a stimulus fails to result in a seizure, the contact between the electrodes and the skin should be checked, and the intensity of the stimulus should be increased by 25 to 100 percent. The clinician can also change the anesthetic agent to minimize increases in the seizure threshold caused by the anesthetic. Additional procedures to lower the seizure threshold include hyperventilation and administration of 500 to 2,000 mg IV of caffeine sodium benzoate 5 to 10 minutes before the stimulus.

Prolonged and Tardive Seizures. Prolonged seizures (seizures lasting more than 180 seconds) and status epilepticus can be terminated either with additional doses of the barbiturate anesthetic agent or with IV diazepam (Valium) (5 to 10 mg). Management of such complications should be accompanied by intubation, because the oral airway is insufficient to maintain adequate ventilation over an extended apneic period. Tardive seizures—that is, additional seizures appearing sometime after the ECT treatment—may develop in patients with preexisting seizure disorders. Rarely, ECT precipitates the development of an epileptic disorder in patients. Such situations should be managed clinically as if they were pure epileptic disorders.

Number and Spacing of Treatments

ECT treatments are usually administered two to three times a week; twice-weekly treatments are associated with less memory impairment than thrice-weekly treatments. In general, the course of treatment of major depressive disorder can take 6 to 12 treatments (although up to 20 sessions are possible); the treatment of manic episodes can take 8 to 20 treatments; the treatment of schizophrenia can take more than 15 treatments; and the treatment of catatonia and delirium can take as few as 1 to 4 treatments. Treatment should continue until the patient achieves what is considered the maximal therapeutic response. Further treatment does not yield any therapeutic benefit, but increases the severity and duration of the adverse effects. The point of maximal improvement is usually thought to occur when a patient fails to continue to improve after two consecutive treatments. If a patient is not improving after 6 to 10 sessions, bilateral placement and high-density treatment (three times the seizure threshold) should be attempted before ECT is abandoned.

Multiple-Monitored Electroconvulsive Therapy. Multiple-monitored ECT (MMECT) involves giving multiple ECT stimuli during a single session, most commonly two bilateral stimuli within 2 minutes. This approach may be warranted in severely ill patients and in those at especially high risk from the anesthetic procedures. MMECT is associated with the most frequent occurrences of serious cognitive adverse effects.

Maintenance Treatment

A short-term course of ECT induces a remission in symptoms but does not, of itself, prevent a relapse. Post-ECT maintenance treatment should always be considered. Maintenance therapy is generally pharmacological, but maintenance ECT treatments (weekly, biweekly, or monthly) have been reported to be effective relapse prevention treatments, although data from large studies are lacking. Indications for maintenance ECT treatments can include rapid relapse after initial ECT, severe symptoms, psychotic symptoms, and the inability to tolerate medications. If ECT was used because a patient was unresponsive to a specific medication, then, following ECT, the patient should be given a trial of a different medication.

Failure of Electroconvulsive Therapy Trial

Patients who fail to improve after a trial of ECT should again be treated with the pharmacological agents that failed in the past. Although the data are primarily anecdotal, many reports indicate that patients who had previously failed to improve while taking an antidepressant drug do improve while taking the same drug after receiving a course of ECT treatments, even if the ECT seemed to be a therapeutic failure. Nonetheless, with the increased availability of drugs that act at diverse receptor sites, it is less often necessary to return to a drug that has failed than it was formerly.

ADVERSE EFFECTS

Contraindications

ECT has no absolute contraindications, only situations in which a patient is at increased risk and has an increased need for close monitoring. Pregnancy is not a contraindication for ECT, and fetal monitoring is generally considered unnecessary unless the pregnancy is high risk or complicated. Patients with space-occupying central nervous system lesions are at increased risk for edema and brain herniation after ECT. If the lesion is small, however, pretreatment with dexamethasone (Decadron) is given, and hypertension is controlled during the seizure and the risk of serious complications minimized for these patients. Patients who have increased intracerebral pressure or are at risk for cerebral bleeding (e.g., those with cerebrovascular diseases and aneurysms) are at risk during ECT because of the increased cerebral blood flow during the seizure. This risk can be lessened, although not eliminated, by controlling the patient's blood pressure during the treatment. Patients with recent myocardial infarctions are another high-risk group, although the risk is greatly diminished 2 weeks after the myocardial infarction and is even further reduced 3 months after the infarction. Patients with hypertension should be stabilized on their antihypertensive medications before ECT is administered. Propranolol (Inderal) and sublingual nitroglycerin can also be used to protect such patients during treatment.

Mortality

The mortality rate with ECT is about 0.002 percent per treatment and 0.01 percent for each patient. These numbers compare favorably with the risks associated with general anesthesia and childbirth. ECT death is usually from cardiovascular complications and is most likely to occur in patients whose cardiac status is already compromised.

Central Nervous System Effects

Common adverse effects associated with ECT are headache, confusion, and delirium shortly after the seizure while the patient is coming out of anesthesia. Marked confusion may occur in up to 10 percent of patients within 30 minutes of the seizure and can be treated with barbiturates and benzodiazepines. Delirium is usually most pronounced after the first few treatments and in patients who receive bilateral ECT or who have coexisting neurological disorders. The delirium characteristically clears within days or a few weeks at the longest.

Memory. The greatest concern about ECT is the association between ECT and memory loss. About 75 percent of all patients given ECT say that the memory impairment is the worst adverse effect. Although memory impairment during a course of treatment is almost the rule, follow-up data indicate that almost all patients are back to their cognitive baselines after 6 months. Some patients, however, complain of persistent memory difficulties. For example, a patient may not remember the events leading up to the hospitalization and ECT, and such autobiographical memories may never be recalled. The degree of cognitive impairment during treatment and the time it takes to return to baseline are related, in part, to the amount of electrical stimulation used during treatment. Memory impairment is most often reported by patients who have experienced little improvement with ECT. Despite the memory impairment, which usually resolves, no evidence indicates brain damage caused by ECT. This subject has been the focus of several brain-imaging studies, using a variety of modalities; virtually all concluded that permanent brain damage is not an adverse effect of ECT. Neurologists and epileptologists generally agree that seizures that last less than 30 minutes do not cause permanent neuronal damage.

Other Adverse Effects of Electroconvulsive Therapy

Fractures often accompanied treatments in the early days of ECT. With routine use of muscle relaxants, fractures of long bones or vertebrae should not occur. Some patients, however, may break teeth or experience back pain because of contractions during the procedure. Muscle soreness can occur in some individuals, but it often results from the effects of muscle depolarization by succinylcholine and is most likely to be particularly troublesome after the first session in a series. This soreness can be treated with mild analgesics, including nonsteroidal anti-inflammatory drugs (NSAIDs). A significant minority of patients experience nausea, vomiting, and headaches following an ECT treatment. Nausea and vomiting can be prevented by treatment with antiemetics at the time of ECT (e.g., metoclopramide [Reglan], 10 mg IV, or prochlorperazine [Compazine],

10 mg IV; ondansetron [Zofran] is an acceptable alternative if adverse effects preclude use of dopamine receptor antagonists).

ECT can be associated with headaches, although this effect is usually readily manageable. Headaches often respond to NSAIDs given in the ECT recovery period. In patients with severe headaches, pretreatment with ketorolac (Toradol) (30 to 60 mg IV), an NSAID approved for brief parenteral use, can be helpful. Acetaminophen (Tylenol), tramadol (Ultram), propoxyphene (Darvon), and more potent analgesia provided by opioids can be used individually or in various combinations (e.g., pretreatment with ketorolac and postseizure management with acetaminophen-propoxyphene) to manage more intractable headache. ECT can induce migrainous headache and related symptoms; sumatriptan (Imitrex) (6 mg SC or 25 mg orally) may be a useful addition to the agents described above. Ergot compounds can exacerbate cardiovascular changes observed during ECT and probably should not be a component of ECT pretreatment.

INVESTIGATIONS IN ELECTRICAL BRAIN STIMULATION TREATMENT

There is interest in continued refinements of ECT techniques. Common themes in these approaches are focusing the treatment spatially to optimize dosing in brain areas associated with putative neural networks involved in depression and other psychopathologies that are indications for ECT, diminishing dosing in areas associated with adverse cognitive effects, and improving the efficiency of a noninvasive electrical stimulus in direction and amplitude, even to a subconvulsive level. This research is parallel to investigations in magnetic stimulation (e.g., repetitive transcranial magnetic stimulation) and to the renaissance of invasive electrical techniques (e.g., vagal nerve stimulation and deep brain stimulation).

▲ 26.2 Other Brain Stimulation Methods

Brain stimulation in psychiatric practice and research uses electrical currents or magnetic fields to alter neuronal firing. There is a growing list of tools capable of eliciting such neuromodulation, each with a different spectrum of action. These tools either apply electrical or magnetic field transcranially or involve the surgical implantation of electrodes to deliver electrical currents to a cranial nerve or to the brain directly. The transcranial techniques include cranial electrical stimulation (CES), electroconvulsive therapy (ECT), transcranial direct current stimulation (tDCS, also called direct current polarization), transcranial magnetic stimulation (TMS), and magnetic seizure therapy (MST). The surgical techniques include cortical brain stimulation (CBS), deep brain stimulation (DBS), and vagus nerve stimulation (VNS).

In 1985, nearly 50 years after the first use of ECT, Anthony Barker and colleagues published on the first use of pulsed magnetic fields to stimulate the brain with a procedure called *TMS.* TMS was initially used in neurology for studies of nerve conduction, but it quickly caught the attention of psychiatrists eager to explore other, less invasive alternatives to ECT. This nonconvulsive stimulation method through TMS is under active study, with some promising results in the treatment of various psychiatric disorders, including depression, anxiety, and schizophrenia, as described by Sarah H. Lisanby, Leann H. Kinnunen, and colleagues in 2002. In the past decade, a convulsive treatment derived from the application of more powerful magnetic stimulation has been under investigation in nonhuman primates and in human studies in both the United States and Europe. The first MST procedure was performed in an animal in 1998 and in a human in 2000. MST is under development as a more focal means of inducing seizures in an attempt to retain the thus-far-unparalleled efficacy of ECT with fewer cognitive side effects.

Two more recent additions to brain stimulation methods, DBS and VNS, were introduced about a decade following the first trials of TMS. Both were first approved by the U.S. Food and Drug Administration (FDA) in 1997 in the realm of treating sequelae of neurological syndromes. DBS was initially approved for the treatment of essential tremor and Parkinson's tremor, whereas VNS was approved for the treatment of epilepsy. Five years later, in 2002, indications for DBS were expanded to include treatment of all symptoms of Parkinson's disease, including tremor, slowness, and stiffness, as well as involuntary movements induced by medications. TMS, DBS, and VNS originated in the field of neurology. Psychiatrists quickly saw the potential for those tools in the treatment of psychiatric conditions, however, and as a result of clinical trials in depression, VNS subsequently received FDA approval for the adjunctive long-term treatment of chronic or recurrent depression in adults. In addition, human studies are under way to validate the efficacy of DBS in the treatment of depression and obsessive-compulsive disorder.

THERAPEUTIC NEUROMODULATION: TREATING PSYCHIATRIC DISORDERS THROUGH BRAIN STIMULATION

Mechanism of Action

Electrical Stimulation—Common Pathway. The brain stimulation modalities just reviewed generate either electrical or magnetic pulses. However, both of these share a common final pathway—they affect the neurons electrically. That electrical effect may either be through the direct application of electricity or through the indirect induction of electricity via magnetic stimulation. The direct forms of electrical stimulation are exemplified in either *transcranial* delivery, as with ECT, CES, and tDCS, or *intracerebral* delivery, as in the case of DBS or direct cortical stimulation (epidural or subdural). The indirect forms of electrical stimulation include TMS and MST, which induce electrical fields in the brain through the application of alternating magnetic fields. Of note, both the epidural and intracerebral modalities are more focal than the transcranial application of electricity because electrodes are placed directly in the neuronal tissue, bypassing the impedance of the scalp and skull. The relatively more contemporary magnetic stimulation methods (TMS and MST) also bypass the impedance of the scalp and skull and are thus likewise more focal. However, magnetic stimulation is in fact an example of an indirect method of electrical brain stimulation, in that the changing magnetic fields from these devices induce electricity in the brain, the latter acting as a conductor, according to the principle first described by Michael Faraday in a law that bears his name and later incorporated into James

Clerk Maxwell's equations, which unify all of electromagnetism. The magnetic modalities achieve their enhanced focality noninvasively, in contrast to the intracerebral and epidural methods, and are thus at the center of intensive research in that they offer the promise of an unparalleled degree of spatial specificity without the need for surgery.

All but one of the brain stimulation modalities described here act by stimulating neurons. The one exception is tDCS, which does not stimulate but rather polarizes. In this sense, the "S" of tDCS is a misnomer. It is more accurate to conceptualize tDCS as exerting a polarizing effect that may alter the likelihood of neuronal firing.

The action of the subconvulsive modalities of stimulation relies on the effects of the repeated stimulation of the targeted neural circuitry. However, in the case of the convulsive modalities (ECT and MST), the action depends on the seizure induced by the stimulation and the effects of repeated seizure induction on brain processes. This is not to say that the form of stimulation that triggers the seizure has no effect on outcome. Indeed, it is well replicated that electrode placement and electrical stimulus parameters have a profound effect on the efficacy and side effects of ECT. Whether the same will be true for MST is under active investigation.

Acute versus Prolonged Effects. Brain stimulation can have immediate or lasting effects. A single electrical pulse delivered at sufficient intensity can induce depolarization, trigger an action potential, release neurotransmitters at the synapse, and result in transsynaptic propagation with subsequent activation of a functional circuit. For example, brain stimulation applied to the hand area of the primary motor cortex may activate the corticospinal tract and induce a muscle twitch in the contralateral hand. Such stimulation can result acutely in the induction of either a positive effect, as in the case of a muscle twitch or visualization of phosphenes, or a disruptive effect, as in the case of visual masking.

Repetitive pulses delivered at fixed frequencies can exert even more powerful effects. Epstein and colleagues described in 1999 how repetitive TMS (rTMS) applied to the language-dominant hemisphere induced an arrest of speech. After termination of the stimulation, speech returned to normal.

Some more invasive brain stimulation modalities, such as DBS or VNS, are programmed to operate chronically, thus extending the acute action for as long as the stimulation is turned on. In the case of DBS, the pulses are typically given continuously at a high frequency, whereas in the case of VNS the pulses are given in trains lasting up to 30 seconds and typically repeated every 5 minutes. The less invasive modalities, such as rTMS, tDCS, CES, and even ECT, presumably require the induction of some form of neuroplasticity for their effect to become lasting.

TRANSCRANIAL MAGNETIC STIMULATION

Definition

TMS is the application of a rapidly changing magnetic field to the superficial layers of the cerebral cortex, which locally induces small electric currents, also referred to as *eddy* currents. This induction was originally discovered by Faraday through his experiments in 1831 and later quantified in Maxwell's equations of electromagnetism. Thus, TMS may be referred to as electrical stimulation without an electrode, in that it uses magnetic fields to indirectly induce electrical pulses. TMS devices deliver strong magnetic pulses via a coil that is held on the scalp. Because magnetic fields are unaffected by the electrical impedance of the scalp and skull, this method of stimulation enables the focal stimulation of smaller areas of the brain than is possible with other noninvasive devices that use either alternating (ECT, CES) or direct (tDCS) electrical current for primary stimulation. TMS is an example of noninvasive stimulation of focal regions of the brain and, as such, can be used for research or therapeutically without the need for anesthesia.

Mechanisms of Action

At sufficient intensity, electrical currents will stimulate neuronal depolarization, which can result in an action potential. For example, when the TMS coil is positioned over the hand area of the cerebral cortex's motor strip, the changing magnetic field generated by the repetitive pulses induces local currents immediately below the site of stimulation that cause the neurons in area M1 to fire. In turn, this action potential propagates through the polysynaptic corticospinal tract and results in a twitch in the contralateral hand muscle. In summary, TMS uses magnetic fields to indirectly induce focal electrical currents in the brain, thereby triggering the firing of functional neuronal circuits that can lead to observable behavioral effects. This effect can be easily demonstrated by single TMS pulses that can be used to map the homunculus simply by moving the TMS coil across the cortical representation of neighboring muscle groups and simultaneously to study the excitability of the corticospinal system.

Single TMS pulses can exert other effects when moved to different cortical areas. When positioned over the primary visual cortex (V1), scotomas, or "blind spots," are often elicited. This illustrates that TMS can transiently disrupt functions.

Activation of motor neurons resulting in a muscle twitch and disruption of visual perception with a single-pulse TMS represent examples of the acute effects of TMS-induced neuronal depolarization, as shown in Table 26.2–1. The effects of single TMS pulses are believed to be immediate and short lived. The muscle twitch as induced by TMS to area M1 is nearly instantaneous, with the hand movement occurring approximately 20 milliseconds after the TMS pulse is applied. The visual masking likewise operates on a similar time scale measured in

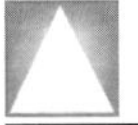

Table 26.2–1
Acute and Prolonged Mechanisms of Action

Acute effects
- Phasic activation of neural circuits
- Observable motor responses (e.g., twitch)
- Temporary disruption (e.g., speech arrest) or facilitation of ongoing processing (e.g., speeds reaction time)

Prolonged effects
- Neuroplasticity
  - ▲ Change in synaptic efficacy, akin to long-term potentiation or depression
  - ▲ Alterations in neurotropic factors
  - ▲ Modulation of cortical excitability
  - ▲ Modulation of functional connectivity

milliseconds. TMS can, however, exert longer-lasting effects when the pulses are repeated at regular intervals in a process of rTMS or when they are paired with other forms of stimulation in which TMS pulses are coupled with electrical stimulation of a peripheral nerve (as in paired associative stimulation [PAS]) or when TMS is paired with audiovisual stimuli, as in the example of classical conditioning of the brain response to TMS. The mechanisms underlying these lasting effects of TMS have been described by various researchers and are thought to be related to neuroplasticity and alterations in synaptic efficacy.

Treatment of psychiatric disorders with rTMS has been informed by attempts to focally alter pathological cortical excitability, believed to be linked to a specific illness. Reduced activity in the left dorsolateral prefrontal cortex (DLPFC) has been implicated in several studies as a physiological correlate of affective disorders. To correct this, numerous studies have applied high frequencies of rTMS, which have been reported to increase excitability, to the left DLPFC in an attempt to normalize activity in this region. In a related approach, some investigators who implicated abnormal interhemispheric balance in activation between the right and left DLPFC applied low-frequency rTMS, which has been reported to be inhibitory, to the right DLPFC in an attempt to normalize this balance.

Side Effects, Interactions with Medications, and Other Risks

Administration of TMS is a noninvasive, relatively benign procedure when applied by a knowledgeable professional to a subject who has been properly evaluated. However, it is not entirely without risk. The most serious known risk of TMS is an unintended seizure. There are several factors that may contribute to seizure risk. Primarily, these include the form of TMS, with single-pulse stimulation less likely to result in a seizure than rTMS, and, in an equally important manner, the dose, which is the combination of treatment parameters including frequency, power, train duration, and intertrain interval. In addition, subject factors can be important, such as the presence of a neurological disorder (epilepsy or a focal brain lesion) or use of seizure-lowering medications.

Single-pulse TMS is generally considered to be of minimal risk when administered to appropriately screened adults without seizure risk factors. On the other hand, rTMS can induce seizures in individuals without predisposing conditions when given at sufficiently high doses.

Patient Selection

Patients who have failed a trial of one or more antidepressant medications or have untoward side effects to medications may be good candidates for TMS. However, given the lower effect size of TMS, for urgent or severely refractory cases, ECT would remain the ultimate gold standard treatment.

Future Directions and Controllable Pulse Shape TMS

TMS and other forms of magnetic stimulation hold a tremendous promise in psychiatric treatment due to their focality and noninvasiveness. However, much research is needed to replicate preliminary findings, improve optimal dosing, establish the patient characteristics that predict response, and examine the influence of concomitant medications on TMS effect. Posttreatment relapse prevention is one of many areas that have to be properly explored. Other vigorously pursued directions are attempts to develop stimulation coils that will allow deeper brain penetration and work on pulse shapes that may be more physiologically optimal for human stimulation.

TRANSCRANIAL DIRECT CURRENT STIMULATION

Definition

tDCS is a noninvasive form of treatment that uses very weak (1 to 3 mA) direct electrical current applied to the scalp. Because direct current (DC) polarizes rather than stimulates with discrete pulses, its action does not appear directly to result in action potential firing in cortical neurons. It is also this DC form of electrical stimulation that distinguishes it from devices that use alternating currents (AC) as found in CES, ECT, VNS, and DBS, which produce discrete pulse stimulation. In addition, because tDCS works via polarization and does not affect action potential firing in cortical neurons, the term *transcranial direct current polarization* is favored by some modern investigators, and both terms appear interchangeably in the literature today. The small device is very portable and usually operated by readily available DC batteries.

Side Effects

There are no known serious adverse effects of tDCS. It is well tolerated, with reported common side effects in the literature listing mostly minimal tingling at the site of stimulation, with a few reported cases of skin irritation.

Mechanism of Action

DC polarizes current, and tDCS is believed to act via the alteration of neuronal membrane polarization, but little is known about the actual mechanism of action of tDCS. Polarization may affect the firing and conductance of neurons by either lowering or raising the threshold of activation. Because tDCS involves the application of low currents to the scalp via cathodal and anodal electrodes, depending on the direction of current flow, polarization can either inhibit (cathodal) or facilitate (anodal) function.

Clinical Studies

Preliminary research suggests that tDCS may enhance certain brain functions independent of mood; however, tDCS technology and its use in psychiatry are in the early stages of exploration. Research is focusing on its potential effectiveness in facilitating recovery from stroke and from certain forms of dementia.

Future Directions

Most of the current tDCS devices use large, saline solution–soaked electrodes. Future device development will most likely investigate electrode shape and contact material to optimize the intended clinical effects and further improve ease of use. However, basic questions of efficacy, indications, and dose–response relationships, as well as predictors of response, will need to be explored first.

CRANIAL ELECTRICAL STIMULATION

Definition

CES, like tDCS, uses a weak (1 to 4 mA) current. However, with CES the current is alternating. It is traditionally applied via saline-soaked, felt-covered electrodes clipped onto the earlobes. Other placement strategies are also being investigated.

Mechanism of Action

The exact mechanism of action has not been elicited, and there is no agreement among researchers on the predominant mode of action. Previous hypotheses proposed that the stimulation with the alternating microcurrent affects the thalamic and hypothalamic brain tissue and facilitates the release of neurotransmitters. Claims have been made that through interaction with cell membranes, the stimulation produces changes in signal transduction associated with classical second-messenger pathways, including calcium channels and cyclic adenosine monophosphate (AMP). There are summary reports that CES causes increases in plasma serotonin, norepinephrine, dopamine, and monoamine oxidase type B (MAO_B) in blood platelets and cerebrospinal fluid (CSF), as well as release of 5-hydroxy-indol-acetic acid (DHEA) and enkephalins and reduction of cortisol and tryptophan. However, most of these reports have not been validated through modern research.

Side Effects

It is believed that the CES stimulation is not harmful, primarily due to its low-voltage power supply (9-V battery) and lack of any reported adverse event by the FDA. Local skin effects, as well as a general feeling of dizziness, have been reported, however, and the use of the device during pregnancy, in those with low blood pressure, or in people who have arrhythmias or pacemakers is not advised by device manufacturers.

Clinical Studies

In a meta-analysis by the Harvard School of Public Health, 18 human clinical trials were examined that used CES to treat depression, anxiety, drug addiction, insomnia, headache, and pain. The overall pooled result showed CES to be better than sham treatment for anxiety at a statistically significant level.

Current Status in Treatment Algorithms, Patient Selection, and Dosing

The use of CES has not been studied sufficiently in the United States, and it does not have a specific place in any algorithm of standard US psychiatric practice.

Future Directions

As with tDCS, basic issues of indications, patient selection, dose–response relationships, and efficacy are under active research and remain to be optimized.

MAGNETIC SEIZURE THERAPY

Definition

MST is a novel form of a convulsive treatment that is under development in several research institutions in the United States and Europe. The treatment uses an alternating magnetic field that crosses the scalp and the calvarium bone unaffected by their high electrical impedance, to in turn induce a more localized electrical current in the targeted regions of the cerebral cortex than is possible with ECT. The aim is to produce a seizure whose focus and patterns of spread may be controlled.

MST is a convulsive treatment, in many ways similar to ECT. It is performed under general anesthesia. It requires approximately the same preparation and infrastructure as ECT. However, MST is given using a modified TMS device, one that can administer higher output than the conventional TMS devices and thus relies on magnetic stimulation, unlike electric stimulation in ECT. The MST procedure is performed under general anesthesia with a muscle relaxant. MST is at the stage of clinical trials and is not FDA approved.

Mechanism of Action

Induction of a seizure is hypothesized to be the underlying event responsible for the likely multiple specific mechanisms of action of MST treatment. As in ECT, these are not fully understood. However, due to its focality, MST appears to represent a tool better suited than ECT to study the mechanisms of action of convulsive therapy through its potential of inducing seizures initiated in different regions of the brain.

Side Effects

Adverse effects from MST, like those of ECT, are largely connected to the risks associated with anesthesia and generalized seizure. In addition, the MST magnetic coil produces a clicking noise that may potentially affect hearing. To mitigate that risk and prevent any cumulative damage, earplugs should be worn by both the patient and members of the treating team. Studies suggest that MST results in less retrograde and anterograde amnesia than ECT, although this result should be replicated in a larger trial.

Current Status in Treatment Algorithms

No clinical algorithms exist for MST, given that it is still an investigational protocol and treatments outside of research are not FDA approved. Assuming that the hypothesis that MST can approach the efficacy of ECT (but with fewer side effects) is correct, this magnetically induced convulsive treatment will play an important role prior to referral for ECT.

Future Directions

MST is a novel treatment in early phases of clinical testing. Clinical treatment variables, including dosing, optimal coil placement, patient selection, and mechanisms of action, are the topics of ongoing and future studies.

VAGUS NERVE STIMULATION

Definition

VNS is the direct, intermittent electrical stimulation of the left cervical vagus nerve via an implanted pulse generator, usually in the left chest wall. The electrode is wrapped around the left vagus nerve in the neck and is connected to the generator subcutaneously.

Mechanisms of Action

The majority of the fibers contained in the left vagus are afferents. It is estimated that as many as 80 percent of these fibers are up-going afferents, and thus chronic stimulation of these nerve fibers predominantly changes activity in the brainstem nuclei such as the nucleus of the tractus solitarius and other neighboring nuclei (e.g., Raphe) that alter serotonergic activity in cortical and limbic structures. In addition, persistent stimulation of the vagal afferents is anticonvulsant, an effect that appears to depend on the norepinephrine-producing locus ceruleus.

Side Effects and Contraindications

To date, reasonably comprehensive literature confirms that VNS is generally well tolerated. The adverse events that are most frequently reported are voice alteration, dyspnea, and neck pain. Besides the risk of perioperative infection, the surgical implantation carries a small risk of vocal cord paralysis, bradycardia, or asystole.

Current Status in Treatment Algorithms

The FDA indicated VNS for the adjunctive long-term treatment of chronic or recurrent depression in patients 18 years or older experiencing a major depressive episode in the setting of unipolar or bipolar disease who have not had an adequate response to four or more adequate antidepressant treatments. Consultation with another clinician experienced with treatment-resistant depression and VNS is recommended.

VNS treatment success rates are lower than those with ECT. Its onset of action is also comparatively slow—typically an approximately 30 percent response rate is observed after 1 year. VNS may be worth considering, therefore, when patients have failed to respond to less invasive treatments, ECT was ineffective, or post-ECT relapse cannot be prevented with less invasive means. VNS might be helpful with longer-term relapse prevention, but results of controlled trials would be useful to guide practice.

Patient Selection

VNS is approved as an adjunctive long-term treatment for chronic or recurrent depressive episodes in adults with a major depressive episode who have not had a satisfactory response to four or more adequate antidepressant trials. The efficacy of VNS in other disorders is unknown.

ECT can be safely used in patients with an implant as long as the VNS generator is turned off during the convulsive treatment. This is needed because of the anticonvulsant effects of VNS. It remains to be studied whether VNS could be useful in relapse prevention post-ECT.

Dosing

The optimal dosing for psychiatric applications of VNS is still largely an area of investigation. The published studies do not identify optimal dosing parameters like time on, time off, frequency, current, or pulse width. However, the epilepsy literature suggests that there is a threshold current for efficacy. Given current knowledge of VNS dosing, electrical current is typically increased up to greater than 1 mA and clinical benefit is assessed over several months. Because the adverse effects of VNS are known to be dose dependent, treatment parameters are often chosen to mitigate specific side effects. For example, lowering pulse width reduces neck pain, allowing patients to tolerate higher currents.

Future Directions

More research is required to establish the dose–response relationships for VNS. Future studies may explore optimal medication strategies to augment responses, test the potential role of VNS for long-term relapse prevention (e.g., after ECT), and study its mechanisms of action.

IMPLANTED CORTICAL STIMULATION

CBS is a novel neurosurgical approach in which electrodes are implanted over the surface of the cortex to provide electrical brain stimulation in a targeted superficial region. This approach is being studied for treatment of conditions like stroke, tinnitus, and treatment-resistant depression.

▲ 26.3 Neurosurgical Treatments and Deep Brain Stimulation

After a long and checkered history, neurosurgical treatments for psychiatric illness have reemerged as a focus of great interest. Many still associate psychiatric neurosurgery with the bygone era of crude freehand "psychosurgery," when prefrontal lobotomy saw wide and indiscriminate use. Those primitive operations, which predated modern psychopharmacology, yielded modest reductions in symptoms but were accompanied by unacceptable adverse effects. Over nearly five decades, techniques, and importantly, procedures and practices have evolved tremendously. First, ablative lesions are now accurately, precisely, and reproducibly placed in specific brain targets stereotactically guided by MRI and specialized software. Alternative methods include radiosurgery, which allows stereotactic lesion placement without craniotomy. Deep brain stimulation (DBS), while requiring craniotomy to implant stimulating electrodes in specific brain targets, is intentionally nonablative and allows flexible and reversible modulation of brain function. Second, strict criteria for patient selection are observed, and the process of determining appropriate candidacy has been formalized.

Currently, surgical intervention is predominantly reserved for patients with severe, incapacitating major depression or obsessive-compulsive disorder (OCD) who have failed an exhaustive array of standard treatments. Surgery is not approved unless a multidisciplinary committee reaches consensus regarding its appropriateness for a given candidate and the patient renders informed consent. Although a large body of clinical data has already been collected that indicates the effectiveness and safety of modern neurosurgical interventions, major centers providing these treatments continue to gather information prospectively, and controlled trials are under way or planned. With these advances in neurosurgical techniques and better-established selection criteria and long-term follow-up procedures, available data suggest that psychiatric neurosurgery yields substantial improvement in symptoms and functioning in approximately 40 to 70 percent of cases, with morbidity and mortality drastically lower than for earlier procedures.

Although lesion procedures have been influenced by theories implicating corticolimbic systems in disordered behavior, they were initially developed largely empirically. Although psychiatric neurosurgery is sometimes criticized for this reason, as for any clinical therapy, the relevant issues are safety and efficacy, not correction of pathophysiological processes that are not yet fully understood. However, in addition to the promise of modern lesion procedures and DBS as clinical treatments, clinicians permit testing of hypotheses derived from the results of lesions or from systematic human neuroimaging. Thus, psychiatric neurosurgery is now developing in a scientific context where translation of data between clinical results to cross-species anatomical, neuroimaging, and physiological studies of neural networks involved a promise to illuminate mechanisms of therapeutic action.

HISTORY

Trephination performed by ancient civilizations probably represents the earliest form of surgical intervention for psychopathology. In 1891, the first formal report of neurosurgical treatment in psychiatry was published, describing bilateral cortical excisions in demented and depressed patients, which yielded mixed results. After four decades in which little progress was made, in 1935 John Fulton and Charles Jacobsen presented their research on primate behavior following frontal cortical ablation. They observed that lobectomized chimpanzees showed reduction in "experimental neurosis" and were less fearful, while retaining an ability to perform complex tasks. Egaz Moniz, a renowned Portuguese neurologist, pioneered prefrontal leukotomy in collaboration with his neurosurgical colleague Almeida Lima. First by using absolute alcohol injections and subsequently by mechanical means with a leukotome, Moniz and Lima performed "psychosurgery" on 20 severely ill institutionalized patients; 14 were said to have exhibited worthwhile improvement. In an era of overflowing asylums and few effective treatments for chronic debilitating psychiatric illness, this mode of therapy was initially enthusiastically embraced, and Moniz won the 1949 Nobel Prize in Medicine or Physiology for this contribution.

From the mid-1930s until the emergence of the phenothiazines in the mid-1950s, these techniques proliferated globally. Walter Freeman, a neuropsychiatrist, was perhaps the most zealous promoter of psychosurgery in the United States. Pioneering a series of freehand procedures to achieve prefrontal lobotomy (i.e., severing the white matter connections between the prefrontal cortex and the rest of the brain), Freeman together with neurosurgeon James Watts reported on their first 200 cases by 1942. Although the benefits of the surgery were highlighted, others acknowledged a significant complication rate, including frontal lobe syndrome, seizures, and even deaths. At its peak, lobotomy was being performed on approximately 5,000 patients per year in the United States alone. A review of the results of 10,365 prefrontal lobotomies performed from 1942 to 1954 in Britain concluded that while 70 percent showed improvement, adverse effects included 6 percent mortality, seizures in 1 percent, and disinhibition syndromes in 1.5 percent. There were widespread reports of blunted personality and socially inappropriate behavior. In the late 1940s and early 1950s, recognition of these risks prompted attempts to develop modified stereotactic surgical procedures that might yield better results. For example, Ernest Spiegel and Henry Wycis, who began stereotactic neurosurgery in humans, reported in the 1940s that dorsomedial thalamotomies improved obsessive-compulsive symptoms. However, with the introduction of chlorpromazine (Thorazine) in 1954, medical management of psychiatric illness became newly possible. Thus, despite the advent of stereotactic neurosurgical techniques and a continued high prevalence of severe, treatment-refractory psychiatric illness, psychiatric neurosurgery was all but abandoned in favor of nonsurgical therapies.

PATIENT SELECTION: INDICATIONS AND CONTRAINDICATIONS

Although limited reports have suggested efficacy across a broad range of psychiatric conditions and research is expanding rapidly, as of this writing the best established indications for psychiatric neurosurgery remain major depression and OCD. In evaluating candidates, several factors are considered:

1. *Primary diagnosis:* The patient must meet clinical criteria for the diagnostic indication, and this disorder should be a primary cause of the patient's debility and suffering.
2. *Severity:* The patient must have chronic, severe, and debilitating illness; duration of the primary illness must exceed 1 year and typically exceeds 5 years. Severity is gauged on standardized instruments (e.g., patients with OCD typically have Yale-Brown Obsessive-Compulsive Scale scores of 25 to 30; patients with major depression typically have Beck Depression Inventory scores of 30 or higher), while debility should be indicated by a low level of functioning (e.g., a Global Assessment of Functioning score of 50 or less) and a poor quality of life.
3. *Adequacy of previous treatment:* Patients must have already undergone an exhaustive array of other available established treatments, which are documented in detail.
4. *Psychiatric comorbidity:* Appropriate treatment must have been rendered for any comorbid psychiatric disorder; the presence of psychoactive substance use or severe personality disorders is considered strong relative contraindications.
5. *Medical comorbidity and surgical fitness:* Structural brain lesions or significant central nervous system injuries are strong contraindications. Medical conditions that increase neurosurgical risks (e.g., cardiopulmonary disease) and age 65 years are relative contraindications for lesion procedures, while for DBS the relative age restriction might be older. A history of past seizures is a risk factor for perioperative seizures after lesion procedures and must be weighed in the

overall risk–benefit assessment (again, data are currently less clear in this regard for psychiatric DBS).

6. *Access to postoperative care:* The psychiatric neurosurgery procedures themselves represent the beginning of a new episode of care. It is crucial that patients have access to adequate postoperative treatment, including a psychiatrist (typically the referring physician) who will accept responsibility for managing the case after discharge. Arrangements for postoperative care (e.g., intensive behavior therapy) should be confirmed ahead of time. Importantly, after lesion procedures, care can generally be delivered in standard treatment settings without the need for highly specialized psychiatric neurosurgery teams. For DBS, access to such teams is essential over the long term. Once implanted, patients require clinical monitoring and device adjustment, which can be intensive and time-consuming, especially early in treatment. Device monitoring and replacements may need to occur on a relatively urgent basis. The continuing costs incurred can be substantial, and adequacy of third-party reimbursement needs to be ensured in advance to the extent possible. After either lesion procedures or DBS, family or significant others may be needed to support and accompany patients to follow-up care, similar to the level of support that is usually necessary during the intensive evaluation process.
7. *Informed consent:* Under no circumstances should psychiatric neurosurgery be performed on patients against their will. The patient must be able and willing to render an informed consent. Formal consent monitoring may be used to ensure that the consent process is adequate. In rare instances, these procedures are performed with assent of the patient and formal consent from a legal guardian. In this context, age less than 18 years also represents a relative contraindication.

POSTOPERATIVE CARE

Immediate postoperative care includes the standard medical and surgical considerations following any stereotactic neurosurgical procedure. Special attention is paid to signs or symptoms of potential surgical complications, including infection, hemorrhage, seizures, or altered mental status. A postoperative MRI should be obtained to document the placement and extent of lesions. Intensive postoperative psychiatric treatment is recommended since the efficacy of the surgery may rely on some synergy between the neurosurgical intervention itself and enhanced response to pharmacological or behavioral therapies. Although dosages of psychotropic medications may be reduced during the immediate perioperative period, the medication regimen should be readjusted as tolerated postoperatively. Moreover, in the case of OCD, intensive behavior therapy should be initiated as soon as possible, preferably within the first month postoperatively.

For DBS, electrode implantation is usually followed by a several-week delay to enable resolution of local edema and stabilization of other factors that might influence the response to stimulation. Then, systematic outpatient adjustment of stimulation parameters is performed before initial settings are determined. This is often a time-consuming process, lasting hours over 1 or more days. Ongoing protocols for DBS entail frequent follow-up, especially during the approximate 6 months after implantation, to enable optimization of stimulation parameters, monitoring of the patient, and coordination of other pharmacological and behavioral therapies.

LESION PROCEDURES

Although numerous approaches have been tried, four lesion procedures have evolved as the safest and most effective for treating psychiatric disorders. All four entail bilateral lesions and are performed using modern stereotactic methods.

Subcaudate Tractotomy

Subcaudate tractotomy was introduced by Geoffrey Knight in Great Britain in 1964 as one of the first attempts to limit adverse effects by restricting lesion size. By targeting the substantia innominata (just inferior to the head of the caudate nucleus), the goal was to interrupt white matter tracts connecting orbitofrontal cortex and subcortical structures. The surgery involved placement of radioactive yttrium-90 seeds at the desired centroid, yielding lesion volumes of approximately 2 cc on each side. Indications for subcaudate tractotomy are major depression, OCD, and other severe anxiety disorders.

Anterior Cingulotomy

Anterior cingulotomy remains the most commonly employed neurosurgical treatment for psychiatric disease in North America. The surgery is conducted under local anesthesia and two or three approximately 1-cc lesions are made on each side by thermocoagulation through bilateral burr holes. The target is within the anterior cingulate cortex (Brodmann areas 24 and 32), at the margin of the white matter bundle known as the cingulum. Originally, the placement of lesions was determined by ventriculography; however, since 1991, anterior cingulotomy has been conducted via MRI guidance. Approximately 40 percent of patients return several months following the first operation for a second procedure to extend the first set of lesions. The indications for anterior cingulotomy include major depression and OCD.

Limbic Leukotomy

Limbic leukotomy was introduced by Desmond Kelly and colleagues in England in 1973. The procedure combines the targets of subcaudate tractotomy and anterior cingulotomy. The lesions have typically been made via thermocoagulation or with a cryoprobe. Historically, the precise placement of the lesions was guided by intraoperative stimulation; pronounced autonomic responses were believed to designate the optimal lesion site. The indications for limbic leukotomy include major depression, OCD, and other severe anxiety disorders. More recently, there is also some evidence that this procedure might be beneficial for repetitive self-injurious behaviors or in the context of severe tic disorders.

Anterior Capsulotomy

Anterior capsulotomy or its newer variant, Gamma Knife (Elekta, Stockholm) capsulotomy, are used in Scandinavia, the United States, Belgium, Brazil, and elsewhere. The procedure places lesions within the anterior limb of the internal capsule, which impinges on the adjacent ventral striatum, thereby interrupting fibers of passage between prefrontal cortex and subcortical nuclei including the dorsomedial thalamus. Although the original anterior capsulotomy procedure is performed using thermocoagulation via burr holes in the skull, over the past 15 years capsulotomy has also been performed using the Gamma Knife as an alternative. This radiosurgical instrument makes craniotomy unnecessary. Typically, gamma capsulotomy lesions are smaller than those induced by thermocapsulotomy, remaining within the ventral portion of the anterior capsule. Hence, the term *gamma ventral capsulotomy* is coming into use to describe this procedure. In contrast to thermocapsulotomy, gamma ventral capsulotomy may be performed as an outpatient procedure, with an overnight hospital stay usually the most that is required. The relative advantages and disadvantages of this radiosurgical approach are the focus of ongoing research, including a current controlled study of gamma ventral capsulotomy for OCD, the first of its kind for a lesion procedure in psychiatry. Some data suggest, unsurprisingly, that the rates of neuropsychiatric adverse effects may be considerably lower for gamma ventral capsulotomy than for earlier procedures in which much larger tissue volumes were lesioned. Indications for anterior capsulotomy include major depression, OCD, and other severe anxiety disorders.

Deep Brain Stimulation

DBS for psychiatric illness is not a new idea, although the devices, surgical techniques, and theoretical models of relevant neurocircuitry have all advanced. The procedure involves placement of small-diameter brain "leads" (e.g., approximately 1.3 mm) with multiple electrode contacts into subcortical nuclei or specific white matter tracts. The surgeon drills burr holes in skull bone under local anesthesia and then places the leads, guided by multimodal imaging and precise stereotactic landmarking. Usually this is done bilaterally. The patient is typically sedated but awake during surgery. Later, the "pacemaker" (also known as an implantable neurostimulator or pulse generator) is implanted subdermally (e.g., in the upper chest wall) and connects it, via extension wires tunneled under the skin, to the brain leads. The goals of DBS are to achieve improved efficacy and more favorable adverse effect profiles in comparison with ablation. Because various combinations of electrodes can be activated, at adjustable polarity, intensity, and frequency, DBS allows more flexible modulation of brain function, referred to as *neuromodulation*. Thus, parameters can be optimized for individual patients, but the process, typically performed by a specially trained psychiatrist in the outpatient setting, can be quite time-consuming and requires attentive, long-term follow-up. In cases where no beneficial settings can be identified despite extensive efforts, the electrodes can be inactivated, and devices may be removed. In that event, devices are usually only partly explanted, with the brain electrodes left in place given the small risk of hemorrhage upon removal. The relative advantages and disadvantages of DBS are the focus of very active research.

TREATMENT OUTCOME

For all four contemporary ablative procedures, outcome cannot be fairly assessed for a considerable period postoperatively, which could extend from 6 months to 2 years. In the first two or three decades of this work, clinical reports usually employed measures of global improvement, such as the Pippard Postoperative Rating Scale, which rates outcomes as follows: (1) symptom free, (2) much improved, (3) slightly improved, (4) unchanged, and (5) worse. Most studies have operationalized significant improvement as categories 1 and 2. In addition, many of the reports employ a measure of symptom severity that is specific to the indication for the procedure (e.g., the Yale-Brown Obsessive-Compulsive Scale for OCD and the Beck Depression Inventory for major depression). The majority of studies focus on one or another of the procedures and are best reviewed according to surgical approach.

Outcome with Subcaudate Tractotomy

Significant improvement was seen in 68 percent of patients with major depression, 50 percent of patients with OCD, and 62.5 percent of patients with other anxiety disorders. Patients with schizophrenia, substance abuse, or personality disorders did poorly. Short-term side effects include transient headache and confusion or somnolence, which typically resolve in less than 1 week. Patients are usually ambulatory by the third postoperative day. Transient disinhibition syndromes were common. In 1994, a large-scale review of 1,300 cases was conducted and concluded that the procedure enables 40 to 60 percent of patients to lead normal or near-normal lives, with a reduction in suicide rate to 1 percent versus 15 percent in a similarly affected control group with major affective disorders.

Outcome with Anterior Cingulotomy

Significant improvement occurred in 62 percent of patients with affective disorders, 56 percent with OCD, and 79 percent with other anxiety disorders. Among patients with unipolar depression, 60 percent responded favorably; among patients with bipolar disorder, 40 percent responded favorably; and among patients with OCD, 27 percent were classified as responders with another 27 percent categorized as possible responders. Short-term side effects include headache, nausea, or difficulty with urination; however, these typically resolve within a few days. Patients are usually ambulatory within 12 hours following the operation and discharged on the third to the fifth postoperative day. Over the past 10 years the practice of treating patients who experience perioperative seizures with chronic anticonvulsant therapy has been discontinued, and no cases of new-onset recurrent seizures have been seen. Although patients have occasionally (5 percent or less) noted transient problems with memory, an independent analysis of 34 patients was performed and demonstrated no significant intellectual or behavioral impairments attributable to anterior cingulotomy; a subsequent study of 57 patients likewise found no evidence for lasting neurological or behavioral adverse effects.

Outcome with Limbic Leukotomy

Significant improvement occurred in 89 percent of patients with OCD, 78 percent with major depression, and 66 percent with other anxiety conditions. Short-term side effects include headache, lethargy or apathy, confusion, and lack of sphincter control, which may last from a few days to a few weeks. In particular, it is common for postoperative confusion to last at least several days, and patients are often not discharged in less than 1 week. There were no seizures and no deaths; however, one patient suffered severe memory loss due to improper lesion placement, and enduring lethargy was present in 12 percent of cases.

Outcome with Anterior Capsulotomy

Thermocapsulotomy. A favorable response occurred in 50 percent of those with OCD and 48 percent of those with major depression. Short-term side effects can include transient headache or incontinence. Postoperative confusion often lasts for up to 1 week. Recovery from gamma capsulotomy is swifter and characterized by less discomfort and virtually no confusion, but side effects from radiation exposure, principally cerebral edema, may be delayed for up to 8 to 12 months. For the open capsulotomy, patients are typically ambulatory in a matter of hours to days following the operation, although the length of hospital stay may be influenced by the duration of confusion. Weight gain has been noted to be a common enduring side effect with a mean increase in mass of 10 percent.

Gamma Ventral Capsulotomy. Gamma capsulotomy was generally well tolerated and effective for patients with otherwise intractable OCD. Adverse events included cerebral edema and headache, small asymptomatic caudate infarctions, and possible exacerbation of preexisting bipolar mania. A therapeutic response, defined conservatively, was seen in 60 percent of over 50 patients receiving the most recent gamma capsulotomy procedure, in which pairs of lesions in the ventral capsule are made bilaterally, impinging on the ventral striatum. Therapeutic benefit was achieved over 1 to 2 years and was essentially stable by 3 years. Adverse effects of gamma ventral capsulotomy include significant radiation-induced edema, appearing months after the procedure, apparently due to a differential sensitivity to radiation that remains poorly understood. Long-term follow-up will be necessary to clarify risks and benefits of gamma ventral capsulotomy. The same applies to any neurosurgery, including lesion procedures and DBS.

Outcomes with DBS

Obsessive-Compulsive Disorder. Over the past 10 years, four groups have collaborated closely on development of DBS at the ventral anterior limb of the internal capsule and adjacent ventral striatum (the VC/VS) for otherwise intractable OCD: Leuven/Antwerp, Butler Hospital/Brown University, the Cleveland Clinic, and the University of Florida. Long-term outcomes of open stimulation in 26 patients showed clinically significant symptom reductions and functional improvement in about two thirds of patients overall. Conservatively defined responses (35 percent or greater reductions on the Yale-Brown Obsessive-Compulsive Scale) were seen in one-third of patients in the initial group, irrespective of study center, while the response rate was over 70 percent in the second and third patient cohorts treated. Development of psychiatric DBS is following the path of stimulation for movement disorders, where several targets have been pursued with therapeutic benefit. As in movement disorders, overlapping or converging effects of DBS at different anatomical sites on the neurocircuitry involved are likely and are a focus of active research. The same reasoning applies to DBS for depression.

Major Depression. A body of functional neuroimaging research implicates the subgenual cingulate cortex as a node in circuits involved in the normal experience of sadness, symptoms of depressive illness, and responses to depression treatments. Chronic DBS for up to 6 months was associated with sustained remission of depression in four of the six patients studied. Another line of research on DBS for depression was prompted by the OCD research discussed above and also by the reported antidepressant effects of anterior capsulotomy on which the VC/VC stimulation target was initially based. The OCD patients, who had very high rates of comorbid depression, characteristically responded to stimulation onset with mood enhancement and reductions in nonspecific as well as OCD-related anxiety. Such effects were accompanied, or even preceded, by improvements in social interaction and daily functioning. Worsening in these same clinical domains was noted in some patients with cessation of VC/VS stimulation. Moreover, DBS-induced changes in mood and nonspecific anxiety often seemed to precede reductions in core OCD symptoms.

Outcome across Contemporary Neurosurgical Procedures

Although the field is developing rapidly, the conclusion reached is that 40 to 70 percent of carefully selected psychiatric patients should meaningfully benefit from contemporary neurosurgical treatment. Twenty-five percent or more might be expected to show outstanding improvement. Responses to ablative procedures have appeared marginally superior for major depression than for OCD generally. The adverse-effect profiles of this group of procedures are influenced by lesion size, the surgical approach, and whether radiosurgical methods (in which the tempo of lesion development is very slow vs. thermocoagulation) are used. But adverse effects are greatly minimized in comparison with procedures of the past. Although minor short-term side effects may be common after some modern ablative procedures, severe or enduring adverse consequences are relatively rare. These can include seizures in about 1 to 5 percent of cases. Although frontal syndromes, confusion, or subtle cognitive deficits can still be seen, overall cognitive function, as indicated by the standard intelligence quotient, is generally enhanced, a finding that has been attributed to the overriding beneficial effects of symptomatic improvement. Psychiatric neurosurgery likely reduces mortality, as evidenced by data on comparative suicide rates. Nonetheless, patients who undergo and fail to benefit from these procedures are at particularly high risk for completed suicide. Therefore, as with any therapy, the potential risks and benefits of psychiatric neurosurgery must be weighed against the potential risks and benefits of undergoing this brand of treatment.

The advent of DBS in psychiatry has created tremendous interest and considerable research activity. This therapy is intentionally nonablative, can be optimized for individual patients, is reversible, and is based on devices that are (to varying degrees) removable. DBS may therefore be accepted by patients who would not choose to undergo lesion procedures (although the reverse is also true). With all of its advantages, DBS requires that patients be treated by highly specialized teams willing and able to provide long-term care. The logistics and expenses involved can represent significant barriers. In contrast, psychiatric care can be delivered in standard treatment settings after lesion procedures. However, although the relative risks of enduring adverse effects after psychiatric DBS remain to be clearly established, at this stage ablative methods appear to carry a greater potential for them. Because rates of adverse outcomes are low when modern lesion procedures are performed at highly experienced centers, there may be a particularly strong rationale for referral of appropriate patients to such expert centers.

27 Child Psychiatry

▲ 27.1 Introduction: Infant, Child, and Adolescent Development

The transactional nature of development in infancy, childhood, and adolescence, consisting of a continuous interplay between biological predisposition and environmental experiences, forms the basis of current conceptualizations of development. There is much evidence that observed developmental outcomes evolve from interactions between particular biological substrates and specific environmental events. For example, the serotonin transporter gene sensitizes a child with early adverse experiences of abuse or neglect to increased risk for later development of a depressive disorder. In addition, the degree of resilience and adaptation, that is, the ability to withstand adversity without negative effects, is likely to be mediated by endogenous glucocorticoids, cytokines, and neurotrophins. Thus, allostasis, the process of achieving stability in the face of adverse environmental events, results from interactions between specific environmental challenges and particular genetic backgrounds that combine to result in a response. It is widely accepted that adverse childhood experiences (ACEs) are likely to alter the trajectory of development in a given individual, and that during early development the brain is especially vulnerable to injury. Future studies may uncover windows of plasticity in older children and adolescents that affect vulnerability as well. Changes in both white matter and gray matter in the brains of adolescents are linked to increased acquisition of subtle social skills. Adolescents' keen abilities, competencies, and interests in a host of technological advances—including the Internet, social media sites such as Facebook, Twitter, and Instagram, and smart phones, to name a few—shed some light on their potential to adapt to new and challenging demands.

PRENATAL, INFANT, AND CHILD

The phases of development described in this section are defined as follows: prenatal is the time frame from conception to 8 weeks; the fetus, from 8 weeks to birth; infancy, from birth to 15 months; the toddler period, from 15 months to 2½ years; the preschool period, from 2½ years to 6 years; and the middle years, from 6 to 12 years.

PRENATAL

Historically, the analysis of human development began with birth. The influence of endogenous and exogenous in utero factors, however, now requires that developmental schemes take intrauterine events into consideration. The infant is not a tabula rasa, a smooth slate upon which outside influences etch patterns. To the contrary, the newborn has already been influenced by myriad factors that have occurred in the safety of the womb, the result of which has produced wide individual differences among infants. For example, the studies of Stella Chess and Alexander Thomas (described later) have demonstrated a wide range of temperamental differences among newborns. Maternal stress, through the production of adrenal hormones, also influences behavioral characteristics of newborns.

The time frame in which the development of the embryo and fetus occurs is known as the prenatal period. After implantation, the egg begins to divide and is known as an embryo. Growth and development occur at a rapid pace; by the end of 8 weeks, the shape is recognizably human, and the embryo has become a fetus.

The fetus maintains an internal equilibrium that, with variable effects, interacts continuously with the intrauterine environment. In general, most disorders that occur are multifactorial—the result of a combination of effects, some of which can be additive. Damage at the fetal stage usually has a more global impact than damage after birth, because rapidly growing organs are the most vulnerable. Boys are more vulnerable to developmental damage than girls are; geneticists recognize that in humans and animals, female fetuses show a propensity for greater biological vigor than male fetuses, possibly because of the second X chromosome in the female.

Prenatal Life

Much biological activity occurs in utero. A fetus is involved in a variety of behaviors that are necessary for adaptation outside the womb. For example, a fetus sucks on thumb and fingers; folds and unfolds its body, and eventually assumes a position in which its occiput is in an anterior vertex position, which is the position in which fetuses usually exit the uterus.

Behavior

Pregnant women are extraordinarily sensitive to prenatal movements. They describe their unborn babies as active or passive, as kicking vigorously or rolling around, as quiet when the mothers are active, but as kicking as soon as the mothers try to rest.

Women usually detect fetal movements 16 to 20 weeks into the pregnancy; the fetus can be artificially set into total body motion by in utero stimulation of its ventral skin surfaces by the 14th week. The fetus may be able to hear by the 18th week, and it responds to loud noises with muscle contractions, movements, and an increased heart rate. Bright light flashed on the abdominal wall of the 20-week pregnant woman causes changes in fetal heart rate and position. The retinal structures begin to function at that time. Eyelids open at 7 months. Smell and taste are also developed at this time, and the fetus responds to substances that may be injected into the amniotic sac, such as contrast medium. Some reflexes present at birth exist in utero: the grasp reflex, which appears at 17 weeks; the Moro (startle) reflex, which appears at 25 weeks; and the sucking reflex, which appears at about 28 weeks.

Nervous System. The nervous system arises from the neural plate, which is a dorsal ectodermal thickening that appears on about day 16 of gestation. By the sixth week, part of the neural tube becomes the cerebral vesicle, which later becomes the cerebral hemispheres.

The cerebral cortex begins to develop by the 10th week, but layers do not appear until the sixth month of pregnancy; the sensory cortex and the motor cortex are formed before the association cortex. Some brain function has been detected in utero by fetal encephalographic responses to sound. The human brain weighs about 350 g at birth and 1,450 g at full adult development, a fourfold increase, mainly in the neocortex. This increase is almost entirely because of the growth in the number and branching of dendrites establishing new connections. After birth, the number of new neurons is negligible. Uterine contractions can contribute to fetal neural development by causing the developing neural network to receive and transmit sensory impulses.

Pruning. Pruning refers to the programmed elimination during development of neurons, synapses, axons, and other brain structures from the original number, present at birth, to a lesser number. Thus, the developing brain contains structures and cellular elements that are absent in the older brain. The fetal brain generates more neurons than it will need for adult life. For example, in the visual cortex, neurons increase in number from birth to 3 years of age, at which point they diminish in number. Another example is that the adult brain contains fewer neural connections than were present during the early and middle years of childhood. Approximately twice as many synapses are present in certain parts of the cerebral cortex during early postnatal life than during adulthood.

Pruning occurs to rid the nervous system of cells that have served their function in the development of the brain. Some neurons, for example, exist to produce neurotrophic or growth factors and are programmed to die—a process called apoptosis—when that function is fulfilled.

The implication of these observations is that the immature brain can be vulnerable in locations that lack sensitivity to injury later on. The developing white matter of the human brain before 32 weeks of gestation is especially sensitive to damage from hypoxic and ischemic injury and metabolic insults. Neurotransmitter receptors located on synaptic terminals are subject to injury from excessive stimulation by excitatory amino acids (e.g., glutamate, aspartate), a process referred to as excitotoxicity. Research is proceeding on the implications of such events in the etiology of child and adult neuropsychiatric disorders such as schizophrenia.

Maternal Stress

Maternal stress correlates with high levels of stress hormones (epinephrine, norepinephrine, and adrenocorticotropic hormone) in the fetal bloodstream, which act directly on the fetal neuronal network to increase blood pressure, heart rate, and activity level. Mothers with high levels of anxiety are more likely to have babies who are hyperactive, irritable, and of low birth weight, and who have problems feeding and sleeping than are mothers with low anxiety levels. A fever in the mother causes the fetus's temperature to rise.

Genetic Disorders

In many cases, genetic counseling depends on prenatal diagnosis. The diagnostic techniques used include amniocentesis (transabdominal aspiration of fluid from the amniotic sac), ultrasound examinations, x-ray studies, fetoscopy (direct visualization of the fetus), fetal blood and skin sampling, chorionic villus sampling, and α-fetoprotein screening. In about 2 percent of women tested, the results are positive for some abnormality, including X-linked disorders, neural tube defects (detected by high levels of α-fetoprotein), chromosomal disorders (e.g., trisomy 21), and various inborn errors of metabolism (e.g., Tay–Sachs disease and lipoidoses).

Some diagnostic tests carry a risk; for instance, about 5 percent of women who undergo fetoscopy miscarry. Amniocentesis, which is usually performed between the 14th and 16th weeks of pregnancy, causes fetal damage or miscarriage in less than 1 percent of women tested. Fully 98 percent of all prenatal tests in pregnant women reveal no abnormality in the fetus. Prenatal testing is recommended for women older than 35 years of age and for those with a family history of a congenital defect.

Parental reactions to birth defects can include feelings of guilt, anxiety, or anger as their worst fears during the pregnancy are realized. Some degree of depression over the loss of the fantasized perfect child may be observed before the parents develop more active coping strategies. Termination of a pregnancy because of a known or suspected birth defect is an option chosen by some women.

Maternal Drug Use

Alcohol. Alcohol use in pregnancy is a major cause of serious physical and mental birth defects in children. Each year, up to 40,000 babies are born with some degree of alcohol-related damage. The National Institute on Drug Abuse (NIDA) reports that 19 percent of pregnant women used alcohol during their pregnancy, the highest rate being among white women.

Fetal alcohol syndrome affects about one-third of all infants born to alcoholic women. The syndrome is characterized by growth retardation of prenatal origin (height, weight); minor anomalies, including microphthalmia (small eyeballs), short palpebral fissures, midface hypoplasia (underdevelopment), a smooth or short philtrum, and a thin upper lip; and central nervous system (CNS) manifestations, including microcephaly (head circumference below the third percentile), a history of delayed development, hyperactivity, attention deficits, learning disabilities, intellectual deficits, and seizures. The incidence of infants born with fetal alcohol syndrome is about 0.5 per 1,000 live births.

Some studies suggest that alcohol use during pregnancy may contribute to attention-deficit/hyperactivity disorder (ADHD). Animal experiments have shown that alcohol reduces the number of active dopamine neurons in the midbrain area, and ADHD is associated with reduced dopaminergic activity in the brain.

Smoking. Smoking during pregnancy is associated with both premature births and below-average infant birth weight. Some reports have associated sudden infant death syndrome (SIDS) with mothers who smoke.

Other Substances. Marijuana (used by 3 percent of all pregnant women) and cocaine (used by 1 percent) are the two most commonly abused illegal drugs, followed by heroin. Chronic marijuana use is associated with low infant birth weight, prematurity, and withdrawal-like symptoms, including excessive crying, tremors, and hyperemesis (severe and chronic vomiting). Crack cocaine use by women during pregnancy has been correlated with behavioral abnormalities such as increased irritability and crying and decreased desire for human contact. Infants born to mothers dependent on narcotics go through a withdrawal syndrome at birth.

Prenatal exposure to various prescribed medications can also result in abnormalities. Common drugs with teratogenic effects include antibiotics (tetracyclines), anticonvulsants (valproate [Depakene], carbamazepine [Tegretol], and phenytoin [Dilantin]), progesterone–estrogens, lithium (Eskalith), and warfarin (Coumadin). Table 27.1–1 outlines the etiologies of malformations that may emerge during the first year of life.

Infancy

The delivery of the fetus marks the start of infancy. The average newborn weighs about 3,400 g (7.5 lb). Small fetuses, defined as those with a birth weight below the 10th percentile for their gestational age, occur in about 7 percent of all pregnancies. At the 26th to the 28th week of gestation, the prematurely born fetus has a good chance of survival. Arnold Gesell described developmental landmarks that are widely used in both pediatrics and child psychiatry. These landmarks outline the sequence of children's motor, adaptive, and personal–social behavior from birth to 6 years (Table 27.1–2).

Premature infants are defined as those with a gestation of less than 34 weeks or a birth weight less than 2,500 g (5.5 lb). Such infants are at increased risk for learning disabilities, such as dyslexia, emotional and behavioral problems, mental retardation, and child abuse. With each 100 g increment of weight, beginning at about 1,000 g (2.2 lb), infants have a progressively better chance of survival. A 36-week-old fetus has less chance of survival than a 3,000 g (6.6 lb) fetus born close to term. The differences between full-term and infants born prematurely are shown in Table 27.1–2.

Postmature infants are defined as infants born 2 weeks or more beyond the expected date of birth. Because pregnancy at term is calculated as extending 40 weeks from the last menstrual period and the exact time of fertilization varies, the incidence of postmaturity is high if based on menstrual history alone. The postmature baby typically has long nails, scanty lanugo, more scalp hair than usual, and increased alertness.

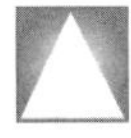

Table 27.1–1
Causes of Human Malformations Observed During the First Year of Life

Suspected Cause	% of Total
Genetic	
Autosomal genetic disease	15–20
Cytogenic (chromosomal abnormalities)	5
Unknown	
Polygenic	
Multifactorial (genetic–environmental interactions)	
Spontaneous error of development	
Synergistic interactions of teratogens	
Environmental	
Maternal conditions: diabetes; endocrinopathies; nutritional deficiencies, starvation; drug and substance addictions	4
Maternal infections: rubella, toxoplasmosis, syphilis, herpes, cytomegalic inclusion disease, varicella, Venezuelan equine encephalitis, parvovirus B19	3
Mechanical problems (deformations): abnormal cord constrictions, disparity in uterine size, and uterine contents	1–2
Chemicals, drugs, radiation, and hyperthermia	<1
Preconception exposures (excluding mutagens and infectious agents)	<1

Reprinted from Brent RL, Beckman DA. Environmental teratogens. *Bull NY Acad Med*. 1990;66:125.

Developmental Milestones in Infants

Reflexes and Survival Systems at Birth. Reflexes are present at birth. They include the rooting reflex (puckering of the lips in response to perioral stimulation), the grasp reflex, the plantar (Babinski) reflex, the knee reflex, the abdominal reflexes, the startle (Moro) reflex and the tonic neck reflex. In normal children, the grasp reflex, the startle reflex, and the tonic neck reflex disappear by the fourth month. The Babinski reflex usually disappears by the 12th month.

Survival systems—breathing, sucking, swallowing, and circulatory and temperature homeostasis—are relatively functional at birth, but the sensory organs are incompletely developed. Further differentiation of neurophysiological functions depends on an active process of stimulatory reinforcement from the external environment, such as persons touching and stroking the infant. The newborn infant is awake for only a short period each day; rapid eye movement (REM) and non-REM sleep are present at birth. Other spontaneous behaviors include crying, smiling, and penile erection in males. Infants 1 day old can detect the smell of their mother's milk, and those 3 days old distinguish their mother's voice.

Language and Cognitive Development. At birth, infants can make noises, such as crying, but they do not vocalize until about 8 weeks. At that time, guttural or babbling sounds occur spontaneously, especially in response to the mother. The persistence and further evolution of children's vocalizations depend on parental reinforcement. Language development occurs in well-delineated stages as outlined in Table 27.1–3.

By the end of infancy (about 2 years), infants have transformed reflexes into voluntary actions that are the building blocks of cognition. They begin to interact with the environment, to experience feedback from their own bodies, and to

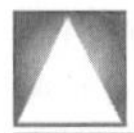

Table 27.1–2
Landmarks of Normal Behavioral Development

Age	Motor and Sensory Behavior	Adaptive Behavior	Personal and Social Behavior
Birth–4 weeks	Hand-to-mouth reflex, grasping reflex Rooting reflex (puckering lips in response to perioral stimulation), Moro reflex (digital extension when startled), sucking reflex, Babinski reflex (toes spread when sole of foot is touched) Differentiates sounds (orients to human voice) and sweet and sour tastes Visual tracking Fixed focal distance of 8 in Makes alternating crawling movements Moves head laterally when placed in prone position	Anticipatory feeding-approach behavior at 4 days Responds to sound of rattle and bell Regards moving objects momentarily	Responsiveness to mother's face, eyes, and voice within first few hours of life Endogenous smile Independent play (until 2 years) Quiets when picked up Impassive face
4 weeks	Tonic neck reflex positions predominate Hands fisted Head sags but can hold head erect for a few seconds Visual fixation, stereoscopic vision (12 weeks)	Follows moving objects to the midline Shows no interest and drops object immediately	Regards face and diminishes activity Responds to speech Smiles preferentially to mother
16 weeks	Symmetrical postures predominate Holds head balanced Head lifted 90 degrees when prone on forearm Visual accommodation	Follows a slowly moving object well Arms activate on sight of dangling object	Spontaneous social smile (exogenous) Aware of strange situations
28 weeks	Sits steadily, leaning forward on hands Bounces actively when placed in standing position	One-hand approach and grasp of toy Bangs and shakes rattle Transfers toys	Takes feet to mouth Pats mirror image Starts to imitate mother's sounds and actions
40 weeks	Sits alone with good coordination Creeps Pulls self to standing position Points with index finger	Matches two objects at midline Attempts to imitate scribble	Separation anxiety manifest when taken away from mother Responds to social play, such as pat-a-cake and peek-a-boo Feeds self-cracker and holds own bottle
52 weeks	Walks with one hand held Stands alone briefly	Seeks novelty	Cooperates in dressing
15 months	Toddles Creeps up stairs		Points or vocalizes wants Throws objects in play or refusal
18 months	Coordinated walking, seldom falls Hurls ball Walks up stairs with one hand held	Builds a tower of three or four cubes Scribbles spontaneously and imitates a writing stroke	Feeds self in part, spills Pulls toy on string Carries or hugs a special toy, such as a doll Imitates some behavioral patterns with slight delay
2 years	Runs well, no falling Kicks large ball Goes up and down stairs alone Fine motor skills increase	Builds a tower of six or seven cubes Aligns cubes, imitating train Imitates vertical and circular strokes Develops original behaviors	Pulls on simple garment Domestic mimicry Refers to self by name Says "no" to mother Separation anxiety begins to diminish Organized demonstrations of love and protest Parallel play (plays side by side but does not interact with other children)
3 years	Rides tricycle Jumps from bottom steps Alternates feet going up stairs	Builds tower of 9 or 10 cubes Imitates a three-cube bridge Copies a circle and a cross	Puts on shoes Unbuttons buttons Feeds self well Understands taking turns
4 years	Walks down stairs one step to a tread Stands on one foot for 5–8 seconds	Copies a cross Repeats four digits Counts three objects with correct pointing	Washes and dries own face Brushes teeth Associative or joint play (plays cooperatively with other children)
5 years	Skips, using feet alternately Usually has complete sphincter control Fine coordination improves	Copies a square Draws a recognizable person with a head, a body, and limbs Counts 10 objects accurately	Dresses and undresses self Prints a few letters Plays competitive exercise games
6 years	Rides two-wheel bicycle	Prints name Copies triangle	Ties shoelaces

Gesesll Developmental Observation (www.gesellinstitute.org); (Thomas, Chess & Birch, 1968).

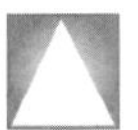

Table 27.1–3
Language Development

Age and Stage of Development	Mastery of Comprehension	Mastery of Expression
0–6 months	Shows startle response to loud or sudden sounds; attempts to localize sounds, turning eyes or head; appears to listen to speakers, may respond with smile; Recognizes warning, angry, and friendly voices; responds to hearing own name	Has vocalizations other than crying; has differential cries for hunger, pain; makes vocalizations to show pleasure; plays at making sounds Babbles (a repeated series of sounds)
7–11 months Attending-to-Language	Shows listening selectivity (voluntary control over responses to sounds); listens to music or singing with interest; recognizes "no," "hot," own name; looks at pictures being named for up to 1 minute; listens to speech without being distracted by other sounds	Responds to own name with vocalizations; imitates the melody of utterances; uses jargon (own language); has gestures (shakes head for no); has exclamation ("oh-oh"); plays language games (pat-a-cake, peekaboo)
12–18 months Single-Word	Shows gross discriminations between dissimilar sounds (bells vs. dog vs. horn vs. mother's or father's voice); understands basic body parts, names of common objects; Acquires understanding of some new words each week; can identify simple objects (baby, ball, etc.) from a group of objects or pictures; understands up to 150 words by age 18 months	Uses single words (mean age of first word is 11 months; by age 18 months, child is using up to 20 words); "Talks" to toys, self, or others using long patterns of jargon and occasional words; approximately 25% of utterances are intelligible; all vowels articulated correctly; initial and final consonants often omitted
12–24 months Two-Word Messages	Responds to simple directions ("Give me the ball") Responds to action commands ("Come here," "Sit down") Understands pronouns (me, him, her, and you) Begins to understand complex sentences ("When we go to the store, I'll buy you some candy")	Uses two-word utterances ("Mommy sock," "all gone," "ball here"); imitates environmental sounds in play ("moo," "mmm, mmm," etc.); refers to self by name, begins to use pronouns; echoes two or more last words of sentences; begins to use three-word telegraphic utterances ("all gone ball," "me go now"); utterances 26–50% intelligible; uses language to ask for needs
24–36 months Grammar Formation	Understands small body parts (elbow, chin, eyebrow); understands family name categories (grandma, baby) Understands size (little one, big one) Understands most adjectives Understands functions (why do we eat, why do we sleep)	Uses real sentences with grammatical function words (can, will, the, and a); usually announces intentions before acting "conversations" with other children, usually just monologues jargon and echolalia gradually drop from speech; increased vocabulary (up to 270 words at 2 years, 895 words at 3 years); speech 50–80% intelligible P, b, m articulated correctly; speech may show rhythmic disturbances
36–54 months Grammar Development	Understands prepositions (under, behind, and between) Understands many words (up to 3,500 at 3 years, 5,500 at 4 years) Understands cause and effect (What do you do when you're hungry? cold?) Understands analogies (Food is to eat, milk is to ____)	Correct articulation of *n, w, ng, h, t, d, k,* and *g;* uses language to relate incidents from the past; uses wide range of grammatical forms: plurals, past tense, negatives, questions; plays with language: rhymes, exaggerates; Speech 90% intelligible, occasional errors in the ordering of sounds within words; able to define words; egocentric use of language rare; can repeat a 12-syllable sentence correctly; some grammatical errors still occur
55 months on True Communication	Understands concepts of number, speed, time, space; understands left and right; understands abstract terms; is able to categorize items into semantic classes	Uses language to tell stories, share ideas, and discuss alternatives; increasing use of varied grammar; spontaneous self-correction of grammatical errors; stabilizing of articulation f, v, s, z, l, r, th, and consonant clusters; speech 100% intelligible

Reprinted from Rutter M, Hersov L, eds. Child and Adolescent Psychiatry. London: Blackwell; 1985, with permission.

become intentional in their actions. By the end of the second year of life, children begin to use symbolic play and language.

Jean Piaget (1896–1980), a Swiss psychologist, observed the growing capacity of young children (including his own) to think and to reason. An outline of the Piaget's stages of cognitive development is presented in Table 27.1–4.

Emotional and Social Development. By the age of 3 weeks, infants imitate the facial movements of adult caregivers. They open their mouths and thrust out their tongues in response to adults who do the same. By the third and fourth months of life, these behaviors are easily elicited. These imitative behaviors are believed to be the precursors of the infant's emotional life. The smiling response occurs in two phases: the first phase is endogenous smiling, which occurs spontaneously within the first 2 months and is unrelated to external stimulation; the second phase is exogenous smiling, which is stimulated from the outside, usually by the mother, and occurs by the 16th week.

Table 27.1–4
Piaget's Stages of Cognitive Development

Period of Development	Cognitive Spatial Stages	Cognitive Achievements
Gestational		Fetus can "learn" sounds and respond differentially to them after birth
Infancy: Birth–2 years	Sensorimotor Includes concepts:	Infants "think" with their eyes, ears, and senses
Birth–1 month	Reflective; egocentric (newer research refutes this)	Newborns can learn to associate stroking with sucking
4–8 months	Secondary circular: looks for objects partially hidden	Newborns can learn to suck to produce certain visual displays or music
8–12 months	Secondary circulation coordinated: peek-a-boo, finds hidden objects	Can remember for 1-month periods Can play with parent by looking for partially hidden objects
12–18 months	Tertiary circular: explores properties and drops objects	Memory improves
18 months–2 years	Mental representation, make-believe play; memory of objects	Body parts used as objects Can stack one object within another Remembers hidden objects Drops objects over crib Knows animal sounds; names objects Knows body parts and familiar pictures Can understand causes not visible
Early Childhood: 2–5 years		
2–7 years	Preoperational Includes concepts: Egocentrism: "I want you to eat this too." Animistic: "I'm afraid of the moon." Lack of hierarchy: "Where do these blocks go?" Centration: "I want it now, not after dinner." Irreversibility: "I don't know how to go back to that room."	Preschoolers use symbols Development of language and make-believe No sign of logic 3-year-olds can count 2–3 objects; know colors and age 4-year-olds can fantasize without concrete props
2–5 years	Transductive reasoning: "We have to go this way because that's the way Daddy goes."	5- to 6-year-olds get humor; understand good and bad; can do some chores 7- to 11-year-olds have good memory; recall; can solve problems
Middle Childhood: 6–11 years		
6 years onward	Concrete operational	Children begin to think logically
7–11 years	Includes concepts: Hierarchical classification—arranges cars by types Reversibility—can play games backward and forward (e.g., checkers, triple kings) Conservation—lose two dimes and look for same Decentration—worry about small details, obsessive Spatial operations—likes models for directions Horizontal decalage e—conservation of weight, logic Transitive inference—syllogisms; compare everything, brand names important	Understand conservation of matter Frozen milk same amount as melted Can organize objects into hierarchies Children seem rational and organized
Adolescence: 11–19 years		
11 years onward	Formal operational Includes concepts: Hypothetical-deductive reasoning; adolescent quick thinking or excuses Imaginary audience—everyone is looking at them Personal fable—inflated opinion of themselves Propositional thinking—logic	Abstraction and reason Can think of all possibilities

The stages of emotional development parallel those of cognitive development. Indeed, the caregiving person provides the major stimulus for both aspects of mental growth. Human infants depend totally on adults for survival. Through warm and predictable interactions, an infant's social and emotional repertoire expands with the interplay of caregivers' social responses (Table 27.1–5).

In the first year, infants' moods are highly variable and intimately related to internal states such as hunger. Toward the second two-thirds of the first year, infants' moods grow increasingly related to external social cues; a parent can get even a hungry infant to smile. When the infant is internally comfortable, a sense of interest and pleasure in the world and in its primary caregivers should prevail. Prolonged separation from the mother (or other primary caregiver) during the second 6 months of life can lead to depression that may persist into adulthood as part of an individual's character.

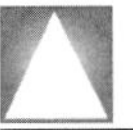

Table 27.1–5
Emotional Development

Stages First Seen	Emotional Skills	Emotional Behavior
Gestational–Infancy: 0–2 years		
0–2 months onward	Love, evoked by touching Fear, evoked by loud noise Rage, evoked by body restrictions Brain pathways for emotion forming	Social smile and joy shown Responds to emotions of others All emotions there
3–4 months onward	Self-regulation of emotions starts; brain pathways of emotion growing	Laughter possible and more control over smiles; anger shown
7–12 months	Self-regulation of emotion grows Increased intensity of basic three	Able to elicit more responsiveness Denies to cope with stress
1–2 years	Shame and pride appear; envy, embarrassment appear Displaces onto other children	Some indications of empathy starting; expressions of feeling: "I like you, Daddy" "I'm sorry" Likes attention and approval; enjoys play alone or next to peers
Early Childhood: 2–5 years		
3–6 years	Can understand causes of many emotions Can begin to find ways for regulating emotions and for expressing them Identifies with adult to cope	Empathy increases with understanding More response and less reaction; self-regulation: "Use your words to say that you are angry with him" Aggression becomes competition By age 5, shows sensitivity to criticism and cares about feelings of others Ego rules until age 6
Middle Childhood: 5–11 years		
7–11 years	Can react to the feelings of others More aware of other's feelings	Empathy becomes altruism: "I feel so bad about their fire, I'm going to give them some of my things" Superego dominates

Temperamental Differences

There are strong suggestions of inborn differences and wide variability in autonomic reactivity and temperament among individual infants. Chess and Thomas identified nine behavioral dimensions, in which reliable differences among infants can be observed (Table 27.1–6).

Most temperamental dimensions of individual children showed considerable stability over a 25-year follow-up period, but some temperamental traits did not persist. This finding was attributed to genetic and environmental effects on personality. A complex interplay exists among the initial characteristics of infants, the mode of parental interactions, and children's subsequent behavior. Observations of the stability and plasticity of certain temperamental traits support the importance of interactions between genetic endowment (nature) and environmental experience (nurture) in behavior.

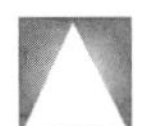

Table 27.1–6
Temperament—Newborn to 6 Years

Dimension	Description
Activity level	Percent of time spent in activities
Distractibility	Degree to which stimuli are allowed to alter behavior
Adaptability	Ease moving into change
Attention span	Amount of time spent on attending
Intensity	Energy level
Threshold of responsiveness	Intensity required for response
Quality of mood	Amount positive compared to amount negative behavior
Rhythmicity	Regulation of functions
Approach/withdrawal	Response to new situations

Attachment

Bonding is the term used to describe the intense emotional and psychological relationship a mother develops for her baby. Attachment is the relationship the baby develops with its caregivers. Infants in the first months after birth become attuned to social and interpersonal interaction. They show a rapidly increasing responsivity to the external environment and an ability to form a special relationship with significant primary caregivers—that is, to form an attachment. Table 27.1–7 lists the commonly observed attachment styles.

Harry Harlow. Harry Harlow studied social learning and the effects of social isolation in monkeys. Harlow placed newborn rhesus monkeys with two types of surrogate mothers—one a wire-mesh surrogate with a feeding bottle and the other a wire-mesh surrogate covered with terry cloth. The monkeys preferred the terry-cloth surrogates, which provided contact and comfort, to the feeding surrogate. (When hungry, the infant monkeys would go to the feeding bottle but then would quickly return to the terry-cloth surrogate.) When frightened, monkeys raised with terry-cloth surrogates showed intense clinging behavior and appeared to be comforted, whereas those raised with wire-mesh surrogates gained no comfort and appeared to be disorganized. The results of Harlow's experiments were widely interpreted as indicating that infant attachment is not simply the result of feeding.

Both types of surrogate-reared monkeys were subsequently unable to adjust to life in a monkey colony and had extraordinary difficulty learning to mate. When impregnated, the female monkeys failed to mother their young. These behavioral peculiarities were attributed to the isolates' lack of mothering in infancy.

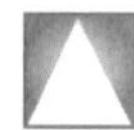

Table 27.1–7
Types of Attachment

Secure Attachment	Children show fewer adjustment problems; however, these children have typically received more consistent and developmentally appropriate parenting for most of their life. The parents of securely attached children are likely better able to maintain these aspects of parenting through a divorce. Given that the family factors that lead to divorce also impact the children, there could be fewer securely attached children in divorcing families.
Insecure/ Avoidant Attachment	Children become anxious, clinging, and angry with the parent. These children typically come from families with adults who were also insecurely attached to their families and, thus, were unable to provide the kind of consistency, emotional responsiveness, and care that securely attached parents could offer. Such parents have a more difficult time with divorce, and are more likely to become rejecting.
Insecure/ Ambivalent Attachment	Children generally are raised with disorganized, neglecting, and inattentive parenting. The parents are even less able to provide stability and psychological strength for them after a divorce and, as a result, the children are even more likely to become clinging but inconsolable in their distress, as well as to act out, suffer mood swings, and become oversensitive to stress.

John Bowlby. John Bowlby studied the attachment of infants to mothers and concluded that early separation of infants from their mothers had severe negative effects on children's emotional and intellectual development. He described attachment behavior, which develops during the first year of life, as the maintenance of physical contact between the mother and child when the child is hungry, frightened, or in distress.

Mary Ainsworth. Mary Ainsworth expanded on Bowlby's observations and found that the interaction between mother and baby during the attachment period influences the baby's current and future behavior significantly. Many observers believe that patterns of infant attachment affect future adult emotional relationships. Patterns of attachment vary among babies; for example, some babies signal or cry less than others. Sensitive responsiveness to infant signals, such as cuddling the baby when it cries, causes infants to cry less in later months. Close bodily contact with the mother when the baby signals for her is also associated with the growth of self-reliance, rather than clinging dependence, as the baby grows older. Unresponsive mothers produce anxious babies.

Ainsworth also confirmed that attachment serves to reduce anxiety. What she called the secured base effect enables a child to move away from the attachment figure and explore the environment. Inanimate objects, such as a teddy bear or a blanket (called the transitional object by Donald Winnicott), also serve as a secure base, one that often accompanies children as they investigate the world. A growing body of literature derived from direct observation of mother–infant interactions and longitudinal studies has expanded on, and refined, Ainsworth's original descriptions. Maternal sensitivity and responsiveness are the main determinants of secure attachment. But when the attachment is insecure, the type of insecurity (avoidant, anxious, or ambivalent) is determined by infant temperament. Overall, male infants are less likely to have secure attachments and are more vulnerable to changes in maternal sensitivity than are female infants.

The attachment of the firstborn child is decreased by the birth of a second, but it is decreased much more when the firstborn is 2 to 5 years of age when the younger sibling is born than when the firstborn is younger than 24 months. Not surprisingly, the extent of the decrease also depends on the mother's own sense of security, confidence, and mental health.

Social Deprivation Syndromes and Maternal Neglect. Investigators, especially René Spitz, have long documented the severe developmental retardation that accompanies maternal rejection and neglect. Infants in institutions characterized by low staff-to-infant ratios and frequent turnover of personnel tend to display marked developmental retardation, even with adequate physical care and freedom from infection. The same infants, placed in adequate foster or adoptive care, exhibit marked acceleration in development.

Fathers and Attachment. Babies become attached to fathers as well as to mothers, but the attachment is different. Generally, mothers hold babies for caregiving, and fathers hold babies for purposes of play. Given a choice of either parent after separation, infants usually go to the mother, but if the mother is unavailable they turn to the father for comfort. Babies raised in extended families or with multiple caregivers are able to establish many attachments.

Stranger Anxiety. A developmentally expected fear of strangers is first noted in infants at about 26 weeks of age, and more fully developed by 32 weeks (8 months). At the approach of a stranger, infants cry and cling to their mothers. Babies exposed to only one caregiver are more likely to have stranger anxiety than babies exposed to a variety of caregivers. Stranger anxiety is believed to result from a baby's growing ability to distinguish caregivers from all other persons.

Separation anxiety, which occurs between 10 and 18 months of age, is related to stranger anxiety but is not identical to it. Separation from the person to whom the infant is attached precipitates separation anxiety. Stranger anxiety, however, occurs even when the infant is in the mother's arms. The infant learns to separate as it starts to crawl and move away from the mother, but the infant constantly looks back and frequently returns to the mother for reassurance.

Margaret Mahler (1897–1985) proposed a theory to describe how young children acquire a sense of identity separate from that of their mothers'. Her theory of separation–individuation was based on observations of the interactions of children and their mothers. Mahler's stages of separation–individuation are outlined in Table 27.1–8.

Infant Care

Clinicians are now beginning to view infants as important actors in the family drama, ones who partly determine its course. Infants' behavior controls mothers' behavior, just as mothers'

Table 27.1–8
Stages of Separation–Individuation Proposed by Mahler

1. Normal autism (birth–2 months).
2. Periods of sleep outweigh periods of arousal in a state reminiscent of intrauterine life.
3. Symbiosis (2–5 months).
4. Developing perceptual abilities gradually enable infants to distinguish the inner from the outer world; mother–infant is perceived as a single fused entity.
5. Differentiation (5–10 months).
6. Progressive neurological development and increased alertness draw infants' attention away from self to the outer world. Physical and psychological distinctiveness from the mother is gradually appreciated.
7. Practicing (10–18 months).
8. The ability to move autonomously increases children's exploration of the outer world.
9. Rapprochement (18–24 months).
10. As children slowly realize their helplessness and dependence, the need for independence alternates with the need for closeness. Children move away from their mothers and come back for reassurance.
11. Object constancy (2–5 years).
12. Children gradually comprehend and are reassured by the permanence of mother and other important people, even when not in their presence.

behavior modulates infants' behavior. A calm, smiling, predictable infant is a powerful reward for tender maternal care. A jittery, irregular, irritable infant tries a mother's patience. When a mother's capacity for giving is marginal, such infant traits may cause her to turn away from her child and thus complicate the child's already-troubled beginnings.

Parental Fit

Parental fit describes how well the mother or father relates to the newborn or developing infant; the idea takes into account temperamental characteristics of both parent and child. Each newborn has innate psychophysiological characteristics, which are known collectively as temperament. Chess and Thomas identified a range of normal temperamental patterns, from the difficult child at one end of the spectrum to the easy child at the other end.

Difficult children, who make up 10 percent of all children, have a hyperalert physiological makeup. They react intensely to stimuli (cry easily at loud noises), sleep poorly, eat at unpredictable times, and are difficult to comfort. Easy children, who make up 40 percent of all children, are regular in eating, eliminating, and sleeping; they are flexible, can adapt to change and new stimuli with a minimum of distress, and are easily comforted when they cry. The other 50 percent of children are mixtures of these two types. The difficult child is harder to raise and places greater demands on the parent than the easy child. Chess and Thomas used the term goodness-of-fit to characterize the harmonious and consonant interaction between a mother and a child in their motivations, capacities, and styles of behavior. Poor fit is likely to lead to distorted development and maladaptive functioning. A difficult child must be recognized, because parents of such infants often have feelings of inadequacy and believe that they are doing something wrong to account for the child's difficulty in sleeping and eating and their problems comforting the child. In addition, most difficult children have emotional disturbances later in life.

Good-Enough Mothering. Winnicott believed that infants begin life in a state of nonintegration, with unconnected and diffuse experiences, and that mothers provide the relationship that enables infants' incipient selves to emerge. Mothers supply a holding environment in which infants are contained and experienced. During the last trimester of pregnancy and for the first few months of a baby's life, the mother is in a state of primary maternal preoccupation, absorbed in fantasies about, and experiences with, her baby. The mother need not be perfect, but she must provide good-enough mothering. She plays a vital role in bringing the world to the child and offering empathic anticipation of the infant's needs. If the mother can resonate with the infant's needs, the baby can become attuned to its own bodily functions and drives that are the basis for the gradually evolving sense of self.

TODDLER PERIOD

The second year of life is marked by accelerated motor and intellectual development. The ability to walk gives toddlers some control over their own actions; this mobility enables children to determine when to approach and when to withdraw. The acquisition of speech profoundly extends their horizons. Typically, children learn to say "no" before they learn to say "yes." Toddlers' negativism is vital to the development of independence, but if it persists, oppositional behavior connotes a problem.

Learning language is a crucial task in the toddler period. Vocalizations become distinct, and toddlers can name a few objects and make needs known in one or two words. Near the end of the second year and into the third year, toddlers sometimes use short sentences. The pace of language development varies considerably from child to child, and although a small number of children are truly late developers, most child experts recommend a hearing test if the child is not making two-word sentences by age 2.

Developmental Milestones in Toddlers

Language and Cognitive Development. Toddlers begin to listen to explanations that can help them tolerate delay. They create new behaviors from old ones (originality) and engage in symbolic activities, for instance, using words and playing with dolls when the dolls represent something, such as a feeding sequence. Toddlers have varied capacities for concentration and self-regulation.

Emotional and Social Development. In the second year, pleasure and displeasure become further differentiated. Social referencing is often apparent at this age; the child looks to parents and others for emotional cues about how to respond to novel events. Toddlers show exploratory excitement, assertive pleasure, and pleasure in discovery and in developing new behavior (e.g., new games), including teasing and surprising or fooling the parent (e.g., hiding). The toddler has capacities for an organized demonstration of love, as when the toddler runs up and hugs, smiles, and kisses the parent at the same time, and of protest when the toddler turns away, cries, bangs, bites, hits, yells, and kicks. Comfort with family and apprehension with strangers may increase. Anxiety appears to be related to disapproval and the loss of a loved caregiver and can be disorganizing.

Sexual Development. Sexual differentiation is evident from birth, when parents start dressing and treating infants differently because of the expectations evoked by sex typing. Through imitation, reward, and coercion, children assume the behaviors that their cultures define as appropriate for their sexual roles. Children exhibit curiosity about anatomical sex. When their curiosity is recognized as healthy and is met with honest, age-appropriate replies, children acquire a sense of the wonder of life and are comfortable with their own roles. If the subject of sex is taboo and children's questions are rebuffed, shame and discomfort may result.

Gender identity, the conviction of being male or female, begins to manifest at 18 months of age and is often fixed by 24 to 30 months. It was once widely believed that gender identity was primarily a function of social learning. John Money reported on children with ambiguous or damaged external genitalia who were raised as the sex opposite to their chromosomal sex. Long-term follow-up of those individuals suggests that the major part of gender identity is innate and that rearing may not affect the genetic diathesis.

Gender role describes the behavior that society deems appropriate for one sex or another, and it is not surprising that significant cultural differences exist. There may be different expectations for boys and girls in what and with whom they play, their tone of voice, the expression of emotions, and how they dress. Nevertheless, some generalizations are possible. Boys are more likely than girls to engage in rough and tumble play. Mothers talk more to girls than to boys, and by the time the child is 2 years of age, fathers generally pay more attention to boys. Many educated, middle-class parents determined to raise nonsexist children are startled to see their children's determined preference for sex-stereotyped toys—girls want to play with dolls, and boys with guns.

Toilet Training. The second year of life is a period of increasing social demands on children. Toilet training serves as a paradigm of the family's general training practices; that is, the parent who is overly severe in the area of toilet training is likely to be punitive and restrictive in other areas also. Control of daytime urination is usually complete by the age of 2½, and control of nighttime urination is usually complete by the age of 4 years, when bowel control is usually accomplished. Since 1900, the pendulum has swung between extremes of permissiveness and control in toilet training. The trend in the United States has been toward delayed training, but in the last few years this trend appears to be shifting back to early training.

Toddlers may have sleep difficulties related to fear of the dark, which can often be managed by using a nightlight. Most toddlers generally sleep about 12 hours a day, including a 2-hour nap. Parents must be aware that children of this age may need reassurance before going to bed and that the average 2-year-old takes about 30 minutes to fall asleep.

Parenting Challenges. In infancy, the major responsibility for parents is to meet the infant's needs in a sensitive and consistent fashion. The parental task in the toddler stage requires firmness about the boundaries of acceptable behavior and encouragement of the child's progressive emancipation. Parents must be careful not to be too authoritarian at this stage; children must be allowed to operate for themselves and to learn from their mistakes and must be protected and assisted when challenges are beyond their abilities.

During the toddler period, children are likely to struggle for the exclusive affection and attention of their parents. This struggle includes rivalry, both with siblings and with one or another parent for the star role in the family. Although children are beginning to be able to share, they do so reluctantly. When the demands for exclusive possession are not resolved effectively, the result is likely to be jealous competitiveness in relationships with peers and lovers. The fantasies aroused by the struggle lead to fear of retaliation and to displacement of fear onto external objects. In an equitable, loving family a child elaborates a moral system of ethical rights. Parents need to balance between punishment and permissiveness and set realistic limits on a toddler's behavior.

PRESCHOOL PERIOD

The preschool period is characterized by marked physical and emotional growth. Generally, between 2 and 3 years of age, children reach half their adult height. The 20 baby teeth are in place at the beginning of the stage, and by the end they begin to fall out. Children are ready to enter school by the time the stage ends at age 5 or 6. They have mastered the tasks of primary socialization—to control their bowels and urine, to dress and feed themselves, and to control their tears and temper outbursts, at least most of the time.

The term preschool for the age group of 2½ to 6 years may be a misnomer; many children are already in school-like settings, such as preschool nurseries and day care centers, where working mothers must often place their children. Preschool education can be valuable, but stressing academic advancement too far beyond a child's capabilities can be counterproductive.

Developmental Milestones in Preschoolers

Language and Cognitive Development. In the preschool period, children's use of language expands, and they use sentences. Individual words have regular and consistent meanings at the beginning of the period, and children begin to think symbolically. In general, however, their thinking is egocentric; they cannot place themselves in the position of another child and are incapable of empathy. Children think intuitively and prelogically and do not understand causal relations.

Emotional and Social Behavior. At the start of the preschool period, children can express such complex emotions as love, unhappiness, jealousy, and envy, both preverbally and verbally. Their emotions are still easily influenced by somatic events, such as tiredness and hunger. Although they still think mostly egocentrically, children's capacity for cooperation and sharing is emerging. Anxiety is related to loss of a person who was loved and depended on and to loss of approval and acceptance. Although still potentially disorganizing, anxiety can be tolerated better than in the past. Four-year-olds are learning to share and to have concern for others. Feelings of tenderness are sometimes expressed. Anxiety over bodily injury and the loss of a loved person's approval is sometimes disruptive.

By the end of the preschool period, children have many relatively stable emotions. Expansiveness, curiosity, pride, and gleeful excitement related to the self and the family are balanced with coyness, shyness, fearfulness, jealousy, and envy. Shame and humiliation are evident. Capacities for empathy and love are developed but are fragile and easily lost if competitive or jealous strivings intervene. Anxiety and fears are related to bodily injury and loss of respect, love, and emerging self-esteem. Guilt feelings are possible.

Children between the ages of 3 and 6 years are aware of their bodies, and of differences between the sexes. In their play, doctor–nurse games allow children to act out their sexual fantasies. Their awareness of their bodies extends beyond the genitalia; they show a preoccupation with illness or injury, so much so that the period has been called "the Band-Aid phase." Every injury must be examined and taken care of by a parent.

Children develop a division between what they want and what they are told to do. The division increases until a gap grows between their set of expanded desires, their exuberance at unlimited growth, and their parents' restrictions; they gradually turn parental values into self-obedience, self-guidance, and self-punishment.

At the end of the preschool stage, the child's conscience is evolving. The development of a conscience sets the tone for the moral sense of "right and wrong." Until about 7 years of age, children typically experience rules as "absolute" and as existing for their own sake. They do not understand that more than one point of view on a moral issue may exist; a violation of the rules calls for absolute retribution—that is, children have the notion of immanent justice.

SIBLING RIVALRY. In the preschool period, children relate to others in new ways. The birth of a sibling (a common occurrence during this time) tests a preschool child's capacity for further cooperation and sharing but may also evoke sibling rivalry, which is most likely to occur at this time. Sibling rivalry depends on child-rearing practice. Favoritism for any reason commonly aggravates such rivalry. Children who get special treatment because they are gifted, are defective in some way, or have a preferred gender are likely to receive angry feelings from their siblings. Experiences with siblings can influence growing children's relationships with peers and authority; for example, a problem may result if the needs of a new baby prevent the mother from attending to a firstborn child's needs. If not handled properly, the displacement of the firstborn can be a traumatic event.

PLAY. In the preschool years, children begin to distinguish reality from fantasy, and play reflects this growing awareness. Pretend games are popular and help test real-life situations in a playful manner. Dramatic play in which children act out a role, such as a housewife or a truck driver, is common. One-to-one play relationships advance to complicated patterns with rivalries, secrets, and two-against-one intrigues. Children's play behavior reflects their level of social development.

Between 2½ and 3 years, children commonly engage in parallel play, solitary play alongside another child with no interaction between them. By age 3, play is often associative, that is, playing with the same toys in pairs or in small groups, but still with no real interaction among them. By age 4, children are usually able to share and engage in cooperative play. Real interactions and taking turns become possible.

Between 3 and 6 years of age, growth can be traced through drawings. A child's first drawing of a human being is a circular line with marks for the mouth, nose, and eyes; ears and hair are added later; arms and stick-like fingers appear next; and then legs appear. Last to appear is a torso in proportion to the rest of the body. Intelligent children can deal with details in their art. Drawings express creativity throughout a child's development: They are representational and formal in early childhood, make use of perspective in middle childhood, and become abstract and affect-laden in adolescence. Drawings also reflect children's body image concepts and sexual and aggressive impulses.

IMAGINARY COMPANIONS. Imaginary companions most often appear during preschool years, usually in children with above-average intelligence and usually in the form of persons. Imaginary companions may also be things, such as toys that are anthropomorphized. Some studies indicate that up to 50 percent of children between the ages of 3 and 10 years have imaginary companions at one time or another. Their significance is not clear, but these figures are usually friendly, relieve loneliness, and reduce anxiety. In most instances, imaginary companions disappear by age 12, but they can occasionally persist into adulthood.

MIDDLE YEARS

The period between age 6 and puberty is often called the middle years. During this time, children enter elementary school. The formal demands for academic learning and accomplishment become major determinants of further personality development.

Developmental Milestones in School-Age Children

Language and Cognitive Development. In the middle years, language expresses complex ideas with relations among several elements. Logical exploration tends to dominate fantasy, and children show an increased interest in rules and orderliness and an increased capacity for self-regulation. During this period, children's conceptual skills develop, and thinking becomes organized and logical. The ability to concentrate is well established by age 9 or 10, and by the end of the period, children begin to think in abstract terms. Improved gross motor coordination and muscle strength enable children to write fluently and draw artistically. They are also capable of complex motor tasks and activities, such as tennis, gymnastics, golf, baseball, and skateboarding.

Recent evidence has shown that changes in thinking and reasoning during the middle years result from maturational changes in the brain. Children are now capable of increased independence, learning, and socialization. Theorists consider moral development a gradual, stepwise process spanning childhood, adolescence, and young adulthood.

In the middle years, both girls and boys make new identifications with other adults, such as teachers and counselors. These identifications may so influence girls that their goals of wanting to marry and have babies, as their mothers did, may be combined with a desire for a career or may be postponed or abandoned entirely.

Girls who cannot identify with their mothers or whose fathers are overly attached may become fixated at about a 6-year-old level; as a result, they may fear men or women or both or become seductively close to them. In either case, such girls may not be seen as normal during the school-age years. A similar situation can occur in boys who have been unable to identify successfully with fathers who were aloof, brutal, or absent. Perhaps his mother prevented a boy from identifying with his father by being overprotective or by binding the son too closely to her. As a result, boys may enter this period with a variety of problems. They may be fearful of men, unsure of their sense of masculinity, or unwilling to leave their mothers (sometimes manifested by a school phobia); they may lack initiative and be unable to master school tasks, thus incurring academic problems.

The school-age period is a time when peer interaction assumes major importance. Interest in relationships outside the family takes precedence over those within the family. Nevertheless, a special relationship exists with the same-sex parent, with whom children identify and who is now an ideal and a role model.

Empathy and concern for others begin to emerge early in the middle years; by the time children are 9 or 10, they have well-developed capacities for love, compassion, and sharing. They have a capacity for long-term, stable relationships with family, peers, and friends, including best friends. Emotions about sexual differences begin to emerge as either excitement or shyness with the opposite sex. School-age children prefer to interact with children of the same sex. Although the middle years have sometimes been referred to as a latency period—a moratorium on psychosexual exploration and play until the eruption of sexual impulses with puberty—it is now recognized that a considerable amount of sexual interest continues through these years. Sex play and curiosity are common, especially among boys, but also among girls. Boys compare genitals and sometimes engage in group or mutual masturbation. An interest in anal humor and toilet jokes is often seen. Children at this age often start using sexual and excretory words as expletives.

BEST FRIEND. Harry Stack Sullivan postulated that a buddy, or best friend, is an important phenomenon during the school years. By about 10 years of age, children develop a close same-sex relationship, which Sullivan believed is necessary for further healthy psychological growth. Moreover, Sullivan believed that the absence of a chum during the middle years of childhood is an early harbinger of schizophrenia.

SCHOOL REFUSAL. Some children refuse to go to school at this time, generally because of separation anxiety. A fearful mother may transmit her own fear of separation to a child, or a child who has not resolved dependence needs panics at the idea of separation. School refusal is usually not an isolated problem; children with the problem typically avoid many other social situations.

Sex Role Development

Persons' sex roles are similar to their gender identity; persons see themselves as male or female. The sex role also involves identification with culturally acceptable masculine or feminine ways of behaving; but changing expectations in society (particularly in the United States) of what constitutes masculine and feminine behavior can create ambiguity.

Parents react differently to their male and female children. Independence, physical play, and aggressiveness are encouraged in boys; dependence, verbalization, and physical intimacy are encouraged in girls. Nowadays, however, boys are encouraged to verbalize their feelings and to pursue interests traditionally associated with girls, whereas girls are encouraged to pursue careers traditionally dominated by men and to participate in competitive sports. As society grows more tolerant in its expectations of the sexes, roles become less rigid, and opportunities for boys and girls enlarge and broaden.

Biologically, boys are more physically aggressive than girls; and parental expectations, particularly the expectations of fathers, reinforce this trait. Differences also exist between boys and girls in the influence of persons outside the family. Girls tend to respond to the expectations and opinions of girls and of teachers of either sex, but to ignore boys. Boys, on the other hand, tend to respond to other boys, but to ignore girls and teachers.

Dreams and Sleep

Children's dreams can have a profound effect on behavior. During the first year of life, when reality and fantasy are not yet fully differentiated, dreams may be experienced as if they were, or could be, true. At age 3, many children believe dreams are shared directly by more than one person, but most 4-year-olds understand that dreams are unique to each person. Children view dreams either with pleasure or, as is most often reported, with fear. The dream content should be seen in connection with children's life experience, developmental stage, mechanisms used during dreaming, and sex.

Disturbing dreams peak when children are 3, 6, and 10 years of age. Two-year-old children may dream about being bitten or chased; at the age of 4, they may have many animal dreams and also dream of persons who either protect or destroy. At age 5 or 6, dreams of being killed or injured, of flying and being in cars, and of ghosts become prominent; the role of conscience, moral values, and increasing conflicts are concerned with these themes. In early childhood, aggressive dreams rarely seem to occur; instead, dreamers are in danger, a state that perhaps reflects children's dependent position. By about the age of 5, children realize that their dreams are not real; before then, they believed them to be real events. By age 7, children know that they create their dreams themselves.

Between the ages of 3 and 6 years, children normally want to keep their bedroom door open or to have a nightlight, so that they can either maintain contact with their parents or view the room in a realistic, nonfearful way. At times, children resist going to sleep to avoid dreaming. Disorders associated with falling asleep, therefore, are often connected with dreaming. Children often create rituals to protect themselves in the withdrawal from the world of reality into the world of sleep. Parasomnias, such as sleepwalking, sleep talking, enuresis (bed-wetting), and night terrors, are common at this age. They usually occur during stage 4 sleep when dreaming is minimal, and they do not indicate emotional trouble or underlying psychopathology. Most children grow out of parasomnias by adolescence.

Periods of REM occur about 60 percent of the time during the first few weeks of life, a period when infants sleep two-thirds of the time. Premature babies sleep even longer than full-term babies, and a greater proportion of their sleep is REM sleep. The sleep–wake cycle of newborns is about 3 hours long. Among adults, the dream-to-sleep ratio is stable: 20 percent of sleeping time is spent dreaming. Even newborns have brain activity similar to that of the dreaming state.

Birth Spacing

For women in the United States, 10 percent of conceptions that lead to live births are considered unwanted, and 20 percent are wanted but considered ill timed.

Children born close together have higher rates of premature or underweight births, and malnutrition; they develop more slowly and are at increased risk of contracting and dying from childhood infectious diseases. Studies have shown when a child is born 3 to 5 years after a previous birth, health risks are reduced for both mother and child. Compared with 24- to 29-month intervals, children born in 36- to 41-month intervals are associated with a 28 percent reduction in stunting and a 29 percent reduction of low birth weight. Women who have children at 27- to 32-month intervals are 1.3 times more likely to avoid anemia, 1.7 times more likely to avoid third-trimester bleeding, and 2.5 times more likely to survive childbirth.

Birth Order

The effects of birth order vary. Firstborn children are often more highly valued and given more attention than subsequent children. Firstborn children appear to be more achievement oriented and motivated to please their parents than subsequent children born to the same parents. Some studies show that people in certain competitive occupational areas, such as architecture, accounting, and engineering, tend to be firstborn children.

Second and third children have the advantage of their parents' previous experience. Younger children also learn from their older siblings. For example, they may show more sophisticated use of pronouns at an earlier age than firstborns did. When children are spaced too closely, however, there may not be enough time for each child. The arrival of new children in the family affects not only the parents but also the siblings. Firstborn children may resent the birth of a new sibling, who threatens their sole claim on parental attention. In some cases, regressive behavior, such as enuresis or thumb-sucking, occurs.

According to Frank Sulloway, firstborn children tend to be conservative and conformists; by contrast, youngest children tend to be independent and rebellious in regard to family and cultural norms. Sulloway found that a high proportion of prominent persons were lastborn children. He ascribes these differences to birth order and suggests that each child develops personality traits to fit an unfilled slot in the family. His findings need to be replicated.

Children and Divorce

Many children live in homes in which divorce has occurred. Approximately 30 to 50 percent of all children in the United States live in homes in which one parent (usually the mother) is the sole head of the household, and 61 percent of all children born in any given year can expect to live with only one parent before they reach the age of 18 years. A child's age at the time of the parents' divorce affects the child's reaction to the divorce. Immediately after a divorce, an increase in behavioral and emotional disorders appears in all age groups. Infants do not understand anything about separation or divorce; however, they do notice changes in their parents' responses to them and may experience changes in their eating or sleeping patterns; have bowel problems; and seem more fretful, fearful, or anxious. Children 3 to 6 years of age may not understand what is happening, and those who do understand often assume that they are somehow responsible for the divorce. Older children, especially adolescents, comprehend the situation and may believe that they could have prevented the divorce had they intervened in some way, but they are still hurt, angry, and critical of their parents' behavior.

Some children harbor the fantasy that their parents will be reunited in the future. Such children may show animosity toward a parent's real or potential new mate because they are faced with the reality that reconciliation between their parents is not taking place. Adaptation to the effects of divorce in children typically takes several years; however, up to about one-third of children from divorced homes may have lasting psychological trauma. Among boys, physical aggression is a common sign of distress. Adolescents tend to spend more time away from the parental home after the divorce. Children who adapt best to divorce are typically in a situation in which both parents make genuine efforts to spend time and relate to the child despite the child's potential anger about the divorce. To facilitate adaptation in children, a divorced couple who are amicable, and avoid arguing with one another is most likely to succeed. Table 27.1–9 lists potential psychological effects of divorce on children.

Stepparents. Although there are many different scenarios that may occur after a divorce and remarriage, several potential

Table 27.1–9
Effects of Divorce on Children

- ▲ Children in homes with absent fathers are more likely to suffer from antisocial personality disorder, child conduct disorder, and attention-deficit hyperactivity disorder.
- ▲ The divorce rate of children of divorced parents doubles that of children from stable families.
- ▲ Children of divorce are far more likely to be delinquent, engage in premarital sex, and bear children out of wedlock during adolescence and young adulthood.
- ▲ Children from divorced homes function more poorly than children from continuously married parents across a variety of domains, including academic achievement, social relations, and conduct problems.
- ▲ Children from divorced homes have more psychological problems than those from homes disrupted by the death of a parent.
- ▲ Children from disrupted marriages experience greater risk of injury, asthma, headaches, and speech defects than children from intact families.
- ▲ Children of divorce tend to be impulsive, irritable, socially withdrawn, lonely, unhappy, anxious, and insecure.
- ▲ Children of divorce, especially boys, are more aggressive than children whose parents stayed married.
- ▲ Suicide rates for children of divorce are much higher than for children from intact families.
- ▲ 20–25% have significant adjustment problems as teenagers.

Data adapted from Americans for Divorce Reform, Arlington, VA. Table by Nitza Jones.

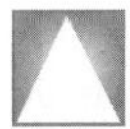

Table 27.1–10
Types of Step-Families

Neo-Traditional Families	▲ Resembles "traditional" families. ▲ Absent biological parent is included at times. ▲ Discipline, boundaries and limits, and expectations are discussed openly. ▲ Family coalitions and "side-taking" are better avoided.
Romantic Families	▲ Expect to be a "traditional family" immediately. ▲ The absent biological parent is expected to disappear and is often criticized. ▲ Stepparent/stepchild difficulties are common. ▲ Stress is unbearable. ▲ Few open and frank discussions about problems.
Matriarchal Families	▲ Run by a highly competent mom and her companion follows. ▲ Companion is a "buddy" to the children, not to the parent. ▲ Birth of a step-sibling causes problems.

scenarios have been outlined in Table 27.1–10. These include: (1) Neo-traditional, (2) Romantic, and (3) Matriarchal. When remarriage occurs, children must learn to adapt to the stepparent and to the "blended" family. Adaptation is often challenging, especially when a child feels that a stepparent is nonsupportive, resents the stepchild, or favors his or her own natural children. Of step-families, 25 percent tend to dissolve within the first 2 years, whereas 75 percent grow to find a new balance in their blended family. A biological child born to a new couple with a stepchild already in the home may receive more attention than the stepchild, leading to of sibling rivalry. After 5 years, about 20 percent of adolescents in step-families suggest that they move out and try living with their other biological parent.

Family Factors in Child Development

Family Stability. Parents and children living under the same roof in harmonious interaction is the expected cultural norm in Western society. Within this framework, childhood development presumably proceeds most expeditiously. Deviations from the norm, such as divorced- and single-parent families, are associated with a broad range of problems in children, including low self-esteem, increased risk of child abuse, and increased incidence of divorce when they eventually marry, and increased incidence of mental disorders, particularly depressive disorders and antisocial personality disorder as adults. Why some children from unstable homes are less affected than others (or even immune to these deleterious effects) is of great interest. Michael Rutter has postulated that vulnerability is influenced by sex (boys are more affected than girls), age (older children are less vulnerable than younger ones), and inborn personality characteristics. For example, children who have a placid temperament are less likely to be victims of abuse within a family than are hyperactive children; by virtue of their placidity, they may be less affected by the emotional turmoil surrounding them.

Adverse Events. It is now well known that significant adverse events, especially in early childhood such as sexual and physical abuse, neglect, or loss of a parent, interact with genetic background in a given child and influences the trajectory of development. For example, as mentioned earlier early severe maltreatment such as sexual abuse increases the risk of multiple psychosocial difficulties and emergence of many psychiatric disorders. Among young maltreated children, those with particular genetics, that is, who have the "short" variant of the serotonin transporter gene (short 5-HTTLPR polymorphism) are significantly more vulnerable to chronic depression in adulthood. This example of specific gene–environment interaction plays an important role in a child's development as well as in the risk for future psychopathology. Current investigations are also seeking insight into what factors lead to resilience in youth who have been exposed to adverse events, yet maintain allostasis, that is, stability in the face of stressful events. Hormones of the adrenal glands, thyroid, gonads, as well as metabolic hormones play a role on the brain's ability to maintain stability upon exposure to stress, and the prefrontal cortex, hippocampus, and amygdala play critical roles in regulating emotionality, aggression, and resilience.

Day Care Centers. The role of day care centers for children is under continuous investigation, and various studies have produced different results. One study found that children placed in day care centers before the age of 5 are less assertive and less effectively toilet trained than home-reared children. Another study found children in day care to be more advanced in social and cognitive development than children who were not in day care. The National Institute of Child Health and Human Development reported that 4½ year olds who had spent more than 30 hours a week in child care were more demanding, more aggressive, and more noncompliant than those raised at home and showed higher cognitive skills, particularly in math and reading. These same children who were tracked through the third grade continued to score higher in math and reading skills but had poorer work habits and social skills. The researchers were careful to note that this behavior was within the normal range, however.

All studies of day care must take into account the quality of both the day care center and the homes from which children come. For example, a child from a disadvantaged home may be better off at a day care center than a child from an advantaged home. Similarly, a woman who wishes to leave the home to work for financial or other reasons and cannot do so may resent being forced to remain in the home in a child-rearing role, which may adversely affect the child.

Parenting Styles. The ways in which children are raised vary considerably between and within cultures. Rutter has clustered the diversity into four general styles. Subsequent research has confirmed that certain styles tend to correlate with certain behavior in the children, although the outcomes are by no means absolute. The authoritarian style, characterized by strict, inflexible rules, can lead to low self-esteem, unhappiness, and social withdrawal. The indulgent–permissive style, which includes little or no limit setting coupled with unpredictable parental harshness, can lead to low self-reliance, poor impulse control, and aggression. The indulgent–neglectful style, one of noninvolvement in the child's life and rearing, puts the child at risk for low self-esteem, impaired self-control, and increased aggression. The authoritative–reciprocal style, marked by firm rules and shared decision-making in a warm, loving environment, is believed to be the style most likely to result in self-reliance, self-esteem, and a sense of social responsibility.

Development and Expression of Psychopathology

The expression of psychopathology in children can be related to both age and developmental level. Specific developmental disorders, particularly developmental language disorders, often are diagnosed in the preschool years. Delayed development of language is a common parental concern. Children who do not use words by 18 months or phrases by 2½ to 3 years may need assessment, particularly if they do not appear to understand normal verbal cues or much language at all. Mild mental retardation or specific learning problems often are not diagnosed until after the child begins elementary school. Disruptive behavior disorder will become apparent at that time as the child begins to interact with peers. Similarly, attention-deficit disorders are only diagnosed when the demands for sustained attention are made in school. Other conditions, particularly schizophrenia and bipolar disorder, are rare in preschool and school-aged children.

ADOLESCENCE

Adolescence, marked by the physiological signs and surging sexual hormones of puberty, is the period of maturation between childhood and adulthood. Adolescence is a transitional period in which peer relationships deepen, autonomy in decision-making grows, and intellectual pursuits and social belonging are sought. Adolescence is largely a time of exploration and making choices, a gradual process of working toward an integrated concept of self. Adolescents can best be described as "works in progress," characterized by increasing ability for mastery over complex challenges of academic, interpersonal, and emotional tasks, while searching for new interests, talents, and social identities. A body of growing literature of the specific mechanisms of brain development in adolescence has increased our understanding of broadening social skills in adolescents, in addition to the three expected developmental changes in adolescence: increased risk taking, increased sexual behavior, and a move toward peer affiliation rather than primary family attachment. The total cortical gray matter is at its peak at about age 11 years in girls and 13 years in boys, which enhances the ability to understand subtle social situations, control impulses, make long range plans, and think ahead. White matter volume increases throughout childhood and adolescence, which may allow for increased "connectivity," thereby enhancing the abilities of adolescents to acquire new competencies, such as those needed to master today's technology.

What Is Normal Adolescence?

The concept of normality in adolescent development refers to the degree of psychological adaptation that is achieved while navigating the hurdles and meeting the milestones characteristic of this period of growth. For up to approximately 75 percent of youth, adolescence is a period of successful adaptation to physical, cognitive, and emotional changes, largely continuous with their previous functioning. Psychological maladjustment, self-loathing, disturbance of conduct, substance abuse, affective disorders, and other impairing psychiatric disorders emerge in approximately 20 percent of the adolescent population.

Adolescent adjustment is continuous with previous psychological function; thus, psychologically disturbed children are at greater risk for psychiatric disorders during adolescence. Adolescents with psychiatric disorders are at increased risk for greater conflicts with families and for feeling alienated from their families. Although up to 60 percent of adolescents endorse occasional distress, or a psychiatric symptom, this group of adolescents functions well academically and with peers and describes themselves as generally satisfied with their lives.

The developmentalist Erik Erikson characterizes the normative task of adolescence as identity versus role confusion. The integration of past experiences with current changes takes place in what Erikson terms ego identity. Adolescents explore various aspects of their psychological selves by becoming fans of heroes, or other well-known musical or political idols. Some adolescents appear consumed by their identification with a particular idol, whereas others are more moderate in their expression. Adolescents who feel accepted by a peer group and are involved in a variety of activities are less likely to become consumed by adoration of an idol. Adolescents who are socially isolated, feel socially rejected, and become overly identified with an idol to the exclusion of all other activities are at greater risk for serious emotional problems and require psychiatric intervention.

Erikson uses the term moratorium to describe that interim period between the concrete thinking of childhood and a more evolved complex ethical development. Erikson defines identity crisis as a normative part of adolescence in which adolescents pursue alternative behaviors and styles and, then, successfully mold these different experiences into a solid identity. A failure to do so would result in identity diffusion, or role confusion, in which the adolescent lacks a cohesive or confident sense of identity. Adolescence is the time to bond with peers, experiment with new beliefs and styles, fall in love for the first time, and explore creative ideas for future endeavors.

Most adolescents go through this developmental process with optimism, develop good self-esteem, maintain good peer relationships, and sustain basically harmonious relationships with their families.

Stages of Adolescence

Early Adolescence. Early adolescence, from 12 to 14 years of age, is the period in which the most striking initial changes are noticed—physically, attitudinally, and behaviorally. Growth spurts often begin in these years for boys, whereas girls may have already had rapid growth for 1 to 2 years. At this stage, boys and girls begin to criticize usual family habits, insist on spending time with peers with less supervision, have a greater awareness of style and appearance, and may question previously accepted family values. A new awareness of sexuality may be displayed by increased modesty and embarrassment with their current physical development or may exhibit itself in an increased interest in the opposite sex.

Early adolescents engage in subtle or overt displays of their growing desire for autonomy, sometimes with challenging behaviors toward authority figures, including teachers and school administrators, and exhibit disdain for rules themselves. At this age, some adolescents begin to experiment with cigarettes, alcohol, and marijuana.

In early adolescence, there is normal variation during which new social behaviors are acquired. Overall, although many early adolescents make new friends and modify their public image, most maintain positive connections to family members, old friends, and their family's values. However, early adolescence has been viewed as a time of overwhelming turmoil, during which there is a dramatic rejection of family, friends, and lifestyle, resulting in a powerful alienation of the adolescent.

Jake, a 13-year-old adolescent, had just started the 8th grade. In the past, he has been a jovial, fun-loving, and cooperative student, but this year he found the school rules increasingly irritating and felt that his teachers were too strict. He had always been a good student while putting in a minimum of work. His older brother Sean, now in 11th grade, had established himself as a compliant, well-liked, and well-behaved student who always put maximal effort into school projects in the same school, so Jake was compared with his brother on a regular basis by many teachers. Jake resented these comparisons because, unlike his brother, whom Jake felt was a "nerd," Jake was more rebellious, took more risks, and made friends with more popular peers. To distinguish himself from his older brother in school and at home, Jake began to challenge the rules at school, stating that they were "stupid" and "meaningless." Jake began to cut classes, to stay out late, and to experiment with alcohol and marijuana. He rejected his best friends from 6th and 7th grade, and began to hang out with peers who were more daring. When Jake was at home, he was able to relate to his older brother Sean only when they played basketball and video games.

Jake's grades began to deteriorate only slightly, but his parents noticed that on his report cards, his effort and behavior were rated as unsatisfactory. During the second month of school, Jake's parents received a phone call that Jake was going to be suspended due to possession of a small amount of marijuana on the school grounds during recess. During a subsequent meeting with the assistant principal and school counselor, Jake argued that the suspension was unfair because his grades were still good, and did not understand why his marijuana possession had triggered a suspension. When confronted with the fact that he had not only broken the school rules, but also violated the law, and that he was fortunate because the school did not involve the police, Jake became angry and continued to insist that he was being treated unfairly. He also blurted out that all of his teachers and his parents favored his older brother Sean, and treated him like a second-class citizen. Jake was suspended for 5 days, but the school indicated that they would report the incident to the police unless Jake and his family initiated immediate counseling.

Jake begrudgingly began psychotherapy and entered into a weekly therapy group specializing in substance use, for teens. Jake's parents also sought therapy to work on becoming more unified in their parenting. Jake remained in psychotherapy for the next 1½ years, during which time his attitude and reasoning style changed and evolved considerably. At age 15, Jake was able to understand why his school had suspended him for possession of marijuana and came to appreciate their willingness to give him the chance to seek counseling, rather than be turned over to the police. Over time, Jake was able to admit the dangers of using drugs, and took responsibility for his ill-advised behaviors. Alcohol and drug use continued to be a focus of his therapy and, by 15, Jake had virtually lost interest in alcohol, and admitted to smoking marijuana rarely at parties. Jake became more open to making friends with a variety of peers, and he disclosed that he liked himself better now than when he was 13. He now treated his brother respectfully when alone or with friends, and he felt that his parents appreciated him for "who he was." *(Courtesy of Caroly S. Pataki, M.D.)*

Middle Adolescence. During the middle phase of adolescence (roughly between the ages of 14 and 16), adolescents' lifestyles may reflect their efforts to pursue their own stated goals of being independent. Their abilities to combine abstract reasoning with realistic decision-making and the application of social judgment are put to the test in this phase of adolescent development. In this phase, sexual behavior intensifies, making romantic relationships more complicated, and self-esteem becomes a pivotal influence on positive and negative risk-taking behaviors.

In this phase of development, adolescents tend to identify with a group of peers who become highly influential in their choices of activities, styles, music, idols, and role models. Adolescents' underestimation of the risks associated with a variety of recreational behaviors and their sense of "omnipotence," mixed with their drive to be autonomous, frequently cause some conflict with parental requests and expectations. For most teens, the process of defining themselves as unique and different from their families can be achieved while still maintaining alliances with family members.

Jenna, a 16-year-old junior in high school, had just gotten her driver's license. She realized that she was lucky to have been given a brand new car at 16, because many of her friends did not yet have cars, she was upset that her parents disapproved of her agreement to drive all of her friends to places that she did not even want to go. Jenna was an attractive and well-liked adolescent who had always been an "A" and "B" student, and she and her family had never had conflicts about school. She played the flute in the school's orchestra, and was not involved in any team sports. Jenna started "going out" with a boy in her grade at school, Brett, who was also 16 years old, shortly after she got her license, and even though they didn't know each other that well, she felt that they had a close relationship. Since he did not yet have a car, she was the "identified driver" whenever they went out or to parties. Jenna was glad about this, because she didn't really like alcohol and was relieved that Brett would not be driving, given that he liked to drink quite a bit at parties. Jenna got along fairly well with her parents, who were considered very "easy-going" by her friends, and she felt that she and her parents had similar values and ideas.

Things were going well until Brett began to pressure her to go further in their sexual relationship. When Jenna told him that she wasn't ready, Brett hounded her more. When the subject of sex had come up with her parents "hypothetically" in the past, they had dismissed the subject, indicating that when it was the right time for her, Jenna would know. Jenna knew that she was not ready to have sex, although many of her classmates were sexually active. Jenna was not an impulsive person and liked to plan things carefully so that they would feel right to her. Jenna realized that she could not agree with Brett's request but she was confident that she could make him understand. One of Jenna's friends suggested that Brett might break up with her if she didn't have sex with him, but Jenna was willing to take that risk. Jenna carefully told Brett that she loved him but she was not yet ready for sex. Jenna was slightly surprised that instead of pressuring her more, or breaking up with her, Brett accepted her decision, in fact, he seemed a little relieved.

Jenna and Brett continued their relationship into their senior year of high school, and, toward the end of her senior year, Jenna desired to be sexually active with him. They decided to go to a community clinic known for its positive attitude toward adolescents, to learn about birth control methods and pick one, without including their parents. Jenna and Brett took the time to learn about a variety of birth control methods and chose to use condoms. When they left the clinic, Jenna and Brett felt closer than they had before, and realized how they had both grown in their relationship. Jenna and Brett both felt that they were doing the right thing. *(Courtesy of Caroly S. Pataki, M.D.)*

Late Adolescence. Late adolescence (between the ages of 17 and 19) is a time when continued exploration of academic pursuits, musical and artistic tastes, athletic participation, and social bonds lead a teen toward greater definition of self and a sense of belonging to certain groups or subcultures within mainstream society. Well-adjusted adolescents can be comfortable with current choices of activities, tastes, hobbies, and friendships, yet remain aware that their "identities" will continue to be refined during young adulthood.

Joey was in his second semester of his freshman year of college, living away from home, and had just turned 18 years of age. He reflected on the fact that he was no longer a "minor" and could make almost any decision for himself without his parents being involved.

Joey felt liberated, but at the same time, he was confused and a little lost. Since 10th grade, Joey had planned to pursue a career in medicine like his father, so he had taken a heavy load of science courses in the first semester, all of which he had despised. This semester, however, he had signed up only for liberal arts classes. He did not mention this to his father. He was now enrolled in classes that ranged from art history to architectural drafting to sociology, philosophy, and music. He had been influenced, he believed, by his roommate Tony, who was in the architecture program, and by his girlfriend, Lisa, who was majoring in studio art.

As the semester progressed, Joey found that his favorite course was the drafting class, just like Tony had predicted. Tony was in a more advanced drafting class than Joey, and Joey couldn't help but wonder whether he liked the drafting class so much because of how much he idolized Tony, or because he really enjoyed the class. He talked this over with Lisa, who suggested that he chill out and not figure out the rest of his life right now. She recommended that he take at least two more semesters of varied classes including those in the architecture curriculum before making a final decision about a career. Joey realized that Lisa's approach to college, and to life was so relaxed, the opposite of his approach, following his parents' pressure to plan ahead, make commitments early, and see them through, regardless of how it felt. Lisa's approach left more room for reflecting on experiences, and then making a choice, rather than jumping into what he was "supposed" to do. Joey took her advice and allowed himself another year to try out majors and then decide on a career. After experiencing courses in many varied subjects, Joey decided that he did truly enjoy architecture and was able to switch his focus from premed to architecture. *(Courtesy of Caroly S. Pataki M.D.)*

Components of Adolescence

Physical Development. Puberty is the process by which adolescents develop physical and sexual maturity, along with reproductive ability. The first signs of the pubertal process are an increased rate of growth in both height and weight. This process begins in girls by approximately 10 years of age. By the age of 11 or 12, many girls noticeably tower over their male classmates, who do not experience a growth spurt, on average, until they reach 13 years of age. By age 13, many girls have experienced menarche, and most have developed breasts and pubic hair.

Wide variation exists in the normal range of onset and timing of pubertal development and its components. A set sequence occurs, however, in the order in which pubertal development proceeds. Thus, secondary sexual characteristics in boys, such as increased length and width of the penis, for example, will occur after the release of androgens from developed enlarged testes.

Sexual maturity ratings (SMR), also referred to as Tanner stages, range from SMR 1 (prepuberty) to SMR 5 (adult). The SMR ratings include stages of genital maturity in boys and breast development in girls, as well as pubic hair development. Table 27.1–11 outlines SMR for boys and girls.

The primary female sex characteristic is ovulation, the release of eggs from ovarian follicles, approximately once every 28 days. When adolescent girls reach SMR 3 to 4, ovarian follicles are producing enough estrogen to result in menarche, the onset of menstruation. When adolescent girls reach SMR 4 to 5, an ovarian follicle matures on a monthly basis and ovulation occurs. Estrogen and progesterone promote sexual maturation, including further development of fallopian tubes and breasts.

For adolescent boys, the primary sex characteristic is the development of sperm by the testes. In boys, sperm development occurs in response to follicle-stimulating hormone acting on the seminiferous tubules within the testes. The pubertal process in boys is marked by the growth of the testes stimulated by luteinizing hormone. An adolescent boy's ability to ejaculate generally emerges within 1 year of reaching SMR 2. Secondary sexual characteristics in boys include thickening of skin, broadening of the shoulders, and the development of facial hair.

Table 27.1–11
Sexual Maturity Ratings for Male and Female Adolescents

Sexual Maturity Rating	Girls	Boys
Stage 1	Preadolescent, papilla elevated No pubic hair	Penis, testes, scrotum preadolescent No pubic hair
Stage 2	Breast bud, small mound; areola diameter increased Sparse long pubic hair, mainly along labia	Penis size same, testes and scrotum enlarged, with scrotal skin reddened Sparse long pubic hair, mainly at the base of penis
Stage 3	Breast and areola larger; no separation of contours Pubic hair darker and coarser; spread over pubic area	Penis elongated, with increased size of testes and scrotum Pubic hair darker and coarser; spread over pubic area
Stage 4	Breast size increased Areola and papilla raised Pubic hair coarse and thickened; covers less area than in adults, does not extend to thighs	Penis increased in length and width Testes and scrotum larger Pubic hair coarse and thickened; covers less area than in adults, does not extend to thighs
Stage 5	Breasts resemble adult female breast; areola has recessed to breast contour Pubic hair increased in density; area extends to thighs	Penis, testes, scrotum appear mature Pubic hair increased in density; area extends to thighs

Cognitive Maturation. Cognitive maturation in adolescence encompasses a wide range of expanded abilities that fall within the global category of executive functions of the brain. These include the transition from concrete thinking to more abstract thinking; an increased ability to draw logical conclusions in scientific pursuits, with peer interactions and in social situations; and new abilities for self-observation and self-regulation. Adolescents acquire increased awareness of their own intellectual, artistic, and athletic gifts and talents; yet it often takes many more years into young adulthood to establish a practical application for these abilities.

The central cognitive change that occurs gradually during adolescence is the shift from concrete thinking (concrete operational thinking, according to Jean Piaget) to the ability to think abstractly (formal operational thinking, in Piaget's terminology). This evolution occurs as an adaptation to stimuli that demand an adolescent to produce hypothetical responses, as well as in response to the adolescent's expanded abilities to provide generalizations from specific situations. The development of abstract thinking is not a sudden epiphany but, rather, a gradual process of expanding logical deductions beyond concrete experiences and achieving the capacity for idealistic and hypothetical thinking based on everyday life.

Adolescents often use an omnipotent belief system that reinforces their sense of immunity from danger, even when confronted with logical risks. Some degree of child-like magical thinking continues to coexist with more mature abstract thinking in many adolescents. Despite the persistence of magical thinking into adolescence, adolescent cognition departs from that of younger children insofar as the increased ability for self-observation and development of strategies to promote strengths and compensate for weaknesses.

One of the important cognitive tasks in adolescence is to identify and gravitate toward those pursuits that seem to match the adolescent's cognitive strengths, in academic courses and in thinking about future aspirations. Piaget believed that cognitive adaptation in adolescence is profoundly influenced by social relationships and the dialogue between adolescents and peers, making social cognition an integral part of cognitive development in adolescence.

Socialization. Socialization in adolescence encompasses the ability to find acceptance in peer relationships, as well as the development of more mature social cognition. The skills to develop a sense of belonging to a peer group are of central importance to a sense of well-being. Being viewed as socially competent by peers is a critical component in building good self-esteem for most early adolescents. Peer influences are powerful and can foster positive social interactions, as well as apply pressure in less socially accepted behaviors or even high-risk behavior. Belonging to a peer group is, in general, a sign of adaptation and a developmentally appropriate step in separating from parents and turning the focus of loyalty toward friends. Children between the ages of 6 and 12 are able to engage in exchanges of ideas and opinions and acknowledge feelings of peers, but the relationships often wax and wane in a discontinuous way on the basis of altercations and good times. Friendships deepen with repeated good times but, for some school-aged children, a variety of peers are often interchangeable—that is, a companion is sought when a given child has free time, rather than out of a desire to spend time with a specific friend. As adolescence ensues, friendships become more individualized, and personal secrets are likely shared with a friend rather than a family member. A comfort level is achieved with one or several early adolescent peers, and the group may "stick together," spending most free time together. In early adolescence, a blend of the above two social modes may emerge, small "cliques" arise, and, even within the cliques, competition and jealousies regarding which dyads are "preferred" or higher ranked within the clique may result in some discontinuities in the relationships. In later adolescence, the peer group solidifies, leading to increased stability in the friendships and a greater mutuality in the quality of the interactions.

Moral Development. Morality is a set of values and beliefs about codes of behavior that conform to those shared by others in society. Adolescents, as do younger children, tend to develop patterns of behaviors characteristic of their family and educational environments and by imitation of specific peers and adults whom they admire. Moral development is not strictly tied to chronological age but, rather, is an outgrowth from cognitive development.

Piaget described moral development as a gradual process parallel to cognitive development, with expanded abilities in differentiating the best interests for society from those of individuals occurring during late adolescence. Preschool children simply follow rules set forth by the parents; in the middle years, children accept rules but show an inability to allow for exceptions; and during adolescence, young persons recognize rules in terms of what is good for the society at large.

Lawrence Kohlberg integrated Piaget's concepts and described three major levels of morality. The first level is preconventional morality, in which punishment and obedience to the parent are the determining factors. The second level is morality of conventional role-conformity, in which children try to conform to gain approval and to maintain good relationships with others. The third and highest level is morality of self-accepted moral principles, in which children voluntarily comply with rules on the basis of a concept of ethical principles and make exceptions to rules in certain circumstances.

Although Kohlberg's and Piaget's notions of moral development focus on a unified theory of cognitive maturation for both sexes, Carol Gilligan emphasizes the social context of moral development leading to divergent patterns in moral development. Gilligan points out that, in women, compassion and the ethics of caring are dominant features of moral decision-making, whereas, for men, predominant features of moral judgments are related more to a perception of justice, rationality, and a sense of fairness.

Self-Esteem. Self-esteem is a measure of one's sense of self-worth based on perceived success and achievements, as well as a perception of how much one is valued by peers, family members, teachers, and society in general. The most important correlates of good self-esteem are one's perception of positive physical appearance and high value to peers and family. Secondary features of self-esteem relate to academic achievement, athletic abilities, and special talents. Adolescent self-esteem is mediated, to a significant degree, by positive feedback received from a peer group and family members, and adolescents often seek out a peer group that offers acceptance, regardless of negative behaviors associated with that group.

Adolescent girls have more of a problem maintaining self-esteem than do boys. Girls continued to rate themselves with generally lower self-esteem into adulthood.

Current Environmental Influences and Adolescence

Adolescent Sexual Behavior. Sexual experimentation in adolescents often begins with fantasy and masturbation in early adolescence followed by noncoital genital touching with the opposite sex or, in some cases, same-sex partners, oral sex with partners, and initiation of sexual intercourse at a later point in development. By high school, most male adolescents report experience with masturbation, and more than half of adolescent girls report masturbation. The balance between healthy adolescent sexual experimentation and emotionally and physically safe sexual practices is one of the major challenges for society.

Estimates vary, but about 50 percent of 9th to 12th grade students reported having had sexual intercourse. The median age at first intercourse is about 16 years for boys and 17 years for girls. Boys generally have more sexual partners than do girls, and boys are less likely than girls to seek emotional attachments with their sexual partners.

FACTORS INFLUENCING ADOLESCENT SEXUAL BEHAVIOR. Factors that affect sexual behavior in adolescents include personality traits, gender, cultural and religious background, racial factors, family attitudes, and sexual education and prevention programs.

Personality factors have been found to be associated with sexual behavior, as well as sexual risk-taking. Higher levels of impulsivity are associated with a younger age at first experience of sexual intercourse; higher number of sexual partners; sexual intercourse without the use of contraception, including condoms; and a history of sexually transmitted disease (STD) (chlamydia).

Historically, male adolescents have initiated sexual intercourse at a younger age than female adolescents. The younger a teenage girl is when she has sex for the first time, the more likely she is to have had unwanted sexual activity. Close to four of ten girls who had first intercourse at 13 or 14 years of age report it was either not voluntary or unwanted. Three of four girls and over half of boys report that girls who have sex do so because their boyfriends want them to. In general, adolescents who initiate sexual intercourse at younger ages are also more likely to have a greater number of sexual partners.

The additive effects of more highly educated families, social and religious youth groups, and school-based educational programs can be credited with a decline in high-risk sexual behavior among adolescents. Responsible sexual behavior among adolescents has been determined as one of the ten leading health indicators for the next decade. The primary reason that teenage girls who have never had intercourse give for abstaining from sex is that having sex would be against their religious or moral values. Other reasons include desire to avoid pregnancy, fear of contracting a STD, and not having met the appropriate partner.

CONTRACEPTIVES. Currently, 98 percent of teenagers 15 to 19 years are using at least one method of birth control. The two most common methods are condoms and birth control pills. STDs, despite use of condoms, are still at high levels in teens. Approximately one in four sexually active teens contracts an STD every year. Approximately half of all new human immunodeficiency virus (HIV) infections occur in people younger than age 25.

PREGNANCY. Each year 750,000 to 850,000 teenage girls younger than age 19 become pregnant. Of this number, 432,000 give birth, a 19 percent decline from 532,000 in 1991; the rest (418,000) obtain abortions. The largest decline in teen pregnancy by race is for black women. Hispanic teen births have declined 20 percent, but continue to have the highest teen birth rates compared with other races.

Teenage pregnancy creates a plethora of health risks for both mother and child. Children born to teenage mothers have a greater chance of dying before the age of 5 years. Those who survive are more likely to perform poorly in school and are at greater risk of abuse and neglect. Teenage mothers are less likely to gain adequate weight during pregnancy, increasing the risk of premature births and low–birth-weight infants. Low–birth-weight babies are more likely to have organs that are not fully developed, resulting in bleeding in the brain, respiratory distress syndrome, and intestinal problems. Teenage mothers are also less likely to seek regular prenatal care and to take recommended daily multivitamins, and they are more likely to smoke, drink, or use drugs during pregnancy. Only one-third of teenage mothers obtain high school diplomas, and only 1.5 percent have a college degree by the age of 30.

The average adolescent mother who cannot care for her child has the child either placed in foster care or raised by the teenager's already overburdened parents or other relatives. Few teenage mothers marry the fathers of their children; the fathers, usually teenagers, cannot care for themselves, much less the mothers of their children. If the two do marry, they usually divorce. Many are more likely to end up on welfare.

ABORTION. Nearly four of ten teen pregnancies end in abortion. Almost all the girls are unwed mothers from low socioeconomic groups; their pregnancies result from sex with boys to whom they felt emotionally attached. Most (61 percent) teenagers elect to have abortions with their parents' consent, but laws of mandatory parental consent put two rights into competition: a girl's claim to privacy and a parent's need to know. Most adults believe that teenagers should have parental permission for an abortion; but when parents refuse to give their consent, most states prohibit parents from vetoing the teenager's decision.

The abortion rate in many European countries tends to be far lower than that in the United States. In the United States, the rate of abortion among girls between the ages of 15 and 19 is about 30 per 1,000 girls, according to the Centers for Disease Control and Prevention. In France, for instance, about 10.5 of every 1,000 girls under the age of 20 had an abortion, according to World Health Organization statistics. The rate of abortion in Germany was 6.8; in Italy, 6.3; and in Spain, 4.5. Britain has a higher rate, 18.5. Family planning experts believe that more sex education and availability of contraceptive devices help keep the number of abortions down. In Holland, where contraceptives are freely available in schools, the teenage pregnancy rate is among the lowest in the world.

Risk-Taking Behavior. Reasonable risk-taking is a necessary endeavor in adolescence, leading to confidence both in forming new relationships and in sports and social situations. High-risk behaviors among adolescents are associated with serious negative consequences, however, and can take many forms, including drug and alcohol use, unsafe sexual practices, self-injurious behaviors, and reckless driving.

Drug Use

ALCOHOL. About 30 percent of 12th graders report having five or more drinks in a row within a 2-week period. The average age when youths first try alcohol is 11 years for boys and 13 years for girls. The national average age at which Americans begin drinking regularly is 15.9 years of age. People ages 18 to 25 show the highest prevalence of binge and heavy drinking. Drunk driving has declined since 2002. Alcohol dependence, along with other drugs, is associated with depression, anxiety, oppositional defiant disorder, antisocial personality disorder, and an increased rate of suicide.

NICOTINE. The number of younger Americans who smoke has declined since 1990; however, the rate of smoking among teenagers is still as high as or higher than that of adults. According to the American Cancer Society, on average more than one of five students has smoked cigarettes. Each day, more than 4,000 teenagers try their first cigarette and another 2,000 become regular, daily smokers. Cigarette smokers are more likely to get into fights, carry weapons, attempt suicide, suffer from mental health problems such as depression, and engage in high-risk sexual behaviors. One of three will eventually die from smoking-related diseases. Cigarettes are the most common type of tobacco used among middle-school students followed by cigars, smokeless tobacco, and pipes.

CANNABIS. Marijuana is the most popular illicit drug, with 14.6 million people using it (6.2 percent of the population), two-thirds being under the age of 18. Its use, however, is slowly declining. About 6 percent of 12th graders report daily use of marijuana.

One of the major reasons for such prevalence of marijuana use among teenagers is because many find that marijuana is easier to get than alcohol or cigarettes. This belief has declined in recent years. Once teenagers are dependent on marijuana, they often tumble into truancy, crime, and depression.

COCAINE. About 13 percent of high school seniors use cocaine exceeding the national average of 3.6 percent. In addition, about 1 percent of 12th graders admit to using phencyclidine (PCP). Crystal methamphetamine (ice) has an annual prevalence in 12th graders of about 2 percent.

OPIOIDS. In recent years, the number of teens using prescription pain relievers for nonmedical reasons has increased. Prescription drug abuse by people ages 18 to 25 has increased 15 percent. Drugs of specific concern are the pain relievers oxycodone (OxyContin) and hydrocodone (Vicodin). OxyContin has gained ground among high school students since its emergence in 2001, with 5 percent of 12th graders, 3.5 percent of 10th graders, and 1.7 percent of 8th graders reporting use. Vicodin was used by 9.3 percent of 12th graders, 6.2 percent of 10th graders, and 2.5 percent of 8th graders.

HEROIN. Heroin use is prevalent among adolescents, although less so than cocaine. The average age of use is 19, but it is used by almost 2 percent of 12th graders, the nasal route (snorting) being the most common method of use.

Violence. Although rates of violent crime have decreased throughout the United States in recent years, violent crimes by young offenders are on the increase. Homicides are the second leading cause of death among persons ages 15 to 25. (Accidents are first; suicides are third.) Black male teenagers are far more likely to be murder victims than are boys from any other racial or ethnic group or girls of any race. The factor most strongly associated with violence among adolescent boys is growing up in a household without a father or father surrogate; this factor aside, race, socioeconomic status, and education show no effect on the propensity toward violence.

BULLYING. Bullying is defined as the use of one's strength or status to intimidate, injure, or humiliate another person of lesser strength or status. It can be categorized as physical, verbal, or social. Physical bullying involves physical injury or threat of injury to someone. Verbal bullying refers to teasing or insulting someone. Social bullying refers to the use of peer rejection or exclusion to humiliate or isolate a victim.

Approximately 30 percent of 6th through 10th grade students are involved in some aspect of moderate-to-frequent bullying, either as a bully, the target of bullying, or both. Approximately 1.7 million children within this age group can be identified as bullies. Boys are more likely to be involved in bullying and violent behavior than girls. Girls tend to use verbal bullying rather than physical.

An estimated 160,000 students miss school each day because of fear of attack or intimidation from peers; some are forced to drop out. Stresses of "victimization" can interfere with student's engagement and learning in school. Children who bully other children are at risk for engaging in more serious violent behaviors, such as frequent fighting and carrying a weapon.

CYBER BULLYING. During the last decade, electronic or internet bullying has become of great concern to adolescents. Cyber bullying is defined broadly, to convey the use of electronic means to intentionally intimidate or harm someone. The reported prevalence of cyber bullying is variable, reports ranging from 1 to 62 percent of youth reporting that they were victims of cyber victimization. A study of about 700 Australian students, recruited at age 10 years, and followed until age 14 to 15 years, found that 15 percent had engaged in cyber bullying, 21 percent had engaged in traditional bullying, and 7 percent had engaged in both. Another study of self-reported information collected from 399 teens in the 8th to 10th grades, found that involvement in cyber bullying, either as a victim or a bully, specifically contributed to the prediction of depressive symptoms and suicidal ideation. This correlation of cyber bullying and depressive symptomatology was found to be stronger than the association of traditional bullying and affective disorder.

GANGS. Gang violence is a problem in various communities throughout the United States. There are 2,000 different youth gangs around the country with more than 200,000 teens and young adults as members. Most members are between the ages of 12 and 24 years, with an average of 17 to 18 years. Gang membership is a brief phase for many teenagers; one-half to two-thirds leave the gang by the 1-year mark. Boys are more likely to join gangs than girls; however, female gang membership may be underrepresented. Female gang members are more likely to be found in small cities and rural areas and tend to be younger than male gang members. Female gang members are also involved in less delinquent or criminal activity than males and commit fewer violent crimes.

WEAPONS. Each day, on average, nearly ten American children younger than the age of 18 years are killed in handgun suicides, homicides, and accidents. Many more are wounded. One in five youths in grades 9 to 12 carries a weapon—knife, gun, or club.

By law, firearms cannot be sold to anyone younger than the age of 18 years. Two-thirds of students in grades 6 to 12 say that they can get a firearm within 24 hours, however. More than 22 million children live in a home with a firearm. In 40 percent of these homes, at least one gun is kept unlocked and 13 percent are kept unlocked and loaded. Two of three students involved in school shootings acquired their guns from their own home or that of a relative. At least 60 percent of suicide deaths in teens involve the use of a handgun.

SCHOOL VIOLENCE. According to the CDC of all youth homicides in 2010 about 2 percent occurred in schools. Approximately 7 percent of teachers report they have been threatened with injury or physically attacked by a student from their school. In addition, among students in grades 9 through 12, about 6 percent reported carrying a weapon on school property on one or more days in the 30 days before the survey.

Many factors can lead to violent acts in teenagers. Some inherited traits include impulsivity, learning difficulties, low IQ, or fearlessness. A correlation also exists between witnessing violent acts and involvement in violence. Children who witness violent acts are more aggressive and grow up more likely to become involved in violence—either as a victimizer or as a victim. Table 27.1–12 lists some of the early and imminent warning signs of school violence.

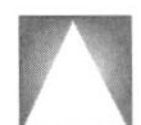

Table 27.1–12
Warning Signs of School Violence

Early Warning Signs
Social withdrawal
Excessive feelings of isolation and being alone
Excessive feelings of rejection
Being a victim of violence
Feelings of being picked on and persecuted
Expression of violence in writings and drawings
Uncontrolled anger
Patterns of impulsive and chronic hitting, intimidating, and bullying behaviors
History of discipline problems
History of violent and aggressive behavior
Intolerance for differences and prejudicial attitudes
Drug and alcohol use
Affiliation with gangs
Inappropriate access to, possession of, and use of firearms
Serious threats of violence

Imminent Warning Signs
Serious physical fighting with peers or family members
Severe destruction of property
Severe rage for seemingly minor reasons
Detailed threats of lethal violence
Possession and/or use of firearms and other weapons
Other self-injurious behaviors or threats of suicide

On April 20, 1999, two teenage boys, ages 17 and 18 years, went on a shooting rampage through Columbine High School of Littleton, Colorado. Armed with shotguns, a semiautomatic rifle, and a pistol, they laughed and hollered as they shot classmates and teachers at point-blank range while hurling homemade explosives. Fifteen were killed, including the 2 gunmen, and 25 were injured.

The gunmen were members of the "trench coat mafia" at the high school, a clique of social misfits who stood out at the school for their gothic style of dress and nihilistic attitude. The two gunmen were obsessed with violent video games and intrigued with Nazi culture, even though one was part Jewish. The date of the attack was picked because it was Adolf Hitler's birthday.

On March 21, 2005, a 16-year-old boy went on a shooting rampage at Red Lake High School on the Red Lake Indian Reservation in far northern Minnesota. He began his shooting spree by killing his grandfather and the grandfather's companion. He then donned his grandfather's police-issue gun belt and bulletproof vest before heading to the school, where he killed a security guard, a teacher, five students, and then himself. About 15 others were injured.

The gunman had a troubled childhood; his father committed suicide in 1997 and his mother suffered head injuries in an auto accident. He expressed admiration for Adolf Hitler on a neo-Nazi website, using the handle "Todesengel," which is German for "Angel of Death." He had bouts of depression, suicide ideation, and was taking fluoxetine (Prozac). He was a member of a clique of about five students known as "The Darkers," who wore black clothes and chains, spiked or dyed their hair, and loved heavy-metal music. The gunman was usually seen in a long black trench coat, eyeliner, and combat boots, and was described as a quiet teenager.

SEXUAL OFFENSE. Adolescents younger than age 18 years account for 20 percent of arrests for all sexual offenses (excluding prostitution), 20 to 30 percent of rape cases, 14 percent of aggravated sexual assault offenses, and 27 percent of child sexual homicides. These adolescent offenders account for the victimization of approximately one-half of boys and one-fourth of girls who are molested or sexually abused. Most instances have involved adolescent male perpetrators.

There appear to be two types of juvenile sex offenders: those who target children and those who offend against peers or adults. The main distinction between the two groups is based on the age difference between the victim and the offender. Table 27.1–13 lists the differences and similarities of these two groups.

Etiological factors of juvenile sex offending include maltreatment experiences, exposure to pornography, substance abuse, and exposure to aggressive role models. A significant number of offending adolescents have a childhood history of physical abuse (25 to 50 percent) or sexual abuse (10 to 80 percent). Half of adolescent offenders lived with both parents and one other juvenile at the time of their offending. Evidence also suggests that most juvenile sex offenders are likely to become adult sex offenders. The most common psychosocial deficits of adolescent sexual offenders include low self-esteem, few social skills, minimal assertive skills, and poor academic performance. The most common psychiatric diagnoses are conduct disorder, substance abuse disorder, adjustment disorder, ADHD, specific phobia, and mood disorders. Male offenders are more often diagnosed with paraphilias and antisocial behavior, whereas female offenders are more likely to be diagnosed with mood disorders and engage in self-mutilation.

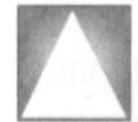

Table 27.1–13
Juvenile Sex Offender Subtypes

Juvenile Offenders Who Sexually Offend against Peers or Adults
Predominantly assault females and strangers or casual acquaintances.
Sexual assaults occur in association with other types of criminal activity (e.g., burglary).
Have histories of nonsexual criminal offenses, and appear more generally delinquent and conduct disordered.
Commit their offenses in public areas.
Display higher levels of aggression and violence in the commission of their sexual crimes.
More likely to use weapons and to cause injuries to their victims.
Juvenile Offenders Who Sexually Offend against Children
Most victims are male and are related to them, either siblings or other relatives.
Almost half of the offenders have had at least one male victim.
The sexual crimes tend to reflect a greater reliance on opportunity and guile than injurious force. This appears to be particularly true when their victim is related to them. These youths may "trick" the child into complying with the molestation, use bribes, or threaten the child with loss of the relationship.
Within the overall population of juveniles who sexually assault children are certain youths who display high levels of aggression and violence. Generally, these are youths who display more severe levels of personality and/or psychosexual disturbances, such as psychopathy, sexual sadism, and so on.
Suffer from deficits in self-esteem and social competency.
Many show evidence of depression.
Characteristics Common to Both Groups
High rates of learning disabilities and academic dysfunction (30–60%).
The presence of other behavioral health problems, including substance abuse, and disorders of conduct (up to 80% have some diagnosable psychiatric disorder).
Observed difficulties with impulse control and judgment.

Prostitution. Teenagers constitute a large portion of all prostitutes, with estimates ranging up to 1 million teenagers involved in prostitution. The average age of a new recruit is 13 years; however, some are as young as 9 years of age. Most adolescent prostitutes are girls, but boys are involved as homosexual prostitutes. Most teenagers who enter a life of prostitution come from broken homes; however, a growing number of teenage prostitutes come from middle- to upper middle-class homes. Many have been victims of rape, or were abused as children. Most teenagers ran away from home and were taken in by pimps and substance abusers; the adolescents themselves then became substance abusers. Twenty-seven percent of teenage prostitution occurs in large cities, and incidents usually take place at an outside location, such as highways, roads, alleys, fields, woods, or parking lots. Teenage prostitutes are at high risk for acquired immunodeficiency syndrome (AIDS), and many (up to 70 percent in some studies) are infected with HIV.

As many as 17,500 individuals are smuggled into the United States each year as "sex slaves." They are brought under the pretenses of a better life and job opportunities, but once they are in the United States, they are forced into prostitution, making little money while traffickers make thousands of dollars from their services. Many times they are raped and abused.

Tattoos and Body Piercing. Body piercing and tattoos have become more prevalent among adolescents since the 1980s. In the general population, approximately 10 to 13 percent of adolescents have tattoos. Of the more than 500 adolescents surveyed in a study, 13.2 percent report at least one tattoo, and 26.9 percent report at least one body piercing, other than in their ear lobe, at some point in their lives. Both tattoos and body piercing are more common in girls than in boys. Adolescents who endorsed possession of at least one tattoo or body piercing are more likely to endorse use of gateway drugs (cigarettes, alcohol, and marijuana), as well as experience with hard drugs (cocaine, crystal methamphetamine, and ecstasy).

▲ 27.2 Assessment, Examination, and Psychological Testing

A comprehensive evaluation of a child is composed of interviews with the parents, the child, and other family members; gathering information regarding the child's current school functioning; and often, a standardized assessment of the child's intellectual level and academic achievement. In some cases, standardized measures of developmental level and neuropsychological assessments are useful. Psychiatric evaluations of children are rarely initiated by the child, so clinicians must obtain information from the family and the school to understand the reasons for the evaluation. In some cases, the court or a child protective service agency may initiate a psychiatric evaluation. Children can be excellent informants about symptoms related to mood and inner experiences, such as psychotic phenomena, sadness, fears, and anxiety, but they often have difficulty with the chronology of symptoms and are sometimes reticent about reporting behaviors that have gotten them into trouble. Very young children often cannot articulate their experiences verbally and do better showing their feelings and preoccupations in a play situation. Assessment of a child or adolescent includes identifying the reasons for referral; assessing the nature and extent of the child's psychological and behavioral difficulties; and determining family, school, social, and developmental factors that may be influencing the child's emotional well-being.

The first step in the comprehensive evaluation of a child or adolescent is to obtain a full description of the current concerns and a history of the child's previous psychiatric and medical problems. This is often done with the parents for school-aged children, whereas adolescents may be seen alone first, to get their perception of the situation. Direct interview and observation of the child is usually next, followed by psychological testing, when indicated.

Clinical interviews offer the most flexibility in understanding the evolution of problems and in establishing the role of environmental factors and life events, but they may not systematically cover all psychiatric diagnostic categories. To increase the breadth of information generated, the clinician may use semistructured interviews such as the *Kiddie Schedule for Affective Disorders and Schizophrenia for School-Age Children* (K-SADS); structured interviews such as the *National Institute for Mental Health Diagnostic Interview Schedule for Children Version IV* (NIMH DISC-IV); and rating scales, such as the *Child Behavior Checklist* and *Connors Parent or Teacher Rating Scale for ADHD.*

It is not uncommon for interviews from different sources, such as parents, teachers, and school counselors, to reflect different or even contradictory information about a given child. When faced with conflicting information, the clinician must determine whether apparent contradictions actually reflect an accurate picture of the child in different settings. Once a complete history is obtained from the parents, the child is examined, the child's current functioning at home and at school is assessed, and psychological testing is completed, the clinician can use all the available information to make a best-estimate diagnosis and can then make recommendations.

Once clinical information is obtained about a given child or adolescent, it is the clinician's task to determine whether criteria are met for one or more psychiatric disorders according to the Fifth Edition of the *Diagnostic and Statistical Manual of Mental Disorders* (DSM-5). This most current version is a categorical classification reflecting the consensus on constellations of symptoms believed to comprise discrete and valid psychiatric disorders. Psychiatric disorders are defined by the DSM-5 as a clinically significant set of symptoms that is associated with impairment in one or more areas of functioning. Whereas clinical situations requiring intervention do not always fall within the context of a given psychiatric disorder, the importance of identifying psychiatric disorders when they arise is to facilitate meaningful investigation of childhood psychopathology.

CLINICAL INTERVIEWS

To conduct a useful interview with a child of any age, clinicians must be familiar with normal development to place the child's responses in the proper perspective. For example, a young child's discomfort on separation from a parent and a school-age child's lack of clarity about the purpose of the interview are both perfectly normal and should not be misconstrued as psychiatric symptoms. Furthermore, behavior that is normal in a child at one age, such as temper tantrums in a 2-year-old, takes on a different meaning, for example, in a 17-year-old.

The interviewer's first task is to engage the child and develop a rapport so that the child is comfortable. The interviewer should inquire about the child's concept of the purpose of the interview and should ask what the parents have told the child. If the child appears to be confused about the reason for the interview, the examiner may opt to summarize the parents' concerns in a developmentally appropriate and supportive manner. During the interview with the child, the clinician seeks to learn about the child's relationships with family members and peers, academic achievement and peer relationships in school, and the child's pleasurable activities. An estimate of the child's cognitive functioning is a part of the mental status examination.

The extent of confidentiality in child assessment is correlated with the age of the child. In most cases, almost all specific information can appropriately be shared with the parents of a very young child, whereas privacy and permission of an older child or adolescent are mandated before sharing information with parents. School-age and older children are informed that if the clinician becomes concerned that any child is dangerous to him- or herself or to others, this information must be shared with parents and, at times, additional adults. As part of a psychiatric assessment of a child of any age, the clinician must determine whether that child is safe in his or her environment and must develop an index of suspicion about whether the child is a victim of abuse or neglect. Whenever there is a suspicion of child maltreatment, the local child protective service agency must be notified.

Toward the end of the interview, the child may be asked in an open-ended manner whether he or she would like to bring up anything else. Each child should be complimented for his or her cooperation and thanked for participating in the interview, and the interview should end on a positive note.

Infants and Young Children

Assessments of infants usually begin with the parents present, because very young children may be frightened by the interview situation; the interview with the parents present also allows the clinician to assess the parent–infant interaction. Infants may be referred for a variety of reasons, including high levels of irritability, difficulty being consoled, eating disturbances, poor weight gain, sleep disturbances, withdrawn behavior, lack of engagement in play, and developmental delay. The clinician assesses areas of functioning that include motor development, activity level, verbal communication, ability to engage in play, problem-solving skills, adaptation to daily routines, relationships, and social responsiveness.

The child's developmental level of functioning is determined by combining observations made during the interview with standardized developmental measures. Observations of play reveal a child's developmental level and reflect the child's emotional state and preoccupations. The examiner can interact with an infant age 18 months or younger in a playful manner by using such games as peek-a-boo. Children between the ages of 18 months and 3 years can be observed in a playroom. Children ages 2 years or older may exhibit symbolic play with toys, revealing more in this mode than through conversation. The use of puppets and dolls with children younger than 6 years of age is often an effective way to elicit information, especially if questions are directed to the dolls, rather than to the child.

School-Age Children

Some school-age children are at ease when conversing with an adult; others are hampered by fear, anxiety, poor verbal skills, or oppositional behavior. School-age children can usually tolerate a 45-minute session. The room should be sufficiently spacious for the child to move around, but not so large as to reduce intimate contact between the examiner and the child. Part of the interview can be reserved for unstructured play, and various toys can be made available to capture the child's interest and to elicit themes and feelings. Children in lower grades may be more interested in the toys in the room, whereas by the sixth grade, children may be more comfortable with the interview process and less likely to show spontaneous play.

The initial part of the interview explores the child's understanding of the reasons for the meeting. The clinician should confirm that the interview was not set up because the child is "in trouble" or as a punishment for "bad" behavior. Techniques that can facilitate disclosure of feelings include asking the child to draw peers, family members, a house, or anything else that comes to mind. The child can then be questioned about the drawings. Children may be asked to reveal three wishes, to describe the best and worst events of their lives, and to name a favorite person to be stranded with on a desert island. Games such as Donald W. Winnicott's "squiggle," in which the examiner draws a curved line and then the child and the examiner take turns continuing the drawing, may facilitate conversation.

Questions that are partially open ended with some multiple choices may elicit the most complete answers from school-age children. Simple, closed (yes or no) questions may not elicit sufficient information, and completely open-ended questions can overwhelm a school-age child who cannot construct a chronological narrative. These techniques often result in a shoulder shrug from the child. The use of indirect commentary—such as, "I once knew a child who felt very sad when he moved away from all his friends"—is helpful, although the clinician must be careful not to lead the child into confirming what the child thinks the clinician wants to hear. School-age children respond well to clinicians who help them compare moods or feelings by asking them to rate feelings on a scale of 1 to 10.

Adolescents

Adolescents usually have distinct ideas about why the evaluation was initiated, and can usually give a chronological account of the recent events leading to the evaluation, although some may disagree with the need for the evaluation. The clinician should clearly communicate the value of hearing the story from an adolescent's point of view and must be careful to reserve judgment and not assign blame. Adolescents may be concerned about confidentiality, and clinicians can assure them that permission will be requested from them before any specific information is shared with parents, except in situations involving danger to the adolescent or others, in which case confidentiality must be sacrificed. Adolescents can be approached in an open-ended manner; however, when silences occur during the interview, the clinician should attempt to reengage the patient. Clinicians can explore what the adolescent believes the outcome of the evaluation will be (change of school, hospitalization, removal from home, removal of privileges).

Some adolescents approach the interview with apprehension or hostility, but open up when it becomes evident that the clinician is neither punitive nor judgmental. Clinicians must be aware of their own responses to adolescents' behavior (countertransference) and stay focused on the therapeutic process even in the face of defiant, angry, or difficult teenagers. Clinicians should set appropriate limits and should postpone or discontinue an interview if they feel threatened or if patients become destructive to property or engage in self-injurious behavior. Every interview should include an exploration of suicidal thoughts, assaultive behavior, psychotic symptoms, substance use, and knowledge of safe sexual practices along with a sexual history. Once rapport has been established, many adolescents appreciate the opportunity to tell their side of the story and may reveal things that they have not disclosed to anyone else.

Family Interview

An interview with parents and the patient may take place first or may occur later in the evaluation. Sometimes, an interview with the entire family, including siblings, can be enlightening. The purpose is to observe the attitudes and behavior of the parents toward the patient and the responses of the children to their parents. The clinician's job is to maintain a nonthreatening atmosphere in which each member of the family can speak freely without feeling that the clinician is taking sides with any particular member. Although child psychiatrists generally function as advocates for the child, the clinician must validate each family member's feelings in this setting, because lack of communication often contributes to the patient's problems.

Parents

The interview with the patient's parents or caretakers is necessary to get a chronological picture of the child's growth and development. A thorough developmental history and details of any stressors or important events that have influenced the child's development must be elicited. The parents' view of the family dynamics, their marital history, and their own emotional adjustment are also elicited. The family's psychiatric history and the upbringing of the parents are pertinent. Parents are usually the best informants about the child's early development and previous psychiatric and medical illnesses. They may be better able to provide an accurate chronology of past evaluations and treatment. In some cases, especially with older children and adolescents, the parents may be unaware of significant current symptoms or social difficulties of the child. Clinicians elicit the parents' formulation of the causes and nature of their child's problems and ask about their expectations for the current assessment.

DIAGNOSTIC INSTRUMENTS

The two main types of diagnostic instruments used by clinicians are diagnostic interviews and questionnaires. Diagnostic interviews are administered to either children or their parents and typically are designed to elicit sufficient information on various aspects of functioning in order to determine whether DSM-5 criteria are met.

Semistructured interviews, or "interviewer-based" interviews, such as K-SADS and the *Child and Adolescent Psychiatric Assessment* (CAPA), serve as guides for the clinician. They help the clinician clarify answers to questions about symptoms. Structured interviews, or "respondent-based" interviews, such as NIMH DISC-IV, the *Children's Interview for Psychiatric Syndromes* (ChIPS), and the *Diagnostic Interview for Children and Adolescents* (DICA), provide a script for the interviewer without interpretation of the patient responses during the interview process. Two other diagnostic instruments, the *Dominic-R* and the *Pictorial Instrument for Children and Adolescents* (PICA-III-R), use pictures as cues along with an accompanying question to elicit information about symptoms, which can be especially useful for young children as well as for adolescents.

Diagnostic instruments aid the collection of information in a systematic way. Diagnostic instruments, even the most comprehensive, however, cannot replace clinical interviews, because clinical interviews are superior in understanding the chronology of symptoms, the interplay between environmental stressors and emotional responses, and developmental issues. Clinicians often find it helpful to combine data from diagnostic instruments with clinical material gathered in a comprehensive evaluation.

Questionnaires can cover a broad range of symptom areas, such as the *Achenbach Child Behavior Checklist,* or they can be focused on a particular type of symptomatology, such as the *Connors Parent Rating Scale for ADHD.*

Semistructured Diagnostic Interviews

Kiddie Schedule for Affective Disorders and Schizophrenia for School-Age Children. The K-SADS can be used for children and adolescents from 6 to 18 years of age. It contains multiple items with some space for further clarification of symptoms. It elicits information on current diagnosis and on symptoms present in the previous year. Another version can also ascertain lifetime diagnoses. This instrument has been used extensively, especially in evaluation of mood disorders, and includes measures of impairment caused by symptoms. The schedule comes in a form for parents to give information about their child and in a version for use directly with the child. The schedule takes about 1 to 1.5 hours to administer. The interviewer should have some training in the field of child psychiatry, but need not be a psychiatrist.

Child and Adolescent Psychiatric Assessment. The CAPA is an "interviewer-based" instrument that can be used for children from 9 to 17 years of age. It comes in modular form so that certain diagnostic entities can be administered without having to give the entire interview. It covers disruptive behavior disorders, mood disorders, anxiety disorders, eating disorders, sleep disorders, elimination disorders, substance use disorders, tic disorders, schizophrenia, posttraumatic stress disorder, and somatization symptoms. It focuses on the 3 months before the interview, called the "primary period." In general, it takes about 1 hour to administer. It has a glossary to help clarify symptoms, and it provides separate ratings for presence and severity of symptoms. The CAPA can be used to obtain information that is applicable to making diagnoses according to the DSM-5. Training is necessary to administer this interview, and the interviewer must be prepared to use some clinical judgment in interpreting elicited symptoms.

Structured Diagnostic Interviews

National Institute of Mental Health Interview Schedule for Children Version IV. The NIMH DISC-IV is a highly structured interview designed to assess more than 30 DSM-IV diagnostic entities administered by trained "laypersons." Although it was formulated to match diagnostic criteria in DSM-IV, information from this interview can be utilized, along with clinical information for diagnoses in DSM-5. It is available in parallel child and parent forms. The parent form can be used for children from 6 to 17 years of age, and the direct child form of the instrument was designed for children from 9 to 17 years of age. A computer scoring algorithm is available. This instrument assesses the presence of diagnoses that have been present within the last 4 weeks, and also within the last year. Because it is a fully structured interview, the instructions serve as a complete guide for the questions, and the examiner need not have any knowledge of child psychiatry to administer the interview correctly.

Children's Interview for Psychiatric Syndromes. The ChIPS is a highly structured interview designed for use by trained interviewers with children from 6 to 18 years of age. It is composed of 15 sections, and it elicits information on psychiatric symptoms as well as psychosocial stressors targeting 20 psychiatric disorders, according to DSM-IV criteria; however, it can also be applied to diagnoses in DSM-5. There are parent and child forms. It takes approximately 40 minutes to administer the ChIPS. Diagnoses covered include depression, mania, ADHD, separation disorder, obsessive-compulsive disorder (OCD), conduct disorder, substance use disorder, anorexia, and bulimia. The ChIPS was designed for use as a screening instrument for clinicians and a diagnostic instrument for clinical and epidemiological research.

Diagnostic Interview for Children and Adolescents. The current version of the DICA was developed in 1997 to assess information resulting in diagnoses according to either DSM-IV or DSM-III-R. This instrument can be used to help obtain information that can be applied to DSM-5 as well. Although the DICA was originally designed to be a highly structured interview, it can now be used in a semistructured format. This means that, although interviewers are allowed to use additional questions and probes to clarify elicited information, the method of probing is standardized so that all interviewers will follow a specific pattern. When using the interview with younger children, more flexibility is built in, allowing interviewers to deviate from written questions to ensure that the child understands the question. Parent and child interviews are expected to be used. The DICA is designed for use with children 6 to 17 years of age and generally takes 1 to 2 hours to administer. It covers externalizing behavior disorders, anxiety disorders, depressive disorders, and substance abuse disorders, among others.

Pictorial Diagnostic Instruments

Dominic-R. The Dominic-R is a pictorial, fully structured interview designed to elicit psychiatric symptoms from children 6 to 11 years of age. The pictures illustrate abstract emotional and behavioral content of diagnostic entities according to the DSM-III-R; however, information gleaned from this instrument can also be applied in conjunction with clinical information to the DSM-5. The instrument uses a picture of a child called "Dominic" who is experiencing the symptom in question. Some symptoms have more than one picture, with a brief story that is read to the child. Along with each picture is a sentence asking about the situation being shown and asking the child if he or she has experiences similar to the one that Dominic is having. Diagnostic entities covered by the Dominic-R include separation anxiety, generalized anxiety, depression and dysthymia, ADHD, oppositional defiant disorder, conduct disorder, and specific phobia. Although symptoms of the preceding diagnoses can be fully elicited from the Dominic-R, no specific provision within the instrument inquires about frequency of the symptom, duration, or age of onset. The paper version of this interview takes about 20 minutes, and the computerized version of this instrument takes about 15 minutes. Trained lay-interviewers can administer this interview. Computerized versions of this interview are available with pictures of a child who is white, black, Latino, or Asian.

Pictorial Instrument for Children and Adolescents. PICA-III-R is composed of 137 pictures organized in modules and designed to cover five diagnostic categories, including disorders of anxiety, mood, psychosis, disruptive disorders, and substance use disorder. It is designed to be administered by clinicians and can be used for children and adolescents ranging from 6 to 16 years of age. The PICA-III-R provides a categorical (diagnosis present or absent) and a dimensional (range of severity) assessment. This instrument presents pictures of a child experiencing emotional, behavioral, and cognitive symptoms. The child is asked, "How much are you like him/her?" and a five-point rating scale with pictures of a person with open arms in increasing degrees is shown to the child to help him or her identify the severity of the symptoms. It takes about 40 minutes to 1 hour to administer the interview. This instrument is currently keyed to the DSM-III-R, but can be used along with clinical information to make diagnoses according to the DSM-5. This assessment can be used to aid in clinical interviews and in research diagnostic protocols.

QUESTIONNAIRES AND RATING SCALES

Achenbach Child Behavior Checklist

The parent and teacher versions of the *Achenbach Child Behavior Checklist* were developed to cover a broad range of symptoms and several positive attributes related to academic and social competence. The checklist presents items related to mood, frustration tolerance, hyperactivity, oppositional behavior, anxiety, and various other behaviors. The parent version consists of 118 items to be rated 0 (not true), 1 (sometimes true), or 2 (very true). The teacher version is similar, but without the items that apply only to home life. Profiles were developed based on normal children of three different age groups (4 to 5, 6 to 11, and 12 to 16).

Such a checklist identifies specific problem areas that might otherwise be overlooked, and it may point out areas in which the child's behavior deviates from that of normal children of the same age group. The checklist is not used specifically to make diagnoses.

Revised Achenbach Behavior Problem Checklist

Consisting of 150 items that cover a variety of childhood behavioral and emotional symptoms, the *Revised Achenbach Behavior Problem Checklist* discriminates between clinic-referred and nonreferred children. Separate subscales have been found to correlate in the appropriate direction with other measures of intelligence, academic achievement, clinical observations, and peer popularity. As with the other broad rating scales, this instrument can help elicit a comprehensive view of a multitude of behavioral areas, but it is not designed to make psychiatric diagnoses.

Connors Abbreviated Parent–Teacher Rating Scale for ADHD

In its original form, the *Connors Abbreviated Parent–Teacher Rating Scale for ADHD* consisted of 93 items rated on a 0 to 3 scale and was subgrouped into 25 clusters, including problems with restlessness, temper, school, stealing, eating, and sleeping. Over the years, multiple versions of this scale were developed and used to aid in systematic identification of children with ADHD. A highly abbreviated form of this rating scale, the *Connors Abbreviated Parent–Teacher Questionnaire,* was developed for use with both parents and teachers by Keith Connors in 1973. It consists of ten items that assess both hyperactivity and inattention.

Brief Impairment Scale

A newly validated 23-item instrument suitable to obtain information on children ranging from 4 years to 17 years, the *Brief Impairment Scale* (BIS) evaluates three domains of functioning: interpersonal relations, school/work functioning, and care/self-fulfillment. This scale is administered to an adult informant about his or her child, does not take long to administer, and provides a global measure of impairment along the above three dimensions. This scale cannot be used to make clinical decisions on individual patients, but it can provide information on the degree of impairment that a given child is experiencing in a certain area.

COMPONENTS OF THE CHILD PSYCHIATRIC EVALUATION

Psychiatric evaluation of a child includes a description of the reason for the referral, the child's past and present functioning, and any test results. An outline of the evaluation is given in Table 27.2–1.

Identifying Data

Identifying data for a child includes the child's gender, age, as well as the family constellation surrounding the child.

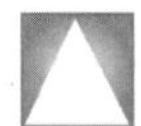

Table 27.2–1
Child Psychiatric Evaluation

Identifying data
- Identified patient and family members
- Source of referral
- Informants

History
- Chief complaint
- History of present illness
- Developmental history and milestones
- Psychiatric history
- Medical history, including immunizations
- Family social history and parents' marital status
- Educational history and current school functioning
- Peer relationship history
- Current family functioning
- Family psychiatric and medical histories
- Current physical examination

Mental status examination
Neuropsychiatric examination (when applicable)
Developmental, psychological, and educational testing
Formulation and summary
DSM-5 diagnosis
Recommendations and treatment plan

History

A comprehensive history contains information about the child's current and past functioning from the child's report, from clinical and structured interviews with the parents, and from information from teachers and previous treating clinicians. The chief complaint and the history of the present illness are generally obtained from both the child and the parents. Naturally, the child will articulate the situation according to his or her developmental level. The developmental history is more accurately obtained from the parents. Psychiatric and medical histories, current physical examination findings, and immunization histories can be augmented with reports from psychiatrists and pediatricians who have treated the child in the past. The child's report is critical in understanding the current situation regarding peer relationships and adjustment to school. Adolescents are the best informants regarding knowledge of safe sexual practices, drug or alcohol use, and suicidal ideation. The family's psychiatric and social histories, and family function are best obtained from the parents.

Mental Status Examination

A detailed description of the child's current mental functioning can be obtained through observation and specific questioning. An outline of the mental status examination is presented in Table 27.2–2. Table 27.2–3 lists components of a comprehensive neuropsychiatry mental status.

Physical Appearance. The examiner should document the child's size, grooming, nutritional state, bruising, head circumference, physical signs of anxiety, facial expressions, and mannerisms.

Parent–Child Interaction. The examiner can observe the interactions between parents and child in the waiting area before the interview and in the family session. The manner in which parents and child converse and the emotional overtones are pertinent.

Separation and Reunion. The examiner should note both the manner in which the child responds to the separation from a parent for an individual interview and the reunion behavior. Either lack of affect at separation and reunion or severe distress on separation or reunion can indicate problems in the parent–child relationship or other psychiatric disturbances.

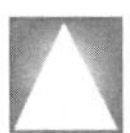

Table 27.2–2
Mental Status Examination for Children

1. Physical appearance
2. Parent–child interaction
3. Separation and reunion
4. Orientation to time, place, and person
5. Speech and language
6. Mood
7. Affect
8. Thought process and content
9. Social relatedness
10. Motor behavior
11. Cognition
12. Memory
13. Judgment and insight

Table 27.2–3
Neuropsychiatric Mental Status Examination[a]

A. General Description
  1. General appearance and dress
  2. Level of consciousness and arousal
  3. Attention to environment
  4. Posture (standing and seated)
  5. Gait
  6. Movements of limbs, trunk, and face (spontaneous, resting, and after instruction)
  7. General demeanor (including evidence of responses to internal stimuli)
  8. Response to examiner (eye contact, cooperation, and ability to focus on interview process)
  9. Native or primary language
B. Language and Speech
  1. Comprehension (words, sentences, simple and complex commands, and concepts)
  2. Output (spontaneity, rate, fluency, melody or prosody, volume, coherence, vocabulary, paraphasic errors, and complexity of usage)
  3. Repetition
  4. Other aspects
    a. Object naming
    b. Color naming
    c. Body part identification
    d. Ideomotor praxis to command
C. Thought
  1. Form (coherence and connectedness)
  2. Content
    a. Ideational (preoccupations, overvalued ideas, and delusions)
    b. Perceptual (hallucinations)
D. Mood and Affect
  1. Internal mood state (spontaneous and elicited; sense of humor)
  2. Future outlook
  3. Suicidal ideas and plans
  4. Demonstrated emotional status (congruence with mood)
E. Insight and Judgment
  1. Insight
    a. Self-appraisal and self-esteem
    b. Understanding of current circumstances
    c. Ability to describe personal psychological and physical status
  2. Judgment
    a. Appraisal of major social relationships
    b. Understanding of personal roles and responsibilities
F. Cognition
  1. Memory
    a. Spontaneous (as evidenced during interview)
    b. Tested (incidental, immediate repetition, delayed recall, cued recall, and recognition; verbal, nonverbal; explicit, implicit)
  2. Visuospatial skills
  3. Constructional ability
  4. Mathematics
  5. Reading
  6. Writing
  7. Fine sensory function (stereognosis, graphesthesia, and two-point discrimination)
  8. Finger gnosis
  9. Right–left orientation
  10. "Executive functions"
  11. Abstraction

[a]Questions should be adapted to the age of the child.
Courtesy of Eric D. Caine, M.D. and Jeffrey M. Lyness, M.D.

Orientation to Time, Place, and Person. Impairments in orientation can reflect organic damage, low intelligence, or a thought disorder. The age of the child must be kept in mind, however, because very young children are not expected to know the date, other chronological information, or the name of the interview site.

Speech and Language. The examiner should evaluate the child's speech and language acquisition. Is it appropriate for the child's age? A disparity between expressive language usage and receptive language is notable. The examiner should also note the child's rate of speech, rhythm, latency to answer, spontaneity of speech, intonation, articulation of words, and prosody. Echolalia, repetitive stereotypical phrases, and unusual syntax are important psychiatric findings. Children who do not use words by age 18 months or who do not use phrases by age 2.5 to 3 years, but who have a history of normal babbling and responding appropriately to nonverbal cues, are probably developing normally. The examiner should consider the possibility that a hearing loss is contributing to a speech and language deficit.

Mood. A child's sad expression, lack of appropriate smiling, tearfulness, anxiety, euphoria, and anger are valid indicators of mood, as are verbal admissions of feelings. Persistent themes in play and fantasy also reflect the child's mood.

Affect. The examiner should note the child's range of emotional expressivity, appropriateness of affect to thought content, ability to move smoothly from one affect to another, and sudden labile emotional shifts.

Thought Process and Content. In evaluating a thought disorder in a child, the clinician must always consider what is developmentally expected for the child's age and what is deviant for any age group. The evaluation of thought form considers loosening of associations, excessive magical thinking, perseveration, echolalia, the ability to distinguish fantasy from reality, sentence coherence, and the ability to reason logically. The evaluation of thought content considers delusions, obsessions, themes, fears, wishes, preoccupations, and interests.

Suicidal ideation is always a part of the mental status examination for children who are sufficiently verbal to understand the questions and old enough to understand the concept. Children of average intelligence who are older than 4 years of age usually have some understanding of what is real and what is make-believe and may be asked about suicidal ideation, although a firm concept of the permanence of death may not be present until several years later.

Aggressive thoughts and homicidal ideation are assessed here. Perceptual disturbances, such as hallucinations, are also assessed. Very young children are expected to have short attention spans and may change the topic and conversation abruptly without exhibiting a symptomatic flight of ideas. Transient visual and auditory hallucinations in very young children do not necessarily represent major psychotic illnesses, but they do deserve further investigation.

Social Relatedness. The examiner assesses the appropriateness of the child's response to the interviewer, general level of social skills, eye contact, and degree of familiarity or withdrawal in the interview process. Overly friendly or familiar behavior may be as troublesome as extremely retiring and withdrawn responses. The examiner assesses the child's self-esteem, general and specific areas of confidence, and success with family and peer relationships.

Motor Behavior. The motor behavior part of the mental status examination includes observations of the child's coordination and activity level and ability to pay attention and carry out developmentally appropriate tasks. It also involves involuntary movements, tremors, motor hyperactivity, and any unusual focal asymmetries of muscle movement.

Cognition. The examiner assesses the child's intellectual functioning and problem-solving abilities. An approximate level of intelligence can be estimated by the child's general information, vocabulary, and comprehension. For a specific assessment of the child's cognitive abilities, the examiner can use a standardized test.

Memory. School-age children should be able to remember three objects after 5 minutes and to repeat five digits forward and three digits backward. Anxiety can interfere with the child's performance, but an obvious inability to repeat digits or to add simple numbers may reflect brain damage, mental retardation, or learning disabilities.

Judgment and Insight. The child's view of the problems, reactions to them, and suggested solutions may give the clinician a good idea of the child's judgment and insight. In addition, the child's understanding of what he or she can realistically do to help and what the clinician can do adds to the assessment of the child's judgment.

Neuropsychiatric Assessment

A neuropsychiatric assessment is appropriate for children who are suspected of having a psychiatric disorder that coexists with neuropsychiatric impairment, psychiatric symptoms that may be caused by neuropsychiatric dysfunction, or a neurologic disorder. Although a neuropsychiatric assessment is not sufficient in most cases to make a psychiatric diagnosis, neuropsychological profiles have been, in some cases correlated with particular psychiatric symptoms and syndromes. For example, neuropsychological differences in executive function, language and memory functions, as well as measures of mood and anxiety, have been found between youth with histories of childhood maltreatment and those without it. The neuropsychiatric evaluation combines information from neurological, neuropsychological testing, and mental status examinations. The neurological examination can identify asymmetrical abnormal signs (hard signs) that may indicate lesions in the brain. A physical examination can evaluate the presence of physical stigmata of particular syndromes in which neuropsychiatric symptoms or developmental aberrations play a role (e.g., fetal alcohol syndrome, Down syndrome). In a study of 119 youth with either early onset schizophrenia or schizoaffective disorder, by Hooper and colleagues significantly high rates of deficits in intellectual function and academic skills were found, and the severity of these deficits was mildly correlated with severity of their psychiatric illness.

A neuropsychiatric examination also includes neurological soft signs and minor physical anomalies. The term *neurological soft signs* was first noted by Loretta Bender in the 1940s in reference to nondiagnostic abnormalities in the neurological examinations of children with schizophrenia. Soft signs do not indicate focal neurological disorders, but they are associated with a wide variety of developmental disabilities and occur frequently in children with low intelligence, learning disabilities, and behavioral disturbances. Soft signs may refer to both behavioral symptoms (which are sometimes associated with brain damage, such as severe impulsivity and hyperactivity), physical findings (including contralateral overflow movements), and a variety of nonfocal signs (e.g., mild choreiform movements, poor balance, mild incoordination, asymmetry of gait, nystagmus, and the persistence of infantile reflexes). Soft signs can be divided into those that are normal in a young child, but become abnormal when they persist in an older child, and those that are abnormal at any age. The *Physical and Neurological Examination for Soft Signs* (PANESS) is an instrument used with children up to the age of 15 years. It consists of 15 questions about general physical status and medical history and 43 physical tasks (e.g., touch your finger to your nose, hop on one foot to the end of the line, and tap quickly with your finger). Neurological soft signs are important to note, but they are not useful in making a specific psychiatric diagnosis.

Minor physical anomalies or dysmorphic features occur with a higher than usual frequency in children with developmental disabilities, learning disabilities, speech and language disorders, and hyperactivity. As with soft signs, the documentation of minor physical anomalies is part of the neuropsychiatric assessment, but it is rarely helpful in the diagnostic process and does not imply a good or bad prognosis. Minor physical anomalies include a high-arched palate, epicanthal folds, hypertelorism, low-set ears, transverse palmar creases, multiple hair whorls, a large head, a furrowed tongue, and partial syndactyl of several toes.

When a seizure disorder is being considered in the differential diagnosis or a structural abnormality in the brain is suspected, electroencephalography (EEG), computed tomography (CT), or magnetic resonance imaging (MRI) may be indicated.

Developmental, Psychological, and Educational Testing

Psychological testing, structured developmental assessments, and achievement testing are valuable in evaluating a child's developmental level, intellectual functioning, and academic difficulties. A measure of adaptive functioning (including the child's competence in communication, daily living skills, socialization, and motor skills) is the most definitive way to determine the level of intellectual disability in a child. Table 27.2–4 outlines the general categories of psychological tests.

Development Tests for Infants and Preschoolers. The *Gesell Infant Scale,* the *Cattell Infant Intelligence Scale, Bayley Scales of Infant Development,* and the *Denver Developmental Screening Test* include developmental assessments of infants as young as 2 months of age. When used with very young infants, the tests focus on sensorimotor and social responses to a variety of objects and interactions. When these instruments are used with older infants and preschoolers, emphasis is placed on language acquisition. The *Gesell Infant Scale* measures development in four areas: motor, adaptive functioning, language, and social.

An infant's score on one of these developmental assessments is not a reliable way to predict a child's future intelligence quotient (IQ) in most cases. Infant assessments are valuable, however, in detecting developmental deviation and mental retardation and in raising suspicions of a developmental disorder. Whereas infant assessments rely heavily on sensorimotor functions, intelligence testing in older children and adolescents includes later-developing functions, including verbal, social, and abstract cognitive abilities.

Intelligence Tests for School-Age Children and Adolescents. The most widely used test of intelligence for school-age children and adolescents is the third edition of the *Wechsler Intelligence Scale for Children* (WISC-III-R). It can be given to children from 6 to 17 years of age and yields a verbal IQ, a performance IQ, and a combined full-scale IQ. The verbal subtests consist of vocabulary, information, arithmetic, similarities, comprehension, and digit span (supplemental) categories. The performance subtests include block design, picture completion, picture arrangement, object assembly, coding, mazes (supplemental), and symbol search (supplemental). The scores of the supplemental subtests are not included in the computation of IQ.

Each subcategory is scored from 1 to 19, with 10 being the average score. An average full-scale IQ is 100; 70 to 80 represents borderline intellectual function; 80 to 90 is in the low average range; 90 to 109 is average; 110 to 119 is high average; and above 120 is in the superior or very superior range. The multiple breakdowns of the performance and verbal subscales allow great flexibility in identifying specific areas of deficit and scatter in intellectual abilities. Because a large part of intelligence testing measures abilities used in academic settings, the breakdown of the WISC-III-R can also be helpful in pointing out skills in which a child is weak and may benefit from remedial education.

The *Stanford–Binet Intelligence Scale* covers an age range from 2 to 24 years. It relies on pictures, drawings, and objects for very young children and on verbal performance for older children and adolescents. This intelligence scale, the earliest version of an intelligence test of its kind, leads to a mental age score as well as an IQ.

The *McCarthy Scales of Children's Abilities* and the *Kaufman Assessment Battery for Children* are two other intelligence tests that are available for preschool and school-age children. They do not cover the adolescent age group.

Long-Term Stability of Intelligence. Although a child's intelligence is relatively stable throughout the school-age years and adolescence, some factors can influence intelligence and a child's score on an intelligence test. The intellectual functions of children with severe mental illnesses and of those from deprived and neglectful environments may decrease over time, whereas the IQs of children with intensively enriched environments, may increase over time. Factors that influence a child's score on a given test of intellectual functioning and, thus, affect the accuracy of the test are motivation, emotional state, anxiety, and cultural milieu. The interactions between cognitive ability and

Table 27.2–4
Commonly Used Child and Adolescent Psychological Assessment Instruments

Test	Age/Grades	Data Generated and Comments
Intellectual ability		
Wechsler Intelligence Scale for Children—Third Edition (WISC-III-R)	6–16	Standard scores: verbal, performance, and full-scale IQ; scaled subtest scores permitting specific skill assessment.
Wechsler Adult Intelligence Scale—(WAIS-III)	16–adult	Same as WISC-III-R.
Wechsler Preschool and Primary Scale of Intelligence—Revised (WPPSI-R)	3–7	Same as WISC-III-R.
Kaufman Assessment Battery for Children (K-ABC)	2.6–12.6	Well-grounded in theories of cognitive psychology and neuropsychology. Allows immediate comparison of intellectual capacity with acquired knowledge. Scores: Mental Processing Composite (IQ equivalent); sequential and simultaneous processing and achievement standard scores: scaled mental processing and achievement subtest scores; age equivalents; percentiles.
Kaufman Adolescent and Adult Intelligence Test (KAIT)	11–85+	Composed of separate Crystallized and Fluid scales. Scores: Composite Intelligence Scale; Crystallized and Fluid IQ; scaled subtest scores; percentiles.
Stanford–Binet, 4th Edition (SB:FE)	2–23	Scores: IQ; verbal, abstract/visual, and quantitative reasoning; short-term memory; standard age.
Peabody Picture Vocabulary Test—III (PPVT-III)	4–adult	Measures receptive vocabulary acquisition; standard scores, percentiles, and age equivalents.
Achievement		
Woodcock–Johnson Psycho-Educational Battery—Revised (W-J)	K–12	Scores: reading and mathematics (mechanics and comprehension), written language, other academic achievement; grade and age scores, standard scores, and percentiles.
Wide Range Achievement Test—3, Levels 1 and 2 (WRAT-3)	Level 1: 1–5 Level 2: 12–75	Permits screening for deficits in reading, spelling, and arithmetic; grade levels, percentiles, stanines, and standard scores.
Kaufman Test of Educational Achievement, Brief and Comprehensive Forms (K-TEA)	1–12	Standard scores: reading, mathematics, and spelling; grade and age equivalents, percentiles, and stanines. Brief Form is sufficient for most clinical applications; Comprehensive Form allows error analysis and more detailed curriculum planning.
Wechsler Individual Achievement Test (WIAT)	K–12	Standard scores: basic reading, mathematics reasoning, spelling, reading comprehension, numerical operations, listening comprehension, oral expression, and written expression. Conormal with WISC-III-R.
Adaptive behavior		
Vineland Adaptive Behavior Scales	Normal: 0–19 Retarded: All ages	Standard scores: adaptive behavior composite and communication, daily living skills, socialization, and motor domains; percentiles, age equivalents, and developmental age scores. Separate standardization groups for normal, visually handicapped, hearing impaired, emotionally disturbed, and retarded.
Scales of Independent Behavior—Revised	Newborn–adult	Standard scores: four adaptive (motor, social interaction/communication, personal living, and community living) and three maladaptive (internalized, asocial, and externalized) areas; General Maladaptive Index and Broad Independence cluster.
Attentional capacity		
Trail Making Test	8–adult	Standard scores, standard deviations, and ranges; corrections for age and education.
Wisconsin Card Sorting Test	6.6–adult	Standard scores, standard deviations, T-scores, percentiles, developmental norms for number of categories achieved, perseverative errors, and failures to maintain set; computer measures.
Behavior Assessment System for Children (BASC)	4–18	Teacher and parent rating scales and child self-report of personality permitting multireporter assessment across a variety of domains in home, school, and community. Provides validity, clinical, and adaptive scales. ADHD component avails.
Home Situations Questionnaire—Revised (HSQ-R)	6–12	Permits parents to rate child's specific problems with attention or concentration. Scores for number of problem settings, mean severity, and factor scores for compliance and leisure situations.
ADHD Rating Scale	6–12	Score for number of symptoms keyed to DSM cutoff for diagnosis of ADHD; standard scores permit derivation of clinical significance for total score and two factors (Inattentive–Hyperactive and Impulsive–Hyperactive).
School Situations Questionnaire (SSQ-R)	6–12	Permits teachers to rate a child's specific problems with attention or concentration. Scores for number of problem settings and mean severity.
Child Attention Profile (CAP)	6–12	Brief measure allowing teachers' weekly ratings of presence and degree of child's inattention and overactivity. Normative scores for inattention, overactivity, and total score.

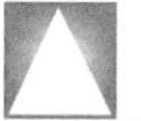

Table 27.2–4
Commonly Used Child and Adolescent Psychological Assessment Instruments (Continued)

Test	Age/Grades	Data Generated and Comments
Projective tests		
Rorschach Inkblots	3–adult	Special scoring systems. Most recently developed and increasingly universally accepted is John Exner's Comprehensive System (1974). Assesses perceptual accuracy, integration of affective and intellectual functioning, reality testing, and other psychological processes.
Thematic Apperception Test (TAT)	6–adult	Generates stories which are analyzed qualitatively. Assumed to provide especially rich data regarding interpersonal functioning.
Machover Draw-A-Person Test (DAP)	3–adult	Qualitative analysis and hypothesis generation, especially regarding subject's feelings about self and significant others.
Kinetic Family Drawing (KFD)	3–adult	Qualitative analysis and hypothesis generation regarding an individual's perception of family structure and sentient environment. Some objective scoring systems in existence.
Rotter Incomplete Sentences Blank	Child, adolescent, and adult forms	Primarily qualitative analysis, although some objective scoring systems have been developed.
Personality tests		
Minnesota Multiphasic Personality Inventory-Adolescent (MMPI-A)	14–18	1992 version of widely used personality measure, developed specifically for use with adolescents. Standard scores: 3 validity scales, 14 clinical scales, additional content, and supplementary scales.
Million Adolescent Personality Inventory (MAPI)	13–18	Standard scores for 20 scales grouped into three categories: Personality styles; expressed concerns; and behavioral correlates. Normed on adolescent population. Focuses on broad functional spectrum, not just problem areas. Measures 14 primary personality traits, including emotional stability, self-concept level, excitability, and self-assurance.
Children's Personality Questionnaire	8–12	Generates combined broad trait patterns including extraversion and anxiety.
Neuropsychological screening tests and test batteries		
Developmental Test of Visual–Motor Integration (VMI)	2–16	Screening instrument for visual motor deficits. Standard scores, age equivalents, percentiles.
Benton Visual Retention Test	6–adult	Assesses presence of deficits in visual–figure memory. Mean scores by age.
Benton Visual Motor Gestalt Test	5–adult	Assesses visual–motor deficits and visual–figural retention. Age equivalents.
Reitan–Indiana Neuropsychological Test Battery for Children	5–8	Cognitive and perceptual–motor tests for children with suspected brain damage.
Halstead–Reitan Neuropsychological Test Battery for Older Children	9–14	Same as Reitan–Indiana.
Luria–Nebraska Neuropsychological Battery: Children's Revision LNNB:C	8–12	Sensory–motor, perceptual, and cognitive tests measuring 11 clinical and 2 additional domains of neuropsychological functioning. Provides standard scores.
Developmental status		
Bayley Scales of Infant Development-Second Edition	16 days–42 months	Mental, motor, and behavior scales measuring infant, development. Provides standard scores.
Mullen Scales of Early Learning	Newborn–5 years	Language and visual scales for receptive and expressive ability. Yields age scores and T scores.

Adapted from Racusin G, Moss N. Psychological assessment of children and adolescents. In: Lewis M, ed. *Child and Adolescent Psychiatry: A Comprehensive Textbook*. Baltimore, MD: Williams & Wilkins; 1991, with permission.

anxiety, and depression and psychosis are complex. One study of 4,405 youth from the Canadian National Longitudinal Study of Children and Youth (NLSCY), by Weeks and colleagues (2013) found that greater cognitive ability was associated with less risk for anxiety and depressive symptoms in youth from 12 to 13 years of age, however, by age 14 to 15 years, cognitive ability had no effect on the odds of anxiety or depression.

Perceptual and Perceptual Motor Tests. The *Bender Visual Motor Gestalt Test* can be given to children between the ages of 4 and 12 years. The test consists of a set of spatially related figures that the child is asked to copy. The scores are based on the number of errors. Although not a diagnostic test, it is useful in identifying developmentally age-inappropriate perceptual performances.

Personality Tests. Personality tests are not of much use in making diagnoses, and they are less satisfactory than intelligence tests with regard to norms, reliability, and validity, but they can be helpful in eliciting themes and fantasies.

The Rorschach test is a projective technique in which ambiguous stimuli—a set of bilaterally symmetrical inkblots—are shown to a child, who is then asked to describe what he or she sees in each. The hypothesis is that the child's interpretation of the vague stimuli reflects basic characteristics of personality. The examiner notes the themes and patterns.

A more structured projective test is the *Children's Apperception Test* (CAT), which is an adaptation of the *Thematic Apperception Test* (TAT). The CAT consists of cards with pictures of animals in scenes that are somewhat ambiguous, but are related to parent–child and sibling issues, caretaking, and other relationships. The child is asked to describe what is happening and to tell a story about the scene. Animals are used because it was hypothesized that children might respond more readily to animal images than to human figures.

Drawings, toys, and play are also applications of projective techniques that can be used during the evaluation of children. Dollhouses, dolls, and puppets have been especially helpful in allowing a child a nonconversational mode in which to express a variety of attitudes and feelings. Play materials that reflect household situations are likely to elicit a child's fears, hopes, and conflicts about the family.

Projective techniques have not fared well as standardized instruments. Rather than being considered tests, projective techniques are best considered as additional clinical modalities.

Educational Tests. Achievement tests measure the attainment of knowledge and skills in a particular academic curriculum. The *Wide-Range Achievement Test-Revised* (WRAT-R) consists of tests of knowledge and skills and timed performances of reading, spelling, and mathematics. It is used with children from 5 years of age to adulthood. The test yields a score that is compared with the average expected score for the child's chronological age and grade level.

The *Peabody Individual Achievement Test* (PIAT) includes word identification, spelling, mathematics, and reading comprehension.

The *Kaufman Test of Educational Achievement,* the *Gray Oral Reading Test-Revised* (GORT-R), and the *Sequential Tests of Educational Progress* (STEP) are achievement tests that determine whether a child has achieved the educational level expected for his or her grade level. Children, whose achievement is significantly lower than expected for their grade level in one or more subjects, often exhibit a specific learning disorder.

Biopsychosocial Formulation. A clinician's task is to integrate all of the information obtained into a formulation that takes into account the biological predisposition, psychodynamic factors, environmental stressors, and life events that have led to the child's current level of functioning. Psychiatric disorders and any specific physical, neuromotor, or developmental abnormalities must be considered in the formulation of etiologic factors for current impairment. The clinician's conclusions are an integration of clinical information along with data from standardized psychological and developmental assessments. The psychiatric formulation includes an assessment of family function as well as the appropriateness of the child's educational setting. A determination of the child's overall safety in his or her current situation is made. Any suspected maltreatment must be reported to the local child protective service agency. The child's overall well-being regarding growth, development, and academic and play activities is considered.

Diagnosis

Structured and semistructured (evidence-based) assessment tools often enhance a clinician's ability to make the most accurate diagnoses. These instruments, described earlier, include the K-SADS, the CAPA, and the NIMH DISC-IV interviews. The advantages of including an evidence-based instrument in the diagnostic process include decreasing potential clinician bias to make a diagnosis without all of the necessary symptoms information, and serving as guides for the clinician to consider each symptom that could contribute to a given diagnosis. These data can enable the clinician to optimize his expertise to make challenging judgments regarding child and adolescent disorders, which may possess overlapping symptoms. The clinician's ultimate task includes making all appropriate diagnoses according to the DSM-5. Some clinical situations do not fulfill criteria for DSM-5 diagnoses, but cause impairment and require psychiatric attention and intervention. Clinicians who evaluate children are frequently in the position of determining the impact of behavior of family members on the child's well-being. In many cases, a child's level of impairment is related to factors extending beyond a psychiatric diagnosis, such as the child's adjustment to his or her family life, peer relationships, and educational placement.

RECOMMENDATIONS AND TREATMENT PLAN

The recommendations for treatment are derived by a clinician who integrates the data gathered during the evaluation into a coherent formulation of the factors that are contributing to the child's current problems, the consequences of the problems, and strategies that may ameliorate the difficulties. The recommendations can be broken down into their biological, psychological, and social components. That is, identification of a biological predisposition to a particular psychiatric disorder may be clinically relevant to inform a psychopharmacologic recommendation. As part of the formulation, an understanding of the psychodynamic interactions between family members may lead a clinician to recommend treatment that includes a family component. Educational and academic problems are addressed in the formulation and may lead to a recommendation to seek a more effective academic placement. The overall social situation of the child or adolescent is taken into account when recommendations for treatment are developed. Of course, the physical and emotional safety of a child or adolescent is of the utmost importance and always at the top of the list of recommendations.

The child or adolescent's family, school life, peer interactions, and social activities often have a direct impact on the child's success in overcoming his or her difficulties. The psychological education and cooperation of a child or adolescent's family are essential ingredients in successful application of treatment recommendations. Communications from clinicians to parents and family members that balance the observed positive qualities of the child and family with the weak areas are often perceived as more helpful than a focus only on the problem areas. Finally, the most successful treatment plans are those developed cooperatively between the clinician, child, and family members during which each member of the team perceives that he or she has been given credit for positive contributions.

▲ 27.3 Intellectual Disability

Intellectual disability, formerly known as *mental retardation,* can be caused by a range of environmental and genetic factors that lead to a combination of cognitive and social impairments. The American Association on Intellectual and Developmental Disability (AAIDD) defines intellectual disability as a disability characterized by significant limitations in both intellectual functioning (reasoning, learning, and problem solving) and in adaptive behavior (conceptual, social, and practical skills) that emerges before the age of 18 years. Wide acceptance of this definition has led to the international consensus that an assessment of both social adaptation and IQ are necessary to determine the level of intellectual disability. Measures of adaptive function assess competency in social functioning, understanding of societal norms, and performance of everyday tasks, whereas measures of intellectual function focus on cognitive abilities. Although individuals with a given intellectual level do not all have identical levels of adaptive function, epidemiologic data suggest that prevalence of intellectual disability is largely determined by intellectual level and a level of adaptive function, which typically corresponds closely with cognitive ability.

In the *Diagnostic and Statistical Manual of Mental Disorders,* Fifth Edition (DSM-5), various levels of severity of intellectual disability are determined on the basis of adaptive functioning, not on IQ scores. This change in emphasis from prior diagnostic manuals has been adopted by DSM-5 because adaptive functioning determines the level of support that is required. Furthermore, IQ scores are less valid in the lower portions of the IQ range. Making a determination of severity level of intellectual disability, according to DSM-5, includes assessment of functioning in a conceptual domain (e.g., academic skills), a social domain (e.g., relationships), and a practical domain (e.g., personal hygiene).

Societal approaches to children with intellectual disability have shifted significantly over time. Historically, in the mid-1800s many children with intellectual disability were placed in residential educational facilities based on the belief that with sufficient intensive training, these children would be able to return to their families and function in society at a higher level. However, the expectation of educating these children in order to overcome their disabilities was not realized. Gradually, many residential programs increased in size, and eventually the focus began to shift from intensive education to more custodial care. Residential settings for children with intellectual disability received their maximal use in the mid-1900s, until public awareness of the crowded, unsanitary, and, in some cases, abusive conditions sparked the movement toward "deinstitutionalization." An important force in the deinstitutionalization of children with intellectual disability was the philosophy of "normalization" in living situations, and "inclusion" in educational settings. Since the late 1960s, few children with intellectual disability have been placed in residences, and the concepts of normalization and inclusion remain prominent among advocacy groups and parents.

The passage of Public Law 94–142 (the Education for all Handicapped Children Act) in 1975 mandates that the public school system provide appropriate educational service to all children with disabilities. The Individuals with Disabilities Act in 1990 extended and modified the above legislation. Currently, provision of public education for all children, including those with disabilities, "within the least restrictive environment" is mandated by law.

In addition to the educational system, advocacy groups, including the Council for Exceptional Children (CEC) and the National Association for Retarded Citizens (NARC), are well-known parental lobbying organizations for children with intellectual disability and were instrumental in advocating for Public Law 94–142. The American Association on Intellectual and Developmental Disabilities, formerly known as The American Association on Intellectual disability (AAMR), is the most prominent advocacy organization in this field. It has been very influential in educating the public about, and in supporting research and legislation relating to intellectual disability.

The AAIDD promotes a view of intellectual disability as a functional interaction between an individual and the environment, rather than a static designation of a person's limitations. Within this conceptual framework, a child or adolescent with intellectual disability is determined to need intermittent, limited, extensive, or pervasive "environmental support" with respect to a specific set of adaptive function domains. These include communication, self-care, home living, social or interpersonal skills, use of community resources, self-direction, functional academic skills, work, leisure, health, and safety.

The United Nations Convention on the Rights of Persons with Disabilities (2006) has created a forum to promote the full social inclusion of people with intellectual disability. Through its recognition and focus on social barriers, this international forum aims to provide protections for individuals with intellectual disability, and to seek more inclusion of those with intellectual disability in social, civic, and educational activities.

NOMENCLATURE

The accurate definition of intellectual disability has been a challenge for clinicians over the centuries. All current classification systems underscore that intellectual disability is based on more than cognitive deficits, that is, it also includes impaired social adaptive function. According to DSM-5, a diagnosis of intellectual disability should be made only when there are deficits in intellectual functioning and deficits in adaptive functioning. Once intellectual disability is recognized, the level of severity is determined by the level of adaptive functional impairment.

CLASSIFICATION

DSM-5 criteria for intellectual disability include significantly subaverage general intellectual functioning associated with concurrent impairment in adaptive behavior, manifested before the age of 18. The diagnosis is made independent of coexisting physical or mental disorders. Table 27.3–1 presents an overview of developmental levels in communication, academic functioning, and vocational skills expected of persons with various degrees of intellectual disability.

If the clinician chooses to use a standardized test of intelligence—which is still common practice—the term *significantly subaverage* is defined as an IQ of approximately 70 or below or two standard deviations below the mean for the particular test. Adaptive functioning can be measured by using a standardized scale, such as the *Vineland Adaptive Behavior Scale.* This scale scores communications, daily living skills, socialization, and motor skills (up to 4 years, 11 months) and generates an adaptive behavior composite that is correlated with the expected skills at a given age.

Approximately 85 percent of individuals who have intellectual disability fall within the DSM-5 mild intellectual disability category. This is typically defined by a Full Scale IQ between 50 and 70 and an adaptive function severity in the mild range.

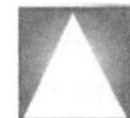

Table 27.3–1
Developmental Characteristics of Intellectual Disability

Level of Intellectual Disability	Preschool Age (0–5 yrs) Maturation and Development	School Age (6–20 yrs) Training and Education	Adult (21 yrs and above) Social and Vocational Adequacy
Profound	Gross disability; minimal capacity for functioning in sensorimotor areas; needs nursing care; constant aid and supervision required	Some motor development present; may respond to minimal or limited training in self-help	Some motor and speech development; may achieve very limited self-care; needs nursing care
Severe	Poor motor development; speech minimal; generally unable to profit from training in self-help; little or no communication skills	Can talk or learn to communicate; can be trained in elemental health habits; profits from systematic habit training; unable to profit from vocational training	May contribute partially to self-maintenance under complete supervision; can develop self-protection skills to a minimal useful level in controlled environment
Moderate	Can talk or learn to communicate; poor social awareness; fair motor development; profits from training in self-help; can be managed with moderate supervision	Can profit from training in social and occupational skills; unlikely to progress beyond second-grade level in academic subjects; may learn to travel alone in familiar places	May achieve self-maintenance in unskilled or semiskilled work under sheltered conditions; needs supervision and guidance when under mild social or economic stress
Mild	Can develop social and communication skills; minimal retardation in sensorimotor areas; often not distinguished from normal until later age	Can learn academic skills up to approximately sixth-grade level by late teens; can be guided toward social conformity	Can usually achieve social and vocational skills adequate to minimal self-support, but may need guidance and assistance when under unusual social or economic stress

Adapted from Mental Retarded Activities of the US Department of Health, Education and Welfare. Washington, DC: US Government Printing Office; 1989:2.

Adaptive function includes skills such as communication, self-care, social skills, work, leisure, and understanding of safety. Intellectual disability is influenced by genetic, environmental, and psychosocial factors. A host of subtle environmental and developmental factors, including subclinical lead intoxication and prenatal exposure to drugs, alcohol, and other toxins have been implicated as contributors to intellectual disability. Certain genetic syndromes associated with intellectual disability such as fragile X syndrome, Down syndrome, and Prader–Willi syndrome, have characteristic patterns of social, linguistic, and cognitive development and typical behavioral manifestations.

DEGREES OF SEVERITY OF INTELLECTUAL DISABILITY

The severity levels of intellectual disability are expressed in DSM-5 as mild, moderate, severe, and profound. "Borderline intellectual functioning," a term previously used to describe individuals with a full-scale IQ in the range of 70 to 80, is no longer described as a diagnosis in DSM-5. The term is used in DSM-5 as a condition that may be the focus of clinical attention; however, no criteria are given.

Mild intellectual disability represents approximately 85 percent of persons with intellectual disability. Children with mild intellectual disability are often not identified until the first or second grade, when academic demands increase. By late adolescence, they often acquire academic skills at approximately a sixth-grade level. Specific causes for the intellectual disability are often unidentified in this group. Many adults with mild intellectual disability can live independently with appropriate support and raise their own families. IQ for this level of adaptive function may typically range from 50 to 70.

Moderate intellectual disability represents about 10 percent of persons with intellectual disability. Most children with moderate intellectual disability acquire language and can communicate adequately during early childhood. They are challenged academically and are often not able to achieve above a second to third grade level. During adolescence, socialization difficulties often set these persons apart, and a great deal of social and vocational support is beneficial. As adults, individuals with moderate intellectual disability may be able to perform semiskilled work under appropriate supervision. IQ for this level of adaptive function may typically range from 35 to 50.

Severe intellectual disability represents about 4 percent of individuals with intellectual disability. They may be able to develop communication skills in childhood and often can learn to count as well as recognize words that are critical to functioning. In this group, the cause for the intellectual disability is more likely to be identified than in milder forms of intellectual disability. In adulthood, persons with severe intellectual disability may adapt well to supervised living situations, such as group homes, and may be able to perform work-related tasks under supervision. IQ in individuals with this level of adaptive function may typically range from 20 to 35.

Profound intellectual disability constitutes approximately 1 to 2 percent of individuals with intellectual disability. Most individuals with profound intellectual disability have identifiable causes for their condition. Children with profound intellectual disability may be taught some self-care skills and learn to communicate their needs given the appropriate training. IQ in individuals with this level of adaptive function may typically be less than 20.

The DSM-5 also includes a disorder called "Unspecified Intellectual Disability" (Intellectual Developmental Disorder), reserved for individuals over the age of 5 years who are difficult to evaluate but are strongly suspected of having intellectual disability. Individuals with this diagnosis may have sensory or physical impairments such as blindness or deafness, or concurrent mental disorders, making it difficult to administer typical assessment tools (e.g., *Bayley Scales of Infant Development* and *Cattell Infant Scale*) to aid in determining adaptive functional impairment.

EPIDEMIOLOGY

The majority of population-based prevalence estimates for intellectual disability in developing countries range from 10 to 15 per 1,000 children. The prevalence of intellectual disability at any one time is estimated to range from 1 to 3 percent of the population in Western societies. The incidence of intellectual disability is difficult to accurately calculate because mild disabilities may be unrecognized until middle childhood. In some cases, even when intellectual function is limited, social adaptive skills may not be challenged until late childhood or early adolescence, and the diagnosis is not made until that time. The highest incidence of intellectual disability is reported in school-age children, with the peak at ages 10 to 14 years. Intellectual disability is about 1.5 times more common among males than females.

COMORBIDITY

Prevalence

Epidemiological surveys indicate that up to two-thirds of children and adults with intellectual disability have comorbid psychiatric disorders; and this rate is several times higher than that in community samples without intellectual disability. The prevalence of psychopathology appears to be correlated with the severity of intellectual disability; the more severe the intellectual disability, the higher the risk for coexisting psychiatric disorders. An epidemiological study found that 40.7 percent of intellectually disabled children between 4 and 18 years of age met criteria for at least one additional psychiatric disorder. The severity of intellectual disability influenced the risk for particular comorbid psychiatric disorders. Disruptive and conduct-disorder behaviors occurred more frequently in those diagnosed with mild intellectual disability, whereas those with more severe intellectual disability were more likely to meet criteria for autism spectrum disorder and exhibited symptoms such as self-stimulation and self-mutilation. Comorbidity of psychiatric disorders with intellectual disability in children in this study was not correlated with age or gender. Children diagnosed with profound intellectual disability were less likely to exhibit comorbid psychiatric disorders.

Psychiatric disorders among persons with intellectual disability are varied, and include mood disorders, schizophrenia, ADHD, and conduct disorder. Children diagnosed with severe intellectual disability have a particularly high rate of comorbid autism spectrum disorder. Approximately 2 to 3 percent of those with intellectual disability meet diagnostic criteria for schizophrenia, which is several times higher than the rate for the general population. Up to 50 percent of children and adults with intellectual disability are found to meet criteria for a mood disorder when instruments such as the *Kiddie Schedule for Affective Disorders and Schizophrenia* (K-SADS), the *Beck Depression Inventory,* and the *Children's Depression Inventory* were used in studies. However, a limitation of these studies is that these instruments have not been standardized within intellectual disability populations. Frequent psychiatric symptoms that occur in children with intellectual disability, outside the context of a full psychiatric disorder, include hyperactivity and short attention span, self-injurious behaviors (e.g., head-banging and self-biting), and repetitive stereotypical behaviors (hand-flapping and toe-walking). In children and adults with milder forms of intellectual disability, negative self-image, low self-esteem, poor frustration tolerance, interpersonal dependence, and a rigid problem-solving style are frequent.

Neurological Disorders

Seizure disorders occur more frequently in individuals with intellectual disability than in the general population, and prevalence rates for seizures increase proportionally to severity level of intellectual disability. A review of psychiatric disorders in children and adolescents with intellectual disability and epilepsy found that approximately one-third had comorbid autism spectrum disorder. The combination of intellectual disability, epilepsy, and autism spectrum disorder has been estimated to occur in 0.07 percent of the general population.

Psychosocial Features

A negative self-image and poor self-esteem are common features of mildly and moderately intellectually disabled persons who are aware of their social and academic differences from others. Given their experience of repeated failure and disappointment in being unable to meet their parents' and society's expectations, they may also be faced with falling progressively behind younger siblings. Communication difficulties further increase their vulnerability to feelings of ineptness and frustration. Inappropriate behaviors, such as withdrawal, are common. The perpetual sense of isolation and inadequacy has been linked to feelings of anxiety, anger, dysphoria, and depression.

ETIOLOGY

Etiological factors in intellectual disability can be genetic, developmental, environmental, or a combination. Genetic causes include chromosomal and inherited conditions; developmental and environmental factors include prenatal exposure to infections and toxins; and environmental or acquired factors include prenatal trauma (e.g., prematurity) and sociocultural factors. The severity of intellectual disability may be related to the timing and duration of a given trauma as well as to the degree of exposure to the CNS. In about three-fourths of persons diagnosed with severe intellectual disability, the etiology is known, whereas the etiology is apparent in up to half of those diagnosed with mild intellectual disability. A study of 100 consecutive children diagnosed with intellectual disability admitted to a clinical genetics unit of a university pediatric hospital reported that in 41 percent of cases, a causative diagnosis was made. No cause is known for three-fourths of persons with IQ ranging from 70 to 80 and variable adaptive functioning. Among chromosomal disorders, Down syndrome and fragile X syndrome are the most common disorders that usually produce at least moderate intellectual disability. A prototype of a metabolic disorder associated with intellectual disability is phenylketonuria (PKU). Deprivation of nutrition, nurturance, and social stimulation can potentially contribute to the development of at least mild forms of intellectual disability. Current knowledge suggests that genetic, environmental, biological, and psychosocial factors work additively in the emergence of intellectual disability.

Genetic Etiological Factors in Intellectual Disability

Single-Gene Causes. One of the most well-known single gene causes of intellectually disability is found in the *FMR1* gene whose mutations cause fragile X syndrome. It is the most common and first X-linked gene to be identified as a direct cause of intellectual disability. Abnormalities in autosomal chromosomes are frequently associated with intellectual disability, whereas aberrations in sex chromosomes can result in characteristic physical syndromes that do not include intellectual disability (e.g., Turner's syndrome with XO and Klinefelter's syndrome with XXY, XXXY, and XXYY variations). Some children with Turner's syndrome have normal to superior intelligence. Agreement exists on a few predisposing factors for chromosomal disorders—among them, advanced maternal age, increased age of the father, and x-ray radiation.

Visible and Submicroscopic Chromosomal Causes of Intellectual Disability. Trisomy 21 (Down syndrome) is a prototype of a cytogenetically visible abnormality that accounts for about two-thirds of the 15 percent of intellectual disability attributable to visible abnormal cytogenetics. Other microscopically visible chromosomal abnormalities associated with intellectual disability include deletions, translocations, and supernumerary marker chromosomes. Typically, microscopic chromosome analysis is able to identify abnormalities of 5 to 10 million base pairs or greater.

Submicroscopic identification requires the use of microarrays that can identify losses of chromosomal segments too small to be picked up by light microscopy. The altered copy number variants (CNVs) in submicroscopic segments of the chromosome have been identified to be associated with up to 13 to 20 percent of cases of intellectual disability. That is, the genes associated with a particular developmental abnormality have been identified to be located in the critical regions of the pathogenic copy number variants.

Genetic Intellectual Disability and Behavioral Phenotype

Specific and predictable behaviors have been found to be associated with certain genetically based cases of intellectual disability. These behavioral phenotypes are defined as a syndrome of observable behaviors that occur with a significantly greater probability than expected among those individuals with a specific genetic abnormality.

Examples of behavioral phenotypes occur in genetically determined syndromes such as fragile X syndrome, Prader–Willi syndrome, and Down syndrome in which specific behavioral manifestations can be expected. Persons with fragile X syndrome have extremely high rates (up to three-fourths of those studied) of ADHD. High rates of aberrant interpersonal behavior and language function often meet the criteria for autistic disorder and avoidant personality disorder. Prader–Willi syndrome is almost always associated with compulsive eating disturbances, hyperphagia, and obesity. Socialization is an area of weakness, especially in coping skills. Externalizing behavior problems—such as temper tantrums, irritability, and arguing—seem to be heightened in adolescence.

Down Syndrome. The etiology of Down syndrome, known to be caused by an extra copy of the entire chromosome 21, makes it one of the more complex disorders. The original description of Down syndrome, first made by the English physician Langdon Down in 1866, was based on physical characteristics associated with subnormal mental functioning. Since then, Down syndrome has been the most investigated, and most discussed, syndrome in intellectual disability. Recent data have suggested that Down syndrome may be more amenable to postnatal interventions to address the cognitive deficits that it produces than was previously thought. Although still in the early stages of animal research, data from experiments with one mouse model, the Ts65Dn, indicates that pharmacologic interventions may influence learning and memory deficits known to occur in Down syndrome.

Phenotypically, children with Down syndrome are observed to have characteristic physical attributes, including slanted eyes, epicanthal folds, and a flat nose.

The etiology of Down syndrome is complicated by the recognition of three types of chromosomal aberrations in Down syndrome:

1. Patients with trisomy 21 (three chromosomes 21, instead of the usual two) represent the overwhelming majority; they have 47 chromosomes, with an extra chromosome 21. The mothers' karyotypes are normal. A nondisjunction during meiosis, occurring for unknown reasons, is held responsible for the disorder.
2. Nondisjunction occurring after fertilization in any cell division results in mosaicism, a condition in which both normal and trisomic cells are found in various tissues.
3. In translocation, a fusion occurs of two chromosomes, usually 21 and 15, resulting in a total of 46 chromosomes, despite the presence of an extra chromosome 21. The disorder, unlike trisomy 21, is usually inherited, and the translocated chromosome may be found in unaffected parents and siblings. The asymptomatic carriers have only 45 chromosomes.

Approximately 6,000 babies are affected with Down syndrome in the United States, which makes the incidence of Down syndrome 1 in every 700 births, or 15 per 10,000 live births. For women older than 32 years of age, the risk of having a child with Down syndrome (trisomy 21) is about 1 in 100 births, but when translocation is present, the risk is about 1 in 3. Most children with Down syndrome are mildly to moderately intellectually disabled, with a minority having an IQ above 50. Cognitive development appears to progress normally from birth to 6 months of age; IQ scores gradually decrease from near normal at 1 year of age to about 30 to 50 as development proceeds. The decline in intellectual function may not be readily apparent. Infant tests may not reveal the full extent of the deficits.

According to anecdotal clinical reports, children with Down syndrome are typically placid, cheerful, and cooperative and adapt easily at home. With adolescence, the picture changes: youth with Down syndrome may experience more social and emotional difficulties and behavior disorders, and there is an increased risk for psychotic disorders.

In Down syndrome, language function is a relative weakness, whereas sociability and social skills, such as interpersonal cooperation and conformity with social conventions, are relative strengths. Children with Down syndrome typically manifest deficits in scanning the environment; they are more likely to focus on a single stimulus, leading to difficulty noticing environmental changes. A variety of comorbid psychiatric disorders emerge in persons with Down syndrome; however, the rates appear to be lower than in children with intellectual disability and autism spectrum disorder.

The diagnosis of Down syndrome is made with relative ease in an older child, but it is often difficult in newborn infants. The most important signs in a newborn include general hypotonia; oblique palpebral fissures; abundant neck skin; a small, flattened skull; high cheekbones; and a protruding tongue. The hands are broad and thick, with a single palmar transversal crease, and the little fingers are short and curved inward. Moro reflex is weak or absent. More than 100 signs or stigmata are described in Down syndrome, but rarely are all found in one person. Commonly occurring physical problems in Down syndrome include cardiac defects, thyroid abnormalities, and gastrointestinal problems. Life expectancy was once drastically limited to about the age of 40; however, currently it is vastly increased, although still not as long as those without intellectual disability.

Down syndrome is characterized by deterioration in language, memory, self-care skills, and problem-solving by the third decade of life. Postmortem studies of individuals with Down syndrome older than age 40 have shown a high incidence of senile plaques and neurofibrillary tangles, similar to those seen in Alzheimer's disease. Neurofibrillary tangles are known to occur in a variety of degenerative diseases, whereas senile plaques seem to be found most often in Alzheimer's disease and in Down syndrome.

Fragile X Syndrome. Fragile X syndrome is the second most common single cause of intellectual disability. The syndrome results from a mutation on the X chromosome at what is known as the fragile site (Xq27.3). The fragile site is expressed in only some cells, and it may be absent in asymptomatic males and female carriers. Much variability is present in both genetic and phenotypic expression. Fragile X syndrome is believed to occur in about 1 of every 1,000 males and 1 of every 2,000 females. The typical phenotype includes a large, long head and ears, short stature, hyperextensible joints, and postpubertal macroorchidism. Associated intellectual disability ranges from mild to severe. The behavioral profile of persons with the syndrome includes a high rate of ADHD, learning disorders, and autism spectrum disorder. Deficits in language function include rapid perseverative speech with abnormalities in combining words into phrases and sentences. Persons with fragile X syndrome seem to have relatively strong skills in communication and socialization; their intellectual functions seem to decline in the pubertal period. Female carriers are often less impaired than males with fragile X syndrome, but females can also manifest the typical physical characteristics and may have mild intellectual disability.

Prader–Willi Syndrome. Prader–Willi syndrome is believed to result from a small deletion involving chromosome 15, occurring sporadically. Its prevalence is less than 1 in 10,000. Persons with the syndrome exhibit compulsive eating behavior and often obesity, intellectual disability, hypogonadism, small stature, hypotonia, and small hands and feet.

Cat's Cry (Cri-du-Chat) Syndrome. Children with cat's cry syndrome have a deletion in chromosome 5. They are typically severely intellectually disabled and show many signs often associated with chromosomal aberrations, such as microcephaly, low-set ears, oblique palpebral fissures, hypertelorism, and micrognathia. The characteristic cat-like cry that gave the syndrome its name is caused by laryngeal abnormalities that gradually change and disappear with increasing age.

Phenylketonuria. PKU was first described by Ivar Asbjörn Fölling in 1934 as an inborn error of metabolism. PKU is transmitted as a simple recessive autosomal Mendelian trait and occurs in about 1 of every 10,000 to 15,000 live births. For parents who have already had a child with PKU, the chance of having another child with PKU is 20 to 25 percent of successive pregnancies. PKU is reported predominantly in persons of North European origin; a few cases have been described in blacks, Yemenite Jews, and Asians. The basic metabolic defect in PKU is an inability to convert phenylalanine, an essential amino acid, to paratyrosine because of the absence or inactivity of the liver enzyme phenylalanine hydroxylase, which catalyzes the conversion. Therefore, PKU is largely preventable with a screening for it, which, if positive, should be followed with a low phenylalanine diet. Two other types of hyperphenylalaninemia have recently been described. One is caused by a deficiency of the enzyme dihydropteridine reductase, and the other to a deficiency of a cofactor, biopterin. The first defect can be detected in fibroblasts, and biopterin can be measured in body fluids. Both these rare disorders carry a high risk of fatality.

Most patients with PKU are severely intellectually disabled, but some are reported to have borderline or normal intelligence. Eczema, vomiting, and convulsions occur in about one-third of all patients. Although the clinical picture varies, typically, children with PKU are reported to be hyperactive and irritable. They frequently exhibit temper tantrums and often display bizarre movements of their bodies and upper extremities, including twisting hand mannerisms. Verbal and nonverbal communication is commonly severely impaired or nonexistent. The children's coordination is poor, and they have many perceptual difficulties.

Currently, the Guthrie inhibition assay is a widely applied screening test using a bacteriological procedure to detect phenylalanine in the blood. In the United States, newborn infants are routinely screened for PKU. Early diagnosis is important, because a low-phenylalanine diet, in use since 1955, significantly improves both behavior and developmental progress. The best results seem to be obtained with early diagnosis and the start of dietary treatment before the child is 6 months of age. Dietary treatment, however, is not without risk. Phenylalanine is an essential amino acid, and its omission from the diet can lead to such severe complications as anemia, hypoglycemia, or edema. Dietary treatment of PKU should be continued indefinitely. Children who receive a diagnosis before the age of 3 months and are placed on an optimal dietary regimen may have normal intelligence. A low-phenylalanine diet does not reverse intellectual disability in untreated older children and adolescents with PKU, but the diet does decrease irritability and abnormal electroencephalography (EEG) changes and does increase social responsiveness and attention span. The parents of children with PKU and some of the children's normal siblings are heterozygous carriers.

Rett Syndrome. Rett syndrome, now diagnosed in the DSM-5 as a form of autism spectrum disorder, is believed to be caused by a dominant X-linked gene. It is degenerative and affects only females. In 1966, Andreas Rett reported on 22 girls with a serious progressive neurological disability. Deterioration in communications skills, motor behavior, and social functioning starts at about 1 year of age. Symptoms include ataxia, facial grimacing, teeth-grinding, and loss of speech. Intermittent hyperventilation and a disorganized breathing pattern are characteristic while the child is awake. Stereotypical hand movements, including hand-wringing, are typical. Progressive gait disturbance, scoliosis, and seizures occur. Severe spasticity is usually present by middle childhood. Cerebral atrophy occurs with decreased pigmentation of the substantia nigra, which suggests abnormalities of the dopaminergic nigrostriatal system.

Neurofibromatosis. Also called *von Recklinghausen's*, neurofibromatosis is the most common of the neurocutaneous syndromes caused by a single dominant gene, which may be inherited or occur as a new mutation. The disorder occurs in about 1 of 5,000 births and is characterized by café au lait spots on the skin and by neurofibromas, including optic gliomas and acoustic neuromas, caused by abnormal cell migration. Mild intellectual disability occurs in up to one-third of those with the disease.

Tuberous Sclerosis. Tuberous sclerosis is the second most common of the neurocutaneous syndromes; a progressive intellectual disability occurs in up to two-thirds of all affected persons. It occurs in about 1 of 15,000 persons and is inherited by autosomal dominant transmission. Seizures are present in all those with intellectual disability, and in two-thirds of those who are not. Infantile spasms may occur as early as 6 months of age. The phenotypic presentation includes adenoma sebaceum and ash-leaf spots that can be identified with a slit lamp.

Lesch–Nyhan Syndrome. Lesch–Nyhan syndrome is a rare disorder caused by a deficiency of an enzyme involved in purine metabolism. The disorder is X-linked; patients have intellectual disability, microcephaly, seizures, choreoathetosis, and spasticity. The syndrome is also associated with severe compulsive self-mutilation by biting the mouth and fingers. Lesch–Nyhan syndrome is another example of a genetically determined syndrome with a specific, predictable behavioral pattern.

Adrenoleukodystrophy. The most common of several disorders of sudanophilic cerebral sclerosis, adrenoleukodystrophy is characterized by diffuse demyelination of the cerebral white matter resulting in visual and intellectual impairment, seizures, spasticity, and progression to death. The cerebral degeneration in adrenoleukodystrophy is accompanied by adrenocortical insufficiency. The disorder is transmitted by a sex-linked gene located on the distal end of the long arm of the X chromosome. The clinical onset is generally between 5 and 8 years of age, with early seizures, disturbances in gait, and mild intellectual impairment. Abnormal pigmentation reflecting adrenal insufficiency sometimes precedes the neurological symptoms, and attacks of crying are common. Spastic contractures, ataxia, and swallowing disturbances are also frequent. Although the course is often rapidly progressive, some patients may have a relapsing and remitting course.

Maple Syrup Urine Disease. The clinical symptoms of maple syrup urine disease appear during the first week of life. The infant deteriorates rapidly and has decerebrate rigidity, seizures, respiratory irregularity, and hypoglycemia. If untreated, maple syrup urine disease is usually fatal in the first months of life, and the survivors have severe intellectual disability. Some variants have been reported with transient ataxia and only mild intellectual disability. Treatment follows the general principles established for PKU and consists of a diet very low in the three involved amino acids—leucine, isoleucine, and valine.

Other Enzyme Deficiency Disorders. Several enzyme deficiency disorders associated with intellectual disability have been identified, and still more diseases are being added as new discoveries are made, including Hartnup disease, galactosemia, and glycogen-storage disease. Table 27.3–2 lists 30 important disorders with inborn errors of metabolism, hereditary transmission patterns, defective enzymes, clinical signs, and relation to intellectual disability.

Acquired and Developmental Factors

Prenatal Period. Important prerequisites for the overall development of the fetus include the mother's physical, psychological, and nutritional health during pregnancy. Maternal chronic illnesses and conditions affecting the normal development of the fetus's CNS include uncontrolled diabetes, anemia, emphysema, hypertension, and long-term use of alcohol and narcotic substances. Maternal infections during pregnancy, especially viral infections, have been known to cause fetal damage and intellectual disability. The extent of fetal damage depends on such variables as the type of viral infection, the gestational age of the fetus, and the severity of the illness. Although numerous infectious diseases have been reported to affect the fetus's CNS, the following maternal illnesses have been identified to increase risk of intellectual disability in the newborn.

RUBELLA (GERMAN MEASLES). Rubella has replaced syphilis as the major cause of congenital malformations and intellectual disability caused by maternal infection. The children of affected mothers may show several abnormalities, including congenital heart disease, intellectual disability, cataracts, deafness, microcephaly, and microphthalmia. Timing is crucial, because the extent and frequency of the complications are inversely related to the duration of the pregnancy at the time of maternal infection. When mothers are infected in the first trimester of pregnancy, 10 to 15 percent of the children are affected, but the incidence rises

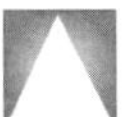

Table 27.3–2
Impairment in Disorders with Inborn Errors of Metabolism

Disorder	Hereditary Transmission	Enzyme Defect	Prenatal Diagnosis	Intellectual Disability	Clinical Signs
I. Lipid Metabolism					
Niemann–Pick disease					
Group A, infantile		Unknown			Hepatomegaly
Group B, adult	AR	Sphingomyelinase	+	±	Hepatosplenomegaly
Groups C and D, intermediate		Unknown	–	+	Pulmonary infiltration
Infantile Gaucher's disease	AR	β-Glucosidase	+	±	Hepatosplenomegaly, pseudobulbar palsy
Tay–Sachs disease	AR	Hexosaminidase A	+	+	Macular changes, seizures, spasticity
Generalized gangliosidosis	AR	β-Galactosidase	+	+	Hepatosplenomegaly, bone changes
Krabbe's disease	AR	Galactocerebroside β-Galactosidase	+	+	Stiffness, seizures
Metachromatic leukodystrophy	AR	Cerebroside sulfatase	+	+	Stiffness, developmental failure
Wolman's disease	AR	Acid lipase	+	–	Hepatosplenomegaly, adrenal calcification, vomiting, diarrhea
Farber's lipogranulomatosis	AR	Acid ceramidase	+	+	Hoarseness, arthropathy, subcutaneous nodules
Fabry's disease	XR	β-Galactosidase	+	–	Angiokeratomas, renal failure
II. Mucopolysaccharide Metabolism					
Hurler's syndrome MPS I	AR	Iduronidase	+	+	?
Hurler's disease II	XR	Iduronate sulfatase	+	+	?
Sanfilippo's syndrome III	AR	Various sulfatases (types A–D)	+	+	Varying degrees of bone changes, hepatosplenomegaly, joint restriction, etc.
Morquio's disease IV	AR	*N*-Acetylgalactosamine-6-sulfate sulfatase	+	–	?
Maroteaux–Lamy syndrome VI	AR	Arylsulfatase B	+	±	?
III. Oligosaccharide and Glycoprotein Metabolism					
I-cell disease	AR	Glycoprotein *N*-acetyl-glucosaminyl-phospho transferase	+	+	Hepatomegaly, bone changes, swollen gingivae
Mannosidosis	AR	Mannosidase	+	+	Hepatomegaly, bone changes, facial coarsening
Fucosidosis	AR	Fucosidase	+	+	Same as above
IV. Amino Acid Metabolism					
Phenylketonuria	AR	Phenylalanine hydroxylase	–	+	Eczema, blonde hair, musty odor
Hemocystinuria	AR	Cystathionine β-synthetase	+	+	Ectopia lentis, Marfan-like phenotype, cardiovascular anomalies
Tyrosinosis	AR	Tyrosine amine transaminase	–	+	Hyperkeratotic skin lesions, conjunctivitis
Maple syrup urine disease	AR	Branched-chain ketoacid decarboxylase	+	+	Recurrent ketoacidosis
Methylmalonic acidemia	AR	Methylmalonyl-CoA mutase	+	+	Recurrent ketoacidosis, hepatomegaly, growth retardation
Propionic acidemia	AR	Propionyl-CoA carboxylase	+	+	Same as above
Nonketotic hyperglycinemia	AR	Glycine cleavage enzyme	+	+	Seizures
Urea cycle disorders	Mostly AR	Urea cycle enzymes	+	+	Recurrent acute encephalopathy, vomiting
Hartnup disease	AR	Renal transport disorder	–	–	None consistent
V. Others					
Galactosemia	AR	Galactose-1-phosphate uridyltransferase	+	+	Hepatomegaly, cataracts, ovarian failure
Wilson's hepatolenticular degeneration	AR	Unknown factor in copper metabolism	–	±	Liver disease, Kayser–Fleischer ring, neurological problems
Menkes' kinky-hair disease	XR	Same as above	+	–	Abnormal hair, cerebral degeneration
Lesch–Nyhan syndrome	XR	Hypoxanthine guanine phosphoribosyltransferase	+	+	Behavioral abnormalities

AR, autosomal recessive transmission; XR, X-linked recessive transmission.
Adapted from Leroy JC. Hereditary, development, and behavior. In: Levine MD, Carey WB, Crocker AC, eds. *Developmental-Behavioral Pediatrics*. Philadelphia, PA: WB Saunders; 1983:315.

to almost 50 percent when the infection occurs in the first month of pregnancy. The situation is often complicated by subclinical forms of maternal infection that go undetected. Maternal rubella can be prevented by immunization.

CYTOMEGALIC INCLUSION DISEASE. In many cases, cytomegalic inclusion disease remains dormant in the mother. Some children are stillborn, and others have jaundice, microcephaly, hepatosplenomegaly, and radiographic findings of intracerebral calcification. Children with intellectual disability from the disease frequently have cerebral calcification, microcephaly, or hydrocephalus. The diagnosis is confirmed by positive findings of the virus in throat and urine cultures and the recovery of inclusion-bearing cells in the urine.

SYPHILIS. Syphilis in pregnant women was once the main cause of various neuropathological changes in their offspring, including intellectual disability. Today, the incidence of syphilitic complications of pregnancy fluctuates with the incidence of syphilis in the general population. Some recent alarming statistics from several major cities in the United States indicate that there is still no room for complacency.

TOXOPLASMOSIS. Toxoplasmosis can be transmitted by the mother to the fetus. It causes mild or severe intellectual disability and, in severe cases, hydrocephalus, seizures, microcephaly, and chorioretinitis.

HERPES SIMPLEX. The herpes simplex virus can be transmitted transplacentally, although the most common mode of infection is during birth. Microcephaly, intellectual disability, intracranial calcification, and ocular abnormalities may result.

HUMAN IMMUNODEFICIENCY VIRUS. Cognitive impairments are well known to be associated with transmission of HIV from mothers to their babies. HIV may have both direct and indirect influences on the developing brain. A subset of infants born infected with HIV may develop progressive encephalopathy, intellectual disabilities, and seizures within the first year of life. Fortunately, over the last two decades, there has been a dramatic decrease in perinatal HIV transmission due to a combination of antiviral agents provided to mothers during pregnancy and delivery, obstetric interventions that reduce risk, and administration of zidovudine (ZDV) as a prophylaxis for 6 weeks to newborns exposed to HIV. In the United States, the highest rate of reported pediatric AIDS occurred in 1992, with 1,700 cases reported compared to less than 50 cases reported annually now. In the United States, fewer than 300 cases of HIV transmission from mother to child were reported in 2005. However, vertical transmission of HIV from mother to child around the world, especially in Africa, is considerable. Most babies born to HIV-infected mothers in the United States are not infected with the virus.

FETAL ALCOHOL SYNDROME. Fetal alcohol syndrome (FAS) results from prenatal alcohol exposure and can lead to a wide range of problems in the newborn. According to the Centers for Disease Control and Prevention, FAS in the United States occurs at a rate ranging from 0.2 to 1.5 per 1,000 live births. FAS is one of the leading preventable causes of intellectual disability and physical disabilities. The typical phenotypic picture of a child with FAS includes facial dysmorphism comprising hypertelorism, microcephaly, short palpebral fissures, inner epicanthal folds, and a short, turned-up nose. Often, the affected children have learning disorders and ADHD, and in some cases intellectual disability. Cardiac defects are also frequent. The entire syndrome occurs in up to 15 percent of babies born to women who regularly ingest large amounts of alcohol. Babies born to women who consume alcohol regularly during pregnancy have a high incidence of ADHD, learning disorders, and intellectual disability without the facial dysmorphism.

PRENATAL DRUG EXPOSURE. Prenatal exposure to opioids, such as heroin, often results in infants who are small for their gestational age, with a head circumference below the tenth percentile and withdrawal symptoms that appear within the first 2 days of life. The withdrawal symptoms of infants include irritability, hypertonia, tremor, vomiting, a high-pitched cry, and an abnormal sleep pattern. Seizures are unusual, but the withdrawal syndrome can be life-threatening to infants if it is untreated. Diazepam (Valium), phenobarbital (Luminal), chlorpromazine (Thorazine), and paregoric have been used to treat neonatal opioid withdrawal. The long-term sequelae of prenatal opioid exposure are not fully known; the children's developmental milestones and intellectual functions may be within the normal range, but they have an increased risk for impulsivity and behavioral problems. Infants prenatally exposed to cocaine are at high risk for low birth weight and premature delivery. In the early neonatal period, they may have transient neurological and behavioral abnormalities, including abnormal results on EEG studies, tachycardia, poor feeding patterns, irritability, and excessive drowsiness. Rather than a withdrawal reaction, the physiological and behavioral abnormalities are a response to the cocaine, which may be excreted for up to a week postnatally.

COMPLICATIONS OF PREGNANCY. Toxemia of pregnancy and uncontrolled maternal diabetes present hazards to the fetus and can potentially result in intellectual disability. Maternal malnutrition during pregnancy often results in prematurity and other obstetrical complications. Vaginal hemorrhage, placenta previa, premature separation of the placenta, and prolapse of the cord can damage the fetal brain by causing anoxia. The use of lithium during pregnancy was recently implicated in some congenital malformations, especially of the cardiovascular system (e.g., Ebstein's anomaly).

Perinatal Period. Some evidence indicates that premature infants and infants with low birth weight are at high risk for neurological and subtle intellectual impairments that may not be apparent until their school years. Infants who sustain intracranial hemorrhages or show evidence of cerebral ischemia are especially vulnerable to cognitive abnormalities. The degree of neurodevelopmental impairment generally correlates with the severity of the intracranial hemorrhage. Recent studies have documented that, among children with very low birth weight (less than 1,000 g), 20 percent had significant disabilities, including cerebral palsy, intellectual disability, autism, and low intelligence with severe learning problems. Very premature children and those who had intrauterine growth retardation were found to be at high risk for developing both social problems and academic difficulties. Socioeconomic deprivation can also affect the adaptive function of these vulnerable infants. Early intervention may improve their cognitive, language, and perceptual abilities.

Acquired Childhood Disorders

Infection. The most serious infections affecting cerebral integrity are encephalitis and meningitis. Measles encephalitis has been virtually eliminated by the universal use of measles vaccine, and the incidence of other bacterial infections of the CNS has been markedly reduced with antibacterial agents. Most episodes of encephalitis are caused by viruses. Sometimes a clinician must retrospectively consider a probable encephalitic component in a previous obscure illness with high fever. Meningitis that was diagnosed late, even when followed by antibiotic treatment, can seriously affect a child's cognitive development. Thrombotic and purulent intracranial phenomena secondary to septicemia are rarely seen today except in small infants.

Head Trauma. The best-known causes of head injury in children that produces developmental handicaps, including seizures, are motor vehicle accidents, but more head injuries are caused by household accidents, such as falls from tables, open windows, and on stairways. Child maltreatment is not infrequently implicated in head traumas or intracranial trauma such as bleeding due to "shaken baby" syndrome.

Asphyxia. Brain damage due to asphyxia associated with near drowning is not an uncommon cause of intellectual disability.

Long-Term Exposures. Long-term exposure to lead is a well-established cause of compromised intelligence and learning skills. Intracranial tumors of various types and origins, surgery, and chemotherapy can also adversely affect brain function.

Environmental and Sociocultural Factors

Mild intellectual disability has been associated with significant deprivation of nutrition and nurturance. Children who have endured these conditions are at risk for a host of psychiatric disorders including mood disorders, post-traumatic stress disorder, and attentional and anxiety disorders. Prenatal environment compromised by poor medical care and poor maternal nutrition may be contributing factors in the development of mild intellectual disability. Teenage pregnancies are at risk for mild intellectual disability in the baby due to the increased risk of obstetrical complications, prematurity, and low birth weight. Poor postnatal medical care, malnutrition, exposure to toxic substances such as lead, and potential physical trauma are additional risk factors for mild intellectual disabilities. Child neglect and inadequate caretaking may deprive an infant of both physical and emotional nurturances, leading to failure to thrive syndromes.

DIAGNOSIS

The diagnosis of intellectual disability can be made after the history is obtained, using information from a standardized intellectual assessment, and a standardized measure of adaptive function indicating that a child is significantly below the expected level in both areas. The severity of the intellectual disability will be determined on the basis of the level of adaptive function. A history and psychiatric interview are useful in obtaining a longitudinal picture of the child's development and functioning. Examination of physical signs, neurological abnormalities, and in some cases, laboratory tests can be used to ascertain the cause and prognosis.

History

The clinician taking the history, which may elucidate pathways to intellectual disability, should pay particular attention to the mother's pregnancy, labor, and delivery; the presence of a family history of intellectual disability; consanguinity of the parents; and known familial hereditary disorders.

Psychiatric Interview

A psychiatric interview of a child or adolescent with intellectual disability requires a high level of sensitivity in order to elicit information at the appropriate intellectual level while remaining respectful of the patient's age and emotional development. The patient's verbal abilities, including receptive and expressive language, can be initially screened by observing the communication between the caretakers and patient. If the patient communicates largely through gestures or sign language, the parents may serve as interpreters. Patients with milder forms of intellectual disability are often well aware of their differences from others and their failures, and may be anxious and ashamed during the interview. Approaching patients with a clear, supportive, concrete explanation of the diagnostic process, particularly patients with sufficiently receptive language ability, may allay anxiety and fears. Providing support and praise in language appropriate to the patient's age and understanding is beneficial. Subtle direction, structure, and reinforcement may be necessary to keep patients focused on the task or topic.

In general, the psychiatric examination of an intellectually disabled child or adolescent should reveal how the patient has coped with stages of development. Frustration tolerance, impulse control, and over-aggressive motor and sexual behavior are important areas of attention in the interview. It is equally important to elicit the patient's self-image, areas of self-confidence, and an assessment of tenacity, persistence, curiosity, and willingness to explore the environment.

Structured Instruments, Rating Scales, and Psychological Assessment

In children and adolescents who have acquired language, one of several standardized instruments that include numerous domains of cognitive function are used. For children aged 6 to 16 years, the Wechsler Intelligence Test for Children is typically administered, and for children aged 3 to 6 years, the Wechsler Preschool and Primary Scale of Intelligence-Revised is commonly used. The Stanford–Binet Intelligence Scale, Fourth Edition, has the advantage that it can be administered to children even younger, starting at age 2 years. The Kaufman Assessment Battery for Children can be used in children aged 2½ to 12½ years, whereas the Kaufman Adolescent and Adult Intelligence Test is applicable to a wide range of ages, from 11 to 85 years. All of the above standardized instruments evaluate cognitive abilities across multiple domains including verbal, performance, memory, and problem solving. Standardized instruments measuring adaptive function (functions of "everyday" life) are based on the construct that adaptive skills increase with age, and that adaptation may vary across different settings such as school, peer relationships, and family life. The Vineland Adaptive Behavior Scales can be used in infants through youth 18 years of age and includes four basic domains including *Communication* (Receptive, Expressive, and Written); *Daily Living Skills* (Personal, Domestic, and Community); *Socialization* (Interpersonal Relations, Play and Leisure, and Coping Skills); *Motor Skills* (Fine and Gross).

Several behavioral rating scales have been developed for the population with intellectual disability. General behavioral ratings scales include the Aberrant Behavior Checklist (ABC) and the Developmental Behavior Checklist (DBC). The Behavior Problem Inventory (BPI) is a good screening instrument for self-injurious, aggressive, and stereotyped behaviors. The Psychopathology Inventory for Mentally Retarded Adults (PIMRA) is utilized to identify the presence of comorbid psychiatric symptoms and disorders.

Examining clinicians can use several screening instruments for developmental and intellectual delay or disability in infants and toddlers. However, controversy over the predictive value of infant psychological tests is heated. Some report the correlation of abnormalities during infancy with later abnormal functioning as very low, and others report it to be very high. The correlation rises in direct proportion to the age of the child at the time of the developmental examination. Some exercises such as copying geometric figures, the *Goodenough Draw-a-Person Test,* the *Kohs Block Test,* and geometric puzzles all may be used as quick screening tests of visual–motor coordination. The *Gesell* and *Bayley scales* and the *Cattell Infant Intelligence Scale* are most commonly used with infants.

The *Peabody Vocabulary Test* is the most widely used vocabulary test solely based on pictures. Other tests often found useful in detecting intellectual disability are the *Bender Gestalt Test* and the *Benton Visual Retention Test.* The psychological evaluation should assess perceptual, motor, linguistic, and cognitive abilities.

Physical Examination

Various parts of the body may demonstrate identifying characteristics of specific perinatal and prenatal events or conditions associated with intellectual disabilities. For example, the configuration and the size of the head may offer clues to a variety of conditions, such as microcephaly, hydrocephalus, or Down syndrome. A patient's facial characteristics, for example, hypertelorism, a flat nasal bridge, prominent eyebrows, epicanthal folds may provide clues to a recognizable syndrome such as FAS. Additional facial characteristics including corneal opacities, retinal changes, low-set and small or misshapen ears, a protruding tongue, and disturbance in dentition may be stigmata of a variety of known syndromes. Facial expression, color and texture of the skin and hair, a high-arched palate, the size of the thyroid gland, and the proportions of a child's trunk and extremities may offer clues for particular syndromes. The circumference of the head should be measured as part of the clinical investigation. Dermatoglyphics may offer another diagnostic tool, because uncommon ridge patterns and flexion creases on the hand are often found in persons who are intellectually disabled. Abnormal dermatoglyphics occur in chromosomal disorders and in persons who were prenatally infected with rubella. Table 27.3–3 lists syndromes with intellectual disability and their behavioral phenotypes.

Neurological Examination

Sensory impairments occur frequently among persons with intellectual disabilities. For example, hearing impairment occurs in 10 percent of persons with intellectual disability, a rate that is four times that of the general population. Visual disturbances can range from blindness to disturbances of spatial concepts, design recognition, and concepts of body image. Seizure disorders occur in about 10 percent of intellectually disabled populations and in one-third of those with severe intellectual disability. Neurological abnormalities increase in incidence and severity in direct proportion to the degree of intellectual disability. Disturbances in motor areas are manifested in abnormalities of muscle tone (spasticity or hypotonia), reflexes (hyperreflexia), and involuntary movements (choreoathetosis). Less disability may also be associated with clumsiness and poor coordination.

CLINICAL FEATURES

Mild intellectual disability may not be recognized or diagnosed in a child until school challenges the child's social and communication skills. Cognitive deficits include poor ability to abstract and egocentric thinking, both of which become more easily evident as a child reaches middle childhood. Children with milder intellectual disabilities may function academically at the high elementary level and may acquire vocational skills sufficient to support themselves in some cases; however, social assimilation may be problematic. Communication deficits, poor self-esteem, and dependence may further contribute to a relative lack of social spontaneity.

Moderate levels of intellectual disability are significantly more likely to be observed at a younger age, since communication skills develop more slowly and social isolation may ensue in the elementary school years. Academic achievement is usually limited to the middle-elementary level. Children with moderate intellectual deficits benefit from individual attention focused on the development of self-help skills. However, these children are aware of their deficits and often feel alienated from their peers and frustrated by their limitations. They continue to require a relatively high level of supervision but can become competent at occupational tasks in supportive settings.

Severe intellectual disability is typically obvious in the preschool years; affected children have minimal speech and impaired motor development. Some language development may occur in the school-age years. By adolescence, if language has not improved significantly, poor, nonverbal forms of communication may have evolved. Behavioral approaches are useful means to promote some self-care, although those with severe intellectual disability generally need extensive supervision.

Children with profound intellectual disability require constant supervision and are severely limited in both communication and motor skills. By adulthood, some speech development may be present, and simple self-help skills may be acquired. Clinical features frequently observed in populations with intellectual disability either in isolation or as part of a mental disorder, include hyperactivity, low frustration tolerance, aggression,

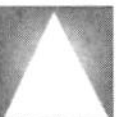

Table 27.3–3
Syndromes with Intellectual Disability and Behavioral Phenotypes

Disorder	Pathophysiology	Clinical Features and Behavioral Phenotype
Down syndrome	Trisomy 21, 95% nondisjunction, approx. 4% translocation; 1/1,000 live births: 1:2,500 in women less than 30 years old, 1:80 over 40 years old, 1:32 at 45 years old; possible overproduction of β-amyloid due to defect at 21q21.1	Hypotonia, upward-slanted palpebral fissures, midface depression, flat wide nasal bridge, simian crease, short stature, increased incidence of thyroid abnormalities and congenital heart disease Passive, affable, hyperactivity in childhood, stubborn; verbal > auditory processing, increased risk of depression, and dementia of the Alzheimer type in adulthood
Fragile X syndrome	Inactivation of *FMR-1* gene at X q27.3 due to CGG base repeats, methylation; recessive; 1:1,000 male births, 1:3,000 female; accounts for 10–12% of intellectual disability in males	Long face, large ears, midface hypoplasia, high arched palate, short stature, macroorchidism, mitral valve prolapse, joint laxity, strabismus Hyperactivity, inattention, anxiety, stereotypies, speech and language delays, IQ decline, gaze aversion, social avoidance, shyness, irritability, learning disorder in some females; mild intellectual disability in affected females, moderate to severe in males; verbal IQ > performance IQ
Prader–Willi syndrome	Deletion in 15q12 (15q11–15q13) of paternal origin; some cases of maternal uniparental disomy; dominant 1/10,000 live births; 90% sporadic; candidate gene: small nuclear ribonucleoprotein polypeptide (SNRPN)	Hypotonia, failure to thrive in infancy, obesity, small hands and feet microorchidism, cryptorchidism, short stature, almond-shaped eyes, fair hair and light skin, flat face, scoliosis, orthopedic problems, prominent forehead and bitemporal narrowing Compulsive behavior, hyperphagia, hoarding, impulsivity, borderline to moderate intellectual disability, emotional lability, tantrums, excess daytime sleepiness, skin picking, anxiety, aggression
Angelman syndrome	Deletion in 15q12 (15q11–15q13) of maternal origin; dominant; frequent deletion of γ-aminobutyric acid (GABA) B-3 receptor subunit, prevalence unknown but rare, estimated 1/20,000–1/30,000	Fair hair and blue eyes (66%); dysmorphic faces including wide smiling mouth, thin upper lip, and pointed chin; epilepsy (90%) with characteristic EEG; ataxia; small head circumference, 25% microcephalic Happy disposition, paroxysmal laughter, hand flapping, clapping; profound intellectual disability; sleep disturbance with nighttime waking; possible increased incidence of autistic features; anecdotal love of water and music
Cornelia de Lange syndrome	Lack of pregnancy associated plasma protein A (PAPPA) linked to chromosome 9q33; similar phenotype associated with trisomy 5p, ring chromosome 3; rare (1/40,000–1/100,000 live births); possible association with 3q26.3	Continuous eyebrows, thin downturning upper lip, microcephaly, short stature, small hands and feet, small upturned nose, anteverted nostrils, malformed upper limbs, failure to thrive Self-injury, limited speech in severe cases, language delays, avoidance of being held, stereotypic movements, twirling, severe to profound intellectual disability
Williams' syndrome	1/20,000 births; hemizygous deletion that includes elastin locus chromosome 7q11–23; autosomal dominant	Short stature, unusual facial features including broad forehead, depressed nasal bridge, stellate pattern of the iris, widely spaced teeth, and full lips; elfinlike facies; renal and cardiovascular abnormalities; thyroid abnormalities; hypercalcemia Anxiety, hyperactivity, fears, outgoing, sociable, verbal skills > visual spatial skills
Cri-du-chat syndrome	Partial deletion 5p; 1/50,000; region may be 5p15.2	Round face with hypertelorism, epicanthal folds, slanting palpebral fissures, broad flat nose, low-set ears, micrognathia; prenatal growth retardation; respiratory and ear infections; congenital heart disease; gastrointestinal abnormalities Severe intellectual disability, infantile catlike cry, hyperactivity, stereotypies, self-injury
Smith–Magenis syndrome	Incidence unknown, estimated 1/25,000 live births; complete or partial deletion of 17p11.2	Broad face; flat midface; short, broad hands; small toes; hoarse, deep voice Severe intellectual disability; hyperactivity; severe self-injury including hand biting, head banging, and pulling out finger- and toenails; stereotyped self-hugging; attention seeking; aggression; sleep disturbance (decreased REM)
Rubinstein–Taybi syndrome	1/250,000, approx. male = female; sporadic; likely autosomal dominant; documented microdeletions in some cases at 16p13.3	Short stature and microcephaly, broad thumb and big toes, prominent nose, broad nasal bridge, hypertelorism, ptosis, frequent fractures, feeding difficulties in infancy, congenital heart disease, EEG abnormalities, seizures Poor concentration, distractible, expressive language difficulties, performance IQ > verbal IQ; anecdotally happy, loving, sociable, responsive to music, self-stimulating behavior; older patients have mood lability and temper tantrums
Tuberous sclerosis complex 1 and 2	Benign tumors (hamartomas) and malformations (hamartias) of central nervous system (CNS), skin, kidney, heart; dominant; 1/10,000 births; 50% TSC 1, 9q34; 50% TSC 2, 16p13	Epilepsy, autism, hyperactivity, impulsivity, aggression; spectrum of intellectual disability from none (30%) to profound; self-injurious behaviors, sleep disturbances

(*continued*)

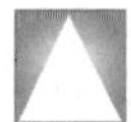

Table 27.3–3
Syndromes with Intellectual Disability and Behavioral Phenotypes (Continued)

Disorder	Pathophysiology	Clinical Features and Behavioral Phenotype
Neurofibromatosis type 1 (NF1)	1/2,500–1/4,000; male = female; autosomal dominant; 50% new mutations; more than 90% paternal NF1 allele mutated; *NFI* gene 17q11.2; gene product is neurofibromin thought to be tumor suppressor gene	Variable manifestations; café au lait spots, cutaneous neurofibromas, Lisch nodules; short stature and macrocephaly in 30–45 Half with speech and language difficulties; 10% with moderate to profound intellectual disability; verbal IQ > performance IQ; distractible, impulsive, hyperactive, anxious; possibly associated with increased incidence of mood and anxiety disorders
Lesch–Nyhan syndrome	Defect in hypoxanthine guanine phosphoribosyl-transferase with accumulation of uric acid; Xq26–27; recessive; rare (1/10,000–1/38,000)	Ataxia, chorea, kidney failure, gout Often severe self-biting behavior; aggression; anxiety; mild to moderate intellectual disability
Galactosemia	Defect in galactose-1-phosphate uridyltransferase or galactokinase or empiramase; autosomal recessive; 1/62,000 births in the U.S.	Vomiting in early infancy, jaundice, hepatosplenomegaly; later cataracts, weight loss, food refusal, increased intracranial pressure and increased risk for sepsis, ovarian failure, failure to thrive, renal tubular damage Possible intellectual disability even with treatment, visuospatial deficits, language disorders, reports of increased behavioral problems, anxiety, social withdrawal, and shyness
Phenylketonuria	Defect in phenylalanine hydroxylase (PAH) or cofactor (biopterin) with accumulation of phenylalanine; approximately 1/11,500 births; varies with geographical location; gene for PAH, 12q22–24.1; autosomal recessive	Symptoms absent neonatally, later development of seizures (25% generalized), fair skin, blue eyes, blond hair, rash Untreated: mild to profound intellectual disability, language delay, destructiveness, self-injury, hyperactivity
Hurler's syndrome	1/100,000; deficiency in α-L- iduronidase activity; autosomal recessive	Early onset; short stature, hepatosplenomegaly; hirsutism, corneal clouding, death before age 10 years, dwarfism, coarse facial features, recurrent respiratory infections Moderate-to-severe intellectual disability, anxious, fearful, rarely aggressive
Hunter's syndrome	1/100,000, X-linked recessive; iduronate sulfatase deficiency; X q28	Normal infancy; symptom onset at age 2–4 years; typical coarse faces with flat nasal bridge, flaring nostrils; hearing loss, ataxia, hernia common; enlarged liver and spleen, joint stiffness, recurrent infections, growth retardation, cardiovascular abnormality Hyperactivity, intellectual disability by 2 years; speech delay; loss of speech at 8–10 years; restless, aggressive, inattentive, sleep abnormalities; apathetic, sedentary with disease progression
Fetal alcohol syndrome	Maternal alcohol consumption (trimester III>II>I); 1/3,000 live births in Western countries; 1/300 with fetal alcohol effects	Microcephaly, short stature, midface hypoplasia, short palpebral fissure, thin upper lip, retrognathia in infancy, micrognathia in adolescence, hypoplastic long or smooth philtrum Mild to moderate intellectual disability, irritability, inattention, memory impairment

Table by BH King, M.D., RM Hodapp, Ph.D., and EM Dykens, Ph.D.

affective instability, repetitive and stereotypic motor behaviors, and self-injurious behaviors. Self-injurious behaviors occur more frequently and with greater intensity in more severe intellectual disability.

Dylan was a full-term infant, the second child born to his 42-year-old mother, a medical technician, and 48-year-old father, a high school basketball coach. The pregnancy was unremarkable, and Dylan's sister, who was 2 years older, was healthy and developing normally. The family lived in a rural town in the Midwest.

Dylan was an extremely fussy, active newborn with extended periods of crying that the pediatrician labeled classic colic. As a newborn, it was noticed that Dylan seemed to have large ears and strabismus, which the pediatrician said would probably resolve spontaneously. At 2 months of age, at a regular pediatric visit, a systolic heart murmur was heard and electrocardiography (ECG) revealed a mitral valve prolapse. Because Dylan was not cyanotic and had no other cardiac symptoms, no treatment was recommended except monitoring. Although Dylan became less fussy over time, he remained very active, did not sleep through the night, and was a picky eater, refusing solid foods.

Milestones were slightly delayed, with Dylan sitting unassisted at 10 months and walking at 18 months. Language was also delayed, and, although his first words appeared at 20 months, Dylan had always made his wants and needs known. Dylan's parents were concerned about his activity level and his developmental delays compared with his sister; however, they were reassured by the pediatrician's sense that boys often develop more slowly than girls in the first 2 years.

When Dylan was 3 years of age, his preschool teacher noted that he was unable to pay attention and he was hyperactive compared to his classmates, prompting his parents to obtain a developmental evaluation. Results showed modest delays in cognitive, linguistic, and motor functioning, with a developmental quotient (DQ) of 74. Dylan was described as inattentive, shy, and anxious, and he had poor eye contact. Enrolled in a special kindergarten, Dylan remained in a combination of special education and mainstreamed classes throughout his academic life.

At 7 years of age, the school psychologist evaluated Dylan and results indicated that he met criteria for a "learning disability" profile. Dylan had an overall IQ of 66, with close to average functioning in short-term memory and pronounced deficits in long-term memory, expressive language, and visual-spatial functioning. Dylan struggled with writing tasks and arithmetic, but loved science. Due to his significant problems with inattention and hyperactivity, Dylan was placed on Concerta, which was beneficial, and titrated up to 54 mg per day. He displayed transient, intense interests in unusual items, such as vacuum cleaners. When Dylan reached the older elementary grades, he began to have more difficulty socially, and he was bullied about being in special education, and teased for his long head and big ears.

As he entered adolescence, Dylan became increasingly anxious, so much so that he occasionally rubbed his hands or rocked, and he "fretted" about day-to-day issues and what would happen next. His long-term sensitivities to loud sounds seemed to wane slightly, but he developed fears of storm clouds and dogs and refused to ride on elevators. He became tearful and upset after his older sister left for a party, and worried that she might have a car accident. Dylan was very shy and would occasionally pace with worry and complain of stomachaches, but he attended school and had a small group of acquaintances in the Special Olympics bowling league. He enjoyed activities that did not involve much talking or sustained attention.

When Dylan was 17 years of age, his parents happened to watch a television documentary on genetic causes of intellectual disability. They were overwhelmed by the similarities between Dylan and some of the people described in the program. They later described the experience as a "jolt." They had always accepted Dylan, quirks and all, and had stopped pushing their doctors for reasons "why" when Dylan was a preschooler. Nevertheless, they immediately called the informational number offered in the show, and within 2 months, they had the genetic tests done that confirmed a diagnosis of fragile X syndrome.

Although Dylan's day-to-day life did not change dramatically after the diagnosis, his parents reported a big difference in their approach to his shyness, restricted interests, and inattention. Dylan was later treated for anxiety with a selective serotonin reuptake inhibitor (SSRI) antidepressant, which decreased his social anxiety and facilitated activities with a few peers. Dylan's parents reported a mixture of feelings at having such a late diagnosis—disappointment in their doctors, relief in finally knowing, and twinges of guilt. They were energized by Dylan's positive responses to treatments for his attentional and anxiety symptoms and were pleased with Dylan's recent increased interest in sharing activities with classmates and peers.

LABORATORY EXAMINATION

Laboratory tests that may elucidate the causes of intellectual disability include chromosomal analysis, urine and blood testing for metabolic disorders, and neuroimaging. Chromosomal abnormalities are the single most known common cause of intellectual disability.

Chromosome Studies

Chromosome analysis is commonly obtained when multiple physical anomalies, developmental delays, and intellectual disability present together. Current techniques are able to mark chromosomal regions with specific fluorescent in situ hybridization (FISH) markers, leading to microscopic deletions being identified in up to 7 percent of persons with moderate to severe intellectual disability. A history of growth retardation, the presence of microcephaly, a family history of intellectual disability, short stature, hypertelorism, and other facial abnormalities increase the risk for finding subtelomeric defects.

Amniocentesis, in which a small amount of amniotic fluid is removed from the amniotic cavity transabdominally at about the 15 weeks of gestation, has been useful in diagnosing prenatal chromosomal abnormalities. Its use is considered when an increased fetal risk exists, such as with increased maternal age. Amniotic fluid cells, mostly fetal in origin, are cultured for cytogenetic and biochemical studies.

Chronic villi sampling (CVS) is a screening technique to determine fetal chromosomal abnormalities. It is done at 8 to 10 weeks of gestation, 6 weeks earlier than amniocentesis is done. The results are available in a short time (hours or days) and, if the result is abnormal, the decision to terminate the pregnancy can be made within the first trimester. The procedure has a miscarriage risk between 2 and 5 percent; the risk in amniocentesis is lower (1 in 200). A noninvasive blood test called materniT21 is a proprietary prenatal test that detects abnormalities of chromosomes 21, 18, 13, X, and Y. It is highly specific for Down syndrome. There is no risk of miscarriage.

Urine and Blood Analysis

Lesch–Nyhan syndrome, galactosemia, PKU, Hurler's syndrome, and Hunter's syndrome are examples of disorders characterized by intellectual disability that can be identified through assays of the appropriate enzyme or organic or amino acids. Enzymatic abnormalities in chromosomal disorders, particularly Down syndrome, promise to become useful diagnostic tools.

Electroencephalography

Electroencephalography is indicated whenever a seizure disorder is considered. "Nonspecific" EEG changes, characterized by slow frequencies with bursts of spikes and sharp or blunt wave complexes, are found with greater frequency among populations with intellectual disability than in the general population; however, these findings do not elucidate specific diagnoses.

Neuroimaging

Neuroimaging studies with populations of intellectually disabled patients using either CT or MRI have found high rates of abnormalities in those patients with microcephaly, significant delay, cerebral palsy, and profound disability. Among patients with intellectual disability, neuroimaging is indicated, accompanying findings that suggest seizures, microcephaly or macrocephaly, loss of previously acquired skills, or neurologic signs such as dystonia, spasticity, or altered reflexes.

Although clinically not diagnostic, neuroimaging studies are currently also utilized to gather data that may eventually uncover biological mechanisms contributing to intellectual disability. Structural MRI, functional MRI (fMRI), and diffusion tensor imaging (DTI) are utilized in current research. For example, current data suggest that individuals with fragile X syndrome and concurrent attentional deficits are also more likely to show aberrant frontal-striatal pathways on MRI than those patients without attentional problems. MRI is also useful to elucidate myelination patterns. MRI studies can also provide a baseline for comparison of a later, potentially degenerative process in the brain.

Hearing and Speech Evaluations

Hearing and speech should be evaluated routinely. Speech development may be the most reliable criterion in investigating intellectual disability. Various hearing impairments often occur in persons who are intellectually disabled, but in some instances hearing impairments can simulate intellectual disability. The commonly used methods of hearing and speech evaluation, however, require the patient's cooperation and, thus, are often unreliable in severely disabled persons.

COURSE AND PROGNOSIS

Although the underlying intellectual impairment does not improve, in most cases of intellectual disability, level of adaptation increases with age and can be influenced positively by an enriched and supportive environment. In general, persons with mild and moderate mental intellectual disabilities have the most flexibility in adapting to various environmental conditions. Comorbid psychiatric disorders negatively impact overall prognosis. When psychiatric disorders are superimposed on intellectual disability, standard treatments for the comorbid mental disorders are often beneficial; however, less robust responses and increased vulnerability to side effects of psychopharmacologic agents are often the case.

DIFFERENTIAL DIAGNOSIS

By definition, intellectual disability must begin before the age of 18. In some cases, severe child maltreatment in the form of neglect or abuse may contribute to delays in development, which can appear to be intellectual disability. However these damages are partially reversible when a corrective, enriched, and stimulating environment is provided in early childhood. Sensory disabilities, especially deafness and blindness, can be mistaken for intellectual disability when a lack of awareness of the sensory deficit leads to inappropriate testing. Expressive and receptive speech disorders may give the impression of intellectual disability in a child of average intelligence, and cerebral palsy may be mistaken for intellectual disability. Chronic, debilitating medical diseases may depress and delay a child's functioning and achievement, despite normal intelligence. Seizure disorders, especially those that are poorly controlled, may contribute to persisting intellectual disability. Specific organic syndromes leading to isolated handicaps, such as failure to read (alexia), failure to write (agraphia), or failure to communicate (aphasia), may occur in a child of normal and even superior intelligence. Children with learning disorders (which can coexist with intellectual disability) experience a delay or failure of development in a specific area, such as reading or mathematics, but they develop normally in other areas. In contrast, children with intellectual disability show general delays in most areas of development.

Intellectual disability and autism spectrum disorder (ASD) often coexist; 70 to 75 percent of those with ASD have an IQ below 70. In addition, epidemiologic data indicate that ASD occurs in approximately 19.8 percent of persons with intellectual disability. Children with ASD have relatively more severe impairment in social relatedness and language than other children with the same level of intellectual disability.

A child younger than the age of 18 years with significant adaptive functional impairment, with an IQ less than 70, who also meets diagnostic criteria for dementia, will receive both a diagnosis of dementia and intellectual disability. However, a child whose IQ drops below 70 after the age of 18 years with newly acquired cognitive impairment will receive only the diagnosis of dementia.

TREATMENT

Interventions for children and adolescents with intellectual disability are based on an assessment of social, educational, psychiatric, and environmental needs. Intellectual disability is associated with a variety of comorbid psychiatric disorders that often require specific treatment, in addition to psychosocial support. Of course, when preventive measures are available, the optimal approach includes primary, secondary, and tertiary interventions.

Primary Prevention

Primary prevention comprises actions taken to eliminate or reduce the conditions that lead to development of intellectual disability, as well as associated disorders. For example, screening babies for PKU, and administrating a low-phenylalanine diet when PKU is present, significantly alters the emergence of intellectual disability in those affected children. Additional primary prevention steps include education of the general public about strategies to prevent intellectual disability, such as abstinence from alcohol during pregnancy; continuing efforts of health professionals to ensure and upgrade public health policies; and legislation to provide optimal maternal and child health care. Family and genetic counseling helps reduce the incidence of intellectual disability in a family with a history of a genetic disorder.

Secondary and Tertiary Prevention

Prompt attention to medical and psychiatric complications of intellectual disability can diminish their course (secondary prevention) and minimize the sequelae or consequent disabilities (tertiary prevention). Hereditary metabolic and endocrine disorders, such as PKU and hypothyroidism, can be treated effectively in an early stage by dietary control or hormone replacement therapy.

Educational Interventions. Educational settings for children with intellectual disability should include a comprehensive program that addresses academics and training in adaptive skills, social skills, and vocational skills. Particular attention should focus on communication and efforts to improve the quality of life.

Behavioral and Cognitive-Behavioral Interventions. The difficulties in adaptation among the intellectual disability populations are widespread and so varied that several interventions alone or in combination may be beneficial. Behavior therapy has been used for many years to shape and enhance social behaviors and to control and minimize aggressive and destructive behaviors. Positive reinforcement for desired behaviors and benign punishment (e.g., loss of privileges) for objectionable behaviors has been helpful. Cognitive therapy, such as dispelling false beliefs and relaxation exercises with self-instruction, has also been recommended for intellectually disabled persons who can follow the instructions. Psychodynamic therapy has been used with patients and their families to decrease conflicts about expectations that result in persistent anxiety, rage, and depression. Psychiatric treatment modalities require modifications that take into consideration the patient's level of intelligence.

Family Education. One of the most important areas that a clinician can address is educating the family of a child or adolescent with intellectual disability about ways to enhance competence and self-esteem while maintaining realistic expectations for the patient. The family often finds it difficult to balance the fostering of independence and the providing of a nurturing and supportive environment for an intellectually disabled child, who is likely to experience some rejection and failure outside the family context. The parents may benefit from continuous counseling or family therapy and should be allowed opportunities to express their feelings of guilt, despair, anguish, recurring denial, and anger about their child's disorder and future. The psychiatrist should be prepared to give the parents all the basic and current medical information regarding causes, treatment, and other pertinent areas (e.g., special training and the correction of sensory defects).

Social Intervention. One of the most prevalent problems among persons with intellectual disability is a sense of social isolation and social skills deficits. Thus, improving the quantity and quality of social competence is a critical part of their care. Special Olympics International is the largest recreational sports program geared for this population. In addition to providing a forum to develop physical fitness, Special Olympics also enhances social interactions, friendships, and (it is hoped) general self-esteem. A recent study confirmed positive effects of the Special Olympics on the social competence of the intellectually disabled adults who participated.

Psychopharmacologic Interventions. Pharmacological approaches to the treatment of behavioral and psychological symptoms in children with intellectual disability follow the paradigms of the evidence-based literature on treatment for all children with psychiatric disorders. However, given the paucity of randomized trials in the childhood intellectual disability population, an empirical approach must also be taken.

COMMON COMORBID PSYCHIATRIC SYMPTOMS AND DISORDERS

Aggression, Irritability, and Self-injurious Behavior. Risperidone has been well documented as an efficacious treatment for irritability (aggression, self-injury, and severe tantrums) in children with ASD by the Research Units on Pediatric Psychopharmacology (RUPP, Autism Network 2002). Risperidone is helpful in treating disruptive behaviors in children with below-average intelligence, and has a good overall safety and tolerability profile. Cognitive testing has demonstrated small but significant improvement in cognitive ability with risperidone use. Children and adolescents with intellectual disability appear to be at higher risk for the development of tardive dyskinesia after use of antipsychotic medications; however, the atypical antipsychotics, including risperidone and clozapine (Clozaril), may provide some relief with a decreased risk of tardive dyskinesia.

There is evidence to support the use of antipsychotic agents in the management of self-injurious behavior (SIB). Although data exist on the efficacy of thioridazine in improving SIB, a "black box" warning regarding QT prolongation with thioridazine has drastically diminished use of this drug, and atypical antipsychotic agents are currently preferred.

Attention-Deficit/Hyperactivity Disorder. Estimates of ADHD and ADHD-like symptoms among children with subaverage intelligence, genetic disorders, and developmental delay are estimated to be significantly higher than rates in the community. Randomized clinical trials of several psychopharmacologic agents have been done in children with subaverage intelligence. These include trials with methylphenidate, clonidine, and risperidone. The existing data for the treatment of ADHD and ADHD-like symptoms in youth with subaverage intelligence and developmental disorders suggest that agents, particularly stimulants used to treat ADHD in typically developing children, provide some degree of benefit to children with intellectual disability and ADHD. However, the occurrence of side effects within this population appears to be greater than in children with ADHD in the community. Thus, recommendations regarding treatment of ADHD in children and adolescents with comorbid ADHD include close monitoring for side effects. Studies of methylphenidate (Ritalin) treatment in those mildly intellectually disabled with ADHD have shown significant improvement in the ability to maintain attention and to stay focused on tasks. Methylphenidate treatment studies have not shown evidence of long-term improvement in social skills or learning. Risperidone also has been found to be beneficial in reducing symptoms of ADHD in this population; however, it may produce an increase in serum prolactin level. It is prudent to begin with a trial of a stimulant medication before the use of antipsychotic agents for the treatment of ADHD symptoms in intellectual disorder. A new extended release methylphenidate oral suspension (Quillivant XR, 2013) is currently available in 25 mg/5 mL preparation, and is taken once daily for the treatment of ADHD in children 6 to 12 years of age.

Amphetamine-based preparations have been shown to be efficacious in treating ADHD in typically developing children; however, it does not appear that these stimulant preparations have been specifically studied in children with intellectual disability. Clonidine has been used clinically in this population, especially to ameliorate hyperactivity and impulsivity. Although there are scant data, clinical ratings by parents and clinicians suggest its efficacy.

Atomoxetine has been shown to be efficacious in children diagnosed with ASD and prominent ADHD features, and it is used clinically in the intellectually disabled population.

Depressive Disorders. The identification of depressive disorders among individuals with intellectual disability requires careful evaluation, since it may be inadvertently overlooked when behavioral problems are prominent. There have been anecdotal reports of disinhibition in response to SSRIs (e.g., fluoxetine

[Prozac], paroxetine [Paxil], and sertraline [Zoloft]) in intellectually disabled individuals with ASD. Given the relative safety of SSRI antidepressants, a trial is indicated when a depressive disorder is diagnosed in a child or adolescent with intellectual disability.

Stereotypical Motor Movements. Antipsychotic medications—historically, haloperidol (Haldol) and chlorpromazine, and currently, the atypical antipsychotics—are used in the treatment of repetitive self-stimulatory behaviors in children with intellectual disability when these behaviors are either harmful to the child or disruptive. Anecdotal reports indicate that these agents may diminish self-stimulatory behaviors; however, there is no improvement seen in adaptive behavior. Obsessive-compulsive symptoms often overlap with the repetitive stereotypical behaviors seen in children and adolescents with intellectual disability, particularly in those with comorbid ASD. SSRIs such as fluoxetine, fluvoxamine (Luvox), paroxetine, and sertraline have been shown to have efficacy in treating obsessive-compulsive symptoms in children and adolescents and may have some efficacy for stereotyped motor movements.

Explosive Rage Behavior. Antipsychotic medications, particularly risperidone, have been shown to be efficacious for the treatment of explosive rage. Systematic controlled studies are indicated to confirm the efficacy of these drugs in the treatment of rage outbursts. β-Adrenergic receptor antagonists (beta-blockers), such as propranolol (Inderal), have been reportedly anecdotally to result in fewer explosive rages in some children with intellectual disability and ASD.

SERVICES AND SUPPORT FOR CHILDREN WITH INTELLECTUAL DISABILITY

Early Intervention

Early intervention programs serve individuals for the first 3 years of life. Such services are generally provided by the state and begin with a specialist visiting the home for several hours per week. Since the passage of Public Law 99–447, the Education of the Handicapped Amendments of 1986, early intervention services for the entire family are emphasized. Agencies are required to develop an Individualized Family Service Plan (IFSP) for each family, which identifies specific interventions to best help the family and child.

School

From ages 3 to 21 years, school is responsible by law to provide appropriate educational services to children and adolescents with intellectual disability in the United States. These mandates were created by the passage of Public Law 94–142, the Education for all Handicapped Children Act of 1975, and expanded with the addition of the Individuals with Disabilities Act (IDEA) of 1990. Through these laws, public schools must develop and provide an individualized educational program for each student with intellectual disability, determined at a meeting designated as the Individualized Education Plan (IEP) with school personnel and the family. The education must be provided for the child in the "least restrictive environment" that will allow the child to learn.

Supports

A wide variety of organized groups and services are available for children with intellectual disability and their families. These include short-term respite care, which allow families a break and is generally set up by state agencies. Other programs include the Special Olympics, which allows children with intellectual disability to participate in team sports and in sports competitions. Many organizations also exist for families who wish to connect with others who have children with intellectual disability.

▲ 27.4 Communication Disorders

Communication disorders range from mild delays in acquiring language to expressive or mixed receptive–expressive disorders, phonological disorders, and stuttering, which may remit spontaneously or persist into adolescence or even adulthood. Language delay is one of the most common very early childhood developmental delays, affecting up to approximately 7 percent of 5-year-olds. The rates of language disorders are understandably higher in preschoolers than in school-age children; rates were reported to be close to 20 percent of 4-year-olds in the Early Language in Victoria Study (ELVS). To communicate effectively, children must have a mastery of multiple aspects of language—that is, the ability to understand and express ideas—using words and speech, and express themselves in vernacular language. In the Fifth Edition of the American Psychiatric Association's *Diagnostic and Statistical Manual of Mental Disorders* (DSM-5), language disorder includes both expressive and mixed receptive–expressive problems. DSM-5 speech disorders include speech sound disorder (formerly known as phonological disorder) and childhood-onset fluency disorder (stuttering). Children with expressive language deficits have difficulties expressing their thoughts with words and sentences at a level of sophistication expected for their age and developmental level in other areas. These children may struggle with limited vocabularies, speak in sentences that are short or ungrammatical, and often present descriptions of situations that are disorganized, confusing, and infantile. They may be delayed in developing an understanding and a memory of words compared with others at their age. Children with language disorder are at higher risk for developing reading difficulties. Current expert consensus considers reading comprehension impairment a form of language impairment, distinct from other reading deficits such as dyslexia.

Language and speech are pragmatically intertwined, despite the distinct categories of language disorders and speech disorders in DSM-5. Language competence spans four domains: phonology, grammar, semantics, and pragmatics. *Phonology* refers to the ability to produce sounds that constitute words in a given language and the skills to discriminate the various phonemes (sounds that are made by a letter or group of letters in a language). To imitate words, a child must be able to produce the sounds of a word. *Grammar* designates the organization of words and the rules for placing words in an order that makes sense in that language. *Semantics* refers to the organization of concepts and the acquisition of words themselves. A child draws from a mental list of words to produce sentences. Children with language impairments exhibit a wide range of difficulties with semantics that include acquiring new words, storage and organization of known words, and word retrieval. Speech and language evaluations that are sufficiently broad to test all of the preceding skill levels will be more accurate in evaluating a child's remedial needs. *Pragmatics* has to do with skill in the actual use of language and the "rules" of conversation, such as pausing so that a listener can answer a question and knowing when to change the topic when a break occurs in a conversation. By age 2 years, toddlers without speech or language delay may know a few words or up to 200 words, and by age 3 years, most children understand the basic rules of language and can converse effectively.

Over the last decade there have been an increasing number of investigative studies of speech and language interventions with positive outcomes identified in numerous areas of language. These include improvements in expressive vocabulary, syntax usage, and overall phonologic development. Most interventions are targeted strategies for the child's particular deficit, and delivered by speech and language therapists.

LANGUAGE DISORDER

Language disorder consists of difficulties in the acquisition and use of language across many modalities, including spoken and written, due to deficits in comprehension or production based on both expressive and receptive skills. These deficits include reduced vocabulary, limited abilities in forming sentences using the rules of grammar, and impairments in conversing based on difficulties using vocabulary to connect sentences in descriptive ways.

Expressive Language Deficits

Expressive language deficits are present when a child demonstrates a selective deficit in expressive language development relative to receptive language skills and nonverbal intellectual function. Infants and young children with typically developing expressive language will laugh and coo by about 6 months of age, babble and verbalize syllables such as dadada or mamama by about 9 months, and by 1 year, babies imitate vocalizations and can often speak at least one word. Expressive speech and language generally continue to develop in a stepwise fashion so that at a year and a half, children typically can say a handful of words, and by 2 years, children generally are combining words into simple sentences. By the age of 2½ years, children can name an action in a picture, and are able to make themselves understood through their verbalizations about half of the time. By 3 years, most children can speak understandably, and are able to name a color and describe what they see with several adjectives. At 4 years, children typically can name at least 4 colors, and can converse understandably. In the early years, prior to entering preschool, the development of proficiency in vocabulary and language usage is highly variable, and influenced by the amount and quality of verbal interactions with family members, and after beginning school, a child's language skills are significantly influenced by the level of verbal engagement in school. A child with expressive language deficits may be identified using the *Wechsler Intelligence Scale for Children III* (WISC-III), in that verbal intellectual level may appear to be depressed compared with the child's overall IQ. A child with expressive language problems is likely to function below the expected levels of acquired vocabulary, correct tense usage, complex sentence constructions, and word recall. Children with expressive language deficits often present verbally as younger than their age. Language disability can be acquired during childhood (e.g., secondary to a trauma or a neurological disorder), although less frequently, or it can be developmental; it is usually congenital, without an obvious cause. Most childhood language disorders fall into the developmental category. In either case, deficits in receptive skills (language comprehension) or expressive skills (ability to use language) can occur. Expressive language disturbance often appears in the absence of comprehension difficulties, whereas receptive dysfunction generally diminishes proficiency in the expression of language. Children with expressive language disturbance alone have better prognoses, and less interference with learning, than children with mixed receptive–expressive language disturbances.

Although language use depends on both expressive and receptive skills, the degree of deficits in a given individual may be severe in one area, and hardly impaired at all in the other. Thus, language disorder can be diagnosed in children with expressive language disturbance in the absence of receptive language problems, or when both receptive and expressive language syndromes are present. In general, when receptive skills are sufficiently impaired to warrant a diagnosis, expressive skills are also impaired. In DSM-5 language disorder is not limited to developmental language disabilities; acquired forms of language disturbances are included. To meet the DSM-5 criteria for language disorder, patients must have scores on standardized measures of expressive or receptive language markedly below those of standardized nonverbal IQ subtests and standardized tests.

Epidemiology. The prevalence of expressive language disturbance decreases with a child's increasing age, and overall it is estimated to be as high as 6 percent in children between the ages of 5 and 11 years of age. Surveys have indicated rates of expressive language as high as 20 percent in children younger than 4 years of age. In school-age children over the age of 11 years, the estimates are lower, ranging from 3 percent to 5 percent. The disorder is two to three times more common in boys than in girls and is most prevalent among children whose relatives have a family history of phonologic disorder or other communication disorders.

Comorbidity. Children with language disorder have above-average rates of comorbid psychiatric disorders. In one large study of children with speech and language disorders, the most common comorbid disorders were ADHD (19 percent), anxiety disorders (10 percent), oppositional defiant disorder, and conduct disorder (7 percent combined). Children with expressive language disorder are also at higher risk for a speech disorder, receptive difficulties, and other learning disorders. Many disorders—such as reading disorder, developmental coordination disorder, and other communication disorders—are associated with expressive language disturbance. Children with expressive language disturbance often have some receptive impairment, although not always sufficiently significant for the diagnosis of language disorder on this basis. Speech sound disorder, formerly known as phonologic disorder, is commonly found in young children with language disorder, and neurologic abnormalities have been reported in a number of children, including soft neurologic signs, depressed vestibular responses, and EEG abnormalities.

Etiology. The specific causes of the expressive components of language disorder are likely to be multifactorial. Scant data are available on the specific brain structure of children with language disorder, but limited MRI studies suggest that language disorders are associated with diminished left–right brain asymmetry in the perisylvian and planum temporale regions. Results of one small MRI study suggested possible inversion of brain asymmetry (right > left). Left-handedness or ambilaterality appears to be associated with expressive language problems with more frequency than right-handedness. Evidence shows that language disorders occur more frequently within some families, and several studies of twins show significant concordance for monozygotic twins with respect to language disorders. Environmental and educational factors are also postulated to contribute to developmental language disorders.

Diagnosis. Language disorder of the expressive disturbance type is diagnosed when a child has a selective deficit in language skills and is functioning well in nonverbal areas. Markedly below-age-level verbal or sign language, accompanied by a low score on standardized expressive verbal tests, is diagnostic of expressive deficits in language disorder. Although expressive language deficits are frequently exhibited in children with autism spectrum disorders, these disturbances also occur frequently in the absence of autism spectrum disorder and are characterized by the following features: limited vocabulary, simple grammar, and variable articulation. "Inner language" or the appropriate use of toys and household objects is present. One assessment tool, the *Carter Neurocognitive Assessment,* itemizes and quantifies skills in areas of social awareness, visual attention, auditory comprehension, and vocal communication even when there are compromised expressive language and motor skills in very young children—up to 2 years of age. To confirm the diagnosis, a child is given standardized expressive language and nonverbal intelligence tests. Observations of children's verbal and sign language patterns in various settings (e.g., school yard, classroom, home, and playroom) and during interactions with other children help ascertain the severity and specific areas of a child's impairment and aid in early detection of behavioral and emotional complications. Family history should include the presence or absence of expressive language disorder among relatives.

Clinical Features. Children with expressive language deficits are vague when telling a story and use many filler words such as "stuff" and "things" instead of naming specific objects.

The essential feature of expressive deficits in language disorder is marked impairment in the development of age-appropriate expressive language, which results in the use of verbal or sign language markedly below the expected level in view of a child's nonverbal intellectual capacity. Language understanding (decoding) skills remain relatively intact. When severe, the disorder becomes recognizable by about the age of 18 months, when a child fails to utter spontaneously or even echo single words or sounds. Even simple words, such as "Mama" and "Dada," are absent from the child's active vocabulary, and the child points or uses gestures to indicate desires. The child seems to want to communicate, maintains eye contact, relates well to the mother, and enjoys games such as pat-a-cake and peek-a-boo. The child's vocabulary is severely limited. At 18 months, the child may be limited to pointing to common objects when they are named.

When a child with expressive language deficits begins to speak, the language impairment gradually becomes apparent. Articulation is often immature; numerous articulation errors occur but are inconsistent, particularly with such sounds as *th, r, s, z, y,* and *l,* which are either omitted or are substituted for other sounds.

By the age of 4 years, most children with expressive language disturbance can speak in short phrases, but may have difficulty retaining new words. After beginning to speak, they acquire language more slowly than do most children. Their use of various grammatical structures is also markedly below the age-expected level, and their developmental milestones may be slightly delayed. Emotional problems involving poor self-image, frustration, and depression may develop in school-age children.

Damien was a friendly, alert, and hyperactive 2-year-old, whose expressive vocabulary was limited to only two words (*mama, daddy*). He used these words one at a time in inappropriate situations. He supplemented his infrequent verbal communications with pointing and other simple gestures to request desired objects or actions. He was unable to communicate for other purposes (e.g., commenting or protesting). Damien appeared to be developing normally in other areas, especially in gross motor skills, although his fine motor skills were also poor. Damien sat, stood, and walked, and played happily with other children, enjoying activities and toys that were appropriate for 2-year-olds. Although he had a history of frequent ear infections, a recent hearing test revealed normal hearing. Despite his expressive limitations, Damien exhibited age-appropriate comprehension for the names of familiar objects and actions and for simple verbal instructions (e.g., "Put that down." "Get your shirt." "Clap your hands."). However, due to his hyperactivity and impulsivity, he often required multiple directions to complete a simple task.

Despite Damien's slow start in language development, his pediatrician had reassured his parents that most of the time, toddlers like Damien spontaneously overcome their initial slow start in language development. Fortunately, Damien's language delay spontaneously remitted by the time he entered preschool at 3½ years of age, although he was diagnosed at that time with attention-deficit/hyperactivity disorder.

Jessica was a sociable, active 5-year-old, who was diagnosed with language disorder. She was well liked in kindergarten despite her language deficits and played with many of her classmates. During an activity in which each student recounted the story of Little Red Riding Hood to her doll, Jessica's classmate's story began: "Little Red Riding Hood was taking a basket of food to her grandmother who was sick. A bad wolf stopped Red Riding Hood in the forest. He tried to get the basket away from her but she wouldn't give it to him."

When it was Jessica's turn, she tried to avoid being picked, but when she could not avoid her turn, Jessica's story sounded quite different. Jessica struggled and came up with: "Riding Hood going to grandma house. Her taking food. Bad wolf in a bed. Riding Hood say, what big ears, and grandma? Hear you, dear. What big eyes, grandma? See you, dear. What big mouth, grandma? Eat you all up!"

Jessica's story was characteristic of expressive language deficits at her age: including short, incomplete sentences; simple sentence structures; omission of grammatical function words (e.g., *is* and *the*) and inflectional endings (e.g., possessives and present tense verbs); problems in question formation; and incorrect use of pronouns (e.g., *her* for *she*). Jessica, however, performed as well as her classmates in understanding the details and plot of the Riding Hood tale, as long as she was not required to retell the story verbally. Jessica also demonstrated adequate comprehension skills in her kindergarten classroom, where she readily followed the teacher's complex, multistep verbal instructions (e.g., "After you write your name in the top left corner of your paper, get your crayons and scissors, put your library books under your chair, and line up at the back of the room.").

Ramon was a quiet, sullen 8-year-old boy whose expressive language problems had improved over time and were no longer obvious in play with peers. His speech now rarely contained the incomplete sentences and grammatical errors that were so evident when he was younger. Ramon's expressive problems, however, were still impairing him in tasks involving abstract use of language, and he was struggling in his third-grade academic work. An example was Ramon's explanation of a recent science experiment: "The teacher had stuff in some jars. He poured it, and it got pink. The other thing made it white." Although each sentence was grammatical, his explanation was difficult to follow, because key ideas and details were vaguely explained. Ramon also showed problems in word finding, and he relied on vague and nonspecific terms, such as *thing, stuff,* and *got.*

In the first and second grades, Ramon had struggled to keep up with his classmates in reading, writing, and other academic skills. By third grade, however, the increasing demands for written work were beyond his abilities. Ramon's written work was characterized by poor organization and lack of specificity. In addition, classmates began to tease him about his difficulties, and he was ashamed of his disability and reacted quite aggressively, often leading to physical fighting. Nonetheless, Ramon continued to show relatively good comprehension of spoken language, including classroom teaching concerning abstract concepts. He also comprehended sentences that were grammatically and conceptually complex (e.g., "The car the truck hit had hubcaps that were stolen. Had it been possible, she would have notified us by mail or by phone.")

Differential Diagnosis. Language disorders are associated with various psychiatric disorders including other learning disorders and ADHD, and in some cases, the language disorder is difficult to separate from another dysfunction. In mixed receptive–expressive language disorder, language comprehension (decoding) is markedly below the expected age-appropriate level, whereas in expressive language disorder, language comprehension remains within normal limits.

In autism spectrum disorders, children often have impaired language, symbolic and imagery play, appropriate use of gesture, or capacity to form typical social relationships. In contrast, children with expressive language disorder become very frustrated with their disorder, and are usually highly motivated to make friends despite their disability.

Children with acquired aphasia or dysphasia have a history of early normal language development; the disordered language had its onset after a head trauma or other neurologic disorder (e.g., a seizure disorder). Children with selective mutism have normal language development. Often these children will speak only in front of family members (e.g., mother, father, and siblings). Children affected by selective mutism are socially anxious and withdrawn outside the family.

Pathology and Laboratory Examination. Children with speech and language disorders should have an audiogram to rule out hearing loss.

Course and Prognosis. The prognosis for expressive language disturbance worsens the longer it persists in a child; prognosis is also dependent on the severity of the disorder. Studies of infants and toddlers who are "late talkers" concur that 50 to 80 percent of these children master language skills that are within the expected level during the preschool years. Most children who are delayed in acquiring language catch up during preschool years. Outcome of expressive language deficits is influenced by other comorbid disorders. If children do not develop mood disorders or disruptive behavior problems, the prognosis is better. The rapidity and extent of recovery depends on the severity of the disorder, the child's motivation to participate in speech and language therapy, and the timely initiation of therapeutic interventions. The presence or absence of hearing loss, or intellectual disability, impedes remediation and leads to a worse prognosis. Up to 50 percent of children with mild expressive language disorder recover spontaneously without any sign of language impairment, but those children with severe expressive speech disorder may persist in exhibiting some symptoms into middle childhood or later.

Current literature shows that children who demonstrate poor comprehension, poor articulation, or poor academic performance tend to continue to have problems in these areas at follow-up 7 years later. An association is also seen between particular language impairment profiles and persistent mood and behavior problems. Children with poor comprehension associated with expressive difficulties seem to be more socially isolated and impaired with respect to peer relationships.

Treatment. The primary goals for early childhood speech and language treatment are to guide children and their parents toward greater production of meaningful language. There are more data to support improvements through speech and language interventions for expressive language deficit in young school-aged children with primary deficits than in preschool children. A recent study investigating Parent–Child Interaction Therapy (PCIT) for school-aged children with expressive language impairment found that PCIT was particularly efficacious in improving a child's verbal initiation, mean length of utterances, and the proportion of child-to-parent utterances. A large-scale randomized trial of a yearlong intervention targeting preschoolers with language delay in Australia found that a community-based program did not affect language acquisition in 2- and 3-year-olds. Given the high rate of spontaneous remission of speech and language deficits in preschoolers, and less than robust responses to s interventions in children that young, speech and language therapy is generally not initiated unless problems persist after the preschool years. Various techniques have been used to help a child improve use of such parts of speech as pronouns, correct tenses, and question forms. Direct interventions use a speech and language pathologist who works directly with the child. Mediated interventions, in which a speech and language professional teaches a child's teacher or parent how to promote therapeutic language techniques, have also been efficacious. Language therapy is often aimed at using words to improve communication strategies and social interactions as well. Such therapy consists of behaviorally reinforced exercises and practice with phonemes (sound units), vocabulary, and sentence construction. The goal is to increase the number of phrases by using block-building methods and conventional speech therapies.

Mixed Receptive and Expressive Deficits

Children with both receptive and expressive language impairment may have impaired ability in sound discrimination, deficits in auditory processing, or poor memory for sound sequences. Children with mixed receptive–expressive disturbance exhibit impaired skills in the expression and reception (understanding and comprehension) of spoken language. The expressive difficulties in these children may be similar to those of children with only expressive language disturbance, which is characterized by limited vocabulary, use of simplistic sentences, and short sentence usage. Children with receptive language difficulties may be experiencing additional deficits in basic auditory processing skills, such as discriminating between sounds, rapid sound changes, association of sounds and symbols, and the memory of sound sequences. These deficits may lead to a whole host of communication barriers for a child, including lack of understanding of questions or directives from others, or inability to follow the conversations of peers or family members. Recognition of mixed expressive–receptive language disturbance may be delayed because of early misattribution of their communication by teachers and parents as a behavioral problem rather than a deficit in understanding.

The essential features of mixed receptive–expressive language disturbance are shown on scores on standardized tests; both receptive (comprehension) and expressive language development scores fall substantially below those obtained from standardized measures of nonverbal intellectual capacity. Language difficulties must be sufficiently severe to impair academic achievement or daily social communication.

Epidemiology. Mixed receptive–expressive language deficits occur less frequently than expressive deficits; however, epidemiologic data are scant regarding specific prevalence rates. Mixed receptive–expressive language disturbance is believed to occur in about 5 percent of preschoolers and to persist in approximately 3 percent of school-age children. It is known to be less common than expressive language disturbance. Mixed receptive–expressive language disorder is believed to be at least twice as prevalent in boys as in girls.

Comorbidity. Children with mixed receptive–expressive deficits are at high risk for additional speech and language disorders, learning disorders, and additional psychiatric disorders. About half of children with these deficits also have pronunciation difficulties leading to speech sound disorder, and about half also have reading disorder. These rates are significantly higher than the comorbidity found in children with only expressive language problems. ADHD is present in at least one-third of children with mixed receptive–expressive language disturbances.

Etiology. Language disorders most likely have multiple determinants, including genetic factors, developmental brain abnormalities, environmental influences, neurodevelopmental immaturity, and auditory processing features in the brain. As with expressive language disturbance alone, evidence is found of familial aggregation of mixed receptive–expressive language deficits. Genetic contribution to this disorder is implicated by twin studies, but no mode of genetic transmission has been proved. Some studies of children with various speech and language disorders have also shown cognitive deficits, particularly slower processing of tasks involving naming objects, as well as fine motor tasks. Slower myelinization of neural pathways has been hypothesized to account for the slow processing found in children with developmental language disorders. Several studies suggest an underlying impairment of auditory discrimination, because most children with the disorder are more responsive to environmental sounds than to speech sounds.

Diagnosis. Children with mixed receptive–expressive language deficits develop language more slowly than their peers and have trouble understanding conversations that peers can follow. In mixed receptive–expressive language disorder, receptive dysfunction coexists with expressive dysfunction. Therefore, standardized tests for both receptive and expressive language abilities must be given to anyone suspected of having language disorder with mixed receptive–expressive disturbance.

A markedly below-expected level of comprehension of verbal or sign language with intact age-appropriate nonverbal intellectual capacity, confirmation of language difficulties by standardized receptive language tests, and the absence of autism spectrum disorder confirm the diagnosis of mixed receptive–expressive language deficits; however, in DSM-5, these deficits are included in the diagnosis of language disorder.

Clinical Features. The essential clinical feature of this language disturbance is significant impairment in both language comprehension and language expression. In the mixed type, expressive impairments are similar to those of expressive language disturbance, but can be more severe. The clinical features of the receptive component of the disorder typically appear before the age of 4 years. Severe forms are apparent by the age of 2 years; mild forms may not become evident until age 7 (second grade) or older, when language becomes complex. Children with language disorder characterized by mixed receptive–expressive disturbance show markedly delayed and below-normal ability to comprehend (decode) verbal or sign language, although they have age-appropriate nonverbal intellectual capacity. In most cases of receptive dysfunction, verbal or sign expression (encoding) of language is also impaired. The clinical features of mixed receptive–expressive language disturbance in children between the ages of 18 and 24 months result from a child's failure to utter a single phoneme spontaneously or to mimic another person's words.

Many children with mixed receptive–expressive language deficits have auditory sensory difficulties and compromised ability to process visual symbols, such as explaining the meaning of a picture. They have deficits in integrating both auditory and visual symbols—for example, recognizing the basic common attributes of a toy truck and a toy passenger car. Whereas at 18 months, a child with expressive language deficits only comprehends simple commands and can point to familiar household objects when told to do so, a child of the same age with mixed receptive–expressive language disturbance typically cannot either point to common objects or obey simple commands. A child with mixed receptive–expressive language deficits may appear to be deaf. He or she responds normally to sounds from the environment, but not to spoken language. If the child later starts to speak, the speech contains numerous articulation errors, such as omissions, distortions, and substitutions of phonemes. Language acquisition is much slower for children with mixed receptive–expressive language disturbance than for other children of the same age.

Children with mixed receptive–expressive language disturbance have difficulty recalling early visual and auditory memories and recognizing and reproducing symbols in proper sequence. Some children with mixed receptive–expressive language deficits have a partial hearing defect for true tones, an increased threshold of auditory arousal, and an inability to localize sound sources. Seizure disorders and reading disorder are more common among the relatives of children with mixed receptive–expressive problems than in the general population.

Pathology and Laboratory Examination. An audiogram is indicated for all children thought to have mixed receptive–expressive language disturbance to rule out or confirm the presence of deafness or auditory deficits. A history of the child and family and observation of the child in various settings help to clarify the diagnosis.

Jenna was a pleasant 2-year-old, who did not yet use any spoken words, and did not respond to simple commands without gestures. She made her needs known with vocalizations and simple gestures (e.g., showing or pointing) such as those typically used by younger children. She seemed to understand the names for only a few familiar people and objects (e.g., *mommy, daddy, cat, bottle,* and *cookie*). Compared with other children of her age, she had a small comprehension vocabulary and showed limited understanding of simple verbal directions (e.g., "Get your doll." "Close your eyes."). Nonetheless, her hearing was normal, and her motor and play skills were developing as expected for her age. She showed interest in her environment and in the activities of the other children at her day care.

Lena was a shy, reserved 5-year-old who grew up in a bilingual home. Lena's parents and older siblings spoke English and Cantonese proficiently. Her grandparents, who lived in the same home, spoke only Cantonese. Lena began to understand and speak both languages much later than her older siblings had. Throughout her preschool years, Lena continued to develop slowly in comprehension and production. At the start of kindergarten, Lena understood fewer English words for objects, actions, and relations than her classmates did. Lena was unable to follow complex classroom instructions, particularly those that involved words for concepts of time (e.g., *tomorrow, before,* or *day*) and space (e.g., *behind, next to,* or *under*). It was also hard for Lena to match one of several pictures to a syntactically complex sentence that she had heard (e.g., "It was not the train she was waiting for." "Because he had already completed his work, he was not kept after school."). Lena played with other children but only rarely tried to speak with them, which led to her being ostracized by her classmates. Lena's attempts at conversations usually broke down, because she misinterpreted what others said or could not express her own thoughts clearly. Consequently, her classmates generally ignored her, preferring instead to play with more verbally competent peers. Lena's infrequent interactions further limited her opportunities to learn and to practice her already weak language skills. Lena also showed limited receptive and expressive skills in Cantonese, as revealed by an assessment conducted with the assistance of a Cantonese interpreter. Nonetheless, her nonverbal cognitive and motor skills were within the normal range for her age. Lena was quite proficient in solving spatial and numerical problems, provided they were presented on paper and not word problems.

Mark received a diagnosis of language disorder, based on mixed receptive–expressive deficits when he was a preschooler. By 7 years of age, he had also received the comorbid diagnoses of reading disorder and ADHD. This combination of language, reading, and attention problems made it virtually impossible for Mark to succeed in school, although he was able to engage his peers during free play. His comprehension and attention difficulties limited his ability to understand and to learn important information, or to follow classroom instructions or discussions. Mark fell further and further behind his classmates. He was also disadvantaged because he could read only a few familiar words. This meant that he was neither motivated nor able to learn academic information outside of the classroom by reading. Mark received tutoring and speech and language interventions, and despite some improvements, he continued to lag behind his classmates academically. Despite his academic problems, however, Mark made friends during sports activities in which he excelled, and continued to show nonverbal intellectual skills within the average range.

Differential Diagnosis. Children with language disorder characterized by mixed receptive–expressive deficits have a deficit in language comprehension as well as in language production. The receptive deficit may be overlooked at first, because the expressive language deficit may be more obvious. In expressive language disturbance alone, comprehension of spoken language (decoding) remains within age norms. Children with speech sound disorder and child-onset fluency disorder (stuttering) have normal expressive and receptive language competence, despite the speech impairments.

Most children with mixed receptive–expressive language disturbance have a history of variable and inconsistent responses to sounds; they respond more often to environmental sounds than to speech sounds (Table 27.4–1). Intellectual disability, selective mutism, acquired aphasia, and autism spectrum disorder should also be ruled out.

Course and Prognosis. The overall prognosis for language disorder with mixed receptive–expressive disturbance is less favorable than that for expressive language disturbance alone. When the mixed disorder is identified in a young child, it is usually severe, and the short-term prognosis is poor. Language develops at a rapid rate in early childhood, and young children with the disorder may appear to be falling behind. In view of the likelihood of comorbid learning disorders and other mental disorders, the prognosis is guarded. Young children with severe mixed receptive–expressive language deficits are likely to have learning disorders in the future. In children with mild versions, mixed disorder may not be identified for several years, and the disruption in everyday life may be less overwhelming than that in severe forms of the disorder. Over the long run, some children with mixed receptive–expressive language disturbance

Table 27.4–1
Differential Diagnosis of Language Disorder

	Hearing Impairment	Intellectual Disability	Autism Spectrum Disorder	Expressive Language Deficits Disturbance	Receptive-Expressive Language Deficits Disturbance	Selective Mutism	Speech Sound Disorder
Language comprehension	–	–	–	+	–	+	+
Expressive language	–	–	–	–	–	Variable	+
Audiogram	–	+	+	+	Variable	+	+
Articulation	–	–	– (Variable)	– (Variable)	– (Variable)	+	–
Inner language	+	+ (Limited)	–	+	+ (Slightly limited)	+	+
Uses gestures	+	+ (Limited)	–	+	+	+ (Variable)	+
Echoes	–	+	+ (Inappropriate)	+	+	+	+
Attends to sounds	Loud or low frequency only	+	–	+	Variable	+	+
Watches faces	+	+	–	+	+	+	+
Performance	+	–	+	+	+	+	+

+, normal; –, abnormal.
Adapted from Dennis Cantwell, M.D. and Lorian Baker, Ph.D., 1991.

achieve close to normal language functions. The prognosis for children who have mixed receptive–expressive language disturbances varies widely and depends on the nature and severity of the damage.

Treatment. A comprehensive speech and language evaluation is recommended for children with mixed receptive–expressive language disturbance, given the complexities of having both deficits. Some controversy exists as to whether remediation of receptive deficits before expressive language provides more efficacy overall. A review of the literature indicates that it is not more beneficial to address receptive deficits before expressive, and in fact, in some cases, remediation of expressive language may reduce or eliminate the need for receptive language remediation. Thus, current recommendations are either to address both simultaneously, or to provide interventions for the expressive component first, and then address the receptive language. Preschoolers with mixed receptive–expressive language problems optimally receive interventions designed to promote social communication and literacy as well as oral language. For children at the kindergarten level, optimal intervention includes direct teaching of key pre-reading skills as well as social skills training. An important early goal of interventions for young children with mixed receptive–expressive language disturbance is the achievement of rudimentary reading skills, in that these skills are protective against the academic and psychosocial ramifications of falling behind early on in reading. Some language therapists favor a low-stimuli setting, in which children are given individual linguistic instruction. Others recommend that speech and language instruction be integrated into a varied setting with several children who are taught several language structures simultaneously. Often, a child with receptive and expressive language deficits will benefit from a small, special educational setting that allows more individualized learning.

Psychotherapy may be helpful for children with mixed language disorder who have associated emotional and behavioral problems. Particular attention should be paid to evaluating the child's self-image and social skills. Family counseling in which parents and children can develop more effective, less frustrating means of communicating may be beneficial.

SPEECH SOUND DISORDER

Children with speech sound disorder have difficulty pronouncing speech sounds correctly due to omissions of sounds, distortions of sounds, or atypical pronunciation. Formerly called phonological disorder, typical speech disturbances in speech sound disorder include omitting the last sounds of the word (e.g., saying *mou* for *mouse* or *drin* for *drink*), or substituting one sound for another (saying *bwu* instead of *blue* or *tup* for *cup*). Distortions in sounds can occur when children allow too much air to escape from the side of their mouths while saying sounds like *sh* or producing sounds like *s* or *z* with their tongue protruded. Speech sound errors can also occur in patterns because a child has an interrupted airflow instead of a steady airflow preventing their words to be pronounced (e.g., *pat* for *pass* or *bacuum* for *vacuum*). Children with a speech sound disorder can be mistaken for younger children because of their difficulties in producing speech sounds correctly. The diagnosis of a speech sound disorder is made by comparing the skills of a given child with the expected skill level of others of the same age. The disorder results in errors in whole words because of incorrect pronunciation of consonants, substitution of one sound for another, omission of entire phonemes, and, in some cases, dysarthria (slurred speech because of incoordination of speech muscles) or dyspraxia (difficulty planning and executing speech). Speech sound development is believed to be based on both linguistic and motor development that must be integrated to produce sounds.

Speech sound disturbances such as dysarthria and dyspraxia are not diagnosed as speech sound disorder if they are known to have a neurological basis, according to DSM-5. Thus, speech sound abnormalities accounted for by cerebral palsy, cleft palate, deafness or hearing loss, traumatic brain injury, or neurological conditions are not diagnosed as speech sound disorder. Articulation difficulties not associated with a neurological condition are the most common components of speech sound disorder in children. Articulation deficits are characterized by poor articulation, sound substitution, and speech sound omission, and give the impression of "baby talk." Typically, these deficits are not caused by anatomical, structural, physiological, auditory, or neurological abnormalities. They vary from mild to severe and result in speech that ranges from completely intelligible to unintelligible.

Epidemiology

Epidemiologic studies suggest that the prevalence of speech sound disorder is at least 3 percent in preschoolers, 2 percent in children 6 to 7 years of age, and 0.5 percent in 17-year-old adolescents. Approximately 7 to 8 percent of 5-year-old children in one large community sample had speech sound production problems of developmental, structural, or neurological origins. Another study found that up to 7.5 percent of children between the ages of 7 and 11 years had speech sound disorders. Of those, 2.5 percent had speech delay (deletion and substitution errors past the age of 4 years) and 5 percent had residual articulation errors beyond the age of 8 years. Speech sound disorders occur much more frequently than disorders with known structural or neurological origin. Speech sound disorder is approximately two to three times more common in boys than in girls. It is also more common among first-degree relatives of patients with the disorder than in the general population. Although speech sound mistakes are quite common in children younger than 3 years of age, these mistakes are usually self-corrected by age 7 years. Misarticulating after the age of 7 years is likely to represent a speech sound disorder. The prevalence of speech sound disorders reportedly falls to 0.5 percent by mid to late adolescence.

Comorbidity

More than half of children with speech sound disorder have some difficulty with language. Disorders most commonly present with speech sound disorders are language disorder, reading disorder, and developmental coordination disorder. Enuresis may also accompany the disorder. A delay in reaching speech milestones (e.g., first word and first sentence) has been reported in some children with speech sound, but most children with the disorder begin speaking at the appropriate age. Children with both speech sound and language disorders are at greatest risk for attentional problems and specific learning disorders. Children with speech sound disorder in the absence of language disorder have lower risk of comorbid psychiatric disorders and behavioral problems.

Etiology

Contributing factors leading to speech disturbance may include perinatal problems, genetic factors, and auditory processing problems. Given the high rates of spontaneous remission in very young children, a maturational delay in the developmental brain process underlying speech has been postulated in some cases. The likelihood of neuronal cause is supported by the observation that children with speech sound disorder are also more likely to manifest "soft neurological signs" as well as language disorder and a higher-than-expected rate of reading disorder. Genetic factors are implicated by data from twin studies that show concordance rates for monozygotic twins that are higher than chance.

Articulation disorders caused by structural or mechanical problems are rare. Articulation problems that are not diagnosed as speech sound disorder may be caused by neurological impairment and can be divided into dysarthria and apraxia or dyspraxia. Dysarthria results from an impairment in the neural mechanisms regulating the muscular control of speech. This can occur in congenital conditions, such as cerebral palsy, muscular dystrophy, or head injury, or because of infectious processes. Apraxia or dyspraxia is characterized by difficulty in the execution of speech, even when no obvious paralysis or weakness of the muscles used in speech exists.

Environmental factors may play a role in speech sound disorder, but constitutional factors seem to make the most significant contribution. The high proportion of speech sound disorder in certain families implies a genetic component in the development of this disorder. Developmental coordination disorder and coordination in the mouth such as in chewing and blowing the nose may be associated.

Diagnosis

The essential feature of speech sound disorder is a child's delay or failure to produce developmentally expected speech sounds, especially consonants, resulting in sound omissions, substitutions, and distortions of phonemes. A rough guideline for clinical assessment of children's articulation is that normal 3-year-olds correctly articulate *m, n, ng, b, p, h, t, k, q,* and *d;* normal 4-year-olds correctly articulate *f, y, ch, sh,* and *z;* and normal 5-year-olds correctly articulate *th, s,* and *r.*

Speech sound disorder cannot be accounted for by structural or neurological abnormalities, and typically, it is accompanied by normal language development.

Clinical Features

Children with speech sound disorder are delayed in, or incapable of, producing accurate speech sounds that are expected for their age, intelligence, and dialect. The sounds are often substitutions—for example, the use of *t* instead of *k*—and omissions, such as leaving off the final consonants of words. Speech sound disorder can be recognized in early childhood. In severe cases, the disorder is first recognized at between 2 and 3 years of age. In less severe cases, the disorder may not be apparent until the age of 6 years. A child's articulation is judged disordered when it is significantly behind that of most children at the same age level, intellectual level, and educational level.

In very mild cases, a single speech sound (i.e., phoneme) may be affected. When a single phoneme is affected, it is usually one that is acquired late in normal language acquisition. The speech sounds most frequently misarticulated are also those acquired late in the developmental sequence, including *r, sh, th, f, z, l,* and *ch.* In severe cases and in young children, sounds such as *b, m, t, d, n,* and *h* may be mispronounced. One or many speech sounds may be affected, but vowel sounds are not among them.

Children with speech sound disorder cannot articulate certain phonemes correctly and may distort, substitute, or even omit the affected phonemes. With omissions, the phonemes are absent entirely—for example, bu for blue, ca for car, or whaa? For what's that? With substitutions, difficult phonemes are replaced with incorrect ones—for example, wabbit for rabbit, fum for thumb, or whath dat? For what's that? With distortions, the correct phoneme is approximated but is articulated incorrectly. Rarely, additions (usually of the vowel uh) occur—for example, puhretty for pretty, what's uh that uh? For what's that?

Omissions are thought to be the most serious type of misarticulating, with substitutions the next most serious, and distortions the least serious type. Omissions, which are most frequent in the speech of young children, usually occur at the ends of words or in clusters of consonants (ka for car, scisso for scissors). Distortions, which are found mainly in the speech of older children, result in a sound that is not part of the speaker's dialect. Distortions may be the last type of misarticulating remaining in the speech of children whose articulation problems have mostly remitted. The most common types of distortions are the lateral slip—in which a child pronounces *s* sounds with the airstream going across the tongue, producing a whistling effect—and the palatal or lisp—in which the *s* sound, formed with the tongue too close to the palate, produces a *ssh* sound effect.

The misarticulating of children with speech sound disorder is often inconsistent and random. A phoneme may be pronounced correctly one time and incorrectly another time. Misarticulating is most common at the ends of words, in long and syntactically complex sentences, and during rapid speech.

Omissions, distortions, and substitutions also occur normally in the speech of young children learning to talk. But, whereas young, normally speaking children soon replace their misarticulating, children with speech sound disorder do not. Even as children with articulation problems grow and finally acquire the correct phoneme, they may use it only in newly acquired words and may not correct the words learned earlier that they have been mispronouncing for some time.

Most children eventually outgrow speech sound disorder, usually by the third grade. After the fourth grade, however, spontaneous recovery is unlikely, and so it is important to try to remediate the disorder before the development of complications. Often, beginning kindergarten or school precipitates the improvement when recovery from speech sound disorder is spontaneous. Speech therapy is clearly indicated for children who have not shown spontaneous improvement by the third or fourth grade. Speech therapy should be initiated at an early age for children whose articulation is significantly unintelligible and who are clearly troubled by their inability to speak clearly.

Children with speech sound disorder may have various concomitant social, emotional, and behavioral problems, particularly when comorbid expressive language problems are present. Children with chronic expressive language deficits and severe articulation impairment are the ones most likely to suffer from psychiatric problems.

Martin was a talkative, likeable 3-year-old with virtually unintelligible speech, despite excellent receptive language skills and normal hearing. Martin's level of expressive language development was difficult to quantify due to his very poor pronunciation. The rhythm and melody of his speech, however, suggested that he was trying to produce multiword utterances, as would be expected at his age. Martin produced only a few vowels (*/ee/*, */ah/*, and */oo/*), some early developing consonants (*/m/, /n/, /d/, /t/, /p/, /b/, /h/, and /w/*), and limited syllables. This reduced sound repertoire made many of his spoken words indistinguishable from one another (e.g., he said *bahbah* for *bottle, baby,* and *bubble,* and he used *nee* for *knee, need,* and *Anita* [his sister]). Moreover, he consistently omitted consonant sounds at the end of words and in consonant cluster sequences (e.g., */tr-/*, */st-/*, */-nt/*, and */-mp/*). Understandably, on occasion Martin reacted with frustration and tantrums to his difficulties in making his needs understood.

Brad was a pleasant, cooperative 5-year-old, who was recognized as early as preschool to have articulation problems, and these persisted into kindergarten. His language comprehension skills and hearing were within normal limits. He showed some mild expressive language problems, however, in the use of certain grammatical features (e.g., pronouns, auxiliary verbs, and past-tense word endings) and in the formulation of complex sentences. He correctly produced all vowel sounds and most of the early developing consonants, but he was inconsistent in his attempts to produce later-developing consonants (e.g., */r/, /l/, /s/, /z/, /sh/, /th/, and ch/*). Sometimes, he omitted them; sometimes, he substituted other sounds for them (e.g., */w/* for */r/* or */f/* for */th/*); occasionally, he even produced them correctly. Brad had particular problems in correctly producing consonant cluster sequences and multisyllabic words. Cluster sequences had omitted or incorrect sounds (e.g., *blue* might be produced as *bue* or *bwue,* and *hearts* might be said as *hots* or *hars*). Multisyllabic words had syllables omitted (e.g., *efant* for *elephant* and *getti* for *spaghetti*) and sounds mispronounced or even transposed (e.g., *aminal* for *animal* and *lemon* for *melon*). Strangers were unable to understand approximately 80 percent of Brad's speech. Brad often spoke more slowly and clearly than usual, however, when he was asked to repeat something, as he often was.

Jane was a hyperactive 8-year-old, with a history of significant speech delay. During her preschool and early school years, she had overcome many of her earlier speech errors. A few late-developing sounds (*/r/, /l/,* and */th/*), however, continued to pose a challenge for her. Jane often substituted */f/* or */d/* for */th/* and produced */w/* for */r/* and */l/*. Overall, her speech was easily understood, despite these minor errors. Nonetheless, she became somewhat aggressive with her peers because of the teasing she received from her classmates about her speech.

Differential Diagnosis

The differential diagnosis of speech sound disorder includes a careful determination of symptoms, severity, and possible medical conditions that might be producing the symptoms. First, the clinician must determine that the misarticulating is sufficiently severe to be considered impairing, rather than a normative developmental process of learning to speak. Second, the clinician must determine that no physical abnormalities account for the articulation errors and must rule out neurological disorders that may cause dysarthria, hearing impairment, mental retardation, and pervasive developmental disorders. Third, the clinician must obtain an evaluation of receptive and expressive language

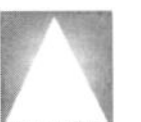

Table 27.4–2
Differential Diagnosis of Speech Sound Disorder

Criteria	Speech Sound Dysfunction Due to Structural or Neurological Abnormalities (Dysarthria)	Speech Sound Dysfunction due to Hearing Impairment	Speech Sound Disorder	Speech Sound Dysfunction Associated with Intellectual Disability Autism Spectrum Disorder Developmental Dysphasia, Acquired Aphasia, or Deafness
Language development	Within normal limits	Within normal limits unless hearing impairment is serious	Within normal limits	Not within normal limits
Examination	Possible abnormalities of lips, tongue, or palate; muscular weakness, incoordination, or disturbance of vegetative functions, such as sucking or chewing	Hearing impairment shown on audiometric testing	Normal	
Rate of speech	Slow; marked deterioration of articulation with increased rate	Normal	Normal; possible deterioration of articulation with increased rate	
Phonemes affected	Any phonemes, even vowels	*f, th, sh,* and *s*	*r, sh, th, ch, dg, j, f, v, s,* and *z* are most commonly affected	

Adapted from Dennis Cantwell, M.D. and Lorian Baker, Ph.D., 1991.

to determine that the speech difficulty is not solely attributable to the above-mentioned disorders.

Neurological, oral structural, and audiometric examinations may be necessary to rule out physical factors that cause certain types of articulation abnormalities. Children with dysarthria, a disorder caused by structural or neurological abnormalities, differ from children with speech sound disorder in that dysarthria is less likely to remit spontaneously and may be more difficult to remediate. Drooling, slow, or uncoordinated motor behavior; abnormal chewing or swallowing; and awkward or slow protrusion and retraction of the tongue indicate dysarthria. A slow rate of speech also indicates dysarthria (Table 27.4–2).

Course and Prognosis

Spontaneous remission of symptoms is common in children whose misarticulating involves only a few phonemes. Children who persist in exhibiting articulation problems after the age of 5 years may be experiencing a myriad of other speech and language impairments so that a comprehensive evaluation may be indicated at that time. Children older than age 5 with articulation problems are at higher risk for auditory perceptual problems. Spontaneous recovery is rare after the age of 8 years. Some debate exists regarding the relationship between articulation problems and reading disorder, or dyslexia. A recent study comparing children with phonological problems only, with children who had dyslexia only, and those with both phonological difficulties and dyslexia concluded that children with both disorders have somewhat distinct profiles and are comorbid disorders rather than one mixed disorder.

Treatment

Two main approaches have been used successfully to improve speech sound difficulties. The first one, the *phonological approach,* is usually chosen for children with extensive patterns of multiple speech sound errors that may include final consonant deletion, or consonant cluster reduction. Exercises in this approach to treatment focus on guided practice of specific sounds, such as final consonants, and when that skill is mastered, practice is extended to use in meaningful words and sentences. The other approach, the *traditional approach,* is utilized for children who produce substitution or distortion errors in just a few sounds. In this approach, the child practices the production of the problem sound while the clinician provides immediate feedback and cues concerning the correct placement of the tongue and mouth for improved articulation. Children who have errors in articulation because of abnormal swallowing resulting in tongue thrust and lisps are treated with exercises that improve swallowing patterns and, in turn, improve speech. Speech therapy is typically provided by a speech-language pathologist, yet parents can be taught to provide adjunctive help by practicing techniques used in the treatment. Early intervention can be helpful, because for many children with mild articulation difficulties, even several months of intervention may be helpful in early elementary school. In general, when a child's articulation and intelligibility are noticeably different than peers by 8 years of age, speech deficits often lead to problems with peers, learning, and self-image, especially when the disorder is so severe that many consonants are misarticulated, and when errors involve omissions and substitutions of phonemes, rather than distortions.

Children with persistent articulation problems are likely to be teased or ostracized by peers and may become isolated and demoralized. Therefore, it is important to give support to children with phonological disorders and, whenever possible, to support prosocial activities and social interactions with peers. Parental counseling and monitoring of child–peer relationships and school behavior can help minimize social impairment in children with speech sound and language disorder.

CHILD-ONSET FLUENCY DISORDER (STUTTERING)

Child-onset fluency disorder (stuttering) usually begins during the first years of life and is characterized by disruptions in the normal flow of speech by involuntary speech motor events. Stuttering can include a variety of specific disruptions of fluency, including sound or syllable repetitions, sound prolongations, dysrhythmic phonations, and complete blocking or unusual pauses between sounds and syllables of words. In severe cases, the stuttering may be accompanied by accessory or secondary attempts to compensate such as respiratory, abnormal voice phonations, or tongue clicks. Associated behaviors, such as eye blinks, facial grimacing, head jerks, and abnormal body movements, may be observed before or during the disrupted speech.

Early intervention is important because children who receive early intervention have been found to be more than 7 times more likely to have full resolution of their stuttering. In severe and some untreated cases, stuttering can become an entrenched pattern that is more challenging to remediate later in life and is associated with significant psychological and social distress. When stuttering becomes chronic, persisting into adulthood, the rates of concurrent social anxiety disorder are reported to be between 40 and 60 percent.

Epidemiology

An epidemiologic survey of 3- to 17-year-olds derived from the United States National Health Interview Surveys reports that the prevalence of stuttering is approximately 1.6 percent. Stuttering tends to be most common in young children and has often resolved spontaneously by the time the child is older. The typical age of onset is 2 to 7 years of age, with 90 percent of children exhibiting symptoms by age 7 years. Approximately 65 to 80 percent of young children who stutter are likely to have a spontaneous remission over time. According to the DSM-5, the rate dips to 0.8 percent by adolescence. Stuttering affects about three to four males for every one female. The disorder is significantly more common among family members of affected children than in the general population. Reports suggest that for male persons who stutter, 20 percent of their male children and 10 percent of their female children will also stutter.

Comorbidity

Very young children who stutter typically show some delay in the development of language and articulation without additional disorders of speech and language. Preschoolers and school-age children who stutter exhibit an increased incidence of social anxiety, school refusal, and other anxiety symptoms. Older children who stutter also do not necessarily have comorbid speech and language disorders, but often manifest anxiety symptoms and disorders. When stuttering persists into adolescence, social isolation occurs at higher rates than in the general adolescent population. Stuttering is also associated with a variety of abnormal motor movements, upper body tics, and facial grimaces. Other disorders that coexist with stuttering include phonological disorder, expressive language disorder, mixed receptive expressive language disorder, and ADHD.

Etiology

Converging evidence indicates that cause of stuttering is multifactorial, including genetic, neurophysiological, and psychological factors that predispose a child to have poor speech fluency. Although research evidence does not indicate that anxiety or conflicts cause stuttering or that persons who stutter have more psychiatric disturbances than those with other forms of speech and language disorders, stuttering can be exacerbated by certain stressful situations.

Other theories about the cause of stuttering include organic models and learning models. Organic models include those that focus on incomplete lateralization or abnormal cerebral dominance. Several studies using EEG found that stuttering males had right hemispheric alpha suppression across stimulus words and tasks; nonstutterers had left hemispheric suppression. Some studies of stutterers have noted an overrepresentation of left-handedness and ambidexterity. Twin studies and striking gender differences in stuttering indicate that stuttering has some genetic basis.

Learning theories about the cause of stuttering include the semantogenic theory, in which stuttering is basically a learned response to normative early childhood disfluencies. Another learning model focuses on classic conditioning, in which the stuttering becomes conditioned to environmental factors. In the cybernetic model, speech is viewed as a process that depends on appropriate feedback for regulation; stuttering is hypothesized to occur because of a breakdown in the feedback loop. The observations that stuttering is reduced by white noise and that delayed auditory feedback produces stuttering in normal speakers lend support to the feedback theory.

The motor functioning of some children who stutter appears to be delayed or slightly abnormal. The observation of difficulties in speech planning exhibited by some children who stutter suggests that higher level cognitive dysfunction may contribute to stuttering. Although children who stutter do not routinely exhibit other speech and language disorders, family members of these children often exhibit an increased incidence of a variety of speech and language disorders. Stuttering is most likely to be caused by a set of interacting variables that include both genetic and environmental factors.

Diagnosis

The diagnosis of childhood-onset fluency disorder (stuttering) is not difficult when the clinical features are apparent and well developed and each of the following four phases (described in the next section) are readily recognized. Diagnostic difficulties can arise when evaluating for stuttering in young children, because some preschool children experience transient dysfluency. It may not be clear whether the nonfluent pattern is part of normal speech and language development or whether it represents the initial stage in the development of stuttering. If incipient stuttering is suspected, referral to a speech pathologist is indicated.

Clinical Features

Stuttering usually appears between the ages of 18 months and 9 years, with two sharp peaks of onset between the ages of 2 to 3.5 years and 5 to 7 years. Some, but not all, stutterers have other speech and language problems, such as phonological disorder and expressive language disorder. Stuttering does not begin suddenly; it typically develops over weeks or months with a repetition of initial consonants, whole words that are usually the first words of a phrase, or long words. As the disorder progresses, the repetitions become more frequent, with consistent stuttering on the most important words or phrases. Even after it develops, stuttering may be absent during oral readings, singing, and talking to pets or inanimate objects.

Four gradually evolving phases in the development of stuttering have been identified:

- ▲ **Phase 1** occurs during the preschool period. Initially, the difficulty tends to be episodic and appears for weeks or months between long interludes of normal speech. A high percentage of recovery from these periods of stuttering occurs. During this phase, children stutter most often when excited or upset, when they seem to have a great deal to say, and under other conditions of communicative pressure.
- ▲ **Phase 2** usually occurs in the elementary school years. The disorder is chronic, with few if any intervals of normal speech. Affected children become aware of their speech difficulties and regard themselves as stutterers. In phase 2, the stuttering occurs mainly with the major parts of speech—nouns, verbs, adjectives, and adverbs.
- ▲ **Phase 3** usually appears after the age of 8 years and up to adulthood, most often in late childhood and early adolescence. During phase 3, stuttering comes and goes largely in response to specific situations, such as reciting in class, speaking to strangers, making purchases in stores, and using the telephone. Some words and sounds are regarded as more difficult than others.
- ▲ **Phase 4** typically appears in late adolescence and adulthood.

Stutterers show a vivid, fearful anticipation of stuttering. They fear words, sounds, and situations. Word substitutions and circumlocutions are common. Stutterers avoid situations requiring speech and show other evidence of fear and embarrassment.

Stutterers may have associated clinical features: vivid, fearful anticipation of stuttering, with avoidance of particular words, sounds, or situations in which stuttering is anticipated; and eye blinks, tics, and tremors of the lips or jaw. Frustration, anxiety, and depression are common among those with chronic stuttering.

Differential Diagnosis

Normal speech dysfluency in preschool years is difficult to differentiate from incipient stuttering. In stuttering occurs more nonfluencies, part-word repetitions, sound prolongations, and disruptions in voice airflow through the vocal track. Children who stutter appear to be tense and uncomfortable with their speech pattern, in contrast to young children who are nonfluent in their speech but seem to be at ease. Spastic dysphonia is a stuttering-like speech disorder distinguished from stuttering by the presence of an abnormal breathing pattern.

Cluttering is a speech disorder characterized by erratic and dysrhythmic speech patterns of rapid and jerky spurts of words and phrases. In cluttering, those affected are usually unaware of the disturbance, whereas, after the initial phase of the disorder, stutterers are aware of their speech difficulties. Cluttering is often an associated feature of expressive language disturbance.

Course and Prognosis

The course of stuttering is often long term, with periods of partial remission lasting for weeks or months and exacerbations occurring most frequently when a child is under pressure to communicate. In children with mild cases, 50 to 80 percent recover spontaneously. School-age children who stutter chronically may have impaired peer relationships as a result of teasing and social rejection. These children may face academic difficulties, especially if they persistently avoid speaking in class. Stuttering is associated with anxiety disorders in chronic cases, and approximately half of individuals with persistent stuttering have social anxiety disorder.

Treatment

Evidence-based treatments for stuttering are emerging in the literature. One such treatment is the Lidcombe Program, which is based on an operant conditioning model in which parents use praise for periods of time in which the child does not stutter, and intervene when the child does stutter to request the child to self-correct the stuttered word. This treatment program is largely administered at home by parents, under the supervision of a speech and language therapist. A second treatment program being investigated in clinical trials is a family-based, parent–child interaction therapy that identifies stressors possibly associated with increased stuttering and aims to diminish these stressors. A third treatment currently under investigation in clinical trials is based on the knowledge that speaking each syllable in time to a particular rhythm has led to diminished stuttering in adults. This treatment program appears to be promising when administered early on, to preschoolers.

Distinct forms of interventions have historically been used in the treatment of stuttering. The first approach, direct speech therapy, targets modification of the stuttering response to fluent-sounding speech by systematic steps and rules of speech mechanics that the person can practice. The other form of therapy for stuttering targets diminishing tension and anxiety during speech. These treatments may utilize breathing exercises and relaxation techniques, to help children slow the rate of speaking and modulate speech volume. Relaxation techniques are based on the premise that it is nearly impossible to be relaxed and stutter in the usual manner at the same time. Current interventions for stuttering use individualized combinations of behavioral distraction, relaxation techniques, and directed speech modification.

Stutterers who have poor self-image, comorbid anxiety disorders, or depressive disorders are likely to require additional treatments with cognitive–behavioral therapy (CBT) and/or pharmacologic agents such as one of the SSRI antidepressants.

An approach to stuttering proposed by the Speech Foundation of America is labeled self-therapy, based on the premise that stuttering is not a symptom, but a behavior that can be modified. Stutterers are told that they can learn to control their difficulty partly by modifying their feelings about stuttering and attitudes toward it and partly by modifying the deviant behaviors associated with their stuttering blocks. The approach includes desensitizing; reducing the emotional reaction to, and fears of, stuttering; and substituting positive action to control the moment of stuttering.

SOCIAL (PRAGMATIC) COMMUNICATION DISORDER

Social (pragmatic) communication disorder is a newly added diagnosis to DSM-5 characterized by persistent deficits in using verbal and nonverbal communication for social purposes in the absence of restricted and repetitive interests and behaviors. Deficits may be exhibited by difficulty in understanding and following social rules of language, gesture, and social context. This may limit a child's ability to communicate effectively with peers, in academic settings, and in family activities. To successfully achieve social and pragmatic communication, a child or adolescent would be expected to integrate gestures, language, and social context of a given interaction to correctly infer its meaning. Thus, the child or adolescent would be able to understand another speaker's "intention" of the communication with verbal and nonverbal cues as well as through an understanding of the environmental and social context of the interaction. One of the reasons that social (pragmatic) communication disorder was introduced into the DSM-5 was to include those children with social communication impairment who do not exhibit restrictive and repetitive interests and behaviors, and therefore do not fulfill the criteria for autism spectrum disorders. Pragmatic communication encompasses the ability to infer meaning in a given communication by not only understanding the words used, but also integrating the phrases into their prior understanding of the social environment. Social (pragmatic) communication disorder is a new disorder; however, the concept of children with social communication deficits without repetitive and restrictive interests and behaviors has been identified for many years, and is often associated with delayed language acquisition and language disorder.

Epidemiology

It is difficult to estimate the prevalence of social (pragmatic) communication disorder. Nevertheless, a body of literature has documented a profile of children who present with these persistent difficulties in pragmatic language, who do not meet criteria for autism spectrum disorder.

Comorbidity

Social (pragmatic) communication disorder is commonly associated with language disorder, consisting of diminished vocabulary for expected age, deficits in receptive skills, as well as impaired ability to use expressive language. ADHD is often concurrent with social (pragmatic) communication disorder. Specific learning disorders with impairments in reading and writing are also commonly comorbid disorders with social (pragmatic) communication disorder. Although some symptoms of social anxiety disorder may overlap with social (pragmatic) communication disorder, the full disorder of social anxiety disorder may emerge comorbidly with social (pragmatic) communication disorder.

Etiology

A family history of communication disorders, autism spectrum disorder, or specific learning disorder all appear to increase the risk for social (pragmatic) communication disorder. This suggests that genetic influences are contributing factors in the development of this disorder. The etiology of social (pragmatic) communication disorder, however, is likely to be multifactorial, and given its frequent comorbidity with both language disorder and ADHD, developmental and environmental influences are likely to also play a role.

Diagnosis

The diagnosis of social (pragmatic) communication disorder can be difficult to distinguish from mild variants of autism spectrum disorder in which repetitive and restricted interests and behaviors are minimal. There have been largely discrepant data regarding how many children previously diagnosed with autism would be excluded from the DSM-5 criteria, which now focus on only two symptom domains: social communication deficits and restricted repetitive interests and behaviors. In one study, only 60.6 percent of children who had previously met the criteria for autistic spectrum disorder in the previous edition of the DSM met DSM-5 criteria for autistic spectrum disorder. However, in another study, up to 91 percent patients with autism continued to meet the same DSM-5 criteria.

The essential features of social (pragmatic) communication disorder are persistently impaired social pragmatic communication resulting in limited effective communication, compromised social relationships, and difficulties with academic or occupational achievement.

Clinical Features

Social (pragmatic) communication disorder is characterized by impaired ability to effectively use verbal and nonverbal communication for social purposes and occurs in the absence of restricted and repetitive interests and behaviors. According to the DSM-5, all of the following features must be present in order to meet diagnostic criteria: (1) Deficits in using appropriate communication such as greeting, or sharing information in a social situation or context. (2) Impaired ability to modulate the tone, level, or vocabulary used in social communication to match the listener and the situation, such as inability to simplify communication when speaking to a young child. (3) Impaired ability in following the rules for conversations such as taking turns or rephrasing a statement for clarification and failure to recognize and respond socially appropriately to verbal and nonverbal feedback. (4) Difficulty understanding things that are not explicitly stated, impaired ability to make inferences, understand humor, or interpret socially ambiguous stimuli. Although the preceding deficits begin in the early developmental period, the diagnosis is rarely made in a child younger than 4 years of age. In milder cases, the difficulties may not become apparent until adolescence when the demands for language and social understanding are increased. The deficits in social communication lead to impairment in function in social situations, in developing relationships, and in family and academic settings.

Differential Diagnosis

The primary diagnostic consideration in social (pragmatic) communication disorder is autism spectrum disorder. The two disorders are most easily distinguished when the prominence of restricted and repetitive interests and behaviors characteristic of autistic spectrum disorder is present. However, in many cases of autism, the restrictive interests and repetitive behaviors manifest more prominently in the early developmental period and are not obvious in older childhood. However, even when these features are not observable, if they are obtained by history, social (pragmatic) communication disorder is not diagnosed, rather autism is the diagnosis. Social (pragmatic) communication disorder is considered only when the restricted interests and repetitive behaviors have never been present. ADHD may overlap with social (pragmatic) communication disorder in social communication disturbance; however, the core features of ADHD are not likely to be confused with autism spectrum disorder. In some cases, however, the two disorders may coexist. Another childhood disorder with socially impairing symptoms that may overlap with social (pragmatic) communication disorder is social anxiety disorder. In social anxiety disorder, however, social communication skills are present, but not manifested in feared social situations. In social (pragmatic) communication disorder, appropriate social communication skills are not present in any setting. Both social anxiety disorder and social (pragmatic) communication disorder may occur comorbidly, however, and children with social (pragmatic) communication disorder may be at higher risk for social anxiety disorder. Finally, intellectual disability may be confused with social (pragmatic) communication disorder, in that social communication skills may be deficits in children with intellectual disability. A diagnosis of social (pragmatic) communication disorder is made only when social communication skills are clearly more severe than the intellectual disability.

Course and Prognosis

The course and outcome of social (pragmatic) communication disorder is highly variable and dependent on both the severity of the disorder and potential interventions administered. By age 5 years, most children demonstrate enough speech and language to be able to discern the presence of deficits in social communication. However, in the milder forms of the disorder, social communication deficits may not be identified until adolescence, when language and social interactions are sufficiently complex that deficits stand out. Many children have significant improvement over time; however, even so, some early pragmatic deficits may cause lasting impairment in social relationships and in academic progress. There is a newly growing body of investigations on therapeutic interventions that may affect future outcome and prognosis of social (pragmatic) communication disorder.

Treatment

There are few data to date to inform an evidence-based treatment for social (pragmatic) communication disorder, or to fully distinguish it from other disorders with overlapping symptoms such as autism spectrum disorder, ADHD, and social anxiety disorder. A randomized controlled trial of a social communication intervention directed specifically at children with social (pragmatic) communication disorder aimed at three areas of communication: (1) social understanding and social interaction; (2) verbal and nonverbal pragmatic skills, including conversation; and (3) language processing, involving making inferences, and learning new words. Although the primary outcome measure in this study did not show significant differences for the intervention group versus the "treatment as usual" group, there were several ratings by parents and teachers that demonstrate potential improvements in social communication skills after a 20-session intensive intervention for social (pragmatic) communication disorder. It is clear that continued investigation is necessary to both validate the preceding results and to promote evidence-based treatments for children with social (pragmatic) communication disorder.

UNSPECIFIED COMMUNICATION DISORDER

Disorders that do not meet the diagnostic criteria for any specific communication disorder fall into the category of unspecified communication disorder. An example is voice disorder, in which the patient has an abnormality in pitch, loudness, quality, tone, or resonance. To be coded as a disorder, the voice abnormality must be sufficiently severe to impair academic achievement or social communication. Operationally, speech production can be broken down into five interacting subsystems, including respiration (airflow from the lungs), phonation (sound generation in the larynx), resonance (shaping of the sound quality in the pharynx and nasal cavity), articulation (modulation of the sound stream into consonant and vowel sounds with the tongue, jaw, and lips), and suprasegmentalia (speech rhythm, loudness, and intonation). These systems work together to convey information, and voice quality conveys information about the speaker's emotional, psychological, and physical status. Thus, voice abnormalities can cover a broad area of communication as well as indicate many different types of abnormalities.

Cluttering is not listed as a disorder in the DSM-5, but it is an associated speech abnormality in which the disturbed rate and rhythm of speech impair intelligibility. Speech is erratic and dysrhythmic and consists of rapid, jerky spurts that are inconsistent with normal phrasing patterns. The disorder usually occurs in children between 2 and 8 years of age; in two-thirds of cases, the patient recovers spontaneously by early adolescence. Cluttering is associated with learning disorders and other communication disorders.

▲ 27.5 Autism Spectrum Disorder

Autism spectrum disorder, previously known as the pervasive developmental disorders, is a phenotypically heterogeneous group of neurodevelopmental syndromes, with polygenic heritability, characterized by a wide range of impairments in social communication and restricted and repetitive behaviors. Prior to the development of the Fifth Edition of the American Psychiatric Association's *Diagnostic and Statistical Manual of Mental Disorders* (DSM-5), autism spectrum disorder was conceptualized as five discrete disorders, including *autistic disorder, Asperger's disorder, childhood disintegrative disorder, Rett syndrome,* and *pervasive developmental disorder not otherwise specified.* Autistic disorder was characterized by impairments in three domains: social communication, restricted and repetitive behaviors, and aberrant language development and usage. A less extensive form of autism spectrum disorder, Asperger's disorder, did not include language impairment as a diagnostic criterion. Recent clinical consensus has shifted the conceptualization of autism spectrum disorder toward a continuum model in which heterogeneity of symptoms is recognized as inherent in the disorder, and core diagnostic impairments are collapsed into two domains: deficits in social communication, and restricted and repetitive behaviors. Aberrant language development and usage is no longer considered a core feature of autism spectrum disorder. This diagnostic change is based, in part, on recent studies in siblings with diagnoses of autistic disorder, suggesting that symptom domains may be transmitted separately, and that aberrant language development and usage is not a defining feature, but an associated feature in some individuals with autism spectrum disorder. Autism spectrum disorder is typically evident during the second year of life, and in severe cases, a lack of developmentally appropriate interest in social interactions may be noted even in the first year. Some studies suggest that a decline in social interaction may ensue between the first and second years of life. However, in milder cases, core impairments in autism spectrum disorder may not be identified for several more years. Although language impairment is not a core diagnostic criterion in autism spectrum disorder, clinicians and parents share concerns about a child who by 12 to 18 months has not developed any language, and delayed language accompanied by diminished social behavior are frequently the heralding symptoms in autism spectrum disorder. In up to 25 percent of cases of autism spectrum disorder, some language develops and is subsequently lost. Autism spectrum disorder in children with normal intellectual function and mild impairment in language function may not be identified until middle childhood when both academic and social demands are increased. Children with autism spectrum disorder often exhibit idiosyncratic intense interest in a narrow range of activities, resist change, and typically do not respond to their social environment in accordance with their peers.

According to the DSM-5, diagnostic criteria for autism spectrum disorder include deficits in social communication and restricted interests, which present in the early developmental period, however, when subtle, may not be identified until several years later. approximately one-third of children meeting the current DSM-5 diagnosis of autism spectrum disorder exhibit intellectual disability (ID).

Of interest is that according to DSM-IV-TR, Rett syndrome or disorder appeared to occur exclusively in females and is characterized by normal development for at least 6 months, followed by stereotyped hand movements, a loss of purposeful motions, diminishing social engagement, poor coordination, and decreasing language use. In the formerly labeled *childhood disintegrative disorder,* development progresses normally for approximately 2 years, after which the child shows a loss of previously acquired skills in two or more of the following areas: language use, social responsiveness, play, motor skills, and bladder or bowel control. The former *Asperger's disorder* is characterized by impairment in social relatedness and repetitive and stereotyped patterns of behavior without a delay or marked aberrant in language development and usage. In Asperger's disorder, cognitive abilities and major adaptive skills are age appropriate, although social communication is impaired. A survey of children undertaken with the former autism spectrum disorders revealed that the average age of diagnosis was 3.1 years for children with autistic disorder, 3.9 years for children diagnosed with pervasive developmental disorder not otherwise specified, and 7.2 years for those youth with Asperger's disorder. Children with autism spectrum disorder who exhibited severe language deficits received an autism spectrum disorder diagnosis, on average, a year earlier than children without impairment in language. Children with autism spectrum disorder who exhibited repetitive behaviors such as hand-flapping, toe-walking, and odd play were also identified with autism spectrum disorder at a younger age than those who did not exhibit such behaviors. The current DSM-5 autism spectrum disorder criteria provide specifiers for severity of the main domains of impairment and also specifiers for the presence or absence of language impairment and intellectual impairment.

HISTORY OF AUTISTIC DISORDER

"Early infantile autism" was described by Leo Kanner in 1943; however, even as early as 1867, the psychiatrist Henry Maudsley had observed a group of very young children with severe mental disorders characterized by marked deviation, delay, and distortion in development. In that era, most serious developmental disturbance in young children was believed to fall within the category of psychoses. Kanner's classic paper "Autistic Disturbances of Affective Contact" coined the term *infantile autism* and provided a clear, comprehensive account of the early childhood syndrome. Kanner described children who exhibited extreme "autistic aloneness"; failure to assume an anticipatory posture; delayed or deviant language development with echolalia and often with pronominal reversal (using you for I); monotonous repetitions of noises or verbal utterances; excellent rote memory; limited range of spontaneous activities, stereotypies, and mannerisms; and anxiously obsessive desire for the maintenance of sameness and dread of change. Socially, Kanner's sample was described as having poor eye contact; awkward relationships; and a preference for pictures and inanimate objects. Kanner suspected that the syndrome was more frequent than it seemed, and suggested that some children with infantile autism may have been misclassified as "mentally retarded" or schizophrenic. Before 1980, children with symptoms of autism spectrum disorder were generally diagnosed with childhood schizophrenia. Over time, it became evident that autism spectrum disorder and schizophrenia were two distinct psychiatric entities. In some cases, however, a child with autism spectrum disorder may develop comorbid schizophrenic disorder later in childhood.

EPIDEMIOLOGY

Prevalence

Autism spectrum disorders have been increasingly diagnosed over the last two decades, with the current prevalence estimated at approximately 1 percent in the United States. Autistic disorder, based on DSM-IV-TR criteria, is believed to occur at a rate of about 8 cases per 10,000 children (0.08 percent). By definition, the onset of autism spectrum disorder is in the early developmental period; however, some cases are not recognized until the child is much older. Because of this delay between onset and diagnosis, the prevalence rates increase with age in young children.

Sex Distribution

Autism spectrum disorder is diagnosed four times more often in boys than in girls. In clinical samples, girls with autism spectrum disorder more often exhibit ID than boys. One potential explanation for this is that girls with autism spectrum disorder without ID may be less likely to be identified, referred clinically, and diagnosed.

ETIOLOGY AND PATHOGENESIS

Genetic Factors

Family and twin studies suggest that autism spectrum disorder has a significant heritable contribution; however, it does not appear to be fully penetrant. Although up to 15 percent of cases of autism spectrum disorder appear to be associated with a known genetic mutation, in most cases, its expression is dependent on multiple genes. Family studies have demonstrated increased rates of autism spectrum disorder in siblings of an index child, as high as 50 percent in some families with two or more children with autism spectrum disorder. Siblings of a child with autism spectrum disorder are also at increased risk for a variety of developmental impairments in communication and social skills, even when they do not meet criteria for autism spectrum disorder.

The concordance rate of autistic disorder in two large twin studies was 36 percent in monozygotic pairs versus 0 percent in dizygotic pairs in one study and about 96 percent in monozygotic pairs versus about 27 percent in dizygotic pairs in the second study. High rates of cognitive impairments, in the nonautistic twin in monozygotic twins with perinatal complications, suggest that contributions of perinatal environmental factors interact with genetic vulnerability differentially in autism spectrum disorder.

The heterogeneity in expression of symptoms in families with autism spectrum disorder suggests that there are multiple patterns of genetic transmission. Studies indicate that both an increase and decrease in certain genetic patterns may be risk factors for autism spectrum disorder. In addition to specific genetic factors, gender plays a strong role in the expression of autism spectrum disorder. Genetic studies have identified two biological systems that are influenced in autism spectrum disorder: the consistent finding of elevated platelet serotonin (5-HT), and the mTOR, that is, mammalian target of rapamycin-linked synaptic plasticity mechanisms, which appear to be disrupted in autism spectrum disorder. These will be discussed further in the next section.

A number of known genetically caused syndromes include autism spectrum disorder as part of a broader phenotype. The most common of these inherited disorders is fragile X syndrome, an X-linked recessive disorder that is present in 2 to 3 percent of individuals with autism spectrum disorder. Fragile X syndrome exhibits a nucleotide repeat in the 5' untranslated region of the *FMNR1* gene, resulting in symptoms of autism spectrum disorder. Children with fragile X syndrome characteristically exhibit ID, gross and fine motor impairments, an unusual facies, macroorchidism, and significantly diminished expressive language ability. Tuberous sclerosis, another genetic disorder characterized by multiple benign tumors, inherited by autosomal dominant transmission, is found with greater frequency among children with autism spectrum disorder. Up to 2 percent of children with autism spectrum disorder also have tuberous sclerosis.

Researchers who screened the DNA of more than 150 pairs of siblings with autism spectrum disorder found evidence of two regions on chromosomes 2 and 7 containing genes that may contribute to autism spectrum disorder. Additional genes hypothesized to be involved in autism spectrum disorder were found on chromosomes 16 and 17.

Biomarkers in Autism Spectrum Disorder

Autism spectrum disorder is associated with several biomarkers, potentially resulting from interactions of genes and environmental factors, which then influence neuronal function, dendrite development, and contribute to altered neuronal information processing. Several biomarkers of abnormal signaling in the 5-HT system, the mTOR-linked synaptic plasticity mechanisms, and alterations of the γ-aminobutyric acid (GABA) inhibitory system may be associated with Autism spectrum disorder.

The first biomarker identified in autism spectrum disorder was elevated serotonin in whole blood, almost exclusively in the platelets. Platelets acquire 5-HT through the process of SERT (serotonin transporter), known to be hereditary, as they pass through the intestinal circulation. The genes that mediate SERT (*SLC64A*) and the 5-HT receptor 5-HT 2A gene (*HTR2A*) are known to be more heritable than autism spectrum disorder, and encode the same protein in the platelets and in the brain. Because 5-HT is known to be involved in brain development, it is possible that the changes in 5-HT regulation may lead to alterations in neuronal migration and growth in the brain.

Both structural and functional neuroimaging studies have suggested specific biomarkers associated with autism spectrum disorder. Several studies found increased total brain volume in children younger than 4 years of age with autism spectrum disorder, whose neonatal head circumferences were within normal limits or slightly below. By about age 5 years, however, 15 to 20 percent of children with autism spectrum disorder developed macrocephaly. Additional studies found confirmatory data in samples of infants who were later diagnosed with autism spectrum disorder, who exhibited normal head circumferences at birth; by 4 years, 90 percent had larger brain volumes than controls, with 37 percent of the autism spectrum disorder group meeting criteria for macrocephaly. In contrast, structural magnetic resonance imaging (sMRI) studies of children with autism spectrum disorder ranging from 5 to 16 years did not find mean values of total brain volume increased. One study followed the size of the amygdala in youth with autism spectrum disorder in the first few years of life, and similarly, found an increased size in the first few years of life, followed by a decrease in size over time. The size of the striatum has also been found in several studies to be enlarged in young children with autism spectrum disorder, with a positive correlation of striatal size with frequency of repetitive behaviors. The dynamic process of the atypical and changing total brain volume observed in children with autism spectrum disorder lends support for the overarching hypothesis that there are sensitive periods or "critical periods" within the brain's plasticity that may be disrupted in ways that may contribute to the emergence of autism spectrum disorder.

fMRI studies have focused on identifying biomarkers, that is, the functional brain correlates of various observed core symptoms in autism spectrum disorder. fMRI studies of children, adolescents, and adults with autism spectrum disorder have employed tasks including face perception, neutral face tasks, "theory of mind" deficits, language and communication impairments, working memory, and repetitive behaviors. fMRI studies have provided evidence that individuals with autism spectrum disorder have a tendency to scan faces differently than controls, in that they focus more on the mouth region of the face rather than on the eye region and rather than scan the entire face multiple times, individuals with autism spectrum disorder focus more on individual features of the face. In response to socially relevant stimuli, researchers have come to the conclusion that individuals with autism spectrum disorder have greater amygdala hyperarousal. In terms of "theory of mind," that is, the ability to attribute emotional states to others, and to oneself, fMRI studies find differences in activation in brain regions such as the right temporal lobe and other areas of the brain known to become activated in controls during tasks involving theory of mind. This difference has been hypothesized by some researchers to represent dysfunction of the mirror neuron system (MNS). Atypical patterns of frontal lobe activation have been found in multiple studies of autism spectrum disorder during face-processing tasks, suggesting that this area of the brain may be critical in social perception and emotional reasoning. Decreased activation in individuals with autism spectrum disorder in the left frontal regions of the brain during memory and language-based tasks led researchers to hypothesize that individuals with autism spectrum disorder utilized more visual strategies during language processing than controls did.

Both sMRI and fMRI research has contributed to demonstrating brain correlates of core impairments observed in individuals with autism spectrum disorder.

Immunological Factors

Several reports have suggested that immunological incompatibility (i.e., maternal antibodies directed at the fetus) may contribute to autistic disorder. The lymphocytes of some autistic children react with maternal antibodies, which raises the possibility that embryonic neural tissues may be damaged during gestation. These reports usually reflect single cases rather than controlled studies, and this hypothesis is still under investigation.

Prenatal and Perinatal Factors

A higher-than-expected incidence of prenatal and perinatal complications seems to occur in infants who are later diagnosed with autism spectrum disorder. The most significant prenatal factors associated with autism spectrum disorder in the offspring are advanced maternal and paternal age at birth, maternal gestational bleeding, gestational diabetes, and first-born baby. Perinatal risk factors for autism spectrum disorder include umbilical cord complications, birth trauma, fetal distress, small for gestational age, low birth weight, low 5-minute Apgar score, congenital malformation, ABO blood group system or Rh factor incompatibility, and hyperbilirubinemia. Many of the obstetrical complications that are associated with risk for autism spectrum disorder are also risk factors for hypoxia, which may be an underlying risk factor itself. There is not sufficient evidence to implicate any one single perinatal or prenatal factor in autism spectrum disorder etiology, and a genetic predisposition to autism spectrum disorder may be interacting with perinatal factors.

Comorbid Neurological Disorders

EEG abnormalities and seizure disorders occur with greater than expected frequency in individuals with autism spectrum disorder. Four percent to 32 percent of individuals with autism spectrum disorder have grand mal seizures at some time, and about 20 to 25 percent show ventricular enlargement on CT scans. Various EEG abnormalities are found in 10 to 83 percent of children with the previously defined autistic disorder, and although no EEG finding is specific to autistic disorder, there is some indication of failed cerebral lateralization. The current consensus is that autism spectrum disorder is a set of behavioral syndromes caused by a multitude of factors acting on the central nervous system.

Psychosocial Theories

Studies comparing parents of children with autism spectrum disorder with parents of normal children have shown no significant differences in child-rearing skills. Kanner's early speculation that parental emotional factors might be implicated as contributing to the development of autism spectrum disorder has been clearly refuted.

CORE SYMPTOMS OF AUTISM SPECTRUM DISORDER

Persistent Deficits in Social Communication and Interaction

Children with autism spectrum disorder characteristically do not conform to the expected level of reciprocal social skills and spontaneous nonverbal social interactions. Infants with autism spectrum disorder may not develop a social smile, and as older babies may lack the anticipatory posture for being picked up by a caretaker. Less frequent and poor eye contact is common during childhood and adolescence compared to other children. The social development of children with autism spectrum disorder is characterized by atypical, but not absent, attachment behavior. Children with autism spectrum disorder may not explicitly acknowledge or differentiate the most important persons in their lives—parents, siblings, and teachers—and on the other hand, may not react as strongly to being left with a stranger compared to others their age. Children with autism spectrum disorder often feel and display extreme anxiety when their usual routine is disrupted. By the time children with autism spectrum disorder reach school age, their social skills may have increased, and social withdrawal may be less obvious, particularly in higher-functioning children. An observable deficit, however, often remains in spontaneous play with peers and in subtle social abilities that promote developing friendships. The social behavior of children with autism spectrum disorder is often awkward and may be inappropriate. In older school-aged children, social impairments may be manifested in a lack of conventional back-and-forth conversation, fewer shared interests, and fewer body and facial gestures during conversations. Cognitively, children with autism spectrum disorder are frequently more skilled in visual-spatial tasks than in tasks requiring skill in verbal reasoning.

One observation of the cognitive style of children with autism spectrum disorder is an impaired ability to infer the feelings or emotional state of others around them. That is, individuals with autism spectrum disorder have difficulty with making attributions about the motivation or intentions of others (also termed "theory of mind") and thus have difficulty developing empathy. The lack of a "theory of mind" produces difficulties interpreting the social behavior of others and leads to a lack of social reciprocation.

Individuals with autism spectrum disorder generally desire friendships, and higher functioning children may be aware that their lack of spontaneity and poor skills in responding to the emotions and feelings of their peers are major obstacles in developing friendships. Children with autism spectrum disorder are often avoided or shunned by peers who expect them to conform to their mainstream activities, and experience their behavior as awkward and alienating. Adolescents and adults with autism spectrum disorder often desire romantic relationships, and for some, their increase in social competence and skills over time enables them to develop long-term relationships.

Restricted, Repetitive Patterns of Behavior, Interests, and Activities

From the first years of life, in a child with autism spectrum disorder, developmentally expected exploratory play is restricted and muted. Toys and objects may not be used typically, instead, are often manipulated in a ritualistic manner, with fewer symbolic features. Children with autism spectrum disorder generally do not show the level of imitative play or abstract pantomime that other children of their age exhibit spontaneously. The activities and play of children with autism spectrum disorder may appear more rigid, repetitive, and monotonous than their peers. Ritualistic and compulsive behaviors are common in early and middle childhood. Children with autism spectrum disorder often seem to enjoy spinning, banging, and watching water flowing. Frank compulsive behaviors are not uncommon among children with autism spectrum disorder, such as lining up objects, and not infrequently a child with autism spectrum disorder may exhibit a strong attachment to a particular inanimate object. Children with autism spectrum disorder who are severely intellectually disabled have increased rates of self-stimulatory and self-injurious behaviors. Stereotypies, mannerisms, and grimacing emerge most frequently when a child with autism spectrum disorder is a less-structured situation. Children with autism spectrum disorder often find transitions and changes intimidating. Moving to a new house, rearranging furniture in a room, or even a change such as eating a meal before a bath when the reverse was the routine may evoke panic, fear, or temper tantrums in a child with autism spectrum disorder.

Associated Physical Characteristics

At first glance, children with autism spectrum disorder do not show any physical signs indicating the disorder. Children with autism spectrum disorder, overall, do exhibit higher rates of minor physical anomalies, such as ear malformations, and others that may reflect abnormalities in fetal development of those organs along with parts of the brain.

A greater than expected number of children with autism spectrum disorder do not show early handedness and lateralization, and remain ambidextrous at an age when cerebral dominance is established in most children. Children with autism spectrum disorder have been observed to have a higher incidence of abnormal dermatoglyphics (e.g., fingerprints) than those in the general population. This finding may suggest a disturbance in neuroectodermal development.

ASSOCIATED BEHAVIORAL SYMPTOMS THAT MAY OCCUR IN AUTISM SPECTRUM DISORDER

Disturbances in Language Development and Usage

Deficits in language development and difficulty using language to communicate ideas are not among the core criteria for diagnosing autism spectrum disorder; however, they occur in a subset of those individuals with autism spectrum disorder. Some children with autism spectrum disorder are not simply reluctant to speak, and their speech abnormalities do not result from lack of motivation. Language deviance, as much as language delay, is characteristic of more severe subtypes of autism spectrum disorder. Children with severe autism spectrum disorder have significant difficulty putting meaningful sentences together, even when they have large vocabularies. When children with autism spectrum disorder whose language was delayed do learn to converse fluently, their conversations may impart information without typical prosody or inflection.

In the first year of life, a typical pattern of babbling may be minimal or absent. Some children with autism spectrum disorder vocalize noises—clicks, screeches, or nonsense syllables—in a stereotyped fashion, without a seeming intent of communication. Unlike most young children who generally have better receptive language skills than expressive ones, children with autism spectrum disorder may express more than they understand. Words and even entire sentences may drop in and out of a child's vocabulary. It is not atypical for a child with autism spectrum disorder to use a word once and then not use it again for a week, a month, or years. Children with autism spectrum disorder may exhibit speech that contains echolalia, both immediate and delayed, or stereotyped phrases that seem out of context. These language patterns are frequently associated with pronoun reversals. A child with autistic disorder might say, "You want the toy" when she means that she wants it. Difficulties in articulation are also common. Many children with autistic disorder use peculiar voice quality and rhythm. About 50 percent of autistic children never develop useful speech. Some of the brightest children show a particular fascination with letters and numbers. Children with autism spectrum disorder sometimes excel in certain tasks or have special abilities; for example, a child may learn to read fluently at preschool age (hyperlexia), often astonishingly well. Very young children with autism spectrum disorder who can read many words, however, have little comprehension of the words read.

Intellectual Disability

About 30 percent of children with autism spectrum disorder function in the intellectually disabled range of intellectual function. Of those, about 30 percent of children function in the mild to moderate range, and about 45 to 50 percent are severely to profoundly intellectually disabled. The IQ scores of autism spectrum disorder children with intellectual impairments tend to reflect most severe problems with verbal sequencing and abstraction skills, with relative strengths in visuospatial or rote memory skills. This finding suggests the importance of defects in language-related functions.

Irritability

Broadly defined, irritability includes aggression, self-injurious behaviors, and severe temper tantrums. These phenomena are commonly encountered in children and adolescents with autism spectrum disorder. Severe temper tantrums may be difficult to subdue, and self-injurious behaviors are often problematic to control. These symptoms are often produced by everyday situations in which these youth are expected to transition from one activity to another, sit in a classroom setting, or remain still when they desire to run around. In children with autism spectrum disorder who are lower functioning and have intellectual deficits, aggression may emerge unexpectedly without an obvious trigger or purpose, and self-injurious behaviors such as head banging, skin picking, and biting oneself may also be noted.

Instability of Mood and Affect

Some children with autism spectrum disorder exhibit sudden mood changes, with bursts of laughing or crying without an obvious reason. It is difficult to learn more about these episodes if the child cannot express the thoughts related to the affect.

Response to Sensory Stimuli

Children with autism spectrum disorder have been observed to over respond to some stimuli and under respond to other sensory stimuli (e.g., to sound and pain). It is not uncommon for a child with autism spectrum disorder to appear deaf, at times showing little response to a normal speaking voice; on the other hand, the same child may show intent interest in the sound of a wristwatch. Some children have a heightened pain threshold or an altered response to pain. Indeed, some children with autism spectrum disorder do not respond to an injury by crying or seeking comfort. Some youth with autism spectrum disorder perseverate on a sensory experience; for example, they frequently hum a tune or sing a song or commercial jingle before saying words or using speech. Some particularly enjoy vestibular stimulation—spinning, swinging, and up-and-down movements.

Hyperactivity and Inattention

Hyperactivity and inattention are both common behaviors in young children with autism spectrum disorder. Lower than average activity level is less frequent; when present, it often alternates with hyperactivity. Short attention span, poor ability to focus on a task, may also interfere with daily functioning

Precocious Skills

Some individuals with autism spectrum disorder have precocious or splinter skills of great proficiency, such as prodigious rote memories or calculating abilities, usually beyond the capabilities of their normal peers. Other potential precocious abilities in some children with autism spectrum disorder include hyperlexia, an early ability to read well (even though they cannot understand what they read), memorizing and reciting, and musical abilities (singing or playing tunes or recognizing musical pieces).

Insomnia

Insomnia is a frequent sleep problem among children and adolescents with autism spectrum disorder, estimated to occur in 44 to 83 percent of school-aged children. Both behavioral and pharmacologic interventions have been applied as interventions. Behavioral interventions (BIs) include modification of parental behavior before and at bedtime, and providing routines that remove reinforcers for remaining awake. Medication interventions have included melatonin, which appears to be a promising agent in doses ranging from 1 mg fast-release to 4 mg controlled-release in the few controlled studies for insomnia in youth with autism spectrum disorder.

Minor Infections and Gastrointestinal Symptoms

Young children with autism spectrum disorder have been reported to have a higher-than-expected incidence of upper respiratory infections and other minor infections. Gastrointestinal symptoms commonly found among children with autism spectrum disorder include excessive burping, constipation, and loose bowel movements. Also seen is an increased incidence of febrile seizures in children with autism spectrum disorder. Some children do not show temperature elevations with minor infectious illnesses and may not show the typical malaise of ill children. In other children, behavior problems and relatedness seem to improve noticeably during a minor illness, and in some, such changes are a clue to physical illness.

ASSESSMENT TOOLS

A standardized instrument that can be very helpful in eliciting comprehensive information regarding autism spectrum disorder is the *Autism Diagnostic Observation Schedule-Generic* (ADOS-G).

Brett was the first of two children born to middle-class parents both in their early 40s after difficult pregnancy, with an induced labor at 36 weeks due to fetal distress. As an infant, Brett was undemanding and relatively placid; he did not have colic, and motor development proceeded appropriately, but language development was delayed. Brett's parents first became concerned about his development when he was 18 months of age and still not speaking; however, upon questioning, they noted that, in comparison to other toddlers in his play group, Brett had seemed less uninterested in social interaction and the social games with toddlers and adults. Stranger anxiety became marked at 18 months, much later compared to the other toddlers in his day care program. Brett would become extremely upset if his usual day care worker was not present and would tantrum until his mother took him home. Brett's pediatrician initially reassured his parents that he was a "late talker"; however, when Brett was 24 months old he was referred for developmental evaluation. At 24 months, motor skills were age appropriate. His language and social development, however, was severely delayed, and he was noted to be resistant to changes in routine and unusually sensitive to aspects of the inanimate environment. Brett's play skills were quite limited, and he played with toys in repetitive and idiosyncratic ways. His younger sister, now 12 months, was beginning to say a few words, and the family history was negative for language and developmental disorders. A comprehensive medical evaluation revealed a normal EEG and CT scan; genetic screening and chromosome analysis were normal as well.

Brett was diagnosed with autism spectrum disorder, and he was enrolled in a special education program in which he gradually began to speak. His speech was extremely literal and characterized by a monotonic voice quality and an occasional pronoun reversal. Brett often spoke and was able to make his needs known; however, his language was odd and the other toddlers did not play with him. Brett pursued mainly solo activities and remained quite isolated. By age 5 years, Brett was quite attached to his mother and often became separation anxious and upset when she went out, exhibiting severe tantrums. Brett also had developed a number of self-stimulatory behaviors in which he engaged, such as waving his fingers in front of his eyes. His extreme sensitivity to change continued over the next few years. Intelligence testing revealed a full-scale IQ in the average range with relative weakness in the verbal subtests compared to the performance subtests. In the 4th grade, Brett began to have serious behavioral problems at school and at home. Brett was unable to complete his class work, would wander around the classroom, and would begin to tantrum when the teacher insisted that he sit in his seat. He would sometimes begin screaming so loudly that he had to be asked to leave the classroom. He would then become upset and throw all of his books off his desk in a rage, sometimes inadvertently hitting other students. It took him up to 2 hours to calm down. At home, Brett would fly into a tantrum if anyone touched his things, and he would become stubborn and belligerent when asked to do anything that he was not expecting. Brett's tantrum behavior continued into middle school, and by the 8th grade, when he was 13 years old, these behaviors became so severe that the school warned his parents that he was becoming unmanageable. Brett was evaluated by a child and adolescent psychiatrist who recommended a social skills group for him and prescribed risperidone, starting with 0.5 mg p.o. b.i.d. and titrating up to 1.5 mg p.o. bid. At that dose, Brett's tantrums were less frequent and less severe. Brett seemed calmer in general, and did not become physically out of control during tantrums. Brett continued in middle school in a combination of special education classes and regular classes. Brett's social skills group was helpful in terms of teaching him how to approach peers in ways that would lead to less rejection. Brett had made some acquaintances, and by the time he started high school, he had acquired two friends who would come to his home and play video games with him. Brett knew that he was different than the other students, but he had trouble articulating what was different about him. Brett continued in high school with a combination of special and regular education and had plans to attend a community college and live at home for the first year. *(Adapted from a case by Fred Volkmar, M.D.)*

DIFFERENTIAL DIAGNOSIS

Disorders to consider in the differential diagnosis of autism spectrum disorder include social (pragmatic) communication disorder, the newly described DSM-5 communication disorder; schizophrenia with childhood onset; congenital deafness or severe hearing disorder; and psychosocial deprivation. It is also difficult to make the diagnosis of autism spectrum disorder because of its potentially overlapping symptoms with childhood schizophrenia, ID syndromes with behavioral symptoms, and language disorders. In view of the many concurrent problems often encountered in autism spectrum disorder, Michael Rutter and Lionel Hersov suggested a stepwise approach to the differential diagnosis.

Social (Pragmatic) Communication Disorder

This disorder is characterized by difficulty in conforming to typical storytelling, understanding the rules of social communication through language, exemplified by a lack of conventional greeting others, taking turns in a conversation, and responding to verbal and nonverbal cues of a listener. Other forms of language impairment may accompany social communication disorder such as delay in learning language or expressive and receptive difficulties. Social communication disorder is found with greater frequency in relatives of individuals with autism spectrum disorder, which increases the difficulty in discriminating this disorder from autism spectrum disorder. Although relationships may be negatively affected by social communication disorder, this disorder does not include restricted or repetitive behaviors and interests, as autism spectrum disorder does.

Childhood Onset Schizophrenia

Schizophrenia is rare in children younger than 12 years and almost nonexistent before the age of 5 years. Characterized by hallucinations or delusions, childhood onset schizophrenia has a lower incidence of seizures and ID and poor social skills. Table 27.5–1 compares autism spectrum disorder and schizophrenia with childhood onset.

Intellectual Disability with Behavioral Symptoms

Children with ID may exhibit behavioral symptoms that overlap with some autism spectrum disorder features. The main differentiating features between autism spectrum disorder and ID are that children with ID syndromes generally display global impairments in both verbal and nonverbal areas, whereas children with autism spectrum disorder are relatively weak in social interactions compared to other areas of performance. Children with ID generally relate verbally and socially to adults and peers in accordance with their mental age, and they exhibit a relatively even profile of limitations.

Language Disorder

Some children with language disorders also have autism spectrum disorder features, which may present a diagnostic challenge. Table 27.5–2 summarizes the major differences between autism spectrum disorder and language disorders.

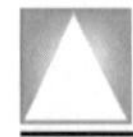

Table 27.5–1
Autism Spectrum Disorder versus Childhood Onset Schizophrenia

Criteria	Autism Spectrum Disorder	Schizophrenia (with Onset before Puberty)
Age of onset	Early developmental period	Rarely under 5 years of age
Incidence	1%	<1 in 10,000
Sex ratio (M:F)	4:1	1.67:1 (slight preponderance of males)
Family history of schizophrenia	Not increased	Likely increased
Prenatal and perinatal complications	Increased	Not increased
Behavioral characteristics	Poor social relatedness; may have aberrant language, speech or echolalia; stereotyped phrases; may have stereotypies, repetitive behaviors	Hallucinations and delusions; thought disorder
Adaptive functioning	Impaired	Deterioration in functioning
Level of intelligence	Wide range, may be intellectually	
Disabled (30%)	Usually within normal range, may be low average normal	
Pattern of IQ	Typical higher performance than verbal	More even
Grand mal seizures	4–32%	Low incidence

Adapted from Magda Campbell, M.D. and Wayne Green, M.D.

Congenital Deafness or Hearing Impairment

Because children with autism spectrum disorder may appear mute or lack language development, congenital deafness and hearing impairment must be considered and ruled out. Differentiating factors include the following: infants with autism spectrum disorder may babble only infrequently, whereas deaf infants often have a history of relatively normal babbling that then gradually tapers off and may stop at 6 months to 1 year of age. Deaf children generally respond only to loud sounds, whereas children with autism spectrum disorder may ignore loud or normal sounds and respond to soft or low sounds. Most importantly, audiogram or auditory-evoked potentials indicate significant hearing loss in deaf children. Deaf children usually seek out nonverbal social communication with regularity and seek social interactions with peers and family members more consistently than children with autism spectrum disorder.

Psychosocial Deprivation

Severe neglect, maltreatment, and lack of parental care can lead children to appear apathetic, withdrawn, and alienated. Language and motor skills may be delayed. Children with these signs generally improve when placed in a favorable and enriched psychosocial environment, but such improvement is not the case with children with autism spectrum disorder.

COURSE AND PROGNOSIS

Autism spectrum disorder is typically a lifelong, albeit heterogeneous, disorder with a highly variable severity and prognosis. Children with autism spectrum disorder and IQs above 70 with average adaptive skills, who develop communicative language by ages 5 to 7 years, have the best prognoses. A longitudinal study comparing symptoms in children with high-IQ autism spectrum disorder at the age of 5 years, with their symptoms at age 13 through young adulthood, found that a small proportion

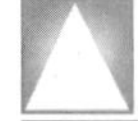

Table 27.5–2
Autism Spectrum Disorder versus Language Disorder

Criteria	Autism Spectrum Disorder	Language Disorder
Incidence	1%	5 of 10,000
Sex ratio (M:F)	4:1	Equal or almost equal sex ratio
Family history of speech delay or language problems	<25% of cases	<25% of cases
Associated deafness	Very infrequent	Not infrequent
Nonverbal communication (e.g., gestures)	Impaired	Actively utilized
Language abnormalities (e.g., echolalia, stereotyped phrases out of context)	Present in a subset	Uncommon
Articulation problems	Infrequent	Frequent
Intellectual level	Impaired in a subset (about 30%)	Uncommon, less frequently severe
Patterns of intelligence quotient (IQ) tests	Typically lower on verbal scores than performance scores	Often verbal scores lower than performance scores
Impaired social communication, restricted and repetitive behaviors	Present	Absent or, if present, mild
Imaginative play	Often impaired	Usually in tact

Adapted from Magda Campbell, M.D. and Wayne Green, M.D.

no longer met criteria for autism spectrum disorder. Most of these youth demonstrated positive changes in communication and social domains over time. Early intensive BIs have been found to provide a profound positive impact on many children with autism spectrum disorder, and in some cases lead to recovery and function in the average range.

The autism spectrum disorder symptom areas that do not seem to improve substantively over time with early BIs are related to ritualistic and repetitive behaviors. However, currently, evidence-based BIs specifically targeting repetitive behaviors may ameliorate them. The prognosis of a given child with autism spectrum disorder is generally improved if the home environment is supportive.

TREATMENT

The goals of treatment for children with autism spectrum disorder are to target core behaviors to improve social interactions, communication, broaden strategies to integrate into schools, develop meaningful peer relationships, and increase long-term skills in independent living. Psychosocial treatment interventions aim to help children with autism spectrum disorder to develop skills in social conventions, increase socially acceptable and prosocial behavior with peers, and to decrease odd behavioral symptoms. In many cases, language and academic remediation are also required. In addition, treatment goals generally include reduction of irritable and disruptive behaviors that may emerge in school and at home and may exacerbate during transitions. Children with ID require developmentally appropriate BIs to reinforce socially acceptable behaviors and encourage self-care skills. In addition, parents of children with autism spectrum disorder often benefit from psychoeducation, support, and counseling in order to optimize their relationships and effectiveness with their children. Comprehensive treatment for autism spectrum disorder including intensive behavioral programs, parent training and participation, and academic/educational interventions have provided the most promising results. Components of these comprehensive treatments include expanding social skills, communication, and language, often through practicing imitation, joint attention, social reciprocity, and play in a directed but child-centered manner. Five randomized controlled trials (RCTs) of early intensive comprehensive BIs targeting core features of autism spectrum disorder in children ranging in age from 2 years to 5 years of age have shown increases in language acquisition, social interactions, and educational achievement at the end of the study period compared to control groups. The study periods ranged from 12 weeks to several years, and the settings were at home, in clinic, or at school. The comprehensive treatment models or adapted versions of them were used either alone or in combinations in these RCTs as described below.

Psychosocial Interventions

Early Intensive Behavioral and Developmental Interventions

1. **UCLA/Lovaas-based Model.** This intensive and manualized intervention primarily utilizes techniques derived from applied behavior analysis, which is administered on a one-to-one basis for many hours per week. A therapist and a child will work on practicing specific social skills, language usage, and other target play skills, with reinforcement and rewards provided for accomplishments and mastery of skills.
2. **Early Start Denver Model (ESDM).** Interventions are administered in naturalistic settings such as in day care, at home, and during play with other children. Parents are typically taught to be co-therapists and provide the training at home while educational settings also provide the interventions. The focus of the interventions is on developing basic play skills and relationship skills, and applied behavior analysis techniques are integrated into the interventions. This approach is focused on training for very young children and is applied within the context of the child's daily routine.
3. **Parent Training Approaches.** This includes *pivotal response training,* in which parents are taught to facilitate social and communication development within the home and during activities by targeting gateway or pivotal social behaviors for mastery by the child with the expectation that once these central social skills were mastered, a natural generalizing of social behaviors would follow. Extensive parent and family components are integrated into this type of intervention. Other parent training approaches focus on language acquisition, and for parents, may be administered at a lower intensity such as weekly; however, once parents are trained, the interventions occur throughout the day with the child. Another example of a parent training approach is the Hanen More Than Words Program.

Social Skills Approaches

1. **Social Skills Training.** Typically provided by therapeutic leaders to children of various ages in a group setting with peers; children are given guided practice in initiating social conversation, greetings, initiating games, and joint attention. Emotion identification and regulation are often included in practice with recognizing and learning how to label emotions in given social situations, learning to attribute appropriate emotional reactions in others, and social problem-solving techniques. The goals are that with practice in the group setting, the child will be able to use the techniques in less-structured settings and internalize strategies to interact positively with peers.

Behavioral Interventions and Cognitive–Behavioral Therapy for Repetitive Behaviors and Associated Symptoms

BEHAVIORAL THERAPY. Applied behavioral analysis has been found to be somewhat effective in reducing some repetitive behaviors in children and adolescents with autism spectrum disorder. Early intervention is recommended for repetitive behaviors that are self-injurious; BIs may need to be combined with pharmacologic treatments to adequately manage the symptoms.

COGNITIVE–BEHAVIORAL THERAPY. There is a significant evidence base from RCTs for the efficacy of CBT for symptoms of anxiety, depression, and obsessive-compulsive disorders in children. There are fewer controlled trials of this treatment in children with autism spectrum disorder, although there are at least two published studies in which CBT was used to treat repetitive behavior in individuals with autism spectrum disorder.

Interventions for Comorbid Symptoms in Autism Spectrum Disorder

1. **Neurofeedback.** This modality has been administered in an attempt to influence symptoms of ADHD, anxiety, and increased social interaction by providing computer games or other games in which the desired behavior is reinforced, while the child wears electrodes that monitor electrical activity in the brain. The aim is to influence brainwave activity to prolong or produce electrical activity present during the desired behaviors. This modality is still under investigation in the treatment of symptoms in autism spectrum disorder.
2. **Management of insomnia in autism spectrum disorder.** Insomnia is a prevalent concern among children and adolescents with autism spectrum disorder, and both behavioral and pharmacologic interventions may be administered to improve this condition. The most common BI for insomnia in autism spectrum disorder is based on changing the parent's behavior first toward the child at bedtime and throughout the night, such that there is a removal of reinforcement and attention for being awake, leading to a gradual extinction of the "staying awake" behavior. Several studies using massage therapy before bedtime in children with autism spectrum disorder between the ages of 2 years and 13 years provided an improvement in falling asleep and a sense of relaxation.

Educational Interventions for Children with Autism Spectrum Disorder

1. **Treatment and Education of Autistic and Communication-related Handicapped children (TEACCH).** Originally developed at the University of North Carolina at Chapel Hill in the 1970s, TEACCH involves structured teaching based on the notion that children with autism spectrum disorder have difficulty with perception, and so this teaching method incorporates many visual supports and a picture schedule to aid in teaching academic subjects as well as socially appropriate responses. The physical environment is arranged to support visual learning, and the day is structured to promote autonomy and social relatedness.
2. **Broad-based approaches.** These educational plans include a blend of teaching strategies that use behavioral analysis and also focus on language remediation. Behavioral reinforcement is provided for socially acceptable behaviors while academic subjects are being taught. TEACCH may also be incorporated into a broader special educational program for autism spectrum disorder.
3. **Computer-based approaches and virtual reality.** Computer-based approaches and virtual reality teaching are centered on using computer-based programs, games, and interactive programs to teach language acquisition and reading skills. This provides the child with a sense of mastery and delivers a behaviorally based instruction in a modality that is appealing for the child. The Let's Face It! program is a computerized game that helps to teach children with autism spectrum disorder to recognize faces. It consists of seven interactive computer games that target changes in facial expression, attention to the eye region of the face, holistic face recognition, and identifying emotional expression. A randomized controlled trial of use of this program with children with autism spectrum disorder provided evidence that after 20 hours of face training with Let's Face It!, compared to the control group, the trained children demonstrated improvement in their ability to focus on the eye region of a face and improved their analytic and holistic face-processing skills. Several studies using virtual reality environments to teach children with autism spectrum disorder social skills and interaction have provided evidence of their value. In one study, a virtual café for children with autism spectrum disorder allowed the children to practice ordering and paying for drinks and food by navigation with the use of a computer mouse.

Psychopharmacological Interventions

Psychopharmacological interventions in autism spectrum disorder are mainly directed at ameliorating impairing associated behavioral symptoms rather than core features of autism spectrum disorder. Target symptoms include irritability, broadly including aggression, temper tantrums and self-injurious behaviors, hyperactivity, impulsivity, and inattention.

Irritability. Two second-generation antipsychotics, risperidone and aripiprazole, have been approved by the Food and Drug Administration (FDA) in the United States for treatment of irritability in individuals with autism spectrum disorder. Risperidone, a high-potency antipsychotic with combined dopamine (D_2) and serotonin (5-HT_2) receptor antagonist properties, has been shown to subdue aggressive or self-injurious behaviors in children with and without autism spectrum disorder. Starting with the National Institutes of Health supported Research Units on Pediatric Psychopharmacology randomized controlled trial of risperidone for treating irritability in autism spectrum disorder in 2002, there have been seven randomized controlled trials, three reanalysis studies, and two add-on studies, which have converged to confirm risperidone as an efficacious pharmacological treatment for irritability in children and adolescents with autism spectrum disorder in doses ranging from 0.5 mg to 1.5 mg. Some of the preschoolers in this study were also receiving intensive behavioral treatments. Risperidone is considered the first-line of medication treatment for children and adolescents with autism spectrum disorder who exhibit severe irritability. Despite its efficacy, risperidone's main side effects of weight gain and increased appetite; metabolic side effects such as hyperglycemia, prolactin elevation, and dyslipidemia; along with other common adverse effects such as fatigue, drowsiness, dizziness, and drooling have limited its use in some individuals. Risperidone should be used with caution in individuals with underlying cardiac abnormalities or hypotension, since risperidone may contribute to orthostatic hypotension. In further continuation studies of risperidone in the treatment of irritability in autism spectrum disorder, persistent efficacy and tolerability were found over a 6-month period, with a rapid return of symptoms in good responders when the risperidone was discontinued. Other drugs studied in the treatment of irritability in autism spectrum disorder include aripiprazole and olanzapine.

Two large studies utilizing aripiprazole in the treatment of tantrums, aggression, and self-injury in children and adolescents with autism spectrum disorder found that aripiprazole was both efficacious and safe. Doses ranged from 5 mg to 15 mg per day. Main side effects included sedation, dizziness, insomnia, akathisia, nausea, and vomiting. Although weight gain was not as pronounced as with risperidone, it was still considered a moderate adverse event, with approximately 1.3 to 1.5 kg gained during an 8-week study period. The weight gain was similar at the lower and higher doses. Olanzapine, which specifically blocks 5-HT_{2A} and D_2 receptors and also blocks muscarinic receptors, has been studied in children and adolescents with autism spectrum disorder for the treatment of irritability with a trend toward a positive response; however, significant weight gain of approximately 3.5 kg occurred. The main side effect was sedation.

Hyperactivity, Impulsivity, and Inattention. Several randomized placebo-controlled trials of methylphenidate have been conducted for the treatment of hyperactivity, impulsivity, and inattention in children and adolescents with autism spectrum disorder. The Research Units of Pediatric Psychopharmacology found methylphenidate to be at least moderately efficacious at doses of 0.25 to 0.5 mg/kg for youth with autism spectrum disorder and ADHD symptoms. Efficacy of methylphenidate in this population was less effective than in children with ADHD without autism spectrum disorder, and children with autism spectrum disorder developed more frequent side effects, including increased irritability, compared to ADHD children. A study of methylphenidate in the treatment of hyperactivity and inattention in preschoolers with autism spectrum disorder found the stimulant safe and relatively efficacious; half of the preschoolers developed side effects including increased stereotypies, gastrointestinal upset, sleep problems, and emotional lability. Among nonstimulants, one double-blind placebo-controlled study of hyperactivity, impulsivity, and inattention using atomoxetine in children with autism spectrum disorder found that it was significantly more effective than placebo. Side effects included sedation, irritability, constipation, and nausea. Clonidine, an α-agonist, has also been studied in children with autism spectrum disorder for the treatment of hyperactivity with mixed results. Guanfacine was also found to be of use in some cases.

Repetitive and Stereotypic Behavior. These core symptoms of autism spectrum disorder have been studied using SSRI antidepressants, second-generation antipsychotics (SGAs), and mood-stabilizing agents such as valproate. One study with fluoxetine found the medication group only slightly better and not significantly better than the placebo group regarding the target symptoms, and another trial with escitalopram found no difference between groups. Risperidone, however, was found to be effective in targeting irritability, and restrictive and repetitive behaviors were improved. One recent study using valproate in a 12-week trial with 55 children with a mean age of 9½ years with autism spectrum disorder found that those who were considered responders with respect to irritability were also found to be spending less time engaging in repetitive behaviors.

Agents Administered for Behavioral Impairment in Autism Spectrum Disorder Based on Open Trials. Quetiapine is an antipsychotic with more potent 5-H_2 than D_2 receptor blocking properties. Although only open-label trials have been done with this agent, it is sometimes tried when risperidone and olanzapine are not efficacious or well tolerated. It has been used in clinical practice at doses ranging from 50 to 200 mg per day. Adverse effects include drowsiness, tachycardia, agitation, and weight gain.

Clozapine has a heterocyclic chemical structure that is related to certain conventional antipsychotics, such as loxapine (Loxitane), although clozapine carries a lower risk of extrapyramidal symptoms. It is not generally used in the treatment of aggression and self-injurious behavior unless those behaviors coexist with psychotic symptoms. The most serious adverse effect is agranulocytosis, which necessitates monitoring white blood cell count weekly during clozapine use. Its use is generally limited to treatment-resistant psychotic patients.

Ziprasidone has receptor-blocking properties at the 5-HT_{2A} and D_2 receptor sites and carries little risk of extrapyramidal and antihistaminic effects. No guidelines exist for its use in autistic children with aggressive and self-injurious behaviors, but it has been used clinically to treat the latter behaviors in children who are treatment resistant. In studies of its use in adults with schizophrenia, dose ranges of 40 to 160 mg were found to be effective. Adverse effects include sedation, dizziness, and lightheadedness. An electrocardiography (ECG) recording is generally obtained before use of this medication.

Lithium (Eskalith) has been shown to be efficacious in children with aggression without autism spectrum disorder, and it is used clinically in the treatment of aggressive or self-injurious behaviors when antipsychotic medications are not effective.

Agents Used for Behavioral Impairment in Autism Spectrum Disorder Without Evidence of Efficacy. A double-blind study investigated the efficacy of amantadine (Symmetrel), which blocks *N*-methyl-D-aspartate (NMDA) receptors, in the treatment of behavioral disturbance, such as irritability, aggression, and hyperactivity, in children with autism. Some researchers have suggested that abnormalities of the glutamatergic system may contribute to the emergence of autism spectrum disorders. High glutamate levels have been found in children with the formerly labeled Rett syndrome. In the amantadine study, 47 percent of children on amantadine were rated "improved" by their parents, and 37 percent of children on placebo were rated "improved" by parents in irritability and hyperactivity, although this difference was not statistically significant. Investigators rated the children on amantadine "significantly improved" with respect to hyperactivity. A double-blind, placebo-controlled study of the efficacy of the anticonvulsant lamotrigine (Lamictal) on hyperactivity in children with autism showed high rates of placebo improvement in ratings of hyperactivity, which were similar to response on the medication.

Clomipramine (Anafranil) has been used in autism spectrum disorder, without RCTs to provide evidence of positive results. Fenfluramine (Pondimin), which reduces blood serotonin levels, has also been used unsuccessfully in the treatment of autism. Improvement does not seem to be associated with a reduction in blood serotonin level. Naltrexone (ReVia), an opioid receptor antagonist, has been investigated without much success, based on the notion that blocking endogenous opioids would reduce autistic symptoms.

Tetrahydrobiopterin, a coenzyme that enhances the action of enzymes, was used in a double-blind placebo-controlled crossover study of 12 children with autistic disorder and low concentrations of spinal tetrahydrobiopterin. The children received a daily dose of 3 mg tetrahydrobiopterin per kilogram during a 6-month period alternating with placebo. Results indicated small, nonsignificant changes in the total scores on the *Childhood*

Autism Rating Scale after 3- and 6-month treatment. Post-hoc analysis of the three core symptoms of autism—social interaction, communication, and stereotyped behaviors—revealed a significant improvement in social interaction score after 6 months of active treatment. A positive correlation was noted between social response and IQ. These results suggest that there is a possible effect of tetrahydrobiopterin on the social functioning of children with autism.

A recent case report suggested that low-dose venlafaxine (Effexor) was efficacious in three adolescents and young adults with autistic disorder with self-injurious behavior and hyperactivity. Dose of venlafaxine used was 18.75 mg per day, and efficacy was reported to be sustained over a 6-month period.

Complementary and Alternative Medicine (CAM) Approaches to Autism Spectrum Disorder

Complementary and alternative medicine is a group of nontraditional treatments that are generally used in conjunction with conventional treatments. Safe interventions that have been applied to target both core and associated behavioral features of autism spectrum disorder with unknown efficacy include the following: music therapy, to promote communication and expression; and yoga, to promote attention and decrease activity level. A biologically based practice that is deemed safe and shown to be efficacious is melatonin, which is effective in reducing sleep-onset latency in children. Other biological practices that are recognized as safe but with unknown efficacy include vitamin C, multivitamins, essential fatty acids, and the amino acids carnosine and carnitine. Secretin has been shown to be ineffective in RCTs in the treatment of autism spectrum disorder.

DISORDERS INCLUDED IN AUTISTIC SPECTRUM DISORDER

The autistic spectrum covers a range of behaviors which, prior to the change in the DSM-5, were listed separately and which are now no longer diagnosed as separate entities in the diagnostic manual. Nevertheless, the descriptive value of these entities remains important, and it may be some time before the disorders described herein disappear from the psychiatric lexicon. In addition, they remain in use in Europe and around the world as useful diagnostic entities and are still coded as separate disorders in ICD-10 as discussed.

International Classification of Diseases, Tenth Edition (ICD-10)

The classification system used in International Classification of Diseases, Tenth Revision (ICD-10), is not congruent with the revisions made in DSM-5 about autistic disorders. ICD-10 still includes separate designations for Rett syndrome, Childhood Disintegrative Disorder, Asperger's Disorder, and Pervasive Development Disorder Not Otherwise Specified (Table 27.5–3). The authors of *Synopsis* believe these subtypes to be clinically useful, and each is described below. The reader should be aware, however, that according to DSM 5, each is subsumed under the rubric of Autism Spectrum Disorder and should so be diagnosed.

Rett Syndrome

In 1965, Andreas Rett, an Australian physician, identified a syndrome in 22 girls who appeared to have developed normally for at least 6 months followed by devastating developmental deterioration. Rett syndrome is a progressive condition that has its onset after some months of what appears to be normal development. Head circumference is normal at birth and developmental milestones are unremarkable in early life. Between 5 and 48 months of age, generally between 6 months and 1 year, head growth begins to decelerate.

Available data indicate a prevalence of 6 to 7 cases of Rett syndrome per 100,000 girls. Originally, it was believed that Rett syndrome occurred only in females, but males with the disorder or syndromes that are very close to this disorder have now been described. Rett syndrome is not fully included within autism spectrum disorder, and if present along with autism spectrum disorder it should be diagnosed as an associated disorder.

Etiology. The cause of Rett syndrome is unknown, although the progressive deteriorating course after an initial normal period is compatible with a metabolic disorder. In some patients with Rett syndrome, the presence of hyperammonemia has led to postulation that an enzyme metabolizing ammonia is deficient, but hyperammonemia has not been found in most patients with Rett syndrome. It is likely that Rett syndrome has a genetic basis. It has been seen primarily in girls, and case reports so far indicate complete concordance in monozygotic twins.

Diagnosis and Clinical Features. During the first 5 months after birth, infants have age-appropriate motor skills, normal head circumference, and normal growth. Social interactions show the expected reciprocal quality. At 6 months to 2 years of age, however, these children develop progressive encephalopathy with a number of characteristic features. The signs often include the loss of purposeful hand movements, which are replaced by stereotypic motions, such as hand-wringing; the loss of previously acquired speech; psychomotor retardation; and ataxia. Other stereotypical hand movements may occur, such as licking or biting the fingers and tapping or slapping. The head circumference growth decelerates and produces microcephaly. All language skills are lost, and both receptive and expressive communicative and social skills seem to plateau at developmental levels between 6 months and 1 year. Poor muscle coordination and an apraxic gait with an unsteady and stiff quality develop.

Associated features include seizures in up to 75 percent of affected children and disorganized EEG findings with some epileptiform discharges in almost all young children with Rett syndrome, even in the absence of clinical seizures. An additional associated feature is irregular respiration, with episodes of hyperventilation, apnea, and breath holding. The disorganized breathing occurs in most patients while they are awake; during sleep, the breathing usually normalizes. Many patients with Rett syndrome also have scoliosis. As the disorder progresses, muscle tone seems to change from an initial hypotonic condition to spasticity to rigidity.

Although children with Rett syndrome may live for well over a decade after the onset of the disorder, after 10 years, many patients are wheelchair-bound, with muscle wasting, rigidity, and

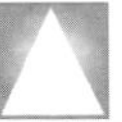

Table 27.5–3
ICD-10 Diagnostic Criteria for Pervasive Developmental Disorders

Childhood Autism

A. Abnormal or impaired development is evident before the age of 3 years in at least one of the following areas:
   1. Receptive or expressive language as used in social communication;
   2. The development of selective social attachments or of reciprocal social interaction;
   3. Functional or symbolic play.

B. A total of at least six symptoms from (1), (2), and (3) must be present, with at least two from (1) and at least one from each of (2) and (3):
   1. Qualitative abnormalities in reciprocal social interaction are manifest in at least two of the following areas:
      a. Failure adequately to use eye-to-eye gaze, facial expression, body posture, and gesture to regulate social interaction;
      b. Failure to develop (in a manner appropriate to mental age, and despite ample opportunities) peer relationships that involve a mutual sharing of interests, activities, and emotions;
      c. Lack of socioemotional reciprocity as shown by an impaired or deviant response to other people's emotions; or lack of modulation of behavior according to social context; or a weak integration of social, emotional, and communicative behaviors;
      d. Lack of spontaneous seeking to share enjoyment, interests, or achievements with other people (e.g., a lack of showing, bringing, or pointing out to other people objects of interest to the individual).
   2. Qualitative abnormalities in communication are manifest in at least one of the following areas:
      a. A delay in, or total lack of, development of spoken language that is not accompanied by an attempt to compensate through the use of gesture or mime as an alternative mode of communication (often preceded by a lack of communicative babbling);
      b. Relative failure to initiate or sustain conversational interchange (at whatever level of language skills is present), in which there is reciprocal responsiveness to the communications of the other person;
      c. Stereotyped and repetitive use of language or idiosyncratic use of words or phrases;
      d. Lack of varied spontaneous make-believe or (when young) social imitative play.
   3. Restricted, repetitive, and stereotyped patterns of behavior, interests, and activities are manifest in at least one of the following areas:
      a. An encompassing preoccupation with one or more stereotyped and restricted patterns of interest that are abnormal in content or focus; or one or more interests that are abnormal in their intensity and circumscribed nature though not in their content or focus;
      b. Apparently compulsive adherence to specific, nonfunctional routines or rituals;
      c. Stereotyped and repetitive motor mannerisms that involve either hand or finger flapping or twisting, or complex whole body movements;
      d. Preoccupations with part-objects or nonfunctional elements of play materials (such as their odor, the feel of their surface, or the noise or vibration that they generate).

C. The clinical picture is not attributable to the other varieties of pervasive developmental disorder: specific developmental disorder of receptive language with secondary socioemotional problems; reactive attachment disorder or disinhibited attachment disorder, mental retardation with some associated emotional or behavioral disorder; schizophrenia of unusually early onset; and Rett syndrome.

Atypical autism

A. Abnormal or impaired development is evident at or after the age of 3 years (criteria as for autism except for age of manifestation).

B. There are qualitative abnormalities in reciprocal social interaction or in communication, or restricted, repetitive, and stereotyped patterns of behavior, interests, and activities. (Criteria as for autism except that it is unnecessary to meet the criteria for number of areas of abnormality.)

C. The disorder does not meet the diagnostic criteria for autism. Autism may be atypical in either age of onset or symptomatology; the two types are differentiated with a fifth character for research purposes. Syndromes that are atypical in both respects should be coded. Atypicality in both ages of onset and symptomatology.

Atypicality in Age of Onset

A. The disorder does not meet Criterion A for autism; that is, abnormal or impaired development is evident only at or after the age of 3 years.

B. The disorder meets Criteria B and C for autism

Atypicality in Symptomatology

A. The disorder meets Criterion A for autism; that is, abnormal or impaired development is evident before the age of 3 years.

B. There are qualitative abnormalities in reciprocal social interactions or in communication, or restricted, repetitive, and stereotyped patterns of behavior, interests, and activities. (Criteria as for autism except that it is unnecessary to meet the criteria for number of areas of abnormality.)

C. The disorder meets Criterion C for autism.

D. The disorder does not fully meet Criterion B for autism.

Atypicality in both Age of Onset and Symptomatology

A. The disorder does not meet Criterion A for autism; that is, abnormal or impaired development is evident only at or after the age of 3 years.

B. There are qualitative abnormalities in reciprocal social interactions or in communication, or restricted, repetitive, and stereotyped patterns of behavior, interests, and activities. (Criteria as for autism except that it is unnecessary to meet the criteria for number of areas of abnormality.)

C. The disorder meets Criterion C for autism.

D. The disorder does not fully meet Criterion B for autism.

Rett Syndrome

A. There is an apparently normal prenatal and perinatal period *and* apparently normal psychomotor development through the first 5 months *and* normal head circumference at birth.

B. There is deceleration of head growth between 5 months and 4 years *and* loss of acquired purposeful hand skills between 5 and 30 months of age that is associated with concurrent communication dysfunction and impaired social interactions and the appearance of poorly coordinated/unstable gait and/or trunk movements.

C. There is severe impairment of expressive and receptive language, together with severe psychomotor retardation.

D. There are stereotyped midline hand movements (such as hand-wringing or "hand-washing") with an onset at or after the time when purposeful hand movements are lost.

(*continued*)

Table 27.5–3
ICD-10 Diagnostic Criteria for Pervasive Developmental Disorders (Continued)

Other Childhood Disintegrative Disorder

A. Development is apparently normal up to the age of at least 2 years. The presence of normal age-appropriate skills in communication, social relationships, play, and adaptive behavior at age 2 years or later is required for diagnosis.

B. There is a definite loss of previously acquired skills at about the time of onset of the disorder. The diagnosis requires a clinically significant loss of skills (not just a failure to use them in certain situations) in at least two of the following areas:
   1. Expressive or receptive language;
   2. Play;
   3. Social skills or adaptive behavior;
   4. Bowel or bladder control;
   5. Motor skills.

C. Qualitatively abnormal social functioning is manifest in at least two of the following areas:
   1. Qualitative abnormalities in reciprocal social interaction (of the type defined for autism);
   2. Qualitative abnormalities in communication (of the type defined for autism);
   3. Restricted, repetitive, and stereotyped patterns of behavior, interests, and activities, including motor stereotypies and mannerisms;
   4. A general loss of interest in objects and in the environment.

D. The disorder is not attributable to the other varieties of pervasive developmental disorder; acquired aphasia with epilepsy; elective mutism; Rett syndrome; or schizophrenia.

Overactive Disorder Associated with Mental Retardation and Stereotyped Movements

A. Severe motor hyperactivity is manifest by at least two of the following problems in activity and attention:
   1. Continuous motor restlessness, manifest in running, jumping, and other movements of the whole body;
   2. Marked difficulty in remaining seated: the child will ordinarily remain seated for a few seconds at most except when engaged in a stereotypic activity (see Criterion B);
   3. Grossly excessive activity in situations where relative stillness is expected;
   4. Very rapid changes of activity so that activities generally last for less than a minute (occasional longer periods spent in highly favored activities do not exclude this, and very long periods spent in stereotypic activities can also be compatible with the presence of this problem at other times).

B. Repetitive and stereotyped patterns of behavior and activity are manifest by at least one of the following:
   1. Fixed and frequently repeated motor mannerisms: these may involve either complex movements of the whole body or partial movements such as hand-flapping;
   2. Excessive and nonfunctional repetition of activities that are constant in form: this may be play with a single object (e.g., running water) or a ritual of activities (either alone or involving other people);
   3. Repetitive self-injury.

C. IQ is less than 50.

D. There is no social impairment of the autistic type, i.e., the child must show at least three of the following:
   1. Developmentally appropriate use of eye gaze, expression, and posture to regulate social interaction;
   2. Developmentally appropriate peer relationships that include sharing of interests, activities, etc.;
   3. Approaches to other people, at least sometimes, for comfort and affection;
   4. Ability to share other people's enjoyment at times; other forms of social impairment, e.g., a disinhibited approach to strangers, are compatible with the diagnosis.

E. The disorder does not meet diagnostic criteria for autism, childhood disintegrative disorder, or hyperkinetic disorders.

Asperger's Syndrome

A. There is no clinically significant general delay in spoken or receptive language or cognitive development. Diagnosis requires that single words should have developed by 2 years of age or earlier and that communicative phrases be used by 3 years of age or earlier. Self-help skills, adaptive behavior, and curiosity about the environment during the first 3 years should be at a level consistent with normal intellectual development. However, motor milestones may be somewhat delayed and motor clumsiness is usual (although not a necessary diagnostic feature). Isolated special skills, often related to abnormal preoccupations, are common, but are not required for diagnosis.

B. There are qualitative abnormalities in reciprocal social interaction (criteria as for autism).

C. The individual exhibits an unusually intense, circumscribed interest or restricted, repetitive, and stereotyped patterns of behavior, interests, and activities (criteria as for autism; however, it would be less usual for these to include either motor mannerisms or preoccupations with part-objects or nonfunctional elements of play materials).

D. The disorder is not attributable to the other varieties of pervasive developmental disorder: simple schizophrenia; schizotypal disorder; obsessive-compulsive disorder; anankastic personality disorder; reactive and disinhibited attachment disorders of childhood.

Other Pervasive Developmental Disorders

Pervasive Developmental Disorder, Unspecified

This is a residual diagnostic category that should be used for disorders which fit the general description for pervasive developmental disorders but in which contradictory findings or a lack of adequate information mean that the criteria for any of the other pervasive developmental disorders codes cannot be met.

virtually no language ability. Long-term receptive and expressive communication and socialization abilities remain at a developmental level of less than 1 year.

Dana was born as a full-term and healthy baby term after an uncomplicated pregnancy. An amniocentesis had been obtained because of advanced maternal age of 40 years, and findings were normal. At birth, Dana received good Apgar scores and her weight, height, and head circumference were all near the 50th percentile. Her development during the first months of life was unremarkable. At approximately 8 months of age, her development seemed to wane, and her interest in the environment, including the social environment, declined. Dana's developmental milestones failed to progress, and she became markedly delayed; she was just starting to walk at her second birthday and had no spoken language. Evaluation at that time revealed that head growth had decelerated. Self-stimulatory behaviors emerged, and in addition, marked cognitive and communicative delays were noted on formal testing. Dana began to lose purposeful hand movements and developed unusual stereotypical hand-washing behaviors. By age 6, her EEG was abnormal and abnormal hand movements were prominent. Subsequently, Dana developed truncal ataxia and breath-holding spells, and motor skills further deteriorated. *(Adapted from Fred Volkmar, M.D.)*

Differential Diagnosis. Rett syndrome shares some features with autism spectrum disorder; however, the two disorders have some predictable differences. In Rett syndrome, there is deterioration of developmental milestones, head circumference, and overall growth, whereas in autism spectrum disorder, aberrant development is usually present from early on. In Rett syndrome, specific and characteristic hand motor movements are always present; in autism spectrum disorder hand mannerisms may or may not appear. Poor coordination, ataxia, and apraxia are predictably part of Rett syndrome; however, individuals with autism spectrum disorder may have unremarkable gross motor function. In Rett syndrome, verbal abilities are usually lost completely, whereas in autism spectrum disorder language is widely variable from markedly aberrant to relatively mildly impaired. Respiratory irregularity is characteristic of Rett syndrome, and seizures often appear early. In autistic disorder, no respiratory disorganization is seen, and seizures do not develop in most patients; when seizures do develop, they are more likely in adolescence than in childhood. For autism spectrum disorder that is associated with another neurodevelopmental disorder such as Rett syndrome, the latter disorder is diagnosed in association with autism spectrum disorder.

Course and Prognosis. Rett syndrome is progressive, and those individuals who live into adolescence and adulthood function at a cognitive and social level equivalent to that in the first year of life.

Treatment. Treatment is symptomatic. Physiotherapy has been beneficial for the muscular dysfunction, and anticonvulsant treatment is usually necessary to control the seizures. Behavior therapy, along with medication, may help control self-injurious behaviors, as it does in the treatment of autistic disorder, and it may help regulate the breathing disorganization.

Childhood Disintegrative Disorder

The previous diagnosis of childhood disintegrative disorder, now included in autism spectrum disorder, is characterized by marked regression in several areas of functioning after at least 2 years of apparently normal development. Childhood disintegrative disorder, also called *Heller's syndrome* and *disintegrative psychosis,* was described in 1908 as a deterioration over several months of intellectual, social, and language function occurring in 3- and 4-year-olds with previously normal function. After the deterioration, the children closely resembled children with autistic disorder.

Epidemiology. Epidemiological data have been complicated by the variable diagnostic criteria used, but childhood disintegrative disorder is estimated to be much less common than the formerly diagnosed autistic disorder. The prevalence has been estimated to occur in about 1 in 100,000 boys. The ratio of boys to girls is estimated to be between 4 and 8 boys to 1 girl.

Etiology. The cause of childhood disintegrative disorder is unknown, but it has been associated with other neurological conditions, including seizure disorders, tuberous sclerosis, and various metabolic disorders.

Diagnosis and Clinical Features. The diagnosis is made based on features that fit a characteristic age of onset, clinical picture, and course. Cases reported have ranged in onset from ages 1 to 9 years, but in most, the onset is between 3 and 4 years. Whereas previously diagnosed as a separate entity, DSM-5 conceives of childhood disintegrative disorder as a subset of autism spectrum disorder. The onset may be insidious over several months or relatively abrupt, with abilities diminishing in days or weeks. In some cases, a child displays restlessness, increased activity level, and anxiety before the loss of function. The core features of the disorder include loss of communication skills, marked regression of reciprocal interactions, and the onset of stereotyped movements and compulsive behavior. Affective symptoms are common, particularly anxiety, as is the regression of self-help skills, such as bowel and bladder control.

To receive the diagnosis, a child must exhibit loss of skills in two of the following areas: language, social, or adaptive behavior; bowel or bladder control; play; and motor skills. Abnormalities must be present in both of the following categories: reciprocal social communication skills, and restricted and repetitive behavior. The main neurological associated feature is seizure disorder.

Ron's early history was within normal limits. By age 2, he was speaking in sentences, and his development appeared to be proceeding appropriately. At 3½ years of age, he abruptly exhibited a period of marked behavioral regression shortly after the birth of a sibling. Ron lost previously acquired skills in communication and was no longer toilet trained. Ron became more withdrawn and less interested in social interaction, exhibiting various self-stimulatory behaviors repeatedly. Comprehensive medical examination failed to reveal any conditions that might account for this developmental regression. Behaviorally, Ron exhibited features of autism spectrum disorder. At follow-up at age 12, he spoke only an occasional single word and had severe mental retardation. *(Adapted from Fred Volkmar, M.D.)*

Differential Diagnosis. The differential diagnosis of the formerly diagnosed childhood disintegrative disorder includes receptive and expressive language disorder, mental retardation with behavioral problems, and Rett syndrome. Childhood disintegrative disorder is characterized by the loss of previously acquired development. Before the onset of childhood disintegrative disorder (occurring at 2 years or older), language has usually progressed to sentence formation. This skill is strikingly different from the premorbid history of even high-functioning patients with autistic disorder, in whom language generally does not exceed single words or phrases before diagnosis of the disorder. Once the disorder occurs, however, those with childhood disintegrative disorder are more likely to have no language abilities than are high-functioning patients with autistic disorder. In Rett syndrome, the deterioration occurs much earlier than in childhood disintegrative disorder, and the characteristic hand stereotypies of Rett syndrome do not occur in childhood disintegrative disorder.

Course and Prognosis. The course of childhood disintegrative disorder is variable, with a plateau reached in most cases, a progressive deteriorating course in rare cases, and some improvement in occasional cases to the point of regaining the ability to speak in sentences. Most patients are left with at least moderate mental retardation.

Treatment. Treatment of childhood disintegrative disorder includes the same components available in the treatment of autistic disorder.

Asperger's Disorder

The former diagnosis of Asperger's disorder is characterized by impairment and oddity of social interaction and restricted interest and behavior. Unlike the former autistic disorder, in Asperger's disorder there are no significant delays in language or cognitive development. In 1944, Hans Asperger, an Austrian physician, described a syndrome that he named "autistic psychopathy." His original description of the syndrome described individuals with normal intelligence who exhibit a qualitative impairment in reciprocal social interaction and behavioral oddities without delays in language development. Asperger's disorder occurs in a wide variety of severities, including cases in which very subtle social cues are missed, but overall social interactions are mastered.

Etiology. Asperger's disorder, a version of autism spectrum disorder, has a complex etiology including genetic contribution and potentially environmental and perinatal contributing factors.

Diagnosis and Clinical Features. The clinical features include at least two of the following indications of qualitative social impairment: markedly abnormal nonverbal communicative gestures, the failure to develop peer relationships at the expected level. Restricted interests and patterns of behavior are present, but when they are subtle, they may not be immediately identified or singled out as different from those of other children. According to DSM-IV-TR, individuals with Asperger's disorder exhibit no language delay, clinically significant cognitive delay, or adaptive impairment. Currently, the clinical phenotype of Asperger's disorder is subsumed within the DSM-5 diagnosis of autism spectrum disorder.

Jared was an only child. Birth, medical, and family histories were unremarkable. His motor development was slightly delayed, but language milestones were within normal limits. His parents became concerned about him at age 4 when he was enrolled in a nursery school and was noted to have difficulties in peer interaction, joining activities, and following the rules that were so pronounced that he could not continue in the program. In grade school, he was enrolled in regular education classes and was noted to have difficulties making friends and playing sports with the other students, and he often played alone and spent time alone at lunch and recess. His greatest difficulties arose in peer interactions—he was viewed as eccentric and did not seem to understand how to interact with peers. At home, he seemed captivated by watching the weather channel on television, which he insisted on watching and pursued with great interest and intensity. On examination at age 13, Jared had markedly restricted and intense interests and exhibited pedantic and odd patterns of communication with a monotonic voice quality. Psychological testing revealed an IQ within the normal range. Formal communication examination revealed age-appropriate skills in receptive and expressive language but marked impairment in pragmatic language skills. *(Adapted from Fred Volkmar, M.D.)*

Differential Diagnosis. The differential diagnosis includes social anxiety disorder, obsessive–compulsive disorder, and schizoid personality disorder. According to the previous DSM-IV-TR, the most obvious characteristics of Asperger's disorder compared to autistic disorder are the absence of language delay and dysfunction. The lack of language delay and impaired use of language were previous requirements for Asperger's disorder; however, social and communication deficits are present. Studies comparing children with Asperger's disorder and autistic disorder found that children with Asperger's disorder were more likely to seek social interaction, and due to their awareness of their impairment sought more vigorously to make friends. Although in this subgroup within autism spectrum disorder significant delay in language is not a feature, some delay in the acquisition of language, and some impairment in verbal communication has been noted in more than one-third of clinical samples.

Course and Prognosis. The factors associated with a good prognosis in this subgroup within autism spectrum disorder are a normal IQ and more competencies in social skills. Reports of some adults diagnosed with Asperger's disorder indicate that their social and communication deficits remain and they continue to relate in an awkward way and appear socially uncomfortable.

Treatment. Treatment of individuals who meet the criteria for the previous Asperger's disorder diagnosis aims to promote social communication and peer relationships. Interventions are initiated with the goal of shaping interactions so that they better match those of peers. Very often children with Asperger's disorder are highly verbal and have excellent academic achievement. The tendency of children and adolescents with Asperger's disorder to rely on rigid rules and routines can become a source of difficulty for them and be an area that requires therapeutic intervention. A comfort with routines, however, can be utilized to foster positive habits that may enhance the social life of a child with Asperger's disorder. Self-sufficiency and problem-solving techniques are often helpful for these individuals in social situations and work settings. Some of the same techniques used for autistic disorder are likely to benefit patients with Asperger's disorder with severe social impairment.

Pervasive Developmental Disorder Not Otherwise Specified

Whereas the DSM-IV-TR defines pervasive disorder not otherwise specified as a condition with severe, pervasive impairment in communication skills or the presence of restricted and repetitive activities and associated impairment in social interactions, DSM-5 conceives of this as encompassed within a diagnosis of autism spectrum disorder.

> Anna was the older of two children. She had been a difficult baby who was not easy to console but her motor and communicative development seemed appropriate. She was socially related and sometimes enjoyed interaction, but she was easily overstimulated. She exhibited some hand flapping behavior, especially when she was excited. Anna's parents sought evaluation when she was 4 years of age because of problems with getting along with other children. At evaluation Anna was found to have language and cognitive function within the normal range. Anna had difficulty relating to her parents as sources of support and comfort. She displayed behavioral rigidity and a tendency to impose routines on social skills. Anna was placed in a special education kindergarten and did well academically, although problems in peer interactions and unusual affective responses persisted. As an adolescent, Anna describes herself as a "loner," who often retreats from others and avoids social interaction and tends to be comfortable with solitary activities. *(Adapted from Fred Volkmar, M.D.)*

Treatment. The treatment approach is identical to that of other autism spectrum disorder. Mainstreaming in school may be possible. Compared with previously diagnosed autistic children, those with the former pervasive developmental disorder not otherwise specified generally have less impairment in language skills and more self-awareness.

▲ 27.6 Attention-Deficit/Hyperactivity Disorder

ADHD is a neuropsychiatric condition affecting preschoolers, children, adolescents, and adults around the world, characterized by a pattern of diminished sustained attention, and increased impulsivity or hyperactivity. Based on family history, genotyping, and neuroimaging studies, there is clear evidence to support a biological basis for ADHD. Although multiple regions of the brain and several neurotransmitters have been implicated in the emergence of symptoms, dopamine continues to be a focus of investigation regarding ADHD symptoms. The prefrontal cortex of the brain has been implicated because of its high utilization of dopamine and its reciprocal connections with other brain regions involved in attention, inhibition, decision-making, response inhibition, working memory, and vigilance. ADHD affects up to 5 to 8 percent of school-aged children, with 60 to 85 percent of those diagnosed as children continuing to meet criteria for the disorder in adolescence, and up to 60 percent continuing to be symptomatic into adulthood. Children, adolescents, and adults with ADHD often have significant impairment in academic functioning as well as in social and interpersonal situations. ADHD is frequently associated with comorbid disorders including learning disorders, anxiety disorders, mood disorders, and disruptive behavior disorders.

The Fifth Edition of the American Psychiatric Association's *Diagnostic and Statistical Manual of Mental Disorders* (DSM-5) has made several changes to the diagnostic criteria of ADHD in youth and in adults. Whereas in the past, ADHD symptoms had to be present by age 7 years, in DSM-5, "several inattentive or hyperactive-impulsive symptoms" must be present by age 12 years. Previously, there were two subtypes: Inattentive and Hyperactive/Impulsive type. In DSM-5, however, subtypes have been replaced by the following three specifiers, which essentially denote the same groups: (1) combined presentation, (2) predominantly inattentive presentation, and (3) predominantly hyperactive/impulsive presentation. Additional changes in DSM-5 include permitting a comorbid ADHD and autism spectrum diagnosis to be made. Finally, in DSM-5, for adolescents 17 years and older and for adults, only five symptoms, rather than six symptoms of either inattention or hyperactivity and impulsivity are required. In addition, to reflect the developmental differences in ADHD across the life span, examples of symptoms have been added to the DSM-5 criteria for ADHD. To confirm a diagnosis of ADHD, impairment from inattention and/or hyperactivity and impulsivity must be present in at least two settings and interfere with developmentally appropriate social or academic functioning.

ADHD has historically been described in the literature using different terminology. In the early 1900s, impulsive, disinhibited, and hyperactive children—many of whom also had neurological damage due to encephalitis—were grouped under the label *hyperactive syndrome.* In the 1960s, a heterogeneous group of children with poor coordination, learning disabilities, and emotional lability, but without specific neurological disorders, were described as having "minimal brain damage"; however, over time, it became clear that this was an inappropriate term. Many hypotheses have been suggested to explain ADHD symptoms including theories of abnormal arousal and poor ability to modulate emotions. This theory was initially supported by the observation that stimulant medications increased sustained attention and improved focus. ADHD is one of the most well-researched childhood psychiatric disorders with strong evidence-based treatments.

EPIDEMIOLOGY

Rates of ADHD have been reported to be 7 to 8 percent in prepubertal elementary school children. Epidemiologic studies suggest that ADHD occurs in about 5 percent of youth including children and adolescents, and about 2.5 percent of adults. The rate of ADHD in parents and siblings of children with ADHD is 2 to 8 times greater than in the general population. ADHD is more prevalent in boys than in girls, with the ratio ranging from 2:1 to as high as 9:1. First-degree biological relatives (e.g., siblings of probands with ADHD) are at high risk for developing ADHD as well as other psychiatric disorders, including disruptive behavior disorders, anxiety disorders, and depressive disorders. Siblings of children with ADHD are also at higher risk than the general population for learning disorders and academic difficulties. The parents of children with ADHD show an increased incidence of substance use disorders. Symptoms of ADHD are often present by age 3 years, but unless they are very severe, the diagnosis is frequently not made until the child is in kindergarten, or elementary school, when teacher information is available comparing the index child peers of the same age.

ETIOLOGY

Data suggest that the etiology of ADHD is largely genetic, with a heritability of approximately 75 percent. ADHD symptoms are the product of complex interactions of neuroanatomical and neurochemical systems evidenced by data from twin and adoption family genetic studies, dopamine transport gene studies, neuroimaging studies, and neurotransmitter data. Most children with ADHD have no evidence of gross structural damage in the CNS. In some cases, contributory factors for ADHD may include prenatal toxic exposures, prematurity, and prenatal mechanical insult to the fetal nervous system. Food additives, colorings, preservatives, and sugar have been proposed as possible contributing causes of hyperactive behavior; however, studies have not confirmed these theories. Neither artificial food coloring nor sugar has been established as a cause of ADHD. There is no clear evidence that omega-3 fatty acids are beneficial in the treatment of ADHD.

Genetic Factors

Evidence for a significant genetic contribution to ADHD has emerged from family studies, which reveal an increased concordance in monozygotic compared to dizygotic twins, as well as a marked increased risk of 2 to 8 times for siblings as well as parents of an ADHD child, compared to the general population. Clinically, one sibling may have predominantly impulsivity/hyperactivity symptoms and others may have predominantly inattention symptoms. Up to 70 percent of children with ADHD meet criteria for a comorbid psychiatric disorder, including learning disorders, anxiety disorders, mood disorder conduct disorders, and substance use disorders. Several hypotheses of the mode of transmission of ADHD have been proposed, including a sex-linked hypothesis, which would explain the significantly increased rates of ADHD in males. Other theories have focused on a model of interaction of multiple genes that produces the various symptoms of ADHD. Numerous investigations continue to identify specific genes involved in ADHD. Cook and colleagues have found an association of the dopamine transporter gene (*DAT1*) with ADHD, although data from other research groups have not confirmed that result. Family studies and population-based studies have found an association between the dopamine 4 receptor seven-repeat allele gene (*DRD4*) and ADHD. Most molecular research on ADHD has focused on genes that influence the metabolism or action of dopamine. Continued investigation is necessary to clarify the complex relationships between multiple interactive genes and the emergence of ADHD.

Neurochemical Factors

Many neurotransmitters are postulated to be associated with ADHD symptoms; however, dopamine is a major focus of clinical investigation, and the prefrontal cortex has been implicated based on its role in attention and regulation of impulse control. Animal studies have shown that other brain regions such as locus ceruleus, which consists predominantly of noradrenergic neurons, also play a major role in attention. The noradrenergic system includes the central system (originating in the locus ceruleus) and the peripheral sympathetic system. Dysfunction in peripheral epinephrine, which causes the hormone to accumulate peripherally, may potentially feed back to the central system and "reset" the locus ceruleus to a lower level. In part, hypotheses regarding the neurochemistry of ADHD have arisen from the predictable effect of medications. Simulants, known to be the most effective medications in the treatment of ADHD, affect both dopamine and norepinephrine, leading to neurotransmitter hypotheses that may include dysfunction in both the adrenergic and dopaminergic systems. Stimulants increase catecholamine concentrations by promoting their release and blocking their uptake.

Neurophysiological Factors

EEG studies in ADHD children and adolescents over the last several decades have found evidence of increased theta activity, especially in the frontal regions. Further studies of youth with ADHD have provided data showing elevated beta activity in their EEG studies. Clarke and colleagues, studying EEG findings in children and adolescents over the last two decades found that those ADHD children with combined type of ADHD were the ones who showed significantly elevated beta activity on EEG, and further studies indicate that these youth also tend to show increased mood lability and temper tantrums. Current investigations of EEG in youth with ADHD have identified behavioral symptom clusters among children with similar EEG profiles.

Neuroanatomical Aspects

Researchers have hypothesized networks within the brain for promoting components of attention including focusing, sustaining attention, and shifting attention. They describe neuroanatomical correlations for the superior and temporal cortices with focusing attention; external parietal and corpus striatal regions with motor executive functions; the hippocampus with encoding of memory traces; and the prefrontal cortex with shifting from one stimulus to another. Further hypotheses suggest that the brainstem, which contains the reticular thalamic nuclei function, is involved in sustained attention. A review of magnetic resonance imaging (MRI), positron emission tomography (PET), and single photon emission computerized tomography (SPECT) suggests that populations of children with ADHD show evidence of both decreased volume and decreased activity in prefrontal regions, anterior cingulated, globus pallidus, caudate, thalamus, and cerebellum. PET scans have also shown that female adolescents with ADHD have globally lower glucose metabolism than both control female and male adolescents without ADHD. One theory postulates that the frontal lobes in children with ADHD do not adequately inhibit lower brain structures, an effect leading to disinhibition.

Developmental Factors

Higher rates of ADHD are present in children who were born prematurely and whose mothers were observed to have maternal infection during pregnancy. Perinatal insult to the brain during early infancy caused by infection, inflammation, and trauma may, in some cases, be contributing factors in the emergence of ADHD symptoms. Children with ADHD have been observed to exhibit nonfocal (soft) neurological signs at higher rates than those in the general population. Reports in the literature indicate that September is a peak month for births of children with ADHD with and without comorbid learning disorders. The implication is that prenatal exposure to winter infections during the first trimester may contribute to the emergence of ADHD symptoms in some susceptible children.

Psychosocial Factors

Severe chronic abuse, maltreatment, and neglect are associated with certain behavioral symptoms that overlap with ADHD including poor attention and poor impulse control. Predisposing factors may include the child's temperament and genetic–familial factors.

DIAGNOSIS

The principal signs of inattention, impulsivity, and hyperactivity may be elicited on the basis of a detailed history of a child's early developmental patterns along with direct observation of the child, especially in situations that require sustained attention. Hyperactivity may be more severe in some situations (e.g., school) and less marked in others (e.g., one-on-one interviews), and may be less obvious in pleasant structured activities (sports). The diagnosis of ADHD requires persistent, impairing symptoms of either hyperactivity/impulsivity or inattention in at least two different settings. For example, most children with ADHD have symptoms in school and at home.

Distinguishing features of ADHD are short attention span and high levels of distractibility for chronological age and developmental level. In school, children with ADHD often exhibit difficulties following instructions and require increased individualized attention from teachers. At home, children with ADHD frequently have difficulty complying with their parents' directions and may need to be asked multiple times to complete relatively simple tasks. Children with ADHD typically act impulsively, are emotionally labile, explosive, lack focus, and are irritable.

Children for whom hyperactivity is a predominant feature are more likely to be referred for treatment earlier than the children whose primarily symptoms are attention deficit. Children with the combined inattentive and hyperactive-impulsive symptoms of ADHD, or predominantly hyperactive-impulsive symptoms of ADHD, are more apt to have a stable diagnosis over time and to exhibit comorbid conduct disorder than those children with inattentive ADHD. Specific learning disorders in the areas of reading, arithmetic, language, and writing occur frequently in association with ADHD. Global developmental assessment must be considered to rule out other sources of inattention.

School history and teachers' reports are critical in evaluating whether a child's difficulties in learning and school behavior are caused primarily by inattention or compromised understanding of the academic material. In addition to intellectual limitations, poor performance in school may result from maturational problems, social rejection, mood disorders, anxiety, or poor self-esteem due to learning disorders. Assessment of social relationships with siblings, peers, and adults, and engagement in free and structured activities may yield valuable diagnostic clues to the presence of ADHD.

The mental status examination in a given child with ADHD who is aware of his or her impairment may reflect a demoralized or depressed mood; however, thought disorder or impaired reality testing is not expected. A child with ADHD may exhibit distractibility and perseveration and signs of visual-perceptual, auditory-perceptual, or language-based learning disorders. A neurological examination may reveal visual, motor, perceptual, or auditory discriminatory immaturity or impairments without overt signs of visual or auditory disorders. Children with ADHD often have problems with motor coordination and difficulty copying age-appropriate figures, rapid alternating movements, right–left discrimination, ambidexterity, reflex asymmetries, and a variety of subtle nonfocal neurological signs (soft signs).

If there are indications of possible absence spells, clinicians should obtain a neurological consultation and an EEG to rule out seizure disorders. A child with an unrecognized temporal lobe seizure focus may have behavior disturbances, which can resemble those of ADHD.

CLINICAL FEATURES

ADHD can have its onset in infancy, although it is rarely recognized until a child is at least toddler age. More commonly, infants with ADHD are active in the crib, sleep little, and cry a great deal.

In school, children with ADHD may attack a test rapidly, but may answer only the first two questions. They may be unable to wait to be called on in school and may respond before everyone else. At home, they cannot be put off for even a minute. Impulsiveness and an inability to delay gratification are characteristic. Children with ADHD are often susceptible to accidents.

The most cited characteristics of children with ADHD, in order of frequency, are hyperactivity, attention deficit (short attention span, distractibility, perseveration, failure to finish tasks, inattention, poor concentration), impulsivity (action before thought, abrupt shifts in activity, lack of organization, jumping up in class), memory and thinking deficits, specific learning disabilities, and speech and hearing deficits. Associated features often include perceptual motor impairment, emotional lability, and developmental coordination disorder. A significant percent of children with ADHD show behavioral symptoms of aggression and defiance. School difficulties, both learning and behavioral, commonly exist with ADHD. Comorbid communication disorders or learning disorders that hamper the acquisition, retention, and display of knowledge complicate the course of ADHD.

Justin was a 9-year-old African American adopted boy who was referred for an evaluation by his 4th grade teacher, who informed his adoptive parents that she was unable to manage Justin's impulsive and aggressive behaviors in the classroom. Justin was attending public school and was in a regular classroom with two resource room periods per day to help him with reading and math. Justin also received speech therapy once a week. Justin had been referred in the past for psychiatric evaluation, but his adoptive parents were opposed to medication so they did not follow through. Justin's adoptive parents knew very little about his biological family other than that his biological mother was known to be a polydrug abuser and was currently incarcerated. Justin was adopted as an infant and his pediatrician had told his adoptive parents that Justin was entirely healthy at birth. However, ever since kindergarten, Justin's teachers had complained that Justin did "not seem to listen," had "poor concentration," and was unable to stay in his seat. Because Justin was an engaging and cute child, his teachers in kindergarten and first grade made accommodations for him in their classrooms despite their complaints. When Justin entered the 2nd grade, however, it became clear that he was struggling with reading and writing, and an individualized educational program (IEP) evaluation was initiated. Justin was provided with resource room periods for remediation during the school day, but Justin continued to have additional problems getting along with his peers during lunch, and even at recess. Justin was often found arguing or fighting with other children who said that he did not know the rules of their games. Justin became angry when he was criticized by his peers and would often push his classmates. At home, Justin's adoptive parents were becoming more and more frustrated with Justin because he seemed to take hours to do a few math problems, and was unable to write a paragraph without a lot of help. Justin would become easily annoyed when frustrated with himself and then run around the house in a silly and disruptive manner. Justin was a good-hearted child who seemed to get along best with children who were younger than he was. Justin did not seem to make any close friends among his classmates, and the teachers indicated that Justin's peers sometimes avoided him because he was too rough during play and he did not follow the rules of their games. Justin had a difficult time waiting his turn and he became easily provoked when he was reprimanded. Consequently, Justin became alienated and often bullied by his classmates. Justin was aware that he was not able to keep up with the classwork, and he told his adoptive parents that he was just "stupid." Although Justin acted in a rambunctious and impulsive manner, he also appeared sad, and one day after a fight with several peers, he told his adoptive parents that he was going to "kill" himself. At this point, Justin's parents became worried and decided that Justin's teacher was right, and they would seek a psychiatric evaluation for Justin. During the initial evaluation with a child and adolescent psychiatrist, Justin was found to be a well-developed, cute, and active child, who appeared distracted and fidgety and somewhat sad. When asked about it, Justin said that he wanted to do "better" in school but that nobody liked him, he was failing his classes, and that he didn't like doing homework. He denied suicidal thoughts and reported that he had only said that to his parents because he was angry at his peers. Justin admitted that it was very difficult for him to understand his school work and impossible to complete his assignments. During the evaluation, several parent and teacher rating scales were obtained. These included The Child Behavior Checklist, and the SNAP Rating Scale. Justin's teacher and parents endorsed similar symptoms including poor organization, inability to follow directions, being forgetful in daily activities, impulsivity, with several episodes of running into the street without looking, blurting things out in the classroom without raising his hand, and recurrent fights with peers. Justin was observed to look dejected in school when he was excluded from play activities by peers, and sullen or angry at home when he was asked to read or do homework. Based on the clinical history, the rating scales and teacher's report, a diagnosis of Attention-Deficit/Hyperactivity Disorder, with the DSM-5 specifier of combined presentation, was made. In addition, Justin was noted to have a mood disorder with depressed mood, which did not qualify for a major depression. A treatment plan was suggested including a behavioral plan allowing Justin to receive rewards for effort on his homework along with a trial of a stimulant medication. After an extensive medical history was obtained and a recent physical examination by his pediatrician did not reveal any systemic illnesses, an EEG was decided upon, mainly because it was not possible to obtain a full medical and cardiac history due to an absence of early medical records, and his adoptive parents did not have access to his birth and neonatal medical records. After obtaining a normal EEG, Justin was started on a trial dose of a short-acting stimulant, methylphenidate (Ritalin) at 10 mg, to determine if he could tolerate a stimulant without any unexpected sensitivities. Justin had no adverse effects and was shortly switched to the long-acting stimulant Concerta, 36 mg which would last between 10 and 12 hours. Justin became more vigilant in class and seemed to be less restless and more focused, and his teacher reported that he was not getting out of his seat as often, although he continued to blurt out in class when he was not called on, and he continued to have difficulty following directions and forgetting things. Because Justin was not experiencing any adverse effects and was still displaying some ADHD symptoms, his Concerta was increased to 54 mg per day. At this dose both his teacher and parents noticed a marked improvement in his ability to sit and finish his classwork and homework. However, he began to have significant problems with insomnia, and was becoming fatigued from not being able to fall asleep until about 2 AM on a nightly basis. The child and adolescent psychiatrist and Justin's parents discussed two options to address the insomnia. One was to add a dose of short-acting clonidine in the evenings to cause a calming effect along with some sedative properties, and the other was to initiate a trial of Daytrana, the methylphenidate transdermal patch, which could be applied to deliver a similar dose of methylphenidate throughout the day, and the patch could be removed at approximately 4 PM or 5 PM to determine which produced the desired effect for the target symptoms for the most optimal amount of time. Because the Daytrana patch may deliver medication for an hour or so after its removal, Justin would need to try several different removal times to find the optimal treatment time. Justin's family and his child psychiatrist determined that it would be the best next step for Justin to try the Daytrana patch rather than add an additional medication to treat his insomnia. Justin was tried on the Daytrana transdermal 20 mg patch and found that if it was removed by 5 PM, he was able to fall asleep within 30 to 45 minutes after getting into bed. Despite some mild erythema around the site of the patch, Justin experienced no other side effects and was glad that he did not have to take pills each morning. It was determined by Justin's parents, teachers, and child and adolescent psychiatrist that Justin's ADHD symptoms were now under much improved control. Justin began to receive better grades and his self-esteem was noticeably increased. However, Justin still had difficulties with peers and felt that he wasn't making as many friends as he wanted. Justin's child psychiatrist suggested that Justin be placed in a weekly social skills group that was led by a psychologist who had experience with group interventions for children with ADHD. This was arranged, and although Justin, at first, did not want to attend, after a few sessions, in which Justin was praised for appropriate interactions with peers within his group, Justin decided that he liked the group, and over time, even invited a few of his peers from the group to his home to play. The combination of the medication and the social skills group resulted in a significant improvement in Justin's ADHD symptoms as well as in the quality of his relationships with peers and even his family. (Adapted from Greenhill LL, Hechtman LI. Attention-Deficit/Hyperactivity Disorder. In: Sadock BJ, Sadock VA, Ruiz P, eds. *Kaplan & Sadock's Comprehensive Textbook of Psychiatry.* 9th ed. Vol 2. Philadelphia, PA: Lippincott Williams & Wilkins; 2009:3571.)

PATHOLOGY AND LABORATORY EXAMINATION

A child being evaluated for ADHD should receive a comprehensive psychiatric and medical history. Prenatal, perinatal, and toddler information should be included in the history. Complications of mother's pregnancy should also be obtained. Medical problems that may produce symptoms overlapping with ADHD include petit mal epilepsy, hearing and visual impairments, thyroid abnormalities, and hypoglycemia. A thorough cardiac history should be taken, including an investigation of the lifetime history of syncope, family history of sudden death, and a cardiac examination of the child. Although it is reasonable to obtain an ECG study prior to treatment, if any cardiac risk factors are present, a cardiology consultation and examination are warranted. No specific laboratory measures are pathognomonic of ADHD.

A continuous performance task, a computerized task in which a child is asked to press a button each time a particular sequence of letters or numbers is flashed on a screen, is not specifically a useful diagnostic tool for ADHD; however, it may be useful in comparing a child's performance before and after medication treatment, particularly at different doses. Children with poor attention tend to make errors of omission—that is, they fail to press the button when the sequence has flashed. Impulsivity is often manifested by errors of commission, in which an impulsive child cannot resist pushing the button, even when the desired sequence has not yet appeared on the screen.

DIFFERENTIAL DIAGNOSIS

A temperamental constellation of high activity level and short attention span, in the normal range for the child's age, and without impairment, should be ruled out. Differentiating these temperamental characteristics from the cardinal symptoms of ADHD before the age of 3 years is difficult, mainly because of the overlapping features of a normally immature nervous system and the emerging signs of visual-motor-perceptual impairments frequently seen in ADHD. Anxiety in a child needs to be evaluated. Anxiety can accompany ADHD as a symptom or comorbid disorder, and anxiety can manifest with overactivity and easy distractibility.

It is not uncommon for a child with ADHD to become demoralized or, in some cases, to develop depressive symptoms in reaction to persistent frustration with academic difficulties and resulting low self-esteem. Mania and ADHD share many core features, such as excessive verbalization, motoric hyperactivity, and high levels of distractibility. In addition, in children with mania, irritability seems to be more common than euphoria. Although mania and ADHD can coexist, children with bipolar I disorder exhibit more waxing and waning of symptoms than those with ADHD. Recent follow-up data for children who met the criteria for ADHD and subsequently developed bipolar disorder suggest that certain clinical features occurring during the course of ADHD predict future mania. Children with ADHD who had developed bipolar I disorder at 4-year follow-up had a greater co-occurrence of additional disorders and a greater family history of bipolar disorders and other mood disorders than children without bipolar disorder.

Frequently, oppositional defiant disorder, or conduct disorder and ADHD may coexist, and when that occurs, both disorders are diagnosed. Specific learning disorders of various kinds must also be distinguished from ADHD; a child may be unable to read or do mathematics because of a learning disorder, rather than because of inattention. ADHD often coexists with one or more learning problems, including deficits in reading, mathematics, or written expression.

COURSE AND PROGNOSIS

The course of ADHD is variable. Symptoms have been shown to persist into adolescence in 60 to 85 percent of cases, and into adult life in approximately 60 percent of cases. The remaining 40 percent of cases may remit at puberty, or in early adulthood. In some cases, the hyperactivity may disappear, but the decreased attention span and impulse-control problems persist. Overactivity is usually the first symptom to remit, and distractibility is the last. ADHD does not usually remit during middle childhood. Persistence is predicted by a family history of the disorder, negative life events, and comorbidity with conduct symptoms, depression, and anxiety disorders. When remission occurs, it is usually between the ages of 12 and 20. Remission can be accompanied by a productive adolescence and adult life, satisfying interpersonal relationships, and few significant sequelae. Most patients with the disorder, however, undergo partial remission and are vulnerable to antisocial behavior, substance use disorders, and mood disorders. Learning problems often continue throughout life.

In about 60 percent of cases, some symptoms persist into adulthood. Those who persist with the disorder may show diminished hyperactivity but remain impulsive and accident-prone. Although the educational attainments of people with ADHD as a group are lower than those of people without ADHD, early employment histories do not differ from those of people with similar educations.

Children with ADHD whose symptoms persist into adolescence are at higher risk for developing conduct disorder. Children with both ADHD and conduct disorder are also at risk for developing substance use disorders. The development of substance abuse disorders among ADHD youth in adolescence appears to be more related to the presence of conduct disorder rather than to ADHD.

Most children with ADHD have some social difficulties. Socially dysfunctional children with ADHD have significantly higher rates of comorbid psychiatric disorders, and experience more problems with behavior in school as well as with peers and family members. Overall, the outcome of ADHD in childhood seems to be related to the degree of persistent comorbid psychopathology, especially conduct disorder, social disability, and chaotic family factors. Optimal outcomes may be promoted by ameliorating children's social functioning, diminishing aggression, and improving family situations as early as possible.

TREATMENT

Pharmacotherapy

Pharmacologic treatment is considered the first line of treatment for ADHD. Central nervous system stimulants are the first choice of agents in that they have been shown to have the greatest efficacy with generally mild tolerable side effects. Stimulants are contraindicated in children, adolescents, and adults with known cardiac risks and abnormalities. In medically healthy youth, however, excellent safety records are documented for short- and sustained-release preparations of methylphenidate (Ritalin, Ritalin-SR, Concerta, Metadate CD, Metadate ER), dextroamphetamine (Dexedrine, Dexedrine spansules, Vyvanse), and dextroamphetamine and amphetamine salt combinations (Adderall, Adderall XR). Newer preparations of methylphenidate include Methylin, a chewable form of methylphenidate; Daytrana, a methylphenidate patch; and dexmethylphenidate, the D-enantiomer (Focalin), and its longer acting form Focalin XR. These newer preparations aim to maximize the target effects and minimize the adverse effects in individuals with ADHD who obtain partial response from methylphenidate or whose dose was limited by side effects. Vyvanse (lisdexamfetamine dimesylate) is a pro-drug of dextroamphetamine, which requires intestinal metabolism in order to reach its active form. Vyvanse is approved by the FDA for children 6 years and older. Vyvanse, inactive until it is metabolized, is a less likely agent to have risks of abuse or overdose. It has side effects and efficacy similar to the other forms of amphetamines used in the treatment of ADHD.

Current strategies favor once a day sustained-release stimulant preparations for their convenience and diminished rebound side effects. Advantages of the sustained-release preparations for children are that one dose in the morning will sustain the effects all day, and the child is no longer required to interrupt his or her school day, as well as the physiologic advantage that the medication is sustained at an approximately even level in the body throughout the day so that periods of rebound and irritability are avoided. Table 27.6–1 contains comparative information on the above medications.

Nonstimulant medications approved by the FDA in the treatment of ADHD include atomoxetine (Strattera), a norepinephrine uptake inhibitor. Unlike the stimulants, Strattera carries with it a "black box" warning for potential increases in suicidal thoughts or behaviors and requires children with ADHD to be monitored for these symptoms, similarly to children who are administered antidepressants. A-agonists including clonidine (Catapres) and guanfacine (Tenex) have also been found to be effective in treating ADHD. The FDA has recently approved the extended-release forms of clonidine (Kapvay) and the extended release form of guanfacine (Intuniv) for the treatment of ADHD in children 6 years and older. Antidepressants, such as bupropion (Wellbutrin, Wellbutrin SR), have been used with variable success in the treatment of ADHD. (Table 27.6–2 contains comparative information on the nonstimulant medications and Table 27.6–3 indicates FDA-approved ages for ADHD medications.)

Stimulant Medications. Methylphenidate and amphetamine preparations are dopamine agonists; however, the precise mechanism of the stimulant's central action remains unknown. Methylphenidate preparations have been shown to be highly effective in up to three-fourths of children with ADHD, with relatively few adverse effects. Concerta, the 10- to 12-hour extended-release OROS (osmotic controlled-release extended delivery system) form of methylphenidate, is administered once daily in the morning and is effective during school hours as well as after school during the afternoon and early evening. Both shorter forms of methylphenidate and Concerta have similar common adverse effects including headaches, stomachaches, nausea, and insomnia. Some children experience a rebound effect, in which they become mildly irritable and appear to be slightly hyperactive for a brief period when the medication wears off. In children with a history of motor tics, some observations must be made as, in some cases, methylphenidate can exacerbate the tics, whereas in other children the tics are unaffected or even improved. Because tics wax and wane, it is important to observe their patterns over some time. Another common concern about

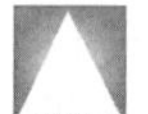

Table 27.6–1
Stimulant Medications in the Treatment of Attention-Deficit/Hyperactivity Disorder (ADHD)

Medication	Preparation (mg)	Approx. Duration (hours)	Recommended Dose
Methylphenidate preparations			
Ritalin	5, 10, 15, 20	3 to 4	0.3–1 mg/kg t.i.d.; up to 60 mg/day
Ritalin-SR	20	8	Up to 60 mg/day
Concerta	18, 36, 54	12	Up to 54 mg/q AM
Metadate ER	10, 20	8	Up to 60 mg/d
Metadate CD	20	12	Up to 60 mg/q AM
Ritalin LA	5, 10, 15, 20	8	Up to 60 mg/day
Methylin	5, 10, 20	3–4	0.3–1 mg/kg t.i.d. up to 60 mg/day
Daytrana Patch	10, 20, 30	12	30 mg/day
Dexmethylphenidate preparation			
Focalin	2.5, 5, 10	3 to 4	Up to 10 mg/day
Focalin XR	5, 10, 20	6 to 8	Up to 20 mg/day
Dextroamphetamine preparations			
Dexedrine	5, 10	3 to 4	0.15 to 0.5 mg/kg b.i.d.; up to 40 mg/day
Dexedrine Spansule	5, 10, 15	8	Up to 40 mg/day
Lisdexamfetamine			
Vyvanse	20, 30, 40, 50, 60, 70	12	Up to 70 mg/d; once daily
Combined Dextroamphetamine/amphetamine salts			
Adderall	5, 10, 20, 30	4 to 6	0.15 to 0.5 mg/kg b.i.d.; up to 40 mg/day
Adderall XR	10, 20, 30	12	Up to 40 mg q AM

t.i.d., three times daily; q, every; b.i.d., twice daily.

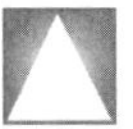

Table 27.6–2
Nonstimulant Medications for Attention-Deficit/Hyperactivity Disorder (ADHD)

Medication	Preparation (mg)	Recommended Dose
Atomoxetine HCl		
Strattera	10, 18, 25, 40	(0.5 to 1.8 mg/kg) 40 to 80 mg/day, may use b.i.d. dosing
Bupropion preparations		
Wellbutrin	75, 100	(3 to 6 mg/kg) 150 to 300 mg/day; up to 150 mg/dose b.i.d.
Wellbutrin SR	100, 150	(3 to 6 mg/kg) 150 to 300 mg/day; up to 150 mg q AM; >150 mg/day, use b.i.d. dosing
α-Adrenergic agonists		
Clonidine (Catapres)	0.1, 0.2, 0.3	up to 0.1 mg t.i.d.
Kapvay (Clonidine Extended release)	0.1, 0.2	0.1–0.2 mg b.i.d.
Guanfacine (Tenex)	1, 2	0.5 to 1.5 mg/day
Intuniv (Guanfacine extended release)	1, 2, 3, 4	Up to 4 mg/day; once daily

b.i.d., twice daily; q, every; t.i.d., three times daily.

use of methylphenidate preparations over long periods is potential growth suppression. During periods of use, methylphenidate is associated with slightly decreased rates of growth, and if used over many years continuously without any drug holidays growth suppression of about several centimeters has been noted. When given "drug holidays" on weekends or summers, children tend to eat more and also make up the growth. The methylphenidate products have been shown to improve ADHD children's scores on tasks of vigilance, such as on math calculation tests, the continuous performance task, and paired associations. Daytrana, a transdermal delivery system designed to release methylphenidate continuously on application of the patch to the skin, has been developed and approved for use in children and adolescents. Advantages of Daytrana include an alternative for children who have difficulties swallowing pills, and that the patch can individualize how many hours per day a given child with ADHD is receiving medication. This is important because a child with ADHD who needs the medication in the late afternoons to do homework but develops insomnia if the medication is still present after dinner, is able to remove the patch at the desired time. Thus, an individualized delivery time may be provided for each child by virtue of how many hours the patch is left on the skin. This is in contrast to oral sustained-release forms of methylphenidate, such as Concerta, in which the release time continues for 12 hours after the pill is swallowed. A double-blind randomized study in children with ADHD, who wore the methylphenidate patch for 12 hours at a time, showed efficacy of the patch preparation doses ranging from patches delivering 0.45 mg per hour to 1.8 mg per hour of methylphenidate. The effectiveness of the patch reached a plateau without much further improvement as dose was increased, but intensive behavioral interventions were

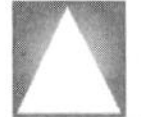

Table 27.6–3
FDA Approval for ADHD Medications

Medication	Generic Name	FDA Approval Age in Years
Methylphenidate		
Concerta	Methylphenidate	6 and older
	(OROS long acting)	6 and older
Ritalin	Methylphenidate	6 and older
Ritalin SR	Methylphenidate (extended release)	6 and older
Ritalin LA	Methylphenidate (long-acting)	6 and older
Metadate ER	Methylphenidate (extended release)	6 and older
Metadate CD	Methylphenidate (extended release)	6 and older
Methylin	Methylphenidate (oral solution and chewable tablet)	6 and older
Daytrana	Methylphenidate (patch)	6 and older
Dexmethylphenidate		
Focalin	Dexmethylphenidate	6 and older
Focalin XR	Dexmethylphenidate (extended release)	6 and older
Dextroamphetamine		
Dexedrine	Dextroamphetamine	3 and older
Amphetamine Salts		
Adderall	Amphetamine	3 and older
Adderall XR	Amphetamine (extended release)	6 and older
Lisdexamfetamine		
Vyvanse	Lisdexamfetamine	6 and older
Nonstimulants		
Strattera	Atomoxetine	6 and older
Alpha Agonists		
Kapvay	Clonidine (extended release)	6–17
Intuniv	Guanfacine (extended release)	6–17

also being administered. A delay in the onset of the transdermal medication effect was approximately an hour. Side effects were similar to oral preparations of methylphenidate. Approximately half of the children exhibited at least minor erythematous reactions to the patch; however, these side effects are usually well tolerated by children on the patch. Dextroamphetamine and dextroamphetamine/amphetamine salt combinations are usually the second drugs of choice when methylphenidate is not effective. Vyvanse is advantageous because it is inactive until it is metabolized.

Nonstimulant Medications. Atomoxetine HCl (Strattera) is a norepinephrine uptake inhibitor approved by the FDA for the treatment of ADHD in children age 6 years and older. The mechanism of action is not well understood, but it is believed to involve selective inhibition of presynaptic norepinephrine transporter. Atomoxetine is well absorbed by the gastrointestinal tract, and maximal plasma levels are reached in 1 to 2 hours after ingestion. It has been shown to be effective for inattention as well as impulsivity in children and in adults with ADHD. Its half-life is approximately 5 hours and it is usually administered twice daily. Most common side effects include diminished appetite, abdominal discomfort, dizziness, and irritability. In some cases, increases in blood pressure and heart rate have been reported. Atomoxetine is metabolized by the cytochrome P450 (CYP) 2D6 hepatic enzyme system. A small fraction of the population are poor metabolizers of CYP 2D6–metabolized drugs and, for those individuals, plasma concentrations of the drug may rise as much as fivefold for a given dose of medication. Drugs that inhibit CYP 2D6, including fluoxetine, paroxetine, and quinidine, may lead to increased plasma levels of this medication. Despite its short half-life, atomoxetine has been shown in a recent study to be effective in reducing symptoms of ADHD in children during the school day when administered once daily. Another recent study of a combination of atomoxetine alone and combined with fluoxetine in the treatment of 127 children with ADHD and symptoms of anxiety or depression suggested that atomoxetine alone can lead to improvements in mood and anxiety. Children who received combined atomoxetine and fluoxetine experienced greater increases in blood pressure and pulse than those who were treated with atomoxetine only.

α-Agonists, short-acting, and the extended-release forms of clonidine hydrochloride (Kapvay) and Guanfacine (Intuniv) are FDA approved for the treatment of ADHD in children and adolescents from 6 to 7 years of age. Kapvay, a centrally acting α-2-adrenergic receptor agonist is believed to exert its effect on the prefrontal cortex, although the mechanism of action is unknown. Kapvay is available in 0.1 mg and 0.2 mg tablets, and is generally used twice daily, once in the morning and once at night, to provide a round-the-clock effect. Kapvay is initiated at 0.1 mg at bedtime and can be increased in increments of 0.1 mg at weekly intervals. The maximal dose recommended is 0.2 mg twice daily. Kapvay is not used interchangeably with the short-acting clonidine. Because Kapvay is an antihypertensive agent, it causes a decrease in blood pressure and heart rate. These vital signs must be monitored in patients, especially during initiation and titration of the dose. Common side effects include somnolence, headache, upper abdominal pain, and fatigue. When Kapvay is tapered, it is recommended to taper no more than 0.1 mg every 3 to 7 days. Intuniv, the extended release preparation of guanfacine, is a once-a-day medication for children between 6 and 17 years of age, available in 1 mg, 2 mg, 3 mg, and 4 mg tabs. Intuniv is a tablet that is swallowed whole, and should be taken with water, milk or other liquids; it is not recommended to take Intuniv with a high-fat meal. Intuniv is typically initiated as a 1 mg tab daily and titrated by 1 mg per day at 1-week intervals. The maximum dose approved is 4 mg per day. As a monotherapy, improvements in ADHD symptoms have been found to occur at 0.05 to 0.08 mg/kg once daily. As an adjunctive treatment, optimal doses are reported to range from 0.05 to 0.12 mg/kg/day. Common side effects for Intuniv include somnolence, sedation, fatigue, nausea, hypotension, insomnia, and dizziness. Heart rate and blood pressure must be monitored as in Kapvay. When discontinuing Intuniv, a gradual taper decreasing by 1 mg every 3 to 7 days is recommended. α-Adrenergic agents including the short- and extended-release preparations of guanfacine and clonidine are sometimes preferred treatments in children with ADHD and comorbid tic disorders that have been exacerbated while the patient was taking stimulants. Bupropion has been shown to be somewhat effective for some children and adolescents in the treatment of ADHD. One multisite, double-blind, placebo-controlled study found a positive result regarding the efficacy of bupropion. No further studies have compared bupropion with other stimulants. The risk of seizure development while on this drug is increased when using doses of greater than 400 mg per day.

Few data confirm the efficacy of SSRIs in the treatment of ADHD, but due to the frequency of comorbid depression and anxiety with ADHD, in cases of comorbidity, the SSRIs are likely to be considered at least in conjunction with a stimulant.

Tricyclic drugs are not recommended in the treatment of ADHD due to potential cardiac arrhythmia effects. The reports of sudden death in at least four children with ADHD who were being treated with desipramine (Norpramin, Pertofrane) have made the tricyclic antidepressants an unlikely choice. Antipsychotics are occasionally introduced to treat refractory severely hyperactive children and adolescents who are significantly dysfunctional. Antipsychotics are generally not chosen in the treatment of ADHD due to the risks of tardive dyskinesia, withdrawal dyskinesia, neuroleptic malignant syndrome, and weight gain.

Modafinil (Provigil), another type of CNS stimulant, originally developed to reduce daytime sleepiness in patients with narcolepsy, has been tried clinically in the treatment of adults with ADHD. Only one randomized, double-blind, placebo-controlled study of the efficacy and safety of modafinil film-coated tablets in approximately 250 adolescents with ADHD showed that 48 percent of those on active treatment were rated as "much" or "very much" improved compared with 17 percent of patients receiving placebo. The dosage range was from 170 to 425 mg administered once daily, titrated to optimal doses based on efficacy and tolerability. Modafinil failed to receive FDA approval based on a Stevens–Johnson skin rash that occurred in a patient during the trial. The most common side effects included insomnia, headache, and decreased appetite.

Venlafaxine has been tried in clinical practice, especially for children and adolescents with combinations of ADHD and depression or anxiety features. No clear empirical evidence supports the use of venlafaxine in the treatment of ADHD.

One open-label report of reboxetine, a selective norepinephrine reuptake inhibitor, in 31 children and adolescents with ADHD who were resistant to methylphenidate treatment suggested that this agent may have efficacy. In this open trial, reboxetine was initiated and maintained at 4 mg per day. Most common side effects included drowsiness, sedation, and gastrointestinal symptoms. Reboxetine and other new agents in this class await controlled studies to further evaluate their potential efficacy.

Treatment of CNS Stimulant Side Effects. CNS stimulants are generally well tolerated, and current consensus is that once a day dosing is preferable for convenience and to minimize rebound side effects. Long-term tolerability of once-daily mixed amphetamine salts has shown mild side effects, most commonly decreased appetite, insomnia, and headache. A variety of strategies have been suggested for children and/or adolescents with ADHD who respond favorably to methylphenidate, but for whom insomnia has become a significant problem. Clinical strategies to manage insomnia include use of diphenhydramine (25 to 75 mg), low dose of trazodone (25 to 50 mg), or the addition of an α-adrenergic agent, such as guanfacine. In some cases, insomnia may attenuate on its own after several months of treatment.

Monitoring Pharmacological Treatment. Stimulant medications have adrenergic effects and cause moderate increases in blood pressure and pulse rate. At baseline, the most recent American Academy of Child and Adolescent Psychiatry (AACAP) practice parameters recommend the following workup before starting use of stimulant medications: physical examination, blood pressure, pulse, weight, and height.

It is recommended that children and adolescents being treated with stimulants have their height, weight, blood pressure, and pulse checked on a quarterly basis and have a physical examination annually. Monitoring starts with the initiation of medication. Because school performance is most markedly affected, special attention and effort should be given to establishing and maintaining a close collaborative working relationship with a child's school personnel. In most patients, stimulants reduce overactivity, distractibility, impulsiveness, explosiveness, and irritability. No evidence indicates that medications directly improve any existing impairments in learning, although, when the attention deficits diminish, children can learn more effectively. In addition, medication can improve self-esteem when children are no longer constantly reprimanded for their behavior. Children treated with medications should be taught the purpose of the medication and given the opportunity to describe any side effects that they may be experiencing.

Psychosocial Interventions

Psychosocial interventions for children with ADHD include psychoeducation, academic organization skills remediation, parent training, behavior modification in the classroom and at home, CBT, and social skills training. Social skills groups, behavioral training for parents of children with ADHD, and behavioral interventions at school and at home have been studied alone and in combination with medication management for ADHD. Evaluation and treatment of coexisting learning disorders or additional psychiatric disorders is important.

When children are helped to structure their environment, their anxiety diminishes. It is beneficial for parents and teachers to work together to develop a concrete set of expectations for the child and a system of rewards for the child when the expectations are met.

A common goal of therapy is to help parents of children with ADHD recognize and promote the notion that, although the child may not "voluntarily" exhibit symptoms of ADHD, he or she is still capable of being responsible for meeting reasonable expectations. Parents should also be helped to recognize that, despite their child's difficulties, every child faces the normal tasks of maturation, including significant building of self-esteem when he or she develops a sense of mastery. Therefore, children with ADHD do not benefit from being exempted from the requirements, expectations, and planning applicable to other children. Parental training is an integral part of the psychotherapeutic interventions for ADHD. Most parental training is based on helping parents develop usable behavioral interventions with positive reinforcement that target both social and academic behaviors.

Group therapy aimed at both refining social skills and increasing self-esteem and a sense of success may be very useful for children with ADHD who have great difficulty functioning in group settings, especially in school. A recent year-long group therapy intervention in a clinical setting for boys with the disorder described the goals as helping the boys improve skills in game playing and feeling a sense of mastery with peers. The boys were first asked to do a task that was fun, in pairs, and then were gradually asked to do projects in a group. They were directed in following instructions, waiting, and paying attention, and were praised for successful cooperation.

Multimodal Treatment Study of Children with ADHD (MTA Study)

The National Institute of Mental Health (NIMH)–supported Multimodal Treatment Study of Children with ADHD (The MTA Cooperative Group, 1999) was a 14-month–long randomized clinical trial involving six clinical sites comparing four treatment strategies. More than 500 children diagnosed with DSM-IV ADHD, combined type, were randomly assigned to (1) systematic medication management utilizing an initial placebo-controlled titration and t.i.d. dosing 7 days per week and monthly 30-minute clinic visits, (2) behavior therapy consisting of 27 sessions of group parent training, eight individual parent sessions, an 8-week summer treatment program, 12 weeks of classroom administered behavior therapy with a half-time aide, and 10 teacher consultation sessions, (3) a combination of medication and behavior therapy, or (4) usual community care. All groups showed improvement over baseline; however, a combination of medication management and behavior therapy led to greater reduction in symptoms in children with ADHD alone or ADHD and *oppositional defiant disorder* than behavior therapy alone or community care. The combination treatment had significantly better outcomes for those children with ADHD and anxiety and/or mood disorders compared to behavioral treatment and community care. Combined treatment but not medication management was superior for improvement in oppositional and aggressive symptoms, anxiety and mood symptoms, teacher rated social skills, parent–child relationships, and reading achievement. Furthermore, mean dose of medication per day was less in the combination group than in the medication-only management group.

Results

A follow-up of the MTA sample at 6 and 8 years revealed that the clinical presentation of the disorder, including severity of ADHD, comorbid conduct disturbance, and intellect were stronger predictors of later functioning than the type of treatment received in childhood during the 14-month study period. Although treatment-related improvements for the children who participated in the MTA study are maintained as long as treatment continues, the differential treatment efficacy appeared to be lost at approximately the 3-year mark.

Overall, the evidence suggests that medication and psychosocial interventions for the combined type of ADHD in childhood provides the broadest benefit in functioning for this population. This is especially pertinent in view of the comorbidity of learning disorders, anxiety, mood disorders, and other disruptive behavior disorders that occur in children with ADHD.

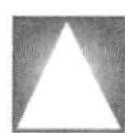

Table 27.6–4
Utah Criteria for Adult Attention-Deficit/Hyperactivity Disorder (ADHD)

I. Retrospective childhood ADHD diagnosis
   A. Narrow criterion: met DSM-IV criteria in childhood by parent interview[a]
   B. Broad criterion: both (1) and (2) are met as reported by patient[b]
      1. Childhood hyperactivity
      2. Childhood attention deficits
II. Adult characteristics: five additional symptoms, including ongoing difficulties with inattentiveness and hyperactivity and at least three other symptoms:
   A. Inattentiveness
   B. Hyperactivity
   C. Mood lability
   D. Irritability and hot temper
   E. Impaired stress tolerance
   F. Disorganization
   G. Impulsivity
III. Exclusions: not diagnosed in presence of severe depression, psychosis, or severe personality disorder

[a]Parent report aided with 10-item Parent Rating Scale of Childhood Behavior.
[b]Patient self-report of retrospective childhood symptoms aided by *Wender Utah Rating Scale.*

UNSPECIFIED ATTENTION-DEFICIT/HYPERACTIVITY DISORDER

The DSM-5 includes Unspecified ADHD as a category for disturbances of inattention or hyperactivity that cause impairment, but do not meet the full criteria for ADHD.

ADULT MANIFESTATIONS OF ADHD

ADHD was historically believed to be a childhood condition resulting in delayed development of impulse control that would be generally outgrown by adolescence. In the last few decades many more adults with ADHD have been identified, diagnosed, and successfully treated. Longitudinal follow-up has shown that up to 60 percent of children with ADHD have persistent impairment from symptoms into adulthood. Genetic studies, brain imaging, and neurocognitive and pharmacological studies in adults with ADHD have replicated findings demonstrated in children with ADHD. Increased public awareness and treatment studies within the last decade have led to widespread acceptance of the need for diagnosis and treatment of adults with ADHD.

Epidemiology

Among adults, evidence suggests an approximate 4 percent prevalence of ADHD in the population. ADHD in adulthood is generally diagnosed by self-report, given the lack of school information and observer information available; therefore, it is more difficult to make an accurate diagnosis.

Etiology

Currently, ADHD is believed to be largely transmitted genetically, and increasing evidence supports this hypothesis, including the genetic studies, twin studies, and family studies outlined in the child and adolescent ADHD section. Brain imaging studies have obtained data suggesting that adults with ADHD exhibit decreased prefrontal glucose metabolism on PET compared with adults without ADHD. It is unclear whether these data reflect the presence of the disorder or a secondary effect of having ADHD over a period of time. Further studies using SPECT have revealed increased dopamine transporter (DAT) binding densities in the striatum of the brain in samples of adults with ADHD. This finding may be understood within the context of treatment for ADHD, in that standard stimulant treatment for ADHD, such as methylphenidate, acts to block DAT activity, possibly leading to a normalization of the striatal brain region in individuals with ADHD.

Diagnosis and Clinical Features

The clinical phenomenology of ADHD features inattention and manifestations of impulsivity prevailing as the core of this disorder. A leading figure in the development of criteria for adult manifestations of ADHD is Paul Wender, from the University of Utah, who began his work on adult ADHD in the 1970s. Wender developed criteria that could be applied to adults (Table 27.6–4) they included a retrospective diagnosis of ADHD in childhood, and evidence of current impairment from ADHD symptoms in adulthood. Furthermore, evidence exists of several additional symptoms that are typical of adult behavior as opposed to childhood behaviors.

In adults, residual signs of the disorder include impulsivity and attention deficit (e.g., difficulty in organizing and completing work, inability to concentrate, increased distractibility, and sudden decision-making without thought of the consequences). Many people with the disorder have a secondary depressive disorder associated with low self-esteem related to their impaired performance and which affects both occupational and social functioning.

Brett was a 26-year-old man convinced by his new wife to seek an evaluation for his distractibility, forgetfulness, and "not listening" after a minor traffic accident. After consulting his mother, Brett reported that in grade school, he was often "in trouble" for talking out of turn, and his mother recalled teachers' reports that Brett often made careless mistakes on tests, forgot his assignments, and had great difficulty sitting still. Although as a young child he was considered gifted intellectually, when he got to the third grade his grades were only average, and he seemed more interested in getting his work done quickly than correctly. Brett was talkative and loud and enjoyed sports, although he was not particularly talented at them. Nevertheless, Brett had acquaintances and superficial friends because he was likeable, funny, and even entertaining. Brett had no idea what he wanted to do when he grew up, and during his senior year in high school, he neglected to finish any of his college applications on time, and ended up attending a community college part-time. During the two years after high school, Brett held down a series of jobs only briefly, including a construction job, a waiter position in a restaurant, and a Fed-Ex driver, and then decided that he wanted to become an actor. Brett went on a series of auditions, but found that he would become distracted and did poorly remembering his lines and even spaced out during readings. Despite that, he was chosen for one commercial. Brett reported that he had never had problems with abuse of drugs or alcohol, and he occasionally drank beer socially. During his evaluation with a child and adolescent psychiatrist, Brett disclosed that his greatest difficulties were with tasks that seemed boring to him. He had difficulty maintaining his attention, was easily distracted, felt restless most of the time, and became frustrated when he was expected to sit still for long periods of time. Brett endorsed 6 inattentive and 5 hyperactive/impulsive symptoms on a DSM ADHD Checklist of current symptoms. Brett met the diagnostic criteria for Adult ADHD, combined type, with a probable onset in childhood. Brett's medical history was negative for all major illnesses, and neither he nor his parents had a history of cardiac abnormalities. He took no prescribed medications. After discussing the situation with his psychiatrist and his wife, Brett decided that he would like to try a stimulant medication. A trial of a once-a-day extended-release formulation of a stimulant medication was selected: Adderall XR 10 mg. At his first follow-up visit, a week later, Brett reported that he felt a slight effect from this medication but it was not enough to improve his functioning, so Brett and his psychiatrist agreed that he would increase his dose to 20 mg per day. At his next follow-up appointment, Brett reported that he had noticed significant improvement in his ability to focus, concentrate, and remember his lines in auditions. In fact, he had just received a small part in an upcoming movie. Brett and his wife were both thrilled with the results, and Brett continued to return monthly for follow up visits. (Adapted from McGough J. Adult manifestations of attention-deficit/hyperactivity disorder. In: Sadock BJ, Sadock VA, Ruiz P, eds. *Kaplan & Sadock's Comprehensive Textbook of Psychiatry.* 9th ed. Philadelphia, PA: Lippincott Williams & Wilkins; 2009:3577.)

Differential Diagnosis

A diagnosis of ADHD is likely when symptoms of inattention and impulsivity are described by adults as a life-long problem, not as episodic events. The overlap of ADHD and hypomania, bipolar II disorder, and cyclothymia is controversial and difficult to sort out retrospectively. Clear-cut histories of discrete episodes of hypomania and mania, with or without periods of depression, are suggestive of a mood disorder rather than a clinical picture of ADHD; however, ADHD may have predated the emergence of a mood disorder in some individuals. In such a case, ADHD and bipolar disorder may be diagnosed comorbidly. Adults with an early history of chronic school difficulties related to paying attention, activity level, and impulsive behavior are generally diagnosed with ADHD, even when a mood disorder occurs later in life. Anxiety disorders can coexist with ADHD, and are less difficult than hypomania to distinguish from it.

Course and Prognosis

The prevalence of ADHD diminishes over time, although at least half of children and adolescents may have the disorder into adulthood. Many children initially diagnosed with ADHD, combined type, exhibit fewer impulsive-hyperactive symptoms as they get older and, by the time they are adults, will meet criteria for ADHD, inattentive type. As with children, adults with ADHD demonstrate higher rates of learning disorders, anxiety disorders, mood disorders, and substance use disorder compared with the general population.

Treatment

Treatment of ADHD in adults targets pharmacotherapy, mainly long-acting stimulants, similar to that used with children and adolescents with ADHD. In adults, only the long-acting stimulants are FDA approved in the treatment of ADHD. Signs of a positive response are an increased attention span, decreased impulsiveness, and improved mood. Psychopharmacological therapy may be needed indefinitely. Clinicians should use standard ways to monitor drug response and patient compliance.

▲ 27.7 Specific Learning Disorder

Specific learning disorder in youth is a neurodevelopmental disorder produced by the interactions of heritable and environmental factors that influence the brain's ability to efficiently perceive or process verbal and nonverbal information. It is characterized by persistent difficulty learning academic skills in reading, written expression, or mathematics, beginning in early childhood, that is inconsistent with the overall intellectual ability of a child. Children with specific learning disorder often find it difficult to keep up with their peers in certain academic subjects, whereas they may excel in others. Academic skills that may be compromised in specific learning disorder include reading single words and sentences fluently, written expression and spelling, and calculation and solving mathematical problems. Specific learning disorder results in underachievement that is unexpected based on the child's potential as well as the opportunity to have learned more. Specific learning disorder in reading, spelling, and mathematics appears to aggregate in families. There is an increased risk of four to eight times in first-degree relatives for reading deficits, and about five to ten times for mathematics deficits, compared to the general population. Specific learning disorder occurs two to three times more often in males than in females. Learning problems in a child or adolescent identified in this manner can establish eligibility for academic services through the public school system.

The American Psychiatric Association's Fifth Edition of the *Diagnostic and Statistical Manual of Mental Disorders* (DSM-5) combines the DSM-IV diagnoses of reading disorder, mathematics disorder, and disorder of written expression and learning disorder not otherwise specified into a single diagnosis: specific learning disorder. Learning deficits in reading, written expression, and mathematics in the DSM-5 are designated using specifiers. DSM-5 notes that the term *dyslexia* is an equivalent term describing a pattern of learning difficulties, including deficits in accurate or fluent word recognition, poor decoding, and poor spelling skills. *Dyscalculia* is noted to be an alternative term referring to a pattern of deficits related to learning arithmetic facts, processing numerical information, and performing accurate calculations.

Specific learning disorder of all types affects approximately 10 percent of youth. This represents approximately half of all public school children who receive special education services in the United States. In 1975, Public Law 94–142 (the Education for All Handicapped Children Act now known as the Individual with Disabilities Education Act [IDEA]) mandated all states to provide free and appropriate educational services to all children. Since that time, the number of children identified with learning disorders has increased, and a variety of definitions of learning disabilities have arisen. To meet the criteria for specific learning disorder, a child's achievement must be significantly lower than expected in one or more of the following: reading skills, comprehension, spelling, written expression, calculation, mathematical reasoning, and/or the learning problems interfere with academic achievement or activities of daily living. It is common for specific learning disorder to include more than one area of skills deficits.

Children with specific learning disorder in the area of reading can be identified by poor word recognition, slow reading rate, and impaired comprehension compared with most children of the same age. Current data suggest that most children with reading difficulties have deficits in speech sound processing skills, regardless of their IQ, and in DSM-5, there is no longer a diagnostic criterion for specific learning disorder comparing the specific deficit to overall IQ. Current consensus is that children with reading impairment have trouble with word recognition and "sounding out" words because they cannot efficiently process and use phonemes (the smaller bits of words that are associated with particular sounds). A recent epidemiologic study found four profiles including (1) weak reading, (2) weak language, (3) weak math, or (4) combined weak math and reading, accounting for 70 percent of children with specific learning impairments. Low scores in short-term memory for speech sounds characterized the profile with weak language, whereas, low speech sound awareness was associated with the weak reading group, but not the weak language group. Finally, in another recent study it was found that the weak math group did not show speech sound deficits.

Severe specific learning disorder may make it agonizing for a child to succeed in school, often leading to demoralization, low self-esteem, chronic frustration, and compromised peer relationships. Specific learning disorder is associated with an increased risk of comorbid disorders, including ADHD, communication disorders, conduct disorders, and depressive disorders. Adolescents with specific learning disorder are at least 1.5 times more likely to drop out of school, approximating rates of 40 percent. Adults with specific learning disorder are at increased risk for difficulties in employment and social adjustment. Specific learning disorder often extends to skills deficits in multiple areas such as reading, writing, and mathematics.

Moderate to high heritability is believed to contribute to specific learning disorder, and furthermore, it appears that many cognitive traits are polygenic. In addition, there is pleiotropy, that is, the same genes may affect skills necessary for diverse learning tasks. Factors such as perinatal injury and specific neurological conditions may contribute to the development of specific learning disorder. Conditions such as lead poisoning, fetal alcohol syndrome, and in utero drug exposure are also associated with increased rates of specific learning disorder.

SPECIFIC LEARNING DISORDER WITH IMPAIRMENT IN READING

Reading impairment is present in up to 75 percent of children and adolescents with specific learning disorder. Students who have learning problems in other academic areas most commonly experience difficulties with reading as well.

Reading impairment is characterized by difficulty in recognizing words, slow and inaccurate reading, poor comprehension, and difficulties with spelling. Reading impairment is often comorbid with other disorders in children, particularly, ADHD. The term *developmental alexia* was historically used to define a developmental deficit in the recognition of printed symbols. This was simplified by adopting the term *dyslexia* in the 1960s. Dyslexia was used extensively for many years to describe a reading disability syndrome that often included speech and language deficits and right–left confusion. Reading impairment is frequently accompanied by disabilities in other academic skills, and the term dyslexia remains as an alternate term for a pattern of reading and spelling difficulties.

Epidemiology

An estimated 4 to 8 percent of youth in the United States have been identified with dyslexia, encompassing a variety of reading, spelling, and comprehension deficits. Three to four times as many boys as girls are reported to have reading impairments in clinically referred samples. In epidemiological samples, however, rates of reading impairments are much closer among boys and girls. Boys with reading impairment are referred for psychiatric evaluation more often than girls due to comorbid ADHD and disruptive behavior problems. No clear gender differential is seen among adults who report reading difficulties.

Comorbidity

Children with reading difficulties are at high risk for additional learning deficits including mathematics and written expression. The DSM-5 language disorder, also known as specific language impairment, has traditionally been viewed as distinct from dyslexia and dyscalculia. Children with language disorder have poor word knowledge, limited abilities to form accurate sentence structure, and impairments in the ability to put words together to produce clear explanations. Children with language disorder may have delayed development of language acquisition, and difficulties with grammar and syntactical knowledge. Specific learning disorder in the areas of reading and mathematics frequently occur comorbidly with language disorder. In one study, it was found that among dyslexic samples, 19 to 63 percent also have language impairment. Conversely, reading impairment has been found in 12.5 to 85 percent of individuals with language disorder. In twin studies, reading impairments were found to be significantly higher in those children with specific learning impairment and in family members of children with the disorder. There are also high rates of comorbidity between reading impairment and mathematics impairment; in some studies the comorbidity has been reported to be up to 60 percent. It appears that children with both reading and math impairment may perform more poorly in mathematics; however, the reading skills of the comorbid children were no different from children who had only reading disorder and not math disorder. Comorbid psychiatric disorders are also frequent, such as ADHD, oppositional defiant disorder, conduct disorders, and depressive disorders, especially in adolescents. Data suggest that up to 25 percent of children with reading impairment may have comorbid ADHD. Conversely, it is estimated that between 15 and 30 percent of children diagnosed with ADHD have specific learning disorder. Family studies suggest that ADHD and reading impairment may share some degree of heritability. That is, some genetic factors contribute to both reading impairment and attentional syndromes. Youth with reading impairments have higher than average rates of depression on self-report measures and experience higher levels of anxiety symptoms than children without specific learning disorder. Furthermore, children with reading impairment are at increased risk for poor peer relationships and exhibit less skill in responding to subtle social cues.

Etiology

Data from cognitive, neuroimaging, and genetic studies suggest that reading impairment is a neurobiological disorder with a significant genetic contribution. It reflects a deficiency in processing sounds of speech sounds, and thus, spoken language. Children who struggle with reading most likely also have a deficit in speech sound processing skills. Children with this deficit cannot effectively identify the parts of words that denote specific sounds, leading to difficulty in recognizing and "sounding out" words. Youth with reading impairment are slower than peers in naming letters and numbers. The core deficits for children with reading impairment include poor processing of speech sounds and deficits in comprehension, spelling, and sounding out words.

Because reading impairment typically includes a language deficit, the left brain has been hypothesized to be the anatomical site of this dysfunction. Several studies using MRI studies have suggested that the planum temporale in the left brain shows less asymmetry than the same site in the right brain in children with both language disorders and specific learning disorder. PET studies have led some researchers to conclude that left temporal blood flow patterns during language tasks differ between children with and without learning disorders. Cell analysis studies suggest that in reading impaired individuals, the visual magnocellular system (which normally contains large cells) contains more disorganized and smaller cell bodies than expected. Studies indicate that 35 to 40 percent of first-degree relatives of children with reading deficits also have reading disability. Several studies have suggested that phonological awareness (i.e., the ability to decode sounds and sound out words) is linked to chromosome 6. Furthermore, the ability to identify single words has been linked to chromosome 15. Impairment in reading and spelling has now been linked to susceptibility loci on multiple chromosomes, including chromosomes 1, 2, 3, 6, 15, and 18. Although a recent research study identified a locus on chromosome 18 as a strong influence on single word reading and phoneme awareness, generalist genes have also been implicated as responsible for learning disorders. Many genes believed to be associated with specific learning disorder, may also influence normal variation in learning abilities. In addition, genes that affect abilities in reading, for example, are hypothesized to also affect written expression and potentially mathematics skills.

Several historical hypotheses about the origin of reading deficits are now known to be untrue. The first myth is that reading impairments are caused by visual–motor problems, or what has been termed *scotopic sensitivity syndrome.* There is no evidence that children with reading impairment have visual problems or difficulties with their visual–motor system. The second false theory is that allergies can cause, or contribute to, reading disability. Finally, unsubstantiated theories have implicated the cerebellar–vestibular system as the source of reading disabilities.

Research in cognitive neuroscience and neuropsychology supports the hypothesis that encoding processes and working memory, rather than attention or long-term memory, are areas of weakness for children with reading impairment. One study found an association between dyslexia and birth in the months of May, June, and July, suggesting that prenatal exposure to a maternal infectious illness, such as influenza, in the winter months may contribute to reading disabilities. Complications during pregnancy and prenatal and perinatal difficulties are common in the histories of children with reading disabilities. Extremely low–birth-weight and severely premature children are at higher risk for specific learning disorder. Children born very preterm have been noted to be at increased risk of minor motor, behavioral, and specific learning disorder.

An increased incidence of reading impairment occurs in intellectually average children with cerebral palsy and epilepsy. Children with postnatal brain lesions in the left occipital lobe, resulting in right visual-field blindness, as well as youth with lesions in the splenium of the corpus callosum that blocks transmission of visual information from the intact right hemisphere to the language areas of the left hemisphere experience reading impairments.

Children malnourished for long periods during early childhood are at increased risk of compromised performance cognition, including reading.

Diagnosis

Reading impairment is diagnosed when a child's reading achievement is significantly below that expected of a child of the same. Characteristic diagnostic features include difficulty recalling, evoking, and sequencing printed letters and words; processing sophisticated grammatical constructions; and making inferences. School failure and ensuing poor self-esteem can exacerbate the problems as a child becomes more consumed with a sense of failure and spends less time focusing on academic work. Students with reading impairment are entitled to an educational evaluation through the school district to determine eligibility for special education services. Special education classification, however, is not uniform across states or regions, and students with identical reading difficulties may be eligible for services in one region, but ineligible in another.

Clinical Features

Children with reading disabilities are usually identified by the age of 7 years (second grade). Reading difficulty may be apparent among students in classrooms where reading skills are expected as early as the first grade. Children can sometimes compensate for reading disorder in the early elementary grades by the use of memory and inference, particularly in children with high intelligence. In such instances, the disorder may not be apparent until age 9 (fourth grade) or later. Children with reading impairment make many errors in their oral reading. The errors are characterized by omissions, additions, and distortions of words. Such children have difficulty in distinguishing between printed letter characters and sizes, especially those that differ only in spatial orientation and length of line. The problems in managing printed or written language can pertain to individual letters, sentences, and even a page. The child's reading speed is slow, often with minimal comprehension. Most children with reading disability have an age-appropriate ability to copy from a written or printed text, but nearly all spell poorly.

Associated problems include language difficulties: discrimination and difficulty in sequencing words properly. A child with reading disorders may start a word either in the middle or at the end of a printed or written sentence. Most children with reading disorder dislike and avoid reading and writing. Their anxiety is heightened when they are confronted with demands that involve printed language. Many children with specific learning disorder who do not receive remedial education have a sense of shame and humiliation because of their continuing failure and subsequent frustration. These feelings grow more intense with time. Older children tend to be angry and depressed and exhibit poor self-esteem.

Jackson, a 10-year-old boy, was referred for evaluation of failing to complete in-class assignments and homework, and failing tests in reading, spelling, and arithmetic. For the past 2 years (grades 5 and 6), he had been attending a special education class every morning in the local community school, based on an assessment from the second grade. A subsequent psychoeducational assessment by a clinical psychologist confirmed reading problems. Jackson was eligible for a full-day special education class, whereupon he started attending a program with eight other students ranging from 6 to 12 years of age.

Clinical interview with his parents revealed a normal pregnancy and neonatal period, and a history of language delay. In preschool and kindergarten, Jackson was reported to have had difficulty with rhyming games and showed a lack of interest in books and preferred to play with construction toys. In the first grade, Jackson had more difficulty learning to read than other boys in his class and continued to have problems pronouncing multisyllabic words (e.g., he said "aminals" for "animals" and "sblanation" for "explanation"). Family history was positive for reading deficits and ADHD. Jackson's father disclosed a history of his own reading problems, and Jackson's older brother, 15 years of age, had ADHD, which was well controlled with stimulant medication. Jackson's parents were concerned about his poor focus in school, and wondered whether he had ADHD. In the clinical interview with Jackson, he rarely made eye contact, mumbled a lot, and struggled to find the right words (e.g., manifested many false starts, hesitations, and nonspecific terms, such as "the thing that you draw ... um ... pencil—no ... um ... lines with"). He admitted to disliking school, adding "Reading is boring and stupid—I'd rather be skateboarding." Jackson complained about how much reading he was given—even in math—and commented, "Reading takes so much time. By the time I figure out a word, I can't remember what I just read and so have to read the stuff again."

Psychoeducational assessment included the Wechsler Intelligence Scale for Children-IV, Clinical Evaluation of Language Fundamentals-IV (CELF-IV), the Wechsler Individual Achievement Test-II, and self-ratings of anxiety, depression, and self-esteem. Results indicated low-average verbal and above average performance IQ, poor word attack and word identification skills (below 12th percentile), poor comprehension (below 9th percentile), poor spelling (below 6th percentile), weak comprehension of oral language (below 16th percentile), elevated but subthreshold scores on the Children's Depression Inventory, and low self-esteem. Although Jackson manifested symptoms of inattention, restlessness, and oppositional behavior (particularly at school), he did not meet criteria for ADHD. Jackson met DSM-5 criteria for specific learning disorder, with deficits in reading and written expression. Recommendations included continuation in special education plus attendance at a summer camp specializing in children with reading disorder, as well as ongoing monitoring of self-esteem and depressive traits.

At 1-year follow-up, Jackson and his parents reported striking improvements in his reading, overall school performance, mood, and self-esteem. Both Jackson and his family felt that the specialized instruction provided during the summer camp was very helpful. The program had provided one-on-one focused and explicit instruction for 1 hour a day for a total of 70 hours. Jackson explained that he had been taught "like a game plan" to read, and challenged the clinician to give him a "really tough long word to read." He demonstrated strategies that he had learned to read the word "unconditionally" and also explained what it meant. To boost his fluency in reading and comprehension, he was provided with assignments to read along with audio-taped versions of books, use of graphic organizers to facilitate reading comprehension, and continued participation in the summer camp reading program. *(Adapted from Rosemary Tannock, Ph.D.)*

Pathology and Laboratory Examination

No specific physical signs or laboratory measures are helpful in the diagnosis of reading deficits. Psychoeducational testing, however, is critical in determining these deficits. The diagnostic battery generally includes a standardized spelling test, written composition, processing and using oral language, design copying, and judgment of the adequacy of pencil use. The reading subtests of the *Woodcock-Johnson Psycho-Educational Battery-Revised,* and the *Peabody Individual Achievement Test-Revised* are useful in identifying reading disability. A screening projective battery may include human-figure drawings, picture-story tests, and sentence completion. The evaluation should also include systematic observation of behavioral variables.

Course and Prognosis

Children with reading disability may gain knowledge of printed language during their first 2 years in grade school, without remedial assistance. By the end of the first grade, many children with reading problems, in fact, have learned how to read a few words; however, by the third grade, keeping up with classmates is exceedingly difficult without remedial educational intervention. When remediation is instituted early, in milder cases, it may not be necessary after the first or second grade. In severe cases and depending on the pattern of deficits and strengths, remediation may be continued into the middle and high school years.

Differential Diagnosis

Reading deficits are often accompanied by comorbid disorders, such as language disorder, disability in written expression, and ADHD. Data indicate that children with reading disability consistently present difficulties with linguistic skills, whereas children with ADHD only, do not. Children with reading disability, without ADHD, however, may have some overlapping deficits in cognitive inhibition, for example, they perform impulsively on continuous performance tasks. Deficits in expressive language and speech discrimination along with reading disorder may lead to a comorbid diagnosis of language disorder. Reading impairment must be differentiated from intellectual disability syndromes in which reading, along with most other skills, are below the achievement expected for a child's chronological age. Intellectual testing helps to differentiate global deficits from more specific reading difficulties.

Poor reading skills resulting from inadequate schooling can be detected by comparing a given child's achievement with classmates on reading performance on standardized reading tests. Hearing and visual impairments should be ruled out with screening tests.

Treatment

Remediation strategies for children with reading impairments focus on direct instruction that leads a child's attention to the connections between speech sounds and spelling. Effective remediation programs begin by teaching the child to make accurate associations between letters and sounds. This approach is based on the theory that the core deficits in reading impairments are related to difficulty recognizing and remembering the associations between letters and sounds. After individual letter-sound associations have been mastered, remediation can target larger components of reading such as syllables and words. The exact focus of any reading program can be determined only after accurate assessment of a child's specific deficits and weaknesses. Positive coping strategies include small, structured reading groups that offer individual attention and make it easier for a child to ask for help.

Children and adolescents with reading difficulties are entitled to an individual education program (IEP) provided by the public school system. Yet, for high school students with persistent reading disorders and ongoing difficulties with decoding and work identification, IEP services may not be sufficient to remediate their problems. A study of students with reading disorders in 54 schools indicated that, at the high school level, specific goals are not adequately met solely through school remediation. It is likely that high schoolers with persisting reading difficulties may have greater benefit from individualized reading remediation.

Reading instruction programs such as the Orton Gillingham and Direct Instructional System for Teaching and Remediation (DISTAR) approaches begin by concentrating on individual letters and sounds, advance to the mastery of simple phonetic units, and then blend these units into words and sentences. Thus, if children are taught to cope with graphemes, they will learn to read. Other reading remediation programs, such as the Merrill program, and the *Science Research Associates, Inc. (SRA) Basic Reading Program,* begin by introducing whole words first and then teach children how to break them down and recognize the sounds of the syllables and the individual letters in the word. Another approach teaches children with reading disorders to recognize whole words through the use of visual aids and bypasses the sounding-out process. One such program is called the *Bridge Reading Program.* The Fernald method uses a multisensory approach that combines teaching whole words with a tracing technique so that the child has kinesthetic stimulation while learning to read the words.

SPECIFIC LEARNING DISORDER WITH IMPAIRMENT IN MATHEMATICS

Children with mathematics difficulties have difficulty learning and remembering numerals, cannot remember basic facts about numbers, and are slow and inaccurate in computation. Poor achievement in four groups of skills have been identified in mathematics disorder: linguistic skills (those related to understanding mathematical terms and converting written problems into mathematical symbols), perceptual skills (the ability to recognize and understand symbols and order clusters of numbers), mathematical skills (basic addition, subtraction, multiplication, division, and following sequencing of basic operations), and attentional skills (copying figures correctly and observing operational symbols correctly). A variety of terms over the years, including *dyscalculia, congenital arithmetic disorder, acalculia, Gerstmann syndrome,* and *developmental arithmetic disorder* have been used to denote the difficulties present in mathematics disorder. Core deficits in dyscalculia are in processing numbers, and good language abilities are skills needed for accurate counting, calculating, and understanding mathematical principles.

Mathematics deficits can, however, occur in isolation or in conjunction with language and reading impairments. According to the DSM-5, the diagnosis of specific learning disorder with impairment in mathematics consists of deficits in arithmetic counting and calculations, has difficulty remembering mathematics facts, and may count on fingers instead. Additional deficits include difficulty with mathematic concepts and reasoning, leading to difficulties in applying procedures to solve quantitative problems. These deficits lead to skills that are substantially below what is expected for the child's chronological age and cause significant interference in academic success, as documented by standardized academic achievement testing.

Epidemiology

Mathematics disability alone is estimated to occur in about 1 percent of school-age children, that is about one of every five children with specific learning disorder. Epidemiological studies have indicated that up to 6 percent of school-age children have some difficulty with mathematics, and prevalence estimates of 3.5 to 6.5 percent have been reported for impairing forms of dyscalculia. Although specific learning disorder overall occurs two to three times more often in males, mathematics deficits may be relatively more frequent in girls than reading deficits. Many studies of learning disorders in children have grouped reading, writing, and mathematics disability together, which makes it more difficult to ascertain the precise prevalence of mathematics disability.

Comorbidity

Mathematics deficits are commonly found to be comorbid, with deficits in both reading and written expression. Children with mathematics difficulties may also be at higher risk for expressive language problems, and developmental coordination disorder.

Etiology

Mathematics deficiency, as with other areas of specific learning disorder, has a significant genetic contribution. High rates of comorbidity with reading deficits have been reported in the range of 17 percent up to 60 percent. One theory proposed a neurological deficit in the right cerebral hemisphere, particularly in the occipital lobe areas. These regions are responsible for processing visual–spatial stimuli that, in turn, are responsible for mathematical skills. This theory, however, has received little support in subsequent neuropsychiatric studies.

Causes of deficits in mathematics are believed to be multifactorial, including genetic, maturational, cognitive, emotional, educational, and socioeconomic factors. Prematurity and very low birth weight are also a risk factor for specific learning disorder, including mathematics. Compared with reading abilities, arithmetic abilities seem to depend more on the amount and quality of instruction.

Diagnosis

The diagnosis of specific learning disorder in mathematics is made when a child's skill in mathematical reasoning, or calculation, remain significantly below what is expected for that child's age, for a period of at least 6 months, even when remedial interventions have been administered. Many different skills contribute to mathematics proficiency. These include linguistic skills, conceptual skills, and computational skills. Linguistic skills involve being able to understand mathematical terms, understand word problems, and translate them into the proper mathematical process. Conceptual skills involve recognition of mathematical symbols and being able to use mathematical signs correctly. Computational skills include the ability to line up numbers correctly and to follow the "rules" of the mathematical operation.

Clinical Features

Common features of mathematics deficit include difficulty learning number names, remembering the signs for addition and subtraction, learning multiplication tables, translating word problems into computations, and performing calculations at the expected pace. Most children with mathematics deficits can be detected during the second and third grades in elementary school. A child with poor mathematics abilities typically has problems with concepts, such as counting and adding even one-digit numbers, compared with classmates of the same age. During the first 2 or 3 years of elementary school, a child with poor mathematics skill may just get by in mathematics by relying on rote memory. But soon, as mathematics problems require discrimination and manipulation of spatial and numerical relations, a child with mathematics difficulties is overwhelmed.

Some investigators have classified mathematics deficiencies into the following categories: difficulty learning to count meaningfully; difficulty mastering cardinal and ordinal systems; difficulty performing arithmetic operations; and difficulty envisioning clusters of objects as groups. Children with mathematics difficulty have trouble associating auditory and visual symbols, understanding the conservation of quantity, remembering sequences of arithmetic steps, and choosing principles for problem-solving activities. Children with these problems are presumed to have good auditory and verbal abilities; however, in many cases, the mathematics deficits may occur in conjunction with reading, writing, and language problems. In these cases, the other deficiencies may compound the impairment of the poor mathematics skill.

Mathematics difficulty, in fact, often coexists with other disorders affecting reading, expressive writing, coordination, and language. Spelling problems, deficits in memory or attention, and emotional or behavioral problems may be present. Young grade-school children may exhibit specific learning problems in reading and writing, and these children should also be evaluated for mathematics deficits. The exact relationship between mathematics deficits and the deficits in language and dyslexia is not clear. Although children with language disorder do not necessarily experience mathematics deficiencies, these conditions often coexist, and both are associated with impairments in decoding and encoding processes.

Lena, an 8-year-old girl, was referred for evaluation of impairing problems in attention and academic achievement, which were first noted in kindergarten but were now causing difficulty at home and school. Lena attended a regular third-grade class in a local public school, which she had been attending since midway through kindergarten.

Lena's history included a mild delay in speech acquisition (e.g., first words at approximately 18 months of age and short sentences at approximately 3 years of age), but otherwise she had no major developmental problems until kindergarten, when her teacher had raised concerns about inattentiveness, difficulty following instructions, and her difficulty in mastering basic number concepts (e.g., inaccurate counting of sets of objects). A speech, language, and hearing assessment completed at the end of kindergarten revealed mild language problems that did not warrant specific intervention. School reports from grades 1 and 2 noted ongoing concerns about inattention, poor reading skills, and difficulty mastering simple arithmetic facts, and "making careless mistakes in copying numbers from the board and in doing addition and subtraction." These problems continued through grade 2, despite some in-school accommodations (e.g., moving Lena's seat closer to the teacher) and modifications (e.g., providing her with printed sheets of arithmetic problems so she did not need to copy them herself). Lena's parents reported a 3-year history of losing things, fidgeting at the dinner table, and difficulty concentrating on games and homework, and forgetting to bring notes to and from school. Psychological assessment included the Wechsler Intelligence Scale for Children-III, Clinical Evaluation of Language Fundamentals-IV,

Comprehensive Test of Phonological Processing, and the Woodcock-Johnson Psycho-Educational Battery–III. Results indicated average intelligence, with relatively weaker performance on tests of perceptual organization, weak phonological (speech sound) awareness, mild deficits in receptive and expressive language, and reading and arithmetic abilities that were well below grade level. Parent and teacher ratings on a standardized behavior questionnaire (Conners' Rating Scales-Long Form) were above clinical threshold for ADHD.

Lena was given a diagnosis of ADHD, predominantly inattentive type, and specific learning disorder with impairment in reading, based on the history, school achievement, and standardized assessment. She did not meet criteria for communication disorder, and it was speculated that her mathematics problems did not cause impairment like her reading disorder and ADHD did. Recommendations included the following: family psychoeducation clarifying the ADHD and specific learning disorder, remedial interventions for reading, and treatment of her ADHD with a long-acting stimulant agent.

At 1-year follow-up, Lena and her parents reported noticeable improvement with inattention, but ongoing problems with reading and more significant deficits in mathematics. Mathematics remediation was added to her weekly schedule. Two years later, when Lena was 11 years of age, her parents called for an "urgent reevaluation" due to a sudden worsening of her difficulties at home and school. Clinical evaluation revealed adequate stimulant treatment response of her ADHD, more marked deficits in reading speed accuracy compared to others her age, and significant deficits in mathematics. Lena's parents reported that she had started lying about having mathematics homework or refused to do it, was suspended from mathematics class twice in the past 3 months because of oppositional behavior, and had failed sixth-grade mathematics. Lena acknowledged disliking and worrying about math: "whenever the teacher starts asking questions and looks in my direction, my mind just goes blank and I feel sort of shaky—it's so bad in tests that I have to leave class to get myself together." At this point, an additional component of anxiety was noted to be contributing to her school impairments. Recommendations were expanded to include increased specific educational remediation for mathematics. At follow-up, Lena reported that the resource teacher had taught her some helpful strategies to address her anxiety about mathematics, as well as ways of classifying word problems and differentiating critical information from irrelevant information. She continued to be a robust responder to long-acting stimulants for her ADHD, and had only minimal difficulties concentrating on homework after school. *(Adapted from case material by Rosemary Tannock, Ph.D.)*

Pathology and Laboratory Examination

No physical signs or symptoms indicate mathematics disorder, but educational testing and standardized measurement of intellectual function are necessary to make this diagnosis. The *Keymath Diagnostic Arithmetic Test* measures several areas of mathematics including knowledge of mathematical content, function, and computation. It is used to assess ability in mathematics of children in grades 1 to 6.

Course and Prognosis

A child with a specific learning disorder in mathematics can usually be identified by the age of 8 years (third grade). In some children, the disorder is apparent as early as 6 years (first grade); in others, it may not be apparent until age 10 (fifth grade) or later. Too few data are currently available from longitudinal studies to predict clear patterns of developmental and academic progress of children classified as having mathematics disorder in early school grades. On the other hand, children with a moderate mathematics disorder who do not receive intervention may have complications, including continuing academic difficulties, shame, poor self-concept, frustration, and depression. These complications can lead to reluctance to attend school, and demoralization about academic success.

Differential Diagnosis

Mathematics deficits must be differentiated from global causes of impaired functioning such as intellectual disability. Arithmetic difficulties in intellectual disability are accompanied by similar impairments in overall intellectual functioning. Inadequate schooling can affect a child's arithmetic performance on a standardized arithmetic test. Conduct disorder or ADHD can occur comorbidly with specific learning disorder in mathematics and, in these cases, both diagnoses should be made.

Treatment

Mathematics difficulties for children are best remediated with early interventions that lead to improved skills in basic computation. The presence of specific learning disorder in reading along with mathematics difficulties can impede progress; however, children are quite responsive to remediation in early grade school. Children with indications of mathematics disorder as early as in kindergarten require help in understanding which digit in a pair is larger, counting abilities, identification of numbers, and remembering sequences of numbers. Flash cards, workbooks, and computer games can be a viable part of this treatment. One study indicated that mathematics instruction is most helpful when the focus is on problem-solving activities, including word problems, rather than only computation. *Project MATH,* a multimedia self-instructional or group-instructional in-service training program, has been successful for some children with mathematics disorder. Computer programs can be helpful and can increase compliance with remediation efforts.

Social skills deficits can contribute to a child's hesitation in asking for help, so a child identified with a mathematics disorder may benefit from gaining positive problem-solving skills in the social arena as well as in mathematics.

SPECIFIC LEARNING DISORDER WITH IMPAIRMENT IN WRITTEN EXPRESSION

Written expression is the most complex skill acquired to convey an understanding of language and to express thoughts and ideas. Writing skills are highly correlated with reading for most children; however, for some youth, reading comprehension may far surpass their ability to express complex thoughts. Written expression in some cases is a sensitive index of more subtle deficits in language usage that typically are not detected by standardized reading and language tests.

Deficits in written expression are characterized by writing skills that are significantly below the expected level for a child's age and education. Such deficits impair the child's academic performance and writing in everyday life. Components of writing disorder include poor spelling, errors in grammar and punctuation, and poor handwriting. Spelling errors are among the most common difficulties for a child with a writing disorder. Spelling mistakes are most often phonetic errors; that is, an erroneous spelling that sounds like the correct spelling. Examples of common spelling errors are: fone for phone, or beleeve for believe.

Historically, dysgraphia (i.e., poor writing skills) was considered to be a form of reading disorder; however, it is now clear that impairment in written expression can occur on its own. Terms once used to describe writing disability include *spelling disorder* and *spelling dyslexia.* Writing disabilities are often associated with other forms of specific learning disorders; however, impaired writing ability may be identified later than other forms because it is generally acquired later than verbal language and reading.

In contrast with the DSM-5, which includes specific learning disorder in written expression, the 10th Edition of the *International Statistical Classification of Diseases and Related Health Problems* (ICD-10) includes a separate specific spelling disorder.

Epidemiology

The prevalence of specific learning disorder with impairment in written expression has been reported to occur in the range of 5 to 15 percent of school-age children. Over time, specific learning disorder remits in many youth, leading to a persistent rate of specific learning disorder of 4 percent in adults. The gender ratio in writing deficits is two to three to one in boys compared with girls. Impaired written expression often occurs along with deficits in reading, but not always.

Comorbidity

Children with impaired writing ability are significantly more likely to have language disorder and impairments in reading and mathematics compared to the general population of youth. ADHD occurs with greater frequency in children with writing disability than in the general population. Youth with specific learning disorder, including writing disability, are at higher risk for social skills difficulties, and some develop poor self-esteem and depressive symptoms.

Etiology

Causes of writing disability are believed to be similar to those of reading disorder, that is, underlying deficits in using the components of language related to letter sounds. Genetic factors are a significant factor in the development of writing disability. Writing difficulties often accompany language disorder, leading an affected child to have trouble with understanding grammatical rules, finding words, and expressing ideas clearly. According to one hypothesis, impairment in written expression may result from combined effects of language disorder, and reading disorder. Hereditary predisposition to writing impairment is supported by the finding that most youth with impaired written expression have first-degree relatives with similar difficulties Children with limited attention spans and high levels of distractibility may find writing an arduous task.

Diagnosis

The DSM-5 diagnosis of specific learning disorder with impairment in written expression is based on a child's poor ability to use punctuation and grammar accurately in sentences, inability to organize paragraphs, or to clearly articulate ideas in writing. Poor performance on composing written text may also include poor handwriting and impaired ability to spell and to place words sequentially in coherent sentences, compared to others of the same age. In addition to spelling mistakes, youth with impaired written expression make grammatical mistakes, such as using incorrect tenses, forgetting words in sentences, and placing words in the wrong order. Punctuation may be incorrect, and the child may have poor ability to remember which words begin with capital letters. Additional symptoms of impaired written expression include the formation of letters that are not legible, inverted letters, and mixtures of capital and lowercase letters in a given word. Other features of writing disorders include poor organization of written stories, which lack critical elements such as "where," "when," and "who" or clear expression of the plot.

Clinical Features

Youth with impairments in written expression struggle early in grade school with spelling words and expressing their thoughts according to age-appropriate grammatical norms. Their spoken and written sentences contain an unusually large number of grammatical errors and poor paragraph organization. Affected children commonly make simple grammatical errors, even when writing a short sentence. For example, despite constant reminders, affected youth frequently fail to capitalize the first letter of the first word in a sentence, and fail to end the sentence with a period. Typical features of impaired written expression include spelling errors, grammatical errors, punctuation errors, poor paragraph organization, and poor handwriting.

In higher grades in school, affected youth's written sentences become more conspicuously primitive, odd, and inaccurate compared to what is expected of students at their grade level. For youth with impaired written expression, word choices are often erroneous and inappropriate, paragraphs are disorganized and not in proper sequence, and spelling accuracy becomes increasingly difficult as their vocabulary becomes larger and more abstract. Associated features of writing impairments may include reluctance to go to school, refusal to do assigned written homework, and concurrent academic difficulties in other areas.

Many children with impaired written expression understandably become frustrated and angry, and harbor feelings of shame and inadequacy regarding poor academic achievement. In some cases, depressive disorders can result from a growing sense of isolation, estrangement, and despair. Young adults with impaired written expression who do not receive remedial intervention continue to have writing skills deficits and a persistent sense of incompetence and inferiority.

Brett, an 11-year-old boy, was referred for evaluation of increasing problems in school over a 2-year period, including failure to complete assigned schoolwork and homework, inattention and oppositional behavior, and deteriorating grades and test scores. At the time of assessment, he was enrolled in a regular fifth-grade class in a public school, which he had been attending since grade 1.

Clinical interview with parents revealed that Brett had a twin brother (monozygotic) with a history of language problems for which he had received speech-language therapy in the preschool years and remedial reading in the primary grades. Brett, however, had not exhibited difficulty in speech or language development, according to parental report and scores on standardized tests of oral language administered in the preschool years. His current and previous school reports indicate that Brett participated well in class discussions and had no difficulty in reading or mathematics; however, his written work was far below grade level. In each of the last 2 years, his teachers had expressed increasing concerns about Brett's refusal to complete written work, failure to hand in homework, daydreaming and fidgeting in class, and withdrawal from class activities. Brett admitted to an increasing dislike of school and especially writing assignments. He explained, "It's writing, writing all day long—even in math and science. I know how to do the problems and the experiments, but I hate having to write it all down—my mind just goes blank." Brett complained "My teacher is always on at me, telling me that I'm lazy and haven't done enough, and that my writing is atrocious. He tells me, I've got a bad attitude—so why would I want to go to school?" Brett and his parents reported that, over the past year, he has been down, increasing frustrated with school, and has refused to do homework. They all agree that Brett has had a few brief episodes of depressed mood.

Testing by a clinical psychologist revealed average to high-average scores on the verbal and performance scales of the Wechsler Intelligence Scale for Children-III and average scores on the reading and arithmetic subtests of the Wide Range Achievement Test-3 (WRAT-3). However, scores on the WRAT-3 spelling subtest were below the 9th percentile, which was significantly below expectations for age and ability. Examination of his spelling errors revealed that, although his spelling was typically phonologically accurate (i.e., could plausibly be pronounced to sound like the target word), it was unacceptable in that he used letter sequences that did not resemble English, regardless of pronunciation (e.g., "houses" was written as "howssis," "phones" was written as "fones," and "exact" was written as "egszakt"). Moreover, his performance was well below age and grade on standardized tests of written expression (TOWL-3), as well as on a brief (5-minute) informal assessment of expository text generation on a favorite topic (e.g., newspaper article on recent sports event). During the 5-minute writing activity, he was observed to frequently stare out of the window, to shift positions and to chew on his pencil, to get up to sharpen his pencil and to sigh when he did put pencil to paper, and to write slowly and laboriously. At the end of 5 minutes, he had produced three short sentences without any punctuation or capitalization that were barely legible, containing several misspellings and grammatical errors, and that were not linked semantically. By contrast, later in the assessment, he described the sporting event with detail and enthusiasm. A speech-language evaluation revealed average scores on standard tests of oral language (Clinical Evaluation of Language Fundamentals-IV), but he was noted to omit sounds or syllables in a multisyllabic word in a nonword repetition test, which has been found to be sensitive to mild residual language impairments and written language impairments.

The clinical team formulated a diagnosis of specific learning disorder with impairment in written expression, based on Brett's inability to compose written text, poor spelling, and grammatical errors, without problems in reading or mathematics or a history of language impairments. He did not meet full diagnostic criteria for any other DSM-5 disorder, including oppositional defiant disorder, ADHD, or mood disorder. Recommendations included the following: psychoeducation, the need for educational accommodations (e.g., provision of additional time for test taking and written assignments, specific educational intervention to facilitate written expression and to teach note taking, and use of specific computer software to support written composition and spelling), and counseling should his depressed mood continue or worsen. *(Adapted from case material from Rosemary Tannock, Ph.D.)*

Pathology and Laboratory Examination

Whereas no physical signs of a writing disorder exist, educational testing is used in making a diagnosis of writing disorder. Diagnosis is based on a child's writing performance being markedly below expected production for his age, as confirmed by an individually administered standardized expressive writing test. Currently available tests of written language include the Test of Written Language (TOWL), the DEWS, and the Test of Early Written Language (TEWL). Evaluation for impaired vision and hearing is recommended.

When impairments in written expression are noted, a child should be administered a standardized intelligence test, such as WISC-R to determine the child's overall intellectual capacity.

Course and Prognosis

Specific learning disorder with impairment in writing, reading, and mathematics often coexist, and additional language disorder may be present as well. A child with all of the above disabilities will likely be diagnosed with language disorder first and impaired written expression last. In severe cases, an impaired written expression is apparent by age 7 (second grade); in less severe cases, the disorder may not be apparent until age 10 (fifth grade) or later. Youth with mild and moderate impairment in written expression fare well if they receive timely remedial education early in grade school. Severely impaired written expression requires continual, extensive remedial treatment through the late part of high school and even into college.

The prognosis depends on the severity of the disorder, the age or grade when the remedial intervention is started, the length and continuity of treatment, and presence or absence of associated or secondary emotional or behavioral problems.

Differential Diagnosis

It is important to determine whether disorders such as ADHD or major depression are interfering with a child's focus and thereby preventing the production of adequate writing in the absence of a specific writing impairment. If true, treatment for the other disorder should improve a child's writing performance. Commonly comorbid disorders with writing disability are language disorder, mathematics disorder, developmental coordination disorder, disruptive behavior disorders, and ADHD.

Treatment

Remedial treatment for writing disability includes direct practice in spelling and sentence writing as well as a review of grammatical rules. Intensive and continuous administration of individually tailored, one-on-one expressive and creative writing therapy appears to effect favorable outcome. Teachers in some special schools devote as much as 2 hours a day to such writing instruction. The effectiveness of a writing intervention depends largely on an optimal relationship between the child and the writing specialist. Success or failure in sustaining the patient's motivation greatly affects the treatment's long-term efficacy. Associated secondary emotional and behavioral problems should be given prompt attention, with appropriate psychiatric treatment and parental counseling.

▲ 27.8 Motor Disorders

27.8a Developmental Coordination Disorder

Developmental coordination disorder is a neurodevelopmental disorder in which a child's fine and/or gross motor coordination is slower, less accurate, and more variable than in peers of the same age. Affecting about 5 to 6 percent of school-age children, 50 percent of children with developmental coordination disorder also have comorbid ADHD or dyslexia. A meta-analysis of recent research on developmental coordination disorder concluded that three general areas of deficits contribute to the disorder: (1) poor predictive control of motor movements; (2) deficits in rhythmic coordination and timing; and (3) deficits in executive functions, including working memory, inhibition, and attention.

Children with developmental motor coordination disorder struggle to perform accurately the motor activities of daily life, such as jumping, hopping, running, or catching a ball. Children with coordination problems may also agonize to use utensils correctly, tie their shoelaces, or write. A child with developmental coordination disorder may exhibit delays in achieving motor milestones, such as sitting, crawling, and walking, because of clumsiness, and yet excel at verbal skills.

Developmental coordination disorder, thus, may be characterized by either clumsy gross and/or fine motor skills, resulting in poor performance in sports and even in academic achievement because of poor writing skills. A child with developmental coordination disorder may bump into things more often than siblings or drop things. In the 1930s, the term *clumsy child syndrome* began to be used in the literature to denote a condition of awkward motor behaviors that could not be correlated with any specific neurological disorder or damage. This term continues to be used to identify imprecise or delayed gross and fine motor behavior in children, resulting in subtle motor inabilities, but often significant social rejection. Gross and fine motor impairment in developmental coordination disorder cannot be explained on the basis of a medical condition, such as cerebral palsy, muscular dystrophy, or a neuromuscular disorder. Currently, certain indications are that perinatal problems, such as prematurity, low birth weight, and hypoxia may contribute to the emergence of developmental coordination disorders. Children with developmental coordination disorder are at higher risk for language and learning disorders. A strong association is seen between speech and language problems and coordination problems, as well as an association of coordination difficulties with hyperactivity, impulsivity, and poor attention span.

Children with developmental coordination disorder may resemble younger children because of their inability to master motor activities typical for their age group. For example, children with developmental coordination disorder in elementary school may not be adept at bicycle riding, skateboarding, running, skipping, or hopping. In the middle school years, children with this disorder may have trouble in team sports, such as soccer, baseball, or basketball. Fine motor skill manifestations of developmental coordination disorder typically include clumsiness using utensils and difficulty with buttons and zippers in the preschool age group. In older children, using scissors and more complex grooming skills, such as styling hair or putting on makeup, is difficult. Children with developmental coordination disorder are often ostracized by peers because of their poor skills in many sports, and they often have long-standing difficulties with peer relationships. Developmental coordination disorder is categorized in the Fifth Edition of the American Psychiatric Association's *Diagnostic and Statistical Manual of Mental Disorders* (DSM-5) as a Motor Disorder, along with stereotypic movement disorder and tic disorders.

EPIDEMIOLOGY

The prevalence of developmental coordination disorder has been estimated at about 5 to 6 percent of school-age children. The male-to-female ratio in school populations tends to show increased rates of the disorder in males, and schools often refer boys at rates that even exceed these ratios for testing and special education evaluations. Reports in the literature of the male-to-female ratio have ranged from 3 to 1 to as high as 7 to 1; however, the most current estimates are approximately two males for every one female.

COMORBIDITY

Developmental coordination disorder is strongly associated with ADHD, specific learning disorder, particularly in reading, as well as language disorder. Children with coordination difficulties have higher than expected rates of language disorder, and studies of children with language disorder report very high rates of "clumsiness." Developmental coordination disorder is also associated, but less strongly, with specific learning disorder with impairment in mathematics, and in written expression. A study of children with developmental coordination disorder reported that, although motor coordination is critical for accuracy in tasks that require speed, poor motor coordination is not directly correlated with degree of inattention. Thus, in children comorbid for ADHD and developmental coordination disorder, children with the most severe ADHD do not necessarily have the worst developmental coordination disorder. Functional neuroimaging, pharmacological, and neuroanatomical studies suggest that motor coordination depends on the integration of sensory input and an action response, not purely through sensorimotor function and higher level thinking. Investigations of comorbid developmental coordination disorder and ADHD are trying to ascertain whether this comorbidity is due to overlapping genetic factors.

Peer relationship problems are common among children with developmental coordination disorders, because of rejection that often occurs along with their poor performance in sports and games that require good motor skill. Adolescents with coordination problems often exhibit poor self-esteem and academic difficulties. Recent studies underscore the importance of attention to both victimization of children and adolescents with developmental motor coordination disorder by peers and the potential resulting damage to self-worth. Children and adolescents with developmental coordination disorder who are bullied have higher rates of poor self-esteem that often deserves clinical attention.

ETIOLOGY

The causes of developmental coordination disorder are believed to be multifactorial, and likely include both genetic and developmental factors. Risk factors postulated to contribute to this disorder include prematurity, hypoxia, perinatal malnutrition, and low birth weight. Prenatal exposure to alcohol, cocaine, and nicotine has also been hypothesized to contribute to both low birth weight and cognitive and behavioral abnormalities. Developmental coordination disorder rates of up to 50 percent have been reported in children born prematurely. Researchers have proposed that the cerebellum may be the neurological substrate for comorbid cases of developmental coordination disorder and ADHD. Neurochemical abnormalities and parietal lobe lesions have also been suggested to contribute to coordination deficits. Studies of postural control, that is, the ability to regain balance after being in motion, indicate that children with developmental coordination disorder who have adequate balance when standing still, are unable to accurately correct for movement, resulting in impaired balance, compared with other children. A study concluded that, in children with developmental coordination disorder, neural signals from the brain to particular muscles involved in balance, are neither being optimally sent or received. These findings have also implicated the cerebellum as a potential anatomical site for the dysfunction of developmental coordination disorder. Two mechanisms of developmental coordination disorder have been hypothesized for the disabilities of the disorder. The first one, called the automatization deficit hypothesis, suggests that, similar to dyslexia, children with developmental coordination disorder have difficulty developing automatic motor skills. The second hypothesis, the internal modeling deficit hypothesis, suggests that children with developmental coordination disorder are unable to perform the typical internal cognitive models that predict the sensory consequences of motor commands. In both scenarios, the cerebellum is believed to play an important role in motor coordination and in developmental coordination disorder.

DIAGNOSIS

The diagnosis of developmental coordination disorder depends on poor performance in activities requiring coordination for a child's age and intellectual level. Diagnosis is based on a history of the child's delay in achieving early motor milestones, as well as on direct observation of current deficits in coordination. An informal screen for developmental coordination disorder involves asking the child to perform tasks involving gross motor coordination (e.g., hopping, jumping, and standing on one foot); fine motor coordination (e.g., finger-tapping and shoelace tying); and hand–eye coordination (e.g., catching a ball and copying letters). Judgments regarding poor performance must be based on what is expected for a child's age. A child who is mildly clumsy, but whose functioning is not impaired, does not qualify for a diagnosis of developmental coordination disorder.

The diagnosis may be associated with below-normal scores on performance subtests of standardized intelligence tests and by normal or above-normal scores on verbal subtests. Specialized tests of motor coordination can be useful, such as the *Bender Visual Motor Gestalt Test,* the *Frostig Movement Skills Test Battery,* and the *Bruininks-Oseretsky Test of Motor Development.* The child's chronological age must be taken into account, and the disorder cannot be caused by a neurological or neuromuscular condition. Examination, however, may occasionally reveal slight reflex abnormalities and other soft neurological signs.

CLINICAL FEATURES

The clinical signs suggesting the existence of developmental coordination disorder are evident as early as infancy in some cases, when a child begins to attempt tasks requiring motor coordination. The essential clinical feature is significantly impaired performance in motor coordination. The difficulties in motor coordination may vary with a child's age and developmental stage (Table 27.8a–1).

In infancy and early childhood the disorder may be manifested by delays in developmental motor milestones, such as turning over, crawling, sitting, standing, walking, buttoning

Table 27.8a–1
Manifestations of Developmental Coordination Disorder

Gross motor manifestations
Preschool age
Delays in reaching motor milestones, such as sitting, crawling, and walking
Balance problems: falling, getting bruised frequently, and poor toddling
Abnormal gait
Knocking over objects, bumping into things, and destructiveness
Primary-school age
Difficulty with riding bikes, skipping, hopping, running, jumping, and doing somersaults
Awkward or abnormal gait
Older
Poor at sports, throwing, catching, kicking, and hitting a ball

Fine motor manifestations
Preschool age
Difficulty learning dressing skills (tying, fastening, zipping, and buttoning)
Difficulty learning feeding skills (handling knife, fork, or spoon)
Primary-school age
Difficulty assembling jigsaw pieces, using scissors, building with blocks, drawing, or tracing
Older
Difficulty with grooming (putting on makeup, blow-drying hair, and doing nails)
Messy or illegible writing
Difficulty using hand tools, sewing, and playing piano

shirts, and zipping up pants. Between the ages of 2 and 4 years, clumsiness appears in almost all activities requiring motor coordination. Affected children cannot hold objects and drop them easily, their gait may be unsteady, they often trip over their own feet, and they may bump into other children while attempting to go around them. Older children may display impaired motor coordination in table games, such as putting together puzzles or building blocks, and in any type of ball game. Although no specific features are pathognomonic of developmental coordination disorder, developmental milestones are frequently delayed. Many children with the disorder also have speech and language difficulties. Older children may have secondary problems, including academic difficulties, as well as poor peer relationships based on social rejection. It has been reported widely that children with motor coordination problems are more likely to have problems understanding subtle social cues and are often rejected by peers. A recent study indicated that children with motor difficulties were found to perform more poorly on scales that measure recognition of static and changing facial expressions of emotion. This finding is likely to be correlated to the clinical observations that children with motor coordination have difficulties in social behavior and peer relationships.

Billy was brought for evaluation of suicidal ideation at 8 years of age, after complaining to his parents that he was being bullied by peers for being "bad" in sports, and that nobody liked him. He only had one friend who also laughed at him sometimes, because he always dropped the ball and he looked "funny" while running. He was so upset about being rejected by peers when he tried to play sports that he refused to go to physical education class. Instead, he voluntarily went to the school counselor's office and stayed there until the period was over. Billy was already irritated because he had been diagnosed with ADHD and was on medication, and on top of that, he had difficulty with reading. Billy became so distraught that one day he told his school counselor that he wanted to kill himself. A developmental history revealed that had been delayed for sitting, which he finally did at 10 months of age, and he could not walk without falling over until 30 months of age. Billy's parents were aware that he was very clumsy, but they believed that he would outgrow that. Even at 8 years of age, Billy's parents reported that, during meals, Billy often spilled his drinks and was quite awkward when he used a fork. Some of his food typically fell off of his fork or spoon before it reached his mouth, and he had great difficulty using a knife and a fork.

A comprehensive assessment of fine and gross motor skills demonstrated the following: Billy was able to hop, but he could not skip without briefly stopping after each step. Billy could stand with both feet together, but was unable to stand on tiptoe. Although Billy could catch a ball, he held a ball bounced to himself at chest level, and was unable to catch a ball bounced to him on the ground from a distance of 15 feet. Billy's agility and coordination were measured with the Bruininks-Oseretsky Test of Motor Development, which revealed functioning levels commensurate with those of an average 6-year-old child.

Billy was referred to a neurologist for a comprehensive evaluation, because he appeared to be generally weak, and his muscles seemed floppy. Neurological evaluation was negative for diagnosable neurological disorders, and his muscle strength was actually found to be normal, despite his appearance. Based on the negative neurological examination and the finding of the Bruininks-Oseretsky Test of Motor Development, Billy was given a diagnosis of developmental coordination disorder. Billy's symptoms included mild hypotonia and fine motor clumsiness.

After the diagnosis of developmental motor coordination was made, in addition to his already diagnosed ADHD and reading disorder, his treatment plan included private sessions with an occupational therapist who used perceptual-motor exercises to improve Billy's fine motor skills, targeting particularly writing and use of utensils. A written request was made for an Individualized Educational Plan (IEP) evaluation from the school with a goal of obtaining an adaptive physical education program. In addition, the request for a reading tutor, and a seat close to the front of the classroom were recommended to maximize his attention. Billy was enrolled in a treatment program using motor imagery training to reduce his clumsiness and improve coordination.

Billy was relieved to be receiving help, especially for his reading and for sports activities, and no longer felt suicidal. Over a period of 3 months of treatment, Billy showed a noticeable improvement in his reading. His mood improved further, especially because he was receiving praise from his teachers and parents. Billy's classmates were not picking on him the way they used to. As Billy began to feel better about himself, he began to play sports informally with his peers, although not competitively. Billy was granted an adaptive physical education program in school, and he was not required to play on teams. Instead, he practiced throwing and catching a ball and playing basketball with a staff member.

Billy continued to show some degree of clumsiness, especially in his fine motor skills over the next few years, yet he was cooperative, with the occupational therapy interventions, his mood was bright, and he demonstrated continual improvement. *(Courtesy of Caroly Pataki, M.D. and Sarah Spence, M.D.)*

DIFFERENTIAL DIAGNOSIS

The differential diagnosis includes medical conditions that produce coordination difficulties (e.g., cerebral palsy and muscular dystrophy). In autism spectrum disorder and intellectual disability, coordination usually does not stand out as a significant deficit compared with other skills. Children with neuromuscular disorders may exhibit more global muscle impairment rather than clumsiness and delayed motor milestones. Neurological examination and workup usually reveal more extensive deficits in neurological conditions than in developmental coordination disorder. Extremely hyperactive and impulsive children may be physically careless because of their high levels of motor activity. Clumsy, gross and fine motor behavior, and ADHD as well as reading difficulties are highly associated.

COURSE AND PROGNOSIS

Historically, it was believed that developmental coordination spontaneously improved over time; however, longitudinal studies have shown that motor coordination problems can persist into adolescence and adulthood. When mild to moderate clumsiness is persistent, some children can compensate by developing interests in other skills. Some studies suggest a more favorable outcome for children who have average or above-average intellectual capacity, in that they come up with strategies to develop friendships that do not depend on physical activities. Clumsiness typically persists into adolescence and adult life. One study following a group of children with developmental coordination problems over a decade found that the clumsy children remained less dexterous, showed poor balance, and continued to be physically awkward. The affected children were also more likely to have both academic problems and poor self-esteem. Children with developmental coordination disorder have also been shown to be at higher risk for obesity, have difficulties with running, and are at greater risk of future cardiovascular diseases.

TREATMENT

Interventions for children with developmental coordination disorder utilize multiple modalities, including visual, auditory, and tactile materials targeting perceptual motor training for specific motor tasks. Two broad categories of interventions are the following: (1) deficit-oriented approaches, including sensory integration therapy, sensorimotor-oriented treatment, and process-oriented treatment; and (2) task-specific interventions, including neuromotor task training and cognitive orientation to daily occupational performance (CO-OP). More recently, motor imagery training has been incorporated into treatment. These approaches involve visual imagery exercises using CD-ROM; they have a broad range of foci, including predictive timing for motor tasks, relaxation and mental preparation, visual modeling of fundamental motor skills, and mental rehearsal of various tasks. This type of intervention is based on the notion that improved internal representation of a movement task will improve a child's actual motor behavior.

The treatment of developmental coordination disorder generally includes versions of sensory integration programs and modified physical education. Sensory integration programs, usually administered by occupational therapists, consist of physical activities that increase awareness of motor and sensory function. For example, a child who bumps into objects often might be given the task of trying to balance on a scooter, under supervision, to improve balance and body awareness. Children who have difficulty writing letters are often given tasks to increase awareness of hand movements. School-based occupational therapies for motor coordination problems in writing include utilizing mechanisms that provide resistance or vibration during writing exercises, to improve grip, and practicing vertical writing on a chalk board to increase arm strength and stability while writing. These programs have been shown to improve legibility of student's writing, but not necessarily speed, because students learn to write with greater accuracy and deliberate letter formation. Currently, many schools also allow and may even encourage children with coordination difficulties that affect writing to use computers to aid in writing reports and long papers.

Adaptive physical education programs are designed to help children enjoy exercise and physical activities without the pressures of team sports. These programs generally incorporate certain sports actions, such as kicking a soccer ball or throwing a basketball. Children with coordination disorder may also benefit from social skills groups and other prosocial interventions. The Montessori technique may promote motor skill development, especially with preschool children, because this educational program emphasizes the development of motor skills. Small studies have suggested that exercise in rhythmic coordination, practicing motor movements, and learning to use word processing keyboards may be beneficial. Parental counseling may help reduce parents' anxiety and guilt about their child's impairment, increase their awareness, and facilitate their confidence to cope with the child.

An investigation of children with developmental coordination disorder showed positive results using a computer game designed to improve ability to catch a ball. These children were able to improve their game score by practicing virtual catching without specific instructions on how to utilize the visual cues. This has implications for treatment, in that certain types of motor task coordination can be positively influenced through the practice of specific motor tasks, even without overt instructions.

27.8b Stereotypic Movement Disorder

Stereotypic movements include a diverse range of repetitive behaviors that usually emerge in the early developmental period, appear to lack a clear function, and sometimes cause interruption in daily life. These movements are typically rhythmic, such as hand flapping, body rocking, hand waving, hair-twirling, lip-licking, skin picking, or self-hitting. Stereotypic movements often appear to be self-soothing or self-stimulating; however, they can result in self-injury in some cases. Stereotypic movements appear to be involuntary; however, they frequently can be suppressed with a concentrated effort. Stereotypic movement disorder occurs with increased frequency in children with ASD and intellectual disability, but they also exist in typically developing children. Stereotypic movements, such as head-banging, face slapping, eye poking, or hand-biting, can cause significant self-harm. Nail-biting, thumb-sucking, and nose-picking are often not included as symptoms of stereotypic movement disorder because they rarely cause impairment. When impairment occurs, however, they can be included in stereotypic movement disorder. Stereotypic movements share several features with tics, including the repetitive, seemingly involuntary, and characteristically identical nature of the movements each time they are displayed. However, distinguishing features of stereotypical movements compared to tics include a younger age of onset, lack of changing anatomical locations, lack of premonitory "urge," and decreased response to medication management.

According to the Fifth Edition of the American Psychiatric Association's *Diagnostic and Statistical Manual of Mental Disorders* (DSM-5), stereotypic movement disorder is characterized by repetitive, seemingly driven, and apparently purposeless motor behavior that interferes with social, academic, or other activities and may result in self-harm.

EPIDEMIOLOGY

Repetitive movements are common in infants and young children, with greater than 60 percent of parents of children between the ages of 2 and 4 years reporting transient emergence of these behaviors. The most common age of onset is in the second year of life. Epidemiologic surveys estimate that up to 7 percent of otherwise typically developing children exhibit stereotypic behaviors. A prevalence of about 15 to 20 percent in children younger than the age of 6 years display stereotypic behavior, with diminishing rates over time. The prevalence of self-injurious behaviors, however, has been estimated to be in the range of 2 to 3 percent among children and adolescents with intellectual disability. Stereotypic movements appear to occur in about twice as many boys as girls. Determining which cases are sufficiently severe to confirm a diagnosis of stereotypic movement disorder may be difficult. Stereotypic behaviors occur in 10 to 20 percent of children with intellectual disability, with increased rates being proportional to level of severity. Self-injurious behaviors frequently occur in genetic syndromes, such as Lesch–Nyhan syndrome, and in children with sensory impairments, such as blindness and deafness.

ETIOLOGY

The etiology of stereotypic movement disorder includes environmental, genetic, and neurobiological factors. Although the neurobiological mechanisms of stereotypic movement disorder have yet to be proven, given their similarity to other involuntary movements, stereotypic movement disorder is hypothesized to originate from the basal ganglia. Dopamine and serotonin are likely to be involved in their emergence. Dopamine agonists tend to induce or increase stereotypic behaviors, whereas dopamine antagonists sometimes decrease them. One study found that 17 percent of typically developing children with stereotypic movement disorder had a first-degree relative with the disorder, and 25 percent had a first- or second-degree relative with stereotypic movement disorder. Transient stereotypic behaviors in very young children can be considered a normal developmental phenomenon. Genetic factors likely play a role in some stereotypic movements, such as the X-linked recessive deficiency of enzymes leading to Lesch–Nyhan syndrome, which has predictable features including intellectual disability, hyperuricemia, spasticity, and self-injurious behaviors. Other minimal stereotypic movements that do not usually cause impairment (e.g., nail-biting) appear to run in families as well. Some stereotypic behaviors seem to emerge or become exaggerated in situations of neglect or deprivation; such behaviors as head-banging have been associated with psychosocial deprivation.

DIAGNOSIS AND CLINICAL FEATURES

The presence of multiple repetitive stereotyped symptoms tends to occur frequently among children with ASD and intellectually disability, particularly when the intellectual disability is severe. Patients with multiple stereotyped movements frequently have other significant mental disorders, including disruptive behavior disorders, or neurological conditions. In extreme cases, severe mutilation and life-threatening injuries can result from self-inflicted trauma.

Head-Banging

Head-banging exemplifies a stereotypic movement disorder that can result in functional impairment. Typically, head-banging begins during infancy, between 6 and 12 months of age. Infants strike their heads with a definite rhythmic and monotonous continuity against the crib or another hard surface. They seem to be absorbed in the activity, which can persist until they become exhausted and fall asleep. The head-banging is often transitory, but sometimes persists into middle childhood. Head-banging that is a component of temper tantrums differs from stereotypic head-banging and ceases after the tantrums and their secondary gains have been controlled.

Nail-Biting

Nail-biting begins as early as 1 year of age and increases in incidence until age 12. Most cases are not sufficiently severe to meet the DSM-5 diagnostic criteria for stereotypic movement disorder. In rare cases, children cause physical damage to the fingers themselves, usually by associated biting of the cuticles, which leads to secondary infections of the fingers and nail beds. Nail-biting seems to occur or increase in intensity when a child is either anxious or stressed. Some of the most severe nail-biting occurs in children with severe or profound intellectual disability, however many nail-biters have no obvious emotional disturbance.

PATHOLOGY AND LABORATORY EXAMINATION

No specific laboratory measures are helpful in the diagnosis of stereotypic movement disorder.

Tim, a 14-year-old with autism spectrum disorder (ASD), and severe intellectual disability was evaluated when he transferred to a new private school for children with ASD. Observed in his classroom, he was noted to be a small boy who appeared younger than his age. He held his hands in his pockets and spun around in place. When offered a toy he took it and manipulated it for a while. When he was prompted to engage in various tasks that required that he take his hands out of his pockets, he began hitting his head with his hands. If his hands were held by the teacher, he hit his head with his knees. He was adept in contorting himself, so that he could hit or kick himself in almost any position, even while walking. Soon, his face and forehead were covered with bruises.

His development was delayed in all spheres, and he never developed language. He lived at home and attended a special educational program. His self-injurious behaviors developed early in life, and, when his parents tried to stop him, he became aggressive. Gradually, he became too difficult to be managed in public school, and, at 5 years of age, he was placed in a special school. The self-abusive and self-restraining (i.e., holding his hands in his pockets) behavior was present throughout his stay there, and, virtually all of the time; he had been tried on several second-generation antipsychotics with only minimal improvement. Although the psychiatrist's notes mentioned some improvement in his self-injurious behavior, it was described as continuing and fluctuating. He was transferred to a new school because of lack of progress and difficulties in managing him as he became bigger and stronger. His intellectual functioning was within the 34 to 40 intelligence quotient (IQ) range. His adaptive skills were poor. He required full assistance in self-care, could not provide even for his own simple needs, and required constant supervision for his safety.

In a few months, Tim settled into the routine in his new school. His self-injurious behavior fluctuated. It was reduced or even absent when he restrained himself by holding his hands in his pockets or inside his shirt or even by manipulating some object with his hands. If left to himself, he could contort himself, while holding his hands inside his shirt. Because the stereotypic self-injurious and self-restraining behavior interfered with his daily activities and education, it became a primary focus of a behavior modification program. For a few months, he did well, especially when he developed a good relationship with a new teacher, who was firm, consistent, and nurturing. With him, Tim could successfully engage in some school tasks. When the teacher left, Tim regressed. To prevent injuries, the staff started blocking his self-hitting with a pillow. He was offered activities that he liked and in which he could engage without resorting to self-injury. After several months, his antipsychotic medication was slowly discontinued, over a period of 11 months, without any behavioral deterioration. *(Adapted from case material from Bhavik Shah, M.D.)*

DIFFERENTIAL DIAGNOSIS

The differential diagnosis of stereotypic movement disorder includes OCD and tic disorders, both of which are exclusionary criteria in DSM-5. Although stereotypic movements can often be voluntarily suppressed, and are not spasmodic, it is difficult to differentiate these features from tics in all cases. A study of stereotyped movements compared with tics found that stereotyped movements tended to be longer in duration, and displayed more rhythmic qualities than tics. Tics seemed to occur more when a child was in an "alone" condition, rather than when the child was in a play condition, whereas stereotypic movements occurred with the same frequency in these two different conditions. Stereotypic movements are often observed to seem self-soothing, whereas tics are often associated with distress.

Differentiating dyskinetic movements from stereotypic movements can be difficult. Because antipsychotic medications can sometimes suppress stereotypic movements, clinicians should note any stereotypic movements before initiating treatment with an antipsychotic agent. Stereotypic movement disorder may be diagnosed concurrently with substance-related disorders (e.g., amphetamine use disorders), severe sensory impairments, central nervous system and degenerative disorders (e.g., Lesch–Nyhan syndrome), and severe schizophrenia.

COURSE AND PROGNOSIS

The duration and course of stereotypic movement disorder vary, and the symptoms may wax and wane. Up to 60 to 80 percent of normal toddlers show transient rhythmic activities that seem purposeful and comforting and tend to disappear by 4 years of age. When stereotypic movements emerge more severely later in childhood they typically range from brief episodes occurring under stress, to an ongoing pattern in the context of a chronic condition, such as ASD or intellectual disability. Even in chronic conditions, stereotypic behaviors may come and go. In many cases, stereotypic movements are prominent in early childhood and diminish as a child gets older.

The severity of the dysfunction caused by stereotypic movements varies with the frequency, amount, and degree of associated self-injury. Children who exhibit frequent, severe, self-injurious stereotypic behaviors have the poorest prognosis. Repetitive episodes of head-banging, self-biting, and eye-poking can be difficult to control without physical restraints. Most nail-biting is benign and often does not meet the diagnostic criteria for stereotypic movement disorder. In severe cases in which the nail beds are repetitively damaged, bacterial and fungal infections can occur. Although chronic stereotypic movement disorders can severely impair daily functioning, several treatments help control the symptoms.

TREATMENT

When stereotypic movements occur in the absence of any other symptoms or disorders, they may not warrant pharmacologic treatment. Treatment modalities yielding the most promising effects include behavioral techniques, such as habit reversal and differential reinforcement of other behavior, as well as pharmacological interventions. A recent report on utilizing both habit reversal (in which the child is trained to replace the undesired repetitive behavior with a more acceptable behavior) and reinforcement for reducing the unwanted behavior, indicated that these treatments had efficacy among 12 typically developing children between 6 and 14 years. One case report detailed a successful habit reversal treatment of a 3-year-old with severe stereotypic movements, which was largely implemented at home by her parents. The estimated change in stereotypic behaviors during regular recorded intervals during treatment diminished from presence in 85 percent of recordings to presence in less than 2 percent of recordings over a period of 4 weeks.

Pharmacological interventions have been used in clinical practice to minimize self-injury in children whose stereotyped movements caused significant harm to their bodies. Small open-label studies have reported benefit of atypical antipsychotics, and case reports have indicated use of SSRIs in the management of self-injurious stereotypies. The dopamine receptor antagonists have been tried most often for treating stereotypic movements and self-injurious behavior. The SSRI agents may be influential in diminishing stereotypies; however, this is still under investigation. Open trials suggest that both clomipramine and fluoxetine may decrease self-injurious behaviors and other stereotypic movements in some patients.

27.8c Tourette's Disorder

Tics are neuropsychiatric events characterized by brief rapid motor movements or vocalizations that are typically performed in response to irresistible premonitory urges. Although frequently rapid, tics may include more complex patterns of movements and longer vocalizations. Converging evidence from many lines of research suggests that the production of tics involves dysfunction in the basal ganglia region of the brain, particularly of dopaminergic transmission in the cortico–striato-thalamic circuits. Because tic disorders are significantly more common in children than in adults, the postulated alterations in dopamine circuitry in many affected children appear to spontaneously improve over time. Tics may be transient or chronic, with a waxing and waning course. Tics typically emerge at age 5 to 6 years of age and tend to reach their greatest severity between 10 and 12 years. About one-half to two-thirds of children with tic disorders will be much improved or in remission by adolescence or early adulthood. Tic disorder is distinguished by the type of tics, their frequency, and the pattern in which they emerge over time. Motor tics most commonly affect the muscles of the face and neck, such as eye-blinking, head-jerking, mouth-grimacing, or head-shaking. Typical vocal tics include throat-clearing, grunting, snorting, and coughing. Tics are repetitive muscle contractions resulting in movements or vocalizations that are experienced as involuntary, although they can sometimes be suppressed voluntarily. Children and adolescents may exhibit tic behaviors that occur after a stimulus or in response to a premonitory internal urge.

The most widely studied and most severe tic disorder is Gilles de la Tourette syndrome, also known as Tourette's disorder. Georges Gilles de la Tourette (1857–1904) first described a patient with a syndrome, which became known as Tourette's disorder in 1885, while he was studying with Jean-Martin Charcot in France. De la Tourette noted a syndrome in several patients that included multiple motor tics, coprolalia, and echolalia. Tics often consist of motions that are used in volitional movements. One-half to two-thirds of children with Tourette's disorder exhibit a reduction in or complete remission of tic symptoms during adolescence. There are many common comorbid psychiatric disorders and behavioral problems likely to emerge along with Tourette's disorder. For example, the relationship between Tourette's disorder, ADHD, and OCD has not been clearly delineated. Epidemiological surveys indicate that more than half of children with Tourette's disorder also meet criteria for ADHD. There appears to be a bidirectional relationship between Tourette's disorder and OCD, with 20 to 40 percent of Tourette's disorder patients meeting full criteria for OCD. First-degree relatives of patients with OCD have been shown to have higher rates of tic disorders compared to the general population. There have been a few small reports suggesting that the obsessive–compulsive symptoms most likely to occur in Tourette's disorder are characteristically related to ordering and symmetry, counting, and repetitive touching, whereas OCD symptoms in the absence of tic disorders are more often associated with fears of contamination and fears of doing harm. Motor and vocal tics are divided into simple and complex types. *Simple motor tics* are those composed of repetitive, rapid contractions of functionally similar muscle groups—for example, eye-blinking, neck-jerking, shoulder-shrugging, and facial-grimacing. Common *simple vocal tics* include coughing, throat-clearing, grunting, sniffing, snorting, and barking. *Complex motor tics* appear to be more purposeful and ritualistic than simple tics. Common *complex motor tics* include grooming behaviors, the smelling of objects, jumping, touching behaviors, echopraxia (imitation of observed behavior), and copropraxia (display of obscene gestures). *Complex vocal tics* include repeating words or phrases out of context, coprolalia (use of obscene words or phrases), palilalia (a person's repeating his or her words), and echolalia (repetition of the last-heard words of others).

Although older children and adolescents with tic disorders may be able to suppress their tics for minutes or hours, young children are often not cognizant of their tics or experience their urges to perform their tics as irresistible. Tics may be attenuated by sleep, relaxation, or absorption in an activity. Tics often disappear during sleep.

EPIDEMIOLOGY

The estimated prevalence of Tourette's disorder ranges from 3 to 8 per 1,000 school-age children. Males are affected between 2 and 4 times more often than females. The unique features of Tourette's disorder in which tics wax and wane and may change in character, frequency, and severity over relatively short periods of time, has made ascertainment of its prevalence challenging. Furthermore, remission of tics is particularly age-dependent in that tics tend to emerge and increase from ages 5 to 10 years of age, and in many cases, decrease in frequency and severity after the age of 10 to 12 years. At age 13 years, however, using stringent criteria, the prevalence rate for Tourette's disorder drops to 0.3 percent. The lifetime prevalence of Tourette's disorder is estimated to be approximately 1 percent.

ETIOLOGY

Genetic Factors

Twin studies, adoption studies, and segregation analysis studies all support a genetic basis, albeit a complex one, for Tourette's disorder. Twin studies indicate that concordance for the disorder in monozygotic twins is significantly greater than that in dizygotic twins. Tourette's disorder and chronic motor or vocal tic disorder are likely to occur in the same families; this lends support to the view that the disorders are part of a genetically determined spectrum. The sons of mothers with Tourette's disorder seem to be at the highest risk for the disorder. Evidence in some families indicates that Tourette's disorder is transmitted in an autosomal dominant fashion. Studies of a long family pedigree suggest that Tourette's disorder may be transmitted in a bilinear mode; that is, Tourette's disorder appears to be inherited through an autosomal pattern in some families, intermediate between dominant and recessive. A study of 174 unrelated probands with Tourette's disorder identified a greater than chance occurrence of a rare sequence variant in SLITRK1, believed to be a candidate gene on chromosome 13q31.

Up to half of all patients with Tourette's disorder also have ADHD, and up to 40 percent of those with Tourette's disorder also have OCD. These frequent comorbidities with Tourette's disorder can lead to a plethora of overlapping symptoms. Family studies have provided compelling evidence for the association between tic disorders and OCD. First-degree relatives of persons with Tourette's disorder are at high risk for the development of Tourette's disorder, chronic motor or vocal tic disorder, and OCD. Current understanding of the genetic bases of Tourette's disorder implicates multiple vulnerability genes that may serve to mediate the type and severity of tics. Candidate genes associated with Tourette's disorder include dopamine receptor genes, dopamine transporter genes, several noradrenergic genes, and serotonergic genes.

Neuroimaging Studies

A functional magnetic resonance imaging (fMRI) study of brain activity 2 seconds before and after a tic, found that paralimbic and sensory association areas were involved. Furthermore, evidence suggests that voluntary tic suppression involves deactivation of the putamen and globus pallidus, along with partial activation of regions of the prefrontal cortex and caudate nucleus. Compelling, but indirect, evidence of dopamine system involvement in tic disorders includes the observations that pharmacological agents that antagonize dopamine (haloperidol [Haldol], pimozide [Orap], and fluphenazine [Prolixin]) suppress tics and that agents that increase central dopaminergic activity (methylphenidate [Ritalin], amphetamines, and cocaine) tend to exacerbate tics. The relation of tics to neurotransmitter systems is complex and not yet well understood; for example, in some cases, antipsychotic medications, such as haloperidol, are not effective in reducing tics, and the effect of stimulants on tic disorders reportedly varies. In some cases, Tourette's disorder has emerged during treatment with antipsychotic medications.

More direct analyses of the neurochemistry of Tourette's disorder have been possible utilizing brain proton magnetic resonance spectroscopy (MRS). Neuroimaging studies using cerebral blood flow in PET and SPECT suggest that alterations of activity may occur in various brain regions in patients with Tourette's disorder compared to controls, including the frontal and orbital cortex, striatum, and putamen. An investigation examining the cellular neurochemistry of patients with Tourette's disorder utilizing MRS of the frontal cortex, caudate nucleus, putamen, and thalamus demonstrated that these patients had a reduced amount of choline and *N*-acetylaspartate in the left putamen along with reduced levels bilaterally in the putamen. In the frontal cortex, patients with Tourette's disorder were found to have lower concentrations of *N*-acetylaspartate bilaterally, lower levels of creatine on the right side, and reduced myoinositol on the left side. These results suggest that deficits in the density of neuronal and nonneuronal cells are present in patients with the disorder. Abnormalities in the noradrenergic system have been implicated in some cases by the reduction of tics with clonidine (Catapres). This adrenergic agonist reduces the release of norepinephrine in the central nervous system and, thus, may reduce activity in the dopaminergic system. Abnormalities in the basal ganglia are known to result in various movement disorders, such as Huntington's disease, and are also implicated as likely sites of disturbance in Tourette's disorder.

Immunological Factors and Postinfection

An autoimmune process and, in particular, one that is secondary to group A beta-hemolytic streptococcal infections was hypothesized as a potential mechanism for the development of tics and obsessive-compulsive symptoms in some cases. Data have been conflicting and controversial, and this mechanism appears to be unlikely as an etiology of Tourette's disorder in most cases. One case-control study found little evidence of the development or exacerbation of tics, or obsessions or compulsions, in children with well-documented and treated group A beta-hemolytic streptococcal infections.

DIAGNOSIS AND CLINICAL FEATURES

A diagnosis of Tourette's disorder depends on a history of multiple motor tics that generally emerge over a period of months or years, and the emergence of at least one vocal tic at some point. According to the American Psychiatric Association's Fifth Edition of the *Diagnostic and Statistical Manual of Mental Disorders* (DSM-5), tics may wax and wane in frequency, but must have persisted for more than a year since the first tic emerged to meet the diagnosis. The average age of onset of tics is between 4 and 6 years of age, although in some cases, tics may occur as early as 2 years of age. The peak age for severity of tics is between 10 and 12 years. To meet diagnostic criteria for Tourette's disorder, the onset must occur before the age of 18 years.

In Tourette's disorder, typically the initial tics are in the face and neck. Over time, the tics tend to occur in a downward progression. The most commonly described tics are those affecting the face and head, the arms and hands, the body and lower extremities, and the respiratory and alimentary systems. In these areas, the tics take the form of grimacing; forehead puckering; eyebrow-raising; eyelid-blinking; winking; nose-wrinkling; nostril-trembling; mouth-twitching; displaying the teeth; biting the lips and other parts; tongue-extruding; protracting the lower jaw; nodding, jerking, or shaking the head; twisting the neck; looking sideways; head-rolling; hand-jerking; arm-jerking; plucking fingers; writhing fingers; fist-clenching; shoulder-shrugging; foot, knee, or toe shaking; walking peculiarly; body writhing; jumping; hiccupping; sighing; yawning; snuffing; blowing through the nostrils; whistling; belching; sucking or smacking sounds; and clearing the throat. Several assessment instruments are currently available that are useful in making diagnoses of tic disorders, including comprehensive self-report assessment tools, such as the *Tic Symptom Self Report* and the *Yale Global Tic Severity Scale,* administered by a clinician (Table 27.8c–1).

Because Tourette's disorder is frequently comorbid with attentional, obsessional, and oppositional behaviors, these symptoms often emerge prior to the tics. In some studies, more

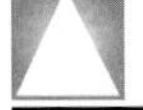

Table 27.8c–1
Clinical Assessment Tools in Tic Disorders

Domain	Type	Reliability and Validity	Sensitive to Change
Tics			
Tic Symptom Self-Report	Parent/self	Good	Yes
Yale Global Tic Severity Scale	Clinician	Excellent	Yes
Attention-Deficit/Hyperactivity Disorder			
Swanson, Nolan, and Pelham-IV	Parent/teacher	Excellent	Yes
Abbreviated Conners' Questionnaire	Parent/teacher	Excellent	Yes
Obsessive-Compulsive Disorder			
Yale-Brown Obsessive Compulsive Scale and Children's Yale-Brown Obsessive Compulsive Scale	Clinician	Excellent	Yes
National Institute of Mental Health Global	Clinician	Excellent	Yes
General			
Child Behavior Checklist	Parent/teacher	Excellent	No

than 25 percent of children with Tourette's disorder received stimulants for a diagnosis of ADHD before receiving a diagnosis of Tourette's disorder. The most frequent initial symptom is an eye-blink tic, followed by a head tic or a facial grimace. Most complex motor and vocal symptoms emerge several years after the initial symptoms. Coprolalia, a very unusual symptom involving shouting or speaking socially unacceptable or obscene words, occurs in less than 10 percent of patients and rarely in the absence of comorbid psychiatric disturbance. Mental coprolalia—in which a patient experiences a sudden, intrusive, socially unacceptable thought or obscene word—occurs more often than coprolalia. In severe cases, physical self-injury has occurred due to tic behaviors.

Jake, age 10 years, came to the Tourette Disorder Clinic for an evaluation of motor tics in the head and neck, occasional coughing and grunting, and a new symptom of throat clearing many times per day. Jake had a past history of ADHD, which included significant hyperactivity, and impulsive and oppositional behavior He is a fifth-grade student in a regular class at the local public school. Before the consultation, parent and teacher ratings, including the *Child Behavior Checklist* (CBCL), *Swanson, Nolan, and Pelham-IV* (SNAP-IV), *Conners' Parent and Teacher Questionnaires, Tic Symptom Self-Report* (TSSR), and medical history survey, were sent to his family. His mother and the classroom teacher rated him well above the norm for hyperactivity, inattention, and impulsiveness. He was failing several subjects in school, often argued with adults, was occasionally aggressive, and had few friends. His tics were rated as moderate.

Jake's mother recalls difficulties with overactivity, oppositional and defiant behaviors and behavior since preschool. At age 5, due to his activity level and argumentative and aggressive behavior, his kindergarten teacher encouraged the family to obtain a psychiatric consultation. Jake's pediatrician made a diagnosis of ADHD and recommended a trial of Concerta (methylphenidate extended-release tablets) at 36 mg per day, which was started at the beginning of the first grade. Within a week of starting medication, Jake's overly active and impulsive behavior showed a dramatic improvement; however, he remained argumentative and oppositional. However, when on his Concerta, Jake was able to stay in his seat and complete his work and was better able to wait his turn on the playground. The next few months went well, however, by early spring, Jake seemed to be returning back to some of his old ways. He was talking out of turn in class, and getting out of his seat, which was disruptive to the class. After an increase in Concerta to 54 mg per day, in the spring of his first-grade year, however, he began showing motor and phonic tics consisting of head-jerking, facial movements, coughing, and grunting. The Concerta was discontinued to see if this made a difference and was immediately stopped and, although the tics transiently decreased, they came back in full force within a month. In hindsight, Jake's mother recalled that Jake had exhibited eye blinking and grunting prior to starting the Concerta, but she had dismissed these events as unimportant and they did not seem to disrupt Jake's daily life.

While Jake was off Concerta during a period when he began middle school in the 6th grade, Jake was disruptive to his classes and he began to be severely teased by several classmates for his impulsivity, frequent motor tics, and loud grunting and throat clearing. Jake became despondent and began to refuse to go to school. At this point, it was decided to place Jake in a special education class. However, after several months of this placement, Jake felt worse about himself, despised school, and begged to be returned to regular classes. At this point Jake's pediatrician made the referral to a child and adolescent psychiatrist at a local university Tourette Disorder Clinic.

During his evaluation at the Tourette Disorder Clinic, Jake was reported to be a healthy child who was the product of an uncomplicated pregnancy, labor, and delivery, and whose developmental milestones were achieved at appropriate times. Intellectual testing completed by the school psychologist revealed a full scale IQ of 105. Jake's mother noted that Jake has had long-standing trouble falling asleep but sleeps through the night. Jake has always been described as argumentative and easily frustrated with frequent outbursts of temper; however, when he is not having a tantrum, his mood is generally upbeat.

Jake was noted by the child and adolescent psychiatrist to be of average height and weight with no dysmorphic features. His speech was rapid in tempo but normal in tone and volume. His speech is coherent and developmentally appropriate, without evidence of thought disorder; however, vocal tics including grunting, coughing, and obvious throat clearing were observed. Jake denied depressed mood or suicidal ideation, although he reported distress about everyday issues such as being teased by peers, not having enough friends, and his poor school performance. Jake also denied recurring worries about contamination or harm coming to him or family members, or fears of acting on unwanted impulses. Other than mild touching habits involving the need to touch objects with each hand three times or in combinations of three, Jake denies repetitive rituals. Several motor tics were also observed during the evaluation session, including blinking, head-jerking, and shoulder tics. Jake was restless and easily distracted throughout the session and often needed assistance with entertaining himself when not directly involved in conversation.

Given the history of enduring motor and phonic tics, confirmed by direct observation, the diagnosis of Tourette's disorder and ADHD, as well as oppositional defiant disorder were confirmed.

Jake and his family attended several sessions with the child and adolescent psychiatrist to learn about the waxing and waning nature of tic symptoms and the natural history of Tourette's Disorder, as well as ADHD. Jake and his family were heartened to hear that, in general, tics tend to be at their maximum around his age, and it was somewhat likely that Jake's tics would lessen over time or possibly fully remit. Jake was referred to a behavioral psychologist specializing in habit reversal training. In this treatment Jake was taught to engage in a behavior physically incompatible with his tic (a competing response) each time he experienced the urge to perform this tic. The competing response for Jake's shoulder tic, which consisted of raising his shoulders up as far as he could, was to gently press his shoulders down and extend his neck each time he felt the urge to engage in this tic. With repeated practice of his competing response, Jake's urge to engage in this tic greatly diminished to the point where he was able to manage the urge without performing the tic. Jake was referred to a child and adolescent psychiatrist who decided to re-start the Concerta at 36 mg per day and titrated it back up to 54 mg per day without worsening of the tics. Jake responded well to his behavioral therapy, and over a period of 8 weeks, he had learned how to become aware of the urges that occurred prior to his tics and to voluntarily replace his usual tics with less-distressing and less-disruptive behaviors.

However, when Jake entered the 7th grade, he had an exacerbation of his motor and vocal tics, and was also touching objects repeatedly throughout the day. Jake again became despondent, not wanting to go to school. It was decided by his psychologist to add relaxation training to his behavioral treatment, and his child and adolescent psychiatrist another medication to his pharmacological regimen. Jake was prescribed risperidone, 0.5 mg per day, which was titrated up to 1 mg twice daily. With the addition of these psychological and pharmacological interventions, Jake became stabilized within a month, and was able to continue in his school and even went to some parties. Jake and his parents understood the waxing and waning nature of his tics, and were hopeful that they would begin to see some decrease in his tic symptoms within the next few years. At follow-up, when Jake was 15 years of age, Jake had minimal tic symptoms; an occasional eye blink and rare throat clearing was all that was observable. Jake was not currently in behavioral treatment; however, over the years, he had, on a few occasions received some booster therapy sessions to brush up on his habit reversal training when he had a minor exacerbation of tics. Jake had been taken off his risperidone a 2 years before without an exacerbation of tics. Jake continued on Concerta 54 mg per day and was well controlled on that dose, was doing well in school, and had become more popular since he had joined the soccer team. *(Adapted from L. Scahill, M.S.N., Ph.D. and J.F. Leckman, M.D.)*

PATHOLOGY AND LABORATORY EXAMINATION

No specific laboratory diagnostic test exists for Tourette's disorder, but many patients with Tourette's disorder have nonspecific abnormal electroencephalographic findings. CT and MRI scans have revealed no specific structural lesions, although about 10 percent of all patients with Tourette's disorder show some nonspecific abnormality on CT scans.

DIFFERENTIAL DIAGNOSIS

Tics must be differentiated from other movements and movement disorders (e.g., dystonic, choreiform, athetoid, myoclonic, and hemiballismic movements) and the neurological diseases that they may characterize (e.g., Huntington's disease, parkinsonism, Sydenham's chorea, and Wilson's disease), as listed in Table 27.8c–2. Tremors, mannerisms, and stereotypic movement disorder (e.g., head-banging or body-rocking) must also be distinguished from tic disorders. Stereotypic movement disorders, including movements such as rocking, hand-gazing, and other self-stimulatory behaviors, seem to be voluntary and often produce a sense of comfort, in contrast to tic disorders. Although tics in children and adolescents may or may not feel controllable, they rarely produce a sense of well-being. Compulsions are sometimes difficult to distinguish from complex tics and may be on the same continuum biologically. Tic disorders may also occur comorbidly with mood disturbances. In a recent survey, the greater the severity of tics, the higher the probability of both aggressive and depressive symptoms in children. When a child experiences an exacerbation of tic symptoms, behavior and mood also seem to deteriorate.

COURSE AND PROGNOSIS

Tourette's disorder is a childhood-onset neuropsychiatric disorder characterized by both motor and vocal tics, which usually emerge in early childhood, with a natural history leading to reduction or complete resolution of tic symptoms in most cases by adolescence or early adulthood. During childhood, individual tic symptoms may decrease, persist, or increase, and old symptoms may be replaced by new ones. Severely afflicted persons may have serious emotional problems, including major depressive disorder. Impairment may also be associated with the motor and vocal tic symptoms of Tourette's disorder; however, in many cases, interference in function is exacerbated by comorbid ADHD and OCD, both of which frequently coexist with the disorder. When the above three disorders are comorbid, severe social, academic, and occupational problems may ensue. Although most children with Tourette's disorder will experience a decline in the frequency and severity of tic symptoms during adolescence, at present, no clinical measures exist to predict which children may have persistent symptoms into adulthood. Children with mild forms of Tourette's disorder often have satisfactory peer relationships, function well in school, and develop adequate self-esteem, and may not require treatment.

TREATMENT

Once a diagnosis of Tourette's disorder is made, psychoeducation is a useful intervention in order for families to gain an understanding of the variability of tics, the natural history of the disorder, and ways to support reduction of stress. It is particularly important for families to be well-informed advocates for their children, since tics may be misinterpreted by an uneducated observer as a child's purposeful misbehavior, rather than a response to an irresistible urge. The need for treatment is based on subjective distress of a child with respect to tics as well as observable disruptions in functioning. In mild cases, children with tic disorders who are functioning well socially and academically may not seek, nor require treatment. In more severe cases, children with tic disorders may be ostracized by peers and have academic work compromised by the disruptive nature of tics, and a variety of interventions including psychosocial, pharmacological, and school based may be considered. A scale to measure tic severity, the *Premonitory Urge for Tics Scale* (PUTS), was examined psychometrically, and found to be internally consistent and correlated with overall tic severity in youth over 10 years of age.

The European clinical guidelines for Tourette's syndrome and other tic disorders summarized and reviewed the evidence-based treatments for Tourette's disorder and developed a consensus for psychosocial and pharmacological treatments. This guideline recommends that both behavioral and pharmacological interventions be considered in more severe cases, with behavioral interventions typically the first line of treatment. Indications for treatment include, but are not limited to, the following clinical presentations. Tics require treatment when they cause social and emotional problems, depression, or isolation. Children who are prone to severe persistent complex motor tics or loud vocal tics may be the objects of bullying and social rejection. In these cases, depressive symptoms commonly result. Tic reduction and psychoeducation to the school may be indicated to preserve healthy social relationships, and to diminish depressive and anxiety symptoms. Tics may also lead to impairment in academic achievement, when school functioning is disrupted. School difficulties in children with Tourette's disorder are not uncommon, and reduction in tics may support increased academic success. Tics may also lead to physical discomfort, based on the repetitive musculoskeletal exertion, especially in relation to head and neck tics. In some children with Tourette's disorder,

Table 27.8c–2
Differential Diagnosis of Tic Disorders

Disease or Syndrome	Age at Onset	Associated Features	Course	Predominant Type of Movement
Hallervorden–Spatz	Childhood–adolescence	May be associated with optic atrophy, club feet, retinitis pigmentosa, dysarthria, dementia, ataxia, emotional lability, spasticity, autosomal recessive inheritance	Progressive to death in 5–20 years	Choreic, athetoid, myoclonic
Dystonia musculorum deformans	Childhood–adolescence	Autosomal recessive inheritance commonly, primarily among Ashkenazi Jews; a more benign autosomal dominant form also occurs	Variable course, often progressive but with rare remissions	Dystonia
Sydenham's chorea	Childhood, usually 5–15 years	More common in females, usually associated with rheumatic fever (carditis elevated ASLO titers)	Usually self-limited	Choreiform
Huntington's disease	Usually 30–50 years, but childhood forms are known	Autosomal dominant inheritance, dementia, caudate atrophy on CT scan	Progressive to death in 10–15 years after onset	Choreiform
Wilson's disease (hepatolenticular degeneration)	Usually 10–25 years	Kayser–Fleischer rings, liver dysfunction, inborn error of copper metabolism; autosomal recessive inheritance	Progressive to death without chelating therapy	Wing-beating tremor, dystonia
Hyperreflexias (including latah, myriachit, jumper disease of Maine)	Generally in childhood (dominant inheritance)	Familial; may have generalized rigidity and autosomal inheritance	Nonprogressive	Excessive startle response; may have echolalia, coprolalia, and forced obedience
Myoclonic disorders	Any age	Numerous causes, some familial, usually no vocalizations	Variable, depending on cause	Myoclonus
Myoclonic dystonia	5–47 years	Nonfamilial, no vocalizations	Nonprogressive	Torsion dystonia with myoclonic jerks
Paroxysmal myoclonic dystonia with vocalization	Childhood	Attention, hyperactive, and learning disorders; movements interfere with ongoing activity	Nonprogressive	Bursts of regular, repetitive clonic (less tonic) movements and vocalizations
Tardive Tourette's disorder syndromes	Variable (after antipsychotic medication use)	Reported to be precipitated by discontinuation or reduction of medication	May terminate after increase or decrease of dosage	Orofacial dyskinesias, choreoathetosis, tics, vocalization
Neuroacanthocytosis	Third or fourth decade	Acanthocytosis, muscle wasting, parkinsonism, autosomal recessive inheritance	Variable	Orofacial dyskinesia and limb chorea, tics, vocalization
Encephalitis lethargica	Variable	Shouting fits, bizarre behavior, psychosis, Parkinson's disease	Variable	Simple and complex motor and vocal tics, coprolalia, echolalia, echopraxia, palilalia
Gasoline inhalation	Variable	Abnormal EEG; symmetrical theta and theta bursts frontocentrally	Variable	Simple motor and vocal tics
Postangiographic complications	Variable	Emotional lability, amnestic syndrome	Variable	Simple motor and complex vocal tics, palilalia
Postinfectious	Variable	EEG: occasional asymmetrical theta bursts before movements, elevated ASLO titers	Variable	Simple motor and vocal tics, echopraxia
Posttraumatic	Variable	Asymmetrical tic distribution	Variable	Complex motor tics
Carbon monoxide poisoning	Variable	Inappropriate sexual behavior	Variable	Simple and complex motor and vocal tics, coprolalia, echolalia, palilalia
XYY genetic disorder	Infancy	Aggressive behavior	Static	Simple motor and vocal tics
XXY and 9_p mosaicism	Infancy	Multiple physical anomalies, mental retardation	Static	Simple motor and vocal tics
Duchenne's muscular dystrophy (X-linked recessive)	Childhood	Mild mental retardation	Progressive	Motor and vocal tics
Fragile X syndrome	Childhood	Mental retardation, facial dysmorphism, seizures, autistic features	Static	Simple motor and vocal tics, coprolalia
Developmental and perinatal disorders	Infancy, childhood	Seizures, EEG and CT abnormalities, psychosis, aggressivity, hyperactivity, Ganser's syndrome, compulsivity, torticollis	Variable	Motor and vocal tics, echolalia

ASLO, Antistreptolysin O; CT, computed tomography; EEG, electroencephalogram.

tics can worsen headaches and migraines. Behavioral and pharmacological interventions can both target tic reductions, which can lead to improved quality of life.

Evidence-Based Behavioral and Psychosocial Treatment

The Canadian guidelines for the evidence-based treatment of tic disorders: behavioral therapy, deep brain stimulation and transcranial magnetic stimulation, and a large multisite randomized controlled trial of "Comprehensive Behavioral Intervention for Tics," (CBIT) both found converging evidence supporting *habit-reversal training* and *exposure and response prevention* as efficacious treatments for tic reduction. In a randomized controlled trial of CBIT, 61 children received habit reversal training as their main component of treatment, and they also received relaxation treatment and a functional intervention to identify situations that worsened or sustained tics and strategies to decrease exposure to these situations. The control group of 65 children received supportive psychotherapy and psychoeducation. After 10 weeks of treatment, the Yale Global Tic Severity Scale Total Tic score was significantly reduced in the behavioral intervention group compared with the control group.

Habit Reversal. The primary components of habit reversal are awareness training, in which the child uses self-monitoring to enhance awareness of tic behaviors and the premonitory urges or sensations indicating that a tic is about to occur. In competing-response training, the patient is taught to voluntarily perform a behavior that is physically incompatible with the tic, contingent on the onset of the premonitory urge or the tic itself, blocking expression of the tic. The competing-response strategy is based on the self-reported observations of patients that tics are performed in response to irresistible premonitory urges to diminish the urge. Because performing the tic satisfies or reduces the premonitory urges, the tics are reinforced, and over time, become repeated entrenched behaviors. Competing-response training is different from voluntary tic suppression in that the patient initiates a voluntary behavior to manage the premonitory urge and thus disrupts the reinforcement of the tic, rather than simply trying to suppress the tic. Successful competing-response training results in significant reduction in premonitory urge intensity or complete elimination of the urge altogether so that tics are no longer provoked. For motor tics, a behavior that is less noticeable may be chosen, whereas for vocal tics, slow rhythmic breathing is the most common voluntary competing response. The competing responses are designed to be performed without disrupting usual activities.

Exposure and Response Prevention. The rationale for this treatment is based on the notion that tics occur as a conditioned response to unpleasant premonitory urges, and since the tics reduce the urge, they become associated with the premonitory urge. Each time the urge is reduced by the tic, their association is further strengthened. Rather than using competing responses, as in habit-reversal training, exposure and response prevention asks the patient to suppress tics for increasingly prolonged periods to break the association between the urges and the tics. Theoretically, if a patient learns to resist performing the tic in response to the urge for long enough periods, the urge may become more tolerable, or attenuate, and the need to perform the tic may diminish.

Many other behavioral interventions such as relaxation training, self-monitoring, bio (neuro) feedback, and cognitive-behavioral treatment (CBT), have not been shown to be efficacious in the reduction of tics on their own; however, some of these strategies may be included in comprehensive treatment programs for children with tic disorders who are receiving habit-reversal training. Habit reversal has been the most extensively researched behavioral treatment for tic disorders; it has been shown to be highly effective, and is currently the first-line behavioral treatment for tic disorders.

Evidence-Based Pharmacotherapy

Several reviews of pharmacological treatments for tics suggest that the following classes of pharmacologic agents have an evidence base for treating tics: typical and atypical antipsychotics; noradrenergic agents; and alternative treatments such as tetrabenazine, topiramate, and tetrahydrocannabinol (THC).

Atypical and Typical Antipsychotic Agents. Risperidone, with its high affinity for dopamine D_2 and serotonin 5-HT_2 receptors, is the most well-studied atypical antipsychotic in the treatment of tics. There is considerable evidence for its efficacy. Multiple randomized, controlled studies in children and adolescents have shown favorable results compared to placebo as well as in head-to-head studies with the typical antipsychotic agents haloperidol and pimozide. Risperidone was associated with fewer adverse events compared to typical antipsychotics; however, it was frequently associated with weight gain, metabolic side effects, and hyperprolactinemia. In a randomized, double-blind, parallel group study of Tourette's disorder comparing risperidone to pimozide, risperidone showed superiority in reducing comorbid obsessive-compulsive symptoms as well as reducing tics. In other randomized clinical trials, efficacy of tic reduction was achieved in studies of children, adolescents, and adults with mean daily doses of 2.5 mg daily with a range of 1 to 6 mg daily.

Haloperidol (Haldol) and pimozide (Orap) are the two most well-investigated and FDA–approved antipsychotic agents in the treatment of Tourette's disorder, although atypical antipsychotics such as risperidone are often chosen as first-line agents due to their safer side-effect profiles. Both haloperidol and pimozide have been shown to be efficacious in multiple randomized clinical trials in the treatment of Tourette's disorder. Both haloperidol and pimozide present significant risks for extrapyramidal side effects; in a long-term naturalistic follow-up study, haloperidol was found to produce more significant acute dyskinesia and dystonia compared to pimozide.

A third typical antipsychotic, fluphenazine, has been used in the United States for many years in the treatment of tic disorders, in the absence of robust data supporting its efficacy. A small controlled study of fluphenazine, trifluphenazine, and haloperidol found similar reductions in tics; however, haloperidol was associated with more extrapyramidal side effects and more sedation. The frequency of sedation, dystonia, and akathisia of typical antipsychotics, probably due to their predominant dopaminergic blockade in the nigrostriatal pathways, limits their use and increases the appeal of the atypical antipsychotics. Risperidone and pimozide were found to be of equal efficacy in one study of children, adolescents, and adults with Tourette's disorder.

Aripiprazole has become a pharmacological agent of interest in the treatment of tic disorders due to its mode of action; in addition to its D_2 receptor antagonistic actions, aripiprazole is also a partial D_2 and 5-HT_{1A} receptor agonist and a 5-HT_{2A} antagonist. A multisite double-blind controlled study of aripiprazole in children with Tourette's disorder in China found a reduction in tic behaviors in about 60 percent of the aripiprazole group compared to about 64 percent reduction in a group treated with tiapride, a benzamide with selective D_2 receptor antagonism. There was no significant difference between the two groups. Although sedation and sleep disturbance are common side effects with aripiprazole, weight gain is less pronounced than with risperidone.

Olanzapine and ziprasidone were shown to be efficacious in the treatment of tic disorders in at least one randomized controlled trial. Sedation and weight gain were prominent side effects with olanzapine, and potential QT prolongation was an issue with ziprasidone. Quetiapine has been suggested as a potentially useful agent in the treatment of tics, with its greater affinity for 5-HT_2 receptors than for D_2 receptors; however, randomized clinical trials are needed. Clozapine, contrary to many other atypical antipsychotics, has not been found to be useful in the treatment of tics.

Noradrenergic Agents. Noradrenergic agents including clonidine and guanfacine, as well as atomoxetine, are frequently used in children as primary treatments or adjunctive treatments for comorbid ADHD and tics. Several studies have provided some evidence for the efficacy of clonidine, an α_2-adrenergic agent, in the treatment of tics in children, adolescents, and adults with tic disorders. The largest randomized trial with oral clonidine compared to placebo found a modest reduction in tics with clonidine. A multisite randomized double-blind placebo-controlled trial using the clonidine patch in the treatment of tic disorders in children found a significant improvement in tic symptoms (about 69 percent) compared to about 47 percent of the children in the control group. Clonidine has generally been used in dosages ranging from 0.05 mg orally three times daily to 0.1 mg four times daily; and guanfacine is usually used in dosages ranging from 1 to 4 mg per day. When used in these dosage ranges, adverse effects of the α-adrenergic agents may include drowsiness, headache, irritability, and occasional hypotension.

Guanfacine has been used frequently to treat children with ADHD successfully, although its efficacy regarding reducing tics is controversial. In one randomized clinical trial treating 34 children with ADHD and tics, guanfacine was found to be superior to placebo in the reduction of tics. In another double-blind placebo-controlled trial of 24 children with Tourette's disorder, guanfacine was not superior to placebo.

Atomoxetine, a selective noradrenaline reuptake inhibitor, was found to reduce both tics and ADHD symptoms in a multicenter industry trial of 148 children. Atomoxetine also reduced both tics and ADHD in a subgroup of patients in this study who were diagnosed with Tourette's disorder. Additional studies are needed to confirm safety and efficacy of atomoxetine in the treatment of children with Tourette's disorder.

In view of the frequent comorbidity of tic behaviors and obsessive-compulsive symptoms or disorders, the SSRIs have been used alone or in combination with antipsychotics in the treatment of Tourette's disorder. Data, thus far, have supported the efficacy of SSRIs in the treatment of OCD, however there have not been controlled trials yet to determine the effect of SSRIs on tic reduction.

Although clinicians must weigh the risks and benefits of using stimulants in cases of severe hyperactivity and comorbid tics, data suggest that methylphenidate does not increase the rate or intensity of motor or vocal tics in most children with hyperactivity and tic disorders.

Alternative Agents: Tetrabenazine, Topiramate, and Tetrahydrocannabinol

TETRABENAZINE. A vesicular monoamine transporter type 2 inhibitor, tetrabenazine depletes presynaptic dopamine and serotonin, and blocks postsynaptic dopamine receptors. There are no randomized clinical trials of this agent in the treatment of Tourette's disorder in children; however, clinical experience suggests that this agent may have benefit in tic reduction. In a follow-up of 2 years of treatment in 77 children and adolescents, one study reports tic reduction improvement in 80 percent of subjects. Side effects of this agent include sedation, parkinsonism, depression, insomnia, anxiety, and akathisia.

TOPIRAMATE. A γ-aminobutyric acid (GABA)ergic drug, used primarily as an anticonvulsant, topiramate was found to be efficacious compared to placebo in reducing tics in a small randomized clinical trial of children and adults with Tourette's disorder. Side effects were minimal. Although this does not confirm its efficacy, GABA-modulating agents require further study in the treatment of tic disorders.

TETRAHYDROCANNABINOL. A suggestion that THC may be safe and efficacious in the treatment of tics, without neuropsychological impairment, is based on a randomized double-blind placebo-controlled trial with 24 patients treated with THC for 6 weeks at doses of up to 10 mg with significant improvement in tic severity. In this trial, reported adverse effects included dizziness, fatigue, and dry mouth. Potential additional side-effects include anxiety, depressive symptoms, tremor, and insomnia. This small trial does not confirm efficacy for this agent in the treatment of tics, rather it raises questions about the potential improvements in treatment-resistant tic disorders using this agent.

In summary, the greatest evidence for the safe and efficacious pharmacological treatment of Tourette's disorder seems to be associated with the atypical antipsychotics, in particular, risperidone. Pharmacological treatment may be combined with and enhanced by a variety of behavioral interventions such as habit reversal and school interventions that may diminish stressful situations in the school environment.

27.8d Persistent (Chronic) Motor or Vocal Tic Disorder

Chronic motor or vocal tic disorder is defined as the presence of either motor tics or vocal tics, but not both. Tics may wax and wane but must have persisted for more than 1 year since the first tic onset to meet the diagnosis for persistent (chronic) motor or vocal tic disorder. According to the Fifth Edition of the American

Psychiatric Association's *Diagnostic and Statistical Manual of Mental Disorders* (DSM-5) criteria, this disorder must have its onset before the age of 18 years. Chronic motor or vocal tic disorder cannot be diagnosed if the criteria for Tourette's disorder have ever been met.

EPIDEMIOLOGY

The rate of chronic motor or vocal tic disorder has been estimated to be 100 to 1,000 times greater than that of Tourette's disorder in school-age children. School-age boys are at highest risk. Although the disorder was once believed to be rare, current estimates of the prevalence of chronic motor or vocal tic disorder range from 1 to 2 percent.

ETIOLOGY

Chronic motor or vocal tic disorder as well as Tourette's disorder tends to aggregate in the same families. Twin studies have found a high concordance for either Tourette's disorder or chronic motor tics in monozygotic twins. This finding supports the importance of hereditary factors in the transmission of tic disorders.

DIAGNOSIS AND CLINICAL FEATURES

The onset of chronic motor or vocal tic disorder typically occurs in early childhood. Chronic vocal tics are considerably rarer than chronic motor tics. Chronic vocal tics, in the absence of motor tics, are typically less conspicuous than the vocal tics in Tourette's disorder. The vocal tics are usually not loud or intense and are not primarily produced by the vocal cords; they consist of grunts or other noises caused by thoracic, abdominal, or diaphragmatic contractions.

DIFFERENTIAL DIAGNOSIS

Chronic motor tics must be differentiated from a variety of other motor movements, including choreiform movements, myoclonus, restless legs syndrome, akathisia, and dystonias. Involuntary vocal utterances can occur in certain neurological disorders, such as Huntington's disease and Parkinson's disease.

COURSE AND PROGNOSIS

Children whose tics emerge between the ages of 6 and 8 years seem to have the best outcomes. Symptoms often last for 4 to 6 years and remit in early adolescence. Children whose tics involve the limbs or trunk may have less prompt remission than those with only facial tics.

TREATMENT

The treatment of chronic motor or vocal tic disorder depends on several factors including the severity and frequency of the tics; the patient's subjective distress; the effects of the tics on school or work, job performance, and socialization; and the presence of any other concomitant mental disorder. Psychotherapy may be indicated to minimize the secondary social difficulties caused by severe tics. Behavioral techniques, particularly habit reversal treatments, are effective in treating chronic motor or vocal tic disorder. When severe, tics may be reduced through the use of atypical antipsychotics such as risperidone. If not effective, typical antipsychotics such as pimozide or haloperidol may be helpful. Behavioral interventions are the first line of treatment.

▲ 27.9 Feeding and Eating Disorders of Infancy or Early Childhood

Feeding and eating disorders of infancy and childhood are characterized by persistent disturbances in eating or eating-related disorders that can lead to significant impairments in physical health and psychosocial functioning. The American Psychiatric Association's Fifth Edition of the *Diagnostic and Statistical Manual of Mental Disorders* (DSM-5) category *Feeding and Eating Disorders* includes three disorders that are often, but not always, associated with infancy and early childhood: pica, rumination disorder, and avoidant/restrictive food intake disorder (formerly known as feeding disorder of infancy or early childhood). These three disorders are discussed in this section. Anorexia nervosa, bulimia nervosa, and binge-eating disorder are more often associated with young adulthood and discussed separately in Chapter 15.

27.9a Pica

Pica is defined as persistent eating of nonnutritive substances. Typically, no specific biological abnormalities account for pica, and in many cases, pica is identified only when medical problems such as intestinal obstruction, intestinal infections, or poisonings arise, such as lead poisoning due to ingestion of lead containing paint chips. Pica is more frequent in the context of ASD or intellectual disability; however, pica is diagnosed only when it is of sufficient severity and persistence to warrant clinical attention. Pica can emerge in young children, adolescents, or adults; however, a minimum of 2 years of age is suggested by DSM-5 in the diagnosis of pica, in order to exclude developmentally appropriate mouthing of objects by infants that may accidentally result in ingestion. Pica occurs in both males and females, and in rare cases, it may be associated with a cultural belief in the spiritual or medicinal benefit of ingesting nonfood substances. In this context, a diagnosis of pica is not made. Among adults, certain forms of pica, including geophagia (clay eating) and amylophagia (starch eating), have been reported in pregnant women.

EPIDEMIOLOGY

The prevalence of pica is unclear. A survey of a large clinic population reported that 75 percent of 12-month-old infants and 15 percent of 2- to 3-year-old toddlers placed nonnutritive substances in their mouth; however, this behavior is developmentally appropriate and typically does not result in ingestion. Pica is more common among children and adolescents with ASD and intellectual disability. It has been reported that up to 15 percent of persons with severe intellectual disability have engaged in pica. Pica appears to affect both sexes equally.

ETIOLOGY

Pica is most often a transient disorder that typically lasts for several months and then remits. In younger children, it is more frequently seen among children with developmental speech and social developmental delays. Among adolescents with pica, a substantial number of them exhibited depressive symptoms and use of substances. Nutritional deficiencies in minerals such as zinc or iron have been anecdotally reported in some instances; however, these reports are rare. For example, cravings for dirt and ice have been reported to be associated with iron and zinc deficiencies, which are corrected by their administration. Severe child maltreatment in the form of parental neglect and deprivation has been reported in some cases of pica. Lack of supervision, as well as adequate feeding of infants and toddlers may increase the risk of pica.

DIAGNOSIS AND CLINICAL FEATURES

Eating nonedible substances repeatedly after 18 months of age is not typical; however, DSM-5 suggests a minimum age of 2 years when making a diagnosis of pica. Pica behaviors, however, may begin in infants 12 to 24 months of age. Specific substances ingested vary with their accessibility, and they increase with a child's mastery of locomotion and the resultant increased independence and decreased parental supervision. Typically, in infants, paint, plaster, string, hair, and cloth are objects that may be ingested, whereas older toddlers and young children with pica may ingest dirt, animal feces, small stones, and paper. The clinical implications can be benign or life-threatening, depending on the objects ingested. Among the most serious complications are lead poisoning (usually from lead-based paint), intestinal parasites after ingestion of soil or feces, anemia and zinc deficiency after ingestion of clay, severe iron deficiency after ingestion of large quantities of starch, and intestinal obstruction from the ingestion of hair balls, stones, or gravel. Except in ASD and intellectual disability, pica often remits by adolescence. Pica associated with pregnancy is usually limited to the pregnancy itself.

Chantal was 2½ years of age when her mother urgently brought her to her pediatrician due to severe abdominal pain and lack of appetite. Chantal's mother complained that she still put everything in her mouth but refused to eat regular food. The pediatrician observed that Chantal to be pale, thin, and withdrawn. She sucked her thumb and quietly looked down while her mother reported that Chantal often chewed on newspapers and put plaster in her mouth.

The medical examination revealed that Chantal was anemic and suffered from lead poisoning. She was admitted to the hospital for treatment, and a child psychiatric consultation was obtained.

Further exploration of the history and the observation of mother and child during feeding and play revealed that Chantal's mother was overwhelmed, caring for five young children and had little affection for Chantal. Chantal's mother was a single mother, living with her five children and four other family members in a three-bedroom apartment in an old housing project. Her 7-year-old daughter had behavior problems, and her 6-year-old and 4-year-old sons were impulsive and hyperactive and required constant supervision. Chantal's 18-month-old sister was an engaging and active little girl, whereas Chantal was withdrawn, and would sit quietly, rocking herself, sucking her thumb, or chewing on newspaper.

The treatment plan included the involvement of social services and protective services to remove any lead paint from the walls in their current apartment, seek better living arrangements for the family, and provide a safe environment for the children. Chantal's mother received guidance in enrolling Chantal in a preschool program, and her older sister and two brothers in an after-school program that provided structure and stimulation, and some respite time for her mother. Chantal, her mother, and her younger sister started family therapy to help their mother's understanding of her children's needs and to increase her positive interactions with Chantal. Once Chantal's mother felt more supported and less overwhelmed, she was able to become more empathic and warm toward Chantal. When Chantal began chewing on paper, her mother was coached to engage her in a play activity rather than screaming at her and grabbing her mouth. Chantal and her mother continued in therapy for a year, during which their relationship gradually became more interactive and warm, while Chantal's chewing behaviors decreased, and even her thumb sucking abated.

PATHOLOGY AND LABORATORY EXAMINATION

No single laboratory test confirms or rules out a diagnosis of pica, but several laboratory tests are useful because pica has sometimes been associated with abnormal levels of lead. Levels of iron and zinc in serum should be determined and corrected if low. In rare cases when this is the etiology, pica may disappear when oral iron and zinc are administered. Hemoglobin level should be determined to rule out anemia.

DIFFERENTIAL DIAGNOSIS

The differential diagnosis of pica includes avoidance of food, anorexia, or rarely iron and zinc deficiencies. Pica may occur in conjunction with failure to thrive, and be comorbid with schizophrenia, ASD, and Kleine–Levin syndrome. In psychosocial dwarfism, a dramatic but reversible endocrinological and behavioral form of failure to thrive, children often show bizarre behaviors, including ingesting toilet water, garbage, and other nonnutritive substances. Lead intoxication may be associated with pica. In children who exhibit pica that warrants clinical intervention, along with a known medical disorder, both disorders should be coded according to DSM-5.

In certain regions of the world and among certain cultures, such as the Australian aborigines, rates of pica in pregnant women are reportedly high. According to DSM-5, however, if such practices are culturally accepted, the diagnostic criteria for pica are not met.

COURSE AND PROGNOSIS

The prognosis for pica is usually good, and typically in children with normal intellectual function, pica generally remits spontaneously within several months. In childhood, pica usually resolves with increasing age; in pregnant women, pica is usually limited to the term of the pregnancy. In some adults with pica, particularly those who also have ASD and intellectual disability, pica can continue for years. Follow-up data on these populations are too limited to permit conclusions.

TREATMENT

The first step in determining appropriate treatment of pica is to investigate the specific situation whenever possible. When pica occurs in the context of child neglect or maltreatment, clearly those circumstances must be immediately corrected. Exposure to toxic substances, such as lead, must also be eliminated. No definitive treatment exists for pica per se; most treatment is aimed at education and behavior modification. Treatments emphasize psychosocial, environmental, behavioral, and family guidance approaches. An effort should be made to ameliorate any significant psychosocial stressors. When lead is present in the surroundings, it must be eliminated or rendered inaccessible or the child must be moved to new surroundings.

When pica persists in the absence of any toxic manifestations, behavioral techniques have been utilized. Positive reinforcement, modeling, behavioral shaping, and overcorrection treatment have been used. Increasing parental attention, stimulation, and emotional nurturance may yield positive results. A study found that pica occurred most frequently in impoverished environments, and in some patients, correcting an iron or zinc deficiency has eliminated pica. Medical complications (e.g., lead poisoning) that develop secondarily to the pica must also be treated.

27.9b Rumination Disorder

Rumination is an effortless and painless regurgitation of partially digested food into the mouth soon after a meal, which is either swallowed or spit out. Rumination can be observed in developmentally normal infants who put their thumb or hand in the mouth, suck their tongue rhythmically, and arch their back to initiate regurgitation. This behavior pattern may be observed in infants who receive inadequate emotional interaction and have learned to soothe and may stimulate themselves through rumination. However, rumination syndromes can be found to occur in children and adolescents, and rumination is considered to a functional gastrointestinal disorder. The pathophysiology of rumination is not well understood; however, it often involves a rise in intragastric pressure, generated by either voluntary or unintentional contraction of the abdominal wall muscles causing movement of gastric contents backup into the esophagus. The onset of the disorder can occur in infancy, childhood, or adolescence. In infants, it typically occurs between 3 and 12 months of age, and once the regurgitation occurs, the food may be swallowed or spit out. Infants who ruminate are characteristically observed to strain with their backs arched and head back to bring the food back into their mouths and appear to find the experience pleasurable. Infants who are "experienced" ruminators are able to bring up the food through tongue movements and may not spit out the food at all, but hold it in their mouths and reswallow it. The disorder is less common in older children, adolescents, and adults. It varies in severity and is sometimes associated with medical conditions, such as hiatal hernia, that result in esophageal reflux. In its most severe form, the disorder can cause malnutrition and be fatal.

The diagnosis of rumination disorder can be made even if an infant has attained a normal weight for his or her age. Failure to thrive, therefore, is not a necessary criterion of this disorder, but it is sometimes a sequela. According to DSM-5, the disorder must be present for at least 1 month after a period of normal functioning, and not better accounted for by gastrointestinal illness, or psychiatric or medical conditions.

Rumination has been recognized for hundreds of years. An awareness of the disorder is important so that it is correctly diagnosed and that unnecessary surgical procedures and inappropriate treatment are avoided. *Rumination* is derived from the Latin word *ruminare,* which means, "to chew the cud." The Greek equivalent is *merycism,* the act of regurgitating food from the stomach into the mouth, rechewing the food, and reswallowing it.

EPIDEMIOLOGY

Rumination is a rare disorder. It seems to be more common among male infants, and emerges between 3 months and 1 year of age. It persists more frequently among children, adolescents, and adults with intellectual disability. Adults with rumination usually maintain a normal weight.

ETIOLOGY

Rumination is associated with high intragastric pressure and the ability to contract the abdominal wall to cause retrograde movement of the gastric contents into the esophagus. Several studies have elucidated other gastrointestinal symptoms such as gastroesophageal reflux that may accompany rumination.

In a study of 2,163 children in Sri Lanka, between the ages of 10 and 16 years, it was found that rumination behaviors were present in 5.1 percent of boys and 5.0 percent of girls. In 94.5 percent of youth who ruminated, the regurgitation occurred in the first hour after the meal, and 73.6 percent reported reswallowing of the regurgitated food, whereas the rest spit it out. Only 8.2 percent of this sample reported daily episodes of regurgitation, whereas 62.7 percent experienced weekly symptoms. Associated gastrointestinal symptoms reported in this sample included abdominal pain, bloating, and weight loss. Approximately 20 percent of youth with rumination in this sample also experienced other gastrointestinal symptoms. Another survey of 147 patients from 5 to 20 years of age found that in their sample, the mean age of onset of rumination was 15 years, and these patients were symptomatic after each meal; 16 percent of this sample met criteria for a psychiatric disorder, 3.4 percent had anorexia or bulimia nervosa, and 11 percent had been treated with a surgical procedure for evaluation of management of their symptoms. Additional gastrointestinal symptoms in this sample included abdominal pain in 38 percent, constipation in 21 percent, nausea in 17 percent, and diarrhea in 8 percent. In some cases, vomiting secondary to gastroesophageal reflux or an acute illness precedes a pattern of rumination that lasts for several months. In many cases, children classified as ruminators are shown to have gastroesophageal reflux or hiatal hernia.

It appears, for some infants, that the rumination behavior is self-soothing or produces a sense of relief, leading to a continuation of behaviors to bring it about. In youth with autism spectrum disorder or intellectual disability, rumination may serve as a self-stimulatory behavior. Overstimulation and tension have also been suggested as contributing factor in rumination. Behaviorists attribute persistent rumination to the positive reinforcement of pleasurable self-stimulation and to the attention a baby receives from others as a consequence of the disorder.

DIAGNOSIS AND CLINICAL FEATURES

The DSM-5 notes that the essential feature of the disorder is repeated regurgitation and rechewing of food for a period of at least 1 month after a period of normal functioning. Partially digested food is brought up into the mouth without nausea, retching, or disgust; on the contrary it may appear to be pleasurable. This activity may be distinguished from vomiting by painless and purposeful movements observable in some infants who induce it. The food is then ejected from the mouth or swallowed. A characteristic position of straining and arching of the back, with the head held back, is observed. The infant makes sucking movements with the tongue and gives the impression of gaining considerable satisfaction from the activity. Usually, the infant is irritable and hungry between episodes of rumination.

Initially, rumination may be difficult to distinguish from the regurgitation that frequently occurs in normal infants. In infants with persistent and frequent rumination behaviors, however, the differences are obvious. Although spontaneous remissions are common, secondary complications can develop, such as progressive malnutrition, dehydration, and lowered resistance to disease. Failure to thrive, with absence of growth and developmental delays in all areas, can occur in the most severe cases. Additional complications may occur if the mother of a given infant with rumination becomes discouraged by the persistent symptoms, viewing it as her feeding failure, as this may lead to more tension and more rumination after feedings.

Luca was 9 months old when he was referred by his pediatrician to a gastroenterologist, and by his gastroenterologist for a psychiatric evaluation due to persistent and frequent rumination. Luca was born full-term and had developed typically until 6 weeks of age, when he began to regurgitate large amounts of milk just after feedings. He was evaluated and diagnosed with gastroesophageal reflux, for which it was recommended to thicken his feedings. Luca responded well to the treatment; his regurgitation was markedly diminished, and he gained weight adequately. Luca continued to do well, and his mother decided to go back to work when Lucas was 8months old. Luca's mother transitioned his care to a young nanny who cared for Luca while she worked. Luca and the nanny seemed to have a warm relationship; however, he started again to regurgitate his meals soon after his mother left the house. The regurgitation seemed to increase in frequency and intensity within 2 weeks of the mother's return to work. At this point, Luca regurgitated after almost every meal, and he was losing weight. Luca was evaluated by a gastroenterologist, and during the barium swallow, his doctor noted that Luca put his hand in his mouth, which seemed to induce the regurgitation. Luca was administered some medication for gastroesophageal reflux; however, he continued to induce regurgitation after meals with increasing frequency, prompting the psychiatric consultation.

Observation of mother and infant during feeding at home revealed that as soon as Luca finished feeding, he purposefully placed his hand in his mouth and induced the regurgitation. When his mother restricted his hand, Luca moved his tongue back and forth in a rhythmic manner until he regurgitated again. Luca engaged in this rhythmic tongue movement repeatedly, even when he could not bring up any more milk, and appeared to be enjoying this behavior.

Due to Luca's poor nutritional state and moderate dehydration, he was admitted to the hospital, and a nasojejunal tube was inserted for feedings. When Luca was awake during feedings, a special duty nurse or his parents played with him and distracted him during attempts to put his hand in his mouth or thrust his tongue rhythmically. Luca became increasingly engaged in this playful activity, and his ruminatory activity decreased accordingly. After 1 week in the hospital, small feedings were started; however, Luca again successfully was able to bring up his food by his rumination activity, and the oral feedings had to be temporarily stopped. At this point, Luca's mother decided to stop working and take Luca home to continue an intensive behavioral "distracting" intervention in order to interrupt his rumination during meals. Luca's mother started small feedings while playing with him during and after feedings, and was able to interest him in other activities, so that he would not ruminate. After 4 weeks of slow increments in his feedings, Luca was able to take all his feedings by mouth without ruminating, and the nasojejunal tube could be removed. Luca and his mother continued to use simulating and distracting activities during and just after meals, which over time became more interesting to Luca than his previous ruminating behavior.

PATHOLOGY AND LABORATORY EXAMINATION

No specific laboratory examination is pathognomonic of rumination disorder; however, rumination disorder is not uncommonly associated with gastrointestinal abnormalities. Clinicians are recommended to evaluate other physical causes of vomiting, such as pyloric stenosis and hiatal hernia, before making the diagnosis of rumination disorder. Rumination disorder can lead to states of malnutrition and dehydration. In very severe cases, laboratory measures of endocrinological function, serum electrolytes, and a hematological workup may determine the need for medical intervention.

DIFFERENTIAL DIAGNOSIS

To make the diagnosis of rumination disorder, clinicians must rule out primary gastrointestinal congenital anomalies, infections, and other medical illnesses that could account for frequent regurgitation. Pyloric stenosis is usually associated with projectile vomiting and is generally evident before 3 months of age, when rumination has its onset. Rumination has been associated with both autism spectrum disorder and intellectual disability in which stereotypic behaviors and eating disturbances are not uncommon. Rumination behavior may occur comorbidly in youth with severe anxiety disorders as well. Rumination disorder may also occur in patients with other eating disorders, such as anorexia nervosa and bulimia nervosa.

COURSE AND PROGNOSIS

Rumination disorder is believed to have a high rate of spontaneous remission. Indeed, many cases of rumination disorder may develop and remit without ever being diagnosed. Limited data are available about the prognosis of rumination disorder in adolescents and adults. Behavioral interventions using habit-reversal techniques may significantly lead to improved prognosis.

TREATMENT

The treatment of rumination disorder is often a combination of education and behavioral techniques. Sometimes, an evaluation of the mother–child relationship reveals deficits that can be influenced by offering guidance to the mother. Behavioral interventions, such as habit-reversal are aimed at reinforcing an alternate behavior that becomes more compelling than the behaviors leading to regurgitation. Aversive behavioral interventions, such as squirting lemon juice into the infant's mouth whenever rumination occurs, have been used in the past to diminish rumination behavior. Although aversive behavioral interventions have been reported anecdotally to be effective in some cases, current recommendations support the use of habit-reversal techniques.

When features of child maltreatment of neglect may have contributed to rumination behaviors in an infant, treatments include improvement of the child's psychosocial environment, increased tender loving care from the mother or caretakers, and psychotherapy for the mother or both parents. Anatomical abnormalities, such as hiatal hernia, are not uncommon, and must be evaluated, in some cases leading to surgical repair. In severe cases in which malnutrition and weight loss have occurred, placement of a jejunal tube may need to be inserted before other treatments can be utilized.

Medication is not a standard part of the treatment of rumination. Case reports, however, cite a variety of medications that have been tried, including metoclopramide (Reglan), cimetidine (Tagamet), and even antipsychotics such as haloperidol (Haldol) have been cited to be helpful according to anecdotal reports. The treatment of adolescents with rumination disorder is often complex and includes a multidisciplinary approach consisting of individual psychotherapy, nutritional intervention, and pharmacologic treatment for the frequent comorbid anxiety and depressive symptoms.

27.9c Avoidant/Restrictive Food Intake Disorder

Avoidant/restrictive food intake disorder, formerly known as feeding disorder of infancy or early childhood, is characterized by a lack of interest in food, or its avoidance based on the sensory features of the food or the perceived consequences of eating. This newly included DSM-5 disorder adds more detail about the nature of the eating problems, and has also been expanded to include adolescents and adults. The disorder is manifested by a persistent failure to meet nutritional or energy needs as evidenced by one or more of the following: significant weight loss or failure to achieve expected weight, nutritional deficiency, dependence on enteral feedings or nutritional supplements, or marked interference with psychosocial functioning. It may take the form of outright food refusal, food selectivity, eating too little, food avoidance, and delayed self-feeding. The diagnosis should not be made in the context of anorexia nervosa or bulimia nervosa, or if caused by a medical condition, by another mental disorder, or by a true lack of available food.

Infants and children with the disorder may be withdrawn, irritable, apathetic, or anxious. Because of the avoidant behavior during feeding, touching and holding between mothers and infants are diminished during the entire feeding process compared with other children. Some reports suggest that food avoidance or restriction may be relatively long-standing; however, in many cases, normal adult functioning is eventually achieved.

EPIDEMIOLOGY

It is estimated that between 15 and 35 percent of infants and young children have transient feeding difficulties. A study of restrictive eating difficulties in Swedish 9-year-olds and 12-year-olds found that restrictive eating problems were present in 0.6 percent of their sample. However, another study of avoidant eating patterns in young children in Germany, found that some degree of avoidance was present in up to 53 percent of children. Thus, avoidant eating behaviors without impairment of nutritional state or psychosocial functioning must be separated from restricted eating disturbances leading to significant functional impairment. A survey of feeding problems in nursery school children revealed a prevalence of 4.8 percent with equal gender distribution. In that study, children with feeding problems exhibited more somatic complaints and mothers of affected infants exhibited increased risk of anxiety symptoms. Data from community samples estimate a prevalence of failure-to-thrive syndromes in approximately 3 percent of infants, with approximately half of those infants exhibiting feeding disorders.

DIFFERENTIAL DIAGNOSIS

The disorder must be differentiated from structural problems with the infants' gastrointestinal tract that may be contributing to discomfort during the feeding process. Because feeding disorders and organic causes of swallowing difficulties often coexist, it is important to rule out medical reasons for feeding difficulties. A study of videofluoroscopic evaluation of children with feeding and swallowing problems revealed that clinical evaluation was 92 percent accurate in identifying those children at increased risk of aspiration. This type of evaluation is necessary before psychotherapeutic interventions in cases where a medical contribution to feeding problems is suspected.

COURSE AND PROGNOSIS

Most infants with feeding disorder who are identified within the first year of life and who receive treatment do not go on to develop malnutrition, growth delay, or failure to thrive. When feeding disorders have their onset later, in children 2 to 3 years of age, growth and development can be affected when the disorder lasts for several months. In older children, or adolescents, the feeding disorder typically interferes with social functioning, until treated. It is estimated that about 70 percent of infants who persistently refuse food in the first year of life continue to have some eating problems during childhood.

Jennifer was 6 months old when she was referred for a psychiatric evaluation because of feeding difficulties, irritability, and poor weight gain since birth. She was small and slight, but she did not appear to be lethargic or malnourished. Her parents were college-educated, and both had pursued their professional careers until Jennifer was born. Although Jennifer was full-term and weighed 7 pounds at birth, she had been unable to be breast feed due to turning away and not ingesting enough milk. When she was 4-weeks-old, Jennifer's mother had reluctantly switched her to bottle feedings because Jennifer was losing weight. Although her intake improved somewhat on bottle feedings, she gained weight very slowly and was still less than 8 pounds at 3 months of age. Since then, she had gained a minimal amount each month to maintain a low but adequate weight. Jennifer's mother appeared tired and described that Jennifer would drink only up to about 6 ounces at a time, or two bites of baby food, and then wiggle and cry; and refuse to continue with the feeding. But after a few hours, she might cry again as if she were hungry. However, she could not settle her into a good rhythm of feeding, and continued attempts to feed her would lead her to cry inconsolably. Jennifer's mother described approximately 10 to 15 attempts at feeding her both liquids and solids in a 24-hour period. Jennifer was reported to be an irritable and fussy infant, who cried multiple times during the day and at night, and woke her family often during the night with her crying. Jennifer's developmental milestones such as sitting up, tracking, and making sounds were within normal limits.

The observation of mother–infant interactions during feeding and play revealed that Jennifer was a very alert and wiggly baby who had difficulty sitting still. While drinking from the bottle she would kick her feet and move around, and if the bottle slipped out of her mouth, she did not try to recapture it. When eating baby foods, she was not interested and her mother had to coax her to open her mouth. This upset Jennifer, and she would start crying. Jennifer's mother reported that she was always anxious during meals, and would try to convince Jennifer to take spoonfuls of baby food while sitting in her high chair. After repeated unsuccessful attempts of adequate feeding, Jennifer and her mother both appeared exhausted and took a break.

The history and examination revealed that Jennifer was a very active and excitable baby who had difficulty keeping calm during feedings. After reviewing the videotape with the mother, the therapist explored ways in which the mother could better facilitate calming Jennifer before and during meals. Using a quiet corner in the house, and singing to Jennifer before meals resulted in Jennifer remaining more calm during meals, and she was able to drink larger amounts of milk, eat more solid foods, and waited longer between meals. This, in turn, relieved her mother's anxiety and helped both to have calmer interactions. *(Adapted by Caroly Pataki, M.D.)*

TREATMENT

Most interventions for feeding disorders are aimed at optimizing the interaction between the mother and infant during feedings and identifying any factors that can be changed to promote greater ingestion. The mother is helped to become more aware of the infant's stamina for length of individual feedings, the infant's biological regulation patterns, and the infant's fatigue level with a goal of increasing the level of engagement between mother and infant during feeding.

A transactional model of intervention has been proposed for infants who exhibit the "difficult" temperamental traits of emotional intensity, stubbornness, lack of hunger cues, and irregular eating and sleeping patterns. The treatment includes education for the parents regarding the temperamental traits of the infant, exploration of the parents' anxieties about the infant's nutrition, and training for the parents regarding changing their behaviors to promote internal regulation of eating in the infant. Parents are encouraged to feed the infant on a regular basis at 3- to 4-hour intervals, and offer only water between meals. The parents are trained to deliver praise to the infant for any self-feeding efforts, regardless of the amount of food ingested. Furthermore, parents are guided to limit any distracting stimulation during meals and give attention and praise to positive eating behaviors rather than intense negative attention to inappropriate behavior during meals. This training process for parents is done in an intense manner within a short period of time. Many parents are able to facilitate improved eating patterns in the infant as a result. If the mother or caregiver is unable to participate in the intervention, it may be necessary to include additional caregivers to contribute to feeding the infant. In rare cases, an infant may require hospitalization until adequate nutrition on a daily basis is accomplished. If an infant tires before ingesting an adequate amount of nutrition, it may be necessary to begin treatment with the placement of a nasogastric tube for supplemental oral feedings.

For older children with failure-to-thrive syndromes, hospitalization and nutritional supplementation may be necessary. Medication is not a standard component of treatment for feeding disorders; however, there are anecdotal reports of preadolescents with failure-to-thrive and feeding disorders who were comorbid for anxiety and mood symptoms and who received enteral nutritional interventions in addition to risperidone (Risperdal), and who were observed to have an increase in oral intake and accelerated weight gain.

▲ 27.10 Elimination Disorders

The developmental milestones of mastering control over bowel and bladder function are complex processes that involve motor and sensory functions, coordinated through frontal lobe activities, and regulated by neurons in the pons and midbrain area. Mastery of bowel and bladder function is achieved over a period of months for the typical toddler. Infants generally void small volumes of urine approximately every hour, commonly stimulated by feeding, and may have incomplete emptying of the bladder. As the infant matures to be a toddler, bladder capacity increases, and between 1 and 3 years of age, cortical inhibitory pathways develop that allow the child to have voluntary control over reflexes that control the bladder muscles. The ability to have muscular control over the bowel occurs even before bladder control for most toddlers, and the assessment of fecal soiling includes determining whether the clinical presentation occurs with or without chronic constipation and overflow soiling. The normal sequence of developing control over bowel and bladder functions is the development of nocturnal fecal continence, diurnal fecal continence, diurnal bladder control, and nocturnal bladder control. Bowel and bladder control develops gradually over time. Toilet training is affected by many factors, such as a child's intellectual capacity and social maturity, cultural determinants, and the psychological interactions between child and parents. The ability to control bowel and bladder functions depends on the maturation of neurobiological systems, so that children with developmental delays may also display delayed continence of bowel and bladder. When children exhibit incontinence of urine or feces on a regular basis, it is troubling to the child and families, and often misunderstood as voluntary misbehavior.

Encopresis (repeated passage of feces into inappropriate places) and enuresis (repeated urination into bed or clothes) are the two elimination disorders described in the Fifth Edition of the American Psychiatric Association's *Diagnostic and Statistical Manual of Mental Disorders* (DSM-5). These diagnoses are not made until after age 4 years, for encopresis, and after age 5 years for enuresis, the ages at which a typically developing child is expected to master these skills. Normal development encompasses a range of time in which a given child is able to devote the attention, motivation, and physiological skills to exhibit competency in elimination processes. Encopresis is characterized by a pattern of passing feces in inappropriate places, such as in clothing or other places, at least once per month for 3 consecutive months, whether the passage is involuntary or intentional. Up to about 80 percent of children with fecal incontinence have associated constipation. A child with encopresis typically exhibits dysregulated bowel function; for example, with infrequent bowel movements, constipation, or recurrent abdominal pain and sometimes pain on defecations. Enuresis is characterized by repeated voiding of urine into clothes or bed, whether the voiding is involuntary or intentional. The behavior must occur twice weekly for at least 3 months or must cause clinically significant distress or impairment socially or academically. The child's chronological or developmental age must be at least 5 years.

27.10a Encopresis

EPIDEMIOLOGY

Encopresis has been estimated to affect 3 percent of 4-year-old and 1.6 percent of 10-year-old children. Incidence rates for encopretic behavior decrease drastically with increasing age. Between the ages of 10 and 12 years, it is estimated to affect 0.75 percent of typically developing children. Globally, community prevalence of encopresis ranges from 0.8 to 7.8 percent. In Western cultures, bowel control is established in more than 95 percent of children by their fourth birthday and in 99 percent by the fifth birthday. Encopresis is virtually absent in youth with normal intellectual function by the age of 16 years. Males are found to from three to six times more likely to have encopresis than females. A significant relation exists between encopresis and enuresis.

ETIOLOGY

Ninety percent of chronic childhood encopresis is considered to be functional. Children with this disorder typically withhold feces by contracting their gluteal muscles, holding their legs together, and tightening their external anal sphincter. In some cases, this is an entrenched behavioral response to previously painful bowel movements due to hard stool, which leads to fear of defecation and withholding behaviors. Encopresis involves an often-complicated interplay between physiological and psychological factors leading to an avoidance of defecation. However, when children chronically hold in bowel movements, the result is often fecal impaction and eventual overflow soiling. This pattern is observed in more than 75 percent of children with encopretic behavior. This common set of circumstances in most children with encopresis supports a behavioral intervention with a focus on ameliorating constipation while increasing appropriate toileting behavior. Inadequate training or the lack of appropriate toilet training may delay a child's attainment of continence.

Evidence indicates that some encopretic children have lifelong inefficient and ineffective sphincter control. Other children may soil involuntarily, either because of an inability to control the sphincter adequately or because of excessive fluid caused by a retentive overflow.

In about 5 to 10 percent of cases, fecal incontinence is caused by medical conditions including abnormal innervation of the anorectal region, ultrashort segment Hirschsprung's disease, neuronal intestinal dysplasia, or spinal cord damage.

One study found encopresis to occur with significantly greater frequency among children with known sexual abuse, and other psychiatric disorders, compared with a sample of healthy children. Encopresis, however, is not a specific indicator of sexual abuse.

It is evident that once a child has developed a pattern of withholding bowel movements, and attempts to defecate have become painful, a child's fear and resistance to changing the pattern are high. Battles with parents who insist that their children attempt to defecate before they are adequately treated may aggravate the condition and cause secondary behavioral difficulties. Children with encopresis who are not promptly treated, however, frequently end up being socially ostracized and rejected. The social consequences of soiling can lead to the development of emotional problems. On the other hand, children with encopresis who clearly can control their bowel function adequately but chronically deposit feces of relatively normal consistency in abnormal places are likely to have preexisting neurodevelopmental problems. Occasionally, a child has a specific fear of using the toilet, leading to a phobia.

Encopresis, in some cases can be considered secondary, that is, emerging after a period of normal bowel habits in conjunction with a disruptive life event, such as the birth of a sibling or a move to a new home. When encopresis manifests after a long period of fecal continence, it may reflect a developmental regressive behavior based on a severe stressor, such as a parental separation, loss of a best friend, or an unexpected academic failure.

Megacolon

Most children with encopresis retain feces and become constipated, either voluntarily or secondary to painful defecation. In some cases, a subclinical preexisting anorectal dysfunction exists that contributes to the constipation. In either case, resulting chronic rectal distention from large, hard fecal masses can cause loss of tone in the rectal wall and desensitization to pressure. Thus, children in this situation become even less aware of the need to defecate, and overflow encopresis occurs, usually with relatively small amounts of liquid or soft stool leaking out.

DIAGNOSIS AND CLINICAL FEATURES

According to DSM-5, encopresis is diagnosed when feces are passed into inappropriate places on a regular basis (at least once a month) for 3 months. Encopresis may be present in children who have bowel control and intentionally deposit feces in their clothes or other places for a variety of emotional reasons. Anecdotal reports have suggested that occasionally encopresis is attributable to an expression of anger or rage in a child whose parents have been punitive or of hostility at a parent. In a case such as this, once a child develops this inappropriate repetitive behavior eliciting negative attention, it is difficult to break the cycle of continuous negative attention. In other children, sporadic episodes of encopresis can occur during times of stress—for example, proximal to the birth of a new sibling—but in such cases, the behavior is usually transient and does not fulfill the diagnostic criteria for the disorder.

Encopresis can also be present on an involuntary basis in the absence of physiological abnormalities. In these cases, a child may not exhibit adequate control over the sphincter muscles, either because the child is absorbed in another activity or because he or she is unaware of the process. The feces may be of normal, near-normal, or liquid consistency. Some involuntary soiling occurs from chronic retaining of stool, which may result in liquid overflow. In rare cases, the involuntary overflow of stool results from psychological causes of diarrhea or anxiety disorder symptoms.

The DSM-5 includes two specifiers to encopresis: *with* constipation and overflow incontinence and *without* constipation and overflow incontinence. To receive a diagnosis of encopresis, a child must have a developmental or chronological level of at least 4 years. If the fecal incontinence is directly related to a medical condition, encopresis is not diagnosed.

Studies have indicated that children with encopresis who do not have gastrointestinal illnesses have high rates of abnormal anal sphincter contractions. This finding is particularly prevalent among children with encopresis with constipation and overflow incontinence who have difficulty relaxing their anal sphincter muscles when trying to defecate. Children with constipation who have difficulties with sphincter relaxation are not likely to respond well to laxatives in the treatment of their encopresis. Children with encopresis without abnormal sphincter tone are likely to improve over a short period.

Jack was a 7-year-old boy with daily encopresis, enuresis, and a history of hoarding behaviors, along with hiding the feces around the house. He lived with his adoptive parents, having been removed from his biological parents at age 3 years because of neglect and physical abuse. He was reported to be cocaine addicted at birth, but was otherwise healthy. Jack's biological mother was a known methamphetamine and alcohol user, and his father had spent time in jail for drug dealing. Jack had always been enuretic at night, and until this year, he had a history of daytime enuresis as well. Jack had a short attention span, was highly impulsive, and had great difficulty staying in his seat at school and remaining on task. He had reading difficulties and was placed in a contained special education classroom because of his disruptive behavior as well as his academic difficulties. Despite experiencing physical abuse, he has not experienced flashbacks or other symptoms that would indicate the presence of posttraumatic stress disorder. Jack was treated for attention-deficit/hyperactivity disorder (ADHD) with good response to methylphenidate (Concerta 36 mg per day).

Jack's adoptive family sought help at a university hospital's outpatient program that had expertise in the behavioral treatments of many psychiatric disorders including encopresis. The treatment program combined use of regular laxatives and a bowel training method with cognitive-behavioral therapy for Jack and for his family. Jack was started on a regimen of daily polyethylene glycol (PEG) solution and was seen by a pediatrician who was able to perform a manual disimpaction under sedation. Following that, Jack was continued on daily PEG solution combined with therapy. He learned to empty his bowel while sitting on the toilet for 10 minutes after each meal, whether or not he felt like he had to go. He soon was eager to stay on this regular bathroom schedule, and felt proud when he was able to have a bowel movement in the toilet. Over a period of 3 months, Jack was noticeably improved, and at 6 months, he was almost completely better. *(Courtesy of Edwin J. Mikkelsen, M.D. and Caroly Pataki, M.D.)*

PATHOLOGY AND LABORATORY EXAMINATION

Although no specific test indicates a diagnosis of encopresis, clinicians must rule out medical illnesses, such as Hirschsprung's disease, before making a diagnosis. It must be determined whether fecal retention is responsible for encopresis with constipation and overflow incontinence; a physical examination of the abdomen is indicated, and an abdominal x-ray can help determine the degree of constipation present. Tests to determine whether sphincter tone is abnormal are generally not conducted in simple cases of encopresis.

DIFFERENTIAL DIAGNOSIS

In encopresis with constipation and overflow incontinence, constipation can begin as early as the child's first year and can peak between the second and fourth years. Soiling usually begins by age 4. Frequent liquid stools and hard fecal masses are found in the colon and the rectum on abdominal palpation and rectal examination. Complications include impaction, megacolon, and anal fissures.

Encopresis with constipation and overflow incontinence is rarely caused by faulty nutrition; structural disease of the anus, rectum, and colon; medicinal adverse effects; or nongastrointestinal medical (endocrine or neurological) disorders. The chief differential medical problem is aganglionic megacolon or Hirschsprung's disease, in which a patient may have an empty rectum and no desire to defecate, but may still have an overflow of feces. The disorder occurs in 1 in 5,000 children; signs appear shortly after birth.

COURSE AND PROGNOSIS

The outcome of encopresis depends on the etiology, the chronicity of the symptoms, and coexisting behavioral problems. In some cases, encopresis is self-limiting, and it rarely continues beyond middle adolescence. Encopresis in children who have contributing physiological factors, such as poor gastric motility and an inability to relax the anal sphincter muscles, is more difficult to treat than that in those with constipation but normal sphincter tone.

Encopresis is a particularly objectionable disorder to family members, who may assume that the behavior is due to "laziness," and family tensions are often high. Peers are intolerant of the developmentally inappropriate behavior and typically taunt and reject a child with encopresis. Many affected children have abysmally low self-esteem and are plagued by constant social rejection. Psychologically, a child may appear blunted toward the symptoms or less frequently, may be entrenched in a pattern of encopresis as a mode of expressing anger. The outcome of encopresis is influenced by a family's willingness and ability to participate in treatment without being overly punitive and by the child's ability and motivation to engage in treatment.

TREATMENT

A typical treatment plan for a child with encopresis includes daily oral administration of laxatives such as PEG at 1 g/kg per day, and often a surgical disimpaction under general anesthesia before maintenance laxatives can be administered. In addition, an ongoing cognitive-behavioral intervention to begin regular attempts to have bowel movements in the toilet, and to diminish anxiety related to bowel movement. By the time a child is brought for treatment, considerable family discord and distress are common. Family tensions about the symptom must be reduced, and a nonpunitive atmosphere established. Similar efforts should be made to reduce the child's embarrassment at school. Many changes of underwear with a minimum of embarrassment should be arranged. Education of the family and correction of misperceptions that a family may have about soiling must occur before treatment. Laxatives are not necessary for children who are not constipated and do have good bowel control, but regular, timed intervals on the toilet may be useful with these children as well.

A report confirms the success of an interactive parent–child family guidance intervention for young children with encopresis based on psychological and behavioral interventions for children younger than 9 years of age.

Supportive psychotherapy and relaxation techniques may be useful in treating the anxieties and other sequelae of children with encopresis, such as low self-esteem and social isolation. Family interventions can be helpful for children who have bowel control but who continue to deposit their feces in inappropriate locations. An optimal outcome occurs when a child achieves a feeling of control over his or her bowel function.

27.10b Enuresis

EPIDEMIOLOGY

The prevalence of enuresis ranges from 5 to 10 percent in 5-year-olds, 1.5 to 5 percent in 9- to 10-year-olds, and about 1 percent in adolescents 15 years and older. The prevalence of enuresis decreases with increasing age. Enuretic behavior is considered developmentally appropriate among young toddlers, precluding diagnoses of enuresis; however, enuretic behavior occurs in 82 percent of 2-year-olds, 49 percent of 3-year-olds, and 26 percent of 4-year-olds on a regular basis.

In the epidemiological Isle of Wight study, investigators reported that 15.2 percent of 7-year-old boys were enuretic occasionally and that 6.7 percent of them were enuretic at least once a week. The study reported that 3.3 percent of girls at the age of 7 years were enuretic at least once a week. By age 10, the overall prevalence of enuresis was reported to be 3 percent. The rate drops drastically for teenagers: a prevalence of 1.5 percent has been reported for 14-year-olds. Enuresis affects about 1 percent of adults.

Although most children with enuresis do not have a comorbid psychiatric disorder, children with enuresis are at higher risk for the development of another psychiatric disorder.

Nocturnal enuresis is about 50 percent more common in boys and accounts for about 80 percent of children with enuresis. Diurnal enuresis is also seen more often in boys who often delay voiding until it is too late. A spontaneous resolution of nocturnal enuresis is about 15 percent per year. Nocturnal enuresis consists of a normal volume of voided urine, whereas when small volumes of urine are voided at night, other medical causes may be present.

ETIOLOGY

Enuresis involves complex neurobiological systems that include contributions from cerebral and spinal cord centers, motor and sensory functions, and autonomic and voluntary nervous systems. Urination is regulated by neurons in the pons and midbrain regions. Bladder detrusor muscle contraction occurs whenever bladder capacity is reached, which can lead to enuresis in a sleeping child. Therefore, excessive volumes of urine produced at night may lead to enuresis at night in children without any physiologic abnormalities. Nighttime enuresis often occurs in the absence of a specific neurogenic cause. Daytime enuresis may develop based on behavioral habits developed over time.

Daytime enuresis may occur in the absence of neurological abnormalities resulting from habitual, voluntary tightening of the external sphincter during urges to urinate. The pattern may be set in a young child who may start out with a normal or overactive detrusor muscle in the bladder, but with repeated attempts to prevent leaking or urination when there is an urge to void. Over time, the sensation of the urge to urinate is diminished and the bladder does not empty regularly, leading to enuresis at night when the bladder is relaxed and can empty without resistance. This immature pattern of urinating can account for some cases of enuresis, especially when the pattern has been in place since early childhood. Most children are not enuretic by intention or even with awareness until after they are wet. Physiological factors often play a role in the development of enuresis, and behavioral patterns are likely to maintain the maladaptive urination. Normal bladder control, which is acquired gradually, is influenced by neuromuscular and cognitive development, socioemotional factors, toilet training, and genetic factors. Difficulties in one or more of these areas can delay urinary continence.

Genetic factors are believed to play a role in the expression of enuresis, given that the emergence of enuresis has been found to be significantly greater in first-degree relatives. A longitudinal study of child development found that children with enuresis were about twice as likely to have concomitant developmental delays as those who did not have enuresis. About 75 percent of children with enuresis have a first-degree relative who has or has had enuresis. A child's risk for enuresis has been found to be more than seven times greater if the father was enuretic. The concordance rate is higher in monozygotic twins than in dizygotic twins. A strong genetic component is suggested, and much can be accounted for by tolerance for enuresis in some families and by other psychosocial factors.

Studies indicate that children with enuresis with a normal anatomical bladder capacity report urge to void with less urine in the bladder than children without enuresis. Other studies report that nocturnal enuresis occurs when the bladder is full because of lower than expected levels of nighttime antidiuretic hormone. This could lead to a higher-than-usual urine output. Enuresis does not appear to be related to a specific stage of sleep or time of night; rather, bed-wetting appears randomly. In most cases, the quality of sleep is normal. Little evidence indicates that children with enuresis sleep more soundly than other children.

Psychosocial stressors appear to precipitate enuresis in a subgroup of children with the disorder. In young children, the disorder has been particularly associated with the birth of a sibling, hospitalization between the ages of 2 and 4 years, the start of school, separation of a family due to divorce, or a move to a new environment.

DIAGNOSIS AND CLINICAL FEATURES

Enuresis is the repeated voiding of urine into a child's clothes or bed; the voiding may be involuntary or intentional. For the diagnosis to be made, a child must exhibit a developmental or chronological age of at least 5 years. According to DSM-5, the behavior must occur twice weekly for a period of at least 3 months or must cause distress and impairment in functioning to meet the diagnostic criteria. Enuresis is diagnosed only if the behavior is not caused by a medical condition. Children with enuresis are at higher risk for ADHD compared with the general population. They are also more likely to have comorbid encopresis. DSM-5 and the 10th revision of *International Statistical Classification of Diseases and Related Health Problems* (ICD-10) break down the disorder into three types: nocturnal only, diurnal only, and nocturnal and diurnal.

PATHOLOGY AND LABORATORY EXAMINATION

No single laboratory finding is pathognomonic of enuresis; but clinicians must rule out organic factors, such as the presence of urinary tract infections, which may predispose a child to enuresis. Structural obstructive abnormalities may be present in up to 3 percent of children with apparent enuresis. Sophisticated radiographic studies are usually deferred in simple cases of enuresis with no signs of repeated infections or other medical problems.

DIFFERENTIAL DIAGNOSIS

To make the diagnosis of enuresis, organic causes of bladder dysfunction must be investigated and ruled out. Organic syndromes, such as urinary tract infections, obstructions, or anatomical conditions are found most often in children who experience both nocturnal and diurnal enuresis combined with urinary frequency and urgency. The organic features include genitourinary pathology—structural, neurological, and infectious—such as obstructive uropathy, spina bifida occulta, and cystitis; other organic disorders that can cause polyuria and enuresis, such as diabetes mellitus and diabetes insipidus; disturbances of consciousness and sleep, such as seizures, intoxication, and sleepwalking disorder, during which a child urinates; and adverse effects from treatment with antipsychotic agents.

COURSE AND PROGNOSIS

Enuresis is often self-limited, and a child with enuresis may have a spontaneous remission. Most children who master the task of control over their bladder gain self-esteem and improved social confidence when they become continent. About 80 percent of affected children have never achieved a year-long period of dryness. Enuresis after at least one dry year usually begins between the ages of 5 and 8 years; if it occurs much later, especially during adulthood, organic causes must be investigated. Some evidence indicates that late onset of enuresis in children is more frequently associated with a concomitant psychiatric difficulty than is enuresis without at least one dry year. Relapses occur in children with enuresis who are becoming dry spontaneously and in those who are being treated. The significant emotional and social difficulties of these children usually include poor self-image, decreased self-esteem, social embarrassment and restriction, and intrafamilial conflict. The course of children with enuresis may be influenced by whether they receive appropriate evaluation and treatment for common comorbid disorders such as ADHD.

TREATMENT

A relatively high rate of spontaneous remission of enuresis occurs over time in childhood; however, in many cases, interventions are necessary because enuresis is causing functional impairment. The first step in any treatment plan is to review appropriate toilet training. If toilet training was not attempted, the parents and the patient should be guided in this undertaking. Record-keeping is helpful in determining a baseline and following the child's progress, and may itself be a reinforcer. A star chart may be particularly helpful. Other useful techniques include restricting fluids before bed and night lifting to toilet train the child. Interventions with alarm therapy, which is triggered by wet underwear, has been a mainstay of treatment for enuresis. Alarm therapy works by alerting a child to respond when voiding begins during sleep. The alarm is a battery-operated device that can be attached to a child's underwear or a mat. The alarm is triggered as soon as voiding begins by emitting a loud noise that awakens the child. The success of this method is based on the child's ability to awaken promptly and respond to the alarm by getting up and voiding in the toilet. A child who can respond optimally is at least 6 or 7 years old. Pharmacological interventions including desmopressin therapy in managing nocturnal enuresis have been shown to be effective in some patients. Desmopressin is a "synthetic analog" of vasopressin, which can be administered as a pill, a sublingual melt, or a nasal spray. Its effect can last up to 8 hours, and it works by reducing urine production at night. This method is optimal when no fluids are ingested in the evening.

Another basic intervention for those children with enuresis and bowel dysfunction is to assess whether chronic constipation is contributing to urinary dysfunction, and to consider increasing dietary fiber to diminish constipation.

Behavioral Therapy

Classic conditioning with the bell (or buzzer) and pad (alarm) apparatus is generally the most effective treatment for enuresis, with dryness resulting in more than 50 percent of cases. Bladder training—encouragement or reward for delaying micturition for increasing times during waking hours—has also been used. Although sometimes effective, this method is decidedly inferior to the bell and pad.

Pharmacotherapy

Medication is considered when enuresis is causing impairment in social, family, and school function and behavioral, dietary, and fluid restriction have not been efficacious. When the problem interferes significantly with a child's functioning, several medications can be considered, although the problem often recurs as soon as medications are withdrawn.

Desmopressin (DDAVP), an antidiuretic compound that is available as an intranasal spray, has shown success in reducing enuresis. Reduction of enuresis has varied from 10 to 90 percent with the use of desmopressin. In most studies, enuresis recurred shortly after discontinuation of this medication. Adverse effects that can occur with desmopressin include headache, nasal congestion, epistaxis, and stomachache. The most serious adverse effect reported with the use of desmopressin to treat enuresis was a hyponatremic seizure experienced by a child.

Reboxetine (Edronax, Vestra), a norepinephrine reuptake inhibitor with a noncardiotoxic side effect profile has recently been investigated as a safer alternative to imipramine in the treatment of childhood enuresis. A trial in which 22 children with enuresis causing social impairment, who had not responded to an enuresis alarm, desmopressin, or anticholinergics were administered 4 to 8 mg of reboxetine at bedtime. Of the 22 children, 13 (59 percent) in this open trial achieved complete dryness with reboxetine alone, or in combination with desmopressin. Side effects were minimal and did not lead to discontinuation of the medication in this trial.

Psychotherapy

Psychotherapy may be useful in dealing with the coexisting psychiatric problems and the emotional and family difficulties that arise secondary to chronic enuresis.

▲ 27.11 Trauma- and Stressor-Related Disorders in Children

27.11a Reactive Attachment Disorder and Disinhibited Social Engagement Disorder

Reactive attachment disorder and disinhibited social engagement disorder are clinical disorders characterized by aberrant social behaviors in a young child that reflect grossly negligent parenting and maltreatment that disrupted the development of normal attachment behavior. A diagnosis of either reactive attachment disorder or disinhibited social engagement disorder is based on the presumption that the etiology is directly linked to the caregiving deprivation experienced by the child. The diagnosis of reactive attachment disorder was first defined in the DSM, Third Edition (DSM-III) in 1980. The formation of this diagnosis is based on the building blocks of attachment theory, which describes the quality of a child's affective relationship with primary caregivers, usually parents. This basic relationship is the product of a young child's need for protection, nurturance, and comfort and the interaction of the parents and child in fulfilling these needs.

Based on observations of a young child and parents during a brief separation and reunion, designated the "strange situation procedure," pioneered by Mary Ainsworth and colleagues, researchers have designated a child's basic pattern of attachment to be characterized as secure, insecure, or disorganized. Children who exhibit secure attachment behavior are believed to experience their caregivers as emotionally available and appear to be more exploratory and well adjusted than children who exhibit insecure or disorganized attachment behavior. Insecure attachment is believed to result from a young child's perception that the caregiver is not consistently available, whereas disorganized attachment behavior in a child is believed to result from experiencing both the need for proximity to the caregiver and apprehension in approaching the caregiver. These early patterns of attachment are believed to influence a child's future capacities for affect regulation, self-soothing, and relationship building. According to the DSM-5, reactive attachment disorder is characterized by a consistent pattern of emotionally withdrawn responses toward adult caregivers, limited positive affect, sadness, and minimal social responsiveness to others, and concomitant neglect, deprivation, and lack of appropriate nurturance from caregivers. It is presumed that reactive attachment disorder is due to grossly pathological caregiving received by the child. The pattern of care may exhibit disregard for a child's emotional or physical needs or repeated changes of caregivers, as when a child is frequently relocated during foster care. Reactive attachment disorder is not accounted for by ASD, and the child must have a developmental age of at least 9 months.

Pathological caretaking can result in two distinct disorders: reactive attachment disorder, in which the disturbance takes the form of the child's constantly failing to initiate and respond to most social interactions in a developmentally normal way; and disinhibited social engagement disorder, in which the disturbance takes the form of undifferentiated, unselective, and inappropriate social relatedness, with familiar and unfamiliar adults.

In disinhibited social engagement disorder, according to DSM-5, a child actively approaches and interacts with unfamiliar adults in an overly familiar way, either verbally or physically. There is diminished checking with or seeking of a known caregiver, and a willingness to go with unfamiliar adults without hesitation. These behaviors in disinhibited social engagement disorder are not accounted for by impulsivity, although socially disinhibited behavior is predominant. These patterns of disinhibited, developmentally inappropriate behaviors are presumed to be caused by pathogenic caregiving. Thus, for both reactive attachment disorder and disinhibited social engagement disorder, aberrant caretaking is presumed to be the predominant cause of the child's inappropriate behaviors. However, there have been cases of less severe disturbances in parenting that may also be associated with young children who exhibit some characteristics of reactive attachment disorder or disinhibited social engagement disorder. The DSM-5 defines reactive attachment disorder as a state of withdrawn inhibited and impaired social behavior in a child, due to severe physical or emotional neglect, and conceptualizes disinhibited social disengagement disorder as a separate disorder, although these two different clinical disorders both stem from emotional and physical neglect by caretakers. In the past, these two clinical entities were conceptualized as subtypes of the same disorder.

These disorders may also result in a picture of failure to thrive, in which an infant shows physical signs of malnourishment and does not exhibit the expected developmental motor and verbal milestones.

EPIDEMIOLOGY

Few data exist on the prevalence, sex ratio, or familial pattern of reactive attachment disorder and disinhibited social engagement disorder. It has been estimated for either one to occur in less than 1 percent of the population. A study of 1,646 children aged 6 to 8 years old living in a deprived sector of urban United Kingdom, found that the prevalence of reactive attachment disorder in this population was 1.4 percent. However, other studies of selected high-risk populations have estimated that about 10 percent of young children with documented neglectful and grossly pathological caregiving exhibit reactive attachment disorder, and up to 20 percent of children in this situation exhibit disinhibited social engagement disorder. In a retrospective report of children in one county of the United States who were removed from their homes because of neglect or abuse before the age of 4 years, 38 percent exhibited signs of either reactive attachment disorder or disinhibited social engagement disorder. Another study established the reliability of the diagnosis by reviewing videotaped assessments of at-risk children interacting with caregivers, along with a structured interview with caregivers. Given that pathogenic care, including maltreatment, occurs more frequently in the presence of general psychosocial risk factors, such as poverty, disrupted families, and mental illness among caregivers, these circumstances are likely to increase the risk of reactive attachment disorder and disinhibited social engagement disorder.

ETIOLOGY

The core features of reactive attachment disorder and disinhibited social engagement disorder are disturbances of normal attachment behaviors. The inability of a young child to develop normative social interactions that culminate in aberrant attachment behaviors in reactive attachment disorder is inherent in the disorder's definition. Reactive attachment disorder and disinhibited social engagement disorder are presumed to be linked to maltreatment of the child, including emotional neglect, physical abuse, or both. Grossly pathogenic care of an infant or young child by the caregiver presumably causes the markedly disturbed social relatedness that is evident. The emphasis is on the unidirectional cause; that is, the caregiver does something inimical or neglects to do something essential for the infant or child. In evaluating a patient for whom such a diagnosis is appropriate, however, clinicians should consider the contributions of each member of the caregiver–child dyad and their interactions. Clinicians should weigh such things as infant or child temperament, deficient or defective bonding, a developmentally disabled child, and a particular caregiver–child mismatch. The likelihood of neglect increases with parental psychiatric disorder, substance abuse, intellectual disability, the parent's own harsh upbringing, social isolation, deprivation, and premature parenthood (i.e., adolescent). These factors compromise parental ability to attend to the needs of the child, as they focus primarily on their own existence rather than on their child. Frequent changes of the primary caregivers, for example, from multiple foster care placements or repeated lengthy hospitalizations, may also lead to impaired attachment. In the general population, a study of 1,600 children found that those children with reactive attachment disorder/disinhibited social engagement disorder showed a constellation of symptoms characterized by early emergence of symptoms eliciting neurodevelopmental examination (ESSENCE). Some of the associated symptoms in children with reactive attachment disorder/disinhibited social engagement disorder include higher risk of failure to gain weight as neonates, feeding difficulty, and poor impulse control. These traits are likely to emerge because of both genetic and environmental factors. The authors found that children with reactive attachment disorder/disinhibited social engagement disorder were more likely to have multiple psychiatric comorbidities, lower IQs compared to the general population, and more behavioral problems. Thus, a broad assessment may be necessary to identify symptoms and disorders associated with reactive attachment disorder/disinhibited social engagement disorder.

DIAGNOSIS AND CLINICAL FEATURES

Children with reactive attachment disorder and disinhibited social engagement disorder may initially be identified by a preschool teacher or by a pediatrician based on direct observation of the child's inappropriate social responses. The diagnoses of reactive attachment disorder and disinhibited social engagement disorder are based partially on documented evidence of pervasive disturbance of attachment due to severe parental neglect, leading to inappropriate social behaviors present before the age of 5 years. The clinical picture varies greatly, depending on a child's chronological and mental ages, but expected social interaction and liveliness are not present. Often, the child is not progressing developmentally or is frankly malnourished. Perhaps the most common clinical picture of an infant with reactive attachment disorder is the nonorganic failure to thrive. Such infants usually exhibit hypokinesis, dullness, listlessness, and apathy, with a poverty of spontaneous activity.

Infants look sad, joyless, and miserable. Some infants also appear frightened and watchful, with a radar-like gaze. Nevertheless, they may exhibit delayed responsiveness to a stimulus that would elicit fright or withdrawal from a normal infant. Infants with failure to thrive and reactive attachment disorder appear significantly malnourished, and many have protruding abdomens. Occasionally, foul-smelling, celiac-like stools are reported. In unusually severe cases, a clinical picture of marasmus appears.

The infant's weight is often below the third percentile and markedly below the appropriate weight for his or her height. If serial weights are available, the weight percentiles may have decreased progressively because of an actual weight loss or a failure to gain weight as height increases. Head circumference is usually normal for the infant's age. Muscle tone may be poor. The skin may be colder and paler or more mottled than skin of a normal child. Laboratory findings may indicate coincident malnutrition, dehydration, or concurrent illness. Bone age is usually retarded. Growth hormone levels are usually normal or elevated, a finding suggesting that growth failure in these children is secondary to caloric deprivation and malnutrition. Cortisol secretion in children with reactive attachment disorder or disinhibited social engagement disorder is lower than in typical developing children. For children with failure to thrive, improvement physically and weight gain generally occur rapidly after they are hospitalized.

Socially, the infants with reactive attachment disorder usually show little spontaneous activity and a marked diminution of both initiative toward others and reciprocity in response to the caregiving adult or examiner. Both mother and infant may be indifferent to separation on hospitalization or to termination of subsequent hospital visits. The infants frequently show none of the normal upset, fretting, or protest about hospitalization. Older infants usually show little interest in their environment. They may not play with toys, even if encouraged; however, they rapidly or gradually take an interest in, and relate to, their caregivers in the hospital.

Psychosocial Dwarfism

Classic psychosocial dwarfism or psychosocially determined short stature is a syndrome that usually first manifest in children 2 to 3 years of age. The children are typically unusually short and have frequent growth hormone abnormalities and severe behavioral disturbances. All of these symptoms result from an inimical caregiver–child relationship. The affectionless character may appear when there is a failure, or lack of opportunity, to form attachments before the age of 2 to 3 years. Children cannot form lasting relationships, and their inability is sometimes accompanied by an inability to obey rules, a lack of guilt, and a need for attention and affection. Children with disinhibited social engagement disorder appear to be overly friendly and familiar with little fear.

A 7-year-old boy was referred by his adoptive parents because of hyperactivity and inappropriate social behavior at school. He had been adopted at 4 years of age, after living most of his life in a Chinese orphanage in which he received care from a rotating shift of caregivers. Although he had been below the 5th percentile for height and weight on arrival, he quickly approached the 15th percentile in his new home. However, his adoptive parents were frustrated by his inability to bond with them. They had initially worried about an intellectual problem, although testing and his capacity to engage almost any adult and many children verbally suggested otherwise. He appeared to be too friendly, talking to anyone and often following strangers willingly. He showed little empathy when others were hurt and yet he would sit on the laps of teachers and students without asking. He was frequently injured because of seemingly reckless behavior, although he had an extremely high tolerance for pain. His parents focused on problem behaviors at home to decrease his impulsive behavior, which improved with much prompting; however, he remained oddly overfriendly at home and in school. The child was diagnosed with disinhibited social engagement disorder. *(Adapted from Neil W. Boris, M.D. and Charles H. Zeanah, Jr., M.D.)*

PATHOLOGY AND LABORATORY EXAMINATION

Although no single specific laboratory test is used to make a diagnosis, many children with reactive attachment disorder have disturbances of growth and development. Thus, establishing a growth curve and examining the progression of developmental milestones may be helpful in determining whether associated phenomena, such as failure to thrive, are present.

DIFFERENTIAL DIAGNOSIS

The differential diagnosis of reactive attachment disorder and disinhibited social engagement disorder must take into account that many other psychiatric disorders may arise in conjunction with maltreatment, including depressive disorders, anxiety disorders, and posttraumatic stress disorders (PTSDs). Psychiatric disorders to consider in the differential diagnosis include language disorders, ASD, intellectual disability, and metabolic syndromes. Children with ASDs are typically well nourished and of age-appropriate size and weight, and are generally alert and active, despite their impairments in reciprocal social interactions. Significant intellectual disability is often present in children with ASD, whereas when intellectual disability occurs with reactive attachment disorder or disinhibited social engagement disorder, it is generally relatively mild. Children with disinhibited social engagement disorder often show comorbid ADHD, PTSD, and language disorder or delay. Furthermore, children with disinhibited social engagement disorder symptoms may have complex neuropsychiatric problems.

COURSE AND PROGNOSIS

Most of the data available on the natural course of children with reactive attachment disorder and disinhibited social engagement disorder come from follow-up studies of children in residential facilities with histories of serious neglect. Findings from these studies suggest that children with reactive attachment disorder, who are later adopted into caring environments, improve in their attachment behaviors and may normalize over time. Children with disinhibited social engagement disorder, however, appear to have more difficulty developing attachments to new caregivers. Children with disinhibited social engagement disorder who exhibit indiscriminate social behavior also tend to have poor peer relationships. The prognosis for children with reactive attachment disorder and disinhibited social engagement disorder is influenced by the duration and severity of the neglect and the degree of impairment that results. Constitutional and nutritional factors interact in children, who may either respond resiliently to treatment or continue to fail to thrive. After a pathological caregiving situation has been recognized, the amount of treatment and rehabilitation that the family receives affects the child. Children who have multiple problems stemming from pathogenic caregiving may recover physically faster and more completely than they do emotionally.

TREATMENT

The first consideration in treating reactive attachment disorder or disinhibited social engagement disorder is a child's safety. Thus, the management of these disorders must begin with a comprehensive assessment of the current level of safety and adequate caregiving. When there is suspicion of maltreatment persisting in the home, the first decision is often whether to hospitalize the child or to attempt treatment while the child remains in the home. If neglect, or emotional, physical, or sexual abuse is suspected, legally, such must be reported to the appropriate law enforcement and child protective services in the area. The child's physical and emotional state and the level of pathological caregiving determine the therapeutic strategy. A determination must be made regarding the nutritional status of the child and the presence of ongoing physical abuse or threat. Hospitalization is necessary for children with malnourishment. Along with an assessment of the child's physical well-being, an evaluation of the child's emotional condition is important. Immediate intervention must address the parents' awareness and capacity to participate in altering the injurious patterns that have heretofore ensued. The treatment team must begin to improve the unsatisfactory relationship between the caregiver and child. This usually requires extensive and intensive intervention and education with the mother or with both parents when possible.

In one study, parents of 120 children between 11.7 and 31.9 months, identified as being at risk for neglect, were randomly assigned to an intervention for at-risk parents called Attachment and Biobehavioral Catch-up (ABC) or to a control intervention. The ABC intervention was designed to decrease frightening behavior toward the infant by parents, and to increase sensitive and nurturing interactions between parents and infant. The intervention was manualized so that parents were specifically guided in how to provide those interactions with their infants. Children were evaluated after 10 sessions, and the 60 children who received the ABC intervention showed significantly lower rates of disorganized attachment (32 percent), and higher rates of secure attachment (52 percent) compared to those who received the control intervention (disorganized attachment 57 percent; secure attachment 33 percent). The authors concluded that parental nurturance and sensitivity can be enhanced by a comprehensive and explicit intervention such as the ABC intervention, and significant improvements in attachment behaviors can be measured in young children after 10 sessions.

The caregiver–child relationship is the basis of the assessment of reactive attachment disorder and disinhibited social engagement disorder symptoms, and the substrate from which to modify attachment behaviors. Structured observations allow a clinician to determine the range of attachment behaviors established with various family members. The clinician may work closely with the caregiver and the child to facilitate greater sensitivity in their interactions. Three basic psychotherapeutic modalities are helpful in promoting positive bonds between children and caregiver. First, a clinician can target the caregiver to promote positive interaction with a child who does not yet have the repertoire to respond positively. Second, a clinician can work with the child and the caregiver together as a dyad to advocate for practicing appropriate positive reinforcement for each other. Through the use of videotapes, parent–child interactions can then be viewed and modifications can be suggested to increase positive engagement. The third modality for clinical intervention is through individual work with the child. Working with the child and caregiver together is often more effective in producing more emotionally meaningful exchanges than working with parent or child individually.

Psychosocial interventions for families in which a child has reactive attachment disorder or disinhibited social engagement disorder include (1) psychosocial support services, including hiring a homemaker, improving the physical condition of the apartment, or obtaining more adequate housing; improving the family's financial status; and decreasing the family's isolation; (2) psychotherapeutic interventions, including individual psychotherapy, psychotropic medications, and family or marital therapy; (3) educational counseling services, including mother–infant or mother–toddler groups, and counseling to increase awareness and understanding of the child's needs and to develop parenting skills; and (4) provisions for close monitoring of the progression of the patient's emotional and physical well-being. Sometimes, separating a child from the stressful home environment temporarily, as in hospitalization, allows the child to break out of the accustomed pattern. A neutral setting, such as the hospital, is the best place to start with families who are genuinely available emotionally and physically for intervention. If interventions are unfeasible or inadequate or if they fail, placement with relatives or in foster care, adoption, or a group home or residential treatment facility must be considered.

27.11b Posttraumatic Stress Disorder of Infancy, Childhood, and Adolescence

PTSD, formerly grouped with anxiety disorders, currently falls under a new chapter in the Fifth Edition of the American Psychiatric Association's *Diagnostic and Statistical Manual of Mental Disorders* (DSM-5) called trauma- and stressor-related disorders, a group comprising disorders in which exposure to a traumatic or stressful event is a diagnostic criterion. PTSD is characterized by a set of symptoms including intrusive memories of the trauma, persistent avoidance of stimuli that are reminders of the traumatic event, persistent negative alterations in cognition and mood, and alterations in arousal, mainly seen as hyperarousal and irritability following the traumatic event. In DSM-5, the traumatic event criterion is defined as exposure to actual or threatened death, serious injury, or sexual violence, whether directly, by witnessing it, learning of a traumatic event to a family member, or experiencing repeated exposures to trauma precipitated by social or natural disasters. Exposure to trauma through electronic media, movies, television, or photographs is excluded from the criteria. In children 6 years or younger, diagnostic criteria fall under the "preschool subtype," in which either persistent avoidance of trauma-evoking stimuli or negative alterations in cognitions suffice as indications for PTSD.

In the United States, the rates of children and adolescents being exposed to violence and traumatic events are extremely high. In a national representative sample of children and adolescents, exposure to a traumatic event was reported to be 60.4 percent, with a lifetime rate ranging from 80 to 90 percent. A significant number of children and adolescents who are exposed to traumatic events, ranging from direct experiences with physical or sexual abuse, domestic violence, motor vehicle accidents, severe medical illnesses, or natural or human-created disasters, will develop PTSD. In children younger than the age of 6 years, spontaneous and intrusive memories may be expressed in play, or occur in frightening dreams; these intrusive thoughts may not be easily identified as related to the traumatic event.

Although posttraumatic stress symptoms have been described in adults for more than a century, PTSD was first officially recognized as a psychiatric disorder in 1980 in the DSM, Third Edition (DSM-III). Recognition of the frequency of PTSD in children and adolescents has increased over the last decade. Reports indicate that up to 6 percent of youth are likely to meet full criteria for PTSD at some point in their development. Developmental factors strongly influence the manifestations of symptoms of PTSD. In children and adolescents, reexperiencing a traumatic event is often observed through play, recurrent nightmares without recall of the traumatic events, and behaviors that reenact the traumatic situation, along with agitation, fear, or disorganization.

EPIDEMIOLOGY

In the United States, it is estimated that approximately 80 percent of individuals have been exposed to at least one traumatic event; however, less than 10 percent of trauma victims develop PTSD. The rates of traumatic events, including assaultive violence, exposure to unexpected deaths, being a witness of trauma to others, and bodily injury, all peak sharply between the ages of 16 to 20 years. PTSD is more common in females than in males throughout the life span mainly due to their increased risk for exposure to traumatic events. In situations of natural disaster, the rates of PTSD in males and females are similar. Lifetime risk for PTSD in the United States ranges from 6.8 to 12.2 percent. A consistent epidemiologic finding in the United States and in other countries is that PTSD is more prevalent in women than in men. Epidemiological studies of children 9 to 17 years of age have found 3-month prevalence rates of PTSD ranging from 0.5 to 4 percent. An epidemiological survey of preschoolers aged 4 to 5 years found a rate of 1.3 percent of PTSD.

Among trauma-exposed samples of persons not referred for treatment, a wide range of 25 to 90 percent have been reported to exhibit the full diagnosis of PTSD. Children exposed chronically to trauma, such as child abuse, or traumas resulting in a broader disruption of entire communities, such as war, have the greatest risk of developing PTSD. In addition to the staggering rate of the full-blown disorder of PTSD among youth, several studies indicate that most children exposed to severe or chronic trauma develop PTSD symptoms sufficiently severe to disrupt functioning, even in the absence of the full diagnosis.

ETIOLOGY

Biological Factors

Risk factors in children for developing PTSD include preexisting anxiety disorders and depressive disorders. A prospective study found that among children exposed to traumatic events, those with anxiety disorders and teacher ratings of externalizing behavior problems by the age of 6 years were at increased risk for PTSD. Furthermore, children with an IQ greater than 115 at the age of 6 years were at lower risk for developing PTSD. In addition, among children exposed to trauma, those who developed PTSD were also at higher risk of developing comorbid disorders such as depression. This suggests that a genetic predisposition for anxiety disorders, as well as a family history indicating increased risk of depressive disorders, may predispose a trauma-exposed child to develop PTSD. Children with PTSD have been found to exhibit increased excretion of adrenergic and dopaminergic metabolites, smaller intracranial volume and corpus callosum, memory deficits, and lower IQs compared with age-matched controls. Adults with PTSD have been found to have an overactive amygdala and decreased hippocampal volume. Whether the above findings are sequelae of PTSD or markers of vulnerability to the disorder remains a focus of investigation.

Psychological Factors

Although the exposure to trauma is the initial etiological factor in the development of PTSD, the enduring symptoms typical of PTSD, such as avoidance of the place where the trauma occurred, can be conceptualized, in part, as the result of both classic and operant conditioning. Extreme physiological responses may accompany fear of a given traumatic event, such as an adolescent who was terrorized by an attack by a group of students near school, who then develops an extreme negative physiological reaction each time he or she is near the school. This is an example of classic conditioning in that a neutral cue (the school) has become paired with an intensely fearful past event. Operant conditioning occurs when a child learns to avoid traumatic reminders to prevent distressing feelings from arising. For example, if a child was in a motor vehicle accident, the child may then refuse to ride in cars altogether to prevent negative physiological reactions and fear from occurring.

Another mechanism in developing and maintaining symptoms of PTSD is through modeling, which is a form of learning. For example, when parents and children are exposed to traumatic events, such as natural disasters, children may emulate parental responses, such as avoidance, withdrawal, or extreme expressions of fear, and "learn" to respond to their own memories of the traumatic event in the same manner.

Social Factors

Family support and reactions to traumatic events in children may play a significant role in the development of PTSD, in that adverse parental emotional reactions to a child's abuse may increase that child's risk of developing PTSD. Lack of parental support and psychopathology among parents—especially maternal depression—have been identified as risk factors in the development of PTSD after a child has been exposed to a traumatic event.

DIAGNOSIS AND CLINICAL FEATURES

For PTSD to ensue, exposure to a traumatic event consisting of either a direct personal experience or witnessing an event involving the threat of death, serious injury, or serious harm must occur. Most common traumatic exposures for children and adolescents include physical or sexual abuse; domestic, school or community violence; being kidnapped; terrorist attacks; motor vehicle or household accidents; or disasters, such as floods, hurricanes, tornadoes, fires, explosions, or airline crashes. A child with PTSD experiences either intrusive memories of the event, recurrent frightening dreams, dissociative reactions including flashbacks in which the child feels as if the traumatic event is recurring, or intense psychological distress when exposed to reminders of the trauma.

Symptoms of PTSD include *reexperiencing* the traumatic event in at least one of the following ways. Children may have intrusive thoughts, memories, or images that spontaneously recur, or body sensations that remind them of the event. In very young children, it is common to observe play that includes elements of the traumatic event, or behaviors, such as sexual behaviors that are not developmentally expected. Children may experience periods during which they either act or feel as though the event is taking place presently; this is a dissociative event usually described by adults as "flashbacks."

Another critical symptom cluster of PTSD is *avoidance,* which in childhood may be displayed by making active physical efforts to avoid the places, people, or situations that would present traumatic reminders of the event. A third cluster of diagnostic criteria for PTSD is negative alterations in cognition and mood following the trauma. In children 6 years or younger, according to DSM-5, negative alterations in cognitions may take the form of socially withdrawn behavior, reduction of expressing positive emotions, diminished interest in play, and feelings of shame, fear, and confusion. In children older than 6 years of age, these may take the form of an inability to remember parts of a traumatic event, that is, *psychological amnesia,* or persistent negative feelings about oneself, including horror, anger, guilt, or shame. After a traumatic event, children may experience a sense of detachment from their usual play activities ("psychological numbing") or a diminished capacity to feel emotions. Older adolescents may express a fear that they expect to die young (sense of foreshortened future).

Other typical responses to traumatic events include symptoms of hyperarousal that were not present before the traumatic exposure, such as difficulty falling asleep or staying asleep; hypervigilance regarding safety and increased checking that doors are locked; or exaggerated startle reaction. In some children, hyperarousal can present as a generalized inability to relax with increased irritability, outbursts, and impaired ability to concentrate.

To meet the diagnostic criteria for PTSD, according to the DSM-5 the symptoms must be present for at least 1 month, and cause distress and impairment in important functional areas of life. When all of the diagnostic symptoms of PTSD are met following the traumatic event, persist for at least 3 days, but resolve within 1 month, acute PTSD is diagnosed. When the full syndrome of PTSD persists beyond 3 months, it is designated as chronic PTSD. In some cases, the PTSD symptoms increase over time, and it is not until more than 6 months have elapsed after the exposure to the trauma that the whole syndrome emerges; in that case, the diagnosis is PTSD, delayed onset.

It is not uncommon for children and adolescents with PTSD to experience feelings of guilt, especially if they have survived the trauma and others in the situation did not. They may blame themselves for the demise of the others and may go on to develop a comorbid depressive episode. Childhood PTSD is also associated with increased rates of other anxiety disorders, depressive episodes, substance use disorders, and attentional difficulties. DSM-5 includes a specifier *With dissociative symptoms,* which can present as either *Depersonalization,* in which there are recurrent experiences of feeling detached, as if outside of one's own body; or *Derealization,* in which the world feels unreal, dreamlike, and distant. A final specifier, *With delayed expression,* indicates that the full diagnostic criteria were not met until 6 months after the traumatic event, although some symptoms may present earlier.

PATHOLOGY AND LABORATORY EXAMINATION

Although reports indicate some alterations in both neurophysiological and neuroimaging studies of children and adolescents with PTSD, no current laboratory tests can help in making this diagnosis.

DIFFERENTIAL DIAGNOSIS

A number of overlapping symptoms are seen between childhood PTSD and presentations of childhood anxiety disorders, such as separation anxiety disorder, OCD or social phobia, in which recurrent intrusive thoughts or avoidant behaviors occur. Children with depressive disorders often exhibit withdrawal and a sense of isolation from peers as well as guilt about life events over which they realistically have no control. Irritability, poor concentration, sleep disturbance, and decreased interest in usual activities can also be observed in both PTSD and major depressive disorder.

Children who have lost a loved one in a traumatic event may go on to experience both PTSD and a major depressive disorder when bereavement persists beyond its expected course. Children with PTSD may also be confused with children who have disruptive behavior disorders, because they often show poor concentration, inattention, and irritability. It is critical to elicit a history of traumatic exposure and evaluate the chronology of the trauma and the onset of the symptoms to make an accurate diagnosis of PTSD.

COURSE AND PROGNOSIS

For some children and adolescents with milder forms of PTSD, symptoms may persist for 1 to 2 years, after which they diminish and attenuate. In more severe circumstances, however, PTSD syndromes persist for many years or decades in children and adolescents, with spontaneous remission in only a portion of them.

The prognosis of untreated PTSD has become an issue of growing concern for researchers and clinicians who have documented a variety of serious comorbidities and psychobiological abnormalities associated with PTSD. In one study, children and adolescents with severe PTSD were at risk for decreased intracranial volume, diminished corpus callosum area, and lower IQs compared to children without PTSD. Children and adolescents with histories of physical and sexual abuse have been found to exhibit higher rates of depression and suicidality themselves and in their offspring as well. This highlights the importance of early recognition and treatment of PTSD that may significantly improve the long-term outcome among youth.

TREATMENT

Trauma-Focused Cognitive-Behavior Therapy

Randomized clinical trials have provided evidence for the efficacy of trauma-focused CBT in the treatment of PTSD in children and adolescents. This treatment is generally administered over 10 to 16 treatment sessions, including nine components itemized in the acronym PRACTICE. Trauma-focused CBT (TF-CBT) as detailed by Cohen, Mannarino, and Deblinger in their text *Treating Trauma and Traumatic Grief in Children and Adolescents* entails the inclusion of gradual exposure to feared stimuli as a critical element. Such stimuli encompass places, people, sounds, and situations. The first component of TF-CBT is *Psychoeducation* regarding the nature of typical emotional and physiological reactions to traumatic events and PTSD. Next, *Parenting Skills* involve sessions focused on guiding parents on providing praise, administering a time out, contingency reinforcement programs, and troubleshooting for specific symptoms in a given child. Component 3 is *Relaxation,* in which children are taught to utilize muscle relaxation, focused breathing, affective modulation, thought-stopping, and other cognitive techniques to diminish feelings of helplessness and distress. Component 4 is *Affective Expression and Modulation,* geared to help children and their parents to identify their feelings, interrupt disturbing thoughts with positive imagery, and teach positive self-talk and social skills building. Component 5 is *Cognitive Coping and Processing,* which deals specifically with reviewing the Cognitive Triangle, in which the relationship between thoughts, feelings, and behaviors is explored. Unhelpful thoughts are challenged with practice. In Component 6, *Trauma Narrative,* the story of the traumatic event and its sequelae are developed over time by the child, with the therapist's support, using a depiction of words, art, or other creative form. Eventually this is shared with the parent. Component 7, *In Vivo Exposure and Mastery of Trauma Reminders,* is a session that reviews with the child how to deal with situations that are a reminder of the trauma and how to maintain control over distressing feelings associated with it. Component 8 is *Conjoint Child–Parent Sessions;* this component may involve several sessions in which the child and parent share their understanding of the process of the therapy and the gains that they have made. Finally, Component 9, *Enhancing Future Safety,* involves sessions that focus on the changes made in the family to ensure the safety of the child. These final sessions also promote healthy communication between the child and the parents.

A variant of TF-CBT for PTSD is called *eye movement desensitization and reprocessing* (EMDR), in which exposure and cognitive reprocessing interventions are paired with directed eye movements. This technique is not as well accepted as the more extensive TF-CBT detailed above.

Cognitive Behavioral Intervention for Trauma in Schools

Cognitive behavioral intervention for trauma in schools (CBITS) is an intervention that administers treatment in the school setting for children who screen positive for PTSD and whose parents agree to treatment in school. It consists of ten weekly group sessions, one to three individual imaginal exposure sessions, two to four optional sessions with parents, and one parent education session. Similar to TF-CBT, CBITS incorporates psychoeducation, relaxation training, cognitive coping skills, gradual exposure to traumatic memories through a narrative, in vivo exposure, and affect modulation, cognitive restructuring, and social problem solving. In one randomized controlled trial, 86 percent of students in the CBITS group reported significantly decreased PTSD symptoms compared to the waitlist controls. Students who received CBITS also reported lower depression scores. Among parents whose children received CBITS treatment, 78 percent reported decreased psychosocial problems in their children. After CBITS treatment, the improvements in both the PTSD and depression symptoms were sustained at 6 months.

Structured Psychotherapy for Adolescents Responding to Chronic Stress

Structured psychotherapy for adolescents responding to chronic stress (SPARCS) consists of a group intervention, generally administered in 16 sessions, with a focus on the needs of adolescents between the ages of 12 and 19 years who have lived with chronic trauma and may also carry a diagnosis of PTSD. SPARCS was tested in a trial of multicultural teens and young adults with moderate or severe trauma exposure. Most of the participants were female, and comprised multiple ethnic groups: 67 percent African American; 12 percent Latino; 21 percent Caucasian. SPARCS demonstrated efficacy in reducing traumatic stress symptoms, mainly in the largest group, the African-American group. SPARCS utilizes cognitive behavioral techniques, and also incorporates many of the components of TF-CBT. In addition, SPARCS includes mindfulness techniques and relaxation.

Trauma Affect Regulation: Guide for Education and Therapy

Trauma affect regulation: Guide for education and therapy (TARGET), an affect regulation therapy, combines CBT components, such as cognitive processing, with affect modulation.

It is administered to adolescents between the ages of 13 and 19 who have been exposed to maltreatment and/or chronic traumatic exposure to such things as community violence or domestic violence. It is generally administered in 12 sessions, which focus on past or current situations. As with SPARCS treatment, gradual exposure may occur in the context of recounting past trauma but is not a core component of the treatment. A randomized trial with 59 delinquent girls aged 13 to 17 years who met full or partial criteria for PTSD found that TARGET reduced anxiety, anger, depression, and PTSD cognitions. TARGET is a promising treatment for girls with histories of delinquency, especially to reduce anger and to enhance optimism and self-efficacy.

Crisis Intervention/Psychological Debriefing

Crisis intervention/psychological debriefing typically consists of several sessions immediately after an exposure to a traumatic event in which a traumatized child or adolescent is encouraged to describe the traumatic event in the context of a supportive environment. Psychoeducation is provided and guidance about the management of initial emotional reactions may be provided. Anecdotal reports suggest that this intervention may be helpful, but no controlled studies have yet provided evidence that this intervention leads to a more positive outcome.

Psychopharmacological Treatment

Several pharmacologic agents have been utilized to treat children and adolescents with PTSD, often focused on diminishing intrusive thoughts, hyperarousal, and avoidance, with some success and mixed results. Given the frequent comorbidity of depressive disorder, anxiety disorders, and behavioral problems associated with PTSD, a multitude of psychopharmacological agents have been utilized to ameliorate symptoms associated with PTSD in youth. Antidepressant agents have been used as adjuncts to psychosocial treatments in youth with PTSD. Despite the fact that sertraline and paroxetine are approved by the FDA in the treatment of PTSD in adults, there is scant evidence to support its use for the core symptoms of PTSD in youth. A randomized controlled trial of TF-CBT plus sertraline compared to TF-CBT plus placebo in 24 children with PTSD found that both groups had significant reduction in PTSD symptoms, with no significant difference between the groups. A multicenter study of 131 children aged 6 to 17 years with PTSD were treated with 10 weeks of sertraline or placebo. Results showed sertraline to be a safe treatment; however, it was not demonstrated to have efficacy compared to placebo. A randomized controlled trial using citalopram did not show superiority of citalopram over placebo in treatment of core PTSD symptoms. There is, however, evidence suggesting that the use of selective serotonin reuptake inhibitors (SSRIs) in traumatized children with burns may be preventive regarding the development of PTSD. Published literature demonstrates that up to 50 percent of children with moderate to severe burns develop PTSD, thus preventive strategies are important. A randomized controlled study of sertraline to prevent PTSD found that children who received sertraline, flexibly dosed between 25 mg and 150 mg per day, had a decrease in parent-reported symptoms of PTSD over 8 weeks compared to a placebo group. Among the child-reported symptoms, however, there was no significant difference between the two groups.

Antiadrenergic agents have been tried to treat dysregulation of the noradrenergic system in adults and youth with PTSD. α_2-agonists such as clonidine and guanfacine, for example, have been used to decrease norepinephrine release, whereas centrally acting β-antagonists such as propranolol, and α_1-antagonists such as prazosin, are hypothesized to improve hyperarousal and intrusive thoughts through attenuation of norepinephrine postsynaptically. In adults, clonidine (Catapres) and propranolol (Inderal) have been used to treat PTSD, especially nightmares and exaggerated startle response, with evidence of improvement. Although there are some data in adults with PTSD to support the use of these agents, data in youth are limited largely to case reports. There is a suggestion that guanfacine may reduce nightmares in children with PTSD and that clonidine may diminish symptoms of reenactment of traumatic events in children. One report of propranolol treatment in 11 pediatric patients with PTSD from sexual or physical abuse with a mean age of 8.5 years, who exhibited agitation and hyperarousal, indicated some decrease in symptoms in 8 of the 11 children studied. Another open study of transdermal clonidine treatment of preschoolers with PTSD suggests that clonidine may be efficacious in this population in decreasing activation and hyperarousal. An additional open trial of oral clonidine with dosage ranges of 0.05 to 0.1 mg twice daily similarly suggests that this medication may provide some relief for the symptoms of hyperarousal, impulsivity, and agitation in young children with PTSD.

Second-generation antipsychotics such as risperidone, olanzapine, quetiapine, ziprasidone, and aripiprazole have been studied in adults with PTSD with mixed results. Risperidone and aripiprazole have both been given FDA approval for use in children and adolescents with aggression, severe behavioral dyscontrol, and severe psychiatric disorders; however, controlled trials have not been done with children with PTSD. A report of three preschool-aged children who exhibited symptoms of acute stress disorder and who had severe thermal burns were reported to improve after being treated with risperidone.

Mood-stabilizing agents including divalproex, carbamazepine, topiramate, and gabapentin have been utilized for adults with PTSD with modest improvement. In children and adolescents with PTSD, one open-label trial of carbamazepine and one trial of divalproex have been undertaken. In the adult carbamazepine trial, all 28 patients were reported to be either asymptomatic or somewhat improved at blood levels of the agent of 10 to 11.5 μg/mL. In the divalproex trial, 12 males who carried diagnoses of conduct disorder comorbid with PTSD were randomly assigned to high- or low-dose divalproex with reported improvement in those receiving the higher doses. Benzodiazepines are often prescribed to treat anxiety symptoms in patients with PTSD, although there are no controlled trials to support their use in youth with PTSD at this time.

Given that many children and adolescents with PTSD have comorbid depressive and anxiety disorders, SSRIs are recommended in the treatment of these coexisting disorders.

▲ 27.12 Mood Disorders and Suicide in Children and Adolescents

27.12a Depressive Disorders and Suicide in Children and Adolescents

Depressive disorders in youth represent a significant public health concern, in that they are prevalent and result in long-term adverse effects on the individual's cognitive, social, and psychological development. These disorders affect approximately 2 to 3 percent of children and up to 8 percent of adolescents, so the need for early identification and access to evidence-based interventions such as CBTs and antidepressant agents, is essential. Although major depression runs in families, with the highest risk in children whose parents experienced early-onset depression, twin studies have demonstrated that major depression is only moderately heritable, approximately 40 to 50 percent, highlighting environmental stressors and adverse events as major contributors to major depressive disorder in youth. The core features of major depression in children, adolescents, and adults bear a striking resemblance; however, clinical presentation is strongly influenced by the developmental level of the child or adolescent. The American Psychiatric Association's *Diagnostic and Statistical Manual of Mental Disorders, Fifth Edition* (DSM-5) utilizes the same criteria for major depressive disorder in youth as in adults, except that for children and adolescents, *irritable mood* may replace a *depressed mood* in the diagnostic criteria.

Most children and adolescents with depressive disorders neither attempt nor complete suicide; however, severely depressed youth often have suicidal ideation, and suicide remains the most serious risk of major depression. Nevertheless, many depressed youth do not ever have suicidal ideation, and many children and adolescents who engage in suicidal behavior do not have a depressive disorder. There is epidemiological evidence to suggest that depressed youth with recurrent active suicidal ideation, including a plan, and who have made prior attempts, are at higher risk to complete suicide, compared to youth who express only passive suicidal ideation.

Mood disorders in children and adolescents have been studied increasingly over the last two decades, culminating in large sample multisite randomized controlled trials (RCTs) such as the Treatment of Adolescent Depression Study (TADS), which provides evidence of the efficacy of both CBT as well as SSRIs. Furthermore, when the preceding modalities are combined, the greatest efficacy is achieved. Increased recognition of depressive disorders in preschool populations has sparked clinicians and researchers to develop psychosocial interventions such as the Parent–Child Interaction Therapy Emotion Development (PCIT-ED), which target treatment specifically for this age group. The expression of disturbed and depressed mood appears to vary with developmental stage. Very young children with major depression are often observed to be sad, listless, or apathetic, even though they may not articulate these feelings verbally. Perhaps surprisingly, mood-congruent auditory hallucinations are not infrequently observed in young children with major depression. Somatic complaints such as headaches and stomachaches, withdrawn and sad appearance, and poor self-esteem are more universal symptoms. Patients in late adolescence with more severe forms of depression often display pervasive anhedonia, severe psychomotor retardation, delusions, and a sense of hopelessness. Symptoms that appear with the same frequency, regardless of age and developmental status, include suicidal ideation, depressed or irritable mood, insomnia, and diminished ability to concentrate.

Developmental issues, however, influence the expression of depressive symptoms. For example, unhappy young children who exhibit recurrent suicidal ideation are rarely able to propose a realistic suicide plan or to carry out such a plan. Children's moods are especially vulnerable to the influences of severe social stressors, such as chronic family discord, abuse and neglect, and academic failure. Many young children with major depressive disorder have histories of abuse, neglect, and families with significant psychosocial burdens such as parental mental illness, substance abuse, or poverty. Children who develop depressive disorders in the midst of acute toxic family stressors may have remission of depressive symptoms when the stressors diminish or when a more nurturing family environment is introduced. Depressive disorders are generally episodic, albeit typically lasting close to a year; however, their onset may be insidious and remain unidentified until significant impairment in peer relationships, deterioration in academic function, or withdrawal from activities emerges. ADHD, oppositional defiant disorder, and conduct disorder are not infrequently comorbid with a major depressive episode. In some cases, conduct disturbances or disorders occur in the context of a major depressive episode and resolve with the resolution of the depressive episode. Clinicians must clarify the chronology of the symptoms to determine whether a given behavior (e.g., poor concentration, defiance, or temper tantrums) was present before the depressive episode and is unrelated to it or whether the behavior is occurring for the first time and is related to the depressive episode.

EPIDEMIOLOGY

Depressive disorders increase in frequency with increasing age in the general population. Mood disorders among preschool-age children are estimated to occur in about 0.3 percent of community samples, and 0.9 percent in clinic settings. The prevalence of major depression in school-age children is 2 to 3 percent. Depression in referred samples of school-age children is found to be the same frequency in boys as in girls, with some surveys indicating a slightly increased rate among boys. In adolescents, prevalence rate of major depression is from 4 to 8 percent and two to three times more likely in females than males. By the age of 18 years, the cumulative incidence of major depression is 20 percent. Children with a family history of major depression in a first-degree relative are about three times more likely to develop the disorder than in those without family histories of affective disorders. The prevalence of persistent depressive disorder in children ranges from 0.6 to 4.6 percent and in adolescence increases to 1.6 to 8 percent. Children and adolescents with persistent depressive disorder have a high likelihood of developing major depressive disorder at some point after 1 year of the persistent depressive disorder. The rate of developing a major depression on top of persistent depressive disorder (double depression) within a 6-month period of persistent depressive disorder is estimated to be about 9.9 percent.

Among psychiatrically hospitalized children and adolescents, the rates of major depressive disorder have been estimated to be close to 20 percent for children and 40 percent for adolescents.

ETIOLOGY

Considerable evidence indicates that major depression in youth is the same fundamental disorder experienced by adults, and that its neurobiology is likely to be an interaction of genetic vulnerability and environmental stressors.

Genetic Studies

Converging evidence suggests that an interaction between genetic susceptibility and environmental stressors contributes to an emerging major depression and is associated with brain volume, especially in the hippocampal region. The serotonin transporter gene and, in particular, the serotonin transporter promoter polymorphism (5-HTTLPR) have become a focus of investigation. Patients with the short S-allele of the serotonin polymorphism who also experienced a significant environmental adverse event such as neglect, developed smaller hippocampal volumes compared to patients with only one of the above risk factors. The S-allele of the polymorphism leads to decreased serotonin (5-HT) reuptake and thus potentially to decreased uptake of serotonin into the brain. A large longitudinal study in New Zealand found that the S-allele of the serotonin transporter gene was associated with early environmental stress and subsequent depression. This study demonstrated a relationship between early environmental stress and subsequent depression in children with one or two short alleles, but not in children with two long alleles. Because the short alleles are less efficient in transcription, this finding suggests that the availability of the transporter gene may provide a marker for vulnerability to depression. The findings that the combination of a decreased volume in the hippocampus is associated with the S-allele of the serotonin transporter gene polymorphism and early adverse events in depression, may represent a mechanism by which the risk of major depression is mediated by both genetics and environmental stressors.

Familiarity

Twin studies have demonstrated that major depression is approximately 40 to 50 percent heritable. There is an increased risk of depression in the children of parents with the disorder, and this risk is further increased for the child when the parents developed depressive disorders at an early age. Studies suggest age-related differences in the heritability of major depression such that in younger children, environmental influences appear to be more dominant and in first episodes in adolescence, heritability may play a larger role. Family studies suggest that for children with a parent with a history of major depressive disorder, the risk of developing an episode of major depressive disorder is doubled, whereas with two depressed parents, the risk of an episode of major depressive disorder quadruples in the offspring before the age of 18 years. Similarly, children with the largest number of severe episodes starting at younger ages exhibit the densest family histories of major depressive disorder.

Neurobiology

Neuroendocrine studies have examined the hypothalamic–pituitary–adrenal axes, the hypothalamic growth hormone, the hypothalamic–pituitary–thyroid, and the hypothalamic–pituitary–gonadal axes, seeking to demonstrate consistent markers in depressed youth. These studies have yielded inconsistent results. For example, depressed prepubertal children secrete significantly more growth hormone during sleep than nondepressed children or youth with other psychiatric disorders. In addition, depressed children secrete significantly less growth hormone in response to insulin-induced hypoglycemia than do nondepressed patients. Both findings appear to persist for months after partial or full remission. Thyroid hormone studies have found lower free total thyroxine (FT_4) levels in depressed adolescents than in a matched control group. These values were associated with normal thyroid-stimulating hormone (TSH). This finding suggests that, although values of thyroid function remain in the normative range, FT_4 levels have shifted downward. These downward shifts in thyroid hormone possibly contribute to the clinical manifestations of depression.

Sleep studies are also inconclusive in depressed children and adolescents. Polysomnography in depressed children have only occasionally shown characteristic sleep markers of adults with major depressive disorder: reduced REM latency and an increased number of REM periods.

Magnetic Resonance Imaging

Neuroimaging studies of depressed youth demonstrate smaller frontal white matter volumes, larger frontal gray matter volumes, and larger lateral ventricle volumes. Depressed youth have been found to have a blunted amygdala response to fearful faces compared to nondepressed children and depressed children have been found to have smaller amygdale volumes compared to healthy controls.

Because twin studies and adoption studies have demonstrated that depression appears to be only 40 to 50 percent heritable, with environmental contributions more predominant in younger children, family and environmental contributions must be examined. Adverse events during childhood such as maltreatment, abuse or neglect, parental death, parental psychiatric illness, substance abuse, parent–child conflict, and lack of family cohesion are all risk factors for childhood depression. Data from twin and genetic studies support the conclusion that the interaction of genetic and environmental factors plays a critical role in depressive disorders, since correlation of adverse life events and depression is stronger in children and adolescents with known genetic susceptibility.

Once a child or adolescent has experienced one major depressive episode, the psychosocial "scars" increase his or her vulnerability for a subsequent episode. The psychosocial impairments in depressed children remain far after recovery from the episode. Among depressed preschoolers, the sooner that adverse life events promoting the depression are identified, the more rapidly interventions may be administered to treat the depression.

DIAGNOSIS AND CLINICAL FEATURES

Major Depressive Disorder

Major depressive disorder in children is diagnosed most easily when it is acute and occurs in a child without previous psychiatric symptoms. Often, however, the onset is insidious, and the disorder occurs in a child who has had several years of difficulties with hyperactivity, separation anxiety disorder, or intermittent depressive symptoms.

According to the DSM-5, diagnostic criteria for a major depressive episode consist of at least five symptoms, for a period of 2 weeks, including either (1) depressed or irritable mood, or (2) a loss of interest or pleasure. Additional symptoms may include failure to make expected weight gains, daily insomnia or hypersomnia, psychomotor agitation or retardation, daily fatigue or loss of energy, feelings of worthlessness or inappropriate guilt, diminished ability to think or concentrate, and recurrent thoughts of death. These symptoms must produce social or academic impairment. To meet the diagnostic criteria for major depressive disorder, the symptoms cannot be due to the direct effects of a substance (e.g., alcohol) or a general medical condition. In contrast to the *Diagnostic and Statistical Manual of Mental Disorders, Fourth Edition, Text Revision* (DSM-IV-TR), in which a diagnosis of major depressive disorder was not made within 2 months of the loss of a loved one, except when marked functional impairment, morbid preoccupation with worthlessness, suicidal ideation, psychotic symptoms, or psychomotor retardation was present, in DSM-5, a diagnosis of major depressive disorder can be made at any time following a loss, even without the preceding symptoms. This change reflects the understanding that grief typically lasts 1 to 2 years, rather than 2 months, and that major depressive disorder may occur in the presence of grief at any time after a loss.

A major depressive episode in a prepubertal child is likely to be manifested by somatic complaints, psychomotor agitation, and mood-congruent hallucinations. Anhedonia is also frequent, but anhedonia, as well as hopelessness, psychomotor retardation, and delusions, are more common in adolescent and adult major depressive episodes than in those of young children. Adults have more problems than depressed children and adolescents with sleep and appetite. In adolescence, negativistic or frankly antisocial behavior and the use of alcohol or illicit substances can occur and may justify the additional diagnoses of oppositional defiant disorder, conduct disorder, and substance abuse or dependence. Feelings of restlessness, irritability, aggression, reluctance to cooperate in family ventures, withdrawal from social activities, and isolation from peers often occur in adolescents. School difficulties are likely. Depressed adolescents may become less attentive to personal appearance and show increased sensitivity to rejection by peers, and in romantic relationships.

Children can be reliable reporters about their emotions, relationships, and difficulties in psychosocial functions. They may, however, refer to depressive feelings in terms of anger, or feeling "mad" rather than sad. Clinicians should assess the duration and periodicity of the depressive mood to differentiate relatively universal, short-lived, and sometimes frequent periods of sadness, usually after a frustrating event, from a true, persistent depressive mood. The younger the child, the more imprecise his or her time estimates are likely to be.

Mood disorders tend to be chronic if they begin early. Childhood onset may be the most severe form of mood disorder and tends to appear in families with a high incidence of mood disorders and alcohol abuse. The children are likely to have such secondary complications as conduct disorder, alcohol and other substance abuse, and antisocial behavior. Functional impairment associated with a depressive disorder in childhood extends to practically all areas of a child's psychosocial world; school performance and behavior, peer relationships, and family relationships all suffer. Only highly intelligent and academically oriented children with no more than a moderate depression can compensate for their difficulties in learning by substantially increasing their time and effort. Otherwise, school performance is invariably affected by a combination of difficulty concentrating, slowed thinking, lack of interest and motivation, fatigue, sleepiness, depressive ruminations, and preoccupations. Depression in a child may be misdiagnosed as a learning disorder. Learning problems secondary to depression, even when longstanding, are corrected rapidly after a child's recovery from the depressive episode.

Children and adolescents with severe forms of major depressive disorder may have hallucinations and/or delusions. Usually, these psychotic symptoms are thematically consistent with the depressed mood, occur with the depressive episode (usually at its worst), and do not include certain types of hallucinations (such as conversing voices and a commenting voice, which are specific to schizophrenia). Depressive hallucinations usually consist of a single voice speaking to the person from outside his or her head, with derogatory or suicidal content. Depressive delusions center on themes of guilt, physical disease, death, nihilism, deserved punishment, personal inadequacy, and (sometimes) persecution. These delusions are rare in prepuberty, probably because of cognitive immaturity, but are present in about half of psychotically depressed adolescents.

Adolescent onset of a mood disorder can be complicated by use of alcohol or drugs. One study found that up to 17 percent of adolescents with depressive disorder received an initial evaluation due to substance abuse.

Persistent Depressive Disorder (Dysthymia)

Persistent depressive disorder, in DSM-5, represents a consolidation of chronic major depressive disorder and what DSM-IV-TR termed dysthymic disorder. In children and adolescents, it consists of a depressed or irritable mood for most of the day, for more days than not, over a period of at least 1 year. DSM-5 notes that in children and adolescents, irritable mood can replace the depressed mood criterion for adults and that the duration criterion is not 2 years but 1 year for children and adolescents. According to the DSM-5 diagnostic criteria, two or more of the following symptoms must accompany the depressed or irritable mood: low self-esteem, hopelessness, poor appetite or overeating, insomnia or hypersomnia, low energy or fatigue, or poor concentration or difficulty making decisions. During the year of the disturbance, these symptoms do not resolve for more than 2 months at a time. In addition, the diagnostic criteria for dysthymic disorder specify that during the first year, no major depressive episode emerges. To meet the DSM-5 diagnostic criteria for persistent depressive disorder, a child must not have a history of a manic or hypomanic episode. Persistent depressive disorder is also not diagnosed if the symptoms occur exclusively during a chronic psychotic disorder or if they are the direct effects of a substance or a general medical condition. DSM-5 provides specifiers for early onset (before 21 years of age) or late onset (after 21 years of age).

A child or adolescent with persistent depressive disorder may have had a major depressive episode before developing persistent depressive disorder; however, it is much more common for a child with persistent depressive disorder for more than 1 year to develop a concurrent episode of major depressive disorder. In this case, both depressive diagnoses apply (double depression). Persistent depressive disorder in youth is known to have an average age of onset that is several years earlier than the typical onset of major depressive disorder. Occasionally, youth fulfill the criteria for persistent depressive disorder, except that their episode does not last for a whole year, or they experience remission from symptoms for more than a 2-month period. These mood presentations in youth may predict additional mood disorder episodes in the future. Current knowledge suggests that the longer, more recurrent, and less directly related to social stress these episodes are, the greater the likelihood of future severe mood disorder. When minor depressive episodes follow a significant stressful life event by less than 3 months, it may be classified as an adjustment disorder.

Cyclothymic Disorder

Cyclothymia is a chronic and fluctuating mood disturbance of hypomanic symptoms and periods of depressive symptoms that do not meet diagnostic criteria for major depressive disorder. The difference in the DSM-5 diagnostic criteria for youth with cyclothymic disorder compared to adults is that a period of 1 year, rather than 2 years, of numerous mood swings is applied. Bipolar II disorder is distinguished from cyclothymia by a history of episodes of major depressive disorder. When an episode of major depressive disorder occurs after a diagnosis of cyclothymia has been present for at least 2 years, a concurrent diagnosis of bipolar II disorder is made.

Bereavement

Bereavement is a state of grief related to the death of a loved one, which presents with an overlap of symptoms characteristic of a major depressive episode. Typical depressive symptoms associated with bereavement include feelings of sadness, insomnia, diminished appetite, and, in some cases, weight loss. Grieving children may become withdrawn and appear sad, and they are not easily drawn into even favorite activities.

In DSM-5, bereavement is not a mental disorder; however, uncomplicated bereavement is included as a category documented with a *v* code, indicating that a normal grief reaction to the loss of a loved one has become a focus of clinical attention. Children in the midst of a typical bereavement period may also meet the criteria for major depressive disorder. Symptoms indicating major depressive disorder exceeding typical bereavement include intense guilt related to issues beyond those surrounding the death of the loved one, preoccupation with death other than thoughts about being dead to be with the deceased person, morbid preoccupation with worthlessness, marked psychomotor retardation, prolonged serious functional impairment, and hallucinations other than transient perceptions of the voice of the deceased person.

The duration of bereavement varies; in children, the duration may depend partly on the support system in place. For example, a child who must be removed from home because of the death of the only parent in the home may feel devastated and abandoned for a long period. Children who lose loved ones may feel a sense of guilt, that the death may have occurred because they were "bad" or did not perform as expected.

Ryan was a 12-year-old 7th grader in middle school who was brought to the emergency room in handcuffs by police after walking into oncoming traffic right after school. Ryan walked in front of a city bus; the driver began honking at the boy who kept walking slowly into the traffic. Two police stationed in their car across the street from the school heard the bus honking and noticed Ryan and confronted him. The police were about to issue the boy a citation for crossing against the red light; however, when they inquired as to why he had crossed against the traffic light he informed them that he was trying to kill himself. The police handcuffed Ryan, placed him in the police car without a struggle and brought him to the local hospital's emergency room. Ryan's mother was contacted and met her son in the emergency room. Ryan was found to be physically intact, without injury, by the emergency room doctors, and psychiatric evaluation was initiated by a team of child psychiatrists including an attending child psychiatrist and two child and adolescent psychiatry residents. Ryan became tearful when asked what had happened, and reported that he had purposefully walked in front of the bus in the hope of being hit by the bus in order to die. Ryan reported that he has been bullied by numerous peers over the last 2 years and is picked on because he is short and overweight. Ryan reported that on this day, a girl in his class had pushed him down and started hitting him and laughing at him. Ryan reported that he had been teased and physically assaulted repeatedly by peers in his grade and that they call him stupid and fat. Ryan has some friends, who usually defend him, but on this day, his friends were not close by and he became desperate. Ryan disclosed, however, that even before this day, he has been consistently sad in school for the past year, and that he has thought about suicide recurrently over the last year, mainly due to feeling ostracized and worthless after being picked on and bullied. Ryan continues to be actively suicidal, disclosing his strong feeling that for him, life is not worth living. Ryan is a relatively good student, earning good grades, especially in math, although he is currently failing history. Upon separate interview with Ryan's mother, she reports that she has no knowledge of any problems that Ryan has been struggling with, and that she feels that Ryan is not depressed, not severely bullied, or seriously unhappy in school, and reports that this must have been a mistake and that she is ready to take him home. Ryan reported that he had previously seen a counselor in school a few times last year when he was bullied, but that he has received no intervention for his depression or his suicidality and that he has not shared these feeling with his family and that he is generally content at home. Ryan has an older brother and a younger brother who are well adjusted. When Ryan and his mother were interviewed together, Ryan was able with some encouragement to let his mother know how depressed, hopeless, and suicidal he feels, and why. Ryan's mother burst into tears and Ryan tried to comfort his mother, although he was crying as well. Ryan was placed on a 72-hour hold for "danger to self," and referred to a children's psychiatric inpatient unit for further evaluation and treatment. A trial of an SSRI antidepressant was recommended as well as psychoeducation and family sessions so that Ryan and his family would reach an understanding about his current psychiatric disorder, and that together they could work on a safe and productive plan for Ryan. Ongoing psychosocial intervention was recommended for Ryan and his family after hospitalization.

PATHOLOGY AND LABORATORY EXAMINATION

No laboratory test is useful in making a diagnosis of a major depression. If a child or adolescent also complains of symptoms of hypothyroidism, that is, dry skin, coldness, lethargy, and so on, then a screening test for thyroid function may be indicated.

Rating scales for depressive symptoms administered by the clinician to the child and parent may be helpful in the evaluation. The Children's Depression Rating Scale-Revised (CDRS-R) is a 17-item instrument administered by the clinician separately to the parent and child or adolescent. The clinician scores a rating for each item using the information from both the parent and the child. The scale assesses affective, somatic, cognitive, and psychomotor symptoms. A cumulative score of 40 is a marker for moderate depression and a score of 45 or greater for significant depression.

DIFFERENTIAL DIAGNOSIS

Substance-induced mood disorder may be difficult to differentiate from other mood disorders until detoxification occurs. Anxiety symptoms and disorders often coexist with depressive disorders. Of particular importance in the differential diagnosis is the distinction between agitated depressive or manic episodes and ADHD, in which the persistent excessive activity and restlessness can cause confusion. Prepubertal children generally do not show classic forms of agitated depression, such as handwringing and pacing. Instead, an inability to sit still, irritability, and frequent temper tantrums are the most common symptoms. Sometimes, the correct diagnosis becomes evident only after remission of the depressive episode.

COURSE AND PROGNOSIS

The course and prognosis of major depression in children and adolescents depends on the severity of illness, the rapidity of interventions, and the degree of response to the interventions. In general, 90 percent of youth recover from a first episode of moderate to severe major depressive disorder within 1 to 2 years. The age of onset, episode severity, and the presence of comorbid disorders also influence course and prognosis. In general, the younger the age of onset, the greater the recurrence of multiple episodes and the presence of comorbid disorders predict a poorer prognosis. The mean length of an untreated episode of major depression in children and adolescents is about 8 to 12 months; the cumulative probability of recurrence is 20 to 60 percent within 2 years and 70 percent by 5 years. The greatest risk for relapse is in the 6 months to 1 year after treatment is discontinued. Depressed children who live in families with high levels of chronic conflict are more likely to have relapses. The relapse rates for childhood major depression into adulthood are also high. In a community sample, 45 percent of adolescents with a history of major depression developed another episode of major depression in early adulthood.

Youth with major depression are at higher risk for the development of future bipolar disorder, compared to adults. Overall estimates of children with an episode of major depression developing bipolar disorder are about 20 to 40 percent. Clinical characteristics of a depressive episode in youth, suggesting the highest risk of developing bipolar I disorder include hallucinations and delusions, psychomotor retardation, and a family history of bipolar illness. In a longitudinal study of prepubertal children with major depression, 33 percent developed bipolar I disorder, whereas 48 percent went on to develop bipolar II or bipolar disorder not otherwise specified by early adulthood.

Depressive disorders are associated with short-term and long-term peer relationship difficulties and complications, compromised academic achievement, and persistently low self-esteem. Persistent depressive disorder has an even more protracted recovery than major depressive disorder; the mean episode length is about 4 years. Early-onset persistent depressive disorder is associated with significant risks of comorbidity with major depressive disorder (70 percent), bipolar disorder (13 percent), and future substance abuse (15 percent). The risk of suicide, which accounts for about 12 percent of adolescent mortalities, is significant among adolescents with depressive disorders.

TREATMENT

The American Academy of Child and Adolescent Psychiatry practice parameters, as well as a consensus of experts who developed the Texas Children's Medication Algorithm Project (TMAP) made evidence-based recommendations for the treatment of children and adolescents with depressive disorders. These include psychoeducation and supportive interventions for youth with mild forms of depression. For youth with moderate to severe depression or recurrent episodes of major depression, with significant impairment and with active suicidal thoughts or behaviors, or psychosis, optimal intervention includes both psychopharmacological and CBT. CBT or interpersonal therapy (IPT) alone may be effective for moderate depression, especially when treatment is continued for 6 months or longer.

Psychiatric Hospitalization

Assessment of suicidal thoughts, behaviors, and past history of suicidal behavior is indicated in evaluating every child or adolescent with major depression. Safety is the most immediate consideration in assessing depression in youth, that is, a determination as to whether immediate psychiatric hospitalization is necessary. Depressed children and adolescents who express suicidal thoughts or behaviors most often require some extended evaluation in the safety of the psychiatric hospital to provide maximal protection from self-destructive impulses and behaviors.

Evidence-Based Treatment Studies

The TADS divided 439 adolescents between 12 and 17 years of age into three treatment groups of 12 weeks, composed of either fluoxetine (Prozac) alone (10 to 40 mg per day), fluoxetine with the same dose range in combination with CBT, or CBT alone. Based on ratings of the CDRS-R combination treatment had significantly superior response rates compared with either treatment alone. Based on CGI scores, at 12 weeks, rates of much or very much improved were 71 percent for the combined treatment group, 60.6 percent for the fluoxetine group, and 43.2 percent for the CBT-alone group; and 34.4 percent for the placebo group. At 12 weeks, combination treatment was rated the optimal strategy in the treatment of adolescent depression. By the end of 9 months of treatment, however, response rates for each group had converged so that response for the combination group was 86 percent, fluoxetine group response was about 81 percent, and CBT-alone group response rate was 81 percent. The long-term effectiveness of treatments for adolescent depression demonstrates that for moderately ill adolescents, fluoxetine, CBT, or the combination is efficacious. However, the addition of CBT to fluoxetine decreased persistent suicidal ideation and potential treatment-related emergence of suicidal ideation.

A second large multicenter randomized placebo-controlled trial, Treatment of SSRI-Resistant Depression in Adolescents (TORDIA), included adolescents with major depression, who had not responded to a 2-month trial with an SSRI antidepressant. In this study, 334 adolescents between 12 and 18 years of age were randomly assigned to a different SSRI agent (either citalopram, paroxetine, or another antidepressant class, venlafaxine) with or without concurrent CBT. The SSRI plus CBT group and the venlafaxine plus CBT group had higher response rates of improvement (54.8 percent) than the group on medications alone (40.5 percent). There were no differences found in the response rates between antidepressant agents.

Psychosocial Interventions

CBT is widely recognized as an efficacious intervention for the treatment of moderately severe depression in children and adolescents. CBT aims to challenge maladaptive beliefs and enhance problem-solving abilities and social competence. A review of controlled cognitive-behavioral studies in children and adolescents revealed that, as with adults, both children and adolescents showed consistent improvement with these methods. Other "active" treatments, including relaxation techniques, were also shown to be helpful as adjunctive treatment for mild to moderate depression. Findings from one large controlled study comparing cognitive-behavioral interventions with non-directive supportive psychotherapy and systemic behavioral family therapy showed that 70 percent of adolescents had some improvement with each of the interventions; cognitive-behavioral intervention had the most rapid effect. Another controlled study comparing a brief course of CBT with relaxation therapy favored the cognitive-behavioral intervention. At a 3- to 6-month follow-up, however, no significant differences existed between the two treatment groups. This effect resulted from relapse in the cognitive-behavioral group, along with continued recovery in some patients in the relaxation group. Factors that seem to interfere with treatment responsiveness include the presence of comorbid anxiety disorder that probably was present before the depressive episode. It has been shown, however, that longer-term CBT is efficacious in the treatment of depression, and has the advantage of mitigating suicidal ideation.

Interpersonal psychotherapy (IPT) focuses on improving depression through a focus on ways in which depression interferes with interpersonal relationships and overcoming these challenges. The four main areas of focus with interpersonal psychotherapy include loss, interpersonal disputes, role transition, and interpersonal deficits. A modification of interpersonal therapy to more specifically address depression for adolescents (IPT-A) includes a focus on separation from parents, authority figures, peer pressures, and dyadic relationships. IPT-A has been studied on an outpatient basis as well as in a school-based clinic setting. A 12-week study of 48 adolescents with major depression randomly assigned to IPT-A or clinical monitoring found that the group receiving IPT-A showed decreased depressive symptoms, increased social functioning, and improved problem solving compared to the other group. In the school-based health clinic, depressed adolescents were randomly assigned to IPT-A or treatment as usual for a period of 16 weeks. Clinic staff were trained and administered the treatment. At the end of 16 weeks, those adolescents receiving IPT-A had greater symptom reduction and improved overall functioning; especially older and more severely depressed adolescents seemed to benefit most significantly.

PCIT-ED for preschool depression, a modification of PCIT historically used in the treatment of disruptive disorders for children, was piloted in an RCT for 54 depressed preschoolers. Fifty-four depressed young children from age 3 to 7 years were randomly assigned to either PCIT-ED or psychoeducation with their caregivers. PCIT-ED was manualized and consists of three modules conducted over 14 sessions in 12 weeks. The core modules of PCIT—Child-Directed Interaction (CDI) and Parent-Directed Interaction (PDI)—were utilized and limited to four sessions each. The focus of these modules is to strengthen the parent–child relationship by coaching parents in positive play techniques, giving effective directives to the child, and responding to disruptive behavior in firm but not punitive ways. The novel portion of the treatment targeting the preschool depression consisted of a 6-week ED module, which focused on helping the parent to be a more effective emotion guide and affect regulator for the child. As part of the ED module, the parent learned to accurately recognize his or her own emotions as well as the child's and serves to help regulate the child's emotions. A psychoeducation control condition, Developmental Education and Parenting Intervention (DEPI) was developed and administered to parents in small group sessions. The DEPI condition was designed to educate parents about child development and emphasized emotional and social development without individual coaching or practice with behavioral techniques as provided in the PCIT-ED group. Primary outcome measures included parent's report of the child's symptoms of depression using a structured instrument, the Preschool-Age Psychiatric Assessment (PAPA), and depression severity was measured pretreatment and posttreatment using parent ratings on the Preschool Feelings Checklist Scale Version (PFC-S) a 20-item checklist. Results revealed that both groups showed significant improvement with particular improvement in the PCIT-ED group with respect to emotion recognition, child executive functioning, and parenting stress. This pilot study indicates that PCIT-ED is a promising novel intervention for preschool depression that deserves further investigation.

Pharmacotherapy

Fluoxetine (Prozac) and escitalopram (Lexapro) have Food and Drug Administration (FDA) approval in the treatment of major depression in adolescents. Three RCTs using fluoxetine with depressed children and adolescents demonstrate its efficacy. Common side effects observed with fluoxetine include headache, gastrointestinal symptoms, sedation, and insomnia.

Short-term randomized clinical trials have demonstrated efficacy of citalopram (Celexa), and sertraline (Zoloft) compared with placebo in the treatment of major depression in children and adolescents.

Sertraline has been shown to provide efficacy in two multicenter, double-blind, placebo-controlled trials of 376 children and adolescents who were treated with sertraline at doses ranging from 50 to 200 mg a day, or placebo. Greater than 40 percent decrease in depression rating scale scores were found in nearly 70 percent of the patients treated with sertraline, compared with 56 percent in the placebo group. Most common side effects are anorexia, vomiting, diarrhea, and agitation.

Citalopram has been demonstrated in one RCT in the United States to be efficacious in 174 children and adolescents treated with citalopram at doses of 20 to 40 mg a day or placebo for 8 weeks. Significantly more of the group on citalopram showed improvement compared with placebo on the CDRS-R. A significantly increased response rate (response defined as less than 28 on CDRS-R) of 35 percent was found in the citalopram group, compared with 24 percent of the placebo group. Common side effects that emerged included headache, nausea, insomnia, rhinitis, abdominal pain, dizziness, fatigue, and flu-like symptoms.

Similar to the literature for adult depression, as many negative as positive study findings have emerged in RCTs of the treatment of childhood and adolescent depression. RCTs to date that have not shown efficacy on primary outcome measures include those using mirtazapine (Remeron), and tricyclic antidepressants. A meta-analysis of SSRI trials in depressed children and adolescents found efficacy of SSRIs compared to placebo with an average response rate of 60 percent for the SSRI compared to 49 percent for placebo.

Starting doses of SSRIs for prepubertal children are lower than doses recommended for adults, and adolescents are generally treated at the same doses recommended for adults.

Venlafaxine (Effexor), which blocks both serotonin and norepinephrine uptake, has been found to be effective in the TORDIA study; however, adverse effects including increased blood pressure have made this agent a second-line choice compared to the SSRIs. Tricyclic antidepressants are not generally recommended for the treatment of depression in children and adolescents due to a lack of proved efficacy along with the potential risk of cardiac arrhythmia associated with their use.

A potential side effect of SSRIs in depressed children is behavioral activation, or induction of hypomanic symptoms. In such situations, the medication should be discontinued to determine whether the activation resolves with discontinuation of the medication, or evolves into a hypomanic or manic episode. Activation due to SSRIs, however, does not necessarily predict a diagnosis of bipolar disorder.

FDA Warning and Suicidality

In September 2004, the FDA received information from their Psychopharmacologic Drug and Pediatric Advisory Committee indicating, based on their review of reported suicidal thoughts and behavior among depressed children and adolescents who participated in randomized clinical trials with nine different antidepressants, an increased risk of suicidality in those children who were on active antidepressant medications. Although no suicides were reported, the rates of suicidal thinking and behaviors were 2 percent for patients on placebo, versus 4 percent among patients on antidepressant medications. The FDA, in accordance with the recommendation of their advisory committees, instituted a "black box" warning to the health professional label of all antidepressant medication indicating the increased risk of suicidal thoughts and behaviors in children and adolescents being treated with antidepressant medications, and the need for close monitoring for these symptoms. Several reviews since 2004, however, concluded that the data do not indicate a significant increase in the risk of suicide or serious suicide attempts after starting treatment with antidepressant drugs.

Duration of Treatment

Based on available longitudinal data and the natural history of major depression in children and adolescents, current recommendations include maintaining antidepressant treatment for 1 year in a depressed child who has achieved a good response, and to then discontinue the medication at a time of relatively low stress for a medication-free period.

Pharmacologic Treatment Strategies for Resistant Depression

Pharmacological recommendations, in accordance with an expert consensus panel that developed the Texas Children's Medication Algorithm Project (TMAP), as well as the TORDIA study in the treatment of children or adolescents who have not responded to treatment with an SSRI agent is to change to another SSRI medication. If a child is not responsive to the second SSRI medication, then either a combination of antidepressants or augmentation strategies may be reasonable choices as well as an antidepressant from another class of medications.

Electroconvulsive Therapy

Electroconvulsive therapy (ECT) has been used for a variety of psychiatric illnesses in adults, primarily severe depressive and manic mood disorders and catatonia. ECT is used rarely for adolescents, although published case reports indicate its efficacy in adolescents with depression and mania. Currently case reports suggest that ECT may be a relatively safe and useful treatment for adolescents who have persistent severe affective disorders, particularly with psychotic features, catatonic symptoms, or persistent suicidality.

SUICIDE

In the United States, suicide is the third leading cause of death among adolescents, after accidental death and homicide. Throughout the world, suicide rarely occurs in children who have not reached puberty. In the last 15 years, the rates of both completed suicide and suicidal ideation rates have decreased among adolescents. This decrease appears to coincide with the increase in SSRI medications prescribed to adolescents with mood and behavioral disturbance.

Suicidal Ideation and Behavior

Suicidal ideation, gestures, and attempts are frequently, but not always, associated with depressive disorders. Reports indicate that as many as half of suicidal individuals express suicidal intentions to a friend or a relative within 24 hours before enacting suicidal behavior.

Suicidal ideation occurs in all age groups and with greatest frequency in children and adolescents with severe mood disorders. More than 12,000 children and adolescents are hospitalized in the United States each year because of suicidal threats or behavior, but completed suicide is rare in children younger than 12 years of age. A young child is hardly capable of designing and carrying out a realistic suicide plan. Cognitive immaturity seems to play a protective role in preventing even children who wish they were dead from committing suicide. Completed suicide occurs about five times more often in adolescent boys than in girls, although the rate of suicide attempts is at least three times higher among adolescent girls than among boys. Suicidal ideation is not a static phenomenon; it can wax and wane with time. The decision to engage in suicidal behavior may be made impulsively without much forethought, or the decision may be the culmination of prolonged rumination.

The method of the suicide attempt influences the morbidity and completion rates, independent of the severity of the intent to die at the time of the suicidal behavior. The most common method of completed suicide in children and adolescents is the use of firearms, which accounts for about two-thirds of all suicides in boys and almost one-half of suicides in girls. The second most common method of suicide in boys, occurring in about one-fourth of all cases, is hanging; in girls, about one-fourth commits suicide through ingestion of toxic substances. Carbon monoxide poisoning is the next most common method of suicide in boys, but it occurs in less than 10 percent; suicide by hanging and carbon monoxide poisoning are equally frequent among girls and account for about 10 percent each. Additional risk factors in suicide include a family history of suicidal behavior, exposure to family violence, impulsivity, substance abuse, and availability of lethal methods. Gender differences in nonfatal suicidal behavior among 9th grade adolescents in a recent survey of students in 100 high schools found that serious suicidal thoughts were reported in 19.8 percent of female students and 10.8 percent of females had made an attempt. In male students, 9.3 percent had a history of suicidal thoughts and 4.9 percent had made an attempt. In this study, female students showed evidence of higher levels of mood and anxiety problems, whereas males had a slightly higher level of disruptive behavior problems. Female students reported higher levels of depression, anxiety, somatic complaints, and increased levels of emotional and behavioral problems than males. In young adolescents, even without meeting full criteria for psychiatric disorders, females report more psychopathology along with higher likelihood of nonfatal suicidal behavior.

Epidemiology

In a study of 9- to 16-year-olds in a 3-month period, passive suicidal thoughts were approximately 1 percent, suicidal ideation with a plan was 0.3 percent, and suicide attempt was 0.25 percent. In adolescents 14 to 18 years, the current rate of suicidal ideation was found to be 2.7 percent and annual incidence was 4.3 percent. Among this population of adolescents, lifetime prevalence of suicide attempt was 7.1 percent with a much higher rate of suicidal behavior for girls than for boys: 10.1 percent compared to 3.8 percent. Completed suicide rates in youth are much less common in children and younger teens 10 to 14 years, with a slighter lower rate of 0.95 per 100,000 for females compared to 1.71 per 100,000 for males. In older adolescents 15 to 19 years of age, completed suicide is considerably lower for females, 3.52 per 100,000 compared to males, 12.65 per 100,000 in the United States in 2004.

Etiology

Universal features in adolescents who resort to suicidal behaviors are the inability to synthesize viable solutions to ongoing problems and the lack of coping strategies to deal with immediate crises. Therefore, a narrow view of the options available to deal with recurrent family discord, rejection, or failure contributes to a decision to commit suicide.

Genetic Factors. Completed suicide and suicidal behavior is two to four times more likely to occur in individuals with a first-degree family member with similar behavior. Evidence of a genetic contribution to suicidal behavior is based on family suicide risk studies and the higher concordance for suicide among monozygotic twins compared to dizygotic twins. Recent studies have investigated the possible contributions of the short allele of the serotonin transporter promoter polymorphism (5-HTTLPT) to suicidal behaviors, although to date, the evidence has not been consistent. Current studies are seeking to investigate correlations between genetic vulnerability and environment and timing interactions as multiple variables that may interact to increase the risk of suicidal behavior.

Biological Factors. A relationship between altered central serotonin with suicide as well as impulsive aggression has been found in children and adolescents, and has been demonstrated in adults. Studies have documented a reduction in the density of serotonin transporter receptors in the prefrontal cortex, and serotonin receptors among individuals with suicidal behaviors. Postmortem studies in adolescents who have completed suicide show the most significant alterations in the prefrontal cortex and hippocampus, brain regions that are also associated with emotion regulation and problem solving. These studies have found altered serotonin metabolites, alteration in 5-HT2a binding and decreased activity of protein kinase A and C. Decreased levels of serotonin metabolite 5-hydroxyindoleacetic acid (5-HIAA) have also been found in the cerebrospinal fluid (CSF) of depressed adults who attempted suicide by violent methods. Meta-analyses suggest an association between the short S-allele of the serotonin transporter promoter gene and depression as well as suicidal behavior, particularly when combined with adverse life events.

Psychosocial Factors. Although severe major depressive illness is the most significant risk factor for suicide, increasing its risk by 20 percent, many severely depressed individuals are not suicidal. A sense of hopelessness, impulsivity, recurrent substance use, and a history of aggressive behavior, have been associated with an increased risk of suicide. A wide range of psychopathological symptoms are associated with exposure to violent and abusive homes. Aggressive, self-destructive, and suicidal behaviors seem to occur with greatest frequency among youth who have endured chronically stressful family lives. The most significant family risk factor for suicidal behavior is maltreatment, including physical and sexual abuse and neglect. The single largest association is between sexual abuse and suicidal behavior. Large community studies have provided data suggesting that youth at risk for suicidal behavior include those who feel disconnected, isolated, or alienated from peers. Sexual orientation is a risk factor, with increased rates of suicidal behavior of two to six times among youth who identify themselves as gay, lesbian, or bisexual. Protective factors mitigating the risk of suicidal behavior are youth who have a strong connection to school and peers even in the face of other risk factors.

Diagnosis and Clinical Features

The characteristics of adolescents who attempt suicide and those who complete suicide are similar and up to 40 percent of suicidal persons have made a previous attempt. Direct questioning of children and adolescents about suicidal thoughts is necessary, because studies have consistently shown that caregivers are frequently unaware of these ideas in their children. Suicidal thoughts (i.e., children talking about wanting to harm themselves) and suicidal threats (e.g., children stating that they want to jump in front of a car) are more common than suicide completion.

Most older adolescents with suicidal behavior meet criteria for one or more psychiatric disorders, often including major depressive disorder, bipolar disorder, and psychotic disorders. Youth with mood disorders in combination with substance abuse and a history of aggressive behavior are at particularly high risk for suicide. The most common precipitating factors in younger adolescent suicide completers appear to be impending disciplinary actions, impulsive behavioral histories, and access to loaded guns, particularly in the home. Adolescents without mood disorders with histories of disruptive and violent, aggressive, and impulsive behavior may be susceptible to suicide during family or peer conflicts. High levels of hopelessness, poor problem-solving skills, and a history of aggressive behavior are risk factors for suicide. A less common profile of an adolescent who completes suicide is one of high achievement and perfectionistic character traits facing a perceived failure, such an academically proficient adolescent humiliated by a poor grade on an examination.

Findings from a World Health Organization mental health survey reveals that a range of psychiatric disorders increase the risk of suicidal ideation across the lifespan. Youth with psychiatric disorders characterized by severe anxiety and poor impulse control are at higher risk to act on suicidal ideation. In psychiatrically disturbed and vulnerable adolescents, suicide behavior may represent impulsive responses to recent stressors. Typical precipitants of suicidal behavior include conflicts and arguments with family members and boyfriends or girlfriends. Alcohol and other substance use can further predispose an already vulnerable adolescent to suicidal behavior. In other cases, an adolescent attempts suicide in anticipation of punishment after being caught by the police or other authority figures for a forbidden behavior.

About 40 percent of youth who complete suicide had previous psychiatric treatment, and about 40 percent had made a previous suicide attempt. A child who has lost a parent by any means before age 13 is at higher risk for mood disorders and suicide. The precipitating factors include loss of face with peers, a broken romance, school difficulties, unemployment, bereavement, separation, and rejection. Clusters of suicides among adolescents who know one another and go to the same school have been reported. Suicidal behavior can precipitate other such attempts within a peer group through identification—so-called copycat suicides. Some studies have found a transient increase in adolescent suicides after television programs in which the main theme was the suicide of a teenager.

The tendency of disturbed young persons to imitate highly publicized suicides has been referred to as *Werther syndrome,* after the protagonist in Johann Wolfgang von Goethe's novel, *The Sorrows of Young Werther.* The novel, in which the hero kills himself, was banned in some European countries after its publication more than 200 years ago because of a rash of suicides by young men who read it; some dressed like Werther before killing themselves or left the book open at the passage describing his death. In general, although imitation may play a role in the timing of suicide attempts by vulnerable adolescents, the overall suicide rate does not seem to increase when media exposure increases. In contrast, direct exposure to peer suicide is associated with increased risk of depression and PTSD rather than suicide.

Treatment

The prognostic significance of suicidal ideation and behaviors in adolescents ranges from relatively low lethality, to high risk for completion. One of the challenges in addressing suicide is to identify children and adolescents with suicidal ideation, and particularly to treat those who have untreated psychiatric disorders, as the risk of completed suicide increases with age, as does the onset of an untreated psychiatric disorder. Adolescents who come to medical attention because of suicidal attempts must be evaluated before determining whether hospitalization is necessary. Pediatric patients who present to the emergency room with suicidal ideation benefit from an intervention that occurs in the emergency room to ensure that the patient is transitioned to outpatient care when hospitalization is not necessary. Those who fall into high-risk groups should be hospitalized until the acute suicidality is no longer present. Adolescents at higher risk include those who have made previous suicide attempts, especially with a lethal method, males older than 12 years of age with histories of aggressive behavior or substance abuse, use of a lethal method, and severe major depressive disorder with social withdrawal, hopelessness, and persistent suicidal ideation.

Relatively few adolescents evaluated for suicidal behavior in a hospital emergency room subsequently receive ongoing psychiatric treatment. Factors that may increase the probability of psychiatric treatment include psychoeducation for the family in the emergency room, diffusing acute family conflict, and setting up an outpatient follow-up during the emergency room visit. Emergency room discharge plans often include providing an alternative if suicidal ideation reoccurs, and a telephone hotline number provided to the adolescent and the family in case suicidal ideation reappears.

Scant data exist to evaluate the efficacy of various interventions in reducing suicidal behavior among adolescents. CBT alone and in combination with SSRIs have been shown to decrease suicidal ideation in depressed adolescents over time in the TADS, a large multisite study; however, these interventions do not work immediately, so safety precautions must be taken for high-risk situations. Dialectical behavior therapy (DBT), a long-term behavioral intervention that can be applied to individuals or groups of patients, has been shown to reduce suicidal behavior in adults, but has yet to be investigated in adolescents. Components of DBT include mindfulness training to improve self-acceptance, assertiveness training, instruction on avoiding situations that may trigger self-destructive behavior, and increasing the ability to tolerate psychological distress. This approach warrants investigation among adolescents.

Given the reduction in completed suicide among adolescents over the last decade, during the same period in which SSRI treatment in the adolescent population has markedly risen, it is possible that SSRIs have been instrumental in this effect. Given the risk of increased rate of suicidal thoughts and behaviors among depressed children and adolescents (indicated in randomized clinical trials with antidepressant medications and leading to the "black box" warning for all antidepressants for depressed youth), close monitoring for suicidality is mandatory for any child or adolescent being treated with antidepressants.

27.12b Early-Onset Bipolar Disorder

Early-onset bipolar disorder has been recognized in children as a rare disorder with greater continuity with its adult counterpart when it occurs in adolescents than in prepubertal children. Over the last decade there has been a significant increase in the diagnosis of bipolar I disorder made in youth referred to psychiatric outpatient clinics and inpatient units. Questions have arisen regarding the phenotype of bipolar disorder in youth, particularly in view of the continuous irritability and mood dysregulation and lack of discrete mood episodes in most prepubertal children who have received the diagnosis. The "atypical" bipolar symptoms among prepubertal children often include extreme mood dysregulation, severe temper tantrums, intermittent aggressive or explosive behavior, and high levels of distractibility and inattention. This constellation of mood and behavior disturbance in the majority of prepubertal children with a current diagnosis of bipolar disorder is nonepisodic, although some fluctuation in mood may occur. The high frequency of the above symptoms in combination with chronic irritability has led to the inclusion of a new mood disorder in youth in the Fifth Edition of the American Psychiatric Association's *Diagnostic and Statistical Manual of Mental Disorders* (DSM-5) called *Disruptive Mood Dysregulation Disorder,* which is discussed in the next section (27.12c). Many children with nonepisodic mood disorders often have past histories of severe ADHD, making the diagnosis of bipolar disorder even more complicated. Family studies of children with ADHD have not revealed an increased rate of bipolar I disorder. Children with "atypical" bipolar disorders, however, are frequently seriously impaired, are difficult to manage in school and at home, and often require psychiatric hospitalization. Longitudinal follow-up studies are under way with groups of children diagnosed with subthreshold bipolar disorders and nonepisodic mood disorders, to determine how many will develop classic bipolar disorder. In one recent study of 140 children with bipolar disorder not otherwise specified (i.e., the presence of distinct manic symptoms but subthreshold for manic episodes), 45 percent developed bipolar I or bipolar II illness over a follow-up period of 5 years. In another study, 84 children who were labeled with "severe mood dysregulation" (i.e., a persistent nonepisodic negative mood along with severe anger outbursts) who also exhibited at least three manic symptoms (either pressured speech, agitation, insomnia, or flight of ideas) plus distractibility (also common to ADHD), followed for approximately 2 years, found that only one child experienced a hypomanic or mixed episode. Although childhood severe mood dysregulation has been found to be common in community samples—one study reported a lifetime prevalence of 3.3 percent in youth 9 to 19 years of age—its relationship to future bipolar disorder remains questionable. A longitudinal community-based study that followed children and adolescents with nonepisodic irritability over a 20-year period, found that these children were at higher risk to develop depressive disorders and generalized anxiety disorder, rather than bipolar disorders over time.

Among adults and older adolescents with bipolar disorder who present with classic manic episodes, a major depressive episode typically precedes a manic episode. A classic manic episode in an adolescent, similar to in a young adult, may emerge as a distinct departure from a preexisting state often characterized by grandiose and paranoid delusions and hallucinatory phenomena. According to DSM-5, the diagnostic criteria for a manic episode are the same for children and adolescents as for adults. The diagnostic criteria for a manic episode include a distinct period of an abnormally elevated, expansive, or irritable mood that lasts at least 1 week or for any duration if hospitalization is necessary. In addition, during periods of mood disturbance, at least three of the following significant and persistent symptoms must be present: inflated self-esteem or grandiosity, decreased need for sleep, pressure to talk, flight of ideas or racing thoughts, distractibility, an increase in goal-directed activity, and excessive involvement in pleasurable activities that may result in painful consequences.

According to the DSM-5, in contrast to DSM-IV-TR, diagnostic criteria for bipolar disorder now include changes in both mood and activity or energy level. Furthermore, whereas previously, full criteria for both mania or hypomania and major depressive disorder were required to make a diagnosis of a *mixed episode,* in DSM-5, this requirement no longer applies; instead a specifier, "with mixed features," has been added. This specifier can be applied to a current manic episode, hypomanic episode, or depressive episode. Thus, for example, to add the "mixed features" specifier to a manic or hypomanic episode, three of the following symptoms must be present during the majority of days of the current or most recent episode of mania or hypomania: prominent depressed mood, diminished interest in most activities, psychomotor retardation nearly every day, fatigue or loss of energy, feelings of excessive guilt or worthlessness, or recurrent thoughts of death. To apply the "with mixed features" specifier to a full major depressive episode, three of the following hypomanic/manic symptoms must be present: elevated or expansive mood, grandiosity, pressured speech or increased speech, flight of ideas, increased energy, or decreased need for sleep.

When mania appears in an adolescent, there is a high incidence of psychotic features including both delusions and hallucinations, which most typically involve grandiose notions about their power, worth, and relationships. Persecutory delusions and flight of ideas are also common. Overall, gross impairment of reality testing is common in adolescent manic episodes. In adolescents with major depressive disorder destined for bipolar I disorder, those at highest risk have family histories of bipolar I disorder and exhibit acute, severe depressive episodes with psychosis, hypersomnia, and psychomotor retardation.

EPIDEMIOLOGY

The prevalence rates of bipolar disorder among youth vary depending on the age group studied, and on whether the diagnostic criteria are applied narrowly, restricting it to discrete mood episodes or more broadly, to include nonepisodic mood and behavioral states. In younger children, bipolar disorder is extremely rare, with no cases of bipolar I disorder identified in children between the ages of 9 and 13 years by the Great Smokey Mountain Study. However, severe mood dysregulation, often a prominent feature in prepubertal children receiving a diagnosis of bipolar disorder, was found in 3.3 percent of an epidemiological sample. In adolescents, bipolar disorder is more frequent, found to range from 0.06 to 0.1 percent of the general population of 16-year-olds in studies using a narrow definition of bipolar I disorder. Prevalence of subthreshold symptoms of bipolar illness was found to be 5.7 percent in one study to at least 10 percent in another. Follow-up studies into adulthood revealed that the subthreshold manic symptoms predicted high levels of impairment with progression to depression and anxiety disorders, not bipolar I or II disorders.

Community use of the diagnosis of bipolar disorder in youth has increased markedly over the last 15 years in both outpatient and inpatient psychiatric settings. A recent survey indicated a 40-fold increase in the diagnosis of bipolar disorder in youth being treated at outpatient clinics from the mid-1990s to the mid-2000s. Furthermore, from 2000 through 2006, the rate of youth hospitalized with a primary diagnosis of bipolar disorder increased from 3.3 per 10,000 to 5.7 per 10,000.

ETIOLOGY

Genetic Factors

Estimates of the heritability of bipolar disorder based on adult twin studies range from approximately 60 to 90 percent, with shared environmental variables accounting for 30 to 40 percent and the nonshared environmental factors accounting for approximately 10 to 20 percent. High rates of bipolar disorder have been reported in the relatives of the narrow phenotype of early-onset bipolar disorder compared to young adult-onset of bipolar disorder. The high rates of comorbid ADHD among children with early-onset bipolar disorder has led to questions regarding the cotransmission of these disorders in family members. However, children with the broader phenotype of bipolar disorder, that is, severe mood dysregulation without episodes of mania, have not been found to have higher rates of bipolar disorder in family members, which suggests that the narrow and broad phenotypes of bipolar disorder may be distinct and separate entities. Nearly 25 percent of adolescent offspring of families with probands with bipolar disorder experienced a mood disorder by the age of 17 years old, compared to 4 percent of controls, with approximately 8 percent representing bipolar I, bipolar II, or bipolar disorder not otherwise specified. Most of the risk in the offspring, therefore, is for unipolar major depressive disorder. Disruptive behavior disorders were not found to be increased, in a longitudinal study, in the offspring of families with a bipolar proband, compared to controls. The combination of ADHD and bipolar disorder is not found as frequently in relatives of children with only ADHD compared with first-degree relatives of children with the combination.

Although bipolar disorder appears to have a significant heritable component, its mode of inheritance remains unknown. A number of research groups have concluded that early-onset bipolar disorder is a more severe form of the illness, characterized by more mixed episodes, greater psychiatric comorbidity, more lifetime psychotic symptoms, poorer response to prophylactic lithium treatment, and a greater heritability. The European collaborative study of early-onset bipolar disorder (France, Germany, Ireland, Scotland, Switzerland, England, and Slovenia) carried out a genome-wide linkage analysis of both the narrow and the broad early-onset bipolar disorder. This group concluded that a genetic factor located in the 2q14 region is either specifically involved in the etiology of early-onset bipolar disorder, or that a gene in this region exerts influence as a modifier of other genes in the development of bipolar disorder in this age group. Other linkage regions that were found by this collaborative did not find specific genome regions that pertained only to the early-onset group of bipolar disorder, suggesting that there may be some genetic factors common to early-onset and adult-onset bipolar disorder. This is consistent with the increased incidence of adult-onset bipolar disorder among siblings of early-onset disease. Further genome-wide studies are needed to elucidate the genetic etiology of early-onset bipolar disorder.

Neurobiological Factors

Converging data suggest that early-onset bipolar disorder is associated with both structural and functional brain alterations in prefrontal cortical and subcortical regions associated with the processing and regulation of emotional stimuli. Structural MRI studies suggest that altered development of white matter and a decreased amygdalar volume are found more frequently in this population than in the general population. fMRI studies are important in that they can identify altered brain function in vulnerable populations such as youth with early-onset bipolar disorder at baseline, and can also be utilized to elucidate functional changes toward normalization in brain functioning after various treatments, and potentially identify pretreatment neural predictors of good response to various treatments.

A recent fMRI study of pediatric bipolar patients documented pretreatment brain activity and posttreatment effects of a trial of risperidone versus divalproex. This double-blind study included 24 unmedicated manic patients with a mean age of 13 years, randomized to either risperidone or divalproex treatment, and 14 healthy controls examined over a 6-week period. Prior to treatment, the patient group showed increased amygdala activity compared to healthy controls, which was poorly controlled by the higher ventrolateral prefrontal cortex (VLPFC) and the dorsolateral prefrontal cortex (DLPFC), which are believed to exert influence on the amygdala to control emotional regulation and processing. Increased amygdala activity at baseline predicted a poorer treatment response to both the risperidone and the divalproex in the patient group. Patients were given an affective color-matching word task involving matching positive words (i.e., happiness, achievement, or success), negative words (i.e., disappointment, depression, or rejection), or neutral words, with one of two colored circles displayed on a screen while fMRI was administered. Greater pretreatment right amygdala activity during a word task with positive and negative words in the risperidone group, and greater pretreatment left amygdala activity with a positive word task in the divalproex group, predicted poor response on the Young Mania Rating Scale. Increased amygdala activity in early-onset bipolar patients is hypothesized to be a potential biomarker predicting resistance and poor treatment response to both risperidone and divalproex.

Neuropsychological Studies

Impairments in verbal memory, processing speed, executive function, working memory, and attention are commonly found in early-onset bipolar disorder. Data suggest that on tasks of working memory, processing speed, and attention, children and adolescents with comorbid bipolar disorder and ADHD demonstrate more pronounced impairments compared with those without ADHD. Other studies found that children with bipolar disorder make a greater number of emotion recognition errors compared with controls. They more frequently identified faces as "angry" when presented with adult faces; however, these errors did not occur when children's faces were shown. Impaired perception of facial expression has also been reported in studies of adults with bipolar disorder.

DIAGNOSIS AND CLINICAL FEATURES

Early-onset bipolar disorder is often characterized by extreme irritability that is severe and persistent, and may include aggressive outbursts and violent behavior. In between outbursts, children with the broad diagnosis may continue to be angry or dysphoric. It is rare for a prepubertal child to exhibit grandiose thoughts or euphoric mood; for the most part, children diagnosed with early-onset bipolar disorder are intensely emotional with a fluctuating but overriding negative mood. Current diagnostic criteria for bipolar disorders in children and adolescents in DSM-5 are the same as those used in adults. The clinical picture of early-onset bipolar disorder, however, is complicated by the prevalence of comorbid psychiatric disorders.

Comorbidity with ADHD

ADHD is the most common comorbid condition among youth with early-onset bipolar disorder and has been reported in up to 90 percent of prepubertal children and up to 50 percent of adolescents diagnosed with bipolar disorder. One of the main sources of diagnostic confusion regarding children with early-onset bipolar disorder is the comorbid ADHD, since the two disorders share many diagnostic criteria, including distractibility, hyperactivity, and talkativeness. Even when the overlapping symptoms are removed from the diagnostic count, a significant percentage of children with bipolar disorder continued to meet the full criteria for ADHD. This implies that both disorders with their own distinct features are present in many cases.

Comorbidity with Anxiety Disorders

Children and adolescents with bipolar disorder have been reported to have higher than expected rates of panic and other anxiety disorders. In youth with the narrow phenotype of bipolar disorders, up to 77 percent have been reported to exhibit an anxiety disorder. Lifetime prevalence of panic disorder was found to be 21 percent among subjects with the broader phenotype of bipolar disorder compared with 0.8 percent in those without mood disorders. Patients diagnosed with bipolar disorder who have comorbid high levels of anxiety symptoms are reported as adults to have higher risks of alcohol abuse and suicidal behavior. On the other hand, children who exhibit the broader phenotype of bipolar disorder are at higher risk to go on to have anxiety disorders as well as depressive disorders.

Jeanie is a 13-year-old adopted teen who was admitted to the hospital after assaulting her adoptive mother, causing bruises on her arms and legs from Jeanie's kicks and punches. Jeanie has had a long history of excessively severe tantrums, which include assaultive and self-injurious behavior since before she was adopted at the age of 3 years. Jeanie had always been a child who was irritable and explosive, with a short fuse, who could blow up with very little provocation, even when things were going her way. Jeanie had become increasingly hard to manage at home, refused to go to school, yelled and screamed for hours on a daily basis, and often hit and kicked her adoptive parents by the time she was 10 years old. Jeannie had been placed in residential treatment for about a year and a half from age 11 and a half to almost 13, where she had been given a diagnosis of bipolar disorder and placed on lithium and citalopram. She was doing so well there after a year that Jeanie's adoptive mother decided to take her home. After a few weeks at home, however, Jeanie began to decompensate, having daily explosive tantrums during which she became aggressive and out of control. On multiple occasions she had hurt herself and her adoptive mother and father. Upon arriving at the hospital, Jeanie was calm by the time she was brought to her hospital room; however, her adoptive mother refused to consider taking her home until she had received a full psychiatric evaluation and something new was done to control Jeanie's unsafe behaviors. Jeanie was initially evaluated by the child and adolescent psychiatrist on-call, after which she was admitted to a pediatric inpatient unit, where she awaited a bed on a psychiatric adolescent inpatient unit. The psychiatrist learned that Jeanie had been born prematurely to a teenage mother and placed in multiple foster homes until she was adopted. Jeanie was a small girl who appeared younger than her stated age, although her demeanor was bossy and pedantic. Jeanie's biological family history was unknown, and although she had at least one stigmata of fetal alcohol syndrome, her IQ was in the average range and there was no other evidence to corroborate this possibility. On mental status examination in the hospital, Jeanie reported that things were fine, that she was not depressed, and that she did not get along with kids her own age but that she had a few friends. Jeanie admitted that she had a bad temper and that she did not remember what she did after she was in a rage. Jeanie's affect was odd, and she seemed to like having the psychiatrist as her audience. Jeanie denied suicidal ideation or past attempts, and she denied having been a danger to herself or her adoptive parents. Jeanie seemed annoyed when she was asked about the reasons for her placement in a residential facility, and she became irritable when questioned about the reasons for her current admission. Jeanie was referred for admission to an adolescent psychiatric inpatient unit with the following recommendations: Jeanie was referred for a trial of an atypical antipsychotic, such as risperidone or olanzapine, and a reconsideration of a return to a more structured school program, either a day program or residential facility. The diagnosis of bipolar disorder remained in question, as she did not meet the narrow phenotype for this disorder.

PATHOLOGY AND LABORATORY EXAMINATION

No specific laboratory indices are currently helpful in making the diagnosis of bipolar disorders among children and adolescents.

DIFFERENTIAL DIAGNOSIS

The most important clinical entities to distinguish from early-onset bipolar disorder are also the disorders with which it is most frequently comorbid. Included are ADHD, oppositional defiant disorder, conduct disorder, anxiety disorders, and depressive disorders.

Although childhood ADHD tends to have its onset earlier than pediatric mania, current evidence from family studies supports the presence of ADHD and bipolar disorders as highly comorbid in children, and the concurrence is not because of the overlapping symptoms that the two disorders share. In a recent study of more than 300 children and adolescents who attended a psychopharmacology clinic and received a diagnosis of ADHD, bipolar disorder was also evident in almost one-third of those children with ADHD who had combined-type and hyperactive-types, and occurred with much less frequency (i.e., in less than 10 percent) in children with ADHD, inattentive-type.

COURSE AND PROGNOSIS

There are several pathways regarding the course and prognosis of children diagnosed with early-onset bipolar disorder. Those who present with severe mood dysregulation at an early age, without discrete mood cycles, are most likely to develop anxiety and depressive disorders as they mature. Youth who present in adolescence with a recognizable manic episode are most likely to continue to meet criteria for bipolar I disorder in adulthood. In both cases, the long-term impairment is considerable.

A longitudinal study of 263 child and adolescent inpatients and outpatients with bipolar disorder followed for an average of 2 years found that approximately 70 percent recovered from their index episode within that period. Half of these patients had at least one recurrence of a mood disorder during this time, more frequently a depressive episode than a mania. No differences were found in the rates of recovery for children and adolescents whose diagnosis was bipolar I disorder, bipolar II disorder, or bipolar disorder not otherwise specified; however, those youth whose diagnosis was bipolar disorder not otherwise specified had a significant longer duration of illness before recovery, with less frequent recurrences once they recovered. About 19 percent of patients changed polarity once per year or less, 61 percent shifted five or more times per year, about half cycled more than ten times per year, and about one-third cycled more than 20 times per year. Predictors of more rapid cycling included lower socioeconomic status (SES), presence of lifetime psychosis, and bipolar disorder not otherwise specified diagnosis. Over the follow-up period, about 20 percent of subjects who were diagnosed with bipolar II disorder converted to bipolar I disorder, and 25 percent of the bipolar disorder not otherwise specified subjects developed bipolar I disorder or bipolar II disorder during the follow-up period.

Similar to the natural history of bipolar disorders in adults, children have a wide range of symptom severity in manic and depressed episodes. The more frequent diagnostic conversions from bipolar II disorder to bipolar I disorder among children and adolescents, compared with adults, highlight the lack of stability of the bipolar II disorder diagnosis in youth. This is also the case with respect to conversion from bipolar disorder not otherwise specified to other bipolar disorders. When bipolar disorder occurs in young children, recovery rates are lower. In addition, a greater likelihood is seen of mixed states and rapid cycling, and higher rates of polarity changes compared with those who develop bipolar disorders in late adolescence or early adulthood.

TREATMENT

Treatment of early-onset bipolar disorder incorporates multimodal interventions including pharmacotherapy, psychoeducation, psychosocial intervention with the family and the child, and school interventions to optimize a child's school adjustment and achievement.

Pharmacotherapy

Two classes of medications—atypical antipsychotics and mood stabilizing agents—are the most well-studied agents that provide efficacy in the treatment of early-onset bipolar disorders. Eight randomized controlled trials have shown efficacy of atypical antipsychotic agents in the treatment of bipolar disorder in youth between the ages of 10 and 17 years. These studies compared an atypical antipsychotic to placebo, or compared an atypical antipsychotic to a mood stabilizer, or added an antipsychotic to a mood-stabilizing agent. The atypical antipsychotics included olanzapine, quetiapine, risperidone, aripiprazole, and ziprasidone. All five of the atypical antipsychotic studies demonstrated significant efficacy in the treatment of early-onset bipolar manic or mixed states. A recent trial comparing quetiapine and valproate found that both were efficacious, but the quetiapine was superior in the speed of its effect. In another trial comparing risperidone and divalproex treatment for bipolar disorder in youth, risperidone was found to have a more rapid improvement and a greater final reduction in manic symptoms compared to divalproex.

Mood-stabilizing agents have been used in open trials and anecdotally with early-onset bipolar illness with little evidence of efficacy at this time. In trials using lithium or divalproex for treatment of early-onset bipolar disorder, responses were less robust compared to results with atypical antipsychotics. Controlled trials have provided some evidence suggesting that lithium is efficacious in the management of aggression behavior disorders. Although lithium has been approved for use in adolescent mania, more research is needed to know if lithium is effective for more classic forms of mania in adolescents. The Collaborative Lithium Trials (CoLT) established a set of protocols to establish the safety and potential efficacy of lithium in youth, and to develop studies to provide evidence-based dosing of lithium for youth. A group of researchers recently studied the first-dose pharmacokinetics of lithium carbonate in youth and found that clearance and volume are correlated with total body weight in youth, and particularly with fat-free mass. Difference in body size was consistent with the pharmacokinetics of lithium metabolism in children and adults. An open-label trial of lamotrigine (Lamictal) in the treatment of bipolar depression among youth provides possible support for its use in children and adolescents.

Current evidence suggests a faster response and more robust effect with atypical antipsychotics compared to mood-stabilizing agents in the treatment of early-onset bipolar disorder. However, given the severity and impairment of bipolar disorder in youth, when only partial recovery is achieved, consideration of adding an additional agent may be necessary.

Psychosocial Treatment

Psychosocial treatment interventions for early-onset bipolar illness have included a family-focused treatment. This treatment consists of several sessions of psychoeducation, then sessions focusing on current stressors and mood management plan, and then several sessions of communication enhancement training and problem-solving skills training. The use of this type of intervention for youth diagnosed with bipolar disorder as well as youth at risk for the disorder by virtue of their family history or subthreshold conditions has been of value. Adjunctive family-focused psychoeducational treatment modified for children and adolescents has been shown to reduce relapse rate. Children and adolescents treated with mood-stabilizing agents in addition to a psychosocial intervention showed improvement in depressive symptoms, manic symptoms, and behavioral disturbance over 1 year.

A year-long trial of a modified Family Focused Treatment-High Risk in youth with bipolar disorder showed significant improvement in mood disturbance, especially depressive mood and hypomania, and improved psychosocial functioning. Family-focused treatment for high-risk youth is a promising intervention that deserves further investigation as a longitudinal follow-up to determine the course of youth at risk to develop bipolar disorder.

27.12c Disruptive Mood Dysregulation Disorder

Disruptive mood dysregulation disorder, a new inclusion in the American Psychiatric Association's *Diagnostic and Statistical Manual of Mental Disorders, Fifth Edition* (DSM-5), is characterized by severe, developmentally inappropriate, and recurrent temper outbursts at least three times per week, along with a persistently irritable or angry mood between temper outbursts. In order to meet diagnostic criteria, the symptoms must be present for at least a year, and the onset of symptoms must be present by the age of 10 years. Children with these symptoms have typically been diagnosed with bipolar disorder, or a combination of oppositional defiant disorder, ADHD and intermittent explosive disorder. Recent longitudinal data suggest, however, that these children do not typically develop classic bipolar disorder in late adolescence or early adulthood. Instead, studies suggest that youth with chronic irritability and severe mood dysregulation are at higher risk for future unipolar depressive disorders and anxiety disorders. Although the initial studies of children and adolescents with severe mood dysregulation included several symptoms of hyperarousal (such as distractibility, physical restlessness, insomnia, racing thoughts, flight of ideas, pressured speech, or intrusiveness), the current DSM-5 diagnostic criteria for disruptive mood dysregulation do not include any hyperarousal criteria. Youths diagnosed with mood dysregulation disorder who also exhibit multiple symptoms of hyperarousal may be comorbid for ADHD.

EPIDEMIOLOGY

Most of the epidemiological data applied to disruptive mood dysregulation disorder was gathered from children and adolescents with severe mood dysregulation, which includes hyperarousal symptoms. Because disruptive mood dysregulation disorder differs from severe mood dysregulation disorder only in the absence of hyperarousal symptoms, the epidemiological data from the severe mood dysregulation disorder studies can be viewed as a useful proxy for disruptive mood dysregulation disorder. Severe mood dysregulation has a lifetime prevalence of 3 percent in children age 9 to 19 years. Within that percentage, males (78 percent) are more prevalent than females (22 percent). The mean age of onset is 5 to 11 years of age.

COMORBIDITY

Disruptive mood dysregulation disorder often co-occurs with other psychiatric disorders. The most common comorbidities are ADHD (94 percent), oppositional defiant disorder (84 percent), anxiety disorders (47 percent), and major depressive disorder (20 percent). The relationship of severe mood dysregulation and disruptive mood dysregulation disorder to bipolar disorder has been a topic of clinical investigation. Youth with severe mood dysregulation and hyperarousal symptoms have been conceptualized as a "broad phenotype" of pediatric bipolar disorder; however, the term "severe mood dysregulation" was utilized by researchers for these youth because it remains unclear whether these youth go on to meet the criteria for a bipolar disorder. Disruptive mood dysregulation disorder is conceptualized as a disorder that is not episodic, and may coexist with ADHD. However, current evidence does not support its continuity with an emerging bipolar disorder.

DIAGNOSIS AND CLINICAL FEATURES

The DSM-5 diagnostic criteria for disruptive mood dysregulation disorder require outbursts that are grossly out of proportion to the situation. These temper outbursts present with verbal rages and/or physical aggression toward people or property, and are inappropriate for the child's developmental level. Temper outbursts occur, on average, three or more times per week, with variations in mood between outbursts. Symptoms must exhibit before the age of 10 years, be present for at least 12 months, and be present within at least two settings (i.e., home and school). The diagnosis is not made for the first time in youth younger than 6 years or older than 18 years. In between temper outbursts, the child's mood is persistently irritable and angry, and this mood is observable by others such as parents, teachers, or peers. There has never been period lasting more than 1 day in which full criteria for a manic or hypomanic episode (except for duration) are fulfilled. The above behaviors do not occur exclusively in the context of an episode of major depression and are not better accounted for by another psychiatric disorder.

Daniel, a 12-year-old 7th grade boy was brought to his pediatrician by his mother, who was exasperated with Daniel's rages and inappropriate tantrums. Daniel was on the floor in the waiting room, pounding his hands on the floor, yelling at his mother "get me out of here!" and crying. His mother had bruises on both legs from Dylan's kicks, and she appeared distressed. Daniel's mother walked into the office, leaving Daniel on the floor in the waiting room and burst into tears. "I can't deal with him anymore." She recounted the problems that Daniel had been having for the last 2 years—Severe recurrent tantrums four to five times/week. "He tantrums like a 6-year-old, and even when he is not having a tantrum, he is perpetually angry and irritable." She reported that Daniel had lost all of his friends due to his short fuse and frequent verbal and physical outbursts. He was almost always irritable, even on his birthday. Daniel's mother wonders whether there is anything physical wrong with him, but physical examination and routine blood tests reveal no abnormalities. Daniel's tantrums had lessened somewhat last summer during the 2-month summer vacation; however, as soon as school resumed, he was back to consistent irritability. After an interview with Daniel, his pediatrician determined that he was not acutely suicidal; however, he required urgent psychotherapeutic intervention. Daniel was referred to a clinical psychologist for cognitive-behavioral treatment, and a child and adolescent psychiatrist for a medication evaluation. Daniel resisted psychotherapy; however, after several sessions, Daniel's parents felt more hopeful than they had in a long time, and learned that Daniel's problems were not "all their fault." Daniel agreed to begin a trial of fluoxetine, which was titrated up to 30 mg over several weeks; and after about a month, it became clear that his irritability had diminished noticeably. Daniel still had many problems with peers, and he still had one or two tantrums per week; however, the tantrums were becoming less prolonged and less intense. Daniel seemed genuinely happy when he was invited to a classmate's birthday party, and he was able to interact successfully with his peers during the party without any conflicts. Daniel continues to benefit from CBT, and he remains on fluoxetine 40 mg a day. Daniel is still described as a "temperamental" boy, but he is doing well in school, has rekindled several friendships, and is able to participate in family gatherings without a major tantrum.

DIFFERENTIAL DIAGNOSIS

Bipolar Disorder

Disruptive mood dysregulation disorder closely resembles the "broad phenotype" of bipolar disorder. Although not episodic, it has been theorized by some clinicians and researchers that the chronic and persistent symptoms of mood disturbance and irritability may be an early developmental presentation of bipolar disorder. Disruptive mood dysregulation; however, does not meet formal diagnostic criteria for mania in bipolar disorder, because irritability in disruptive mood dysregulation disorder is chronic and nonepisodic.

Oppositional Defiant Disorder

Disruptive mood dysregulation disorder is similar to oppositional defiant disorder in that they both include irritability, temper outbursts, and anger. Many patients with disruptive mood dysregulation disorder meet the criteria for oppositional defiant disorder; however, most patients with oppositional defiant disorder do not meet the criteria for disruptive mood dysregulation disorder. Oppositional defiant disorder includes symptoms of annoyance and defiance that are not found in disruptive mood dysregulation disorder. Disruptive mood dysregulation disorder requires that irritable outbursts be present in at least two settings, whereas oppositional defiant disorder requires that they be present in only one setting.

COURSE AND PROGNOSIS

Disruptive mood dysregulation disorder is a chronic disorder. Longitudinal studies thus far have shown that patients with disruptive mood dysregulation disorder in childhood have a high risk of progressing to major depressive disorder, dysthymic disorder, and anxiety disorders over time.

TREATMENT

The current treatment of disruptive mood dysregulation is based on symptomatic interventions, in view of the fact that its etiology is not well understood at this time. If disruptive mood dysregulation disorder is confirmed to resemble unipolar depression and anxiety disorders in its pathophysiology, and it is often comorbid with ADHD, then SSRIs and stimulants would likely be the pharmacological agents of first choice. However, if the pathophysiology of disruptive mood dysregulation disorder is similar to that of bipolar disorder, then first-line treatments for youth would include atypical antipsychotic agents and mood stabilizers. There are scant treatment studies of disruptive mood dysregulation disorder in the current literature. One controlled trial of youths with symptoms of severe mood dysregulation and ADHD symptoms who did not respond to stimulants, responded to divalproex (Depakote) combined with behavioral psychotherapy compared to placebo and behavioral psychotherapy. There are treatment studies underway of youth who exhibit symptoms of severe mood dysregulation utilizing an SSRI plus a stimulant compared to a stimulant and placebo.

Psychosocial interventions such as cognitive-behavioral psychotherapy are likely to be an essential component of treatment for youth with disruptive dysregulation disorder, and psychosocial interventions targeting children diagnosed with bipolar disorder may be beneficial.

27.12d Oppositional Defiant Disorder

Disruptive behaviors, especially oppositional patterns and aggressive behaviors, are among the most frequent reasons for children and adolescents to be referred for psychiatric evaluation. Demonstration of impulsive and oppositional behaviors are developmentally normative in young children; many youth who continue to display excessive patterns in middle childhood will find other forms of expression as they mature and will no longer demonstrate these behaviors in adolescence or adulthood. The origin of stable patterns of oppositional defiant behavior is widely accepted as a convergence of multiple contributing factors, including biological, temperamental, learned, and psychological conditions. Risk factors for the development of aggressive behavior in youth include childhood maltreatments such as physical or sexual abuse, neglect, emotional abuse, and overly harsh and punitive parenting. The American Psychiatric Association's *Diagnostic and Statistical Manual of Mental Disorders, Fifth Edition* (DSM-5) has divided oppositional defiant disorder into three types: Angry/Irritable Mood, Argumentative/Defiant Behavior, and Vindictiveness. A child may meet diagnostic criteria for oppositional defiant disorder with a 6-month pattern of at least four symptoms from the three types above. Angry/Irritable children with oppositional defiant disorder often lose their tempers, are easily annoyed, and feel irritable much of the time. Argumentative/Defiant children display a pattern of arguing with authority figures, and adults such as parents, teachers, and relatives. Children with this type of oppositional defiant disorder actively refuse to comply with requests, deliberately break rules, and purposely annoy others. These children often do not take responsibility for their actions, and often blame others for their misbehavior. Children with the Vindictive type of oppositional defiant disorder are spiteful, and have shown vindictive or spiteful actions at least twice in 6 months to meet diagnostic criteria.

Oppositional defiant disorder is characterized by enduring patterns of negativistic, disobedient, and hostile behavior toward authority figures, as well as an inability to take responsibility for mistakes, leading to placing blame on others. Children with oppositional defiant disorder frequently argue with adults and become easily annoyed by others, leading to a state of anger and resentment. Children with oppositional defiant disorder may have difficulty in the classroom and with peer relationships, but generally do not resort to physical aggression or significantly destructive behavior.

In contrast, children with conduct disorder engage in severe repeated acts of aggression that can cause physical harm to themselves and others and frequently violate the rights of others.

In oppositional defiant disorder, a child's temper outbursts, active refusal to comply with rules, and annoying behaviors exceed expectations for these behaviors for children of the same age. The disorder is an enduring pattern of negativistic, hostile, and defiant behaviors in the absence of serious violations of the rights of others.

EPIDEMIOLOGY

Oppositional and negativistic behavior, in moderation, is developmentally normal in early childhood and adolescence. Epidemiological studies of negativistic traits in nonclinical populations found such behavior in 16 to 22 percent of school-age children. Although oppositional defiant disorder can begin as early as 3 years of age, it typically is noted by 8 years of age and usually not later than early adolescence. Oppositional defiant disorder has been reported to occur at rates ranging from 2 to 16 percent with increased rates reported in boys before puberty, and an equal sex ratio reported after puberty. The prevalence of oppositional defiant behavior in males and females diminishes in youth older than 12 years of age.

ETIOLOGY

The most dramatic example of normal oppositional behavior peaks between 18 and 24 months, the "terrible twos," when toddlers behave negativistically as an expression of growing autonomy. Pathology begins when this developmental phase persists abnormally, authority figures overreact, or oppositional behavior recurs considerably more frequently than in most children of the same mental age. Among the criteria included in oppositional defiant disorder, irritability appears to be the one most predictive of later psychiatric disorders, whereas the other elements may be considered components of temperament.

Children exhibit a range of temperamental predispositions to strong will, strong preferences, or great assertiveness. Parents who model more extreme ways of expressing and enforcing their own will may contribute to the development of chronic struggles with their children that are then reenacted with other authority figures. What begins for an infant as an effort to establish self-determination may become transformed into an exaggerated behavioral pattern. In late childhood, environmental trauma, illness, or chronic incapacity, such as mental retardation, can trigger oppositionality as a defense against helplessness, anxiety, and loss of self-esteem. Another normative oppositional stage occurs in adolescence as an expression of the need to separate from the parents and to establish an autonomous identity.

Classic psychoanalytic theory implicates unresolved conflicts as fueling defiant behaviors targeting authority figures. Behaviorists have observed that in children, oppositionality may be a reinforced, learned behavior through which a child exerts control over authority figures; for example, if having a temper tantrum when a request or demand is made of the child coerces the parents to withdraw their request, then tantrum behavior becomes strongly reinforced. In addition, increased parental attention during a tantrum can reinforce the behavior.

DIAGNOSIS AND CLINICAL FEATURES

Children with oppositional defiant disorder often argue with adults, lose their temper, and are angry, resentful, and easily annoyed by others at a level and frequency that is outside of the expected range for their age and developmental level. Frequently, youth with oppositional defiant disorder actively defy adults' requests or rules and deliberately annoy other persons. They tend to blame others for their own mistakes and misbehavior, more often than is appropriate for their developmental age. Manifestations of the disorder are almost invariably present in the home, but they may not be present at school or with other adults or peers. In some cases, features of the disorder from the beginning of the disturbance are displayed outside the home; in other cases, the behavior starts in the home, but is later displayed outside. Typically, symptoms of the disorder are most evident in interactions with adults or peers whom the child knows well. Thus, a child with oppositional defiant disorder may not show signs of the disorder when examined clinically. Although children with oppositional defiant disorder may be aware that others disapprove of their behavior, they may still justify it as a response to unfair or unreasonable circumstances. The disorder appears to cause more distress to those around the child than to the child.

Chronic oppositional defiant disorder or irritability almost always interferes with interpersonal relationships and school performance. These children are often rejected by peers, and may become isolated and lonely. Despite adequate intelligence, they may do poorly or fail in school, due to their lack of cooperation, poor participation, and inability to accept help. Secondary to these difficulties are low self-esteem, poor frustration tolerance, depressed mood, and temper outbursts. Adolescents who are ostracized may turn to alcohol and illegal substances as a modality to fit in with peers. Children who are chronically irritable often develop mood disorders in adolescence or adulthood.

PATHOLOGY AND LABORATORY EXAMINATION

No specific laboratory tests or pathological findings help diagnose oppositional defiant disorder. Because some children with oppositional defiant disorder become physically aggressive and violate the rights of others as they get older, they may share some characteristics with people with high levels of aggression, such as low CNS serotonin.

DIFFERENTIAL DIAGNOSIS

Oppositional behaviors are both normal and adaptive within an expected range at specific developmental stages. Periods of normative negativism must be distinguished from oppositional defiant disorder. Developmentally appropriate oppositional behavior is neither considerably more frequent nor more intense than that seen in other children of the same mental age. Oppositional defiant disorder must be distinguished from disruptive mood dysregulation disorder in so far as they are both characterized by chronic irritability and inappropriate temper outbursts. According to the DSM-5, oppositional defiant disorder cannot be diagnosed in the presence of disruptive mood dysregulation disorder. (See Section 27.12c for a further discussion of disruptive mood dysregulation disorder.)

Oppositional defiant behavior occurring temporarily in reaction to a stressor should be diagnosed as an adjustment disorder. When features of oppositional defiant disorder appear during the course of conduct disorder, schizophrenia, or a mood disorder, the diagnosis of oppositional defiant disorder should not be made. Oppositional and negativistic behaviors can also be present in ADHD, cognitive disorders, and mental retardation. Whether a concomitant diagnosis of oppositional defiant disorder should be made depends on the severity, pervasiveness, and duration of such behavior. Some young children who receive a diagnosis of oppositional defiant disorder go on in several years to meet the criteria for conduct disorder. Some investigators believe that the two disorders may be developmental variants of each other, with conduct disorder being the natural progression of oppositional defiant behavior when a child matures. Most children with oppositional defiant disorder, however, do not later meet the criteria for conduct disorder, and up to one-fourth of children with oppositional defiant disorder may not meet the diagnosis several years later.

The subtype of oppositional defiant disorder that tends to progress to conduct disorder is one in which aggression is prominent, for example, the Angry/Irritable type and the Vindictive type. Many children who have ADHD and oppositional defiant disorder develop conduct disorder before the age of 12 years. Many children who develop conduct disorder have a history of oppositional defiant disorder. Overall, the current consensus is that two subtypes of oppositional defiant disorder may exist. One type, which is likely to progress to conduct disorder, includes certain symptoms of conduct disorder (e.g., fighting, bullying). The other type, which is characterized by less aggression and fewer antisocial traits, does not progress to conduct disorder. However, in either case, when both oppositional defiant disorder and conduct disorder are present, according to DSM-5, they may be diagnosed concurrently.

Jackson, age 8 years, was brought to the clinic for evaluation of irritability, negativity, and defiant behavior by his mother. She complained that he had frequent prolonged tantrums, triggered by not "getting his way." Jackson's mother described the tantrums as consisting of shouting, cursing, crying, slamming doors, and sometimes throwing books or objects on the floor. Jackson had been having troubles in school as well and his teacher had reported to the family that he seemed to have a habit of provoking other students as well as the teacher by making noises, rocking in his seat, and whistling in class. Recently, at home, Jackson was kicking his foot against his mother's chair and she asked him to stop. He looked at her and continued to kick her chair until she became angry and sent him to his room. He then started yelling and stated that he wasn't doing anything and that his mother was just picking on him. Jackson's mother reports that she has given up on asking him to help with chores, because it inevitably results in an argument. Jackson appears sullen and irritable on interview. He insists that his problems are all his mother's fault and she is always nagging him unfairly. During the interview with his mother, he interrupted her several times, to say that she was lying and to contradict her story. Despite Jackson's behavioral problem he has been able to succeed academically and scores highly on standardized tests. His mother reports that Jackson used to have some friends in kindergarten, but as he has gotten older, he has lost almost all of his friends because he has difficulty sharing his things and tends to be bossy. Jackson's mother reports that ever since his sister was born when he was 2 years old, he has been aggressive and rivalrous toward her. Jackson's parents separated and divorced when he was 3. He has had no contact with his father since then. Jackson's mother was depressed for a year after the divorce until she sought treatment. She has always felt guilty that his father is not in his life, and Jackson blames her for not having his father around. She believes his behaviors have become worse since she recently started dating again.

COURSE AND PROGNOSIS

The course of oppositional defiant disorder depends on the severity of the symptoms and the ability of the child to develop more adaptive responses to authority. The stability of oppositional defiant disorder varies over time, with approximately 25 percent of children with the disorder no longer meeting diagnostic criteria. Persistence of oppositional defiant symptoms poses an increased risk of additional disorders, such as mood disorders, conduct disorder, and substance use disorders. Positive outcomes are more likely for intact families who can modify their own expression of demands and give less attention to the child's argumentative behaviors.

An association exists between oppositional defiant disorder and ADHD, as well as with mood disorders. In children who have a long history of aggression and oppositional defiant disorder, there is a greater risk of the development of conduct disorder and later substance use disorders. Parental psychopathology, such as antisocial personality disorder and substance abuse, appears to be more common in families with children who have oppositional defiant disorder than in the general population, which creates additional risks for chaotic and troubled home environments. The prognosis for oppositional defiant disorder in a child depends somewhat on family functioning and the development of comorbid psychopathology.

TREATMENT

The primary treatment of oppositional defiant disorder is family intervention using both direct training of the parents in child management skills and careful assessment of family interactions. The goals of this intervention are to reinforce more prosocial behaviors and to diminish undesired behaviors at the same time. Cognitive behavioral therapists emphasize teaching parents how to alter their behavior to discourage the child's oppositional behavior by diminishing attention to it, and encourage appropriate therapy focuses on selectively reinforcing and praising appropriate behavior and ignoring or not reinforcing undesired behavior.

Children with oppositional defiant behavior may also benefit from individual psychotherapy in which they role play and "practice" more adaptive responses. In the therapeutic relationship, the child can learn new strategies to develop a sense of mastery and success in social situations with peers and families. In the safety of a more "neutral" relationship, children may discover that they are capable of less provocative behavior. Often, self-esteem must be restored before a child with oppositional defiant disorder can make more positive responses to external control. Parent–child conflict strongly predicts conduct problems; patterns of harsh physical and verbal punishment particularly evoke the emergence of aggression in children. Replacing harsh, punitive parenting and increasing positive parent–child interactions may positively influence the course of oppositional and defiant behaviors.

27.12e Conduct Disorder

Aggressive patterns of behavior are among the most frequent reasons for children and adolescents to be referred for psychiatric intervention. Although demonstration of impulsive behaviors is developmentally normative in children, many youth who continue to display excessive patterns of aggression in middle childhood generally require intervention. Children who develop enduring patterns of aggressive behaviors that begin in early childhood and violate the basic rights of peers and family members, however, may be destined for an entrenched pattern of conduct-disordered behaviors over time. Controversy remains as to whether a set of "voluntary" behaviors can constitute a valid psychiatric disorder, or may be better accounted for as maladaptive responses to adverse events, harsh or punitive parenting, or a threatening environment. Longitudinal studies have demonstrated that, for some youth, early patterns of disruptive behavior may become a lifelong pervasive repertoire culminating in adult antisocial personality disorder. The etiology of enduring patterns of aggressive behavior is widely accepted as a convergence of multiple contributing factors, including biological, temperamental, learned, and psychological conditions. Risk factors for the development of aggressive behavior in youth include childhood maltreatment such as physical or sexual abuse, neglect, emotional abuse, and overly harsh and punitive parenting. Chronic exposure to violence in the media including television, video games, and music videos has been shown to promote lower levels of empathy in children, which may add a risk factor for the development of aggressive behavior.

Conduct disorder is an enduring set of behaviors in a child or adolescent that evolves over time, usually characterized by aggression and violation of the rights of others. Youth with conduct disorder often demonstrate behaviors in the following four categories: physical aggression or threats of harm to people, destruction of their own property or that of others, theft or acts of deceit, and frequent violation of age-appropriate rules. Conduct disorder is associated with many other psychiatric disorders including ADHD, depression, and learning disorders. It is also associated with certain psychosocial factors, including childhood maltreatment, harsh or punitive parenting, family discord, lack of appropriate parental supervision, lack of social competence, and low socioeconomic level. The American Psychiatric Association's DSM-5 criteria require three persistent specific behaviors of 15 conduct disorder symptoms listed, over the past 12 months, with at least one of them present in the past 6 months. Conduct disorder symptoms include bullying, threatening, or intimidating others, and staying out at night despite parental prohibition. DSM-5 also specifies that when truancy from school is a symptom, it begins before 13 years of age. The disorder may be diagnosed in a person older than 18 years only if the criteria for antisocial personality disorder are not met. DSM-5 includes specifiers denoting the severity of the disorder, including "mild" in which there are few conduct problems in excess of those needed to make the diagnosis and behaviors cause only minor harm to others. In "moderate" cases, symptoms exceed the minimum; however, there is less confrontation that may cause harm to individuals than in "severe" cases. According to DSM-5, the "severe" level shows many conduct problems in excess of the minimal diagnostic criteria or conduct problems that cause considerable harm to others. DSM-5 has also added the following specifier: "With limited prosocial emotions." To qualify for this specifier, the individual must show a persistent interpersonal and emotional pattern that can be characterized by at least two of the following: (1) lack of remorse or guilt, (2) callous lack of empathy, (3) unconcerned about performance, (4) shallow or deficient affect. Individuals with conduct disorder who qualify for this specifier are more likely to have childhood-onset type and meet the criteria for a "severe" disorder. Children with conduct disorder engage in severe repeated acts of aggression that can cause physical harm to themselves and others and frequently violate the rights of others. Children with conduct disorder usually have behaviors characterized by aggression to persons or animals, destruction of property, deceitfulness or theft, and multiple violations of rules, such as truancy from school. These behavior patterns cause distinct difficulties in school life as well as in peer relationships. Conduct disorder has been divided into three subtypes, based on the age of onset of the disorder. Childhood-onset subtype, in which at least one symptom has emerged repeatedly before age 10 years; adolescent-onset type, in which no characteristic persistent symptoms were seen until after age 10 years; and unspecified-onset, in which age of onset is unknown. Although some young children show persistent patterns of behavior consistent with violating the rights of others or destroying property, the diagnosis of conduct disorder in children appears to increase with age. Epidemiological surveys indicate that geographic locations representing a broad range of different cultures are not associated with significant variability in prevalence rates of either oppositional defiant disorder or conduct disorder. A longitudinal study of population density and antisocial behaviors in youth found no relationship in children 4 to 13 years of age between conduct problems and density of living area. However, higher rates of conduct problems were self-reported by youth of 10 to 17 years who lived in higher-density communities.

EPIDEMIOLOGY

Estimated prevalence rates of conduct disorder in the United States range from 6 to 16 percent for males, and from 2 to 9 percent for females. Ratio of conduct disorder in males compared to females ranges from 4:1 to as much as 12:1. Conduct disorder occurs with greater frequency in the children of parents with antisocial personality disorder and alcohol dependence than in the general population. The prevalence of conduct disorder and antisocial behavior is associated with socioeconomic factors, as well as parental psychopathology.

ETIOLOGY

A meta-analysis of longitudinal studies indicates that the most important risk factors that predict conduct disorder include impulsivity, physical or sexual abuse or neglect, poor parental supervision and harsh and punitive parental discipline, low IQ, and poor school achievement.

Parental Factors

Harsh, punitive parenting characterized by severe physical and verbal aggression is associated with the development of children's maladaptive aggressive behaviors. Chaotic home conditions are associated with conduct disorder and delinquency. Divorce itself is not necessarily a risk factor, but the persistence of hostility, resentment, and bitterness between divorced parents may be the more important contributor to maladaptive behavior. Parental psychopathology, child abuse, and negligence often contribute to conduct disorder. Sociopathy, alcohol dependence, and substance abuse in the parents are associated with conduct disorder in their children. Parents may be so negligent that a child's care is shared by relatives or assumed by foster parents. Many such parents were scarred by their own upbringing and tend to be abusive, negligent, or engrossed in getting their own personal needs met.

Studies indicate that parents of children with conduct disorder have high rates of serious psychopathology, including psychotic disorders. Data show that children who exhibit a pattern of aggressive behavior have frequently been exposed to physically or emotionally harsh parenting.

Genetic Factors

A study of more than 6,000 male, female, and opposite sex twins found that genetic and environmental factors accounted for proportionally the same amount of variance in males and females. Genetic, and/or shared environmental factors exert different effects on males and females in childhood conduct disorder, but by adulthood, the gender-specific influences on antisocial behavior are no longer apparent. The sex-specific effects on antisocial behavior in youth along with the replicated finding of a potential role for the X-linked monoamine oxidase A gene in the etiology of antisocial behavior leads to the need for further genetic investigation of conduct disorder on the X chromosome and for analyses of these behaviors to be done separately by gender.

Sociocultural Factors

Youth residing in geographic areas with greater population density report increased rates of aggression and delinquency. Unemployed parents, lack of a supportive social network, and lack of positive participation in community activities seem to predict conduct disorder. Associated findings that may influence the development of conduct disorder in urban areas are increased exposure to and prevalence of substance use. A survey of alcohol use and mental health in adolescents found that weekly alcohol use among adolescents is associated with increased delinquent and aggressive behavior. Significant interactions between frequent alcohol use and age indicated that those adolescents with weekly alcohol use at younger ages were most likely to exhibit aggressive behaviors and mood disorders. Although drug and alcohol use does not cause conduct disorder, it increases the risks associated with it. Drug intoxication itself can also aggravate the symptoms. Thus, all factors that increase the likelihood of regular substance use may, in fact, promote and expand the disorder.

Psychological Factors

Poor emotion regulation among youth is associated with higher rates of aggression and conduct disorder. Emotion regulation is associated with social competence and can be observed even in children of preschool age. Those children with greater degrees of emotion dysregulation exhibit higher levels of aggression. Poor modeling of impulse control and the chronic lack of having their own needs met lead to a less well-developed sense of empathy.

Neurobiological Factors

Neuroimaging studies utilizing MRI have used voxel-based morphometry methods to compare structural brain differences between children with conduct disorder compared to normal controls. Studies have reported that children with conduct disorder had decreased gray matter in limbic brain structures, and in the bilateral anterior insula and left amygdala compared to healthy controls. A study investigated structural brain differences in children comorbid for oppositional defiant disorder or conduct disorder and ADHD compared to those with ADHD alone, and normal controls. Findings included decreased gray matter in ADHD and ADHD comorbid for oppositional defiant disorder or conduct disorder compared to controls in regions including bilateral temporal and occipital cortices, and the left amygdala.

Neurotransmitter studies in children with conduct disorder, suggest low level of plasma dopamine β-hydroxylase, an enzyme that converts dopamine to norepinephrine, leading to a hypothesis of decreased noradrenergic functioning in conduct disorder. Other studies of conduct-disordered juvenile offenders have found high plasma serotonin levels in blood. Evidence indicates that blood serotonin levels correlate inversely with levels of 5-HIAA in the CSF and that low 5-HIAA levels in CSF correlate with aggression and violence.

Neurologic Factors

An electroencephalography (EEG) study investigating resting frontal brain electrical activity, emotional intelligence, aggression, and rule breaking in 10-year-old children found that aggressive children had significantly greater relative right frontal brain activity at rest compared with nonaggressive children. Frontal resting brain electrical activity has been hypothesized to reflect the ability to regulate emotion. Boys tended to show lower emotional intelligence than girls and greater aggressive behavior than girls. No relationship, however, was found between emotional intelligence and pattern of frontal EEG activation.

Child Abuse and Maltreatment

Evidence shows that children chronically exposed to violence, physical or sexual abuse, and neglect, particularly at a young age, are at high risk for demonstrating aggression. A study of female caregivers exposed to intimate partner violence revealed a strong association with offspring aggression and mood disturbance. Severely abused children and adolescents tend to be hypervigilant; in some cases, they misperceive benign situations as directly threatening and respond defensively with violence. Not all expressed aggressive behavior in adolescents is synonymous with conduct disorder; however, youth with a repetitive pattern of hypervigilance and violent responses are likely to violate the rights of others.

Comorbid Factors

ADHD and conduct disorder are often found to coexist, with ADHD often predating the development of conduct disorder, and not infrequently substance abuse. CNS injury, dysfunction, or damage predisposes a child to impulsivity and behavioral disturbances, which sometimes evolve into conduct disorder.

DIAGNOSIS AND CLINICAL FEATURES

Conduct disorder does not develop overnight, instead, many symptoms evolve over time until a consistent pattern develops that involves violating the rights of others. Very young children are unlikely to meet the criteria for the disorder, because they are not developmentally able to exhibit the symptoms typical of older children with conduct disorder. A 3-year-old does not break into someone's home, steal with confrontation, force someone into sexual activity, or deliberately use a weapon that can cause serious harm. School-age children, however, can become bullies, initiate physical fights, destroy property, or set fires.

The average age of onset of conduct disorder is younger in boys than in girls. Boys most commonly meet the diagnostic criteria by 10 to 12 years of age, whereas girls often reach 14 to 16 years of age before the criteria are met.

Children who meet the criteria for conduct disorder express their overt aggressive behavior in various forms. Aggressive antisocial behavior can take the form of bullying, physical aggression, and cruel behavior toward peers. Children may be hostile, verbally abusive, impudent, defiant, and negativistic toward adults. Persistent lying, frequent truancy, and vandalism are common. In severe cases, destructiveness, stealing, and physical violence often occur. Some adolescents with conduct disorder make little attempt to conceal their antisocial behavior. Sexual behavior and regular use of tobacco, liquor, or illicit psychoactive substances begin unusually early for such children and adolescents. Suicidal thoughts, gestures, and acts are frequent in children and adolescents with conduct disorder who are in conflict with peers, family members, or the law and are unable to problem-solve their difficulties.

Some children with aggressive behavioral patterns have impaired social attachments, as evinced by their difficulties with peer relationships. Some may befriend a much older or younger person or have superficial relationships with other antisocial youngsters. Many children with conduct problems have poor self-esteem, although they may project an image of toughness. They may lack the skills to communicate in socially acceptable ways and appear to have little regard for the feelings, wishes, and welfare of others. Children and adolescents with conduct disorders often feel guilt or remorse for some of their behaviors, but try to blame others to stay out of trouble.

Many children and adolescents with conduct disorder suffer from the deprivation of having few of their dependency needs met and may have had either overly harsh parenting or a lack of appropriate supervision. The deficient socialization of many children and adolescents with conduct disorder can be expressed in physical violation of others and, for some, in sexual violation of others. Severe punishments for behavior in children with conduct disorder almost invariably increases their maladaptive expression of rage and frustration rather than ameliorating the problem.

In evaluation interviews, children with aggressive conduct disorders are typically uncooperative, hostile, and provocative. Some have a superficial charm and compliance until they are urged to talk about their problem behaviors. Then, they often deny any problems. If the interviewer persists, the child may attempt to justify misbehavior or become suspicious and angry about the source of the examiner's information and perhaps bolt from the room. Most often, the child becomes angry with the examiner and expresses resentment of the examination with open belligerence or sullen withdrawal. Their hostility is not limited to adult authority figures, but is expressed with equal venom toward their age-mates and younger children. In fact, they often bully those who are smaller and weaker. By boasting, lying, and expressing little interest in a listener's responses, such children reveal their lack of trust in adults to understand their position.

Evaluation of the family situation often reveals severe marital disharmony, which initially may center on disagreements about management of the child. Because of a tendency toward family instability, parent surrogates are often in the picture. Children with conduct disorder are more likely to be unplanned or unwanted babies. The parents of children with conduct disorder, especially the father, have higher rates of antisocial personality disorder or alcohol dependence. Aggressive children and their family show a stereotyped pattern of impulsive and unpredictable verbal and physical hostility. A child's aggressive behavior rarely seems directed toward any definable goal and offers little pleasure, success, or even sustained advantages with peers or authority figures.

In other cases, conduct disorder includes repeated truancy, vandalism, and serious physical aggression or assault against others by a gang, such as mugging, gang fighting, and beating. Children and adolescents who become part of a gang often have troubled age-appropriate friendships. They may protect their own gang members, and refrain from informing on them due to fear of the consequences to themselves. In many cases, gang members have a history of early childhood behavioral and psychiatric problems, physical abuse and/or exposure to parental violence. They develop a delinquent peer group, usually in preadolescence or during adolescence. Also present in the history is some evidence of early problems, such as marginal or poor school performance, mild behavior problems, anxiety, and depressive symptoms. Family histories of adolescent gang members are often positive for psychiatric disorders in parents, substance use and time spent incarcerated. Patterns of paternal discipline are rarely ideal and can vary from harshness and excessive strictness to inconsistency or relative absence of supervision and control. The mother has often protected the child from the consequences of early mild misbehavior, but does not seem to encourage delinquency actively. Delinquency, also called juvenile delinquency, is most often associated with conduct disorder but can also result from other psychological or neurological disorders.

Violent Video Games and Violent Behavior

Longitudinal studies corroborate the contribution of media violence including video gaming in middle-school children with the expression of aggression in those adolescents. A review of the literature of the effect of violent video games on children and adolescents revealed that violent video game playing is related to aggressive affect, physiologic arousal, and aggressive behaviors. It stands to reason that the degree of exposure to violent games and the more restriction of activity would be related to a greater preoccupation with violent themes.

PATHOLOGY AND LABORATORY EXAMINATION

No specific laboratory test or neurological pathology helps make the diagnosis of conduct disorder. Some evidence indicates that amounts of certain neurotransmitters, such as serotonin in the CNS, are low in some persons with a history of violent or aggressive behavior toward others or themselves. Whether this association is related to the cause, or is the effect, of violence or is unrelated to the violence is not clear.

DIFFERENTIAL DIAGNOSIS

Disturbances of conduct, including impulsivity and aggression, may occur in many childhood psychiatric disorders, ranging from ADHD, to oppositional defiant disorder, to disruptive mood dysregulation disorder, to major depression, to bipolar disorder, specific learning disorders, and psychotic disorders. Therefore, clinicians must obtain a comprehensive history of the chronology of the symptoms to determine whether the conduct disturbance is a transient or an enduring pattern. Isolated acts of aggressive behavior do not justify a diagnosis of conduct disorder; an entrenched pattern must be present. The relationship of conduct disorder to oppositional defiant disorder is still under debate. Historically, oppositional defiant disorder has been conceptualized as a mild precursor of conduct disorder, without the violation of rights, likely to be diagnosed in younger children who may be at risk for conduct disorder. Children who progress from oppositional defiant disorder to conduct disorder over time, maintain their oppositional characteristics, and some evidence indicates that the two disorders are independent. Currently, in the DSM-5, oppositional defiant disorder and conduct disorder are considered distinct, and they may be diagnosed comorbidly. Many children with oppositional defiant disorder do not develop conduct disorder, and conduct disorder emerging in adolescence is not necessarily preceded by oppositional defiant disorder. The main distinguishing clinical feature between these two disorders is that in conduct disorder, the basic rights of others are violated, whereas in oppositional defiant disorder, hostility and negativism fall short of seriously violating the rights of others.

Mood disorders are often present in children who exhibit irritability and aggressive behavior. Both major depressive disorder and bipolar disorders must be ruled out, but the full syndrome of conduct disorder can occur and be diagnosed during the onset of a mood disorder. Substantial comorbidity exists of conduct disorder and depressive disorders. A recent report concludes that the high correlation between the two disorders arises from shared risk factors for both disorders rather than a causal relation. Thus, a series of factors, including family conflict, negative life events, early history of conduct disturbance, level of parental involvement, and affiliation with delinquent peers, contribute to the development of affective disorders and conduct disorder. This is not the case with oppositional defiant disorder, which cannot be diagnosed if it occurs exclusively during a mood disorder.

ADHD and learning disorders are commonly associated with conduct disorder. Usually, the symptoms of these disorders predate the diagnosis of conduct disorder. Substance abuse disorders are also more common in adolescents with conduct disorder than in the general population. Evidence indicates an association between fighting behaviors as a child and substance use as an adolescent. Once a pattern of drug use is formed, this pattern may interfere with the development of positive mediators, such as social skills and problem-solving, which could enhance remission of the conduct disorder. Thus, once substance abuse develops, it may promote continuation of the conduct disorder. OCD also frequently seems to coexist with disruptive behavior disorders. All the disorders described here should be noted when they co-occur. Children with ADHD often exhibit impulsive and aggressive behaviors that may not meet the full criteria for conduct disorder.

Damien, age 12 years, was referred for psychiatric evaluation after being picked up by police for truancy, and running away from home. Damien explained that he just wanted to get out of his house and go see his friends. He doesn't like to be at home because his mother tries to tell him what to do. Damien's mother says that he left and stayed out overnight multiple times in the past year, but that he usually returns the next morning. She complains that he is constantly in trouble. He has shoplifted on several occasions that she knows of, the first time at age 8 years. She suspects that he also steals from neighbors or school. The police have been involved on many occasions including truancy, staying out all night, stealing from a neighborhood store, and smoking marijuana. Damien has a quick temper, and his mother knows he was involved in several fights over the past year in the neighborhood. Damien is particularly cruel to his younger brother, constantly taunting and teasing him. Damien's mother stated that he lies constantly, sometimes for no apparent reason. When he was 6 years of age, he was fascinated with fire and set several small fires at home, fortunately with no serious injury or damage. Damien's mother was tearful when she disclosed that Damien is just like his no-good father and that she wished she never had him. Damien initially refused to answer questions, and turned away scowling, but gradually began to talk. Damien presented a tough image with an indifferent attitude toward the interviewer. Damien denied any abuse at home, saying that he ran off because he was bored. However, upon further questioning, Damien admitted that his mother's previous boyfriend who was in the home when Damien was between 6 and 8 years of age used to hit him with a belt when he got out of line. Damien justified his own behaviors as just having fun. He explained the fights as being provoked by the others and denied the use of any weapons, although he bragged about breaking the nose of another youth. Damien's school records indicate that an Individualized Educational Plan (IEP) was required when he was in the 2nd grade, and he was evaluated for symptoms of ADHD when he was in 1st grade. Methylphenidate (Ritalin) was prescribed; however, the family did not continue with treatment, and he is currently on no medication. Damien is currently in 6th grade special education classes, having failed and repeated 5th grade. Damien's grades are failing, and he may have to repeat 6th grade. Damien admits to truancy on several occasions this year in addition to his problems with completing schoolwork. His previous evaluation indicates that child protective services evaluated the family for possible neglect when he was 5 years of age after he and his brother were found barefoot on the street late one evening without his mother in sight. Apparently, Damien's family was referred for counseling and never attended. Both of Damien's parents have a history of drug and alcohol abuse. Damien's birth was unplanned, and his mother used drugs during pregnancy. His parents separated soon after his birth, and his mother returned to live with her parents briefly. Damien and his mother moved to live with her boyfriend when Damien was 1 year of age after she became pregnant with his younger sister. Damien's mother's relationship ended within a year, and only Damien, his mother, and his sister live in their apartment. Damien's mother has worked several different jobs, and Damien wonders if she has a drinking problem.

COURSE AND PROGNOSIS

The course and prognosis for children with conduct disorder is most guarded in those who have symptoms at a young age, exhibit the greatest number of symptoms, and the most severe, and express them most frequently. This finding is true partly because those with severe conduct disorder seem to be most vulnerable to comorbid disorders later in life, such as mood disorders and substance use disorders. A longitudinal study found that, although assaultive behavior in childhood and parental criminality predict a high risk for incarceration later in life, the diagnosis of conduct disorder per se was not correlated with imprisonment. The best prognosis is predicted for mild conduct disorder in the absence of coexisting psychopathology and the presence of normal intellectual functioning.

TREATMENT

Psychosocial Interventions

Early sustained preventive interventions can significantly alter the course and prognosis of aggressive behavior when it is administered starting at kindergarten age. A screening program used with kindergarteners predicted lifetime disruptive behavior disorder by the age of 18 years, with the highest-risk group demonstrating an 82 percent chance of a disruptive behavior diagnosis without intervention. A prevention program, the *Fast Track Preventive Intervention,* randomized 891 kindergarteners to either a 10-year prevention program or a control condition. The 10-year intervention included parent behavior management, child social cognitive skills, reading, home visiting, mentoring, and classroom curricula. The children in the Fast Track Intervention were substantially prevented from the development of conduct disorder during the 10-year period and for 2 years thereafter.

A meta-analysis of controlled trials of CBT programs indicates that CBT can result in significant reductions in conduct-disordered symptoms in children and adolescents. CBT treatment interventions that are proven to be efficacious include the following.

Kazdin's Problem-Solving Skills Training (PSST) in which a 12-week sequential program helps children develop problem-solving solutions when faced with conflictual situations. Assignments called "supersolvers" provide vignette situations in which children can practice these techniques. A companion program, Parent Management Training (PMT) can be added to the intervention, but PSST can be effective even without the parent component. Another CBT-based intervention, the Incredible Years (IY), targeting young children from 3 to 8 years, is administered over 22 weeks and delivers sessions to the child and has a parent training component and a teacher training. Another CBT-based intervention is the Anger Coping Program, an 18-session intervention for school-aged children in the grades 4 to 6 focused on a child's increased development of emotion recognition and regulation, and managing anger. Anger-coping strategies include distraction, self-talk, perspective taking, goal setting, and problem-solving.

Overall, treatment programs have been more successful in decreasing overt symptoms of conduct, such as aggression, than the covert symptoms, such as lying or stealing. Treatment strategies for young children that focus on increasing social behavior and social competence are believed to reduce aggressive behavior. A study of 548 third graders administered a school-based intervention instead of a regular health curriculum in several public schools in North Carolina, called *Making Choices: Social Problem Solving Skills for Children* (MC) program along with supplemental teacher and parent components. Compared with third graders receiving the routine health curriculum, children exposed to the MC program were rated lower on the posttest social and overt aggression, and higher on social competence. In addition, they scored higher on an information-processing skills posttest. These findings support the notion that school-based prevention programs have the potential to strengthen social and emotional skills and diminish aggressive behavior among normal populations of school-age children. School settings can also use behavioral techniques to promote socially acceptable behavior toward peers and to discourage covert antisocial incidents.

Psychopharmacologic Interventions

Efficacy of psychopharmacologic interventions includes several placebo-controlled studies of risperidone for aggression in youth associated with disruptive behavior disorders, and/or mental retardation. In addition, risperidone has been found to be superior to placebo in reducing aggressive behavior in a large 6-month placebo-substitution study. One randomized double-blind placebo-controlled trial with quetiapine also showed efficacy for aggressive behavior. Early studies of antipsychotics, most notably haloperidol (Haldol), reported decreased aggressive and assaultive behaviors in children with a variety of psychiatric disorders. Atypical antipsychotics risperidone (Risperdal), olanzapine (Zyprexa), quetiapine (Seroquel), ziprasidone (Geodon), and aripiprazole (Abilify) have generally replaced the older antipsychotics in clinical practice due to their comparable efficacy and improved side-effect profiles. Side effects of second-generation antipsychotics include sedation, increased prolactin levels (with risperidone use) and extrapyramidal symptoms, including akathisia. In general, however, the atypical antipsychotics appear to be well tolerated. A study of divalproex in youth with conduct disorder showed that those who responded most robustly exhibited aggression characterized by agitation, dysphoria, and distress. Although early trials suggested that carbamazepine (Tegretol) was useful to control aggression, a double-blind, placebo-controlled study did not show superiority of carbamazepine over placebo in decreasing aggression. A pilot study found that clonidine (Catapres) may decrease aggression. The SSRIs, including fluoxetine (Prozac), sertraline (Zoloft), paroxetine (Paxil), and citalopram (Celexa), are used clinically to target symptoms of impulsivity, irritability, and mood lability, which frequently accompany conduct disorder. Conduct disorder often coexists with ADHD, learning disorders, and, over time, mood disorders and substance-related disorders; thus, the treatment of concurrent disorders must also be addressed.

▲ 27.13 Anxiety Disorders of Infancy, Childhood, and Adolescence

Anxiety disorders are among the most common disorders in youth, affecting 10 to 20 percent of children and adolescents. Although observable anxiety behaviors mark normative development in infants, anxiety disorders in childhood predict a wide range of psychological difficulties in adolescence including additional anxiety disorders, panic attacks, and depressive disorders. Fear is an expected response to real or perceived threat; however, anxiety is the anticipation of future danger. Anxiety disorders are characterized by recurrent emotional and physiological arousal in response to excessive perceptions of perceived threat or danger. Anxiety disorders commonly found in youth include separation anxiety disorder, generalized anxiety disorder, social anxiety disorder, and selective mutism. Anxiety is classified into disorders based on how it is experienced, the situations that trigger it, and the course that it tends to follow.

27.13a Separation Anxiety Disorder, Generalized Anxiety Disorder, and Social Anxiety Disorder (Social Phobia)

Separation anxiety disorder, generalized anxiety disorder, and social anxiety disorder in children are often considered together in the evaluation process and differential diagnosis, and in developing treatment strategies, because they are highly comorbid and have overlapping symptoms. A child with separation anxiety disorder, generalized anxiety disorder, or social anxiety disorder has a 60 percent chance of having at least one of the other two disorders as well. Of children with one of the above anxiety disorders, 30 percent have all three of them. Children and adolescents may also have additional comorbid anxiety disorders such as specific phobia or panic disorder. Separation anxiety disorder, generalized anxiety disorder, and social anxiety disorder are distinguished from each other by the types of situations that elicit the excessive anxiety and avoidance behaviors.

SEPARATION ANXIETY DISORDER

Separation anxiety is a universal human developmental phenomenon emerging in infants younger than 1 year of age and marking a child's awareness of a separation from his or her mother or primary caregiver. Normative separation anxiety peaks between 9 and 18 months and diminishes by about 2½ years of age, enabling young children to develop a sense of comfort away from their parents in preschool. Separation anxiety or stranger anxiety most likely evolved as a human response that has survival value. The expression of transient separation anxiety is also normal in young children entering school for the first time. Approximately 15 percent of young children display intense and persistent fear, shyness, and social withdrawal when faced with unfamiliar settings and people. Young children with this pattern of significant behavioral inhibition are at higher risk for the development of separation anxiety disorder, generalized anxiety disorder, and social phobia. Behaviorally inhibited children, as a group, exhibit characteristic physiological traits, including higher than average resting heart rates, higher morning cortisol levels than average, and low heart rate variability. Separation anxiety disorder is diagnosed when developmentally inappropriate and excessive anxiety emerges related to separation from the major attachment figure. According to the American Psychiatric Association's *Diagnostic and Statistical Manual of Mental Disorders, Fifth Edition* (DSM-5), separation anxiety disorder is characterized by a level of fear or anxiety regarding separation from their parents or primary caregiver, which is beyond developmental expectations. Furthermore, there may be a pervasive worry that harm will come to a parent upon separation, which leads to extreme distress, and sometimes nightmares. The DSM-5 requires the presence of at least three symptoms related to excessive worry about separation from a major attachment figure for a period of at least 4 weeks. The worries often take the form of refusal to go to school, fears and distress on separation, repeated complaints of physical symptoms such as headaches and stomachaches when separation is anticipated, and nightmares related to separation issues.

GENERALIZED ANXIETY DISORDER

Children with generalized anxiety disorder have significant distress in activities of daily life often focused on the child's fears of incompetence in many areas, including school performance and in social settings. In addition, children with generalized anxiety disorder, according to DSM-5, experience at least one of the following symptoms: restlessness, being easily fatigued, "mind going blank," irritability, muscle tension, or sleep disturbance. Children with generalized anxiety disorder tend to feel fearful in multiple settings and expect more negative outcomes when faced with academic or social challenges, compared with peers. Children and adolescents with generalized anxiety disorder may experience symptoms of autonomic hyperarousal such as tachycardia, shortness of breath, or dizziness, and are more likely than nonanxious youth to experience sweating, nausea, or diarrhea when they become anxious. Children and adolescents with generalized anxiety disorder tend to be overly concerned about potential natural disasters such as earthquakes or floods, and these worries can interfere with their daily activities. Finally, children and adolescents with generalized anxiety disorder are continuously worried about the quality of their performance in academics, sports, and other activities, and often seek excessive reassurance about their performance.

SOCIAL ANXIETY DISORDER (SOCIAL PHOBIA)

Children who experience intense discomfort and distress in social situations and are impaired by their fear of scrutiny or humiliation are given the diagnosis of social anxiety disorder. Their distress may be expressed in the form of crying, tantrums, avoidance, freezing, or even becoming "mute" in these situations. According to DSM-5, this disorder is characterized by consistent anxiety and distress in almost all social situations. Any situation in which the child feels exposed to possible scrutiny by others can provoke fear or anxiety, and the child will often try to avoid these feared social situations. Children must experience the anxiety in the presence of peers, not only with adults, in order to receive the diagnosis. A child or adolescent with social anxiety disorder may exhibit the performance only type, which targets a specific type of performing, such as fear of public speaking. The performance only type typically manifests in school or academic settings in which public presentations must be performed, such as in front of classmates in school.

Social anxiety disorder has significant implications for future accomplishments, since it is associated with lower levels of satisfaction in leisure activities, increased rates of school dropout, less productivity in the workplace as adults, and increased rates of remaining single. Despite the significant impairment caused by social anxiety disorder, up to half of individuals with the disorder do not receive treatment.

EPIDEMIOLOGY

The prevalence of anxiety disorders has varied with the age group of the children surveyed and the diagnostic instruments used. Lifetime prevalence of any anxiety disorder in children and adolescents ranges from 10 to 27 percent. Anxiety disorders are common in preschoolers as well, and follow a similar epidemiologic profile as in older children. An epidemiologic survey using the *Preschool-Age Psychiatric Assessment* (PAPA) found that 9.5 percent of preschoolers met criteria for any anxiety disorder, with 6.5 percent exhibiting generalized anxiety disorder, 2.4 percent meeting criteria for separation anxiety disorder, and 2.2 percent meeting criteria for social phobia. Separation anxiety disorder is estimated to be about 4 percent in children and young adolescents. Separation anxiety disorder is more common in young children than in adolescents and has been reported to occur equally in boys and girls. The onset may occur during preschool years, but is most common in children 7 to 8 years of age. The rate of generalized anxiety disorder in school-age children is estimated to be approximately 3 percent, the rate of social phobia is 1 percent, and the rate of simple phobias is 2.4 percent. In adolescents, lifetime prevalence for panic disorder was found to be 0.6 percent; the prevalence for generalized anxiety disorder was 3.7 percent.

ETIOLOGY

Biopsychosocial Factors

Evidence for the influences of parental psychopathology and parenting styles on the emergence of anxiety disorders in childhood has been found in multiple investigations. Longitudinal studies have found that parental overprotection has been associated with an increased risk of the development of anxiety disorders in children, and insecure parent–child attachment is associated with higher than expected rates of anxiety disorders in childhood. It is also well known that maternal depression and anxiety have led to an increased risk for anxiety and depression in children. Psychosocial factors in conjunction with a child's temperament influences the degree of separation anxiety evoked in situations of brief separation and exposure to unfamiliar environments. The temperamental trait of shyness and withdrawal in unfamiliar situations has been shown to be associated with a higher risk of developing separation anxiety disorder, generalized anxiety disorder, social anxiety disorder, or all three during childhood and adolescence.

External life stresses often coincide with development of the disorder. The death of a relative, a child's illness, a change in a child's environment, or a move to a new neighborhood or school is frequently noted in the histories of children with separation anxiety disorder. In a vulnerable child, these changes probably intensify anxiety.

Neurophysiological correlations are found with behavioral inhibition (extreme shyness); children with this constellation are shown to have a higher resting heart rate and an acceleration of heart rate with tasks requiring cognitive concentration. Additional physiological correlates of behavioral inhibition include elevated salivary cortisol levels, elevated urinary catecholamine levels, and greater papillary dilation during cognitive tasks.

Neuroimaging studies of adolescents with anxiety show an increased activation of the amygdala compared to nonanxious adolescents when presented with anxiety-provoking stimuli. Furthermore, anxious adolescents maintain the hyperactivation of the amygdala over time, rather than showing an attenuation of the effect as in nonanxious adolescents. Structural studies of the amygdala in adolescents with anxiety have led to conflicting results, some studies finding increased amygdala volumes, whereas other studies finding decreased amygdala volumes.

Social Learning Factors

Fear, in response to a variety of unfamiliar or unexpected situations, may be unwittingly communicated from parents to children by direct modeling. If a parent is fearful, the child will probably have a phobic adaptation to new situations, especially to a school environment. There are much data to suggest that overprotective parenting promotes increased interpersonal sensitivity in healthy children, and increases the risk of social anxiety disorder in children with behavioral inhibition or other anxiety disorders such as separation anxiety disorder. Some parents appear to teach their children to be anxious by overprotecting them from expected dangers or by exaggerating the dangers. For example, a parent who cringes in a room during a lightning storm teaches a child to do the same. A parent who is afraid of mice or insects conveys the affect of fright to a child. Conversely, a parent who becomes angry with a child when the child expresses fear of a given situation, for example, when exposed to animals, may promote a phobic concern in the child by exposing the child to the intensity of the anger expressed by the parent. Social learning factors in the development of anxiety reactions are magnified when parents have anxiety disorders themselves. These factors may be pertinent in the development of separation anxiety disorder as well as in generalized anxiety disorder and social phobia. A recent study found no association between psychosocial hardships, such as ongoing family conflict, and behavioral inhibition among young children. It appears that temperamental predisposition to anxiety disorders emerges as a highly heritable constellation of traits, and is not created by psychosocial stressor.

Genetic Factors

Genetic studies suggest that genes account for at least one-third of the variance in the development of anxiety disorders. Heritability for anxiety disorders in children and adolescents ranges from 36 to 65 percent, with the highest estimates found in younger children with anxiety disorders. Two heritable characteristics—behavioral inhibition (the tendency toward fear and withdrawal in new situations) and physiological hyperarousal—have both been found to impart significant risk factors for future development of an anxiety disorder. However, although the temperamental constellation of behavioral inhibition, excessive shyness, the tendency to withdraw from unfamiliar situations, and the eventual emergence of anxiety disorders have a genetic contribution, one-third to two-thirds of young children with behavioral inhibition do not appear to go on to develop anxiety disorders.

Family studies have shown that the offspring of adults with anxiety disorders are at an increased risk of having an anxiety disorder themselves. Separation anxiety disorder and depression in children overlap, and the presence of an anxiety disorder increases the risk of a future episode of a depressive disorder. Current consensus on the genetics of anxiety disorders suggests that what is inherited is a general predisposition toward anxiety, causing heightened levels of arousal, emotional reactivity, and increased negative affect, all of which increase the risk of developing separation anxiety disorder, generalized anxiety disorder, and social phobia.

DIAGNOSIS AND CLINICAL FEATURES

Separation anxiety disorder, generalized anxiety disorder, and social phobia are highly related in children and adolescence because, in most children, overlapping symptoms as well as comorbid disorders emerge. Generalized anxiety disorder is the most common anxiety disorder among youth, more common in adolescents than in younger children; in almost one-third of these cases, a child with generalized anxiety disorder also exhibits separation anxiety disorder and social anxiety disorder.

Diagnostic criteria for separation anxiety disorder, according to the DSM-5, include three of the following symptoms for at least 4 weeks: persistent and excessive worry about losing, or possible harm befalling, major attachment figures; persistent and excessive worry that an untoward event can lead to separation from a major attachment figure; persistent reluctance or refusal to go to school or elsewhere because of fear of separation; persistent and excessive fear or reluctance to be alone or without major attachment figures at home or without significant adults in other settings; persistent reluctance or refusal to go to sleep without being near a major attachment figure or to sleep away from home; repeated nightmares involving the theme of separation; repeated complaints of physical symptoms, including headaches and stomachaches, when separation from major attachment figures is anticipated; and recurrent excessive distress when separation from home or major attachment figures is anticipated or involved. The following case history demonstrates separation anxiety disorder along with autonomic arousal symptoms.

Jake was a 9-year-old boy who was referred for outpatient evaluation by his family physician. He refused to sleep in his room alone at night and exhibited violent tantrums each morning in order to avoid going to school. Jake expressed recurrent fears that something bad would happen to his mother. He worried that she would get into a car accident or that there would be a fire at home and his mother would be killed. Developmental history revealed that Jake was anxious and irritable as an infant and toddler. He had trouble adjusting to babysitters in the preschool years. There was a history of panic disorder, with agoraphobia in the mother and major depression in his father. Jake became more concerned and territorial over his mother when his father left the family, and his mother became depressed. Jake always kept track of his mother's whereabouts and insisted that she stay at home.

Nighttime was a particularly difficult time at home. When Jake's mother tried to get Jake to remain in his room, Jake would whine and cry and insist that his mother lie in bed with him until he fell asleep. He also expected his mother to be in the master bedroom across the hall from his room throughout the evening. Jake's mother reported that each evening her son would get up and peek through the crack in the master bedroom door, as frequently as every 10 minutes, to be certain that she was still there. Jake reported frequent nightmares that his mother was killed and that monsters prevented him from rescuing his mother, taking him away from his family forever.

During the daytime, Jake would shadow his mother around the house. Jake would agree to play a game with his sister in the lower level of the house only if his mother was close by. When Jake's mother went upstairs, he would interrupt the game and follow her upstairs. He refused to sleep at a friend's house. Frequently, at home as the evening progressed, Jake described a queasy sensation in his stomach mixed with feelings of sadness.

On school days, Jake usually complained of stomachaches and tried to stay home. Jake appeared distressed and panicky and would become violent when his mother attempted to drop him off at school. Once at school, he seemed calmer and less distressed, but frequently was seen in the nurse's office, complaining of nausea and seeking to be sent home. *(Adapted from case material from Gail A. Bernstein, M.D. and Anne E. Layne, Ph.D.)*

The essential feature of separation anxiety disorder is extreme anxiety precipitated by separation from parents, home, or other familiar surroundings, whereas in generalized anxiety disorder, fears are extended to negative outcomes for all kinds of events, including academic, peer relationship, and family activities. In generalized anxiety disorder, a child or adolescent experiences at least one recurrent physiological symptom, such as restlessness, poor concentration, irritability, or muscle tension. In social phobia, the child's fears peak during performance situations involving exposure to unfamiliar people or situations. Children and adolescents with social phobia have extreme concerns about being embarrassed, humiliated, or negatively judged. In each of the preceding anxiety disorders, the child's experience can approach terror or panic. The distress is greater than that normally expected for the child's developmental level and cannot be explained by any other disorder. Morbid fears, preoccupations, and ruminations characterize separation anxiety disorder. Children with anxiety disorders overestimate the probability of danger and the likelihood of negative outcome. Children with separation anxiety disorder and generalized anxiety disorder become overly fearful that someone close to them will be hurt or that something terrible will happen to them or their families, especially when they are away from important caring figures. Many children with anxiety disorders are preoccupied with health and worry that their families or friends will become ill. Fears of getting lost, being kidnapped, and losing the ability to be in contact with their families is predominant among children with separation anxiety disorder.

Adolescents with anxiety disorders may not directly express their worries; however, their behavior patterns often reflect either separation anxiety or other anxiety if they exhibit discomfort about leaving home, engage in solitary activities because of fears about how they will perform in front of peers, or have distress when away from their families. Separation anxiety disorder in children is often manifested at the thought of travel or in the course of travel away from home. Children may refuse to go to camp, a new school, or even a friend's house. Frequently, a continuum exists between mild anticipatory anxiety before separation from an important figure and pervasive anxiety after the separation has occurred. Premonitory signs include irritability, difficulty eating, whining, staying in a room alone, clinging to parents, and following a parent everywhere. Often, when a family moves, a child displays separation anxiety by intense clinging to the mother figure. Sometimes, geographical relocation anxiety is expressed in feelings of acute homesickness or psychophysiological symptoms that break out when the child is away from home or is going to a new country. The child yearns to return home and becomes preoccupied with fantasies of how much better the old home was. Integration into the new life situation may become extremely difficult. Children with anxiety disorders may retreat from social or group activities and express feelings of loneliness because of their self-imposed isolation.

Sleep difficulties are frequent in children and adolescents with any anxiety disorder or in severe separation anxiety; a child or adolescent may require having someone remain with him or her until he or she falls asleep. An anxious child may awaken and go to a parent's bed or even sleep at the parents' door in an effort to diminish anxiety. Nightmares and morbid fears may be expressions of anxiety.

Associated features of most anxiety disorders include fear of the dark and imaginary worries. Children may have the feeling that eyes are staring at them and monsters are reaching out for them in their bedrooms. Children with separation anxiety disorder, generalized anxiety disorder, and social anxiety disorder often complain of somatic symptoms and may be more sensitive to changes in their bodies compared to youth without anxiety disorders. Children with separation anxiety disorder, generalized anxiety disorder, or social anxiety disorder are often more emotionally sensitive than peers and more easily brought to tears. Frequent somatic complaints accompanying anxiety disorders include gastrointestinal symptoms, nausea, vomiting, and stomachaches; unexplained pain in various parts of the body; sore throats; and flu-like symptoms. Older children and adolescents typically complain of somatic experiences classically reported by adults with anxiety, such as cardiovascular and respiratory symptoms—palpitations, dizziness, faintness, and feelings of strangulation. Physiological signs of anxiety are a part of the diagnostic criteria for generalized anxiety disorder, but they are more often also experienced by children with separation anxiety and social phobia than the general population. The following case history demonstrates a young adolescent with generalized anxiety disorder.

Rachel was a 13-year-old girl referred for an evaluation by her pediatrician based on her chronic gastrointestinal complaints without any organic illness. On interview, Rachel appeared withdrawn and meek but responsive to questions. She endorsed a number of worries that included concerns about her health, her parents' safety, her school performance, and her peer relationships. Rachel's greatest worries were related to her health and safety. Rachel's mother reported that Julie had recently been very reluctant to play outside, because she feared she would contract Lyme disease from a tick bite or West Nile virus from a mosquito bite. Rachel was also very distressed by news reports about catastrophic events locally and around the world (e.g., kidnapping, crime, terrorism). Rachel was described by her family and teachers as overly conscientious about her schoolwork and as often being concerned about adult matters (e.g., finances, parents' job security). Symptoms that accompanied Rachel's worries primarily involved stomach pain and problems falling asleep. Rachel tended to be quite perseverative; repetitively verbalizing her worries even after reassurance was given. Rachel admitted that she worried for hours each day and could not "turn off" her worried thoughts.

Rachel was the product of a normal pregnancy and delivery. Her medical history was unremarkable, with the exception of frequent gastrointestinal pain since kindergarten. Julie was described as irritable and difficult to soothe as an infant. Developmental milestones were met within normal limits. She was described as very obedient and had no history of externalizing behavior problems. She was very concerned about her academic performance from an early age and earned A's with an occasional B. Rachel was somewhat shy in social situations but well-liked by her peers. Family history included depression in her maternal grandmother and a maternal history of generalized anxiety disorder, social anxiety, and separation anxiety disorder as a child. Rachel had two younger siblings who were high achievers and without notable problems. *(Adapted from case material from Gail A. Bernstein, M.D. and Anne E. Layne, Ph.D.)*

The next case history demonstrates an adolescent with multiple anxiety and depressive disorders.

Kate is a 15-year-old 10th grader who lives with her biological parents and two sisters, age 9 and 14 years. Kate is a very articulate teen who has always been a good student, although she never volunteers answers in school unless she is called on by her teachers. She gets along well with her sisters when at home, but ever since she entered high school in the 9th grade year, she declines invitations to go to friends' homes, has turned down opportunities to go to parties, and has even stopped going on outings with her sisters to the neighborhood mall and the movies. Kate reports that she gets too nervous, and blushes when she is with friends outside of the classroom at school because she can't think of anything to say to them. She reports that she is embarrassed to go shopping or to the movies with her sisters because they often run into neighborhood peers along the way, stop to chat, and this makes her feel "stupid," because even though she is the oldest, she does not say anything, and believes that her sisters' friends will laugh at her shyness. Recently, one of her former best friends confronted her about why she had stopped "hanging out" with her friends. Kate had stopped eating lunch with her friends in school because she felt humiliated when they would talk about their weekend plans and even when they invited her to join, she would just look the other way and ignore the conversation. Kate had become isolated, even in school, and admitted to her sister that she was lonely. Kate was brought for an evaluation after her younger sister commented to her mother that Kate spent all of her time alone whenever her sisters saw their friends, and that she looked sad and stressed out whenever she was around peers. Kate was down, always in poor spirits and had stopped interacting with her sisters even at home, and her sisters were often out with their own friends. On rare occasions Kate's younger sister had invited Kate to parties or to friend's homes, but Kate had declined and burst into tears.

Kate was evaluated by a child psychiatrist who made the diagnoses of social anxiety disorder, generalized anxiety disorder, and major depression and recommended a combination of treatment options, including cognitive-behavioral therapy (CBT) and a trial of a selective serotonin reuptake inhibitor (SSRI), fluoxetine. Kate and her family decided to try the medication first. Kate was started on 10 mg of fluoxetine and over the next month was titrated to a dose of 20 mg. By the third week of the medication trial, Kate was noticeably less resistant to going out with her sisters to places where they were likely to encounter peers. Her sisters noticed that she did not seem as stressed and started to occasionally sit with peers at lunch in the school cafeteria. She stated that she did not feel as self-conscious as she used to in class and was willing to go to a friend's house. She still declined to go to a birthday party of a peer that she didn't know very well. Kate continued on the same medication and within 2 months, she was significantly less anxious in social situations. She complained occasionally of a stomachache, but tolerated the medication well. Her family was impressed when she requested they plan a birthday party for her 16th birthday and decided to invite 10 friends.

PATHOLOGY AND LABORATORY EXAMINATION

No specific laboratory measures help in the diagnosis of separation anxiety disorder, generalized anxiety disorder, or social anxiety disorder.

DIFFERENTIAL DIAGNOSIS

The presence of separation anxiety is a developmentally expected feature in a young child and often does not represent an impairing condition, thus clinical judgment must be used in distinguishing normal anxiety from separation anxiety disorder in this age group. In older school-age children, a child experiencing more than normal distress is apparent when school is refused on a regular basis. For children who resist school, it is important to distinguish whether fear of separation, general worry about performance, or more specific fears of humiliation in front of peers or the teacher are driving the resistance. In many cases in which anxiety is the primary symptom, all three of the above-feared scenarios come into play. In generalized anxiety disorder, anxiety is not primarily focused on separation.

When depressive disorders occur in children, possible comorbidities such as separation anxiety disorder should be evaluated as well. A comorbid diagnosis of separation anxiety disorder and depressive disorder should be made when the criteria for both disorders are met; the two diagnoses often coexist. Panic disorder with agoraphobia is uncommon before 18 years of age; the fear is of being incapacitated by a panic attack rather

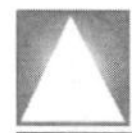

Table 27.13a–1
Common Characteristics in Childhood Anxiety Disorders

Criteria	Separation Anxiety Disorder	Social Anxiety Disorder	Generalized Anxiety Disorder
Minimum duration to establish diagnosis	At least 4 weeks	Persistent, typically at least 6 months	At least 6 months
Age of onset	Not specified	Not specified	Not specified
Precipitating stressors	Separation from home or attachment figures	Social situations with peers or specific	Pressure for any type of performance, activities which are scored, school performance
Peer relationships	Good when no separation is involved	Tentative, overly inhibited	May appear overly eager to please, peers sought out for reassurance
Sleep	Reluctance or refusal to sleep away from home or not near attachment figure	May experience insomnia	Often difficulty falling asleep
Psychophysiological symptoms	Stomachaches, headaches nausea, vomiting, palpitations, dizziness when anticipating separation	May exhibit blushing, inadequate eye contact, soft voice, or rigid posture	Stomachaches, nausea, lump in the throat, shortness of breath, dizziness, palpitations when anticipating performing an activity
Differential diagnosis	GAD, Soc AD, major depressive disorder, panic disorder with agoraphobia, PTSD, oppositional defiant disorder	GAD, Soc AD, major depressive disorder, dysthymic disorder, selective mutism, agoraphobia	SAD, Soc AD, attention-deficit/hyperactivity disorder, obsessive-compulsive disorder, major depressive disorder, PTSD

GAD, generalized anxiety disorder; Soc AD, social anxiety disorder; PTSD, posttraumatic stress disorder.
Adapted from Sidney Werkman, M.D.

than of separation from parental figures. School refusal is a frequent symptom in separation anxiety disorder, but is not pathognomonic of it. Children with other diagnoses, such as specific phobias, or social anxiety disorder, or fear of failure in school because of learning disorder, may also lead to school refusal. When school refusal occurs in an adolescent, the severity of the dysfunction is generally greater than when it emerges in a young child. Similar and distinguishing characteristics of childhood separation anxiety disorder, generalized anxiety disorder, and social anxiety disorder are presented in Table 27.13a–1.

COURSE AND PROGNOSIS

The course and the prognosis of separation anxiety disorder, generalized anxiety disorder, and social anxiety disorder are varied and are related to the age of onset, the duration of the symptoms, and the development of comorbid anxiety and depressive disorders. Young children who can maintain attendance in school, after-school activities, and peer relationships generally have a better prognosis than children or adolescents who refuse to attend school and withdraw from social activities. The large multisite randomized clinical trial, CAMS, provided acute treatment for children and adolescents with one or more anxiety disorders with sertraline medication alone, CBT alone, or both together, and found that predictors of future remission included younger age of initiation of treatment, lower severity of anxiety, absence of a comorbid depressive or anxiety disorder, and the absence of social anxiety disorder as the primary anxiety disorder being treated. A follow-up study of children and adolescents with mixed anxiety disorders over a 3-year period reported that up to 82 percent no longer met criteria for the anxiety disorder at follow-up. Of the group followed, 96 percent of those with separation anxiety disorder were remitted at follow-up. Most children who recovered did so within the first year. Early age of onset and later age at diagnosis were factors in this study that predicted slower recovery. Close to one-third of the group studied, however, had developed another psychiatric disorder within the follow-up period, and 50 percent of these children developed another anxiety disorder. Studies have shown a significant overlap between separation anxiety disorder and depressive disorders. In cases with multiple comorbidities, the prognosis is more guarded. Longitudinal data indicate that some children with severe school refusal continue to resist attending school into adolescence and remain impaired for many years.

TREATMENT

The treatment of child and adolescent separation anxiety disorder, generalized anxiety disorder, and social anxiety disorder are often considered together, given the frequent comorbidity and overlapping symptomatology of these disorders. A multimodal comprehensive treatment approach usually includes psychotherapy, most often CBT, family education, family psychosocial intervention, and pharmacological interventions, such as SSRIs. The best evidence-based treatments for childhood anxiety disorders include CBT and SSRIs. The comparative efficacy of CBT, SSRI medication, and their combination (CBT + SSRI) in the treatment of childhood anxiety disorders was investigated in the National Institute of Mental Health (NIMH)–funded CAMS. This double-blind, placebo-controlled, multisite study included 488 children and adolescents with separation anxiety disorder, generalized anxiety disorder, or social anxiety disorder, who were randomly assigned to be treated with either CBT alone, SSRI medication (sertraline) alone, both CBT and sertraline, or placebo. After an acute treatment phase of 12 weeks, those in the combined CBT + sertraline group had an 80.7 percent response rate of much or very much improved on the clinical global improvement (CGI) rating. Response rates for the CBT-only and sertraline-only groups were 59.7 percent and 54.9 percent, respectively. Placebo response was 23.7 percent. Over time, during open follow-up, the combination of CBT plus sertraline continued to provide the most efficacy. All three treatments—CBT, sertraline, and their combination—were superior to placebo, and thus effective treatments in childhood anxiety, but combined treatment was most likely to help children and adolescents with anxiety disorders. A trial of CBT may be applied first, if available, when a child is able to function sufficiently to engage in daily activities while obtaining this treatment. For a child with severe impairment, however, a combination of treatments is recommended. BT is widely accepted as first-line evidence-based treatment for childhood anxiety disorders. A meta-analysis reviewed 16 randomized controlled trials of CBT for childhood anxiety disorders and found CBT to be consistently superior to a wait list control group or a psychological placebo group. Exposure-based CBT has received the most empiric support among psychotherapeutic interventions for anxiety disorders in youth and has been shown to be superior to wait list control groups in reducing impairment and symptoms of anxiety.

Several psychosocial interventions have been designed specifically for anxiety disorders in young children. A randomized clinical trial of CBT for 4- to 7-year-old children was administered via a manualized intervention called "Being Brave: A Program for Coping with Anxiety for Young Children and Their Parents." This manual was loosely modeled after the manualized Coping Cat program. The intervention utilized a combination of parent-only sessions and child-and-parent sessions. Response rate, measured as much or very much improved on the CGI scale for anxiety, was 69 percent among completers versus 32 percent of the wait-list controls. The treated children showed significantly better CGI improvement on social anxiety disorder, separation anxiety disorder, and specific phobia, but not on generalized anxiety disorder. This treatment, a developmentally modified parent–child CBT, shows promise in young children.

Coaching approach behavior and Leading by Modeling (the CALM program) is an intervention aimed at treating anxiety disorders in children younger than 7 years of age, who are too young to effectively engage in traditional CBT. The CALM program draws on previous work with children aged 2 to 7 years through interventions that target a child's undesired behavior by modifying parents' behavior, called PCIT. The CALM program is a 12-session manual-based intervention that provides live, individualized coaching via a bug-in-the-ear receiver worn by the parent during sessions. It incorporates exposure tasks and promotes "brave" behavior with parent coaching. A pilot study using the CALM program with nine patients with a mean age of 5.4 years found that all treatment completers (seven patients and families) were rated as global responders, and all but one showed functional improvement. Adapting the PCIT model for anxiety disorders in young children appears to be a promising approach to treating anxiety in early childhood.

A meta-analysis of randomized controlled trials of antidepressant agents for childhood anxiety provides evidence that multiple SSRIs, including fluvoxamine (Luvox), fluoxetine (Prozac), sertraline (Zoloft), and paroxetine (Paxil) are efficacious in the treatment of childhood anxiety. Based on this evidence, SSRIs are the first choice of medication in the treatment of anxiety disorders in children and adolescents.

A large, multisite investigation by the NIMH (Research Units in Pediatric Psychopharmacology [RUPP]) confirmed the safety and efficacy of fluvoxamine in the treatment of childhood separation anxiety disorder, generalized anxiety disorder, and social phobia. This double-blind, placebo-controlled study of 128 children and adolescents revealed that 76 percent of children in the group treated with fluvoxamine showed significant improvement compared with 29 percent of those in the placebo group. Response to medication was noticeable after only 2 weeks of treatment. Fluvoxamine dosages ranged from 50 to 250 mg per day in children and up to 300 mg per day in adolescents. Children and adolescents with less comorbid depressive symptoms had the best response. Children and adolescents who responded to this medication were continued on fluvoxamine for a period of 6 months, and almost all of them continued to be responders at the 6-month mark.

Several other randomized clinical trials have also supported the efficacy of SSRIs in the treatment of child and adolescent anxiety disorders. A randomized, controlled trial found fluoxetine, at a dose of 20 mg per day, to be safe and effective for children with these disorders, with minor side effects including gastrointestinal distress, headache, and drowsiness. In addition, a randomized clinical trial for the treatment of generalized anxiety disorder in children lends support for the efficacy of sertraline (Zoloft). Finally, a large industry randomized clinical trial of paroxetine (Paxil) in the treatment of children with social phobia found that paroxetine was associated with response in 78 percent of children treated. Paroxetine was utilized at a dosage range of 10 to 50 mg per day.

The FDA has placed a "black box" warning on antidepressants, including all of the SSRI agents, used in the treatment of any childhood disorder, because of concerns about increased suicidality; however, no individual childhood anxiety study has found a statistically significant increase in suicidal thoughts or behaviors.

Tricyclic drugs are not currently recommended due to their potentially serious cardiac adverse effects. β-Adrenergic receptor antagonists, such as propranolol (Inderal), and buspirone (BuSpar) have been used clinically in children with anxiety disorders, but currently no data support their efficacy. Diphenhydramine (Benadryl) may be used in the short term to control sleep disturbances in children with anxiety disorders. Open trials and one double-blind, placebo-controlled study suggested that alprazolam (Xanax), a benzodiazepine, may help to control anxiety symptoms in separation anxiety disorder. Clonazepam (Klonopin) has been studied in open trials and may be useful in controlling symptoms of panic and other anxiety symptoms.

Although SSRIs and CBT alone and in combination have demonstrated efficacy in the treatment of anxiety disorders in youth, approximately 20 to 35 percent of children and adolescents with anxiety disorders do not appear to benefit. Several novel agents have been suggested as potential treatments, some based on their effect on the *N*-methyl-D-aspartate (NMDA) system. For example, D-cycloserine (DCS), currently FDA approved in the treatment of pediatric tuberculosis, is a partial receptor agonist of the NMDA system and is hypothesized to augment the benefits of exposure treatment for phobias. Some evidence suggests that DCS may increase the speed of exposure interventions; however, long-term gains have not been proven. Riluzole is an antiglutamatergic agent that decreases glutamatergic transmission by inhibiting glutamate release and inactivation of sodium channels in cortical neurons, and blocking GABA reuptake. Due to its antiglutamatergic effects, Riluzole has been postulated to provide augmentation in the treatment of OCD and generalized anxiety disorder. Another agent, memantine, an NMDA receptor antagonist, with FDA approval in the treatment of Alzheimer's disease, has been hypothesized to decrease anxiety due to its influence on the glutamatergic system. Published case reports have provided mixed results.

Although most childhood anxiety disorders wax and wane over time, school refusal associated with separation anxiety disorder can be viewed as a psychiatric emergency. A comprehensive treatment plan involves the child, the parents, and the child's peers and school. Family interventions are critical in the management of separation anxiety disorder, especially in children who refuse to attend school, so that firm encouragement of school attendance is maintained while appropriate support is also provided. When a return to a full school day is overwhelming, a program should be arranged so the child can progressively increase the time spent at school. Graded contact with an object of anxiety is a form of behavior modification that can be applied to any type of separation anxiety. Some severe cases of school refusal require hospitalization. Cognitive-behavioral modalities include exposure to feared separations and cognitive strategies, such as coping self-statements aimed at increasing a sense of autonomy and mastery.

In summary, evidence-based treatments for anxiety disorders have focused SSRIs and CBT. SSRIs have been shown to be both safe and efficacious in the treatment of childhood anxiety disorders; however, in severe disorders, the evidence suggests that optimal treatment is to provide both CBT and SSRI antidepressant agents simultaneously.

27.13b Selective Mutism

Selective mutism, believed to be related to social anxiety disorder, although an independent disorder, is characterized in a child by persistent lack of speaking in one or more specific social situations, most typically, the school setting. A child with selective mutism may remain completely silent or near silent, in some cases only whispering in a school setting. Although selective mutism often begins before age 5 years, it may not be apparent until the child is expected to speak or read aloud in school. Current conceptualization of selective mutism highlights a convergence of underlying social anxiety, along with an increased likelihood of speech and language problems leading to the failure to speak in certain situations. Typically, children with the disorder are silent during stressful situations, whereas some may verbalize almost inaudibly single-syllable words. Despite an increased risk for delayed speech and language acquisition in children with selective mutism, children with this disorder are fully capable of speaking competently when not in a socially anxiety-producing situation. Some children with the disorder will communicate with eye contact or nonverbal gestures but not verbally when at school. Otherwise, children with selective mutism speak fluently at home and in many familiar settings. Selective mutism is believed to be related to social anxiety disorder because of its expression primarily in selective social situations.

EPIDEMIOLOGY

The prevalence of selective mutism varies with age, with younger children at increased risk for the disorder. According to the DSM-5, the point prevalence of selective mutism using clinic or school samples has been found to range between 0.03 and 1 percent, depending on whether a clinical or community sample is studied. A large epidemiologic survey in the United Kingdom reported a prevalence rate of selective mutism to be 0.69 percent in children 4 to 5 years of age, which dropped to 0.8 percent near the end of the same academic year. Another survey in the United Kingdom identified 0.06 percent of 7-year-olds as having selective mutism. Young children are more vulnerable to the disorder than older ones. Selective mutism appears to be more common in girls than in boys. Clinical reports suggest that many young children spontaneously "outgrow" this disorder as they get older; the longitudinal course of the disorder remains to be studied.

ETIOLOGY

Genetic Contribution

Selective mutism may have many of the same etiologic factors leading to the emergence of social anxiety disorder. In contrast to other childhood anxiety disorders, however, children with selective mutism are at greater risk for delayed onset of speech or speech abnormalities that may be contributory. However, in addition to the speech and language factor, one survey found that 90 percent of children with selective mutism met diagnostic criteria for social phobia. These children showed high levels of social anxiety without notable psychopathology in other areas, according to parent and teacher ratings. Thus, selective mutism may not represent a distinct disorder, but may be better conceptualized as a subtype of social phobia. Maternal anxiety, depression, and heightened dependence needs are often noted in families of children with selective mutism, similar to families with children who exhibit other anxiety disorders.

Parental Interactions

Maternal overprotection and anxiety disorders in parents may exacerbate interactions that unwittingly reinforce selective mutism behaviors. Children with selective mutism usually speak freely at home, and only exhibit symptoms when under social pressure either in school or other social situations. Some children seem predisposed to selective mutism after early emotional or physical trauma; thus, some clinicians refer to the phenomenon as *traumatic mutism* rather than selective mutism.

Speech and Language Factors

Selective mutism is conceptualized as an anxiety-based refusal to speak; however, a higher than expected proportion of children with the disorder have a history of speech delay. An interesting finding suggests that children with selective mutism are at higher risk for a disturbance in auditory processing, which may interfere with efficient processing of incoming sounds. For the most part, however, speech and language problems in children with selective mutism are subtle and cannot account for the diagnosis of selective mutism.

DIAGNOSIS AND CLINICAL FEATURES

The diagnosis of selective mutism is not difficult to make after it is clear that a child has adequate language skills in some environments but not in others. The mutism may have developed gradually or suddenly after a disturbing experience. The age of onset can range from 4 to 8 years. Mute periods are most commonly manifested in school or outside the home; in rare cases, a child is mute at home but not in school. Children who exhibit selective mutism may also have symptoms of separation anxiety disorder, school refusal, and delayed language acquisition. Because social anxiety is almost always present in children with selective mutism, behavioral disturbances, such as temper tantrums and oppositional behaviors, may also occur in the home. Compared to children with other anxiety disorders, except social anxiety disorder, children with selective mutism tend to have less social competence and more social anxiety.

Janine is a 6-year-old Chinese-American first-grade girl who lives with her biological mother, father, and siblings. Janine's parents reported a 2-year history of not speaking at school, beginning in kindergarten, or to any children or adults outside of her family, despite speaking normally at home. At home, she reportedly is animated and quite talkative with her immediate family and a few young cousins as well. Although she speaks to adult relatives outside of her immediate family, her communication is often limited to one-word responses to their questions. By her parents' report, Janine also exhibits extreme social anxiety, to the point of "freezing" in certain situations when attention is focused on her. At the time of her evaluation, Janine had not received prior treatment. Janine speaks fluent English, as well as Mandarin, and, according to her parents, met all developmental milestones on time and appears to have above-average intelligence. They also reported that Janine enjoys dancing, singing, and imaginative play with her sisters.

During initial evaluation, Janine failed to make eye contact or respond verbally to the intake clinician. Janine's parents reported that this behavior is typical of her when in a new situation but that she communicates nonverbally and makes eye contact with most people once she "gets to know them." On request, Janine's parents provided a videotaped recording of Janine playing at home with her sisters. In the video, Janine was animated and was speaking spontaneously and fluently without obvious impairment. Janine received diagnoses of selective mutism and social anxiety disorder. CBT was recommended at this time.

CBT was initiated and the therapist instructed Janine and her mother to come up with lists of easy, medium, and most difficult "speaking" situations and lists of small, medium, and large rewards. These lists then became the basis for assignments for exposures and reinforcement for speaking tasks that gradually increased in difficulty. BT sessions included time with Janine and her mother together to review past and future assignments and time with Janine and the therapist alone.

When treatment began, Janine did not communicate at all verbally or nonverbally with the therapist. The therapist gradually developed a rapport with Janine utilizing less stressful tasks such as whispering to her mother with the therapist in the corner, then nodding yes or no, pointing, whispering to a stuffed animal, whispering to her mother while facing the therapist, and eventually responding to the therapist directly. The therapist used animal puppets to enable Janine to "warm up" without talking directly to the therapist. After three sessions, Janine began to speak to the therapist in a quiet whisper. Janine received stickers for completing each speaking assignment, and, after filling up the sticker charts, she received rewards (a small toy or treat from reward list).

Janine was also given assignments that involved her teacher and classmates. These were implemented in gradual fashion and included waving to the teacher, playing an audiotape of her saying "hello" to the teacher, whispering "hello" to the teacher, speaking "hello" to the teacher in a regular voice, and so on. After approximately 14 sessions, Janine succeeded in speaking a complete sentence in front of the class when called on and spoke to her teacher in front of several other students.

During the last few sessions, Janine's mother took an increasingly active role in assigning and following up on speaking assignments. When Janine entered the 2nd grade it took only a few days for her to speak to her teacher and to most peers in class. After completion of therapy, Janine's mother continued to monitor Janine's speaking behaviors and to promote speaking in new situations by encouraging (and rewarding) Janine's gradual successes with novel people and situations. *(Adapted from case material from Lindsey Bergman, Ph.D. and John Piacentini, Ph.D.)*

PATHOLOGY AND LABORATORY EXAMINATION

No specific laboratory measures are useful in the diagnosis or treatment of selective mutism.

DIFFERENTIAL DIAGNOSIS

Differential diagnosis of children who are silent in social situations emphasizes ruling out communications disorder, ASD, and social anxiety disorder, which may be diagnosed comorbidly. Once it is confirmed that the child is fully capable of speaking in certain situations, which are comfortable, but not in school and other social situations, an anxiety-related disorder comes to mind. Shy children may exhibit a transient muteness in new, anxiety-provoking situations. These children often have histories of not speaking in the presence of strangers and of clinging to their mothers. Most children who are mute on entering school improve spontaneously and may be described as having transient adaptation shyness. Selective mutism must also be distinguished from mental retardation, pervasive developmental disorders, and expressive language disorder. In these disorders, the symptoms are widespread, and no one situation exists in which the child communicates normally; the child may have an inability, rather than a refusal, to speak. In mutism secondary to conversion disorder, the mutism is pervasive. Children introduced into an environment in which a different language is spoken may be reticent to begin using the new language. Selective mutism should be diagnosed only when children also refuse to converse in their native language and when they have gained communicative competence in the new language but refuse to speak it.

COURSE AND PROGNOSIS

Children with selective mutism are often excessively shy during preschool years, but the onset of the full disorder is usually not evident until age 5 or 6 years. Many very young children with early symptoms of selective mutism in a transitional period when entering preschool have a spontaneous improvement over a number of months and never fulfill criteria for the disorder. A common pattern for a child with selective mutism is to speak almost exclusively at home with the nuclear family but not elsewhere, especially not at school. Consequently, a child with selective mutism may have academic difficulties, or even failure due to a lack of participation. Children with selective mutism are typically shy, anxious, and at increased risk for a depressive disorder. Many children with early-onset selective mutism remit with or without treatment. Recent data suggest that fluoxetine (Prozac) may influence the course of selective mutism, and treatment enhances recovery. Children in whom the disorder persists often have difficulty forming social relationships. Teasing and scapegoating by peers may cause them to refuse to go to school. Some children with any form of severe social anxiety are characterized by rigidity, compulsive traits, negativism, temper tantrums, and oppositional and aggressive behavior at home. Other children with the disorder tolerate the feared situation by communicating with gestures, such as nodding, shaking the head, and saying "Uh-huh" or "No." In one follow-up study, about one-half of children with selective mutism improved within 5 to 10 years. Children who do not improve by age 10 years appear to have a long-term course and a worse prognosis. As many as one-third of children with selective mutism, with or without treatment, may develop other psychiatric disorders, particularly other anxiety disorders and depression.

TREATMENT

A multimodal approach using psychoeducation for the family, CBT, and SSRIs as needed is recommended. Preschool children may also benefit from a therapeutic nursery. For school-age children, individual CBT is recommended as a first-line treatment. Family education and cooperation are beneficial. Published data on the successful treatment of children with selective mutism is scant, yet solid evidence indicates that children with social anxiety disorder respond to various SSRIs and, currently, CBT treatments are under investigation in a multisite, randomized placebo-controlled trial of children with anxiety disorders.

A recent report of 21 children with selective mutism treated in an open trial with fluoxetine suggested that this medication may be effective for childhood selective mutism. Reports have confirmed the efficacy of fluoxetine in the treatment of adult social phobia and in at least one double-blind, placebo-controlled study using fluoxetine with children with mutism. A large NIMH-funded study of anxiety disorders in children and adolescents called Research Units in Pediatric Psychopharmacology (RUPP), has shown distinct superiority of fluvoxamine over placebo in the treatment of a variety of childhood anxiety disorders. Children with selective mutism may benefit similarly to those with social phobia given the current belief that it is a subgroup of social phobia. SSRI medications that have been shown in randomized, placebo-controlled trials to have benefit in the treatment of children with social phobia include fluoxetine (20 to 60 mg per day), fluvoxamine (Luvox; 50 to 300 mg per day), sertraline (Zoloft; 25 to 200 mg per day), and paroxetine (Paxil; 10 to 50 mg per day).

▲ 27.14 Obsessive-Compulsive Disorder in Childhood and Adolescence

Childhood OCD is characterized by recurrent intrusive thoughts associated with anxiety or fear and/or repetitive purposeful mental or behavioral actions aimed at reducing fears and tensions caused by obsessions. Data suggest that up to 25 percent of cases of OCD have their onset by 14 years of age. The overall clinical presentation of OCD in youth is similar to that in adults; however, compared to adults, children and adolescents with OCD more often do not consider their obsessional thoughts or repetitive behaviors to be unreasonable. In milder cases of OCD, a trial of CBT is recommended as an initial intervention. OCD in youth is often treated successfully with SSRIs or CBT alone, or in combination. The results of a large-scale, randomized, placebo-controlled study called the Pediatric OCD Treatment Study (POTS), demonstrated that the greatest rates of remission in pediatric OCD are achieved with a combination of both serotonergic agents and CBT treatment.

The American Psychiatric Association's *Diagnostic and Statistical Manual of Mental Disorders, Fifth Edition* (DSM-5) removed OCD from its former category of Anxiety Disorders and placed it in a new category called Obsessive-Compulsive and Related Disorders, with related disorders such as trichotillomania (hair pulling disorder), hoarding disorder, body dysmorphic disorder, and excoriation (skin picking) disorder. Nevertheless the relationship between OCD and other anxiety disorders remains significant and supported by research.

EPIDEMIOLOGY

OCD is common among children and adolescents, with a point prevalence of about 0.5 percent and a lifetime prevalence of 2 to 4 percent. The rate of OCD among youth rises exponentially with increasing age, with rates of 0.3 percent in children between the ages of 5 and 7 years, rising to rates between 0.6 and 1 percent among teens. According to the DSM-5, the prevalence of OCD in the United States is 1.2 percent, with a slightly higher rate in females. Rates of OCD among adolescents are greater than those for schizophrenia or bipolar disorder. Among young children with OCD there appears to be a slight male predominance, which diminishes with age.

ETIOLOGY

Genetic Factors

Genetic factors have been estimated to contribute significantly to the development of OCD in early-onset illness. The rate of OCD among first-degree relatives of children and adolescents who develop OCD is ten times greater than for the general population. Twin studies have shown that the concordance rates for OCD is higher for monozygotic twins (0.57) than for dizygotic twins (0.22); however, nongenetic factors play a role that may be equal to or greater than genetic contributions in some cases. OCD is a heterogeneous disorder that has been recognized for decades to run in families. In addition, the presence of subclinical symptom constellations in family members appears to breed true. Genetic linkage studies have revealed evidence of susceptibility loci on chromosomes 1q, 3q, 6q, 7p, 9p, 10p, and 15q. The OCD collaborative genetics study found that the *Sapap3* gene was associated with grooming disorders and may be a promising candidate gene for OCD. There is evidence that the glutamate receptor–modulating genes may also be associated with and play a role in the emergence of OCD. Family studies have suggested a relationship between OCD and tic disorders such as Tourette's syndrome. OCD and tic disorders are believed to share susceptibility factors, which may include both genetic and nongenetic factors.

Neuroimmunology

Immunological contributions to the emergence of OCD have been hypothesized to be related to an inflammatory process in the basal ganglia associated with an immune response to a systemic infection that may trigger OCD and tics. A prototype of this hypothesis has been the controversial association of OCD symptoms in a small subgroup of children and adolescents following documented exposure to or infection with *group A β-hemolytic streptococcus* (GABHS). Under this hypothesis, cases of infection-triggered OCD have been termed Pediatric Autoimmune Neuropsychiatric Disorders Associated with Streptococcus (PANDAS), and are believed to parallel an autoimmune process leading to a movement disorder much like Sydenham's chorea following rheumatic fever. Some evidence from MRI studies has documented a proportional relationship between the size of the basal ganglia and the severity of OCD symptoms in a small sample. GABHS may be one of many physiological stressors that can lead to an increase or emergence of OCD or tics; however, a prospective longitudinal study of youth with PANDAS followed over a 2-year period found no evidence of a temporal association between GABHS infections and OCD symptom exacerbations in children who met the criteria for PANDAS. The presentation of OCD in children and adolescents due to acute exposure to GABHS represents a minority of OCD cases in youth and remains controversial.

Neurochemistry

The evidence that SSRIs diminish symptoms of OCD, along with findings of altered sensitivity to the acute administration of 5-hydroxytryptamine (5-HT) agonists in individuals with OCD, supports the probability of serotonin's role in OCD. In addition, the dopamine system is believed to be influential in OCD, especially in light of the frequent comorbidity of OCD with tic disorders in childhood. Clinical observations have indicated that obsessions and compulsions may be exacerbated during the treatment of ADHD (another frequent OCD comorbidity) with stimulant agents. Dopamine antagonists administered along with SSRIs may augment effectiveness of SSRIs in the treatment of OCD. Evidence suggests that multiple neurotransmitter systems may play a role in OCD.

Neuroimaging

Both CT and MRI of untreated children and adults with OCD have revealed smaller volumes of basal ganglia segments compared to normal controls. A meta-analysis of voxel-based morphometry (VBM) to assess gray matter density compared 343 OCD patients with 318 healthy controls, and found that gray matter density in OCD patients was smaller in parietofrontal cortical regions (including the supramarginal gyrus, the dorsolateral prefrontal cortex, and the orbitofrontal cortex), but larger in the basal ganglia (the putamen) and anterior prefrontal cortex compared to healthy controls. Increased gray matter volume in the basal ganglia of patients with OCD has been reported in other studies as well. These structural abnormalities in the prefrontal–basal ganglia are likely to be integrally involved in the pathophysiology of OCD. It is not clear whether the increases in gray matter in individuals with OCD occur before or after the symptoms emerge. In children, evidence suggests that thalamic volume is increased. Adult studies have provided evidence of hypermetabolism of frontal cortical–striatal–thalamocortical networks in untreated individuals with OCD. Of interest, imaging studies before and after treatment have revealed that both medication and behavioral interventions lead to a reduction of orbit frontal and caudate metabolic rates in children and adults with OCD.

DIAGNOSIS AND CLINICAL FEATURES

Children and adolescents with obsessions or compulsions are often referred for treatment due to the excessive time that they devote to their intrusive thoughts and repetitive rituals. For some children, their compulsive rituals are perceived as reasonable responses to their extreme fears and anxieties. Nevertheless, they are aware of their discomfort and inability to carry out usual daily activities in a timely manner due to the compulsions, such as getting ready to leave their homes to go to school each morning.

The most commonly reported obsessions in children and adolescents include extreme fears of contamination—exposure to dirt, germs, or disease—followed by worries related to harm befalling themselves, family members, or fear of harming others due to losing control over aggressive impulses. Also commonly reported are obsessional needs for symmetry or exactness, hoarding, and excessive religious or moral concerns. Typical compulsive rituals among children and adolescents involve cleaning, checking, counting, repeating behaviors, or arranging items. Associated features in children and adolescents with OCD include avoidance, indecision, doubt, and a slowness to complete tasks. In most cases of OCD among youth, obsessions and compulsions are present. According to the DSM-5, diagnosis of OCD is identical to that of adults, with the note that young children may not be able to articulate the aims of their compulsions in diminishing their anxiety. The DSM-5 has also added the following specifiers: with good, fair, poor, or absent insight; that is, the greater the belief in the OCD obsessions and compulsions, the poorer the insight. An additional specifier indicates whether the individual has a current or past history of a tic disorder. Many children and adolescents who develop OCD have an insidious onset and may hide their symptoms as long as possible so that their rituals will not be challenged or disrupted. A minority of children, particularly males with early onset may have a rapid unfolding of multiple symptoms within a few months. OCD is commonly found to be comorbid with anxiety disorders, ADHD, and tic disorders, especially Tourette's syndrome. Children with comorbid OCD and tic disorders are more likely to exhibit counting, arranging, or ordering compulsions and less likely to manifest excessive washing and cleaning compulsions. The high comorbidity of OCD, Tourette's syndrome, and ADHD has led investigators to postulate a common genetic vulnerability to all three of these disorders. It is important to search for comorbidity in children and adolescents with OCD so that optimal treatments can be administered.

Jason, a 12-year-old boy in the sixth grade, was brought for evaluation by his parents, who expressed concerns over his repeated questions and anxiety regarding developing acquired immunodeficiency syndrome (AIDS). Jason was a high-functioning and well-adjusted boy who abruptly began to exhibit extremely disruptive behaviors related to his fears of AIDS approximately 2 to 3 months before the evaluation. Jason's new behaviors included relentless concerns about contracting illness, washing rituals, repeated expressions of uncertainty over his own behavior, seeking reassurance, repeating rituals, and avoidance.

Specifically, Jason repeatedly expressed his fear and belief that he was exposed to human immunodeficiency virus (HIV) through exposure to multiple strangers who were infected. For example, while riding in the car, if Jason saw a stranger from the window who appeared to him to be poor or ill kempt, he experienced a surge of extreme anxiety and obsessively agonized about whether the stranger could have AIDS and had exposed him to it. Despite his parents' reassurances about his safety and lack of exposure to illness, Jason insisted on vigorously washing himself for approximately one hour each time he reached home after being out. Jason continually expressed doubts about his own behavior. He often asked his parents, "Did I use the s___ word? Did I use the f___ word?" Reassurance was only slightly calming. Jason, previously an excellent student, began to lose the ability to focus on schoolwork. While reading passages from assigned materials, Jason frequently experienced severe anxiety, wondering if he had missed a word or misunderstood the sentence, and proceeded to reread the material. Completing a page of written material began to take Jason 30 to 60 minutes. Over several weeks, he was less and less able to complete assignments, following which, he became very distressed over his deteriorating grades.

During Jason's evaluation, his family history suggested that Jason's older sister had experienced a period in which she too had similar but milder anxieties, with less interference in functioning, and she had never received any treatment for those symptoms.

At the intake interview, Jason presented as a preoccupied and sad boy who was cooperative with questioning. He did not volunteer much information, and he allowed his parents to recount the extent of his symptoms. Jason believed that his relentless concerns were well founded, and that he required repeated reassurance from his parents in order to continue his daily activities. Jason met full diagnostic criteria for OCD. Symptoms of depression were present but not sufficient for major depressive disorder.

CBT was initiated; however, Jason was so fearful of deviating from his rituals that he was unable to participate fully in his treatment, and he became despondent about his future. Jason refused to go to school due to his increasing distress associated with reading and his shame regarding his diminishing academic performance. Given his limited progress during the first 2 months of CBT, fluoxetine (Prozac) was added and increased up to 40 mg per day. Over a 3-week period some improvement was noted, and Jason was more amenable to cooperating with his CBT treatment. CBT and SSRI treatment was continued over the next 3 months on a regular basis. Over time, Jason finally began to show some flexibility with his rituals, and he was able to decrease the amount of time he spent with rituals. Once he had found some relief from his symptoms, Jason was able to focus more on his schoolwork and his family life. Follow-up over the next year was positive; Jason had maintained his gains from treatment, with only minimal interference from residual OCD symptoms. Jason's academic achievement improved, he was able to engage in activities with friends, and he spent almost no time preoccupied with obsessional thoughts of illness and cleansing rituals. *(Adapted from a case courtesy of James T. McCracken, M.D.)*

PATHOLOGY AND LABORATORY EXAMINATION

No specific laboratory measures are useful in the diagnosis of OCD.

Even when the onset of obsessions or compulsions appears to be associated with a recent infection with GABHS, antigens, and antibodies to the bacteria do not indicate a causal relationship between GABHS and OCD.

DIFFERENTIAL DIAGNOSIS

Developmentally appropriate rituals in the play and behavior of young children should not be confused with OCD in that age group. Preschoolers often engage in ritualistic play and request a predictable routine such as bathing, reading stories, or selecting the same stuffed animal at bedtime, to promote a sense of security and comfort. These routines allay developmentally normal fears and lead to reasonable completion of daily activities. On the other hand, obsessions or compulsions are driven by extreme fears, and they significantly interfere with daily function because of the excessive time that they consume and the extreme distress that ensues when they are interrupted. The rituals of preschoolers generally become less rigid by the time they enter grade school, and school-age children do not typically experience a surge of anxiety when they encounter small changes in their routine.

Children and adolescents with generalized anxiety disorder, separation anxiety disorder, and social phobia experience intense worries that are often expressed repeatedly; however, these are mundane compared to obsessions, which are often so extreme that they appear bizarre. A child with generalized anxiety disorder typically worries repeatedly about performance on academic examinations, whereas a child with OCD may experience repeated intrusive thoughts that he may harm someone he loves. The compulsions of OCD are not present in other anxiety disorders; however, children with ASDs often display repetitive behaviors that may resemble OCD. In contrast with the rituals of OCD, children with ASD are not responding to anxiety, but are more often exhibiting stereotyped behaviors that are self-stimulating or self-comforting.

Children and adolescents with tic disorders such as Tourette's syndrome may display complex repetitive compulsive behaviors similar to the compulsions seen in OCD. Children and adolescents with tic disorders, in fact, are at higher risk for the development of concurrent OCD.

Severe OCD symptoms may be difficult to distinguish from delusional symptoms, especially when the obsessions and compulsions are bizarre in nature. In most adults, and often in youth with OCD, despite an inability to control their obsessions or resist completing compulsions, insight into their lack of reasonableness is preserved. That is, an individual's conviction in their beliefs often does not reach delusional intensity. When insight is present, and underlying anxiety can be described, even in the face of significant dysfunction due to bizarre obsessions and compulsion, the diagnosis of OCD is suspect.

COURSE AND PROGNOSIS

OCD with an onset in childhood and adolescence is most often a chronic, waxing, and waning disorder with variability in severity and outcome. Follow-up studies suggest that up to 40 to 50 percent of children and adolescents recover from OCD with minimal residual symptoms. A study of childhood OCD treatment with sertraline resulted in close to 50 percent of participants experiencing complete remission, and partial remission in another 25 percent with a follow-up time of 1 year. Predictors of the best outcome were in those children and adolescents without comorbid disorders, including tic disorders and ADHD. A study of 142 children and adolescents with OCD followed over a period of 9 years at the Maudsley Hospital in England found 41 percent to have a persistence of OCD, with 40 percent exhibiting an additional psychiatric diagnosis at follow-up. The main predictor for persistent OCD was duration of illness at the time of initial assessment. Approximately half of the follow-up group was still receiving treatment, and half believed that they needed continued treatment.

Neuropsychological functioning may also play a role in outcome and prognosis. A study of 63 youth with OCD who completed the Rey–Osterrieth Complex Figure (ROCF) along with specific subtests of the *Wechsler Intelligence Scale for Children, Third Edition* (WISC-III), found that 5-minute recall accuracy from the ROCF was positively correlated with response to treatment, particularly CBT. These findings imply that poorer performance on the ROCF and poor response to CBT may be in part due to executive functioning difficulties and that treatment may need to be modified to account for these obstacles.

Overall, the prognosis is hopeful for most children and adolescents with mild to moderate OCD. In about 10 percent of cases, OCD may represent a prodrome of a psychotic disorder in children and adolescents. In youth with subthreshold OCD symptoms, there is a high risk of developing of the full OCD disorder within a period of 2 years. Childhood OCD has been shown to be responsive to available treatments, resulting in improvement, if not complete remission, in the majority of cases.

TREATMENT

CBT and SSRIs have both been shown to be efficacious treatments for OCD in youth. CBT geared toward children of varying ages is based on the principle of developmentally appropriate exposure to the feared stimuli coupled with response prevention, leading to diminishing anxiety over time on exposure to feared situations. CBT manuals have been developed to ensure that developmentally appropriate interventions are made and that comprehensive education is provided to the child and parents.

Treatment guidelines for children and adolescents with mild to moderate OCD recommend a trial of CBT prior to initiating medication. However, the POTS, a multisite National Institute of Health (NIH)–funded investigation of sertraline and CBT each alone, and in combination, for the treatment of childhood-onset OCD, revealed that the combination was superior to either treatment alone. Each treatment alone also provided encouraging levels of response. Mean daily dose of sertraline was 133 mg/day in the group administered the combination treatment, and 170 mg/day for the sertraline alone group. Improvement with pharmacologic intervention of childhood OCD usually occurs within 8 to 12 weeks of treatment. Most children and adolescents who experienced a remission with acute treatment using SSRIs were still responsive over a period of a year. Among youth with OCD who obtain partial response to a therapeutic trial of SSRI treatment, augmentation with a short-term OCD-specific CBT leads to a significantly greater response. Evidence shows that higher treatment expectations by patients and families are linked to better treatment response, greater compliance with home-based CBT assignments, less drop out of treatment, and reduced impairment.

In addition to individual CBT, both family and group CBT interventions have been shown to be efficacious in the treatment of childhood OCD. Family CBT (FCBT) intervention in the treatment of OCD in youth has been shown to increase response rates. A controlled comparison of FCBT and psychoeducation and relaxation (PRT) in 71 families of children with OCD showed that clinical remission rates in the FCBT group were significantly higher than those in the PRT group. The FCBT treatment reduced parent involvement and accommodation in their affected child's symptoms, which led to decreased symptomatology.

A randomized controlled study investigating web-camera delivered FCBT (W-CBT) compared to a waitlist condition assigned 31 families to one of the above conditions. Assessments were conducted immediately before and after treatment and at 3-month follow-up for the W-CBT group. The W-CBT group was superior to the waitlist control group on all primary outcome measures, with large effect sizes. Eighty-one percent of the W-CBT group responded compared to 13 percent of the waitlist group. The gains were maintained at the 3-month follow-up assessment. The authors conclude that W-CBT may be efficacious in the treatment of OCD in youth and may be a promising tool for future dissemination.

Exposure and response prevention (ERP), a common strategy within CBT already shown to be effective on an individual basis for OCD, was studied in a group format in youth with OCD in a community-based program. Group-based ERP was found to be effective in reducing OCD symptom severity and depressive symptoms, but not anxiety symptoms, in a naturalistic treatment setting for children with OCD and comorbid anxiety and/or depressive features.

Robust evidence of SSRI efficacy for OCD in youth has been shown through multiple randomized clinical trials. A meta-analysis of 13 studies of SSRIs, including sertraline, fluvoxamine, fluoxetine, and paroxetine have provided evidence of efficacy of SSRIs with a moderate effect size. A randomized controlled clinical trial of citalopram versus fluoxetine in youth with OCD found that citalopram was as safe and effective as fluoxetine for the treatment of OCD in children and adolescents. There have been no apparent differences in the rate of response for the individual SSRIs.

Currently, three SSRIs: sertraline (at least 6 years), fluoxetine (at least 7 years), and fluvoxamine (at least 8 years), as well as clomipramine (at least 10 years), have received FDA approval for the treatment of OCD in youth. The "black box" warning for antidepressants used in children for any disorder, including OCD is applicable, so that close monitoring for suicidal ideation or behavior is mandated when these agents are used in the treatment of childhood OCD.

Typical side effects that emerge with the use of SSRIs include insomnia, nausea, agitation, tremor, and fatigue. Dosage ranges for the various SSRIs found to have efficacy in randomized clinical trials are the following: fluoxetine (20 to 60 mg), sertraline (50 to 200 mg), fluvoxamine (up to 200 mg), and paroxetine (up to 50 mg).

Clomipramine was the first antidepressant studied in the treatment of OCD in childhood and the only tricyclic antidepressant that has FDA approval for the treatment of anxiety disorders in childhood. Clomipramine was found to be efficacious in doses up to 200 mg, or 3 mg/kg, whichever is less, and may be chosen for children or adolescents who cannot tolerate other SSRIs due to insomnia, significant appetite suppression, or activation. Nevertheless, clomipramine is not recommended as a first-line treatment due to its greater potential risks compared to other SSRIs, including cardiovascular risk of hypotension and arrhythmia, and seizure risk.

Pediatric patients with OCD who respond only partially to medications tend to have at least moderate to severe OCD symptoms, high ratings of global impairment and significant comorbidity even after their partial response to an adequate trial of medication. Augmentation strategies with medications to enhance serotonergic effects, such as with atypical antipsychotics (e.g., risperidone) have demonstrated increased response when partial response has been achieved with SSRIs. Aripiprazole augmentation in 39 adolescents with OCD who did not respond to two trials of monotherapy with SSRIs led to 59 percent of patients being rated as improved or very much improved. Patients who responded to aripiprazole were less impaired at baseline in functional impairment but not in clinical severity of their OCD. Aripiprazole final mean dose was 12.2 mg per day. This agent may be effective for pediatric OCD and warrants further controlled trials.

Given the lack of data on discontinuation, recommendations for maintaining medication such as stabilization, education about relapse risk, and tapering medication during the summer are likely in order to minimize academic compromise in case of relapse. For children and adolescents with more severe or multiple episodes of significant exacerbation of symptoms, treatment for more than a year is recommended. Overall, efficacy of treatment for children and adolescents with OCD is high with choices of SSRIs and CBT.

▲ 27.15 Early-Onset Schizophrenia

Early-onset schizophrenia comprises childhood-onset and adolescent-onset schizophrenia. Childhood-onset schizophrenia is a very rare and virulent form of schizophrenia now recognized as a progressive neurodevelopmental disorder. Childhood onset is characterized by a more chronic course, with severe social and cognitive consequences and increased negative symptoms compared to adult-onset schizophrenia. Childhood-onset schizophrenia is defined by an onset of psychotic symptoms before the age of 13 years, believed to represent a subgroup of patients with schizophrenia with an increased heritable etiology, and evidence of widespread abnormalities in the development of brain structures including the cerebral cortex, white matter, hippocampus, and cerebellum. Children diagnosed with childhood-onset schizophrenia have higher than normal rates of premorbid developmental abnormalities that appear to be nonspecific markers of abnormal brain development. Early-onset schizophrenia is defined as an onset of disease before the age of 18 years, including childhood-onset as well as adolescent-onset schizophrenia. Early-onset schizophrenia is associated with severe clinical course, poor psychosocial functioning, and increased severity of brain abnormality. Despite the more severe course, current evidence supports the efficacy of both psychosocial and pharmacological interventions in the management of childhood-onset and, particularly, adolescent-onset schizophrenia.

Children with childhood-onset schizophrenia have been shown to have more significant deficits in measures of IQ, memory, and tests of perceptuomotor skills compared with adolescent-onset schizophrenia. Increased impairment in childhood-onset schizophrenia of cognitive measures such as IQ, working memory, and perceptuomotor skills such deficits may be premorbid markers of illness, rather than sequelae, of the disorder. Although cognitive impairments are greater in younger patients with schizophrenia, clinical presentation of schizophrenia remains remarkably similar across the ages, and the diagnosis of childhood-onset schizophrenia is continuous with that in adolescents and adults, with one exception: in childhood-onset schizophrenia a failure to achieve expected social and academic functioning may replace deterioration in functioning. According to the American Psychiatric Association's *Diagnostic and Statistical Manual of Mental Disorders, Fifth Edition* (DSM-5), the diagnosis of schizophrenia includes an "active phase" of the illness, consisting of at least one of the following three symptoms: delusions, hallucinations, or disorganized speech, and at least one additional symptom present most of the time for a month. The additional symptom may be another one of the preceding three, or one of the following two symptoms: grossly disorganized or catatonic behavior, or negative symptoms (i.e., diminished emotional expression or avolition). In the active phase, symptoms are present for a significant amount of time during a single month and cause impairment. To meet full criteria for schizophrenia, continuous signs of disturbance must persist for at least 6 months. Social, academic, or occupational impairment must be present. In contrast to previous diagnostic criteria, the subtypes of schizophrenia (paranoid, disorganized, catatonic, undifferentiated, and residual) have been eliminated due to their lack of diagnostic validity and reliability. Instead, an eight-symptom "Clinician-Rated Dimensions of Psychosis Symptom Severity" scale for determining severity of psychosis across many psychotic illnesses is included in Section III of the DSM-5. Symptom domains rated in this scale include the following: hallucinations, delusions, disorganized speech, abnormal psychomotor behavior, negative symptoms (restricted emotional expression or avolition), impaired cognition, depression, and mania.

HISTORICAL PERSPECTIVE

Before the 1960s, the term *childhood psychosis* was applied to a heterogeneous group of children, many of whom exhibited ASD symptoms without hallucinations and delusions. In the late 1960s and 1970s, reports of children with evidence of a profound psychotic disturbance very early in life included observations of intellectual disabilities, social deficits, and severe communication and language impairments, and no family history of schizophrenia. Children whose psychoses emerged after the age of 5 years, however, more often exhibited auditory hallucinations, delusions, inappropriate affect, thought disorder, normal intellectual function, and a positive family history of schizophrenia.

In the 1980s, schizophrenia with childhood onset was formally separated from what was then termed autistic disorder, and currently termed ASD. The distinction of childhood schizophrenia from ASD reflected evidence accrued during the 1960s and 1970s showing a divergent clinical picture, family history, age of onset, and course between the two disorders. However, even after the separation of the disorders, controversy and confusion remained as to the distinctiveness in the long-term courses of these disorders. First, research documented a small group of children with ASD who developed schizophrenia in later childhood or adolescence. Second, many children with childhood-onset schizophrenia exhibit neurodevelopmental abnormalities, some of which are also evident in children with ASD. Children with ASD and those with childhood-onset schizophrenia are typically impaired in multiple areas of adaptive functioning from relatively early in life. However, in ASD, the onset is almost always before 3 years of age, whereas the onset of childhood-onset schizophrenia occurs before the age of 13 years, but most often is not recognizable in children until after the age of 3 years. Childhood-onset schizophrenia is significantly less frequent than adolescent-onset or onset in young adulthood, and few reports document cases of schizophrenia onset before 5 years of age. According to the DSM-5, schizophrenia can be diagnosed in the presence of ASD, provided that the diagnosis of schizophrenia is specifically differentiated from ASD.

EPIDEMIOLOGY

The frequency of childhood-onset schizophrenia is reported to be less than one case in about 40,000 children, whereas among adolescents between the ages of 13 and 18 years, the frequency of schizophrenia is increased by a factor of at least 50. Schizophrenia with childhood onset resembles the more severe, chronic, and treatment-refractory adult-onset schizophrenic subgroups, in that the same core phenomenological features are present; however, in childhood-onset schizophrenia, extremely high rates of comorbidities are present, including ADHD, depressive disorders, anxiety disorders, speech and language disorders, and motor disturbances. In adolescents, the prevalence of schizophrenia is estimated to be 50 times that in younger children, with probable rates of 1 to 2 per 1,000. Boys seem to have a slight preponderance among children diagnosed with schizophrenia, with an estimated ratio of about 1.67 boys to 1 girl. Boys often become identified at a younger age than girls do. Schizophrenia rarely is diagnosed in children younger than 5 years of age. The prevalence of schizophrenia among the parents of children with schizophrenia is about 8 percent, which is about twice the prevalence in the parents of patients with adult-onset schizophrenia.

ETIOLOGY

Childhood-onset schizophrenia is a neurodevelopmental disorder in which complex interactions between genes and the environment are presumed to result in abnormal early brain development. The consequences of the aberrant brain development in schizophrenia may not be fully evident until adolescence or early adulthood; however, data support the hypothesis that white matter abnormalities and disturbances in myelination in childhood, lead to abnormal connectivity between brain regions. The aberrant connectivity in various regions of the brain is believed to be an important contributing factor in the psychotic symptoms and cognitive deficits in childhood-onset schizophrenia.

Genetic Factors

Estimates of heritability for childhood-onset schizophrenia have been as high as 80 percent. The precise mechanisms of transmission of schizophrenia are still not well understood. Schizophrenia is known to be up to eight times more prevalent among first-degree relatives of those with schizophrenia than in the general population. Adoption studies of patients with adult-onset schizophrenia have shown that schizophrenia occurs in the biological relatives, not the adoptive relatives. Additional genetic evidence is supported by higher concordance rates for schizophrenia in monozygotic twins than in dizygotic twins. Higher rates of schizophrenia have been established among relatives of those with childhood-onset schizophrenia than in the relatives of those with adult-onset schizophrenia.

Endophenotype Markers for Childhood-Onset Schizophrenia

Currently, no reliable method can identify persons at the highest risk for schizophrenia in a given family. Neurodevelopmental abnormalities and higher-than-expected rates of neurological soft signs and impairments in sustaining attention and in strategies for information processing appear among children at high risk. Increased rates of disturbed communication styles are found in family members of individuals with schizophrenia. Reports have documented higher-than-expected neuropsychological deficits in attention, working memory, and premorbid IQ among children who later develop schizophrenia and its spectrum disorders.

Magnetic Resonance Imaging Studies

A National Institute of Mental Health (NIMH) prospective study of more than 100 patients with childhood-onset schizophrenia and their typically developing siblings has demonstrated progressive loss of gray matter, delayed and disrupted white matter growth, and a decline in cerebellar volume in those with childhood-onset schizophrenia. Although siblings of children with childhood-onset schizophrenia also showed some of these brain disruptions, the gray matter abnormalities were normalized over time in the siblings, indicating a protective mechanism in siblings that was not present in those children with childhood-onset schizophrenia. Furthermore, the hippocampal volume loss across the age span appears to be static among children with childhood-onset schizophrenia. An MRI NIMH study of more than 100 children with childhood-onset schizophrenia and their typically developing siblings, studied for about two decades, documented that in childhood-onset schizophrenia, progressive brain gray matter loss occurs continuously over time. This gray matter shrinkage occurs with ventricular increases, with a pattern of loss originating in the parietal region and proceeding frontally to dorsolateral prefrontal and temporal cortices, including superior temporal gyri. Studies of childhood-onset schizophrenia at the NIMH provided evidence that early loss of parietal gray matter followed by frontal and parietal gray matter loss is more pronounced in childhood-onset schizophrenia than in schizophrenia with later onset. Other research utilized diffusion tensor images from children with childhood-onset schizophrenia versus controls and found increased diffusivities in the posterior corona radiata in children with childhood-onset schizophrenia, which implicated abnormal connectivity with the parietal lobes. These results contrasted with findings among subjects with later onset of schizophrenia in whom there were more abnormalities in the frontal lobes.

DIAGNOSIS AND CLINICAL FEATURES

All of the symptoms included in adult-onset schizophrenia may be manifest in children and adolescents with the disorder. However, youth with schizophrenia are more likely to have a premorbid history of social rejection, poor peer relationships, clingy withdrawn behavior, and academic trouble than those with adult-onset schizophrenia. Some children with schizophrenia evaluated in middle childhood have early histories of delayed motor milestones and language acquisition similar to some symptoms of ASD.

The onset of schizophrenia in childhood is frequently insidious, starting with inappropriate affect or unusual behavior; it may take months or years for a child to meet all of the diagnostic criteria for schizophrenia.

Auditory hallucinations commonly occur in children with schizophrenia. The voices may reflect an ongoing critical commentary, or command hallucinations may instruct children to harm or kill themselves or others. Hallucinatory voices may sound human or animal, or "bizarre," for example, identified as "a computer in my head," martians, or the voice of someone familiar, such as a relative. The childhood-onset schizophrenia project at the NIMH found high rates across all hallucination modalities. However, there were unexpectedly high rates of tactile, olfactory, and visual hallucinations among this study group of patients with childhood-onset schizophrenia. Visual hallucinations were associated with lower IQ and earlier age at onset of disease. Visual hallucinations are often frightening; affected children may "see" images of the devil, skeletons, scary faces, or space creatures. Transient phobic visual hallucinations occur in severely anxious or traumatized children who do not develop major psychotic disorders. Visual, tactile, and olfactory hallucinations may be a marker of more severe psychosis.

Delusions occur in up to half of children and adolescents with schizophrenia, in various forms, including persecutory, grandiose, and religious. Delusions increase in frequency with increased age. Blunted or inappropriate affect appears almost universally in children with schizophrenia. Children with schizophrenia may giggle inappropriately or cry without being able to explain why. Formal thought disorders, including loosening of associations and thought blocking, are common features among youth with schizophrenia. Illogical thinking and poverty of thought are also often present. Unlike adults with schizophrenia, children with schizophrenia do not have poverty of speech content, but they speak less than other children of the same intelligence and are ambiguous in the way they refer to persons, objects, and events. The communication deficits observable in children with schizophrenia include unpredictably changing the topic of conversation without introducing the new topic to the listener (loose associations). Children with schizophrenia also exhibit illogical thinking and speaking and tend to underuse self-initiated repair strategies to aid in their communication. When an utterance is unclear or vague, normal children attempt to clarify their communication with repetitions, revision, and more detail. Children with schizophrenia, on the other hand, fail to aid communication with revision, fillers, or starting over. These deficits may be conceptualized as negative symptoms in childhood schizophrenia.

Although core phenomena for schizophrenia seem to be universal across the age span, a child's developmental level significantly influences the presentation of the symptoms. Delusions of young children are less complex, therefore, than those of older children, for example, age-appropriate content, such as animal imagery and monsters, is likely to be a source of delusional fear in young children. According to the DSM-5, a child with schizophrenia may experience deterioration of function, along with the emergence of psychotic symptoms, or the child may never achieve the expected level of functioning.

A 12-year-old 6th grade boy named Ian, with a longstanding history of social isolation, academic problems, and temper outbursts began to develop concerns that his parents might be poisoning his food. Over the next year, his symptoms progressed with increased suspiciousness and fearfulness, preoccupation with food, and beliefs that Satan was trying to communicate with him. Ian also appeared to be responding to auditory hallucinations that he believed were coming from the radio and television, which he found frightening and commanded him to harm his parents. Ian had also been informing his mother that their food had a strange smell and that's why he thought it was poisoned, and at night, he would see frightening figures in his room. During this time, his parents also observed bizarre behaviors, including talking and yelling to himself, perseverating about devils and demons, and finally, assaulting family members because he thought they were evil. On one occasion, Ian was found to be scratching himself with a kitchen knife in an effort to "please God." No predominant mood symptoms emerged, and there was no history of substance abuse found.

Developmentally, Ian was the product of a full-term pregnancy complicated by a difficult labor and forceps delivery. His early motor and speech milestones were each delayed by about 6 months; however, his pediatrician reassured his parents that this was within the limits of normal development. As a younger child, Ian tended to be quiet and socially awkward. His intellectual function was tested and was found to be in the average range; however, academic achievement testing was consistently below grade level. Ian remained lonely and isolated, and he had great difficulty making friends.

Ian has had no medical problems and his immunizations were up to date.

Ian's family psychiatric history was significant for depression in a maternal aunt and a completed suicide in a maternal great-grandparent.

Ian was sent by ambulance to the hospital for the first time from school when he tried to jump off a balcony on the second story of his school, in response to auditory hallucinations commanding him to kill himself. During his hospitalization his parents reluctantly consented to a trial of risperidone for him, and he was titrated up to 3 mg per day. His auditory hallucinations were moderately improved after 2 weeks of treatment; however, he continued to be suspicious and mistrustful of his physicians and family. Ian's family was very confused as to what had caused Ian's serious symptoms, and the hospital treatment team met with his parents multiple times during his hospitalization to reassure them that they had not caused his illness and that; their continued support might improve his chances of improvement. After discharge from the hospital, 30 days later, Ian was placed in a special education program, in a nonpublic school, and he was assigned a psychotherapist who met regularly with him individually and with his family. At the time of discharge from the hospital, Ian's symptoms had moderately improved, although he still had auditory hallucinations intermittently. Over the next 5 years subsequent to the onset of his illness, Ian had many exacerbations of his psychosis and he was hospitalized nine times, including placement in a long-term residential program. Ian had received trials of olanzapine, quetiapine, and aripiprazole, each of which seemed to lead to improvement for a period of time, after which he was no longer responsive to the medications. Ian continued to receive individual cognitive behavioral therapy and family therapy, and his family was very supportive. Even with these interventions, Ian's mental status continued to display tangential and disorganized thinking, paranoid delusions, loose associations, perseverative speech patterns, and a flat, at times inappropriate, affect. He had periods of time in which he resorted to pacing and muttering to himself, with no social interaction with others unless initiated by adults. Finally, Ian achieved significant improvement after being placed on clozapine (Clozaril) therapy, although he remained mildly symptomatic. *(Adapted from a case by Jon M. McClellan, M.D.)*

PATHOLOGY AND LABORATORY EXAMINATIONS

No specific laboratory tests are diagnostically specific for childhood-onset schizophrenia. EEG studies have not been helpful in distinguishing children with schizophrenia from other children. Although data exist to suggest that hyperprolinemia is associated with the risk of schizoaffective disorder due to an alteration on chromosome 22q11, no association of hyperprolinemia with childhood-onset schizophrenia has been identified.

DIFFERENTIAL DIAGNOSIS

One of the significant challenges in making a diagnosis of childhood-onset schizophrenia is that very young children who report hallucinations, apparent thought disorders, language delays, and poor ability to differentiate reality from fantasy may be manifesting phenomena better accounted for by other disorders such as posttraumatic stress disorder, or sometimes developmental immaturity, none of which evolve into a major psychotic illness.

Nevertheless, the differential diagnosis of childhood-onset schizophrenia includes ASD, bipolar disorders, depressive psychotic disorders, multicomplex developmental syndromes, drug-induced psychosis, and psychosis caused by organic disease states. Children with childhood-onset schizophrenia have been shown to have frequent comorbidities, including ADHD, oppositional defiant disorder, and major depression. Children with schizotypal personality disorder have some traits in common with children who meet diagnostic criteria for schizophrenia. Blunted affect, social isolation, eccentric thoughts, ideas of reference, and bizarre behavior can be seen in both disorders; however, in schizophrenia, overt psychotic symptoms, such as hallucinations, delusions, and incoherence, must be present at some point. Hallucinations alone, however, are not evidence of schizophrenia; patients must show either a deterioration of function or an inability to meet an expected developmental level to warrant the diagnosis of schizophrenia. Auditory and visual hallucinations can appear as self-limited events in nonpsychotic young children who are experiencing extreme stress or anxiety related to unstable home lives, abuse, or neglect or in children experiencing a major loss.

Psychotic phenomena are common among children with major depressive disorder, in which both hallucinations and, less commonly, delusions may occur. The congruence of mood with psychotic features is most pronounced in depressed children, although children with schizophrenia may also seem sad. The hallucinations and delusions of schizophrenia are more likely to have a bizarre quality than those of children with depressive disorders. In children and adolescents with bipolar I disorder, it often is difficult to distinguish a first episode of mania with psychotic features from schizophrenia if the child has no history of previous depressions. Grandiose delusions and hallucinations are typical of manic episodes, but clinicians often must follow the natural history of the disorder to confirm the presence of a mood disorder. ASDs share some features with schizophrenia, most notably, difficulty with social relationships, an early history of delayed language acquisition, and ongoing communication deficits. However, hallucinations, delusions, and formal thought disorder are core features of schizophrenia and are not expected features of ASD. ASD is usually diagnosed by 3 years of age, whereas schizophrenia with childhood onset can rarely be diagnosed before 5 years of age.

Among adolescents, alcohol and other substance abuse sometimes can result in a deterioration of function, psychotic symptoms, and paranoid delusions. Amphetamines, lysergic acid diethylamide (LSD), and PCP may lead to a psychotic state. A sudden, flagrant onset of paranoid psychosis may suggest substance-induced psychotic disorder. Medical conditions that can induce psychotic features include thyroid disease, systemic lupus erythematosus, and temporal lobe disease.

COURSE AND PROGNOSIS

Important predictors of the course and outcome of childhood and early-onset schizophrenia include the child's premorbid level of functioning, the age of onset, IQ, response to psychosocial and pharmacological interventions, degree of remission after the first psychotic episode, and degree of family support. Early age at onset, and children with comorbid developmental delays, learning disorders, lower IQ, and premorbid behavioral disorders, such as ADHD and conduct disorder, are less treatment responsive and likely to have the most guarded prognoses. Predictors of a poorer course of childhood-onset schizophrenia include family history of schizophrenia, young age and insidious onset, developmental delays and lower level of premorbid function, and chronic or length of first psychotic episode. Psychosocial and family stressors are known to influence the relapse rate in adults with schizophrenia, and high expression of negative emotion (EE) likely affects children with childhood-onset schizophrenia as well.

An important factor in outcome is the accuracy and stability of the diagnosis of schizophrenia. One study reported that one-third of children who received an initial diagnosis of schizophrenia were later diagnosed with bipolar disorder in adolescence. Children and adolescents with bipolar I disorder may have a better long-term prognosis than those with schizophrenia. The NIMH-funded Treatment of Early-Onset Schizophrenia reported outcome of neurocognitive functioning in 8- to 19-year-old youth with schizophrenia or schizoaffective disorders, who participated in a randomized double-blind clinical trial comparing molindone, olanzapine, and risperidone. The three medication groups yielded no group differences in neurocognitive functioning over a year; however, when data from the three groups were combined, a significant modest improvement was observed in several domains of neurocognitive functioning. The authors concluded that antipsychotic intervention in youth with early-onset schizophrenia spectrum disorders led to modest improvement in neurocognitive function.

TREATMENT

The treatment of childhood-onset schizophrenia requires a multimodal approach, including psychoeducation for families, pharmacological interventions, psychotherapeutic interventions, social skills interventions, and appropriate educational placement. A recent randomized controlled trial investigated the effectiveness of several psychosocial interventions on youth in an early prodromal stage, characterized by changes in cognitive and social behavior. The interventions, termed integrated psychological interventions, specifically included CBT, group skills training, cognitive remediation therapy, multifamily psychoeducation, and supportive counseling on the prevention of psychosis. Of interest, the integrated psychological intervention was shown to be more effective than standard treatments in delaying the onset of psychosis over a 2-year follow-up period. These results sparked interest in the potential utility of psychosocial interventions to mediate psychosis, and to alter relapse rate and severity of illness over time. Children with childhood-onset schizophrenia may have less robust responses to antipsychotic medications than adolescents and adults. Family education and ongoing therapeutic family interventions are critical to maintain the maximum level of support for the patient. Monitoring the most appropriate educational setting for a child with childhood-onset schizophrenia is essential, especially in view of the frequent social skill deficits, attention deficits, and academic difficulties that often accompany childhood-onset schizophrenia.

Pharmacotherapy

Second-generation antipsychotics (SGAs), serotonin-dopamine antagonists (SDAs), are current mainstay pharmacological treatments for children and adolescents with schizophrenia, having largely replaced the conventional antipsychotics, that is, dopamine receptor antagonists, due to their more favorable side-effect profiles. Current data include six randomized clinical trials in youth investigating the efficacy of SGAs for early-onset schizophrenia, with limited support for one agent over the others. Although clozapine, a serotonin receptor antagonist with some dopamine (D_2) antagonism, which is hypothesized to be more effective in reducing positive and negative symptoms, has been shown to be highly effective in adults with treatment-refractory schizophrenia, it remains a choice of last resort in youth, based on its serious side effects. To date, however, evidence from multisite randomized clinical trials supports some efficacy of risperidone, olanzapine, aripiprazole, and clozapine in the treatment of childhood- and adolescent-onset schizophrenia. Two randomized clinical trials using risperidone in adolescents with schizophrenia found risperidone at doses up to 3 mg per day to be superior to placebo. A multisite randomized 6-week controlled trial of olanzapine in adolescents with schizophrenia found that it was more efficacious than placebo. A randomized controlled trial of aripiprazole at two fixed doses found that it was superior to placebo in the treatment of positive symptoms of adolescent schizophrenia; however, more than 40 percent of subjects in the active medication group did not achieve remission. Finally, clozapine has been demonstrated to be more effective than haloperidol in improving both positive and negative symptoms in treatment-resistant schizophrenia in youth. More recently, a study compared clozapine to high doses of olanzapine and found that response rates were about twice as great for clozapine as olanzapine (66 vs. 33 percent) when response was defined by a 30 percent or greater reduction in symptoms on the Brief Psychiatric Rating Scale and improvement on the Clinical Global Impression Scale. The Treatment of Early-Onset Schizophrenia Spectrum Disorders Study compared the efficacy of risperidone and olanzapine with those of molindone, a mid-potency conventional antipsychotic. In this study, lacking a placebo group, each of these agents provided a similar therapeutic effect; however, fewer than half of the patients responded optimally. Despite the limited randomized controlled studies of second-generation antipsychotics for the treatment of schizophrenia in youth, the FDA is progressively approving the use of these agents for pediatric schizophrenia and bipolar illness. In 2007, the FDA approved the use of risperidone and aripiprazole for the treatment of schizophrenia in 13- to 17-year-olds. The use of olanzapine and quetiapine were approved by the FDA in 2009 in the treatment of schizophrenia in 13- to 17-year-olds.

A double-blind, randomized 8-week controlled trial compared the efficacy and safety of olanzapine to clozapine in childhood-onset schizophrenia. Children with childhood-onset schizophrenia who were resistant to at least two previous treatments with antipsychotics were randomized to treatment for 8 weeks with either olanzapine or clozapine followed by a 2-year open-label follow-up. Using the *Clinical Global Impression of Severity of Symptoms Scale and Schedule for the Assessment of Negative/Positive Symptoms,* clozapine was found to be associated with a significant reduction in all outcome measures, whereas olanzapine showed improvement on some measures but not on all. The only statistically significant measure in which clozapine was superior to olanzapine was in alleviating negative symptoms, compared with baseline. Clozapine was associated with more adverse events, such as lipid abnormalities and a seizure in one patient.

Several studies have provided evidence that risperidone, a benzisoxazole derivative, is as effective as the older high-potency conventional antipsychotics, such as haloperidol (Haldol), and causes less frequent severe side effects, in the treatment of schizophrenia in older adolescents and adults. Published case reports and limited larger controlled studies have supported the efficacy of risperidone in the treatment of psychosis in children and adolescents. Risperidone has been reported to cause weight gain and dystonic reactions and other extrapyramidal adverse effects in children and adolescents. Olanzapine is generally well tolerated with respect to extrapyramidal adverse effects compared with conventional antipsychotics and risperidone, but it is associated with moderate sedation and significant weight gain.

Psychosocial Interventions

Psychosocial interventions aimed at family education and patient and family support are recognized as critical components of the treatment plan for childhood-onset schizophrenia. Although there are not yet randomized controlled trials of psychosocial interventions in children and adolescents with schizophrenia, family therapy, psychoeducation, and social skills training have been shown to lead to improved clinical symptoms in young adults with a first episode of schizophrenia, and reviews of the adult literature support the benefit of CBT, and cognitive remediation as adjunctive treatments to pharmacologic agents in adults. Psychotherapists who work with children with schizophrenia must take into account a child's developmental level in order to support the child's reality testing and be sensitive to the child's sense of self. Long-term supportive family interventions and cognitive behavioral and remediation interventions combined with pharmacotherapy are likely to be the most effective approach to early-onset schizophrenia.

▲ 27.16 Adolescent Substance Abuse

Substance use is a public health concern among American youth. The most common substances used by adolescents in the United States are tobacco, alcohol, and marijuana. Adolescent substance use and abuse, however, includes a wider range of substances, including cocaine, heroin, inhalants, PCP, LSD, dextromethorphan, anabolic steroids and various club drugs, 3,4-methylenedioxymethamphetamine (MDMA or Ecstasy), flunitrazepam (Rohypnol), gamma-hydroxybutyrate (GHB), and ketamine (Ketalar). It is estimated that approximately 20 percent of 8th graders in the United States have tried illicit drugs and about 30 percent of 10th through 12th graders have used an illicit substance. Alcohol remains the most common substance used and abused by adolescents. Binge drinking occurs in about 6 percent of adolescents, and teens with alcohol use disorders are at greater risk of problems with other substances as well.

The American Psychiatric Association's *Diagnostic and Statistical Manual of Mental Disorders, Fifth Edition* (DSM-5), in contrast to the previous *Diagnostic and Statistical Manual of Mental Disorders, Fourth Edition, Text Revision* (DSM-IV-TR), does not separate the diagnoses of substance abuse from substance dependence. Instead, the DSM-5 provides criteria for substance use disorder, accompanied by criteria for intoxication, withdrawal, and substance-induced disorders. The previous DSM-IV-TR criterion of recurrent substance-related legal problems has been deleted in the DSM-5, and a new criterion, craving, or a strong desire or urge to use a substance, has been added. In the DSM-5, a threshold of two or more criteria must be present. Cannabis withdrawal and caffeine withdrawal are new disorders in the DSM-5. The combined substance use criteria including both abuse and withdrawal phenomena may strengthen the validity of the disorder in adolescents, and the elimination of the criterion for "legal problems" is also an appropriate change for adolescents, since this is less common for younger adolescents and for adolescent females who use substances. Two recent commentaries raise concerns regarding the application of DSM-5 criteria to adolescents with respect to the symptom of tolerance, particularly to alcohol, that may occur across the board, and may be developmentally normal for adolescents who use alcohol but for whom there is no clinical impairment, and for withdrawal symptoms, which may have clinical significance but is only moderately associated with level of severity of substance use.

Many risk and protective factors influence the age of onset and severity of substance use among adolescents. Psychosocial risk factors mediating the development of substance use disorders include parent modeling of substance use, family conflict, lack of parental supervision, peer relationships, and individual stressful life events. Protective factors that mitigate substance use among adolescents include variables such as a stable family life, strong parent–child bond, consistent parental supervision, investment in academic achievement, and a peer group that models prosocial family and school behaviors. Interventions that diminish risk factors are likely to mitigate substance use.

Approximately one of five adolescents has used marijuana or hashish. Approximately one-third of adolescents have used cigarettes by age 17 years. Studies of alcohol use among adolescents in the United States have shown that by 13 years of age, one-third of boys and almost one-fourth of girls have tried alcohol. By 18 years of age, 92 percent of males and 73 percent of females reported trying alcohol, and 4 percent reported using alcohol daily. Of high school seniors, 41 percent reported using marijuana; 2 percent reported using the drug daily.

Drinking among adolescents follows adult demographic drinking patterns: The highest proportion of alcohol use occurs among adolescents in the northeast; whites are more likely to drink than are other groups; among whites, Roman Catholics are the least likely nondrinkers. The four most common causes of death in persons between the ages of 10 and 24 years are motor vehicle accidents (37 percent), homicide (14 percent), suicide (12 percent), and other injuries or accidents (12 percent). Of adolescents treated in pediatric trauma centers, more than one-third are treated for alcohol or drug use.

Studies considering alcohol and illicit drug use by adolescents as psychiatric disorders have demonstrated a greater prevalence of substance use, particularly alcoholism, among biological children of alcoholics than among adopted youth. This finding is supported by family studies of genetic contributions, by adoption studies, and by observing children of substance users reared outside the biological home.

Numerous risk factors influence the emergence of adolescent substance abuse. These include parental belief in the harmlessness of substances, lack of anger control in families of substance abusers, lack of closeness and involvement of parents with children's activities, maternal passivity, academic difficulties, comorbid psychiatric disorders such as conduct disorder and depression, parental and peer substance use, impulsivity, and early onset of cigarette smoking. The greater the number of risk factors, the more likely it is that an adolescent will be a substance user.

EPIDEMIOLOGY

Alcohol

The Centers for Disease Control and Prevention Youth Risk Behavior Survey found that 72.5 percent of high school students had tried at least one alcoholic drink, and 24.2 percent reported an episode of heavy drinking in the month preceding the survey. Findings from the Monitoring the Future Survey suggest that about 39 percent of adolescents have used alcohol before the 8th grade. Another survey found that drinking was a significant problem for 10 to 20 percent of adolescents. Drinking was reported by 70 percent of 8th grade students: 54 percent reported drinking within the past year, 27 percent reported having gotten drunk at least once, and 13 percent reported binge drinking in the 2 weeks before the survey. By the 12th grade, 88 percent of high school students reported drinking, and 77 percent drank within the past year; 5 percent of 8th grade students, 1.3 percent of 10th grade students, and 3.6 percent of 12th grade students reported daily alcohol use. In the age range of 13 to 17 years, in the United States, reports indicate there are 3 million problem drinkers and 300,000 adolescents with alcohol dependence. The gap between male and female alcohol consumers is narrowing.

Marijuana

For the last two decades, marijuana has been one of the most widely used drugs by young people in developed countries, and recently it has become highly used globally. The United Nations Office on Drugs and Crime estimated that marijuana was used by 3.9 percent of people worldwide between 15 and 64 years of age. Marijuana is the most commonly used illicit drug among high school students in the United States. It is estimated that about 10 percent of those who try marijuana become daily users, and 20 to 30 percent become weekly users. Marijuana has been termed a "gateway drug," because the strongest predictor of future cocaine use is frequent marijuana use during adolescence. Of 8th grade, 10th grade, and 12th grade students, 10, 23, and 36 percent, respectively, report using marijuana, a slight decrease from the year preceding the survey. Of 8th grade, 10th grade, and 12th grade students, 0.2, 0.8, and 2 percent, respectively, report daily marijuana use. Prevalence rates for marijuana are highest among Native American males and females; these rates are nearly as high in white males and females and Mexican American males. The lowest annual rates are reported by Latin American females, African American females, and Asian American males and females.

Cocaine

The annual cocaine use reported by high school seniors decreased more than 30 percent between 1990 and 2000. Currently, about 0.5 percent of 8th grade students, 1 percent of 10th grade students, and 2 percent of 12th grade students are estimated to have used cocaine. The prevalence rates for crack cocaine use, however, is increasing and is most common among those between the ages of 18 and 25.

Crystal Methamphetamine

Crystal methamphetamine, or "ice," was at a relative low level of use in adolescence about one decade ago of 0.5 percent, and has steadily increased to a recent rate of 1.5 percent among 12th graders.

Opioids

A survey of 7,374 high school seniors found that 12.9 percent reported nonmedical use of opioids. Of users, more than 37 percent reported intranasal administration of prescription opioids.

Lysergic Acid Diethylamide

LSD is reportedly used by 2.7 percent of 8th grade students, 5.6 percent of 10th grade students, and 8.8 percent of 12th grade students. Of 12th grade students, 0.1 percent report daily use. The current LSD rates are lower than rates of LSD use during the past two decades.

3,4-Methylenedioxymethamphetamine

The popularity of MDMA has increased over the last decade, and current rates of use in the United States are in the range of about 5 percent for 10th graders and 8 percent for 12th graders, despite that the perceived harmfulness of this drug has increased over the last decade to almost 50 percent among 12th graders. Accidental adolescent deaths have been associated with the use of MDMA.

Gamma-Hydroxybutyrate

Gamma-hydroxybutyrate, a club drug, has been found in surveys to have an annual prevalence rate of 1.1 percent for 8th graders, 1.0 percent rate for 10th graders, and a 1.6 percent rate of use for 12th graders.

Ketamine (Ketalar)

Ketamine, another club drug, was found recently to have a rate of 1.3 percent annual prevalence for 8th graders, 2.1 percent for 10th graders, and 2.5 percent rate for 12th graders.

Flunitrazepam (Rohypnol)

Flunitrazepam (Rohypnol), a third club drug, has been found to have an annual prevalence rate of about 1 percent for all high school grades combined.

Anabolic Steroids

Despite reported knowledge of the risks of anabolic steroids among high school students, surveys over the last 5 years found rates of anabolic steroid use to be 1.6 percent among 8th graders and 2.1 percent among 10th graders. Up to 45 percent of 10th and 12th graders reported knowledge of the risks of anabolic steroids; however, over the last decade it appears that high school seniors reported less disapproval of their use.

Inhalants

The use of inhalants in the form of glue, aerosols, and gasoline is relatively more common among younger than older adolescents. Among 8th grade, 10th grade, and 12th grade students, 17.6, 15.7, and 17.6 percent, respectively, report using inhalants; 0.2 percent of 8th grade students, 0.1 percent of 10th grade students, and 0.2 percent of 12th grade students report daily use of inhalants.

Multiple Substance Use

Among adolescents enrolled in substance abuse treatment programs, 96 percent are polydrug users; 97 percent of adolescents who abuse drugs also use alcohol.

ETIOLOGY

Genetic Factors

The concordance for alcoholism is reportedly higher among monozygotic than dizygotic twins. Considerably fewer studies have been conducted of families of drug abusers. One twin study of drug users showed that the drug abuse concordance for male monozygotic twins was twice that for dizygotic twins. Studies of children of alcoholics reared away from their biological homes have shown that these children have about a 25 percent chance of becoming alcoholics.

Psychosocial Factors

Among adolescents, substance use, particularly marijuana use, is strongly influenced by peers, and especially for those adolescents who report using marijuana for relaxation, the drug is used to escape from stress, and as a social activity. There are data to suggest, however, that marijuana use is also associated with both social anxiety disorder and depressive symptoms. Among young adolescents who start using alcohol, tobacco, and marijuana at an early age, data suggest that they often come from families with low parental supervision. The risk of early initiation of substances is greatest for children below 11 years of age. Increased parental supervision during middle childhood years may diminish drug and alcohol sampling and ultimately diminish the risk of using marijuana, cocaine, or inhalants in the future.

Comorbidity

Rates of alcohol and marijuana use are reportedly higher in relatives of youth with depression and anxiety disorders. On the other hand, mood disorders are common among those with alcoholism. Evidence indicates another strong link between early antisocial behavior, conduct disorder, and substance abuse. Substance abuse can be viewed as one form of behavioral deviance that, unsurprisingly, is associated with other forms of social and behavioral deviance. Early intervention with children who show early signs of social deviance and antisocial behavior may conceivably impede the processes that contribute to later substance abuse.

Comorbidity, the occurrence of more than one substance use disorder or the combination of a substance use disorder and another psychiatric disorder, is common. It is important to know about all comorbid disorders, which may show differential responses to treatment. Surveys of adolescents with alcoholism show rates of 50 percent or higher for additional psychiatric disorders, especially mood disorders. A recent survey of adolescents who used alcohol found that more than 80 percent met criteria for another disorder. The disorders most frequently present were depressive disorders, disruptive behavior disorders, and drug use disorders. These rates of comorbidity are even higher than those for adults. The diagnosis of alcohol abuse or dependence was likely to follow, rather than precede, other disorders; that a large proportion of adolescents with alcoholism have a previous childhood disorder may have both etiological and treatment implications. In this survey, the onset of alcohol disorders did not systematically precede drug abuse or dependence. In 50 percent of cases, alcohol use followed drug use. Alcohol use may be a gateway to drug use, but is not in most cases. The presence of other psychiatric disorders was associated with an earlier onset of alcohol disorder, but it did not seem to indicate a more protracted course of alcoholism.

DIAGNOSIS AND CLINICAL FEATURES

According to the DSM-5, substance-related disorders include the following three categories: substance use, substance intoxication, and substance withdrawal disorder. Whereas in DSM-IV-TR, substance abuse and dependence were two separate categories, in DSM-5, they are combined in one diagnosis called substance use disorder.

Substance use refers to a maladaptive pattern of substance use leading to clinically significant impairment or distress, manifest by one or more of the following symptoms within a 12-month period: recurrent substance use in situations that causes physical danger to the user, recurrent substance use in the face of obvious impairment in school or work situations, recurrent substance use despite resulting legal problems, or recurrent substance use despite social or interpersonal problems.

Substance intoxication refers to the development of a reversible, substance-specific syndrome caused by use of a substance. Clinically significant maladaptive behavioral or psychological changes must be present.

Substance withdrawal refers to a substance-specific syndrome caused by the cessation of, or reduction in, prolonged substance use. The substance-specific syndrome causes clinically significant distress or impairs social or occupational functioning.

Two new disorders in DSM-5 include Cannabis withdrawal disorder and caffeine withdrawal disorder.

The diagnosis of alcohol or drug use in adolescents is made through careful interview, observations, laboratory findings, and history provided by reliable sources. Many nonspecific signs may point to alcohol or drug use, and clinicians must be careful to corroborate hunches before jumping to conclusions. Substance use can be viewed on a continuum with experimentation (the mildest use), regular use without obvious impairment, abuse, and finally, dependence. Changes in academic performance, nonspecific physical ailments, and changes in relationships with family members, changes in peer group, unexplained phone calls, or changes in personal hygiene may indicate substance use in an adolescent. Many of these indicators, however, also can be consistent with the onset of depression, adjustment to school, or the prodrome of a psychotic illness. It is important, therefore, to keep the channels of communication with an adolescent open when substance use is suspected.

Nicotine

Nicotine is one of the most addictive substances known; it involves cholinergic receptors, and enhancing acetylcholine, serotonin, and β-endorphin release. Young teens who smoke cigarettes are also exposed to other drugs more frequently than nonsmoking peers.

Alcohol

Alcohol use in adolescents rarely results in the sequelae observed in adults with chronic use of alcohol, such as withdrawal seizures, Korsakoff's syndrome, Wernicke's aphasia, or cirrhosis of the liver. One report, however, has stated that adolescent exposure to alcohol may result in diminished hippocampal brain volume. Because the hippocampus is involved with attention, it is conceivable that adolescent alcohol use could result in compromised cognitive function, especially with respect to attention.

Marijuana

The short-term effects of the active ingredient in marijuana, THC, include impairment in memory and learning, distorted perception, diminished problem-solving ability, loss of coordination, increased heart rate, anxiety, and panic attacks. Abrupt cessation of heavy marijuana use by adolescents has been reported to result in a withdrawal syndrome characterized by insomnia, irritability, restlessness, drug craving, depressed mood, and nervousness followed by anxiety, tremors, nausea, muscle twitches, increased sweating, myalgia, and general malaise. Typically, the withdrawal syndrome begins 24 hours after the last use, peaks at 2 to 4 days, and diminishes after 2 weeks. Marijuana use has been associated with increased risk of psychiatric disorders. Poor cognitive functioning has been associated with chronic marijuana use, although it is not clear whether marijuana impairs cognitive function. Deficits in verbal learning, memory, and attention have been reported in chronic marijuana users, and both acute and chronic marijuana use is associated with changes in cerebral blood flow to certain brain regions, which can be detected by positron emission tomography. Functional imaging studies suggest that there is less activity in brain regions involved with attention and memory in chronic marijuana users. A 15-year follow-up of 50,465 Swedish males in the military reported that participants who had used marijuana by 18 years of age were 2.4 times more likely to develop schizophrenia. Risks associated with chronic marijuana use include higher rates of motor vehicle accidents, impaired respiratory function, increased risk of cardiovascular disease, and potential increased risk for psychotic symptoms and disorders.

Cocaine

Cocaine can be sniffed or snorted, injected, or smoked. *Crack* is the term given to cocaine after it has been changed to a free base for smoking. Cocaine's effects include constriction of peripheral blood vessels, dilated pupils, hyperthermia, increased heart rate, and hypertension. High doses or prolonged use of cocaine can induce paranoid thinking. There is immediate risk of death secondary to cardiac arrest or from seizures followed by respiratory arrest. In contrast to stimulants used to treat ADHD, such as methylphenidate, cocaine quickly crosses the blood–brain barrier and moves off the dopamine transporter within 20 minutes; methylphenidate remains bound to dopamine for long periods.

Heroin

Heroin, a derivative of morphine, is produced from a poppy plant. Heroin usually appears as a white or brown powder that can be snorted, but more commonly, it is used intravenously. Withdrawal symptoms include restlessness, muscle and bone pain, insomnia, diarrhea and vomiting, cold flashes with goose bumps, and kicking movements. Withdrawal occurs within a few hours after use; symptoms peak between 48 and 72 hours later and remit within about a week.

Club Drugs

Adolescents who frequent nightclubs, raves, bars, or music clubs also frequently use MDMA, GHB, Rohypnol, and ketamine. GHB, Rohypnol (a benzodiazepine), and ketamine (an anesthetic) are primarily depressants and can be added to drinks without detection because they are often colorless, tasteless, and odorless. The Drug-Induced Rape Prevention and Punishment Act was passed after these drugs were found to be associated with date rape. MDMA is a derivative of methamphetamine, a synthetic with both stimulant and hallucinogenic properties. MDMA can inhibit serotonin and dopamine reuptake. MDMA can result in dry mouth, increased heart rate, fatigue, muscle spasm, and hyperthermia.

Lysergic Acid Diethylamide

LSD is odorless, colorless, and has a slightly bitter taste. Higher doses of LSD can produce visual hallucinations and delusions and, in some cases, panic. The sensations experienced after ingestion of LSD usually diminish after 12 hours. Flashbacks can occur up to 1 year after use. LSD can produce tolerance; that is, after multiple uses, more is needed to provide the same degree of intoxication.

Substance use is related to a variety of high-risk behaviors, including early sexual experimentation, risky driving, destruction of property, stealing, "heavy metal" or alternative music, and, occasionally, preoccupation with cults or Satanism. Although none of these behaviors necessarily predicts substance use, at the extreme, these behaviors reflect alienation from the mainstream of developmentally expected social behavior. Adolescents with inadequate social skills may use a substance as a modality to join a peer group. In some cases, adolescents begin their substance use at home with their parents, who also use substances to enhance their social interactions. Although no evidence indicates what determines a typical adolescent user of alcohol or drugs, many substance users seem to have underlying social skills deficits, academic difficulties, and less than optimal peer relationships.

TREATMENT

Interventions for substance use disorders in adolescents first require effective screening and identification of those teens in need of treatment. Once a substance use disorder has been identified in a teen, a variety of treatment options can be sought.

In accordance with the goals of the U.S. Substance Abuse Mental Health Services Administration (SAMHSA), a school-based alcohol and drug Screening, Brief Intervention, and Referral to Treatment (SBIRT) has been initiated in a study with 629 adolescents ages 14 to 17 years in 13 participating high schools in New Mexico. Initially, school-based health centers provided substance use screenings for all students who were seen in the clinic for any reason. Once identified, substance using adolescents were offered either brief intervention by clinic staff (85.1 percent of those identified), whereas 14.9 percent received brief treatment or referral to treatment. The brief intervention was based on motivational interviewing, with the goal of helping the student to gain motivation for behavioral change, and being referred for more intensive treatment if needed. Students who received the intervention, regardless of the severity of their substance use, reported decreases in self-reported drinking to intoxication at the 6-month follow-up. Furthermore, students who reported drug use, self-reported decreased use at follow-up. Alcohol use was reported by 42 percent of the student participants, and alcohol intoxication was reported by 37 percent. Eighty-five percent of study participants who reported drug use, reported only marijuana use in the month prior to entering the study. The frequency of alcohol and marijuana as the most predominant substances in this age group is consistent with epidemiological data. Overall, this school-based intervention had the advantage of being easily accessible to adolescents and provided a graded option for treatment according to the severity of the substance use. This study suggests that school-based programs for identifying and providing brief interventions for high school students is viable and merits further study.

Treatment of substance use disorders in adolescents is designed to directly prevent the substance use behaviors and to provide education for the patient and family and to address cognitive, emotional, and psychiatric factors that influence the substance use in a variety of settings such as a residential milieu, group, and individual psychosocial session.

One validated instrument used as a guide for clinicians in the treatment of adolescent substance use designates levels of care appropriate for the symptoms. This instrument called the *Child and Adolescent Levels of Care Utilization Services* (CALOCUS) outlines six levels of care:

Level 0: Basic services (prevention)

Level 1: Recovery maintenance (relapse prevention)

Level 2: Outpatient (once per week visits)

Level 3: Intensive outpatient (two or more visits per week)

Level 4: Intensive integrated services (day treatment, partial hospitalization, wraparound services)

Level 5: Nonsecure, 24-hour medically monitored service (group home, residential treatment facility)

Level 6: Secure 24-hour medical management (inpatient psychiatric or highly programmed residential facility)

Treatment settings that serve adolescents with alcohol or drug use disorders include inpatient units, residential treatment facilities, halfway houses, group homes, partial hospital programs, and outpatient settings. Basic components of adolescent alcohol or drug use treatment include individual psychotherapy, drug-specific counseling, self-help groups (Alcoholics Anonymous [AA], Narcotics Anonymous [NA], Alateen, Al-Anon), substance abuse education and relapse prevention programs, and random urine drug testing. Family therapy and psychopharmacological intervention may be added.

Before deciding on the most appropriate treatment setting for a particular adolescent, a screening process must take place in which structured and unstructured interviews help to determine the types of substances being used and their quantities and frequencies. Determining coexisting psychiatric disorders is also critical. Rating scales are typically used to document pretreatment and posttreatment severity of abuse. The *Teen Addiction Severity Index* (T-ASI), the *Adolescent Drug and Alcohol Diagnostic Assessment* (ADAD), and the *Adolescent Problem Severity Index* (APSI) are several severity-oriented rating scales. The T-ASI is broken down into dimensions that include a family function, school or employment status, psychiatric status, peer social relationships, and legal status.

After most of the information about substance use and the patient's overall psychiatric status has been obtained, a treatment strategy must be chosen and an appropriate setting must be determined. Two very different approaches to the treatment of substance abuse are embodied in the Minnesota model and the multidisciplinary professional model. The Minnesota model is based on the premise of AA; it is an intensive 12-step program with a counselor who functions as the primary therapist. The program uses self-help participation and group processes. Inherent in this treatment strategy is the need for adolescents to admit that substance use is problematic and that help is necessary. Furthermore, they must be willing to work toward altering their lifestyle to eradicate substance use. The multidisciplinary professional model consists of a team of mental health professionals that usually is led by a physician. Following a case-management model, each member of the team has specific areas of treatment for which he or she is responsible. Interventions may include CBT, family therapy, and pharmacological intervention. This approach usually is suited for adolescents with comorbid psychiatric diagnoses.

Cognitive-behavioral approaches to psychotherapy for adolescents with substance use generally require that adolescents be motivated to participate in treatment and refrain from further substance use. The therapy focuses on relapse prevention and maintaining abstinence.

Psychopharmacological interventions for adolescent alcohol and drug users are still in their early stages. The presence of mood disorders clearly indicates the need for antidepressants, and generally, the SSRIs are the first line of treatment. Occasionally, an intervention is made to substitute the illicit drug with another drug that is more amenable to the treatment situation; for example, using methadone instead of heroin. Adolescents are required to have documented attempts at detoxification and consent from an adult before they can enter such a treatment program.

Peter, a 16-year-old 11th grader, was admitted to substance abuse treatment for the second time, following a relapse and threats of suicide. He was initially admitted to an adolescent psychiatric inpatient unit following a serious suicide attempt. Peter reported a longstanding history of ADHD, but he had been a good student and not had any difficulties until middle school. Peter reported an onset of substance use at age 13 years, rapid progression in substance involvement since age 14 years, and then current use of marijuana on a daily basis, drinking alcohol up to five times each week, and experimentation with a variety of substances, such as LSD and Ecstasy. After being discharged from the psychiatric hospital, Peter attended teen group sessions focusing on his substance use problems. Family sessions led to the realization that Peter's mother had been depressed for some time, and she entered into her own treatment. Peter was improving with respect to his substance use; however, his depressive symptoms increased following 4 weeks of abstinence. Peter was started on fluoxetine (Prozac). After the medication was titrated to 30 mg, he remained on it for a month at which time he showed improvement in mood and treatment compliance. Peter continued to attend the teen AA meetings and outpatient therapy. Family conflict soon recurred, however, and Peter became noncompliant with outpatient treatment, medication, and meetings. He resumed old relationships with substance using peers and relapsed into daily marijuana use and occasional alcohol use. *(Courtesy of Oscar G. Bukstein, M.D.)*

Efficacious treatments for cigarette smoking cessation include nicotine-containing gum, patches, or nasal spray or inhaler. Bupropion (Zyban) aids in diminishing cravings for nicotine and is beneficial in the treatment of smoking cessation.

Because comorbidity influences treatment outcome, it is important to pay attention to other disorders, such as mood disorders, anxiety disorders, conduct disorder, or ADHD during the treatment of substance use disorders.

▲ 27.17 Child Psychiatry: Other Conditions

27.17a Attenuated Psychosis Syndrome

Attenuated Psychosis Syndrome (APS) is a new diagnostic category included in the American Psychiatric Association's *Diagnostic and Statistical Manual of Mental Disorders, Fifth Edition* (DSM-5) as a condition for further study. It is a syndrome characterized by subthreshold psychotic symptoms, less severe than those found in psychotic disorders, but which are often present in prodromal psychotic states.

Debate and controversy among clinicians and researchers have surrounded the inclusion of APS in the DSM-5. There are those who believe that the identification and treatment of a prodromal syndrome of a psychotic disorder would either delay or diminish the severity of the future psychotic illness. And, there are others who believe that identification of a prodromal syndrome, which may rarely if ever progress to a full psychotic illness, would lead to unnecessary exposure to antipsychotic agents with unpredictable and possibly harmful effects. There is agreement, however, that patients with subthreshold prodromal psychotic symptoms are often impaired and are in need of psychological and psychiatric intervention.

A recent meta-analysis reported that the rate of onset of psychotic disorders in those patients with prodromal psychotic symptoms was 18 percent at 6 months, 22 percent at 1 year, 29 percent at 2 years, and 36 percent at 3 years. In a follow-up study it was found that of those with prodromal symptoms who went on to develop a threshold psychotic illness, 73 percent met criteria for schizophrenia.

In children and adolescents, psychotic symptoms are not necessarily a hallmark of a threshold psychotic disorder compared to adults. For example, in 50 percent of children with major depressive episodes, psychotic symptoms were present. In addition, epidemiological studies have found that globally, auditory hallucinations occur in 9 to 21 percent of children and in 8.4 percent of adolescents. Thus, in youth, the association between subthreshold psychotic symptoms and the emergence of future psychotic illness may not be a reliable predictor. Nevertheless, identification and follow-up of youth with APS may provide an increased understanding of the longitudinal significance of these symptoms.

ETIOLOGY

Genetic Factors

Family studies have demonstrated that genetic factors influence vulnerability for schizophrenia spectrum disorders and other psychotic disorders. To the extent that APS and schizophrenia are related, genetic contributions are likely to be significant. Adoption and twin studies have confirmed that monozygotic twins have about a 50 percent concordance rate for schizophrenia compared to dizygotic twins who have a concordance rate of about 10 percent. In addition, adopted children of parents with schizophrenia do not have higher rates of schizophrenia; but biological children of schizophrenic parents do. However, genetic factors do not account fully for the emergence of schizophrenia spectrum disorders, since there is only a 50 percent concordance of exhibiting these disorders among monozygotic twins. Environmental factors also play an important role.

Environmental Factors

Early environmental factors that increase the risk of developing schizophrenia include fetal malnutrition, hypoxia at birth, and possibly prenatal infections. Other environmental factors include trauma, stress, social adversity, and isolation. Finally, gene–environment interactions may influence an individual's sensitivity to adverse environmental events.

DIAGNOSIS

Attenuated psychosis syndrome, according to DSM-5, is based on the presence of at least one of the following: delusions, hallucinations, or disorganized speech, which causes functional impairment. Although the symptoms may not have progressed to full psychotic severity, they must have been present at least once per week for 1 month, and must have emerged or worsened in the past year. The symptoms must cause impairment and warrant clinical attention.

Attenuated delusions are described as either suspiciousness, persecutory, or grandiose, resulting in a lack of trust in others, and a sense of danger. Attenuated delusions, in contrast to delusions of threshold illness, may lead to loosely organized beliefs about hostile intentions of others, or danger; however, the delusions are not as fixed as they become in full blown psychotic illness. Attenuated hallucinations include altered sensory perceptions such as perception of murmurs, rumblings, or shadows that are disturbing; but they can be challenged, and skepticism about their reality is likely to be present. Disorganized communication or speech may be displayed as vague, or confused explanations, or circumstantial or tangential communication. When severe, but still in the attenuated range, thought blocking or loose associations may emerge; however, in contrast to psychotic illness, redirection is possible, and a logical conversation is typically achieved. Although impairment is present in APS, the individual retains an awareness and insight into the mental changes that are occurring.

TREATMENT

A recent review of the literature on treatment trials with patients at ultra-high-risk for psychosis found that early intervention with both psychological interventions and pharmacological agents can reduce symptoms and either delay or prevent the onset of a full psychotic illness. Other studies, however, found mixed results for early psychological or pharmacological interventions to prevent the onset of psychotic illness. One study found that most patients who became frankly psychotic did so within a few months after joining the study, making it difficult to determine if these patients were already exhibiting early signs of onset of schizophrenia when identified as prodromal.

A variety of treatment approaches have been used including treatment with risperidone, olanzapine, omega-3 polyunsaturated fatty acid (ω-3PUFA), CBT, cognitive therapy (CT), and one using an integrated psychological intervention (IPI) including cognitive approaches, psychoeducation, and social skills intervention. A review of treatment effectiveness in APS found that receiving treatment was associated with lower risk of psychotic illness at 1 year, 2 years, and 3 years. Given the limited data, however, it is not clear which interventions are most efficacious. Therefore, until additional treatment trials provide efficacy data, the safest choices for the treatment of APS includes psychological interventions rather than the use of antipsychotic agents. In summary, APS identifies a group of patients with psychotic-like phenomena that warrant interventions in order to improve their distress and functional levels. Further study is needed, however, to determine the relationship between APS and the development of schizophrenia and other psychotic illnesses.

27.17b Academic Problem

Academic underachievement or failure is a major public health concern in youth, affecting between 10 and 20 percent of youth, with long-ranging associations with high-risk behaviors and poorer adjustment in early adulthood. The DSM-5 includes the category *Academic or Educational Problem* in the section "other conditions that may be a focus of clinical attention," since school failure requires clinical intervention and influences a child's level of overall functioning.

An investigation of the effects of students' perception of support from parents, teachers, and peers showed a correlation with adolescent academic achievement. That is, adolescents' perception of support from their teachers and parents was directly related to their academic achievement, whereas perceived peer support was indirectly related to actual academic achievement, it contributed to an adolescent's overall perception of support, which was correlated to achievement.

Academic difficulties and externalizing behavior problems have been found to coexist at higher rates than would be expected by chance. This association has been found in both clinical and epidemiological samples. A longitudinal study of academic underachievement and behavior problems in school-aged children from 1st grade to 6th grade found that the combination of academic and behavior problems in the 1st grade predicted continued academic difficulties and behavioral problems 5 years later. This combination was more frequently seen in boys than in girls, beginning with the 1st grade. This is also true for children with reading difficulties, attentional problems, and behavioral problems.

Behavioral choices and life events can exacerbate academic problems in the absence of learning disorder and can interfere with lessening academic failures. For example, once a student perceives that he or she is falling behind academically, a greater temptation is to replace academic pursuits with other activities, such as drug use. A recent study assessed the level of, and deterioration in, academic achievement in relation to initiation of marijuana use among young teens. In a sample of rural teens, 36 percent of boys and 23 percent of girls initiated use of marijuana by the end of the 9th grade and that deteriorating academic performance was a significant predictor of initiating marijuana use. The hypothesis remaining to be tested is whether timely intervention to improve academic standing would lower the risk of beginning drug use.

The DSM-5 Academic and Educational problem category is used when a child or adolescent is having significant academic difficulties that are not caused by a specific learning disorder or communication disorder or directly related to a psychiatric disorder. Nevertheless, intervention is necessary because the child's achievement in school is significantly impaired, and this has an impact on the well-being of the child and may negatively influence concurrent psychiatric disorders.

ETIOLOGY

Many risk factors may play a role in academic underachievement or failure, including genetic factors, and developmental factors such as premature birth, as well as environmental factors such as level of maternal education. Very preterm children exhibit difficulties in working memory, which is a crucial ability and skill in learning new information and developing academic skills.

Children and adolescents troubled by social isolation, identity issues, or extreme shyness may withdraw from full participation in academic activities. Academic problems may be the result of a confluence of multiple contributing factors and may occur in adolescents who were previously high academic achievers. School is the main social and educational venue for children and adolescents. Success and acceptance in the school setting depend on children's physical, cognitive, social, and emotional adjustment. Children and adolescents' competency in general coping with developmental tasks are reflected in their academic and social success in school.

Anxiety can play a major role in interfering with children's academic performance. Anxiety can hamper their ability to perform well on tests, to speak in public, and to ask questions when they do not understand something. Depressed youth also may withdraw from academic pursuits; they require specific interventions to improve their academic performance and to treat their depression. Youth consumed by family problems, such as financial troubles, marital discord in their parents, and mental illness in family members, may be distracted and unable to attend to academic tasks.

Cultural and economic background can play a role in how well accepted a child feels in school and can affect the child's academic achievement. Familial socioeconomic level, parental education, race, religion, and family functioning can influence a child's sense of fitting in and can affect preparation to meet school demands.

Schools, teachers, and clinicians can share insights about how to foster productive and cooperative environments for all students in a classroom. Teachers' expectations about their students' performance influence these performances. Teachers serve as agents whose varying expectations can shape the differential development of students' skills and abilities. Such conditioning early in school, especially when negative, can disturb academic performance. A teacher's affective response to a child, therefore, can prompt the appearance of an academic problem. Most important is a teacher's humane approach to students at all levels of education, including medical school.

DIAGNOSIS

This category can be used when an academic or educational problem is the focus of clinical attention or has an impact on the individual's diagnosis, treatment, or prognosis. Problems to be considered include illiteracy or low-level literacy; lack of access to schooling owing to unavailability or unattainability; problems with academic performance (e.g., failing school examinations, receiving failing marks, or grades) or underachievement (below what would be expected given the individual's intellectual capacity); discord with teachers, school staff, or other students; and any other problems related to education and/or literacy.

A 15-year-old 10th grade boy, Greg, with a history of prematurity and ADHD, was called to a meeting with his parents and school counselor due to his 12-week report card reflecting failure in two classes, and Cs and Ds in the rest. Until the end of 9th grade, Greg was a B and C student, and he had been stabilized for many years on his treatment for ADHD. In the 10th grade, however, since the beginning of the semester, Greg had not been able to keep up. His counselor had also noticed insidiously increasing isolative behavior for the past 2 months; previous evaluation of ADHD had included a full intellectual evaluation, which showed his full-scale intelligence quotient (IQ) to be 100 and revealed no specific areas of academic weakness. Discussion with his parents and school counselor revealed that Greg had become upset when his parents had announced that they would be separating. Greg had not been doing his homework, and felt that school was no longer relevant for his social life or future. After getting behind in his classes in the first 6 weeks of the semester, Greg stopped trying, feeling overwhelmed and demoralized. It was decided that Greg would be given accommodations from his teachers so that he could pass his classes without having to hand in every assignment that had long passed. Greg would receive daily tutoring, and was referred for a psychiatric evaluation to determine the severity of his mood disorder.

TREATMENT

The initial step in determining a useful intervention for an academic problem is an evaluation of educational problems and psychosocial issues. Identifying and addressing family-, school-, and peer-related stressors are critical. An individualized evaluation may be indicated so that specific educational accommodations can be applied.

In children with poor working memory, that is, a poor ability to store and retrieve information, learning and academic achievement is often impeded. Children with ADHD, as well as children born prematurely, often exhibit difficulties in working memory. In an effort to improve working memory in very preterm children, a computerized working memory training program (Cogmed) is being evaluated, consisting of 25 sessions of 35 minutes each, to be administered at home. Participants will undergo a baseline cognitive assessment, and then be randomized to either an adaptive or placebo version of Cogmed.

Psychosocial intervention may be applied successfully for scholastic difficulties related to poor motivation, poor self-concept, and underachievement. In some cases, on the other hand, excessive hours spent in extracurricular activities, such as mandatory practices for multiple high school sports can result in compromised academic achievement. Early efforts to relieve academic problems are critical: Sustained problems in learning and school performance frequently are compounded and precipitate severe difficulties. Feelings of anger, frustration, shame, loss of self-respect, and helplessness—emotions that most often accompany school failures—damage self-esteem emotionally and cognitively, disabling future performance and clouding expectations for success. Generally, children with academic problems require either school-based intervention or individual attention.

Tutoring on an individual and frequent basis is an effective technique for increasing academic production and is typically included in a comprehensive educational program. Tutoring has proved of value in preparing for standardized multiple-choice examinations, such as the *Scholastic Aptitude Test* (SAT), as well as for increasing academic achievement in daily school subjects. Taking examinations, either school-based or standardized examinations repetitively and using relaxation skills are techniques of great value in diminishing interference of test anxiety.

27.17c Identity Problem

The normative developmental process for an adolescent was conceptualized by the developmentalist Erik Erikson as an adolescent "crisis of identity." The transition between a childhood identity and the process of accepting a more mature sense of self is the resolution of the "crisis." Consolidation of identity encompasses cognitive, psychodynamic, psychosexual, neurobiological, and cultural development. As identity is confirmed in adolescence, a sense of self-sameness and continuity over time unfolds. The notion of an *identity crisis* in adolescence gained widespread attention by clinicians and the popular media during the late 1960s and early 1970s, when many adolescents displayed rejection of mainstream cultural values and ideas and demonstrated alternative lifestyles. The concept of *identity disorder* as a psychiatric diagnosis was embraced in the 1980s when the DMS-III was devised, as a disorder usually first evident in childhood. It was meant to include adolescents who presented with "severe subjective distress regarding uncertainty about a variety of issues relating to identity" to the point where they became impaired.

Identity problem is not currently conceptualized as a psychiatric disorder; rather it refers to uncertainty about issues, such as goals, career choice, friendships, sexual behavior, moral values, and group loyalties. An identity problem can cause severe distress for a young person and can lead a person to seek psychotherapy or guidance; however, it is not included in the DSM-5. It sometimes occurs in the context of such mental disorders as mood disorders, psychotic disorders, and borderline personality disorder. A study examining Intolerance of Uncertainty (IU), that is, the tendency to react negatively to uncertain situations, in 191 adolescents found that IU is correlated with adolescent social anxiety, worry, and to a lesser extent, depression.

EPIDEMIOLOGY

No reliable information is available regarding overall prevalence; however, factors increasing risk for identity problems include psychiatric disorders, psychosocial difficulties, and the pressures of assimilation as an ethnic minority into mainstream society.

ETIOLOGY

The causes of identity problems often are multifactorial and include the pressures of dysfunctional families, the influences of coexisting mental disorders, and the degree to which adolescents feel integrated into their school and family environments. In general, adolescents with social skills deficits, major depressive disorder, psychotic disorders, and other mental disorders report feeling alienated from their peer group and family members, and experience some turmoil. Children who have had difficulty mastering expected developmental tasks all along are likely to have difficulty with the pressure to establish a well-defined identity during adolescence. Erikson used the term *identity versus role diffusion* to describe the developmental and psychosocial tasks challenging adolescents to incorporate past experiences and present goals into a coherent sense of self.

CLINICAL FEATURES

The essential features of identity problem seem to revolve around the question, "Who am I?" Conflicts are experienced as irreconcilable aspects of the self that the adolescent cannot integrate into a coherent identity. As Erikson described identity problem, youth manifests severe doubting and an inability to make decisions, a sense of isolation, inner emptiness, a growing inability to relate to others, disturbed sexual functioning, a distorted time perspective, a sense of urgency, and the assumption of a negative identity. The associated features frequently include marked discrepancy between the adolescent's self-perception and the views that others have of the adolescent; moderate anxiety and depression that are usually related to inner preoccupation, rather than external realities; and self-doubt and uncertainty about the future, with either difficulty making choices or impulsive experiments in an attempt to establish an independent identity. Adolescents with identity problem may join "outcast" cult-like groups. A study examining relationships of social context and identity of high-risk Hispanic adolescents found that school problems and identity confusion among these adolescents were related to behavioral problems and risk-taking behaviors including alcohol use, illicit drug use, and sexual risk-taking behaviors.

DIFFERENTIAL DIAGNOSIS

Identity problems must be differentiated from sequelae of a mental disorder (e.g., borderline personality disorder, schizophreniform disorder, schizophrenia, or a mood disorder). At times, what initially seems to be an identity problem may be the prodromal manifestations of one of these disorders. Intense, but normal, conflicts associated with maturing, such as adolescent turmoil and midlife crisis may be confusing, but they usually are not associated with marked deterioration in school, in vocational or social functioning, or with severe subjective distress. Considerable evidence indicates that adolescent turmoil often is not a phase that is outgrown but an indication of true psychopathology.

COURSE AND PROGNOSIS

The onset of identity problem most frequently occurs in late adolescence, as teenagers separate from the nuclear family and attempt to establish an independent identity and value system. The onset usually is characterized by a gradual increase in anxiety, depression, regressive phenomena (e.g., loss of interest in friends, school, and activities), irritability, sleep difficulties, and changes in eating habits. The course usually is relatively brief, as developmental lags respond to support, acceptance, and the provision of a psychosocial moratorium.

Extensive prolongation of adolescence with continued identity problem can lead to the chronic state of role diffusion, which may indicate a disturbance of early developmental stages and the presence of borderline personality disorder, a mood disorder, or schizophrenia. An identity problem usually resolves by the mid-20s. If it persists, the person with the identity problem may have difficulty with career commitments and lasting attachments.

Jenna, an 8-year-old girl, was adopted in Taiwan at 10 months of age by a white Midwestern couple. As she grew, her vulnerability to separations became increasingly more pronounced. Jenna developed school refusal, and would exhibit outbursts of rage and misbehavior when she was forced to go to school. She pleaded with her mother to care for the many aches and pains that plagued her.

By the time she reached adolescence, Jenna had an entrenched habit of cutting and self-mutilating. She responded to frustration, separations, or perceived threats of abandonment by cutting herself or burning herself with cigarette lighters. Eventually, she was able to verbalize the multiple functions that self-injury served for her. She noted that she was able to stay home from school, be in the company of her mother, and avoided the stresses of peer interactions. Jenna and her mother began a course of psychotherapy in which Jenna learned that she would still need to attend school, regardless of her cutting behavior, and her mother learned to provide incentives for Jenna to diminish her maladaptive behaviors. Over time, Jenna became more flexible and realized that she was harming herself, and not others around her. Jenna was able to return to school, and with the help of her therapist, she was able to discontinue her self-injurious behaviors and focus on succeeding in school and with her peers. *(Adapted from Efrain Bleiberg, M.D.)*

TREATMENT

Considerable consensus exists among clinicians that adolescents experiencing identity problems may respond to brief psychosocial intervention. Individual psychotherapy directed toward encouraging growth and development usually is considered the therapy of choice. Adolescents with identity problems often feel developmentally unprepared to deal with the increasing demands for social, emotional, and sexual independence. Issues of separation and individuation from their families can be challenging and overwhelming. Enlisting the concepts outlined by Erikson with regard to adolescent development, psychotherapy may include discussion of adolescent exploration (active search among alternatives for activities and friendships that fit) and commitment (demonstrated investment) in activities that promote independence and autonomy. Treatment is aimed at helping these adolescents develop a sense of competence and mastery about necessary social and vocational choices. A therapist's empathic acknowledgment of an adolescent's struggle can be helpful in the process.

▲ 27.18 Psychiatric Treatment of Children and Adolescents

27.18a Individual Psychotherapy

Individual psychotherapy with children and adolescents generally begins by establishing rapport through developmentally appropriate psychoeducation regarding the target symptoms and disorders to be addressed. As a rule, the younger the child, the more extensively family members participate in the treatment. Even among adolescents, family members are often directly involved in some components of the treatment in order to achieve the maximum benefit. In recent years, randomized clinical trials have provided a body of literature to support the efficacy of cognitive-behavioral psychotherapy for a wide range of childhood psychiatric disorders including OCD, anxiety disorders, and depressive disorders. Additional therapeutic approaches including supportive, psychodynamic, and more recently, mindfulness-based stress reduction (MBSR), mindful meditation, and yoga are sometimes incorporated into psychosocial treatments, creating an "eclectic" mixture. The initial goal of any psychotherapeutic strategy is to establish a working relationship with the child or adolescent. In general, successful individual psychotherapeutic interventions with youth also necessitate establishing a therapeutic rapport with parents. To establish a therapeutic relationship with a child of any age requires knowledge of normal development as well as an understanding of the context in which the symptoms emerged. Individual psychotherapy with children focuses on improving adaptive skills as well as diminishing specific symptomatology. Most children do not seek psychiatric treatment; typically, they are brought to a psychotherapist due to symptoms noted by a family member, schoolteacher, or, pediatrician. Children often believe that they are being taken for treatment because of their *misbehavior* or as a punishment for *wrongdoing.*

Children and adolescents are the most accurate informants of their own thoughts, feelings, moods, and perceptual experiences; however, external behavior problems are often more accurately identified by parents or teachers. Psychotherapists for children frequently function as their advocates in interactions with schools, after-school programs, and community organizations. Individual psychotherapy with a child often takes place in conjunction with family therapy, group therapy, educational remediation, and psychopharmacological interventions.

PSYCHOTHERAPEUTIC TECHNIQUES AND UNDERLYING THEORIES

Cognitive-Behavioral Therapy

CBT is an amalgam of behavioral therapy and cognitive psychology. It emphasizes how children may use thinking processes and cognitive modalities to reframe, restructure, and solve problems. A child's distortions are addressed by generating alternative ways of dealing with problematic situations. Cognitive-behavioral strategies have been shown in multiple studies to be effective in the treatment of child and adolescent mood disorders, OCD, and anxiety disorders. A recent study compared a family-focused CBT, the "Building Confidence Program," with traditional child-focused CBT, with minimal family involvement for children with anxiety disorders. Both interventions included coping skills training and in vivo exposure, but the family CBT intervention also included parent communication training. Compared with the child-focused CBT, family CBT was associated with greater improvement on independent evaluators' ratings and parent reports of child anxiety, but not on children's self-reports of improvement. Family-focused CBT has also been used in the treatment of pediatric bipolar disorder with promising results.

One of the limiting factors in providing CBT to children with OCD, anxiety disorders, and depressive disorders is the lack of sufficient numbers of trained child and adolescent cognitive-behavioral therapists. A recent study addressed the feasibility of combining a CBT via clinic-plus-Internet treatment. Children who received the clinic-plus-Internet treatment showed significantly greater reductions in anxiety from pretreatment to posttreatment, and maintained gains for a period of 12 months compared with children who received no active treatment, but were on a wait list. The Internet treatment was acceptable to families and dropout rate was minimal.

Psychoanalysis and Psychoanalytic Therapy

Child Psychoanalysis. Child psychoanalysis, an intensive, uncommon form of psychoanalytic psychotherapy, involves three to four sessions a week and places an emphasis on unconscious resistance and defenses. In this approach, therapists anticipate unconscious resistance and allow transference manifestations to mature to a full transference neurosis, through which neurotic conflicts are ultimately resolved. Interpretations of dynamically relevant conflicts are emphasized in psychoanalytic descriptions, and elements that are predominant in other types of psychotherapies are included. In all psychotherapy, children should derive support from a consistently understanding and accepting relationship with their therapists. Remedial educational guidance is provided when necessary.

In classic psychoanalytic theory, exploratory psychotherapy is applicable to patients of all ages and involves reversing the evolution of psychopathological processes. A principal difference noted with advancing age is a sharpening distinction between psychogenetic and psychodynamic factors. The younger the child, the more the genetic and dynamic forces are intertwined. The development of pathological processes generally is believed to begin with experiences that have proved to be particularly significant to children and to have affected them adversely. Although in one sense the experiences were real, in another sense, they may have been misinterpreted or imagined. In any event, to children, these were traumatic experiences that caused unconscious complexes. Being inaccessible to conscious awareness, the unconscious elements readily escape rational adaptive maneuvers and are subject to pathological misuse of adaptive and defensive mechanisms. The result is the development of conflicts leading to distressing symptoms, character attitudes, or patterns of behavior that constitute the emotional disturbance.

Psychoanalytic Psychotherapy. Psychoanalytic psychotherapy, a modified form of psychoanalysis, is expressive and exploratory and endeavors to reverse the evolution of emotional disturbance through reenacting and desensitizing traumatic events. This is achieved by having children freely express thoughts and feelings in an interview-play situation. Ultimately, therapists help patients understand feelings that they may have avoided, as well as fears and wishes that have been self-defeating.

Behavioral Therapy

All behavior, whether adaptive or maladaptive, is a consequence of the same basic principles of behavior acquisition and maintenance. Behavior is either learned or unlearned. What renders behavior abnormal or disturbed is its social significance. Although theories and their derivative therapeutic intervention techniques have become increasingly complex over the years, all learning can be subsumed in two global basic mechanisms. One is classic *respondent conditioning,* akin to Ivan Pavlov's famous experiments, and the second is *operant instrumental learning,* which is associated with B. F. Skinner; the latter is also basic to both Edward Thorndike's law of effect, which is about the influence of reinforcing consequences of behavior, and to Sigmund Freud's pain–pleasure principle. Behavior therapy assigns the highest priority to the immediate precipitants of behavior and deemphasizes remote underlying causal determinants that are important in the psychoanalytic tradition.

Respondent conditioning theory asserts that only two types of abnormal behavior exist: behavioral deficits that result from a failure to learn, and deviant maladaptive behavior that is a consequence of learning inappropriate things. Such concepts have always been an implicit part of the rationale underlying all child psychotherapy. Intervention strategies derive much of their success, particularly with children, from rewarding previously unnoticed good behavior, thereby highlighting it, and making it occur more frequently than in the past.

Family Therapy

Family therapies have been influenced by conceptual contributions from systems theory, communications theory, object relations theory, social role theory, ethology, and ecology. The core premise entails the idea of a family as a self-regulating, open system that possesses its own unique history and structure. This structure is constantly evolving as a consequence of dynamic interaction between the family's mutually interdependent systems and persons who share a complementarity of needs. From this conceptual foundation, a wealth of ideas has emerged under rubrics such as family development, life cycle, homeostasis, functions, identity, values, goals, congruence, symmetry, myths, and rules; roles, such as spokesperson, symptoms-bearer, scapegoat, affect barometer, pet, persecutor, victim, arbitrator, distractor, saboteur, rescuer, breadwinner, disciplinarian, and nurturer; structure, such as boundaries, splits, pairings, alliances, coalitions, enmeshed, and disengaged; and double bind, scapegoating, and mystification. Increasingly, appreciation of the family system sometimes explains why a minute therapeutic input at a critical junction may result in far-reaching changes.

Justin was a 14-year-old boy from a middle-class family enrolled in the 9th grade at a public school. He was brought in by his parents for treatment of a long-standing history of shyness and anxiety in social situations, which was more evident now that most of his peers were getting together after school and he was spending his weekends alone. Evaluation revealed social anxiety disorder as the primary disorder. Justin was initially resistant to treatment despite his wish to feel more comfortable with other people and in social situations with peers. After much discussion and some pressure from his parents, Justin began to attend a cognitive-behavioral group treatment for adolescents with social anxiety. Justin became mildly agitated each time he was scheduled for a session; however, once he arrived, he was able to participate. He began, a 16-session course of treatment combining education, cognitive restructuring, behavioral exposure, relapse prevention, and four sessions of parent involvement. As treatment progressed, Justin increased his visibility at school, and even attended a school football game with a few peers. Justin told his therapist that he wanted to go to the next school dance but was afraid that he would be embarrassed and would have to go home before the dance was over. The therapists designed several exposures whereby the various things that could happen at a dance were presented to Justin, including being offered alcohol or drugs, having a good time dancing, being left alone or ignored by his friends, or being turned down if he asked a girl to dance with him. As it turned out, Justin's few school acquaintances ignored him and left him at the dance. Justin, prepared for this less-than-desired outcome in his group experience, asked two girls to dance, and forced himself to interact with other peers. To his surprise, despite his shyness, one girl agreed to dance with him. He considered the evening a success. Justin subsequently went to another social event with a new group of peers who seemed more accepting of him. In Justin's case, the importance of practicing responses to potential rejections in the safety of his treatment group was crucial to his success at the dance, and it increased his motivation to continue treatment. Through his treatment, Justin became more and more appropriately prepared, through behavioral exposure and practice, to handle what might previously have been awkward and discouraging situations. *(Adapted from a case contributed by Anne Marie Albano, Ph.D.)*

Tim was a 3-year-old child, developing normally and quite verbal, until he started preschool, at which time he suddenly refused to speak at all outside his home. Tim had begun preschool shortly after his parents had separated and his father had left the home. Prior to his parents' separation, Tim was highly verbal and developmentally ahead of many children his age in language skill. Although he was observed constantly in preschool, he was never "caught" speaking to peers. He was described as a compliant child who didn't smile as easily as the other children, who played with others and followed requests without problem but would not speak. During his psychiatric evaluation, it was revealed that Tim enjoyed eating Froot Loops in a favorite cup as a treat. Treatment was designed to provide incentive for speaking through the delivery of a reinforcement of high value, the Froot Loops. Hence, Froot Loops became available only in the preschool and the therapist's office and, temporarily, were not available in his home. The therapist enacted a process of graduated shaping of communication behaviors—first nonverbal and then vocal noises—and trained the preschool teacher to do the same. Froot Loop boxes were kept in full view of Tim at all times during the initial phase of treatment and, when he was "caught" gazing at the box, the therapist or teacher would prompt Tim for acknowledgment that he wanted the treat. Pointing, looking, and nodding in their direction resulted in receiving four Froot Loops. Next, Tim was asked to make a sound or ask for the Froot Loop to receive the reward. This step was accomplished as he grunted and eventually said, "Loop." Finally, prompts to ask for the Froot Loops in a sentence were enacted, and Tim complied with this demand. This phase of treatment took 2 days at the preschool and 2 hours of therapy to accomplish. Eventually, the boxes of Froot Loops were removed from the environments, but the teacher kept the cereal with her to deliver four Loops whenever Tim made sounds or spoke in school. This shaping procedure took an additional 3 days to result in Tim speaking to the teacher and peers, albeit in short sentences. The treat was faded—that is, delivered on a variable ratio schedule of every three to eight times that he spoke, to promote further speaking and decrease the association with the treat. By the end of the second week of training, Tim was speaking at the level he had achieved prior to his parents' separation. Tim's parents were cautioned to allow Tim to speak for himself in social situations (e.g., order his own food at a restaurant, say hello to others, make his own requests before providing a treat) as a way of relapse prevention. *(Adapted from a case contributed by Anne Marie Albano, Ph.D.)*

Jenna was a 13-year-old teen with a family history of anxiety and depression. Her parents brought her to treatment because of recurrent obsessions involving contamination and germs, with corresponding compulsions during which she had convinced her parents to check her food, while she washed her hands repeatedly until they became raw and bleeding. Evaluation revealed a fear that, unless her parents checked her food for bugs or germs, the meal was likely contaminated. Jenna's parents, attempting to ease her fear, would physically pull apart her food and examine it to her satisfaction, often spending upward of 1 hour before each meal. However, this process caused much distress and discord between Jenna and her family. Jenna's hand washing had generalized to almost every daily activity—after opening a door, reading a book, using a pencil, or touching any object that she deemed dirty. Jenna's evaluation led to a recommendation of behavioral therapy utilizing exposure and response prevention. This consisted of formulating a hierarchy of her obsessions and compulsions, from the least upsetting (checking food prepared by her mother) to the most upsetting (touching something that was wet or slimy and then touching her mouth). Systematically, the therapist engaged Jenna first in a series of imaginal exposures to a scene (e.g., you take a bite of hamburger and something tastes gritty to you and you realize that your mom did not check the burger) until her anxiety dropped to an acceptable level. The drop in anxiety typically took approximately 25 minutes. Next, the scene was enacted in vivo, whereby foods were introduced with "contaminants" in them (e.g., putting pieces of uncooked rice into the burger to mimic "grit"), and Jenna ate the food without having her parents check. As treatment progressed, Jenna learned that her chronic fear of becoming sick was not likely to occur. Similarly, washing rituals were addressed by having her touch items with various substances coating them and then touching her face and mouth. Jenna's treatment entailed a 14-session program during which her parents were taught to assist her with these exposures in the home. Her parents were also instructed to refrain from engaging in her rituals. Relapse prevention plans were added to expand her range of food choices and situational contexts (cafeterias, food stands, restaurants) for exposure. By the end of treatment, Jenna was eating without the need for checking and with minimal anxiety. Moreover, she was engaging in a wide range of activities without the need to wash after touching each object. *(Adapted from a case contributed by Anne Marie Albano, Ph.D.)*

Supportive Psychotherapy

Supportive psychotherapy is particularly helpful in enabling a well-adjusted youngster to cope with emotional turmoil engendered by a crisis. It also is used to treat disturbances related to traumatic experiences, losses, mild mood disorders, and mild forms of anxiety.

A 6-year-old boy was brought for treatment because of long-standing severe aggression and destruction of property. In addition to an evaluation for medication, the child was seen in twice-weekly psychoanalytically oriented psychotherapy. The beginning sessions were marked by the repeated need to set limits and contain the child's aggressive behaviors. Two months into treatment, he began to pump himself up, roar, and announce that he was "the Incredible Hulk." He would then proceed to stomp around the play therapy room, attempting to destroy the toys. The therapist then suggested, "You know you can't really *be* the Hulk. You can *pretend* that you are the Hulk, and then maybe we can play this together." After a number of similar exchanges, the child gradually allowed the therapist to join in the game with him. Over the next 6 months, the boy was able to modulate his behavior in that he was able to "play the part" of the Hulk, but without destroying property, and limiting himself to actions that were less aggressive. He was able to understand that he could pretend to be the Hulk without literally trying to be the Hulk. *(Adapted from a case contributed by David L. Kaye, M.D.)*

Combined Psychodynamic and Behavioral Therapy. Probably the most vivid examples of the integration of psychodynamic and behavioral approaches are demonstrated in the milieu of child and adolescent inpatient, residential, and partial hospital or intensive outpatient treatment programs. Behavioral change is initiated in these settings, and its repercussions are explored concurrently in individual psychotherapeutic sessions, so that the action in one arena and the information stemming from it augment and illuminate what transpires in the other arena.

Alternative and Complementary Psychosocial Interventions: Mindfulness-Based Stress Reduction, Mindfulness Meditation, and Yoga. MBSR, a psychoeducational training program leading to applying the practice of mindfulness into everyday life was studied in adolescent psychiatric outpatients. Mindfulness practices focus on paying sustained attention to moment-to-moment stimuli without engaging in cognitive judgments or self-criticism, and promoting an attitude of acceptance. In adults, this practice has been shown to facilitate improved coping and decrease symptoms of anxiety, stress, and in some cases, self-harming behaviors. The current study was a trial of approximately 100 adolescents aged 14 to 18, with heterogeneous diagnoses, who were randomized to a waitlist control group receiving treatment as usual (TAU), which consisted of individual or group therapy, or to manualized sessions of MBSR for 2 hours per week for 8 weeks. The MBSR group was led by trained instructors who facilitated the use of mindfulness practices by the participants during formal sessions and encouraged practice at home as well. The participants were tested diagnostically at the end of the 8-week study period and again at 3 months following the end of the study. The results found that both the MBSR and the TAU groups reported significantly reduced anxiety, depressive, and somatization symptoms, and improved self-esteem; but only the MBSR group reported significant declines in perceived stress, obsessive symptoms, and interpersonal problems. Furthermore, although more than 45 percent of the MBSR group showed changes in diagnoses at the end of the study (such as no longer meeting criteria for a mood disorder) none of the TAU group was found to have remitted from a diagnosis.

Mindfulness meditation practices have been applied in various forms to a multitude of psychiatric conditions including mood disorders, chronic pain syndromes, anxiety disorder, and ADHD. Mindfulness, according to Kabat-Zinn, is characterized by paying complete attention to the present moment without judgment, with an ability to be aware of inner and outer experiences in the present. There are many forms of meditation which incorporate mindfulness, and both MBSR, and Mindfulness-Based Cognitive Therapy (MBCT) developed by Teasdale, can be considered forms of mindfulness meditation. There is evidence based on neuroimaging studies that mindfulness meditation can induce specific brain states. One study indicated that Vipassana meditation is associated with activation of the rostral anterior cingulate cortex as well as the dorsal medial prefrontal cortex. There is evidence to suggest that mindfulness meditations can improve attention, and that these changes may lead to clinically important improvements.

Yoga originated in ancient India, and while there are many varieties, key components include physical postures, controlled breathing, deep relaxation, and meditation. Randomized controlled trials using yoga have provided evidence of its benefit as an adjunctive intervention in mild depression, sleep disturbance, and attention problems. Clinical trials comparing yoga to cooperative game playing or physical exercises in children with ADHD found moderate improvements in ADHD symptoms when yoga was added as an adjunct to medication. There is some evidence suggesting that yoga may be beneficial as an adjunctive intervention for mild depression, even in the absence of medication and potentially for schizophrenia, as an adjunct to medication.

THE ROLE OF PLAY

Observing play and engaging in play with children can be extremely informative in assessing developmental abilities, and in understanding sensitive situations. This is particularly relevant for young children, and for children who have experienced trauma, which is difficult to describe in words.

Although the choices of play material vary among therapists, the following equipment can constitute a well-balanced playroom or play area: multigenerational families of dolls of various races; dolls representing special roles and feelings, such as police officer, doctor, and soldier; dollhouse furnishings with or without a dollhouse; toy animals; puppets; paper, crayons, paint, and blunt-ended scissors; a sponge-like ball; clay or something comparable; tools such as rubber hammers, rubber knives, and guns; building blocks, cars, trucks, and airplanes; and eating utensils. The toys should enable children to communicate through play. Therapists should avoid fragile objects that can break easily, that can result in physical injury to a child, or that can increase a child's guilt.

Psychotherapy with children and adolescents generally is more directed and active than it is with adults. Children usually cannot synthesize histories of their own lives, but they are excellent reporters of their current internal states. Even with adolescents, a therapist often takes an active role, is somewhat less open-ended than with adults, and offers more direction and advocacy than with adults.

Nurturing and maintaining a therapeutic alliance may require educating children about the process of therapy. Another educational intervention may entail assigning labels to affects that have not been part of a youngster's experience.

The temptation for therapists to offer themselves as a quasi-parent role model for children may stem from helpful educational attitudes toward children. Although this may sometimes be an appropriate therapeutic strategy, therapists should not lose sight of the potential pitfalls of engaging in a highly parental role with their child and adolescent patients.

PARENTS AND FAMILY MEMBERS

Parents and family members are involved in child psychotherapy to varying degrees. For preschool-age children, the entire therapeutic effort may be directed toward the parents, without any direct treatment of the child. At the other extreme, children can be treated in psychotherapy without any parental involvement beyond the payment of fees and transporting the child to the therapy sessions. Most practitioners, however, prefer to maintain an alliance with parents to obtain additional information about the child.

Probably the most frequent parental arrangements are those developed in child guidance clinics—that is, parent guidance focused on the child or the parent–child interaction and therapy for the parents' own individual needs concurrent with the child's therapy. Parents may be seen by their child's therapist or by someone else. Recently, increasing efforts have been made to shift the focus from the child as the primary patient to the child as the family's emissary to the clinic. In such family therapy, all or selected members of the family are treated simultaneously as a family group. Although the preferences of specific clinics and practitioners for either an individual or a family therapeutic approach may be unavoidable, the final decision regarding which therapeutic strategy or combination to use should be derived from the clinical assessment.

CONFIDENTIALITY

The issue of confidentiality takes on greater meaning as children grow older. Very young children are unlikely to be as concerned about this issue as are adolescents. Confidentiality usually is preserved unless a child is believed to be in danger or to be a danger to someone else. In other situations, a child's permission usually is sought before a specific issue is raised with parents. Advantages exist to creating an atmosphere in which children can feel that all words and actions are viewed by therapists as simultaneously both serious and tentative. In other words, children's communications do not bind therapists to a commitment; nevertheless, they are too important to be communicated to a third party without a patient's permission. Although such an attitude may be implied, sometimes therapists should explicitly discuss confidentiality with children. Most of what children do and say in psychotherapy is common knowledge to the parents.

The therapist should try to enlist parents' cooperation in respecting the privacy of children's therapeutic sessions. The respect is not always readily honored, because parents are naturally curious about what transpires, and they may be threatened by a therapist's apparently privileged position.

Routinely reporting to a child the essence of communications with third parties about the child underscores the therapist's reliability and respect for the child's autonomy. In certain treatments, the report can be combined with soliciting the child's guesses about these transactions. A therapist also may find it fruitful to invite children, particularly older children, to participate in discussions about them with third parties.

INDICATIONS

Psychotherapy usually is indicated for children with psychiatric symptoms or disorders that interfere with their ability to function at home and in school, and causes significant distress. A developmental perspective always informs psychosocial interventions with a given child, so that it matches that child's cognitive function and emotional maturity. If a psychotherapy situation is not effective, it is important to determine whether the therapist and patient are poorly matched, whether the type of psychotherapy is inappropriate to the nature of the problems, and whether the child is cognitively inappropriate for the treatment.

27.18b Group Psychotherapy

Therapeutic groups for children and adolescents are varied in terms of problems addressed, age of patients, group structure, and therapeutic approach implemented. Group formats have been used to treat a broad range of clinical symptoms, including anger-management for aggressive children and adolescents, social skills improvement, support groups for survivors of childhood sexual abuse, and other traumatic events such as the September 11th World Trade Center tragedy. In addition, groups have also been settings for the treatment of adolescents with social anxiety and OCD, and youth with depressive disorders. Groups have successfully used cognitive-behavioral techniques to treat childhood anxiety disorders, adolescents with substance abuse, and youth with specific learning disorders. Support groups for youth exposed to loss have provided evidence of efficacy, including data from a study investigating the benefits of a psychotherapy group for adolescent survivors of homicide victims. Group therapies can be utilized with children of all ages using developmentally appropriate formats. The groups can focus on behavioral, educational, and social skills and psychodynamic issues. The mode in which the group functions depends on children's developmental levels, intelligence, and problems to be addressed. In behaviorally oriented and cognitive-behavioral groups, the group leader is a directive, active participant who facilitates prosocial interactions and desired behaviors. In groups using psychodynamic approaches, the leader may monitor interpersonal interactions less actively than in behavior therapy groups.

Gathering children and adolescents into groups may lead to greater psychological impact than treating them individually. A number of factors, described by Irving Yalom, may contribute to the effectiveness of groups. These factors include the following theoretical components:

Hope: Hope may be generated by gathering with others who are experiencing similar difficulties and by observing others actively mastering the problems.

Universality: Children and adolescents with psychiatric disorders often feel isolated and alienated from peers. Working together in groups may diffuse the isolation and help children and adolescents view their disorder as only a small part of their overall identity.

Imparting Information: Children and adolescents are familiar with a format of gaining new information in a group setting, such as in school. The group therapy format provides an opportunity to reinforce learning when the child or adolescent "helps" or demonstrates what he or she has learned to peers.

Altruism: Helping other peers in a group setting by supporting them and identifying with their struggles can improve a child or adolescent's self-esteem and help them gain a sense of mastery over their own issues.

Improved Social Skills: Group therapy is a safe format in which children and adolescents with poor social skills can improve their interpersonal and communication abilities under the supervision of a leader and with peers who also benefit from the practice scenarios.

Groups can be highly effective modalities to provide peer feedback and support to children who are either socially isolated or unaware of their effects on their peers. Groups with very young children generally are highly structured by the leader and use imagination and play to foster socially acceptable peer relationships and positive behavior. Therapists must be keenly aware of the level of children's attention span and the need for consistency and limit setting. Leaders of preschool-age groups can model supportive adult behavior in meaningful ways for children who have been deprived or neglected. School-age children's groups can be single sex or include both boys and girls. School-age children are more sophisticated in verbalizing their feelings than preschoolers, but they also benefit from structured therapeutic games. Children of school age need frequent reminders about rules, and they are quick to point out infractions of the rules to each other. Interpersonal skills can be addressed nicely in group settings with school-age children.

Same-sex groups are often used among adolescents. Physiological changes in early adolescence and the new demands of high school lead to stress that may be ameliorated when groups of same-age peers compare and share. In older adolescence, groups more often include both boys and girls. Even with older adolescents, the leader often uses structure and direct intervention to maximize the therapeutic value of the group. Adolescents who are feeling dejected or alienated may find a special sense of belonging in a therapy group.

Keith was a high-functioning, 14-year-old boy diagnosed with autism spectrum disorder. Keith was an awkward-looking adolescent who seemed younger than his chronological age. His academic level was above average, but his social development was odd. His pedantic speaking style contributed considerably to his social isolation, particularly after starting 7th grade. He was referred to a group of adolescents with social skills problems in order to improve his ability to make friends and have more successful social interactions. Initially, Keith limited his participation to monosyllabic answers to direct questions, and then he would go back to reading a book on the history of Napoleon, his favorite subject and object of fascination. Group members chose to ignore him after a while. Over a period of several weeks, his interest in the book seemed to abate. Keith brought it, but it remained unopened on his lap. He would make an occasional remark, which was often not related to the topic of conversation. The other adolescents in the group seemed to respect his "differentness"; however, it was still difficult to have successful social interactions. Two months later a very shy 13-year-old boy joined the group. After a few sessions Keith developed an unexpected interest in the newer member and sat near him and encouraged him to interact with the group. Soon Keith was not bringing a book any longer and was more involved with group members. In response to the group leader's guidance and practice exercises in the group, Keith learned to respond to social cues in a more appropriate manner, and although he continued having morbid preoccupations with power and a fascination with Napoleon, he was able to converse with group members about more pertinent social topics. Keith's increasing social skills and greater interest in people was clinically evident. Social skills practice within the group became a most significant tool to help Keith with his interpersonal interactions in school and with his family. *(Adapted from a case contributed by Alberto C. Serrano, M.D.)*

PRESCHOOL-AGE AND EARLY SCHOOL-AGE GROUPS

Work with a preschool-age group usually is structured by a therapist through the use of a particular technique, such as puppets or artwork. In therapy with puppets, children project their fantasies onto the puppets in the same way as in ordinary play. Here, the group aids the child less by interaction with other members than by action with the puppets.

In play group therapy, the emphasis rests on children's interactional qualities with each other and with the therapist in the permissive playroom setting. A therapist should be a person who can allow children to produce fantasies verbally and in play but who can also use active restraint when children undergo excessive tension. The toys are the traditional ones used in individual play therapy. The children use the toys to act out aggressive impulses and to relive their home difficulties with group members and with the therapist. The children selected for group treatment have a common social hunger and need to be like their peers and be accepted by them. Selected children usually include those with phobias, effeminate boys, shy and withdrawn children, and children with disruptive behavior disorders.

Modifications of these criteria have been used in group psychotherapy for autistic children, parent group therapy, and art therapy. A modification of group psychotherapy has been used for toddlers with physical disabilities who show speech and language delays. The experience of twice-weekly group activities involves mothers and children in a mutual teaching–learning setting. This experience has proved effective for mothers who received supportive psychotherapy in the group experience; their formerly hidden fantasies about their children emerged and were dealt with therapeutically.

SCHOOL-AGE GROUPS

Activity group psychotherapy is based on the idea that corrective experiences in a therapeutically conditioned environment may increase appropriate social interactions between children and with adults. The format uses interview techniques, verbal explanations of fantasies, group play, work, and other communications. In this type of group psychotherapy, children verbalize in a problem-oriented manner, with the awareness that problems brought them together and that the group aims to change them. They report dreams, fantasies, daydreams, and unpleasant experiences.

Therapists vary in their use of time, co-therapists, food, and materials. Most groups meet after school for at least 1 hour, although other group leaders prefer a 90-minute session. Some therapists serve food during the last 10 minutes; others prefer serving times when the children are together for talking. Food, however, does not become a major feature and is never central to the group's activities.

PUBERTAL AND ADOLESCENT GROUPS

Group therapy methods similar to those used in younger-age groups can be modified to apply to pubertal children, who are often grouped monosexually. Their problems resemble those of late latency-age children, but they (especially the girls) are also beginning to feel the effects and pressures of early adolescence. Groups offer help during a transitional period; they seem to satisfy the social appetite of preadolescents, who compensate for feelings of inferiority and self-doubt by forming groups. This therapy takes advantage of the influence of the socialization process during these years. Because pubertal children experience difficulties in conceptualizing, pubertal therapy groups tend to use play, drawing, psychodrama, and other nonverbal modes of expression. The therapist's role is active and directive.

Activity group psychotherapy has been the recommended group therapy for pubertal children who do not have significantly disturbed personality patterns. The children, usually of the same sex and in groups of not more than eight, freely engage in activities in a setting especially designed and planned for its physical and environmental characteristics. Samuel Slavson, a pioneer in group psychotherapy, pictured the group as a substitute family in which the passive, neutral therapist becomes the surrogate for parents. The therapist assumes various roles, mostly in a nonverbal manner, as each child interacts with the therapist and other group members. Currently, however, therapists tend to see the group as a form of peer group, with its attendant socializing processes, rather than a reenactment of the family.

Late adolescents, 16 years of age and older, often may be included in groups of adults. Group therapy has been useful in the treatment of substance-related disorders. Combined therapy (the use of group and individual therapy) also has been used successfully with adolescents.

OTHER GROUP SITUATIONS

Groups are also helpful in more focused treatments, such as specific social skills training for children with ADHD, cognitive-behavioral group interventions for depressed children, and for children with bereavement problems or eating disorders. In these more specialized groups, the issues are more specific, and actual tasks (as in social skills groups) can be practiced within the group. Some residential and day treatment units use group psychotherapy techniques. Group psychotherapy in schools for underachievers and children from low socioeconomic levels has relied on reinforcement and on modeling theory, in addition to traditional techniques, and has been supplemented by parent groups.

In controlled conditions, residential treatment units have been used for specific studies in group psychotherapy, such as behavioral contracting. Behavioral contracting with reward–punishment reinforcement provides positive reinforcements among preadolescent boys with severe concerns in basic trust, low self-esteem, and dependence conflicts. Somewhat akin to formal residential treatment units are social group work homes. For children who undergo many psychological assaults before placement, supportive group psychotherapy offers ventilation and catharsis, but more often it succeeds in letting children become aware of the enjoyment of sharing activities and developing skills.

Public schools—also a structured environment, although not usually considered the best site for group psychotherapy—have been used by several workers. Group psychotherapy as group counseling readily lends itself to school settings. One such group used gender- and problem-homogeneous selection for groups of six to eight students, who met once a week during school hours over 2 to 3 years.

INDICATIONS

Many indications exist for the use of group psychotherapy as a treatment modality. Some indications are situational; a therapist may work in a reformatory setting, in which group psychotherapy seems to reach adolescents better than individual treatment does. Another indication is time economics; more patients can be reached in a given time by the use of groups than by individual therapy. Group therapy best helps a child at a given age and developmental stage and with a given type of problem. In young age groups, children's social hunger and their potential need for peer acceptance help determine their suitability for group therapy. Criteria for unsuitability are controversial and have been loosened progressively.

PARENT GROUPS

In group psychotherapy, as in most treatment procedures for children, parental difficulties can present obstacles. Sometimes, uncooperative parents refuse to bring a child or to participate in their own therapy. The extreme of this situation reveals itself when severely disturbed parents use a child as their channel of communication to work out their own needs. In such circumstances, a child is in the unfortunate position of receiving positive group experiences that seem to create havoc at home.

Parent groups, therefore, can be a valuable aid to group psychotherapy for their children. A recent study of a cognitive-behavioral group intervention for parents to learn how to utilize therapeutic interventions with their anxiety disordered children suggested that parent groups to teach these skills can be successfully utilized with their children. Parents of children in therapy often have difficulty understanding their children's ailments, discerning the line of demarcation between normal and pathological behavior, relating to the medical establishment, and coping with feelings of guilt. Parent groups assist in these areas and help members formulate guidelines for action.

27.18c Residential, Day, and Hospital Treatment

Inpatient, partial hospital, and residential treatment are designed for the management of acute stabilization, stepdown care, and longer-term management of children and adolescents with psychiatric disorders. Given the limited number of psychiatric inpatient units for children and adolescents, however, intensive outpatient programs and partial hospital treatment programs are often used for children with severe psychiatric disorders. Partial hospital programs are increasingly being offered by managed care companies as alternatives to hospitalization to contain treatment cost. These programs are designed to serve the needs of children and adolescents with severe disorders who require immediate psychosocial and/or pharmacological interventions, but who may not meet the acuity criteria of "medical necessity" for hospitalization. Residential treatment centers are appropriate settings for children and adolescents with psychiatric disorders who require a highly structured and supervised setting for several months or longer. Such settings provide a stable, consistent environment with a high level of psychiatric monitoring that is less intensive than in a hospital. Children and adolescents with serious psychiatric disturbances are sometimes admitted to residential facilities due to family situations in which appropriate supervision and parenting are impossible.

Dan was a 16-year-old adolescent boy with a long history of depression and multiple suicide attempts. He was admitted to a local adolescent psychiatric inpatient unit after for a life-threatening suicide attempt. At the end of the first week of hospitalization, Dan's family's managed care company refused continued coverage, since they determined that he was no longer an acute suicide risk. Dan was remorseful about his recent suicide attempt and was determined not to repeat his self-destructive behavior. However, due to continued serious depressive symptoms and chronic family dysfunction, the inpatient treatment team did not feel that Dan was ready to be discharged to weekly outpatient treatment. Dan was transferred to a partial hospital program affiliated with the inpatient unit. Over the course of Dan's 8-week treatment, he developed a strong therapeutic alliance with his individual therapist, and the psychoeducation provided to the family resulted in the beginning of meaningful changes. The partial hospital program child psychiatrist met with Dan regularly, managed his medication, and collaborated with his therapist to manage his suicidal ideation. At the end of 8 weeks, Dan's depressive symptoms were decreased, and he was safely transitioned to outpatient therapy and returned to school successfully. The partial hospital program allowed for a safe transition from full hospitalization with continued consolidation of progress in a highly structured system. *(Adapted from case material courtesy of Laurel J. Kiser, Ph.D., M.B.A., Jerry Heston M.D., and David Pruitt, M.D.)*

Mark was an 8-year-old boy referred to a rural community mental health center for evaluation and treatment. Mark presented with extreme irritability, labile mood, tantrums, and physical violence toward his peers and adults. Even when he was not having a tantrum, he seemed discontent and irritated and had a short fuse. He had received multiple school suspensions and was at risk for expulsion. His family psychiatric history was positive for schizophrenia in his maternal grandmother. Upon finishing his outpatient psychiatric evaluation, the clinician recommended participation in a newly established partial hospital/day treatment program that used a behavioral management program close to Mark's elementary school. The clinician also recommended a trial of fluoxetine to determine whether Mark's irritability would be ameliorated, and individual therapy, social skills group, and family therapy.

During Mark's 6-month participation in the day program, his behavioral management program extended into the classroom setting as well as in therapeutic activities. His daily goals included increasing compliance, decreasing anger outbursts, and decreasing physical aggression. He was able to improve peer relations while receiving immediate feedback and direct instruction on social skills in a group setting and also in his individual therapy. Each staff member was able to consistently apply behavior management principles in their domain areas. Mark's parents actively participated in family therapy sessions and parent conferences. Mark seemed to be benefitting from the fluoxetine and was less irritable. Although he still had occasional outbursts, they were milder and shorter. Mark was gradually transitioned to half a day in a regular classroom setting, and he remained the other half day in the day program. After 8 more weeks of this transition, he was able to return to his public school. *(Adapted from case material courtesy of Laurel J. Kiser, Ph.D., M.B.A., Jerry Heston, M.D., and David Pruitt, M.D.)*

HOSPITALIZATION

Psychiatric hospitalization is necessary when a child or adolescent is contemplating or exhibiting dangerous behaviors directed at him- or herself or toward others. The most frequent reasons for psychiatric hospitalization among youth include suicidal thoughts or behavior, and aggressive and assaultive behaviors. Safety, stabilization, and initiation of effective treatment are the main goals of hospitalization. In some cases, psychiatric hospitalization may be a given child's first experience of a stable, safe environment. Hospitals are often the most appropriate places to initiate a new psychopharmacological agent, especially when side effects are prevalent, to provide around-the-clock observations of a child's behavior. Children who have been maltreated often show remission of certain symptoms by virtue of being removed from a stressful and abusive environment. Given the frequency of uncontrollable aggression as the trigger for many psychiatric admissions among youth, inpatient units must provide safe and effective ways to defuse and stabilize aggressive and violent acts. Placing a child or adolescent on the verge of a violent act in a contained room away from the rest of the milieu is one method of de-escalating a potentially violent situation. Both restraint and seclusion have been considered therapeutic interventions for youth who cannot control aggressive impulses, but given the rare but reported deaths of patients by asphyxiation during restraint procedures, there have been efforts to reduce this intervention. However, seclusion and restraint cannot be abandoned until another form of intervention is found to be highly effective. In some cases, psychopharmacological interventions, that is, "chemical restraint," has been utilized to defuse acutely dangerous situations on an inpatient unit. Optimally, identifying and recognizing antecedents of aggressive behaviors and intervening before the aggression is enacted is the goal. Inpatient care is a setting for initiation and stabilization of treatment with the expectation that children or adolescents will not pose a danger to themselves or others when discharged.

PARTIAL HOSPITAL

In most cases, children and adolescents who attend partial hospital, or day treatment programs, have serious mental disorders and might warrant psychiatric hospitalization without the program's support. Family therapy, group and individual psychotherapy, psychopharmacology, behavioral management programs, and special education are integral parts of these programs. Partial hospital programs are excellent alternatives for children and adolescents who require more intensive support, monitoring, and supervision than is available in the community, but who can live successfully at home if they receive the proper level of intervention.

The concept of daily comprehensive therapeutic experiences that do not require removing children from their homes or families is derived partly from experiences with a therapeutic nursery school. The main advantages of partial hospital programs are that children remain with their families and the families can be more involved in day treatment than they are in residential or hospital treatment. Partial hospital also is much less expensive than residential treatment. At the same time, the risks of day treatment include a child's relative social isolation and confinement to a narrow band of social contacts in the program's disturbed peer population.

Indications

The primary indication for a partial hospital plan is the need for a more structured, intensive, and specialized treatment program than can be provided on an outpatient basis. At the same time, the home in which the child is living should be able to provide an environment that is at least not destructive to the child's development. Children who are likely to benefit from day treatment may have a wide range of diagnoses, including autistic disorder, conduct disorder, ADHD, and mental retardation. Exclusion symptoms include behavior that is likely to be destructive to the children themselves or to others under the treatment conditions. Therefore, some children who threaten to run away, set fires, attempt suicide, hurt others, or significantly disrupt the lives of their families while they are at home are not suitable for day treatment.

Programs

Ingredients that lead to a successful partial hospital program include clear administrative leadership, team collaboration, open communication, and an understanding of children's behavior.

A major function of child-care staff in partial hospital programs is to provide positive experiences and a structure that enables the children and their families to internalize controls and to function better than in the past. Because the ages, needs, and range of diagnoses of children who may benefit from some form of day treatment vary, many day treatment programs have been developed. Some programs specialize in the special educational and structured environmental needs of mentally retarded children. Others offer therapeutic efforts designed to treat children with autism and schizophrenia. Still other programs provide the total spectrum of treatment usually found in full residential treatment, of which they may be an extension. Children may move from one part of the program to another and may be in residential treatment or partial hospital according to their needs. A school program is always a major component of partial hospital treatment. Attempts have been made to analyze the treatment outcome of partial hospitalization. Many different dimensions exist to analyze the overall benefits of such programs; assessment of level of improvement in clinical status, academic progress, peer relationships, community interactions (legal difficulties), and family relationships are some pertinent areas to measure. In a follow-up 1 year after discharge from a partial hospital program, comparison of patients at admission and 1-year postdischarge showed statistically significant improvement in clinical symptoms on each subscale of the *Child Behavior Checklist,* except for sex problems. Improvements were found in mood, somatic complaints, attention problems, thought problems, delinquent behavior, and aggressive behavior. The assessment of long-term effectiveness of day treatment is fraught with difficulties, and may differ when measuring a child's maintenance of gains, a therapist's view of psychological gains, or cost-to-benefit ratios.

The lessons learned from day treatment programs have encouraged mental health disciplines to have services follow children, rather than have separate programs, which result in discontinuity of care. The experiences of partial hospital programs for psychiatric conditions of children and adolescents have also encouraged pediatric hospitals and departments to adopt models that promote continuity of care for children with chronic physical illness.

RESIDENTIAL TREATMENT

Children in residential treatment often have combinations of severe psychiatric disorders and severely troubled families who cannot adequately care for their children. In some cases, a child or adolescent requires a more structured environment than is possible at home. In other cases, a family is unable to oversee a child's psychiatric treatment due to their own psychiatric illness, substance abuse, or medical debilitation. In cases of child abuse or neglect, a family does not provide a safe and nurturing environment for a child. When families are available and motivated, their participation is strongly encouraged while their children are in residential treatment. The aim is to enable them to reunite with their children and care for them at home in the future.

Staff and Setting

Staffing patterns include various combinations of child-care workers, teachers, social workers, psychiatrists, pediatricians, nurses, and psychologists; therefore, residential treatment can be very expensive. The Joint Commission on the Mental Health of Children made the following structural and setting recommendations:

In addition to space for therapy programs, there should be facilities for a first-rate school and a rich evening activity program, and there should be ample space for play, both indoors and out. Facilities should be small, seldom exceeding 60 patients in capacity with a limit of 100 patients, and they should make provisions for children to live in small groups. The centers should be located near the families they serve and should be readily accessible by public transportation. They should be located for ready access to special medical and educational services and to various community resources, including consultants. The centers should be open institutions whenever possible; locked buildings, wards, or rooms should be required only rarely. In designing residential programs, the guiding principle should be that children should be removed from their normal life settings the least possible distance in space, in time, and in the psychological texture of the experience.

Indications

Most children who are referred for residential treatment have had multiple evaluations by professionals, such as school psychologists, outpatient psychotherapists, juvenile court officials, or state welfare agency staff. Attempts at outpatient treatment and foster home placement usually precede residential treatment. Sometimes, the severity of a child's problems or the inability of a family to provide for the child's needs prohibits sending a child home. Many children sent to residential treatment centers have disruptive behavior problems in addition to other problems, including mood disorders and psychotic disorders. In some cases, serious psychosocial problems, such as physical or sexual abuse, neglect, indigence, or homelessness, necessitate out-of-home placement. The age range of the children varies among institutions, but most children are between 5 and 15 years of age. Boys are referred more frequently than girls.

An initial review of data enables the intake staff to determine whether a particular child is likely to benefit from the treatment program; often, for every child accepted for admission, three are rejected. The next step usually is interviews with the child and the parents by various staff members, such as a therapist, a group-living worker, and a teacher. Psychological testing and neurological examinations are given, when indicated, if they have not already been performed. The child and parents should be prepared for these interviews.

Milieu

Most of a child's time in a residential treatment setting is spent in the milieu. The staff consists of clinicians and care workers who offer a structured environment that forms a therapeutic milieu; the environment places boundaries and limitations on the children. Tasks are defined within the limits of children's abilities; incentives, such as additional privileges, encourage them to progress rather than regress. In milieu therapy, the environment is structured, limits are set, and a therapeutic atmosphere is maintained.

The children often select one or more staff members with whom to form a relationship; through this relationship, they express, consciously and unconsciously, many of their feelings about their parents. The child-care staff should be trained to recognize such transference reactions and to respond to them in a way that differs from the children's expectations, which are based on their previous or even current relationships with their parents. This requires an awareness of countertransference in staff members.

To maintain consistency and balance, the group-living staff members must communicate freely and regularly with each other and with the other professional and administrative staff members of the residential setting, particularly the children's teachers and therapists. Behavior modification principles are typically embedded into the daily program for children in residential settings. A recent study examined the association between use of antipsychotic medication and seclusion/restraint (S/R) frequency in the management of acute aggressive behavior in adolescents in residential facilities. Adolescents who were in the moderate and high groups for having S/R were significantly more likely to have changes in antipsychotic medication and receive higher doses of medication. However, even with high doses, their rates of S/R continued to be frequent. These findings bring into question the efficacy of antipsychotic agents for managing acute aggression in residential settings.

Education

Children in residential treatment frequently have severe learning disorders, disruptive behavior, and ADHD. Usually, the children cannot function in a regular community school and consequently need a special on-grounds school. A major goal of the on-grounds school is to motivate children to learn. The educational process in residential treatment is complex; Table 27.18c–1 shows its components.

Therapy

Most residential facilities use a basic behavior modification program to set guidelines and to give the residents a concrete sense of how to earn privileges. These behavioral programs range in detail and intensity. Some programs operate with level systems that are associated with privileges and responsibilities. Some programs use a token economy system in which residents earn points for appropriate behavior and for meeting specific goals. Most programs include basic tasks of living as well as specific therapeutic goals for the residents.

Psychotherapy offered in these programs generally is supportive and oriented toward reunion with the family when possible. Insight-oriented psychotherapy is included when it can be used by a resident.

Parents

Concomitant work with parents is essential. Children usually have a strong tie to at least one parent, no matter how disturbed the parent may be. Sometimes, a child idealizes the parent, who repeatedly fails the child. Other times, the parent has an ambivalent or unrealistic expectation that the child will return home. In some instances, the parent must be helped to enable the child to live in another setting when it is in the child's best interest. Most residential treatment centers offer individual or group therapy for parents, couples, or marital therapy, and in some cases, conjoint family therapy.

DAY TREATMENT

The concept of daily comprehensive therapeutic experiences that do not require removing children from their homes or families is derived partly from experiences with a therapeutic nursery school. Day hospital programs for children were then developed, and the number of programs continues to grow. The main advantages of day treatment are that children remain with their families and the families can be more involved in day

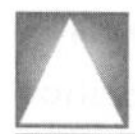

Table 27.18c–1
Education Process in Residential Treatment

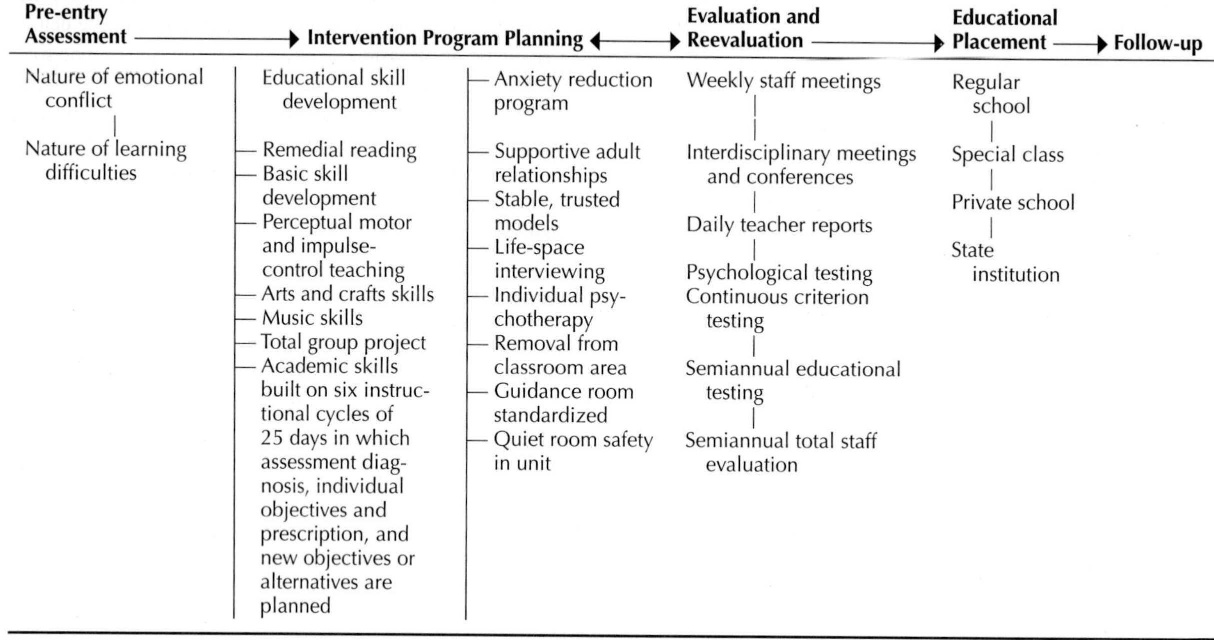

Pre-entry Assessment →	Intervention Program Planning ↔		Evaluation and Reevaluation →	Educational Placement →	Follow-up
Nature of emotional conflict | Nature of learning difficulties	Educational skill development — Remedial reading — Basic skill development — Perceptual motor and impulse-control teaching — Arts and crafts skills — Music skills — Total group project — Academic skills built on six instructional cycles of 25 days in which assessment diagnosis, individual objectives and prescription, and new objectives or alternatives are planned	— Anxiety reduction program — Supportive adult relationships — Stable, trusted models — Life-space interviewing — Individual psychotherapy — Removal from classroom area — Guidance room standardized — Quiet room safety in unit	Weekly staff meetings | Interdisciplinary meetings and conferences | Daily teacher reports | Psychological testing Continuous criterion testing | Semiannual educational testing | Semiannual total staff evaluation	Regular school | Special class | Private school | State institution	

Courtesy of Melvin Lewis, M.B., B.S. (London), F.R.C.Psych., D.C.H.

treatment than they are in residential or hospital treatment. Day treatment also is much less expensive than residential treatment. At the same time, the risks of day treatment are a child's social isolation and confinement to a narrow band of social contacts in the program's disturbed peer population.

Indications

The primary indication for day treatment is the need for a more structured, intensive, and specialized treatment program than can be provided on an outpatient basis. At the same time, the home in which the child is living should be able to provide an environment that is at least not destructive to the child's development. Children who are likely to benefit from day treatment may have a wide range of diagnoses, including autistic disorder, conduct disorder, ADHD, and mental retardation. Exclusion symptoms include behavior that is likely to be destructive to the children themselves or to others under the treatment conditions. Therefore, some children who threaten to run away, set fires, attempt suicide, hurt others, or significantly disrupt the lives of their families while they are at home may not be suitable for day treatment.

Programs

The same ingredients that lead to a successful residential treatment program apply to day treatment. These ingredients include clear administrative leadership, team collaboration, open communication, and an understanding of children's behavior. Indeed, having a single agency offer both residential and day treatment has advantages.

A major function of child-care staff in day treatment for psychiatrically disturbed children is to provide positive experiences and a structure that enables the children and their families to internalize controls and to function better than in the past regarding themselves and the outside world. Again, the methods used are essentially similar to those in full residential treatment programs.

Because the ages, needs, and range of diagnoses of children who may benefit from some form of day treatment vary, many day treatment programs have been developed. Some programs specialize in special educational and structured environmental needs of mentally retarded children. Others offer special therapeutic efforts required to treat children with autism and schizophrenia. Still other programs provide the total spectrum of treatment usually found in full residential treatment, of which they may be a part. Children may move from one part of the program to another and may be in residential treatment or day treatment according to their needs. The school program always is a major component of day treatment, and psychiatric treatment varies according to a child's needs and diagnosis.

Results

Recently, attempts have been made to analyze the treatment outcome of day treatment and partial hospitalization. Many different dimensions exist to analyzing overall benefits of such programs. Assessment of level of improvement in clinical status, academic progress, peer relationships, community interactions (legal difficulties), and family relationships are some pertinent areas to measure. In a recent follow-up 1 year after discharge from a partial hospital program, comparison of patients at admission and 1-year postdischarge showed statistically significant improvement in clinical symptoms on each subscale of the *Child Behavior Checklist,* except for sex problems. These improvements were in mood symptoms, somatic complaints, attention problems, thought problems, delinquent behavior, and aggressive behavior. The assessment of long-term effectiveness of day treatment is fraught with difficulties, from the point of view of a child's maintenance of gains, a therapist's view of psychological gains, or cost-to-benefit ratios.

At the same time, the advantage of day treatment has encouraged further development of programs. Moreover, the lessons learned from day treatment programs have moved mental health disciplines toward having services follow children, rather than perpetuating discontinuities of care. The experiences of day treatment for psychiatric conditions of children and adolescents have also encouraged pediatric hospitals and departments to adopt a model that promotes continuity of care for the medical treatment of children with chronic physical illnesses.

27.18d Pharmacotherapy

Over the last decade, increasing evidence has emerged regarding the efficacy and safety of psychopharmacological agents to treat child and adolescent psychiatric disorders. Randomized placebo-controlled trials have confirmed the short-term efficacy of SSRIs, for depressive disorders, anxiety, and OCD; SGAs for psychosis and aggression; and multiple CNS stimulants for ADHD. Published data support the short-term efficacy and safety of fluoxetine, sertraline, fluvoxamine, and escitalopram in the treatment of youth depression, anxiety disorders, and OCD.

First-line evidence-based treatment for ADHD, has preferentially shifted toward long-acting stimulant medications, including methylphenidate preparations (Concerta) and amphetamine and amphetamine salt preparations (Adderall XR).

Significant progress in the field has been made through multisite, NIMH-funded research comparing types of treatment with treatment combinations of pharmacological interventions and psychosocial treatments, for disorders including OCD and major depressive disorders, and anxiety disorders. Studies repeatedly found that cognitive-behavioral psychotherapy in combination with an SSRI has advantages over either alone. Another area of progress has been evidence-based treatment of ADHD in younger age groups. The NIMH Preschooler with ADHD Treatment Study (PATS) was the first multisite study of ADHD preschool children, treated first with a parent training component and followed, if necessary, by administration of methylphenidate. This regimen was found to be effective and safe.

Double-blind, placebo-controlled studies have provided evidence for the efficacy of fluoxetine, sertraline, and escitalopram treatment for depressive disorders in youth, and the FDA has approved both fluoxetine and escitalopram in the treatment of adolescent depression. Fluoxetine, sertraline, and fluvoxamine have been shown to have positive results based on RCTs in the treatment of OCD in youth. Although the FDA has not yet approved SSRIs in the treatment of child and adolescent anxiety, positive RCTs exist for fluoxetine, sertraline, paroxetine, and fluvoxamine in the treatment of youth anxiety.

In 2004, the FDA released a statement on the recommendation of the Psychopharmacologic Drugs and Pediatric Advisory Committees of a "black box" warning relating to an increased risk for suicidality in pediatric patients for all antidepressant medications. The advisory committees came to the conclusion that an increased risk of suicidal behaviors existed, although there were no suicides completed among the data reviewed. All of the antidepressant medications must include the "black box" warning for pediatric patients regardless of whether they have been studied in pediatric populations. Currently, the SGAs, also known as SDAs, have generally replaced the conventional antipsychotics (dopamine receptor antagonists) in the treatment of psychotic disorders and for aggressive behavior management.

THERAPEUTIC CONSIDERATIONS

As psychopharmacologic interventions for childhood psychiatric disorders have gained an evidence base, establishing a therapeutic alliance, identifying and monitoring target symptoms, and promoting medication compliance are important components of successful clinical outcomes. Teamwork between the child, parents, and psychiatrist is critical in successful treatment of childhood disorders with psychopharmacologic agents.

An evaluation for psychopharmacotherapy must first include an assessment of a child's psychopathology and physical condition to rule out any predisposition for side effects (Table 27.18d–1). An assessment of the child's caregivers focuses on their ability to provide a safe, consistent environment in which a clinician can conduct a drug trial. The physician must consider the risk-to-benefit ratio and must explain it to the patient, if he or she is old enough, and to the child's caregivers and others (e.g., child welfare workers) who may be involved in the decision to medicate.

The clinician must obtain baseline ratings before medicating. Behavioral rating scales help objectify the child's response to medication. The physician generally starts at a low dose and titrates upward on the basis of the child's response and the appearance of adverse effects. Optimal drug trials cannot be rushed (e.g., by insurance-imposed, inadequately short hospital stays or by infrequent outpatient visits), nor can drug trials be prolonged by the physician's insufficient contact with the patient and the caregivers. The success of drug trials often hinges on the physician's daily accessibility.

CHILDHOOD PHARMACOKINETICS

Compared with adults, children have greater hepatic capacity, more glomerular filtration, and less fatty tissue. Thus, stimulants, antipsychotics, and tricyclic drugs are eliminated more rapidly by children than by adults; lithium (Eskalith) may also be eliminated more rapidly, and children may be less able to store drugs in their fat. Because of children's quick elimination, the half-lives of many medications may be shorter in children than in adults.

Table 27.18d–1
Diagnostic Processes of Biological Therapy

1. Diagnostic evaluation
2. Symptom measurement
3. Risk–benefit ratio analysis
4. Periodic reevaluation
5. Termination and tapered drug withdrawal

Little evidence indicates that clinicians can predict a child's blood level from the dosage or a treatment response from the plasma level. Relatively low serum levels of haloperidol seem to be adequate to treat Tourette's disorder in children. No correlation is seen between the methylphenidate (Ritalin) serum level and a child's response. The data are incomplete and conflicting about major depressive disorder and serum levels of tricyclic drugs. Serum level is related to response for tricyclic drugs in the treatment of enuresis.

With lithium therapy, a ratio of lithium concentration in saliva to that in serum can be established for a child by averaging three to four individual ratios. The average ratio can then be used to convert subsequent saliva levels to serum levels and, thus, avoid some venipuncture in children who are stressed by blood tests. As with serum levels, regular clinical monitoring for adverse effects is necessary. Table 27.18d–2 lists representative agents, their indications, dosages, adverse reactions, and monitoring requirements.

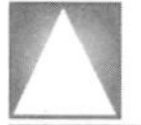

Table 27.18d–2
Pharmacologic Agents for Psychiatric Disorders in Children Adolescents

Drug	Indications	Dosage	Adverse Reactions
Antipsychotics Risperidone (Risperdal) Olanzapine (Zyprexa) Quetiapine (Seroquel) Aripiprazole (Abilify) Ziprasidone (Geodon) Clozapine (Clozaril) Haloperidol (Haldol)	Psychosis; agitation self-injurious behaviors aggression Tics Clozapine-refractory schizophrenia in adolescents	Risperidone 1–4 mg per day Olanzapine 2.5–10 mg per day Quetiapine 25–500 mg per day Aripiprazole 2–20 mg per day Ziprasidone up to 160 mg per day Clozapine <600 mg per day Haloperidol up to 10 mg per day	Sedation, weight gain, hypotension, lowered seizure threshold, constipation, extrapyramidal symptoms, jaundice, agranulocytosis, dystonic reaction, tardive dyskinesia Hyperprolactinemia **Monitor** Blood pressure, CBC, LFTs, prolactin Clozapine: weekly WBC
Stimulants Dextroamphetamine and Amphetamine (Dexedrine spansule) Mixed Amphetamine Salts (Adderall) FDA approved for 3 years and older Adderall XR Lisdexamfetamine (Vyvanse) Methylphenidate Ritalin Ritalin SR Concerta	ADHD hyperactivity, impulsivity, and inattentiveness Narcolepsy	Dextroamphetamine 5–40 mg per day 0.25 mg/kg/dose FDA max 40 mg per day 5–40 mg per day Or 0.25 mg/kg/dose FDA approved max 40 mg per day 5–30 mg per day FDA approved max 30 mg per day 20–70 mg per day FDA approved max 70 mg per day Methylphenidate—10–60 mg per day or up to 0.5 mg/kg per dose FDA approved max 60 mg per day FDA approved max 54 mg per day for children; 72 mg per day for adolescents	Insomnia, anorexia, weight loss (possibly growth delay), rebound hyperactivity, headache, tachycardia, precipitation, or exacerbation of tic disorders
Daytrana patch Focalin XR		FDA approved max 30 mg per day patch worn 9 hours per day FDA approved max 20 mg per day	Skin irritation
Nonstimulants Atomoxetine (Straterra)	ADHD	Begin with 0.5 mg/kg up to 1.4 mg/kg or 100 mg, whichever is less	Abdominal pain, loss of appetite
Mood stabilizers Lithium—antiaggression properties	Studies support use in MR and CD for aggressive and self-injurious behaviors; can be used for same in PDD; also indicated for early-onset bipolar disorder	600–2,100 mg in two or three divided doses; keep blood levels to 0.4–1.2 mEq/L	Nausea, vomiting, polyuria, headache, tremor, weight gain, hypothyroidism Experience with adults suggests renal function monitoring
Divalproex (Depakote)	Bipolar disorder, aggression	Up to about 20 mg/kg per day; therapeutic blood level range appears to be 50–100 μg/mL	Monitor CBC count and LFTs for possible blood dyscrasias and hepatotoxicity Nausea, vomiting, sedation, hair loss, weight gain, possibly polycystic ovaries

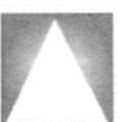

Table 27.18d–2
Pharmacologic Agents for Psychiatric Disorders in Children Adolescents (Continued)

Drug	Indications	Dosage	Adverse Reactions
Antidepressants			
Tricyclic antidepressants clomipramine (Anafranil)	Major depressive disorder, separation anxiety disorder, bulimia nervosa, enuresis; sometimes used in ADHD, sleepwalking disorder, and sleep terror disorder Clomipramine is effective in childhood OCD and sometimes in PDD	Eventually combine in one dose, which is usually 50–100 mg before sleep Clomipramine—start at 50 mg per day; can raise to not more than 3 mg/kg per day or 200 mg per day	Dry mouth, constipation, tachycardia, arrhythmia
Selective serotonin reuptake inhibitors—fluoxetine (Prozac), sertraline (Zoloft), fluvoxamine (Luvox), paroxetine (Paxil), citalopram (Celexa)	OCD, anxiety disorders, depressive disorders, bulimia	Less than adult dosages	Nausea, headache, nervousness, insomnia, dry mouth, diarrhea, drowsiness, disinhibition
Bupropion (Wellbutrin)	ADHD	Start 50 mg and titrate up to between 100 and 250 mg per day	Disinhibition, insomnia, dry mouth, gastrointestinal problems, tremor, seizures
Anxiolytics			
Benzodiazepines			
Clonazepam (Klonopin)	Panic disorder, generalized anxiety disorder	0.5–2.0 mg per day	Drowsiness, disinhibition
Alprazolam (Xanax)	Separation anxiety disorder	Up to 1.5 mg per day	Drowsiness, disinhibition
Buspirone (BuSpar)	Various anxiety disorders	15–90 mg per day	Dizziness, upset stomach
α_2-Adrenergic receptor agonists			
Clonidine (Catapres)	ADHD, Tourette's disorder, aggression	Up to 0.4 mg per day	Bradycardia, arrhythmia, hypertension, withdrawal hypotension
Guanfacine (Tenex)	ADHD	0.5–3.0 mg per day	Same as with clonidine plus headache, stomachache
β-Adrenergic receptor antagonist (beta blocker)			
Propranolol (Inderal)	Explosive aggression	Start at 20–30 mg per day, and titrate	Monitor for bradycardia, hypotension, bronchoconstriction Contraindicated in asthma and diabetes
Other agents			
Desmopressin (DDAVP)	Nocturnal enuresis	20–40 μg intranasally	Headache, nasal congestion, hyponatremic seizures (rare)

Table by Richard Perry, M.D.

STIMULANT AGENTS, ATOMOXETINE, AND α-AGONIST AGENTS

Stimulant pharmacologic agents remain the primary treatment for ADHD in children, adolescents, and adults. Multiple studies support the efficacy of stimulant medications for ADHD. Current practice is leaning toward more use of once-a-day, long-acting preparations of stimulants such as methylphenidate, amphetamine, and amphetamine salts, and dex-methylphenidate (Focalin LA). The most frequently researched and used stimulant is methylphenidate. Dextroamphetamine (Dexedrine) has comparable efficacy and, unlike methylphenidate, is approved by the FDA for children 3 years of age and older; the starting age for methylphenidate is 6 years. The amphetamine, Adderall, combines dextroamphetamine and amphetamine salts. The extended-release preparations, such as Concerta and Adderall XR, have the advantages of coverage of symptoms throughout the school day without the necessity of taking another dose, as well as a more continuous delivery of medication. Stimulants reduce hyperactivity, inattentiveness, and impulsivity in about 75 percent of children with ADHD. The effects are not paradoxical, because normal children respond similarly. The dose-related adverse effects of stimulants are listed in Table 27.18d–3.

The methylphenidate transdermal patch (Daytrana) is approved by the FDA for the treatment of ADHD in children 6 to 12 years of age. Daytrana comes in patches that can deliver

Table 27.18d–3
Common Dose-Related Side Effects of Stimulants

Insomnia
Decreased appetite
Irritability or nervousness
Weight loss

15 mg, 20 mg, and 30 mg when worn for 9 hours per day. The medication begins to have its effects on the target symptoms of ADHD approximately 2 hours after the patch is placed, and continues to deliver medication throughout the wear time. Given that its active ingredient is methylphenidate, the side effects are generally the same as those for methylphenidate, except for the potential skin irritation that may emerge from wearing the patch. The patch should not be worn in the presence of a heating pad or electric blanket because heat increases the rate of methylphenidate delivery into the skin. Patients with glaucoma or known hypersensitivity to methylphenidate products should not begin treatment with Daytrana. Daytrana has the advantages of being able to deliver medication until the patch is removed and, for children who are unable to swallow pills, Daytrana offers a unique administration option.

Lisdexamfetamine dimesylate (LDX), sold as Vyvanse, is a pro-drug of dextroamphetamine upon cleavage of the lysine portion of the molecule. LDX was created to be longer lasting than dextroamphetamine and less likely to become a drug of abuse because it requires enzymes to convert it to dextroamphetamine. LDX has been approved by the FDA for the treatment of ADHD in children 6 to 12 years of age as well as in adults with ADHD. In contrast to Adderall, which contains approximately 75 percent dextroamphetamine, LDX comprises the dextro enantiomer only. In trials, LDX has also been shown to be effective and safe in the treatment of adolescents with ADHD. Similar to other stimulant agents, the most common side effects of LDX were decreased appetite, headache, insomnia, decreased weight, and irritability.

Recent studies support the use of atomoxetine (Strattera), a norepinephrine reuptake inhibitor, as an efficacious nonstimulant treatment for ADHD in children and adolescents. Atomoxetine is well absorbed after ingestion and reaches its maximal plasma concentration after about 1 to 2 hours. Common side effects of atomoxetine include abdominal discomfort, decreased appetite, dizziness, and irritability. Rarely, minor increases in blood pressure and heart rate have been noted. Atomoxetine is metabolized by the cytochrome P450 (CYP) 2D6 hepatic enzyme system, and a fraction of the population (about 7 percent of Caucasians and 2 percent of African Americans) are poor metabolizers, which may increase the plasma half-life by about fivefold. When combined with other medications that inhibit CYP 2D6, such as fluoxetine and paroxetine, diminished metabolism of atomoxetine can occur, and the dose may need to be decreased. Atomoxetine is generally initiated at 0.5 mg/kg given once per day and increased to a therapeutic dose ranging between 1.4 and 1.8 mg/kg, either in one dose or in two divided doses.

SECOND-GENERATION ANTIPSYCHOTICS AND CONVENTIONAL ANTIPSYCHOTIC AGENTS

The SGAs represent a major advance in the pharmacological treatment of schizophrenia in children and adolescents, as well as in adults. The atypical antipsychotic agents have largely replaced traditional antipsychotics because of their more favorable side-effect profiles, greater effectiveness for negative symptomatology, and mood-stabilizing effects. Although the SGAs are generally recommended currently as first-line agents in the treatment of psychotic disorders in children and adolescents, only one controlled NIMH trial has been conducted using an atypical agent in the treatment of schizophrenia for youth. This study examined clozapine and found it to be superior to haloperidol for treating positive and negative symptoms of schizophrenia in 21 youth. The serious drawbacks of clozapine, however, limit it as a first-line agent for this disorder. In the NIMH trial, five participants developed significant neutropenia, and two experienced seizures. Clozapine is generally used only for treatment-resistant schizophrenia.

Open label trials in youth with schizophrenia have suggested efficacy of other atypical antipsychotic agents such as olanzapine, risperidone, and quetiapine. Case reports have suggested that ziprasidone is effective. One of the main side effects of the atypical antipsychotic agents is significant weight gain. A newer atypical agent, aripiprazole awaits clinical trials to confirm its potential to be an efficacious and more weight neutral agent for the treatment of childhood psychoses. Although conventional antipsychotics, such as haloperidol, loxapine (Loxitane), and thioridazine (Mellaril) have been shown to be significantly superior to placebo in the treatment of psychosis in youth, given their side-effect profiles they are typically chosen as first-line treatments. Schizophrenia with onset in late adolescence is treated, as is adult-onset schizophrenia.

Aggressive, explosive, and assaultive behaviors associated with disruptive behavior disorders, psychotic disorders, and PTSDs have been treated with antipsychotic agents with varying reports of success. RCTs with several atypical antipsychotics, such as risperidone, olanzapine, quetiapine (Seroquel), and aripiprazole (Abilify), have provided evidence of effectiveness for behavioral improvement, with fewer long-term adverse effects than typical antipsychotics.

When conduct disorder is associated with ADHD, a trial of a stimulant is indicated; stimulants are faster acting than atypical antipsychotics or mood-stabilizing agents used in clinical practice to control dangerously aggressive behaviors.

The management of severe aggression, disruptive behavior, and ADHD remains a challenge. Combinations of antipsychotics with mood-stabilizing agents or stimulants are sometimes used in treatment-resistant cases, although few studies attest to the efficacy or safety of drug combinations. Newer "atypical" antipsychotic medications—SDAs—such as risperidone, olanzapine, clozapine (Clozaril), ziprasidone (Geodon), and aripiprazole have enabled a wider range of treatment-resistant patients to benefit from neuroleptic treatment. The SDAs are believed to relieve both the positive and negative symptoms of schizophrenia and to produce less risk of extrapyramidal adverse effects and less potential for the development of tardive dyskinesia. Nevertheless, all antipsychotics pose some risk of extrapyramidal adverse effects and tardive dyskinesia. One challenge in obtaining optimal pharmacological treatment for children is to decrease maladaptive behaviors while promoting productive academic functioning. To this end, clinicians must consider adverse effects of medication that result in cognitive "dulling." Certain pharmacological agents used in pediatric populations are associated with a specific disorder or with target symptoms that appear in several disorders. For example, haloperidol was shown in past studies to be effective in the treatment of Tourette's disorder, but it has also been used to control severe aggression. The high-potency antipsychotics haloperidol and pimozide (Orap) still have the greatest body of evidence as effective medications for Tourette's disorder, although they also have considerable drawbacks. Pimozide prolongs the QT interval and, thus, requires ECG monitoring. Clonidine, a presynaptic α-adrenergic blocking agent, is less effective than either of the above-mentioned antipsychotics, but has the advantage of avoiding the risk for tardive dyskinesia; sedation is a frequent side effect of clonidine.

Tic disorders often coexist with ADHD in children and adolescents. Stimulant use is controversial; it can precipitate tics and should be avoided in these patients, although recent studies indicate that the prohibition may not be totally warranted. Clonidine sometimes reduces tics in both ADHD and the comorbid cases.

SELECTIVE SEROTONIN REUPTAKE INHIBITOR ANTIDEPRESSANTS AND OTHER ANTIDEPRESSANTS

SSRI antidepressants have been found in randomized clinical trials to have efficacy in the treatment of childhood anxiety disorders, depressive disorders, and OCD. A substantial evidence base exists for the efficacy of SSRIs in the treatment of separation anxiety, generalized anxiety disorder, and social phobia in children and adolescents. Thus, SSRIs are currently recommended as first-line medications in the treatment of childhood anxiety. Separation anxiety disorder, generalized anxiety disorder, and social phobia are often studied together because they so commonly coexist. A given child with one of the preceding anxiety disorders has a 60 percent chance of having a second one, and in 30 percent of cases, all three are comorbid. Alprazolam (Xanax) may be helpful in separation anxiety disorder, but randomized clinical trials are still needed.

The SSRIs currently are the drugs of choice in the pharmacological treatment of depressive disorders in children and adolescents. Given the FDA placement of the "black box" warning on all antidepressants used in children and adolescents because of the slightly increased risk of suicidal behaviors, close monitoring of suicidal ideation and behavior is imperative. Although most side effects of SSRIs are tolerable, anecdotal recent reports indicate occasional SSRI-induced apathy in children and adolescents. Previously, clomipramine proved effective in diminishing obsessions and compulsions in children and adolescents and was generally well tolerated. However, the SSRIs have a more favorable adverse-effect profile and appear to be as effective as clomipramine.

MOOD-STABILIZING AGENTS

Classic mania in children and adolescents is treated as it is treated in adults. Use of lithium in treating adolescent mania has been supported in many open trials. Divalproex is used frequently to treat bipolar disorder in children and adolescents. A recent double-blind, randomized pilot study comparing quetiapine (400 to 600 mg a day) or divalproex (serum level 80 to 120 mg/mL) in a trial lasting approximately 1 month, found that quetiapine is at least as effective as divalproex in treating acute manic symptoms. Reduction of symptoms occurred more quickly with quetiapine compared with divalproex. Lithium has been shown in multiple investigations to reduce aggression in conduct disorder, and propranolol (Inderal) has been chosen as an agent to control aggression in open trials, although no evidence supports its use in children and adolescents. Carbamazepine (Tegretol) has not been shown to be effective in controlling aggression in child and adolescent conduct disorders.

Table 27.18d–4 summarizes the effects of drugs on cognitive tests of learning functions. In children with learning disorders who have attention problems, even in the absence of meeting full criteria for ADHD, methylphenidate facilitates performance on several standard cognitive, psycholinguistic, memory, and vigilance tests, but does not improve children's academic achievement ratings or teacher ratings. Cognitive impairment from psychotropic drugs, especially antipsychotics, may be an even greater problem for persons who are mentally retarded than for those with learning disorders.

BENZODIAZEPINES

Sleep terror disorder and sleepwalking disorder occur in the transition from deep delta-wave sleep (stages 3 and 4) to light sleep. Benzodiazepines may be effective in these disorders. They work by reducing both delta-wave sleep and arousals between sleep stages. The medications should be used temporarily and only in severe cases, because tolerance to the medications develops. Cessation of these medications can lead to severe rebound worsening of the disorders, and reducing delta sleep in children may have deleterious effects; thus, behavioral approaches are preferred for these disorders.

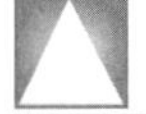

Table 27.18d–4
Effects of Psychotropic Drugs on Cognitive Tests of Learning Functions[a]

	Test Function					
Drug Class	**Continuous Performance Test (Attention)**	**Matching Familiar Figures (Impulsivity)**	**Paired Associates (Verbal Learning)**	**Porteus Maze (Planning Capacity)**	**Short-Term Memory[a]**	**WISC (Intelligence)**
Stimulant	↑	↑	↑	↑	↑	↑
Antidepressant	↑	0	0	0	0	0
Antipsychotic	↑↓	0	↓	↓	↓	0

↑, Improved; ↑↓, inconsistent; ↓, worse; 0, no effect.
[a]Various tests, digit span, word recall, etc.
Adapted from Amar MG. Drugs, learning and the psychotherapies. In: Werry JS, ed. *Pediatric Psychopharmacology: The Use of Behavior Modifying Drugs in Children*. New York: Brunner/Mazel; 1978:356.

Patients with early-onset panic disorder and panic attacks have benefited from clonazepam (Klonopin) in several open trials.

DESMOPRESSIN

Desmopressin (DDAVP) is effective in about 50 percent of patients with intractable enuresis. Improvements with DDAVP range from diminished wetting with less urine volume, to complete cessation of bedwetting. Desmopressin has been used intranasally in dosages of 10 to 40 mg a day. When used over months, nasal discomfort can occur, and water retention is potentially a problem. Patients who respond with full dryness should continue to take the medication for several months to prevent relapses. Desmopressin is now available in oral tablets, and a controlled multicenter study found equal efficacy between intranasal and oral administration of desmopressin in the treatment of enuresis. A dose of 400 mg of oral desmopressin was the study condition associated with greater effectiveness than the lower 200 mg used.

ADVERSE EFFECTS AND COMPLICATIONS

Antidepressants

Adverse effects related to antidepressants have diminished significantly since SSRI antidepressants have been widely accepted as first-line treatments for depressive disorders in children and adolescents. Tricyclics are rarely recommended because of the significant risks of dangerous adverse effects. The adverse effects of tricyclics for children usually are similar to those for adults and result from the drugs' anticholinergic properties. These effects include dry mouth, constipation, palpitations, tachycardia, loss of accommodation, and sweating. The most serious adverse effects in children are cardiovascular; diastolic hypertension is more common and postural hypotension occurs more rarely than in adults. ECG changes are most likely seen in children receiving high doses. Slowed cardiac conduction (PR interval greater than 0.20 seconds or QRS interval greater than 0.12 seconds) may necessitate lowering the dosage. FDA guidelines limit dosages to a maximum of 5 mg/kg a day. The drugs can be toxic in an overdose, and in small children, ingestion of 200 to 400 mg can be fatal. When the dosage is lowered too rapidly, withdrawal effects occur, mainly gastrointestinal symptoms—cramping, nausea, and vomiting—and sometimes apathy and weakness.

Antipsychotics

The SGAs have generally replaced the conventional antipsychotics as first-line agents in the treatment of all psychotic disorders in children and adolescents. Historically, the best-studied antipsychotics given to pediatric age groups are chlorpromazine (Thorazine) and haloperidol. High-potency and low-potency antipsychotics are thought to differ in their adverse-effect profiles. The phenothiazine derivatives (chlorpromazine and thioridazine) have the most pronounced sedative and atropinic actions, whereas the high-potency antipsychotics are commonly believed to be associated with extrapyramidal reactions, such as parkinsonian symptoms, akathisia, and acute dystonias. The risk of tardive dyskinesia in relation to antipsychotics leads to caution in the use of drugs. Tardive dyskinesia, which is characterized by persistent abnormal involuntary movements of the tongue, face, mouth, or jaw and sometimes the extremities, is a known hazard when giving antipsychotics to patients of all age groups. No known treatment is effective. Because transient choreiform movements of the extremities and trunk are common after abrupt discontinuation of antipsychotics, clinicians must distinguish these symptoms from persistent dyskinesia.

27.18e Psychiatric Treatment of Adolescents

Adolescence, biologically beginning with puberty, is a period in which social, intellectual, and sexual development take place alongside specific brain processes that enhance teens' abilities for increased abstract reasoning and greater sensitivity to social nuances. However, the developmental brain processes are spread over many years, and maturation is subject to individual variation. Inherent in development is continuing change; however, most adolescents adapt to changes gradually, and their path toward greater autonomy and independence is not characterized by perpetual crises and struggle. Milestones achieved by adolescents during their developmental journey to adulthood are typically reached without overwhelming strife or intervention. However, psychiatric treatment is indicated for an adolescent who develops a disturbance of thought, affect, or behavior that disrupts normal functioning. In adolescents, disruption of functioning influences eating, sleeping, and school function, as well as relationships with family and peers. A variety of serious psychiatric disorders, including schizophrenia, bipolar disorder, eating disorders, and substance abuse typically have their onset during adolescence. In addition, the risk for completed suicide drastically increases in adolescence. Although some degree of stress is virtually universal in adolescence, most teenagers who do not develop serious mental disorders cope well with environmental demands. Teenagers with preexisting mental disorders often experience exacerbations during adolescence and may become frustrated, alienated, and demoralized.

Clinicians and parents seeking a window into an adolescent's viewpoint should be sensitive to their self-perceptions. A range of emotional maturity exists in teens of the same chronological age. Issues characteristic of adolescence are related to new evolving identities, the development of sexual activity, and developing plans to meet future life goals.

DIAGNOSIS

Adolescents can be assessed with a focus on general progress in accomplishing the tasks of individuating and developing a sense of autonomy. For many adolescents in today's culture, school performance and peer relationship successes are the primary barometers of healthy functioning. Adolescents with normative intellectual function who are deteriorating academically, or teens who become isolated from peers, are typically experiencing significant psychological disturbance, which merits investigation.

Questions to be asked regarding adolescents' stage-specific tasks are the following: What degree of separation from their parents have they achieved? What sort of identities are evolving? How do they perceive their past? Do they perceive themselves as responsible for their own development or only the passive recipients of their parents' influences? How do they perceive themselves with regard to the future, and how do they anticipate their future responsibilities for themselves and others? Can they think about the varying consequences of different ways of living? How do they express their sexual and affectionate interests? These tasks occupy the lives of all adolescents and normally are performed at different times.

Adolescents' family and peer relationships must be evaluated. Do they perceive and accept both "good and bad" qualities in their parents? Do they feel comfortable with their peers and romantic partners as "separate persons" with needs that may not completely match their own?

Respect and acceptance of an adolescent's subcultural and ethnic background are essential.

INTERVIEWS

Adolescent patients and their parents should be interviewed separately in a comprehensive psychiatric evaluation. Other family members also may be included, depending on their involvement in the teenager's life and difficulties. Clinicians often prefer to see the adolescent first, however; in order to develop a rapport with the adolescent and promote being an advocate for the adolescent and avoid the appearance of being the parents' agent. In psychotherapy with an older adolescent, the therapist and the parents usually have little contact after the initial part of the therapy, because ongoing contact inhibits the adolescent's desire to open up.

Interview Techniques

Adolescents may feel pressured by their parents to receive psychiatric treatment and may at first be defensive, or appear guarded. Clinicians must establish themselves as trustworthy and helpful adults to promote a therapeutic alliance. They should encourage adolescents to tell their own stories, without interrupting to check discrepancies; such a tactic may make the therapist seem correcting and disbelieving. Clinicians should ask patients for explanations and theories about what happened. Why did these behaviors or feelings occur? When did things change? What caused the identified problems to begin when they did?

Sessions with adolescents generally follow the adult model; the therapist sits across from the patient. In early adolescence, however, board games may help to stimulate conversation in an otherwise quiet, anxious patient.

Language is crucial. Even when a teenager and a clinician come from the same socioeconomic group, their language use is seldom the same. Psychiatrists should use their own language, explain any specialized terms or concepts, and ask for an explanation of unfamiliar in-group jargon or slang. Many adolescents do not talk spontaneously about illicit substances and suicidal tendencies but do respond honestly to a therapist's questions. A therapist may need to ask specifically about each substance and the amount and frequency of its use.

The sexual histories and current sexual activities of adolescents are increasingly important pieces of information for adequate evaluation. The nature of adolescents' sexual behavior often is a vignette of their whole personality structures and ego development, but a long time may elapse in therapy before adolescents begin to talk about their sexual behavior.

A 15-year-old adolescent male was referred for a psychiatric evaluation by his high school counselor when he disclosed that he was late to school each day because it took him 3 hours to get ready in the mornings. Even after he finally got to school, he often missed classes and was found in the bathroom. In speaking to his counselor, he further disclosed that he had developed a number of bedtime and morning rituals that took longer and longer to complete because if he did them incorrectly, he had to repeat them. They included checking the locks on the windows and doors, placing objects in the "right" places on his dresser, and repeating a prayer 16 times. He also revealed that when in the bathroom, he had to wash his hands a certain way and dry them "just so," or he feared something terrible would happen. He had not wanted his parents to know about his difficulties, and he often told them that he had headaches or stomachaches, which made him late. However, he did explain some of his difficulties to his parents during the course of his psychiatric evaluation. His evaluation revealed significant OCD and social phobia. Treatment was initiated, including use of fluoxetine, an SSRI; CBT; and problem-solving family therapy. Over the course of 6 months, his OCD responded well to the combination of medications and CBT, and he was relieved that his family learned ways of helping him both at home and in school. *(Adapted from case material courtesy of Eugene V. Beresin, M.D. and Steven C. Schlozman, M.D.)*

A 14-year-old girl, one of the stars of her high school gymnastic team, began increasing her daily exercise and restricting her diet after her coach indicated that she should lose a few pounds. She became fixated on the size of her thighs and belly, and once she started losing weight, she found that she was not satisfied and wanted to lose a few more pounds. Over the next four months she lost so much weight that her coach and pediatrician no longer allowed her to participate in athletics. Although she was heartbroken about being restricted from gymnastics and planned to eat enough to be able to participate again with her team, she was unable to gain weight, and continued to lose more. She became increasingly terrified of getting fat and secretly exercised any chance she could. She was a perfectionist in academics as well as in gymnastics. She had started her menses 6 months previously, but after she lost a significant amount of weight, her menses stopped. She was seen by a therapist and she and her parents agreed to a meal plan that would result in weight gain, but her family was baffled because she continued to lose more weight. Finally, when it became clear that she was not able to gain weight under the supervision of her family and her outpatient therapist, she was hospitalized, and the diagnosis of anorexia nervosa, was established. After a 30-day hospitalization with a modest weight gain, she was stepped down to a partial hospital program in which she was supervised for all of her meals, and went home at night. She remained in this program for 8 weeks, and was able to gain 1 to 2 pounds per week. As part of this program, her weight was monitored twice weekly, her vital signs were monitored, and she participated in family therapy, individual psychodynamic psychotherapy, and weekly meetings with a nutritionist. In her psychotherapy, over the course of the next year, she was able to understand that her anorexia had served to prevent her from separating from her parents and kept her close to home and isolated from her peers. She learned that she was slower to mature than many of her peers and felt unable to cope with the social pressures of being a high school student. Over time, she was able to maintain her weight and began to socialize with friends whom she hadn't seen for many months. When she was able to maintain an optimal weight she was thrilled to be able to resume her athletics, and she began to develop closer friendships. *(Adapted from case material courtesy of Eugene V. Beresin, M.D. and Steven C. Schlozman, M.D.)*

TREATMENT

Psychiatric treatment of an adolescent can occur in numerous venues and modalities. Treatment can take place in individual or group settings, and can include interventions that are pharmacological (when indicated), psychosocial, and from an environmental perspective. The best choices for treatment must take into account the characteristics of the individual adolescent and the family or social milieu. Adolescents' striving for autonomy may complicate problems of compliance with therapy and may result in the need for stabilization in inpatient settings, whereas this level of care might not be necessary at a different stage of life. The following discussion is less a set of guidelines than a brief summary of what each treatment modality can or should offer.

Individual Psychotherapy

Individual psychosocial modalities with an evidence base for efficacy with adolescents include cognitive-behavioral treatments for diagnoses of anxiety disorders, mood disorders, and OCD. Interpersonal therapy is a technique that has been used to treat mood disorders in adolescents. Few adolescent patients are trusting or open without considerable time and testing of therapists, and it is helpful to anticipate the testing period by letting patients know that it is expected and is natural and healthy. Pointing out the likelihood of therapeutic problems—for instance, impatience and disappointment with the psychiatrist, with the therapy, with the time required, and with the often intangible results—may help keep problems under control. Therapeutic goals should be stated in terms that adolescents understand and value. Although they may not see the point in exercising self-control, enduring dysphoric emotions, or forgoing impulsive gratification, they may value feeling more confident than in the past and gaining more control over their lives and the events that affect them.

Typical adolescent patients need a relationship with a therapist they can perceive as a real person, whom they feel respected by and they can trust. The therapist may seem like another parent in some respects, since adolescents still need appropriate guidance, especially in situations of high-risk behaviors. Thus, a professional who is impersonal and anonymous is a less useful model than one who can accept and respond rationally to an angry challenge or confrontation without fear or false conciliation—one that can impose limits and controls when adolescents cannot—can admit mistakes and ignorance, and can openly express the gamut of human emotions.

Combined Pharmacotherapy and Psychotherapy

Current evidence suggests that for many psychiatric disorders, optimal treatment includes a combination of psychosocial and psychopharmacological interventions. Randomized clinical trials have provided evidence of the superiority of CBT in combination with SSRIs in the treatment of mood disorders, OCD, and anxiety disorders, to name a few.

ADHD is often comorbid with additional disorders, thus, although the Multimodal Treatment Study of Children with ADHD (MTA) found that psychosocial interventions did not add to the efficacy of stimulant treatments for the core symptoms of ADHD, it is important to consider that other concurrent disorders that affect overall functioning often require psychosocial treatments. Advances in drug development have widened the choice of medications to treat mood disorders (e.g., SSRIs) and schizophrenia (e.g., SGAs, including risperidone [Risperdal], olanzapine [Zyprexa], and clozapine [Clozaril]). Although these medications have been used to treat psychiatric disorders in adolescents, more research is required to determine their efficacy and safety profiles for treatment of adolescent psychopathology.

A 17-year-old girl complained of recurrent episodes of rapid heartbeat, sweating, trembling, and a fear that she was "going crazy." Her first episode had occurred in her high school cafeteria during a "college night" event, when multiple college representatives were displaying their college's information packets. After running out of the cafeteria, she stood outside of her school and the episode gradually dissipated over a period of about 15 minutes. Although she was a little nervous about going back to school the next day, she did not have another episode. She had almost forgotten about the episode, when it happened again, and even more intensely, when she was shopping at the mall and talking about college applications with her friends. After this episode, she became fearful of going out alone to the shopping mall. She was at the beginning of her senior year in high school, considering her options for college and was planning to take her SAT for the last time. Her parents wanted her to maintain the family tradition and pressured her to try for the same college from which her mother graduated. She was not opposed to applying to her mother's alma mater, but was very angry and upset about her parents' pressure on her to make a commitment to this school as her first choice. She became irritable and tearful, and she was experiencing several panic attacks per week, all of which indicated that she needed to get some help. She was evaluated by a psychiatrist and started on Lexapro (escitalopram) to alleviate the panic disorder symptoms, as well as weekly psychotherapy. The psychotherapy focused on the patient's conflicts with her parents, highlighting her chronic concern that she could not meet parental expectations and fears of her independence. Medication appeared to reduce symptoms of tachycardia, tremulousness, decreased her irritability, and diminished her preoccupation with lack of competence. Psychotherapy and medication were both maintained for the next 8 months during her last year in high school. *(Adapted from case material courtesy of Cynthia R. Pfeffer, M.D.)*

Group Psychotherapy

In many ways, group psychotherapy is a natural setting for adolescents. Most teenagers are more comfortable with peers than with adults. A group diminishes the sense of unequal power between the adult therapist and the adolescent patient. Participation varies, depending on an adolescent's readiness. Not all interpretations and confrontations should come from the parent-figure therapist; group members often are adept at noticing symptomatic behavior in each other, and adolescents may find it easier to hear and consider critical or challenging comments from their peers.

Group psychotherapy usually addresses interpersonal and current life issues. Some adolescents, however, are too fragile for group psychotherapy or have symptoms or social traits that are too likely to elicit peer group ridicule; they need individual therapy to attain sufficient ego strength to struggle with peer relationships. Conversely, other adolescents must resolve interpersonal issues in a group before they can tackle intrapsychic issues in the intensity of one-on-one therapy.

Family Therapy

Family therapy is the primary modality when adolescents' difficulties mainly reflect a dysfunctional family (e.g., teenagers with school refusal, runaways). The same may be true when developmental issues, such as adolescent sexuality and striving for autonomy, trigger family conflicts or when family pathology is severe, as in cases of incest and child abuse. In these instances, adolescents usually need individual therapy as well, but family therapy is mandatory if an adolescent is to remain in the home or return to it. Serious character pathology, such as that underlying antisocial and borderline personality disorders, often develops from highly pathogenic early parenting. Family therapy is strongly indicated whenever possible for such disorders, but most authorities consider it adjunctive to intensive individual psychotherapy when individual psychopathology has become so internalized that it persists regardless of the current family status.

Inpatient Treatment

Residential treatment schools often are preferable for long-term therapy, but hospitals are more suitable for emergencies, although some adolescent inpatient hospital units also provide educational, recreational, and occupational facilities for long-term patients. Adolescents whose families are too disturbed or incompetent, who are dangerous to themselves or others, who are out of control in ways that preclude further healthy development, or who are seriously disorganized require, at least temporarily, the external controls of a structured environment.

Long-term inpatient therapy is the treatment of choice for severe disorders that are considered wholly or largely psychogenic in origin, such as major ego deficits that are caused by early massive deprivation and that respond poorly or not at all to medication. Severe borderline personality disorder, for example, regardless of the behavioral symptoms, requires a full-time corrective environment in which regression is possible and safe and in which ego development can take place. Psychotic disorders in adolescence often require hospitalization; however, psychotic adolescents often respond to appropriate medication well enough that therapy is feasible in an outpatient setting, except during exacerbations. Adolescent patients with schizophrenia who exhibit a long-term deteriorating course may require hospitalization periodically.

Day Hospitals

In day hospitals, which have become increasingly popular, adolescents spend the day in class, individual and group psychotherapy, and other programs, but they go home in the evenings. Day hospitals are less expensive than full hospitalization and usually are preferred by patients.

CLINICAL PROBLEMS

Atypical Puberty

Pubertal changes that occur 2.5 years earlier or later than the average age are within the normal range. Body image is so important to adolescents, however, that extremes of the norm may be distressing to some, either because markedly early maturation subjects them to social and sexual pressures for which they are unready or because late maturation makes them feel inferior and excludes them from some peer activities. Medical reassurance, even if based on examination and testing to rule out pathophysiology, may not suffice. An adolescent's distress may show as sexual or delinquent acting out, withdrawal, or problems at school that are sufficiently serious to warrant therapeutic intervention. Therapy also may be prompted by similar disturbances in some adolescents who fail to achieve peer-valued stereotypes of physical development despite normal pubertal physiology.

Substance-Related Disorders

Some experimentation with psychoactive substances is almost ubiquitous among adolescents, especially if this category of behavior includes alcohol use. Most adolescents, however, do not become abusers, particularly of prescription drugs and illegal substances. Any regular substance abuse represents disturbance. Substance abuse sometimes is self-medication against depression or schizophrenic deterioration and sometimes it signals a character disorder in teenagers whose ego deficits render them unequal to the stresses of puberty and the tasks of adolescence. Some substances, including cocaine, have a physiologically reinforcing action that acts independent of preexisting psychopathology. When substance abuse covers an underlying illness or is a maladaptive response to current stresses or disturbed family dynamics, treatment of the underlying cause may diminish the substance use; in most cases of significant abuse, however, the drug-taking behavior typically requires intervention. Substance abuse treatments typically include a 12-step program with behavioral monitoring to accomplish sobriety as well as the ability to verbalize regarding the motivations for substance use. These philosophies are adapted to inpatient, intensive outpatient, and once-a-week outpatient treatment.

Suicide

Suicide is the third leading cause of death among adolescents. Many hospital admissions of adolescents result from suicidal ideation or behavior. Among adolescents who are not psychotic, the highest suicidal risks occur in those who have a history of parental suicide, who are unable to form stable attachments, who display impulsive behavior, and who abuse alcohol or other substances. Many adolescents who complete suicide have backgrounds that include longstanding family conflict and social problems since early childhood and the escalation of subjective distress under the pressure of a sudden perceived conflict or loss. Early childhood loss of parents also can increase the risk of depression in adolescence. Adolescents who are susceptible to rapid and extreme mood swings and a history of impulsive behavior are at greater risk of responding to despair with impulsive suicide attempts. Abuse of alcohol and other substances are known added risks for suicidal behavior in adolescents with suicidal ideations. The developmentally predictable "omnipotent" attitudes of adolescents may cloud the immediate sense of permanence of death and result in impulsive self-destructive behavior in adolescents.

During a psychiatric evaluation of an adolescent with suicidal thoughts, plans and past attempts must be discussed directly when the concern arises and information is not volunteered. Recurring suicidal thoughts should be taken seriously, and a clinician must evaluate the imminent clinical danger requiring inpatient hospitalization versus an adolescent's ability to engage in an agreement or contract mandating that the adolescent will seek help before engaging in self-destructive behavior. Adolescents typically are honest in their refusal of such agreements, and, in such cases, hospitalization is indicated. Hospitalization of a suicidal adolescent by a clinician is an act of serious, protective concern.

▲ 27.19 Child Psychiatry: Special Areas of Interest

27.19a Forensic Issues in Child Psychiatry

Forensic evaluations of youth span a broad spectrum of situations and settings, including child custody during a parental divorce, trauma and abuse situations, and juvenile offender evaluations pertaining to juvenile and criminal court cases. Child and adolescent psychiatrists are increasingly being sought out by patients and attorneys for evaluations and expert opinions related to child sexual and physical abuse, to criminal behaviors perpetrated by minors, and to evaluate the relations between traumatic life events and the emergence of psychiatric symptoms in children and adolescents. As more youth enter the juvenile justice system, an increasing need exists for forensic psychiatrists with expertise in evaluation and treatment for detainees and committed youths.

The specific tasks and role of a child and adolescent psychiatric forensic evaluator are distinctly different from a child and adolescent psychiatrist doing a clinical evaluation and clinical treatment intervention. In clinical settings, child mental health professionals provide psychotherapy, medication evaluations, and advocacy for youth with psychiatric diagnoses. As a forensic child psychiatric evaluator, however, the main task is to be an expert, to report objective psychiatric findings related to the questions asked. Two essential characteristics of a forensic evaluator, in contrast to a clinician are (1) the relationship between the evaluator and the patient is not therapeutic, rather, it is information seeking, and (2) there are clear limits of confidentiality in this situation, that is, the information disclosed during a forensic evaluation may be brought to court, or to an attorney, or to whomever initiated the evaluation.

Society's view of children and their rights has evolved dramatically. In 1980, the AACAP published a code of ethics that was developed to publicly endorse the ethical standards of this discipline. The code is based on the assumption that children are vulnerable and unable to take adequate care of themselves; as they mature, however, their capacity to make judgments of, and choices about, their well-being develops as well. The code has several caveats: From the standpoint of child and adolescent psychiatrists, issues of consent, confidentiality, and professional responsibility must be seen in the context of overlapping and potentially conflicting rights of children, parents, and society.

Confidentiality, or intensive trust, refers to the relationship between two persons with respect to the "entrustment of secrets." Until the 1970s, little attention was paid to issues of confidentiality pertaining to minors. In 1980, among the items in the *AACAP Code of Ethics,* six principles were related to confidentiality. Breaches and limits of confidentiality can be obtained in cases of child abuse or maltreatment or for purposes of appropriate education. Although unnecessary with a child or adolescent, consent for disclosure should be obtained when possible. In 1979, the American Psychiatric Association (APA) stated that a child 12 years of age could give consent for disclosure of confidential information and, with the exception of safety issues, a minor's consent is required for disclosure of information to others, including the child's parents. According to the *AACAP Code of Ethics,* the consent of a minor is not required for disclosure of confidential information. Specific ages for consent are not addressed in the code. Child and adolescent psychiatrists often face the dilemma of weighing the potential benefits and possible harm in sharing information obtained confidentially from a child with the child's parents. Although the smoothest transition occurs when the child and the physician agree that certain information can be shared, in many situations that border on "dangerousness to the child or others," the child or adolescent does not agree to share the information with a parent or another responsible adult. Among adolescents, these secrets that are sometimes shared with a psychiatrist may involve drug or alcohol use, unsafe sex practices, or a thrill-seeking act that places the adolescent in danger. A psychiatrist may choose to work with the child or adolescent toward agreeing to share confidential information when it is determined by the treating psychiatrist that the probable outcome would be beneficial. The initial treatment contract, however, limits confidentiality to situations of "danger" to the child or others.

CHILD CUSTODY

Child custody evaluations by child and adolescent psychiatrists may be initiated by divorcing parents who cannot come to an agreement regarding custody of their children, or can be requested by an attorney. Attorneys are most likely to seek child custody evaluations when allegations are made of parental incompetence, or issues of alleged physical or sexual abuse arise. Comprehensive custody evaluations by mental health professionals may play a significant role in successful negotiations of custody by parents without the necessity of proceeding to a trial.

The evolution of child custody decision-making has been influenced by increasing awareness and recognition of the rights of children and women, as well as by a broadening perspective on the developmental and psychological needs of the children involved. Historically, children were considered to be their fathers' property. At the beginning of the 20th century, the "tender years" doctrine became the standard for determining child custody. According to this doctrine, the relationship between mother and infant, later generalized to mother and child, is responsible for the optimal emotional development of the child; the doctrine thus supported custody decisions in the mother's favor in most cases. With this doctrine as its guide, psychological issues in developing children became an acceptable dimension to consider in the determination of custody. In controversial and unclear cases, psychological expert testimony began to be accepted as a valuable part of child custody decision-making.

The "best interest of the child" standard replaced the "tender years" doctrine and expanded considerations of the optimal parent to include assessing issues of emotional climate, safety, and educational and social opportunities for the children. The "best interest of the child" grew from the movement to support legislation about the rights of children in the areas of compulsory education, child labor laws, and child abuse and neglect protection laws. Therefore, although "best interest" standards have broadened the dimensions considered in evaluating which parent is best able to serve the best interest of the child, how to measure these qualities in a parent remains vague. In view of the lack of clarity regarding what specific parameters in a parent best correspond to the interest of the child, child and adolescent psychiatrists have increasingly been asked to help make decisions by defining relevant psychological conditions in parents and in the relationships between parents and children.

Psychiatric evaluators may be asked to give an opinion about child custody at various points during the separation and divorce process. Sometimes, a psychiatric evaluation is requested by the parents before any legal action occurs. When the parents and an evaluator can agree on custody decisions before the legal process, a court is likely to go along with these decisions rather than launch an additional investigation. A psychiatric evaluation may be ordered by the court or by the attorneys representing the feuding parents. In such cases, an evaluator is faced with two disgruntled parents, who often are consumed by their mutual conflict to the point that neither is willing to compromise, even in the child's interest. The advantage in such cases, however, is that evaluators represent the court and can act as advocate for the child without the same pressures that an evaluator hired by only one parent faces. A psychiatric evaluation also may be initiated by a *guardian ad litem,* an attorney who is appointed by the court to represent the child. Psychiatric evaluators also may be requested to give an opinion about custody during a mediation process. Mediation is a legal process that usually involves one attorney and one evaluator. Because mediation can occur outside the judicial system, some families may prefer it to going through a trial. In addition to custody, psychiatric evaluators often are asked to give opinions about visitation.

In undertaking a custody evaluation, an evaluator is expected to determine the best interests of the child while keeping in mind the standard elements that the court considers. These considerations include the wishes of the parents and the child; relationships with significant others in the child's life; the child's adjustment to the current home, school, and community; the psychiatric and physical health of all parties; and the level of conflict and potential danger to the child under the care of either parent. A psychiatric evaluator must maintain his or her role as an advocate for the best interest of the child and does not consider the fairest outcome for parents. The psychiatric evaluator conducts a series of interviews, often including at least one separate interview with each parent and the child alone and one interview with the child and both parents. The evaluator may obtain a written waiver of confidentiality from all parties because he or she may have made disclosures to opposing attorneys and in court before the judge. The evaluator uses direct questioning as well as observations of the relationships between the child and each parent. The age and developmental needs of the child are considered in making a judgment regarding which parent may better serve the child's interests. As part of the psychiatric assessment of the child custody evaluation, the evaluator determines the need for psychiatric treatment of any of the parties involved.

The child custody evaluation generally is provided in a written report. This document is not confidential and can be used in court. The report contains a description of the relationship between the child and parents, the capabilities of the parents, and finally, the custody recommendations. In view of data supporting the importance of continuing a relationship with both parents in most cases, it is recommended that joint custody be considered before other options. When sufficient cooperation exists to negotiate for joint custody, the best interests of the child often are served. Joint custody may not be the best option for a child when the relationship of the child with either parent is jeopardized and undermined by the other. The next most frequent choice when joint custody is not advisable is full custody by one parent with visitation rights for the other parent. The parent awarded full custody should be able to support the visitations and relationship with the noncustodial parent. In custody disputes involving a biological parent and a nonbiological parent, the biological parent generally has the right to custody unless he or she is shown to be unable to provide for the child. After the custody evaluation has been submitted in writing, the results must be communicated to the parents, the child, and possibly their respective attorneys. The evaluator may be called on to testify in court, and the parties can use the custody evaluation to mediate other areas of their dispute.

Many complications can occur in an ongoing bitter dispute between divorcing or divorced parents. Both true and false allegations of psychiatric illness, drug or alcohol abuse, or sexual or physical abuse are not uncommon during custody battles. The evaluator must be prepared to verify any allegations and to carefully discuss their effects on custody and visitation. Evidence suggests that markedly elevated numbers of unfounded allegations of child sexual abuse occur during the course of custody disputes.

Tremain, age 9 years, has been in a therapeutic foster home for 2 years, having been removed from his home along with his younger sister, due to profound neglect, as well as physical abuse. Although he is receiving cognitive-behavioral therapy, medication, and a social skills group, he remains volatile, and typically becomes more aggressive and regressed after weekly supervised visits with his mother. Tremain's sister has been reunited with their mother, and his guardian *ad litem* requests that a child psychiatrist perform a forensic evaluation to determine whether visits should continue. She reviews extensive records, evaluates each parent, obtains history from them and the foster parent, and then observes a visit. Tremain's little sister totally dominates the visit, and her mother is at a loss to control her aggressive and hyperactive behavior. Tremain is passive and clingy with his mother. According to the social work supervisor, this is a fairly typical visit. When the child and adolescent psychiatrist meets individually with Tremain, he expresses concern that his sister is probably being abused at home, and he likes to check on her during these visits. Tremain wants to go home, but he says that his mother has too many problems to take care of him. Tremain has developed a positive relationship with his foster father and, in contrast, has little to say about his biological mother. The child and adolescent psychiatrist recommends a psychiatric evaluation of the sister, but Tremain's mother does not follow through. The child and adolescent psychiatrist recommends cutting visits back to monthly, but Tremain's anxiety and aggressive behavior persist around these limited visits. It also becomes apparent that Tremain's mother is not up to the demands of caring for two special-needs children, as she is having difficulty containing her little daughter. The child and adolescent psychiatrist recommends delaying efforts at parental reunification however, maintaining contact between Tremain, his mother, and his sister. *(Adapted from case material from Diane H. Schetky, M.D.)*

JUVENILE OFFENDERS

According to the AACAP Practice Parameter for Child and Adolescent Forensic Evaluations, at least 2.7 million youth younger than 18 years are arrested each year in the United States, and more than 1 million youth will have a formal interaction with the juvenile justice system. Historically, a separate juvenile court system in the United States occurred by statute in the state of Illinois in the late 1800s. Its mandate was to rehabilitate rather than to punish. Despite the protective intentions of the legal system, children and adolescents involved in the juvenile justice system are at high risk for multiple psychiatric disorders and suicidal thoughts and behavior. The omission of various constitutional safeguards, such as the rights to counsel, confrontation, and cross-examination of an accuser, eventually led to criticism and disillusionment with this system. Juvenile offenders of small and significant crimes often were sent to state-run residential programs that were criticized for being overcrowded, neglectful, and frankly abusive. Despite the strong sentiment to increase due process protection for juveniles rather than pretrial, trial, and sentencing, the juvenile court system includes intake, adjudication, and disposition. The intake is a determination of whether probable cause exists that the youth committed a crime. A youth who confesses may be diverted from the court system altogether at this time, and appropriate plans for rehabilitation can be made in a community setting. For more serious crimes or when juveniles deny perpetrating a crime, the process continues. Juveniles must be represented by counsel, and an attorney is provided if the family cannot afford to provide its own. Unlike adult court, in juvenile court, guilt or innocence is determined by a judge, not a jury. The case is argued by a prosecuting attorney and a defense attorney, and the judge is bound by the same standards as in adult court; that is, a judgment of delinquency requires proof beyond a reasonable doubt. When the charge is substantiated and the judgment is for delinquency, the juvenile is an "adjudicated delinquent." Disposition must next be determined. Dispositions include a wide range of options, from placement in youth correctional facilities, to residential treatment settings, to psychiatric hospitalizations for further evaluation. *Delinquent acts* refer to ordinary crimes committed by juveniles; *status offenses* refer to behaviors that would not be criminal if perpetrated by adults, such as truancy, running away, or drinking alcohol. Sometimes, youths who are believed to have committed a serious crime are turned over (receive a waiver) to adult criminal court.

DEVELOPMENTAL IMMATURITY VERSUS JUVENILE COMPETENCE TO STAND TRIAL

A growing body of research is elucidating the significance of "developmental immaturity" on the capacity of children and young adolescents' competency to stand trial. Starting in the 1960s, the Supreme Court mandated a series of due process rights in juvenile court proceedings including the rights to notice of charges, an adversarial hearing with representation by counsel, the ability to cross-examine witnesses, and a trial transcript. Furthermore, juveniles have the right to a hearing prior to being transferred to adult court, and use of the standard of proof beyond a reasonable doubt to sustain a delinquency petition; however, there is no mention of the right to be competent to stand trial in delinquency proceedings. In the 1960 landmark case *Dusky v. United States,* the Supreme Court established a minimum national standard for competency in criminal proceedings for adults. This standard mandates that in order for a defendant to be competent to stand trial, he or she must possess "sufficient present ability to consult with his lawyer with a reasonable degree of rational understanding and a rational as well as factual understanding of the proceedings against him." Thus, there is no legal requirement for juveniles to be competent to participate in delinquency proceedings; however, many states have adopted their own competency standards for their juvenile courts. This is critical insofar as research suggests that developmental level has a definite impact on a child or early adolescent's understanding of legal concepts, and long-term implications of legal decisions, and thereby influences their competency to stand trial. The following two U.S. Supreme Court rulings have provided legal stipulations pertaining to the limitations of developmental immaturity and legal culpability. (1) In the case, *Roper v. Simmons* (2005), a successful argument was made that, among other reasons, but including a juvenile's normative immaturity, including impulsive decision making, susceptibility to peer pressure, and transitory behavior patterns, youth younger than 18 years of age should be excluded from the death penalty. (2) In 2010, in the case *Graham v. Florida,* using the developmental information that fueled the exclusion of minors from the death penalty, the

Court ruled that a life sentence without parole for a juvenile offender (with the exclusion of homicide cases), constituted cruel and unusual punishment.

In one study using vignettes to elicit responses from children and adolescents pertaining to competent participation in legal proceedings, findings included that children 11 to 13 years were less able to recognize risks and long-term consequences associated with their decisions and were more likely than adults to accept plea agreements; whereas youths up to 15 years also demonstrated greater compliance with authority figures in their decision making, compared to adults. Researchers in this field have concluded that due to developmental status alone, young juveniles are at greater risk to make poor decisions on their own behalf in the context of working with their own attorneys.

There are many factors that may influence a juvenile's competency, and several are essential in a competency evaluation of a juvenile, including: (1) age, with special consideration in any child of 12 years or younger; (2) developmental stage with respect to judgment, reasoning, responsibility, risk perception, suggestibility, temperance (seeking advice rather than acting without the facts), and future orientation; (3) assessment of mental disorder and intellectual level.

MENTAL HEALTH NEEDS OF YOUTH IN THE JUVENILE JUSTICE SYSTEM

Youth in the juvenile justice system are at extremely high risk for psychiatric disturbance, and unmet mental health needs have reached such high proportions that they are of public health concern. Adolescents in juvenile justice residential facilities not only have higher rates of psychiatric disorders, including depression, substance use, and suicidal behavior, but they are also significantly more likely to have been victims of physical and sexual abuse, educational failure, and family conflict. A survey of 991 youth at an initial juvenile justice intake revealed high levels of suicidal ideation with recent attempts more common in females, and youth with major depression or substance use disorders, and those who were violent offenders. Few studies, however, have documented the needs of juveniles in residential facilities and the medical and psychiatric care available. A recent study collected data from the U.S. Department of Justice censuses of all public and private juvenile justice facilities in the United States: The Juvenile Residential Facilities Census (JRFC) and the Census of Juveniles in Residential Placement (CJRP) investigated data on death rates of youth under the age of 21 years who had been charged with, or adjudicated for, an offense and are housed in that facility because of the offense. In the 2-year period, a total of 62 deaths of youth occurred. The leading cause of death was from suicide (20 cases), followed by accidents (17 cases), illness (14 cases), and homicides by nonresidents (6 cases). No deaths resulted from AIDS, homicide by another resident, or an injury that occurred before placement. The risk for death of youth in juvenile justice facilities was found to be 8 percent higher than the death rate for the general population of adolescents aged 15 to 19 years. Above all, the risk for suicide is clearly increased in the juvenile justice facility compared with the general population, indicating a significant need for increased mental health evaluation and treatment in this population.

FORENSIC ASPECTS OF SCHOOL BULLYING

The forensic aspects of school bullying have increased over the last two decades, particularly in the wake of the serious incidents of school violence that took place in the mid-1990s such as the Columbine school shootings. The responsibilities of schools to protect students and safeguard against injury have extended from a *duty* to care, to a *duty* to protect. Bullying is typically observed in four different realms: physical, relational, verbal, and cyberbullying. Forensic evaluations often begin with a referral from an attorney, the court, or a family. After obtaining a comprehensive history of the youths involved in a reported bullying incident, the evaluator is tasked with determining if the alleged bullying has had a negative impact on the mental health and well-being of the victim. In some cases, investigators have reported findings of increased suicidality in the bully as well as the victim. One study reported that victims of cyberbullying attempt suicide twice as often as other youth.

THE RELATIONSHIPS BETWEEN TRAUMA, ABUSE, AND VIOLENT DELINQUENCY

Child and adolescent psychiatrists are frequently sought out to evaluate children or adolescents who have been exposed to a traumatic or adverse life event and are exhibiting a variety of violent and delinquent behaviors. The child and adolescent psychiatrist may be asked to determine whether a child or adolescent is experiencing PTSD or whether a given set of symptoms is likely to have been caused by exposure to the adverse life event. It is clear from surveys of delinquent adolescents that there is a relationship between PTSD, previous histories of trauma and abuse, and aggressive behavior. Some researchers argue that evidence supports a trauma-related psychopathology in youth that evolves into aggressive behavior, and often into delinquency. It appears that brain circuits that monitor "threat response," that is, circuits that run from the medial nucleus of the amygdala to the medial hypothalamus and to the periaqueductal gray matter, are overly reactive in reactive/affective/defensive/impulsive aggression (RADI, also referred to as "hot" aggression), as well as in planned or predatory aggression (PIP, also referred to as "cold" aggression). Particularly in RADI, structures may have become dysregulated by traumatic emotional activation, resulting in a lack of subtle differentiation between emotions such as sadness, anger, and fear. The result is that any stress is perceived as a threat, and activates the "defense" system, leading to the flight or fight decisions. The final response seems to be "fight," a response triggered during abusive or life-threatening situations in which escape seems impossible.

In another study, a cognitive mechanism for the link between abusive parenting and violent delinquency is offered. In this retrospective study of 112 adolescents (male 90; female 22), ages 12 to 19 years who were incarcerated in a juvenile detention facility pending criminal charges, participants completed questionnaires pertaining to exposure to abusive and nonabusive discipline, expressed and converted shame, and violent delinquency. The authors defined shame as a state in which negative attributions of the self and self-blame are made as a result of perceived failure in meeting their own expected standards. Higher levels of shame have been found among youth exposed to trauma. Converted shame is an expression of externalizing blame to others so that hostility is directed away from oneself, and decreases one's own sense of responsibility for something negative, such as abuse. Converted shame can serve as a self-protective attribution. The findings of this study led to subjects' responses, which fell into four groups: (1) Low shame, and low blaming of others, (2) Converters: low shame and high blaming of others, (3) Expressers: high shame, and low blaming of others, and (4) High shame and high blaming of others. Subjects who were in group 2 (low shame and high blaming of others) had significantly more exposure to abusive parenting, and exhibited significantly more violent delinquent behaviors than those in group 3 (high shame, low blaming of others). Thus, although converting shame is "meant" to be self-protective, and a potentially adaptive response to consistent abusive parenting, those adolescents who strongly blamed others appeared to develop more violent delinquency. The authors considered the violent delinquency a pathological response to trauma.

Dr. Sullivan is called by a defense attorney to review discovery material in a case that alleges permanent harm and suffering in 6-year-old Travis, who is alleged to have been sexually abused at age 3 in his day care center. Dr. Lane, the forensic expert for the plaintiff, has evaluated the child and performed psychological testing of him and concluded that the boy's conduct problems are all related to the alleged abuse, which the child has difficulty recalling. His early history on the boy is cursory, however, and he has little information about the mother, who is a single parent, and he did not review medical records. In her thorough review of discovery material, Dr. Sullivan learns that Travis has witnessed extensive domestic violence and his mother's rape, shown signs of hyperactivity since age 2, and has exhibited much anxiety related to his mother's safety and several separations from her at times when she was unable to care for him owing to depression. Travis also has had delayed language development. Dr. Lane, at the time of his deposition, was asked why he had not asked about these matters. He said he considered the mother's personal life a private matter and did not see its relevance to the litigation. Dr. Sullivan, when deposed, points out that many other factors beside the alleged abuse might account for Tony's behavioral problems. *(Adapted from case material from Diane H. Schetky, M.D.)*

27.19b Adoption and Foster Care

According to the U.S. Department of Health and Human Services, 408,425 children and adolescents were in foster care in the United States in 2010. Most children entering foster care have experienced multiple traumatic events including neglect, or abuse, which are typically the precipitant for their removal from their biological parents. One study estimated that 26 percent of children in the United States will experience a traumatic event by the age of 4 years. Over the last decade, specifically between the years 2000 and 2010, the number of evaluations for suspected child maltreatment has increased by 17 percent, according to another study.

Foster care is intended to be temporary out-of-home care, provided by the welfare system, for children and adolescents whose immediate families are unable to care for them. Given the severity of the pathology of vulnerable parents; however, care is often needed for many months and years. In 1997, President Clinton signed the Adoption and Safe Families Act, a law designed to improve provisions for child safety, to decrease the length of time that a child remains in foster care without long-term planning, and to limit the amount of time in which a biological parent has to undergo rehabilitation to 12 months. An additional law was added to allocate federal funds for independent living assistance for adolescents and young adults aged 16 to 21 years to assist them in transitioning to independent living.

EPIDEMIOLOGY AND DEMOGRAPHICS OF FOSTER CARE

The number of children entering foster care due to maltreatment has risen in the last decade by 19 percent. Of those children who entered foster care, there was an increase of 60 percent in the number who were identified as emotionally disturbed. In the United States, one of the most common scenarios of children being placed in foster care involves parental substance abuse, which leads to inability of the parent to care for their children. The National Center on Addiction and Substance Abuse of Columbia University reported that seven of ten abused or neglected children had parents with substance abuse. Furthermore, children in foster care were more often being raised by a single mother prior to placement compared to children in the community.

Minority children are overrepresented in the foster care population. In a study utilizing birth records and child protective service (CPS), black children were more than twice as likely to be referred due to maltreatment, be substantiated as victims of maltreatment, and enter the foster care system before age 5 years, compared to white children. However, low socioeconomic black children had a lower rate of referral, substantiation, and placement in foster care than socioeconomically similar white children. Among Latinos, children of U.S.-born mothers were significantly more likely to have involvement with CPS, compared to Latino children of foreign-born mothers. However, after adjusting for socioeconomic factors, the relative risk of referral, substantiation, and entry into the foster care system was significantly higher for all Latino children than for white children. Approximately 38 percent of children in the foster care system are African American, more than three times their representation in the general population. Whites make up approximately 48 percent, and Hispanics make up almost 15 percent of foster children; 55 to 69 percent are girls, and 83.4 percent enter foster care at a mean age of 3 years. Children placed in care as infants are more likely to stay in care. Those younger than 5 years of age currently comprise the fastest growing segment of the foster care population. Studies reveal that up to 62 percent of foster children had prenatal drug exposure.

NEEDS OF FOSTER CARE CHILDREN

Children entering foster care have enormous mental health needs; more than 80 percent of them have developmental, emotional, or behavioral problems. It is estimated that up to 70 percent of these children have diagnosable psychiatric disorders. In addition, according to one study, quality of life (QOL) is significantly poorer among children in the foster care system than children in the general community. Children and adolescents living in residential care rated their QOL as poorer than those living with foster families. Up to 50 percent of foster care children exhibit depressive symptoms, and self-reports of anxiety problems occur in about 36 percent. QOL is adversely affected by the presence of mental health problems, and those youth with greater mental health difficulties rated their QOL as poorer whether in residential facilities or foster placement. In a review of the literature, psychiatric disorders found with increased frequency in foster youth were ADHD, PTSD, conduct disorders, attachment disorders, substance abuse, depression, and eating disorders.

In addition to high rates of psychiatric disorders, foster care youth are referred to pediatric clinics more frequently due to multiple health problems compared to community youth. Growth abnormalities (including failure to thrive), neurological abnormalities, neuromuscular disorders, language disorders, cognitive delays, and asthma are prevalent. Health care costs in foster care youth are six to ten times that of matched non–foster-care peers. Among children 0 to 5 years of age, approximately 25 percent are seriously emotionally damaged; attachment disorders are increasingly diagnosed. Foster care children use the full range of mental health services: outpatient, acute inpatient, day treatment, partial hospitalization, and residential treatment. Adolescents in foster care are at increased risk for substance abuse, teenage pregnancies, and STDs, including HIV. With public health care increasingly adopting a managed health care system, which is designed to limit care, grave concern exists that the provision and delivery of services to this medically and psychiatrically vulnerable population may be seriously compromised.

KINSHIP CARE FOR FOSTER CHILDREN

More states are recognizing kinship care as an alternative placement option and are authorizing licensing and reimbursement to kinship caregivers who are generally female (mostly maternal grandmothers), of low income, of low education, and of minority status. Currently, nationwide, approximately 23 percent of African American children are in foster kinship care. It is unknown just how many children are in informal kinship care within the African American population, which has had a long cultural tradition of taking in children of family members who are unable to care for their offspring. The few studies available indicate that outcomes, although mixed, are somewhat more positive than for those children in nonkinship care. Children reportedly receive more positive regard from caregivers in kinship care, and a consistent outcome, when it works, is that it provides more stability than nonrelative foster care. Most foster children have consistently said that they would rather be with a family member than stay in the system. When foster children feel embraced by their families of origin, and the latter can provide appropriate nurturance and access to good therapeutic services, the foster children's sense of identity and belonging is less disrupted. However, no demonstrable difference is seen in the need for mental health, medical, and special educational services for these children.

THERAPEUTIC FOSTER CARE

Therapeutic foster care (TFC) has emerged as a cost-effective alternative to the more restrictive *residential treatment center* (RTC). Therapeutic effectiveness is mixed. TFC is designed to provide nurturing family-based care with specialized treatment interventions from an interdisciplinary treatment team. Therapeutic foster parents are meant to be the agents of therapeutic change, functioning as *extenders* of the clinical treatment team. Because of the children's special needs, therapeutic foster parents must have more extensive training than other foster parents, receive a higher reimbursement, and receive more intensive monitoring, supervision, and support from the foster care agency. Although the concept of TFC is promising, good outcome data do not show consistent success. Several models exist, but implementation that shows fidelity to empirically tested models is often spotty. Some models have proved too expensive and complicated to implement in the real-world setting. The concept of professional therapeutic parents, who are paid competitive full-time wages to care for special needs foster children, holds promise as an alternative to current prevailing practice. Clinical practice demonstrates that, when adequate and appropriate intensive in-home services with good case management is provided in a well-managed foster care setting, children can show significant gains.

CULTURAL COMPETENCE

Anna McPhatter defines *cultural competence* as the ability to use knowledge and cultural awareness to design psychosocial interventions that support and sustain healthy client–system functioning within a cultural context that is meaningful to the client. Because American society is still significantly encumbered by racial conflicts, some children have been denied placement with families of a different race, and have ended up in long-term foster care rather than in a permanent adoption placement. The Association of Black Social Workers went on record as opposing transracial placement of African American children. In 1978, the Indian Child Welfare Act transferred to Tribal Courts the power to make placement decisions about Native American children to reverse the practice of placement in non–Native American homes. Adoption studies have shown that it is not inherently harmful for children to be cross-racially adopted. Congress has passed legislation, the Multiethnic Placement Act of 1994, facilitating transracial adoptions, while maintaining the language of cultural awareness in placement decisions. The need for cultural sensitivity, respect, and a capacity to facilitate a foster child's cultural development and identity are well acknowledged. These issues must be addressed in training providers of foster care services.

PSYCHOLOGICAL ISSUES IN FOSTER CARE CHILDREN

Family risk factors including alcohol and drug abuse in parents, parental neglect and abuse, and cognitive or mental or physical health problems in parents, as well as low socioeconomic status and low social support, are strongly associated with a child being placed out of the home. Psychiatric and behavior problems in the child may also contribute to being placed out of the home. Among children who return home, 40 percent reenter the foster care system. These children struggle with issues of abandonment, neglect, rejection, and physical, emotional, and sexual maltreatment. The child's age, home environment, and the specific reasons for going into placement affect the emotional issues that the child must handle. Early abandonment and neglect can lead to anaclitic depression. Attachment issues are prevalent in this young population, because there has been no opportunity to form secure attachments with consistent nurturing figures in early life.

Foster children are often unprepared for separations, which can be abrupt and repeated in the current foster care climate. Early separation from the primary caretaker is considered a major trauma for a child and sets the stage for vulnerability to subsequent trauma. Those children who bounce from foster home to foster home have their capacity to form enduring emotional attachments compromised; trust becomes a lifelong challenge.

Children who have experienced traumatic physical and sexual abuse often become mistrustful, hypervigilant, aggressive, impulsive, oppositional, and avoidant as they attempt to negotiate a world that they experience as threatening, hostile, and uncaring. When a child's early developmental period is spent in a psychosocial environment of trauma, aggression, and lack of empathy from adults, the psychological seeds are sown for later violence against the self and others. A wide range of behavior problems is likely to emerge in foster care children given their early family experiences. A pervasive problem is one of dysregulation: dysregulation of behavior, emotions and affect, attention, and sleep. The empirical data on the neurobiology of maltreatment on the developing brain reveals that stress hormones play an important role in adaptation and coping, and that these capacities are compromised in varying degrees of severity in abused and neglected children. The data also show that, because of the developmental plasticity of the brain, appropriate early intervention can induce remediation and repair at the neurobiological level.

Nick, a 5-year-old, was placed in foster care because of maternal substance abuse and inability to take care of her child. When seen for a psychiatric evaluation, it was noted that all of his primary teeth were full of dental cavities. The foster mother was asked about dental care, and she responded that the dentist had said that he would wait until the teeth had fallen out, because they were his first set of teeth and did not require intervention. This response aroused suspicion that neglect in the foster family was exacerbating Nick's hyperactive and aggressive behaviors. A neglect report was made and the investigation revealed that Nick was not only neglected, but was also being physically abused in that foster care placement. Subsequent to removal and placement with a nurturing and responsible foster family, Nick has shown considerable emotional stabilization, does well academically and socially, and is now being adopted by that family. *(Adapted from case material Marilyn B. Benoit, M.D., Steven L. Nickman, M.D., and Alvin Rosenfeld, M.D.)*

FAMILY PRESERVATION

Family preservation has come under increasing scrutiny in the last decade. Estimates on the percentage of children who are reportedly reunited vary from 66 to 90 percent. Philosophically, family reunification appears to be the right thing to do, yet approximately 40 percent of reunified children reenter out-of-home care. The field needs discriminating criteria that would identify psychosocial profiles of families that could best benefit from family preservation services. In 1996, the Child Welfare League of America (CWLA) acknowledged the failure of family preservation efforts and requested that child welfare policy makers rethink the current use of intensive family preservation. Recent research has validated poor outcomes with family preservation. Hopes are that the Adoption and Safe Families Act of 1997 will give child welfare agencies the opportunity to step back from the myopic view of family preservation and to consider the needs of the child as the major priority. The AACAP and the CWLA jointly launched a national effort to address the mental health needs of children in foster care. This effort is supported by a broad-based coalition of agencies that are all stakeholders in foster care. The coalition proposes that the foster care system be child focused, but inclusive of the biological and foster families in intervention planning on the child's behalf if families are to be preserved.

One case of a 7-year-old boy who was in foster care for 2 years is illustrative of why some family preservation efforts fail. When James was returned to his biological mother, she was in a new marriage with a new baby. Her husband was new to parenting. The family was financially strapped and lived under harsh conditions. James' mother completed the required parenting course for resuming custody of her child, and seemed pleased to have him back with her; however, no supports were put in place to assist this young couple financially or with any family therapy, psychoeducation, or case management interventions. Frequent and increasingly urgent calls to the child welfare family reunification services were made to seek respite and financial help, but this was not possible. The outcome for James was that he was reabused and had to reenter the foster care system.

This outcome represents a failure of the system, but also translates into a debilitated family, with a profound sense of failure. *(Adapted from case material from Marilyn B. Benoit, M.D., Steven L. Nickman, M.D., and Alvin Rosenfeld, M.D.)*

FOSTER CARE OUTCOMES AND RESEARCH INITIATIVES

The overall quality of available outcome studies is poor. Some patterns, however, recur across studies. Several studies reveal that 15 to 39 percent of the homeless are foster care graduates, who are also overrepresented among adult substance abusers and clients in the criminal justice system. It is likely that the reasons that initially precipitated the child's foster care placement contributed to the negative adult outcomes. Studies indicate that children entering care who have been victimized, who have substance-abusing parents or parents with major mental illness or high criminality, or both, and who come from homes with a high degree of domestic violence are at greater risk of having poor outcomes. Research on early maltreatment indicates that the influence of maltreatment on brain development can be profound over the life span. Developmental disabilities occur in more than 50 percent of the foster care population. Children returned to their families of origin typically have fared worse than those who have remained in long-term placement.

Several studies report findings indicating that multiple placements and poor parental involvement consistently lead to negative outcomes. Federal mandate requires states to maintain a tracking system for children in foster care. New reporting systems, the Adoption and Foster Care Analysis and Reporting System (AFCARS) and the Statewide Automated Child Welfare Information System (SACWIS), are available nationwide. States are being monitored for compliance with their use, and continued federal funds are contingent on the implementation of these information systems. Because foster care placement is the result of psychosocial environmental failure, fixing the existing system requires more than good information systems. Integration of sound, theory-driven, child-focused, family-centered services, collaboratively funded by multiple governmental agencies, is essential. Through the use of longitudinal, research-based performance measures, reliable data are emerging. The NIMH has funded some research focusing on foster care children and youth. The complexity of the impact of ever-changing psychosocial variables makes this type of research challenging. Despite that, it must be done if welfare dollars are to be spent doing the right thing for needy children and their families. In 2004, in a groundbreaking study, the Pew Commission on Children in Foster Care made sweeping recommendations to overhaul the system, stating that "children deserve more from our child welfare system."

HISTORY OF ADOPTION

Adoption has existed in different forms throughout history. In ancient Babylonia, it provided for the transmission of property or artisan's skills, whereas, in the Roman Empire, it was often used to elevate the status of an adult protégé. In some Pacific islands, adoption of young children formed part of an exchange system between related clans. Concerns expressed by adopted persons about not knowing their roots are as ancient as they are contemporary. Euripides' *Ion* contains a touching dialogue between a woman in search of the child she had given up years before and a young priest of Apollo, who does not know that he is the woman's son and says that the only mother he knows is Apollo's priestess.

Historically, *closed adoptions* were common practice. That was done to ensure the sealed identities of birth and adoptive parents and was believed to be in the best interests of adopted children. That practice is now considered flawed; contemporary, although still controversial, thinking is that most adoptees should grow up knowing their adoption status, as well as the identities of their birth parents. Currently, adoptees, as well as many birth parents and adoptive parents, increasingly have shared interests in legislation that affects the open or closed status of birth records and the placement of children in families. The phrase *adoption triad* has come to stand for these shared interests. Several other organizations represent each of these three groups, and those organizations often have divergent agendas. Since the 1980s, adoption practice has been profoundly affected by federal legislation.

EPIDEMIOLOGY OF ADOPTION

Estimates suggest that between 2.5 and 3.5 percent of children in the United States are adopted, with more than 2 percent adopted by nonrelatives, and about 1.5 percent in relative adoptions, which include stepparents. Foster care children who are adopted account for about 15 percent of all adopted children. Approximately 125,000 children are adopted each year, in a variety of scenarios. Infants may be relinquished by their biological parents at birth and adopted through private agencies. These adoptions are increasingly "open," with some continued contact with biological parents. About 50,000 babies are adopted in this manner each year. Another 50,000 children are adopted through the child welfare system, and these children have often been exposed to multiple foster home placements before they are adopted. These adoptees range in age, with more than half of them being older than 6 years of age, and the majority of them having experienced significant early abuse or neglect.

INTERNATIONAL ADOPTION

International adoptions have been growing over the last two decades. Each year more than 20,000 children are adopted from overseas, and many of these are transracial adoptions. More than 17,000 children were adopted from Guatemala, for example, in the last two decades. In the Guatemalan adoptees, the mean age was 1.5 years and the children had previously resided in orphanages, foster homes, or mixed-care settings. Investigation of the health records of international adoptees who were evaluated in an international adoption specialty clinic in the United States revealed that younger children at the time of adoption have better growth, language development, cognitive skills, and competence in activities of daily living compared to children who were older at the time of adoption. Among children matched for age, gender, and time from adoption to evaluation, those who were previously living in foster care were observed to have higher cognitive scores and improved growth compared to children who had resided in orphanages. These findings support the priority of adoptive placement at younger ages and that foster care has benefits over orphanage care.

EARLY CHILDHOOD VERSUS LATE ADOPTION

Data suggest that earlier age adoption predicts better outcome than adoption in middle or late childhood. A recent prospective study examined factors related to successful outcome in public adoption of children ranging in age from 5 to 11 years of age. Prospective data were collected from domestic adoptions in the United Kingdom at the first year, and 6 years later on 108 adoptees who were placed primarily because of situations involving childhood abuse and neglect. Outcome was assessed by the disruption rate and measures of psychological adaptation. At the adolescent follow-up, 23 percent of the adoption placements had been disrupted, 49 percent were continuing with positive adaptations, and 28 percent were ongoing but with significant conflicts. Four factors contributed independently to the risk of disruptions: older age at placement, report of being singled out and rejected by siblings, time in care, and greater degree of behavioral problems. Given that almost half of the placements were ongoing, it is apparent that later childhood age of adoption can also be successful; assessment of the constellation of the adoptive families, and of the children's behavioral problems, may determine the likelihood of positive outcome for school-aged child adoptees.

BIRTH PARENTS: SEARCH AND REUNION

The increasing trend toward open adoption allows the opportunity for adoptees to more easily search and successfully find their birth parents. Many adoptive parents choose open adoptions in the belief that they can experience a greater connection with the child if they have some relationship with the birth mother. Some adoptees want to develop an ongoing relationship with birth parents, but many who search are satisfied to meet birth parents without further correspondence. Outcomes of reunions with birth parents vary widely. In some cases, especially when the birth parents are well functioning and welcoming toward their child, the adoptee may experience a sense of relief and joy in knowing that their birth mother is no longer vulnerable.

27.19c Child Maltreatment, Abuse, and Neglect

Child maltreatment includes all types of abuse and neglect and is a major public health concern in the United States. The Centers for Disease Control and Prevention (CDC) estimate that one in every five children in the United States has been a victim of child maltreatment. Among the CDC's estimates of maltreated children, in 2012 for which the latest figures are available, 18 percent were victims of physical abuse, 9 percent were victims of sexual abuse, 78 percent were victims of neglect, and 12 percent experienced emotional abuse. Estimates of children maltreated in the United States each year are close to 1 million, and the annual number of deaths caused by abuse or neglect is reported to be about 1,500. A majority of child neglect and abuse occurs in infancy and early childhood, negatively impacting overall brain development, and disrupting time-sensitive developmental brain processes. A growing body of research suggests that child maltreatment potentially results in long-term damage in the neuroendocrine system, cell loss, and delays in myelination in the hippocampus and prefrontal cortex, as well as a chronic inflammatory state independent of clinical comorbidities.

The National Longitudinal Study on Adolescent Health investigated the prevalence, risk factors, and health consequences of maltreatment in 12,118 adolescents. Maltreated adolescents retrospectively reported the most common experiences were being left home alone as a child, (reported by 41.5 percent of the sample), physical assault (reported by 28.4 percent), physical neglect (reported by 11.8 percent), and sexual abuse (reported by 4.5 percent). Each type of maltreatment was associated with at least eight of the ten adolescent health risks examined, including self-report of depression, regular alcohol use, binge drinking, marijuana use, overweight status, generally "poor" health, inhalant use, and aggressive behaviors, including fighting and hurting others. Clearly, the effects of self-reported maltreatment had far ranging and long-lasting associations with multiple detrimental consequences.

The identification, management, and treatment of child maltreatment require cooperative efforts between professionals, including primary care physicians, emergency room staff, law enforcement, attorneys, social service staff, and mental health professionals. Perpetrators typically deny abuse or neglect and maltreated children often fear disclosure of their abuse or neglect.

DEFINITIONS

DSM-5

The *Diagnostic and Statistical Manual of Mental Disorders, Fifth Edition* (DSM-5) lists Child Maltreatment and Neglect in the section "Other Conditions That May Be a Focus of Clinical Attention." The presence of Child physical abuse, Child sexual abuse, Child neglect, and Child psychological abuse can be coded as confirmed or suspected and as an Initial encounter or a Subsequent encounter. Under a subcategory of "other circumstances related to" each form of child maltreatment or neglect, five "V" coded clinical situations related to maltreatment can be coded. These include the following: (1) encounter for mental health services for victim of child maltreatment by parent; (2) encounter for mental health services for victim of nonparental child maltreatment; (3) personal history (past history) of childhood maltreatment; (4) encounter for mental health services for perpetrator of parental child maltreatment; and (5) encounter for mental health services for perpetrator of nonparental child maltreatment.

Federal Law

The Child Abuse Prevention and Treatment Act was passed in 1974 and has been amended several times, most recently in 2003. In federal law, *child abuse* and *neglect* mean, at a minimum, any recent act or failure to act on the part of a parent or caretaker that results in death, serious physical or emotional harm, or sexual abuse or exploitation. It also includes an act or failure to act that presents an imminent risk of serious harm. In federal law, *sexual abuse* means the employment, use, persuasion, inducement, enticement, or coercion of any child to engage in or to assist any other person to engage in any sexually explicit conduct (or simulation of such conduct for the purpose of producing a visual depiction of such conduct) or the rape (and in cases of caretaker or interfamilial relationships, statutory rape), molestation, prostitution, or other forms of sexual exploitation of children or incest with children.

State Law

A large mass of legal definitions and guidelines exists at the state level. The legal definitions of terms related to the maltreatment of children vary from one jurisdiction to another, so clinicians should be aware of the definitions used in their own locale. The following generic definitions are used in this section.

Neglect

Neglect, the most prevalent form of child maltreatment, is the failure to provide adequate care and protection for children. Children can be harmed by malicious or ignorant withholding of physical, emotional, and educational necessities. Neglect includes failure to feed children adequately and to protect them from danger. Physical neglect includes abandonment, expulsion from home, disruptive custodial care, inadequate supervision, and reckless disregard for a child's safety and welfare. Medical neglect includes refusal, delay, or failure to provide medical care. Educational neglect includes failure to enroll a child in school and allowing chronic truancy.

Physical Abuse

Physical abuse can be defined as any act that results in a nonaccidental physical injury, such as beating, punching, kicking, biting, burning, and poisoning. Some physical abuse is the result of unreasonably severe corporal punishment or unjustifiable punishment. Physical abuse can be organized by damage to the site of injury: skin and surface tissue, the head, internal organs, and skeletal.

Emotional Abuse

Emotional or *psychological abuse* occurs when a person conveys to children that they are worthless, flawed, unloved, unwanted, or endangered. The perpetrator may spurn, terrorize, ignore, isolate, or berate the child. Emotional abuse includes verbal assaults (e.g., belittling, screaming, threats, blaming, or sarcasm), exposing the child to domestic violence, overpressuring through excessively advanced expectations, and encouraging or instructing the child to engage in antisocial activities. The severity of emotional abuse depends on (1) whether the perpetrator actually intends to inflict harm on the child and (2) whether the abusive behaviors are likely to cause harm to the child. Some authors believe that the terms *emotional* or *psychological abuse* should not be used and that *verbal abuse* more accurately describes the pathological behavior of the caregiver.

Sexual Abuse

Sexual abuse of children refers to sexual behavior between a child and an adult or between two children when one of them is significantly older or uses coercion. The perpetrator and the victim may be of the same sex or the opposite sex. The sexual behaviors include touching breasts, buttocks, and genitals, whether the victim is dressed or undressed; exhibitionism; fellatio; cunnilingus; and penetration of the vagina or anus with sexual organs or objects. Sexual abuse can involve behavior over an extended time or a single incident. Developmental factors must be considered in assessing whether sexual activities between two children are abusive or normative. In addition to the forms of inappropriate sexual touching, *sexual abuse* also refers to sexual exploitation of children, for instance, conduct or activities related to pornography depicting minors and promoting or trafficking in prostitution of minors.

Ritual Abuse

Cult-based *ritual abuse,* which includes satanic ritual abuse, is physical, sexual, or psychological abuse that involves bizarre or ceremonial activity that is religiously or spiritually motivated. Typically, multiple perpetrators abuse multiple victims over an extended period. Ritual abuse is a controversial concept; some professionals believed in the 1990s that ritual abuse was a common, horrible phenomenon in society, whereas others were skeptical about most allegations and descriptions of ritual abuse.

Perpetrators of Abuse

Some lack of consistency is seen in who may be defined as an *abuse perpetrator.* Usually, a person must be a parent or designated caregiver to be charged with neglect, physical abuse, or emotional abuse. Another adult (e.g., a stranger) who injures a child would be charged with battery, not with child abuse. On the other hand, a caretaker or any other person could be charged with child sexual abuse. State laws vary in this regard.

ETIOLOGY

Physical Abuse

Although child abuse occurs at all socioeconomic levels, it is highly associated with poverty and psychosocial stress, parental substance abuse, and mental illness. Child maltreatment is strongly correlated with less parental education, underemployment, poor housing, welfare reliance, and single parenting. Child abuse tends to occur more often in families characterized by domestic violence, social isolation, parental mental illness, and drug and alcohol abuse. The probability of maltreatment may be increased by risk factors in the child such as prematurity, intellectual disability, and physical handicap. In addition, the risk of child abuse increases in families with many children.

Sexual Abuse

Social, cultural, physiological, and psychological factors all contribute to the breakdown of the incest taboo. Incestuous behavior has been associated with alcohol abuse, overcrowding, increased physical proximity, and rural isolation that prevent adequate extrafamilial contacts. Some communities may be more tolerant of incestuous behavior. Major mental disorders and intellectual deficiency have been described in some perpetrators of incest and sexual abuse.

CLINICAL FEATURES

Maltreated children manifest a variety of emotional, behavioral, and somatic reactions. These psychological symptoms are neither specific nor pathognomonic: The same symptoms can occur without any history of abuse. The psychological symptoms manifested by abused children and the behaviors of abusive parents can be organized into clinical patterns. Although it may be helpful to note whether a particular case falls into one of these patterns, which in itself is not diagnostic of child abuse.

Physically Abused Children

In many cases, the physical examination and radiological evaluation show evidence of repeated suspicious injuries. Abused children display behaviors that should arouse the suspicions of the health professional. For example, these children may be unusually fearful, docile, distrustful, and guarded. On the other hand, they may be disruptive and aggressive. They may be wary of physical contact and show no expectation of being comforted by adults, they may be on the alert for danger and continually size up the environment, and they may be afraid to go home.

The literature regarding the psychological consequences of physical abuse and neglect indicates a wide range of effects: affect dysregulation, insecure and atypical attachment patterns, impaired peer relationships involving increased aggression or social withdrawal, and academic underachievement. Physically abused children exhibit a range of psychopathology; including depression, conduct disorder, ADHD, oppositional defiant disorder, dissociation, and PTSD.

Physically Abusive Parents

Abusive parents often feel significant guilt, and may delay seeking help for the child's injuries, fearful that the child will be taken away. Often the history of how a child sustained injuries given by the parents is implausible or incompatible with the physical findings. Parents may blame a sibling or claim that the children injured themselves. The characteristics of abusive parents often include a history of abuse in their own early lives, a lack of empathy for the child, unrealistic expectations of the child, and an impaired parent–child attachment.

Katie, 3 years of age, had been exhibiting new negative and aggressive behavior at preschool beginning 3 months after the birth of her brother. Katie's teacher observed her increased irritability and aggression, at times pushing other children, and she had recently hit a classmate with a wooden block, causing a laceration of the child's lip. When Katie's teacher took her aside to talk about her behavior, she noticed several bruises on Katie's arms and face. When her teacher asked Katie how she had gotten the bruises, Katie replied "my mommy's boyfriend gets mad at me and hits me with his belt." The teacher reported suspected child abuse to Child Protective Services. Katie's teacher also called her mother to let her know what was happening, and suggested that they take Katie for a psychiatric evaluation.

Katie's baby brother was colicky and slept only for short periods of time throughout the day and night. He stopped crying only when his mother held him. Her mother, therefore, had little time for Katie, and the mother's boyfriend was left to take care of Katie on evenings after day care and on weekends. He began to drink more than usual and became increasingly irritable. Katie's mother and her boyfriend often argued, and Katie had seen her mother physically pushed and threatened by her boyfriend. Katie, who was a bright, curious, and talkative child, had tried to be helpful by asking to hold the baby. When refused, however, Katie became upset and would lie on the floor and have a tantrum. Katie began to have difficulty falling asleep and awoke repeatedly during the night. Katie's mother's boyfriend would become extremely angry when Katie would wake him up, and often told her to shut up and slapped her when she told him that she couldn't go back to sleep. On many occasions, he responded to her tantrums or repeated demands for attention by hitting her with his belt.

Child Protective Services suggested that mother's boyfriend voluntarily move out, and no longer spend time alone with Katie caring for her, which he did begrudgingly, and Katie and her mother began a family therapy program that included parenting training for Katie's mother and, a behavioral program to help Katie with her tantrums. Katie's mother's boyfriend attended Alcoholics Anonymous (AA) meetings and stopped drinking. He was able to control his anger, and was allowed to visit the home, as long as Katie's mother was present. Within the next three months, Katie's aggressive behavior had ceased, and she was less irritable and was no longer having tantrums. She was doing well with peers, was sleeping through the night, and was no longer afraid to be at home. *(Adapted from case material from William Bernet, M.D.)*

Sexually Abused Children

A variety of symptoms, behavioral changes, and diagnoses sometimes occur in sexually abused children: anxiety symptoms, dissociative reactions and hysterical symptoms, depression, disturbances in sexual behaviors, and somatic complaints.

Anxiety Symptoms. Anxiety symptoms include fearfulness, phobias, insomnia, nightmares that directly portray the abuse, somatic complaints, and PTSD.

Dissociative Reactions and Hysterical Symptoms. The child may exhibit periods of amnesia, daydreaming, trancelike states, hysterical seizures, and symptoms of dissociative identity disorder.

Depression. Depression may be manifested by low self-esteem and suicidal and self-mutilative behaviors.

Disturbances in Sexual Behaviors. Some sexual behaviors are particularly suggestive of abuse, such as masturbating with an object, imitating intercourse, and inserting objects into the vagina or anus. Sexually abused children may display sexually aggressive behavior toward others. Other sexual behaviors are less specific, such as showing genitals to other children and touching the genitals of others. A younger child may manifest age-inappropriate sexual knowledge. In contrast to these overly sexualized behaviors, the child may avoid sexual stimuli through phobias and inhibitions.

Somatic Complaints. Somatic complaints include enuresis, encopresis, anal and vaginal itching, anorexia, bulimia, obesity, headache, and stomachache.

These symptoms are not pathognomonic. Nonabused children may exhibit any of these symptoms and behaviors. For example, normal, nonabused children commonly exhibit sexual behaviors, such as masturbating, displaying their genitals, and trying to look at people who are undressing.

Approximately one-third of sexually abused children have no apparent symptoms. Many adults who were abused as children have no significant abuse-related symptoms. On the other hand, the following factors tend to be associated with more severe symptoms in the victims of sexual abuse: greater frequency and duration of abuse, sexual abuse that involved force or penetration, and sexual abuse perpetrated by the child's father or stepfather. Other factors associated with poorer prognosis are the child's perception of not being believed, family dysfunction, and lack of maternal support. Also, multiple investigatory interviews appear to increase symptoms.

Intrafamilial Sexual Abuse

Incest can be defined strictly as sexual relations between close blood relatives, that is, between a child and the father, uncle, or sibling. Because of increased reporting, sibling incest is an area of growing concern. In its broader sense, incest includes sexual intercourse between a child and a stepparent or stepsibling. Although father–daughter incest is the most common form, incest can also involve father and son, mother and daughter, and mother and son.

Intrafamilial sexual abuse and other sexual abuse that occurs over a period of time are characterized by a particular pattern or sequence of steps. Victims of sexual abuse recount a gradual progression of boundary violations by the perpetrator, starting with tiny invasions and escalating to serious, overwhelming intrusions. Healthy, self-confident children rebuff the intrusions directly (via temper tantrums and verbal disagreements) or indirectly (through silence and distancing maneuvers) or by adopting any strategy that causes the offender to refrain.

Sexual abuse that occurs over a period of time evolves through five phases: engagement, sexual interaction, secrecy, disclosure, and suppression.

Engagement Phase. The perpetrator induces the child into a special relationship. The daughter in father–daughter incest has frequently had a close relationship with her father throughout her childhood and may be pleased at first when he approaches her sexually.

Sexual Interaction Phase. The sexual behaviors progress from less to more intrusive forms of abuse. As the behavior continues, the abused daughter becomes confused and frightened, because she never knows whether her father will be parental or sexual. If the victim tells her mother about the abuse, the mother may not be supportive. The mother often refuses to believe her daughter's reports or refuses to confront her husband with her suspicions. Because the father provides special attention to a particular daughter, her brothers and sisters may distance themselves from her.

Secrecy Phase. The perpetrator threatens the victim not to tell. The father, fearful that his daughter may expose their relationship and often jealously possessive of her, interferes with the girl's development of normal peer relationships.

Disclosure Phase. The abuse is discovered accidentally (when another person walks into the room and sees it), through the child's reporting it to a responsible adult, or when the child is brought for medical attention and an alert clinician asks the right questions.

Suppression Phase. The child often retracts the statements of the disclosure because of family pressure or because of the child's own mental processes. That is, the child may perceive that violent or intrusive attention is synonymous with interest or affection. Many incest survivors rally around their perpetrators, seeking to capture any modicum of tenderness or interest. At times, affection for the perpetrator outweighs the facts of abuse, and children recant their statements about sexual assault, regardless of substantiated evidence of molestation.

A family with a comfortable financial situation lived in a pleasant, clean house in a nice neighborhood, but they had no friends. Their four teenagers never had visitors. One day, the oldest girl, 17 years of age, went to the police and told them that she had a baby at home and that her own father was the father of the baby. The teen said that her father had been having sexual relations with her for more than 4 years and that he was now doing the same with her younger sisters. The mother admitted suspecting the situation for years, but she had not reported it to the authorities for fear of losing her husband and her children. *(Courtesy of William Bernet, M.D.)*

Extrafamilial Sexual Abuse

Of course, sexual abuse is not limited to incest. Children can be abducted and sexually abused by strangers. A perpetrator may observe a playground and may identify a child who is not closely supervised. A pedophile may molest this child and hundreds of other children before he or she is apprehended. For the child, this is usually a single, isolated experience.

On the other hand, children can be repeatedly abused by trusted adults, such as teachers, counselors, family friends, and clergy. In this scenario, the pedophilic perpetrator grooms the child over a period of time. He or she gains the friendship of children through enjoyable activities and gifts, introduces sexual activities that may seem innocent and even pleasurable, and progresses to more intrusive activities. The pedophile encourages secrecy.

A solo sex ring is a form of child sexual abuse that involves one adult perpetrator and multiple child victims, who may know about each other's sexual activities with the perpetrator. A sex ring may also involve multiple perpetrators and multiple victims.

Neurobiological and Health Consequences of Child Maltreatment

Current data document long-term physical and mental health consequences of child physical abuse, sexual abuse, emotional abuse, and neglect. Severe physical abuse and repeated sexual abuse cause changes in the child's developing brain that persist into adulthood. A review of 20 studies concluded that child maltreatment is associated with future increased levels of inflammatory markers such as increased C-reactive protein (CRP), fibrinogen, and proinflammatory cytokines. The association of child maltreatment with an increased state of inflammatory markers in adulthood is a robust finding. However, it is not clear how this occurs, and how it impacts functioning. According to the CDC, and the Child Maltreatment report, long-term consequences of child maltreatment lead to increased risk of multiple physical illnesses and high-risk behaviors such as alcoholism and drug abuse, which in turn can lead to depression, unemployment, and unstable relationships. Physical abuse, emotional abuse, and neglect are strongly related to future depressive disorders, anxiety disorders, eating disorders, suicidal behaviors, drug use, and risky sexual behavior. Child maltreatment is also associated with a host of physical conditions and illnesses, including ischemic heart disease, liver disease, adolescent pregnancy, chronic obstructive pulmonary disease, fetal death, and skeletal fractures. Studies have demonstrated that adults with childhood histories of maltreatment are at higher risk for abnormalities on MRI of the brain that indicate reduced size of the adult hippocampus. These abnormalities are more pronounced on the left side of the brain. Deficient integration exists between the left and right hemispheres, manifested by reduced size of the corpus callosum. These neurobiological effects of child maltreatment probably mediate the behavioral and psychological symptoms that follow abuse, such as increased aggressiveness, heightened autonomic arousal, depression, and memory problems.

EVALUATION PROCESS

The evaluation of a child or adolescent who may have been physically or sexually abused depends on its circumstances and context. Practitioners must consider whether they are conducting a forensic evaluation, which has legal implications and may ultimately be used in court, or a clinical evaluation, which is done for a therapeutic purpose. A forensic evaluation emphasizes collecting accurate and complete data to determine—as objectively as possible—what happened to the child. Was the injury an accident, was it self-inflicted, or was it a result of parental abuse? Was the child actually sexually abused, or was he or she indoctrinated to believe that he or she was abused? The data collected in a forensic evaluation must be preserved in a reliable manner through audiotape, videotape, or detailed notes. The results of the forensic evaluation are organized into a report that is read by attorneys, a judge, and others. The emphasis in a therapeutic evaluation is to assess psychological strengths and weaknesses, to make a clinical diagnosis, to develop a treatment plan, and to lay the foundation for continuing psychotherapy. The clinician is also interested in determining what happened to the child, but it is not as essential to distinguish facts from fantasies. Compared with the forensic evaluation, the psychotherapist does not need to keep such detailed records and ordinarily does not prepare a report for court.

In addition to distinguishing a forensic examination from a therapeutic consultation, a number of factors can affect the evaluation of a child who was abused or may have been abused: whether one is a pediatrician in an emergency department or a child psychiatrist in an office, whether a parent or another person is suspected of the abuse, the severity of the abuse and the victim's relationship to the perpetrator, whether physical signs of abuse are obvious or absent, the age and gender of the child, and the degree of anxiety, defensiveness, anger, or mental disorganization that the child exhibits. Often, the examiner must be creative and persistent.

From the psychiatric perspective, the interview is usually the primary source of information, and the physical examination is secondary. In practice, children who may have been neglected or sexually abused are interviewed first and are later given a physical examination and other tests. A child who has been physically abused is more likely to have a physical examination that may be followed by a psychiatric interview.

When the child is brought to the emergency room, a detailed and spontaneous account of the injury should be obtained promptly from parents or other caregivers before secondary details and rationalizations cloud the information provided. The interviewer should allow the caregiver to explain, to expound, to derail, or to detour the story line. An abuser or codependent parent may claim to have happened on the injured child in a coma or bleeding from some unknown trauma or to have noticed significant bruising, burns, or a crooked extremity while bathing the child. Comparing the parents' histories can provide valuable insight into how power is wielded in the family unit.

A one-month-old baby girl was transferred from a rural hospital to a university medical center because of a reported near sudden infant death syndrome (SIDS). The child was unresponsive and required mechanical ventilation. A nuclear magnetic resonance imaging (MRI) study revealed bilateral subdural hematomas, subarachnoid hemorrhage, and hemorrhage in the parenchyma of the brain. An X-ray skeletal survey showed two posterior rib fractures. An ophthalmologist observed extensive retinal hemorrhages. After the child was admitted to the Pediatric Intensive Care Unit, the child abuse consultant interviewed the parents separately. The mother, 28 years of age, said that she had recently started a new job. The baby was perfectly fine when she left her in the care of her live-in boyfriend, the child's biological father. The father, 24 years of age, said that when he checked on the baby, he found her not breathing, blue, and unresponsive. He ran to report this to a neighbor and then called 911. The child abuse consultant suggested to the father that the baby must have been injured in some way and asked whether the father had any explanation for this injury. The father said, "I shook the baby after I found her not breathing." The consultant concluded that severe child abuse had occurred in the form of shaken baby syndrome. The consultant notified child protective services and the local police department, so that they could initiate and coordinate their investigation. *(Courtesy of William Bernet, M.D.)*

Suspected Sexual Abuse

The examiner should consider the possibility that the parents are not telling the truth. This situation is more complex, however, than suspected physical abuse. For example, the mother may wish to avoid the discovery of father–daughter incest by blaming the child's genital injury on another child or a stranger. In another scenario, the mother may concoct an allegation of incest when the child had never been abused at all. The first version protects a father who is guilty; the second version implicates a father who is innocent.

The examiner should determine how the allegation originally arose and what subsequent statements were made. Determine the emotional tone of the first disclosure (e.g., whether the disclosure arose in the context of a high level of suspicion of abuse). Determine the sequence of previous examinations, the techniques used, and what was reported. Try to determine whether the previous interviews may have distorted the child's recollections. If possible, review transcripts, audiotapes, and videotapes of earlier interviews. Seek a history of overstimulation, prior abuse, or other traumas. Consider other stressors that could account for the child's symptoms. The examiner should also ask about exposure to other possible male and female perpetrators.

In Either Case

Whether physical or sexual abuse is involved, a pertinent psychosocial history should be collected and organized, including the following:

1. Symptoms and behavioral changes that sometimes occur in abused children.
2. Confounding variables, such as psychiatric disorder or cognitive impairment, that may need to be considered.
3. Family's attitude toward discipline, sex, and modesty.
4. Developmental history from birth through periods of possible trauma to the present.
5. Family history, such as earlier abuse of or by the parents, substance abuse by the parents, spouse abuse, and psychiatric disorder in the parents.
6. Underlying motivation and possible psychopathology of adults involved.

Collateral Information

The evaluator should consider requesting collateral information from the following people, after obtaining authorizations: protective services, school personnel, other caregivers (e.g., babysitters), other family members (e.g., siblings), the pediatrician, and police reports.

Child Interview

Several structured and semistructured interview protocols have been developed that were designed to maximize the amount of accurate information and to minimize mistaken or false information provided by children. These approaches include the *Cognitive Interview,* which encourages witnesses to search their memories in various ways, such as recalling events forward and then backward. The *Step-Wise Interview* is a funnel approach that starts with open-ended questions and, if necessary, moves to more specific questions. The interview protocol developed at the National Institute of Child Health and Human Development (NICHD) includes a series of phases and makes use of detailed interview scripts.

Although these protocols may be particularly important in a forensic context, experienced clinicians endorse flexibility and consistent good-hearted behavior by the interviewer. As with seeing any patient, the evaluator must size up the situation and use techniques that are likely to help the youngster become comfortable and communicative. One victim might need a favorite object (e.g., a teddy bear or a toy truck); another might need to have a particular person included in the interview. Some children are comfortable talking; others prefer to draw pictures. An unrelated joke, a shared cookie, or a picture on the evaluator's wall may lead to a disclosure of abuse. Important comments might be made while chatting during the break time, instead of during the structured interviews.

GENOTYPE AND MALTREATMENT: RISK AND PROTECTIVE FACTORS

Two studies of Caucasian males have provided evidence that particular genotypes with high levels of monoamine oxidase A (MAOA) seem to protect against the malignant impact of childhood maltreatment on the development of conduct disorder and antisocial behavioral patterns. Subjects in a prospective cohort design involving court-substantiated cases of child abuse and neglect and matched comparison groups were followed into adulthood. A composite index of violent and antisocial behavior (VASB) was created based on arrest record, self-report, and diagnostic information. Genotypes associated with high levels of MAOA activity were correlated with less risk of violent and antisocial behavior in later life for Caucasians, but this effect was not found for non-Caucasians. This result was not replicated in a group of adolescents with respect to the development of adolescent conduct disorder. Further studies are needed to understand the possible links between genotypes of high levels of MAOA and potential behavioral outcomes.

TREATMENT AND PREVENTION STRATEGIES

The immediate strategic intervention is to ensure the child's safety, which may require the child's removal from an abusive or neglectful home environment. Physicians are among a group of professionals who are mandated by law to report suspected child abuse or neglect to the local protective services agency.

Several evidence-based psychotherapies now exist in the treatment of childhood abuse and neglect. These include Multisystemic Therapy for Child Abuse and Neglect (MST–CAN), Parent–Child Interaction Therapy (PCIT), adapted for children who have been physically abused, and Combined Parent–Child Cognitive Behavioral Therapy (CPC–CBT).

MST–CAN uses a home-based model in which therapists come to the home to involve families in a highly monitored positive interactional approach toward their physically abused children. Parents receive support and guidance to care for their children in a less harsh, nonneglectful manner. This approach has been shown to reduce behavioral problems in the children, while increasing parental understanding of meeting their children's needs in a safe environment.

PCIT consists of combined treatment for parents and children in which parenting is coached directly by the therapist and practiced in sessions with parents and children together. Typically, therapists observe parent–child interactions through a one-way mirror and coach parents during the live interaction using a radio earphone. This model is based on the premise that changing parent–child interaction patterns will break the cycle of parent and child behaviors that maintain abusive behavior, and replace it with more nurturing and supportive interactions. Although PCIT has been shown to be effective, additional treatments are likely to be needed for parents with mental health problems such as depression or substance use.

CPC–CBT is designed to help parents to develop more positive strategies with their children and to help children to cope more effectively with their past abuse and to learn more positive interactions with parents. Therapeutic techniques used with parents include motivational interviewing, psychoeducation, adaptive coping skills, and better problem solving when difficult situations arise. Therapeutic strategies used with children focus on the development of positive coping, anger management, and gradual exposure through the use of a developmentally appropriate trauma narrative. Parents and children participate together in sessions in which the parent is able to convey complete responsibility for their abusive behavior, and then, the parent and child collaborate on a new joint family plan that promotes safety and more positive relationships. Therapeutic sessions with the child and parent together appear to add to the effectiveness of treatment.

Children who have been maltreated are at increased risk for further maltreatment according to studies of child victims of abuse and maltreatment. Studies have shown that four factors were most consistently identified as predictors of future maltreatment: number of previous episodes of maltreatment; neglect as the form of maltreatment; parental conflict; and parental psychiatric illness. Maltreated children were found to be about six times more likely to experience recurrent maltreatment, and the risk of recurrence was highest within 30 days of the index experience. This underscores the importance of a careful examination of the protective factors in the home environment and the early initiation of therapeutic sessions.

27.19d Impact of Terrorism on Children

In recent years, exposure to mass trauma and terrorism has become an increasing concern regarding the well-being of youth. Mass trauma has occurred directly and by witness through highly publicized traumatic events globally and in the United States, pertaining to terrorism, war, mass killings, and natural disasters.

On April 15, 2013, the first major terrorist attack in the United States since 9/11 occurred at the finish line of the Boston Marathon in the mid-afternoon. Two "improvised explosive devices" (IEDs), that is, homemade bombs, detonated 8 minutes apart in the middle of a densely packed crowd of thousands of marathon runners and bystanders, killing three people and injuring about 264 others. Within moments after the blasts, the crowd's panic and chaos turned to purposeful attention to help others get to emergency medical teams arriving on the scene. Courageously, bystanders ran toward others to give aid rather than dispersing away from the scene in all directions. Runners tore off their own shirts to apply pressure to fellow runners who were bleeding, or to use them as tourniquets. Boston's emergency response medical teams worked quickly, efficiently, and tirelessly to transport injured runners to hospitals and into operating rooms in order to save limbs, and stop bleeding. The fact that almost all the injured were saved is a tribute to the emergency preparedness and collaboration of law enforcement, medical, and surgical teams carrying out an emergency plan that they had previously been briefed on, as a matter of course.

Additional situations in which youth are exposed to severe trauma and terror involve armed conflict around the world, multiple mass school shootings that have taken place across the United States in recent years, and hurricanes, devastating storms, and tsunamis. Of course, more than a decade ago, the youth in the United States experienced the large-scale domestic terrorist attack on September 11, 2001, on the World Trade Center in New York City and the Pentagon in Washington, DC.

There is an increasing body of literature on the impact of terrorism on children as well as a variety of other forms of trauma. One predominant and near universal symptom in children in response to these stimuli is anxiety. Young children may cling excessively to their parents, whereas older children may become preoccupied with fear about unrelated issues. Some youth express overt anger, and others experience a sense of hopelessness, lack of control, and/or depression. Severe traumas, such as experiencing a terrorist event, may be more likely to result in posttraumatic stress syndromes among exposed youth, compared to less severe forms of trauma. The number of traumas experienced by a child, degree of family support provided after the exposure, and the reactions of parents are all important factors in a child's reaction.

According to a national survey after the terrorist attack of September 11th, stress reactions to that disaster were increased by watching repeated media coverage of those events. A similar study evaluating the impact of media versus direct exposure to collective trauma, on acute stress response was undertaken 2 to 4 weeks after the Boston Marathon bombings through surveying 846 people from Boston, 941 people from New York City, and 2,888 people through Internet means. Direct exposure, defined as being at or near the bombings, was compared to media exposure, including footage on television and bombing related stories on the radio, in print, online, and other social media coverage. Because acute stress responses appear within weeks of a traumatic event, this study was able to capture acute stress difference between the two groups. The study found that trauma related to media exposure was associated with acute stress reactions in people from all over the United States who were not directly exposed to the event in Boston. Furthermore, respondents reporting exposure to media coverage of the bombings for 6 or more hours daily in the week following the bombings were nine times more likely to report high acute stress than those who had minimal exposure to media coverage of the events. In fact, the group who engaged in extensive media coverage had higher levels of acute stress than respondents who had direct exposure in Boston, but who had minimal exposure to media coverage of the bombings. These findings suggest that prolonged media exposure to collective traumatic events may have a strong negative impact on psychological symptoms and acute stress syndromes. However, the study noted substantial resilience in the surveyed population. Researchers have suggested that the effectiveness of Boston's medical and law enforcement teams in response to the terrorist bombings may have promoted some degree of resilience in the population.

A unique aspect of exposure to terrorist-related trauma, as well as school shootings, is the psychological effects of knowing that the trauma was both consciously and purposely perpetrated, and yet also random. The random nature of terrorist attacks appears to lead to especially adverse reactions in children. School shootings are among the most tragic of traumatic events involving youth. On December 14, 2012, in the village of Sandy Hook, in Newtown, Connecticut, a 20-year-old male in black clothing carrying his mother's rifle, shot his way through a glass window at the front of the Sandy Hook Elementary School, rampaged the school, shooting and killing 20 first-grade students from multiple classrooms and 6 school personnel, and then shot and killed himself. He had shot and killed his mother before arriving at the school. The psychological impact of this massacre on children who survived is moderated by age, gender, and family reactions. Younger children appear to be at higher risk for PTSD, somatic symptoms, depression, and distress than older children and adolescents. Gender also has been found to influence behavioral symptoms after exposure to severe trauma or terrorism, with girls experiencing higher levels of posttraumatic stress syndromes and depression, while boys exhibit more external behavior problems.

Although the United States has launched a series of initiatives in response to the threats and consequences of terrorism in the form of an act of Congress in 2002 called the Public Health Security and Bioterrorism Preparedness and Response Act, children and adolescents continue to view media exposure to terrorist events throughout the world that reinforces a sense of danger.

The concept of terrorist acts is characterized by three distinct features: (1) they produce a societal atmosphere of extreme danger and fear, (2) they inflict significant personal harm and destruction, and (3) they undermine the expectation of citizens that the state is able to protect them.

Child and adolescent reactions to exposure to terrorism are mediated by numerous factors, including personal appraisal of

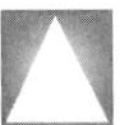

Table 27.19d–1
Experience of Danger Consequent to Terrorist Acts

Objective Features	Subjective Features
Actualized threat	Disruption of protective shield
Realistic threats	Appraisals of threat
False alarms	Fears of recurrence
Hoaxes	Living with uncertainty
Official risk communication, media coverage, and personal exchanges of information	Ongoing worries about significant others
Heightened security	Modulation of information exposure
Mobilization of prevention and response capabilities	Safety and protective behaviors
Attribution of responsibility	Anxious and restrictive behaviors
Evacuation and rescue efforts	Aggressive and reckless behaviors
Military mobilization	Categorization over discrimination of threat—risk of intolerance
War	Themes of heroism and patriotism
Additional dangers, terrorist acts, and personal tragedies	Political ideology
	Changes in spiritual schema
	Parental demoralization

Courtesy of Robert S. Pynoos, M.D. M.P.H., Merritt D. Schreiber, Ph.D., Alan M. Steinberg Ph.D., and Betty Pfefferbaum, M.D., J.D.

persisting danger, the likelihood of recurrent attack, and the perception of the relative safety of one's family and close friends. Children's responses to terrorist exposure are influenced by how their parents cope with the trauma and resulting turmoil and how well they understand the situation. PTSD has been studied in adolescents, with and without learning disabilities, who have been exposed to terror attacks. Findings from this study revealed that personal exposure to terror, past personal life-threatening events, and history of anxiety all contributed to the development of posttraumatic stress reactions. In addition, adolescents with learning disabilities who had difficulties in cognitively processing the traumatic events were at higher risk of developing PTSD when this was combined with the other high-risk factors, such as being personally exposed to the traumatic events.

Table 27.19d–1 identifies the relationship between objective features of danger and subjective features related to exposure to terrorist acts.

The following summarizes data collected after the terrorist attack of the World Trade Center on September 11, 2001.

SEPTEMBER 11, 2001 ATTACKS

The U.S. Department of Education, through Project SERV, supported the New York City Board of Education in conducting a needs assessment of New York City schoolchildren. A total of 8,000 randomly selected students were surveyed 6 months after the September 11, 2001 attacks. Striking differences were seen among students in the vicinity of Ground Zero as compared with students in the rest of the city, in exposure to smoke and dust, fleeing for safety, problems getting home, and smelling smoke in the days and weeks after September 11. Approximately 70 percent of all children, however, were exposed to one of these factors. Interpersonal exposure through direct victimization of a family member was greater among children attending schools outside the Ground Zero vicinity as compared with those attending school in this area. Media exposure was extensive and prolonged. Signs of heightened security were visible throughout the city. The study used several scales of the *Diagnostic Interview Schedule for Children* (DISC). Three sets of findings stand out from this study. First a significant degree of persistent separation anxiety was seen, especially among school-age children, but also among adolescents. Second, reflecting an age-related vulnerability to incident-specific new fears (e.g., subways and buses) and avoidant behavior of school-age children, a nearly 25 percent rate of agoraphobia was reported among 4th- and 5th-graders. Care must be taken, however, not to misrepresent *incident-specific new fears* as agoraphobia, because the course of recovery and intervention strategies may differ. Third, an enormous reservoir of prior traumatic experiences (more than one-half of the total sample) was associated with severity of current PTSD symptoms, emphasizing the need to attend to prior trauma in conducting needs assessments, surveillance, and intervention strategies. Other risk factors, in addition to younger age, included female gender and Hispanic ethnicity. The finding of age-related increases in rates of conduct disorder also needs to be interpreted in light of adolescent response to an ecology of danger in which overly aggressive, reckless, and risk-taking behaviors are well documented and associated with posttraumatic stress reactions. A major strength of this study was the inclusion of self-reported impairment as well as symptoms, setting an important standard for future studies.

J. Stuber and colleagues conducted a telephone survey of a random sample of adult residents of Manhattan 1 to 2 months after the September 11th attacks. The sample included more than 100 parents who were asked to describe the experiences and reactions of their children. Not surprisingly, given the time of the incident, most children were at school or day care when the disaster occurred. Many of the parents recalled concern about their children's safety at the time, and most were not reunited with their children for more than 4 hours. More than 20 percent of the parents studied reported that their children had received counseling related to the disaster. Receiving counseling was associated with male gender, parental posttraumatic stress, and having at least one sibling living in the household.

Also using parent report in a New York City telephone survey, researchers assessed predictors of posttraumatic stress reactions in children between the ages of 4 and 17 years, 4 to 5 months after the attacks. Almost 20 percent of children were reported by their parents to have experienced severe or very severe posttraumatic stress reactions, and approximately two-thirds had moderate posttraumatic stress reactions. Parental reactions and viewing three or more graphic images of the disaster on television were associated with severe or very severe posttraumatic stress reactions in children. Another study reported that 27 percent of children with severe or very severe posttraumatic stress reactions received some mental health care 4 to 5 months after September 11th.

Two surveys of representative samples of adults were conducted after the September 11th attacks; the first between 4 and 5 months and the second between 6 and 9 months after the attacks. Behavior problems were related to the child's race or ethnicity, family income, living in a single-parent household, disaster event experiences, and parental reactions to the attacks.

The results of these surveys were examined in light of findings from a representative survey conducted before September 11th. The rate of behavior problems was lower in the first post-September 11th survey (4 to 6 months after the attacks) than rates in the pre-September 11th survey, but problems returned to pre-September 11th levels by the second post-September 11th study (6 to 9 months after the attacks). Consistent with findings in studies of Hurricane Andrew, these results suggest that behavior problems may decrease in the months after a disaster or that parents may be insensitive to them, but that they return to predisaster levels over time.

Media coverage of the September 11th attacks brought renewed debate about its impact, especially on children, even children with no direct exposure. One study reported extensive exposure to television coverage in children throughout the nation, using a representative survey of adults conducted in the first days after the attacks. Approximately one-third of the parents surveyed attempted to limit or to prevent their children's viewing, but, among those whose parents made no attempt to restrict viewing, the number of hours of disaster coverage watched was related to the number of reported stress symptoms.

Using a web-based, nationally representative sample of adults, another study examined distress in children 1 to 2 months after the attacks by asking parents if their children were upset by the events. Among the children perceived as most upset, 20 percent had trouble sleeping, 30 percent were irritable or easily upset, and 27 percent feared separation from their parents. The mean age of children perceived as most upset was 11 years, with no statistically significant gender differences. The proportion of parents reporting at least one child upset did not differ by community in analysis of data from the New York City metropolitan area, Washington, DC, other major metropolitan areas, and the rest of the country.

A strength of these surveys was their examination of representative samples, but earlier work points to concern about assessing children by interviewing their parents. Furthermore, as with the Oklahoma City studies, the samples were composed mainly of indirectly exposed children, and the clinical significance of the findings is unclear.

Nine-year-old Jason endured the traumatic loss of his father on the first plane into the World Trade Center. Jason's father was on board American Airlines Flight No. 11 on a business trip. Jason and his siblings were preparing to leave for school when he, his mother and his siblings learned of the event. Jason watched his mother nearly collapse when she confirmed the presence of his father aboard the aircraft. Jason observed the recurring video segments of the second plane crashing into the second tower several times that morning before his mother limited television access. Jason, the oldest child in his family, had enjoyed an exceptionally close relationship with his father.

Almost immediately after the terrorist attacks, Jason's mother became worried that he was despondent, suicidal and unable to function, just preoccupied with the grisly nature of his father's death. He was becoming increasingly agitated as he talked constantly about the gruesome way that his father had died. Jason's mother sought immediate psychological treatment for him, during which he began to ask a continual series of questions about his father's death, including aspects of burning, fragmentation, pain, blood, and the exact moment of his father's deaths in comparison with what he had initially observed on television. This became the main theme of Jason's early treatment, in which he ruminated (i.e., whether his father had been "blown up in a thousand pieces" and the sequence of fire, burning, pain, and death). Jason developed nightmares within days in which he awakened and called for his mother at least three times a night. Jason was unwilling to discuss the content of his dreams with his mother, given his observations of her own serious distress. Jason began to express fears that the "hijackers" would hurt his mother and siblings. He became focused on the concept that "half our freedom is gone," and he was concerned that one-half of New York City was destroyed. He was preoccupied with enacting in play, repetitive crashing down of creating the World Trade Center. Although after 3 months, he was able to resume sleeping through the night, he reported new troubling dreams with themes of ghosts "popping out" and "everyone is killed, and then I'm killed." This worsened after the onset of the war in Afghanistan, and his mother had to constantly reassure him that the war was not near their home.

Jason told his therapist of his wish that could find a time machine and be transported back in time on board his father's flight before it crashed. While his therapist could fly the plane, he would overpower the "hijackers" and throw them off the plane, and then the plane would land safely in Boston. Jason continued his wish that after landing, his father and the other passengers tell him "thank you," and be very happy. After expressing his wish verbally, he appeared to be somewhat comforted and he began to recall many positive activities with his father, and a series of happy, highly detailed memories of his father, which then caused him to suddenly become tearful with profound sadness at the realization that these would be no more.

In therapy, Jason alternately expressed rage and anger and confusion about the actions of "Osama Bin Laden." Over many months, Jason was able to remember and speak about the good things he remembered about his father without immediately breaking down in tears. Jason became a helpful big brother, who often tried to care for his younger siblings, and his mother often told him how proud she was of him. *(Adapted from Robert S. Pynoos, M.D. M.P.H., Merritt D. Schreiber, Ph.D., Alan M. Steinberg, Ph.D., Betty Pfefferbaum, M.D., and J.D.)*

To respond to the mental health needs of children and adolescents who have been exposed to terrorism either through personal experience or through exposure to media depicting world-wide terrorism, the adverse psychological reactions listed in Table 27.19d–2 must be considered.

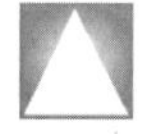

Table 27.19d–2
Psychological Disorders Associated with Terrorism

Acute stress disorder
PTSD
Depression
Anxiety
Separation anxiety disorder
Agoraphobia
Phobic disorders
Bereavement
Somatization
Irritability
Dissociative reactions
Sleep disturbances
Diminished self-esteem
Deterioration in school performance
Distress when exposed to traumatic reminders
Substance abuse

COMPONENTS OF MECHANISMS FOR RECOVERY FROM EXPOSURE TO TERRORISM

In order to begin the process of recovery from exposure to mass trauma, an assessment of a child's current coping must be done. Numerous instruments to measure coping exist. These include COPE, a self-report questionnaire which has 52 items that can be used with children, adolescents and adults; Children's Coping Strategies Checklist (CCSC), a self-report questionnaire with 45 general coping items used with children 9 to 13 years of age; and How I Coped Under Pressure (HICIPS), which has 45 event-specific questions for children in the 4th to 6th grade. Once this assessment has been determined, the next steps can be taken to begin the road to recovery.

Perception of Safety

The notion of perceived safety is an important protective factor as well as a component of recovery for a child, adolescent, or adult who has been exposed to terrorism. A recent report of symptoms of PTSD, depression, and perceived safety in disaster workers 2 weeks after the September 11th terrorist attacks found that lower perceived safety was associated with increased symptoms of hyperarousal and intrusive fearful thoughts, but not avoidance. An expected diminished sense of safety was found in those individuals who had personally been in greater physical danger, or who had worked with dead bodies compared with others who were physically less exposed. To regain a sense of security, reestablishment of a perception of safety is a necessary first step.

Reestablishment or Maintenance of Daily Routines

Although it is clearly not always possible to maintain usual daily routines amidst war or exposure to terrorism, a study of Israeli adolescents found that those whose families were able to maintain their usual activities, such as attending school and family functions, were at lower risk for the development of posttraumatic reactions.

Proactive Interventions to Enhance Resilience

Perceived personal resilience has been shown to be protective against symptoms of posttraumatic stress development. Proactive interventions aimed at enhancing a sense of personal resilience and an ability to cope with the stressful situation may serve to decrease the risk of psychiatric symptoms after exposure to terrorism. Interventions may include regaining a sense of perceived safety through reestablishing routines, altruistic tasks, family preparedness planning, and parental expression of security.

28 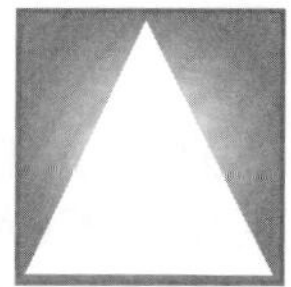

Adulthood

INTRODUCTION

For most of the history of developmental psychology, the predominant theory held that development ended with childhood and adolescence. Adults were considered to be finished products in whom the ultimate developmental states had been reached. Beyond adolescence, the developmental point of view was relevant only insofar as success or failure to reach adult levels or to maintain them determined the maturity or immaturity of the adult personality.

In contradistinction were the long-recognized ideas that adult experiences, such as pregnancy, marriage, parenthood, and aging, had an obvious and significant impact on mental processes and experience in the adult years. This view of adulthood suggests that the patient, of any age, is still in the process of ongoing development, as opposed to merely being in possession of a past that influences mental processes and is the primary determinant of current behavior. Although the debate continues, the idea that development continues throughout life is increasingly accepted.

Development in adulthood, as in childhood, is always the result of the interaction among body, mind, and environment, never exclusively the result of any one of the three variables. Most adults are forced to confront and adapt to similar circumstances: establishing an independent identity, forming a marriage or other partnership, raising children, building and maintaining careers, and accepting the disability and death of one's parents.

In modern Western societies, adulthood is the longest phase of human life. Although the exact age of consent varies from person to person, adulthood can be divided into three main parts: young or early adulthood (ages 20 to 40), middle adulthood (ages 40 to 65), and late adulthood or old age.

YOUNG ADULTHOOD (20 TO 40 YEARS OF AGE)

Usually considered to begin at the end of adolescence (about age 20) and to end at age 40, early adulthood is characterized by peaking biological development, the assumption of major social roles, and the evolution of an adult self and life structure. The successful passage into adulthood depends on satisfactory resolution of childhood and adolescent crises.

During late adolescence, young persons generally leave home and begin to function independently. Sexual relationships become serious, and the quest for intimacy begins. The 20s are spent, for the most part, exploring options for occupation and marriage or alternative relationships and making commitments in various areas.

Early adulthood requires choosing new roles (e.g., husband, father) and establishing an identity congruent with those new roles. It involves asking and answering the questions "Who am I?" and "Where am I going?" The choices made during this time may be tentative; young adults may make several false starts.

Transition from Adolescence to Young Adulthood

The transition from adolescence to young adulthood is characterized by real and intrapsychic separation from the family of origin and the engagement of new, phase-specific tasks (Table 28–1). It involves many important events, such as graduating from high school, starting a job or entering college, and living independently. During these years, the individual resolves the issue of childhood dependency sufficiently to establish self-reliance and begins to formulate new, young-adult goals that eventually result in creation of new life structures that promote stability and continuity.

Developmental Tasks

Establishing a self that is separate from parents is a major task of young adulthood. For most individuals, the emotional detachment from parents that takes place in adolescence and young adulthood is followed by a new inner definition of themselves as comfortably alone and competent, able to care for themselves in the real world. This shift away from the parents continues long after marriage, and parenthood results in the formation of new relationships that replace the progenitors as the most important individuals in the young adult's life.

Psychological separation from the parents is followed by synthesis of mental representations from the childhood past and the young-adult present. The psychological separation from parents in adolescence has been called the *second individuation,* and the

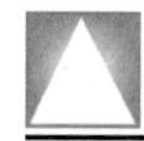

Table 28–1
Development Tasks of Young Adulthood

To develop a young-adult sense of self and other: the third individuation
To develop adult friendships
To develop the capacity for intimacy; to become a spouse
To become a biological and psychological parent
To develop a relationship of mutuality and equality with parents while facilitating their midlife development
To establish an adult work identity
To develop adult forms of play
To integrate new attitudes toward time

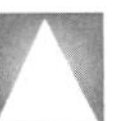

Table 28–2
Psychological Development Concepts

Concept	Definition	Example
Transition	The bridge between two successive stages	Late adolescence
Normative crisis	A period of rapid change or turmoil that strains a person's adaptive capacities	Midlife crisis
Stage	Period of consolidation of skills and capacities	Mature adulthood
Plateau	Period of developmental stability	Adulthood up to midlife
Rite of passage	Social ritual that facilitates a transition	Graduation; marriage

Adapted from Wolman T, Thompson T. Adult and later-life development. In: Stoudemire A, ed. *Human Behavior*. Philadelphia, PA: Lippincott-Raven; 1998.

continued elaboration of these themes in young adulthood has been called the *third individuation*. The continuous process of elaboration of self and differentiation from others that occurs in the developmental phases of young (20 to 40 years of age) and middle (40 to 65 years of age) adulthood is influenced by all important adult relationships.

A number of different models have been proposed for understanding adult development. They are all theoretical and somewhat idealized. They all use metaphors to describe complex social, psychological, and interpersonal interactions. The models are heuristic: They provide a conceptual framework for thinking about common important experiences. They are descriptive rather than prescriptive; that is, they provide a useful way of looking at what many persons do, not a formula for what all persons should do. Some of the terms and concepts commonly used are explained in Table 28–2. These periods involve individuation that is, leaving the family of origin and becoming one's own man or woman, passing through midlife, and preparing in middle adulthood for the transition into late adulthood.

Work Identity. The transition from learning and play to work may be gradual or abrupt. Socioeconomic group, gender, and race affect the pursuit and development of particular occupational choices. Blue-collar workers generally enter the workforce directly after high school; white-collar workers and professionals usually enter the workforce after college or professional school. Depending on choice of career and opportunity, work may become a source of ongoing frustration or an activity that enhances self-esteem. Symptoms of job dissatisfaction are a high rate of job changes, absenteeism, mistakes at work, accident proneness, and even sabotage.

Unemployment. The effects of unemployment transcend those of loss of income; the psychological and physical tolls are enormous. The incidence of alcohol dependence, homicide, violence, suicide, and mental illness rises with unemployment. One's core identity, which is often tied to occupation and work, is seriously damaged when a job is lost, whether through firing, attrition, or early or sometimes even regular retirement.

A young adult female patient had greatly enjoyed her 5 years in college and only reluctantly accepted a job with a large real estate firm. During college, she had had limited interest in her appearance, and she began work in clothing borrowed from family and friends. She scoffed when her boss began to criticize her dress and gave her an advance to buy an upscale wardrobe, but she then began to enjoy the fine clothing and the respect engendered by her appearance and position. As her income began to rise, work became a source of pleasure and self-esteem and the way to acquire some of the trappings of adulthood. *(Courtesy of Calvin Colarusso, M.D.)*

Developing Adult Friendships. In late adolescence and young adulthood, before marriage and parenthood, friendships are often the primary source of emotional sustenance. Roommates, apartment mates, sorority sisters, and fraternity brothers, as indicated by the names used to describe them, are substitutes for parents and siblings, temporary stand-ins until more permanent replacements are found.

The emotional needs for closeness and confidentiality are largely met by friendships. All major developmental issues are discussed with friends, particularly those in similar circumstances. As marriages occur and children are born, the central emotional importance of friendships diminishes. Some friendships are abandoned at this point, because the spouse objects to the friend, recognizing at some level that they are competitors. Gradually, there is movement toward a new form of friendship, couples friendships. They reflect the newly committed status but are more difficult to form and to maintain, because four individuals must be compatible, not just two.

As children begin to move out of the family into the community, parents follow. Dance classes and Little League games provide the progenitors with a new focus and the opportunity to make friends with others who are at the same point developmentally and who are receptive to the formation of relationships that help explain, and cushion, the pressures of young adult life.

Sexuality and Marriage. The developmental shift from sexual experimentation to the desire for intimacy is experienced in young adulthood as an intense loneliness, resulting from the awareness of an absence of committed love similar to that experienced in childhood with their parents. Brief sexual encounters in short-lived relationships no longer significantly boost self-esteem. Increasingly, the desire is for emotional involvement in a sexual context. The young adult who fails to develop the capacity for intimate relationships runs the risk of living in isolation and self-absorption in midlife.

For most individuals in Western culture, the experience of intimacy increases the desire for marriage. Most persons in the United States marry for the first time in their mid- to late 20s. The median age of first marriage has been rising steadily since 1950 for both men and women, and the number of persons who never marry has been increasing. Today, approximately 50 percent of all adults age 18 and older are not married, compared with only 28 percent in 1960. The proportion of 30- to 34-year-olds who never married has almost tripled, and the proportion of never-married 35- to 39-year-olds doubled.

INTERRACIAL MARRIAGE. Mixed-race marriages were banned in 19 states until a U.S. Supreme Court decision in 1967. In

1970, such marriages accounted for only 2 percent of all marriages. The trend has been steadily upward. Currently, interracial marriages account for about 1.5 million marriages in the United States.

Despite the trend toward more interracial marriages, they still remain a small proportion of all marriages. Most persons are more likely to marry someone from the same racial and ethnic background. Marriages between Hispanic whites and non-Hispanic whites and between Asians and whites are more common than those between blacks and whites.

SAME-SEX MARRIAGE. Same-sex marriage is recognized as legal by many states in the United States and by the U.S. Supreme Court, as well as in several countries around the world (e.g., France and Denmark). It differs from same-sex civil unions granted by states, which do not provide the same federal protection or benefits as marriage. No reliable estimates are available for the number of same-sex marriages in the United States; however, in 2013 it was estimated to be about 80,000. There is growing consensus in the United States and around the world that homosexual persons should be allowed the same marital rights and privileges as heterosexuals. Same-sex marriage can be subject to more stress than heterosexual marriage because of continued prejudice toward such unions among certain conservative political or religious groups who oppose such unions.

MARITAL PROBLEMS. Although marriage tends to be regarded as a permanent tie, unsuccessful unions can be terminated, as indeed they are in most societies. Nevertheless, many marriages that do not end in separation or divorce are disturbed. In considering marital problems, clinicians are concerned with both the persons involved and with the marital unit itself. How any marriage works relates to the partner selected, the personality organization or disorganization of each, the interaction between them, and the original reasons for the union. Persons marry for a variety of reasons—emotional, social, economic, and political, among others. One person may look to the spouse to meet unfulfilled childhood needs for good parenting. Another may see the spouse as someone to be saved from an otherwise unhappy life. Irrational expectations between spouses increase the risk of marital problems.

MARRIAGE AND COUPLES THERAPY. When families consist of grandparents, parents, children, and other relatives living under the same roof, assistance for marital problems can sometimes be obtained from a member of the extended family with whom one or both partners have rapport. With the contraction of the extended family in recent times, however, this source of informal help is no longer as accessible as it once was. Similarly, religion once played a more important role than it does now in the maintenance of family stability. Wise religious leaders are available to provide counseling, but they are not sought out to the extent they once were, which reflects the decline in religious influence among large segments of the population. Formerly, both the extended family and religion provided guidance for couples in distress and also prevented dissolution of marriages by virtue of the social pressures that the extended family and religion exerted on couples to stay together. As family, religious, and societal pressures have been relaxed, legal procedures for relatively easy separation and divorce have expanded. Concurrently, the need for formalized marriage counseling services has developed.

Marital therapy is a form of psychotherapy for married persons in conflict with each other. A trained person establishes a professional contract with the patient-couple and, through definite types of communication, attempts to alleviate the disturbance, to reverse or change maladaptive patterns of behavior, and to encourage personality growth and development.

In *marriage counseling,* only a particular conflict related to the immediate concerns of the family is discussed; marriage counseling is conducted much more superficially by persons with less psychotherapeutic training than is marital therapy. *Marital therapy* places greater emphasis on restructuring the interaction between the couple, including, at times, exploration of the psychodynamics of each partner. Both therapy and counseling emphasize helping marital partners cope effectively with their problems.

Parenthood. Parenthood intensifies the relationship between the new parents. Through their physical and emotional union, the couple has produced a fragile, dependent being. This recognition expands their internal images of each other to include thoughts and feelings emanating from the role of parent. As they live together as a family, the lovers' relationship to each other changes. They become parents relating to one another and to their children.

Parent–child problems do arise, however. In addition to the economic burden of raising a child (estimated to be more than $250,000 for a middle-class family whose child goes to college), there are emotional costs. Children may reawaken conflicts that parents themselves had as children, or children may have chronic illnesses that challenge families' emotional resources. In general, men have been more concerned with their work and occupational advancement than with child rearing, and women have been more concerned about their role as mothers than with advancement in their occupation, but this emphasis is changing dramatically for both sexes. A small, but growing, number of couples are choosing to split a job (or work at two part-time jobs) and share child-rearing duties.

Parenting has been described as a continuing process of letting go. Children must be allowed to separate from parents and, in some cases, must be encouraged to do so. Letting go involves separation from children who are starting school. School phobias and school refusal syndromes that are accompanied by extreme separation anxiety may have to be dealt with. Often, a parent who cannot let go of a child accounts for this situation; some parents want their children to remain tightly bound to them emotionally. Family therapy that explores these dynamics may be needed to resolve such problems.

As children get older and enter adolescence, the process of establishing identity assumes great importance. Peer relationships become crucial to a child's development, and overprotective parents who keep a child from developing friendships or having the freedom to experiment with friends that the parents disapprove of can interfere with the child's passage through adolescence. Parents need not refrain from exerting influence over their children; guidance and involvement are crucial. But they must recognize that adolescents especially need parental approval; although rebellious on the surface, adolescents are much more tractable than they appear, provided parents are not overbearing or generally punitive.

SINGLE-PARENT FAMILIES. More than 10 million single-parent families exist with one or more children under the age of 18; of these families, 20 percent are single-parent homes in which a woman is the sole head of the household. The increase in number of single-parent families has risen almost 200 percent since 1980.

ALTERNATIVE LIFESTYLE PARENTING. Single, partnered, and married homosexual men and women are choosing to raise children. In most cases, such children are obtained through adoption. Some, however, may be born to a lesbian woman through artificial insemination or obtained from a willing mother surrogate. The number of such family units is increasing. The data about the development of children in these homes indicate that they are at no greater risk for emotional problems (or for a homosexual orientation) than children raised in conventional households.

ADOPTION. Since the turn of the century, adoption or foster placement has replaced institutional care as the preferred way to raise children who are neglected, unwanted, or abandoned. Many couples who are unable to conceive (and some couples who already have children) turn to adoption.

In addition to the full range of normal parent–child developmental issues, adoptive parents face special problems. They must decide how and when to tell the child about the adoption. They must deal with the child's possible desire for information about his or her biological parents. Adopted children are more likely to develop conduct disorders, problems with drug abuse, and antisocial personality traits. It is unclear whether these problems result from the process of adoption or whether parents who give up children for adoption are more likely to pass along a genetic predisposition for these behaviors.

With widespread use of birth control and access to safe abortions, the number of infants available for adoption has declined steeply. Wealthy parents may prefer to arrange for private adoption rather than wait many uncertain years for an institutional adoption. (In private adoptions, a biological mother is paid for her legal and medical expenses but not for the baby. Baby selling is a felony in all states.) International adoptions (especially from Bosnia, Latin America, eastern Europe, and China) have also become more common. Questionable regulation in these countries has raised concern that some infants put up for adoption in poor countries may not be orphans but are being sold by destitute mothers.

MIDDLE ADULTHOOD (40 TO 65 YEARS OF AGE)

Middle adulthood is the golden age of adulthood, similar to the latency years in childhood, but much longer. Physical health, emotional maturity, competence and power in the work situation, and gratifying relationships with spouse, children, parents, friends, and colleagues all contribute to a normative sense of satisfaction and well-being. With regard to occupation, many persons begin to experience the gap between early aspirations and current achievements. They may wonder whether the lifestyle and the commitments they chose in early adulthood are worth continuing; they may feel that they would like to live their remaining years in a different, more satisfying way, without knowing exactly how. As children grow up and leave home, parental roles change, and persons redefine their roles as husbands and wives.

Important gender-specific changes occur in middle adulthood. Many women who no longer need to nurture young children can release their energy into independent pursuits that require assertiveness and a competitive spirit, traits that were traditionally considered masculine. Alternatively, men in middle adulthood may develop qualities that enable them to express their emotions and recognize their dependency needs, traits that were traditionally considered feminine. With the new balance of the masculine and the feminine, a person may now be able to relate more effectively to someone of the other sex than in the past. For a further discussion of adoption see Section 27.19b.

Transition from Young to Middle Adulthood

The transition from young adulthood to middle adulthood is slow and gradual, with no sharp physical or psychological demarcation. The aging process picks up speed and becomes a powerful organizing influence on intrapsychic life, but the change is gradual, unlike during adolescence. Mental change is experienced in a similar fashion, slow and imperceptible, without a sense of disruption.

Development in young adulthood is embedded in close relationships. Intimacy, love, and commitment are related to the mastery of the relationships most immediate to personal experience. The transition from young adulthood to middle age includes widening concern for the larger social system and differentiation of one's own social, political, and historical system from others. Authors have described middle adulthood in terms of generativity, self-actualization, and wisdom.

Developmental Theorists

Robert Butler described several underlying themes in middle adulthood that appear to be present regardless of marital and family status, gender, or economic level (Table 28–3). These themes include aging (as changes in bodily functions are noticed in middle adulthood); taking stock of accomplishments and setting goals for the future; reassessing commitments to family, work, and marriage; dealing with parental illness and death; and attending to all the developmental tasks without losing the capacity to experience pleasure or to engage in playful activity.

Erik Erikson. Erikson described middle adulthood as characterized either by generativity or by stagnation. Erikson defined *generativity* as the process by which persons guide the oncoming generation or improve society. This stage includes having and raising children, but wanting or having children does not ensure generativity. A childless person can be generative by (1) helping others, (2) being creative, and (3) contributing to society. Parents must be secure in their own identities to raise children successfully: They cannot be preoccupied with themselves and act as if they were, or wished to be, the child in the family.

To be *stagnant* means that a person stops developing. For Erikson, stagnation was anathema, and he referred to adults without any impulses to guide the new generation or to those who produce children but don't care for them as being "within a cocoon of self-concern and isolation." Such persons are in great

Table 28–3
Features Salient to Middle Adulthood

Issues	Positive Features	Negative Features
Prime of life	Responsible use of power; maturity; productivity	Winner–loser view; competitiveness
Stock taking: what to do with the rest of one's life	Possibility; alternatives; organization of commitments; redirection	Closure; fatalism
Fidelity and commitments	Commitment to self, others, career, society; filial maturity	Hypocrisy; self-deception
Growth-death (to grow is to die); juvenescence and rejuvenation fantasies	Naturality regarding body, time	Obscene or frenetic efforts (e.g., to be youthful); hostility and envy of youth and progeny; longing
Communication and socialization	Matters understood; continuity; picking up where left off; large social network; rootedness of relationships, places, and ideas	Repetitiveness; boredom; impatience; isolation; conservatism; confusion; rigidity

Adapted from Robert N. Butler, M.D.

danger. Because they are unable to negotiate the developmental tasks of middle adulthood, they are unprepared for the next stage of the life cycle, old age, which places more demands on the psychological and physical capacities than all the preceding stages.

George Vaillant. In his longitudinal study of 173 men who were interviewed at 5-year intervals after they graduated from Harvard, Vaillant found a strong correlation between physical and emotional health in middle age. In addition, those with the poorest psychological adjustment during college years had a high incidence of physical illness in middle age. No single factor in childhood accounted for adult mental health, but an overall sense of stability in the parental home predicted a well-adjusted adulthood. A close sibling relationship during college years was correlated with emotional and physical well-being in middle age. In another study, Vaillant found that childhood and adult work habits were correlated, and that adult mental health and good interpersonal relationships were associated with the capacity to work in childhood. Vaillant's studies are ongoing and represent the longest continuous study of adulthood ever performed.

Calvin Colarusso and Robert Nemiroff. On the basis of their experience as clinicians and psychoanalysts, Calvin Colarusso and Robert Nemiroff propose a broad theoretical foundation for adult development by suggesting that the developmental process is basically the same in the adult as in the child because, like the child, the adult is always in the midst of an ongoing dynamic process, continually influenced by a constantly changing environment, body, and mind. Whereas child development focuses primarily on the formation of psychic structure, adult development is concerned with the continuing evolution of existing psychic structure and with its use. Although the fundamental issues of childhood continue in altered form as central aspects of adult life, attempts to explain all adult behavior and pathology in terms of the experiences of childhood are considered reductionistic. The adult past must be taken into account in understanding adult behavior in the same way that the childhood past is considered. The aging body is understood to have a profound influence on psychological development in adulthood, as is the growing midlife recognition and acceptance of the finiteness of time and the inevitability of personal death.

Developing Midlife Friendships

Unlike friendships in latency and adolescence and, to some extent, in young adulthood, midlife friendships do not usually have the sense of urgency or the need for frequent or nearly constant physical presence of the friend. Midlife individuals have neither the need to build new psychic structure (as do latency-age children and adolescents) nor the pressing need to find new relationships (as do young adults). They may have many sources of gratification available through relationships with spouse, children, and colleagues.

> As their firstborn sons progressed through high school, two women in their mid-40s became fast friends. In addition to raising money for the school activities in which their sons were involved, thus maintaining a close involvement with the boys, they spent many hours talking about the boys' activities, girlfriends, and plans for college. Their husbands, who liked each other, became acquaintances, not friends. They directed their own feelings about their sons into other relationships. After the boys left for college, the intensity of the friendship diminished, tending to peak again during vacation periods. *(Courtesy of Calvin Colarusso, M.D.)*

Because of their unique position in the life cycle, midlife adults are easily able to initiate and sustain friendships with individuals of different ages, as well as chronological peers. In the face of a disrupted marriage or intimacy or the pressure of other midlife developmental themes, friendships may quickly become vehicles for the direct expression of impulses.

Reappraising Relationships. Midlife is a time of serious reappraisal of marriage and committed relationships. In the process, individuals struggle with the question of whether to settle for what they have or to search for greater perfection with a new partner. For some, the conflict rages internally and is kept from others; others express it through actions that take the form of affairs, trial separations, and divorce.

Recent research on happy marriage indicates that these couples, despite internal and real conflict, have found or achieved a special *goodness-of-fit* between their individual needs, wishes, and expectations. In the eyes of these couples, marital success is based on the ongoing, successful engagement of a number of psychological tasks. Among the most important are providing a safe place for conflict and difference, holding a double vision of the other, and maintaining a satisfying sexual life.

The decision to leave a longstanding, committed relationship has great consequences, not only for the two individuals involved, but also for their friends and loved ones. The effect on children, in particular, is especially profound, extending far beyond childhood. The effects on the abandoned spouse, parents, and close relatives may be nearly as severe.

Various forms of therapeutic intervention, such as marital counseling, individual psychotherapy, and psychoanalysis, can be extremely effective in helping uncertain individuals decide what to do or in helping those who leave deal with the consequences of their decision on the abandoned partner, children, and other loved ones. Problems relating to intimacy, love, and sex can occupy a prominent position in an outpatient practice.

The four case studies presented here by Calvin Colarusso, M.D., illustrate some of the issues described above.

A couple in their late 50s sought treatment in order to make a decision about their marriage. Both had been unhappy for years and wanted to divorce, feeling that they had to act now while there was still time to begin new relationships that would fulfill them. Their concerns were for their children and grandchildren. How would they react? Would they respect their decision to end a relationship of more than 30 years or attempt to stop the separation? As the work progressed, they decided that seeking happiness in the hopefully 20 or 30 years that they had left to live had to come ahead of the feelings of their loved ones. The fact that their decision was a mutual one was the determining factor in the gradual acceptance by their family members of the divorce.

A 43-year-old patient, Mr. S, was continually preoccupied with his marriage during this 4-year psychoanalysis. Sexually inhibited during adolescence, he "married the only girl in the world who knew less about sex than I did." Both were virgins on their wedding night. As the marriage progressed, the couple gradually developed a "satisfactory" sex life, but the patient always wondered what he had missed. As his sexual inhibitions were explored Mr. S's sense of having "missed out on a lot of opportunities" lead to visits to massage parlors and prostitutes. Eventually such behavior ceased because of the recognition that his wife was a wonderful mother and loving wife and not the cause of the lack of sexual experience that he brought into the marriage. "I'll always feel that I missed out when I was young, but I've got so much going for me now, I'm not going to mess it up over something that I can't change."

A 38-year-old woman entered therapy after her husband discovered that she was having sexual relations with men in their early and middle 20s. She explained that she loved her husband but he seemed to take her for granted. He no longer made her feel attractive and wanted. As the therapy progressed it became clear that she felt that as long as she could attract younger men she was still young and sexually desirable. Struggling with the early signs of physical aging, the realization that the young men were only using her to satisfy their own sexual needs was sobering and distressing. As she began to see that such behavior was self-destructive, she approached her husband about starting marital therapy.

Fifty-year-old Mrs. T left her "wonderful" husband because "I've missed something. I just have to get out on my own." Married at 18 years of age, "after going from my parents' home to his home," she recognized that her rage at her husband for "not being all the other men I could have married, for closing off all the living I could have done" was irrational but uncontrollable. "I have to live on my own for a while, to see if I can do it, before it's too late." Fully intending to return to her husband, she continued exploring the infantile and adult issues that precipitated the separation, leaving the future of the marriage in doubt.

Sexuality

Whereas the young adult is preoccupied with developing the capacity for intimacy, the midlife individual is focused on maintaining intimacy in the face of deterring physical, psychological, and environmental pressures. In a longstanding relationship, these pressures include real and imaginary concerns about diminished sexual capability, emotional withdrawal because of preoccupation with developmental tasks, and the realistic pressures related to work and providing for dependent children and, sometimes, elderly parents as well. In relationships that begin in midlife, the maintenance of intimacy can be compromised by the absence of a common past, age and generational differences in interests and activities, and the difficulties involved in forming a stepfamily.

For sexual intimacy to continue, the participants must (1) accept the appearance of the partner's middle-aged body, (2) continue to find it sexually stimulating, and (3) accept the normative changes that occur in sexual functioning. For those who master these developmental issues, the partner's body remains sexually stimulating. Diminished sexual ability is compensated for by feelings of love and tenderness generated over the years by a satisfying relationship. Those who cannot accept the changes in the partner's body or their own stop having sex, begin affairs, or leave the relationship, usually in search of a younger partner.

Normative changes in midlife sexual functioning include diminished sexual drive and an increase in mechanical problems. Men have greater difficulty getting and sustaining erections and experience a longer refractory period after ejaculation. Because of diminished estrogen production, women experience a thinning of the vaginal mucosa, a decrease in secretions, and fewer contractions at the time of orgasm. Women do not reach their sexual prime until their mid-30s; consequently, they have a greater capacity for orgasm in middle adulthood than in young adulthood. Women, however, are more vulnerable than men to narcissistic blows to their self-esteem as they lose their youthful appearance, which is overvalued in today's society. During middle adulthood, they may feel less sexually desirable than in early adulthood and, thus, feel less entitled to an adequate sex life. An inability to deal with changes in body image prompts many women and men to undergo cosmetic surgery in an effort to maintain their youthful appearance.

The demands of raising children interfere with the privacy and emotional equilibrium required for intimacy, as do the pressures and responsibilities of work. Fatigue and diminished interest are common denominators in these circumstances. Patients with deeply rooted problems with sexuality or relationships may use aging, work, and relationships with children or elderly parents as a means of rationalizing their conflicts and refusing to analyze them.

Climacterium

Middle adulthood is the time of the male and female climacterium, the period in life characterized by decreased biological and physiological functioning. For women, the menopausal period is considered the climacterium, and it may start anywhere from the 40s to the early 50s. Bernice Neugarten studied this period and found that more than 50 percent of women described menopause as an unpleasant experience, but a significant portion believed that their lives had not changed in any significant way, and many women experienced no adverse effects. Because they no longer had to worry about becoming pregnant, some women report feeling sexually freer after menopause than before its onset. Generally, the female climacterium has been stereotyped as a sudden or radical psychophysiological experience, but it is more often a gradual experience as estrogen secretion decreases with changes in the flow, timing, and eventual cessation of the menses. Vasomotor instability (hot flashes) can occur, and menopause can extend over several years. Some women experience anxiety and depression, but women who have a history of poor adaptation to stress are more predisposed to the menopausal syndrome.

For men, the climacterium has no clear demarcation; male hormones stay fairly constant through the 40s and 50s and then begin to decline. Nevertheless, men must adapt to a decline in biological functioning and overall physical vigor. About age 50, a slight decrease in healthy sperm and seminal fluid occurs; not sufficient, however, to preclude insemination. Coincident with the decreased testosterone level may be fewer and less firm erections and decreased sexual activity generally. Some men experience a so-called midlife crisis during this period. The crisis can be mild or severe, characterized by a sudden drastic change in work or marital relationships, severe depression, increased use of alcohol or drugs, or a shift to an alternate lifestyle.

Midlife Transition and Crisis

The *midlife transition* has been defined as an intense reappraisal of all aspects of life precipitated by the growing recognition that life is finite and approaching an end. It is characterized by mental turmoil, not action. For most people, the reappraisal results in decisions to keep most life structures, such as marriages and careers, which have been painstakingly built over time. When major changes are made, they are thoughtful and considered, even when they include major shifts, such as divorce or a job change. The developmentally aware clinician recognizes that every patient in this age group is engaged in a midlife transition (whether the patient is talking about it or not) and facilitates the process by making it conscious and verbal.

A true *midlife crisis* is a major, revolutionary turning point in life, involving changes in commitments to career or spouse, or both, and accompanied by significant, ongoing emotional turmoil for the individual and others. It is an upheaval of major proportions. A period of internal agitation is followed by a flurry of impulsive actions; for example, leaving spouse and children, becoming involved with a new sexual partner, and quitting a job, all within days or weeks of each other. Although unrecognized warning signs may have existed, those who are left behind are often shocked by the suddenness and abruptness of the change.

Efforts by family members or therapists to get the individual to stop and to reconsider usually fall on deaf ears. The overwhelming need is to avoid anyone who counsels restraint and to ignore therapists who recommend examining motivations and feelings before making such major decisions. Usually, in the midst of the crisis, the therapist is left with the painful job of helping those who have been left to deal with their shock and grief.

Empty-Nest Syndrome

Another phenomenon described in middle adulthood has been called the *empty-nest syndrome,* a depression that occurs in some men and women when their youngest child is about to leave home. Most parents, however, perceive the departure of the youngest child as a relief rather than a stress. If no compensating activities have been developed, particularly by the mother, some parents become depressed. This is especially true of women whose predominant role in life has been mothering or of couples who decided to stay in an otherwise unhappy marriage "for the sake of the children."

Other Tasks of Middle Adulthood

As persons approach the age of 50, they clearly define what they want from work, family, and leisure. Men who have reached their highest level of advancement in work may experience disillusionment or frustration when they realize they can no longer anticipate new work challenges. For women who have invested themselves completely in mothering, this period leaves them with no suitable identity after the children leave home. Sometimes, social rules become rigidly established; lack of freedom in lifestyle and a sense of entrapment can lead to depression and a loss of confidence. Also unique financial burdens can occur in middle age, produced by pressures to care for aged parents at one end of the spectrum and children at the other end.

Daniel Levinson described a transitional period between the ages of 50 and 55 during which a developmental crisis may occur when persons feel incapable of changing an intolerable life structure. Although no single event characterizes the transition, the physiological changes that begin to appear may have a dramatic effect on a person's sense of self. For example, a person may experience a decrease in cardiovascular efficiency that accompanies aging. Chronological age and physical infirmity are not linear, however; those who exercise regularly, who do not smoke, and who eat and drink in moderation can maintain their physical health and emotional well-being.

Middle adulthood is when persons frequently feel overwhelmed by too many obligations and duties, but it is also a time of great satisfaction for most persons. They have developed a wide array of acquaintances, friendships, and relationships, and the satisfaction they express about their network of friends predicts positive mental health. Some social ties, however, may be a source of stress when demands either cannot be met or assault a person's self-esteem. Power, leadership, wisdom, and understanding are most generally possessed by persons who are middle aged, and if their health and vitality remain intact, it is truly the prime of life.

DIVORCE

Divorce is a major crisis of life. Spouses often grow, develop, and change at different rates; one spouse may discover that the other is not the same as when they first married. In truth, both partners have changed and evolved, not necessarily in complementary directions. Frequently, one spouse blames a third person for alienation of affections and refuses to examine his or her own role in the marital problems. Certain aspects of marital deterioration and divorce seem to be related to specific qualities of middle life—need for change, weariness with acting responsibly, fear of facing up to oneself.

Types of Separation

Paul Bohannan, an anthropologist with expertise in marriage and divorce, described the types of separations that take place at the time of divorce.

Psychic Divorce. In psychic divorce, the love object is given up, and a grief reaction about the death of the relationship occurs. Sometimes a period of anticipatory mourning sets in before the divorce. Separating from a spouse forces a person to become autonomous, to change from a position of dependence. The separation may be difficult to achieve, especially if both are used to being dependent on each other (as normally happens in marriage) or if one was so dependent as to be afraid or incapable of becoming independent. Most persons report such feelings as depression, ambivalence, and mood swings at the time of divorce. Studies indicate that recovery from divorce takes about 2 years; by then, the ex-spouse may be viewed neutrally, and each spouse accepts his or her new identity as a single person.

Legal Divorce. Legal divorce involves going through the courts so that each of the parties is remarriageable. Of divorced women and divorced men, 75 percent and 80 percent, respectively, remarry within 3 years of divorce. No-fault divorce, in which neither person is judged to be the guilty party, has become the most widely used legal mechanism for divorce.

Economic Divorce. Economic divorce involves major concerns to the division of the couple's property between them and economic support for the wife. Many men who are ordered by the courts to pay alimony or child support flout the law and create a major social problem.

Community Divorce. The social network of the divorced couple changes markedly. A few relatives and friends are retained from the community and new ones are added. The task of meeting new friends is often difficult for divorced persons, who may realize how dependent they were on their spouses for social exchanges.

Coparental Divorce. Coparental divorce is the separation of a parent from the child's other parent. Being a single parent differs from being a married parent.

Custody

The parental right doctrine is a legal concept that awards custody to the more fit natural parent and attempts to ensure that the best interests of the child are served. In the past, mothers were almost always awarded custody, but custody is now given to fathers in about 15 percent of cases. Custodial fathers are likely to be white, married, older, and better educated than custodial mothers. Women who are granted custody have a better chance of being awarded child support and of actually receiving payment than do men who are granted custody. Nevertheless, women who receive payments still have lower incomes than men who receive payment.

The types of custody include *joint custody,* in which a child spends equal time with each parent, an increasingly common practice; *split custody,* in which siblings are separated and each parent has custody of one or more of the children; and *single custody,* in which the children live solely with one parent and the other parent has rights of visitation that may be limited in some way by the court. Child support payments are more likely to be made when parents have joint custody or when the noncustodial parent is given visitation rights.

Problems can surface in the parent–child relationship with the custodial or the noncustodial parent. The absence of the noncustodial parent in the home represents the reality of the divorce, and the custodial parent may become the target of the child's anger about the divorce. The parent under such stress may not be able to deal with the child's increased needs and emotional demands.

The noncustodial parent must cope with limits placed on time spent with the child. This parent loses the day-to-day gratification and the responsibilities involved with parenting. Emotional distress is common in parent and child. Joint custody offers a solution with some advantages, but it requires substantial maturity on the part of the parents and can present some problems. Parents must separate their child-rearing practices from their postdivorce resentments, and they must develop a spirit of cooperation about rearing the child. They must also be able to tolerate frequent communication with the ex-spouse.

Reasons for Divorce

Divorce tends to run in families and rates are highest in couples who marry as teenagers or come from different socioeconomic backgrounds. Every marriage is psychologically unique and so is each divorce. If a person's parents were divorced, he or she may choose to resolve a marital problem in the same way, through divorce. Expectations of the spouse may be unrealistic: One partner may expect the other to act as an all-giving mother or a magically protective father. The parenting experience places the greatest strain on a marriage. In surveys of couples with and without children, those without children reported getting more pleasure from their spouse than those with children. Illness in the child creates the greatest strain of all, and more than 50 percent of marriages in which a child has died through illness or accident end in divorce.

Other causes of marital distress are problems about sex and money. Both areas may be used as a means of control, and withholding sex or money is a means of expressing aggression. Also, less social pressure to remain married currently exists. As discussed above, the easing of divorce laws and the declining influence of religion and the extended family make divorce an acceptable course of action today.

Intercourse Outside of Marriage. Adultery is defined as voluntary sexual intercourse between a married person and someone other than his or her spouse. For men, the first extramarital affair is often associated with the wife's pregnancy, when coitus may be interdicted. Most of these incidents are kept secret from the spouse and, if known, rarely account for divorce. Nevertheless, the infidelity can serve as the catalyst for basic dissatisfactions in the marriage to surface, and these problems may then lead to its dissolution. Adultery may decline, as potentially fatal sexually transmitted diseases such as acquired immune deficiency syndrome (AIDS) serve as sobering deterrents.

ADULT MATURITY

Success and happiness in adulthood are made possible by achieving a modicum of maturity—a mental state, not an age. The capacity for maturity, however, is a direct outgrowth of the engagement and mastery of the developmental tasks of young and middle adulthood. From a developmental perspective, maturity can be defined as a mental state found in healthy adults that is characterized by detailed knowledge of the parameters of human existence, a sophisticated level of self-awareness based on an honest appraisal of one's own experience within those basic parameters, and the ability to use this intellectual and emotional knowledge and insight caringly in relation to one's self and others.

The achievement of maturity in midlife leads to emergence of the capacity for wisdom. Those who possess wisdom have learned from the past and are fully engaged in life in the present. Just as important, they anticipate the future and make the necessary decisions to enhance prospects for health and happiness. In other words, a philosophy of life has been developed that includes understanding and acceptance of the person's place in the order of human existence. Unfortunately, the joys of midlife do not last forever. Old age lies ahead. Although the hope and statistical expectation is for many years of mental competence and independence, physical and mental decline, increased dependence, and, eventually, death must be anticipated. Late adulthood has its own great pleasure, when there is a focus on continued mental and physical activity, a dominant preoccupation with the present and the future, and involvement with and facilitation of the young. Then, death can be met with feelings of satisfaction and acceptance, the natural end point of human existence that follows a life lived and well loved.

29

Geriatric Psychiatry

INTRODUCTION

For many individuals, the passage from youth to old age is mirrored by a shift from the pursuit of wealth to the maintenance of health. In late adulthood, the aging body increasingly becomes a central concern, replacing the midlife preoccupations with career and relationships. This is so because of normal diminution in function, altered physical appearance, and the increased incidence of physical illness. Despite these occurrences, the body in late adulthood can still be a source of considerable pleasure and can convey a sense of competence, particularly if attention is paid to regular exercise, healthy diet, adequate rest, and preventive maintenance medical care. The normal state in the aged is physical and mental health, not illness and debilitation. The developmental tasks of late adulthood that lead to mental health are listed in Table 29–1.

Old age, or late adulthood, usually refers to the stage of the life cycle that begins at age 65. Gerontologists—those who study the aging process—divide older adults into two groups: young-old, ages 65 to 74; and old-old, ages 75 and beyond. Some use the term oldest old to refer to those over 85. Older adults can also be described as well-old (persons who are healthy) and sick-old (persons who have an infirmity that interferes with functioning and requires medical or psychiatric attention). The health needs of older adults have grown enormously as the population ages, and geriatric physicians and psychiatrists play major roles in treating this population.

DEMOGRAPHICS

The number of individuals over age 65 is rapidly expanding. In 1900, for example, 4 percent of the US population was older than 65 years. By 2012, it was 43.1 million, and by 2050, it is projected to be about 83.7 million. That increase far exceeds the general population growth—10-fold compared with just over 3-fold between 1900 and 2000—and is projected to continue (e.g., 2.5 times vs. just over 1.5 times between 1990 and 2050) (Table 29–2).

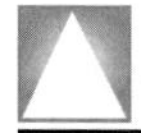

Table 29–1
Developmental Tasks of Late Adulthood

To maintain the body image and physical integrity
To conduct the life review
To maintain sexual interests and activities
To deal with the death of significant loved ones
To accept the implications of retirement
To accept the genetically programmed failure of organ systems
To divest oneself of the attachment to possessions
To accept changes in the relationship with grandchildren

The life expectancy for women at birth is projected to continue to exceed that for men by 7 years until 2050. By 2050, the composition of the US population by age and sex is estimated to differ markedly from that today. Such changes are bound to influence income and marital statistics, the percentage of elderly persons living alone or in long-term care facilities, and other aspects of the social network. A summary of demographic highlights of the aged is given in Table 29–3.

The accuracy of these projections, however, depends on the accuracy of other predications such as birth rates, immigration, and emigration—all of which are more difficult to gauge for the future than the remaining variables, death rates, or life expectancies. Projections concerning life expectancy, for example, can change substantially within a single decade.

BIOLOGY OF AGING

The aging process, or senescence (from the Latin *senescere,* "to grow old"), is characterized by a gradual decline in the functioning of all of the body's systems—cardiovascular, respiratory, genitourinary, endocrine, and immune, among others. But the belief that old age is invariably associated with profound intellectual and physical infirmity is a myth. Many older persons retain their cognitive abilities and physical capacities to a remarkable degree.

An overview of the biological changes that accompany old age is given in Table 29–4. The various decrements listed do not occur in a linear fashion in all systems. Not all organ systems deteriorate at the same rate, nor do they follow a similar pattern of decline for all persons. Each person is genetically endowed with one or more vulnerable systems, or a system may become vulnerable because of environmental stressors or intentional misuse, such as excessive ultraviolet exposure, smoking, or alcohol use. Moreover, not all organ systems deteriorate at the same time. Any one of a number of organ systems begins to deteriorate, and this deterioration then leads to illness or death.

Aging generally means the aging of cells. In the most commonly held theory, each cell has a genetically determined life span during which it can replicate itself a limited number of times before it dies. Structural changes occur in cells with age. In the central nervous system (CNS), for example, age-related cell changes occur in neurons, which show signs of degeneration. In senility (characterized by severe memory loss and a loss of intellectual functioning), signs of degeneration are much

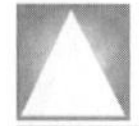

Table 29–2
Aging Population of the United States: 1900–2050

			Population, in Millions and as a Percentage of Total Population				
Year	**Median Age**	**Mean Age**	**All Ages**	**65 and Over**		**85 and Over**	
			(N)	(N)	(%)	(N)	(%)
1900			76.0	3.1	4.1	0.1	0.1
1950			150.1	12.3	8.2	0.6	0.4
1990			248.7	31.1	12.5	3.0	1.2
2000	35.7	36.5	276.2	35.3	12.8	4.3	1.6
2010	37.2	37.8	300.4	40.1	13.3	6.0	2.0
2030	38.5	39.9	350.0	70.2	20.1	8.8	2.5
2050	38.1	40.3	392.0	80.1	20.4	18.9	4.8

Population: U.S. Bureau of the Census. Current Population Reports, Special Studies, P23-190, 65+ in the United States. Washington, DC: U.S. Government Printing Office; 1996.
Mean/Median Age, 2000–2050: Day JC. Population projections of the United States by age, sex, race and Hispanic origin: 1995 to 2050. In: U.S. Bureau of the Census, Current Population Reports, P25-1130. Washington, DC: U.S. Government Printing Office; 1996.

more severe. An example is the neurofibrillary degeneration seen most commonly in dementia of the Alzheimer's type.

Structural changes and mutations in deoxyribonucleic acid (DNA) and ribonucleic acid (RNA) are also found in aging cells; these have been attributed to genotypic programming, x-rays, chemicals, and food products, among others. Probably no single cause of aging exists, and all areas of the body are affected to some degree. Genetic factors have been implicated in disorders that commonly occur in older persons, such as hypertension, coronary artery disease, arteriosclerosis, and neoplastic disease. Family studies indicate inheritance factors for breast and stomach cancer, colon polyps, and certain mental disorders of old age. Huntington's disease shows an autosomal dominant mode of inheritance with complete penetrance. The average age of onset is between 35 and 40 years, but cases have occurred as late as 70 years.

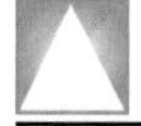

Table 29–3
Demographic Highlights of the Aged

- ▲ The older population (65+) numbered 4.04 million in 2010, an increase of 5.4 million for 15.3 since 2000.
- ▲ The number of Americans aged 45–64—who will reach 65 over the next two decades—increased by 31% during this decade.
- ▲ Over one in every eight, or 13.1%, of the population is an older American.
- ▲ Persons reaching age 65 have an average life expectancy of an additional 18.8 years (20 years for females and 17.3 for males).
- ▲ Older women outnumber older men at 23 million older women to 17.5 million older men.
- ▲ In 2010, 20% of persons 65+ were minorities—8.4% were African American.[a] Persons of Hispanic origin (who may be of any race) represented 6.9% of the older population. About 3.5% were Asian or Pacific Islanders,[a] and less than 1% were American Indian or Native Alaskan.[a] In addition, 0.8% of persons 65+ identified themselves as being of two or more races.
- ▲ Older men were much more likely to be married than older women—72% of men vs. 42% of women. In 2010, 40% older women were widows.
- ▲ About 29% (11.3 million) of noninstitutionalized older persons live alone (8.1 million women, 3.2 million men).
- ▲ Almost half of older women (47%) age 75+ live alone.
- ▲ About 485,000 grandparents aged 65 or more had the primary responsibility for their grandchildren who lived with them.
- ▲ The population 65 and over has increased from 35 million in 2000 to 40 million in 2010 (a 15% increase) and is projected to increase up to 55 million in 2020 (a 36% increase for that decade).
- ▲ The 85+ population is projected to increase from 5.5 million in 2010 and then 6.6 million in 2020 (19%) for that decade.
- ▲ Minority populations have increased from 5.7 million in 2000 (16.3% of the elderly population) to 8.1 million in 2010 (20% of the elderly) and are projected to increase to 13.1 million in 2020 (24% of the elderly).
- ▲ The median income of older persons in 2010 was $25,704 for males and $15,072 for females. Median money income (after adjusting for inflation) of all households headed by older people fell 1.5% (not statistically significant) from 2009 to 2010. Households containing families headed by person 65+ reported a median income in 2010 of $45,763.
- ▲ The major sources of income as reported by older persons in 2009 were Social Security (reported by 87% of older persons), income from assets (reported by 53%), private pensions (reported by 28%), government employee pensions (reported by 14%), and earnings (reported by 26%).
- ▲ Social Security constituted 90% or more of the income received by 35% of beneficiaries in 2009 (22% married couples and 43% of nonmarried beneficiaries).
- ▲ Almost 3.5 million elderly persons (9.0%) were below the poverty level in 2010. This poverty rate is not statistically different from the poverty rate in 2009 (8.9%). During 2011, the U.S. Census Bureau also released a new Supplemental Poverty Measure (SPM) that takes into account regional variations in the living costs, noncash benefits received, and nondiscretionary expenditures but does not replace the official poverty measure. The SPM shows a poverty level for older persons of 15.9%, an increase of over 75% over the official rate of 9% mainly due to medical out-of-pocket expenses.
- ▲ About 11% (3.7 million) of older Medicare enrollees received personal care from a paid or unpaid source in 1999.

[a]Principal source data for the profile are from the U.S. Census Bureau, the National Center for Health Statistics, and the Bureau of Labor Statistics. The profile incorporates the latest data (2010) available but not all items are updated on an annual basis.

Table 29–4
Biological Changes Associated with Aging

Cellular Level
- Change in cellular DNA (deoxyribonucleic acid) and RNA (ribonucleic acid) structures: intracellular organelle degeneration
- Neuronal degeneration in central nervous system, primarily in superior temporal precentral and inferior temporal gyri; no loss in brainstem nuclei
- Receptor sites and sensitivity altered
- Decreased anabolism and catabolism of cellular transmitter substances
- Intercellular collagen and elastin increase

Immune System
- Impaired T-cell response to antigen
- Increase in function of autoimmune bodies
- Increased susceptibility to infection and neoplasia
- Leukocytes unchanged, T lymphocytes reduced
- Increased erythrocyte sedimentation (nonspecific)

Musculoskeletal
- Decrease in height because of shortening of spinal column (2-in loss in both men and women from the second to the seventh decades)
- Reduction in lean muscle mass and muscle strength; deepening of thoracic cage
- Increase in body fat
- Elongation of nose and ears
- Loss of bone matrix, leading to osteoporosis
- Degeneration of joint surfaces may produce osteoarthritis
- Risk of hip fracture is 10–25% by age 90
- Continual closing of cranial sutures (parietomastoidsuture does not attain complete closure until age 80)
- Men gain weight until about age 60, then lose; women gain weight until age 70, then lose

Integument
- Graying of hair results from decreased melanin production in hair follicles (by age 50, 50% of all persons male and female are at least 50% gray; pubic hair is last to turn gray)
- General wrinkling of skin
- Less active sweat glands
- Decrease in melanin
- Loss of subcutaneous fat
- Nail growth slowed

Genitourinary and Reproductive
- Decreased glomerular filtration rate and renal blood flow
- Decreased hardness of erection, diminished ejaculatory spurt
- Decreased vaginal lubrication
- Enlargement of prostate
- Incontinence

Special Senses
- Thickening of optic lens, reduced peripheral vision
- Inability to accommodate (presbyopia)
- High-frequency sound hearing loss (presbycusis)—25% show loss by age 60, 65% by age 80
- Yellowing of optic lens
- Reduced acuity of taste, smell, and touch
- Decreased light-dark adaption

Neuropsychiatric
- Takes longer to learn new material, but complete learning still occurs
- Intelligence quotient (IQ) remains stable until age 80
- Verbal ability maintained with age
- Psychomotor speed declines

Memory
- Tasks requiring shifting attentions performed with difficulty
- Encoding ability diminishes (transfer of short- to long-term memory and vice versa)
- Recognition of right answer on multiple-choice tests remains intact
- Simple recall declines

Neurotransmitters
- Norepinephrine decreases in central nervous system
- Increased monoamine oxidase and serotonin in brain

Brain
- Decrease in gross brain weight, about 17% by age 80 in both sexes
- Widened sulci, smaller convolutions, gyral atrophy
- Ventricles enlarge
- Increased transport across blood–brain barrier
- Decreased cerebral blood flow and oxygenation

Cardiovascular
- Increase in size and weight of heart (contains lipofuscin pigment derived from lipids)
- Decreased elasticity of heart valves
- Increased collagen in blood vessels
- Increased susceptibility to arrhythmias
- Altered homeostasis of blood pressure
- Cardiac output maintained in absence of coronary heart disease

Gastrointestinal (GI) System
- At risk for atrophic gastritis, hiatal hernia, diverticulosis
- Decreased blood flow to gut, liver
- Diminished saliva flow
- Altered absorption from GI tract (at risk for malabsorption syndrome and avitaminosis)
- Constipation

Endocrine
- Estrogen levels decrease in women
- Adrenal androgen decreases
- Testosterone production declines in men
- Increase in follicle-stimulating hormone (FSH) and luteinizing hormone (LH) in postmenopausal women
- Serum thyroxine (T_4) and thyroid-stimulating hormone (TSH) normal, triiodothyronine (T_3) reduced
- Glucose tolerance test result decreases

Respiratory
- Decreased vital capacity
- Diminished cough reflex
- Decreased bronchial epithelium ciliary action

Longevity

Longevity has been studied since the beginning of recorded history and has always been a topic of great interest. The research about longevity reveals that a family history of longevity is the best indicator of a long life; of persons who live past 80, half of their fathers also lived past 80. Nevertheless, many conditions leading to a shortened life can be prevented, ameliorated, or delayed with effective intervention. Heredity is but one factor—one beyond a person's control. Predictors of longevity that are within a person's control include regular medical checkups, minimal or no caffeine or alcohol consumption, work gratification, and a perceived sense of the self as being socially useful in an altruistic role, such as spouse, teacher, mentor, parent, or grandparent. Healthy eating and adequate exercise are also associated with health and longevity.

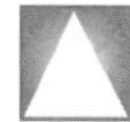

Table 29–5
Projected Life Expectancy at Birth and Age 65, by Sex: 1990–2050 (in Years)

	At Birth			At Age 65		
Year	Men	Women	Difference	Men	Women	Difference
1990	72.1	79.0	6.9	15.0	19.4	4.4
2000	73.5	80.4	6.9	15.7	20.3	4.6
2010	74.4	81.3	6.9	16.2	21.0	4.8
2020	74.9	81.8	6.9	16.6	21.4	4.8
2030	75.4	82.3	6.9	17.0	21.8	4.8
2040	75.9	82.8	6.9	17.3	22.3	5.0
2050	76.4	83.3	6.9	17.7	22.7	5.0

Data from U.S. Bureau of the Census, Washington, DC.

Life Expectancy

In the United States, the average life expectancy of both sexes has increased in every decade—from 48 years in 1900 to 77.4 years for men and 82.2 years for women in 2013. The projected life expectancy at birth and at age 65 is indicated in Table 29–5. Changes in morbidity and mortality have also occurred. Over the past 30 years, for example, a 60 percent decline has occurred in mortality from cerebrovascular disease and a 30 percent decline in mortality from coronary artery disease. In contrast, mortality from cancer, which rises steeply with age, has increased, especially cancer of the lung, colon, stomach, skin, and prostate.

The oldest old, persons over 85 years of age, is the most rapidly growing segment of the older population. Over the past 25 years, the population of all older persons increased by 100 percent, compared with 45 percent for the entire US population, but the increase for the 85 and older group exceeded 275 percent. It is expected that by 2050, the oldest old will make up about 25 percent of the elderly population and 5 percent of the total population in the United States.

The leading causes of death among older persons are heart disease, cancer, and stroke. Accidents are among the leading causes of death of persons over 65. Most fatal accidents are caused by falls, pedestrian incidents, and burns. Falls are most commonly the result of cardiac arrhythmias and hypotensive episodes.

Some gerontologists consider death in very old persons (over 85) to result from an aging syndrome characterized by diminished elastic-mechanical properties of the heart, arteries, lungs, and other organs. Death results from trivial tissue injuries that would not be fatal to a younger person; accordingly, senescence is viewed as the cause of death.

Ethnicity and Race

The proportion of older persons in the black, Hispanic, and Asian populations is smaller than that in the white population, but it is increasing rapidly. By 2050, 20 percent of older persons will be nonwhite. The proportion of older persons who are Hispanic will increase from 4 percent to approximately 14 percent over the same period. According to the U.S. Census Bureau, Hispanic refers to persons "whose origins are Mexican, Puerto Rican, Cuban, Central or South American, and other Hispanic or Latino, regardless of race."

Sex Ratios

On average, women live longer than men and are more likely than men to live alone. The number of men per 100 women decreases sharply from ages 65 to 85.

Geographic Distribution

The most populous states have the largest number of older persons. California has the most (3.3 million), followed by New York, Pennsylvania, Texas, Michigan, Illinois, Florida, and Ohio, each with more than 1 million. States with high proportions of older persons include Pennsylvania, Florida, Nebraska, and North Dakota. The high proportion in Florida is owing to those who move into the state for retirement; in the others, because of young persons moving out.

Exercise, Diet, and Health

Diet and exercise play a role in preventing or ameliorating chronic diseases of older persons, such as arteriosclerosis and hypertension. Hyperlipidemia, which correlates with coronary artery disease, can be controlled by reducing body weight, decreasing the intake of saturated fat, and limiting the intake of cholesterol. Increasing the daily intake of dietary fiber can also help decrease serum lipoprotein levels. A daily intake of 1 oz (about 30 mL) of alcohol has been correlated with longevity and elevated high-density lipoproteins (HDL). Studies have also clearly demonstrated that statin drugs that reduce cholesterol have a dramatic effect on reducing cardiovascular disease in persons with diet-resistant or exercise-resistant hyperlipidemia.

Low salt intake (less than 3 g a day) is associated with a lowered risk of hypertension. Hypertensive geriatric patients can often correct their condition by moderate exercise and decreased salt intake without the addition of drugs.

A regimen of daily moderate exercise (walking for 30 minutes a day) has been associated with a reduction in cardiovascular disease, decreased incidence of osteoporosis, improved respiratory function, the maintenance of ideal weight, and a general sense of well-being. Exercise has been shown to improve strength and function even among the very old. In many cases, a disease process has been reversed and even cured by diet and exercise, without additional medical or surgical intervention.

Table 29–6 lists the biological changes associated with diet and exercise. A comparison with Table 29–2 reveals that almost

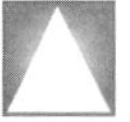

Table 29–6
Positive and Healthy Physiological Effects of Exercise and Nutrition

Increases
Strength of bones, ligaments, and muscles
Muscle mass and body density
Articular cartilage thickness
Skeletal muscle ATP (adenosine triphosphatase), CRP (C-reactive protein), K+ (potassium), and myoglobin
Skeletal muscle oxidative enzyme content and mitochondria
Skeletal muscle arterial collaterals and capillary density
Heart volume and weight
Blood volume and total circulating hemoglobin
Cardiac stroke volume
Myocardial contractility
Maximal CO_2 (A-V)
Maximal blood lactate concentration
Maximal pulmonary ventilation
Maximal respiratory work
Maximal oxygen diffusing capacity
Maximal exercise capacity as measured by the maximal oxygen intake, exercise time, and distance
Serum high-density lipoprotein concentration
Anaerobic threshold
Plasma insulin concentration with submaximal exercise
Decreases
Heart rate at rest and during submaximal exercise
Blood lactate concentration during submaximal exercise
Pulmonary ventilation during submaximal work
Respiratory quotient during submaximal work
Serum triglyceride concentration
Body fatness
Serum low-density lipoprotein concentration
Systolic blood pressure
Core temperature threshold for initiation of sweating
Sweat sodium and chloride content
Plasma epinephrine and norepinephrine with submaximal exercise
Plasma glucagon and growth hormone concentrations with submaximal exercise
Relative hemoconcentration with submaximal exercise in the heat

Reprinted from Buskirk ER. In: White PL, Monderka T, eds. *Diet and Exercise: Synergism in Health Maintenance*. Chicago: American Medical Association; 1982:133.

every biological change associated with aging is positively affected by diet and exercise.

STAGE THEORIES OF PERSONALITY DEVELOPMENT

Early personality theorists proposed that development was completed by the end of childhood or adolescence. One of the first development theorists to propose that personality continues to develop and grow over the life span was Erik Erikson. Erikson believed that development proceeded through a series of psychosocial stages, each with its own conflict that is resolved by the individual with greater or lesser success. Erikson termed the crisis of the last epoch of life integrity versus despair and believed that successful resolution of this crisis involved a process of life review and achieving a sense of peace and wisdom through coming to terms with how one's life was lived. For example, Erikson proposed that successful resolution of this crisis would be characterized by a sense of having lived one's life well, whereas a less successful resolution would be characterized by feeling that life was too short, that one did not choose wisely, and bitterness that one will not have a chance to live life over.

Several studies have attempted to validate aspects of Erikson's theory. In one study, a sample of more than 400 men was studied prospectively, and the highest Eriksonian life stage each achieved was rated according to data gathered on the circumstances of his life. For example, if a man had achieved independence from his family of origin and was self-sufficient but was unable to develop an intimate relationship, the highest life stage achieved would be the identity stage, not the intimacy stage. This study found that Eriksonian stages are passed through in sequential order, although often not at the same age for every individual, and that the stages are surprisingly universal in populations that are ethnically and socioeconomically diverse.

A longitudinal study of approximately 500 subjects from two age cohorts found that the earlier age cohort scored significantly higher on integrity than the later age cohort, and scores for both age cohorts on integrity had declined significantly by the final time of testing. These data suggest that the conflict of integrity versus despair may have a more favorable outcome in earlier age cohorts than in later ones, raising the possibility that changing societal values have had a negative impact on the struggle for integrity. Another study found that wisdom, a construct related to integrity, bore a stronger relation to life satisfaction in elderly adults than other variables, including finances, health, and living situation.

A survey of theories of development in old age is given in Table 29–7.

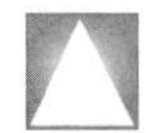

Table 29–7
Old Age Developmental Theorists

Sigmund Freud	Increasing control of the ego and id with aging results in increased autonomy. Regression may permit primitive modes of functioning to reappear.
Erik Erikson	The central conflict in old age is between integrity, the sense of satisfaction people feel reflecting on a life lived productively, and despair, the sense that life has little purpose or meaning. Contentment in old age comes only with getting beyond narcissism and into intimacy and generativity.
Heinz Kohut	Old people must continually cope with narcissistic injury as they attempt to adapt to the biological, psychological, and social losses associated with the aging process. The maintenance of self-esteem is a major task of old age.
Bernice Neugarten	The major conflict of old age relates to giving up the position of authority and evaluating achievements and former competence. It is a time of reconciliation with others and resolution of grief over the death of others and the approaching death of self.
Daniel Levinson	Ages 60–65 is a transition period ("the late adult transition"). People who are narcissistic and too heavily invested in body appearance are liable to become preoccupied with death. Creative mental activity is a normal and healthy substitute for reduced physical activity.

Table 29–8
Top Ten Chronic Conditions for People 65+, by Age and Race (Number per 1,000 People)

	Age				Race (65+)		
Condition	**65+**	**45–64**	**65–74**	**75+**	**White**	**Black**	**Black as of White**
Arthritis	483.0	253.8	437.3	554.5	483.2	522.6	108
Hypertension	380.6	229.1	383.8	375.6	367.4	517.7	141
Hearing impairment	286.5	127.7	239.4	360.3	297.4	174.5	59
Heart disease	278.9	118.9	231.6	353.0	286.5	220.5	77
Cataracts	156.8	16.1	107.4	234.3	160.7	139.8	87
Deformity or orthopedic impairment	155.2	155.5	141.4	177.0	156.2	150.8	97
Chronic sinusitis	153.4	173.5	151.8	155.8	157.1	125.2	80
Diabetes	88.2	58.2	89.7	85.7	80.2	165.9	207
Visual impairment	81.9	45.1	69.3	101.7	81.1	77.0	95
Varicose veins	78.1	57.8	72.6	86.6	80.3	64.0	80

Data from National Center for Health Statistics, Washington, DC.

PERSONALITY OVER THE LIFE SPAN: STABILITY OR CHANGE?

Although Erikson and other stage theorists focused on unique developmental tasks and stages central to each phase of life, other theorists focused on defining core personality traits within the individual and determining their course over the life span. For example, do those who are gregarious or extroverted during early childhood and adolescence remain extroverted through midlife and old age? Several well-designed longitudinal studies that have followed individuals over periods ranging from 10 to 50 years have found strong evidence for stability in five basic personality traits: extroversion, neuroticism, agreeableness, openness to experience, and conscientiousness. Some studies found slight decreases in extroversion and slight increases in agreeableness as individuals move into the oldest-old category, which contrasts with early theories that proposed that personality rigidifies as individuals age.

Is the fact that personality appears to have considerable stability over time inconsistent with the basic tenets of stage theories? Perhaps not. It may be that although individuals are consistent over time in their basic personality structure, the themes and conflicts with which they struggle change considerably over the life span, from concerns about developing identity and a stable sense of self, to finding a life partner, to issues related to life review, as hypothesized by the stage theories. In addition, in developing theories about personality change, few studies have examined the impact of significant historical events on personality; thus, the ways in which these events may result in personality change have not been studied systematically.

PSYCHOSOCIAL ASPECTS OF AGING

Social Activity

Healthy older persons usually maintain a level of social activity that is only slightly changed from that of earlier years. For many, old age is a period of continued intellectual, emotional, and psychological growth. In some cases, however, physical illness or the death of friends and relatives may preclude continued social interaction. Moreover, as persons experience an increased sense of isolation, they may become vulnerable to depression. Growing evidence indicates that maintaining social activities is valuable for physical and emotional well-being. Contact with younger persons is also important. Old persons can pass on cultural values and provide care services to the younger generation and thereby maintain a sense of usefulness that contributes to self-esteem.

Ageism

Ageism, a term coined by Robert Butler, refers to discrimination toward old persons and to the negative stereotypes about old age that are held by younger adults. Old persons may themselves resent and fear other old persons and discriminate against them. In Butler's scheme, persons often associate old age with loneliness, poor health, senility, and general weakness or infirmity. The experience of older persons, however, does not consistently support this attitude. For example, although 50 percent of young adults expect poor health to be a problem for those over 65 years old, 75 percent of persons 65 to 74 years of age describe their health as good. Two-thirds of persons 75 and older feel the same way. Health problems, when they do exist, more often involve chronic than acute conditions. More than four of five persons over the age of 65 have at least one chronic condition (Table 29–8).

Good health, however, is not the sole determinant of a good quality of life in old age. Surveys of old persons show that social contacts are at least as highly valued. In fact, the factors affecting good aging appear to be multidimensional. Aging "robustly" means considering aging in terms of productive involvement, affective status, functional status, and cognitive status. These four indicators are only minimally correlated. The most robustly aging individuals report greater social contact, better health and vision, and fewer significant life events in the past 3 years than their less robustly aging counterparts. A linear, age-related decrease occurs in robustness, but it can still be found among the oldest old.

George Vaillant followed up a group of Harvard freshmen into old age and found the following about emotional health at age 65: Having been close to brothers and sisters during college correlated with emotional well-being; undergoing early traumatic life experiences, such as the death of a parent or parental divorce, did not correlate with poor adaptation in old age; being depressed at some point between ages 21 and 50 predicted emotional problems at age 65; and possessing the personality traits of pragmatism and dependability as a young adult was associated with a sense of well-being at age 65.

Transference

Several forms of transference, some of them unique to adulthood, are present in older adults. First is the well-recognized parental transference, in which the patient reacts to the therapist as a child to a parent. Peer or sibling transference, expressions of experiences from a variety of nonparental relationships, is also common. In this form of transference, the patient looks to the therapist to share experiences with siblings, spouses, friends, and associates. At first, therapists may be surprised by older patients' ability to ignore their age in creating such transferences.

In son or daughter transference, quite common in middle-aged individuals and the elderly, the therapist is cast in the role of the patient's child, grandchild, or son-in-law or daughter-in-law. The themes expressed in this form of transference are multiple and often center on defenses against dependency feelings, activity and dominance versus passivity and submission, and attempts to rework unsatisfying aspects of relationships with children before time runs out. Finally, sexual transferences in older individuals are frequent and intense, and the therapist needs to be able to accept them and manage his or her countertransference responses.

Countertransference

Older individuals are dealing with illness and signs of aging, the loss of spouses and friends, and the constant awareness of time limitation and the nearness of death. These are painful issues that are just beginning to come into focus for younger therapists who would prefer not to confront them with great intensity on a daily basis.

A second source of countertransference responses centers on the older patient's sexuality. The presence of a vivid fantasy life, masturbation, and intercourse are disconcerting in and of themselves if the therapist has not had much experience in working with individuals who are the same age as their parents and grandparents. Consider the experience presented in the case study of a 31-year-old female therapist who was treating a 62-year-old man.

Early in the treatment process, Mr. E's sexual feelings emerged. His well-groomed appearance and adolescent-like nervousness caused the therapist discomfort. Her concern was how to engender respect and develop a therapeutic alliance with a patient who approached each session as a date, particularly because he was old enough to be her grandfather. At first shocked by his open expression of sexual interest in her, with the help of supervision and her own therapy, she was able to recognize that she and the patient had similar conflicts to resolve, despite the 30-year age difference between them. She had hoped that Mr. E would be "all grown up," devoid of issues that she was grappling with also. She came to recognize that failure to help him understand the relation between his past and still vibrant sexuality would do the patient a great disservice and would spring from her a lack of understanding of late-life sexual development and her countertransference reaction to him based on her conflicted attitudes toward the sexuality of her parents and grandparents. *(Courtesy of Calvin A. Colarusso, M.D.)*

Socioeconomics

The economics of old age is of paramount importance to older persons themselves and to society at large. The past 30 years have seen a dramatic decline in the proportion of the US elderly population who are poor, primarily as a result of the availability of Medicare, Social Security, and private pensions. In 1959, 35.2 percent of persons over 65 lived below the poverty line, but by 2012 this figure had declined to 9.1 percent. Persons over age 65 make up 12 percent of the population, but they include only 9 percent of those living at low socioeconomic levels. Women are more likely than men to be poor. Income sources vary for persons age 65 and older. Despite overall economic gains, many older persons are so preoccupied by money worries that their enjoyment of life is lessened. Obtaining proper medical care may be especially difficult when personal funds are not available or are insufficient.

Medicare (Title 18) provides both hospital and medical insurance for those over age 65. About 150 million medical bills are reimbursed under the Medicare program each year; but only about 40 percent of all medical expenses incurred by older persons are covered under Medicare. The rest is paid by private insurance, state insurance, or personal funds. Some services—such as outpatient psychiatric treatment, skilled nursing care, physical rehabilitation, and preventive physical examinations—are covered minimally or not at all.

In addition to Medicare, the Social Security program pays benefits to persons over age 65 (over age 67 in 2027) and pays benefits at reduced rates from age 62 on. To qualify for benefits, a person must have worked long enough to become insured: A worker must have worked for 10 years to be eligible for benefits. Benefits are also paid to widows, widowers, and dependent children if those receiving benefits or contributing to Social Security die (survivor benefits). Social Security is not a pension scheme but a pay-as-you-go income supplement to prevent mass destitution among older persons. Benefits are paid by those currently working to those who are retired. Serious difficulties for Social Security are forecast for the next three decades, when the number of baby boomers reaching old age will greatly exceed the number of younger workers paying into the plan.

Retirement

For many older persons, retirement is a time for the pursuit of leisure and for freedom from the responsibility of previous working commitments. For others, it is a time of stress, especially when retirement results in economic problems or a loss of self-esteem. Ideally, employment after age 65 should be a matter of choice. With the passage of the Age Discrimination in Employment Act of 1967 and its amendments, forced retirement at age 70 has been virtually eliminated in the private sector, and it is not legal in federal employment.

Most of those who retire voluntarily reenter the workforce within 2 years, for a variety of reasons, including negative reactions to being retired, feelings of being unproductive, economic hardship, and loneliness. The amount of time spent in retirement has increased as the life span has nearly doubled since 1900. Currently, the number of years spent in retirement is almost equal to the number of years spent working.

Sexual Activity

The frequency of orgasm, from coitus or masturbation, decreases with age in men and women. The most important factors in determining the level of sexual activity with age are the health and survival of the spouse, one's own health, and the level of past sexual activity. Although some degree of declining sexual interest and function is inevitable with age, social and cultural factors appear to be more responsible for the sexual changes observed than for the psychological changes of aging per se. Although satisfying sexual activity is possible for the reasonably healthy elderly, many do not actualize this potential. The widely held notion that the elderly are essentially asexual is often a self-fulfilling prophecy.

Long-Term Care

Many older persons who are infirm require institutional care. Although only 5 percent are institutionalized in nursing homes at any one time, about 35 percent of older persons require care in a long-term facility at some time during their lives. Older nursing home residents are mainly widowed women and about 50 percent are over age 85.

Nursing home care costs are not covered by Medicare; they range from $20,000 to $1 million a year. About 20,000 long-term nursing care institutions are available in the United States, this is not enough to meet the need. Those older persons who do not require skilled nursing care can be managed in other types of health-related facilities, such as centers they attend during the daytime hours, but the need for care far exceeds the availability of such centers.

Outside institutions, care for older persons is provided by their children (primarily their daughters and daughters-in-law), their wives, and other women. More than 50 percent of these women caregivers also work in jobs outside the home, and about 40 percent also care for their own children. In general, women end up as caregivers more often than men because of cultural and societal expectations. According to the American Association of Retired Persons, daughters with jobs spend an average of 12 hours a week providing care and currently spend about $150 a month for travel, telephone calls, special foods, and medication for older persons.

PSYCHIATRIC PROBLEMS OF OLDER PERSONS

Despite the ubiquity of loss in old age, the prevalence of major depressive disorder and dysthymia is actually less than in younger age groups. Several explanations for this phenomenon have been proposed: rarity of late-onset depression, higher mortality among persons with depression, and a general decrease in disorders caused by emotional upheavals or substance abuse in older persons. Depression in old persons is often accompanied by physical symptoms or cognitive changes that may mimic dementia.

The incidence of suicide among older persons is high (40 per 100,000 population) and is highest for older white men. The suicide of older persons is perceived differently by surviving friends and family members on the basis of gender: Men are thought to have been physically ill, and women are thought to have been mentally ill.

The relation between good mental and good physical health is clear in older persons. Adverse effects on the course of chronic medical illness are correlated with emotional problems. The following section will discuss the psychiatric problems in older persons.

PSYCHIATRIC EXAMINATION OF THE OLDER PATIENT

Psychiatric history taking and the mental status examination of older adults follow the same format as for younger adults; however, because of the high prevalence of cognitive disorders in older persons, psychiatrists must determine whether a patient understands the nature and purpose of the examination. When a patient is cognitively impaired, an independent history should be obtained from a family member or caretaker. The patient still should be seen alone—even in cases of clear evidence of impairment—to preserve the privacy of the doctor–patient relationship and to elicit any suicidal thoughts or paranoid ideation, which may not be voiced in the presence of a relative or nurse.

When approaching the examination of the older patient, it is important to remember that older adults differ markedly from one another. The approach to examining the older patient must take into account whether the person is a healthy 75-year-old who recently retired from a second career or a frail 96-year-old who just lost the only surviving relative with the death of the 75-year-old care-giving daughter.

Psychiatric History

A complete psychiatric history includes preliminary identification (name, age, sex, marital status), chief complaint, history of the present illness, history of previous illnesses, personal history, and family history. A review of medications (including over-the-counter medications) that the patient is currently using or has used in the recent past is also important.

Patients older than age 65 often have subjective complaints of minor memory impairments, such as forgetting persons' names and misplacing objects. Minor cognitive problems also can occur because of anxiety in the interview situation. These age-associated memory impairments are of no significance; the term *benign senescent forgetfulness* has been used to describe them.

A patient's childhood and adolescent history can provide information about personality organization and give important clues about coping strategies and defense mechanisms used under stress. A history of learning disability or minimal cerebral dysfunction is significant. The psychiatrist should inquire about friends, sports, hobbies, social activity, and work. The occupational history should include the patient's feelings about work, relationships with peers, problems with authority, and attitudes toward retirement. The patient also should be questioned about plans for the future. What are the patient's hopes and fears?

The family history should include a patient's description of parents' attitudes and adaptation to their old age and, if applicable, information about the causes of their deaths. Alzheimer's disease is transmitted as an autosomal dominant trait in 10 to 30 percent of the offspring of parents with Alzheimer's disease; depression and alcohol dependence also run in families. The patient's current social situation should be evaluated. Who cares for the patient? Does the patient have children? What are the characteristics of the patient's parent–child relationships? A financial history helps the psychiatrist evaluate the role of economic hardship in the patient's illness and to make realistic treatment recommendations.

The marital history includes a description of the spouse and the characteristics of the relationship. If the patient is a widow or a widower, the psychiatrist should explore how grieving was handled. If the loss of the spouse occurred within the past year, the patient is at high risk for an adverse physical or psychological event.

The patient's sexual history includes sexual activity, orientation, libido, masturbation, extramarital affairs, and sexual symptoms (e.g., impotence and anorgasmia). Young clinicians may have to overcome their own biases about taking a sexual history: Sexuality is an area of concern for many geriatric patients, who welcome the chance to talk about their sexual feelings and attitudes.

Mental Status Examination

The mental status examination offers a cross-sectional view of how a patient thinks, feels, and behaves during the examination. With older adults, a psychiatrist may not be able to rely on a single examination to answer all of the diagnostic questions. Repeat mental status examinations may be needed because of fluctuating changes in the patient's family.

General Description. A general description of the patient includes appearance, psychomotor activity, attitude toward the examiner, and speech activity.

Motor disturbances (e.g., shuffling gait, stooped posture, "pill rolling" movements of the fingers, tremors, and body asymmetry) should be noted. Involuntary movements of the mouth or tongue may be adverse effects of phenothiazine medication. Many depressed patients seem to be slow in speech and movement. A mask-like facies occurs in Parkinson's disease.

The patient's speech may be pressured in agitated, manic, and anxious states. Tearfulness and overt crying occur in depressive and cognitive disorders, especially if the patient feels frustrated about being unable to answer one of the examiner's questions. The presence of a hearing aid or another indication that the patient has a hearing problem (e.g., requesting repetition of questions) should be noted.

The patient's attitude toward the examiner—cooperative, suspicious, guarded, ingratiating—can give clues about possible transference reactions. Because of transference, older adults can react to younger physicians as if the physicians were parent figures, despite the age difference.

Functional Assessment. Patients older than 65 years of age should be evaluated for their capacity to maintain independence and to perform the activities of daily life, which include toileting, preparing meals, dressing, grooming, and eating. The degree of functional competence in their everyday behaviors is an important consideration in formulating a treatment plan for these patients.

Mood, Feelings, and Affect. Suicide is a leading cause of death of older persons, and an evaluation of a patient's suicidal ideation is essential. Loneliness is the most common reason cited by older adults who consider suicide. Feelings of loneliness, worthlessness, helplessness, and hopelessness are symptoms of depression, which carries a high risk for suicide. Nearly 75 percent of all suicide victims suffer from depression, alcohol abuse, or both. The examiner should specifically ask the patient about any thoughts of suicide: Does the patient feel life is no longer worth living? Does the patient think he or she would be better off dead or, when dead, would no longer be a burden to others? Such thoughts—especially when associated with alcohol abuse, living alone, recent death of a spouse, physical illness, and somatic pain—indicate a high suicidal risk.

Disturbances in mood states, most notably depression and anxiety, can interfere with memory functioning. An expansive or euphoric mood may indicate a manic episode or may signal a dementing disorder. Frontal lobe dysfunction often produces *witzelsucht,* which is the tendency to make puns and jokes and then laugh aloud at them.

The patient's affect may be flat, blunted, constricted, shallow, or inappropriate, all of which can indicate a depressive disorder, schizophrenia, or brain dysfunction. Such affects are important abnormal findings, although they are not pathognomonic of a specific disorder. Dominant lobe dysfunction causes *dysprosody,* an inability to express emotional feelings through speech intonation.

Perceptual Disturbances. Hallucinations and illusions by older adults can be transitory phenomena resulting from decreased sensory acuity. The examiner should note whether the patient is confused about time or place during the hallucinatory episode; confusion points to an organic condition. It is particularly important to ask the patient about distorted body perceptions. Because hallucinations can be caused by brain tumors and other focal pathology, a diagnostic workup may be indicated. Brain diseases cause perceptive impairments; agnosia, the inability to recognize and interpret the significance of sensory impressions, is associated with organic brain diseases. The examiner should note the types of agnosia—the denial of illness (anosognosia), the denial of a body part (atopognosia), or the inability to recognize objects (visual agnosia) or faces (prosopagnosia).

Language Output. The language output category of the geriatric mental status examination covers the aphasias, which are disorders of language output related to organic lesions of the brain. The best described are nonfluent or Broca's aphasia, fluent or Wernicke's aphasia, and global aphasia, a combination of fluent and nonfluent aphasias. In nonfluent or Broca's aphasia, the patient's understanding remains intact, but the ability to speak is impaired. The patient cannot pronounce "Methodist Episcopalian." Words are generally mispronounced and speech may be telegraphic. A simple test for Wernicke's aphasia is to point to some common objects—such as a pen or a pencil, a doorknob, and a light switch—and ask the patient to name them. The patient also may be unable to demonstrate the use of simple objects, such as a key and a match (ideomotor apraxia).

Visuospatial Functioning. Some decline in visuospatial capability is normal with aging. Asking a patient to copy figures or a drawing may be helpful in assessing the function. A neuropsychological assessment should be performed when visuospatial functioning is obviously impaired.

Thought. Disturbances in thinking include neologisms, word salad, circumstantiality, tangentially, loosening of associations, flight of ideas, clang associations, and blocking. The loss of the ability to appreciate nuances of meaning (abstract thinking) may be an early sign of dementia. Thinking is then described as concrete or literal.

Thought content should be examined for phobias, obsessions, somatic preoccupations, and compulsions. Ideas about suicide or homicide should be discussed. The examiner should determine whether delusions are present and how such delusions affect the patient's life. Delusions may be present in nursing home patients and may have been a reason for admission. Ideas of reference or of influence should be described. Patients who are hard of hearing can be classified mistakenly as paranoid or suspicious.

Sensorium and Cognition. *Sensorium* concerns the functioning of the special senses; *cognition* concerns information processing and intellect. The survey of both areas, known as the neuropsychiatric examination, consists of the clinician's assessment and a comprehensive battery of psychological tests.

CONSCIOUSNESS. A sensitive indicator of brain dysfunction is an altered state of consciousness in which the patient does not seem to be alert, shows fluctuations in levels of awareness, or seems to be lethargic. In severe cases, the patient is somnolescent or stuporous.

ORIENTATION. Impairment in orientation to time, place, and person is associated with cognitive disorders. Cognitive impairment often is observed in mood disorders, anxiety disorders, factitious disorders, conversion disorder, and personality disorders, especially during periods of severe physical or environmental stress. The examiner should test for orientation to place by asking the patient to describe his or her present location. Orientation to person may be approached in two ways: Does the patient know his or her own name, and are nurses and doctors identified as such? Time is tested by asking the patient the date, the year, the month, and the day of the week. The patient also should be asked about the length of time spent in a hospital, during what season of the year, and how the patient knows these facts. Greater significance is given to difficulties concerning person than to difficulties of time and place, and more significance is given to orientation to place than to orientation to time.

MEMORY. Memory usually is evaluated in terms of immediate, recent, and remote memory. Immediate retention and recall are tested by giving the patient six digits to repeat forward and backward. The examiner should record the result of the patient's capacity to remember. Persons with unimpaired memory usually can recall six digits forward and five or six digits backward. The clinician should be aware that the ability to do well on digit-span tests is impaired in extremely anxious patients. Remote memory can be tested by asking for the patient's place and date of birth, the patient's mother's name before she was married, and names and birthdays of the patient's children.

In cognitive disorders, recent memory deteriorates first. Recent memory assessment can be approached in several ways. Some examiners give the patient the names of three items early in the interview and ask for recall later. Others prefer to tell a brief story and ask the patient to repeat it verbatim. Memory of the recent past also can be tested by asking for the patient's place of residence, including the street number, the method of transportation to the hospital, and some current events. If the patient has a memory deficit, such as amnesia, careful testing should be performed to determine whether it is retrograde amnesia (loss of memory before an event) or anterograde amnesia (loss of memory after the event). Retention and recall also can be tested by having the patient retell a simple story. Patients who confabulate make up new material in retelling the story.

INTELLECTUAL TASKS, INFORMATION, AND INTELLIGENCE. Various intellectual tasks can be presented to estimate the patient's fund of general knowledge and intellectual functioning. Counting and calculation can be tested by asking the patient to subtract 7 from 100 and to continue subtracting 7 from the result until the number 2 is reached. The examiner records the responses as a baseline for future testing. The examiner can also ask the patient to count backward from 20 to 1 and can record the time necessary to complete the exercise.

The patient's fund of general knowledge is related to intelligence. The patient can be asked to name the president of the United States, to name the three largest cities in the United States, to give the population of the United States, and to give the distance from New York to Paris. The examiner must take into account the patient's educational level, socioeconomic status, and general life experience in assessing the results of some of these tests.

READING AND WRITING. It may be important for the clinician to examine the patient's reading and writing and to determine whether the patient has a specific speech deficit. The examiner may have the patient read a simple story aloud or write a short sentence to test for a reading or writing disorder. Whether the patient is right handed or left handed should be noted.

JUDGMENT. *Judgment* is the capacity to act appropriately in various situations. Does the patient show impaired judgment? What would the patient do on finding a stamped, sealed, addressed envelope in the street? What would the patient do if he or she smelled smoke in a theater? Can the patient discriminate? What is the difference between a dwarf and a boy? Why are couples required to get a marriage license?

Neuropsychological Evaluation

A thorough neuropsychological examination includes a comprehensive battery of tests that can be replicated by various examiners and can be repeated over time to assess the course of a specific illness. The most widely used test of current cognitive functioning is the Mini-Mental State Examination (MMSE), which assesses orientation, attention, calculation, immediate and short-term recall, language, and the ability to follow simple commands. The MMSE is used to detect impairments, follow the course of an illness, and monitor the patient's treatment responses. It is not used to make a formal diagnosis. The maximal MMSE score is 30. Age and educational level influence cognitive performance as measured by the MMSE.

The assessment of intellectual abilities is performed with the Wechsler Adult Intelligence Scale-Revised (WAIS-R), which gives verbal, performance, and full-scale intelligence quotient (IQ) scores. Some test results, such as those of vocabulary tests, hold up as aging progresses; results of other tests, such as tests of similarities and digit-symbol substitution, do not. The performance part of the WAIS-R is a more sensitive indicator of brain damage than the verbal part.

Visuospatial functions are sensitive to the normal aging process. The Bender Gestalt Test is one of a large number of instruments used to test visuospatial functions; another is the Halstead–Reitan Battery, which is the most complex battery of tests covering the entire spectrum of information processing and cognition. Depression, even in the absence of dementia, often impairs psychomotor performance, especially visuospatial functioning and timed motor performance. The Geriatric Depression Scale is a useful screening instrument that excludes somatic complaints from its list of items. The presence of somatic complaints on a rating scale tends to confound the diagnosis of a depressive disorder.

Medical History. Elderly patients have more concomitant, chronic, and multiple medical problems and take more medications than younger adults; many of these medications can influence their mental status. The medical history includes all major illnesses, traumata, hospitalizations, and treatment interventions. The psychiatrist should also be alert to underlying medical illness. Infections, metabolic and electrolyte disturbances, and myocardial infarction and stroke may first be manifested by psychiatric symptoms. Depressed mood, delusions, and hallucinations may precede other symptoms of Parkinson's disease by many months. On the other hand, a psychiatric disorder can also cause such somatic symptoms as weight loss, malnutrition, and inanition of severe depression.

Careful review of medications (including over-the-counter medications, laxatives, vitamins, tonics, and lotions) and even substances recently discontinued is extremely important. Drug effects can be long lasting and may induce depression (e.g., antihypertensives), cognitive impairment (e.g., sedatives), delirium (e.g., anticholinergics), and seizures (e.g., neuroleptics). The review of medications must include sufficient detail to identify misuse (overdose, underuse) and relate medication use to special diets. A dietary history is also important; deficiencies and excesses (e.g., protein, vitamins) can influence physiological function and mental status.

EARLY DETECTION AND PREVENTION STRATEGIES

Many age-related illnesses develop insidiously and gradually progress over the years. The most common cause of late-life cognitive impairment, Alzheimer's disease, is characterized neuropathologically by a gradual accumulation of neuritic plaques and neurofibrillary tangles in the brain. Clinically, a progression of cognitive decline is seen, which begins with mild memory loss and ends with severe cognitive and behavioral deterioration.

Because it will likely be easier to prevent neural damage than to repair it once it occurs, investigators are developing strategies for early detection and prevention of age-related illnesses, such as Alzheimer's disease. Considerable progress has been made in the detection component of this strategy, using brain imaging technologies, such as positron emission tomography (PET) and functional magnetic resonance imaging (fMRI), in combination with genetic risk measures. With these approaches, subtle brain changes can now be detected that progress and can be followed over time. Such surrogate markers allow clinical scientists to track disease progression and to test novel treatments designed to decelerate brain aging. Clinical trials of cholinesterase inhibitor drugs, anticholesterol drugs, anti-inflammatory drugs, and others (e.g., vitamin E) are in progress to determine if such treatments delay the onset of Alzheimer's disease or the progression of brain metabolic or cognitive decline.

Novel approaches to measuring the physical evidence of Alzheimer's disease, the plaques and tangles in the cerebral cortex, have been successful in initial studies and will likely facilitate the testing of innovative treatments designed to rid the brain of these pathognomonic lesions. Scientists may not be able to cure Alzheimer's disease in its advanced stages, but they may be able to delay its onset effectively, thus helping patients live longer without the debilitating manifestations of the disease, including cognitive decline.

MENTAL DISORDERS OF OLD AGE

The National Institute of Mental Health's Epidemiologic Catchment Area (ECA) program has found that the most common mental disorders of old age are depressive disorders, cognitive disorders, phobias, and alcohol use disorders. Older adults also have a high risk for suicide and drug-induced psychiatric symptoms. Many mental disorders of old age can be prevented, ameliorated, or even reversed. Of special importance are the reversible causes of delirium and dementia; if not diagnosed accurately and treated in a timely fashion, however, these conditions can progress to an irreversible state requiring a patient's institutionalization. Table 29–9 lists the general cognitive domains assessed in a neuropsychological evaluation, with the tests used to measure that skill and a description of the specific behaviors measured by each test. The tests listed in the table constitute a comprehensive test battery generally appropriate for use with a geriatric population. Use of a comprehensive battery is preferable for confident determination of the presence and type of dementia or other cognitive disorder in elderly persons; in some circumstances, however, administering a several-hour battery is not possible.

Several psychosocial risk factors also predispose older persons to mental disorders. These risk factors include loss of social roles, loss of autonomy, the deaths of friends and relatives, declining health, increased isolation, financial constraints, and decreased cognitive functioning.

Many drugs can cause psychiatric symptoms in older adults. These symptoms can result from age-related alterations in drug absorption, a prescribed dosage that is too large, not following instructions and taking too large a dose, sensitivity to the medication, and conflicting regimens presented by several physicians. Almost the entire spectrum of mental disorders can be caused by drugs.

Dementing Disorders

Only arthritis is a more common cause of disability among adults age 65 and older than dementia, a generally progressive and irreversible impairment of the intellect, the prevalence of which increases with age. About 5 percent of persons in the

Table 29–9
Cognitive Domains

Gross cognitive functioning
Mini-Mental State Examination: *orientation, repetition, following commands, naming, constructional skill, written expression, memory, mental flexibility, and calculations*
Intelligence
Wechsler Adult Intelligence Scale-Revised (WAIS-R) or Wechsler Intelligence Scale-III (WAIS-III): *verbal and nonverbal intelligence*
Basic attention
WAIS-R or WAIS-III Digit Span: *repetition of digits forward and backward*
Information-processing speed
WAIS-R or WAIS-III Digit Symbol: *rapid graphomotor tracking*
Trailmaking Part A: *rapid graphomotor tracking*
Stroop A and B: *rapid word reading and color naming*
Motor dexterity
Finger tapping: *right and left index finger dexterity*
Language
Boston Naming Test: *word retrieval*
WAIS-R or WAIS-III Vocabulary: *vocabulary range*
Visual perceptual/spatial
WAIS-R or WAIS-III Picture Completion: *visual perception*
WAIS-R or WAIS-III Block Design: *constructional ability*
Rey–Osterrieth Complex Figure: *paper-and-pencil copy of complex design*
Beery Developmental Test of Visual Motor Integration: *paper-and-pencil copy of simple-to-complex designs*
Learning and memory
An 8- to 10-item word list learning task: *learning and recall of rote verbal information*
Wechsler Memory Scale-Revised (WMS-R) or Wechsler Memory Scale-III (WMS-III)
Logical Memory subtest: *immediate and delayed recall of paragraph information*
Visual Reproduction subtest: *immediate and delayed recall of visual designs*
Rey–Osterrieth Complex Figure 3-minute delayed recall: *delayed recall of complex design*
Executive functions
Trailmaking Part B: *rapid alternation between tasks*
Stroop C: *inhibition of an overlearned response*
Wisconsin Card Sorting Test: *categorization and mental flexibility*
Verbal fluency (FAS and category): *rapid word generation*
Design fluency: *rapid generation of novel designs*

Courtesy of Kyle Brauer Boone, Ph.D.

United States older than age 65 have severe dementia, and 15 percent have mild dementia. Of persons older than age 80, about 20 percent have severe dementia. Known risk factors for dementia are age, family history, and female sex.

In contrast to intellectual disability, the intellectual impairment of dementia develops over time—that is, previously achieved mental functions are lost gradually. The characteristic changes of dementia involve cognition, memory, language, and visuospatial functions, but behavioral disturbances are common as well and include agitation, restlessness, wandering, rage, violence, shouting, social and sexual disinhibition, impulsiveness, sleep disturbances, and delusions. Delusions and hallucinations occur during the course of the dementias in nearly 75 percent of patients.

Cognition is impaired by many conditions, including brain injuries, cerebral tumors, acquired immune deficiency syndrome (AIDS), alcohol, medications, infections, chronic pulmonary diseases, and inflammatory diseases. Although dementias associated with advanced age typically are caused by primary degenerative CNS disease and vascular disease, many factors contribute to cognitive impairment; in older persons, mixed causes of dementia are common.

About 10 to 15 percent of all patients who exhibit symptoms of dementia have potentially treatable conditions. The treatable conditions include systemic disorders, such as heart disease, renal disease, and congestive heart failure; endocrine disorders, such as hypothyroidism; vitamin deficiency; medication misuse; and primary mental disorders, most notably depressive disorders.

Depending on the site of the cerebral lesion, dementias are classified as cortical and subcortical. A subcortical dementia occurs in Huntington's disease, Parkinson's disease, normal pressure hydrocephalus, vascular dementia, and Wilson's disease. The subcortical dementias are associated with movement disorders, gait apraxia, psychomotor retardation, apathy, and akinetic mutism, which can be confused with catatonia. Table 29–10 lists some potentially reversible conditions that may resemble dementia. The cortical dementias occur in dementias of the Alzheimer's type, Creutzfeldt–Jakob disease (CJD), and Pick's disease, which frequently manifest aphasia, agnosia, and apraxia. In clinical practice, the two types of dementias overlap and, in most cases, an accurate diagnosis can be made only by autopsy. Human prion diseases result from coding mutations in the prion protein gene

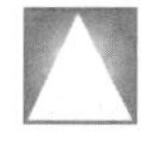

TABLE 29–10
Some Potentially Reversible Conditions That May Resemble Dementia

Substance
Anticholinergic agents
Antihypertensives
Antipsychotics
Corticosteroids
Digitalis
Narcotics
Nonsteroidal anti-inflammatory agents
Phenytoin
Polypharmacotherapy
Sedative hypnotics
Psychiatric Disorders
Anxiety
Depression
Mania
Delusional (paranoid) disorders
Metabolic and Endocrine Disorders
Addison's disease
Cushing's syndrome
Hepatic failure
Hypercarbia (chronic obstructive pulmonary disease)
Hypernatremia
Hyperparathyroidism
Hyperthyroidism
Hypoglycemia
Hyponatremia
Hypothyroidism
Renal failure
Volume depletion
Miscellaneous Conditions
Fecal impaction
Hospitalization
Impaired hearing or vision

Courtesy of Gary W. Small, M.D.

(*PRNP*) and may be inherited, acquired, or sporadic. They include familial CJD, Gerstmann–Sträussler–Scheinker syndrome, and fatal familial insomnia. These are inherited as autosomal dominant mutations. The acquired diseases include kuru and iatrogenic CJD. Kuru was an epidemic prion disease of the Fore people of Papua, New Guinea, caused by cannibalistic funeral rituals, which peaked in incidence in the 1950s. Iatrogenic disease is rare and is caused, for example, by the use of contaminated dura mater and corneal grafts and treatment with human cadaveric pituitary-derived growth hormone and gonadotropin. Sporadic CJD accounts for 85 percent of the human prion diseases and occurs worldwide, with a uniform distribution and an incidence of about 1 in 1 million per annum, with a mean age at onset of 65 years. It is exceedingly rare in individuals under 30 years of age.

Depressive Disorders

Depressive symptoms are present in about 15 percent of all older adult community residents and nursing home patients. Age itself is not a risk factor for the development of depression, but being widowed and having a chronic medical illness are associated with vulnerability to depressive disorders. Late-onset depression is characterized by high rates of recurrence.

The common signs and symptoms of depressive disorders include reduced energy and concentration, sleep problems (especially early morning awakening and multiple awakenings), decreased appetite, weight loss, and somatic complaints. The presenting symptoms may be different in older depressed patients from those seen in younger adults because of an increased emphasis on somatic complaints in older persons. Older persons are particularly vulnerable to major depressive episodes with melancholic features, characterized by depression, hypochondriasis, low self-esteem, feelings of worthlessness, and self-accusatory trends (especially about sex and sinfulness) with paranoid and suicidal ideation. A geriatric depression scale is given in Table 29–11.

Cognitive impairment in depressed geriatric patients is referred to as the *dementia syndrome of depression* (pseudodementia), which can be confused easily with true dementia. In true dementia, intellectual performance usually is global, and impairment is consistently poor; in pseudodementia, deficits in attention and concentration are variable. Compared with patients who have true dementia, patients with pseudodementia are less likely to have language impairment and to confabulate; when uncertain, they are more likely to say "I don't know"; and their memory difficulties are more limited to free recall than to recognition on cued recall tests. Pseudodementia occurs in about 15 percent of depressed older patients, and 25 to 50 percent of patients with dementia are depressed.

Schizophrenia

Schizophrenia usually begins in late adolescence or young adulthood and persists throughout life. Although first episodes diagnosed after age 65 are rare, a late-onset type beginning after age 45 has been described. Women are more likely to have a late onset of schizophrenia than men. Another difference between early-onset and late-onset schizophrenia is the greater prevalence of paranoid schizophrenia in the late-onset type. About 20 percent of persons with schizophrenia show no active symptoms by age 65; 80 percent show varying degrees of impairment. Psychopathology becomes less marked as patient's age.

The residual type of schizophrenia occurs in about 30 percent of persons with schizophrenia. Its signs and symptoms include emotional blunting, social withdrawal, eccentric behavior, and illogical thinking. Delusions and hallucinations are uncommon. Because most persons with residual schizophrenia cannot care for themselves, long-term hospitalization is required.

Older persons with schizophrenic symptoms respond well to antipsychotic drugs. Medication must be administered judiciously, and lower-than-usual dosages often are effective for older adults.

Delusional Disorder

The age of onset of delusional disorder usually is between ages 40 and 55, but it can occur at any time during the geriatric

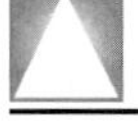

Table 29–11
Geriatric Depression Scale (Short Version)

Answers indicating depression are boldfaced. Each answer counts one point; scores greater than 5 indicate probable depression.

1. Are you basically satisfied with your life?	Yes/No
2. Have you dropped many of your activities and interests?	Yes/No
3. Do you feel that your life is empty?	Yes/No
4. Do you often get bored?	Yes/No
5. Are you in good spirits most of the time?	Yes/No
6. Are you afraid that something bad is going to happen to you?	Yes/No
7. Do you feel happy most of the time?	Yes/No
8. Do you often feel helpless?	Yes/No
9. Do you prefer to stay at home, rather than going out and doing new things?	Yes/No
10. Do you feel you have more problems with memory than most?	Yes/No
11. Do you think it is wonderful to be alive now?	Yes/No
12. Do you feel pretty worthless the way you are now?	Yes/No
13. Do you feel full of energy?	Yes/No
14. Do you feel that your situation is hopeless?	Yes/No
15. Do you think that most people are better off than you are?	Yes/No

Special Instructions. The scale can be used as a self-rating or observer-rated metric. It has also been used as an observer-rated scale in mildly demented subjects.

From Yesavage JA. Geriatric depression scale. *Psychopharmacol Bull.* 1988;24:709, with permission.

period. Delusions can take many forms; the most common are persecutory—patients believe that they are being spied on, followed, poisoned, or harassed in some way. Persons with delusional disorder may become violent toward their supposed persecutors. Some persons lock themselves in their rooms and live reclusive lives. Somatic delusions, in which persons believe they have a fatal illness, also can occur in older persons. In one study of persons older than 65 years of age, pervasive persecutory ideation was present in 4 percent of persons sampled.

Among those who are vulnerable, delusional disorder can occur under physical or psychological stress and can be precipitated by the death of a spouse, loss of a job, retirement, social isolation, adverse financial circumstances, debilitating medical illness or surgery, visual impairment, and deafness. Delusions also can accompany other disorders—such as dementia of the Alzheimer's type, alcohol use disorders, schizophrenia, depressive disorders, and bipolar I disorder—which need to be ruled out. Delusional syndromes also can result from prescribed medications or be early signs of a brain tumor. The prognosis is fair to good in most cases; best results are achieved through a combination of psychotherapy and pharmacotherapy.

A late-onset delusional disorder called *paraphrenia* is characterized by persecutory delusions. It develops over several years and is not associated with dementia. Some workers believe that the disorder is a variant of schizophrenia that first becomes manifest after age 60. Patients with a family history of schizophrenia show an increased rate of paraphrenia.

Anxiety Disorders

Anxiety disorders usually begin in early or middle adulthood, but some appear for the first time after age 60. An initial onset of panic disorder in older persons is rare but can occur. The ECA study determined that the 1-month prevalence of anxiety disorders in persons age 65 and older is 5.5 percent. By far the most common disorders are phobias (4 to 8 percent). The rate for panic disorder is 1 percent.

The signs and symptoms of phobia in older adults are less severe than those that occur in younger persons, but the effects are equally, if not more, debilitating for older patients. Existential theories help explain anxiety when no specifically identifiable stimulus exists for a chronically anxious feeling. Older persons must come to grips with death. The person may deal with the thought of death with a sense of despair and anxiety, rather than with equanimity and Erikson's "sense of integrity." The fragility of the autonomic nervous system in older persons may account for the development of anxiety after a major stressor. Because of concurrent physical disability, older persons react more severely to PTSD than younger persons.

Obsessive-Compulsive Disorders

Obsessions and compulsions may appear for the first time in older adults, although older adults with obsessive-compulsive disorder (OCD) usually had demonstrated evidence of the disorder (e.g., being orderly, perfectionistic, punctual, and parsimonious) when they were younger. When symptomatic, patients become excessive in their desire for orderliness, rituals, and sameness. They may become generally inflexible and rigid and have compulsions to check things again and again. OCD (in contrast to obsessive-compulsive personality disorder) is characterized by ego-dystonic rituals and obsessions and may begin late in life.

Somatic Symptom Disorders

Disorders characterized by physical symptoms resembling medical diseases are relevant to geriatric psychiatry because somatic complaints are common among older adults. More than 80 percent of persons over 65 years of age have at least one chronic disease—usually arthritis or cardiovascular problems. After age 75, 20 percent have diabetes and an average of four diagnosable chronic illnesses that require medical attention.

Hypochondriasis is common in persons over 60 years of age, although the peak incidence is in those 40 to 50 years of age. The disorder usually is chronic, and the prognosis guarded. Repeated physical examinations help reassure patients that they do not have a fatal illness, but invasive and high-risk diagnostic procedures should be avoided unless medically indicated.

Telling patients that their symptoms are imaginary is counterproductive and usually engenders resentment. Clinicians should acknowledge that the complaint is real, that the pain is really there and perceived as such by the patient, and that a psychological or pharmacological approach to the problem is indicated.

Alcohol and Other Substance Use Disorder

Older adults with alcohol dependence usually give a history of excessive drinking that began in young or middle adulthood. They usually are medically ill, primarily with liver disease, and are either divorced, widowed, or are men who never married. Many have arrest records and are numbered among the homeless persons. A large number have chronic dementing illness, such as Wernicke's encephalopathy or Korsakoff's syndrome. Of nursing home patients, 20 percent have alcohol dependence.

Over all, alcohol and other substance use disorders account for 10 percent of all emotional problems in older persons, and dependence on such substances as hypnotics, anxiolytics, and narcotics is more common in old age than is generally recognized. Substance-seeking behavior characterized by crime, manipulativeness, and antisocial behavior is rarer in older than in younger adults. Older patients may abuse anxiolytics to allay chronic anxiety or to ensure sleep. The maintenance of chronically ill cancer patients with narcotics prescribed by a physician produces dependence, but the need to provide pain relief takes precedence over the possibility of narcotic dependence and is entirely justified.

The clinical presentation of older patients with alcohol and other substance use disorders varies and includes confusion, poor personal hygiene, depression, malnutrition, and the effects of exposure and falls. The sudden onset of delirium in older persons hospitalized for medical illness is most often caused by alcohol withdrawal. Alcohol abuse also should be considered in older adults with chronic gastrointestinal problems.

Older persons may misuse over-the-counter substances, including nicotine and caffeine. Over-the-counter analgesics are used by 35 percent of older persons, and 30 percent use laxatives. Unexplained gastrointestinal, psychological, and metabolic problems should alert clinicians to over-the-counter substance abuse.

Sleep Disorders

Advanced age is the single most important factor associated with the increased prevalence of sleep disorders. Sleep-related phenomena reported more frequently by older than by younger adults are sleeping problems, daytime sleepiness, daytime napping, and the use of hypnotic drugs. Clinically, older persons experience higher rates of breathing-related sleep disorder and medication-induced movement disorders than younger adults.

In addition to altered regulatory and physiological systems, the causes of sleep disturbances in older persons include primary sleep disorders, other mental disorders, general medical disorders, and social and environmental factors. Among the primary sleep disorders, dyssomnias are the most frequent, especially primary insomnia, nocturnal myoclonus, restless legs syndrome, and sleep apnea. Of the parasomnias, rapid eye movement (REM) sleep behavior disorder occurs almost exclusively among elderly men. The conditions that commonly interfere with sleep in older adults also include pain, nocturia, dyspnea, and heartburn. The lack of a daily structure and of social or vocational responsibilities contributes to poor sleep.

As a result of the decreased length of their daily sleep–wake cycle, older persons without daily routines, especially patients in nursing homes, may experience an advanced sleep phase, in which they go to sleep early and awaken during the night.

Even modest amounts of alcohol can interfere with the quality of sleep and can cause sleep fragmentation and early morning awakening. Alcohol can also precipitate or aggravate obstructive sleep apnea. Many older persons use alcohol, hypnotics, and other CNS depressants to help them fall asleep, but data show that these persons experience more early morning awakening than trouble falling asleep. When prescribing sedative-hypnotic drugs for older persons, clinicians must monitor the patients for unwanted cognitive, behavioral, and psychomotor effects, including memory impairment (anterograde amnesia), residual sedation, rebound insomnia, daytime withdrawal, and unsteady gait.

Changes in sleep structure among persons over 65 years of age involve both REM sleep and nonrapid eye movement (NREM) sleep. The REM changes include the redistribution of REM sleep throughout the night, more REM episodes, shorter REM episodes, and less total REM sleep. The NREM changes include the decreased amplitude of delta waves, a lower percentage of stages 3 and 4 sleep, and a higher percentage of stages 1 and 2 sleep. In addition, older persons experience increased awakening after sleep onset.

Much of the observed deterioration in the quality of sleep in older persons is caused by the altered timing and consolidation of sleep. For example, with advanced age, persons have a lower amplitude of circadian rhythms, a 12-hour sleep-propensity rhythm, and shorter circadian cycles.

SUICIDE RISK

Elderly persons have a higher risk for suicide than any other population. The suicide rate for white men over the age of 65 is five times higher than that of the general population. One-third of elderly persons reports loneliness as the principal reason for considering suicide. Approximately 10 percent of elderly individuals with suicidal ideation report financial problems, poor medical health, or depression as reasons for suicidal thoughts. Suicide victims differ demographically from individuals who attempt suicide. About 60 percent of those who commit suicide are men; 75 percent of those who attempt suicide are women. Suicide victims, as a rule, use guns or hang themselves, whereas 70 percent of suicide attempters take a drug overdose, and 20 percent cut or slash themselves. Psychological autopsy studies suggest that most elderly persons who commit suicide have had a psychiatric disorder, most commonly depression. Psychiatric disorders of suicide victims, however, often do not receive medical or psychiatric attention. More elderly suicide victims are widowed and fewer are single, separated, or divorced than is true of younger adults. Violent methods of suicide are more common in the elderly, and alcohol use and psychiatric histories appear to be less frequent. The most common precipitants of suicide in older individuals are physical illness and loss, whereas problems with employment, finances, and family relationships are more frequent precipitants in younger adults. Most elderly persons who commit suicide communicate their suicidal thoughts to family or friends before the act of suicide.

Older patients with major medical illnesses or a recent loss should be evaluated for depressive symptomatology and suicidal ideation or plans. Thoughts and fantasies about the meaning of suicide and life after death may reveal information that the patient cannot share directly. There should be no reluctance to question patients about suicide, because no evidence indicates that such questions increase the likelihood of suicidal behavior.

OTHER CONDITIONS OF OLD AGE

Vertigo

Feelings of vertigo or dizziness, a common complaint of older adults, cause many older adults to become inactive because they fear falling. The causes of vertigo vary and include anemia, hypotension, cardiac arrhythmia, cerebrovascular disease, basilar artery insufficiency, middle ear disease, acoustic neuroma, benign postural vertigo, and Ménière's disease. Most cases of vertigo have a strong psychological component, and clinicians should ascertain any secondary gain from the symptom. The overuse of anxiolytics can cause dizziness and daytime somnolence. Treatment with meclizine (Antivert), 25 to 100 mg daily, has been successful in many patients with vertigo.

Syncope

The sudden loss of consciousness associated with syncope results from a reduction of cerebral blood flow and brain hypoxia. A thorough medical workup is required to rule out the potential causes. Causes of syncope are listed in Table 29–12.

Hearing Loss

About 30 percent of persons over age 65 have significant hearing loss (presbycusis). After age 75, that figure rises to 50 percent. The causes vary. Clinicians should be sensitive to hearing loss in patients who complain they can hear but cannot understand what

Table 29–12
Causes of Syncope

Cardiac Disorders
Anatomical/valvular
Aortic stenosis
Mitral prolapse and regurgitation
Hypertrophic cardiomyopathy
Myxoma
Electrical
Tachyarrhythmia
Bradyarrhythmia
Heart block
Sick sinus syndrome
Functional
Ischemia and infarct
Situational Hypotension
Dehydration (diarrhea, fasting)
Orthostatic hypotension
Postprandial hypotension
Micturition, defecation, coughing, swallowing
Abnormal Cardiovascular Reflexes
Carotid sinus syndrome
Vasovagal syncope
Drugs
Vasodilators
Calcium channel blockers
Diuretics
β-blockers
Central Nervous System Abnormalities
Cerebrovascular insufficiency
Seizures
Metabolic Abnormalities
Hypoxemia
Hypoglycemia or hyperglycemia
Anemia
Pulmonary Disorders
Chronic obstructive pulmonary disease
Pneumonia
Pulmonary embolus

is being said or who ask that questions be repeated. Most elderly persons with hearing loss can be treated with hearing aids.

Elder Abuse

An estimated 10 percent of persons above 65 years of age are abused. Elder abuse is defined by the American Medical Association as "an act or omission which results in harm or threatened harm to the health or welfare of an elderly person." Mistreatment includes abuse and neglect—physically, psychologically, financially, and materially. Sexual abuse does occur. Acts of omission include withholding food, medicine, clothing, and other necessities.

Family conflicts and other problems often underlie elder abuse. The victims tend to be very old and frail. They often live with their assailants, who may be financially dependent on the victims. Both the victim and the perpetrator tend to deny or minimize the presence of abuse. Interventions include providing legal services, housing, and medical, psychiatric, and social services.

SPOUSAL BEREAVEMENT

Demographic data suggest that 51 percent of women and 14 percent of men over the age of 65 will be widowed at least once. Spousal loss is among the most stressful of all life experiences. As a group, older adults appear to have a more favorable outcome than expected following the death of a spouse. Depressive symptoms peak within the first few months after a death, but decline significantly within a year. A relationship exists between spousal loss and subsequent mortality. Elderly survivors of spouses who committed suicide are especially vulnerable, as are those with psychiatric illness.

PSYCHOPHARMACOLOGICAL TREATMENT OF GERIATRIC DISORDERS

Certain guidelines should be followed regarding the use of all drugs in older adults. A pretreatment medical evaluation is essential, including an electrocardiogram (ECG). It is especially useful to have the patient or a family member bring in all currently used medications, because multiple drug use could be contributing to the symptoms.

Most psychotropic drugs should be given in equally divided doses three or four times over a 24-hour period. Older patients may not be able to tolerate a sudden rise in drug blood level resulting from one large daily dose. Any changes in blood pressure and pulse rate and other side effects should be watched. For patients with insomnia, however, giving the major portion of an antipsychotic or antidepressant at bedtime takes advantage of its sedating and soporific effects. Liquid preparations are useful for older patients who cannot, or will not, swallow tablets. Clinicians should frequently reassess all patients to determine the need for maintenance medication, changes in dosage, and development of adverse effects. If a patient is taking psychotropic drugs at the time of the evaluation, the clinician should discontinue these medications, if possible, and, after a washout period, reevaluate the patient during a drug-free baseline state.

Adults over 65 years of age use the greatest number of medications of any age group; 25 percent of all prescriptions are written for them. Adverse drug reactions caused by medications result in the hospitalization of nearly 250,000 persons in the United States each year. Psychotropic drugs are among the most commonly prescribed, along with cardiovascular and diuretic medications; 40 percent of all hypnotics dispensed in the United States each year are to those older than 75 years of age, and 70 percent of older persons use over-the-counter medications, compared with only 10 percent of young adults.

Principles

The major goals of the pharmacological treatment of older persons are to improve the quality of life, maintain persons in the community, and delay or avoid their placement in nursing homes. Individualization of dosage is the basic tenet of geriatric psychopharmacology.

Alterations in drug dosages are required because of the physiological changes that occur as persons age. Renal disease is associated with decreased renal clearance of drugs; liver disease results in a decreased ability to metabolize drugs; cardiovascular disease and reduced cardiac output can affect both renal and hepatic drug clearance; and gastrointestinal disease and decreased gastric acid secretion influence drug absorption. As a person ages, the ratio of lean to fat body mass also changes. With normal aging, lean body mass decreases and body fat increases. Changes in the ratio of lean to fat body mass that accompany aging affect the distribution of drugs. Many lipid-soluble psychotropic drugs are distributed more widely in fat than in lean tissue, so a drug's action can be unexpectedly prolonged in older persons. Similarly, changes in end-organ or receptor-site sensitivity must be taken into account. In older persons, the increased risk of orthostatic hypotension from psychotropic drugs is related to reduced functioning of blood pressure–regulating mechanisms.

As a general rule, the lowest possible dose should be used to achieve the desired therapeutic response. Clinicians must know the pharmacodynamics, pharmacokinetics, and biotransformation of each drug prescribed and the effects of the interaction of the drug with other drugs that a patient is taking. An adage in geriatric medicine regarding the use of drugs is: Start low, go slow.

PSYCHOTHERAPY FOR GERIATRIC PATIENTS

The standard psychotherapeutic interventions—such as insight-oriented psychotherapy, supportive psychotherapy, cognitive therapy, group therapy, and family therapy—should be available to geriatric patients. According to Sigmund Freud, persons older than 50 years are not suited for psychoanalysis because their mental processes lack elasticity. In the view of many who followed Freud, however, psychoanalysis is possible after age 50. Advanced age certainly limits plasticity of the personality, but as Otto Fenichel stated, "It does so in varying degrees and at very different ages so that no general rule can be given." Insight-oriented psychotherapy may help remove a specific symptom, even in older persons. It is of most benefit when patients have possibilities for libidinal and narcissistic gratification, but it is contraindicated if it would bring only the insight that life has been a failure and that the patient has no opportunity to make up for it.

Common age-related issues in therapy involve the need to adapt to recurrent and diverse losses (e.g., the deaths of friends and loved ones), the need to assume new roles (e.g., the adjustment to retirement and the disengagement from previously defined roles), and the need to accept mortality. Psychotherapy helps older persons to deal with these issues and the emotional problems surrounding them and to understand their behavior and the effects of their behavior on others. In addition to improving interpersonal relationships, psychotherapy increases self-esteem and self-confidence, decreases feelings of helplessness and anger, and improves the quality of life.

Psychotherapy helps relieve tensions of biological and cultural origins and helps older persons work and play within the limits of their functional status and as determined by their past training, activities, and self-concept in society. In patients with impaired cognition, psychotherapy can produce remarkable gains in both physical and mental symptoms. In one study conducted in an old-age home, 43 percent of the patients receiving psychotherapy showed less urinary incontinence, improved gait, greater mental alertness, improved memory, and better hearing than before psychotherapy.

Therapists must be more active, supportive, and flexible in conducting therapy with older than with younger adults, and they must be prepared to act decisively at the first sign of an incapacity that requires the active involvement of another physician, such as an internist, or that requires consulting with, or enlisting the aid of, a family member.

Older persons usually seek therapy for a therapist's unqualified and unlimited support, reassurance, and approval. Patients often expect a therapist to be all powerful, all knowing, and able to effect a magical cure. Most patients eventually recognize that the therapist is human and that they are engaged in a collaborative effort. In some cases, however, the therapist may have to assume the idealized role, especially when the patient is unable or unwilling to test reality effectively. With the help of the therapist, the patient deals with problems that had been avoided previously. As the therapist offers direct encouragement, reassurance, and advice, the patient's self-confidence increases as conflicts are resolved.

30

End-of-Life Issues

30.1 Death, Dying, and Bereavement

DEATH AND DYING

Definitions

The terms *death* and *dying* require definition: Whereas *death* may be considered the absolute cessation of vital functions, *dying* is the process of losing these functions. Dying may also be seen as a developmental concomitant of living, a part of the birth-to-death continuum. Living may entail numerous mini-deaths—the end of growth and its potential, health-compromising illnesses, multiple losses, decreasing vitality and growing dependency with aging, and dying. Dying, and the individual's awareness of it, imbues humans with values, passions, wishes, and the impetus to make the most of time.

Two terms that have been used with increased frequency in recent years refer to the quality of living as death comes near. A *good death* is one that is free from avoidable distress and suffering for patients, families, and caregivers and is reasonably consistent with clinical, cultural, and ethical standards. A *bad death,* in contrast, is characterized by needless suffering, a dishonoring of the patient or family's wishes or values, and a sense among participants or observers that norms of decency have been offended.

Uniform Determination of Death Act

The President's Commission for the Study of Ethical Problems in Medicine and Biomedical and Behavioral Research published its definition of death in 1981. Working with the American Bar Association, the American Medical Association (AMA), and the National Conference of Commissioners on Uniform State Laws, the Commission established that one who has sustained either (1) irretrievable cessation of circulatory and respiratory functions or (2) irretrievable cessation of all functions of the entire brain, including the brainstem, is dead. Determination of death must be in accordance with accepted medical standards.

Generally accepted criteria for determining brain death require a series of neurological and other assessments. For children, special guidelines apply. They generally specify two assessments separated by an interval of at least 48 hours for those between the ages of 1 week and 2 months, 24 hours for those between the ages of 2 months and 1 year, and 12 hours for older children; additional confirmatory tests may also be advisable under some circumstances. Brain death criteria are normally not applied to infants younger than 7 days. Table 30.1–1 lists the clinical criteria for brain death in adults and children.

Legal Aspects of Death

According to law, physicians must sign the death certificate, which attests to the cause of death (e.g., congestive heart failure or pneumonia). They must also attribute the death to natural, accidental, suicidal, homicidal, or unknown causes. A medical examiner, coroner, or pathologist must examine anyone who dies unattended by a physician and perform an autopsy to determine the cause of death. In some cases, a psychological autopsy is performed: A person's sociocultural and psychological background is examined retrospectively by interviewing friends, relatives, and doctors to determine whether a mental illness, such as a depressive disorder, was present. For example, a determination can be made that a person died because he or she was pushed (murder) or because he or she jumped (suicide) from a high building. Each situation has clear medical and legal implications.

Table 30.1–1
Clinical Criteria for Brain Death in Adults and Children

Coma
Absence of motor responses
Absence of pupillary responses to light and pupils at midposition with respect to dilatation (4–6 mm)
Absence of corneal reflexes
Absence of caloric responses
Absence of gag reflex
Absence of coughing in response to tracheal suctioning
Absence of sucking and rooting reflexes
Absence of respiratory drive at a Pa_{CO_2} that is 60 or 20 mm Hg above normal baseline values
Interval between two evaluations, according to patient's age
Term to 2 months old, 48 hours
>2 months to 1 year old, 24 hours
>1 year to <18 years old, 12 hours
≥18 years old, interval optional
Confirmatory tests
Term to 2 months old, two confirmatory tests
>2 months to 1 year old, one confirmatory test
>1 year to <18 years old, optional
≥18 years old, optional

Pa_{CO_2}, partial pressure of arterial carbon dioxide.
Reprinted from Wijdicks EFM. The diagnosis of brain death. *N Engl J Med.* 2001;344:1216.

Stages of Death and Dying

Elisabeth Kübler-Ross, a psychiatrist and thanatologist, made a comprehensive and useful organization of reactions to impending death. A dying patient seldom follows a regular series of responses that can be clearly identified; no established sequence is applicable to all patients. Nevertheless, the following five stages proposed by Kübler-Ross are widely encountered.

Stage 1: Shock and Denial. On being told that they are dying, persons initially react with shock. They may appear dazed at first and then may refuse to believe the diagnosis; they may deny that anything is wrong. Some persons never pass beyond this stage and may go from doctor to doctor until they find one who supports their position. The degree to which denial is adaptive or maladaptive appears to depend on whether a patient continues to obtain treatment even while denying the prognosis. In such cases, physicians must communicate to patients and their families, respectfully and directly, basic information about the illness, its prognosis, and the options for treatment. For effective communication, physicians must allow for patients' emotional responses and reassure them that they will not be abandoned.

Stage 2: Anger. Persons become frustrated, irritable, and angry at being ill. They commonly ask, "Why me?" They may become angry at God, their fate, a friend, or a family member; they may even blame themselves. They may displace their anger onto the hospital staff members and the doctor, whom they blame for the illness. Patients in the stage of anger are difficult to treat. Doctors who have difficulty understanding that anger is a predictable reaction and is really a displacement may withdraw from patients or transfer them to other doctors' care.

Physicians treating angry patients must realize that the anger being expressed cannot be taken personally. An empathic, nondefensive response can help defuse patients' anger and can help them refocus on their own deep feelings (e.g., grief, fear, loneliness) that underlie the anger. Physicians should also recognize that anger may represent patients' desire for control in a situation in which they feel completely out of control.

Stage 3: Bargaining. Patients may attempt to negotiate with physicians, friends, or even God; in return for a cure, they promise to fulfill one or many pledges, such as giving to charity and attending church regularly. Some patients believe that if they are good (compliant, nonquestioning, cheerful), the doctor will make them better. The treatment of such patients involves making it clear that they will be taken care of to the best of the doctor's abilities and that everything that can be done will be done, regardless of any action or behavior on the patients' part. Patients must also be encouraged to participate as partners in their treatment and to understand that being a good patient means being as honest and straightforward as possible.

Stage 4: Depression. In the fourth stage, patients show clinical signs of depression—withdrawal, psychomotor retardation, sleep disturbances, hopelessness, and, possibly, suicidal ideation. The depression may be a reaction to the effects of the illness on their lives (e.g., loss of a job, economic hardship, helplessness, hopelessness, and isolation from friends and family), or it may be in anticipation of the loss of life that will eventually occur. A major depressive disorder with vegetative signs and suicidal ideation may require treatment with antidepressant medication or electroconvulsive therapy (ECT). All persons feel some sadness at the prospect of their own death, and normal sadness does not require biological intervention. But major depressive disorder and active suicidal ideation can be alleviated and should not be accepted as normal reactions to impending death. A person who suffers from major depressive disorder may be unable to sustain hope, which can enhance the dignity and quality of life and even prolong longevity. Studies have shown that some terminally ill patients can delay their death until after a loved one's significant event, such as graduation of a grandson from college.

Stage 5: Acceptance. In the stage of acceptance, patients realize that death is inevitable, and they accept the universality of the experience. Their feelings can range from a neutral to a euphoric mood. Under ideal circumstances, patients resolve their feelings about the inevitability of death and can talk about facing the unknown. Those with strong religious beliefs and a conviction of life after death sometimes find comfort in the ecclesiastical maxim, "Fear not death; remember those who have gone before you and those who will come after."

Near-Death Experiences

Near-death descriptions are often strikingly similar, involving an out-of-body experience of viewing one's body and overhearing conversations, feelings of peace and quiet, hearing a distant noise, entering a dark tunnel, leaving the body behind, meeting dead loved ones, witnessing beings of light, returning to life to complete unfinished business, and a deep sadness on leaving this new dimension. This pattern of sensations and perceptions is usually described as peaceful and loving; it feels real to participants, who distinguish it from dreams or hallucinations. These experiences provoke sweeping lifestyle changes, such as fewer material concerns, a heightened sense of purpose, a belief in God, joy of life, compassion, less fear of death, an enhanced approach to life, and intense feelings of love. In a similar vein, hospice nurses have described experiences among terminally ill patients of visions that may include a sense of presence of departed loved ones, of spiritual beings, of a bright light, or of being in a particular place, often described with a sense of warmth and love. Although such "visions" do not readily lend themselves to scientific investigation and thus are not legitimized, patients may benefit from discussing them with clinicians. A term to describe this experience is *unio mystica,* which refers to an oceanic feeling of mystic unity with an infinite power.

Life Cycle Considerations about Death and Dying

The clinical diversity of death-related attitudes and behaviors between children and adults has its roots in developmental factors and age-dependent differences in causes of death. As opposed to adults, who usually die from chronic illness, children are apt to die from sudden, unexpected causes. Almost half of the children who die between the ages of 1 and 14 years and nearly 75 percent of those who die in late adolescence and early adulthood die from accidents, homicides, and suicides. With their characteristics of violence, suddenness, and mutilation, such unnatural causes of death are special stressors for grieving survivors. Bereaved parents and siblings of dead young children and teenagers often feel victimized and traumatized by their losses; their grief reactions resemble posttraumatic stress disorder (PTSD). Devastating family disruptions can occur, and surviving siblings risk having their emotional needs put on the back burner, ignored, or completely unnoticed.

Children. Children's attitudes toward death mirror their attitudes toward life. Although they share with adolescents, adults, and elderly adults similar fears, anxieties, beliefs, and attitudes about dying, some of their interpretations and reactions are age specific. None welcome it without ambivalence, and all temper their acceptance with healthy doses of denial and avoidance. Dying children are often aware of their condition and want to discuss it. They often have more sophisticated views about dying than their medically well counterparts, engendered by their own failing health, separations from parents, subjection to painful procedures, and the deaths of hospital chums.

At the preschool, preoperational stage of cognitive development, death is seen as a temporary absence, incomplete and reversible, like departure or sleep. Separation from the primary caretaker(s) is the main fear of preschool-age children. This fear surfaces as an increase in nightmares, more aggressive play, or concern about the deaths of others rather than in direct discourse. Terminally ill children may assume responsibility for their death, feeling guilty for dying. Preschool children may be unable to relate the treatment to the illness, instead viewing treatment as punishment and family separation as rejection. They need reassurance that they are loved, have done nothing wrong, are not responsible for their illness, and will not be abandoned.

School-age children manifest concrete-operational thinking and recognize death as a final reality. They, however, view death as something that happens to old people, not to them. Between the ages of 6 and 12 years, children have active fantasies of violence and aggression, often dominated by themes of death and killing. School-age children ask questions about serious illness and death if encouraged to do so; however, if they receive cues that the subject is taboo, they may withdraw and participate less fully in their care. Facilitating open discussion and updating children with important information, including prognostic changes, can be very helpful. In addition, children may need help coping with peers and school demands. Teachers should be informed and updated. Classmates may need education and assistance to help them understand the situation and respond appropriately.

Adolescents. Capable of formal cognitive operations, adolescents understand that death is inevitable and final but may not accept that their own death is possible. The major fears of dying teenagers parallel those of all teenagers—losing control, being imperfect, and being different. Concerns about body image, hair loss, or loss of bodily control can generate great resistance to continuing treatment. Alternating emotions of despair, rage, grief, bitterness, numbness, terror, and joy are common. The potential for withdrawal and isolation is great because teenagers may equate parental support with loss of independence or may deny their fears of abandonment by actually repulsing friendly gestures. Teenagers must be included in all decision-making processes surrounding their deaths. Many are capable of great courage, grace, and dignity in facing death.

Adults. Some of the most often expressed fears of adult patients entering hospice care, listed in the approximate order of frequency, include fears of (1) separation from loved ones, homes, and jobs; (2) becoming a burden to others; (3) losing control; (4) what will happen to dependents; (5) pain or other worsening symptoms; (6) being unable to complete life tasks or responsibilities; (7) dying; (8) being dead; (9) the fears of others (reflected fears); (10) the fate of the body; and (11) the afterlife. Problems in communication arise out of trepidation, making it important for those involved in health care to provide environments of trust and safety in which people can begin to talk about uncertainties, anxieties, and concerns.

Late-age adults often accept that their time has come. Their main fears include long, painful, and disfiguring deaths; prolonged vegetative states; isolation; and loss of control or dignity. Elderly patients may talk or joke openly about dying and sometimes welcome it. In their 70s and beyond, they rarely harbor illusions of indestructibility—most have already had several close calls: Their parents have died, and they have gone to funerals for friends and relatives. Although they may not be happy to die, they can be reconciled to it.

According to Erik Erikson, the eighth and final stage in the life cycle brings a sense of either integrity or despair. As elderly adults enter the last phase of their lives, they reflect on their pasts. When they have taken care of their affairs, have been relatively successful, and have adapted to the triumphs and disappointments of life, they can look back with satisfaction and only a few regrets. Integrity of the self allows people to accept inevitable disease and death without fear of succumbing helplessly. If elderly individuals look back on life as a series of missed opportunities or personal misfortunes, however, they feel a sense of bitter despair, a preoccupation with what might have been if only this or that had happened. Then death is fearsome because it symbolizes emptiness and failure.

Management

Caring for a dying patient is highly individual. Caretakers need to deal with death honestly, tolerate wide ranges of affects, connect with suffering patients and bereaved loved ones, and resolve routine issues as they arise. Although each therapeutic relationship between a patient and health provider has a uniqueness derived from the patient's and health provider's gender, constitution, life experience, age, stage of life, resources, faith, culture, and other considerations, major themes confront all health providers caring for dying patients.

BEREAVEMENT, GRIEF, AND MOURNING

Bereavement, grief, and *mourning* are terms that apply to the psychological reactions of those who survive a significant loss. Grief is the subjective feeling precipitated by the death of a loved one. The term is used synonymously with mourning, although, in the strictest sense, mourning is the process by which grief is resolved; it is the societal expression of postbereavement behavior and practices. Bereavement literally means the state of being deprived of someone by death and refers to being in the state of mourning. Regardless of the fine points that differentiate these terms, the experiences of grief and bereavement have sufficient similarities to warrant a syndrome that has signs, symptoms, a demonstrable course, and an expected resolution.

Normal Bereavement Reactions

The first response to loss, *protest,* is followed by a longer period of *searching* behavior. As hope to reestablish the attachment bond diminishes, searching behaviors give way to *despair* and *detachment* before bereaved individuals eventually *reorganize* themselves around the recognition that the lost person will not return. Although the bereaved ultimately learn to accept the reality of the death, they also find psychological and symbolic ways of keeping the memory of the deceased person very much alive. Grief work allows the survivor to redefine his or her relationship to the deceased person and to form new but enduring ties.

Duration of Grief

Most societies mandate modes of bereavement and time for grieving. In contemporary America, bereaved individuals are expected to return to work or school in a few weeks, to establish equilibrium within a few months, and to be capable of pursuing new relationships within 6 months to 1 year. Ample evidence suggests that the bereavement process does not end within a prescribed interval; certain aspects persist indefinitely for many otherwise high-functioning, normal individuals.

The most lasting manifestation of grief, especially after spousal bereavement, is loneliness. Often present for years after the death of a spouse, loneliness may, for some, be a daily reminder of the loss. Other common manifestations of protracted grief occur intermittently. For example, a man who has lost his wife may experience elements of acute grief every time he hears her name or sees her picture on the nightstand. Usually, these reactions become increasingly short lived over time, dissipating within minutes, and become tinged with positive and pleasant affects. Such bittersweet memories may last a lifetime. Thus, most grief does not fully resolve or permanently disappear; rather, grief becomes circumscribed and submerged only to reemerge in response to certain triggers.

Anticipatory Grief

In *anticipatory grief,* grief reactions are brought on by the slow dying process of a loved one through injury, illness, or high-risk activity. Although anticipatory grief may soften the blow of the eventual death, it can also lead to premature separation and withdrawal while not necessarily mitigating later bereavement. At times, the intensification of intimacy during this period may heighten the actual sense of loss even though it prepares the survivor in other ways.

Anniversary Reactions

When the trigger for an acute grief reaction is a special occasion, such as a holiday or birthday, the rekindled grief is called an *anniversary reaction.* It is not unusual for anniversary reactions to occur each year on the same day the person died or, in some cases, when the bereaved individual becomes the same age the deceased person was at the time of death. Although these anniversary reactions tend to become relatively mild and brief over time, they can be experienced as the reliving of one's original grief and prevail for hours or days.

Mourning

From earliest history, every culture records its own beliefs, customs, and behaviors related to bereavement. Specific patterns include rituals for mourning (e.g., wakes or Shiva), for disposing of the body, for invocation of religious ceremonies, and for periodic official remembrances. The funeral is the prevailing public display of bereavement in contemporary North America. The funeral and burial service acknowledge the real and final nature of the death, countering denial; they also garner support for the bereaved, encouraging tribute to the dead, uniting families, and facilitating community expressions of sorrow. If cremation replaces burial, ceremonies associated with dissemination of the ashes perform similar functions. Visits, prayers, and other ceremonies allow for continuing support, coming to terms with reality, remembering, emotional expression, and concluding unfinished business with the deceased. Several cultural and religious rituals provide purpose and meaning, protect the survivors from isolation and vulnerability, and set limits on grieving. Subsequent holidays, birthdays, and anniversaries serve to remind the living of the dead and may elicit grief as real and fresh as the original experience; over time, these anniversary grieving's become attenuated but often remain in some form.

Bereavement

Because bereavement often evokes depressive symptoms, it may be necessary to demarcate normal grief reactions from major depressive disorder (Table 30.1–2). In the fifth edition of the *Diagnostic and Statistical Manual of Mental Disorders* (DSM-5), a new condition has been proposed for further study called persistent complex bereavement disorder to account for bereavement that lasts for more than 1 year. This disorder may resemble symptoms of a major depressive episode, which is characterized by severe functional impairment and includes morbid preoccupation with worthlessness, suicidal ideation, psychotic symptoms, or psychomotor retardation. This is discussed further below.

Complicated Bereavement

Complicated bereavement has a confusing array of terms to describe it—*abnormal, atypical, distorted, morbid, traumatic,* and *unresolved,* to name a few types. Three patterns of complicated, dysfunctional grief syndromes have been identified—chronic, hypertrophic, and delayed grief. These are not diagnostic categories within DSM-5 but are descriptive syndromes that, if present, may be prodromata of a major depressive disorder.

Chronic Grief. The most common type of complicated grief is chronic grief, often highlighted by bitterness and idealization of the dead person. Chronic grief is most likely to occur when the relationship between the bereaved and the deceased had been extremely close, ambivalent, or dependent or when

Table 30.1–2
Differentiating the Depressive Symptoms Associated with Bereavement from Major Depression

Bereavement	Major Depressive Disorder
Symptoms may meet syndromal criteria for major depressive episode, but the survivor rarely has morbid feelings of guilt and worthlessness, suicidal ideation, or psychomotor retardation	Any symptoms as defined by DSM-5
Considers self bereaved	May consider self weak, defective, or bad
Dysphoria often triggered by thoughts or reminders of the deceased	Dysphoria is often autonomous and independent of thoughts or reminders of the deceased
Onset is within the first 2 months of bereavement	Onset at any time
Duration of depressive symptoms is less than 2 months	Depression often becomes chronic, intermittent, or episodic
Functional impairment is transient and mild	Clinically significant distress or impairment
No family or personal history of major depression	Family or personal history of major depression

social supports are lacking and friends and relatives are not available to share the sorrow over the extended period of time needed for most mourners.

Hypertrophic Grief. Most often seen after a sudden and unexpected death, bereavement reactions are extraordinarily intense in hypertrophic grief. Customary coping strategies are ineffectual to mitigate anxiety, and withdrawal is frequent. When one family member is experiencing a hypertrophic grief reaction, disruption of family stability can occur. Hypertrophic grief frequently takes on a long-term course, albeit one attenuated over time.

Delayed Grief. Absent or inhibited grief when one normally expects to find overt signs and symptoms of acute mourning is referred to as delayed grief. This pattern is marked by prolonged denial; anger and guilt may complicate its course.

Traumatic Bereavement. Traumatic bereavement refers to grief that is both chronic and hypertrophic. This syndrome is characterized by recurrent, intense pangs of grief with persistent yearning, pining, and longing for the deceased; recurrent intrusive images of the death; and a distressing admixture of avoidance and preoccupation with reminders of the loss. Positive memories are often blocked or excessively sad, or they are experienced in prolonged states of reverie that interfere with daily activities. A history of psychiatric illness appears to be common in this condition, as is a very close, identity-defining relationship with the deceased person.

Medical or Psychiatric Illnesses Associated with Bereavement. Medical complications include exacerbations of existing diseases and vulnerability to new ones; fear for one's health and more trips to the doctor; and an increased mortality rate, especially in men. The highest relative mortality risk is found immediately after bereavement, particularly from ischemic heart disease. The greatest effect of bereavement on mortality is for men younger than 65 years. Higher mortality rates in bereaved men than in bereaved women are due to increases in the relative risk of death by suicide, accident, cardiovascular disease, and some infectious diseases. In widows, the relative risk of death from cirrhosis and suicide may increase. In both sexes, bereavement appears to exacerbate health-compromising behaviors, such as increased alcohol consumption, smoking, and the use of over-the-counter medications.

Psychiatric complications of bereavement include an increased risk for major depressive disorder, prolonged anxiety, panic, and a posttraumatic stress–like syndrome; increased alcohol, drug, and cigarette consumption; and an increased risk of suicide. Because of their psychosocial, emotional, and cognitive immaturity, bereaved children may be especially vulnerable to psychopathology.

Bereavement and Depression. Although symptoms overlap, grief can be distinguished from a full depressive episode. Most bereaved individuals experience intense sadness, but only a few meet DSM-5 criteria for major depressive episode. Grief is a complex experience in which positive emotions take their place beside the negative ones. Grief is fluid and changing, an evolving state in which emotional intensity gradually lessens and positive, comforting aspects of the lost relationship come to the fore. Pangs of grief are stimulus bound, related to internal and external reminders of the deceased person. This differs from depression, which is more pervasive and characterized by much difficulty experiencing self-validating, positive feelings. Grief is a fluctuating state with individual variability, in which cognitive and behavioral adjustments are progressively made until the bereaved individual can hold the deceased person in a comfortable place in memory and a satisfying life can be resumed. By contrast, major depressive episode consists of a recognizable and stable cluster of debilitating symptoms accompanied by a protracted, enduring low mood. Major depressive episode tends to be persistent and associated with poor work and social functioning, pathological psychoneuroimmunological function, and other neurobiological changes, unless treated.

Bereavement and Posttraumatic Stress Disorder. Unnatural and violent deaths, such as homicide, suicide, or death in the context of terrorism, are much more likely to precipitate PTSD in surviving loved ones than are natural deaths. In such circumstances, themes of violence, victimization, and volition (i.e., the choice of death over life, as in the case of suicide) are intermixed with other aspects of grief, and traumatic distress marked by fear, horror, vulnerability, and disintegration of cognitive assumptions ensues. Disbelief, despair, anxiety symptoms, preoccupation with the deceased person and the circumstances of the death, withdrawal, hyperarousal, and dysphoria are more intense and more prolonged than they are under nontraumatic circumstances, and an increased risk may exist for other complications. Although treatment studies in survivors of sudden death are few and far between, most experts agree that initial attention should be focused on traumatic distress, that a role is seen for both pharmacotherapy and psychotherapy, and that self-help support groups can be enormously beneficial.

Biological Perspectives

Grief is both a physiological and an emotional response. During acute grief (as with other stressful events), persons may experience disruption of biological rhythms. Grief is also accompanied by impaired immune functioning, including decreased lymphocyte proliferation and impaired functioning of natural killer cells. Whether the immune changes are clinically significant has not been established, but the mortality rate for widows and widowers following the death of a spouse is higher than that in the general population. Widowers appear to be at risk longer than widows.

Phenomenology of Grief. Bereavement reactions include intense feeling states; invoke a variety of coping strategies; and lead to alterations in interpersonal relationships, biopsychosocial functioning, self-esteem, and world view that can last indefinitely. Manifestations of grief reflect the individual's personality, previous life experiences, and past psychological history; the significance of the loss; the nature of the bereaved person's relationship with the deceased person; the existing social network; intercurrent life events; health; and other resources. Despite individual variations in the bereavement process, investigators have proposed grieving process models, which include at least three partially overlapping phases or states: (1) initial shock, disbelief, and denial; (2) an intermediate period of acute discomfort and social withdrawal; and (3) a culminating period of restitution and reorganization. As with Kübler-Ross' stages of dying, the grieving stages do not prescribe a correct course of grief; rather, they are general guidelines describing an overlapping and fluid process that varies with the survivors (Table 30.1–3).

Table 30.1–3
Phases of Grief

Shock and denial (minutes, days, weeks)
Disbelief and numbness
Searching behaviors: pining, yearning, and protest
Acute anguish (weeks, months)
Waves of somatic distress
Withdrawal
Preoccupation
Anger
Guilt
Lost patterns of conduct
Restless and agitated
Aimless and amotivational
Identification with the bereaved
Resolution (months, years)
Have grieved
Return to work
Resume old roles
Acquire new roles
Reexperience pleasure
Seek companionship and love of others

LIFE CYCLE PERSPECTIVES ABOUT BEREAVEMENT

Bereavement During Childhood and Adolescence

Approximately 4 percent of North American children lose one or both parents by the age of 15 years; sibling death is the second most commonly experienced bereavement. Grief reactions are colored by developmental levels and concepts of death and may not resemble adult reactions. Children may display minimal grief at time of death and experience the full effect of the loss later. Grieving children may not withdraw and dwell on the person who died, but instead, may throw themselves into activities. Indifference, anger, or misbehavior may be displayed rather than sadness; behaviors can be erratic and labile. Strong feelings of anger and fears of abandonment or death may show up in the behavior of grieving children. Children often play death games as a way of working out their feelings and anxieties. These games are familiar to the children and provide safe opportunities to express their feelings. Although they may seem to show grief only occasionally and briefly, in reality, a child's grief often lasts longer than that of an adult.

Mourning in children may need to be addressed again and again as the child gets older. Children will think about the loss repeatedly, especially during important times in their lives, such as going to camp, graduating from school, getting married, or giving birth to their own children. A child's grief can be influenced by his or her age, personality, developmental stage, earlier experiences with death, and relationship with the deceased person. The surroundings, cause of death, and family members' ability to communicate with one another and to continue as a family after the death can also affect grief. The child's ongoing need for care, his or her opportunity to share feelings and memories, the parent's ability to cope with stress, and the child's steady relationships with other adults are other factors that may influence grief. Even older children frequently feel abandoned or rejected when a parent dies and may show hostility toward the deceased or the surviving parent, now perceived as one who might also "abandon" them. They may feel responsible because of earlier misbehavior or because they said or wished that that person would die at some time.

Children younger than 2 years may show loss of speech or diffuse distress. Children younger than 5 years are apt to respond with eating, sleeping, and bowel and bladder dysfunctions. Strong feelings of sadness, fear, and anxiety can occur, but these feelings are not persistent and tend to alternate between longer lasting normal states. School-age children may become phobic or hypochondriacal, withdrawn, or pseudomature, and school performance and peer relations often suffer. Adolescents, as with adults, run the gamut in expressing bereavement, ranging from behavioral problems, somatic symptoms, and erratic moods to stoicism. Whereas adolescent boys losing a parent may become delinquent, girls may turn to a sexual pattern for comfort and reassurance. Behavioral disturbances and depression are common at all ages. Rates of depressive episodes in bereaved children and adolescents are as high as in bereaved adults.

Bereaved children must be treated with respect to their own levels of emotional and cognitive maturity. They need to be told that the death is real and irreversible and that they are blameless. Feelings and concerns should be expressed, and questions should be invited and answered with simplicity, candor, and clarity. Children, as with adults, need rituals to commemorate their loved ones; attendance at the funeral and participation in mourning may be beneficial first steps.

Bereavement During Adulthood

No consensus exists on which type of loss is associated with the most severe reactions. Although the death of a spouse is often ranked as the most stressful life event, some have argued that losing a child is even more profound. The death of a child is a special sorrow, a lifelong loss for surviving mothers, fathers, brothers, sisters, grandparents, and other family members. A child's death is a life-altering experience. The deaths of parents and siblings in adult life have not achieved much systematic study, but they are generally considered relatively mild compared with the loss of a spouse or child.

Grief appears most intense for the mother in late perinatal losses (stillbirths or neonatal deaths rather than miscarriages) and often is reexperienced during subsequent pregnancies. Sudden infant death syndrome is particularly problematic in that the death is sudden and unexpected. Parents may experience extra guilt or blame each other, often resulting in subsequent marital difficulties.

The surviving family members, friends, or lovers of individuals who have died from acquired immunodeficiency syndrome (AIDS) are uniquely challenged. The illness carries with it the stigmata of the illness itself and of the gay community in general; it carries with it caretakers' fears of contracting the illness; and it is most prevalent in people who are in the prime of life. Asymptomatic infection may permit the infected person and those close to him or her time to adapt to the diagnosis. When a person who is human immunodeficiency virus (HIV) positive begins to manifest symptoms of opportunistic infection or associated cancer, however, the illness again becomes a threat. Coping with the emotional reality is arduous and complex. Often caretakers, as well as HIV-positive patients, wish for death, which can evoke feelings of guilt. For bereaved lovers, their own HIV status, multiple losses, and other concurrent stressors can complicate recovery. Gay men who have lost lovers to AIDS may be more depressed, consider suicide more often, and be more vulnerable to illicit drug use than are other bereaved individuals.

Elderly adults face more losses than individuals at other phases of the life cycle, and intense loneliness may be a lasting memorial to those who have died. For highly impaired elders who lose a spouse they depended on for daily functions or who was their sole source of companionship, bereavement reactions are profound.

Grief Therapy

Persons in normal grief seldom seek psychiatric help because they accept their reactions and behavior as appropriate. Accordingly, a bereaved person should not routinely see a psychiatrist or psychologist unless a markedly divergent reaction to the loss is noted. For example, under usual circumstances, a bereaved person does not make a suicide attempt; if someone seriously contemplates suicide, psychiatric intervention is indicated.

When professional assistance is sought, it usually involves a request for sleeping medication from a family physician. A mild sedative to induce sleep may be useful in some situations, but antidepressant medication or antianxiety agents are rarely indicated in normal grief. Bereaved persons may have to go through the mourning process, however painful it is, for successful resolution to occur. Narcotizing patients with drugs interferes with the normal process that ultimately can lead to a favorable outcome.

Because grief reactions can develop into a depressive disorder or pathological mourning, specific counseling sessions for bereaved individuals are often valuable. Grief therapy is an increasingly important skill. In regularly scheduled sessions, grieving persons are encouraged to talk about feelings of loss and about the person who has died. Many bereaved persons have difficulty recognizing and expressing angry or ambivalent feelings toward a deceased person, and they must be reassured that these feelings are normal.

Grief therapy need not be conducted only on a one-to-one basis; group counseling is also effective. Self-help groups also have great value in certain cases. About 30 percent of widows and widowers report that they become isolated from friends, withdraw from social life, and thus experience feelings of isolation and loneliness. Self-help groups offer companionship, social contacts, and emotional support; they eventually enable their members to reenter society in a meaningful way. Bereavement care and grief therapy have been most effective with widows and widowers. The necessity for this therapy stems, in part, from the contraction of the family unit; extended family members are no longer available to provide the needed emotional support and guidance during the mourning period.

▲ 30.2 Palliative Care

Psychological symptoms are nearly universal at the end of life. Psychiatric syndromes occur with an increased but definable frequency and have a different age and gender distribution. For example, anxiety and depression are as common in men as in women. Psychiatric classification remains an important framework on which to base clinical observations, but it was not designed with dying patients in mind. Hence, for such patients, it is pragmatically useful to think of a few syndromes for which this exists. The most common ones are anxiety states, depressive states, and confusional states. These frequently coexist and overlap. Rarely, specific phobias of needles, enclosures, and the like may interfere with comfort and should be addressed, adapting the usual treatments to the patient's medical status. Occasionally, an emotional crisis or exacerbation of symptoms can be identified as an adjustment disorder, but it is occurring against the backdrop of other serious symptoms, so technically it does not meet diagnostic criteria. However, this should not prevent the consultant from identifying the precipitating factor and defusing the response in the usual ways. Major psychotic disorders become submerged by the increasing symptomatology of the active dying process and only require specific attention when the patient is not actively dying and when the psychotic symptoms are clearly separate from and superimposed on the symptoms of the illness.

PREVALENCE

Much of the research on prevalence has been done in cancer and AIDS and shows a marked increase of psychiatric conditions near the end of life. Severe depressive symptoms rose from

25 to 77 percent in a sample of hospitalized cancer patients, although stricter criteria find 15 percent with major depression and another 15 percent having severe depressive symptoms. The prevalence of delirium rises from a range of 25 to 40 percent to as high as 85 percent with increasingly advanced disease. The association of psychiatric symptoms with pain was demonstrated in one of several consistent studies in which 39 percent of patients with a psychiatric diagnosis reported significant pain compared with 19 percent for those without a psychiatric diagnosis. In a sample of inpatients with AIDS, 65 percent had an organic mental disorder, and 27 percent had major depression. The financial cost of psychiatric disorders can be inferred from a study in which patients with a psychiatric diagnosis remained in the hospital 60 days longer than those without a psychiatric diagnosis.

Most commonly, terminally ill patients demonstrate an intertwining of anxiety and depression. These are difficult to tease apart, and the term *negative affect* has been suggested to define them as a symptom complex. It is hard not to feel grief at what is being lost and fear about the ultimate unknown. Individuals whose deep faith in an afterlife animates their spirit are an exception, and, even among them, many describe coexisting regret at the loss of their temporal life and its furnishings.

GENERAL TREATMENT PRINCIPLES

Because improved quality of life is the primary goal, pharmacological treatment and any other measures that bring symptom relief should be instituted rapidly while an integrated plan for psychological and family interventions is being designed and set into motion. Psychiatric syndromes in this group are often secondary to medical conditions; hence, an etiological diagnosis often yields useful clues to prevention and improved management. It should be sought simultaneously as long as the search is in line with treatment goals.

ANXIETY IN PATIENTS WITH ADVANCED DISEASE

Anxiety can be the presenting symptom for almost all medical disorders and can occur as a side effect from many medications. However, in patients with advanced disease, it usually presents with somatic symptoms, such as restlessness, hyperactivity, tachycardia, gastrointestinal (GI) distress, nausea, insomnia, shortness of breath, numbness, or tremor. It lowers the threshold for pain, worsens functional impairment, and increases the distress experienced in all comorbid conditions. It often interferes with the patient's ability to cooperate with other treatments or to relate optimally with loved ones. Patients refer to fear, worry, apprehension, or ruminations more often than to anxiety per se.

Mr. S, a 50-year-old physical therapist with newly diagnosed advanced lung cancer, was noted by his family to be anxious to the point of having panic symptoms when his wife would leave his bedside to attend to chores. He would start hyperventilating, would feel short of breath, would become restless and unable to concentrate on anything, and would be overwhelmed with morbid ruminations about his future. He was upset and felt guilty at having become overly dependent on his wife. He was taught relaxation and breathing exercises and was treated with clonazepam (Klonopin), which brought about a marked resolution of his anxiety. Mr. S felt more relaxed, less anxious, and more resilient and became able to withstand periods of solitude without difficulty. *(Courtesy of Marguerite Lederberg, M.D.)*

DEPRESSION IN PATIENTS WITH ADVANCED DISEASE

Depressive symptoms are also common in advanced disease and are associated with the same existential factors found with anxiety. Studies have found a prevalence ranging from 9 percent, using the strictest criteria, to 58 percent, with less demanding ones. Risk factors include a previous history or a family history. Having a way of differentiating somatic effects of disease from the neurovegetative criteria of major depression is especially daunting in terminally ill patients.

Table 30.2–1 describes the Endicott Substitution Criteria, which have been found to perform as well as the DSM criteria for depression and go further in that they also reflect the clinical observation that classically described depressive thoughts and feelings are not universal in terminally ill patients and, when present, reflect depression just as they do in physically healthy patients.

Although there are not many studies on the treatment of depression in terminally ill individuals, the available studies and a large body of clinical experience with medically ill patients show that the pharmacological treatment of depression can be useful even when definable medical causes exist and even in the last days of life.

A patient with diabetes and end-stage renal disease who had been on dialysis for 2 years was diagnosed with depression with marked insomnia and was started on 15 mg by mouth every day of mirtazapine, which helped her sleep immediately and showed an antidepressant effect within 3 weeks. Four weeks later, she was admitted to the hospital in congestive heart failure for what was to be her terminal admission. She did not wish to give up the antidepressant but now felt oversedated and wished that she could be more alert during the day to interact with her loved ones. She was started on methylphenidate 5 mg by mouth twice daily, after which she was more alert, engaged, and communicative with her family. On her death, her family was grateful to have been able to connect with her until the end.

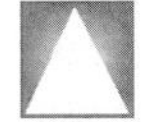

Table 30.2–1
Endicott Substitution Criteria for Depression

Physical Somatic Symptoms	Psychological Symptom Substitute
Changes in appetite or weight, or both	Tearfulness, depressed appearance
Sleep disturbance	Social withdrawal, decreased talkativeness
Fatigue, loss of energy	Brooding, self-pity, pessimism
Memory and concentration deficits, indecisiveness	Lack of reactivity

CONFUSIONAL STATES IN PATIENTS WITH ADVANCED DISEASE

The prevalence of delirium rises to 85 percent in patients with advanced disease. If one includes the last hours of life, it nears 100 percent unless the patient lapses rapidly into coma or dies of an acute event, such as pulmonary embolus. Acute events are always unexpected and traumatize the survivors even though they knew full well that the patient was near the end of life. Some patients slip into an irreversible coma, leaving families in a bedside vigil, which may actually give them a period of adaptation before the final instant of death. However, for some 75 to 85 percent of patients, death is associated with a period of delirium.

Patients frequently experience some disorientation, impaired memory, concentration, and altered arousal as they become increasingly ill. These symptoms may remain mild or may be the harbingers of full delirium. Clinicians should be aware that mild and early signs of delirium are often mistaken for depression, anxiety, and poor coping.

A psychiatric consultation was sought to evaluate depression in a 56-year-old practicing attorney with pancreatic cancer. His moderately severe back pain was being treated with morphine. The patient was noted by the inpatient staff to be more withdrawn, disengaged, and quiet, making poor eye contact and sleeping most of the day.

On examination, the psychiatric consultant found Mr. K to have disturbed arousal and to be mildly confused and disoriented. His speech was slow and his thought process disorganized. Mr. K admitted to intermittently experiencing visual hallucinations that he had been too embarrassed to report earlier to the nursing staff.

Mr. K was diagnosed with a hypoactive delirium secondary to opioid medications. He was treated with a low dose of olanzapine, 2.5 mg at bedtime. Mr. K's sensorium improved dramatically. He became alert, fully oriented, and better related, without any perceptual disturbances or thought disorder. This was accomplished without needing to decrease his much needed pain medications.

DISEASE-SPECIFIC CONSIDERATIONS

Different illnesses bring special issues. For example, a patient on dialysis can opt for death three times a week and is more vulnerable to acting on feelings of depression, anger, hopelessness, and reactions to family neglect or conflict. Patients with cancer must acknowledge possible death while hoping for a cure or remission. Treatment decisions in the face of disease that is less and less treatable become increasingly difficult and can cause acute anxiety. Stem cell transplant patients experience high levels of anxiety and depression because they are getting a last chance with high stakes and high risks. The availability of organ transplants has created a large population of patients who wait knowing that they may die while waiting for a cure that could be just around the corner. Neurodegenerative disorders are associated with increasing physical disability and dependence. When there is associated loss of cognitive faculties, the problems may be behavioral. Otherwise, depression is a frequent, although not inevitable, problem. Many patients state that they will not tolerate complete immobility and dependence, yet when the time comes, they go on life supports and stay on them. It has been shown in several settings that as patients become sicker, they accept an increasingly limited quality of life as worth living and opt for more onerous, less promising treatments if they offer even a small chance of help.

PATIENT–FAMILY UNIT

The intensity of family relationships becomes even greater during the terminal period. The response of family members can be a conspiracy of silence. Nothing is sadder than a bedside where family members are tense and silent because they want to protect the patient by not talking about dying and the patient is tense and silent because he or she is protecting the family by not talking about things that will upset them. Instead of closeness, expressions of gratitude, apologies, reminiscences, and farewells, there is distance, and the patient is dying alone even though he or she is physically surrounded by others.

The psychiatrist can use family sessions to open patient–family dialogues. He or she can identify discrepant views of the illness, can deal with conflicts regarding treatment, and can explore concerns regarding an absent member, all of which undermine patient support and medical management. A major crisis, such as the imminent loss of a member, destabilizes the family structure, creating an opportunity for the psychiatrist to promote adaptive change and reconstitution. *Family-centered grief therapy,* which initially includes the patient and continues after the patient's death, provides a natural setting for such interventions.

When an older adolescent dropped out of college to take over her dying mother's duties, the family subtly discouraged her return to school after her mother's death. Psychiatric intervention allowed the patient to play a part in reorganizing family roles in a way that made it more possible for her daughter to continue her studies.

DECISION POINTS, ADVANCE DIRECTIVES, PROXIES, AND SURROGATES

This section reviews transitions and decisions that characterize the end of life.

Transition to Palliative Care

The transition to palliative care is not always clear. As soon as a diagnosis of an incurable disease is made, cure is no longer the goal of care. However, if death is distant or even if some life extension can still be obtained, the patient and family focus on this positive goal. The physician is under no illusion about the future but has the delicate task of promoting short-term gains without obliterating the awareness of what lies ahead. Only when the nearness of death is acknowledged can thoughtful decisions be made about palliative care.

Where to Die?

Unattended Deaths. Many traumatic or unexpected deaths become known from a catastrophic phone call. The patient is gone, but the traumatized family needs help to absorb the loss, to cope with the circumstances, and to come to some kind of closure. It is not realized how much the experience of living through the illness, the death, and the funeral rites is crucial to the normal resolution of the mourning process.

A totally unexpected death, even an understandable one, such as a heart attack, leaves an aching sense of unfinished business over and above the expected grief. If the person was the victim of a crime, obsessive thoughts may be difficult to repress, and grief may turn to unquenchable anger with profound psychological disruption. It is also difficult, if not impossible, for survivors to make peace with suicide.

Emergency departments, police departments, and religious and community institutions should be equipped with a list of referral resources to help survivors of traumatic deaths. Psychiatric input can include program development and consultation to a wide range of professionals and individuals. Families must be helped to construct their own ritual whereby they acknowledge to themselves and others the finality of their loss and perhaps create a place, if not a grave, around which to center their memorializing.

Attended Deaths. Patients can die in an acute hospital, in nursing homes, in hospices, and at home, with or without hospice support.

Most patients still die in acute care hospitals, having received active care until shortly before they die. This may occur because death is sudden or because the family or patient needed to be in a place where "everything is being done." Fortunately, a growing number of hospitals have palliative care teams that provide appropriate care in the acute hospital setting.

Many patients die in nursing homes without the benefit of special care. This unfortunate situation could be remedied by bringing formal hospice care into nursing homes, but funding sources and turf issues need to be settled before it can become routine practice.

Inpatient hospice care was the first model of care to be developed and is warmly remembered by grateful families whose multiple human needs and those of their loved one had been met in ways that they had not been trained to expect. As hospice gained acceptance, the insufficiency of inpatient beds encouraged the development of home hospice. Its existence has, in turn, encouraged more families to elect to keep dying patients at home.

In a home hospice program, the patient is evaluated and accepted in the usual manner but stays at home. The patient and family receive extensive instruction about what to expect. They are helped to obtain necessary materials, taught how to use them, and helped to obtain as much home help as they need. All the while, they receive medical supervision, nursing care, and emotional support with 24-hour phone availability and routine daily contacts.

Without this kind of help, a good death at home can be difficult to achieve. With it, patients feel safe from the abandonment that is so commonly feared, and families feel safe from the terror of an unmanageable event. The families of these patients work hard, but they are more likely to feel competent and in control. They experience more of a sense of achievement and less of the gnawing sense of inadequacy that is otherwise common.

CARING FOR THE DYING PATIENT

Marguerite S. Lederberg, M.D., at Memorial Sloan-Kettering Cancer Center in New York makes the following observation:

A dying human being whose physical, social, emotional, and spiritual needs are being effectively attended to seldom demands to be helped to commit suicide, and the family members—given proper help and support—derive a deep sense of peace from having helped their loved one to die feeling loved and secure.

Table 30.2–2
Risk Factors for the Development of Aversive Reactions in Physicians

The physician:
- Identifies with the patient: looks, profession, age, character, and so on
- Identifies the patient with someone in his or her own life.
- Is currently dealing with a sick family member.
- Is recently bereaved or dealing with unresolved loss or grief issues.
- Feels professionally insecure.
- Is fearful of death and disability.
- Is unconsciously reflecting feelings felt or expressed by the patient or family.
- Cannot tolerate high and protracted levels of ambiguity or uncertainty.
- Carries a psychiatric diagnosis, such as depression or substance abuse.

Adapted from Meier DE, Back AL, Morrison RS. The inner life of physicians and care of the seriously ill. *JAMA*. 2001;286:3007–3014.

One of the most important tasks for a physician caring for a dying patient is to determine when the time for curative care has ceased. It is only then that palliative care can begin. Some physicians are so upset by death that they are reluctant to use palliative methods; rather, they continue to treat the patient knowing that efforts are futile. Or they resort to using so-called heroic methods that do not prevent death and that may produce needless suffering. Ideally, physicians should strive to extend life and decrease suffering; at the same time, they must accept death as a defining characteristic of life. Some physicians, however, have developed dysfunctional attitudes about death, which have been reinforced throughout their lives by their experiences and training. It has been postulated that doctors are more frightened of death than members of other professional groups and that many enter the study of medicine so they may gain control of their own mortality using the defense mechanism of intellectualization. Risk factors that can interfere with a physician's ability to care optimally for dying patients are listed in Table 30.2–2. These factors range from over identifying with the patient to being fearful of death as mentioned.

Physicians able to deal with death and dying are able to communicate effectively in several areas: diagnosis and prognosis, the nature of terminal illness, advance directives about life-sustaining treatment, hospice care, legal and ethical issues, grief and bereavement, and psychiatric care. In addition, palliative care physicians must be skilled in pain management, especially in the use of powerful opioids—the gold standard of drugs used for pain relief. In 1991, the American Board of Pain Medicine was established to ensure that physicians treating patients in pain were both qualified to do so and were kept up to date on the latest advances in the field.

COMMUNICATION

After a diagnosis and prognosis have been made, physicians need to talk to the patient and the patient's family. Formerly, doctors subscribed to a conspiracy of silence, believing that their patient's chances for recovery would improve if they knew less because news of impending death might bring despair. The current practice is now one of honesty and openness toward patients; in fact, the question is not whether to tell the patient but when and how. In 1972, the American Hospital Association drafted the Patient's Bill of Rights, declaring that patients have the "right to obtain complete, current information regarding diagnosis, treatment and prognosis in terms the patient can be reasonably expected to understand."

Breaking Bad News

When breaking news of impending death to the patient, as when relating any bad news, diplomacy and compassion should be the guiding principles. Often, bad news is not completely related during one meeting but rather is absorbed gradually over a series of separate conversations. Advance preparations, including scheduling sufficient time for the visit; researching pertinent information, such as test results and facts about the case; and even arranging furniture appropriately can only make the patient feel more comfortable.

If possible, these conversations should take place in a private, suitable space with the patient on equal terms with the physician (i.e., the patient dressed and the physician seated). If it is possible and desired by the patient, the patient's spouse or partner should be present. The treating physician should explain the current situation to the patient in clear, simple language even when speaking to highly educated patients. Information may need to be repeated or additional meetings may be necessary to communicate all of the information. A gentle, sensible approach will help modulate the patient's own denial and acceptance. At no time should physicians take their patient's angry comments personally, and they should never criticize the patient's response to the bad news.

Physicians can signal their availability for honest communication by encouraging and answering questions from patients. Estimates on how long a patient has to live are usually inaccurate and thus should not be given, or given with that caveat. Also, physicians should make it clear to their patients that they are willing to see them through until death occurs. Ultimately, physicians must choose how much information to give and when on the basis of each patient's needs and capacities.

The same general approaches apply as physicians seek to comfort members of the patient's family. Helping family members deal with feelings about the patient's illness can be just as important as comforting the patient because family members are often the main source of emotional support for patients.

Telling the Truth

Tactful honesty is the doctor's most important aid. Honesty, however, need not preclude hope or guarded optimism. It is important to be aware that if 85 percent of patients with a particular disease die in 5 years, 15 percent are still alive after that time. The principles of doing good and not doing harm inform the decision of whether to tell the patient the truth. In general, most patients want to know the truth about their condition. Various studies of patients with malignancies show that 80 to 90 percent want to know their diagnosis.

Doctors, however, should ask patients how much they want to know because some persons do not want to know all the facts about their illness. Such patients, if told the truth, deny that they ever were told, and they cannot participate in end-of-life decisions, such as the use of life-sustaining equipment. The patients who openly request that they not be given "bad news" are often those who most fear death. Physicians should deal with these fears directly, but if the patient still cannot bear to hear the truth, someone closely related to the patient must be informed.

Informed Consent

In the United States, informed consent is legally required for both conventional and experimental treatment. Patients must be given sufficient information about their diagnosis, prognosis, and treatment options to make knowledgeable decisions. This includes discussion of potential risks and benefits, available alternative treatments, and the results of not receiving treatment. This approach may come at some psychological cost; severe anxiety and occasional psychiatric decompensation can occur when patients feel overburdened by demands to make decisions. Nevertheless, patients respond best to doctors who explain the various options in detail. Physicians must be prepared to deal with difficult questions posed by patients.

End-of-life discussions are challenging, especially because they can influence how patients make informed choices.

TERMINAL CARE DECISIONS

Modern society is poorly equipped to cope with the life-and-death decisions spawned by technology. When it first emerged, cardiopulmonary resuscitation was enthusiastically supported by the medical profession. It was endowed with magical power and eventually became a ritualized rite rather than an optional medical treatment. That practice played into the therapeutic activism characteristic of many physicians. By the end of the 20th century, however, a countermovement began. First, the right to refuse treatment was established, largely because of synergy between the consumer movement and the bioethics movement, with its emphasis on patient autonomy. Next, the legality of do not resuscitate (DNR) orders and the moral equivalence of stopping and not starting treatment were established. The medical profession was less enthusiastic than the public about these changes, perhaps because practitioners know too well the emotional ambiguities that surround death and must repeatedly experience them.

Brain Death and Persistent Vegetative State

In an attempt to deal with these ambiguities, the concept of brain death emerged. Brain death is associated with the loss of higher brain functions (e.g., cognition) and all brainstem function (e.g., pupillary and reflex eye movement), respiration, and gag and corneal reflexes. Determination of brain death is a generally accepted criterion for death. Some clinicians advocate an absence of brain waves on electroencephalography (EEG) to confirm the diagnosis.

Persistent vegetative state was defined by the American Academy of Neurology as a condition in which no awareness exists of self or environment associated with severe neurological damage (Table 30.2–3). Medical treatment provides no benefits to patients in a persistent vegetative state and after the diagnosis is established, DNR and do not intubate (DNI) orders can be followed and life-sustaining methods (e.g., feeding tubes, ventilators) can be removed.

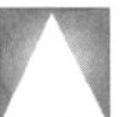

Table 30.2–3
Persistent Vegetative State

No evidence of awareness of self or environment; no interaction with others
No meaningful response to stimuli
No receptive or expressive language
Return of sleep–wake cycles, arousal, even smiling, frowning, yawning
Preserved brainstem or hypothalamic autonomic functions to permit survival
Bowel and bladder incontinence
Variably preserved cranial nerve and spinal reflexes

In 1976, the case of Karen Quinlan made international headlines when her parents sought the assistance of a judge to discontinue the use of a ventilator in their daughter, who was in a persistent vegetative state. Ms. Quinlan's physician had refused her parents' request to remove the ventilator because, they said, they feared that they might be held civilly or even criminally liable for her death. The New Jersey Supreme Court ruled that competent persons have a right to refuse life-sustaining treatment and that this right should not be lost when a person becomes incompetent. Because the Court believed that the physicians were unwilling to withdraw the ventilator because of the fear of legal liability, not precepts of medical ethics, it devised a mechanism to grant the physicians prospective legal immunity for taking this action. Specifically, the New Jersey Supreme Court ruled that after a prognosis, confirmed by a hospital ethics committee, that "no reasonable possibility of a patient returning to a cognitive, sapient state," exists, life-sustaining treatment can be removed, and no one involved, including the physicians, can be held civilly or criminally responsible for the death.

The publicity surrounding the Quinlan case motivated two independent developments: It encouraged states to enact "living will" legislation that provided legal immunity to physicians who honored patients' written "advance directives" specifying how they would want to be treated if they ever became incompetent, and it encouraged hospitals to establish ethics committees that could attempt to resolve similar treatment disputes without going to court. (Annas GJ. "Culture of life" politics at the bedside. *N Eng J Med.* 2005;352:16.)

Advance Directives

Advance directives are wishes and choices about medical intervention when the patient's condition is considered terminal. Advance directives, which are legally binding in all 50 states, include three types: living will, health care proxy, and DNR and DNI orders.

Living Will. In a living will, a patient who is mentally competent gives specific instructions that doctors must follow when the patient cannot communicate them because of illness. These instructions may include rejection of feeding tubes, artificial airways, and any other measures to prolong life.

Health Care Proxy. Also known as *durable power of attorney,* the health care proxy gives another person the power to make medical decisions if the patient cannot do so. That person, also known as the surrogate, is empowered to make all decisions about terminal care on the basis of what he or she thinks the patient would want.

Do Not Resuscitate and Do Not Intubate Orders. These orders prohibit doctors from attempting to resuscitate (DNR) or intubate (DNI) the patient who is in extremis. DNR and DNI orders are made by the patient who is competent to do so. They can be made part of the living will or expressed by the health care proxy. A sample advance directive that incorporates both a living will and a health care proxy is given in Table 30.2–4.

The Uniform Rights of the Terminally Ill Act, drafted by the National Conference on Uniform State Laws, was approved and recommended for enactment in all states. This act authorizes an adult to control the decisions regarding the administration of life-sustaining treatment by executing a declaration instructing a physician to withhold or to withdraw life-sustaining treatment if the person is in a terminal condition and cannot participate in medical treatment decisions. In 1991, the Federal Patient Self-Determination Act became law in the United States and required that all health care facilities (1) provide each patient admitted to a hospital with written information about the right to refuse treatment, (2) ask about advance directives, and (3) keep written records of whether the patient has an advance directive or has designated a health care proxy.

Today, patients who have left no advance directives or who are legally incompetent to do so have access to hospital ethics committees that hold active legal and ethical debates about these issues. These ethics committees are also of help to doctors, who can gain both legal and moral support when recommending that no further treatment occur. It is much easier for all parties, however, if the patient has advance directives or a proxy. Ideally, physicians should initiate discussions with patients about advance directives and proxies early even while the patient is healthy. The patient should be reminded that these early formulations can be modified but that even having preliminary advance directives will ensure that treating physicians observe the patient's wishes in the event of an emergency.

CARING FOR THE FAMILY

Family members play an important role as caregivers to terminally ill patients and have needs of their own that often go unrecognized. Their responsibilities can be overwhelming, especially if only one family member is available or if family members themselves are infirm or elderly. Table 30.2–5 lists some family caregiving tasks. Many of these tasks require long hours of work or supervision that can lead to physical and emotional fatigue. One study of caregivers reports that 25 to 30 percent lost their jobs and more than half moved to lower paying jobs to accommodate the need for flexibility. The highest stress level was found in families who cared for a terminally ill patient at home, especially when death occurs in the home, and realized in retrospect that they would have preferred an environment in which death occurs in the presence of skilled caretakers.

DYING AT HOME

Depending on the patient's wishes and the nature of his or her disease, the choice to die at home is one that should be explored. Although it is more burdensome on a family than dying in a hospital or hospice, death at home can be a welcome alternative for the patient and family seeking to spend quality time together. A

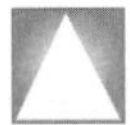

Table 30.2–4
Advance Directive Living Will and Health Care Proxy[a]

Death is a part of life. It is a reality like birth, growth, and aging. I am using this advance directive to convey my wishes about medical care to my doctors and other people looking after me at the end of my life. It is called an advance directive because it gives instructions in advance about what I want to happen to me in the future. It expresses my wishes about medical treatment that might keep me alive. I want this to be legally binding.

If I cannot make or communicate decisions about my medical care, those around me should rely on this document for instructions about measures that could keep me alive.

I do not want medical treatment (including feeding and water by tube) that will keep me alive if:

▲ I am unconscious and there is no reasonable prospect that I will ever be conscious again (even if I am not going to die soon in my medical condition), or

▲ I am near death from an illness or injury with no reasonable prospect of recovery.

I do want medicine and other care to make me more comfortable and to take care of pain and suffering. I want this even if the pain medicine makes me die sooner.

I want to give some extra instructions: [*Here list any special instructions, e.g., some people fear being kept alive after a debilitating stroke. If you have wishes about this, or any other condition, please write them here.*]

The legal language in the box that follows is a health care proxy. It gives another person the power to make medical decisions for me.

I name. __________ who __________ lives at, __________ phone number __________, __________, to make medical decisions for me if I cannot make them myself. This person is called a health care "surrogate," "agent," "proxy," or "attorney in fact." This power of attorney shall become effective when I become incapable of making or communicating decisions about my medical care. This means that this document stays legal when and if I lose the power to speak for myself, for instance, if I am in a coma or have Alzheimer's disease.

My health care proxy has power to tell others what my advance directive means. This person also has power to make decisions for me based either on what I would have wanted, or, if this is not known, on what he or she thinks is best for me.

If my first choice health care proxy cannot or decides not to act for me, I name __________, address __________, phone number __________, as my second choice.

I have discussed my wishes with my health care proxy and with my second choice if I have chosen to appoint a second person. My proxy(ies) has(have) agreed to act for me.

I have thought about this advance directive carefully. I know what it means and want to sign it. I have chosen two witnesses, neither of whom is a member of my family, nor will inherit from me when I die. My witnesses are not the same people as those I named as my health care proxies. I understand that this form should be notarized if I use the box to name (a) health care proxy(ies).

Signature __________

Date __________

Address __________

Witness's __________ signature __________

Witness's printed name __________

Address __________

Witness's signature __________

Witness's printed name __________

Address __________

Notary [to be used if proxy is appointed] __________

[a]The reader should be advised that this sample is one of many directives available.
From Choice in Dying, Inc.—the National Council for the Right to Die.

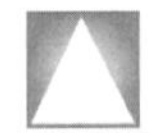

Table 30.2–5
Tasks of Family Members of Dying Individuals

1. Administering medications
2. Dealing with adverse effects of medications
3. Providing help with, or actually performing, activities of daily living
4. Changing wound dressing
5. Managing ambulatory infusion pumps or other equipment
6. Providing symptom management (e.g., for pain, nausea and vomiting, shortness of breath, seizures, and terminal agitation)
7. Notifying the nurse or doctor when they are needed
8. Shopping for needed items and picking up prescriptions
9. Providing a presence and companionship
10. Attending to spiritual and religious needs
11. Carrying out advance directives
12. Managing financial matters

home care team can assess a home for its suitability and suggest ways to facilitate activities of daily living, including modifications to furniture; hospital bed leasing; and installation of assistive devices, such as handrails and commodes. The family's care can be supplemented with house calls by physicians, nurses, therapists, and chaplains. In any case, the family must know what their responsibilities are and must be well prepared to care for the patient. Recently, hospice home care was approved by Medicare and is being more widely used.

Family therapy sessions allow family members to explore feelings about death and dying. They serve as a forum in which anticipatory grief and mourning can take place. The ability to share feelings can be cathartic, especially if guilt is involved. Family members often have to deal with feelings of guilt about past interactions with the dying patient. Family sessions also help to achieve consensus about the patient's advance directives. If family members disagree about the patient's wishes, the medical staff may be unable to act. In such cases, legal action may be needed to resolve family disputes about what course of action to pursue.

PALLIATIVE CARE

Palliative care is the most important part of end-of-life care. It refers to providing relief from the suffering caused by pain or other symptoms of terminal disease. Although this is most commonly associated with analgesic drug administration, many other medical interventions and surgical procedures fall under the umbrella of palliative care because they can make the patient more comfortable. Monitors and their alarms, peripheral and central lines, phlebotomy, measurement of signs, and even supplemental oxygen are usually discontinued to allow the patient to die peacefully. Relocating the patient to a quiet, private room (as opposed to an intensive care unit) and allowing family members to be present is another very important palliative care modality.

The shift from active, curative treatment to palliative care is sometimes the first tangible sign that the patient will die, a transition that is emotionally difficult for everyone concerned about the patient to accept. The discontinuation of machines and measurements, which up until this point have been an integral part of the hospital experience, can be extremely disconcerting to the patient, family members, and even other physicians. Indeed, if these parties are not active in planning this transition, it can easily seem that persons have given up on the patient.

Because of this difficulty, palliative care is sometimes avoided altogether (i.e., curative treatment is continued until the patient dies). This approach is likely to cause problems if it is adopted merely to avoid the reality of impending death. A well-negotiated transition to palliative care often decreases anxiety after the patient and family go through an appropriate anticipatory grief reaction. Furthermore, a positive emotional outcome is much more likely if the physician and staff project a conviction that palliative care will be an active, involved process, without hint of withdrawal or abandonment. When this does not occur or when the family cannot tolerate the transition, the ensuing stress frequently results in a need for psychiatric consultation.

> A 36-year-old physician with end-stage leukemia was seen in psychiatric consultation because he reported seeing the "angel of death" at the foot of his hospital bed. He described the experience as frightening and inexplicable. The consultant asked the patient, "Are you afraid that you are going to die?" That was the first time anyone had mentioned death or dying in any context to the patient. He welcomed the opportunity to talk openly about his fears to the medical staff and to his family and eventually died a peaceful death.

Psychiatric consultation is indicated for patients who become severely anxious, suicidal, depressed, or overtly psychotic. In each instance, appropriate psychiatric medication can be prescribed to provide relief. Patients who are suicidal do not always have to be transferred to a psychiatric service. An attendant or nurse can be assigned to the patient on a 24-hour basis (one-on-one coverage). In such instances, the relationship that develops between the observer and the patient may have therapeutic overtones, especially with patients whose depression is related to a sense of abandonment. Patients who are terminal and who are at high risk for suicide are usually in pain. When pain is relieved, suicidal ideation is likely to diminish. A careful evaluation of suicide potential is required for all patients. A premorbid history of past suicide attempts is a high risk factor for suicide in terminally ill patients. In patients who become psychotic, impaired cognitive function secondary to metastatic lesions to the brain must always be considered. Such patients respond to antipsychotic medications, and psychotherapy may also be of use.

PAIN MANAGEMENT

Types of Pain

Dying patients are subject to several different kinds of pain, summarized in Table 30.2–6. The distinctions are important because they call for different treatment strategies; whereas somatic and visceral pain are responsive to opiates, neuropathic and sympathetically maintained pain may require adjuvant medications in addition to opiates. Most patients with advanced cancer, for example, have more than one kind of pain and require complex treatment regimens.

Treatment of Pain

It cannot be overemphasized that pain management should be aggressive, and treatment should be multimodal. In fact, a good pain regimen may require several drugs or the same drug used in different ways and administered via different routes. For example, intravenous morphine can be supplemented by self-administered oral "rescue" doses, or a continuous epidural drip can be supplemented by bolus intravenous doses. Transdermal patches may provide baseline concentrations in patients for whom intravenous or oral intake is difficult. Patient-controlled analgesia systems for intravenous opiate administration result

Table 30.2–6
Types of Pain

Nociceptive pain	
Somatic pain	Usually, but not always constant, aching, gnawing, and well localized (e.g., bone metastases)
Visceral pain	Usually, but not always constant, deep, squeezing, poorly localized, with possible cutaneous referral (e.g., pleural effusion leading to deep chest pain, diaphragmatic irritation referred to the shoulder)
Neuropathic pain	Burning dysesthetic pain with shock-like paroxysms associated with direct damage to peripheral receptors, afferent fibers, or the central nervous system, leading to loss of central inhibitory modulation and spontaneous firing (e.g., phantom limb pain; can involve sympathetic somatic afferents)
Psychogenic pain	Variable characteristics secondary to psychological factors in the absence of medical factors; rare as a pure phenomenon in patients with cancer but often an additional factor in the presence of organic pain

Courtesy of Marguerite S. Lederberg, M.D. and Jimmie C. Holland, M.D.

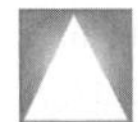

Table 30.2–7
Opioid Analgesics for Management of Pain

Drug and Equianalgesic Dose Relative Potency	Dose (mg IM or oral)	Plasma Half-Life (hr)[a]	Starting Oral Dose[b] (mg)	Available Commercial Preparations
Morphine	10 IM 60 oral	3–4	30–60	Oral: tablet, liquid, slow-release tablet Rectal: 5–30 mg Injectable: SC, IM, IV, epidural, intrathecal
Hydromorphone	1.5 IM 7.5 oral	2–3	2–18	Oral: tablets: 1, 2, 4 mg Injectable: SC, IM, IV 2 mg/mL, 3 mg/mL, and 10 mg/mL
Methadone	10 IM 20 oral	12–24	5–10	Oral: tablets, liquid Injectable: SC, IM, IV
Levorphanol	2 IM 4 oral	12–16	2–4	Oral: tablets Injectable: SC, IM, IV
Oxymorphone	1	2–3	NA	Rectal: 10 mg Injectable: SC, IM, IV
Heroin	5 IM 60 oral	3–4	NA	NA
Meperidine	75 IM 300 oral	3–4 (normeperidine 12–16)	75	Oral: tablets Injectable: SC, IM, IV
Codeine	130 oral 200 oral	3–4	60	Oral: tablets in combination with acetylsalicylic acid, acetaminophen, liquid
Oxycodone[c]	15 oral 30 oral	—	5	Oral: tablets, liquid, oral formulation in combination with acetaminophen (tablet and liquid) and aspirin (tablet)

IM, intramuscular; IV, intravenous; NA, not applicable; SC, subcutaneous.
[a]The time of peak analgesia in nontolerant patients ranges from ½ to 1 hour and the duration from 4 to 6 hours. The peak analgesic effect is delayed, and the duration is prolonged after oral administration.
[b]Recommended starting IM doses; the optimal dose for each patient is determined by titration, and the maximal dose is limited by adverse effects.
[c]A long-acting sustained-release form of oxycodone (OxyContin) has been abused by drug addicts, and its use has been criticized because of this; however, it is a very useful preparation available in 10-, 20-, 40-, and 160-mg doses that need to be taken once every 12 hours. It is used as a maintenance therapy for severe persistent pain.
Adapted from Foley K. Management of cancer pain. In: DeVita VT, Hellman S, Rosenberg SA, eds. *Cancer: Principles and Practice of Oncology*. 4th ed. Philadelphia, PA: JB Lippincott; 1993:936.

in better pain relief with lower amounts dispensed than in staff-administered dosing.

Opioids commonly cause delirium and hallucinations. A frequent mechanism of psychotoxicity is the accumulation of drugs or metabolites whose durations of analgesia are shorter than their plasma half-lives (morphine, levorphanol [Levo-Dromoran], and methadone [Dolophine]). Use of drugs such as hydromorphone (Dilaudid), which have half-lives closer to their analgesic duration, can relieve the problem without loss of pain control. Cross-tolerance is incomplete between opiates; hence, several should be tried in any patient with the dosage lowered when switching drugs. Table 30.2–7 lists opioid analgesics.

The benefits of maintenance analgesia administration in terminally ill patients compared with as-needed administration cannot be overemphasized. Maintenance dosing improves pain control, increases drug efficiency, and relieves patient anxiety, but as-needed orders allow pain to increase while waiting for the drug to be given. Moreover, as-needed analgesia administration perversely sets up the patient for staff complaints about drug-seeking behavior. Even when maintenance treatment is used, extra doses of medication should be available for breakthrough pain, and repeated use of these medications should signal the need to raise the maintenance dose. Depending on their previous experiences with opioid analgesics and their weight, it is not unusual for some patients to require 2 g or more of morphine per day for relief of symptoms.

Knowing doses of different drugs and different routes of administration is important to avoid accidental under medication. For example, when changing a patient from intramuscular to oral morphine use, the intramuscular dose must be multiplied by 6 to avoid causing the patient pain and provoking drug-seeking behavior. Many adjuvant drugs used for pain are psychotropics with which psychiatrists are familiar, but in some cases, their analgesic effect is separate from their primary psychotropic effect. Commonly used adjuvants include antidepressants, mood stabilizers (e.g., gabapentin) phenothiazines, butyrophenones, antihistamines, amphetamines, and steroids. They are particularly important in neuropathic and sympathetically maintained pain, for which they can be the mainstay of treatment.

Other developments in pain management include more intrusive procedures, such as nerve blocks or the use of continuous epidural infusions. Additionally, radiation therapy, chemotherapy, and even surgical resection can be considered as pain management modalities in palliative care. Short courses of radiotherapy or chemotherapy can be used to shrink tumors or manage metastatic lesions that cause pain or impairment. In patients with end-stage Hodgkin's disease, for example, systemic chemotherapy can improve the patient's quality of life by decreasing tumor burden. Surgical resection of invasive tumors, most notably breast carcinomas, can be useful for the same reason.

PALLIATION OF OTHER SYMPTOMS

Symptom management is a high priority in palliative care. Patients are often more concerned about the day-to-day distress of their symptoms than they are about their impending death,

Table 30.2–8
Common End-of-Life Symptoms/Signs

Symptom/Sign	Comments	Management/Care
Cachexia	All terminal disease states are associated with cachexia secondary to anorexia and dehydration	Feeding tubes useful in some cases; small sips of water of help
Delusions	Common in terminal state	Antipsychotic medication useful
Delirium/ Confusion	Occurs in nearly 90% of all terminal patients but is reversible in over 50%	Can be reversed if cause is found and treatable; may respond to antipsychotic and/or pain medication
Depression or anxiety	Psychological factors, e.g., fear of death, abandonment and/or physiological factors, e.g., pain, hypoxia	Antianxiety and antidepressant medication of use; opioids have strong antianxiety effects
Dysphagia	Seen in neurological disease, e.g., multiple sclerosis, amyotrophic lateral sclerosis	Attention to oral care, e.g., ice chips, lip balm; adjust to upright position when feeding
Dyspnea or cough	Associated with severe anxiety; fear of suffocation in extreme case; common in lung cancer patients	Opioids, supplemental oxygen, bronchodilators of use
Fatigue	Most common occurrence in terminal illness	Psychostimulants can be used for relief
Incontinence	Associated with radiation induced fistulas	Keep patient clean and dry; use indwelling or condom catheter if necessary
Nausea or vomiting	Side effect of radiation and chemotherapy	Antiemetics, e.g., metoclopramide, prochlorperazine; marijuana of use
Loss of skin integrity	Decubiti most common on weight-bearing areas	Turn body frequently; elbow and hip pads; inflating mattresses
Pain	Pain medications can be administered orally, sublingually, by injection or infusion, or via skin patch	Opioids are the gold standard

Data from National Coalition on Health Care (NCHC) and the Institute for Health Care Improvement (IHI). Promises to Keep: Changing the Way We Provide Care at the End of Life, release, October 12, 2000.

which may not be as real to them. Table 30.2–8 lists common end-of-life symptoms. A comprehensive approach to palliation involves attending to these end-of-life symptoms as well as pain. Sources of distress include psychiatric symptoms, such as anxiety, and physical symptoms. Foremost among physical symptoms are those involving the GI system, including diarrhea, constipation, anorexia, nausea, vomiting, and bowel obstruction. Other important symptoms include insomnia, confusion, mouth sores, dyspnea, cough, pruritus, decubitus ulcers, and urinary frequency or incontinence. Caretakers should follow these symptoms closely and establish appropriate early and aggressive care for these symptoms before they become burdensome.

An effective treatment for nausea and vomiting associated with chemotherapy is the use of Δ-tetrahydrocannabinol (THC), the active ingredient of marijuana. Oral synthetic cannabinoid, dronabinol (Marinol) is used in 1- to 2-mg doses every 8 hours. The use of marijuana cigarettes to deliver THC is believed to be more effective than pills. Proponents say that its absorption is faster and antiemetic properties are more potent via the pulmonary system. Repeated attempts to legalize marijuana cigarettes for medical use have met with only limited success in this country.

> A 47-year-old man with incurable lung cancer who had been treated unsuccessfully with chemotherapy and radiotherapy had been suffering from intractable dyspnea for 1 week. His family, nursing, and other staff were increasingly upset by his difficulty breathing and his pleas for relief. The attending physician refused to prescribe anything stronger than codeine. The palliative care team at the hospital intervened at the family's request. Relief was obtained with the use of 5 to 10 mg of an intravenous bolus of morphine every 15 minutes. When the patient became comfortable, a continuous drip of intravenous morphine was instituted, complemented by subcutaneous morphine as needed.

The American Medical Association supports the position that patients with a terminal condition require substantial doses of opioids on a regular basis and should not be denied drugs for fear of producing physical dependence. A similar view is endorsed in *Goodman and Gilman's the Pharmacological Basis of Therapeutics* as follows:

The physician should not wait until the pain becomes agonizing; no patient should ever wish for death because of a physician's reluctance to use adequate amounts of effective opioids. Accordingly, physicians who treat the terminally ill should not be intimidated by legal oversight.

This is especially important because the Drug Enforcement Administration (DEA) is considering examining the prescribing practices of physicians who care for terminally ill patients. In a strongly worded editorial (*New England Journal of Medicine,* January 5, 2006), the DEA was criticized for its involvement in what constitutes acceptable medical practice for dying patients because the DEA's federal mandate is limited to combating criminal substance abuse, not monitoring the care of dying patients. Physicians must be vigilant and forceful in protecting their rights to administer opioids to treat patients for intractable pain.

HOSPICE CARE

In 1967, the founding of St. Christopher's Hospice in England by Cicely Saunders launched the modern hospice movement. Several factors in the 1960s propelled the development of hospices, including concerns about inadequately trained physicians, inept terminal care, gross inequities in health care, and neglect of elderly adults. Life expectancy had increased, and heart disease and cancer were becoming more common. Saunders emphasized an interdisciplinary approach to symptom control, care of the patient and family as a unit, the use of volunteers, continuity of care (including home care), and follow-up with family members after a patient's death. The first hospice in the United States, Connecticut Hospice, opened in 1974. By 2000, more than 3,000 hospices were open in the United States. Round-the-clock pain control with opioids is an essential component of hospice management. In 1983, Medicare began reimbursing hospice care. Medicare hospice guidelines emphasize home care, with benefits provided for a broad spectrum of physician, nursing, psychosocial, and spiritual services at home or, if necessary, in a hospital or nursing home. To be eligible, the patient must be physician certified as having 6 months or less to live. By electing hospice care, patients agree to receive palliative rather than curative treatment. Many hospice programs are hospital-based, sometimes in separate units and sometimes in the form of hospice beds interspersed throughout the facility. Other program models include free-standing hospices and programs, hospital-affiliated hospices, nursing home hospice care, and home care programs. Nursing homes are the site of death for many elderly patients with incurable chronic illness, yet dying nursing home residents have limited access to palliative and hospice care. Families generally express satisfaction with their personal involvement in hospice care. Savings with hospice care vary, but home care programs generally cost less than conventional institutional care, particularly in the final months of life. Hospice patients are less likely to receive diagnostic studies or such intensive therapy as surgery or chemotherapy; however, a new trend is to allow treatment programs to continue while the patient remains in the hospice. Hospice care is a proven, viable alternative for patients who elect a palliative approach to terminal care. In addition, hospice goals of dignified, comfortable death for terminally ill patients and care for patients and families together have been increasingly adopted in mainstream medicine.

NEONATAL AND INFANT END-OF-LIFE CARE

Advances in reproductive medicine have increased the number of infants born prematurely as well as the number of multiple births. These advances have increased the need for life-sustaining methods of care and have made decisions about when to use palliative care more complex. Some bioethicists believe that withholding life-sustaining interventions is appropriate under certain circumstances; others maintain that life-sustaining methods should not be used at all. An extensive study of attitudes among neonatologists about end-of-life decisions found no consensus about if and when to terminate life.

Most decisions to forego life-sustaining procedures for newborns concern those whose death is imminent. Even if their future quality of life is determined to be bleak, most physicians believe that some life is better than no life at all. Physicians who support withholding intensive care consider the following quality-of-life issues: (1) extent of bodily damage (e.g., severe neurological impairment), (2) the burden that a disabled child will place on the family, and (3) the ability of the child to derive some pleasure from existence (e.g., having an awareness of being alive and being able to form relationships).

The American Academy of Pediatrics permits nontreatment decisions for newborns when the infant is irreversibly comatose or when treatment would be futile and only prolong the process of dying. These standards do not permit the parents to have any input in the decision-making process. In a well-publicized case in England in 2000, it was decided to surgically separate conjoined twins knowing that one would die as a result of the procedure and despite the objections of the parents, who believed that nature should take its course even if that led to the death of both infants. Neonatal end-of-life decisions remain in a state of limbo. No clear-cut criteria exist about which patients should receive intensive care and which should receive palliative care.

CHILD END-OF-LIFE CARE

After accidents, cancer is the second most common cause of death in children. Although many childhood cancers are treatable, palliative care is necessary for children with cancers that are not. Children require more support than adults in coping with death. On average, a child does not view death as permanent until the age of about 10 years; before that, death is viewed as a sleep or separation. Therefore, children should be told only what they can understand; if they are capable, they should be involved in the decision-making process about treatment plans. Assurances that patients are pain free and physically comfortable are just as important for children as they are for adults.

A unique aspect of end-of-life care in children involves addressing their fear of being separated from their parents. It is helpful to have parents participate in end-of-life care tasks within their capacities. Family sessions with the child in attendance allow feelings to emerge and questions to be answered.

SPIRITUAL ISSUES

There is increasing awareness of the importance of this area to patients, families, and many staff members as well. Several studies have shown that religious beliefs are often associated with mature and active coping methods, and the field of psychological and spiritual interfaces in terminally ill patients is spawning a whole new area of psychological research within the traditional medical establishment. The psychiatric consultant should inquire about faith, its meaning, associated religious practices, and impact on the coping response. It can be a source of strength or guilt at all stages of the disease, ranging from the earliest "What did I do to cause this?" through "Will God give me only what I can carry?" to the poignant life review of the late stage. It is often a primary factor in the reactions to suicidality and in attitudes toward terminal care decisions. Mental health professionals should deal with these areas in an unself-conscious and noncondescending manner and work to help patients fully integrate this aspect of their personality into their current crisis. The professional should also work in harmony with the patient's spiritual guide if one is available. Sometimes an experienced, effective chaplain working with the appropriate patient can achieve positive results more directly than any psychotherapy. The following case exemplifies how creative pastoral care can relieve suffering.

A young woman was admitted to a hospice in a terminal state. She was experiencing a severe depression, which she attributed to not being able to see her oldest daughter receive her first communion. Arrangements were made for a ceremonial communion for her daughter to take place at the hospice. After the ceremony, the patient's mood improved markedly as one of her fears was alleviated and a religious need was satisfied. As her mood improved, she was able to address other unresolved issues and have quality visits with her children in her remaining days. (From O'Neil MT. Pastoral care. In: Cimino JE, Brescia MJ, eds. *Calvary Hospital Model for Palliative Care in Advanced Cancer.* Bronx, NY: Palliative Care Institute; 1998, with permission.)

ALTERNATIVE AND COMPLEMENTARY MEDICINE

Many patients, when they are told they are terminally ill, seek alternative treatments, ranging from innocuous programs aimed at enhancing general health to more aggressive, harmful, or fraudulent regimens. Although most patients combine the alternative and the traditional, a substantial number favor complementary medicine as the only treatment for their disease.

Complementary methods to cure terminal illness, especially cancer, emphasize a holistic approach, involving purification of the body, detoxification through internal cleansing, and attention to nutritional and emotional well-being. Despite their widespread appeal, not one of these methods has been demonstrated to cure cancer or prolong life, yet all have strong followings bolstered by anecdotal accounts of their efficacy. The popular metabolic therapy attributes cancer and other potentially fatal illnesses to toxins and waste materials accumulating in the body; treatment is based on reversing this process by diet, vitamins, minerals, enzymes, and colonic irrigations. Another approach includes macrobiotic diets or megavitamins to enhance the body's capacity to destroy malignancy. In 1987, the National Research Council recommended minimizing carcinogenic substances and fat in the diet and increasing whole-grain, fruit, and vegetable consumption as preventive guidelines. Psychological approaches cite maladaptive personality and coping styles as contributors to fatal diseases; treatment consists of shaping a positive attitude. Spiritual approaches aim at achieving harmony between the patient and nature. Some groups use spirituality as a way to ward off illness, which is sometimes seen as an external evil to be exorcised. Immunotherapies have gained popularity in recent years; cancer is attributed to a defective immune system, and restoration of immunocompetency is seen as the cure. Many patients find increased strength to endure the suffering of terminal illness with the help of alternative medicine even though the course of the disease may not be affected.

▲ 30.3 Euthanasia and Physician-Assisted Suicide

EUTHANASIA

From the Greek term for good death, *euthanasia* means compassionately allowing, hastening, or causing the death of another. Generally, someone resorts to euthanasia to relieve suffering, maintain dignity, and shorten the course of dying when death is inevitable. Euthanasia can be *voluntary* if the patient has requested it or *involuntary* if the decision is made against the patient's wishes or without the patient's consent. Euthanasia can be *passive*—simply withholding heroic lifesaving measures—or *active*—deliberately taking a person's life. Euthanasia assumes that the intent of the physician is to aid and abet the patient's wish to die.

Arguments for euthanasia revolve around patient autonomy and dignified dying. One of the most dramatic ways patients can exercise their right to self-determination is by asking that life-sustaining treatment to be withdrawn. If the patient is mentally competent, physicians must respect such wishes. Proponents of active, voluntary euthanasia argue that the same rights should be extended to patients who are not on life-sustaining treatment but also choose to have their physicians help them die.

Opponents of euthanasia also provide strong ethical and medical justification for their position. First, active euthanasia, even if the patient voluntarily requests it, is a form of killing and should never be sanctioned. Second, many patients who request aid in dying may be suffering from depression, which, when treated, will change the patient's mind about wanting to die.

Most medical, religious, and legal groups in the United States are against euthanasia. Both the American Psychiatric Association (APA) and the AMA condemn active euthanasia as illegal and contrary to medical ethics; however, few individuals have been convicted of euthanasia. Most physicians and medical groups in other parts of the world also oppose legalizing euthanasia. In the United Kingdom, for example, the British Medical Association believes that euthanasia is "alien to the traditional ethos and moral focus of medicine" and, if legalized, "would irrevocably change the context of health care for everyone, but especially for the most vulnerable."

The World Medical Association issued the following declaration on euthanasia in October 1987:

Euthanasia, that is, the act of deliberately ending the life of a patient, even at his own request or at the request of his close relatives, is unethical. This does not prevent the physician from respecting the will of a patient to allow the natural process of death to follow its course in the terminal phase of sickness.

Again, in 2002, the World Medical Association reissued a resolution condemning euthanasia as "unethical" and urging all doctors and medical associations to refrain from the practice.

Similarly, the New York State Committee on Bioethical Issues issued a statement declaring its opposition to euthanasia. The committee stated that the physician's obligation to relieve pain and suffering and to promote the dignity and autonomy of dying patients in their care, including providing effective palliative treatment, even though it may occasionally hasten death. Physicians, however, should not perform active euthanasia or participate in assisted suicide. The Committee believed that support, comfort, respect for patient autonomy, good communication, and adequate pain control would dramatically decrease the demand for euthanasia and assisted suicide. They argued that the societal risks of involving physicians in medical interventions to cause a patient's death were too great to condone active euthanasia or physician-assisted suicide. In response to shifting public opinion and lobbying groups with different views, state laws that banned physician-assisted death in Washington State and New York were sent to the United States Supreme Court, challenging the constitutionality of these prohibitions. In June

1997, the Court unanimously held that terminally ill patients do not have the right to physician aid in dying. The ruling, however, left room for continuing debate and future policy initiatives at the state level.

PHYSICIAN-ASSISTED SUICIDE

In the United States, most of the debate centers on physician-assisted suicide rather than on euthanasia. Some have argued that physician-assisted suicide is a humane alternative to active euthanasia in that the patient maintains more autonomy, remains the actual agent of death, and may be less likely to be coerced. Others believe that the distinctions are capricious in that the intent in both cases is to bring about a patient's death. Indeed, it may be difficult to justify providing a lethal dose of medication to a terminally ill patient (physician-assisted suicide) while ignoring the desperate pleas of another patient who may be even more ill and distressed but who cannot complete the act because of problems with swallowing, dexterity, or strength.

Several degrees are seen to which a physician may assist the suicidal patient to end his or her life. Physician-assisted suicide can involve providing information on ways of committing suicide, supplying a prescription for a lethal dose of medication or a means of inhaling a lethal amount of carbon monoxide, or perhaps even providing a suicide device that the patient can operate.

The controversy over physician-suicide came to national attention surrounding the activities of retired pathologist Jack Kevorkian, who, in 1989, provided his suicide machine to a 54-year-old woman with probable Alzheimer's disease. After the woman killed herself with his device, Kevorkian was charged with first-degree murder. The charges were later dismissed because Michigan had no law against physician-assisted suicide. Since that first case, Kevorkian assisted in several more suicides, often for persons he met on only a few occasions and frequently for persons who did not have a terminal illness. Claiming to have helped more than 130 people take their lives, Kevorkian was sent to prison in 1999, was released in 2006, and died in 2011. His attorneys and followers applauded his courage in easing pain and suffering; his detractors countered that he was a serial mercy killer. Opponents of Kevorkian's methods charged that, without safeguards, consultations, and thorough psychiatric evaluations, patients may search out suicide not because of terminal illness or intractable pain but because of untreated depressive disorders. They argued that suicide rarely occurs in the absence of psychiatric illness. Finding more effective treatments for pain and depression, rather than inventing more sophisticated devices to help desperate patients kill themselves, defines compassionate and effective physician care.

In 1994, Oregon passed a ballot initiative legalizing physician-assisted suicide (Death with Dignity Act), making Oregon the first state in the United States to permit assisted suicides (Table 30.3–1). An assessment of the first 4 years revealed the following: Patients dying from physician-assisted suicide represent approximately 8 of 10,000 deaths. The most common underlying illnesses were cancer, amyotrophic lateral sclerosis, and chronic lower respiratory disease. The three most common end-of-life concerns were loss of autonomy (85 percent), a decreasing ability to participate in activities that made life enjoyable (77 percent), and losing control of bodily functions (63 percent). Eighty percent of the patients were enrolled in hospice programs, and 91 percent died at home. The prescribing physician was present in 52 percent of the cases.

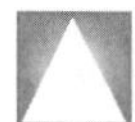

Table 30.3–1
Oregon's Assisted Suicide Law

The patient must be terminally ill and expected to die within 6 months; mentally competent; fully informed about his or her diagnosis, prognosis, risks, and alternatives, such as comfort care; and be making a voluntary choice.
A second doctor must agree that the patient is terminally ill, acting on his or her own free will, fully informed, and capable of making health care decisions.
If either doctor thinks that the patient is suffering from any form of mental illness that could affect his or her judgment, they must refer the patient for counseling.
The patient must make one written request and two spoken requests.
The doctor must ask the patient to tell the next of kin, but the patient may decide not to do so.
The patient is free to change his or her mind at any time.
There is a 15-day waiting period between the patient making the request and the doctor writing the prescription.
All information must be written down in the medical records.
Only people who normally live in Oregon may use the Act.
Mercy killing, lethal injection, and active euthanasia are not permitted.
Pharmacists must be told of the prescribed medication's ultimate use.
Physicians, pharmacists, and health care systems are under no obligation to participate in the Death with Dignity Act.

In 2001, Attorney General John Ashcroft attempted to prosecute Oregon doctors who helped terminally ill patients die, claiming that doctor-assisted suicide is not a legitimate medical purpose. The case was brought to the Supreme Court, which in 2006 supported the Oregon law and said the "authority claimed by the attorney general is both beyond his expertise and incongruous with the statutory purposes and design." Since 2001, three other states—Washington (2008), Montana (2009), and Vermont (2011)—have passed laws similar to the one in Oregon.

Despite the abhorrence that many physicians and medical ethicists express regarding physician-assisted suicide, poll after poll shows that as many as two-thirds of Americans favor the legalization of physician-assisted suicide in certain circumstances, and evidence even indicates that the formerly uniform opposition to physician-assisted suicide within the medical community has eroded. Consistent with their positions on active euthanasia, the AMA, APA, and American Bar Association, however, continue to oppose physician-assisted suicide. Recently, the American College of Physicians–American Society of Internal Medicine (ACP–ASIM) expressed its commitment to improving care for patients at the end of life while recommending against legalization of physician-assisted suicide. The ACP–ASIM believes physician-assisted suicide raises serious ethical concerns, undermines the physician–patient relationship and the trust necessary to sustain it, alters the medical profession's role in society, and endangers the values American society places on life, especially on the lives of disabled, incompetent, and vulnerable individuals.

The American Association of Suicidology in its 1996 *Report of the Committee on Physician-Assisted Suicide and Euthanasia* concluded that involuntary euthanasia can never be condoned; the report also stated, however, that "intolerable, prolonged suffering of persons in extremis should never be insisted upon, against their wishes, in single-minded efforts to preserve life at all cost." This position acknowledges that patients can die as a result of treatment given to them for the explicit purpose of relieving suffering, but death associated with palliative care differs greatly from physician-assisted suicide in that death is not the goal of treatment and is not intentional.

HOW TO DEAL WITH REQUESTS FOR SUICIDE

To help guide clinicians facing requests for physician-assisted suicide, the AMA's Institute for Ethics has proposed the following eight-step clinical protocol:

1. Evaluation of the patient for depression or other psychiatric conditions that could cause disordered thought.
2. Evaluation of the patient's "decision-making competence."
3. Discussion with the patient about his or her goals for care
4. Evaluation and response to the patient's "physical, mental, social, and spiritual suffering."
5. Discussion with the patient about the full range of treatment and care options.
6. Consultation by the attending physician with other professional colleagues.
7. Assurance that care plans chosen by the patient are being followed, including removal of unwanted treatment and the provision of adequate pain and symptom relief.
8. Discussion with the patient explaining why physician-assisted suicide is to be avoided and why it is not compatible with the principled nature of the care protocol.

Psychiatrists view suicide as an irrational act that is the product of mental illness, usually depression. In almost every case in which a patient asks to be put to death, a triad exists of depression associated with an incurable medical condition that causes the patient intolerable pain. In these instances, every effort should be made to provide antidepressants or psychostimulants for depression and opioids for pain. Psychotherapy, spiritual counseling, or both may also be needed. In addition, family therapy to help with the stress of dealing with a dying patient may be necessary. Family therapy is also useful because some patients may ask to be put to death because they do not wish to be a burden to their families; others may feel coerced by their families into believing that they are, or will be, a burden and may choose death as a result. Currently, no professional codes countenance euthanasia or assisted suicide in the United States. Therefore, psychiatrists must stand on the side of responsible rescue and treatment.

A distinction also is needed between major depression and suffering. The nature of suffering has not been sufficiently studied by psychiatrists. It remains the province of theologians and philosophers. Suffering is a complex mix of spiritual, emotional, and physical factors that transcends pain and other symptoms of terminal illness. Physicians are more skilled at dealing with depression than with suffering. Anatole Broyard, who chronicled his own death in his book *Intoxicated by My Illness,* wrote the following:

> I see no reason or need for my doctor to love me nor would I expect him to suffer with me. I wouldn't demand a lot of my doctor's time; I just wish he would brood on my situation for perhaps five minutes, that he would give me his whole mind just once, be bonded with me for a brief space, survey my soul as well as my flesh, to get at my illness, for each man is ill in his own way.

FUTURE DIRECTIONS

Advances in technology bring more complex medical, legal, moral, and ethical controversies regarding life, death, euthanasia, and physician-assisted suicide. Some forms of euthanasia have found a place in modern medicine, and expansion of the boundaries of patients' rights and their ability to choose the way they live and die are inevitable. Both patients and physicians need to be better educated about depression, pain management, palliative care, and quality of life. Medical schools and residency training programs need to give the topics of death, dying, and palliative care the attention they deserve. Society must ensure that economics, ageism, and racism do not get in the way of adequate and humane management of patients with chronic terminal illnesses. Finally, national health care policy must provide adequate insurance coverage, home care, and hospice services to all appropriate patients. If these mandates are followed, the argument for physician assistance in dying will lose much of its impact.

31

Public Psychiatry

INTRODUCTION

The subject area of public psychiatry embodies a fundamental core of experience and tradition. In the context of the reexamination of American health care initiated by the effect of managed care and the health care reform, the experience of public psychiatry is poised to serve as the foundation for a transformation of behavioral health care.

The term *public* can refer to psychiatric programs, treatment, or institutions paid for by public funds or as objects of public policy, whether paid for or not. The traditional concept of public psychiatry has been expanded to include medical and psychosocial initiatives directed for the public good, whether funded by public or private funds, and directed in particular to those who are economically disadvantaged.

The care and treatment offered under public psychiatry are delivered in a variegated mosaic of inpatient and community-based services that are more or less integrated into a coherent network sponsored by public agencies. Funding for public psychiatric services tends to be provided by federally legislated appropriations that are passed through state, county, and municipal government agencies (such as departments of mental health; substance use treatment services; children, youth, and family services; and public health, social services, education, adult corrections, and juvenile justice agencies). Ultimately, most public psychiatry and community services are provided by not-for-profit community mental health, substance use treatment, child guidance, or health care organizations that either are funded by or subcontracted to government agencies. Thus, the very existence of public and community psychiatric services and the policies and resources determining how they are delivered are extremely dependent on legislative mandates and fiscal appropriations from all levels of public government.

CONTEMPORARY PUBLIC AND COMMUNITY PSYCHIATRY

There are five themes around which the discussion of contemporary public and community psychiatry is structured: public health, public agencies, evidence-based psychiatry, roles for psychiatrists, and delivery systems.

Public Health

Public health is not simply publicly funded health care but is rather a specific discipline and tradition. It is a complicated field that historically has been defined negatively by the dominance of *personal health,* that is, the health care delivery systems that take care of individual patients. Until the advent of managed care in the 1990s, U.S. health care was an industry organized largely in terms of individual doctor-entrepreneurs. Each jurisdiction uniquely defined and organized its public health programs, and the particular pattern of personal health practices had substantial influence—hence the wide variation in public health programs. Nonetheless, as a discipline and tradition, public health's mission is to assure the conditions in which people can be healthy. Public health consists of organized community efforts aimed at the prevention of disease and the promotion of health. It involves many disciplines but rests on the scientific core of epidemiology. It provides an essential template for contemporary public and community psychiatry.

The Surgeon General's report on mental health underscored the necessity of a public health approach to care and rehabilitation for people experiencing mental illness that is "broader in focus than medical models that concentrate on diagnosis and treatment." Although diagnosis and treatment are core areas of expertise for all psychiatrists, the Surgeon General recommended that even when psychiatric diagnosis or treatment is the primary focus for practitioners, researchers, or educators, they should ground their professional activities in a vision and knowledge base that is "*population-based*... encompass[ing] a focus on epidemiologic surveillance, health promotion, disease prevention, and access to services." These fundamental public health functions define the public health perspective in public and community psychiatry. In the discussion that follows, these four public health components are framed in current terms of health care reform to define a coherent "public health" strategy for public and community psychiatry.

Health Promotion

Psychiatric professionals can contribute substantially to the promotion of public health by working with primary health care professionals and educators to identify and provide frontline treatment and referrals to adults and children who have undetected psychiatric symptoms, subthreshold syndromes, and psychiatric disorders. Collaborative care models bring psychiatric professionals into primary care and school settings as consultants for medical, nursing, and education professionals who work in those settings, as well as for educators and direct treatment providers to at-risk or psychiatrically impaired individuals.

Furthermore, people with identified mental illness or addictive disorders can benefit from enhanced physical and mental health care, as well as from the alleviation or management of psychiatric symptoms. Achieving or regaining physical or mental health (i.e., recovery) depends not only on genetic and biological factors but also on a person's or family's access to social and psychological resources and integration into supportive social networks. Illness management (also known as *disease management* or *chronic illness care management*) is a framework that has been adapted from medicine to guide mental health professionals in delivering services that go beyond traditional diagnostic treatment to promote the health and recovery of people with mental illness or addiction. *Illness management* has been defined as "professional-based interventions designed to help people collaborate with professionals in the treatment of their mental illness, reduce their susceptibility to relapses, and cope more effectively with their symptoms… [to] improve self-efficacy and self-esteem and to foster skills that help people pursue their personal goals." A number of approaches to illness management have been scientifically and clinically evaluated and have been found to enhance standard psychiatric treatment.

Prevention. Psychiatric disorders most often follow a course over time that begins with an often lengthy period in which prodromal or subthreshold symptoms or functional problems precede the full onset of a disorder with marked impairment. Intervention with adults, adolescents, or children who are not clinically impaired but who are at high risk (e.g., owing to a family history of psychiatric or addictive disorders or exposure to extreme stressors, such as violence, neglect, or the modeling of antisocial behavior) or who are manifesting preclinical symptoms or functional problems (e.g., periodic or pervasive dysphoria, problems with separation from caregivers, or involvement with deviant peers) is an approach to prevention that has been found to be cost effective because it targets a relatively small group of individuals in a timely manner.

Application of the traditional public health concepts of *primary, secondary,* and *tertiary psychiatry* has been confusing in psychiatry. *Primary prevention* involves addressing the root causes of illness with healthy individuals, with a goal of preventing illness before it occurs. *Secondary prevention* involves the early identification and early treatment of individuals with acute or subclinical disorders or *high-risk* persons to reduce morbidity. *Tertiary prevention* attempts to reduce the effects of a disorder on an individual through rehabilitation and chronic illness care management. The Institute of Medicine, in an effort to clarify different aspects of prevention, developed a classification system with three different categories. *Universal* interventions are those intended for the general public, such as immunizations or media campaigns providing information about illnesses, early warning signs, and resources for health promotion and timely treatment. *Selective* interventions focus on individuals at higher-than-average risk (e.g., persons with prodromal symptoms or a family history of psychiatric disorders) to reduce morbidity by enhancing resilience and preventing the onset of illness. *Indicated interventions* target individuals who are experiencing impairment as a result of illness as early as possible in the course of the illness, to reduce the burden of the illness on the individual, family, community, and treatment system. Psychiatric services most often take the form of indicated interventions, but the smaller number of psychiatric practitioners and researchers who conduct and evaluate selective or universal interventions in public and community settings is making a substantial contribution to the larger health of society.

Prevention interventions have been found to be effective with adults with a variety of risk factors or preclinical problems. For example, women who have been raped are less likely to develop posttraumatic stress disorder (PTSD) if they receive a five-session cognitive-behavioral treatment than if their recovery is left to chance. Men and women identified with subthreshold symptoms of depression by primary care medical providers are more likely to remain free from the full syndrome of depression if their standard medical treatment is enhanced by learning skills for coping actively with depressive symptoms or stressors. Prevention with adults must be judiciously designed to address the specific factors that place a person at risk for illness or that enhance the person's ability to cope effectively. For example, brief supportive meetings with people who have experienced a traumatic stressor (e.g., a mass disaster or life-threatening accident) tend to have little benefit and may inadvertently intensify posttraumatic stress, whereas a focused cognitive-behavioral approach to teaching skills for coping with traumatic memories and stress symptoms has been shown to be effective in preventing posttraumatic stress and depressive disorders with adult and child disaster or accident survivors.

A number of prevention programs have been developed and evaluated to address physical and mental health risks in childhood and adolescence, incorporating several elements that influence intervention effectiveness. Their broad and systematic implementation, however, has been halting. A number of states have made an effort to implement *school-based* interventions involving teachers and the peer group. These tend to be more effective than programs exclusively relying on intervening with parents or children alone. Such interventions in middle childhood have been successful in influencing peer group norms regarding alcohol and substance use, violence and bullying, and depression, thus achieving the dual outcome of reducing immediate initiation of alcohol and substance use and increasing the long-term support within the peer group for sustained abstinence into adolescence. Thus, systems-based *multimodal* interventions simultaneously targeting and developing enhanced relationships among the child, peer group, school personnel, parents, and the wider community tend to be most effective as universal or selected approaches to early prevention of what otherwise may become lifelong behavioral, legal, academic, and addictive problems.

Access to Effective Mental Health Care. Access is a serious problem for most people with severe mental illness or addictions. In the United States, the National Comorbidity Study (NCS) and the National Comorbidity Study-Replication (NCS-R) found that fewer than 40 percent of people with severe psychiatric disorders had received any mental health treatment in the previous year, and fewer than one in six (15 percent) had received minimally adequate mental health services. Young adults, African Americans, people residing in certain geographical areas, people with psychotic disorders, and patients treated by medical but not mental health providers were at highest risk for inadequate psychiatric treatment. Although income was not a predictor of inadequate treatment, it is likely that many of the people who did not receive adequate mental health services were uninsured or had insufficient insurance coverage for mental health conditions and had no viable source of mental health care other than through a medical provider or clinic or in the public mental health system.

Even when mental illness is identified, people with socioeconomic adversities often do not, or cannot, get adequate mental health services in their communities. For example, although it is estimated that more than 200,000 incarcerated adults in the United States have psychiatric disorders, few were detected or received treatment until they reached jail or prison. Federal and state correctional systems have instituted mental health screening and treatment programs to address psychiatric disorders as a health problem for incarcerated adults and to manage the problematic behavior that can occur in controlled settings as a result of mental illness. On returning to the community, the vast majority of prisoners with psychiatric disorders cease to receive more than minimal mental health services: A recent study found that fewer than one in six (16 percent—strikingly similar to the NCS finding) received steady mental health services, and only 1 in 20 with addictions received steady substance abuse recovery services. Thus, access to mental health and addiction treatment services is far better *in prison* than in the community! This has caused great concern because of the possibility that correctional facilities may be a de facto system of care for low-income people (often of minority backgrounds) with serious mental illness.

Evidence of serious and pervasive barriers to accessing mental health care can be found in several social crises. Poor children and adults increasingly are deferring physical and mental health care until illnesses become chronic and severe and then often do not know or cannot gain entry into any setting for services except public hospital emergency departments. Children with severe psychiatric or behavioral disorders are being held in emergency department facilities for days and even weeks because the staff cannot locate any treatment facilities with an appropriate level of care that have an opening or are willing to take the child as a patient (or accept the child or family's insurance coverage or lack thereof). People who cannot afford private services thus face daunting obstacles when seeking appropriate mental health care as a result of a serious underfunding of practitioners and programs. The economic forces and public policy dilemmas driven by the ever-increasing cost of health care bear directly on the field of public psychiatry, as well as the lives of tens or hundreds of thousands of people who do not receive adequate care.

Psychiatry and Public Agencies

Psychiatry's relationship to public sector agencies has, with some specific exceptions, been one of detachment because of the dominance of the private practice models before the advent of managed care and also largely because of the nature and structure of U.S. social welfare programs. This is a divide that often begins during academic preparation, in that many psychiatry training programs eschew meaningful rotations in public sector settings. In contrast to most industrial nations in which comprehensive social welfare reforms have been initiated, U.S. social welfare programs grew incrementally and categorically, that is, one category of service at a time. Large-scale initiatives, such as President Johnson's War on Poverty, have been implemented in piecemeal fashion by fragmented federal, state, and local government bureaucracies and have been vastly reduced through subsequent initiatives, such as the recent changes in federal regulations to "end welfare as we know it." Various social service agencies have been created through a process and set of alliances that has been called the *iron triangle.* Advocates form an organization to champion a particular cause, such as blindness, developmental disabilities, primary care, or mental health, among others. They find key legislative sponsors who advance the cause through legislation and appropriation. This creates a bureaucracy and bureaucrats that join the alliance. Through successive legislative sessions, the alliance of advocates, lawmakers, and bureaucrats builds a stronger and stronger categorical agency, for example, adults and families with dependent children or people with biologically based, severe mental illness. From the 1930s through the end of the 20th century, U.S. social welfare agencies were created on this pattern: The system has resulted in generous funding and hopeless fragmentation of services at local service delivery levels in which each agency depends on separate funding silos that also deliver conflicting rules and regulations.

It has been said that "mental health is not a place." Psychiatrists have a role at the receiving end of every categorical silo because the clients of each categorical agency experience mental illness or various addictions. Services for children with severe emotional, mental, or behavioral disturbances are a dramatic case. Five categorical agencies—child welfare, education, primary health, substance abuse, and juvenile justice—all have a responsibility to care for these children (and, indirectly, for their caregivers, including parents and families). Especially for the children with the most severe disabilities, the protective service worker taking a child into court, the special education teacher working day to day with the child, the juvenile probation officer, the substance abuse counselor, and the child's pediatrician all need the consultation and support of a skilled psychiatrist. The situation is similar for adults with severe mental illness, for whom case managers, vocational rehabilitation counselors, basic needs benefits specialists, social workers, psychotherapists, substance abuse counselors, parole or probation officers, legal conservators, visiting nurses, peer specialists, and physicians all may be mandated to deliver services.

Workforce Influences on Contemporary Practice

Shortages in the ranks of psychiatry have been well documented historically, and some project this to continue. However, as the field of psychiatry connects with its science and evidence base (e.g., neuroscience, genetics, pharmacology, outcomes science) while retaining its strength in the meaningful connection with patients and their families, some would argue that the reversal of the shortage trend has begun. The Decade of the Brain in the 1990s and the Decade of the Mind begun in the 2000s sponsored by the National Institutes of Health (NIH) contributed to this change. Medical students are increasingly stimulated to enter the field by recognizing the importance of psychiatry to health care in general, realizing that this is still a field in which the practitioner (and by extension the interdisciplinary team) is an instrument of change through integration of contemporary knowledge, skillful learned interactions with patients, and a willingness to commit to providing value. The national aggregate numbers, however, cannot adequately capture the extreme variations that exist geographically: Rural and frontier sites are dramatically more likely to experience shortages than more urban environments.

Because subsets of the public sector populations have special needs, responses to their needs have to be correspondingly tailored:

- ▲ Children and family needs are expressed differently than those for adults and require different responses.
- ▲ Mental illnesses have culturally driven ways of presenting, and interventions must be culturally competent.
- ▲ Issues of language (including American Sign Language with hearing-impaired individuals) can complicate diagnosis and treatment.
- ▲ The rapidly expanding elderly population will pose significant new challenges for effective treatment.

Just these few examples suggest the sophistication with which education and training must be engineered to meet the existing and changing demands of people in need of services.

Contemporary Evidence Base for Effective Public and Community Psychiatry

Since the 1980s, several structured interventions have been developed to address the gap between what historically has been taught in most psychiatry training programs—typically, an office-, clinic-, or hospital-based approach focusing on diagnoses and pharmacotherapy supplemented by psychotherapy—and the competencies required to deliver or to support the delivery of the full array of psychiatric rehabilitation services. Public and community approaches to psychiatric rehabilitation involve not only pharmacotherapy but also an array of complementary services that must be coordinated to assist people with severe mental illness or behavioral disorders and their families and support systems to manage symptoms, to access and use resources effectively, and to gain the greatest degree of autonomy in the least restrictive setting possible. The competences required to effect these interventions go beyond the scope of psychiatry, thus requiring that psychiatrists effectively collaborate with other rehabilitation and mental health specialists. Although psychiatrists rarely implement the educational, resource linkage, and psychotherapy interventions involved in these protocols, it is essential that the psychiatrist become aware of and be able to reinforce these interventions. Hence, familiarity with the manuals that describe how to implement these interventions with fidelity is strongly advised—and increasingly incorporated into psychiatry training.

Evidence-Based Manualized Interventions for Child Psychiatric Rehabilitation. Children with severe emotional disturbance and adolescents with severe behavioral disorders traditionally have been removed from their families and placed in restrictive psychiatric or juvenile justice settings (e.g., psychiatric inpatient wards, residential group homes, and juvenile detention centers). These placements separate the child from the natural family, school, peer group, and community environments, which may provide some benefit by reducing the child's exposure to addiction, conflict, violence, or deviant behavior. However, the placements also deprive the child and family of the opportunity to build better relationships with one another and with other children, families, teachers, and community groups. The second key ingredient to effective public and community child psychiatry comprises interventions that complement pharmacotherapy. Since the 1970s, several rehabilitative approaches for children with severe disorders (and their families) have been developed, tested, and disseminated in replicable manuals and training programs.

Implementation of evidence-based practices is not always easy and rarely occurs even in clinics and practice groups that are well trained and motivated to use evidence-based treatment models, given that most current systems of payment and service delivery were not designed to accommodate or support the use of science-based interventions such as those highlighted here. In addition, evidence-based dissemination and implementation strategies must be deliberately designed to support the initial adoption and sustained use of evidence-based mental health treatment models. For example, a recent study of the implementation of one of the most widely disseminated evidence-based mental health interventions for children and families, multisystemic therapy (MST), demonstrated that initial training yielded a very positive early rate of adoption of the program with good fidelity to the model, but only teams that were provided with regular ongoing supervision and support (for supervisors as well as therapists) from expert consultants were able to sustain the initial successes.

Roles of Psychiatrists in Public and Community Psychiatry Multidisciplinary Teams

Psychiatrists in the public sector rarely work in isolation. Most often, psychiatrists work within a team that includes professionals from several disciplines (e.g., psychology, social work, nursing, occupational therapy, rehabilitation or addiction counseling, social services, housing, and employment specialists) and nondegreed direct care workers (e.g., bachelor's degree–level counselors or case managers, high school graduate indigenous outreach workers, peer-support specialists, and family advocates), each of whom brings unique skills and experience to address the varied needs of people with severe and persistent mental illnesses. The team, rather than any single provider, assumes responsibility for the ongoing care of each patient across the many levels of services and often for many years. Its success is based on effective communication. Every communication should be explicitly focused on the *client's* (i.e., patient and family) *stated goals,* as well as on the team's technical and logistical issues, to maximize the client's motivation to participate actively and productively in all services by ensuring that the services truly are patient centered and collaborative.

Psychiatrists play three primary roles on multidisciplinary psychiatric rehabilitation teams: Conducting psychiatric evaluations, providing pharmacotherapy, and serving as the team's medical director (and, at times, as the administrative supervisor or team leader).

Psychiatric Evaluation and Diagnosis. In public and community settings and populations no less than in any other practice setting or patient population, the sine qua non is a thorough evaluation of all relevant history and systems and an accurate diagnosis. The goal of evaluation and diagnosis is to develop the most clinically effective individualized approach to treatment and rehabilitation for each patient. Psychiatric evaluations in public and community settings must include a careful review of the individual's psychosocial strengths and resources. The focus on strengths and resources often is lost or obscured when systemic factors (e.g., eligibility regulations for governmentally funded services or benefits) emphasize disability or limit the individual's or family's access to services or benefits (e.g., welfare-to-work regulations that place time or other eligibility restrictions on types of temporary aid, such as food stamps or vouchers for household supplies or housing).

Pharmacotherapy. The psychiatrist's most visible role usually is providing pharmacotherapy. The most difficult challenge in public sector mental health settings often is not the technical formulation of an effective medication regimen but instead the arranging of a plan of care so that the patient reliably follows the prescribed regimen (i.e., *adherence* or *compliance*). A recent review of interventions designed to enhance adherence to psychotropic medication regimens by patients with schizophrenia found that education alone often was the only strategy used even though it was less effective than approaches that focus on "concrete problem solving," "motivational techniques," and "reminders, self-monitoring tools, cues, and reinforcements" or that provide "an array of supportive and rehabilitative community-based services." Thus, although the psychiatrist must address technical medical issues accurately to formulate diagnoses and to establish an effective psychotropic regimen, effective pharmacotherapy depends heavily on providing—directly, in encounters with patients, or indirectly, by working closely with nonpsychiatric mental health professionals and nondegreed care workers—practical assistance to patients to enable them to anticipate and to manage the psychosocial stressors or problems that can render even the most technically sound medication regimen completely ineffective as a result of nonadherence by the patient.

Team Leadership. The psychiatrist also often plays a leadership role as the project or program medical director—with the attendant responsibilities of monitoring the medical safety and well-being of all patients and establishing or supporting management and clinical procedures that support quality of care and a cohesive treatment team. As the team leader or simply as a team member, the psychiatrist serves as a role model for compassionate and professional behavior in relation not only to patients but also to all other team members. Formal or informal leadership is especially important when psychiatry residents and medical students work on a team as a training experience. The team psychiatrist serves not only as a mentor and a role model for the core aspects of psychiatric practice but also to demonstrate the values and skills necessary to integrate psychiatry within the framework of multimodal community-based longitudinal psychosocial interventions.

Psychiatrists who work with persons with severe mental illness and who wish to contribute as key members or leaders of their teams must go beyond their prescription pads to acquire knowledge, attitudes, and skills congruent with contemporary practice guidelines for psychiatric rehabilitation; give respect and support to multidisciplinary team members and gain their respect and support in return; cope with large caseloads; collaborate with agencies and programs to ensure continuity, consistency, and coordination of care; and value the roles and expertise of staff who provide case management, supported employment, skills training, and family and housing supports. If psychiatrists can incorporate these attitudes and skills, they can expect reciprocity and cohesion from other team members, and clients will benefit. Surveys of psychiatrists in the public sector indicate that those who embrace the rehabilitation perspective by expanding their roles to be consultants and teachers for patients, families, trainees, and colleagues from other mental health disciplines are more satisfied professionally than those who focus on diagnosis and treatment alone.

New Paradigms. Virtually all health care should be integrated and coordinated to deliver effective, rational, and cost-efficient care. The broader, contemporary definition of care must include public health. In fact, linking public health models with acute care management, which, in turn, is coupled with chronic illness care management, rehabilitation, or recovery models, represents the continuum for an integrated system.

However, this continuum is insufficient without four other components: (1) the application of new research to improve care and the application of bench-to-bedside models to translational research, (2) meaningful involvement of patients and families in a shared decision-making paradigm, (3) integration with primary and specialty care systems, and (4) the development of the clinical system as a system of advocacy. Training preprofessionals in such a model is one approach to introduce meaningful and sustained change to health care and its delivery and is already operational in some systems.

New Models for Service Delivery and Treatment

Organized Systems of Care. The focus of reform has moved increasingly to coherent, efficient, and accountable delivery systems. The basic idea of the *system of care* for children with serious emotional disturbances can be described in two ways—in terms of interagency structures and in terms of clinical processes. Five categorical agencies in a given community form a *strong consortium* that targets a specific population of children (and their families) to whose needs none of the agencies can adequately respond on their own. The consortium agencies commit themselves to treat the child and family with a *common plan of care* and to find ways to pool their resources to do so appropriately. This often requires that in the central bureaucracies at the state level, a parallel interagency commitment be in place that supports the local system of care initiative, resolves any regulatory conflicts that may arise, and gives permission to innovative aspects of the delivery system. The collaborative interagency structure provides the resources and the flexibility for effective clinical work.

From the viewpoint of *clinical processes,* the system of care provides a full enactment of the traditional clinical practice that meets the requirements of medical quality assurance. What is different is that it is carried out in home and community settings, and it involves participants from different disciplines—child welfare, special education, and juvenile justice—in one standardized treatment methodology. The center of the system of care is the *child and family team* that is made up of the child and family, clinicians and agency representatives involved in the case, and significant supportive individuals identified by the child and family. Current issues are reviewed—strengths, problems, and needs—diagnostic issues are considered, clinical goals are articulated, and appropriate treatment strategies are identified. The expected outcome of each intervention is specified, and progress toward it is systematically charted. The system of care requires a full array of flexible services. The essential *starters* include clinical diagnostic services, care coordination or case management, crisis intervention services, and a flexible essential supportive service—child care specialists who can be assigned to support the child and family in any situation. Systems of care that have been particularly effective have relied on substantial community organization and collaboration or innovative funding models, or both, that blend or braid funding streams to focus on clear assignment of responsibility for a particular child and family, as well as adequate resources.

The basic model for community support for adults was called *assertive community treatment* (ACT). ACT was implemented with multidisciplinary teams with psychiatrists, nurses, psychologists, social workers, psychiatric aides, and paraprofessionals. The ACT team would assume the care of a designated number of adult patients with serious and persistent mental illness and would be available around the clock, 7 days a week. The team would help find housing, manage money, organize household routines, find social contacts, find work, and support the individual's adjustment to workplace settings. Concurrently, medications would be managed and help provided to facilitate an individual adjusting to community living. At the heart of the program was the basic clinical process that developed and maintained an individualized treatment plan, which was constantly adjusted to the changing needs of each client. The ACT model has been modified in various ways as it has been implemented in different states. Innovative funding models have been developed in several states by using bundled rates and case rates, which make it easier to implement and to sustain than traditional fee-for-service payment systems.

In contemporary managed care terms, ACT teams are *disease and disability management models* that assign accountability to provider systems that may not assume risk in managing community support of persons with disabling conditions. The National Alliance on Mental Illness (NAMI) has developed program models and protocols for the Program for Assertive Community Treatment (PACT) to encourage public agencies to contract for ACT services.

Effective Treatment Models. The previous discussions have outlined the various treatment models that have been introduced since the 1980s in the effort to establish an evidence base for the effectiveness of specific interventions and approaches to care. The attention to *evidence-based* treatment models has been a response to the call for quality and accountability for service outcomes demanded from health care services in general by purchasers and policy makers and part of an effort to cope with the difficulties of evaluating service delivery models or systems of care.

The movement to evidence-based services is necessary to break down components of the service delivery system to determine the relative effectiveness of specific service interventions using the evaluative tools and methods that are available. Eventually, the case will be made to address the larger policy questions concerning the value of coherent and rationally organized service delivery in mitigating the effects of mental disability on the development of the child and enabling the recovery process for adults with serious and persistent mental illness.

Chronic Illness Care Model: Psychiatry in the Context of Primary Care. Finally, the care of persons with long-term mental health problems is included in innovative developments in the provision of primary health care for persons with chronic illnesses (http://www.improvingchroniccare.org). The Health Resources Services Administration (HRSA), the federal agency responsible for the community health centers or Federally Qualified Health Centers (FQHCs), has adopted the chronic illness care model in its training and technical assistance efforts for community health centers. The model grows out of the current concern for quality of care and accountability for health care delivery systems for effective outcomes. Depression management is one of the four chronic health conditions that the HRSA has selected for its training collaborative.

The model begins with the assumption that the health care delivery system is part of a community context and must be responsive in its interactions with the community. Four areas of focus are essential in implementing the model in the health care delivery system: self-management support, delivery system design, decision support, and clinical tracking system. *Self-management support* gives patients a central role in determining their care, fostering a sense of responsibility for their health. Patients collaborate with the primary care team to establish goals, create treatment plans, and solve problems along the way. *Delivery system design* requires a reorganization of the way in which the health system operates, so that up-to-date information about a given patient is centralized, follow-up responsibility is assigned as a standard procedure, and so on. *Decision support* requires that treatment decisions are based on explicit, proven practice guidelines supported by at least one defining study. Guidelines are discussed with patients and providers, and treatment team members are constantly trained in the latest proven methods. Finally, *clinical tracking systems* track individual patients and populations of patients with similar problems. These systems must be practical and operational—able to check an individual's treatment at any point to confirm that the treatment conforms to recommended guidelines. The real integration of psychiatric care into primary care is an important innovation to consider that would improve physical health care for individuals with psychiatric disorders and eliminate the separation imposed by placing individuals with psychiatric problems into community mental health centers.

THE ROLE OF PUBLIC AND COMMUNITY PSYCHIATRY IN TWENTY-FIRST CENTURY HEALTH CARE

Public psychiatry emerged historically as an attempt to provide humane care for people with severe mental disabilities who did not have the resources to be protected from the stigma and approbation that shielded the so-called "eccentrics" and "black sheep" fortunate enough to have been born into the wealthier social strata. Community psychiatry evolved as an answer to concerns that public psychiatric treatment was a de facto form of marginalization and oppression, if not inhumane exile and imprisonment, of economically disadvantaged persons with mental illness. The great ideas of public psychiatry (e.g., providing compassionate respite and meaningful social and vocational rehabilitation) and community psychiatry (e.g., preserving social ties while providing evidence-based treatment) often are lost in the competition for scarce economic and political resources that faces every mental health, medical, and human service profession and organization in the early 21st century. The spirit and skills of advocacy that sparked the development and continue to characterize the best practices of public and community psychiatry, as well as the dedication to bring demonstrably effective services to the people who are most in need but are least served, have never been more needed by the entire mental health field.

32 ▲

Forensic Psychiatry and Ethics in Psychiatry

▲ 32.1 Forensic Psychiatry

The word *forensic* means belonging to the courts of law, and at various times, psychiatry and the law converge. Forensic psychiatry covers a broad range of topics that involve psychiatrists' professional, ethical, and legal duties to provide competent care to patients; the patients' rights of self-determination to receive or refuse treatment; court decisions, legislative directives, governmental regulatory agencies, and licensure boards; and the evaluation of those charged with crimes to determine their culpability and ability to stand trial. Finally, the ethical codes and practice guidelines of professional organizations and their adherence also fall within the realm of forensic psychiatry.

MEDICAL MALPRACTICE

Medical malpractice is a tort, or civil wrong. It is a wrong resulting from a physician's negligence. Simply put, negligence means doing something that a physician with a duty to care for the patient should not have done or failing to do something that should have been done as defined by current medical practice. Usually, the standard of care in malpractice cases is established by expert witnesses. The standard of care is also determined by reference to journal articles; professional textbooks, such as the *Comprehensive Textbook of Psychiatry;* professional practice guidelines; and ethical practices promulgated by professional organizations.

To prove malpractice, the plaintiff (e.g., patient, family, or estate) must establish by a preponderance of evidence that (1) a doctor–patient relationship existed that created a *duty* of care, (2) a *deviation* from the standard of care occurred, (3) the patient was *damaged,* and (4) the deviation *directly* caused the damage.

These elements of a malpractice claim are sometimes referred to as the *four Ds* (duty, deviation, damage, direct causation).

Each of the four elements of a malpractice claim must be present or there can be no finding of liability. For example, a psychiatrist whose negligence is the direct cause of harm to an individual (physical, psychological, or both) is not liable for malpractice if no doctor–patient relationship existed to create a duty of care. Psychiatrists are not likely to be sued successfully if they give advice on a radio program that is harmful to a caller, particularly if a caveat was given to the caller that no doctor–patient relationship was being created. No malpractice claim will be sustained against a psychiatrist if a patient's worsening condition is unrelated to negligent care. Not every bad outcome is the result of negligence. Psychiatrists cannot guarantee correct diagnoses and treatments. When the psychiatrist provides due care, mistakes may be made without necessarily incurring liability. Most psychiatric cases are complicated. Psychiatrists make judgment calls when selecting a particular treatment course among the many options that may exist. In hindsight, the decision may prove wrong but not be a deviation in the standard of care.

In addition to negligence suits, psychiatrists can be sued for the intentional torts of assault, battery, false imprisonment, defamation, fraud or misrepresentation, invasion of privacy, and intentional infliction of emotional distress. In an intentional tort, wrongdoers are motivated by the intent to harm another person or realize, or should have realized, that such harm is likely to result from their actions. For example, telling a patient that sex with the therapist is therapeutic perpetrates a fraud. Most malpractice policies do not provide coverage for intentional torts.

Negligent Prescription Practices

Negligent prescription practices usually include exceeding recommended dosages and then failing to adjust the medication level to therapeutic levels, unreasonable mixing of drugs, prescribing medication that is not indicated, prescribing too many drugs at one time, and failing to disclose medication effects. Elderly patients frequently take a variety of drugs prescribed by different physicians. Multiple psychotropic medications must be prescribed with special care because of possible harmful interactions and adverse effects.

Psychiatrists who prescribe medications must explain the diagnosis, risks, and benefits of the drug within reason and as circumstances permit (Table 32.1–1). Obtaining competent informed consent can be problematic if a psychiatric patient has diminished cognitive capacity because of mental illness or chronic brain impairment; a substitute health care decision maker may need to provide consent.

Informed consent should be obtained each time a medication is changed and a new drug is introduced. If patients are injured because they were not properly informed of the risks and consequences of taking a medication, sufficient grounds may exist for a malpractice action.

The question is often asked: How frequently should patients be seen for medication follow-up? The answer is that patients

Table 32.1–1
Informed Consent: Reasonable Information to Be Disclosed

Although there exists no consistently accepted standard for information disclosure for any given medical or psychiatric situation, as a rule of thumb, five areas of information are generally provided:

1. Diagnosis—description of the condition or problem
2. Treatment—nature and purpose of proposed treatment
3. Consequences—risks and benefits of the proposed treatment
4. Alternatives—viable alternatives to the proposed treatment, including risks and benefits
5. Prognosis—projected outcome with and without treatment

Table by RI Simon, M.D.

should be seen according to their clinical needs. No stock answer about the frequency of visits can be given. The longer the time interval between visits, however, the greater the likelihood of adverse drug reactions and clinical developments. Patients taking medications should probably not go beyond 6 months for follow-up visits. Managed care policies that do not reimburse for frequent follow-up appointments can result in a psychiatrist prescribing large amounts of medications. The psychiatrist is duty bound to provide appropriate treatment to the patient, quite apart from managed care or other payment policies.

Other areas of negligence involving medication that have resulted in malpractice actions include failure to treat adverse effects that have, or should have, been recognized; failure to monitor a patient's compliance with prescription limits; failure to prescribe medication or appropriate levels of medication according to the treatment needs of the patient; prescribing addictive drugs to vulnerable patients; failure to refer a patient for consultation or treatment by a specialist; and negligent withdrawal of medication treatment.

Split Treatment

In split treatment, the psychiatrist provides medication, and a nonmedical therapist conducts the psychotherapy. The following vignette illustrates a possible complication.

> A psychiatrist provided medications for a depressed 43-year-old woman. A master's level counselor saw the patient for outpatient psychotherapy. The psychiatrist saw the patient for 20 minutes during the initial evaluation and prescribed a tricyclic drug, and the patient was prescribed sufficient drugs for follow-up in 3 months. The psychiatrist's initial diagnosis was recurrent major depression. The patient denied suicidal ideation. Appetite and sleep were markedly diminished. The patient had a long history of recurrent depression with suicide attempts. No further discussions were held between the psychiatrist and the counselor, who saw the patient once a week for 30 minutes in psychotherapy. Within 3 weeks, after a failed romantic relationship, the patient stopped taking her antidepressant medication, started to drink heavily, and committed suicide with an overdose of alcohol and antidepressant drugs. The counselor and psychiatrist were sued for negligent diagnosis and treatment.

Psychiatrists must do an adequate evaluation, obtain prior medical records, and understand that no such thing as a partial patient exists. Split treatments are potential malpractice traps because patients can "fall between the cracks" of fragmented care. The psychiatrist retains full responsibility for the patient's care in a split treatment situation. This does not preempt the responsibility of the other mental health professionals involved in the patient's treatment. Section V, annotation 3 of the *Principles of Medical Ethics with Annotations Especially Applicable to Psychiatry,* states: "When the psychiatrist assumes a collaborative or supervisory role with another mental health worker, he/she must expend sufficient time to assure that proper care is given."

In managed care or other settings, a marginalized role of merely prescribing medication apart from a working doctor–patient relationship does not meet generally accepted standards of good clinical care. The psychiatrist must be more than just a medication technician. Fragmented care in which the psychiatrist only dispenses medication while remaining uninformed about the patient's overall clinical status constitutes substandard treatment that may lead to a malpractice action. At a minimum, such a practice diminishes the efficacy of the drug treatment itself or may even lead to the patient's failure to take the prescribed medication.

Split-treatment situations require that the psychiatrist remain fully informed of the patient's clinical status as well as the nature and quality of treatment the patient is receiving from the nonmedical therapist. In a collaborative relationship, the responsibility for the patient's care is shared according to the qualifications and limitations of each discipline. The responsibilities of each discipline do not diminish those of the other disciplines. Patients should be informed of the separate responsibilities of each discipline. The psychiatrist and the nonmedical therapist must periodically evaluate the patient's clinical condition and requirements to determine whether the collaboration should continue. On termination of the collaborative relationship, both parties treating the patient should inform the patient either separately or jointly. In split treatments, if the nonmedical therapist is sued, the collaborating psychiatrist will likely be sued also and vice versa.

Psychiatrists who prescribe medications in a split-treatment arrangement should be able to hospitalize a patient if it becomes necessary. If the psychiatrist does not have admitting privileges, prearrangements should be made with other psychiatrists who can hospitalize patients if emergencies arise. Split treatment is increasingly used by managed care companies and is a potential malpractice minefield.

PRIVILEGE AND CONFIDENTIALITY

Privilege

Privilege is the right to maintain secrecy or confidentiality in the face of a subpoena. Privileged communications are statements made by certain persons within a relationship—such as husband–wife, priest–penitent, or doctor–patient—that the law protects from forced disclosure on the witness stand. The right of privilege belongs to the patient, not to the physician, so the patient can waive the right.

Psychiatrists, who are licensed to practice medicine, may claim medical privilege, but privilege has some qualifications. For example, privilege does not exist at all in military courts, regardless of whether the physician is military or civilian and whether the privilege is recognized in the state in which the court martial takes place.

In 1996, the United States Supreme Court recognized a psychotherapist–patient privilege in *Jaffee v. Redmon*. Emphasizing the important public and private interests served by the psychotherapist–patient privilege, the Court wrote:

Because we agree with the judgment of the state legislatures and the Advisory Committee that a psychotherapist–patient privilege will serve a "public good transcending the normal predominant principle utilizing all rational means for ascertaining truth"... we hold that confidential communications between a licensed psychotherapist and her patients in the course of diagnosis or treatment are protected from compelled disclosure under Rule 501 of the Federal Rules of Evidence.

Confidentiality

A long-held premise of medical ethics binds physicians to hold secret all information given by patients. This professional obligation is called *confidentiality*. Confidentiality applies to certain populations and not to others; a group that is within the circle of confidentiality shares information without receiving specific permission from a patient. Such groups include, in addition to the physician, other staff members treating the patient, clinical supervisors, and consultants.

A subpoena can force a psychiatrist to breach confidentiality, and courts must be able to compel witnesses to testify for the law to function adequately. A subpoena ("under penalty") is an order to appear as a witness in court or at a deposition. Physicians usually are served with a *subpoena duces tecum*, which requires that they also produce their relevant records and documents. Although the power to issue subpoenas belongs to a judge, they are routinely issued at the request of an attorney representing a party to an action.

In bona fide emergencies, information may be released in as limited a way as feasible to carry out necessary interventions. Sound clinical practice holds that a psychiatrist should make the effort, time allowing, to obtain the patient's permission anyway and should debrief the patient after the emergency.

As a rule, clinical information may be shared with the patient's permission—preferably written permission, although oral permission suffices with proper documentation. Each release is good for only one piece of information, and permission should be reobtained for each subsequent release, even to the same party. Permission overcomes only the legal barrier, not the clinical one; the release is permission, not obligation. If a clinician believes that the information may be destructive, the matter should be discussed, and the release may be refused, with some exceptions.

Third-Party Payers and Supervision. Increased insurance coverage for health care is precipitating a concern about confidentiality and the conceptual model of psychiatric practice. Today, insurance covers about 70 percent of all health care bills; to provide coverage, an insurance carrier must be able to obtain information with which it can assess the administration and costs of various programs.

Quality control of care necessitates that confidentiality not be absolute; it also requires a review of individual patients and therapists. The therapist in training must breach a patient's confidence by discussing the case with a supervisor. Institutionalized patients who have been ordered by a court to get treatment must have their individualized treatment programs submitted to a mental health board.

Discussions about Patients. In general, psychiatrists have multiple loyalties: to patients, to society, and to the profession. Through their writings, teaching, and seminars, they can share their acquired knowledge and experience and provide information that may be valuable to other professionals and to the public. It is not easy to write or talk about a psychiatric patient, however, without breaching the confidentiality of the relationship. Unlike physical ailments, which can be discussed without anyone's recognizing the patient, a psychiatric history usually entails a discussion of distinguishing characteristics. Psychiatrists have an obligation not to disclose identifiable patient information (and, perhaps, any descriptive patient information) without appropriate informed consent. Failure to obtain informed consent could result in a claim based on breach of privacy, defamation, or both.

Internet and Social Media. It is imperative that psychiatrists and other mental health professionals be aware of the legal implications of discussing patients over the Internet. Internet communications about patients are not confidential, are subject to hacking, and are open to legal subpoenas. Some psychiatrists have blogged about patients thinking they were sufficiently disguised only to find that they were recognized by others, including the involved patient. Some professional organizations have electronic mailing lists in which they ask advice about patients from their colleagues or make referrals and in so doing provide detailed information about the patient that can easily be traced. Similarly, using social media to communicate about patients is equally risky.

Child Abuse. In many states, all physicians are legally required to take a course on child abuse for medical licensure. All states now legally require that psychiatrists, among others, who have reason to believe that a child has been the victim of physical or sexual abuse make an immediate report to an appropriate agency. In this situation, confidentiality is decisively limited by legal statute on the grounds that potential or actual harm to vulnerable children outweighs the value of confidentiality in a psychiatric setting. Although many complex psychodynamic nuances accompany the required reporting of suspected child abuse, such reports generally are considered ethically justified.

HIGH-RISK CLINICAL SITUATIONS

Tardive Dyskinesia

It is estimated that at least 10 to 20 percent of patients and perhaps as high as 50 percent of patients treated with neuroleptic drugs for more than 1 year exhibit some tardive dyskinesia. These figures are even higher for elderly patients. Despite the possibility for many tardive dyskinesia–related suits, relatively few psychiatrists have been sued. In addition, patients who develop tardive dyskinesia may not have the physical energy and psychological motivation to pursue litigation. Allegations of negligence involving tardive dyskinesia are based on a failure to evaluate a patient properly, a failure to obtain informed consent, a negligent diagnosis of a patient's condition, and a failure to monitor.

Suicidal Patients

Psychiatrists may be sued when their patients commit suicide, particularly when psychiatric inpatients kill themselves. Psychiatrists are assumed to have more control over inpatients, making the suicide preventable.

The evaluation of suicide risk is one of the most complex, dauntingly difficult clinical tasks in psychiatry. Suicide is a rare event. In our current state of knowledge, clinicians cannot accurately predict when or if a patient will commit suicide. No professional standards exist for predicting who will or will not commit suicide. Professional standards do exist for assessing suicide risk, but at best, only the degree of suicide risk can be judged clinically after a comprehensive psychiatric assessment.

A review of the case law on suicide reveals that certain affirmative precautions should be taken with a suspected or confirmed suicidal patient. For example, failing to perform a reasonable assessment of a suicidal patient's risk for suicide or implement an appropriate precautionary plan will likely render a practitioner liable. The law tends to assume that suicide is preventable if it is foreseeable. Courts closely scrutinize suicide cases to determine if a patient's suicide was foreseeable. *Foreseeability* is a deliberately vague legal term that has no comparable clinical counterpart, a common-sense rather than a scientific construct. It does not (and should not) imply that clinicians can predict suicide. Foreseeability should not be confused with preventability, however. In hindsight, many suicides seem preventable that were clearly not foreseeable.

Violent Patients

Psychiatrists who treat violent or potentially violent patients may be sued for failure to control aggressive outpatients and for the discharge of violent inpatients. Psychiatrists can be sued for failing to protect society from the violent acts of their patients if it was reasonable for the psychiatrist to have known about the patient's violent tendencies and if the psychiatrist could have done something that could have safeguarded the public. In the landmark case *Tarasoff v. Regents of the University of California,* the California Supreme Court ruled that mental health professionals have a duty to protect identifiable, endangered third parties from imminent threats of serious harm made by their outpatients. Since then, courts and state legislatures have increasingly held psychiatrists to a fictional standard of having to predict the future behavior (dangerousness) of their potentially violent patients. Research has consistently demonstrated that psychiatrists cannot predict future violence with any dependable accuracy.

The duty to protect patients and endangered third parties should be considered primarily a professional and moral obligation and, only secondarily, a legal duty. Most psychiatrists acted to protect both their patients and others threatened by violence long before *Tarasoff.*

If a patient threatens harm to another person, most states require that the psychiatrist perform some intervention that might prevent the harm from occurring. In states with duty-to-warn statutes, the options available to psychiatrists and psychotherapists are defined by law. In states offering no such guidance, health care providers are required to use their clinical judgment and act to protect endangered third persons. Typically, a variety of options to warn and protect are clinically and legally available, including voluntary hospitalization, involuntary hospitalization (if civil commitment requirements are met), warning the intended victim of the threat, notifying the police, adjusting medication, and seeing the patient more frequently. Warning others of danger, by itself, is usually insufficient. Psychiatrists should consider the *Tarasoff* duty to be a national standard of care, even if they practice in states that do not have a duty to warn and protect.

Tarasoff I. This issue was raised in 1976 in the case of *Tarasoff v. Regents of University of California* (now known as *Tarasoff I*). In this case, Prosenjiit Poddar, a student and a voluntary outpatient at the mental health clinic of the University of California, told his therapist that he intended to kill a student readily identified as Tatiana Tarasoff. Realizing the seriousness of the intention, the therapist, with the concurrence of a colleague, concluded that Poddar should be committed for observation under a 72-hour emergency psychiatric detention provision of the California commitment law. The therapist notified the campus police, both orally and in writing, that Poddar was dangerous and should be committed.

Concerned about the breach of confidentiality, the therapist's supervisor vetoed the recommendation and ordered all records relating to Poddar's treatment destroyed. At the same time, the campus police temporarily detained Poddar but released him on his assurance that he would "stay away from that girl." Poddar stopped going to the clinic when he learned from the police about his therapist's recommendation to commit him. Two months later, he carried out his previously announced threat to kill Tatiana. The young woman's parents thereupon sued the university for negligence.

As a consequence, the California Supreme Court, which deliberated the case for the unprecedented time of about 14 months, ruled that a physician or a psychotherapist who has reason to believe that a patient may injure or kill someone warn the potential victim.

The discharge of the duty imposed on the therapist to warn intended victims against danger may take one or more forms, depending on the case. Therefore, stated the court, it may call for the therapist to notify the intended victim or others likely to notify the victim of the danger, to notify the police, or to take whatever other steps are reasonably necessary under the circumstances.

The *Tarasoff I* ruling does not require therapists to report a patient's fantasies; instead, it requires them to report an intended homicide, and it is the therapist's duty to exercise good judgment.

Tarasoff II. In 1982, the California Supreme Court issued a second ruling in the case of *Tarasoff v. Regents of University of California* (now known as *Tarasoff II*), which broadened its earlier ruling extending the duty to warn to include the duty to protect.

The *Tarasoff II* ruling has stimulated intense debates in the medicolegal field. Lawyers, judges, and expert witnesses argue the definition of protection, the nature of the relationship between the therapist and the patient, and the balance between public safety and individual privacy.

Clinicians argue that the duty to protect hinders treatment because a patient may not trust a doctor if confidentiality is not maintained. Furthermore, because it is not easy to determine whether a patient is sufficiently dangerous to justify long-term incarceration, unnecessary involuntary hospitalization may occur because of a therapist's defensive practices.

As a result of such debates in the medicolegal field, since 1976, the state courts have not made a uniform interpretation of the *Tarasoff II* ruling (the duty to protect). Generally, clinicians should note whether a specific identifiable victim seems to be in imminent and probable danger from the threat of an action contemplated by a mentally ill patient; the harm, in addition to being imminent, should be potentially serious or severe. Usually, the patient must be a danger to another person and not to property; the therapist should take clinically reasonable action.

HOSPITALIZATION

All states provide for some form of involuntary hospitalization. Such action usually is taken when psychiatric patients present a danger to themselves or others in their environment to the extent that their urgent need for treatment in a closed institution is evident. Certain states allow involuntary hospitalization when patients are unable to care for themselves adequately.

The doctrine of *parens patriae* allows the state to intervene and to act as a surrogate parent for those who are unable to care for themselves or who may harm themselves. In English common law, *parens patriae* ("father of his country") dates to the time of King Edward I and originally referred to a monarch's duty to protect the people. In U.S. common law, the doctrine has been transformed into a paternalism in which the state acts for persons who are mentally ill and for minors.

The statutes governing hospitalization of persons who are mentally ill generally have been designated commitment laws, but psychiatrists have long considered the term to be undesirable. *Commitment* legally means a warrant for imprisonment. The American Bar Association and the American Psychiatric Association (APA) have recommended that the term *commitment* be replaced by the less offensive and more accurate term *hospitalization,* which most states have adopted. Although this change in terminology does not correct the punitive attitudes of the past, the emphasis on hospitalization is in keeping with psychiatrists' views of treatment rather than punishment.

Procedures of Admission

Four procedures of admission to psychiatric facilities have been endorsed by the American Bar Association to safeguard civil liberties and to make sure that no person is railroaded into a mental hospital. Although each of the 50 states has the power to enact its own laws on psychiatric hospitalization, the procedures outlined here are gaining much acceptance.

Informal Admission. Informal admission operates on the general hospital model, in which a patient is admitted to a psychiatric unit of a general hospital in the same way that a medical or surgical patient is admitted. Under such circumstances, the ordinary doctor–patient relationship applies, with the patient free to enter and to leave, even against medical advice.

Voluntary Admission. In cases of voluntary admission, patients apply in writing for admission to a psychiatric hospital. They may come to the hospital on the advice of a personal physician, or they may seek help on their own. In either case, patients are admitted if an examination reveals the need for hospital treatment. The patient is free to leave, even against medical advice.

Temporary Admission. Temporary admission is used for patients who are so senile or so confused that they require hospitalization and are not able to make decisions on their own and for patients who are so acutely disturbed that they must be admitted immediately to a psychiatric hospital on an emergency basis. Under the procedure, a person is admitted to the hospital on the written recommendation of one physician. After the patient has been admitted, the need for hospitalization must be confirmed by a psychiatrist on the hospital staff. The procedure is temporary because patients cannot be hospitalized against their will for more than 15 days.

Involuntary Admission. Involuntary admission involves the question of whether patients are suicidal and thus a danger to themselves or homicidal and thus a danger to others. Because these persons do not recognize their need for hospital care, the application for admission to a hospital may be made by a relative or a friend. After the application is made, the patient must be examined by two physicians, and if both physicians confirm the need for hospitalization, the patient can then be admitted.

Involuntary hospitalization involves an established procedure for written notification of the next of kin. Furthermore, the patients have access at any time to legal counsel, who can bring the case before a judge. If the judge does not think that hospitalization is indicated, the patient's release can be ordered.

Involuntary admission allows a patient to be hospitalized for 60 days. After this time, if the patient is to remain hospitalized, the case must be reviewed periodically by a board consisting of psychiatrists, nonpsychiatric physicians, lawyers, and other citizens not connected with the institution. In New York State, the board is called the Mental Health Information Service.

Persons who have been hospitalized involuntarily and who believe that they should be released have the right to file a petition for a writ of habeas corpus. Under law, a writ of habeas corpus can be proclaimed by those who believe that they have been illegally deprived of liberty. The legal procedure asks a court to decide whether a patient has been hospitalized without due process of law. The case must be heard by a court at once, regardless of the manner or the form in which the motion is filed. Hospitals are obligated to submit the petitions to the court immediately.

RIGHT TO TREATMENT

Among the rights of patients, the right to the standard quality of care is fundamental. This right has been litigated in highly publicized cases in recent years under the slogan of "right to treatment."

In 1966, Judge David Bazelon, speaking for the District of Columbia Court of Appeals in *Rouse v. Cameron,* noted that the purpose of involuntary hospitalization is treatment and concluded that the absence of treatment draws into question the constitutionality of the confinement. Treatment in exchange for liberty is the logic of the ruling. In this case, the patient was discharged on a writ of habeas corpus, the basic legal remedy to ensure liberty. Judge Bazelon further held that if alternative treatments that infringe less on personal liberty are available, involuntary hospitalization cannot take place.

Alabama Federal Court Judge Frank Johnson was more venturesome in the decree he rendered in 1971 in *Wyatt v. Stickney.* The *Wyatt* case was a class-action proceeding brought under newly developed rules that sought not release but treatment. Judge Johnson ruled that persons civilly committed to a mental institution have a constitutional right to receive such individual treatment as will give them a reasonable opportunity to be cured or to have their mental condition improved. Judge Johnson set out minimal requirements for staffing, specified physical facilities, and nutritional standards and required individualized treatment plans.

The new codes, more detailed than the old ones, include the right to be free from excessive or unnecessary medication; the right to privacy and dignity; the right to the least restrictive environment; the unrestricted right to be visited by attorneys, clergy, and private physicians; and the right not to be subjected to lobotomies, electroconvulsive treatments, and other procedures without fully informed consent. Patients can be required to perform therapeutic tasks but not hospital chores unless they volunteer for them and are paid the federal minimum wage. This requirement is an attempt to eliminate the practice of peonage, in which psychiatric patients were forced to work at menial tasks, without payment, for the benefit of the state.

In a number of states today, medication or electroconvulsive therapy cannot be forcibly administered to a patient without first obtaining court approval, which may take as long as 10 days.

RIGHT TO REFUSE TREATMENT

The right to refuse treatment is a legal doctrine that holds that, except in emergencies, persons cannot be forced to accept treatment against their will. An emergency is defined as a condition in clinical practice that requires immediate intervention to prevent death or serious harm to the patient or another person or to prevent deterioration of the patient's clinical state.

In the 1976 case of *O'Connor v. Donaldson,* the Supreme Court of the United States ruled that harmless mentally ill patients cannot be confined against their will without treatment if they can survive outside. According to the Court, a finding of mental illness alone cannot justify a state's confining persons in a hospital against their will. Instead, involuntarily confined patients must be considered dangerous to themselves or others or possibly so unable to care for themselves that they cannot survive outside. As a result of the 1979 case of *Rennie v. Klein,* patients have the right to refuse treatment and to use an appeal process. As a result of the 1981 case of *Roger v. Oken,* patients have an absolute right to refuse treatment, but a guardian may authorize treatment.

Questions have been raised about psychiatrists' ability to accurately predict dangerousness to self or others and about the risk to psychiatrists, who may be sued for monetary damages if persons who are involuntarily hospitalized are thereby deprived of their civil rights.

CIVIL RIGHTS OF PATIENTS

Because of several clinical, public, and legal movements, criteria for the civil rights of persons who are mentally ill, apart from their rights as patients, have been both established and affirmed.

Least Restrictive Alternative

The principle holds that patients have the right to receive the least restrictive means of treatment for the requisite clinical effect. Therefore, if a patient can be treated as an outpatient, commitment should not be used; if a patient can be treated on an open ward, seclusion should not be used.

Although apparently fairly straightforward on first reading, difficulty arises when clinicians attempt to apply the concept to choose among involuntary medication, seclusion, and restraint as the intervention of choice. Distinguishing among these interventions on the basis of restrictiveness proves to be a purely subjective exercise fraught with personal bias. Moreover, each of these three interventions is both more and less restrictive than each of the other two. Nevertheless, the effort should be made to think in terms of restrictiveness when deciding how to treat patients.

Visitation Rights

Patients have the right to receive visitors and to do so at reasonable hours (customary hospital visiting hours). Allowance must be made for the possibility that, at certain times, a patient's clinical condition may not permit visits. This fact should be clearly documented, however, because such rights must not be suspended without good reason.

Certain categories of visitors are not limited to the regular visiting hours; these include a patient's attorney, private physician, and members of the clergy—all of whom, broadly speaking, have unrestricted access to the patient, including the right to privacy in their discussions. Even here, a bona fide emergency may delay such visits. Again, the patient's needs come first. Under similar reasoning, certain noxious visits may be curtailed (e.g., a patient's relative bringing drugs into the ward).

Communication Rights

Patients should generally have free and open communication with the outside world by telephone or mail, but this right varies regionally to some degree. Some jurisdictions charge the hospital administration with a responsibility for monitoring the communications of patients. In some areas, hospitals are expected to make available reasonable supplies of paper, envelopes, and stamps for patient's use.

Specific circumstances affect communication rights. A patient who is hospitalized in relation to a criminal charge of making harassing or threatening phone calls should not be given unrestricted access to the telephone, and similar considerations apply to mail. As a rule, however, patients should be allowed private telephone calls, and their incoming and outgoing mail should not be opened by hospital staff members.

Private Rights

Patients have several rights to privacy. In addition to confidentiality, they are allowed private bathroom and shower space,

Table 32.1–2
Indications and Contraindications for Seclusion and Restraint

Indications
Prevent clear, imminent harm to the patient or others
Prevent significant disruption to treatment program or physical surroundings
Assist in treatment as part of ongoing behavior therapy
Decrease sensory overstimulation[a]
Patient's voluntary reasonable request
Contraindications
Extremely unstable medical and psychiatric conditions[b]
Delirious or demented patients who are unable to tolerate decreased stimulation[b]
Overtly suicidal patients[b]
Patients with severe drug reactions or overdoses or who require close monitoring of drug dosages[b]
For punishment or convenience of staff

[a]Seclusion only.
[b]Unless close supervision and direct observation are provided.
Data from The Psychiatric Uses of Seclusion and Restraint (Task Force Report No. 22). Washington, DC: American Psychiatric Association.

secure storage space for clothing and other belongings, and adequate floor space per person. They also have the right to wear their own clothes and to carry their own money.

Economic Rights

Apart from special considerations related to incompetence, psychiatric patients generally are permitted to manage their own financial affairs. One feature of this fiscal right is the requirement that patients be paid if they work in the institution (e.g., gardening or preparing food). This right often creates tension between the valid therapeutic need for activity, including jobs, and exploitative labor. A consequence of this tension is that valuable occupational, vocational, and rehabilitative therapeutic programs may have to be eliminated because of the failure of legislatures to supply the funding to pay wages to patients who participate in these programs.

SECLUSION AND RESTRAINT

Seclusion and restraint raise complex psychiatric legal issues. Seclusion and restraint have both indications and contraindications (Table 32.1–2). Seclusion and restraint have become increasingly regulated over the past decade.

Legal challenges to the use of restraints and seclusion have been brought on behalf of institutionalized persons with psychiatric illnesses or cognitive disabilities. Typically, these lawsuits do not stand alone but are part of a challenge to a wide range of alleged abuses.

Generally, courts hold, or consent decrees provide, that restraints and seclusion be implemented only when a patient creates a risk of harm to self or others and no less restrictive alternative is available. Table 32.1–3 lists additional restrictions.

INFORMED CONSENT

Lawyers representing an injured claimant now invariably add to a claim of negligent performance of procedures (malpractice) an informed consent claim as another possible area of liability.

Table 32.1–3
Restrictions for Seclusion and Restraint

Restraints and seclusion can be implemented only when a patient creates a risk of harm to self or others and no less restrictive alternative is available.
Restraint and seclusion can only be implemented by a written order from an appropriate medical official.
Orders are to be confined to specific, time-limited periods.
A patient's condition must be regularly reviewed and documented.
Any extension of an original order must be reviewed and reauthorized.

Ironically, this is one claim under which the requirement of expert testimony may be avoided. The usual claim of medical malpractice requires the litigant to produce an expert to establish that the defendant physician departed from accepted medical practice. But in a case in which the physician did not obtain informed consent, the fact that the treatment was technically well performed, was in accord with the generally accepted standard of care, and effected a complete cure is immaterial. As a practical matter, however, unless the treatment had adverse consequences, a complainant will not get far with a jury in an action based solely on an allegation that the treatment was performed without consent.

In the case of minors, the parent or guardian is legally empowered to give consent to medical treatment. By statute, most states, however, list specific diseases and conditions that a minor can consent to have treated—including venereal disease, pregnancy, substance dependence, alcohol abuse, and contagious diseases. In an emergency, a physician can treat a minor without parental consent. The trend is to adopt the so-called mature minor rule, which allows minors to consent to treatment under ordinary circumstances. As a result of the Supreme Court's 1967 *Gault* decision, all juveniles must now be represented by counsel, must be able to confront witnesses, and must be given proper notice of any charges. Emancipated minors have the rights of an adult when it can be shown that they are living as adults with control over their own lives.

Consent Form

The basic elements of a consent form should include a fair explanation of the procedures to be followed and their purposes, including identification of any procedures that are experimental, a description of any attendant discomforts and risks reasonably to be expected, a description of any benefits reasonably to be expected, a disclosure of any appropriate alternative procedures that may be advantageous to the patient, an offer to answer any inquiries concerning the procedures, and an instruction that the patient is free to withdraw patient consent and to discontinue participation in the project or activity at any time without prejudice.

Some theorists have suggested that the form can be replaced by a standardized discussion that covers the issues noted above and a progress note that documents that the issues were discussed.

CHILD CUSTODY

The action of a court in a child custody dispute is now predicated on the child's best interests. The maxim reflects the idea that a natural parent does not have an inherent right to be named a custodial parent, but the presumption, although a bit eroded, remains in favor of the mother in the case of young children. As a rule, the courts presume that the welfare of a child of tender years generally is best served by maternal custody when the mother is a good and fit parent. The best interest of the mother may be served by naming her as the custodial parent because a mother may never resolve the effects of the loss of a child, but her best interest is not to be equated ipso facto with the best interest of the child. Care and protection proceedings are the court's interventions in the welfare of a child when the parents are unable to care for the child.

More fathers are asserting custodial claims. In about 5 percent of all cases, fathers are named custodians. The movement supporting women's rights also is enhancing the chances of paternal custody. With more women going to work outside the home, the traditional rationale for maternal custody has less force today than it did in the past.

Currently, every state has a statute allowing a court, usually a juvenile court, to assume jurisdiction over a neglected or abused child and to remove the child from parental custody. It usually orders that the care and custody of the child be supervised by the welfare or probation department.

TESTAMENTARY AND CONTRACTUAL CAPACITY AND COMPETENCE

Psychiatrists may be asked to evaluate patients' testamentary capacities or their competence to make a will. Three psychological abilities are necessary to prove this competence. Patients must know the nature and the extent of their bounty (property), the fact that they are making a bequest, and the identities of their natural beneficiaries (spouse, children, and other relatives).

When a will is being probated, one of the heirs or another person may challenge its validity. A judgment in such cases must be based on a reconstruction, using data from documents and from expert psychiatric testimony, of the testator's mental state at the time the will was written. When a person is unable to, or does not exercise the right to, make a will, the law in all states provides for the distribution of property to the heirs. If there are no heirs, the estate goes to the public treasury.

Witnesses at the signing of a will, who might include a psychiatrist, may attest that the testator was rational at the time the will was executed. In unusual cases, a lawyer may videotape the signing to safeguard the will from attack. Ideally, persons who are thinking of making a will and believe that questions might be raised about their testamentary competence hire a forensic psychiatrist to perform a dispassionate examination antemortem to validate and record their capacity.

An incompetence proceeding and the appointment of a guardian may be considered necessary when a family member is spending the family's assets and the property is in danger of dissipation, as in the case of patients who are elderly, have cognitive disabilities, are dependent on alcohol, or have psychosis. At issue is whether such persons are capable of managing their own affairs. A guardian appointed to take control of the property of one deemed incompetent, however, cannot make a will for the ward (the incompetent person).

Competence is determined on the basis of a person's ability to make a sound judgment—to weigh, to reason, and to make reasonable decisions. Competence is task specific, not general; the capacity to weigh decision-making factors (competence) often is best demonstrated by a person's ability to ask pertinent and knowledgeable questions after the risks and the benefits have been explained. Although physicians (especially psychiatrists) often give opinions on competence, only a judge's ruling converts the opinion into a finding; a patient is not competent or incompetent until the court so rules. The diagnosis of a mental disorder is not, in itself, sufficient to warrant a finding of incompetence. Instead, the mental disorder must cause an impairment in judgment for the specific issues involved. After they have been declared incompetent, persons are deprived of certain rights: they cannot make contracts, marry, start a divorce action, drive a vehicle, handle their own property, or practice their professions. Incompetence is decided at a formal courtroom proceeding, and the court usually appoints a guardian who will best serve a patient's interests. Another hearing is necessary to declare a patient competent. Admission to a mental hospital does not automatically mean that a person is incompetent.

Competence also is essential in contracts because a contract is an agreement between parties to do a specific act. A contract is declared invalid if, when it was signed, one of the parties was unable to comprehend the nature and effect of his or her act. The marriage contract is subject to the same standard and thus can be voided if either party did not understand the nature, duties, obligations, and other characteristics entailed at the time of the marriage. In general, however, the courts are unwilling to declare a marriage void on the basis of incompetence.

Whether competence is related to wills, contracts, or the making or breaking of marriages, the fundamental concern is a person's state of awareness and capacity to comprehend the significance of the particular commitment made.

Durable Power of Attorney

A modern development that permits persons to make provisions for their own anticipated loss of decision-making capacity is called a *durable power of attorney.* The document permits the advance selection of a substitute decision maker who can act without the necessity of court proceedings when the signatory becomes incompetent through illness or progressive dementia.

CRIMINAL LAW

Competence to Stand Trial

The Supreme Court of the United States stated that the prohibition against trying someone who is mentally incompetent is fundamental to the US system of justice. Accordingly, the Court, in *Dusky v. United States,* approved a test of competence that seeks to ascertain whether a criminal defendant "has sufficient present ability to consult with his lawyer with a reasonable degree of rational understanding—and whether he has a rational as well as factual understanding of the proceedings against him."

Competence to Be Executed

One of the new areas of competence to emerge in the interface between psychiatry and the law is the question of a person's competence to be executed. The requirement for competence in this area is believed to rest on three general principles. First, a person's awareness of what is happening is supposed to heighten the retributive element of the punishment. Punishment is meaningless unless the person is aware of it and knows the punishment's purpose. Second, a competent person who is about to be executed is believed to be in the best position to make whatever peace is appropriate with his or her religious beliefs, including confession and absolution. Third, a competent person who is about to be executed preserves, until the end, the possibility (admittedly slight) of recalling a forgotten detail of the events or the crime that may prove exonerating.

The need to preserve competence was supported recently in the Supreme Court case of *Ford v. Wainwright.* But no matter the outcome of legal struggles with this question, most medical bodies have gravitated toward the position that it is unethical for any clinician to participate, no matter how remotely, in state-mandated executions; a physician's duty to preserve life transcends all other competing requirements. Major medical societies, such as the American Medical Association (AMA), believe that doctors should not participate in the death penalty. A psychiatrist who agrees to examine a patient slated for execution may find the person incompetent on the basis of a mental disorder and may recommend a treatment plan, which, if implemented, would ensure the person's fitness to be executed. Although room exists for a difference of opinion regarding whether or not a psychiatrist should become involved, the authors of this text believe such involvement to be wrong.

Criminal Responsibility

According to criminal law, committing an act that is socially harmful is not the sole criterion of whether a crime has been committed. Instead, the objectionable act must have two components: voluntary conduct (*actus reus*) and evil intent (*mens rea*). An evil intent cannot exist when an offender's mental status is so deficient, so abnormal, or so diseased to have deprived the offender of the capacity for rational intent. The law can be invoked only when an illegal intent is implemented. Neither behavior, however harmful, nor the intent to do harm is, in itself, a ground for criminal action.

M'Naghten Rule. The precedent for determining legal responsibility was established in 1843 in the British courts. The so-called M'Naghten rule, which, until recently, has determined criminal responsibility in most of the United States, holds that persons are not guilty by reason of insanity if they labored under a mental disease such that they were unaware of the nature, the quality, and the consequences of their acts or if they were incapable of realizing that their acts were wrong. Moreover, to absolve persons from punishment, a delusion used as evidence must be one that, if true, would be an adequate defense. If the delusional idea does not justify the crime, such persons are presumably held responsible, guilty, and punishable. The M'Naghten rule is known commonly as the right–wrong test.

The M'Naghten rule derives from the famous M'Naghten case of 1843. When Daniel M'Naghten murdered Edward Drummond, the private secretary of Robert Peel, M'Naghten had been suffering from delusions of persecution for several years, had complained too many persons about his "persecutors," and finally had decided to correct the situation by murdering Robert Peel. When Drummond came out of Peel's home, M'Naghten shot Drummond, mistaking him for Peel. The jury, as instructed under the prevailing law, found M'Naghten not guilty by reason of insanity. In response to questions about what guidelines could be used to determine whether a person could plead insanity as a defense against criminal responsibility, the English chief judge wrote:

1. To establish a defense on the ground of insanity, it must be clearly proved that, at the time of committing the act, the party accused was laboring under such a defect of reason, from disease of the mind, as not to know the nature and quality of the act he was doing, or if he did know it, he did not know he was doing what was wrong.
2. Where a person labors under partial delusions only and is not in other respects insane and as a result commits an offense, he must be considered in the same situation regarding responsibility as if the facts with respect to which the delusion exists were real.

According to the M'Naghten rule, the question is not whether the accused knows the difference between right and wrong in general; rather, it is whether the defendant understood the nature and the quality of the act and whether the defendant knew the difference between right and wrong with respect to the act—that is, specifically whether the defendant knew the act was wrong or perhaps thought the act was correct, a delusion causing the defendant to act in legitimate self-defense.

Jeffery Dahmer killed 17 young men and boys between June 1978 and July 1991. Most of his victims were either homosexual or bisexual. He would meet and select his prey at gay bars or bathhouses and then lure them by offering them money for posing for photographs or simply to enjoy some beer and videos. Then he would drug them, strangle them, masturbate on the body or have sex with the corpse, dismember the body, and dispose of it. Sometimes he would keep the skull or other body parts as souvenirs.

On July 13, 1992, Dahmer changed his plea to guilty by means of insanity. That Dahmer could plan his murders and systematically dispose of the bodies convinced the jury, however, that he was able to control his behavior. All of the testimony bolstered the notion that, as with most serial killers, Dahmer knew what he was doing and knew right from wrong. Finally, the jury did not accept the defense that Dahmer experienced a mental illness to the degree that it had disabled his thinking or behavioral controls. Dahmer was sentenced to 15 consecutive life terms or a total of 957 years in prison. He was killed by an inmate on November 28, 1994.

Irresistible Impulse. In 1922, a committee of jurists in England reexamined the M'Naghten rule. The committee suggested broadening the concept of insanity in criminal cases to include the irresistible impulse test, which rules that a person charged with a criminal offense, is not responsible for an act if the act was committed under an impulse that the person was unable to resist because of mental disease. The courts have chosen to interpret this concept in such a way that it has been called the *policeman-at-the-elbow law.* In other words, the court grants an impulse to be irresistible only when it can be determined that the accused would have committed the act even if a policeman had been at the accused person's elbow. To most psychiatrists, this interpretation is unsatisfactory because it covers only a small, special group of those who are mentally ill.

Durham Rule. In the case of *Durham v. United States,* Judge Bazelon handed down a decision in 1954 in the District of Columbia Court of Appeals. The decision resulted in the product rule of criminal responsibility, namely that an accused person is not criminally responsible if his or her unlawful act was the product of mental disease or mental defect. In the Durham case, Judge Bazelon expressly stated that the purpose of the rule was to get good and complete psychiatric testimony. He sought to release the criminal law from the theoretical straitjacket of the M'Naghten rule, but judges and juries in cases using the *Durham* rule became mired in confusion over the terms *product, disease,* and *defect.* In 1972, some 18 years after the rule's adoption, the Court of Appeals for the District of Columbia, in *United States v. Brawner,* discarded the rule. The court—all nine members, including Judge Bazelon—decided in a 143-page opinion to throw out its *Durham* rule and to adopt in its place the test recommended in 1962 by the American Law Institute in its model penal code, which is the law in the federal courts today.

Model Penal Code. In its model penal code, the American Law Institute recommended the following test of criminal responsibility: Persons are not responsible for criminal conduct if, at the time of such conduct, as a result of mental disease or defect, they lacked substantial capacity either to appreciate the criminality (wrongfulness) of their conduct or to conform their conduct to the requirement of the law. The term *mental disease or defect* does not include an abnormality manifest only by repeated criminal or otherwise antisocial conduct.

Subsection 1 of the American Law Institute rule contains five operative concepts: mental disease or defect, lack of substantial capacity, appreciation, wrongfulness, and conformity of conduct to the requirements of law. The rule's second subsection, stating that repeated criminal or antisocial conduct is not, of itself, to be taken as mental disease or defect, aims to keep the sociopath or psychopath within the scope of criminal responsibility.

Guilty but Mentally Ill. Some states have established an alternative verdict of guilty but mentally ill. Under guilty but mentally ill statutes, this alternative verdict is available to the jury if the defendant pleads not guilty by reason of insanity. Under an insanity plea, four outcomes are possible: not guilty, not guilty by reason of insanity, guilty but mentally ill, and guilty.

The problem with guilty but mentally ill is that it is an alternative verdict without a difference. It is basically the same as finding the defendant just plain guilty. The court must still impose a sentence on the convicted person. Although the convicted person supposedly receives psychiatric treatment, if necessary, this treatment provision is available to all prisoners.

OTHER AREAS OF FORENSIC PSYCHIATRY

Emotional Damage and Distress

A rapidly rising trend in recent years is to sue for psychological and emotional damage, both secondary to physical injury or as a consequence of witnessing a stressful act and from the suffering endured under the stress of such circumstances as concentration camp experiences. The German government heard many of these claims from persons detained in Nazi camps during World War II. In the United States, the courts have moved from a conservative to a liberal position in awarding damages for such claims. Psychiatric examinations and testimony are sought in these cases, often by both the plaintiffs and the defendants.

Recovered Memories

Patients alleging recovered memories of abuse have sued parents and other alleged perpetrators. In a number of instances, the alleged victimizers have sued therapists who, they claim, negligently induced false memories of sexual abuse. In an about-face, some patients have recanted and joined forces with others (usually their parents) to sue therapists.

Courts have handed down multimillion dollar judgments against mental health practitioners. A fundamental allegation in these cases is that the therapist abandoned a position of neutrality to suggest, persuade, coerce, and implant false memories of childhood sexual abuse. The guiding principle of clinical risk management in recovered memory cases is maintenance of therapist neutrality and establishment of sound treatment boundaries. Table 32.1–4 lists the risk management principles that should be considered when evaluating or treating a patient who recovers memories of abuse in psychotherapy.

Worker's Compensation

The stresses of employment can cause or accentuate mental illness. Patients are entitled to be compensated for their job-related disabilities or to receive disability retirement benefits. A psychiatrist is often called on to evaluate such situations.

Table 32.1–4
Risk Management Principles for Cases of Recovered Memories of Abuse in Psychotherapy

1. Maintain therapist neutrality: Do not suggest abuse.
2. Stay clinically focused: Provide adequate evaluation and treatment for patients presenting problems and symptoms.
3. Carefully document the memory recovery process.
4. Manage personal bias and countertransference.
5. Avoid mixing treater and expert witness roles.
6. Closely monitor supervisory and collaborative therapy relationships.
7. Clarify nontreatment roles with family members.
8. Avoid special techniques (e.g., hypnosis or sodium amobarbital [Amytal]) unless clearly indicated; obtain consultation first.
9. Stay within professional competence: Do not take cases that you cannot handle.
10. Distinguish between narrative truth and historical truth.
11. Obtain consultation in problematic cases.
12. Foster patient autonomy and self-determination: Do not suggest lawsuits.
13. In managed care settings, inform patients with recovered memories that more than brief therapy may be required.
14. When making public statements, distinguish personal opinions from scientifically established facts.
15. Stop and refer, if uncomfortable with a patient who is recovering memories of childhood abuse.
16. Do not be afraid to ask about abuse as part of a competent psychiatric evaluation.

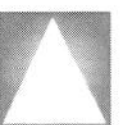

Table 32.1–5
Sexual Exploitation: Legal and Ethical Consequences

Civil lawsuit
Negligence
Loss of consortium
Breach-of-contract action
Criminal sanctions (e.g., statutory, adultery, sexual assault, rape)
Civil action for intentional tort (e.g., battery, fraud)
License revocation
Ethical sanctions
Dismissal from professional organizations

Table by RI Simon, M.D.

Civil Liability

Psychiatrists who sexually exploit their patients are subject to civil and criminal actions in addition to ethical and professional licensure revocation proceedings. Malpractice is the most common legal action (Table 32.1–5).

▲ 32.2 Ethics in Psychiatry

Ethical guidelines and a knowledge of ethical principles help psychiatrists avoid *ethical conflicts* (which can be defined as tension between what one wants to do and what is ethically right to do) and think through *ethical dilemmas* (conflicts between ethical perspectives or values).

Ethics deal with the relations between people in different groups and often entail balancing rights. *Professional ethics* refer to the appropriate way to act when in a professional role. Professional ethics derive from a combination of morality, social norms, and the parameters of the relationship people have agreed to have.

PROFESSIONAL CODES

Most professional organizations and many business groups have codes of ethics that reflect a consensus about the general standards of appropriate professional conduct. The AMA's *Principles of Medical Ethics* and the APA's *Principles of Medical Ethics with Annotations Especially Applicable to Psychiatry* articulate ideal standards of practice and professional virtues of practitioners. These codes include exhortations to use skillful and scientific techniques; to self-regulate misconduct within the profession; and to respect the rights and needs of patients, families, colleagues, and society.

BASIC ETHICAL PRINCIPLES

Four ethical principles that psychiatrists ought to weigh in their work are respect for autonomy, beneficence, nonmaleficence, and justice. At times, they are in conflict, and decisions must be made concerning how to balance them.

Respect for Autonomy

Autonomy requires that a person act intentionally after being given sufficient information and time to understand the benefits, risks, and costs of all reasonable options. It may mean honoring an individual's right not to hear every detail and even choosing someone else (e.g., family or doctor) to decide the best course of treatment.

Psychiatrists need to provide patients with a rational understanding of their disorder and options for treatment. Patients need conceptual understanding; the psychiatrist should not simply state isolated facts. Patients also need time to think and to talk with friends and family about their decision. Finally, if a patient is not in a state of mind to make decisions for himself or herself, the psychiatrist should consider mechanisms for alternative decision making, such as guardianship, conservators, and health care proxy.

A young adult experienced a schizophrenic episode in which his religious fervor turned into psychotic delusions. After being involuntarily hospitalized because he became suicidal, he insistently refused medication, claiming that his physicians were trying to poison him. His psychiatrist decided to respect his refusal of medication as long as his suicidal tendencies could be controlled. As his mental suffering became more intense, in 1 week the patient changed his mind about medication and agreed to try it. The therapeutic relationship with his psychiatrist deepened, and the patient left the hospital willing to continue with both antipsychotic medication and psychotherapy. Although not all cases work out so well, this one illustrates the benefits of negotiation about treatment even when hospitalization is involuntary.

Beneficence

The requirement for psychiatrists to act with beneficence derives from their fiduciary relationship with patients and the profession's belief that they also have an obligation to society. As a result of the role obligation of trust, psychiatrists must heed their patients' interests, even to the neglect of their own.

The expression of the principle is paternalism, the use of the psychiatrist's judgment about the best course of action for the patient or research subject. *Weak paternalism* is acting beneficently when the patient's impaired faculties prevent an autonomous choice. *Strong paternalism* is acting beneficently despite the patient's intact autonomy.

Guidelines have been proposed for permitting beneficence to overrule patient autonomy; when the patient faces substantial harm or risk of harm, the paternalistic act is chosen that ensures the optimal combination of maximal harm reduction, low added risk, and minimal necessary infringement on patient autonomy.

Nonmaleficence

To adhere to the principle of nonmaleficence (*primum non nocere* or *first, do no harm*), psychiatrists must be careful in their decisions and actions and must ensure that they have had adequate training for what they do. They also need to be open to seeking second opinions and consultations. They need to avoid creating risks for patients by an action or inaction.

Justice

The concept of justice concerns the issues of reward and punishment and the equitable distribution of social benefits. Relevant issues include whether resources should be distributed equally to those in greatest need, whether they should go to where they can have the greatest impact on the well-being of each individual served, or to where they will ultimately have the greatest impact on society.

SPECIFIC ISSUES

From a practical point of view, several specific issues most frequently involve psychiatrists. These include (1) sexual boundary violations, (2) nonsexual boundary violations, (3) violations of confidentiality, (4) mistreatment of the patient (incompetence, double agentry), and (5) illegal activities (insurance, billing, insider stock trading).

Sexual Boundary Violations

For a psychiatrist to engage a patient in a sexual relationship is clearly unethical. Furthermore, legal sanctions against such behavior make the ethical question moot. Various criminal law statutes have been used against psychiatrists who violate this ethical principle. Rape charges may be, and have been, brought against such psychiatrists; sexual assault and battery charges also have been used to convict psychiatrists.

In addition, patients who have been victimized sexually by psychiatrists and other physicians have won damages in malpractice suits. Insurance carriers for the APA and the AMA no longer insure against patient–therapist sexual relations, and the carriers exclude liability for any such sexual activity.

The issue of whether sexual relations between an ex-patient and a therapist violate an ethical principle, however, remains controversial. Proponents of the view "Once a patient, always a patient" insist that any involvement with an ex-patient—even one that leads to marriage—should be prohibited. They maintain that a transferential reaction that always exists between the patient and the therapist prevents a rational decision about their emotional or sexual union. Others insist that, if a transferential reaction still exists, the therapy is incomplete and that as autonomous human beings, ex-patients should not be subjected to paternalistic moralizing by physicians. Accordingly, they believe that no sanctions should prohibit emotional or sexual involvements by ex-patients and their psychiatrists. Some psychiatrists maintain that a reasonable time should elapse before such a liaison. The length of the "reasonable" period remains controversial: Some have suggested 2 years. Other psychiatrists maintain that any period of prohibited involvement with an ex-patient is an unnecessary restriction. *The Principles,* however, states: "Sexual activity with a current or *former* patient is unethical."

Although not spelled out in *The Principles,* sexual activity with a patient's family member is also unethical. This is most important when the psychiatrist is treating a child or adolescent. Most training programs in child and adolescent psychiatry emphasize that the parents are patients too and that the ethical and legal proscriptions apply to parents (or parent surrogates) as well as to the child. Nevertheless, some psychiatrists misunderstand this concept. Sexual activity between a doctor and a patient's family member is also unethical.

An egregious example of a sexual boundary violation was reported in the *Medical Board of California Action Report* (July 2006) of a psychiatrist who had a 7-year affair with a patient who had schizophrenia. The doctor not only had sex with the patient but also had her procure prostitutes with whom he and the patient had group sex. He paid for their services by providing them with prescriptions for controlled substances and went so far as to bill Medi-Cal for these encounters as group therapy. The physician's license was revoked, and he was also criminally convicted of fraud.

Nonsexual Boundary Violations

The relationship between a doctor and a patient for the purposes of providing and obtaining treatment is what is usually called the *doctor–patient relationship.* That relationship has both boundaries around it and boundaries within it. Either person may cross the boundary.

Not all boundary crossings are boundary violations. For example, a patient may say to a doctor at the end of an hour, "I have left my money at home, and I need a dollar to get my car out of the garage. Will you lend me a dollar until next time?" The patient has invited the doctor to cross the doctor–patient boundary and set up a lender–borrower relationship as well. Depending on the doctor's theoretical orientation, the clinical situation with the patient, and other factors, the doctor may elect to cross the boundary. Whether the boundary crossing is also a boundary violation is debatable. A *boundary violation* is a boundary crossing that is exploitative. It gratifies the doctor's needs at the expense of the patient. The doctor is responsible for preserving the boundary and for ensuring that boundary crossings are held to a minimum and that exploitation does not occur.

A resident in psychiatry was admonished by her psychotherapy supervisor to never, under any circumstances, accept a gift from a patient. In the course of treating a young girl with schizophrenia, she was offered a Christmas gift (a cotton scarf), which she refused to accept, explaining as gently as possible that it was not permitted by the "rules of the hospital." The next day the patient attempted suicide. She experienced the resident's refusal to accept the gift as a profound rejection (to which patients with schizophrenia are exquisitely sensitive), which she could not tolerate. The case illustrates the need to understand the dynamics of gift giving and the transferential meaning to the patients of rejecting (or accepting) the gift.

The story (possibly apocryphal) is told of how Freud, who was an inveterate cigar smoker, was offered a box of difficult-to-find Havana cigars by a patient during the course of his analysis. Freud accepted the cigars and then proceeded to ask his patient to explore his motivations in offering the gift. Freud's reasons for accepting the cigars are more obvious than the patient's unconscious motivation for giving them, about which no information is available.

Harm to the patient is not a component of a boundary violation. For example, using information supplied by the patient (e.g., a stock tip) is an unethical boundary violation, although no obvious harm may come to the patient. For purposes of discussion, nonsexual boundary violations may be grouped into several arbitrary (overlapping and not mutually exclusive) categories.

Business. Almost any business relationship with a former patient is problematic, and almost any business relationship with a current patient is unethical. Naturally, the circumstance and location may play a significant role in this admonition. In a rural area or a small community, a doctor might be treating the only pharmacist (or plumber or couch upholsterer) in town; then when doing business with the pharmacist–patient, the doctor tries to keep boundaries in check. Ethical psychiatrists try to avoid doing business with a patient or a patient's family member or asking a patient to hire one of their family members. Ethical psychiatrists avoid investing in a patient's business ad collaborating with a patient in a business deal.

Ideological Issues. Ideological issues can cloud judgment and may lead to ethical lapses. Any clinical decision should be based on what is best for the patient; the psychiatrist's ideology should play as little a part as possible in such a decision. A psychiatrist who is consulted by a patient with an illness should tell the patient what forms of treatment are available to treat the illness and allow the patient to decide on a course of treatment. Naturally, psychiatrists should recommend the treatment that they feel is in the best interest of the patient, but ultimately, the patient should be free to choose.

Social. The particular locale and circumstances must be considered in any discussion of the behavior of an ethical psychiatrist in social situations. The overarching principle is that the boundaries of the psychiatrist–patient relationship should be respected. Furthermore, if options exist, they should be exercised in favor of the patient. Problems often arise in treatment situations when friendships develop between the psychiatrist and the patient. Objectivity is compromised, therapeutic neutrality is impaired, and factors outside the consciousness of either party may play a destructive role. Such friendship should be avoided during treatment. Similarly, psychiatrists should not treat their social friends for the same set of reasons. Obviously, in an emergency, a person does what a person must.

Financial. For psychiatrists who practice in the private sector, dealing with the patient about money is a part of treatment. Issues surrounding setting the fee, collecting the fee, and other financial matters are grist for the mill. Even so, ethical concerns must be observed. *The Principles* advises the doctor on such matters as charging for missed appointments and other contractual problems. Ethics complaints against doctors are frequently precipitated by financial issues; thus, the doctor must recognize the power that these issues have in the therapeutic relationship. Because the psychotherapeutic relationship is so much like a social relationship—the office looks like a living room; the doctor wears regular clothes; some patients might, without recognizing it, assume that a friendship exists that forgives payment of a fee. When the bill is presented, feelings, even though they are unconscious, are ruffled. The idea that psychiatric services are dispensed in a contractual context cannot be sufficiently emphasized. Early in their careers, psychiatrists are often reluctant to discuss fees openly out of a sense of embarrassment over discussing money or a sense of protecting the patient.

How an ethical psychiatrist handles the situation when a patient temporarily or permanently runs out of money is important. Many options are available—some more problematic than others. The psychiatrist can certainly lower the fee, but caution is needed because a fee lowered to the point where the treatment is not somehow being compensated may evoke countertransference resentment. The number of patients being seen at a reduced fee is a similar consideration. Running up a bill can also be a problem. Is there an expectation of eventually being paid? Is the hypertrophic bill a sham? The frequency of sessions may have to be altered. Any psychiatrist who sees private patients will definitely face these problems.

Confidentiality

Confidentiality refers to the therapist's responsibility not to release information learned in the course of treatment to third parties. *Privilege* refers to the patient's right to prevent disclosure of information from treatment in judicial hearings. Psychiatrists must maintain confidentiality because it is an essential ingredient of psychiatric care; it is a prerequisite for patients to be willing to speak freely to therapists. Violating confidentiality by gossiping embarrasses people and violates nonmaleficence. Violation of confidentiality also breaks the promise that a psychiatrist has explicitly or implicitly made to keep material confidential.

Confidentiality must also give way to the responsibility to protect others when a patient makes a credible threat to harm someone. The situation becomes complicated when the risk is not to a particular individual, such as when a doctor is impaired or someone's mental state adversely affects his or her performance of a dangerous job, such as police work, firefighting, or use of dangerous machinery. Erosion has also arisen from the demands of an insurance company for detailed information. Patients must be told that information may be released to insurance companies, but they do not need to be warned that information concerning abuse of a child or threat to themselves or others needs to be reported.

Various settings exist in which patient data can be used to some degree. The general rule for doing so is to disclose only that information that is truly necessary. In teaching, research, and supervision, patients' names or information that might allow others to identify them should not be unnecessarily released. In ward rounds and case conferences, in which patient material is presented, attendees should be reminded that what they hear should not be repeated.

Confidentiality endures after death, with the ethical obligation to withhold information unless the next of kin provides consent. A subpoena is not automatic license to release the entire record. A psychiatrist can petition the judge for an in-camera (private) review to define what precise information must be disclosed.

Ethics in Managed Care

Psychiatrists have certain responsibilities toward patients treated in managed care settings, including the responsibilities to disclose all treatment options, exercise appeal rights, continue emergency treatment, and cooperate reasonably with utilization reviewers.

Responsibility to Disclose. Psychiatrists have a continuing responsibility to the patient to obtain informed consent for treatments or procedures. All treatment options should be fully disclosed, even those not covered under the terms of a managed care plan. Most states have enacted legislation making gag rules illegal that limit information about treatment provided to patients under managed care.

Responsibility to Appeal. The AMA Council on Ethical and Judicial Affairs states that physicians have an ethical obligation to advocate for any care that they believe will materially benefit their patients, regardless of any allocation guidelines or gatekeeper directives.

Responsibility to Treat. Physicians are liable for failure to treat their patients within the defined standard of care. The treating physician has sole responsibility to determine what is medically necessary. Psychiatrists must be careful not to discharge suicidal or violent patients prematurely merely because continued coverage of benefits is not approved by a managed care company.

Responsibility to Cooperate with Utilization Review. The psychiatrist should cooperate with utilization reviewers' requests for information on proper authorization from the patient. When benefits are denied, it is important to understand and follow grievance procedures carefully; return telephone calls from review agencies; and provide documented, solid justification for continued treatment.

With the advent of managed care and the need to send periodic progress reports and documentation of signs and symptoms to third-party reviewers to pay for treatment, some psychiatrists may diminish or exaggerate symptomatology. The following case report and discussion illustrates the ethical difficulties psychiatrists face in dealing with managed care.

Mrs. P admitted herself to the hospital because she was afraid she might kill herself. She was experiencing a major depressive episode, but she improved markedly during the first weeks on Dr. A's ward. Although Dr. A believed that Mrs. P was no longer suicidal, he thought she would benefit greatly from continued hospitalization. Because he knew that Mrs. P could not afford to pay for hospitalization and that the insurance company would pay only if the patient was suicidally depressed, he decided not to document Mrs. P's improvement. He noted in the chart that "the patient continues to have a risk of suicide."

Does Dr. A engage in a form of deception? Yes, he intentionally misleads by what he writes and what he omits writing in the chart. Although what he writes is true in some literal sense, his statement is misleading in the context of treatment. Mrs. P is not suicidally depressed in the way that she was.

What Dr. A omits from the chart is also deceptive. Whether a particular omission is deceptive depends, in part, on the roles and expectations of the people involved. Not telling a colleague that one dislikes his tie is not a deception. It is simply tact unless the role or relationship involves the expectation that one offers a candid opinion. Dr. A's case is different. His professional role is to document the patient's course and the expectation is that he will note any significant improvement. Thus, his failure to document Mrs. P's progress accurately is a kind of deception.

The second and more difficult question is whether deception is justified in this instance. The answer to that question depends on the reasons for the deception, the reasons against it, and the alternatives available. The reasons for this deception are obvious. Dr. A's aim and primary obligation is to help the patient. He believes that Mrs. P would benefit greatly from continued hospitalization that she cannot afford. He may also believe that it is unfair for the insurance company to refuse to pay for inpatient treatment of nonsuicidal depression and that his deception rectifies that unfair practice.

Important reasons also exist against this deception. The first concerns honesty and social trust. It is a good thing if people can rely on what others say and write. Without some honesty and trust, many social exchanges and practices would be impossible. Deception, even for beneficent purposes, has real potential to damage social trust. A risk exists that deception may damage people's trust in the profession of psychiatry and even patients' trust in their psychiatrists. Damage to trust may, in turn, compromise treatment.

The second reason concerns future medical treatment. If Mrs. P seeks medical treatment in the future, the physicians who attend her will read the misleading notes. If they believe that the notes are an accurate account of the previous treatment, they may suggest an inappropriate treatment for the present problem. Even if they have doubts about the accuracy of the notes in her chart, they are deprived of an accurate history and report. In either case, the prior deception can hinder treatment.

The third reason concerns obligations and coverage policies. Dr. A seems to ignore the obligation that he has to the population that is covered by the insurance policy. He shifts a burden onto this population by forcing the insurance company to pay for treatment that it did not agree to cover. Perhaps the insurance company should pay for inpatient treatment in cases such as Mrs. P's; perhaps its policies are unreasonable and unfair. However, Dr. A's deception does not challenge the insurance company and pressure it to change its policy, nor does his deception encourage patients and their families to contest the company's policies. The use of deception simply circumvents, in an ad hoc way, a policy that should be challenged and discussed.

Dr. A also seems to ignore his obligation to future patients. By introducing an inaccuracy into the chart, he compromises the value of medical records research. His deception works, in a small way, to deprive future patients of the benefit of research that relies on medical records.

Whether the deception is justified depends on both the weight of the reasons for and against the deception and the available alternatives. One alternative is to tailor the chart. Another alternative is to describe Mrs. P's response accurately and to discharge her to outpatient care. However, a third alternative exists. Dr. A can accurately document the patient's course and can recommend continued hospitalization. He can petition the insurance company for coverage. If the insurance company decides not to approve further inpatient care for the patient, Dr. A can appeal that decision. This alternative is more time consuming, and nothing guarantees that it will succeed, but it avoids all the problems associated with the use of deception.

Impaired Physicians

A physician may become impaired as the result of psychiatric or medical disorders or the use of mind-altering and habit-forming substances (e.g., alcohol and drugs). Many organic illnesses can interfere with the cognitive and motor skills required to provide competent medical care. Although the legal responsibility to report an impaired physician varies, depending on the state, the ethical responsibility remains universal. An incapacitated physician should be reported to an appropriate authority, and the reporting physician is required to follow specific hospital, state, and legal procedures. A physician who treats an impaired physician should not be required to monitor the impaired physician's progress or fitness to return to work. This monitoring should be performed by an independent physician or group of physicians who have no conflicts of interest.

The Office of Professional Medical Conduct (OPMC) in New York State regulates the practice of medicine by investigating illegal or unethical practice by physicians and other health professionals, such as physician assistants. Similar regulatory agencies exist in other states. Professional misconduct in New York State is defined as one of the following:

1. Practicing fraudulently and with gross negligence or incompetence
2. Practicing while the ability to practice is impaired
3. Being habitually drunk or being dependent on, or a habitual user of, narcotics or a habitual user of other drugs having similar effects
4. Immoral conduct in the practice of the profession
5. Permitting, aiding, or abetting an unlicensed person to perform activities requiring a license
6. Refusing a client or patient service because of creed, color, or national origin
7. Practicing beyond the scope of practice permitted by law
8. Being convicted of a crime or being the subject of disciplinary action in another jurisdiction

Professional misconduct complaints derive mainly from the public in addition to insurance companies, law enforcement agencies, and doctors, among others.

New York State has established a program called Committee for Physician Health (CPH) in which impaired physicians receive appropriate treatment for their condition without losing their medical license as long as they comply with a treatment program. For example, a physician addicted to opioids or alcohol might be hospitalized to safely withdraw from the drugs and then move to a sober house for further rehabilitation that would involve intensive individual and group psychotherapy, mandatory supervised drug testing and careful oversight by CPH. The physician must be compliant for 5 years during which time he or she may gradually return to practice under supervision. The program has rehabilitated many physicians successfully.

Physicians in Training

It is unethical to delegate authority for patient care to anyone who is not appropriately qualified and experienced, such as a medical student or a resident, without adequate supervision from an attending physician. Residents are physicians in training and, as such, must provide a good deal of patient care. Within a healthy, ethical teaching environment, residents and medical students may be involved with, and responsible for, the day-to-day care of many ill patients, but they are supervised, supported, and directed by highly trained and experienced physicians. Patients have the right to know the level of training of their care providers and should be informed about the resident's or medical student's level of training. Residents and medical students should know and acknowledge their limitations and should ask for supervision from experienced colleagues as necessary.

Physician Charter of Professionalism

In 2001, a movement to clarify the concept of "professionalism" was begun by the American Board of Internal Medicine. A set of principles called the *Physician Charter of Professionalism* was developed, which describes what it means for physicians to perform at their highest and most ethical level. Table 32.2–1

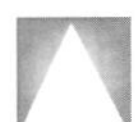

Table 32.2–1
Physician Charter of Professionalism

Fundamental Principles

- ▲ **Primacy of patient welfare.** Altruism contributes to the trust central to doctor–patient relationships. Market forces, societal pressures, and administrative exigencies must not compromise this principle.
- ▲ **Patient autonomy.** Physicians must be honest with patients and empower them to make informed decisions about treatment.
- ▲ **Social justice.** Physicians should work actively to eliminate discrimination in health care, whether based on race, gender, socioeconomic status, ethnicity, religion, or any other social category.

A Set of Commitments

- ▲ **Professional competence.** Physicians must be committed to lifelong learning. The profession as a whole must strive to see that all of its members are competent.
- ▲ **Honesty with patients.** Physicians must ensure that patients are completely and honestly informed before consenting to a treatment; they must be empowered to decide about the course of therapy. Physicians should also acknowledge that medical errors that injure patients sometimes occur. If a patient is injured through error, he or she should be informed promptly because failure to do so seriously compromises patient and societal trust.
- ▲ **Patient confidentiality.** Fulfilling the commitment to confidentiality is more pressing now than ever before given the widespread use of electronic information systems for compiling patient data.
- ▲ **Maintaining appropriate relations with patients.** Physicians should never exploit patients for any sexual advantage, personal financial gain, or other private purpose.
- ▲ **Improving quality of care.** This commitment entails both maintaining clinical competence and working collaboratively with other professionals to reduce medical error, increase patient safety, minimize overuse of health care resources, and optimize the outcomes of care.
- ▲ **Improving access to care.** Physicians must individually and collectively strive to reduce barriers to equitable health care.
- ▲ **Just distribution of finite resources.** Physicians should be committed to working with other physicians, hospitals, and payers to develop guidelines for cost-effective care. The physician's professional responsibility for appropriate allocation of resources requires scrupulous avoidance of superfluous tests and procedures.
- ▲ **Scientific knowledge.** Physicians have a duty to uphold scientific standards, to promote research, and to create new knowledge and ensure its appropriate use.
- ▲ **Maintaining trust by managing conflicts of interest.** Physicians have an obligation to recognize, disclose to the general public, and address conflicts of interest. Relationships between industry and opinion leaders should be disclosed.
- ▲ **Professional responsibilities.** Physicians are expected to participate in the process of self-regulation, including remediation and discipline of members who have failed to meet professional standards.

lists the principles and commitments of professional behaviors in the *Physician Charter of Professionalism* to which all physicians (including psychiatrists) are expected to adhere.

A summary of ethical issues discussed in this section is presented in a question-and-answer format in Table 32.2–2.

Military Psychiatry

Psychiatrists in the military face unique ethical problems because confidentiality does not exist under the military code of conduct.

Health Insurance Portability and Accountability Act

The Health Insurance Portability and Accountability Act (HIPAA) was passed in 1996 to address the medical delivery system's mounting complexity and its rising dependence on electronic communication. The act orders that the Federal Department of Health and Human Services (HHS) develop rules protecting the transmission and confidentiality of patient information, and all units under HIPAA must comply with such rules.

The Privacy Rule, administered by the Office of Civil Rights (OCR) at HHS, protects the confidentiality of patient information (Table 32.2–3).

Table 32.2–2
Ethical Questions and Answers

Topic	Question	Answer
Abandonment	How can psychiatrists avoid being charged with patient abandonment on retirement?	Retiring psychiatrists are not abandoning patients if they provide their patients with sufficient notice and make every reasonable effort to find follow-up care for the patients.
	Is it ethical to provide only outpatient care to a seriously ill patient who may require hospitalization?	This could constitute abandonment unless the outpatient practitioner or agency arranges for their patients to receive inpatient care from another provider.
Bequests	A dying patient bequeaths his or her estate to his or her treating psychiatrist. Is this ethical?	No. Accepting the bequest seems improper and exploitational of the therapeutic relationship. However, it may be ethical to accept a token bequest from a deceased patient who named his or her psychiatrist in the will without that psychiatrist's knowledge.
Competency	Is it ethical for psychiatrists to perform vaginal examinations? Hospital physical examinations?	Psychiatrists may provide nonpsychiatric medical procedures if they are competent to do so and if the procedures do not preclude effective psychiatric treatment by distorting the transference. Pelvic examinations carry a high risk of distorting the transference and would be better performed by another clinician.
	Can ethics committees review issues of physician competency?	Yes. Incompetency is an ethical issue.
Confidentiality	Must confidentiality be maintained after the death of a patient?	Yes. Ethically, confidences survive a patient's death. Exceptions include protecting others from imminent harm or proper legal compulsions.
	Is it ethical to release information about a patient to an insurance company?	Yes, if the information provided is limited to that which is needed to process the insurance claim.
	Can a videotaped segment of a therapy session be used at a workshop for professionals?	Yes, if informed, uncoerced consent has been obtained, anonymity is maintained, the audience is advised that editing makes this an incomplete session, and the patient knows the purpose of the videotape.
	Should a physician report mere suspicion of child abuse in a state requiring reporting of child abuse?	No. A physician must make several assessments before deciding whether to report suspected abuse. One must consider whether abuse is ongoing, whether abuse is responsive to treatment, and whether reporting will cause potential harm. Check specific statutes. Make safety for potential victims the top priority.
Conflict of interest	Is there a potential ethical conflict if a psychiatrist has both psychotherapeutic and administrative duties in dealing with students or trainees?	Yes. You must define your role in advance to the trainees or students. Administrative opinions should be obtained from a psychiatrist who is not involved in a treatment relationship with the trainee or student.
Diagnosis without examination	Is it ethical to offer a diagnosis based only on review of records to determine, for insurance purposes, if suicide was the result of illness?	Yes.
	Is it ethical for a supervising psychiatrist to sign a diagnosis on an insurance form for services provided by a supervisee when the psychiatrist has not examined the patient?	Yes, if the psychiatrist ensures that proper care is given and the insurance form clearly indicates the role of supervisor and supervisee.

Table 32.2–2
Ethical Questions and Answers (Continued)

Topic	Question	Answer
Exploitation (also see Bequests)	What constitutes exploitation of the therapeutic relationship?	Exploitation occurs when the psychiatrist uses the therapeutic relationship for personal gain. This includes adopting or hiring a patient as well as sexual or financial relationships.
Fee splitting	What is fee splitting?	Fee splitting occurs when one physician pays another for a patient referral. This would also apply to lawyers giving a forensic psychiatrist referrals in exchange for a percentage of the fee. Fee splitting may occur in an office setting if the psychiatrist takes a percentage of his or her office mates' fees for supervision or expenses. Costs for such items or services must be arranged separately. Otherwise, it would appear that the office owner could benefit from referring patients to a colleague in the office. Fee splitting is illegal.
Informed consent	Is it ethical to refuse to divulge information about a patient who has agreed to give this information to those requesting it?	No. It is the patient's decision, not the therapist's.
	Is informed consent needed when presenting or writing about case material?	Not if the patient is aware of the supervisory or teaching process and confidentiality is preserved.
Moonlighting	Can psychiatric residents ethically "moonlight"?	They can if their duties are not beyond their ability, if they are properly supervised, and if the moonlighting does not interfere with their residency training.
Reporting	Should psychiatrists expose or report unethical behavior of a colleague or colleagues? Can a spouse bring an ethical complaint?	Psychiatrists are obligated to report colleagues' unethical behavior. A spouse with knowledge of unethical behavior can bring an ethical complaint as well.
Research	How can ethical research be performed with subjects who cannot give informed consent?	Consent can be given by a legal guardian or via a living will. Incompetent persons have the right to withdraw from the research project at any time.
Retirement	See Abandonment.	
Supervision	What are the ethical requirements when a psychiatrist supervises other mental health professionals?	The psychiatrist must spend sufficient time to ensure that proper care is given and that the supervisee is not providing services that are outside the scope of his or her training. It is ethical to charge a fee for supervision.
Taping and recording	Can videotapes of patient interviews be used for training purposes on a national level (e.g., workshops, board exam preparation)?	Appropriate and explicit informed consent must be obtained. The purpose and scope of exposure of the tape must be emphasized in addition to the resulting loss of confidentiality.

Table by Eugene Rubin, M.D. Data derived from the American Medical Association's Principles of Medical Ethics.

Table 32.2–3
Patients' Rights under the Privacy Rule

Physicians must give the patient a written notice of his or her privacy rights; the privacy policies of the practice; and how patient information is used, kept, and disclosed. A written acknowledgment should be taken from the patient verifying that he or she has seen such notice.

Patients should be able to obtain copies of their medical records and to request revisions to those records within a stated amount of time (usually 30 days). Patients do not have the right to see psychotherapy notes.

Physicians must provide the patient with a history of most disclosures of their medical history on request. Some exceptions exist. The APA Committee on Confidentiality has developed a model document for this requirement.

Physicians must obtain authorization from the patient for disclosure of information other than for treatment, payment, and health care operations (these three are considered to be routine uses, for which consent is not required). The APA Committee on Confidentiality has developed a model document for this requirement.

Patients may request another means of communication of their protected information (e.g., request that the physician contact them at a specific phone number or address).

Physicians cannot generally limit treatment to obtaining patient authorization for disclosure of their information for nonroutine uses.

Patients have the right to complain about Privacy Rule violations to the physician, their health plan, or to the Secretary of HHS.

APA, American Psychiatric Association; HHS, Department of Health and Human Services.

33

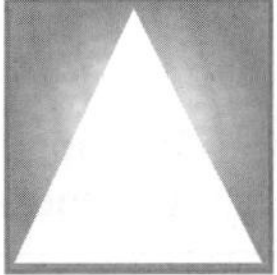

World Aspects of Psychiatry

Mental disorders are highly prevalent in all regions of the world and represent a major source of disability and social burden worldwide. Treatments for all of these disorders are available and have been found to be efficacious in both developed and developing countries. However, mental disorders are remarkably undertreated worldwide, especially in low-income countries. National mental health policies are lacking in several countries, especially low-income ones. Resources for mental health care are scarce and unequally distributed. World psychiatry focuses on these and other issues such as the stigma attached to mental disorders, the relationships between mental and physical diseases, and the ethics of mental health care.

PREVALENCE AND BURDEN OF MENTAL DISORDERS WORLDWIDE

The World Health Organization (WHO) estimates that more than 25 percent of individuals worldwide develop one or more mental disorders during their lifetime. Among people seen by primary health care professionals, more than 20 percent have one or more current mental disorders. In a study carried out by the WHO at 14 sites in Africa, Asia, the Americas, and Europe, the average current prevalence of any mental disorder was 24 percent, without consistent differences between low- and high-income countries. The most common diagnoses were those of depression (average, 10.4 percent) and generalized anxiety disorder (average, 7.9 percent). Female rates were 1.89 times higher than male rates for depression, but male rates were higher for alcohol-related disorders, so that there was no sex difference in the proportion of people having at least one mental disorder. Physical ill health and educational disadvantage were both significantly associated with a diagnosis of mental disorder.

To quantify the burden of the various diseases and injuries, the WHO, in collaboration with the Harvard School of Public Health and the World Bank, introduced the disability-adjusted life year (DALY). DALYs for a given disease or injury are the sum of the years of life lost due to premature mortality plus the years lost due to disability for incident cases of that disease or injury in the general population. In the original estimates for the year 1990, mental and neurological disorders accounted for 10.5 percent of the total DALYs lost due to all diseases and injuries. The estimate for the year 2000 was 12.3 percent, with two mental disorders (depression- and alcohol-use disorders) and suicide ranking in the top 20 causes of DALYs for all ages.

More recent estimates found that mental and neurological disorders accounted for 13.5 percent of all DALYs in the world (27.4 percent in high-income countries, 17.7 percent in middle-income countries, and 9.1 percent in low-income countries).

According to the updated estimates for the future, mental and neurological disorders will account for 14.4 percent of all DALYs in the world and 25.4 percent of those due to noncommunicable diseases. Depression will rank number 2 in the percentage of total DALYs in that year (5.7 percent), following HIV/AIDS and preceding ischemic heart disease (Table 33–1). It will be number 1 in high-income countries (9.8 percent), number 2 in middle-income countries (6.7 percent), and number 3 in low-income countries (4.7 percent).

The WHO estimates that one of four families worldwide has at least one member with a mental disorder. The objective and subjective burden related to caring for people with severe mental disorders (in terms of disruption of family relationships; constraints in social, leisure, and work activities; financial difficulties; negative effect on physical health; feelings of loss, depression, and embarrassment in social situations; and the stress of coping with disturbing behaviors) has been reported to be substantial and significantly higher than that related to caring for people with long-term physical diseases such as diabetes and heart, kidney, or lung diseases. Cross-cultural differences have been reported in some dimensions of family burden.

Suicide is among the 10 leading causes of death for all ages in most of the countries for which information is available. In some countries (e.g., China), it is the leading cause of death for people between 15 and 34 years of age.

According to WHO estimates, about 900,000 people die from suicide worldwide each year. In 2020, approximately 1.53 million

Table 33–1
Leading Causes of Disability-Adjusted Life Year Worldwide as Estimated for the Year 2030

Disease or Injury	Percent of Total
1. HIV/AIDS	12.1
2. Unipolar depressive disorders	5.7
3. Ischemic heart disease	4.7
4. Road traffic accidents	4.2
5. Perinatal conditions	4.0
6. Cerebrovascular disease	3.9
7. Chronic obstructive pulmonary disease	3.1
8. Lower respiratory infections	3.0
9. Hearing loss, adult onset	2.5
10. Cataracts	2.5

From Mathers CD, Loncar D. Projection of global mortality and burden of disease from 2002 to 2030. *PLoS Med.* 2006;3:2011.

people will die from suicide worldwide based on current trends, and 10 to 20 times more people will attempt suicide. Reported suicide rates vary considerably across countries; for instance, annual suicide rates of 48.0 to 79.3 per 100,000 have been reported in many Eastern and Central European countries, and rates of less than 4.0 per 100,000 have been found in Islamic and several Latin American countries. More than 85 percent of suicides are reported to occur in low- or middle-income countries, but this figure may represent an underestimate due to the low reliability of official statistics in those countries: When surveillance with validated verbal autopsy was used in South India, the observed rates for suicide exceeded official national estimates 10-fold. In the Asia-Pacific region, 300,000 cases of suicide per year are estimated to occur by self-poisoning with pesticides.

Suicide rates are higher in men than in women (3.2:1 in 1950, 3.6:1 in 1995, and an estimated 3.9:1 in 2020). China is the only country where suicide rates in women are consistently higher than those in men, especially in rural areas. Over the past few decades, suicide rates have been reported to be stable worldwide, but a rising trend among young men of ages 15 to 19 years has been observed. A systematic review covering 15,629 cases in the general population worldwide estimated that 98 percent of those who committed suicide had a diagnosable mental disorder, with mood disorders accounting for 35.8 percent, substance-related disorders for 22.4 percent, personality disorders for 11.6 percent, and schizophrenia for 10.6 percent of cases.

TREATMENT GAP AND PROJECTED POPULATION-LEVEL TREATMENT EFFECTIVENESS WORLDWIDE

The efficacy of pharmacological and psychosocial treatments for mood, anxiety, psychotic, and substance-related disorders has been convincingly proved by clinical trials carried out in low- and middle-income, as well as in high-income, countries. However, the treatment gap is substantial for all mental disorders worldwide, particularly in low-income countries.

In the World Mental Health Surveys, failure and delays in treatment seeking were generally greater in low-income countries, older cohorts, men, and cases with earlier ages of onset. The earlier treatment contact of people with mood disorders might be partly due to the fact that these disorders have been targeted by educational campaigns and primary care quality improvement programs in several countries.

RESOURCES FOR MENTAL HEALTH CARE WORLDWIDE

According to the *Mental Health Atlas 2005,* only 62.1 percent of countries worldwide—accounting for 68.3 percent of the world population—have a mental health policy (i.e., a document of the government or ministry of health specifying the goals for improving the mental health situation of the country, the priorities among those goals, and the main directions for attaining them). A mental health policy is present in 58.8 percent of low-income and 70.5 percent of high-income countries. In Africa, only 50 percent of countries have a mental health policy. In Southeast Asia, only 54.5 percent of countries have a mental health policy, and 76.4 percent of the population is not covered by such a policy (Table 33–2).

Table 33–2
Presence of a Mental Health Policy in the Countries of Each Region of the World Health Organization

WHO Region	Percent of Countries	Percent Population Coverage
Africa	50.0	69.4
Americas	72.7	64.2
Eastern Mediterranean	72.7	93.8
Europe	70.6	89.1
Southeast Asia	54.5	23.6
Western Pacific	48.1	93.8

From World Health Organization: Mental Health Atlas 2005. Geneva: World Health Organization; 2005.

Community care facilities exist in only 68.1 percent of the countries (51.7 percent of low-income and 93 percent of high-income countries). Only 60.9 percent of the countries report providing treatment facilities for severe mental disorders at the primary care level (55.2 percent of low-income and 79.5 percent of high-income countries). About one-fourth of low-income countries do not provide even basic antidepressant medications in primary care settings. In many others, the supply does not cover all regions of the country or is very irregular. Because medicines are often not available in health care facilities, patients and families are forced to pay for them out of pocket.

Whereas 61.5 percent of European countries spend more than 5 percent of their health budget on mental health care, 70 percent of countries in Africa and 50 percent of countries in Southeast Asia spend less than 1 percent. Out-of-pocket payment is the most important method of financing mental health care in 38.6 percent of countries in Africa and 30 percent of countries in Southeast Asia, but it is not the primary method of financing mental health care in any European country (Table 33–3). All countries with out-of-pocket payment as the dominant method of financing mental health care belong to low-income or lower middle-income categories, but almost all countries with social insurance as the dominant method of financing belong to high-income or upper middle-income categories.

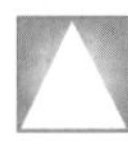

Table 33–3
Countries in Which Out-of-Pocket Payment Is the Most Common Method of Financing Mental Health Care in Each Region of the World Health Organization

WHO Region	Percent of Countries
Africa	38.6
Americas	12.9
Eastern Mediterranean	15.8
Europe	0
Southeast Asia	30.0
Western Pacific	18.5

From World Health Organization: Mental Health Atlas 2005. Geneva: World Health Organization; 2005.

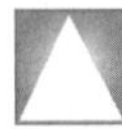

Table 33–4
Median Number of Mental Health Professionals per 100,000 Population in Each Region of the World Health Organization

WHO Region	Psychiatrists	Psychiatric Nurses	Psychologists Working in Mental Health
Africa	0.04	0.20	0.05
Americas	2.00	2.60	2.80
Eastern Mediterranean	0.95	1.25	0.60
Europe	9.80	24.80	3.10
Southeast Asia	0.20	0.10	0.03
Western Pacific	0.32	0.50	0.03

From World Health Organization: Mental Health Atlas 2005. Geneva: World Health Organization; 2005.

The median number of psychiatrists per 100,000 population ranges from 0.04 in Africa and 0.2 in Southeast Asia to 9.8 in Europe (Table 33–4). It is 0.1 in low-income countries compared with 9.2 in high-income countries. Two-thirds of low-income countries have less than one psychiatrist per 100,000 population. Chad, Eritrea, and Liberia (with populations of 9, 4.2, and 3.5 million, respectively) each have just one psychiatrist per 100,000 population. Afghanistan, Rwanda, and Togo (with populations of 25, 8.5, and 5 million, respectively) each have just two psychiatrists per 100,000 population. Large-scale migration of psychiatrists from low- and middle-income to high-income countries, as part of the larger picture of migration of health professionals in general, has been consistently documented. India and some sub-Saharan African countries are the most important contributors to the mental health workforce in the United Kingdom, although the United Kingdom has 110 psychiatrists per million population, but India has 2 per million and sub-Saharan Africa less than 1 per million. The median number of psychologists working in mental health care per 100,000 population ranges from 0.03 in Southeast Asia and 0.05 in Africa to 3.1 in Europe. Approximately 69 percent of low-income countries have less than one psychologist per 100,000 population. The median number of psychiatric nurses per 100,000 population ranges from 0.1 in Southeast Asia and 0.2 in Africa to 24.8 in Europe.

From these figures, it is clear that resources for mental health care are grossly inadequate compared with the needs, and that inequalities across countries are substantial, especially between low- and high-income countries. Moreover, resources tend to be concentrated in urban areas, especially in low-income countries, leaving vast regions without any form of mental health care.

Even worse is the situation concerning child and adolescent mental health care. According to the WHO, only 7 percent of countries worldwide have a specific child and adolescent mental health policy. In less than one-third of all countries it is possible to identify an institution or a governmental entity with an overall responsibility for child mental health. School-based services are almost exclusively present in high-income countries, and even in Europe only 17 percent of countries have a sufficient number of these services. There are no pediatric beds for mental health care identified in low-income countries, but such beds are identified in 50 percent of high-income countries. In all African countries outside South Africa, fewer than 10 psychiatrists could be found who were trained to work with children. In European countries, the number of child psychiatrists ranges from one per 5,300 to one per 51,800. In more than 70 percent of countries worldwide, there is no list of essential psychotropic medications for children. In 45 percent of countries worldwide, psychostimulants are either prohibited or unavailable for use in children with attention-deficit/hyperactivity disorder.

PRINCIPLES FOR MENTAL HEALTH PROGRAM DEVELOPMENT AND BARRIERS TO CHANGE WORLDWIDE

According to the WHO, the development of mental health programs worldwide should be guided by the following principles: (1) providing treatment in primary care; (2) making psychotropic medications available; (3) giving care in the community; (4) educating the public; (5) involving communities, families, and consumers; (6) establishing national policies and legislations; (7) developing human resources; (8) linking with other relevant sectors; (9) monitoring community mental health; and (10) supporting more research.

The guiding principles proposed for the prevention of suicide worldwide include: (1) reducing access to means of suicide (e.g., pesticides, firearms), (2) treating people with mental disorders, (3) improving media portrayal of suicide, (4) training primary health care personnel, (5) implementing school-based programs, and (6) developing hotlines and crisis centers.

The most significant barriers to the implementation of the foregoing principles worldwide, according to the WHO, include the following: (1) some stakeholders may be resistant to the changes; (2) health authorities may not believe in the effectiveness of mental health interventions; (3) there may be no consensus among the country's stakeholders about how to formulate or implement the new policy; (4) financial and human resources may be scarce; (5) other basic health priorities may compete with mental health care for funding; (6) primary care teams may feel overburdened by their workload and refuse to accept the introduction of the new policy; and (7) many mental health specialists may not want to work in community facilities or with primary care teams, preferring to remain in hospitals. The suggested solutions include: (1) adopting an "all-winners approach" that ensures that the needs of all stakeholders are taken into account, (2) developing pilot projects and evaluating their effect on health and consumer satisfaction, (3) asking for technical reports from international experts, (4) focusing the implementation of the mental health policy on a demonstration area and performing cost-effectiveness studies, (5) linking mental health programs to other health priorities, and (6) showing primary care practitioners that people with mental disorders are already a hidden part of their burden and that the burden will decrease if these disorders are identified and treated.

STIGMATIZING ATTITUDES TOWARD PEOPLE WITH MENTAL DISORDERS

Stigmatizing attitudes toward people with mental disorders are widespread in the general public and even among mental health professionals. Although it has been suggested that stigma may be less severe in Asian and African countries, a study carried out in India within the stigma program of the World Psychiatric Association (WPA), in which 463 persons with schizophrenia and 651 family members were interviewed in four cities, reported that two-thirds of the respondents had experienced discrimination. Women and people living in urban areas were more stigmatized. Whereas men experienced greater discrimination in the job area, women experienced more problems in the family and social areas.

Unlike people with physical disabilities, those with mental disorders are often perceived by the public to be in control of their disabilities and responsible for causing them. The view that "weakness," "laziness," or "lack of willpower" contributes to the development of mental disorders has been reported in several countries, including Turkey, Mongolia, and South Africa. The stigmatization of people with mental disorders may result in public avoidance, systematic discrimination, and reduced help-seeking behavior. In a survey carried out in 1996 in a probability sample of 1,444 adults in the United States, more than half of the respondents reported to be unwilling to spend an evening socializing with, work next to, or have a family member marry a person with mental illness. Although most countries have some provision for disability benefits, people with mental illness are often specifically excluded from such entitlements. Moreover, mental disorders are frequently not considered in social and private insurance schemes for health care. Shame is reported to be one of the main barriers from seeking help for mental disorders in both developed and developing countries.

Strategies for addressing stigmatization of people with mental disorders have been subdivided into three groups: protest, education, and contact. There is some evidence that protest campaigns may be effective in reducing stigmatizing behaviors against people with mental disorders. Education may promote a better understanding of mental illness, and educated people may be less likely to endorse stigma and discrimination. An inverse relationship between having contact with a person with mental illness and endorsing stigmatizing behaviors has been documented.

RELATIONSHIPS BETWEEN MENTAL AND PHYSICAL DISEASES

Mortality due to physical illness is significantly increased in people with severe mental disorders compared with the general population. In a follow-up study carried out in the United Kingdom, the standardized mortality ratio (SMR) for natural causes in people with schizophrenia was 2.32 (i.e., death was more than twice higher than in the general population). The SMR for causes "avoidable by appropriate treatment" was 4.68. The highest SMRs were those for endocrine, nervous, respiratory, circulatory, and gastrointestinal diseases. Increased nonsuicide all-cause mortality has also been reported for bipolar disorder (SMR 1.9 for men and 2.1 for women) and dementia (relative risk [RR] 2.63; 95 percent confidence interval [CI] 2.17 to 3.21). A meta-analysis of 15 population-based studies of the effect of a diagnosis of depression on subsequent all-cause mortality yielded a pooled odds ratio of 1.7 (CI 1.5 to 2.0). Evidence from low-income countries is limited, but a large population study conducted in Ethiopia found high mortality rates for major depression (SMR 3.55, 95 percent CI 1.97 to 6.39) and schizophrenia (almost 5 percent per year).

The prevalence of several physical diseases is increased in people with mental disorders compared with the general population. In a study carried out in the United States, people with psychotic disorders were found to be more likely than other people to develop diabetes, hypertension, heart disease, asthma, gastrointestinal disorders, skin infections, malignant neoplasms, and acute respiratory disorders. The rate was increased even when only patients without a concomitant substance use disorder were considered. In a study conducted in Nigeria, 55.2 percent of persons with schizophrenia-spectrum disorders referred for the first time to a psychiatric clinic had at least one physical disease, but in persons with neurotic disorders, the rate was 11.8 percent. A strong prospective association has been documented between depression and coronary heart disease outcomes, including fatal myocardial infarction; on the other hand, the incidence of depression is increased after myocardial infarction, especially in the first month after the event. Depression also increases the risk for type 2 diabetes. In South Asia, an association between maternal perinatal depression and infant malnutrition and stunting at 6 months has been repeatedly reported.

People with severe mental disorders are at increased risk of contracting HIV infection, although prevalence rates vary substantially worldwide. A large multicenter study conducted in sub-Saharan Africa, Asia, Latin America, Europe, and the United States reported a higher prevalence of depressive disorder among symptomatic HIV-seropositive people than in asymptomatic HIV-seropositive cases and seronegative control participants. Evidence from both developed and developing countries shows that adherence to highly active antiretroviral therapy (HAART) is negatively affected by depression, cognitive impairment, and substance abuse.

In a study carried out in the United Kingdom, people with severe mental illness were significantly more likely to be obese (body mass index [BMI] higher than 30) and morbidly obese (BMI higher than 40) than the general population: The respective figures were 35.0 versus 19.4 percent and 3.7 versus 1.3 percent. When these figures were broken down by age and sex, 28.7 percent of men with severe mental illness between 18 and 44 years of age were obese compared with 13.6 percent in the general population and 3.7 versus 0.4 percent were morbidly obese. Even more striking were the figures concerning women of the same age: 50.6 versus 16.6 percent and 7.4 versus 2.0 percent, respectively.

In a meta-analysis of worldwide studies, a highly significant association between schizophrenia and current smoking was confirmed: The weighted average odds ratio was 5.9; it was 7.2 in men and 3.3 in women. The association remained significant when controls with severe mental illness were used (odds ratio, 1.9).

Heavy smoking and high nicotine dependence were also more frequent in people with schizophrenia than in the general population.

The quality of physical health care received by patients with severe mental illness is often worse than the general population. A study conducted in the United States found that adverse events during medical and surgical hospitalizations were significantly more frequent in patients with schizophrenia than in the other people, including infections due to medical negligence, postoperative respiratory failure, postoperative deep venous thrombosis or pulmonary embolism, and postoperative sepsis. All of these adverse events were associated with significantly increased odds of admission to an intensive care unit and of death.

The decreased access of people with mental disorders to medical services has been related to several factors concerning the health care system. The effect of lack of insurance and cost of care is well documented. In a study carried out in the United States, people with mental disorders were twice as likely as those without mental disorders to have been denied insurance because of a pre-existing condition (odds ratio, 2.18). Having a mental disorder conferred a greater risk of having delayed seeking care because of cost (odds ratio, 1.76) and of having been unable to obtain needed medical care (odds ratio, 2.30).

Even when people with mental illness are seen by a doctor, their physical diseases often remain undiagnosed. Primary care providers may misperceive the medical complaints of people with mental disorders as "psychosomatic" or be unskilled, or feel uncomfortable in dealing with this population. An underlying stigmatization may be involved. Moreover, during hospitalizations in medical and surgical wards, health care professionals may not be experienced in dealing with the special needs of patients with schizophrenia, may minimize or misinterpret their somatic symptoms, and may make an inappropriate use of restraints or sedative drugs, or fail to consider possible interactions of psychotropic drugs with other medications. On the other hand, many psychiatrists are unable or unwilling to perform physical and even neurological examinations or are not up to date on the management of even common physical diseases.

To address this situation, the first step is raising awareness of the problem among mental health care professionals, primary care providers, and patients with schizophrenia and their families. Education and training of mental health professionals and primary care providers is a further essential step. Mental health professionals should be trained to perform at least basic medical tasks. They should be educated about the importance of recognizing physical illness in people with severe mental disorders and encouraged to become familiar with the most common reasons for underdiagnosis or misdiagnosis of physical illness in these patients. On the other hand, primary care providers should overcome their reluctance to treat people with severe mental illness and learn effective ways to interact and communicate with them; it is not only an issue of knowledge and skills but also, most of all, one of attitudes.

Another essential step is the development of an appropriate integration between mental health and physical health care. A well-identified professional should be responsible for physical health care in each person with a severe mental disorder. Mental health services should be able to provide at least a standard routine assessment of their patients to identify or at least suspect the presence of physical health problems. Guidelines about the management of patients receiving antipsychotic drugs should be known and applied by all mental health services. Patients should be involved as much as possible; for instance, mental health professionals should encourage patients to monitor and chart their weight. Dietary and exercise programs should be routinely provided by mental health services. Flexible smoking cessation programs, which have shown some degree of success, could be considered in some settings.

ETHICAL ISSUES IN MENTAL HEALTH CARE

The protection and promotion of the human rights of people with mental disorders are emerging as a priority worldwide. In 1991, the United Nations (UN) issued Resolution 46/119 for the Protection of Persons with Mental Illness and the Improvement of Mental Health Care. In that resolution, the human rights of people with mental disorders and their right to treatment were codified for the first time in a UN document. The 25 principles covered the following areas: definition of mental illness; protection of confidentiality; standards of care and treatment, including involuntary admission and consent to treatment; rights of persons with mental disorders in mental health facilities; protection of minors; provision of resources for mental health facilities; role of community and culture; review mechanisms providing for the protection of the rights of offenders with mental disorders; and procedural safeguards protecting rights of persons with mental disorders. National governments were invited to promote the principles of the resolution by appropriate legislative, juridical, administrative, educational, and other provisions. However, violations of the human rights of people with mental disorders are still reported in many countries, and in a substantial number of low- and middle-income countries, patients in mental hospitals are physically restrained or secluded for long periods.

In Latin America, an influential document has been the Declaration of Caracas, adopted in 1990 by the Regional Conference on Restructuring Psychiatric Care in Latin America, which states that resources, care, and treatment for people with mental disorders should safeguard their dignity and human and civil rights, and strive to maintain its people in their communities. The declaration also states that mental health legislation should safeguard the human rights of people with mental disorders and that services should be organized so that these rights can be enforced.

In Africa, the Banjul Charter on Human and People's Rights, a legally binding document supervised by the African Commission on Human and People's Rights, in Article 5 addresses the right to respect for the dignity inherent in human beings and the prohibition of all forms of degradation, including cruel, inhuman, or degrading treatment.

According to the WHO, mental health legislation should cover the following issues: access to basic mental health care, least restrictive care, informed consent to treatment, voluntary and involuntary admission to treatment, competence issues, periodical review mechanism, confidentiality, rehabilitation, accreditation of professionals and facilities, and rights of families and caregivers. Specific legislation in the field of mental health is present in 74 percent of low-income countries versus 92.7 percent of high-income countries.

In 1996, the WPA released the Madrid Declaration, which contains the ethical principles by which all national psychiatric societies are expected to abide. The declaration includes seven general guidelines focusing on the aims of psychiatry: (1) psychiatrists must serve patients by providing the best therapy available, consistent with accepted scientific knowledge and ethical principles, and should devise therapeutic interventions that are the least restrictive to the freedom of the patient; (2) it is the duty of psychiatrists to keep abreast of scientific developments of their specialty and to convey updated knowledge to others; (3) the patient should be accepted as a partner by right in the therapeutic process, and the therapist–patient relationship must be based on mutual trust and respect, to allow the patient to make free and informed decisions; (4) treatment must always be in the best interest of the patient, and no treatment should be provided against the patient's will, unless withholding treatment would endanger life of the patient or those who surround him or her; (5) when psychiatrists are requested to assess a person, it is their duty to inform the person being assessed about the purpose of the intervention; (6) information contained in the therapeutic relationship should be kept confidential and used exclusively for the purpose of improving the mental health of the patient; and (7) because psychiatric patients are particularly vulnerable research subjects, extra caution should be taken to safeguard their autonomy, as well as their mental and physical integrity.

INTERNATIONAL ORGANIZATIONS ACTIVE IN THE MENTAL HEALTH FIELD

Many international organizations are active in the mental health field. They include the WHO, which is the world's leading public health agency; some professional associations, among which the largest is the WPA, representing the psychiatric profession worldwide; and several organizations with a membership of users and families (such as the World Fellowship for Schizophrenia and the Global Alliance of Mental Illness Advocacy Networks [GAMIAN]) or of both mental health professionals and users and families (such as the World Federation for Mental Health [WFMH]).

The WHO is a UN agency with 192 member states, grouped into six regions (Africa, the Americas, European Mediterranean, Europe, Southeast Asia, and Western Pacific). It has a Department of Mental Health and Substance Abuse at its headquarters in Geneva and advisors for mental health in each of its regional offices. Its main functions are direction and coordination of international health work and technical cooperation with countries. Among the numerous recent WHO activities in the mental health field, of special interest is the release of the *World Health Report 2001* and the development of the report *Mental Health: New Understanding, New Hope,* which was completely devoted to mental health. It provided a summary of the current and projected impact of mental disorders and of the principles of mental health policy and service provision, as well as a set of recommendations for future action that can be adapted to the needs and resources of the various countries. Project Atlas aims to collect information on mental health resources across the world. Global and regional analyses of those resources were first published in 2001 and updated in 2005. Volumes focusing on resources for child and adolescent mental health and on psychiatric education and training worldwide (the latter in collaboration with the WPA) were released in 2005.

The WPA is an association of national psychiatric societies aimed at increasing knowledge and skills necessary for work in the field of mental health and care for the mentally ill. Its member society's number 134, spans 122 countries and represents more than 200,000 psychiatrists. The WPA organizes the World Congress of Psychiatry every 3 years. It also organizes international and regional congresses and meetings, and thematic conferences. It has 65 scientific sections, which are aimed at disseminating information and promoting collaborative work in specific domains of psychiatry. It has produced several educational programs and series of books and consensus statements (including the Declaration of Madrid on ethical principles for psychiatric practice). It has an official journal, *World Psychiatry,* which is produced in English, Spanish, and Chinese and is indexed in PubMed and Current Contents and reaches more than 33,000 psychiatrists worldwide.

The WFMH is a multidisciplinary advocacy and education organization aimed at promoting the advancement of mental health awareness, prevention, advocacy, and best-practice recovery-focused interventions worldwide. Among its activities is the organization of the World Mental Health Day, observed every year on October 10, each time with a different theme.

FUTURE PERSPECTIVES

Several statements have been made by various groups and organizations about priorities for future action in the mental health field at the international level. Of special interest is a document produced by 39 leaders that comprises the so-called Lancet Global Mental Health Group's policies. In this document, five main goals are identified: (1) placing mental health on the public health priority agenda, (2) improving the organization of mental health services, (3) integrating the availability of mental health into general health care, (4) developing human resources for mental health, and (5) strengthening public mental health leadership.

Among the strategies proposed to place mental health on the public health priority agenda are the development and use of uniform and clearly understandable messages for mental health advocacy and the education of decision makers within governments and donor agencies on the evidence concerning the public health significance of mental disorders and the cost-effectiveness of mental health care. Strategies suggested to improve the organization of mental health services include, among others, the provision of incentive arrangements to overcome vested interests blocking change and the organization of international technical support to learn from countries that have experienced successful mental health reform. To integrate the availability of mental health in general health care, it is proposed that mental health professionals be appointed and trained specifically for supporting and supervising primary health care staff. To promote the development of human resources for mental health, it is suggested that the professional and specialist workforce be increased and diversified and that the quality of mental health training be improved to ensure that it is practical and occurs also in community or primary care settings.

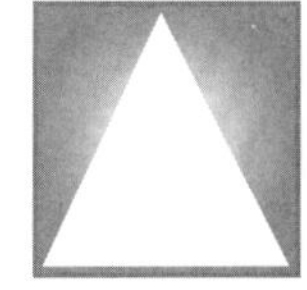

Glossary of Signs and Symptoms in Psychiatry*

Signs are objective; symptoms are subjective. Signs are the clinician's observations, such as noting a patient's agitation; symptoms are subjective experiences, such as a person's complaint of feeling depressed. In psychiatry, signs and symptoms are not as clearly demarcated as in other fields of medicine; they often overlap. Because of this, disorders in psychiatry are often described as syndromes—a constellation of signs and symptoms that together make up a recognizable condition. Schizophrenia, for example, is more often viewed as a syndrome than as a specific disorder. This concept is expressed in the use of the terms *schizophrenic spectrum* or *the group of schizophrenias,* and in the use of the term *autism spectrum disorder.*

GLOSSARY OF SIGNS AND SYMPTOMS

abreaction A process by which repressed material, particularly a painful experience or a conflict, is brought back to consciousness; in this process, the person not only recalls but also relieves the repressed material, which is accompanied by the appropriate affective response.

abstract thinking Thinking characterized by the ability to grasp the essentials of a whole, to break a whole into its parts, and to discern common properties. To think symbolically.

abulia Reduced impulse to act and to think, associated with indifference about consequences of action. Occurs as a result of neurological deficit, depression, and schizophrenia.

acalculia Loss of ability to do calculations; not caused by anxiety or impairment in concentration. Occurs with neurological deficit and learning disorder.

acataphasia Disordered speech in which statements are incorrectly formulated. Patients may express themselves with words that sound like the ones intended but are not appropriate to the thoughts, or they may use totally inappropriate expressions.

acathexis Lack of feeling associated with an ordinarily emotionally charged subject; in psychoanalysis, it denotes the patient's detaching or transferring of emotion from thoughts and ideas. Also called *decathexis.* Occurs in anxiety, dissociative, schizophrenic, and bipolar disorders.

acenesthesia Loss of sensation of physical existence.

acrophobia Dread of high places.

acting out Behavioral response to an unconscious drive or impulse that brings about temporary partial relief of inner tension; relief is attained by reacting to a present situation as if it were the situation that originally gave rise to the drive or impulse. Common in borderline states.

aculalia Nonsense speech associated with marked impairment of comprehension. Occurs in mania, schizophrenia, and neurological deficit.

adiadochokinesia Inability to perform rapid alternating movements. Occurs with neurological deficit and cerebellar lesions.

adynamia Weakness and fatigability, characteristic of neurasthenia and depression.

aerophagia Excessive swallowing of air. Seen in anxiety disorder.

affect The subjective and immediate experience of emotion attached to ideas or mental representations of objects. Affect has outward manifestations that may be classified as restricted, blunted, flattened, broad, labile, appropriate, or inappropriate. *See also* **mood.**

ageusia Lack or impairment of the sense of taste. Seen in depression and neurological deficit.

aggression Forceful, goal-directed action that may be verbal or physical; the motor counterpart of the affect of rage, anger, or hostility. Seen in neurological deficit, temporal lobe disorder, impulse-control disorders, mania, and schizophrenia.

agitation Severe anxiety associated with motor restlessness.

agnosia Inability to understand the import or significance of sensory stimuli; cannot be explained by a defect in sensory pathways or cerebral lesion; the term has also been used to refer to the selective loss or disuse of knowledge of specific objects because of emotional circumstances, as seen in certain schizophrenic, anxious, and depressed patients. Occurs with neurological deficit. For types of agnosia, see the specific term.

agoraphobia Morbid fear of open places or leaving the familiar setting of the home. May be present with or without panic attacks.

agraphia Loss or impairment of a previously possessed ability to write.

ailurophobia Dread of cats.

akathisia Subjective feeling of motor restlessness manifested by a compelling need to be in constant movement; may be seen as an extrapyramidal adverse effect of antipsychotic medication. May be mistaken for psychotic agitation.

akinesia Lack of physical movement, as in the extreme immobility of catatonic schizophrenia; may also occur as an extrapyramidal effect of antipsychotic medication.

akinetic mutism Absence of voluntary motor movement or speech in a patient who is apparently alert (as evidenced by eye movements). Seen in psychotic depression and catatonic states.

alexia Loss of a previously possessed reading facility; not explained by defective visual acuity. *Compare with* **dyslexia.**

alexithymia Inability or difficulty in describing or being aware of one's emotions or moods; elaboration of fantasies associated with depression, substance abuse, and posttraumatic stress disorder.

algophobia Dread of pain.

alogia Inability to speak because of a mental deficiency or an episode of dementia.

ambivalence Coexistence of two opposing impulses toward the same thing in the same person at the same time. Seen in schizophrenia, borderline states, and obsessive-compulsive disorders (OCDs).

amimia Lack of the ability to make gestures or to comprehend those made by others.

amnesia Partial or total inability to recall past experiences; may be organic (*amnestic disorder*) or emotional (*dissociative amnesia*) in origin.

amnestic aphasia Disturbed capacity to name objects, even though they are known to the patient. Also called anomic aphasia.

anaclitic Depending on others, especially as the infant on the mother; anaclitic depression in children results from an absence of mothering.

analgesia State in which one feels little or no pain. Can occur under hypnosis and in dissociative disorder.

anancasm Repetitious or stereotyped behavior or thought usually used as a tension-relieving device; used as a synonym for obsession and seen in obsessive-compulsive (anankastic) personality.

androgyny Combination of culturally determined female and male characteristics in one person.

anergia Lack of energy.

anhedonia Loss of interest in and withdrawal from all regular and pleasurable activities. Often associated with depression.

anomia Inability to recall the names of objects.

anorexia Loss or decrease in appetite. In *anorexia nervosa,* appetite may be preserved, but the patient refuses to eat.

anosognosia Inability to recognize a physical deficit in oneself (e.g., patient denies paralyzed limb).

anterograde amnesia Loss of memory for events subsequent to the onset of the amnesia; common after trauma. *Compare with* **retrograde amnesia.**

anxiety Feeling of apprehension caused by anticipation of danger, which may be internal or external.

apathy Dulled emotional tone associated with detachment or indifference; observed in certain types of schizophrenia and depression.

aphasia Any disturbance in the comprehension or expression of language caused by a brain lesion. For types of aphasia, see the specific term.

aphonia Loss of voice. Seen in conversion disorder.

apperception Awareness of the meaning and significance of a particular sensory stimulus as modified by one's experiences, knowledge, thoughts, and emotions. *See also* **perception.**

appropriate affect Emotional tone in harmony with the accompanying idea, thought, or speech.

apraxia Inability to perform a voluntary purposeful motor activity; cannot be explained by paralysis or other motor or sensory impairment. In *constructional apraxia,* a patient cannot draw two- or three-dimensional forms.

astasia abasia Inability to stand or to walk in a normal manner, even though normal leg movements can be performed in a sitting or lying down position. Seen in conversion disorder.

astereognosis Inability to identify familiar objects by touch. Seen with neurological deficit. *See also* **neurological amnesia.**

asthenopia Pain or discomfort of the eyes, for example, pressure, grittiness.

asyndesis Disorder of language in which the patient combines unconnected ideas and images. Commonly seen in schizophrenia.

ataxia Lack of coordination, physical or mental. (1) In neurology, refers to loss of muscular coordination. (2) In psychiatry, the term *intrapsychic ataxia* refers to lack of coordination between feelings and thoughts; seen in schizophrenia and in severe OCD.

atonia Lack of muscle tone. *See* **waxy flexibility.**

attention Concentration; the aspect of consciousness that relates to the amount of effort exerted in focusing on certain aspects of an experience, activity, or task. Usually impaired in anxiety and depressive disorders.

auditory hallucination False perception of sound, usually voices, but also other noises, such as music. Most common hallucination in psychiatric disorders.

aura (1) Warning sensations, such as automatisms, fullness in the stomach, blushing, and changes in respiration; cognitive sensations; and mood states usually experienced before a seizure. (2) A sensory prodrome that precedes a classic migraine headache.

autistic thinking Thinking in which the thoughts are largely narcissistic and egocentric, with emphasis on subjectivity rather than objectivity, and without regard for reality; used interchangeably with autism and dereism. Seen in schizophrenia and autistic disorder.

automatism A state following a seizure in which the person performs movements or actions without being aware of what is happening.

behavior Sum total of the psyche that includes impulses, motivations, wishes, drives, instincts, and cravings, as expressed by a person's behavior or motor activity. Also called *conation.*

bereavement Feeling of grief or desolation, especially at the death or loss of a loved one.

bizarre delusion False belief that is patently absurd or fantastic (e.g., invaders from space have implanted electrodes in a person's brain). Common in schizophrenia. In nonbizarre delusion, content is usually within the range of possibility.

blackout Amnesia experienced by alcoholics about behavior during drinking bouts; usually indicates reversible brain damage.

blocking Abrupt interruption in train of thinking before a thought or idea is finished; after a brief pause, the person indicates no recall of what was being said or was going to be said (also known as *thought deprivation* or *increased thought latency*). Common in schizophrenia and severe anxiety.

blunted affect Disturbance of affect manifested by a severe reduction in the intensity of externalized feeling tone; one of the fundamental symptoms of schizophrenia, as outlined by Eugen Bleuler.

bradykinesia Slowness of motor activity, with a decrease in normal spontaneous movement.

bradylalia Abnormally slow speech. Common in depression.

bradylexia Inability to read at normal speed.

bruxism Grinding or gnashing of the teeth, typically occurring during sleep. Seen in anxiety disorder.

carebaria Sensation of discomfort or pressure in the head.

catalepsy Condition in which persons maintain the body position into which they are placed; observed in severe cases of catatonic schizophrenia. Also called *waxy flexibility* and *cerea flexibilitas. See also* **command automatism.**

cataplexy Temporary sudden loss of muscle tone, causing weakness and immobilization; can be precipitated by a variety of emotional states and is often followed by sleep. Commonly seen in narcolepsy.

catatonic excitement Excited, uncontrolled motor activity seen in catatonic schizophrenia. Patients in a catatonic state may suddenly erupt into an excited state and may be violent.

catatonic posturing Voluntary assumption of an inappropriate or bizarre posture, generally maintained for long periods of time. May switch unexpectedly with catatonic excitement.

catatonic rigidity Fixed and sustained motoric position that is resistant to change.

catatonic stupor Stupor in which patients ordinarily are well aware of their surroundings.

cathexis In psychoanalysis, a conscious or unconscious investment of psychic energy in an idea, concept, object, or person. *Compare with* **acathexis.**

causalgia Burning pain that may be organic or psychic in origin.

cenesthesia Change in the normal quality of feeling tone in a part of the body.

cephalagia Headache.

cerea flexibilitas Condition of a person who can be molded into a position that is then maintained; when an examiner moves the person's limb, the limb feels as if it were made of wax. Also called *catalepsy* or *waxy flexibility.* Seen in schizophrenia.

chorea Movement disorder characterized by random and involuntary quick, jerky, purposeless movements. Seen in Huntington's disease.

circumstantiality Disturbance in the associative thought and speech processes in which a patient digresses into unnecessary details and inappropriate thoughts before communicating the central idea. Observed in schizophrenia, obsessional disturbances, and certain cases of dementia. *See also* **tangentiality.**

clang association Association or speech directed by the sound of a word rather than by its meaning; words have no logical connection; punning and rhyming may dominate the verbal behavior. Seen most frequently in schizophrenia or mania.

claustrophobia Abnormal fear of closed or confining spaces.

clonic convulsion An involuntary, violent muscular contraction or spasm in which the muscles alternately contract and relax. Characteristic phase in grand mal epileptic seizure.

clouding of consciousness Any disturbance of consciousness in which the person is not fully awake, alert, and oriented. Occurs in delirium, dementia, and cognitive disorder.

cluttering Disturbance of fluency involving an abnormally rapid rate and erratic rhythm of speech that impedes intelligibility; the affected individual is usually unaware of communicative impairment.

cognition Mental process of knowing and becoming aware; function is closely associated with judgment.

coma State of profound unconsciousness from which a person cannot be roused, with minimal or no detectable responsiveness to stimuli; seen in injury or disease of the brain, in systemic conditions such as diabetic ketoacidosis and uremia, and in intoxications with alcohol and other drugs. Coma may also occur in severe catatonic states and in conversion disorder.

coma vigil Coma in which a patient appears to be asleep but can be aroused (also known as *akinetic mutism*).

command automatism Condition associated with catalepsy in which suggestions are followed automatically.

command hallucination False perception of orders that a person may feel obliged to obey or unable to resist.

complex A feeling-toned idea.

complex partial seizure A seizure characterized by alterations in consciousness that may be accompanied by complex hallucinations (sometimes olfactory) or illusions. During the seizure, a state of impaired consciousness resembling a dream-like state may occur, and the patient may exhibit repetitive, automatic, or semipurposeful behavior.

compulsion Pathological need to act on an impulse that, if resisted, produces anxiety; repetitive behavior in response to an obsession or performed according to certain rules, with no true end in itself other than to prevent something from occurring in the future.

conation That part of a person's mental life concerned with cravings, strivings, motivations, drives, and wishes as expressed through behavior or motor activity.

concrete thinking Thinking characterized by actual things, events, and immediate experience rather than by abstractions; seen in young children, in those who have lost or never developed the ability to generalize (as in certain cognitive mental disorders), and in schizophrenic persons. *Compare with* **abstract thinking.**

condensation Mental process in which one symbol stands for a number of components.

confabulation Unconscious filling of gaps in memory by imagining experiences or events that have no basis in fact, commonly seen in amnestic syndromes; should be differentiated from lying. *See also* **paramnesia.**

confusion Disturbances of consciousness manifested by a disordered orientation in relation to time, place, or person.

consciousness State of awareness, with response to external stimuli.

constipation Inability to defecate or difficulty in defecating.

constricted affect Reduction in intensity of feeling tone that is less severe than that of blunted affect.

constructional apraxia Inability to copy a drawing, such as a cube, clock, or pentagon, as a result of a brain lesion.

conversion phenomena The development of symbolic physical symptoms and distortions involving the voluntary muscles or special sense organs; not under voluntary control and not explained by any physical disorder. Most common in conversion disorder, but also seen in a variety of mental disorders.

convulsion An involuntary, violent muscular contraction or spasm. *See also* **clonic convulsion** *and* **tonic convulsion.**

coprolalia Involuntary use of vulgar or obscene language. Observed in some cases of schizophrenia and in Tourette's syndrome.

coprophagia Eating of filth or feces.

cryptographia A private written language.

cryptolalia A private spoken language.

cycloplegia Paralysis of the muscles of accommodation in the eye; observed, at times, as an autonomic adverse effect (anticholinergic effect) of antipsychotic or antidepressant medication.

decompensation Deterioration of psychic functioning caused by a breakdown of defense mechanisms. Seen in psychotic states.

déjà entendu Illusion that what one is hearing one has heard previously. *See also* **paramnesia.**

déjà pensé Condition in which a thought never entertained before is incorrectly regarded as a repetition of a previous thought. *See also* **paramnesia.**

déjà vu Illusion of visual recognition in which a new situation is incorrectly regarded as a repetition of a previous experience. *See also* **paramnesia.**

delirium Acute reversible mental disorder characterized by confusion and some impairment of consciousness; generally associated with emotional lability, hallucinations or illusions, and inappropriate, impulsive, irrational, or violent behavior.

delirium tremens Acute and sometimes fatal reaction to withdrawal from alcohol, usually occurring 72 to 96 hours after the cessation of heavy drinking; distinctive characteristics are marked autonomic hyperactivity (tachycardia, fever, hyperhidrosis, and dilated pupils), usually accompanied by tremulousness, hallucinations, illusions, and delusions. Called *alcohol withdrawal delirium* in the text revision of the fourth edition of the *Diagnostic and Statistical Manual of Mental Disorders. See also* **formication.**

delusion False belief, based on incorrect inference about external reality, that is firmly held despite objective and obvious contradictory proof or evidence and despite the fact that other members of the culture do not share the belief.

delusion of control False belief that a person's will, thoughts, or feelings are being controlled by external forces.

delusion of grandeur Exaggerated conception of one's importance, power, or identity.

delusion of infidelity False belief that one's lover is unfaithful. Sometimes called *pathological jealousy.*

delusion of persecution False belief of being harassed or persecuted; often found in litigious patients who have a pathological tendency to take legal action because of imagined mistreatment. Most common delusion.

delusion of poverty False belief that one is bereft or will be deprived of all material possessions.

delusion of reference False belief that the behavior of others refers to oneself or that events, objects, or other people have a particular and unusual significance, usually of a negative nature; derived from idea of reference, in which persons falsely feel that others are talking about them (e.g., belief that people on television or radio are talking to or about the person). *See also* **thought broadcasting.**

delusion of self-accusation False feeling of remorse and guilt. Seen in depression with psychotic features.

dementia Mental disorder characterized by general impairment in intellectual functioning without clouding of consciousness; characterized by failing memory, difficulty with calculations, distractibility, alterations in mood and affect, impaired judgment and abstraction, reduced facility with language, and disturbance of orientation. Although irreversible when it is due to underlying progressive degenerative brain disease, dementia may be reversible if the cause can be treated.

denial Defense mechanism in which the existence of unpleasant realities is disavowed; refers to keeping out of conscious awareness any aspects of external reality that, if acknowledged, would produce anxiety.

depersonalization Sensation of unreality concerning oneself, parts of oneself, or one's environment that occurs under extreme stress or fatigue. Seen in schizophrenia, depersonalization disorder, and schizotypal personality disorder.

depression Mental state characterized by feelings of sadness, loneliness, despair, low self-esteem, and self-reproach; accompanying signs include psychomotor retardation or, at times, agitation, withdrawal from interpersonal contact, and vegetative symptoms, such as insomnia and anorexia. The term refers to a mood that is so characterized or a mood disorder.

derailment Gradual or sudden deviation in train of thought without blocking; sometimes used synonymously with *loosening of association.*

derealization Sensation of changed reality or that one's surroundings have altered. Usually seen in schizophrenia, panic attacks, and dissociative disorders.

dereism Mental activity that follows a totally subjective and idiosyncratic system of logic and fails to take the facts of reality or experience into consideration. Characteristic of schizophrenia. *See also* **autistic thinking.**

detachment Characterized by distant interpersonal relationships and lack of emotional involvement.

devaluation Defense mechanism in which a person attributes excessively negative qualities to self or others. Seen in depression and paranoid personality disorder.

diminished libido Decreased sexual interest and drive. (Increased libido is often associated with mania.)

dipsomania Compulsion to drink alcoholic beverages.

disinhibition (1) Removal of an inhibitory effect, as in the reduction of the inhibitory function of the cerebral cortex by alcohol. (2) In psychiatry, a greater freedom to act in accordance with inner drives or feelings and with less regard for restraints dictated by cultural norms or one's superego.

disorientation Confusion; impairment of awareness of time, place, and person (the position of the self in relation to other persons). Characteristic of cognitive disorders.

displacement Unconscious defense mechanism by which the emotional component of an unacceptable idea or object is transferred to a more acceptable one. Seen in phobias.

dissociation Unconscious defense mechanism involving the segregation of any group of mental or behavioral processes from the rest of the person's psychic activity; may entail the separation of an idea from its accompanying emotional tone, as seen in dissociative and conversion disorders. Seen in dissociative disorders.

distractibility Inability to focus one's attention; the patient does not respond to the task at hand but attends to irrelevant phenomena in the environment.

doubling The feeling that one has a double who is similar in looks, actions, and feelings. Also known as *Doppelgänger* phenomenon.

dread Massive or pervasive anxiety, usually related to a specific danger.

dreamy state Altered state of consciousness, likened to a dream situation, that develops suddenly and usually lasts a few minutes; accompanied by visual, auditory, and olfactory hallucinations. Commonly associated with temporal lobe lesions.

drowsiness State of impaired awareness associated with a desire or inclination to sleep.

dysarthria Difficulty in articulation—the motor activity of shaping phonated sounds into speech—not in word finding or in grammar.

dyscalculia Difficulty in performing calculations.

dysgeusia Impaired sense of taste.

dysgraphia Difficulty in writing.

dyskinesia Difficulty in performing movements. Seen in extrapyramidal disorders.

dyslalia Faulty articulation caused by structural abnormalities of the articulatory organs or impaired hearing.

dyslexia Specific learning disability syndrome involving an impairment of the previously acquired ability to read; unrelated to the person's intelligence. *Compare with* **alexia.**

dysmetria Impaired ability to gauge distance relative to movements. Seen in neurological deficit.

dysmnesia Impaired memory.

dyspareunia Physical pain in sexual intercourse, usually emotionally caused and more commonly experienced by women; may also result from cystitis, urethritis, or other medical conditions.

dysphagia Difficulty in swallowing.

dysphasia Difficulty in comprehending oral language (*reception dysphasia*) or in trying to express verbal language (*expressive dysphasia*).

dysphonia Difficulty or pain in speaking.

dysphoria Feeling of unpleasantness or discomfort; a mood of general dissatisfaction and restlessness. Occurs in depression and anxiety.

dysprosody Loss of normal speech melody (*prosody*). Common in depression.

dystonia Extrapyramidal motor disturbance consisting of slow, sustained contractions of the axial or appendicular musculature; one movement often predominates, leading to relatively sustained postural deviations; acute dystonic reactions (facial grimacing and torticollis) are occasionally seen with the initiation of antipsychotic drug therapy.

echolalia Psychopathological repeating of words or phrases of one person by another; tends to be repetitive and persistent. Seen in certain kinds of schizophrenia, particularly the catatonic types.

echopraxia The person imitates the clinician's actions even when asked not to do so.

ego-alien Denoting aspects of a person's personality that are viewed as repugnant, unacceptable, or inconsistent with the rest of the personality. Also called *ego-dystonia. Compare with* **ego-syntonic.**

egocentric Self-centered; selfishly preoccupied with one's own needs; lacking interest in others.

ego-dystonic *See* **ego-alien.**

egomania Morbid self-preoccupation or self-centeredness. *See also* **narcissism.**

ego-syntonic Denoting aspects of a personality that are viewed as acceptable and consistent with that person's total personality. Personality traits are usually ego-syntonic. *Compare with* **ego-alien.**

eidetic image Unusually vivid or exact mental image of objects previously seen or imagined.

elation Mood consisting of feelings of joy, euphoria, triumph, and intense self-satisfaction or optimism. Occurs in mania when not grounded in reality.

elevated mood Air of confidence and enjoyment; a mood more cheerful than normal but not necessarily pathological.

emotion Complex feeling state with psychic, somatic, and behavioral components; external manifestation of emotion is *affect.*

emotional insight A level of understanding or awareness that one has emotional problems. It facilitates positive changes in personality and behavior when present.

emotional lability Excessive emotional responsiveness characterized by unstable and rapidly changing emotions.

encopresis Involuntary passage of feces, usually occurring at night or during sleep.

enuresis Incontinence of urine during sleep.

erotomania Delusional belief, more common in women than in men, that someone is deeply in love with them (also known as *de Clérambault syndrome*).

erythrophobia Abnormal fear of blushing.

euphoria Exaggerated feeling of well-being that is inappropriate to real events. Can occur with drugs such as opiates, amphetamines, and alcohol.

euthymia Normal range of mood, implying absence of depressed or elevated mood.

evasion Act of not facing up to, or strategically eluding, something; consists of suppressing an idea that is next in a thought series and replacing it with another idea closely related to it. Also called *paralogia* and *perverted logic.*

exaltation Feeling of intense elation and grandeur.

excited Agitated, purposeless motor activity uninfluenced by external stimuli.

expansive mood Expression of feelings without restraint, frequently with an overestimation of their significance or importance. Seen in mania and grandiose delusional disorder.

expressive aphasia Disturbance of speech in which understanding remains, but the ability to speak is grossly impaired; halting, laborious, and inaccurate speech (also known as *Broca's, nonfluent,* and *motor aphasias*).

expressive dysphasia Difficulty in expressing verbal language; the ability to understand language is intact.

externalization More general term than *projection* that refers to the tendency to perceive in the external world and in external objects elements of one's personality, including instinctual impulses, conflicts, moods, attitudes, and styles of thinking.

extroversion State of one's energies being directed outside oneself. *Compare with* **introversion.**

false memory The recollection and belief by the patient of an event that did not actually occur. In *false memory syndrome,* persons erroneously believe that they sustained an emotional or physical (e.g., sexual) trauma in early life.

fantasy Daydream; fabricated mental picture of a situation or chain of events. A normal form of thinking dominated by unconscious material that seeks wish fulfillment and solutions to conflicts; may serve as the matrix for creativity. The content of the fantasy may indicate mental illness.

fatigue A feeling of weariness, sleepiness, or irritability after a period of mental or bodily activity. Seen in depression, anxiety, neurasthenia, and somatoform disorders.

fausse reconnaissance False recognition, a feature of paramnesia. Can occur in delusional disorders.

fear Unpleasurable emotional state consisting of psychophysiological changes in response to a realistic threat or danger. *Compare with* **anxiety.**

flat affect Absence or near absence of any signs of affective expression.

flight of ideas Rapid succession of fragmentary thoughts or speech in which content changes abruptly and speech may be incoherent. Seen in mania.

floccillation Aimless plucking or picking, usually at bedclothes or clothing, commonly seen in dementia and delirium.

fluent aphasia Aphasia characterized by inability to understand the spoken word; fluent but incoherent speech is present. Also called *Wernicke's, sensory,* and *receptive aphasias.*

folie à deux Mental illness shared by two persons, usually involving a common delusional system; if it involves three persons, it is referred to as *folie à trois,* etc. Also called *shared psychotic disorder.*

formal thought disorder Disturbance in the form of thought rather than the content of thought; thinking characterized by loosened associations, neologisms, and illogical constructs; thought process is disordered, and the person is defined as psychotic. Characteristic of schizophrenia.

formication Tactile hallucination involving the sensation that tiny insects are crawling over the skin. Seen in cocaine addiction and delirium tremens.

free-floating anxiety Severe, pervasive, generalized anxiety that is not attached to any particular idea, object, or event. Observed particularly in anxiety disorders, although it may be seen in some cases of schizophrenia.

fugue Dissociative disorder characterized by a period of almost complete amnesia, during which a person actually flees from an immediate life situation and begins a different life pattern; apart from the amnesia, mental faculties and skills are usually unimpaired.

galactorrhea Abnormal discharge of milk from the breast; may result from the endocrine influence (e.g., prolactin) of dopamine receptor antagonists, such as phenothiazines.

generalized tonic–clonic seizure Generalized onset of tonic–clonic movements of the limbs, tongue biting, and incontinence followed by slow, gradual recovery of consciousness and cognition; also called *grand mal seizure.*

global aphasia Combination of grossly nonfluent aphasia and severe fluent aphasia.

glossolalia Unintelligible jargon that has meaning to the speaker but not to the listener. Occurs in schizophrenia.

grandiosity Exaggerated feelings of one's importance, power, knowledge, or identity. Occurs in delusional disorder and manic states.

grief Alteration in mood and affect consisting of sadness appropriate to a real loss; normally, it is self-limited. *See also* **depression** *and* **mourning.**

guilt Emotional state associated with self-reproach and the need for punishment. In psychoanalysis, refers to a feeling of culpability that stems from a conflict between the ego and the superego (conscience). Guilt has normal psychological and social functions, but special intensity or absence of guilt characterizes many mental disorders, such as depression and antisocial personality disorder, respectively. Psychiatrists distinguish shame as a less internalized form of guilt that relates more to others than to the self. *See also* **shame.**

gustatory hallucination Hallucination primarily involving taste.

gynecomastia Female-like development of the male breasts; may occur as an adverse effect of antipsychotic and antidepressant drugs because of increased prolactin levels or anabolic-androgenic steroid abuse.

hallucination False sensory perception occurring in the absence of any relevant external stimulation of the sensory modality involved. For types of hallucinations, see the specific term.

hallucinosis State in which a person experiences hallucinations without any impairment of consciousness.

haptic hallucination Hallucination of touch.

hebephrenia Complex of symptoms, considered a form of schizophrenia, characterized by wild or silly behavior or mannerisms, inappropriate affect, and delusions and hallucinations that are transient and unsystematized Hebephrenic schizophrenia is now called *disorganized schizophrenia.*

holophrastic Using a single word to express a combination of ideas. Seen in schizophrenia.

hyperacusis Increased sensitivity to sound.

hyperactivity Increased muscular activity. The term is commonly used to describe a disturbance found in children that is manifested by constant restlessness, overactivity, distractibility, and difficulties in learning. Seen in *attention-deficit/hyperactivity disorder* (ADHD).

hyperalgesia Excessive sensitivity to pain. Seen in somatoform disorder.

hyperesthesia Increased sensitivity to tactile stimulation.

hypermnesia Exaggerated degree of retention and recall. It can be elicited by hypnosis and may be seen in certain prodigies; also may be a feature of OCD, some cases of schizophrenia, and manic episodes of bipolar I disorder.

hyperphagia Increase in appetite and intake of food.

hyperpragia Excessive thinking and mental activity. Generally associated with manic episodes of bipolar I disorder.

hypersomnia Excessive time spent asleep. May be associated with underlying medical or psychiatric disorder or narcolepsy, may be part of the Kleine–Levin syndrome, or may be primary.

hyperventilation Excessive breathing, generally associated with anxiety, which can reduce blood-carbon dioxide concentration and can produce lightheadedness, palpitations, numbness, tingling periorally and in the extremities, and, occasionally, syncope.

hypervigilance Excessive attention to and focus on all internal and external stimuli; usually seen in delusional or paranoid states.

hypesthesia Diminished sensitivity to tactile stimulation.

hypnagogic hallucination Hallucination occurring while falling asleep, not ordinarily considered pathological.

hypnopompic hallucination Hallucination occurring while awakening from sleep, not ordinarily considered pathological.

hypnosis Artificially induced alteration of consciousness characterized by increased suggestibility and receptivity to direction.

hypoactivity Decreased motor and cognitive activity, as in psychomotor retardation; visible slowing of thought, speech, and movements. Also called *hypokinesis.*

hypochondria Exaggerated concern about health that is based not on real medical pathology, but on unrealistic interpretations of physical signs or sensations as abnormal.

hypomania Mood abnormality with the qualitative characteristics of mania but somewhat less intense. Seen in cyclothymic disorder.

idea of reference Misinterpretation of incidents and events in the outside world as having direct personal reference to oneself; occasionally observed in normal persons, but frequently seen in paranoid patients. If present with sufficient frequency or intensity or if organized and systematized, these misinterpretations constitute delusions of reference.

illogical thinking Thinking containing erroneous conclusions or internal contradictions; psychopathological only when it is marked and not caused by cultural values or intellectual deficit.

illusion Perceptual misinterpretation of a real external stimulus. *Compare with* **hallucination.**

immediate memory Reproduction, recognition, or recall of perceived material within seconds after presentation. *Compare with* **long-term memory** *and* **short-term memory.**

impaired insight Diminished ability to understand the objective reality of a situation.

impaired judgment Diminished ability to understand a situation correctly and to act appropriately.

impulse control Ability to resist an impulse, drive, or temptation to perform some action.

inappropriate affect Emotional tone out of harmony with the idea, thought, or speech accompanying it. Seen in schizophrenia.

incoherence Communication that is disconnected, disorganized, or incomprehensible. *See also* **word salad.**

incorporation Primitive unconscious defense mechanism in which the psychic representation of another person or aspects of another person are assimilated into oneself through a figurative process of symbolic oral ingestion; represents a special form of introjection and is the earliest mechanism of identification.

increased libido Increase in sexual interest and drive.

ineffability Ecstatic state in which persons insist that their experience is inexpressible and indescribable and that it is impossible to convey what it is like to one who never experienced it.

initial insomnia Falling asleep with difficulty; usually seen in anxiety disorder. *Compare with* **middle insomnia** *and* **terminal insomnia.**

insight Conscious recognition of one's condition. In psychiatry, it refers to the conscious awareness and understanding of one's psychodynamics and symptoms of maladaptive behavior; highly important in effecting changes in the personality and behavior of a person.

insomnia Difficulty in falling asleep or difficulty in staying asleep. It can be related to a mental disorder, can be related to a physical disorder or an adverse effect of medication, or can be primary (not related to a known medical factor or another mental disorder). *See also* **initial insomnia, middle insomnia,** *and* **terminal insomnia.**

intellectual insight Knowledge of the reality of a situation without the ability to use that knowledge successfully to effect an adaptive change in behavior or to master the situation. *Compare with* **true insight.**

intelligence Capacity for learning and ability to recall, to integrate constructively, and to apply what one has learned; the capacity to understand and to think rationally.

intoxication Mental disorder caused by recent ingestion or presence in the body of an exogenous substance producing maladaptive behavior by virtue of its effects on the central nervous system (CNS). The most common psychiatric changes involve disturbances of perception, wakefulness, attention, thinking, judgment, emotional control, and psychomotor behavior; the specific clinical picture depends on the substance ingested.

intropunitive Turning anger inward toward oneself. Commonly observed in depressed patients.

introspection Contemplating one's mental processes to achieve insight.

introversion State in which a person's energies are directed inward toward the self, with little or no interest in the external world.

irrelevant answer Answer that is not responsive to the question.

irritability Abnormal or excessive excitability, with easily triggered anger, annoyance, or impatience.

irritable mood State in which one is easily annoyed and provoked to anger. *See also* **irritability.**

jamais vu Paramnestic phenomenon characterized by a false feeling of unfamiliarity with a real situation that one has previously experienced.

jargon aphasia Aphasia in which the words produced are neologistic, that is, nonsense words created by the patient.

judgment Mental act of comparing or evaluating choices within the framework of a given set of values for the purpose of electing a course of action. If the course of action chosen is consonant with reality or with mature adult standards of behavior, judgment is said to be *intact* or *normal;* judgment is said to be *impaired* if the chosen course of action is frankly maladaptive, results from impulsive decisions based on the need for immediate gratification, or is otherwise not consistent with reality as measured by mature adult standards.

kleptomania Pathological compulsion to steal.

la belle indifférence Inappropriate attitude of calm or lack of concern about one's disability. May be seen in patients with conversion disorder.

labile affect Affective expression characterized by rapid and abrupt changes unrelated to external stimuli.

labile mood Oscillations in mood between euphoria and depression or anxiety.

laconic speech Condition characterized by a reduction in the quantity of spontaneous speech; replies to questions are brief and unelaborated, and little or no unprompted additional information is provided. Occurs in major depression, schizophrenia, and organic mental disorders. Also called *poverty of speech.*

lethologica Momentary forgetting of a name or proper noun. *See* **blocking.**

lilliputian hallucination Visual sensation that persons or objects are reduced in size; more properly regarded as an illusion. *See also* **micropsia.**

localized amnesia Partial loss of memory; amnesia restricted to specific or isolated experiences. Also called *lacunar amnesia* and *patch amnesia.*

logorrhea Copious, pressured, coherent speech; uncontrollable, excessive talking; observed in manic episodes of bipolar disorder. Also called *tachylogia, verbomania,* and *volubility.*

long-term memory Reproduction, recognition, or recall of experiences or information that was experienced in the distant past. Also called remote memory. *Compare with* **immediate memory** *and* **short-term memory.**

loosening of associations Characteristic schizophrenic thinking or speech disturbance involving a disorder in the logical progression of thoughts, manifested as a failure adequately to communicate verbally; unrelated and unconnected ideas shift from one subject to another. *See also* **tangentiality.**

macropsia False perception that objects are larger than they really are. *Compare with* **micropsia.**

magical thinking A form of dereistic thought; thinking similar to that of the preoperational phase in children (Jean Piaget), in which thoughts, words, or actions assume power (e.g., to cause or to prevent events).

malingering Feigning disease to achieve a specific goal, for example, to avoid an unpleasant responsibility.

mania Mood state characterized by elation, agitation, hyperactivity, hypersexuality, and accelerated thinking and speaking (flight of ideas). Seen in bipolar I disorder. *See also* **hypomania.**

manipulation Maneuvering by patients to get their own way; characteristic of antisocial personalities.

mannerism Ingrained, habitual involuntary movement.

melancholia Severe depressive state. Used in the term *involutional melancholia* as a descriptive term and also in reference to a distinct diagnostic entity.

memory Process whereby what is experienced or learned is established as a record in the CNS (registration), where it persists with a variable degree of permanence (retention) and can be recollected or retrieved from storage at will (recall). For types of memory, see **immediate memory, long-term memory,** and **short-term memory.**

mental disorder Psychiatric illness or disease whose manifestations are primarily characterized by behavioral or psychological impairment of function, measured in terms of deviation from some normative concept; associated with distress or disease, not just an expected response to a particular event or limited to relations between a person and society.

mental retardation Subaverage general intellectual functioning that originates in the developmental period and is associated with impaired maturation and learning and social maladjustment. Retardation is commonly defined in terms of intelligence quotient (IQ): mild (between 50 and 55 to 70), moderate (between 35 and 40 to between 50 and 55), severe (between 20 and 25 to between 35 and 40), and profound (below 20 to 25).

metonymy Speech disturbance common in schizophrenia in which the affected person uses a word or phrase that is related to the proper one but is not the one ordinarily used; for example, the patient speaks of consuming a *menu* rather than a *meal,* or refers to losing the *piece of string* of the conversation, rather than the thread of the conversation. *See also* **paraphasia** *and* **word approximation.**

microcephaly Condition in which the head is unusually small as a result of defective brain development and premature ossification of the skull.

micropsia False perception that objects are smaller than they really are. Sometimes called *lilliputian hallucination. Compare with* **macropsia.**

middle insomnia Waking up after falling asleep without difficulty and then having difficulty in falling asleep again. *Compare with* **initial insomnia** *and* **terminal insomnia.**

mimicry Simple, imitative motion activity of childhood.

monomania Mental state characterized by preoccupation with one subject.

mood Pervasive and sustained feeling tone that is experienced internally and that, in the extreme, can markedly influence virtually all aspects of a person's behavior and perception of the world. Distinguished from affect, the external expression of the internal feeling tone. For types of mood, see the specific term.

mood-congruent delusion Delusion with content that is mood appropriate (e.g., depressed patients who believe that they are responsible for the destruction of the world).

mood-congruent hallucination Hallucination with content that is consistent with a depressed or manic mood (e.g., depressed patients hearing voices telling them that they are bad persons and manic patients hearing voices telling them that they have inflated worth, power, or knowledge).

mood-incongruent delusion Delusion based on incorrect reference about external reality, with content that has no association to mood or is mood inappropriate (e.g., depressed patients who believe that they are the new Messiah).

mood-incongruent hallucination Hallucination not associated with real external stimuli, with content that is not consistent with depressed or manic mood (e.g., in depression, hallucinations not involving such themes as guilt, deserved punishment, or inadequacy; in mania, not involving such themes as inflated worth or power).

mood swings Oscillation of a person's emotional feeling tone between periods of elation and periods of depression.

motor aphasia Aphasia in which understanding is intact, but the ability to speak is lost. Also called *Broca's, expressive,* and *nonfluent aphasias.*

mourning Syndrome following loss of a loved one, consisting of preoccupation with the lost individual, weeping, sadness, and repeated reliving of memories. *See also* **bereavement** *and* **grief.**

muscle rigidity State in which the muscles remain immovable; seen in schizophrenia.

mutism Organic or functional absence of the faculty of speech. *See also* **stupor.**

mydriasis Dilation of the pupil; sometimes occurs as an autonomic (anticholinergic) or atropine-like adverse effect of some antipsychotic and antidepressant drugs.

narcissism In psychoanalytic theory, divided into primary and secondary types: *primary narcissism,* the early infantile phase of object relationship development, when the child has not differentiated the self from the outside world, and all sources of pleasure are unrealistically recognized as coming from within the self, giving the child a false sense of omnipotence; *secondary narcissism,* when the libido, once attached to external love objects, is redirected back to the self. *See also* **autistic thinking.**

needle phobia The persistent, intense, pathological fear of receiving an injection.

negative signs In schizophrenia: flat affect, alogia, abulia, and apathy.

negativism Verbal or nonverbal opposition or resistance to outside suggestions and advice; commonly seen in catatonic schizophrenia in which the patient resists any effort to be moved or does the opposite of what is asked.

neologism New word or phrase whose derivation cannot be understood; often seen in schizophrenia. It has also been used to mean a word that has been incorrectly constructed but whose origins are nonetheless understandable (e.g., *headshoe* to mean *hat*), but such constructions are more properly referred to as *word approximations.*

neurological amnesia (1) Auditory amnesia: loss of ability to comprehend sounds or speech. (2) Tactile amnesia: loss of ability to judge the shape of objects by touch. *See also* **astereognosis.** (3) Verbal amnesia: loss of ability to remember words. (4) Visual amnesia: loss of ability to recall or to recognize familiar objects or printed words.

nihilism Delusion of the nonexistence of the self or part of the self; also refers to an attitude of total rejection of established values or extreme skepticism regarding moral and value judgments.

nihilistic delusion Depressive delusion that the world and everything related to it have ceased to exist.

noeisis Revelation in which immense illumination occurs in association with a sense that one has been chosen to lead and command. Can occur in manic or dissociative states.

nominal aphasia Aphasia characterized by difficulty in giving the correct name of an object. *See also* **anomia** *and* **amnestic aphasia.**

nymphomania Abnormal, excessive, insatiable desire in a woman for sexual intercourse. *Compare with* **satyriasis.**

obsession Persistent and recurrent idea, thought, or impulse that cannot be eliminated from consciousness by logic or reasoning; obsessions are involuntary and ego-dystonic. *See also* **compulsion.**

olfactory hallucination Hallucination primarily involving smell or odors; most common in medical disorders, especially in the temporal lobe.

orientation State of awareness of oneself and one's surroundings in terms of time, place, and person.

overactivity Abnormality in motor behavior that can manifest itself as psychomotor agitation, hyperactivity (hyperkinesis), tics, sleepwalking, or compulsions.

overvalued idea False or unreasonable belief or idea that is sustained beyond the bounds of reason. It is held with less intensity or duration than a delusion but is usually associated with mental illness.

panic Acute, intense attack of anxiety associated with personality disorganization; the anxiety is overwhelming and accompanied by feelings of impending doom.

panphobia Overwhelming fear of everything.

pantomime Gesticulation; psychodrama without the use of words.

paramnesia Disturbance of memory in which reality and fantasy are confused. It is observed in dreams and in certain types of schizophrenia and organic mental disorders; it includes phenomena such as *déjà vu* and *déjà entendu,* which may occur occasionally in normal persons.

paranoia Rare psychiatric syndrome marked by the gradual development of a highly elaborate and complex delusional system, generally involving persecutory or grandiose delusions, with few other signs of personality disorganization or thought disorder.

paranoid delusions Includes persecutory delusions and delusions of reference, control, and grandeur.

paranoid ideation Thinking dominated by suspicious, persecutory, or grandiose content of less than delusional proportions.

paraphasia Abnormal speech in which one word is substituted for another, the irrelevant word generally resembling the required one in morphology, meaning, or phonetic composition; the inappropriate word may be a legitimate one used incorrectly, such as *clover* instead of *hand,* or a bizarre nonsense expression, such as *treen* instead of *train.* Paraphasic speech may be seen in organic aphasias and in mental disorders such as schizophrenia. *See also* **metonymy** *and* **word approximation.**

parapraxis Faulty act, such as a slip of the tongue or the misplacement of an article. Freud ascribed parapraxes to unconscious motives.

paresis Weakness or partial paralysis of organic origin.

paresthesia Abnormal spontaneous tactile sensation, such as a burning, tingling, or pins-and-needles sensation.

perception Conscious awareness of elements in the environment by the mental processing of sensory stimuli; sometimes used in a broader sense to refer to the mental process by which all kinds of data—intellectual, emotional, and sensory—are meaningfully organized. *See also* **apperception.**

perseveration (1) Pathological repetition of the same response to different stimuli, as in a repetition of the same verbal response to different questions. (2) Persistent repetition of specific words or concepts in the process of speaking. Seen in cognitive disorders, schizophrenia, and other mental illness. *See also* **verbigeration.**

phantom limb False sensation that an extremity that has been lost is, in fact, present.

phobia Persistent, pathological, unrealistic, intense fear of an object or situation; the phobic person may realize that the fear is irrational but, nonetheless, cannot dispel it. For types of phobias, see the specific term.

pica Craving and eating of nonfood substances, such as paint and clay.

polyphagia Pathological overeating.

positive signs In schizophrenia: hallucinations, delusions, and thought disorder.

posturing Strange, fixed, and bizarre bodily positions held by a patient for an extended time. *See also* **catatonia.**

poverty of content of speech Speech that is adequate in amount but conveys little information because of vagueness, emptiness, or stereotyped phrases.

poverty of speech Restriction in the amount of speech used; replies may be monosyllabic. *See also* **laconic speech.**

preoccupation of thought Centering of thought content on a particular idea, associated with a strong affective tone, such as a paranoid trend or a suicidal or homicidal preoccupation.

pressured speech Increase in the amount of spontaneous speech; rapid, loud, accelerated speech, as occurs in mania, schizophrenia, and cognitive disorders.

primary process thinking In psychoanalysis, the mental activity directly related to the functions of the id and characteristic of unconscious mental processes; marked by primitive, prelogical thinking and by the tendency to seek immediate discharge and gratification of instinctual demands. Includes thinking that is dereistic, illogical, magical; normally found in dreams, abnormally in psychosis. *Compare with* **secondary process thinking.**

projection Unconscious defense mechanism in which persons attribute to another those generally unconscious ideas, thoughts, feelings, and impulses that are in themselves undesirable or unacceptable, as a form of protection from anxiety arising from an inner conflict; by externalizing whatever is unacceptable, they deal with it as a situation apart from themselves.

prosopagnosia Inability to recognize familiar faces that is not due to impaired visual acuity or level of consciousness.

pseudocyesis Rare condition in which a nonpregnant patient has the signs and symptoms of pregnancy, such as abdominal distention, breast enlargement, pigmentation, cessation of menses, and morning sickness.

pseudodementia (1) Dementia-like disorder that can be reversed by appropriate treatment and is not caused by organic brain disease. (2) Condition in which patients show exaggerated indifference to their surroundings in the absence of a mental disorder; also occurs in depression and factitious disorders.

pseudologia phantastica Disorder characterized by uncontrollable lying in which patients elaborate extensive fantasies that they freely communicate and act on.

psychomotor agitation Physical and mental overactivity that is usually nonproductive and is associated with a feeling of inner turmoil, as seen in agitated depression.

psychosis Mental disorder in which the thoughts, affective response, ability to recognize reality, and ability to communicate and relate to others are sufficiently impaired to interfere grossly with the capacity to deal with reality; the classical characteristics of psychosis are impaired reality testing, hallucinations, delusions, and illusions.

psychotic (1) Person experiencing psychosis. (2) Denoting or characteristic of psychosis.

rationalization An unconscious defense mechanism in which irrational or unacceptable behavior, motives, or feelings are logically justified or made consciously tolerable by plausible means.

reaction formation Unconscious defense mechanism in which a person develops a socialized attitude or interest that is the direct antithesis of some infantile wish or impulse that is harbored consciously or unconsciously. One of the earliest and most unstable defense mechanisms, closely related to repression; both are defenses against impulses or urges that are unacceptable to the ego.

reality testing Fundamental ego function that consists of tentative actions that test and objectively evaluate the nature and limits of the environment; includes the ability to differentiate between the external world and the internal world and accurately to judge the relation between the self and the environment.

recall Process of bringing stored memories into consciousness. *See also* **memory.**

recent memory Recall of events over the past few days.

recent past memory Recall of events over the past few months.

receptive aphasia Organic loss of ability to comprehend the meaning of words; fluid and spontaneous, but incoherent and nonsensical, speech. *See also* **fluent aphasia** *and* **sensory aphasia.**

receptive dysphasia Difficulty in comprehending oral language; the impairment involves comprehension and production of language.

regression Unconscious defense mechanism in which a person undergoes a partial or total return to earlier patterns of adaptation; observed in many psychiatric conditions, particularly schizophrenia.

remote memory Recall of events in the distant past.

repression Freud's term for an unconscious defense mechanism in which unacceptable mental contents are banished or kept out of consciousness; important in normal psychological development and in neurotic and psychotic symptom formation. Freud recognized two kinds of repression: (1) repression proper, in which the repressed material was once in the conscious domain, and (2) primal repression, in which the repressed material was never in the conscious realm. *Compare with* **suppression.**

restricted affect Reduction in intensity of feeling tone that is less severe than in blunted affect but clearly reduced. *See also* **constricted affect.**

retrograde amnesia Loss of memory for events preceding the onset of the amnesia. *Compare with* **anterograde amnesia.**

retrospective falsification Memory becomes unintentionally (unconsciously) distorted by being filtered through a person's present emotional, cognitive, and experiential state.

rigidity In psychiatry, a person's resistance to change, a personality trait.

ritual (1) Formalized activity practiced by a person to reduce anxiety, as in OCD. (2) Ceremonial activity of cultural origin.

rumination Constant preoccupation with thinking about a single idea or theme, as in OCD.

satyriasis Morbid, insatiable sexual need or desire in a man. *Compare with* **nymphomania.**

scotoma (1) In psychiatry, a figurative blind spot in a person's psychological awareness. (2) In neurology, a localized visual field defect.

secondary process thinking In psychoanalysis, the form of thinking that is logical, organized, reality oriented, and influenced by the demands of the environment; characterizes the mental activity of the ego. *Compare with* **primary process thinking.**

seizure An attack or sudden onset of certain symptoms, such as convulsions, loss of consciousness, and psychic or sensory disturbances; seen in epilepsy and can be substance induced. For types of seizures, see the specific term.

sensorium Hypothetical sensory center in the brain that is involved with clarity of awareness about oneself and one's surroundings, including the ability to perceive and to process ongoing events in light of past experiences, future options, and current circumstances; sometimes used interchangeably with *consciousness.*

sensory aphasia Organic loss of ability to comprehend the meaning of words; fluid and spontaneous, but incoherent and nonsensical, speech. *See also* **fluent aphasia** *and* **receptive aphasia.**

sensory extinction Neurological sign operationally defined as failure to report one of two simultaneously presented sensory stimuli, despite the fact that either stimulus alone is correctly reported. Also called *sensory inattention.*

shame Failure to live up to self-expectations; often associated with a fantasy of how the person will be seen by others. *See also* **guilt.**

short-term memory Reproduction, recognition, or recall of perceived material within minutes after the initial presentation. *Compare with* **immediate memory** *and* **long-term memory.**

simultanagnosia Impairment in the perception or integration of visual stimuli appearing simultaneously.

somatic delusion Delusion pertaining to the functioning of one's body.

somatic hallucination Hallucination involving the perception of a physical experience localized within the body.

somatopagnosia Inability to recognize a part of one's body as one's own (also called *ignorance of the body* and *autotopagnosia*).

somnolence Pathological sleepiness or drowsiness from which one can be aroused to a normal state of consciousness.

spatial agnosia Inability to recognize spatial relations.

speaking in tongues Expression of a revelatory message through unintelligible words; not considered a disorder of thought if associated with practices of specific Pentecostal religions. *See also* **glossolalia.**

stereotypy Continuous mechanical repetition of speech or physical activities; observed in catatonic schizophrenia.

stupor (1) State of decreased reactivity to stimuli and less than full awareness of one's surroundings; as a disturbance of consciousness, it indicates a condition of partial coma or semicoma. (2) In psychiatry, it is used synonymously with *mutism* and does not necessarily imply a disturbance of consciousness; in *catatonic stupor,* patients are ordinarily aware of their surroundings.

stuttering Frequent repetition or prolongation of a sound or syllable, leading to markedly impaired speech fluency.

sublimation Unconscious defense mechanism in which the energy associated with unacceptable impulses or drives is diverted into personally and socially acceptable channels; unlike other defense mechanisms, it offers some minimal gratification of the instinctual drive or impulse.

substitution Unconscious defense mechanism in which a person replaces an unacceptable wish, drive, emotion, or goal with one that is more acceptable.

suggestibility State of uncritical compliance with influence or of uncritical acceptance of an idea, belief, or attitude; commonly observed among persons with hysterical traits.

suicidal ideation Thoughts or act of taking one's life.

suppression Conscious act of controlling and inhibiting an unacceptable impulse, emotion, or idea; differentiated from repression in that repression is an unconscious process.

symbolization Unconscious defense mechanism in which one idea or object comes to stand for another because of some common aspect or quality in both; based on similarity and association; the symbols formed protect the person from the anxiety that may be attached to the original idea or object.

synesthesia Condition in which the stimulation of one sensory modality is perceived as sensation in a different modality, as when a sound produces a sensation of color.

syntactical aphasia Aphasia characterized by difficulty in understanding spoken speech, associated with gross disorder of thought and expression.

systematized delusion Group of elaborate delusions related to a single event or theme.

tactile hallucination Hallucination primarily involving the sense of touch. Also called *haptic hallucination.*

tangentiality Oblique, digressive, or even irrelevant manner of speech in which the central idea is not communicated.

tension Physiological or psychic arousal, uneasiness, or pressure toward action; an unpleasurable alteration in mental or physical state that seeks relief through action.

terminal insomnia Early morning awakening or waking up at least 2 hours before planning to wake up. *Compare with* **initial insomnia** *and* **middle insomnia.**

thought broadcasting Feeling that one's thoughts are being broadcast or projected into the environment. *See also* **thought withdrawal.**

thought disorder Any disturbance of thinking that affects language, communication, or thought content; the hallmark feature of schizophrenia. Manifestations range from simple blocking and mild circumstantiality to profound loosening of associations, incoherence, and delusions; characterized by a failure to follow semantic and syntactic rules that is inconsistent with the person's education, intelligence, or cultural background.

thought insertion Delusion that thoughts are being implanted in one's mind by other people or forces.

thought latency The period of time between a thought and its verbal expression. Increased in schizophrenia (*see* **blocking**) and decreased in mania (*see* **pressured speech**).

thought withdrawal Delusion that one's thoughts are being removed from one's mind by other people or forces. *See also* **thought broadcasting.**

tic disorders Predominantly psychogenic disorders characterized by involuntary, spasmodic, stereotyped movement of small groups of muscles; seen most predominantly in moments of stress or anxiety, rarely as a result of organic disease.

tinnitus Noises in one or both ears, such as ringing, buzzing, or clicking; an adverse effect of some psychotropic drugs.

tonic convulsion Convulsion in which the muscle contraction is sustained.

trailing phenomenon Perceptual abnormality associated with hallucinogenic drugs in which moving objects are seen as a series of discrete and discontinuous images.

trance Sleep-like state of reduced consciousness and activity.

tremor Rhythmical alteration in movement, which is usually faster than one beat a second; typically, tremors decrease during periods of relaxation and sleep and increase during periods of anger and increased tension.

true insight Understanding of the objective reality of a situation coupled with the motivational and emotional impetus to master the situation or change behavior.

twilight state Disturbed consciousness with hallucinations.

unconscious (1) One of three divisions of Freud's topographic theory of the mind (the others being the conscious and the preconscious) in which the psychic material is not readily accessible to conscious awareness by ordinary means; its existence may be manifest in symptom formation, in dreams, or under the influence of drugs. (2) In popular (but more ambiguous) usage, any mental material not in the immediate field of awareness. (3) Denoting a state of unawareness, with lack of response to external stimuli, as in a coma.

undoing Unconscious primitive defense mechanism, repetitive in nature, by which a person symbolically acts out in reverse something unacceptable that has already been done or against which the ego must defend itself; a form of magical expiatory action, commonly observed in OCD.

unio mystica Feeling of mystic unity with an infinite power.

vegetative signs In depression, denoting characteristic symptoms such as sleep disturbance (especially early-morning awakening), decreased appetite, constipation, weight loss, and loss of sexual response.

verbigeration Meaningless and stereotyped repetition of words or phrases, as seen in schizophrenia. Also called *cataphasia. See also* **perseveration.**

vertigo Sensation that one or the world around one is spinning or revolving; a hallmark of vestibular dysfunction, not to be confused with dizziness.

visual agnosia Inability to recognize objects or persons.

visual amnesia *See* **neurological amnesia.**

visual hallucination Hallucination primarily involving the sense of sight.

waxy flexibility Condition in which a person maintains the body position into which he or she is placed. Also called *catalepsy.*

word approximation Use of conventional words in an unconventional or inappropriate way (metonymy or of new words that are developed by conventional rules of word formation) (e.g., *handshoes* for *gloves* and *time measure* for *clock*); distinguished from a *neologism,* which is a new word whose derivation cannot be understood. *See also* **paraphasia.**

word salad Incoherent, essentially incomprehensible mixture of words and phrases commonly seen in far-advanced cases of schizophrenia. *See also* **incoherence.**

xenophobia Abnormal fear of strangers.

zoophobia Abnormal fear of animals.

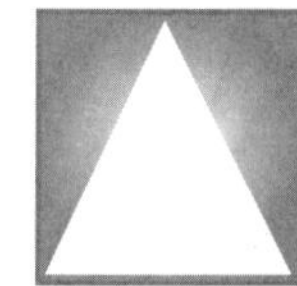

Index

Note: Page number followed by t indicates table only.

C

E

G

O

P

Q

R